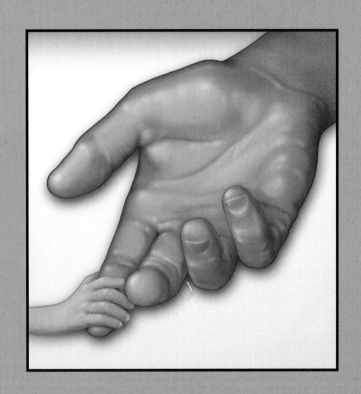

Pediatric Surgery

Pediatric Surgery

SIXTH EDITION

VOLUME ONE

Jay L. Grosfeld, MD
Lafayette Page Professor and Chairman Emeritus
Department of Surgery, Indiana University School of Medicine
Surgeon-in-Chief and Director of Pediatric Surgery Emeritus, Riley Hospital for Children
Indianapolis, Indiana

James A. O'Neill, Jr., MD
John Clinton Foshee Distinguished Professor of Surgery
Former Chairman, Section of Surgical Sciences, Former
Chairman, Department of Surgery, Surgeon-in-Chief Emeritus
Vanderbilt University Medical Center
Nashville, Tennessee

Arnold G. Coran, MD
Professor of Pediatric Surgery
University of Michigan Medical School
Former Surgeon-in-Chief
C.S. Mott Children's Hospital
Ann Arbor, Michigan

Eric W. Fonkalsrud, MD
Professor and Emeritus Chief of Pediatric Surgery
David Geffen School of Medicine at UCLA
Department of Surgery
Los Angeles, California

Anthony A. Caldamone, MD, FAAP
Associate Editor, Urology Section
Professor of Surgery (Urology) and Pediatrics
Brown University School of Medicine
Chief of Pediatric Urology, Hasbro Children's Hospital
Providence, Rhode Island

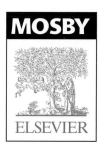

MOSBY

ELSEVIER

MOSBY
ELSEVIER

1600 John F. Kennedy Blvd.
Ste 1800
Philadelphia, PA 19103-2899

PEDIATRIC SURGERY
Copyright © 2006 by Mosby, Inc.

ISBN-13: 978-0-323-02842-4
ISBN-10: 0-323-02842-X
Volume 1 PN 999603772X
Volume 2 PN 9996037789

Notice

Knowledge and best practice in this field are constantly changing. As new research and experience broaden our knowledge, changes in practice, treatment and drug therapy may become necessary or appropriate. Readers are advised to check the most current information provided (i) on procedures featured or (ii) by the manufacturer of each product to be administered, to verify the recommended dose or formula, the method and duration of administration, and contraindications. It is the responsibility of the practitioner, relying on their own experience and knowledge of the patient, to make diagnoses, to determine dosages and the best treatment for each individual patient, and to take all appropriate safety precautions. To the fullest extent of the law, neither the Publisher nor the Editors assumes any liability for any injury and/or damage to persons or property arising out or related to any use of the material contained in this book.

The Publisher

Library of Congress Cataloging-in-Publication Data
Pediatric surgery.— 6th ed. / edited by Jay L. Grosfeld ...[et al.].
    p. ; cm.
    Includes bibliographical references and index.
    ISBN 0-323-02842-X
    1.Children—Surgery. I. Grosfeld, Jay L.
    [DNLM: 1. Surgical Procedures, Operative—Child. 2. Surgical Procedures,
Operative—Infant. WO 925 P371 2006]
RD137.P42 2006
617.9'8- -dc22   2005049600

Acquisitions Editor: Judith Fletcher
Senior Developmental Editor: Janice Gaillard
Publishing Services Manager: Tina K. Rebane
Senior Project Manager: Linda Lewis Grigg
Design Direction: Gene Harris
Cover Designer: Gene Harris

To our wives
Margie, Susan, Peggy, and Susi.
To our children and grandchildren for giving
us the time and providing the sensitivity
and support to prepare these volumes.
To children everywhere who have suffered
from congenital and acquired surgical conditions
and have provided the experience and inspired us.

Contributors

Mark C. Adams, MD, FAAP
Professor of Urology and Pediatrics, Vanderbilt
University School of Medicine; Pediatric Urologist,
Monroe Carell Jr. Children's Hospital at Vanderbilt,
Nashville, Tennessee
Magaureter and Prune-Belly Syndrome

N. Scott Adzick, MD
C. Everett Koop Professor of Pediatric Surgery,
University of Pennsylvania School of Medicine;
Surgeon-in-Chief, The Children's Hospital of
Philadelphia, Philadelphia, Pennsylvania
Cysts of the Lungs and Mediastinum

Craig T. Albanese, MD
Professor of Surgery, Pediatrics, and Obstetrics and
Gynecology, and Chief, Division of Pediatric Surgery,
Department of Surgery, Stanford Hospital & Clinics,
Stanford; John A. and Cynthia Fry Gunn Director of
Surgical Services, Lucile Packard Children's Hospital
at Stanford, Palo Alto, California
Necrotizing Enterocolitis

Fred Alexander, MD
Associate Professor of Surgery, Cleveland Clinic Lerner
School of Medicine of Case Western Reserve University;
Staff Surgeon, Cleveland Clinic Foundation, Cleveland,
Ohio
Crohn's Disease

R. Peter Altman, MD
Professor of Surgery, Columbia University College of
Physicians and Surgeons; Surgeon-in-Chief, Morgan
Stanley Children's Hospital of New York Presbyterian,
New York, New York
The Jaundiced Infant: Biliary Atresia

Richard J. Andrassy, MD
Denton A. Cooley Professor and Chairman, Department
of Surgery, University of Texas Medical School at
Houston; Executive Vice President of Clinical Affairs
and Associate Dean for Clinical Affairs, University of
Texas at Houston, Houston, Texas
Rhabdomyosarcoma

Walter S. Andrews, MD
Professor of Surgery, University of Missouri–Kansas City
School of Medicine; Director, Transplantation Program,
Children's Mercy Hospital, Kansas City, Missouri
Gallbladder Disease and Hepatic Infections

Harry Applebaum, MD
Clinical Professor of Surgery, David Geffen School of
Medicine at UCLA; Head, Division of Pediatric Surgery,
Kaiser Permanente Medical Center, Los Angeles, California
Duodenal Atresia and Stenosis—Annular Pancreas

Marjorie J. Arca, MD
Assistant Professor of Surgery, Medical College of
Wisconsin; Attending Surgeon, Children's Hospital of
Wisconsin, Milwaukee, Wisconsin
Atresia, Stenosis, and Other Obstructions of the Colon

Robert M. Arensman, MD
Professor of Surgery, Louisiana State University School
of Medicine; Attending Surgeon, Ochsner Clinic
Foundation, New Orleans, Louisiana
Gastrointestinal Bleeding

James B. Atkinson, MD
Professor and Chief, Division of Pediatric Surgery,
Department of Surgery, David Geffen School of
Medicine at UCLA, Los Angeles, California
Liver Tumors

Richard G. Azizkhan, MD, PhD(Hon)
Professor of Surgery and Pediatrics, Lester Martin Chair
of Pediatric Surgery, and Vice Chair, Department of
Surgery, University of Cincinnati College of Medicine;
Surgeon-in-Chief and Director, Division of Pediatric
Surgery, Cincinnati Children's Hospital Medical Center,
Cincinnati, Ohio
Teratomas and Other Germ Cell Tumors

Anwar Baban, MD
Laboratory of Molecular Genetics, Gaslini Children's
Hospital, Genoa, Italy
*Hirschsprung's Disease and Related Neuromuscular Disorders
of the Intestine*

Douglas C. Barnhart, MD, MSPH
Assistant Professor, Departments of Surgery and
Pediatrics, University of Alabama at Birmingham
School of Medicine; Attending Surgeon, The Children's
Hospital of Alabama, Birmingham, Alabama
Biopsy Techniques for Children with Cancer

Robert H. Bartlett, MD
Professor of Surgery, University of Michigan Medical
School, Ann Arbor, Michigan
Extracorporeal Life Support for Cardiopulmonary Failure

Laurence S. Baskin, MD
Professor of Urology, University of California,
San Francisco, School of Medicine; Chief, Pediatric
Urology, UCSF Children's Hospital at UCSF Medical
Center, San Francisco, California
Hypospadias

Spencer W. Beasley, MB, ChB, MS
Clinical Professor of Pediatrics and Surgery,
Christchurch School of Medicine and Health Sciences,
University of Otago; Chief of Child Health Services,
Division of Child Health, and Clinical Director,
Paediatric Surgery, Christchurch Hospital,
Christchurch, New Zealand
Torticollis

Michael L. Bentz, MD, FAAP, FACS
Professor of Surgery, Pediatrics, and Plastic Surgery, and
Chairman, Division of Plastic Surgery, University of
Wisconsin School of Medicine and Public Health; Chief
of Plastic Surgery, University of Wisconsin Hospital and
Clinics, Madison, Wisconsin
Hand, Soft Tissue, and Envenomation Injuries

Victor E. Boston, MD, FRCSI, FRCSEng, FRCSEd
Honorary Senior Lecturer, Department of Surgery,
The Queen's University of Belfast Faculty of Medicine;
The Royal Belfast Hospital for Sick Children, Belfast,
Northern Ireland
Ureteral Duplication and Ureteroceles

Scott C. Boulanger, MD, PhD
Assistant Professor of Surgery, Division of Pediatric
Surgery, University of Mississippi Medical Center School
of Medicine, Jackson, Mississippi
Inguinal Hernias and Hydroceles

Edward L. Bove, MD
Professor of Surgery, University of Michigan Medical
School; Head, Section of Cardiac Surgery, C.S. Mott
Children's Hospital, Ann Arbor, Michigan
Congenital Heart Disease and Anomalies of the Great Vessels

Mary L. Brandt, MD
Professor and Vice Chair, Michael E. DeBakey
Department of Surgery, Baylor College of Medicine,
Texas Children's Hospital, Houston, Texas
Disorders of the Breast

John W. Brock III, MD
Professor of Urologic Surgery, Vanderbilt University
School of Medicine; Director, Pediatric Urology,
Vanderbilt Medical Center; Surgeon in Chief,
Monroe Carell Jr. Children's Hospital at Vanderbilt,
Nashville, Tennessee
Bladder Exstrophy

Rebeccah L. Brown, MD
Assistant Professor of Clinical Surgery and Pediatrics,
University of Cincinnati College of Medicine; Associate
Director of Trauma Services, Cincinnati Children's
Hospital Medical Center, Cincinnati, Ohio
Genitourinary Tract Trauma

Marybeth Browne, MD
Surgical Resident, McGaw Medical Center of
Northwestern University, Chicago, Illinois
Gastrointestinal Bleeding

Terry L. Buchmiller, MD
Formerly Assistant Professor of Surgery, Weill Medical
College of Cornell University of New York, New York;
Currently Assistant Professor of Surgery, Harvard
Medical School; Assistant in Surgery, Children's
Hospital Boston, Boston, Massachusetts
The Jaundiced Infant: Biliary Atresia

Ronald W. Busuttil, MD, PhD
Professor and Executive Chairman,
Department of Surgery, David Geffen School of
Medicine at UCLA; Chief, Division of Liver and
Pancreas Transplantation, Dumont-UCLA Liver Cancer
Center; Director, Pfleger Liver Institute, UCLA Medical
Center, Los Angeles, California
Liver Transplantation

Michelle S. Caird, MD
Lecturer, Department of Orthopaedic Surgery,
Alfred Taubman Health Care Center,
University of Michigan, Ann Arbor, Michigan
Musculoskeletal Trauma

Anthony A. Caldamone, MD, FAAP
Professor of Surgery (Urology) and Pediatrics,
Brown University School of Medicine;
Chief of Pediatric Urology, Hasbro Children's Hospital,
Providence, Rhode Island
*Renal Infection, Abscess, Vesicoureteral Reflux, Urinary Lithiasis,
and Renal Vein Thrombosis*

Darrell A. Campbell, Jr., MD
Professor of Surgery, University of Michigan Medical
School; Chief of Clinical Affairs, University of Michigan
Health System, Ann Arbor, Michigan
Renal Transplantation

Donna A. Caniano, MD
Professor of Surgery and Pediatrics, The Ohio State
University College of Medicine and Public Health;
Surgeon-in-Chief, Children's Hospital, Columbus,
Ohio
Ethical Considerations

Michael G. Caty, MD
Associate Professor of Surgery and Pediatrics, University
at Buffalo School of Medicine and Biomedical Science;
Surgeon-in-Chief, Women and Children's Hospital of
Buffalo, Buffalo, New York
Adrenal Tumors

Dai H. Chung, MD
Associate Professor of Surgery and Pediatrics, The
University of Texas Medical Branch School of Medicine
at Galveston; Chief, Section of Pediatric Surgery, UTMB
Children's Hospital, Galveston, Texas
Burns

Robert E. Cilley, MD
Professor of Surgery and Pediatrics, Penn State College of Medicine; Chief, Division of Pediatric Surgery, Milton S. Hershey Medical Center, Hershey, Pennsylvania
Disorders of the Umbilicus

Paul M. Colombani, MD
Professor of Surgery, Pediatrics, and Oncology, and Robert Garrett Professor of Surgery, Johns Hopkins University School of Medicine; Chief, Division of Pediatric Surgery, Johns Hopkins Medicine; Pediatric Surgeon-in-Charge, Johns Hopkins Hospital, Baltimore, Maryland
Surgical Implications Associated with Bone Marrow Transplantation

Joel D. Cooper, MD
Professor of Surgery, University of Pennsylvania School of Medicine; Chief, Division of Thoracic Surgery, Hospital of the University of Pennsylvania, Philadelphia, Pennsylvania
Lung Transplantation

Arnold G. Coran, MD
Professor of Pediatric Surgery, University of Michigan Medical School, Ann Arbor, Michigan
Nutritional Support; Congenital Anomalies of the Esophagus; Hirschsprung's Disease and Related Neuromuscular Disorders of the Intestine; Abnormalities of the Female Genital Tract

Robin T. Cotton, MD
Professor of Otolaryngology, University of Cincinnati School of Medicine; Director, Pediatric Otolaryngology–HNS, Cincinnati Children's Hospital Medical Center, Cincinnati, Ohio
Lesions of the Larynx, Trachea, and Upper Airway

Michael C. Dalsing, MD
Professor of Surgery and Director, Section of Vascular Surgery, Indiana University School of Medicine, Indianapolis, Indiana
Venous Disorders in Childhood

Alan Daneman, MBBCh, BSc, FRANZCR, FRCPC
Professor of Radiology, University of Toronto Faculty of Medicine; Staff Radiologist, Hospital for Sick Children, Toronto, Ontario, Canada
Intussusception

Andrew M. Davidoff, MD
Associate Professor, Department of Surgery and Pediatrics, University of Tennessee School of Medicine; Chief, Division of General Pediatric Surgery, St. Jude Children's Research Hospital, Memphis, Tennessee
Principles of Pediatric Oncology, Genetics of Cancer, and Radiation Therapy

Richard S. Davidson, MD
Associate Professor, University of Pennsylvania School of Medicine; Attending Surgeon, Children's Hospital of Philadelphia and Shrener's Hospital, Philadelphia
Musculoskeletal Trauma

Romano T. DeMarco, MD
Assistant Professor of Urologic Surgery, Division of Pediatric Urology, Vanderbilt University School of Medicine, Nashville, Tennessee
Bladder Exstrophy

Daniel A. DeUgarte, MD
Pediatric Surgery Fellow, University of Michigan Medical School and C.S. Mott Children's Hospital, Ann Arbor, Michigan
Liver Tumors

Eric Devaney, MD
Assistant Professor of Surgery, University of Michigan Medical School; Attending Surgeon, C.S. Mott Children's Hospital, Ann Arbor, Michigan
Congenital Heart Disease and Anomalies of the Great Vessels

William Didelot, MD
Professor of Pediatric Orthopaedics, Indiana University School of Medicine; Staff Surgeon, Riley Hospital for Children, Indianapolis, Indiana
Major Congenital Orthopedic Deformitites

John W. DiFiore, MD
Clinical Assistant Professor of Surgery, Case School of Medicine; Staff Pediatric Surgeon, Children's Hospital at Cleveland Clinic, Cleveland, Ohio
Respiratory Physiology and Care

Patrick A. Dillon, MD
Assistant Professor of Surgery, Washington University in St. Louis School of Medicine; Attending Surgeon, St. Louis Children's Hospital, St. Louis, Missouri
Gastrointestinal Tumors

Peter W. Dillon, MD
Professor of Surgery and Pediatrics, Penn State College of Medicine; Vice Chair, Department of Surgery, and Chief, Division of Pediatric Surgery, Penn State Children's Hospital, Hershey, Pennsylvania
Congenital Diaphragmatic Hernia and Eventration

Patricia K. Donahoe, MD
Marshall K. Bartlett Professor of Surgery, Harvard Medical School; Director, Pediatric Surgical Research Laboratories and Chief, Pediatric Surgical Services Emerita, Massachusetts General Hospital, Boston
Ambiguous Genitalia

James C. Y. Dunn, MD, PhD
Assistant Professor of Surgery, David Geffen School of Medicine at UCLA; Attending Surgeon, Mattel Children's Hospital at UCLA, Los Angeles, California
Appendicitis

Simon Eaton, BSc, PhD
Senior Lecturer in Pediatric Surgery and Metabolic Biochemistry, Department of Pediatric Surgery, Institute of Child Health, University College London, London, United Kingdom
Neonatal Physiology and Metabolic Considerations

Martin R. Eichelberger, MD
Professor of Surgery and Pediatrics, George Washington University School of Medicine and Health Sciences; Director, Emergency Trauma, Burn Service, and Senior Attending, Pediatric Surgery Service, Children's National Medical Center; President and CEO, Safe Kids Worldwide, Washington, DC
Accident Victims and Their Emergency Management

Sigmund H. Ein, MDCM, FRCSC, FAAP, FACS
Associate Professor of Surgery, Adjunct Clinical Faculty, Department of Surgery, University of Toronto Faculty of Medicine; Honorary Staff Surgeon, Division of General Surgery, The Hospital for Sick Children, Toronto; Courtesy Staff, Department of Surgery, Lakeridge Health Corporation, Oshawa, Ontario, Canada
Intussusception

Carolyn Ells, RTT, PhD
Assistant Professor of Medicine, McGill University Faculty of Medicine; Clinical Ethicist, Sir Mortimer B. Davis Jewish General Hospital, Montreal, Quebec, Canada
Ethical Considerations

Barry L. Eppley, MD, DMD
Professor of Plastic Surgery, Indiana University School of Medicine, Indianapolis, Indiana
Cleft Lip and Palate

Mary E. Fallat, MD
Professor of Surgery, and Director, Division of Pediatric Surgery, University of Louisville; Chief of Surgery, Kosdir Children's Hospital, Louisville, Kentucky
Ovarian Tumors

Diana L. Farmer, MD
Professor of Clinical Surgery, Pediatrics and Obstetrics, Gynecology, and Reproductive Medicine, University of California, San Francisco, School of Medicine; Surgeon-in-Chief, UCSF Children's Hospital, San Francisco, California
Cysts of the Lungs and Mediastinum

Douglas G. Farmer, MD
Associate Professor of Surgery, David Geffen School of Medicine at UCLA; Director, Intestinal Transplantation, Dumont-UCLA Transplant Center, Los Angeles, California
Liver Transplantation; Intestinal Transplantation

Steven J. Fishman, MD
Professor of Surgery, Harvard University Medical School; Senior Associate in Surgery, Children's Hospital Boston, Boston, Massachusetts
Vascular Anomalies: Hemangiomas and Malformations

Alan W. Flake, MD
Professor of Surgery and Obstetrics and Gynecology, University of Pennsylvania School of Medicine; Director, Children's Institute for Surgical Science, The Children's Hospital of Philadelphia, Philadelphia, Pennsylvania
Molecular Clinical Genetics and Gene Therapy

Robert P. Foglia, MD
Associate Professor of Surgery and Division Chief, Pediatric Surgery, Washington University in St. Louis School of Medicine; Surgeon-in-Chief, St. Louis Children's Hospital, St. Louis, Missouri
Gastrointestinal Tumors

Eric W. Fonkalsrud, MD
Professor of Surgery, David Geffen School of Medicine at UCLA; Emeritus Chief of Pediatric Surgery, UCLA Medical Center, Los Angeles, California
Ulcerative Colitis; Lymphatic Disorders

Henri R. Ford, MD
Vice-Chair and Visiting Professor of Surgery, Keck School of Medicine of USC; Surgeon-in-Chief and Vice President, Surgery, and Medical Director, Burtie Green Bettingen Surgery Center, Children's Hospital Los Angeles, Los Angeles, California
Sepsis and Related Considerations

Stephanie M. P. Fuller, MD
Clinical Fellow, Division of Cardiothoracic Surgery, The Children's Hospital of Philadelphia and Thomas Jefferson University Hospital, Philadelphia, Pennsylvania
Heart Transplantation

Victor F. Garcia, MD
Professor of Surgery, University of Cincinnati College of Medicine; Director of Trauma Services, Cincinnati Children's Hospital Medical Center, Cincinnati, Ohio
Genitourinary Tract Trauma; Bariatric Surgery in Adolescents

John M. Gatti, MD
Assistant Professor of Surgery and Urology, University of Missouri–Kansas City School of Medicine; Director of Minimally Invasive Urology, Children's Mercy Hospital of Kansas City, Kansas City, Missouri
Abnormalities of the Urethra, Penis, and Scrotum

Michael W. L. Gauderer, MD
Professor of Surgery and Pediatrics (Greenville), University of South Carolina School of Medicine, Columbia; Adjunct Professor of Bioengineering, Clemson University, Clemson; Chief, Division of Pediatric Surgery, Children's Hospital, Greenville Hospital System, Greenville, South Carolina
Stomas of the Small and Large Intestine

James D. Geiger, MD
Associate Professor of Surgery, University of Michigan Medical School; Staff Surgeon, C.S. Mott Children's Hospital, Ann Arbor, Michigan
Biopsy Techniques for Children with Cancer

Keith E. Georgeson, MD
Professor of Surgery, University of Alabama at Birmingham School of Medicine; Chief of Pediatric Surgery, The Children's Hospital of Alabama, Birmingham, Alabama
Gastroesophageal Reflux Disease

Cynthia A. Gingalewski, MD
Assistant Professor of Surgery and Pediatrics,
George Washington University School of Medicine and
Health Science; Pediatric Surgeon, Children's National
Medical Center, Washington, DC
Other Causes of Intestinal Obstruction

Kenneth I. Glassberg, MD
Professor of Urology, Columbia University College of
Physicians and Surgeons; Director, Division of Pediatric
Urology, Morgan Stanley Children's Hospital of
New York–Presbyterian, New York, New York
Renal Agenesis, Dysplasia, and Cystic Disease

Philip L. Glick, MD, MBA
Professor of Surgery, Pediatrics, and Obstetrics and
Gynecology, University of Buffalo School of Medicine
and Biomedical Sciences; Executive Director,
Miniature Access Surgery Center (MASC),
Women and Children's Hospital of Buffalo, Buffalo,
New York
Inguinal Hernias and Hydroceles

Sherilyn A. Gordon, MD
Assistant Professor of Surgery, Division of Liver and
Pancreas Transplantation, David Geffen School of
Medicine at UCLA, Los Angeles, California
Intestinal Transplantation

Tracy C. Grikscheit, MD
Senior Fellow in Pediatric Surgery, Children's Hospital
and Regional Medical Center and University of
Washington School of Medicine, Seattle,
Washington
The Impact of Tissue Engineering in Pediatric Surgery

Jay L. Grosfeld, MD
Lafayette Page Professor of Pediatric Surgery Emeritus,
Indiana University School of Medicine; Surgeon-
in-Chief Emeritus, Riley Hospital for Children,
Indianapolis, Indiana
*Neuroblastoma; Jejunoileal Atresia and Stenosis; Abnormalities
of the Female Genital Tract*

Angelika C. Gruessner, MS, PhD
Associate Professor of Surgical Science,
University of Minnesota Medical School, Minneapolis,
Minnesota
Pancreas and Islet Cell Transplantation

Rainer W. G. Gruessner
Professor of Surgery, University of Minnesota Medical
School, Minneapolis, Minnesota
Pancreas and Islet Cell Transplantation

Philip C. Guzzetta, Jr., MD
Professor of Surgery and Pediatrics, George Washington
University School of Medicine and Health Sciences;
Interim Chief of Pediatric Surgery, Children's National
Medical Center, Washington, DC
Nonmalignant Tumors of the Liver

Carroll M. Harmon, MD, PhD,
Associate Professor of Surgery, University of Alabama
at Birmingham School of Medicine; Attending Surgeon,
Children's Hospital, Birmingham, Alabama
Congenital Anomalies of the Esophagus

Michael R. Harrison, MD
Professor of Surgery, Pediatrics, and Obstetrics,
Gynecology, and Reproductive Sciences, University of
California, San Francisco, School of Medicine; Director,
Fetal Treatment Center, UCSF Children's Hospital and
Medical Center, San Francisco, California
The Fetus as a Patient

Andrea A. Hayes-Jordan, MD
Assistant Professor of Surgery and Pediatrics, University
of Texas Medical School at Houston and M.D.
Anderson Cancer Center; Pediatric Surgeon,
Memorial Hermann Children's Hospital and
M.D. Anderson Cancer Center, Houston, Texas
Lymph Node Disorders

Stephen R. Hays, MD, MS, FAAP
Assistant Professor of Anesthesiology and Pediatrics,
Vanderbilt University School of Medicine; Director,
Pediatric Pain Services, Vanderbilt Children's Hospital,
Nashville, Tennessee
Pediatric Anesthesia

John H. Healey, MD
Professor of Orthopaedic Surgery, Weill Medical
College of Cornell University; Chief of Orthopaedic
Surgery, Memorial Sloan-Kettering Cancer Center,
New York, New York
Bone Tumors

**W. Hardy Hendren III, MD, FACS, FAAP, FRCS
(Irel&Engl), FRCPS(Glasgow), DSc(Drexel),
MD(HonCausa) Université Aix Marseilles**
Robert E. Gross Distinguished Professor of Surgery,
Harvard Medical School; Chief of Surgery Emeritus,
Children's Hospital Boston; Honorary Surgeon,
Massachusetts General Hospital, Boston, Massachusetts
Megaureter and Prune-Belly Syndrome

Bernhard J. Hering, MD
Assistant Professor of Surgery,
University of Minnesota Medical School;
Associate Director, Diabetes Institute for
Immunology and Transplantation, University of
Minnesota Medical Center, Fairview, Minneapolis,
Minnesota
Pancreas and Islet Cell Tranplantation

David N. Herndon, MD
Professor of Surgery and Pediatrics and Jesse H. Jones
Distinguished Chair in Burn Surgery, University of
Texas Medical Branch School of Medicine at Galveston;
Chief of Staff and Director of Research, Shriners Burns
Hospital, Galveston, Texas
Burns

Ronald B. Hirschl, MD
Professor of Surgery, University of Michigan Medical
School; Head, Section of Pediatric Surgery, and
Surgeon-in-Chief, C.S. Mott Children's Hospital,
Ann Arbor, Michigan
Extracorporeal Life Support for Cardiopulmonary Failure

George W. Holcomb III, MD, MBA
Katharine Berry Richardson Professor of Surgery,
University of Missouri–Kansas City School of Medicine;
Surgeon-in-Chief, Children's Mercy Hospital,
Kansas City, Missouri
Gallbladder Disease amd Hepatic Infections

Charles B. Huddleston, MD
Professor of Surgery, Washington University in St. Louis
School of Medicine; Chief, Pediatric Cardiothoracic
Surgery, and Surgical Director, Lung Transplant
Program, St. Louis Children's Hospital, St. Louis, Missouri
Lung Transplantation

Raymond J. Hutchinson, MS, MD
Professor of Pediatrics, University of Michigan
Medical School; Director of Clinical Services,
Pediatric Hematology/Oncology, C.S. Mott
Children's Hospital, Ann Arbor, Michigan
Surgical Implications of Hematologic Disease

**John M. Hutson, MD(Monash), MD(Melb),
FRACS, FAAP(Hon)**
Professor of Pediatric Surgery, Department of
Pediatrics, University of Melbourne Faculty of
Medicine, Melbourne; Director of General Surgery,
Royal Children's Hospital, Parkville, Victoria, Australia
Undescended Testis, Torsion, and Varicocele

Thomas Inge, MD, PhD
Associate Professor of Surgery and Pediatrics, University
of Cincinnati College of Medicine; Surgical Director,
Comprehensive Weight Management Program, Cincinnati
Children's Hospital Medical Center, Cincinnati
Bariatric Surgery in Adolescents

Vincenzo Jasonni, MD
Professor of Pediatric Surgery, University of Genoa
Medical School; Surgeon-in-Chief and Chair of Pediatric
Surgery, Gaslini Children's Hospital, Genoa, Italy
*Hirschsprung's Disease and Related Neuromuscular Disorders
of the Intestine*

Nishwan Jibri, MD
Department of Pediatric Surgery, Gaslini Children's
Hospital, Genoa, Italy
*Hirschsprung's Disease and Related Neuromuscular Disorders
of the Intestine*

Byron D. Joyner, MD
Associate Professor of Urology, University of
Washington School of Medicine; Residency Director,
University of Washington Urology Program, and
Faculty/Staff, Children's Hospital and Regional Medical
Center, Seattle, Washington
Ureteropelvic Junction Obstruction

Martin Kaefer, MD
Associate Professor, Department of Urology,
Indiana University School of Medicine; Pediatric
Urologist, Riley Children's Hospital, Indianapolis,
Indiana
Disorders of Bladder Function

Henry K. Kawamoto, Jr., MD, DDS
Clinical Professor of Surgery, Department of
Surgery, Division of Plastic Surgery, David Geffen
School of Medicine at UCLA; Director,
Craniofacial Surgery, UCLA Medical Center,
Los Angeles, California
Craniofacial Anomalies

Robert M. Kay, MD
Associate Professor of Orthopedic Surgery,
Keck School of Medicine of USC; Orthopedic Surgeon,
Children's Hospital Los Angeles, Los Angeles,
California
Bone and Joint Infections

Kosmas Kayes, MD
Staff Surgeon, Riley Hospital for
Children and St. Vincent
Children's Hospital,
Indianapolis, Indiana
Major Congenital Orthopedic Deformities

Mark L. Kayton, MD
Assistant Member, Memorial Sloan-Kettering Cancer
Center; Assistant Attending Surgeon, Division of
Pediatric Surgery, Memorial Hospital, New York,
New York
*Surgical Implications Associated with Bone Marrow
Transplantation*

Robert E. Kelly, Jr., MD, FACS, FAAP
Associate Professor of Clinical Surgery and Pediatrics,
Eastern Virginia Medical School, Children's Hospital of
the King's Daughters, Norfolk, Virginia
The Nuss Procedure for Pectus Excavatum [Chapter 59]

Stephen S. Kim, MD
Assistant Professor of Surgery, University of Washington
School of Medicine; Attending, Division of Pediatric
Surgery, Children's Hospital and Regional Medical
Center, Seattle, Washington
Necrotizing Enterocolitis

Michael D. Klein, MD
Arvin I. Philippart Chair and Professor of Surgery,
Wayne State University School of Medicine;
Surgeon-in-Chief, Children's Hospital of Michigan,
Detroit, Michigan
Congenital Defects of the Abdominal Wall

Giannoula Klement, MD
Instructor in Pediatrics (Hematology-Oncology),
Harvard University Medical School; Assistant in
Pediatrics, Children's Hospital Boston, Boston,
Massachusetts
Vascular Anomalies: Hemangiomas and Malformations

Matthew J. Krasin, MD
Assistant Member and Radiation Oncologist, St. Jude
Children's Research Hospital, Memphis, Tennessee
*Principles of Pediatric Oncology, Genetics of Cancer,
and Radiation Therapy*

Thomas M. Krummel, MD, FACS
Professor in Surgery, Stanford University School of
Medicine; Service Chief, Surgery, Stanford Hospital &
Clinics, Stanford; Susan B. Ford Surgeon-in-Chief,
Lucile Packard Children's Hospital at Stanford,
Palo Alto, California
New and Emerging Surgical Technologies and the Process of Innovation

Jean-Martin Laberge, MD, FRCSC, FACS
Professor of Surgery, McGill University Faculty of
Medicine; Director, Division of Pediatric General
Surgery, The Montreal Children's Hospital,
Montreal, Quebec, Canada
Infections and Diseases of the Lungs, Pleura, and Mediastinum

Ira S. Landsman, MD
Associate Professor of Anesthesiology and Pediatrics,
Vanderbilt University School of Medicine; Director,
Division of Pediatric Anesthesia, Vanderbilt Children's
Hospital, Nashville, Tennessee
Pediatric Anesthesia

Michael P. La Quaglia, MD
Professor of Surgery, Weill Medical College of Cornell
University; Chief, Pediatric Surgical Service, Memorial
Sloan-Kettering Cancer Center, New York, New York
Hodgkin's Disease and Non-Hodgkin's Lymphoma

Stanley T. Lau, MD
Pediatric Surgery Fellow, Women and Children's
Hospital of Buffalo, Buffalo, New York
Adrenal Tumors

Steven L. Lee, MD
Regional Pediatric Surgeon, Kaiser Permanente,
Los Angeles Medical Center, Los Angeles, California
Duodenal Atresia and Stenosis—Annular Pancreas

Joseph L. Lelli, Jr., MD
Assistant Professor of Surgery, Wayne State Medical
School; Pediatric Surgeon, The Children's Hospital of
Michigan, Detroit, Michigan
Polypoid Diseases of the Gastrointestinal Tract

Marc A. Levitt, MD
Assistant Professor of Surgery and Pediatrics, University
of Cincinnati College of Medicine; Associate Director,
Colorectal Center for Children, Cincinnati Children's
Hospital Medical Center, Cincinnati, Ohio
Anorectal Malformations

Harry Lindahl, MD, PhD
Lecturer in Pediatrics, University of Helsinki School of
Medicine; Chief of Pediatric Surgery, Hospital for
Children and Adolescents, Helsinki; University Central
Hospital, Helsinki, Finland
Esophagoscopy and Diagnostic Techniques

Thom E. Lobe, MD
Professor of Surgery and Pediatrics, University of
Tennessee School of Medicine, Memphis, Tennessee;
Pediatric Surgeon, Blank Children's Hospital,
Des Moines, Iowa
Other Soft Tissue Tumors

Randall T. Loder, MD
Garceau Professor of Orthopaedic Surgery, Indiana
University School of Medicine; Director of Pediatric
Orthopaedics, Riley Hospital for Children,
Indianapolis, Indiana
Amputations in Children

Thomas G. Luerssen, MD
Professor of Neurological Surgery, Indiana University
School of Medicine; Chief, Pediatric Neurosurgery
Service, Riley Hospital for Children, Indianapolis,
Indiana
Central Nervous System Injuries

Jeffrey R. Lukish, MD
Associate Professor of Surgery and Pediatrics,
Uniformed Services University of the Health Sciences
F. Edward Hébert School of Medicine, Bethesda,
Maryland; Chief, Division of Pediatric Surgery, and
Attending Pediatric Surgeon, The National Naval
Medical Center and Walter Reed Army Medical Center,
Washington, DC
Accident Victims and Their Emergency Management

Dennis P. Lund, MD
Chairman, Division of General Surgery,
University of Wisconsin-Madison, and Surgeon-in-Chief,
UW Children's Hospital, Madison, Wisconsin
Alimentary Tract Duplications

Mary Beth Madonna, MD
Assistant Professor of Surgery, Northwestern University
Feinberg School of Medicine; Attending Surgeon,
Children's Memorial Hospital and John H. Stroger,
Jr. Hospital of Cook County, Chicago, Illinois
Gastrointestinal Bleeding

John C. Magee, MD
Associate Professor of Surgery, University of Michigan
Medical School; Director, Adult and Pediatric Renal
Transplantation, and Director, Pediatric Liver
Transplantation, University of Michigan Health System,
Ann Arbor, Michigan
Renal Transplantation

Giuseppe Martucciello, MD
Associate Professor of Pediatric Surgery,
Faculty of Medicine, University of Genoa, Genoa,
and University of Pavia, Pavia; Director, and
Surgeon-in-Chief, Department of Pediatric Surgery,
IRCCS Scientific Institute Policlinico San Matteo,
Pavia, Italy
*Hirschsprung's Disease and Related Neuromuscular Disorders of the
Intestine*

Stephen J. Mathes, MD
Professor of Surgery and Head, Division of Plastic and Reconstructive Surgery, University of California, San Francisco, School of Medicine, San Francisco, California
Congenital Defects of the Skin, Connective Tissues, Muscles, Tendons, and Hands

Eugene D. McGahren III, MD
Associate Professor of Surgery and Pediatrics, University of Virginia School of Medicine; Pediatric Surgeon, University of Virginia Health System, Charlottesville, Virginia
Laryngoscopy, Bronchoscopy, and Thoracoscopy; Ascites

Leslie T. McQuiston, MD, FAAP
Staff Pediatric Urologist, Urology Associates of North Texas, Cook Children's Hospital, Fort Worth, Texas
Renal Infection, Abscess, Vesicoureteral Reflux, Urinary Lithiasis, and Renal Vein Thrombosis

Peter Metcalfe, MD, FRCSC
Pediatric Urology Fellow, Indiana University School of Medicine and Riley Hospital for Children, Indianapolis, Indiana
Incontinent and Continent Urinary Diversion

Alastair J. W. Millar, MBChB(Cape Town), FRCS, FRACS, FCS(SA), DCh
Honorary Professor, Paediatric Transplantation and Hepatopancreaticobiliary Surgery, University of Birmingham; Consultant, Paediatric Liver and Intestinal Transplantation and Hepatopancreaticobiliary Surgery, Birmingham Children's Hospital, Birmingham, United Kingdom
Caustic Strictures of the Esophagus

Eugene Minevich, MD, FACS, FAAP
Assistant Professor of Surgery, Cincinnati Children's Hospital Medical Center, Cincinnati, Ohio
Structural Disorders of the Bladder, Augmentation

Edward P. Miranda, MD
Professor of Surgery, Division of Plastic Surgery, University of California, San Francisco, School of Medicine, San Francisco, California
Congenital Defects of the Skin, Connective Tissues, Muscles, Tendons, and Hands

Michael E. Mitchell, MD
Professor of Urology, University of Washington School of Medicine; Chief, Pediatric Urology, Children's Hospital and Regional Medical Center, Seattle, Washington
Ureteropelvic Junction Obstruction

Takeshi Miyano, MD, PhD
Professor, Department of Pediatric Surgery, Juntendo University School of Medicine; Director, Juntendo University Hospital, Tokyo, Japan
The Pancreas

Delora Mount, MD, FACS, FAAP
Assistant Professor of Surgery and Pediatrics, University of Wisconsin School of Medicine and Public Health; Chief of Pediatric Plastic Surgery, University of Wisconsin Hospital and Clinics; Director, Craniofacial Anomalies Clinic, American Family Children's Hospital, Madison, Wisconsin
Hand, Soft Tissue, and Envenomation Injuries

Pierre Mouriquand, MD
Professor of Pediatric Urology, Claude-Bernard University Medical School; Head, Department of Pediatric Urology, Debrousse Hospital, Lyon, France
Renal Fusions and Ectopia

Noriko Murase, MD
Associate Professor of Surgery, University of Pittsburgh School of Medicine, Pittsburgh, Pennsylvania
Principles of Transplantation

J. Patrick Murphy, MD
Professor of Surgery, University of Missouri–Kansas City School of Medicine; Chief, Urology Section, Children's Mercy Hospital of Kansas City, Kansas City, Missouri
Abnormalities of the Urethra, Penis, and Scrotum

Saminathan S. Nathan, MD
Director, Musculoskeletal Oncology Service, Department of Orthopaedics, National University Hospital, Singapore, Singapore
Bone Tumors

Kurt D. Newman, MD
Professor of Surgery and Pediatrics, George Washington University School of Medicine and Health Sciences; Surgeon-in-Chief, Children's National Medical Center; Executive Director, Joseph E. Robert, Jr. Center for Surgical Care, Washington, DC
Lymph Node Disorders

Alp Numanoglu, MD, FCS(SA)
Senior Lecturer in Paediatric Surgery, University of Cape Town School of Child and Adolescent Health; Senior Specialist, Department of Paediatric Surgery, Red Cross Children's Hospital, Institute of Child Health, Cape Town, South Africa
Caustic Strictures of the Esophagus

Donald Nuss, MB, ChB, FRCS(C), FACS, FAAP
Professor of Clinical Surgery and Pediatrics, Eastern Virginia Medical School; Children's Hospital of the King's Daughters, Norfolk, Virginia
The Nuss Procedure for Pectus Excavatum [Chapter 59]

Richard Ohye, MD
Assistant Professor of Surgery, University of Michigan Medical School; Surgical Director, Pediatric Cardiac Transplantation, and Director, Pediatric Cardiovascular Surgery Fellowship Program, C.S. Mott Children's Hospital, Ann Arbor, Michigan
Congenital Heart Disease and Anomalies of the Great Vessels

Keith T. Oldham, MD
Professor of Surgery, Medical College of Wisconsin;
Surgeon-in-Chief, Children's Hospital of Wisconsin,
Milwaukee, Wisconsin
Atresia, Stenosis, and Other Obstructions of the Colon

James A. O'Neill, Jr., MD, MA(Hon)
J.C. Foshee Professor and Chairman Emeritus,
Section of Surgical Sciences, Vanderbilt University
School of Medicine; Surgeon-in-Chief Emeritus,
Vanderbilt University Medical Center, Nashville,
Tennessee
*Choledochal Cyst; Bladder and Cloacal Exstrophy; Conjoined Twins;
Arterial Disorders*

Evelyn Ong, MBBS, BSc, FRCS(Eng)
Joint Royal College of Surgeons of England/British
Association of Paediatric Surgeons Research Fellow;
Department of Paediatric Surgery, Institute of Child
Health, University College London; Clinical Research
Fellow, Great Ormond Street Hospital for Children
NHS Trust, London, United Kingdom
Neonatal Physiology and Metabolic Considerations

William L. Oppenheim, MD
Professor of Orthopedic Surgery, David Geffen School
of Medicine at UCLA; Director of Pediatric
Orthopedics, UCLA Medical Center; Consultant,
Shriners Hospital of Los Angeles, Los Angeles,
California
Bone and Joint Infections

H. Biemann Othersen, Jr., MD
Professor of Surgery and Pediatrics and Emeritus Head,
Division of Pediatric Surgery, Medical University of
South Carolina College of Medicine; Attending Surgeon,
MUSC Children's Hospital, Charleston, South Carolina
Wilms' Tumor

Mikki Pakarinen, MD, PhD
Consultant Pediatric Surgeon, Hospital for Children
and Adolescents, University of Helsinki Medical Faculty,
Helsinki, Finland
Other Disorders of the Anus and Rectum, Anorectal Function

Keshav Pandurangi, MD
Vascular Surgery Fellow, Indiana University
School of Medicine, Indianapolis, Indiana
Venous Disorders in Childhood

Richard H. Pearl, MD, FACS, FAAP, FRCSC
Professor of Surgery and Pediatrics, University of
Illinois College of Medicine at Peoria; Surgeon-in-Chief,
Children's Hospital of Illinois, Peoria, Illinois
Abdominal Trauma

Alberto Peña, MD
Professor of Surgery and Pediatrics, University of
Cincinnati College of Medicine; Director, Colorectal
Center for Children, Cincinnati Children's Hospital
Medical Center, Cincinnati, Ohio
Anorectal Malformations

Rafael V. Pieretti, MD
Chief, Section of Pediatric Urology,
Department of Pediatric Surgery,
Massachusetts General Hospital, Boston, Massachusetts
Ambiguous Genitalia

Agostino Pierro, MD, FRCS(Eng), FRCS(Ed), FAAP
Nuffield Professor of Paediatric Surgery and Head of
Surgery Unit, Institute of Child Health, University
College London; Consultant Paediatric Surgeon, Great
Ormond Street Hospital for Children NHS Trust,
London, United Kingdom
Neonatal Physiology and Metabolic Considerations

William P. Potsic, MD, MMM
Professor of Otorhinolaryngology–Head and Neck
Surgery, University of Pennsylvania School of Medicine;
Director, Division of Otolaryngology, and Vice Chair for
Clinical Affairs, The Children's Hospital of
Philadelphia, Philadelphia, Pennsylvania
Otolaryngologic Disorders

Pramod S. Puligandla, MD, MSc, FRCSC
Assistant Professor of Surgery and Pediatrics,
McGill University Faculty of Medicine; Attending Staff,
Division of Pediatric Surgery and Pediatric Critical Care
Medicine, The Montreal Children's Hospital of the
McGill University Health Center, Montreal,
Quebec, Canada
Infections and Diseases of the Lungs, Pleura, and Medistinum

Devin P. Puapong, MD
Senior Surgical Resident, Kaiser Permanente Medical
Center, Los Angeles, California
Duodenal Atresia and Stenosis—Annular Pancreas

Prem Puri, MS, FRCS, FRCS(Edin), FACS
Professor of Paediatrics, University College Dublin;
Consultant Paediatric Surgeon and Director of
Research, Children's Research Centre, Our Lady's
Hospital for Sick Children, Crumlin, Dublin, Ireland
Intestinal Neuronal Dysplasia

Judson G. Randolph, MD
Professor of Surgery Emeritus, George Washington
University School of Medicine and Health Sciences;
Former Surgeon-in-Chief, Children's National Medical
Center, Washington, DC
A Brief History of Pediatric Surgery

Frederick J. Rescorla, MD
Professor of Surgery, Indiana University School of
Medicine; Surgeon-in-Chief, Riley Hospital for
Children, Indianapolis, Indiana
The Spleen

Jorge Reyes, MD
Professor of Surgery, University of Washington School
of Medicine; Chief, Division of Transplant Surgery,
University of Washington Medical Center,
Seattle, Washington
Principles of Transplantation

Richard R. Ricketts, MD
Professor of Surgery, Emory University School of
Medicine; Chief, Division of Pediatric Surgery,
Children's Health Care of Atlanta at Egleston,
Atlanta, Georgia
Mesenteric and Omental Cysts

Richard C. Rink, MD
Robert A. Garrett Professor of Pediatric Urologic
Research and Professor of Urology, Indiana University
School of Medicine; Chief, Pediatric Urology,
Riley Hospital for Children, Indianapolis, Indiana
Incontinent and Continent Urinary Diversion

Risto J. Rintala, MD
Professor of Pediatric Surgery, University of Helsinki
Medical Faculty; Chief, General Pediatric Surgery,
Hospital for Children and Adolescents, Helsinki,
Finland
Other Disorders of the Anus and Rectum, Anorectal Function

Albert P. Rocchini, MD
Professor of Pediatrics and Director of Pediatrics
Cardiology, University of Michigan Redical School;
Director of Pediatric Cardiology, University of Michigan
Hospital, Ann Arbor
Neonatal Cardiovascular Physiology and Care

Heinz Rode, M Med(Chir), FCS(SA), FRCS(Edin)
Professor of Paediatric Surgery, University of Cape
Town School of Child and Adolescent Health;
Head of Pediatric Surgery, Red Cross Children's
Hospital, Institute of Child Health, Cape Town,
South Africa
Caustic Strictures of the Esophagus

Bradley M. Rodgers, MD
Professor of Surgery and Pediatrics, University of
Virginia School of Medicine; Chief, Division of
Pediatric Surgery, Department of Surgery, University
of Virginia Medical Center; Chief, Children's Surgery,
UVA Children's Hospital, Charlottesville, Virginia
Laryngoscopy, Bronchoscopy, and Thoracoscopy

A. Michael Sadove MD, MS
James Harbaugh Professor of Surgery (Plastic),
Indiana University School of Medicine;
Chief of Plastic Surgery, Riley Hospital for Children,
Indianapolis; Chairman of Surgery, Clarian North
Medical Center, Carmel, Indiana
Cleft Lip and Palate

Bob H. Saggi, MD
Assistant Professor of Surgery, Department of Surgery,
Division of Immunology and Organ Transplantation,
University of Texas Medical School at Houston;
Staff Surgeon, Memorial Hermann Hospital,
Houston, Texas
Liver Transplantation

Arthur P. Sanford, MD
Assistant Professor of Surgery, The University of
Texas Medical Branch School of Medicine at Galveston;
Staff Physician, Shriners Burns Hospital,
Galveston, Texas
Burns

L. R. Scherer III, MD
Associate Professor of Clinical Medicine, Indiana
University School of Medicine; Director of Trauma,
Riley Hospital for Children, Indianapolis,
Indiana
Peptic Ulcer and Other Conditions of the Stomach

Jay J. Schnitzer, MD, PhD
Associate Professor of Surgery,
Harvard Medical School; Associate Visiting Surgeon,
Massachusetts General Hospital, Boston, Massachusetts
Ambiguous Genitalia

Marshall Z. Schwartz, MD
Professor of Surgery and Pediatrics, Drexel University
College of Medicine; Director, Pediatric Surgery
Research Laboratory, and Surgical Director,
Pediatric Renal Transplantation, St. Christopher's
Hospital for Children, Philadelphia, Pennsylvania
Hypertrophic Pyloric Stenosis

Robert C. Shamberger, MD
Robert E. Gross Professor of Surgery, Harvard Medical
School; Chief, Department of Surgery, Children's
Hospital Boston, Boston, Massachusetts
Congenital Chest Wall Deformities

Nina L. Shapiro, MD
Associate Professor of Surgery/Pediatric
Otolaryngology, David Geffen School of Medicine at
UCLA; Attending Surgeon, UCLA Medical Center,
Los Angeles, California
Salivary Glands

Curtis A. Sheldon, MD
Professor, University of Cincinnati College of Medicine;
Professor and Director (Pediatric Urology),
Cincinnati Children's Hospital Medical Center,
Cincinnati, Ohio
Structural Disorders of the Bladder, Augmentation

Stephen J. Shochat, MD
Professor of Surgery and Pediatrics, University of
Tennessee School of Medicine; Surgeon-in-Chief and
Chairman, Department of Surgery, St. Jude Children's
Research Hospital, Memphis, Tennessee
Tumors of the Lung

Michael A. Skinner, MD
Associate Professor of Surgery and Pediatric Surgery,
Duke University School of Medicine, Durham,
North Carolina
Surgical Diseases of the Thyroid and Parathyroid Glands

C. D. Smith, MD, MS
Associate Professor of Surgery and Pediatrics,
Medical University of South Carolina College of
Medicine; Attending, Division of Pediatric Surgery,
MUSC Medical Center, Charleston, South Carolina
Cysts and Sinuses of the Neck

Jodi L. Smith, MD, PhD
Assistant Professor of Neurological Surgery,
Department of Neurological Surgery, Indiana University
School of Medicine; Pediatric Neurosurgeon,
Riley Hospital for Children, Indianapolis,
Indiana
*Management of Neural Tube Defects, Hydrocephalus,
Refractory Epilepsy, and Central Nervous System Infections*

Samuel D. Smith, MD
Professor of Surgery, University of Arkansas for
Medical Sciences College of Medicine; Chief of
Pediatric Surgery, Arkansas Children's Hospital,
Little Rock, Arkansas
Disorders of Intestinal Rotation and Fixation

Charles L. Snyder, MD
Associate Professor of Surgery, University of
Missouri–Kansas City School of Medicine,
Kansas City, Missouri; Clinical Assistant Professor of
Surgery, University of Kansas School of Medicine,
Kansas City, Kansas; Director of Clinical Research,
The Children's Mercy Hospital, Kansas City,
Missouri
Meckel's Diverticulum

**Lewis Spitz, MBChB, MD(Hon), PhD, FRCS, FRCPCH,
FAAP(Hon), FCS(SA)(Hon)**
Emeritus Nuffield Professor of Pediatric Surgery,
Institute of Child Health, University College London;
Consultant Paediatric Surgeon, Great Ormond Street
Hospital, London, United Kingdom
Esophageal Replacement

Thomas L. Spray, MD
Professor of Surgery, University of Pennsylvania School
of Medicine; Chief, Division of Cardiothoracic Surgery,
and Alice Langdon Warner Endowed Chair in Pediatric
Cardiothoracic Surgery, The Children's Hospital of
Philadelphia, Philadelphia, Pennsylvania
Heart Transplantation

Thomas E. Starzl, MD, PhD
Distinguished Service Professor of Surgery,
University of Pittsburgh School of Medicine;
Director Emeritus, Thomas E. Starzl Transplantation
Institute, Pittsburgh, Pennsylvania
Principles of Transplantation

Charles J. H. Stolar, MD
Professor of Surgery and Pediatrics, Columbia
University College of Physicians and Surgeons; Chief,
Pediatric Surgery, Morgan Stanley Children's Hospital
of New York–Presbyterian, New York, New York
Congenital Diaphragmatic Hernia and Eventration

Phillip B. Storm, MD
Assistant Professor of Neurosurgery, University of
Pennsylvania School of Medicine; Attending
Neurosurgeon, Hospital of the University of
Pennsylvania and The Children's Hospital of
Philadelphia, Philadelphia, Pennsylvania
Brain Tumors

Steven Stylianos, MD
Professor of Surgery, University of Miami Leonard
M. Miller School of Medicine; Chief, Department of
Pediatric Surgery, Miami Children's Hospital,
Miami, Florida
Abdominal Trauma

Wendy T. Su, MD
Fellow, Pediatric Surgical Service, Memorial
Sloan-Kettering Cancer Center, New York, New York
Hodgkin's Disease and Non-Hodgkin's Lymphoma

Riccardo Superina, MD, CM, FRCSC, FACS
Professor of Surgery, Northwestern University,
Director, Transplant Surgery, Children's Memorial
Hospital, Chicago, Illinois
Portal Hypertension

David E. R. Sutherland, MD, PhD
Professor of Surgery, University of Minnesota Medical
School; Head, Transplant Division, and Director,
Diabetes Institute for Immunology and Transplantation,
University of Minnesota Medical Center, Fairview,
Minneapolis, Minnesota
Pancreas and Islet Cell Transplantation

Leslie N. Sutton, MD
Professor of Neurosurgery, University of Pennsylvania
School of Medicine; Chairman, Division of Pediatric
Neurosurgery, The Children's Hospital of Philadelphia,
Philadelphia, Pennsylvania
Brain Tumors

Edward P. Tagge, MD
Professor of Surgery and Pediatrics, Division of
Pediatric Surgery, Medical University of South Carolina
College of Medicine; Attending Surgeon, MUSC
Children's Hospital, Charleston, South Carolina
Wilms' Tumor

Daniel H. Teitelbaum, MD
Professor of Surgery, University of Michigan Medical
School; Pediatric Surgeon, C.S. Mott Children's
Hospital, Ann Arbor, Michigan
*Nutritional Support; Hirschsprung's Disease and Related
Neuromuscular Disorders of the Intestine*

Claire L. Templeman, MD
Assistant Professor of Clinical Gynecology and Surgery,
Keck School of Medicine at USC; Pediatric Surgeon,
Children's Hospital Los Angeles, Los Angeles,
California
Ovarian Tumors

Gonca Topuzlu Tekant, MD
Associate Professor of Pediatric Surgery,
Istanbul University School of Medicine;
Pediatric Surgeon, Cerrahpasa Medical Faculty,
Istanbul, Turkey
Gastroesophageal Reflux Disease

Joseph J. Tepas III, MD
Professor of Surgery and Pediatrics, University of
Florida College of Medicine;
Staff Physician, Shands Jacksonville,
Jacksonville, Florida
Vascular Injuries

Patrick B. Thomas, MD
Pediatric Surgery Fellow, Texas Children's Hospital,
Baylor College of Medicine, Houston, Texas
Wilms' Tumor

Dana Mara Thompson, MD, MS
Associate Professor of Otorhinolaryngology,
Mayo Graduate School of Medicine;
Attending, Otorhinolaryngology Department,
Mayo Clinic, Rochester, Minnesota
Lesions of the Larynx, Trachea, and Upper Airway

Juan A. Tovar, MD, PhD
Professor of Surgical Pediatrics, Department of
Pediatrics, Universidad Autonoma de Madrid;
Head, Department of Pediatric Surgery,
Hospital Universitario LaPaz, Madrid, Spain
Disorders of Esophageal Function

Jeffrey S. Upperman, MD, MA
Assistant Professor of Surgery, Keck School of
Medicine of USC; Attending Surgeon, Children's
Hospital Los Angeles, Los Angeles, California
Sepsis and Related Considerations

Joseph P. Vacanti, MD
John Homans Professor of Surgery, Harvard Medical
School; Chief, Pediatric Surgery, Massachusetts
General Hospital, Boston, Massachusetts
The Impact of Tissue Engineering in Pediatric Surgery

Dennis W. Vane, MD, MS, MBA
Professor of Surgery, University of Vermont College
of Medicine; Chair, Pediatric Surgery, and Vice-Chair,
Clinical Affairs, Department of Surgery,
Fletcher Allen Health Care, Burlington,
Vermont
Child Abuse and Birth Injuries

Mirjana Vustar, MD
Assistant Professor of Anesthesiology and Pediatrics,
Vanderbilt University School of Medicine; Director,
Pediatric Anesthesia Education, Vanderbilt Children's
Hospital, Nashville, Tennessee
Pediatric Anesthesia

Brad W. Warner, MD
Professor of Surgery and Pediatrics, University of
Cincinnati College of Medicine; Attending Surgeon and
Director of Surgical Research, Division of Pediatric
General and Thoracic Surgery, Cincinnati Children's
Hospital Medical Center, Cincinnati, Ohio
Short-Bowel Syndrome

Thomas R. Weber, MD
Professor of Surgery, Saint Louis University School
of Medicine; Director, Pediatric Surgery, Cardinal
Glennon Children's Hospital, St. Louis, Missouri
Esophageal Rupture and Perforation

David E. Wesson, MD
Professor of Surgery and Chief, Division of Pediatric
Surgery, Baylor College of Medicine; Chief,
Pediatric Surgery Service, Texas Children's
Hospital, Houston, Texas
Thoracic Injuries

Karen W. West, MD
Professor of Surgery, Indiana University School of
Medicine; Director of ECMO, Riley Hospital for
Children, Indianapolis, Indiana
Primary Peritonitis

Ralph F. Wetmore, MD
Professor of Otorhinolaryngology–Head and Neck
Surgery, University of Pennsylvania School of Medicine;
Senior Surgeon, The Children's Hospital of
Philadelphia, Philadelphia, Pennsylvania
Otolaryngologic Disorders

Eugene Wiener, MD
Professor, Department of Surgery (Pediatric), University
of Pittsburgh School of Medicine; Executive
Vice President and Chief Medical Officer, Children's
Hospital of Pittsburgh, Pittsburgh, Pennsylvania
Testicular Tumors

Jay M. Wilson, MD
Associate Professor of Surgery, Harvard
Medical School; Attending, Children's Hospital Boston,
Boston, Massachusetts
Respiratory Physiology and Care

Russell K. Woo, MD
Instructor in Surgery, Department of Surgery,
Stanford University School of Medicine;
Staff Physician, Stanford Hospital and Clinic, Stanford,
and Lucile Packard Children's Hospital at Stanford,
Palo Alto, California
*New and Emerging Surgical Technologies and
the Process of Innovation*

Hsi-Yang Wu, MD
Assistant Professor of Urology, University of Pittsburgh
School of Medicine; Director of Pediatric Urology
Research, Children's Hospital of Pittsburgh,
Pittsburgh, Pennsylvania
Testicular Tumors

Elizabeth Yerkes, MD
Assistant Professor of Urology,
Feinberg School of Medicine at Northwestern
University; Attending Urologist, Children's Memorial
Hospital, Chicago, Illinois
Incontinent and Continent Urinary Diversion

Daniel G. Young, MBChB, FRCS(Edin, Glasg), DTM&H
Honorary Senior Research Fellow, University of
Glasgow; Former Head (Retired), Department of
Surgical Pediatrics, Royal Hospital for Sick Children,
Glasgow, United Kingdom
A Brief History of Pediatric Surgery

Moritz M. Ziegler, MD
Professor of Surgery, Division of Pediatric Surgery,
University of Colorado School of Medicine;
Surgeon-in-Chief, The Children's Hospital, Denver,
Colorado
Meconium Ileus

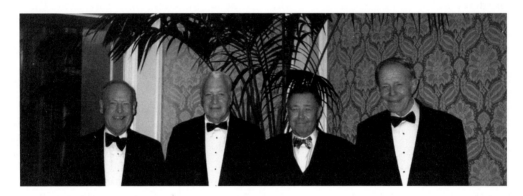

The senior editors (from left to right): James A. O'Neill, Jr., Jay L. Grosfeld, Arnold G. Coran, and Eric W. Fonkalsrud.

Preface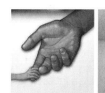

The first edition of **Pediatric Surgery** was published by Year Book Medical Publishers in 1962, with Drs. Kenneth Welch, William Mustard, Mark Ravitch, Clifford Benson, and William Snyder serving as the initial Editorial Board. The project was conceived to meet the need for a comprehensive work on pediatric surgery, with the heaviest concentration focused in the traditional fields of general, thoracic, and urologic surgery. Numerous contributors participated in the development of this new textbook that would for the next 44 years be known worldwide as the leading comprehensive resource in the field of children's surgery. Four additional editions of the textbook have been published since that time.

It has been 8 years since the fifth edition of the book was published in 1998. In the interim, we have experienced a veritable explosion of new scientific information, characterized by the elucidation of the human genome, development of tissue engineering, and introduction of other new technologies that have clearly impacted methods of diagnosis and how we treat our patients.

The sixth edition has an international flair and contains 133 chapters prepared by contributors from the United States, Canada, Europe, Asia, Australia, New Zealand, and Africa. It was the intent of the editors to include expert contributors with a significant or unique experience in their respective areas of interest so that all of the chapters would comply with the goal of providing current and practical information that was very well referenced in a modern comprehensive and authoritative text. A significant number of new authors and coauthors participated in this effort. Among the new contributions is a chapter concerning the history of pediatric surgery, providing a brief background of the origins of our profession in the United Kingdom, United States, and Asia. Other new chapters include material on molecular clinical genetics and gene therapy, the impact of tissue engineering in pediatric surgery, new and emerging technologies in surgical science, principles of pediatric oncology/genetics and radiation therapy, small bowel transplantation, and adolescent bariatric surgery.

All the other chapters were significantly changed, updated, and often expanded with the addition of numerous recent references. Some examples include the current status of the fetus as a patient; congenital chest wall deformities, which now includes up-to-date information on the Nuss procedure; pediatric anesthesia; ethical and legal considerations; the genetics of Hirschsprung disease; new information on short bowel syndrome (i.e., the Step procedure); and the inclusion of minimally invasive surgical techniques (laparoscopy, thoracoscopy) embedded within each chapter where appropriate.

Other major revisions and updated material are included. In Part I: neonatal physiology and metabolic considerations, respiratory physiology and care, neonatal cardiovascular physiology and care, extracorporeal life support and cardiopulmonary failure, sepsis and related conditions, hematologic disorders, and nutrition; Part II: trauma (including burn care); Part III: major tumors of childhood; Part IV: organ transplantation (liver, lung, heart, pancreas, kidney, and surgical implications of bone marrow transplantation), which was also reorganized and updated with the new protocols and information regarding contemporary care techniques and outcomes; Part V: conditions affecting the head and neck; Part VI: thoracic conditions (including esophageal atresia and tracheo-esophageal fistula, along with various other esophageal conditions, lung cysts, congenital diaphragmatic hernia, and others); Part VII: a very wide spectrum of common congenital and acquired abdominal conditions (including hernias, abdominal wall defects, intestinal atresia, meconium ileus, Hirschsprung's disease, anorectal malformations, duplications, inflammatory bowel disease, biliary atresia, choledochal cyst, pancreatic conditions, spleen, portal hypertension and others); Part VIII: genitourinary disorders; and Part IX: special areas of pediatric surgery (conjoined twins, congenital heart disease, hand and soft tissue, orthopedic, neurologic, and vascular disorders). Many of the chapters are well illustrated and enhanced with the use of charts, tables, radiographic images, photographs of gross pathology and histology, and operative techniques.

The Editorial Board for the sixth edition is composed of Drs. Jay L. Grosfeld, James A. O'Neill, Jr., Eric W. Fonkalsrud, and Arnold G. Coran. All four were members of the editorial group for the fifth edition. The initial editorial responsibility for chapter assignments was evenly distributed among the four senior editors. We are grateful to Dr. Anthony A. Caldamone, who ably served as the section editor for Part VIII, genitourinary disorders. Dr. Grosfeld served as chairman of the board and, as lead editor, was the final reviewer of the entire manuscript. We are indebted to the editors who preceded us in the prior five editions who set the standard that we have tried to uphold for the sixth edition of *Pediatric Surgery*.

The editors wish to thank our administrative assistants and secretaries Karen Jaeger, Donna Bock, Gale Fielding, Cheryl Peterson, and Carol Simmons, who in addition to their usual responsibilities, were willing to support us in completing this effort. We recognize this would not have been accomplished without them and appreciate their many contributions. We also express our sincere appreciation and thanks to many contributors from around the world who have played an important role in the preparation of the sixth edition. We are grateful for their willingness to share their knowledge and expertise and for complying with the specified format of the textbook in a timely manner that allowed us to meet production deadlines.

We are also grateful to the Elsevier/Mosby publishing staff for their support and cooperation in maintaining a high standard in the development and preparation of the sixth edition. We wish to recognize Ms. Janice Gaillard, Senior Developmental Editor, and Faith Voit, Freelance Editor, who prepared the manuscript for production;

Judith Fletcher, Publishing Director; and Ms. Linda Grigg, Senior Project Manager, who guided this book throughout the production process.

The photograph of the senior editors was taken in April 2005 during a meeting of the American Surgical Association. The editors have viewed their work in preparing the sixth edition of *Pediatric Surgery* as a labor of love, and we express our hope that the textbook will provide a valued special resource to practicing pediatric surgeons, those in training, and other professionals who care for infants and children. It is our hope that this textbook will serve as a resource that will benefit future generations of children affected with surgical illness thoughout the world.

THE EDITORS

Contents

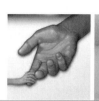

Color
Plates

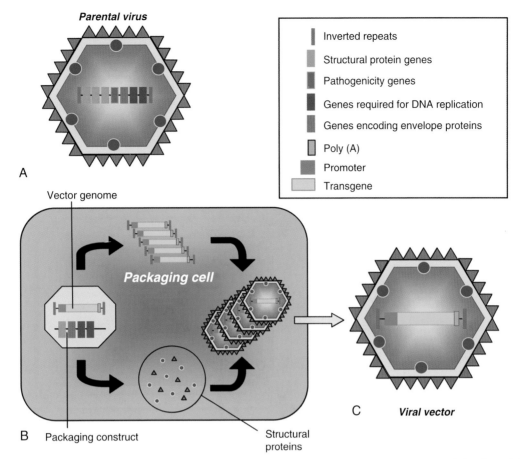

Parental virus

A

Inverted repeats
Structural protein genes
Pathogenicity genes
Genes required for DNA replication
Genes encoding envelope proteins
Poly (A)
Promoter
Transgene

Vector genome

Packaging cell

C   *Viral vector*

B   Packaging construct

Structural proteins

Figure 2–3   Requirements for the creation of a generic viral vector. *A,* The basic machinery of a chosen parental virus is used, including genes encoding specific structural protein genes, envelope proteins, and proteins required for DNA replication, but not genes encoding proteins conferring pathogenicity. *B,* The vector is assembled in a packaging cell. A packaging (helper) construct, containing genes derived from the parental virus, can be delivered as a plasmid or helper virus or stably integrated into the chromatin of the packaging cell. Pathogenicity functions and sequences required for encapsidation are eliminated from the helper construct so that it cannot be packaged into a viral particle. In contrast, the vector genome contains the transgenic expression cassette flanked by inverted terminal repeats and *cis*-acting sequences that are required for genome encapsidation. Viral structural proteins and proteins required for replication of the vector DNA are expressed from the packaging construct, and the replicated vector genomes are packaged into the virus particles. *C,* The viral vector particles are released from the packaging cell and contain only the vector genome.

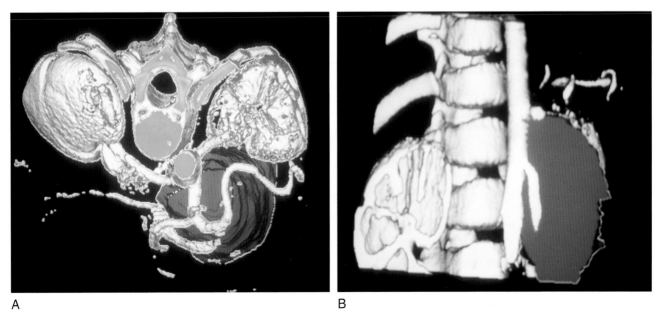

A   B

Figure 28–6   Helical computed tomography scan with three-dimensional reconstruction of a neuroblastoma arising near the celiac axis. *A,* Anterior view indicates that the tumor does not involve the branches of the celiac axis. *B,* Lateral view demonstrates that the superior mesenteric artery passes through the tumor.

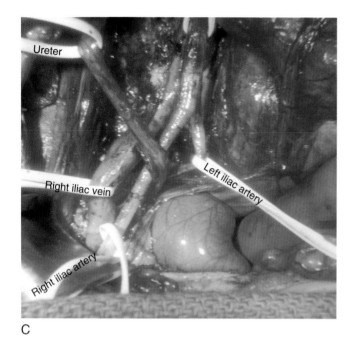

C

Figure 28–10 *C,* Photograph of the operative field after resection of a right-sided pelvic neuroblastoma. Note the vascular loops placed around the iliac arteries, right iliac vein, and ureter to facilitate a safe dissection.

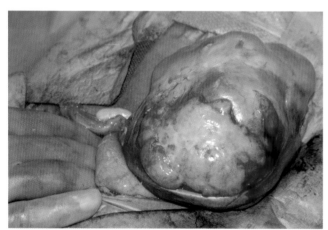

A

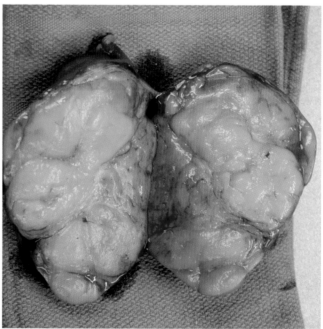

B

Figure 36–7 *A,* This encapsulated mass from a 5-year-old girl with acute abdominal pain proved to be a dysgerminoma. The child's contralateral tube and ovary are seen to the left of the tumor. A small portion of the ipsilateral tube and uterus were in the surgical specimen but uninvolved with tumor. *B,* The cut surface of the tumor is characterized by lobules divided by thin, fibrous septae.

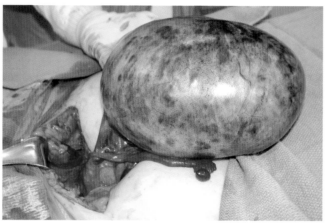

A

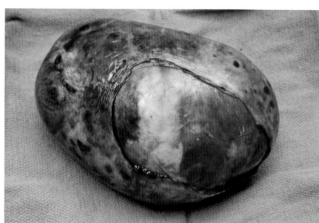

B

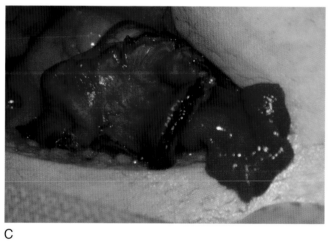

C

Figure 36–9 *A*, Large ovarian dermoid tumor in a 14-year-old girl with acute severe abdominal pain upon awakening. The fallopian tube is seen below the tumor. *B*, After tumor excision, the surface where the cyst was peeled away from the ovary can be seen. *C*, Ovarian tissue (*left*) and fallopian tube (*right*) remaining after cyst removal.

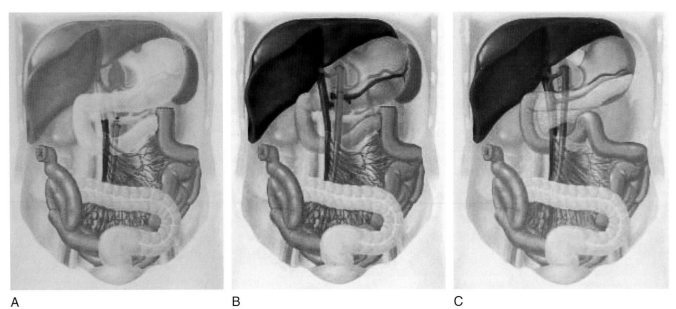

Figure 46–2 *A,* Isolated intestinal graft. *B,* Combined liver-intestinal graft. *C,* Multivisceral graft. (From Fishbein TM, Gondolesi GE, Kaufman SS: Intestinal transplantation for gut failure. Gastroenterology 2003;126:1615.)

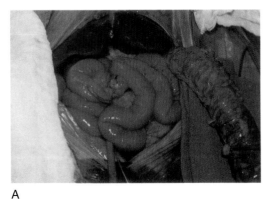

A

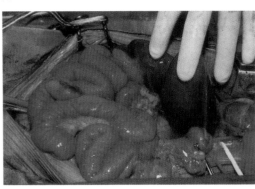

B

Figure 46–4 Operative approach to a multivisceral donor. *A,* The round and falciform ligaments have been divided and the liver completely mobilized. In addition, the left colon has been mobilized to the splenic flexure, the terminal ileum has been stapled (*left lower corner*), and the aortic cannula has been positioned. *B,* The aortic cannula is in position with the supraceliac aorta encircled with umbilical tape (*lower right*). The donor is prepared for systemic heparin, cross-clamping, and organ perfusion. (From Yersiz H, Renz J, Histaki G, et al: Multivisceral and isolated intestinal procurement techniques. Liver Transpl 2003;9:881.)

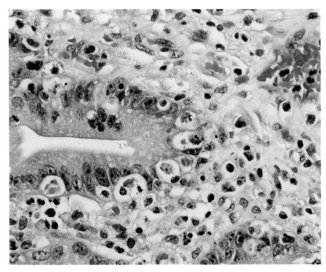

Figure 46–6 Histologic features of intestinal allograft acute cellular rejection, including crypt distortion with apoptosis and an extensive inflammatory infiltrate.

Part I

GENERAL

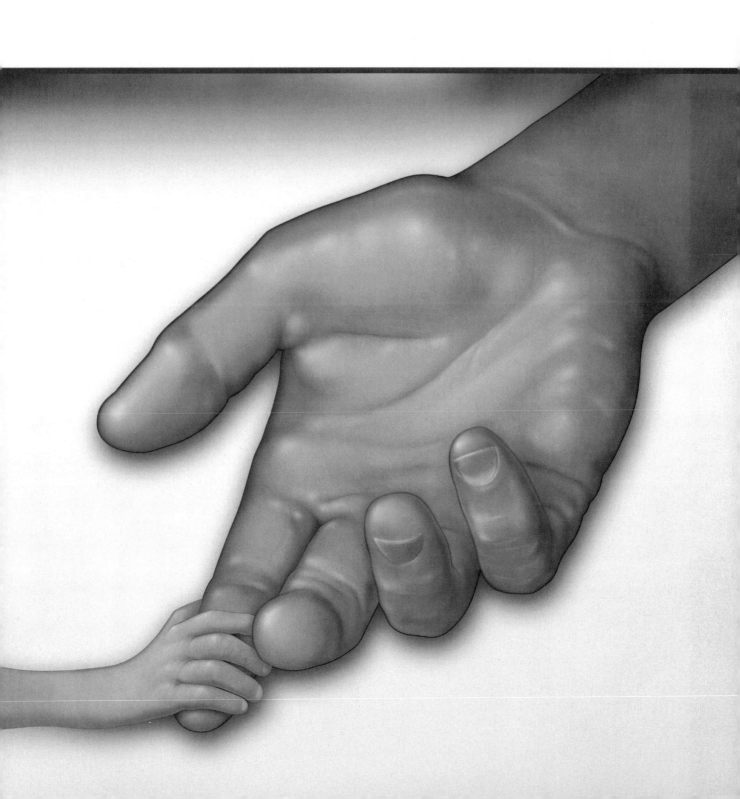

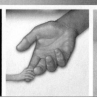
A Brief History of Pediatric Surgery

Judson Randolph and Daniel G. Young

NORTH AMERICA

United States

The clinical practice of pediatric surgery had a rather haphazard start, but any recounting of the development of pediatric surgery in the United States must begin with William E. Ladd (Fig. 1-1). Born in 1880, Ladd graduated from Harvard College in 1903 and from Harvard Medical School in 1906. He also studied with several well-known Boston surgeons of the day. It was not until after World War I that Ladd, undoubtedly influenced by the Halifax disaster, began to spend increasing amounts of time ministering to the surgical needs of infants and children at Boston Children's Hospital. In 1927, at age 47, Ladd was named surgeon-in-chief at Children's Hospital.

The first practitioner of *pure* pediatric surgery in the United States was Dr. Herbert Coe of Seattle. He came east to observe the activities at Children's Hospital in Boston, where Ladd was occasionally present in the operating room. Coe went home to Seattle and in 1919 established the first exclusive practice of pediatric surgery in the United States (Ladd did not give up his adult work until 1927).

If Ladd can be considered the godfather of pediatric surgery in the United States, then his primary pupil, Dr. Robert E. Gross, was destined to become its guru. Born in 1905 and raised in Baltimore, Gross was the son of a piano maker. His father had young Bob work with a fellow craftsman in the hope that he would learn fine movements and detailed craftsmanship. In fact, he did. At Carlton College, Gross was headed for a career in chemistry. However, in his senior year, after reading Cushing's biography of Sir William Osler, he sought admission to Harvard Medical School and was accepted. He graduated in 1931 with an excellent record but did not obtain the surgical internship he coveted, so he entered the Harvard training program in pathology under Dr. S. Burt Wohlbach (Fig. 1-2). His subsequent work on surgical problems was highly influenced by his background in pathology.

In the combined training program in surgery at the Peter Bent Brigham Hospital and Children's Hospital,

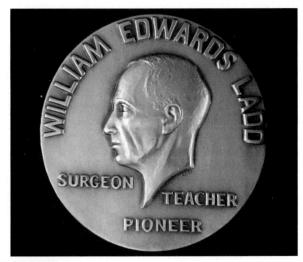

Figure 1–1 The Ladd Medal, awarded by the Surgical Section of the American Academy of Pediatrics for achievement in pediatric surgery.

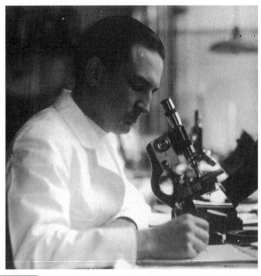

Figure 1–2 Robert E. Gross at his microscope during his residency in pathology at Harvard, 1932.

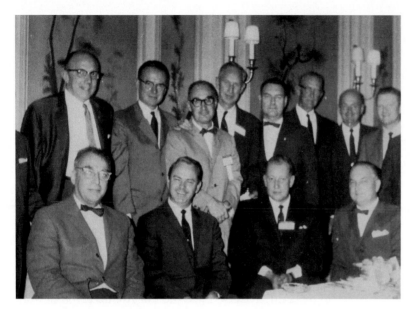

Figure 1–3 A group of North American surgeons attending a meeting of the British Association of Paediatric Surgeons, circa 1964. Front row (left to right): Mark Ravitch, Robert G. Allen, Harvey Beardmore (a Canadian), and Robert E. Gross. Back row (left to right): Lawrence K. Pickett, H. William Clatworthy, Hugh Lynn, Alexander Bill, C. Everett Koop, Willis Potts, Dan Cloud, and George Dorman.

Gross's genius began to emerge. He was always more of a mechanic than a physiologist. His observations in postmortem studies of children who had died of subacute bacterial endocarditis, originating in the patent ductus arteriosus, stimulated him to seek a surgical solution. First with pathologic specimens, then in the animal laboratory, Gross developed a carefully crafted technique for dividing the ductus. Finally in 1938 he selected as his first surgical candidate an 8-year-old girl who was dying from her patent ductus. Her recovery and subsequent course were highly gratifying.

When Gross performed this startling clinical triumph, he was 33 years old and an assistant resident in surgery at Brigham Hospital. This widely acclaimed event was a landmark in terms of addressing a clinical problem in the research laboratory and then bringing the solution to the operating room. After completing his surgical residency in 1939, Gross accepted Ladd's invitation to join him on the staff at Children's Hospital. Thereafter, Gross was instrumental in compiling Ladd's enormous experience in abdominal surgery in infants and children, and in 1941 they published a seminal textbook, *The Abdominal Surgery of Infants and Children*. In this remarkable text, the Ladd operation for malrotation of the intestine (initially described in 1936) and other unique approaches to the operative correction of anomalies in newborn infants were cataloged.

After Ladd's retirement, Gross was appointed surgeon-in-chief at Boston Children's Hospital. He also became the second incumbent of the William E. Ladd Chair in Children's Surgery, established under the aegis of Harvard Medical School in 1941.

Dr. Ovar Swenson, another surgeon at Children's Hospital, made some stellar contributions to pediatric surgery, particularly with regard to unraveling the dilemma of Hirschsprung's disease and defining its surgical solution. In 1950 he accepted the post of surgeon-in-chief at the Boston Floating Hospital, which was part of Tuft's Medical School.

During the 1940s, first under Ladd and then under Gross, a number of subsequently well-known pediatric surgeons received training at Children's Hospital (Fig. 1-3). Most notable were Dr. C. Everett Koop, who came to observe the surgical service for 7 months in 1946, and Dr. Willis Potts of Chicago, who also visited in 1946. After his stay in Boston, Koop returned to Philadelphia and began his long and prominent tenure as pediatric surgeon and professor at the University of Pennsylvania, based at the Children's Hospital of Philadelphia. Potts returned to Chicago and established an equally strong children's surgical program at Children's Memorial Hospital, which trained many outstanding pediatric surgeons.

Also in the circle of leading pediatric surgeons who benefited from their time at Boston Children's Hospital was Dr. H. William Clatworthy, the last resident trained by Ladd and the first trained by Gross. In 1950 Clatworthy began his distinguished career as surgeon in chief at the Columbus Children's Hospital at Ohio State University. Dr. Tague Chisholm left Boston in 1946 and joined Dr. Oswald Wyatt in Minneapolis. Dr. Alexander Bill also completed his training in Boston, including a significant role in the laboratory research that led to Swenson's operation for Hirschsprung's disease. He then joined Coe in 1947 at Children's Orthopedic Hospital in Seattle. Dr. Luther Longino, a taciturn surgeon from Arkansas, finished his residency under Gross in 1948 and stayed on as Gross's number-two departmental associate, where he remained for 20 years teaching legions of residents the technical aspects of surgery.

With vision and relentless energy, Coe badgered officials of the American Academy of Pediatrics until they created a Surgical Section in 1948.[17] Coe envisioned the newly created section as a national forum for pediatric surgeons to gather, exchange information, and gain recognition as a new force in American surgery.

By 1950, in addition to the structured program at Children's Hospital in Boston, one could acquire training in children's surgery as a preceptor, or as a 1- or

2-year fellow, at Chicago Memorial Children's Hospital under Potts, the Philadelphia Children's Hospital under Koop, the Boston Floating Hospital under Swenson, the Babies' Hospital in New York under a new program directed by Dr. Thomas Santulli, or the Children's Hospital of Los Angeles under Dr. William Snyder. In addition, there were well-established programs in Toronto and Montreal, Canada.[6] The output of many of these training programs was sporadic, and the graduates demonstrated a variety of experience—some with cardiac surgical training, some with urologic training, but all with broad experience in general pediatric surgery.

With the publication of his book, *The Surgery of Infancy and Childhood*, in 1953, Gross codified the specialty of pediatric surgery in North America. This masterful text described in meticulous detail Boston Children's Hospital's experience in general pediatric surgery, cardiac surgery, and urology.

In the United States and Canada the 1950s saw an increasing output of children's surgeons from a variety of training programs. Many of these graduates entered private practice. Concomitantly, and belatedly, there was a flurry of activity as children's hospitals sought trained pediatric surgeons to direct their surgical departments. Similarly, medical schools began to realize the necessity of adding to their faculties' surgeons who were specially trained in the surgical diseases of infants and children.

A watershed event in pediatric surgical education occurred in 1965. With great foresight, Clatworthy asked the Surgical Section of the American Academy of Pediatrics to form an Education Committee to evaluate the current educational processes of pediatric surgeons in the United States and Canada. Although the committee's primary mandate was the evaluation of existing training programs, it also made recommendations for basic principles and requirements for the education of pediatric surgeons. Originally, 11 programs in the United States and 2 in Canada were recommended by the committee as meeting the standards set forth in the Clatworthy report.

A number of important events coalesced to substantiate pediatric surgery as a bona fide surgical specialty in North America.[16] It occurred to Dr. Stephen Gans that the specialty required its own journal. With the aid of Koop as editor in chief, the *Journal of Pediatric Surgery* was born in 1966. In 1969 a chance meeting between Drs. Lucian Leape and Thomas Boles resulted in the concept of a new surgical society that would be unencumbered by any attachments to other associations, such as the American Academy of Pediatrics. The idea quickly took hold and, with a number of prominent founding members, the American Pediatric Surgical Association was launched in 1970, with Gross as its first president. Additional training programs, which had been carefully evaluated by the Clatworthy committee, were imposing a standard curriculum of pediatric surgical education.

Several requests that the American Board of Surgery establish a special board in pediatric surgery had been unsuccessful during the 1950s and 1960s. However, with the backing of a new independent surgical organization, inspected and standardized training programs, a journal devoted to the specialty, and insinuations into the curricula of general surgical training programs across the land,

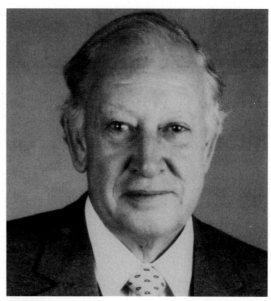

Figure 1–4 Harvey Beardmore, distinguished Canadian pediatric surgeon, fifth president of the American Pediatric Surgical Association, and leader in persuading the American Board of Surgery to grant a Certificate of Special Competence in Pediatric Surgery.

all that was lacking was a spokesperson to approach the American Board of Surgery again.[10] This role fell to Dr. Harvey Beardmore of Montreal (Fig. 1-4), a genial, diplomatic, highly intelligent, and persuasive individual. Beardmore, armed with the facts, succeeded where others had failed. The American Board of Surgery received the carefully prepared petition and in 1975 granted a new Certificate of Special Competence in Pediatric Surgery to be awarded to all qualified applicants.

Research undergirding the specialty of pediatric surgery first took the form of clinical advances in the 1930s and 1940s.[16] Ladd's operation for malrotation was a signal event. Gross's innovations involving the great vessels around the heart—the ductus, coarctation of the aorta, and vascular ring deformities—all deserve mention. Concomitantly, Blalock's triumph with the systemic-pulmonary shunt for babies with tetralogy of Fallot was another landmark. Potts's direct aortic–pulmonary artery shunt accomplished similar physiologic results but required a special clamp. When Potts and Smith developed such a clamp with many delicate teeth to hold a pulsatile vessel securely but gently, they implemented a technical advance that remains useful today in all aspects of vascular surgery. To bridge the gap in long, narrow coarctations, Gross devised the use of freeze-dried, radiated aortic allografts and demonstrated their long-term clinical function. This observation was the foundation for the development of all peripheral vascular surgery, making it a discovery worthy of international recognition. In addition, Swenson's meticulous studies of aganglionic megacolon, followed by his careful adaptation of Hochenegg's operation for removal of the rectum, has helped thousands of children with Hirschsprung's disease.

Research in biology affecting adult surgical patients also began to be commingled with research specifically adapted to children. Studies of body composition as defined by Francis D. Moore were adapted to infants by Rowe, Moore, Artz, Moncrief, and Pruitt added to our knowledge of burn care, which was then used by one of their primary pupils, James O'Neill, to treat burned children. Stanley Dudrick, pioneer with Drs. Rhoads and Wilmore in the use of intravenous nutrition to sustain surgical patients, has created the science of surgical nutrition, saving countless patients of all ages. Bartlett instituted extended extracorporeal oxygenation for infants with temporary inadequate lung function; this technique has now been expanded into important lifesaving techniques for older children and adults. Exquisitely precise care of trauma patients from beginning to end, originally espoused by Cowley and now adapted in child care by Haller, Eichelberger, O'Neill, Tepas, and many others, has allowed the survival of many children who would otherwise have been lost to the ravages of injury.

The awe-inspiring field of transplantation led by Murray, Starzl, Shumway, and many others continues to open new avenues of treatment in an ever-expanding number of diseases in patients of all ages. Jackson of Richmond, followed by DeLorimier in San Francisco, began experimenting with fetal surgery. DeLorimier's prize student, Harrison, and his disciples are now pursuing clinical investigations into the practicalities of this new form of surgical therapy.

Fundamental fetal research is under way in the laboratories of Dr. Patricia Donohoe as she investigates the growth factors influencing embryologic development. Her work has led to the defining of müllerian inhibitory substance, which influences sexual development. Among the many interlinking studies of malignant diseases affecting adults and children, none is more important or has more potential than the work of Judah Folkman of Boston Children's Hospital. Folkman discovered the angiogenesis of malignant tumors, which led him to postulate and search for methods of using antiangiogenesis as a cancer inhibitor. Thus, a whole new science has been created in the field of oncology.

Today, major advances in clinical pediatric surgery, education, and research continue to unfold based on the achievements of the past, and many of these contributions are extending to adult surgery as well.

Canada

As events in children's surgery were unfolding in the United States, Canadian pediatric surgery was experiencing a parallel evolution, primarily at three major institutions. Dr. Alexander Forbes, an orthopedic surgeon, played a key role at the Montreal Children's Hospital from 1904 to 1929. Dr. Dudley Ross, who led the Department of Surgery at Montreal Children's Hospital from 1937 to 1954, was largely responsible for establishing a modern children's surgical unit in the province of Quebec. In 1948 Ross reported the first successful rescue in Canada of a baby with esophageal atresia.[4] Following Ross, Dr. David Murphy served as chief of pediatric surgery and director of the emerging pediatric surgical training program from 1954 to 1974. He was ably assisted by Dr. Herbert Owen, Dr. Gordon Karn, and his first trainee (1954),

Dr. Harvey Beardmore, who went on to establish an international reputation. Beardmore served as chief of surgery at Montreal Children's Hospital during the 1970s and was followed by Dr. Frank Guttman from 1981 to 1994.

In Toronto, the Hospital for Sick Children was established in 1875 by Mrs. Samuel McMaster (whose husband founded McMaster University).[5] As in the United States, surgeons who treated adults answered the call for pediatric surgery at the end of the 19th and beginning of the 20th centuries. Perhaps the most distinguished Toronto surgeon was Dr. W. Edward Gallie, who served as chief surgeon at the Hospital for Sick Children from 1921 to 1929. Gallie was named to the chair in surgery at the University of Toronto, where he established the Gallie surgical training program. In Canada the Gallie School of Surgery became the equivalent of that at Johns Hopkins, led by Dr. William Halsted. With the expansion of Gallie's responsibilities, he relinquished his role as chief of pediatric surgery to Dr. Donald Robertson, an adventuresome thoracic surgeon who held the post until 1944, retiring almost concomitantly with Ladd in Boston. Dr. Arthur Lemesurer, an inventive plastic surgeon, began a general pediatric surgical training program that produced, beginning in 1949, Clinton Stephens, James Simpson, Robert Salter, Phillip Ashmore, Donald Marshall, and Stanley Mercer, to name the most illustrious graduates, all of whom would become leaders in the field of pediatric surgery throughout Canada.

In 1956 Dr. Alfred Farmer was chosen surgeon-in-chief at Toronto's Hospital for Sick Children and immediately formed several specialty surgical divisions, including one for general pediatric surgery. It was a landmark stroke, according to Dr. Clinton Stephens, which allowed separate specialty leadership under the wise direction of Dr. Stewart Thomson from 1956 to 1966 and Stephens himself from 1966 to 1976 (S. Ein, personal communication). During these 2 decades there was a prodigious output in clinical work and clinical research and an impressive roster of graduating trainees. The tradition of excellence in all aspects of pediatric surgery was expanded with the appointment in 1977 of Dr. Robert Filler.

A third children's hospital, the Hospital Sainte-Justine in Montreal, has also contributed richly to children's surgery. Founded in 1907 by Mrs. Justine Lacoste-Beau-Bien, the hospital was combined with the Francophone Obstetrical Unit of Montreal, creating one of the largest maternal and child care centers in North America. Dr. Pierre-Paul Collin came to the hospital in 1954, bringing thoracic surgical experience and a commitment to child care. He trained a number of Canada's latter-day leaders in pediatric surgery, including Frank Guttman, Herve Blanchard, Saleem Yazbeck, and Jean-Martin LaBerge.

From these three key surgical centers, leadership and progress spread across the provinces with the same comprehensive effect seen in the United States.

UNITED KINGDOM

Jean-Jacques Rousseau, the Swiss-French philosopher and moralist, commented in the mid-18th century, "One half of the children born die before their eighth year.

That is Nature's law; why try to contradict it?" This attitude pervaded 18th-century thought. The development of pediatric surgery did not occur until much later, despite the observation that "surgeons and apothecaries are oftener called to cure children than many physicians of greater eminence."

Pediatrics began to occupy the thoughts of doctors and the general population with the development of many foundling hospitals in Britain and elsewhere in Europe. The best known of these in Britain still exists as the Coram Foundation.[13] It was originally established in Holborn, London (1739), close to the current location of the Hospital for Sick Children on Great Ormond Street. Like many other institutions of its kind, although it was called a hospital, it was more of a care home than a treatment center. Hospitals for children, as we understand them today, evolved in the 19th century.

In Europe the major landmark in the development of children's hospitals, and in the evolution of pediatric surgery, was the establishment of the Hôpital des Enfants Malades in Paris in 1802. This 200-bed unit provided treatment for children with medical or surgical disorders. Children younger than 7 years were not allowed admission to other hospitals in Paris. Subsequently, there was a steady movement toward establishing children's hospitals in the main cities in Europe.

In 1852 the Hospital for Sick Children (HSC) opened its doors in a converted house on Great Ormond Street.[7] This hospital was the brainchild of Dr. Charles West, aided by Dr. Bence Jones. West's philosophy was that children with diseases of a medical nature required special facilities and attention, but that those with surgical disorders (at the time, mostly trauma related) could be treated in general hospitals. This attitude took a long time to die from the minds of some pediatricians and is still in evidence in some parts of the world.

West opposed the appointment of a surgeon to the staff of the HSC, but the board disagreed and appointed G. D. Pollock. Pollock soon resigned and was replaced in 1853 by Athol Johnson. Johnson's insight into the scope of surgery for children was presented in three long papers published in the *British Medical Journal* in 1861.[9] T. Holmes, who followed Johnson, published his 37-chapter book, *Surgical Treatment of the Diseases of Infancy and Childhood*, in 1868.[8] Although the specialty of pediatrics, let alone pediatric surgery, had not yet developed, it is clear that surgery for children was already a special field.

Pediatrics in the 19th century was split. One approach was the pattern established in Paris, whereby children were treated in hospitals specially oriented toward children's care. The alternative was the West approach, common in Britain in the second half of the 19th century.[11] There, a number of children's hospitals, such as those in Birmingham and Edinburgh, were established to provide medical treatment but not surgery for children. Around the same time, Charles Dickens,[12] a vital supporter of the HSC, clearly believed in the importance of special facilities for all children who needed hospitalization. Some centers recognized the special requirements of children with surgical disorders. For example, at the Royal Hospital for Sick Children in Glasgow (RHSC), established after a 21-year gestation period, the board

appointed equal numbers of medical specialists and surgical specialists.[19] Laypeople appear to have understood the importance of both medical and surgical services for children.

The latter part of the 19th century saw a major expansion in surgery for children owing to the development of ether and chloroform anesthesia in midcentury and the gradual acceptance of antiseptic surgery. Although carbolic acid had been used earlier, English surgeon Joseph Lister gave the main impetus to the concept of antiseptic surgery. After qualifying in London, he developed his antiseptic approach in Glasgow before moving to Edinburgh and then to King's College, London. One of Lister's young assistants in Glasgow was William Macewen (later Sir William), known as the father of neurosurgery and one of the original surgeons appointed to the RHSC.

In Scotland, where pediatric care was generally ahead of the rest of Britain, the Royal Edinburgh Hospital for Sick Children (REHSC) opened in 1860. It was not until 1887, however, that the board decided to set aside a ward for surgical patients and to use the sewing room as an operating theater.[14] Joseph Bell (president of the Royal College of Surgeons of Edinburgh), Sir Harold Styles (who performed pyloromyotomy the year before Conrad Ramstedt), Sir John Fraser (author of a widely used two-volume textbook, *Surgery of Childhood*), and James J. Mason Brown (also a president of the Royal College of Surgeons of Edinburgh and author of a book titled *Surgery of Childhood*) were the senior surgeons from 1887 to 1964. It is of interest that Gertrude Hertzfeld held a surgical appointment at the REHSC from 1919 to 1947—one of the few women surgeons of that era.

Back in the 19th century, training in pediatric surgery, independent of general surgery, was given in Glasgow. The syllabus of lectures at St. Mungo College in Glasgow is extensive, and an example from 1889-1890 is shown in Table 1-1. A similar 15-lecture course was given on medical diseases.

Soon after these hospitals opened, their boards recognized the need for the development of dispensaries or outpatient departments. In Manchester, the dispensary actually preceded the hospital at Pendelbury. These dispensaries handled many surgical patients, and much of what is called pediatric surgery was done there. One of the most outstanding surgeons of that generation was James Nicoll, who reported 10 years of his work in 1909,[15] one of more than 100 of his publications. He is now known as the Father of Day Surgery, but the title of pediatric surgeon was equally merited, although only part of his time was devoted to children's surgery (Table 1-2). He performed pyloromyotomy with success in the late 19th century in a somewhat different fashion from Styles and Ramstedt.

Although invited to take charge of one of the two surgical units in 1914, Nicoll rejected the offer because he would have been required to give up his adult practice. He preferred the less prestigious position of dispensary surgeon to that of visiting surgeon. The board of the RHSC had decided that physicians or surgeons appointed to the hospital had to devote all their professional time to the treatment of children; the board might grant an exception for some specific work, but it had to

TABLE 1-1 St. Mungo College Syllabus: 1889-1890

Surgical Diseases of Children

Lecturer: James A. Adams, MD, FFPSG, Assistant Surgeon to the Royal Infirmary

The course will be delivered during the summer session at 11:30 am, on Tuesdays and Thursdays, and will include a consideration of the following subjects:

1. The management of infants and children during illness
2. Diathesis—hemorrhagic, tuberculosis, struma, rachitis, etc.
3. Syphilis
4. Fractures
5. Dislocations
6. Affections of the joints
7. Diseases of periosteum and bone
8. Glandular disease—cervical, axillary, femoral, Hodgkin's disease
9. Congenital malformations—harelip, cleft palate, spina bifida and encephalocele, talipes, wry neck, imperforate anus and rectum, malformations of foot and hand
10. Tumors—innocent, malignant, congenital
11. Diphtheria—laryngitis, croup, tracheotomy and its alternatives
12. Burns—scalds, subsequent deformities
13. Diseases of the spinal column—caries, angular and lateral curvature
14. Empyema—hydrothorax
15. Paralysis—pseudohypertrophic, tetany, spastic paralysis, neuroninesis, etc.
16. Genitourinary affections—extroversion of the bladder, hypospadias, phimosis, paraphimosis, masturbation, hermaphroditism, calculus, lithotomy, lithotrity, incontinence of urine
17. Hernia
18. Abdominal diseases—peritonitis, obstruction, tabes, tumors, rectum and anus
19. Organs of special sense
20. Aural disease—its influence on intracranial abscess
21. Foreign bodies in eye, ear, nose, etc.

TABLE 1-2 Types of Outpatient Operations Performed by James Nicholl, Royal Hospital for Sick Children, Glasgow: 1899-1908*

Tuberculosis
Talipes
Harelip and cleft palate
Mastoid empyema
Spina bifida
Fracture
Pyloric stenosis

*In this 10-year period, 7392 of 8988 operations were done by Nicholl.

be secondary to the surgeon's duties at the children's hospital. Clearly, an outside practice was undesirable.

Alex MacLennan was first appointed a dispensary surgeon at the RHSC in 1902, then a visiting surgeon in 1914. In 1919 the University of Glasgow was given money to establish both a medical and a surgical lectureship, the first academic appointments in the specialty in Britain. MacLennan was appointed Barclay lecturer in surgical and orthopedic diseases of children at the University of Glasgow in 1919 and continued in this post until he retired in 1938. His particular interest was in orthopedics; his successor, Matthew White, appointed to the dispensary in 1924, visiting surgeon in 1930, and Barclay lecturer in 1938, was a thoracic and abdominal surgeon. Wallace Dennison and Dan Young were among the other surgeons who later filled these posts.

Meantime, in Edinburgh, the children's surgical services and the adult services remained closely associated until Mason Brown became the chief. Contrary to the statement that "Scotland had paediatric surgeons for a long time, but they practiced only children's surgery until an adult job became vacant,"[18] surgeons at the children's hospitals in both Edinburgh and Glasgow refused to accept prestigious posts in adult surgery because they were dedicated to their children's work. The archives of these institutions record these facts.

To many, pediatric surgery was a development that took place shortly after the Second World War. Contributing to that development were other factors, such as the introduction of the National Health Service in Britain, providing "free" treatment for all individuals irrespective of age or social circumstance. Developments unrelated to medicine, such as the plastics industry and many other technical innovations in the mid-20th century, allowed great strides, particularly in neonatal surgery. A closer look, however, shows that pediatric surgery had been developing over many decades, although the first surgical pediatric "clubs"—the Scottish Surgical Paediatric Club and the Surgical Section of the American Academy of Pediatrics—were established in 1948.[1,2,17]

Developments in the specialty were closely related to committed individuals. Denis Browne, an Australian initially appointed to the HSC in London in 1924, spent his professional life committed to pediatric surgery. In London and elsewhere in England, general surgeons who were interested in pediatric surgery carried on their pediatric practices in the cities, along with their adult practices. Financial considerations were no doubt important, because few were able to sustain themselves on a pediatric surgical practice alone, irrespective of their desire. Browne was the first surgeon in London to confine himself to pediatric surgery. He developed a large number of admirers and disciples over the years. He was widely known, and his tall stature made him easily recognizable. All who knew him would agree that he had a somewhat dominating and domineering manner and did not easily accept contradiction of his views or theories. Browne's longtime colleague James Crooks called him an "intellectual adventurer, a rebel and a cynic." Even a few days before his death, Browne was "still the supreme egotist."[3] His faithful secretary recounts that when she attempted to get Browne to tone down some of his letters, a friend told her, "You must be crazy! It has taken DB all his life to build this reputation for rudeness and you come along at the eleventh hour to wreck it."[20]

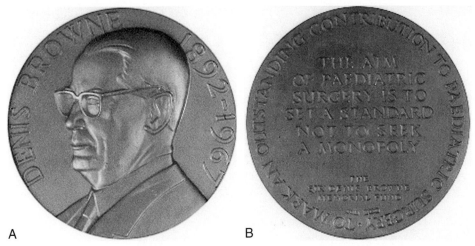

Figure 1-5 Denis Browne Gold Medal. *A*, Front of the medal. *B*, Back of the medal, which reads, "The aim of paediatric surgery is to set a standard not to seek a monopoly."

One of us (Young) worked as his last assistant in his private work and found him stimulating and straightforward. The Denis Browne Gold Medal remains a memento of his presence and clearly demonstrates his views (Fig. 1-5).

After the Second World War, many surgeons from overseas spent some time in the United Kingdom; the majority visited the HSC, where they came under the influence of Browne and some of the other surgeons mentioned. Many subsequently established internationally recognized centers on many continents. Jannie Louw, Douglas Stephens, Durham Smith, and Christian Barnard are a few examples.

Browne's major interest was in the structural anomalies, and he achieved widespread recognition for his advocacy of intrauterine pressure contributing to or causing such anomalies. He had as contemporaries and senior colleagues at the HSC such men as L. Barrington-Ward and T. Twistington Higgins, surgeons of considerable stature, so it was in his latter days that he emerged as the dominant surgeon at Grand Ormond Street. It was Higgins who initially held discussions in London that led to the formation of the British Association of Paediatric Surgeons; Browne was then the senior surgeon at the HSC and became the association's first and longest-serving president. In his latter years in the National Health Service, his colleagues included George McNab (introducer of the Holter valve for hydrocephalus), David Waterston (early pediatric cardiac surgeon), and Sir David Innes Williams (doyen pediatric urologist of Britain). Each of these outstanding men made contributions to the development of pediatric surgery.

Many other developments were also taking place. Andrew Wilkinson and others such as Ole Knutrud from Oslo were studying infant metabolism. Isabella Forshall (later joined by Rickham) was a caring surgeon who established an excellent clinical service, although she made no major scientific contributions. Her 1959 Christmas card pictured a number of prominent individuals at the British Association of Paediatric Surgeons' meeting (Fig. 1-6).

In summary, the history of pediatric surgery on the east side of the Atlantic reveals a division in approach through much of the 19th and 20th centuries. In recent decades, there has been less divergence, but each society has come up with its own solutions to the steadily improving care of infants and children requiring surgery. The past 50 years have seen many changes, and the more recent details are covered in individual chapters.

ASIA

Space constraints prevent a full recounting of the development of pediatric surgery in Asia.* However, it must be acknowledged that the worldwide literature is replete with contributions from Japan, China, Taiwan, and other Asian sources. Zhang in China survived the Cultural Revolution to emerge as that nation's father figure in children's surgery, and there is now a new generation of surgeons.

Pediatric surgery in Japan did not develop until some years after World War II. The first generation of pediatric surgeons appeared in the early 1950s: Ueda in Osaka, Suruga at Juntendo University in Tokyo, Kasai in Sendai, and Ikeda in Fukuoka. Suruga performed the first operation for intestinal atresia in 1952, and Kasai performed the first hepatoportoenterostomy for biliary atresia in 1955. The first children's hospital was the National Children's Hospital in Tokyo, established in 1965. The first Department of Pediatric Surgery was established at Juntendo University in Tokyo in 1968 by Suruga; today, training programs exist in nearly all the major university centers. The Japanese Society of Pediatric Surgeons and its journal were established in 1964, paralleling developments in other parts of the world. The second generation of pediatric surgeons includes Okamoto and

---

*The information in this section was provided by Professor Takeshi Miyano, Juntendo University, Tokyo, Japan.

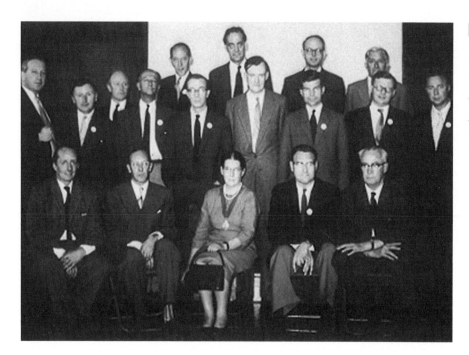

Figure 1–6 Isabella Forshall's 1959 Christmas card. Seated (left to right): D. Waterston, M. Grob, I. Forshall, C. Koop, and D. Browne. Standing: H. Beardmore, R. Zachary, I. Kirkland, T. Ehrenpries, W. Dennison, H. Johnson, A. Wilkinsoon, A. Jolleys, J. Bentley, B. Smyth, V. Swain, H. Nixon, and B. O'Donnell. Missing from the photo is G. McNab.

Okada in Osaka; Akiyama, Tsuchida, and Miyano in Tokyo; Ohi in Sendai; and Suita in Fukuoka. All these individuals have made seminal contributions in the fields of nutrition, biliary and pancreatic disease, oncology, and intestinal disorders.

In recent decades, laboratories and clinical centers in Asia, particularly in Japan, have generated exciting new information in the clinical and basic biologic sciences that continues to enrich the field of children's surgery. Pediatric surgery has truly become internationalized in terms of clinical developments, education, and research, and the future looks promising.

REFERENCES

1. Bisset W, Carachi R: The forerunner in the north: The Scottish Paediatric Surgical Society. J Pediatr Surg 2003;37(Suppl 7):2-6.
2. Campbell JR: History of the Section of Surgery, the American Academy of Pediatrics: The second 25 years. J Pediatr Surg 1999;34(Suppl 1):19-98.
3. Crooks J: In Nixon HH, Waterston DJ, Wink CSA (eds): Selected Writings of Sir Denis Browne. Farnborough, Inkon Printers, 1983, p 1.
4. Delaure NC: Thoracic Surgery in Canada. Toronto, BC Decker, 1989.
5. Ein S: History of the Division of General Surgery at HSC, Toronto. Unpublished manuscript.
6. Glick PL, Azizkhan RG: A Genealogy of North American Pediatric Surgery. St Louis, Quality Medical Publishing, 1997.
7. Higgins TT: Great Ormond Street, 1852-1952. London, Odhams Press, 1952.
8. Holmes T: Surgical Treatment of the Diseases of Infancy and Childhood. London, Longmans, Green, Reader & Dyer, 1868.
9. Johnson A: Surgery of childhood. BMJ 1861;1:1-4, 41-47, 61-63.
10. Johnson DG: Excellence and search of recognition. J Pediatr Surg 1986;22:1019-1031.
11. Lomax EMR: Small and Special: The Development of Hospitals for Children in Victorian Britain. London, Wellcome Institute for the History of Medicine, 1996.
12. Markel H: Charles Dickens' work to help establish Great Ormond Street Hospital, London. Lancet 1999;354:6357.
13. McLure RK: Coram's Children. New Haven, Conn, Yale University Press, 1981.
14. Minutes of the Board of the Royal Edinburgh Hospital for Sick Children, 1887.
15. Nicoll JH: Surgery of infancy. BMJ 1909;2:753-754.
16. Randolph JG: The first of the best. J Pediatr Surg 1985;20:580-591.
17. Randolph JG: History of the Section of Surgery, the American Academy of Pediatrics: The first 25 years. J Pediatr Surg 1999;34(Suppl 1):3-18.
18. Rickham PP: Jpn J Paediatr Surg 2002;38:210-233.
19. Robertson E: The Yorkhill Story. Glasgow, Robert MacLehose & Co, 1972.
20. Waterman R: In Nixon HH, Waterston DJ, Wink CSA (eds): Selected Writings of Sir Denis Browne. Farnborough, Inkon Printers, 1983, p15.

Chapter 2

Molecular Clinical Genetics and Gene Therapy

Alan W. Flake

The topics of this chapter are broad in scope and outside the realm of a classic core education in pediatric surgery. However, both molecular genetics and gene therapy will be of increasing clinical importance in all medical specialties, including pediatric surgery, in the near future. A few conservative predictions include improvements in the diagnostic accuracy and prediction of phenotype, the development of new therapeutic options for many disorders, and the optimization of pharmacotherapy based on patient genotype, but there are many other possible uses. The goal here is to provide an overview of recent developments that are relevant or potentially relevant to pediatric surgery.

MOLECULAR CLINICAL GENETICS

Although hereditary disease has been recognized for centuries, only relatively recently has heredity become the prevailing explanation for numerous human diseases. Before the 1970s, physicians considered genetic diseases to be relatively rare and irrelevant to clinical care. With the advent of rapid advances in molecular genetics, we currently recognize that genes are critical factors in virtually all human diseases. Although an incomplete indicator, McKusick's *Mendelian Inheritance in Man* has grown from about 1500 entries in 1965 to 10,000 in 2000, documenting the acceleration of knowledge in human genetics.[44] Even disorders that were once considered to be purely acquired, such as infectious diseases, are now recognized to be influenced by genetic mechanisms of inherent vulnerability and genetically driven immune system responses.

Despite this phenomenal increase in genetic information and the associated insight into human disease, there remains a wide gap between the identification of genotypic abnormalities that are linked to phenotypic manifestations in humans and any practical application to patient treatment. With the notable exceptions of genetic counseling and prenatal diagnosis, molecular genetics presently has little impact on the daily practice of medicine or, more specifically, on the practice of pediatric surgery. The promise of molecular genetics cannot be denied, however. Identifying the fundamental basis of human disorders and of individual responses to environmental, pharmacologic, and disease-induced perturbations is the first step toward understanding the downstream pathways that may have a profound impact on clinical therapy. The ultimate application of genetics would be the correction of germline defects for affected individuals and their progeny. Although germline correction remains a future fantasy fraught with ethical controversy,[56] there is no question that molecular genetics will begin to impact clinical practice in myriad ways within the next decade. A comprehensive discussion of the field of molecular genetics is beyond the scope of this chapter, and there are many sources of information on the clinical genetics of pediatric surgical disorders.

Human Molecular Genetics and Pediatric Surgical Disease

The rapid identification of genes associated with human disease has revolutionized the field of medical genetics, providing more accurate diagnostic, prognostic, and potentially therapeutic tools. However, increased knowledge is always associated with increased complexity. Whereas the classic model assumed that the spread of certain traits in families is associated with the transmission of a single molecular defect—with individual alleles segregating into families according to Mendel's laws—today's model recognizes that very few phenotypes can be satisfactorily explained by a mutation at a single gene locus. The phenotypic diversity recognized in disorders that were once considered monogenic has led to a reconceptualization of genetic disease. Although mendelian models are useful for identifying the primary cause of familial disorders, they appear to be incomplete as models of the true physiologic and cellular nature of defects.[15,66,71] Numerous disorders that were initially

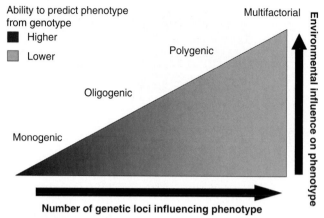

Figure 2-1 Conceptual continuum of modern molecular genetics. The genetic characterization of a disorder depends on (1) whether a major locus makes a dominant contribution to the phenotype, (2) the number of loci that influence the phenotype, and (3) the presence and extent of environmental influence on phenotype. The farther toward the right a disorder lies, the greater the complexity of the genetic analysis and the less predictive genotype is of phenotype.

characterized as monogenic are proving to be either caused or modulated by the action of a small number of loci. These disorders are described as oligogenic disorders, an evolving concept that encompasses a large spectrum of phenotypes that are neither monogenic nor polygenic. In contrast to polygenic or complex traits—which are thought to result from poorly understood interactions between many genes and the environment—oligogenic disorders are primarily genetic in etiology but require the synergistic action of mutant alleles at a small number of loci. One can look at modern molecular genetics as a conceptual continuum between classic mendelian and complex traits (Fig. 2-1). The position of any given disorder along this continuum depends on three main variables: (1) whether a major locus makes a dominant contribution to the phenotype, (2) the number of loci that influence the phenotype, and (3) the presence and extent of environmental influence on phenotype.

Disease-Specific Examples of Changing Concepts in Molecular Genetics

Monogenic Disorders

Cystic fibrosis (CF) is an example of a disorder close to the monogenic end of the continuum, but it also illustrates the complexity of the genetics of some disorders, even when a mutation of a major locus is the primary determinant of phenotype. On the basis of the observed autosomal recessive inheritance in families, the gene *CFTR* (cystic fibrosis transmembrane conductance regulator) was first mapped in humans to chromosome 7q31.2.[68] Once the *CFTR* gene was cloned,[62] it was widely anticipated that mutation analyses might be sufficient to predict the clinical outcome of patients. However, analyses of *CFTR* mutations in large and ethnically diverse

cohorts indicated that this assumption was an oversimplification of the true genetic nature of this phenotype, particularly with respect to the substantial phenotypic variability observed in some CF patients. For instance, although *CFTR* mutations show a degree of correlation with the severity of pancreatic disease, the severity of the pulmonary phenotype—which is the main cause of mortality—is difficult to predict.[1,16,45] Realization of the limitations of a pure monogenic model prompted an evaluation of more complex inheritance schemes. This led to the mapping of a modifier locus for the intestinal component of CF in both human and mouse.[63,73] Further phenotypic analysis led to the discovery of several other loci linked to phenotype, including (1) the association of low-expressing mannose-binding lectin (*MBL*; also known as *MBL2*) alleles, human leukocyte antigen (*HLA*) class II polymorphisms, and variants in tumor necrosis factor-α (*TNFα*) and transforming growth factor-β-1 (*TGFβ1*) with pulmonary aspects of the disease[5,6,21,30]; (2) the correlation of intronic nitric oxide synthase 1 (*NOS1*) polymorphisms with variability in the frequency and severity of microbial infections[22]; and (3) the contribution of mucin 1 (*Muc1*) to the gastrointestinal aspects of the CF phenotype in mice (Fig. 2-2).[55] Recently, further layers of complexity have been discovered for both *CFTR* and its associated phenotype. First, heterozygous CF mutations have been associated with susceptibility to rhinosinusitis, an established polygenic trait.[69] Second, and perhaps more surprising, a recent study reported that some patients with a milder CF phenotype do not have any mutations in *CFTR*. This indicates that the hypothesis that *CFTR* gene dysfunction is requisite for the development of CF might not be true.[23]

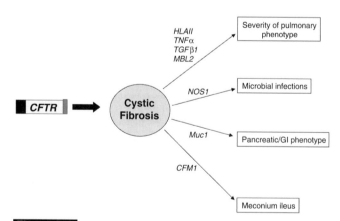

Figure 2-2 Complexity in monogenic diseases. Mutations in the cystic fibrosis transmembrane conductance regulator (*CFTR*) almost always cause the cystic fibrosis (CF) phenotype. Owing to modification effects by other genetic factors, the presence and nature of mutations at the *CFTR* locus cannot predict the phenotypic manifestation of the disease. Therefore, although CF is considered a mendelian recessive disease, the phenotype in each patient depends on a discrete number of alleles at different loci. *CFM1*, cystic fibrosis modifier 1; GI, gastrointestinal; HLAII, major histocompatibility complex class II antigen; *MBL2*, mannose-binding lectin (protein C) 2; *Muc1*, mucin 1; *NOS1*, nitric oxide synthase 1; *TGFβ1*, transforming growth factor-β-1; *TNF*α, tumor necrosis factor-α encoding gene.

Oligogenic Disorders

Recent developments in defining the molecular genetics of Hirschsprung's disease (HD) exemplify a relatively new concept in genetics—the oligogenic disorder. Although mathematical analyses of oligogenicity are beyond the scope of this discussion,[18,47] it is important to recognize that modifications of traditional linkage approaches are useful tools for the study of oligogenic diseases, especially if a major locus that contributes greatly to the phenotype is known. In the case of HD, two main phenotypic groups can be distinguished on the basis of the extent of aganglionosis: short-segment HD (S-HD) and the more severe long-segment HD (L-HD). Autosomal dominant inheritance with incomplete penetrance has been proposed for L-HD, whereas complex inheritance that involves an autosomal recessive trait has been observed in S-HD. Oligogenicity has been established in both HD variants by virtue of several factors: a recurrence risk that varies from 3% to 25%, depending on the length of aganglionosis and the sex of the patient; heritability values close to 100%, which indicates an exclusively genetic basis; significant clinical variability and reduced penetrance; and nonrandom association of hypomorphic changes in the endothelin receptor type B (*EDNRB*), with rearranged during transfection (*RET*) polymorphisms and HD.[54,57] So far, a combination of linkage, positional cloning studies, and functional candidate gene analyses has identified eight HD genes (Table 2-1),[2] of which the proto-oncogene *RET* is thought to be the main predisposing locus,[4,39] particularly in families with a high incidence of L-HD.[20]

The nonmendelian transmission of HD has hindered the identification of predisposing modifier loci by conventional linkage approaches. When these approaches (parametric and nonparametric linkage studies) were carried out on a group of 12 L-HD families, very weak linkage was observed on 9q31. However, based on the hypothesis that only milder *RET* mutations could be associated with another locus, families were categorized according to the *RET* mutational data. Significant linkage on 9q31 was detected when families with potentially weak *RET* mutations were analyzed independently,[39] indicating that mild *RET* alleles, in conjunction with alleles at an unknown gene on chromosome 9, might be required for pathogenesis. The mode of inheritance in S-HD has proved to be more complex than in L-HD, requiring further adjustments to the linkage strategies. Recently, the application of model-free linkage, without assumptions about the number and inheritance mode of segregating factors, showed that a three-locus segregation was both necessary and sufficient to manifest S-HD, with *RET* being the main locus, and that the transmission of susceptibility alleles was additive.[20]

The inheritance patterns observed in disorders such as HD illustrate the power of both expanded models of disease inheritance that account for reduced penetrance and phenotypic variability and the ability of these models to genetically map loci involved in oligogenic diseases—a first step toward identifying their underlying genes. More important, the establishment of nonmendelian models caused a change of perception in human genetics, which in turn accelerated the discovery of oligogenic traits.

Polygenic or Complex Disorders

Polygenic or complex disorders are thought to result from poorly understood interactions between many genes and the environment. An example of a polygenic

TABLE 2-1 Genes Associated with Hirschsprung's Disease and Relationship to Associated Anomalies

Gene	Gene Locus	Gene Product	Inheritance	Population Frequency (%)	Associated Anomalies	Incidence in HD (%)
RET	10q11.2	Coreceptor for GDNF	AD	17-38 (S-HD) 70-80 (L-HD) 50 (familial) 15-35 (sporadic)	CCHS MEN2A MEN2B	1.8-1.9 2.5-5.0 Unknown
GDNF	5p12-13.1	Ligand for RET and GFRα-1	AD	<1*	CCHS	1.8-1.9
NTN	19p13.3	Ligand for RET and GFRα-2	AD	<1*	Unknown	—
GFRα-1	10q26	Coreceptor for GDNF	Unknown	†	Unknown	—
EDNRB	13q22	Receptor for EDN3	AD/AR	3-7	Waardenburg's syndrome	Unknown
EDN3	20q13.2-13.3	Ligand for EDNRB	AD/AR	5	CCHS Waardenburg's syndrome	1.8-1.9 Unknown
ECE-1	1p36.1	EDN3 processing gene	AD	<1	Unknown	—
SOX10	22q13.1	Transcription factor	AD	<1	Waardenburg's syndrome type 4	Unknown

*Limited data available.

† No mutations detected thus far in humans, but associated with HD in mice.

AD, autosomal dominant; AR, autosomal recessive; CCHS, congenital central hypoventilation syndrome (Ondine's curse); ECE-1, endothelin-converting enzyme-1; EDNRB, endothelin receptor B; EDN3, endothelin-3; GDNF, glial cell line–derived neurotrophic factor; GFRα-1, GDNF family receptor α-1; HD, Hirschsprung's disease; L-HD, long-segment HD; MEN, multiple endocrine neoplasia; NTN, *neurturin*; RET, rearranged during transfection; S-HD, short-segment HD; SOX, Sry-like HMG bOX.

disorder relevant to pediatric surgery is hypertrophic pyloric stenosis (HPS). The genetic cause of HPS has long been recognized, with frequent familial aggregation, a concordance rate of 25% to 40% in monogenetic twins, a recurrence rate of 10% for males and 2% for females born after an affected child, and a ratio of risk of 18 for first-degree relatives compared with the general population.[46] However, this risk is considerably less than would be predicted based on mendelian patterns of inheritance.[10] In addition, HPS has been reported as an associated feature in multiple defined genetic syndromes,[9,35,36,59,67] chromosomal abnormalities,[12,27,29,60,70] and anecdotally with many other defects,[24,31,37,42,72] suggesting a polygenic basis. Although the molecular genetic basis of HPS remains poorly defined, a likely common final pathway causing the disorder is altered expression of neural nitric oxide synthase (nNOS) within the pyloric muscle.[51] A detailed analysis of the molecular mechanisms of this alteration has been published, describing a reduction of messenger RNA (mRNA) expression of nNOS exon 1c, with a compensatory up-regulation of nNOS exon 1f variant mRNA in HPS.[51] DNA samples of 16 HPS patients and 81 controls were analyzed for nNOS exon 1c promoter mutations and single nucleotide polymorphism (SNP). Sequencing of the 5′-flanking region of exon 1c revealed mutations in 3 of 16 HPS tissues, whereas 81 controls showed the wild-type sequence exclusively. Carriers of the A allele of a previously uncharacterized nNOS exon 1c promoter SNP (-84G/A SNP) had an increased risk of developing HPS (odds ratio, 8.0; 95% confidence interval, 2.5 to 25.6), which could indicate that the -84G/A promoter SNP alters expression of nNOS exon 1c or is in linkage dysequilibrium with a functionally important sequence variant elsewhere in the nNOS transcription unit and therefore may serve as an informative marker for a functionally important genetic alteration. The observed correlation of the -84G/A SNP with an increased risk for the development of HPS is consistent with a report showing a strong correlation of a microsatellite polymorphism in the *nNOS* gene with a familial form of HPS.[13] However, the -84G/A SNP does not account for all HPS cases; therefore, other components of the nitric oxide–dependent signal transduction pathway or additional mechanisms and genes may be involved in the pathogenesis of HPS. This is in accordance with other observations suggesting a multifactorial cause of HPS.[46] In summary, genetic alterations in the nNOS exon 1c regulatory region influence expression of the *nNOS* gene and may contribute to the pathogenesis of HPS, but there are likely numerous other genes that contribute to the development of HPS as well as predispose to environmental influences in this disorder.

These examples provide insight into the complexity of current models of molecular genetics and illustrate the inadequacy of current methods of analysis to fully define genetic causes of disease, particularly polygenic disorders. The majority of pediatric surgical disorders currently fall into the category of undefined multifactorial inheritance, which is even less well understood than the genetic categories described. In these disorders, no causative, predisposing, or influencing gene loci have been identified. Isolated regional malformations are presumed

to result from interactions between the environment and the actions of multiple genes. Multifactorial inheritance is characterized by the presence of a greater number of risk genes within a family. The presumption of a genetic basis of the anomalies is based on recurrence risk. The recurrence risks in multifactorial inheritance disorders, although generally low, are higher than in the general population; they are increased further if more than one family member is affected, if there are more severe malformations in the proband, or if the parents are closely related. Beyond these generalizations, genetics can provide little specific information about this category of disorder.

Utility of Molecular Genetics in Clinical Pediatric Surgery

Genetic Counseling and Prenatal Diagnosis

As mentioned earlier, there is still a gap between genotypic understanding of a disorder and direct application to clinical treatment. The exceptions are in the areas of genetic counseling and prenatal diagnosis. Pediatric surgeons are likely to require some knowledge of molecular genetics as their role in prenatal counseling of parents continues to increase. Molecular genetics can supply specific information about an affected fetus by providing genotypic confirmation of a phenotypic abnormality, a phenotypic correlate for a confirmed genotype, and, in many instances, the recurrence risk for subsequent pregnancies and the need for concern (or lack thereof) about other family members. Once again, HD is an example of how molecular genetics can be valuable in genetic counseling.[8,64] The generalized risk to siblings is 4% and increases as the length of involved segment increases. In HD associated with known syndromes, genetic counseling may focus more on prognosis related to the syndrome than on recurrence risk. In isolated HD, a more precise risk table can be created. Risk of recurrence of the disease is greater in relatives of an affected female than of an affected male. Risk of recurrence is also greater in relatives of an individual with long-segment compared with short-segment disease. For example, the recurrence risk in a sibling of a female with aganglionosis beginning proximal to the splenic flexure is approximately 23% for a male and 18% for a female, whereas the recurrence risk in a sibling of a male with aganglionosis beginning proximal to the splenic flexure is approximately 11% for a male and 8% for a female. These risks fall to 6% and lower for siblings of an individual with short-segment disease. Prenatal diagnosis is possible if the mutation within the family is known. However, because the penetrance of single gene mutations is low (except for *SOX10* mutations in Waardenburg's syndrome), the clinical usefulness of prenatal diagnosis is limited.

More commonly, a general knowledge of genetics can allow accurate counseling of recurrence risk and reassurance for parents of an affected fetus diagnosed with a multifactorial inheritance defect, the most common circumstance involving prenatal consultation with a pediatric surgeon. Pediatric surgeons should also be aware of the value of genetic evaluation of abortus tissue in cases of multiple anomalies when, after counseling, the parents choose to terminate the pregnancy. It is a disservice to the family not to send the fetus to an appropriate center for a detailed gross examination and a state-of-the-art molecular genetic assessment when appropriate.

As molecular genetics increasingly characterizes the genes responsible for specific disorders, their predisposing and modifier loci, and other genetic interactions, a better ability to predict the presence and severity of specific phenotypes will inevitably follow. This will allow prenatal counseling to be tailored to the specific fetus and lead to improved prognostic accuracy, giving parents the opportunity to make more informed prenatal choices.

Postnatal Treatment

In the future, molecular genetics will allow specific therapies to be optimized for individual patients. This may range from specific pharmacologic treatments for individual patients based on genotype and predicted pharmacologic response to anticipation of propensities for specific postoperative complications, such as infection or postoperative stress response. Of course, the ultimate treatment for an affected individual and their progeny would be to correct the germline genetic alteration responsible for a specific phenotype. Although there are many scientific and ethical obstacles to overcome before considering such therapy, it is conceivable that a combination of molecular genetics and gene transfer technologies could correct a germline mutation, replacing an abnormal gene by the integration of a normal gene and providing the ultimate preventive therapy. Although the state of gene transfer technology is far from this level of sophistication, progress in the past 3 decades can only be described as astounding. The next section provides an overview of the current state of gene transfer and its potential application for therapy.

GENE THERAPY

Gene therapy continues to be embroiled in controversy, its seemingly unlimited potential obscured by repeated disappointments and, more recently, adverse events. The year 2000 brought the first clinical gene therapy success—treatment of X-linked severe combined immune deficiency (XSCID)[11]—only to have this dramatic achievement undermined by the occurrence of leukemia in two patients. This and other adverse events threaten to overshadow the substantial progress made in gene transfer technology in recent years. Slowly but surely, methods for gene transfer are being developed that will have greater safety, specificity, and efficacy than ever before. Although complex issues remain to be solved, it is likely that successful gene therapy strategies will be developed and proved within the next few years. The technology of gene transfer can be divided into viral vector-based gene transfer and nonviral gene transfer. Because of the limited scope of this chapter and the limited efficiency of nonviral-based gene transfer thus far, only the current state of viral-based gene transfer is reviewed.

Viral Vectors for Gene Transfer

Viruses are highly evolved biologic machines that efficiently penetrate hostile host cells and exploit the host's cellular machinery to facilitate their replication. Ideally, viral vectors harness the viral infection pathway but avoid the subsequent replicative expression of viral genes that causes toxicity. This is traditionally achieved by deleting some or all of the coding regions from the viral genome but leaving intact those sequences that are needed for the vector function, such as elements required for the packaging of viral DNA into virus capsid or the integration of vector DNA into host chromatin. The chosen expression cassette is then cloned into the viral backbone in place of those sequences that were deleted. The deleted genes encoding proteins involved in replication or capsid or envelope proteins are included in a separate packaging construct. The vector genome and packaging construct are then cotransfected into packaging cells to produce recombinant vector particles (Fig. 2-3).

Given the diversity of therapeutic strategies and disease targets involving gene transfer, it is not surprising that a large number of vector systems have been devised. Although there is no single vector suitable for all applications, certain characteristics are desirable for all vectors if they are to be clinically useful: (1) the ability to be reproducibly and stably propagated, (2) the ability to be purified to high titers, (3) the ability to mediate targeted delivery (i.e., to avoid widespread vector dissemination), and (4) the ability to achieve gene delivery and expression without harmful side effects. There are presently five main classes of vectors that, at least under specific circumstances, satisfy these requirements: oncoretroviruses, lentiviruses, adeno-associated viruses (AAVs), adenoviruses, and herpesviruses. Table 2-2 compares the general characteristics of these vectors.

Oncoretroviruses and lentiviruses are "integrating," that is, they insert their genomes into the host cellular chromatin. Thus, they share the advantage of persistent gene expression. Nonintegrating viruses can achieve persistent gene expression in nondividing cells, but integrating vectors are the tools of choice if stable genetic alteration needs to be maintained in dividing cells. It is important to note, however, that stable transcription is not guaranteed by integration and that transgene expression from integrated viral genomes can be silenced over time.[53] Oncoretroviruses and lentiviruses differ in their ability to penetrate an intact nuclear membrane. Whereas retroviruses can transduce only dividing cells, lentiviruses can naturally penetrate nuclear membranes and can transduce nondividing cells, making them particularly useful for stem cell targeting applications.[19,74] Because of this difference, lentivirus vectors are superseding retrovirus vectors for most applications. Both types of vector, because of their ability to integrate, share the potential hazard of alteration of the host cell genome.

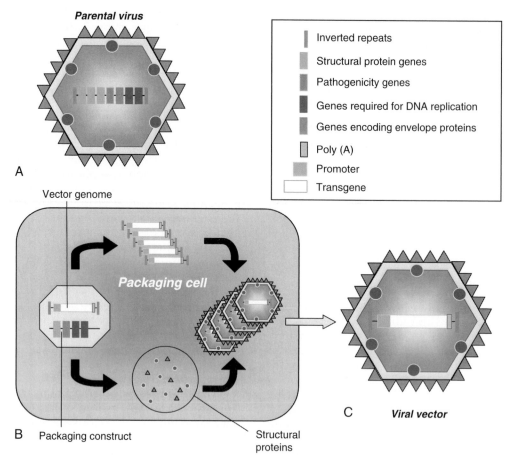

Figure 2–3 Requirements for the creation of a generic viral vector. *A,* The basic machinery of a chosen parental virus is used, including genes encoding specific structural protein genes, envelope proteins, and proteins required for DNA replication, but not genes encoding proteins conferring pathogenicity. *B,* The vector is assembled in a packaging cell. A packaging (helper) construct, containing genes derived from the parental virus, can be delivered as a plasmid or helper virus or stably integrated into the chromatin of the packaging cell. Pathogenicity functions and sequences required for encapsidation are eliminated from the helper construct so that it cannot be packaged into a viral particle. In contrast, the vector genome contains the transgenic expression cassette flanked by inverted terminal repeats and *cis*-acting sequences that are required for genome encapsidation. Viral structural proteins and proteins required for replication of the vector DNA are expressed from the packaging construct, and the replicated vector genomes are packaged into the virus particles. *C,* The viral vector particles are released from the packaging cell and contain only the vector genome. (*See color plate.*)

This could lead to the undesirable complications of human germline alteration or insertional mutagenesis, particularly important considerations for pediatric or fetal gene therapy.[56] Nevertheless, these vectors have proved most efficient for long-term gene transfer into cells in rapidly proliferative tissues and for stem cell–directed gene transfer.

Nonintegrating vectors include adenovirus, AAV, and herpesvirus vectors. Adenovirus vectors have the advantages of broad tropism, moderate packaging capacity, and high efficiency, but they carry the usually undesirable properties of high immunogenicity and consequent short duration of gene expression. Modifications of adenovirus vectors to reduce immunogenicity and further increase the transgene capacity have consisted primarily of deletion of "early" (E1–E4) viral genes that encode immunogenic viral proteins responsible for the cytotoxic immune response.[3,38] The most important advance,

however, has been the development of helper-dependent adenoviruses (HD-Ads) that are deleted of all viral genes, thus eliminating the immune response to adenoviral-associated proteins.[48] These vectors may ultimately be most valuable for long-term gene transfer in tissues with very low rates of cell division, such as muscle or brain.

AAV is a helper-dependent parvovirus that, in the presence of adenovirus or herpesvirus infection, undergoes a productive replication cycle. AAV vectors are single-strand DNA vectors and represent one of the most promising vector systems for safe long-term gene transfer and expression in nonproliferating tissues. AAV is the only vector system for which the wild-type virus has no known human pathogenicity, adding to its safety profile. In addition, the small size and simplicity of the vector particle make systemic administration of high doses of vector possible without eliciting an acute inflammatory response or other toxicity. Although the majority of the

TABLE 2–2 Five Main Viral Vector Groups

Vector Type	Coding Material	Packaging Capacity (kb)	Tissue Tropism	Vector Genome	Advantages	Disadvantages
Retrovirus	RNA	8	Only dividing cells	Integrated	Persistent gene transfer in dividing cells	Requires cell division; may induce oncogenesis
Lentivirus	RNA	8	Broad, including stem cells	Integrated	Integrates into nondividing cells; persistent gene transfer	Potential for oncogenesis
HSV-1	dsDNA	40	Neural	Episomal	Inflammatory response; limited tropism	Large packaging capacity; strong tropism for neurons
AAV	ssDNA	<5	Broad	Episomal (90%) Integrated (<10%)	Noninflammatory; nonpathogenic	Small packaging capacity
Adenovirus	dsDNA	8 30*	Broad	Episomal	Extremely efficient gene transfer in most tissues	Capsid-mediated potent immune response; transient expression in dividing cells

*Helper dependent.
AAV, adeno-associated vector; ds, double-strand; HSV-1; herpes simplex virus-1; ss, single-strand.

AAV vector genome after transduction remains episomal, an approximately 10% rate of integration has been observed.[50] There are two primary limitations of AAV vectors. The first is the need to convert a single-strand DNA genome into a double strand, limiting the efficiency of transduction. Recently this obstacle has been overcome by the development of double-strand vectors that exploit a hairpin intermediate of the AAV replication cycle.[43] Although these vectors can mediate a 10- to 100-fold increase in transgene expression in vitro and in vivo, they can package only 2.4 kb of double-strand DNA, limiting their therapeutic usefulness. This relates to the second primary limitation of AAV vectors, which is limited packaging capacity (4.8 kb of single-strand DNA). One approach to address this limitation is to split the expression cassette across two vectors, exploiting the in vivo concatemerization of rAAV genomes. This results in reconstitution of a functional cassette after concatemerization in the cell nucleus.[17,49] Finally, an approach that has become common for enhancing or redirecting the tissue tropism of AAV vectors is to pseudotype the vectors with capsid proteins from alternative serotypes of AAV.[58] Although most rAAV vectors have been derived from AAV2, eight distinct AAV serotypes have been identified thus far, all of which differ in efficiency for transduction of specific cell types. AAV vectors have proved particularly useful for muscle, liver, and central nervous system directed gene transfer.

Herpes simplex virus (HSV-1) vectors are the largest and most complex of all currently used vector systems. Their primary advantages are a very large packaging capacity (up to 40 kb) and their strong neurotropism, allowing lifelong expression in sensory neurons. This has made neuropathologic disorders a primary target for HSV-1-mediated gene transfer.

Clinically Relevant Challenges in Gene Transfer

Recent adverse events demonstrate the potential for disaster when using vector-based gene transfer. Major initiatives must be undertaken to delineate the potential complications of gene transfer with specific vectors to convince physicians and the public of their safety for future clinical trials. Nevertheless, because of the potential benefit, continued efforts to develop safe and efficacious strategies for clinical gene transfer are warranted.

One of the primary obstacles to successful gene therapy continues to be the host immune response. The intact immune system is highly capable of activation against viral vectors using the same defense systems that combat wild-type infections. Viral products or new transgene encoded proteins are recognized as foreign and are capable of activating an immune response of variable intensity. Adenovirus vectors are the most immunogenic of all the viral vector types and induce multiple components of the immune response, including cytotoxic T-lymphocyte responses, humoral virus-neutralizing responses, and potent cytokine-mediated inflammatory responses.[7] Great progress has been made in reducing T-cell responses against adenoviral antigens by the development of HD-Ad vectors that are deleted of all adenoviral genes. These vectors have demonstrated reduced immunogenicity with long-term phenotypic correction of mouse models and negligible toxicity.[14,34] However, even HD-Ad vectors or less immunogenic vector systems such as AAV or lentivirus vectors can induce an immunologic response to capsid proteins or to novel transgene encoded proteins, a potentially limiting problem in a large number of human protein deficiency disorders caused by a null mutation. Thus, the application of gene transfer technology to many human disorders may require the development of effective and nontoxic strategies for tolerance induction.

Another major area of interest that may improve the safety profile of future viral vector-based gene transfer is specific targeting to affected tissues or organs. Whereas wild-type virus infections are generally restricted to those tissues that are accessible through the route of transmission, recombinant vectors are not subject to the same physical limitations. The promiscuity of viral vectors is a significant liability, because systemic or even local administration of a vector may lead to unwanted vector uptake by many different cell types in multiple organs. For instance, lack of adenovirus vector specificity was directly linked to the induction of a massive systemic immune response that resulted in a gene therapy–related death in 1999.[7] Because many of the toxic effects of viral vector-based gene transfer are directly related to dose, increasing the efficiency with which viral vectors infect specific cell populations should reduce viral load and improve safety.

There are a variety of promising methods to achieve the targeting of viral vectors for specific organs or cell types. Perhaps the simplest approach is vector pseudotyping, which has been performed for retrovirus, lentivirus, and AAV vectors. By changing the capsid envelope proteins to alternative viral types or serotypes, a portfolio of vectors with different tropisms can be generated.[40] Another approach is the conjugation of capsid proteins to molecular adapters such as bispecific antibodies with specific receptor binding properties.[33,61] A third approach is to genetically engineer the capsid proteins themselves to alter their receptor binding (i.e., to abolish their normal receptor binding) or to encode a small peptide ligand for an alternative receptor.[28] These and other approaches, when combined with the appropriate use of tissue-specific promoters, may significantly reduce the likelihood of toxicity from viral-based gene therapy.

Another important obstacle to human gene therapy—particularly fetal gene therapy—is the potential for insertional mutagenesis when using integrating vectors. Until recently, this risk was considered extremely low to negligible, based on the assumption that oncogenesis requires multiple genetic lesions and the fact that induced cancer had not been observed in any of the hundreds of patients treated with retrovirus vectors in the many gene therapy trials. However, recently 2 of 11 patients treated in an otherwise successful trial[11,25] of retroviral gene therapy for XSCID developed a leukemia disorder.[26] Evidence suggests that this was caused by retroviral genome insertion in or near the oncogene *LM02*. These concerns have been further heightened by evidence that retroviral genes are not randomly inserted, as previously believed; rather, they preferentially integrate into transcriptionally active genes.[65] Although such events may be more likely to occur under the unique selective influences of XSCID, it is clear that the risk of insertional mutagenesis can no longer be ignored. Approaches designed to neutralize cells expressing transgene if and when an adverse event occurs, such as engineering suicide genes into the vector, are one option, but this would also neutralize any therapeutic effect. More exciting approaches are based on site-specific integration—for instance, taking advantage of site-integration machinery of bacteriophage φX31.[52] This is undoubtedly only one of many approaches that will use site-specific integration in the future and should, if successful, negate the risk of insertional mutagenesis.

Finally, a critical issue for in vivo gene transfer with integrating vectors in individuals of reproductive age is the potential for germline transmission, with alteration of the human genome. The risk of this event is poorly defined at present and is most likely extremely low, although in some circumstances (e.g., fetal gene transfer), it could be increased.[56] Although still not technically possible, the intentional site-specific correction of defects in the germline would be the ultimate in gene therapy. However, even if the technology becomes available, the intentional alteration of the human genome raises profound ethical and societal questions that will need to be thoroughly addressed before its application. The considerations are similar to those for insertional mutagenesis, so many of the approaches mentioned earlier for gene targeting and reduction of the potential for insertional mutagenesis are applicable here as well.

Overview of the Current Status of Gene Transfer

At present it is clear that viral vectors are the best available vehicle for efficient gene transfer into most tissues. Several gene therapy applications have shown promise in early-phase clinical trials. Although the adverse events noted in the XSCID trial have dampened enthusiasm, this still represents the first successful treatment of a disease by gene therapy. The treatment of hemophilia B using rAAV is also promising.[32,41] The next few years are likely to bring advances in the treatment of certain types of cancer using conditionally replicating oncolytic viruses and in the treatment of vascular and coronary artery disease using viral vectors that express angiogenic factors. In the future, new disease targets are likely to become approachable through the fusion of viral vector-mediated gene transfer with other technologies such as RNA interference, a powerful tool to achieve gene silencing. Such vectors could be useful in developing therapy for a range of diseases, such as dominantly inherited genetic disorders, infectious diseases, and cancer. Advances in the understanding of viral vector technology and DNA entry into cells and nuclei will likely lead to the development of more efficient nonviral vector systems that may rival viral vectors in efficiency and have superior safety. Gene vector systems of the future may be very different from those in use today and will ultimately provide efficient delivery of target-specific, regulated, transgene expression for an appropriate length of time.

REFERENCES

1. Acton JD, Wilmott RW: Phenotype of CF and the effects of possible modifier genes. Paediatr Respir Rev 2001;2: 332-339.
2. Amiel J, Lyonnet S: Hirschsprung disease, associated syndromes, and genetics: A review. J Med Genet 2001;38:729-739.

3. Andrews JL, Kadan MJ, Gorziglia MI, et al: Generation and characterization of E1/E2a/E3/E4-deficient adenoviral vectors encoding human factor VIII. Mol Ther 2001;3:329-336.
4. Angrist M, Kauffman E, Slaugenhaupt SA, et al: A gene for Hirschsprung disease (megacolon) in the pericentromeric region of human chromosome 10. Nat Genet 1993;4:351-356.
5. Arkwright PD, Laurie S, Super M, et al: TGF-beta(1) genotype and accelerated decline in lung function of patients with cystic fibrosis. Thorax 2000;55:459-462.
6. Aron Y, Polla BS, Bienvenu T, et al: HLA class II polymorphism in cystic fibrosis: A possible modifier of pulmonary phenotype. Am J Respir Crit Care Med 1999;159:1464-1468.
7. Assessment of adenoviral vector safety and toxicity: Report of the National Institutes of Health Recombinant DNA Advisory Committee. Hum Gene Ther 2002;13:3-13.
8. Badner JA, Sieber WK, Garver KL, Chakravarti A: A genetic study of Hirschsprung disease. Am J Hum Genet 1990;46:568-580.
9. Balci S, Ercal MD, Onol B, et al: Familial short rib syndrome, type Beemer, with pyloric stenosis and short intestine, one case diagnosed prenatally. Clin Genet 1991;39:298-303.
10. Carter CO, Evans KA: Inheritance of congenital pyloric stenosis. J Med Genet 1969;6:233-254.
11. Cavazzana-Calvo M, Hacein-Bey S, de Saint Basile G, et al: Gene therapy of human severe combined immunodeficiency (SCID)-X1 disease. Science 2000;288:669-672.
12. Cekada S, Kilvain S, Brajenovic-Milic B, et al: Partial trisomy 13q22→qter and monosomy 18q21→qter as a result of familial translocation. Acta Paediatr 1999;88:675-678.
13. Chung E, Curtis D, Chen G, et al: Genetic evidence for the neuronal nitric oxide synthase gene (NOS1) as a susceptibility locus for infantile pyloric stenosis. Am J Hum Genet 1996;58:363-370.
14. DelloRusso C, Scott JM, Hartigan-O'Connor D, et al: Functional correction of adult mdx mouse muscle using gutted adenoviral vectors expressing full-length dystrophin. Proc Natl Acad Sci U S A 2002;99:12979-12984.
15. Dipple KM, McCabe ER: Modifier genes convert "simple" mendelian disorders to complex traits. Mol Genet Metab 2000;71:43-50.
16. Drumm ML: Modifier genes and variation in cystic fibrosis. Respir Res 2001;2:125-128.
17. Duan D, Yue Y, Yan Z, Engelhardt JF: A new dual-vector approach to enhance recombinant adeno-associated virus-mediated gene expression through intermolecular cis activation. Nat Med 2000;6:595-598.
18. Feingold E: Regression-based quantitative-trait-locus mapping in the 21st century. Am J Hum Genet 2002;71:217-222.
19. Follenzi A, Ailles LE, Bakovic S, et al: Gene transfer by lentiviral vectors is limited by nuclear translocation and rescued by HIV-1 pol sequences. Nat Genet 2000;25:217-222.
20. Gabriel SB, Salomon R, Pelet A, et al: Segregation at three loci explains familial and population risk in Hirschsprung disease. Nat Genet 2002;31:89-93.
21. Garred P, Pressler T, Madsen HO, et al: Association of mannose-binding lectin gene heterogeneity with severity of lung disease and survival in cystic fibrosis. J Clin Invest 1999;104:431-437.
22. Grasemann H, Knauer N, Buscher R, et al: Airway nitric oxide levels in cystic fibrosis patients are related to a polymorphism in the neuronal nitric oxide synthase gene. Am J Respir Crit Care Med 2000;162:2172-2176.
23. Groman JD, Meyer ME, Wilmott RW, et al: Variant cystic fibrosis phenotypes in the absence of CFTR mutations. N Engl J Med 2002;347:401-407.
24. Gupta AK, Berry M: Recessive polycystic kidney disease and congenital hypertrophic pyloric stenosis. Pediatr Radiol 1991;21:160.
25. Hacein-Bey-Abina S, Le Deist F, Carlier F, et al: Sustained correction of X-linked severe combined immunodeficiency by ex vivo gene therapy. N Engl J Med 2002;346:1185-1193.
26. Hacein-Bey-Abina S, von Kalle C, Schmidt M, et al: A serious adverse event after successful gene therapy for X-linked severe combined immunodeficiency. N Engl J Med 2003;348:255-256.
27. Heller A, Seidel J, Hubler A, et al: Molecular cytogenetic characterisation of partial trisomy 9q in a case with pyloric stenosis and a review. J Med Genet 2000;37:529-532.
28. Hidaka C, Milano E, Leopold PL, et al: CAR-dependent and CAR-independent pathways of adenovirus vector-mediated gene transfer and expression in human fibroblasts. J Clin Invest 1999;103:579-587.
29. Hodgson SV, Berry AC, Dunbar HM: Two brothers with an unbalanced 8;17 translocation and infantile pyloric stenosis. Clin Genet 1995;48:328-330.
30. Hull J, Thomson AH: Contribution of genetic factors other than CFTR to disease severity in cystic fibrosis. Thorax 1998;53:1018-1021.
31. Kaplan BS, Gordon I, Pincott J, Barratt TM: Familial hypoplastic glomerulocystic kidney disease: A definite entity with dominant inheritance. Am J Med Genet 1989;34:569-573.
32. Kay MA, Manno CS, Ragni MV, et al: Evidence for gene transfer and expression of factor IX in haemophilia B patients treated with an AAV vector. Nat Genet 2000;24:257-261.
33. Khare PD, Liao S, Hirose Y, et al: Tumor growth suppression by a retroviral vector displaying scFv antibody to CEA and carrying the iNOS gene. Anticancer Res 2002;22:2443-2446.
34. Kim IH, Jozkowicz A, Piedra PA, et al: Lifetime correction of genetic deficiency in mice with a single injection of helper-dependent adenoviral vector. Proc Natl Acad Sci U S A 2001;98:13282-13287.
35. Konig R, Fuchs S, Kern C, Langenbeck U: Simpson-Golabi-Behmel syndrome with severe cardiac arrhythmias. Am J Med Genet 1991;38:244-247.
36. Krantz ID, McCallum J, DeScipio C, et al: Cornelia de Lange syndrome is caused by mutations in NIPBL, the human homolog of *Drosophila melanogaster* Nipped-B. Nat Genet 2004;36:631-635.
37. Liede A, Pal T, Mitchell M, Narod SA: Delineation of a new syndrome: Clustering of pyloric stenosis, endometriosis, and breast cancer in two families. J Med Genet 2000;37:794-796.
38. Lusky M, Christ M, Rittner K, et al: In vitro and in vivo biology of recombinant adenovirus vectors with E1, E1/E2A, or E1/E4 deleted. J Virol 1998;72:2022-2032.
39. Lyonnet S, Bolino A, Pelet A, et al: A gene for Hirschsprung disease maps to the proximal long arm of chromosome 10. Nat Genet 1993;4:346-350.
40. MacKenzie TC, Kobinger GP, Kootstra NA, et al: Efficient transduction of liver and muscle after in utero injection of lentiviral vectors with different pseudotypes. Mol Ther 2002;6:349-358.
41. Manno CS, Chew AJ, Hutchison S, et al: AAV-mediated factor IX gene transfer to skeletal muscle in patients with severe hemophilia B. Blood 2003;101:2963-2972.

42. Martucciello G, Torre M, Pini Prato A, et al: Associated anomalies in intestinal neuronal dysplasia. J Pediatr Surg 2002;37:219-223.

43. McCarty DM, Monahan PE, Samulski RJ: Self-complementary recombinant adeno-associated virus (scAAV) vectors promote efficient transduction independently of DNA synthesis. Gene Ther 2001;8:1248-1254.

44. McKusick VA: Mendelian Inheritance in Man: A Catalog of Human Genes and Genetic Disorders, 12th ed. Baltimore, Johns Hopkins University Press, 1998.

45. Mickle JE, Cutting GR: Genotype-phenotype relationships in cystic fibrosis. Med Clin North Am 2000;84:597-607.

46. Mitchell LE, Risch N: The genetics of infantile hypertrophic pyloric stenosis: A reanalysis. Am J Dis Child 1993;147:1203-1211.

47. Moore JH, Williams SM: New strategies for identifying gene-gene interactions in hypertension. Ann Med 2002; 34:88-95.

48. Morsy MA, Caskey CT: Expanded-capacity adenoviral vectors—the helper-dependent vectors. Mol Med Today 1999;5:18-24.

49. Nakai H, Storm TA, Kay MA: Increasing the size of rAAV-mediated expression cassettes in vivo by intermolecular joining of two complementary vectors. Nat Biotechnol 2000;18:527-532.

50. Nakai H, Yant SR, Storm TA, et al: Extrachromosomal recombinant adeno-associated virus vector genomes are primarily responsible for stable liver transduction in vivo. J Virol 2001;75:6969-6976.

51. Ohshiro K, Puri P: Pathogenesis of infantile hypertrophic pyloric stenosis: Recent progress. Pediatr Surg Int 1998;13:243-252.

52. Olivares EC, Hollis RP, Chalberg TW, et al: Site-specific genomic integration produces therapeutic factor IX levels in mice. Nat Biotechnol 2002;20:1124-1128.

53. Pannell D, Osborne CS, Yao S, et al: Retrovirus vector silencing is de novo methylase independent and marked by a repressive histone code. EMBO J 2000;19:5884-5894.

54. Parisi MA, Kapur RP: Genetics of Hirschsprung disease. Curr Opin Pediatr 2000;12:610-617.

55. Parmley RR, Gendler SJ: Cystic fibrosis mice lacking Muc1 have reduced amounts of intestinal mucus. J Clin Invest 1998;102:1798-1806.

56. Prenatal gene transfer: Scientific, medical, and ethical issues: A report of the Recombinant DNA Advisory Committee. Hum Gene Ther 2000;11:1211-1229.

57. Puffenberger EG, Hosoda K, Washington SS, et al: A missense mutation of the endothelin-B receptor gene in multigenic Hirschsprung's disease. Cell 1994;79:1257-1266.

58. Rabinowitz JE, Rolling F, Li C, et al: Cross-packaging of a single adeno-associated virus (AAV) type 2 vector genome into multiple AAV serotypes enables transduction with broad specificity. J Virol 2002;76:791-801.

59. Ramirez-Gomara A, Castejon-Ponce E, Martinez-Martinez M, et al: [Smith-Lemli-Opitz syndrome type II: Neonatal diagnosis and review of the most interesting clinical features]. Rev Neurol 2002;34:946-950.

60. Repetto GM, Wagstaff J, Korf BR, Knoll JH: Complex familial rearrangement of chromosome 9p24.3 detected by FISH. Am J Med Genet 1998;76:306-309.

61. Reynolds PN, Nicklin SA, Kaliberova L, et al: Combined transductional and transcriptional targeting improves the specificity of transgene expression in vivo. Nat Biotechnol 2001;19:838-842.

62. Riordan JR, Rommens JM, Kerem B, et al: Identification of the cystic fibrosis gene: Cloning and characterization of complementary DNA. Science 1989;245:1066-1073.

63. Rozmahel R, Wilschanski M, Matin A, et al: Modulation of disease severity in cystic fibrosis transmembrane conductance regulator deficient mice by a secondary genetic factor. Nat Genet 1996;12:280-287.

64. Russell MB, Russell CA, Niebuhr E: An epidemiological study of Hirschsprung's disease and additional anomalies. Acta Paediatr 1994;83:68-71.

65. Schroder AR, Shinn P, Chen H, et al: HIV-1 integration in the human genome favors active genes and local hotspots. Cell 2002;110:521-529.

66. Scriver CR, Waters PJ: Monogenic traits are not simple: Lessons from phenylketonuria. Trends Genet 1999;15: 267-272.

67. Sponseller PD, Sethi N, Cameron DE, Pyeritz RE: Infantile scoliosis in Marfan syndrome. Spine 1997;22:509-516.

68. Tsui LC, Buchwald M, Barker D, et al: Cystic fibrosis locus defined by a genetically linked polymorphic DNA marker. Science 1985;230:1054-1057.

69. Wang X, Moylan B, Leopold DA, et al: Mutation in the gene responsible for cystic fibrosis and predisposition to chronic rhinosinusitis in the general population. JAMA 2000;284:1814-1819.

70. Webb AL, Sturgiss S, Warwicker P, et al: Maternal uniparental disomy for chromosome 2 in association with confined placental mosaicism for trisomy 2 and severe intrauterine growth retardation. Prenat Diagn 1996;16: 958-962.

71. Weiss KM: Is there a paradigm shift in genetics? Lessons from the study of human diseases. Mol Phylogenet Evol 1996;5:259-265.

72. Yamamoto Y, Oguro N, Nara T, et al: Duplication of part of 9q due to maternal 12;9 inverted insertion associated with pyloric stenosis. Am J Med Genet 1988;31:379-384.

73. Zielenski J, Corey M, Rozmahel R, et al: Detection of a cystic fibrosis modifier locus for meconium ileus on human chromosome 19q13. Nat Genet 1999;22:128-129.

74. Zufferey R, Nagy D, Mandel RJ, et al: Multiply attenuated lentiviral vector achieves efficient gene delivery in vivo. Nat Biotechnol 1997;15:871-875.

Chapter 3

The Impact of Tissue Engineering in Pediatric Surgery

Tracy C. Grikscheit and Joseph P. Vacanti

Extirpative surgery often requires reconstruction to replace the purpose and appearance of the excised tissue. In the case of congenital defects, a tissue deficit may already exist. The goal of tissue engineering and organ fabrication is to create living replacement organs and tissues, with the proposed advantages of more exact replacement and better durability related to cellular proliferation and autologous repair. These techniques are beginning to make the transition from the laboratory to the operating room, providing a better proxy for appearance and function in patients affected by congenital anomalies or resection.

Early attempts by surgeons to substitute for either function or cosmesis include those detailed in the *Sushruta Samhita* from around 6 BC, describing rhinoplasty using a forehead flap, and various wooden and metal prostheses mentioned in the Talmud. Modern progress has embraced both these approaches, developing multiple procedures that rely on either the substitution of tissues, as in the transfer of a toe to replace a finger, or the use of a manufactured substitute such as Dacron aortic grafts. The limitations of native substitution lie in the dilemma of prioritizing the value of various tissues and the trade-off that must be made. In pediatric surgery, there is a fairly limited supply of donor tissue that remains inherently different from the tissue it replaces. Manufactured substitution also has acknowledged problems: material failure, increased rates of infection, and the immune system's destruction of foreign material. In addition, nonliving material does not grow with the patient or adapt to changing circumstances, so pediatric patients may need to undergo multiple operations with increasing levels of complexity. Neither approach can solve the replacement of composite tissues.

Organ transplantation, a modern version of native tissue substitution, has demonstrated that functional replacement can be lifesaving, but there are obstacles, including a limited supply and a long list of associated morbidities.

The resilience of surgical therapy is of particular concern in pediatric surgery, where the surgical outcome may be measured over decades and the surgical reconstruction is subjected to higher levels of activity and physiologic change. In addition, in some congenital defects, the amount of available donor tissue may be insufficient, and prosthetic material may not approximate the functional and cosmetic requirements of the missing tissue, including growth.

Solutions to problems in the surgical treatment of children with short-bowel syndrome, craniofacial defects, and congenital heart defects are imminent. Human application of tissue-engineered skin and cartilage has already occurred. We look forward to significant advances in vascular substitutes and intestinal replacement and progress with the solid organs, which have proved to be the most elaborate systems to replicate.

TECHNIQUES AND PRINCIPLES OF TISSUE ENGINEERING

Monolayer cell culture is a well-defined science, but organizing cell combinations into complex, three-dimensional functional structures relies on numerous relationships between the structure given to the cells and the cells assembled on the structure. After defining the cellular components and the structure of the engineered organ, adding adequate vascularization and directing the symphony of cell signaling found in normal tissues are the greatest challenges.

The manifold approaches to tissue engineering can be broadly reduced to in vitro and in vivo designs. All have attempted to provide an underlying support or scaffold for the cells, a proper population of cells, and a substitute for the extracellular matrix. Interactions between cells and extracellular matrix require cell migration, proliferation, differentiation, and apoptosis, which are all critical functions for a tissue-engineered construct.[60]

In vitro models have usually relied on the formation of a bioreactor system or cell patterning for monolayer co-culture studies.[20,42,58,101] Bioreactors are dynamic tissue culture devices that range from simple mechanical designs to more complex systems with oxygen exchange, defined flow rates, and electrical and mechanical stimulation. The tissue engineering of less complex tissues such as cell sheets requires only a simple method of exchange of growth medium to the engineered construct that avoids stasis. Spinner flasks or rotating vessels are examples.[22]

More complex bioreactors have been designed to furnish stretch to skeletal muscle cultures,[94] shear to endothelial cells,[96] and compression to chondrocytes.[12] There is good evidence that cell-polymer constructs grown in vitro under physiologic conditions that are closer to those found in vivo, including strain and pericellular nutrient flow, result in improved cell morphology, growth characteristics, and metabolic activity.[55,68,81] Studies of chondrocytes grown on polyglycolic acid constructs in cultures subjected to hydrodynamic forces show that cell proliferation rates are nearly 50% greater, there are 60% more glycosaminoglycans, and 125% more collagen in the extracellular matrix is regenerated.[4,32]

Other in vitro models for tissue engineering include cell patterning in either monolayer or three-dimensional culture. Defined tissue architectures yield more predictable patterns of growth and differentiation. In the case of more complex organs, such as the liver, co-culture in tissue-specific media is emerging as a necessity for successful designs.[5] Photolithography has been used to generate alternating domains of *N*-(2-aminoethyl)-3-aminopropyl-trimethoxysilane and dimethyldichlorosilane to preferentially seed human bone-derived cells to the former domains, mediated through vitronectin.[58] High-resolution patterns of poly-L-lysine were used in micrometer scale microcontact printing to align cultured neurons,[42] adhered via microcontact printing of specific oligopeptides.[101] Constraint of cell spreading and nonrandom co-cultures of cells more closely replicate the three-dimensional organized architecture of human tissues.[58] Topographic cues may be just as important as some biologic signals.

A highly promising intersection of microfabrication engineering and improved in vitro tissue culture systems is resulting in the development of smaller, smarter bioreactors in which microfluidics, mass transfer, nutrition extraction, and cell growth can all be studied with known cellular architecture and standardized microfabrication to the micrometer scale.[8,9,20,44] As described later in the section on tissue engineering of the liver, this approach may be critical for complex organs.

In vivo studies have used animals as a complex bioreactor, with composite constructs implanted into vascularized spaces such as the omentum, mesentery, interscapular fat pad, or latissimus dorsi, where an endogenous blood supply can participate in angiogenesis.[93] A substitute for the extracellular matrix in the form of a scaffold is implanted after cell loading onto the construct.[52] Prevascularization of polymer sponges, by implanting a construct days to weeks before adding cells, can increase cell survival rates.[87]

In one of the earlier in vivo models, liver, intestine, and pancreas parenchymal cells were implanted on biodegradable polymers after 4 days of in vitro culture, resulting in viable cells, mitotic figures, and vascularization of the growing cell mass.[93] One polymer used in this report was a 90-10 copolymer of glycolide and lactide, produced commercially as Vicryl. With the recent explosion of available biomaterials, researchers have successfully used an increasing variety of scaffolds, including small intestinal submucosa as a small-caliber venous graft with hepatocyte transplantation, anastomosed between the portal vein and the inferior vena cava.[49] Additional success with calcium alginate gels, commercially available surfactants, agarose, fibrin glue, and microfabricated biodegradable materials illustrates the necessity of collaboration between chemical and tissue engineers.[1,35,36,95]

A combination of in vitro and in vivo approaches has solved some simple tissue engineering problems and will continue to be important for autologous tissue removal, augmentation in the laboratory, and eventual in vivo replacement.

CARTILAGE AND BONE TISSUE ENGINEERING

Structural defects characterize many congenital and acquired problems encountered by pediatric surgeons. Some pioneering treatments have capitalized on in situ tissue engineering, such as distraction osteogenesis followed by bone grafting to treat Treacher Collins syndrome.[57] In the 1960s, Tessier performed wide mobilization of large segments of the skull and translocation of the eyes in the case of Apert and Crouzon syndromes.[83]

To supplement these pioneering approaches, tissue engineers have sought to generate greater quantities of bone and cartilage. This began with the observation that chondrocytes harvested from the articular surfaces differentiated in culture to cartilage, whereas chondrocytes from periosteum initially resembled cartilage but progressed in culture to form new bone.[92]

A relatively simple tissue, cartilage has a limited spontaneous regenerative capacity after destruction.[24,26,59] Repair of major articular cartilaginous defects occurs through the formation of fibrocartilaginous tissue, with a different biochemistry and biomechanical profile from native cartilage.[39] Osteoarthritis with pain and decreased function can result from inadequate repair.[18] In 1988 Vacanti et al. produced new hyaline cartilage from bovine chondrocytes on a polymer scaffold.[90]

In subsequent studies using nonwoven polyglycolic acid mesh or copolymers of polyglycolic acid and polylactic acid, the constructs could be made into predetermined shapes.[90] This led to the formation of cartilage in the shape of a human ear[88] and a temporomandibular joint disk,[66] as well as cartilage shaped specifically to substitute for worn articular cartilage in meniscus replacement.[38] Tissue-engineered cartilage has also been used as a structural mass for nipple reconstruction in pigs[14] and to close cranial defects in animals.[53] Cartilaginous tubes lined with respiratory epithelium have been produced and implanted as a tracheal replacement,[69,91] and formed cilia were seen on some epithelial cells at 3 weeks.[69]

The tissue engineering of bone originated in cartilage tissue engineering, with the transfer of bovine periosteal cells to polyglycolic acid scaffolds and implantation into

Group I

Group II

Group III

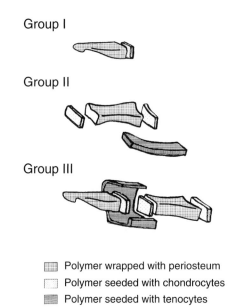

▦ Polymer wrapped with periosteum
▢ Polymer seeded with chondrocytes
▦ Polymer seeded with tenocytes

Figure 3–1 Three different types of composite tissue structures composing a tissue-engineered finger. The structures were constituted in vitro by suturing to create models of a distal phalanx (Group I), a middle phalanx (Group II), and a distal interphalangeal joint (Group III). The sutured tissues were then implanted subcutaneously in athymic mice. (From Isogai N, Landis W, Kim TH, et al: Formation of phalanges and small joints by tissue-engineering. J Bone Joint Surg Am 1999;81:306-316.)

athymic mice. These constructs stained for osteocalcin and showed focal points of bone formation on microscopic evaluation. These constructs were then implanted to repair parietal, frontal, and temporal cranial bone defects in nude rats; polymer without cells was used as a control.[89] Bony repair with the tissue-engineered constructs was observed, compared with no change in the cranial defects in the control group. Similarly, this technique has been applied to femoral shaft defects fixed with plates to maintain a critical gap. Nonunion was observed in the control group, and exuberant callus formation was seen in the tissue-engineered group.

A combination of tissue-engineered bone and cartilage has been used to create a finger replacement.[41] Three types of bovine cells—periosteum, chondrocytes, and tenocytes—seeded on copolymers of polyglycolic acid and poly-L-lactic acid formed a composite tissue resembling a joint (Fig. 3-1). The parts were assembled and sutured together in the form of a distal phalanx, middle phalanx, and distal interphalangeal joint. This assembly was then implanted subcutaneously in athymic mice. At 20 weeks, the shape and histology of a human phalange with a joint were preserved, with mature articular cartilage, subchondral bone, and a tenocapsule. Bone and cartilage tissue engineering is promising for joint reconstruction and to address the complex congenital anomalies that pediatric orthopedic surgeons must contend with.

CARDIOVASCULAR TISSUE ENGINEERING

Each year in the United States 5 to 8 of every 1000 live births result in a child with congenital cardiac malformations,

including valvular disorders.[17] Pediatric surgical treatment of congenital heart defects commonly requires nonautologous conduits or valves.[56,71] In the early 1960s more than 40% of valve replacements were composed of bovine or porcine tissue preserved by glutaraldehyde.[71] Tissue replacement valves avoid the problems of mechanical valves, including systemic thromboembolism and thrombotic occlusion,[21] but they still have a 50% to 60% reoperation rate at 10 years for prosthesis-associated problems, including structural and nonstructural dysfunction, progressive deterioration (calcific and noncalcific), and infection.[21,33] Additionally, the most commonly used replacement tissue valves have limited durability due to progressive deterioration.[71]

The perfect replacement valve would be a nonobstructive, nonthrombotic, self-repairing tissue valve that grows with the patient and remodels in response to in vivo stimuli.[71] These criteria are unchanged from those originally outlined by Harken et al. in 1962.[34] A one-time repair would be invaluable for pediatric patients, who currently may require numerous operations over a lifetime.

The tissue-engineered heart valve has been approached using traditional methods of tissue engineering. Seeded cells on a scaffold construct were tried first with a decellularized xenogeneic valve, then later on pure polymer molded to the proper form.[2,62,72] In the first studies, human endothelial cells from the saphenous vein were seeded on porcine aortic valves treated with Triton detergent to remove the native cells and leave the extracellular matrix as the cellular support.[2] Implanted as pulmonary valve replacements in sheep, the valves were hemodynamically functional and showed no calcification at harvest.[2] Similar results were achieved with a composite bioprosthesis sutured from various leaflets and conduit, again decellularized before seeding.[62]

Engineering a polymer scaffold, rather than destroying the cells of an existing valve and repopulating it, was crucial to achieve a living valve that could possibly grow. As the autologous cells populate the polymer scaffold, which then biodegrades, the cells also secrete an extracellular matrix to retain mechanical strength.[76] Initial studies of polyglycolic acid scaffolds seeded with sheep endothelial cells and myofibroblasts, implanted after resection of the native right posterior leaflet of the pulmonary valve in sheep, resulted in no stenosis and appropriate cellular architecture and matrix formation.[72] When the implanted cells were labeled with a cellular marker, the leaflets increased collagen content and added elastin, and the original cells persisted, again with demonstrable valve function by echocardiography.[10]

The addition of mechanical bioreactors that increasingly stress the engineered valve and improved polymer scaffolds (polyhydroxyalkanoate) resulted in a pulmonary valve with minimal regurgitation, no thrombus formation, laminated fibrous tissue, and increased extracellular matrix.[76] Engineered valves grown under mechanical stress with approximated systolic pulse pressure[77] function in vivo for up to 5 months and resemble native valves in terms of matrix formation, histology, and biomechanics.

Although some of Harken's criteria have been met by the tissue-engineered valves, and the critical ability to grow with the host may be met as well, the valves need to be tested and succeed in the aortic position, because this is the most frequently diseased, studied, and replaced valve.[71]

VASCULAR TISSUE ENGINEERING

In addition to valvular repair, a second factor in many pediatric congenital cardiac defects is the development of an adequate conduit, for which homografts or prosthetic materials have been used. These do not grow and functionally degenerate through calcification and tissue ingrowth, leading to multiple surgical replacements. Smaller vessels, those less than 6 mm, cannot be satisfactorily constructed from textile or expanded polytetrafluoroethylene (PTFE) and must be bypassed with autologous arteries and veins, with a limited supply for multiple operations.[86]

Given these drawbacks, tissue engineering is a logical strategy for small and large vessel replacements. In February 2001 the first human use of a tissue-engineered vessel was reported by Shin'oka et al. (Fig. 3-2) in a 4-year-old girl who had previously undergone a Fontan procedure and pulmonary artery angioplasty at age 3 years 3 months for a single right ventricle and pulmonary atresia.[73] Subsequent angiography revealed total occlusion of the right intermediate pulmonary artery. A 2-cm autologous segment of peripheral vein was harvested and its cells isolated and expanded in culture to 12×10^6 cells at 8 weeks. A tube of polycaprolactone and polylactic acid copolymer in a 1:1 weight ratio reinforced with woven polyglycolic acid served as a scaffold for the seeded cells, which were implanted 10 days after seeding to reconstruct the occluded pulmonary artery. After 7 months of follow-up, no complications were noted.

Tissue engineering of the vasculature began in 1978, when Herring successfully isolated endothelial cells from veins and transplanted them on synthetic scaffolds.[98] Several scientists improved the function and architecture of the tissue by alternating seeding protocols, scaffold composition, and culture conditions. In 1998 Shin'oka et al. cultured ovine arterial and venous endothelial cells in similar conditions to the human replacement and replaced a 2-cm segment of pulmonary artery in lambs.[74] The acellular control was thrombosed, whereas the engineered tissue had a luminal endothelial layer, collagen, and elastin and was nonthrombosed at explant.[74] Similarly, a construct seeded with ovine venous cells on a different polymer (poly-4-hydroxybutyrate) and sutured to the pulmonary artery in patch augmentation resulted in increased proteoglycans, elastin, and collagen and remained patent.[78] Polyhydroxyalkanoate and polyglycolic acid copolymer seeded with ovine arterial cells also resulted in a patent patch graft, and the mechanical stress-strain curve began to approximate that of native vessel over time.[75]

Improved conduit strength, viability, and durability will likely develop with improved understanding of cell-cell and cell-polymer interactions, leading to the regeneration of an architecture that includes extracellular matrix, a smooth lining of endothelial cells at the luminal surface, and collagen and elastin fibers. Use of tissue fragments to seed constructs that contain multiple cell types, including bone marrow, has been reported to accelerate graft healing and preclude intimal hyperplasia.[61] Similarly, improvements in the polymer characteristics have enhanced the rate and quality of vessel development.[75,100]

INTESTINAL TISSUE ENGINEERING

Of the morbid conditions associated with bowel resection, short-bowel syndrome is the most devastating. It is characterized by progressive weight loss, malnutrition, vitamin deficiency, and infections associated with the vascular access commonly used to support patients with this syndrome.[99] Short-bowel syndrome typically ensues when less than one third of normal small intestine remains after massive resection or surgical treatment of a number of intestinal problems. Although there are some surgical innovations for the treatment of this syndrome, including bowel transplantation,[13] reversed segments,[19] recirculating loops,[84] and tapering and lengthening procedures to encourage intestinal mucosa to proliferate,[65,97] there is no perfect surgical solution. Intestinal transplantation has had some early success but is not widely available. Initial work in the tissue engineering of intestine included autologous patches of serosa or vascularized pedicles, which had mixed success.[7,51,54] This was also performed with patches consisting of polymer, AlloDerm, and SIS, the collagenous submucosa of the intestine.[3,15,40] Tissue engineering offers an attractive alternative with

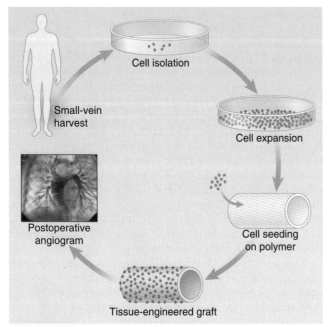

Figure 3–2 Basic tissue-engineering technique. Cells from native vein were isolated and expanded in vitro and seeded on a biodegradable polymer scaffold to form a tissue-engineered pulmonary artery that was subsequently implanted in a child, with good results. (From Shin'oka T, Imai Y, Ikada Y: Transplantation of a tissue engineered pulmonary artery [letter to the editor]. N Engl J Med 2001;344:532-533.)

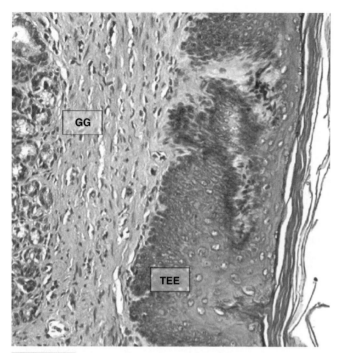

Figure 3–3 Tissue-engineered esophagus (TEE) at the gastro-esophageal junction, with engineered esophagus (EE) and native stomach with gastric glands (GG) in close approximation. (From Grikscheit T, Ochoa ER, Srinivasan A, et al: Tissue-engineered esophagus: Experimental substitution by onlay patch or interposition. J Thorac Cardiovasc Surg 2003;126:537-544.)

the goal of replacing the intestine before establishing a connection to the native intestinal lumen.

Beginning with the observation that fetal intestine transplanted on polymer scaffolds showed proliferation and intestinal morphogenesis,[93] the production of tissue-engineered intestine has expanded in the rat model from small intestine alone to include engineered stomach, gastroesophageal junction, esophagus, and colon (Figs. 3-3 and 3-4).[27-29,31] The generation of a composite

tissue resembling small intestine generated from intestinal cells heterotopically transplanted as organoid units was first reported in 1998.[16] Organoid units are taken from full-thickness harvests of intestine and purified through surgical dissection, enzymatic digestion, and trituration before differential centrifugation. Products from this preparation—the organoid units—are loaded on 2-mm nonwoven cylindrical polymers made of polyglycolic acid and coated with polylactic acid before implantation into the omentum. Although the implanted polymer initially must be subjected to a low oxygen tension, angiogenesis occurs. The growth of the engineered bowel reflects polarization of the epithelial cells to face inward toward the lumen of the cyst, with appropriate reconstitution of the other layers of the intestinal wall, including muscle and nerve. Substantial vascularization accompanies the growth.[16]

Long-term follow-up after anastomosis of tissue-engineered small intestine to native jejunum after 75% small bowel resection in male Lewis rats revealed weight gain, bowel patency, and statistically significant increases in the engineered intestine size.[45,48] When used as a "rescue" following massive small bowel resection, animals with tissue-engineered small intestine regained weight at a more rapid rate, up to their preoperative weights; animals without the engineered intestine foundered.[30] Investigation of the immune system of the anastomosed small bowel indicates that the neomucosal immune cell population is a function of exposure to luminal antigens and time of harvest.[64] In anastomosed tissue-engineered small intestinal mucosa harvested at 20 weeks, the density and topographic distribution of immune cell subsets were identical to that of normal jejunum. Epithelial messenger RNA expression topography of SGLT1, a bowel sodium-glucose cotransporter, is also regenerated in anastomosed engineered small intestine, as is DCT1, an iron transporter; however, vascular endothelial growth factor and basic fibroblast growth factor levels are different from those of native intestine.[25,82] The distribution patterns of these transporters indicate that the engineered intestine repeats the pattern of native jejunum,

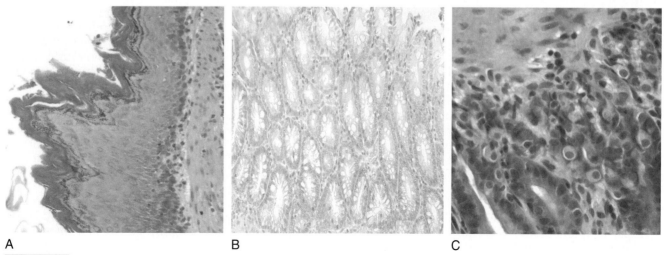

A   B   C

Figure 3–4 Tissues engineered in the Lewis rat model. *A,* Tissue-engineered esophagus (original magnification ×20). *B,* Tissue-engineered colon (original magnification ×20). *C,* Tissue-engineered stomach. Note the large lucent parietal cells and glandular structure. (Courtesy of Dr. T. Grikscheit.)

underlining the therapeutic potential of this conduit for patients who lack small bowels.

With refinements of the organoid protocol for engineered intestine, larger amounts have been created with larger surface areas, and engineered colon, stomach, and esophagus can be generated (see Fig. 3-3).[30] More than 20 times the volume of the implanted polymer can be produced.[27,30] Tissue-engineered colon functioned as a replacement in Lewis rats for 41 days, with maintenance of sodium levels, fluid absorption, generation of stool short-chain fatty acids, prolonged transit time, and architecture that included ganglion cells and authentic colon histology.[27,29] Tissue-engineered esophagus has been used both as a patch and as an interposition graft in rats in preliminary studies (see Fig. 3-3).[28] In the case of tissue-engineered stomach, the idea of exact replacement has been extended in a series of studies showing that a tissue-engineered gastroesophageal junction can be prepared, as well as an antrum alone, and either young or old rats can be the autologous donors.[31] The tissue stains appropriately for gastrin, has parietal cells, and has the exact architecture of native stomach. The tissue-engineered stomach can be labeled with a viral protein (green fluorescent protein) for later identification, opening the door for future transfections for "designer intestine"; for example, tissue-engineered colon could be transfected with SGLT1 to allow it to absorb sugars.[31]

Engineered intestinal replacement is central to the treatment of many critical pediatric surgical diseases and may significantly impact patient care in the coming decade, with improved surface area, transporter function, immune characteristics, and architecture. Large animal studies have begun in some laboratories, with the successful growth of a small amount of tissue-engineered small intestine and stomach in one.

LIVER REPLACEMENT AND TISSUE ENGINEERING

The liver is a complex and indispensable organ that provides vital functions, including metabolism, excretion, detoxification, storage, and phagocytosis. Global failure of this organ with acute or chronic liver dysfunction accounts for the death of 30,000 Americans each year, with acute failure mortality rates exceeding 80%.[85] Chronic failure is the sixth leading cause of death in the United States and ranks eighth in economic costs among major illnesses. Currently, the only definitive treatment for severe hepatic failure is orthotopic liver transplantation, with 3000 of these procedures performed annually. Attempts to tissue-engineer a liver for replacement have included direct cellular injection or transplantation on polymer constructs, with or without hepatotrophic stimulation; the development of extracorporeal bioartificial liver (BAL) devices; and new three-dimensional microfabricated constructs intended to be intracorporeal.

Tissue engineering of the liver initially began with cell transplantation after the observation that orthotopic liver transplantation might not be necessary when the replacement of selected populations of cells could treat the liver function deficiencies.[68] The Promethean

regeneration of the liver made the idea of hepatocyte transplantation more attractive.

In early studies, when hepatocytes were injected into the portal veins of Gunn rats deficient in uridine diphosphate glucuronyltransferase, they maintained a lower bilirubin level than control animals injected with saline.[55] Hepatocyte injection into the portal vein or peritoneal cavity was performed after inducing liver failure with dimethylnitrosamine.[81] Rats that received the injection of hepatocytes lived significantly longer than those in the control group. Hepatocellular injections into the spleen, pancreas, and peritoneal cavity retained functional capacity in several studies and were also noted to migrate. Hepatitis B virus surface antigen–producing hepatocytes, introduced ectopically, were noted to migrate to the pancreas, lung, and spleen while maintaining function.[32] The limitation of this approach is the overall functional capacity of the injected cells, which decreases over time. Migration and attrition contribute to the failure to develop a discrete liver mass.

Tissue-engineered liver mass has increased by concurrent hepatotrophic stimulation and improved cellular selection. Hepatotrophic stimulation, which exists in patients with hepatic failure receiving tissue-engineered liver therapies, has been reproduced by partial hepatectomy, portacaval shunting, and injection of liver toxins. Following liver resection, it is well known that the remaining liver rapidly proliferates with multiple growth stimuli, including epidermal growth factor, hepatocyte growth factor, insulin, and glucagon.[11] The increased amounts of these factors in portal blood have led to the approach of portacaval shunting in host animals when tissue-engineered constructs are implanted into the mesentery or omentum, to give the construct a rich supply of trophic factors. Hepatectomy and portacaval shunting at the time of construct implantation result in increased proliferation of transplanted hepatocytes, longer cell survival, better organization, and higher levels of bilirubin clearance in Gunn rats.[46,70,87]

Cellular transplantation, even with maximal hepatotrophic stimulation, does not yet deliver adequate hepatocellular mass to detoxify the plasma of a human patient in fulminant hepatic failure. Therefore, a tissue-engineered liver may provide temporary liver function replacement in the form of an extracorporeal BAL device or, more recently, a microfabricated intracorporeal device. The goals of an extracorporeal BAL are to serve as a bridge to transplantation, reducing postoperative morbidity and mortality,[79] as well as to support acute liver failure patients while liver regeneration occurs or those who are ineligible for transplant secondary to concomitant disease.

Experimental models of rat, porcine, or human-derived hepatocyte cell lines in a tissue-engineered scaffold-cell combination have been used to detoxify the blood of patients in fulminant hepatic failure.[43,80] In a device that has undergone trials in human patients with hepatic failure, porcine hepatocytes bound to collagen-coated microcarriers in dialysis membranes are attached extracorporeally.[67]

Despite the development of stable hepatocyte culture systems, including collagen sandwich and double gel systems, prolonged plasma exposure to the hepatocyte cultures in microfabricated bioreactors produces significant accumulations of intracellular triglyceride droplets, leading to a severe reduction in cellular function. The current life span of the BAL is hours to days, which must be improved for long-term therapy. In more recent investigations, co-cultured hepatocytes and nonparenchymal cells were more tolerant of the plasma milieu.[6]

The premise of co-culture in liver cell culture originated with the observation that mesenchymal cells of the umbilical and vitelline veins induce the endodermal "liver bud" to proliferate, branch, and differentiate in utero.[37] The adult liver provides a scaffold for many complex cell-cell interactions (biliary ductal, Kupffer, sinusoidal endothelial cells, and hepatocytes), which allow coordinated organ function. These interactions imply an essential role for cell signaling between mesenchymal and parenchymal tissue compartments.

The cellular physiology of the liver is complex, and the life span of mature hepatocytes, although lengthened with improvements in culture conditions, is measured in weeks.

Coupled with modern advances in microfabrication, observations about cellular co-culture may lead to an implantable tissue-engineered liver. Vascular ingrowth into transplanted constructs may never be adequate for a complex organ such as the liver, however. Therefore, our laboratory has sought to build a vascular system down to the level of the capillary itself, and then add the parenchyma of complex organs.[9] A de novo vascular system could be used as a template for any thick and complex tissue such as the heart, liver, or kidney, all of which rely on extensive vascularization, exceeding the limits of host ingrowth alone.[9]

Ordered arrays of channels for hepatocytes with regionally designed cell adhesion properties were first created using three-dimensional printing,[50,63] which couples computer design with polymer fabrication, expelling liquid polymer onto dry, powdered polymer through a machine analogous to an ink-jet printer. As the layers of solidified polymer are built up, complex three-dimensional structures can be formed with high resolution. Therefore, channels for blood supply and cellular support can be designed and fabricated.

FUTURE DIRECTIONS: BETTER STRUCTURES, BETTER CELLS

With the advent of microelectrical mechanical systems (MEMS), also used in inertial guidance and navigation,[9] silicon micromachining has been used to form an improved scaffold for vascular networks. Trench patterns are etched on silicon and Pyrex templates with resolution to 10 µm in patterns that replicate a vascular network (Fig. 3-5). Endothelial cells and hepatocytes cultured on the MEMS template remain viable and proliferative, producing albumin.[9] The monolayers can then be lifted and formed into a three-dimensional structure. Stacking these layers could incorporate a biliary system and increase the available surface area of any vascularized tissue and its parenchyma added to the system.

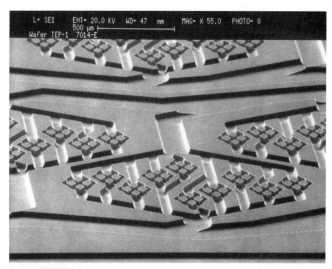

Figure 3-5 Optical micrograph of a portion of a capillary network etched into a silicon wafer using a microelectrical mechanical system. (Courtesy of Dr. J. Borenstein.)

Further studies have confirmed that microfabrication technology can be used to form large sheets of living tissue and that micromachining luminal surfaces for endothelial cells allows ordered co-culture (Fig. 3-6).[9] The lifted organized layers have been implanted as a permanent graft.

Coupled with these advances is the search for a more appropriate cellular population, which may include a mixed culture on a novel scaffold. Improved micromachined templates are already being made in collaboration with Draper Laboratories at the Massachusetts Institute of Technology, with mathematical modeling of the expected microfluidics and nutritional transfer. With the solution to the problem of vascularizing complex organs,

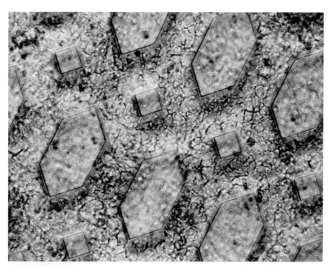

Figure 3-6 Endothelial cells grown on Vitrogen-coated (30 µg/mL) Pyrex wafers after 4 days in culture. (From Kaihara S, Borenstein J, Koka R, et al: Silicon micromachining to tissue engineer branched vascular channels for liver fabrication. Tissue Eng 2000;6:105-117.)

many difficult tissue-engineering targets could finally be within reach.

An evident extension of the tissue-engineering armamentarium is the future use of stem cells or pluripotent cell lines, which involves ethical and political issues that must be addressed. Of note, the majority of tissue-engineering solutions revolve around autologous or syngeneic cells rather than direct stem cell application. The number of projects employing mesenchymal stem cells has rapidly increased, and some in the field have pursued amniotic fluid as a source of mesenchymal stem cells for fetal tissue engineering.[47] In addition, fetal tissues, including chondrocytes for chest wall reconstruction, have been harvested from the lamb fetus, expanded in the laboratory until the birth of the animal, and then implanted at that time, with structural replacement noted up to 10 weeks after implantation.[23] Most tissue-engineering strategies that rely on non–stem cell–based approaches likely make use of the progenitors found in the tissues used, so stem cells have been used in tissue engineering without being clearly identified. It is interesting to note that these cells, already somewhat differentiated, are adequate for the production of many tissues.

The rapid metamorphosis of tissue engineering has occurred primarily through creative collaboration among engineers, chemists, surgeons, physicists, biologists, and scientists in a number of other disciplines, with true progress being made through simultaneous advances in materials, cellular physiology, and surgical application. The evolution of bioreactor devices, including those that stress the cells to approximate physiologic conditions, has also led to better tissues. The combination of mechanical engineering, tissue engineering, and surgical research represents the future of tissue engineering for general and pediatric surgical problems.

REFERENCES

1. Atala A, Cima LG, Kim W, et al: Injectable alginate seeded with chondrocytes as a potential treatment for vesicoureteral reflux. J Urol 1993;150:745-747.
2. Bader A, Schilling T, Tebken OE, et al: Tissue engineering of heart valves—human endothelial cell seeding of detergent acellularized porcine valves. Eur J Cardiothorac Surg 1998;14:279-284.
3. Badylak S, Meurling S, Chen M, et al: Resorbable bioscaffold for esophageal repair in a dog model. J Pediatr Surg 2000;35:1097-1103.
4. Balis UJ, Behnia K, Dwarakanath B, et al: Oxygen consumption characteristics of porcine hepatocytes. Metab Eng 1999;1:49-62.
5. Bhatia SN, Balis UJ, Yarmush ML, et al: Probing heterotypic cell interactions: Hepatocyte function in microfabricated co-cultures. J Biomater Sci Polym Ed 1998;9:1137-1160.
6. Bhatia SN, Yarmush ML, Toner M: Controlling cell interactions by micropatterning in co-cultures: Hepatocytes and 3T3 fibroblasts. J Biomed Mater Res 1997;34:189-199.
7. Binnington HB, Tumbleson ME, Ternberg JL: Use of jejunal neomucosa. Surgery 1982;91:293-300.
8. Borenstein JT, Gerrish ND, Currie MT, et al: New ultra-hard etch-stop layer for high precision micromachining. Proceedings of the 12th IEEE International Conference on Micro Electro Mechanical System, MEMS, 1999, Orlando, Fla, pp 205-210.
9. Borenstein JT, Terai H, King KR, et al: Microfabrication technology for vascularized tissue engineering. Biomed Microdevices 2002;4:167-175.
10. Breuer CK, Shin'oka T, Tanel RE, et al: Tissue engineering lamb heart valve leaflets. Biotech Bioeng 1996;50:562-567.
11. Bucher NLR: Liver regeneration: An overview. J Gastroenterol Hepatol 1991;6:615-624.
12. Buckley MJ, Banes AJ, Jordan R: Effects of mechanical strain on osteoblasts in vitro. J Oral Maxillofac Surg 1998; 48:276-282.
13. Bueno J, Ohwada S, Kocoshis S, et al: Factors impacting the survival of children with intestinal failure referred for intestinal transplantation. J Pediatr Surg 1999;34:27-33.
14. Cao YL, Lach E, Kim TH, et al: Tissue engineered nipple reconstruction. Plast Reconstr Surg 1998;102:2293-2298.
15. Chen MK, Badylak SF: Small bowel tissue engineering using small intestinal submucosa as a scaffold. J Surg Res 2001;99:352-358.
16. Choi RS, Pothoulakis C, Kim BS, et al: Studies of brush border enzymes, basement membrane components, and electrophysiology of tissue-engineered neointestine. J Pediatr Surg 1998;33:991-997.
17. Clark EB: Epidemiology of congenital cardiovascular malformations. In Emmanouilides GC, Riemenschneider TA, Allan HD, Gutesell HP (eds): Moss and Adams' Heart Disease in Infants, Children, and Adolescents. Baltimore, Williams & Wilkins, 1995, pp 60-70.
18. Davis MA, Ettinger WH, Neuhaus JM, et al: The association of knee injury and obesity with unilateral and bilateral osteoarthritis of the knee. Am J Epidemiol 1989;130: 278-288.
19. Diego MD, Miguel E, Lucen CM, et al: Short gut syndrome: A new surgical technique and ultrastructural study of the liver and the pancreas. Arch Surg 1982;117:789-795.
20. Folch A, Ayon A, Hurtado O, et al: Molding of deep polydimethylsiloxane microstructures for microfluidics and biological applications. J Biomech Eng 1999;121:28-34.
21. Fowler VG, Durack DT: Infective endocarditis. Curr Opin Cardiol 1994;9:389-400.
22. Freed LE, Vunjak-Novakovic G: Microgravity tissue engineering in vitro. Cell Dev Biol 1997;33:381-385.
23. Fuchs JR, Terada S, Hannouche D, et al: Fetal tissue engineering: Chest wall reconstruction. J Pediatr Surg 2003; 38:1188-1193.
24. Fuller JA, Chadially FN: Ultrastructural observations on surgically produced partial thickness defects in articular cartilage. Clin Orthop 1972;86:193-205.
25. Gardner-Thorpe J, Grikscheit TC, Ito H, et al: Angiogenesis in tissue-engineered small intestine. Tissue Eng 2003;9: 1255-1261.
26. Ghadially FN, Thomas I, Oryschak AF, et al: Long term results of superficial defects in articular cartilage: A scanning electron microscope study. J Pathol 1977;121:213-217.
27. Grikscheit TC, Ochoa ER, Ramsanahie A, et al: Tissue-engineered large intestine resembles native colon with appropriate in vitro physiology and architecture. Ann Surg 2003;238:35-41.
28. Grikscheit T, Ochoa ER, Srinivasan A, et al: Tissue-engineered esophagus: Experimental substitution by onlay patch or interposition. J Thorac Cardiovasc Surg 2003;126:537-544.
29. Grikscheit TC, Ogilvie JB, Ochoa ER, et al: Tissue-engineered colon exhibits function in vivo. Surgery 2002;132:200-204.
30. Grikscheit TC, Siddique A, Ochoa E, et al: Tissue-engineered small intestine improves recovery after massive small bowel resection. Ann Surg (in press).

31. Grikscheit T, Srinivasan A, Vacanti JP: Tissue-engineered stomach: A preliminary report of a versatile in vivo model with therapeutic potential. J Pediatr Surg 2003;38:1305-1309.

32. Gupta S, Aragona E, Vemuru RP, et al: Permanent engraftment and function of hepatocytes delivered to the liver: Implications for gene therapy and liver repopulation. Hepatology 1991;14:144-149.

33. Hammermeister KE, Sethi GK, Henderson WG, et al: A comparison in men 11 years after heart valve replacement with a mechanical valve or bioprosthesis. Veterans Affairs Cooperative Study on Valvular Heart Disease. N Engl J Med 1993;328:1289-1296.

34. Harken DF, Taylor WJ, LeFemine AA, et al: Aortic valve replacement with a caged ball valve. Am J Cardiol 1962;9: 292-299.

35. Hendrickson DA, Nixon AJ, Grande DA, et al: Chondrocyte-fibrin matrix transplants for resurfacing extensive auricular cartilage defects. J Orthop Res 1994;12:485-497.

36. Homminga GN, Buma P, Koot HW, et al: Chondrocyte behavior in fibrin glue in vitro. Acta Orthop Scand 1993;64:441-445.

37. Houssaint E: Differentiation of the mouse hepatic primordium: An analysis of tissue interactions in hepatocyte differentiation. Cell Differ 1990;9:269-279.

38. Ibarra C, Janetta C, Vacanti CA, et al: Tissue engineered meniscus: A potential new alternative to allogeneic meniscus transplantation. Transplant Proc 1997;29:986-988.

39. Ibarra C, Langer R, Vacanti JP: Tissue engineering: Cartilage, bone, and muscle. Yearbook of Cell and Tissue Transplantation 1996/1997. Netherlands, Kluwer Academic Publishers, 1996, pp 235-245.

40. Isch JA, Engum SA, Ruble CA, et al: Patch esophagoplasty using AlloDerm as a tissue scaffold. J Pediatr Surg 2001; 36:266-268.

41. Isogai N, Landis W, Kim TH, et al: Formation of phalanges and small joints by tissue-engineering. J Bone Joint Surg Am 1999;81:306-316.

42. James CD, Davis R, Meyer M, et al: Aligned microcontact printing of micrometer scale poly-L-lysine structures for controlled growth of cultured neurons on planar microelectrode arrays. IEEE Trans Biomed Eng 2000;47:17-21.

43. Jauregui HO, Gann KL: Mammalian hepatocytes as a foundation for treatment in human liver failure. J Cell Biochem 1991;45:359-365.

44. Kaihara S, Borenstein J, Koka R, et al: Silicon micromachining to tissue engineered branched vascular channels for liver fabrication. Tissue Eng 2000;6:105-117.

45. Kaihara S, Kim SS, Kim BS, et al: Long-term follow-up of tissue engineered intestine after anastomosis to native small bowel. Transplantation 2000;69:1927-1932.

46. Kaufmann PM, Sano K, Uyama S, et al: Heterotopic hepatocyte transplantation: Assessing the impact of hepatotrophic stimulation. Transplant Proc 1994;26:2240-2241.

47. Kaviani A, Guleserian K, Perry TE, et al: Fetal tissue engineering from amniotic fluid. J Am Coll Surg 2003;196:592-597.

48. Kim SS, Kaihara S, Benvenuta M, et al: Regenerative signals for tissue engineered small intestine. Transplant Proc 1999;31:657-660.

49. Kim SS, Kaihara S, Benvenuta MS, et al: Small intestinal submucosa as a small-caliber venous graft: A novel model for hepatocyte transplantation on synthetic biodegradable polymer scaffolds with direct access to the portal venous system. J Pediatr Surg 1999;34:124-128.

50. Kim SS, Utsunomiya H, Koski JA, et al: Survival and function of hepatocytes on a novel three-dimensional synthetic biodegradable polymer scaffold with an intrinsic network of channels. Ann Surg 1998;228:8-13.

51. Kobold EE, Thal AP: A simple method for management of experimental wounds of the duodenum. Surg Gynecol Obstet 1963;116:340-344.

52. Lanza RP, Langer R, Vacanti J: Principles of Tissue Engineering. San Diego, Calif, Academic Press, 2000.

53. Lee IW, Vacanti JP, Yoo J, et al: A tissue engineering approach for dural and cranial grafts. Paper presented at Congress of Neurological Surgeons, 1997, New Orleans.

54. Lillemoe KD, Berry WR, Harmon JW, et al: Use of vascularized abdominal wall pedicle flaps to grow small bowel neomucosa. Surgery 1982;91:293-300.

55. Matas AJ, Sutherland DER, Stefes MW, et al: Hepatocellular transplantation for metabolic deficiencies: Decrease in plasma bilirubin in Gunn rats. Science 1976;192:892-894.

56. Mayer J: Uses of homograft conduits for right ventricle to pulmonary artery connections in the neonatal period. Semin Thorac Cardiovasc Surg 1995;7:130-132.

57. McCarthy JG: Lengthening the human mandible by gradual distraction. Plast Reconstr Surg 1992;89:1-8.

58. McFarland CD, Thomas CH, DeFilippis C, et al: Protein adsorption and cell attachment to patterned surfaces. Biomed Mater Res 2000;49:200-210.

59. Meachim G: The effect of scarification on articular cartilage in the rabbit. J Bone Joint Surg Br 1963;45:150-161.

60. Mooney DJ, Langer RS: Engineering biomaterials for tissue engineering: The 10-100 micron size scale. In Bronzino JD (ed): The Biomedical Engineering Handbook. Boca Raton, Fla, CRC Press, 1995.

61. Noishiki Y, Yamane Y, Okoshi T, et al: Choice, isolation, and preparation of cells for bioartificial vascular grafts. Artif Organs 1998;22:50-62.

62. O'Brien MF, Goldstein S, Walsh S, et al: The synergraft valve: A new acellular (nongluteraldehyde-fixed) tissue heart valve for autologous recellularization: First experimental studies before implantation. Semin Thorac Cardiovasc Surg 1999;11:194-200.

63. Park A, Wu B, Griffith LG: Integration of surface modification and 3D fabrication techniques to prepare patterned poly(L-lactide) substrates allowing regionally selective cell adhesion. J Biomater Sci Polym Ed 1998;9:89-110.

64. Perez A, Grikscheit TC, Ashley SW, et al: Tissue engineered small intestine: Ontogeny of the immune system. Transplantation 2002;74:619-623.

65. Pokorny WJ, Fowler CJ: Isoperistaltic intestinal lengthening for short bowel syndrome. Surg Gynecol Obstet 1991;172:39-43.

66. Puelacher WC, Wisser J, Vacanti CA, et al: Temporomandibular joint disc replacement made by tissue-engineered growth of cartilage. J Oral Maxillofac Surg 1994;52:1172-1177.

67. Rozga J, Williams F, Ro M-S, et al: Development of a bioartificial liver: Properties and function of hollow-fibre module inoculated with liver cells. Hepatology 1993;17:258-265.

68. Russell PS: Selective transplantation. Ann Surg 1985;201:255-262.

69. Sakata J, Vacanti CA, Schloo B, et al: Tracheal composite tissue engineered from chondrocytes, tracheal epithelial cells, and synthetic degradable scaffolding. Transplant Proc 1994;26:3309-3310.

70. Sano K, Cusick RA, Lee H, et al: Regenerative signals for heterotrophic hepatocyte transplantation. Transplant Proc 1996;28:1857-1858.

71. Schoen FJ, Levy RJ: Tissue heart valves: Current challenges and future research perspectives. J Biomed Mater Res 1999;47:439-465.

72. Shin'oka T, Breuer CK, Tanel RE, et al: Tissue engineering heart valves: Valve leaflet replacement study in a lamb model. Ann Thorac Surg 1995;60:S513-S516.

73. Shin'oka T, Imai Y, Ikada Y: Transplantation of a tissue engineered pulmonary artery [letter to the editor]. N Engl J Med 2001;344:532-533.

74. Shin'oka T, Shum-Tim D, Ma PX, et al: Creation of viable pulmonary artery autografts through tissue engineering. J Thorac Cardiovasc Surg 1998;115:536-545.

75. Shum-Tim D, Stock U, Hrkach J, et al: Tissue engineering of autologous aorta using a new biodegradable polymer. Ann Thorac Surg 1999;68:2298-2304.

76. Sodian R, Hoerstrup SP, Sperline JS, et al: Early in vivo experience with tissue-engineered trileaflet heart valves. Circulation 2000;102:III22-III29.

77. Stock UA, Nagashima M, Khalil PN, et al: Tissue engineered valved conduits in the pulmonary circulation. J Thorac Cardiovasc Surg 2000;119:732-740.

78. Stock UA, Sakamoto T, Hatsuoka S, et al: Patch augmentation of the pulmonary artery with bioabsorbable polymers and autologous cell seeding. J Thorac Cardiovasc Surg 2000;120:1158-1167.

79. Sussman N, Kelly J: The artificial liver. Sci Am Sci Med 1995;3:68-77.

80. Sussman N, Kelly J: Temporary liver support: Theory, practice, predictions. Xenop 1995;3:63-67.

81. Sutherland DER, Numata M, Matas AJ, et al: Hepatocellular transplantation in acute liver failure. Surgery 1977;82:124-132.

82. Tavakkolizadeh A, Stephen AE, Kaihara S, et al: Epithelial transporter mRNA expression topography in the tissue-engineered small intestine. Transplantation 2003;75:181-185.

83. Tessier P: Osteotomies totales de la face: Syndrome de Crouzon, Syndrome d'Alpert, Oxycephalies, Scaphocephalies, Turricephalies. Ann Chir Plast Esthet 1967;12:273-286.

84. Thompson JS, Vanderhoot JA, Antonson DL, et al: Comparison of techniques for growing small bowel neomucosa. J Surg Res 1984;36:401-406.

85. Trey C, Burns DG, Saunders SJ: Treatment of hepatic coma by exchange blood transfusion. N Engl J Med 1966;274:473-481.

86. Tu JV, Pashos CL, Naylor CD, et al: Use of cardiac procedures and outcomes in elderly patients with myocardial infarction in the United States and Canada. N Engl J Med 1997;336:1500-1505.

87. Uyama S, Kaufmann PM, Takeda T, et al: Delivery of whole liver-equivalent hepatocyte mass using polymer devices and hepatotrophic stimulation. Transplantation 1993;55:932-935.

88. Vacanti CA, Cima LG, Ratkowski D, et al: Tissue engineered growth of new cartilage in the shape of a human ear using synthetic polymers seeded with chondrocytes. Mat Res Soc Symp Proc 1992;252:367-373.

89. Vacanti CA, Kim WS, Mooney D: Tissue engineered composites of bone and cartilage using synthetic polymers seeded with two cell types. Orthop Trans 1993;18:276.

90. Vacanti CA, Langer R, Schloo B, et al: Synthetic polymers seeded with chondrocytes provide a template for new cartilage formation. Plast Reconstr Surg 1991;87:753-759.

91. Vacanti CA, Paige KT, Kim WS, et al: Experimental tracheal replacement using tissue engineered cartilage. J Pediatr Surg 1994;29:201-204.

92. Vacanti CA, Upton J: Tissue engineered morphogenesis of cartilage and bone by means of cell transplantation using synthetic biodegradable polymer matrices. Clin Plast Surg 1994;21:445-462.

93. Vacanti JP, Morse MA, Saltzmann M, et al: Selective cell transplantation using bioabsorbable artificial polymers as matrices. J Pediatr Surg 1988;23:3-9.

94. Vandenburgh H, Del Tatto M, Shansky J, et al: Tissue engineered skeletal muscle organoids for reversible gene therapy. Hum Gene Ther 1997;7:2195-2200.

95. Wakitani S, Kimura T, Hirooka A, et al: Repair of rabbit articular surfaces with allograft chondrocytes embedded in collagen gel. J Bone Joint Surg Br 1989;71:74-80.

96. Wang DL, Wung BS, Peng YC, et al: Mechanical strain increases endothelin-1 gene expression via protein kinase C pathway in human endothelial cells. J Cell Physiol 1996;163:400-406.

97. Weber TR, Vane DW, Grosfeld JL: Tapering enteroplasty in infants with bowel atresia and short gut. Arch Surg 1982;117:684-688.

98. Williams SK: Endothelial cell transplantation. Cell Transplant 1995;4:401-410.

99. Wilmore DW, Byrne TA, Persinger RL: Short bowel syndrome: New therapeutic approaches. Curr Probl Surg 1997;34:389-444.

100. Yue X, van der Lei B, Schakenraad JM, et al: Smooth muscle seeding in biodegradable grafts in rats: A new method to enhance the process of arterial wall regeneration. Surgery 1988;103:206-212.

101. Zhang S, Yan L, Altman M, et al: Biological surface engineering: A simple system for cell pattern formation. Biomaterials 1999;20:1213-1220.

Chapter 4

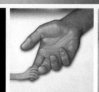

Advanced and Emerging Surgical Technologies and the Process of Innovation

Russell K. Woo and Thomas M. Krummel

"Change is inevitable. Change is constant" (Benjamin Disraeli). From the eons of evolutionary change that gifted *Homo sapiens* with an opposable thumb, to the minute-to-minute changes of the neonatal surgical patient, change and the adaptive response to change define either success or failure.

The development and use of tools and technologies remain a distinguishing characteristic of the human race. The first hunter-gatherers created, built, and modified tools to the demands of a specific task. In much the same fashion, the relentless development and use of surgical tools and technologies have defined both our craft and our care since the first bone needles were used in prehistoric times.

This chapter endeavors to highlight the advanced and emerging surgical technologies that shape the present and direct future changes. A framework to facilitate both thought and action about the innovations to come is presented. Finally, the surgeon's role in the ethical process of innovation is discussed.

As advances in surgical technologies have occurred, our field has moved forward, often in quantum leaps. A thoughtful look around our operating rooms, interventional suites, critical care units, and even teaching facilities is cause to reflect on our use and even dependence on tools and technologies. Clamps, catheters, retractors, energy sources, and monitors fill these spaces and facilitate and enhance surgeons' capabilities in the process of diagnosis, imaging, physiologic care, molecular triage, and performance of surgical procedures. Surgeons constantly function as users of technology; thus, a fundamental understanding underpins its thoughtful use. Administration of a drug without understanding the mechanism and side effects would be regarded as malpractice. A similar case must be made for the use of surgical tools and technologies.

New technologies result from an endless cycle through which innovation occurs. Such a cycle may begin with a fundamental research discovery or begin at the bedside with an unsolved patient problem. Frequently, innovation requires a complex interplay of both. Surgeons are uniquely positioned and privileged to contribute to and even define this cycle. A patient with an unsolvable problem is a constant reminder of our responsibility to advance our field. Theodore Kocher's success in thyroid surgery was enabled by his toothed modification of existing clamps to facilitate thyroid operations. Dr. Thomas Fogarty's development of the balloon catheter began as a surgical assistant while witnessing both the failures and disastrous consequences of extensive arteriotomies for extraction of emboli. His simple, brilliant concept has arguably created the entire field of catheter-based manipulation. Dr. John Gibbon's successful construction of a heart-lung machine was initially motivated by a patient with an unsolved problem of pulmonary emboli and the need for surgical extraction. Although his original intention has been eclipsed by Lazar Greenfield's suction embolectomy catheter and venacaval filter and dwarfed by the utility of the heart-lung machine in cardiac surgery, the story remains the same. Unresolved problems and a surgeon determined to find a solution have led to countless innovations that have changed our field forever. The surgeon's role must extend outside the operating room. Surgeons must remain aware and connected to the tools and techniques of diagnosis, monitoring, and education. Mark M. Ravitch, extraordinary pediatric surgeon, innovator, and one of the most literate surgeons of the 20th century, described surgery as an intellectual discipline characterized by operative procedures but, most important, defined as an attitude or responsibility toward care of the sick. Dr. Ravitch's contribution to the development of stapling devices deserves enormous credit.[203]

A surgical operation can be defined as "an act performed with instruments or by the hands of a surgeon." This definition implies an image and a manipulation; the manipulation implies an energy source. Historically we

TABLE 4-1 Surgical Operation—Image and Manipulation

Image	Manipulation
Direct visual	2 hands direct
Video image	2 hands, long tools
	Robots
Ultrasound	Cold, thermal
Computed tomography	Radiofrequency
Magnetic resonance imaging	Photodynamic energy
	Focused ultrasound energy

have regarded the "image" to be that of a direct visual image and the "manipulation" to be performed with the direct contact of two hands or surgical tools. The laparoscopic revolution has taught us that the image can be a video image and the manipulation can be performed by two hands with long tools. Now these long tools are occasionally attached to surgical robots. Our notion about the image has come to include ultrasound (US), computed tomography (CT), and magnetic resonance imaging (MRI), and the manipulation can include such sources as cold, heat, radiofrequency (RF), and photodynamic or chemical energy. Extracorporeal shock wave lithotripsy is an important urologic example of this principle applied to renal calculi. How will the "image" and "manipulation" exist in the future (Table 4-1)?

DIAGNOSTIC TECHNOLOGIES

Accurate evaluation of surgical disease has always been a vital aspect of surgical practice and always precedes surgery. Whether in the clinic, in the emergency department, or at the bedside, precise assessment defines surgical judgment and care. A thorough history and detailed physical examination will forever remain the foundation of assessment; however, the thoughtful addition of adjunctive imaging studies has considerably enhanced the evaluation of surgical patients. Driven by advancements in medicine, engineering, and biology, these studies entail increasingly sophisticated technologies that may provide more detailed anatomic, functional, and even molecular information in the future.

Over the past 3 decades, the introduction and improvement of US, CT, and MRI techniques have revolutionized the clinical evaluation of surgical disease. The fine anatomic data provided have facilitated the accurate diagnosis of a wide variety of conditions. Functional imaging techniques, such as positron emission tomography (PET) and functional MRI (fMRI), have been developed to provide accurate and often real-time biologic or physiologic information. In the field of pediatric surgery, these imaging modalities may be used in the diagnosis of disease, for preoperative surgical planning, and for postoperative evaluation. This section provides an overview of the imaging modalities used in pediatric surgery, with a focus on emerging techniques and systems.

Ultrasound

US imaging has become a truly invaluable tool in the evaluation of pediatric surgical patients. Providing anatomic as well as real-time functional information, US has unique attributes that have made it particularly useful, including relatively low cost, portability, flexibility, and safety inasmuch as no ionizing radiation is used. For these reasons, this section will focus on US imaging and highlight emerging advances in its technology and practice, including three-dimensional (3-D) US imaging, US contrast imaging, and US harmonic imaging.

US uses the emission and reflection of sound waves to construct images of body structures. It operates on the same principle as active SONAR—a sound beam is projected by the US probe into the body, and based on the time to "hear" the echo, the distance to a target structure can be calculated.[123] In the body, sound waves are primarily reflected at tissue interfaces, with the strength of the returning echoes mainly correlating with tissue properties. Advantages of US imaging include lack of ionizing radiation, real-time imaging with motion, and relatively fast procedure times.[213]

In modern US devices, numerous transducer elements are placed side by side in the transducer probe. The majority of devices currently use linear or sector scan transducers. These transducers consist of 64 to 256 piezoelectric elements arranged in a single row that allow the transducer to interrogate a single slice of tissue whose thickness is correlated to the thickness of the transducer elements.[123] This information is then used to construct real-time, dynamic, two-dimensional (2-D) images. Color, power, and pulsed wave Doppler imaging techniques are enhancements of this technology that allow color or graphic visualization of motion.[213] Conventional Doppler imaging provides information on flow velocity and direction of flow by tracking scattering objects in a region of interest.[61] In contrast, power Doppler displays the power of the Doppler signal and is a more sensitive method in terms of signal-to-noise ratio and low-flow detection.[172]

In pediatric surgery, US imaging is widely used in the evaluation of appendicitis, testicular torsion, intussusception, hypertrophic pyloric stenosis, biliary and pancreatic conditions, and pelvic pathology.[54,74] In addition, US is a powerful and relatively safe tool for the prenatal diagnosis of congenital anomalies such as abdominal wall defects, diaphragmatic hernia, sacrococcygeal teratoma, cystic adenomatoid malformation, pulmonary sequestration, neural tube defects, obstructive uropathy, facial clefting, and twin-twin syndrome.[163] Sonographic guidance is also vital in performing more invasive prenatal diagnostic techniques such as amniocentesis and fetal blood sampling.[163]

Ultrasound and Fetal Surgery

Prenatal US provided the first view of the developing fetus, helped define the natural history of the fetus with an anomaly, and suggested prenatal interventional strategies.[85] US evaluation has become an increasingly important noninvasive modality for diagnosing and characterizing diseases that are amenable to fetal surgical intervention.[237] Today, fetal surgical techniques are used in selected centers to perform a variety of procedures, including surgical repair of myelomeningocele, resection of sacrococcygeal teratoma in fetuses with nonimmune hydrops, resection of an enlarging congenital cystic adenomatoid malformation that is not amenable to thoracoamniotic shunting, and tracheal clip occlusion for severe left congenital diaphragmatic hernia.[42,45] Sonography currently remains the modality of choice for fetal diagnosis and treatment because of its safety and real-time capabilities. In addition, US imaging is vital to the postoperative care and follow-up of fetal surgical patients in utero.

Three-Dimensional Ultrasound

Although 2-D ultrasound systems have improved dramatically over the past 30 years, 2-D images require experienced interpretation. These images represent one cross section, or slice, of the target anatomy and thus require interpretation to mentally reconstruct the 3-D picture. Given these limitations, 3-D US systems that provide volumetric instead of cross-sectional images have recently been developed and have seen increased use for many applications.

The first reported clinical use of a 3-D US system occurred in 1986 when Baba succeeded in obtaining 3-D fetal images by processing 2-D images on a minicomputer (*http://www.ob-ultrasound.net/history-3D.html*). Since then, multiple 3-D US systems have been developed to provide more detailed and cohesive anatomic information. These multislice or volumetric images are generally acquired by one of two techniques: (1) utilization of a 2-D array in which a transducer with multiple element rows is used to capture multiple slices at once and render a volume from real 3-D data and (2) utilization of a one-dimensional phased array to acquire several 2-D slices over time. The resultant images are then fused by the US computer's reconstruction algorithm.

The 3-D information acquired via these techniques is then used to reconstruct and display a 3-D image by maximal signal intensity processing, volume rendering, or surface rendering. When these 3-D images are displayed in real-time fashion, they have the ability to provide both anatomic and functional information. An example is the evaluation of cardiac function with real-time US. Real-time, 3-D US is sometimes referred to as four-dimensional US (including the dimension of time), although it is still essentially providing a 3-D image. A 3-D US view of a fetus in utero is presented in Figure 4-1.

In the field of pediatric and fetal surgery, these 3-D US systems have been used for detailed prenatal evaluation of congenital anomalies. Dyson et al. prospectively scanned 63 patients with 103 anomalies via both 2-D and 3-D US techniques. Each anomaly was reviewed to determine whether 3-D US data were either advantageous, equivalent, or disadvantageous when compared with 2-D US images. The 3-D US images provided additional information in 51% of the anomalies, provided equivalent information in 45% of the anomalies, and were disadvantageous in 4%. Specifically, 3-D US techniques were most helpful in evaluating fetuses with facial anomalies, hand

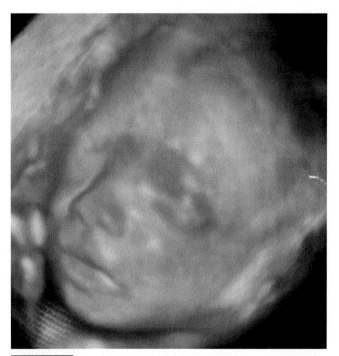

Figure 4–1 Three-dimensional ultrasound image of a fetal face. (From Tonni G, Centini G, Rosignoli L: Prenatal screening for fetal face and clefting in a prospective study on low-risk population: Can 3- and 4-dimensional ultrasound enhance visualization and detection rate? Oral Surg, Oral Med Oral Pathol Oral Radiol Endod 2005;100:420.

and foot abnormalities, and axial spine and neural tube defects. Overall, 3-D US imaging offered diagnostic advantages in about half the selected cases studied and had a significant effect on patient management in 5% of cases. They concluded that 3-D US was a powerful adjunctive tool to 2-D US in the prenatal evaluation of congenital anomalies.[52]

Chang et al. reported several series in which 3-D US techniques were used to effectively evaluate fetal organ volumes. They used 3-D US to accurately estimate fetal lung volume for the evaluation of pulmonary hypoplasia,[30] cerebellar volume,[27,28] heart volume,[31] adrenal gland volume,[29] and liver volume.[32] In all these studies, 3-D US images provided more accurate data than 2-D images did.[32]

In addition to prenatal evaluation, 3-D US systems have been used to image the ventricular system in neonates and infants to aid in the preoperative planning of neuroendoscopic interventions.[104,105] Similarly, these systems have seen relatively extensive use in the area of transthoracic echocardiographic imaging for the evaluation of congenital cardiac anomalies.[122,137] Cannon et al. studied the ability of 3-D US to guide basic surgical tasks in a simulated endoscopic environment.[25] They found that 3-D US imaging guided these tasks more efficiently and more accurately than 2-D US imaging did.[25] 3-D US systems allow the visualization of complex structures in a more intuitive manner than possible with 2-D systems. In addition, they appear to enable more precise measurements of volume and the relative orientation of structures.[222] As technology improves, the use of such systems in the field of pediatric surgery is likely to increase.

Ultrasound Contrast Imaging and Ultrasound Harmonic Imaging

In addition to 3-D US, significant advancements have occurred in US contrast imaging and harmonic imaging. US contrast imaging techniques are currently used for the visualization of intracardiac blood flow in order to evaluate structural anomalies of the heart.[225] US contrast agents are classified as free gas bubbles or encapsulated gas bubbles. These gas bubbles exhibit a unique resonance phenomenon when isonified by a US wave. They exhibit a frequency-dependent volume pulsation that makes the resonating bubble behave as a source of sound, not just a reflector of it.[61] New methods are being developed to enhance the contrast effect, including harmonic imaging, harmonic power Doppler imaging, pulse inversion imaging, release-burst imaging, and subharmonic imaging.[61] As these methods improve, US contrast imaging may provide clinicians with more detailed perfusion imaging of the heart, as well as tumors, arteriovenous malformations, and other conditions. Figure 4-2 depicts a US image of the left ventricle with the use of microbubble contrast.

Interest in US harmonic imaging occurred in 1996 after Burns observed harmonics generated by US contrast agents.[21] Since then, significant development has occurred in utilization of the harmonic properties of sound waves to improve the quality of US images. Sound waves are the sum of different component frequencies— the fundamental frequency (first harmonic) and harmonics, which are integral multiples of the fundamental frequency. The combination of the fundamental frequency and its specific harmonics gives a signal its unique characteristics. Harmonics are generated by the tissue itself; when US contrast agents are used, harmonics are generated by reflections from the injected agent and not by reflections from tissue.[221]

Whereas the fundamental frequency consists of echoes produced by tissue interfaces and differences in tissue properties, the harmonics are generated by the tissue itself. In this manner, harmonic intensity increases with

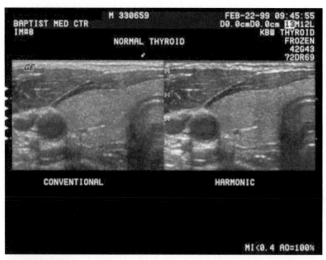

Figure 4-3 Conventional versus ultrasound harmonic imaging.

depth up to the point at which natural tissue attenuation overcomes this effect. In contrast, the intensity of the fundamental frequency is attenuated linearly with depth.[221]

Tissue harmonic imaging takes advantage of these properties by using the harmonic signals that are generated by tissue and filtering out the fundamental echo signals that are generated by the transmitted acoustic energy.[60] Such filtering theoretically leads to an improved signal-to-noise ratio and contrast-to-noise ratio. Additional benefits of US harmonic imaging include improved spatial resolution, better visualization of deep structures, and a reduction in artifacts produced by US contrast agents.[29] Figure 4-3 compares an image obtained by US harmonic imaging and one obtained by standard 2-D US.

Computed Tomography

CT was invented in 1972 by British engineer Godfrey Hounsfield of EMI Laboratories, England, and independently by the South African–born physicist Allan Cormack of Tufts University, Massachusetts. Since then, the medical use of CT imaging has become widespread. Currently, advances in technology have improved the speed, comfort, and image quality. Recent advances such as multidetector CT (MDCT) and volumetric reconstruction, or 3-D CT, may be particularly valuable in the care of pediatric surgical patients. This section provides a brief overview of CT imaging with focus on MDCT and volumetric imaging and their implications in pediatric surgery.

Multidetector Computed Tomography

CT uses a tightly arranged strip of radiation emitters and detectors circled around a patient to obtain a 2-D map of x-ray attenuation values. Numerical regression techniques are then used to turn this list of attenuation values into a 2-D slice image. CT has undergone several major developments since its introduction.

Introduced in the early 1990s, single-detector helical or spiral CT scanning revolutionized diagnostic CT imaging by

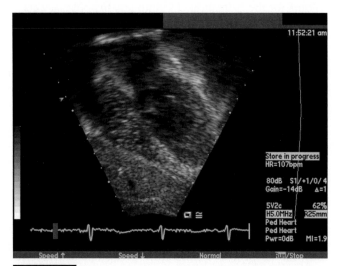

Figure 4-2 Ultrasound contrast echocardiogram demonstrating microbubbles in the right heart. (Courtesy of the Lucille Packard Children's Hospital Echocardiography Laboratory.)

using slip rings to allow for continuous image acquisition.[127] Before this development, the table and patient were moved in stepwise fashion after the acquisition of each image slice, a process that resulted in relatively long scanning times. Helical CT scanners use slip ring technology that allows the tube and detector to continually rotate around the patient. When combined with continuous table motion through the rotating gantry, speed is significantly improved. The improved speed of helical CT scanners enabled the acquisition of large volumes of data in a single breath hold, which has facilitated widespread pediatric use.

Helical CT has improved over the past 8 years, with faster gantry rotation, more powerful x-ray tubes, and improved interpolation algorithms.[183] However, the greatest advance has been the recent introduction of MDCT scanners. In contrast to single–detector row CT, MDCT uses multiple parallel rows of detectors that spiral around the patient simultaneously. Currently capable of acquiring four channels of helical data at the same time, MDCT scanners are significantly faster than single-detector helical CT scanners. This has profound implications on the clinical application of CT imaging, especially in pediatric patients, where the issues of radiation exposure and patient cooperation are magnified. Fundamental advantages of MDCT in comparison to earlier modalities include substantially shorter acquisition times, retrospective creation of thinner or thicker sections from the same raw data, and improved 3-D rendering with diminished helical artifacts.[183]

In the pediatric population, MDCT provides a number of advantages over standard helical CT, including a shortened or decreased need for sedation, a reduction in patient movement artifact, and a potential for more optimal contrast enhancement over a greater portion of the anatomic site. The volumetric data acquired also provide for the ability to perform multiplanar reconstruction, which can be an important problem-solving tool. MDCT has increasingly been used for pediatric trauma, pediatric tumors, evaluation of solid abdominal parenchymal organ masses, suspected abscess or inflammatory disorders,[63] and evaluation of abdominal pain.[49] Callahan et al. used MDCT to evaluate children with appendicitis and reduced the total number of hospital days, negative laparotomy rate, and cost per patient.[24] In addition, MDCT may be useful in identifying alternative diagnoses of pediatric abdominal pain, including bowel, ovarian, and urinary tract pathologies[49] (Fig. 4-4).

Similarly, MDCT may be valuable in the evaluation of urolithiasis and inflammatory bowel disease (IBD). MDCT has gained acceptance as a primary modality for the evaluation of children with abdominal pain and hematuria in whom urolithiasis is suspected.[49] CT findings of urolithiasis include visualization of radiopaque stones, dilatation of the ureter or collecting system, asymmetric enlargement of the kidney, and perinephric stranding.[49] Another condition in which CT is increasingly being used is IBD in children.[49] In the evaluation of these patients, CT may be superior to fluoroscopy in demonstrating inflammatory changes within the bowel, as well as extraluminal manifestations of IBD such as abscess.[49]

In the chest, MDCT has been used in children with infections, for detection and surveillance, and for evaluation of congenital abnormalities of the lung, mediastinum,

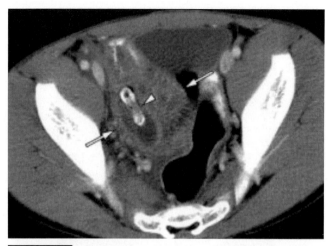

Figure 4–4 Multidetector computed tomogram of an 8-year-old boy with appendicitis. The *arrows* point to an inflammatory mass in the right lower quadrant with a possible appendicolith (*arrowhead*).

and heart. In particular, MDCT may be useful in the assessment of bronchopulmonary foregut malformation in which sequestration is a consideration.[62] The use of MDCT has been particularly valuable for evaluation of the pediatric cardiovascular system.[47] Assessment of cardiovascular conditions such as aortic aneurysms, dissections, and vascular rings may be significantly better than with echocardiography. Finally, MDCT is advantageous in the quantitative evaluation of patients with chest wall deformities because it allows for lower doses of radiation.[49]

Three-Dimensional Computed Tomography

Postacquisition processing of individual studies for the creation of 3-D CT reconstructions has been enabled by MDCT. These 3-D reconstructions are of value in the preoperative planning for complex surgical procedures. Although 3-D CT has been available for almost 20 years, the quality, speed, and affordability of these techniques have only recently improved enough to result in their incorporation in routine clinical practice.[100] Currently, four main visualization techniques are used in CT reconstruction laboratories to create 3-D CT images: multiplanar reformation, maximum intensity projections, shaded surface displays, and volume rendering. Multiplanar reformation and maximum intensity projections are limited to external visualization, whereas shaded surface displays and volume rendering allow for immersive or internal visualization such as virtual endoscopy.[183]

3-D CT is beneficial in the preoperative planning of pediatric craniofacial, vascular, and spinal operations. Specifically, 3-D CT is used to evaluate maxillofacial fractures,[58] craniofacial abnormalities (Fig. 4-5), and vascular malformations. 3-D CT has been useful in the planning of hemivertebra excision procedures for thoracic and thoracolumbar congenital deformities.[87]

A particularly interesting application of 3-D CT is the creation of "virtual endoscopy" images. The interior surface of luminal structures such as the bowel, airways, blood vessels, and urinary tract is reconstructed.[183] Virtual endoscopy using 3-D CT may be useful in the

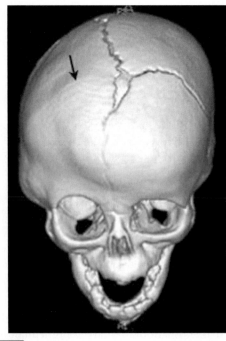

Figure 4–5 Three-dimensional computed tomographic T recon-struction of an infant skull showing premature closure of the right coronal suture (*arrow*).

diagnosis of small bowel tumors, lesions that are often difficult to detect with standard modalities[100] (Fig. 4-6).

Magnetic Resonance Imaging

The first MRI examination on a human was performed in 1977 by Drs. Damadian, Minkoff, and Goldsmith. This initial

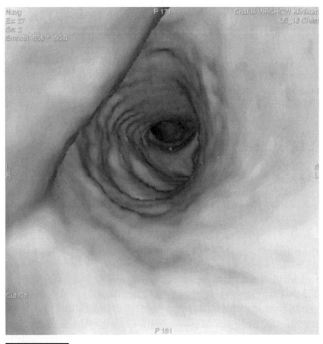

Figure 4–6 Virtual endoscopy.

examination took 5 hours to produce one relatively poor-quality image. Since then, technologic enhancements have improved the resolution and speed of MRI. Today, MRI is able to provide unparalleled noninvasive images of the human body. Newer MRI systems currently allow images to be obtained at subsecond intervals, thereby facilitating fast, near real-time MRI. MRI techniques are now being developed to provide functional information on the physiologic state of the body. This section provides a brief overview of MRI with a focus on recent technologic advances such as ultrafast MRI and fMRI.

MRI creates images by using a strong uniform magnetic field to align the spinning hydrogen protons of the human body. An RF pulse is then applied and causes some of the protons to absorb the energy and spin in a different direction. When the RF pulse is turned off, the protons realign and release their stored energy. This release of energy gives off a signal that is detected, quantified, and sent to a computer. Because different tissues respond to the magnetic field and RF pulse in a different manner, they give off variable energy signals. These signals are then used to create an image via mathematical algorithms.

Ultrafast MRI

The first major development in high-speed MRI occurred in 1986 with introduction of the gradient-echo pulse sequence technique (GRE), which can decrease practical scan times to as short as 10 seconds. In addition to increasing the patient throughput of MRI scanners, the faster scan times significantly increased the application of MRI to body regions (e.g., the abdomen) where suspended respiration could eliminate most motion-related image distortions.[53,226] Since then, GRE techniques have undergone iterations and further developments, and subsecond scan times have been achieved. Currently, ultrafast MRI sequences are able to obtain high-resolution scans in times as fast as one tenth of a second. These ultrafast MRI techniques have revolutionized the practical application of MRI in clinical medicine by reducing motion artifact. It has enabled newer, dynamic imaging modalities, including cardiac MRI, fetal MRI, and physiologic imaging techniques such as diffusion perfusion scanning (potentially valuable in the assessment of cerebral viability during stroke) and fMRI.

Ultrafast MRI provides a significant advantage in the care of children. Most traditional MRI protocols require 30 to 40 minutes, during which the patient must remain still.[199] For many children, sedation, general anesthesia, and even muscular blockade are often required to enable them to remain motionless long enough for a study to be completed. These were major impediments in performing MRI in children. Ultrafast MRI significantly reduces this requirement, thereby not only minimizing the potential side effects of sedation during routine MRI studies but also allowing the use of MRI to study high-risk infants who cannot be adequately sedated or paralyzed.[243]

In addition, ultrafast MRI significantly reduces the motion artifacts that occur in the abdomen and thorax as a result of normal respiratory and peristaltic movements. This is accomplished by achieving scan times that are rapid enough to be completed during a breath hold and fast relative to normal abdominal motion. Ultrafast MRI has been particularly useful in decreasing the smearing artifact associated with the use of oral contrast agents during MRI of the intestinal tract.[81] Moreover, by decreasing motion artifact and enabling fast image acquisition, ultrafast MRI protocols have enabled the practical application of cardiac MRI and fetal MRI. Fetal MRI is currently being used to better identify and characterize fetal brain and spine abnormalities.[73,174]

Functional MRI

fMRI is a rapidly evolving imaging technique that uses blood flow differences in the brain to provide in vivo images of neuronal activity. First described just over 10 years ago, fMRI has seen widespread clinical and research application in the adult population. fMRI is founded on two basic physiologic assumptions regarding neuronal activity and metabolism. Specifically, it assumes that neuronal activation induces an increase in local glucose metabolism associated with an increase in local cerebral blood flow. By detecting small changes in local blood flow, fMRI techniques are able to provide a "functional" image of brain activity. Currently, the most commonly used technique is known as "blood oxygen level–dependent" (BOLD) contrast, which uses blood as an internal contrast medium.[48] BOLD imaging takes advantage of small differences in the magnetic properties of oxygenated and deoxygenated hemoglobin. Because neuronal activation is followed by increased and relatively excessive local cerebral blood flow, more oxygenated hemoglobin appears in the venous capillaries of activated regions of the brain. These differences are detected as minute distortions in the magnetic field by fMRI and can be used to create a functional image of brain activity.[236]

In the pediatric population, fMRI requires significant subject preparation to have the child remain still in the scanner for the duration of the study. Various preparation techniques have been described for decreasing the anxiety and uncertainty that a child might experience regarding the study, including presession educational videos, tours with members of the radiology staff, and practice runs. Unlike anatomic MRI, patients undergoing fMRI cannot be sedated or anesthetized because this influences neuronal activity.

At this time, the use of fMRI in the pediatric population is still in its earliest stages. However, fMRI holds tremendous promise in the evaluation of central nervous system organization and development, characterization of brain plasticity, and evaluation and understanding of neurobehavioral disorders.[236] In addition, current clinical applications of fMRI include the delineation of eloquent cortex near a space-occupying lesion and determination of the dominant hemisphere for language. These clinical applications are designed to provide preoperative functional information before a planned neurosurgical procedure.[236]

Positron Emission Tomography

PET is an increasingly used imaging technology that provides information on the functional status of the human body. First developed in 1973 by Hoffman, Ter-Pogossian, and Phelps at Washington University, PET is now one of the most commonly performed nuclear medicine studies.[94] Although CT, MRI, and US techniques provide detailed information regarding the patient's anatomy, PET provides information on the current metabolic state of the patient's tissues.[107] In this manner, PET is often able to detect metabolic changes indicative of a pathologic state before anatomic changes can be visualized.

PET imaging is based on the detection of photons released when positron-emitting radionuclides undergo annihilation with electrons.[209] These radionuclides are created by bombarding target material with protons that have been accelerated in a cyclotron.[209] Positron-emitting radionuclides are then used to synthesize radiopharmaceuticals that are part of biochemical pathways in the human body. The most commonly used example is a fluorinated analogue of glucose, 2-deoxy-2-[18F] fluorodeoxyglucose (FDG). Like glucose, FDG is phosphorylated by the intracellular enzyme hexokinase.[219] In its phosphorylated form, FDG does not cross cell membranes and therefore accumulates within metabolically active cells. In this manner, PET imaging with FDG provides information on the glucose utilization of different body tissues.[107,219]

To be detected, FDG is synthesized with 18F, a radioisotope with a half-life of 110 minutes. The synthesis process begins by accelerating negatively charged hydrogen ions in a cyclotron until they gain approximately 8 MeV of energy. The orbital electrons from these hydrogen ions are then removed by passing them through a carbon foil. The resultant high-energy protons are next directed toward a target chamber that contains stable 18O-enriched water. The protons undergo a nuclear reaction with the 18O-enriched water to form hydrogen 18F-fluoride. The reaction is detailed in the following equation[107]:

$$H_2(^{18}O) + {}^1H + Energy \rightarrow H_2(^{18}F)$$

18F is an unstable radioisotope that decays by β+ emission or electron capture and emits a neutrino (ν) and a positron (β+). The emitted positrons are then annihilated with electrons to release energy in the form of photons, which are detected by modern PET scanners. The detectors in PET scanners are scintillation crystals coupled to photomultiplier tubes. Currently, most PET scanners use crystals composed of bismuth germinate, cerium-doped lutetium oxyorthosilicate, or cerium-doped gadolinium silicate. Because PET scanning uses unstable radioisotopes, PET probes must be synthesized immediately before a PET study. This drawback limits the immediate and widespread availability of PET imaging because the studies must therefore be scheduled in advance. FDG is a convenient probe because its half-life of 110 minutes allows it to be transported from a remote cyclotron to a PET scanner in enough time to perform a typical whole-body PET imaging study (≥30 minutes).

In a typical PET study, the radiopharmaceutical agent is administered intravenously. The patient is imaged by the PET scanner, which measures the radioactivity (photon emission as previously described) throughout the body and creates 3-D pictures or images of tissue function. Currently, PET imaging is used extensively in the evaluation and monitoring of tumors of the lung, colon, breast, lymph nodes, and skin.[193] PET imaging has been used to facilitate tumor diagnosis, localization, and staging, monitoring of antitumor therapy, tumor tissue characterization, radionuclide therapy, and screening for tumor recurrence.[202,212] Though nonspecific, FDG is often used because malignant cells generally display increased glucose utilization with up-regulation of hexokinase activity.

PET imaging has also been used to assess the activity of noncancerous tissues to provide information regarding their viability or metabolic activity. In adults, PET scans are often used to determine the viability of cardiac tissue to decide whether a patient would benefit from coronary bypass grafting.[75,76] Recently, this application has been extended to the pediatric population to assess cardiac function after arterial switch operations with suspected myocardial infarction.[177] Similarly, PET scans can visualize viability of brain tissue to make prognostic determinations after stroke.[173] Finally, PET imaging has been used to identify regions of abnormal activity in brain tissue and as such can help localize seizure foci or diagnose functional disorders such as Parkinson's disease and Alzheimer's disease.[157,158]

Although PET imaging provides important functional information regarding the metabolic activity of human tissues, it often provides relatively imprecise images when compared with traditional anatomic imaging modalities. It may be difficult to use during preoperative planning because it does not accurately correlate the area of suspicion with detailed anatomic information. Recently, combined PET/CT scanners have been developed that simultaneously perform PET scans and high-resolution CT scans.[192] Introduced only 5 years ago, these scanners provide functional information obtained from the PET scan and accurately map it to the fine anatomic detail of the CT scan[220] (Fig. 4-7).

In the field of pediatric surgery, PET/CT scanning represents a new imaging modality with tremendous potential in regard to preoperative planning and postoperative follow-up. However, several issues specific to the pediatric population make the implementation of PET imaging challenging, including the need for fasting, intravenous access, bladder catheterization, sedation, and clearance from the urinary tract.[109,180] Currently, the clinical application of combined PET/CT imaging in children has not been extensively studied. However, the combination of functional information with fine anatomic data provides obvious advantages with respect to surgical planning and will probably play a larger role in surgical practice in the future.

Molecular Imaging

US, CT, MRI, and PET are established technologies that are commonly used in the care of pediatric patients. Although these technologies provide detailed anatomic and even functional information, their clinical application has yet to provide information at the cellular/molecular level. In contrast to these classic imaging modalities, a new field termed "molecular imaging" probes the molecular abnormalities that are the basis of disease rather than imaging the end effects of these alterations. Molecular imaging is a rapidly growing research discipline that combines molecular and cell biology with noninvasive imaging technologies.[233] The goal of this new field is to develop techniques and assays for imaging physiologic events and pathways in living organisms at the cellular/molecular level, particularly pathways that are key targets in specific disease processes. The development and application of molecular imaging will someday probably affect patient care by elucidating the molecular processes underlying disease and lead to early detection of molecular changes that represent "predisease" states.[91]

Molecular imaging can be defined as the in vivo characterization and measurement of biologic processes at the cellular and molecular level. From a simplistic standpoint, molecular imaging consists of two basic elements: (1) molecular probes whose concentration, activity, or luminescence (or any combination of these properties) is changed by the specific biologic process under investigation and (2) a means by which to monitor these probes.[15,145] At the current time, most molecular probes are either radioisotopes that emit detectable radioactive signals or light or near-infrared–emitting molecules. In general, probes are considered either direct binding probes or indirect binding probes. Radiolabeled antibodies designed to facilitate the imaging of cell-specific surface antigens or epitopes are commonly used examples of direct binding probes. Similarly, radiolabeled oligonucleotide antisense probes developed to specifically hybridize with target mRNA or proteins for the purpose of direct, in vivo imaging are more recent examples.[38] Radiolabeled oligonucleotides represent complementary sequences to a small segment of target mRNA or DNA and therefore allow direct imaging of endogenous gene expression at the transcriptional level. Finally, positron-emitting analogues of dopamine, used to image the dopamine receptors of the brain, are other types of direct binding probes.

Whereas direct binding probes assist in imaging the amount or concentration of their targets, indirect probes reflect the activities of their macromolecular targets. Perhaps the most widely used example of an indirect binding probe is the hexokinase substrate FDG. The most common probe used in clinical PET imaging, FDG has been used for neurologic, cardiovascular, and oncologic investigations. Systemically administered FDG is accessible to essentially all tissues.

The use of reporter transgene technology is another powerful example of molecular imaging with indirect binding probes. Reporter genes are nucleic acid sequences that encode easily assayed proteins. Such reporter genes have long been used in molecular biology and genetics studies to investigate intracellular properties and events such as promoter function/strength, protein trafficking, and gene delivery. Via molecular imaging techniques, reporter genes have now been used to analyze gene delivery, immune cell therapy, and the in vivo efficacy of inhibitory mRNA in animal models.[191] In vivo bioluminescent imaging using firefly or *Rinella* luciferase and fluorescent optical imaging using green fluorescent protein or DsRed are optical imaging examples of this technique.

In the field of immunology and immunotherapy research, Costa et al. transduced the autoantigen-reactive

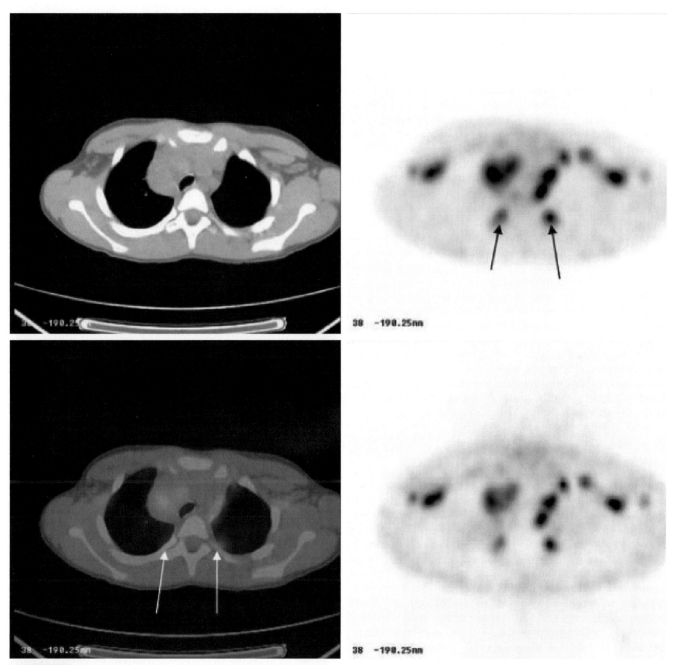

Figure 4-7   Combined PET/CT images (axial) through the upper part of the chest of a 7-year-old girl with necrotizing granuloma. Multiple sites of ^{18}F-FDG avid axillary lymph nodes and multiple foci within the mediastinal mass are visualized. (From Kaste SC: Issues specific to implementing PET-CT for pediatric oncology: What we have learned along the way. Pediatr Radiol 2004;34:205.)

CD4+ T-cell population specific for myelin basic protein with a retrovirus that encoded a dual reporter protein composed of green fluorescent protein and luciferase along with a 40-kDa monomer of interleukin-12 as a therapeutic protein.[44] Bioluminescent imaging techniques were then used to monitor the migratory patterns of the cells in an animal model of multiple sclerosis. Bioluminescent imaging demonstrated that the immune cells that would typically cause destruction of myelin trafficked to the central nervous system in symptomatic animals. Furthermore, they found that CD4+ T-cell expression

of the interleukin-12 immune modulator resulted in a clinical reduction in disease severity.[44]

Similarly, Vooijs et al. generated transgenic mice in which activation of luciferase expression was coupled to deletion of the retinoblastoma (*Rb*) tumor suppressor gene.[230] Loss of *Rb* triggered the development of pituitary tumors in their animal model, which allowed them to monitor tumor onset, progression, and response to therapy in individual animals by repeated imaging of luciferase activity with charge-coupled devices.[230] Although optical imaging techniques are commonly used, reporter genes can also encode for extracellular or intracellular receptors or transporters that bind or transport a radiolabeled or paramagnetic probe, thereby allowing for PET-, single-photon emission computed tomography (SPECT)-, or MRI-based molecular imaging. The second major element of molecular imaging is the imaging modality/technology itself. Direct and indirect binding probes can be radiolabeled to allow for nuclear-based in vivo imaging of a desired cellular/molecular event or process by PET or SPECT imaging. In fact, micro-PET and micro-SPECT systems have been developed specifically for molecular imaging studies in animal models. Similarly, optical imaging techniques such as bioluminescent imaging, near-infrared spectroscopy, visible light imaging with sensitive charge-coupled devices, and intravital imaging can be used with optically active probes to visualize desired cellular events. Finally, anatomic imaging modalities such as MRI, CT, and US have all been adopted for use in animal-based molecular imaging studies.

At this time, the field of molecular imaging is largely experimental, with significant activity in the laboratory and little current clinical application. However, molecular imaging research has been focused on investigating the molecular basis of clinical disease states and their potential treatments. Currently, molecular imaging techniques are being used to investigate the mechanisms surrounding apoptosis, angiogenesis, tumor growth and development, and gene therapy.

DNA Microarrays

The descriptive term *genomics* acknowledges the shift from a desire to understand the actions of single genes and their individual functions to a more integrated understanding of the simultaneous actions of multiple genes and the subsequent effect exerted on cellular behavior. DNA microarrays, or gene chips, are a recent advance that allow for the simultaneous assay of thousands of genes.[17] Microarray technology has been applied to redefine the biologic behavior of tumors, cross-species genomic comparisons, and large-scale analyses of gene expression in a variety of conditions. In essence, it represents a new form of patient and disease triage, *molecular triage*.

THERAPEUTIC TECHNOLOGIES

A surgical operation requires two key elements: an "image" or, more broadly, information regarding the anatomy of interest; and "manipulation" of the patient's tissue to achieve the goal of a therapeutic effect. Classically, the "image" is obtained through the eyes of the surgeon and the "manipulation" is performed with the surgeon's hands and simple, traditional surgical instruments. During the past several decades, this paradigm has been broadened by technologies that enhance these two fundamental elements.

As opposed to standard line-of-sight vision, an "image" may now be obtained through an operating microscope, a flexible endoscope, or a laparoscope. The endoscope may be monocular or binocular to provide 2-D or 3-D

visualization. These technologies provide the surgeon with high-quality, magnified images of anatomic areas that may be inaccessible with the naked eye. Similarly, surgical "manipulation" of tissue may be accomplished with a catheter, flexible endoscope, or longer laparoscopic instruments. Furthermore, devices such as staplers, electrocautery, ultrasonic energy tools, and RF emitters are used to manipulate and affect tissue with a therapeutic goal. These technologies have changed the way surgical procedures are performed; they have enabled and even created fields such as laparoscopic surgery, interventional endoscopy, and catheter-based intervention. In addition to these advances, several emerging technology platforms promise to further broaden this definition of surgery, including stereotactic radiosurgery and surgical robotics. This section presents a review of several of these technologies with a focus on the current status of hemostatic and tissue ablative instruments, stereotactic radiosurgery, and surgical robotics.

Hemostatic and Tissue Ablative Instruments

Hand-held energy devices designed to provide hemostasis and ablate tissue are widely used surgical technologies. Since the first reports concerning electrosurgery in the 1920s, multiple devices and forms of energy have been developed to minimize blood loss, including monopolar and bipolar electrocautery, ultrasonic dissectors, argon beam coagulators, cryotherapy, and infrared coagulators. This section provides a broad overview of the various hemostatic and tissue ablative devices with a focus on their principles of operation and techniques of use.

Monopolar Electrocautery

Although the concept of applying an electrical current to living tissue has been reported as far back as the late 16th century, the practical application of electrocautery in surgery did not begin to develop until the early 1900s. In 1908, Lee deForest developed a high-frequency generator that was capable of delivering a controlled cutting current. However, this device used expensive vacuum tubes and had very limited clinical application. In the 1920s, W. T. Bovie developed a low-cost spark-gap generator. The potential of this device for use in surgery was recognized by Harvey Cushing during a demonstration in 1926, and the first practical electrosurgery units were soon in use.

Energy Sources

Electrocautery

The application of high-frequency alternating current is now known variously as electrocautery, electrosurgery, or simply "the Bovie." The current can be delivered through either a unipolar or a bipolar mechanism. In the unipolar application, the current is delivered by a generator via an application electrode, travels through the patient's body, and returns to a grounding pad. Without a grounding pad the patient would suffer a thermal burn injury wherever the current seeks reentry. The area of contact is critical because heat is inversely related to the size of the application device. Accordingly, the tip of the device is typically small to generate heat efficiently, and the returning electrode is large to broadly disperse energy. Three other settings are pertinent: the frequency of the current (power setting), the activation time, and the characteristics of the waveform produced by the generator (intermittent or continuous).

In the "cut" mode, heat is generated quickly with minimal lateral spread. As a result, the device separates tissue without significant coagulation of underlying vessels. In the "coagulation" mode, the device generates less heat at a slower frequency with larger lateral thermal spread. As a consequence, tissue is desiccated and vessels become thrombosed.

Bipolar cautery creates a short circuit between the grasping tips of the instruments; thus, the circuit is completed through the grasped tissue between the tips. Because heat develops only within the short-circuited tissue, there is less lateral thermal spread and the mechanical advantage of tissue compression, as well as thermal coagulation.

Argon Beam Coagulator

The argon beam coagulator creates an electric circuit between the tip of the probe and the target tissue through a flowing stream of ionized argon gas. The electrical current is conducted to the tissue via the argon gas and produces thermal coagulation. The flow of the argon gas improves visibility and disperses any surface blood, thereby enhancing coagulation. Its applications in hepatic surgery are unparalleled.

Surgical Lasers

Lasers (i.e., light amplification by stimulated emission of radiation) are devices that produce an extremely intense and nearly nondivergent beam of monochromic radiation, usually in the visible region. When focused at close range, laser light is capable of producing intense heat with resultant coagulation. Lateral spread is minimal, and critically, the laser beam can be delivered through a fiber-optic system.

Based on power setting and the photon chosen, depth can be controlled. Penetration depth within tissue is most shallow with the argon laser, intermediate with the carbon dioxide (CO_2) laser, and greatest with the neodymium-yttrium aluminum garnet (Nd-YAG) laser. Photosensitizing agents provide an additional targeting advantage. The degree of absorption and thus destruction depends on the wavelength selected and the absorptive properties of the tissue based on density, fibrosis, and vascularity.

Photodynamic Therapy

A novel application of light energy is used in photodynamic therapy. A photosensitizer that is target cell specific is administered and subsequently concentrated in the tissue to be eradicated. The photosensitizing agent may then be activated with a light energy source to induce tissue destruction. Applications have been widespread.[209] Metaplastic cells, in particular, in Barrett's esophagus, may also be susceptible.[185]

Ultrasound

In addition to the diagnostic use of US at low frequency, delivery of high-frequency US can be used to separate and coagulate tissue. Focused acoustic waves are now used extensively in the treatment of renal calculi as extracorporeal shock wave lithotripsy. The focused energy produces a shock wave that results in fragmentation of the stones to a size that can be spontaneously passed.

Harmonic Scalpel

When US energy at very high frequency (55,000 Hz) is used, tissue can be separated with minimal peripheral damage. Such high-frequency energy creates vibration, friction, heat, and ultimately, tissue destruction.

High-Intensity Focused Ultrasound

When high-intensity US energy from multiple beams is focused at a point on a target tissue, heating and thermal necrosis result. None of the individual US beams are of sufficient magnitude to cause injury; only at the focus point does thermal injury result. As a result, subcutaneous nodules may be targeted without injury to skin, or nodules within the parenchyma of a solid organ may be destroyed without penetrating the surface. Thus far, however, the focal point is extremely small, which has limited its use.

Cavitation Devices

The CUSA, a cavitation US aspirator, uses lower-frequency US energy with concomitant aspiration. Fragmentation of high–water content tissue allows for parenchymal destruction while highlighting vascular structures and permitting their precise coagulation.

Radiofrequency Energy

High-frequency alternating current (350 to 500 kHz) may be used for tissue division, vessel sealing, or tissue ablation. Application of this energy source heats the target tissue and causes protein denaturization and necrosis. A feedback loop sensor discontinues the current at a selected point, thereby minimizing collateral damage. Its targeted use in modulating the lower esophageal sphincter for the treatment of reflux has been reported.[223]

Microwave Energy

Microwave energy (2450 MHz) can be delivered via a probe to a target tissue. This rapidly alternating electrical signal produces heat and thus coagulation necrosis.

Cryotherapy

At the other end of the temperature spectrum, cold temperatures destroy tissue with a cycle of freezing and thawing—ice crystal formation in the freezing phase and disruption during the thawing phase. Thus far this modality has less utility because high vascular flow, especially in tumors, tends to siphon off the cold.

Image Guidance Systems

Recent developments in computation technology have fundamentally enhanced the role of medical imaging, from diagnostics described previously to computer-assisted surgery (CAS). During the last decade, medical imaging methods have grown from their initial use as physically based models of human anatomy to applied computer vision and graphic techniques for planning and analyzing surgical procedures. With rapid advances in high-speed computation, the task of assembling and visualizing clinical data has been greatly facilitated, thus creating new opportunities for real-time, interactive computer applications during surgical procedures.[40,142,197,212] This area of development, termed image-guided surgery, has slowly evolved into a field best called information-guided therapy (IGT) because it involves the use of a variety of data sources to implement the best therapeutic intervention. Such therapeutic interventions could conceivably range from biopsy, to simulation of tissue, to direct implantation of medication, to radiotherapy. Common to all these highly technical interventions is the need to precisely intervene with the therapeutic modality at a specific point.

However, the effective utilization of biomedical engineering, computation, and imaging concepts for IGT has not reached its full potential. Significant challenges remain in the development of basic scientific and mathematical frameworks that form the foundation for improving therapeutic interventions through the application of relevant information sources.

Significance

As stated in the National Institutes of Heath 1995 *Support for Bioengineering Research Report* (*http://grants.nih.gov/grants/becon/externalreport.html*), an appropriate use of technology would be to replace traditional invasive procedures with noninvasive techniques. The current interest in research in CAS, or IGT, can be attributed in part to considerable clinical interest in the well-recognized benefits of minimal access surgery (MAS), while remaining cognizant of its limitations.

Image-based surgical guidance, on the other hand, addresses these limitations. Image-guided surgical navigational systems have now become the standard of care for cranial neurosurgical procedures in which precise localization within and movement through the brain are of utmost importance.

Patient-specific image data sets such as CT or MRI, once correlated with fixed anatomic reference points, or fiducials, can provide surgeons with detailed spatial information about the region of interest. Surgeons can then use these images to precisely target and localize pathologies. Intraoperative computer-assisted imaging improves the surgeon's ability to follow preoperative plans by showing location and optimal direction. Thus, the addition of CAS provides the advantages of MAS with the added benefits of greater precision and an increased likelihood of complete and accurate resection. The junction between CAS and MAS presents research opportunities and challenges for imaging scientists and surgeons everywhere.

General Requirements

Patient-Specific Models

Unlike simulation, IGT requires that modeling data be matched specifically to the patient being treated because standard fabricated models based on typical anatomy are inadequate during actual surgical procedures on a specific patient. Patient-specific images can be generated preoperatively (e.g., by CT or MRI) or intraoperatively (e.g., by US or conventional radiography).

High Image Quality

IGT depends on spatially accurate models. Images require exceptional resolution in order to portray realistic and consistent information.

Real-Time Feedback

Current systems make the surgeon wait while new images are being segmented and updated. Thus, fast dynamic feedback is needed, and the latencies associated with visualization segmentation and registration should be minimized.

High Accuracy and Precision

A recent American Association of Neurological Surgeons survey of 250 neurosurgeons[177] disclosed that surgeons had little tolerance for error (1 to 2 mm accuracy in general, and 2 to 3 mm for spinal and orthopedic applications). All elements of visualization, registration, and tracking must be accurate and precise, with special attention paid to errors associated with intraoperative tissue deformation.

Repeatability and Robustness

IGT systems must be able to automatically incorporate a variety of data so that algorithms work consistently and reliably in any situation.

Correlation of Intraoperative Information with Preoperative Images

This requirement is a key area of interest to biomedical engineers and is especially critical for compensation of tissue deformation. Whether produced by microscopes, endoscopes, fluoroscopes, electrical recordings, physiologic simulation, or other imaging techniques, preoperative and intraoperative images and information need to be incorporated into and correlated by the surgical guidance system.

Intuitive Machine and User Interfaces

The most important part of any IGT system is its usability. The surgeon's attention must be focused on the patient and not on the details of the computational model.

Stereotactic Radiosurgery

Whereas laparoscopy has been the dominant arena for recent technologic development in general surgery, other surgical disciplines have used alternative minimally invasive solutions that follow the surgical theme of "image" and "manipulation" highlighted in this chapter. For example, endovascular interventions such as percutaneous coronary angioplasty, drug-eluting coronary stents, and aortic stent grafts have revolutionized the management of cardiovascular disease.[8,22,23] In the field of otolaryngology and neurosurgery, computerized image guidance systems have been used to accurately correlate intraoperatively encountered structures with preoperative images.[112,113] The discipline of stereotactic radiosurgery takes the concepts underlying image-guided surgery one step further.

Stereotactic radiosurgery uses precision targeting and large numbers of crossfired, highly collimated beams of high-energy ionizing radiation to noninvasively ablate tissue. Conceptualized in the 1950s by the Swedish neurosurgeon Lars Leksell, this technology has been used to treat/ablate a variety of benign and malignant intracranial lesions without an incision.[119] Lesioning of normal brain tissue such as the trigeminal nerve (trigeminal neuralgia), thalamus (tremor), and epileptic foci (intractable seizures) is an important clinical application of this technology.[34] Meanwhile, numerous studies have demonstrated that radiosurgery is an important treatment option for many otolaryngologic conditions, including skull base and head and neck tumors.[4,9,16,66] Most recently, radiosurgical techniques have been applied to the treatment of extracranial diseases, such as spinal tumors and lesions of the thoracic and abdominal cavities.[215,216] Many of the newest applications of stereotactic radiosurgery fall under the traditional realm of general surgery, including lung, liver, and pancreatic cancer.[78,152,154,171,175,206,224,235] As the scientific understanding and clinical practice of radiosurgery develop, such technology may become an increasingly valuable, minimally invasive option for treating a range of pediatric general surgical diseases. The purpose of this section is to review the principles and current application of stereotactic radiosurgery in children. In addition, this section will highlight the relatively new application of stereotactic radiosurgery to extracranial sites, with a focus on emerging scientific and technologic directions.

Radiobiology

Since Roentgen's discovery of x-rays in 1895, scientists and clinicians have studied the effects of ionizing radiation on biologic tissue, a field termed *radiobiology*. In 1906, Bergonié and Tribondeau performed experiments in which it was shown that immature, dividing cells were damaged at lower radiation doses than were mature, nondividing cells.[12] Their observations led to formation of the Bergonié-Tribondeau law, which states that ionizing radiation is more effective against cells that are undifferentiated and actively mitotic.[12] Subsequent generations of research have substantiated this law and further refined our current understanding of the biologic basis for radiotherapy.[19,117,119,198]

Both charged particles (alpha particles, proton beams, or electron beams) and high-energy light beams (gamma rays or x-rays) produce either direct or indirect damage to the DNA of target cells.[83] The densely ionizing nature of particulate radiation causes direct damage to cellular DNA. In contrast, the mechanism of action for most high-energy photon beams (x-rays) is ejection of electrons (radiolysis) from the cell's constituent molecules (mostly water).[82,124] The ejected electrons can damage DNA directly and cause the formation of cell-damaging free radicals. The later entity may combine with other free radicals to form new molecules, such as hydrogen peroxide, that are toxic to vital cellular structures (membranes and lysozymes). These free radicals also have the potential to secondarily damage chromosomal DNA. There are a number of molecular mechanisms for such injury after high-energy irradiation: one involves loss of a nitrogenous base, a second involves damage to the hydrogen bond between the two strands of the DNA molecule, and a third involves damage to the DNA backbone.[82,124]

Damage to a single strand of a DNA molecule is of little consequence because it is usually reparable. However, if the effects of a radiation beam are sufficiently concentrated, two nearby single-strand breaks can produce an uncorrectable double-strand break.[176] During subsequent cycles of cell division, a critical level of genomic instability may lead to cell inactivation.[196] This postmitotic model for cell death is the prevailing mode, although apoptotic cell death may also occur if the damage to DNA initiates p53- and Bcl-2–dependent mechanisms. These mechanisms can begin a cascade that results in the activation of effector caspases, thereby targeting multiple critical cellular death substrates.[228] In addition, radiation damage may affect the rate of cell division and thus result in a delay (of cell division) and an accompanying decrease in the cell population. Finally, interphase death may occur if radiation kills the cells during the G_1, S, or G_2 phase. Cells are most radiosensitive during the G_2 and M phases.[228]

The amount of cellular damage induced by a particular form of radiation is related to the radiation's linear energy transfer (LET). LET describes the amount of energy that is transferred from the radiation beam to the tissue that it is directed through; it is calculated by dividing the energy deposited in kiloelectron volts by the distance traveled in micrometers.[82,83] X-rays and gamma rays are classified as having low LET because their electrons distribute over a greater distance in tissue. The LET level of radiation is important because equal doses of radiation with different LET levels produce a different biologic response. The term "relative biologic response" describes a measure of the comparative biologic effect between the more damaging heavy-particle and x-ray beams.[82]

Various physical, chemical, and biologic factors can influence the sensitivity of a given cell's response to radiation. The important physical factors that influence the cellular response include the LET level and the dose rate of radiation.[198] Optimal LET is approximately 160 keV/μm, which produces the highest level of double-strand DNA breaks. Meanwhile, a higher dose rate of radiation prevents cells from repairing sublethal chromosomal damage.

Certain chemical factors termed radiosensitizers and radioprotectants modulate the effectiveness of radiation. The most potent radiosensitizer, oxygen, promotes the formation of indirectly damaging free radicals.[198] Hypoxic cells, as often seen in larger malignant tumors, are resistant to radiation.

Two vital biologic factors underlying the cellular response to high-energy radiation are the phase in the cell cycle and the capacity of a cell to repair sublethal damage. Cells in the G_2 and M phases are the most sensitive. Cells exposed to the same cumulative dose of radiation but undergoing multiple exposures in a process termed fractionation will have a higher survival rate than will cells exposed to the entire dose in one fraction or session.[117] This phenomenon stems from a cell's ability to repair sublethal damage before subsequent radiation exposure, and it forms an important theoretical basis for the effectiveness of radiosurgery.[117]

Radiotherapy and Fractionation

Radiation therapy, or *radiotherapy*, refers to the use of ionizing radiation for the treatment of pathologic disorders. The use of radiation to cure cancer was first reported in 1899, soon after Roentgen's discovery of x-rays in 1895.[35] In the 1930s, Coutard described the practice of "fractionation," which refers to the division of a total dose of radiation into multiple smaller doses, typically given on a daily basis.[35] Fractionation is a bedrock principle that underlies the field of radiotherapy.[117,118] By administering radiation in multiple daily fractions over the course of several weeks, it is possible to irradiate a tumor with a higher total dose while relatively sparing the surrounding normal tissue from the most injurious effects of treatment. The effect of radiation on tissues is dependent on several factors, commonly referred to as the four R's: repopulation, redistribution, repair, and reoxygenation.[218] Repopulation refers to the division and consequent multiplication of surviving cells in the tumor and adjacent normal tissue. Ideally, the only repopulation that would occur after treatment would be that of adjacent normal tissue. Redistribution refers to the death of cells in their radiosensitive phase (G_2 and M) and survival of cells in the S phase. Ideally, radiation is administered when tumor cells are in their radiosensitive phase and the adjacent normal tissue is in the less sensitive S phase of the cell cycle. Repair of sublethal damage between fractionated doses of radiation is dependent on oxygen.[218] Tumor cells are hypoxic and therefore less able to repair their DNA. Furthermore, oxygen is important in the free radical mechanism that radiation uses to kill a tumor. The manner in which tumor cells gain access to oxygen and become more radiosensitive between treatments is called reoxygenation. Although the exact mechanism is unclear, hypoxic regions of a tumor often tend to become better oxygenated, and therefore more radiosensitive, over a prolonged period. This phenomenon can make fractionated treatment more effective than single-dose radiotherapy under some clinical circumstances.[218] Overall, fractionation is an extremely important concept in radiotherapy inasmuch as standard techniques expose both normal and pathologic tissue to irradiation. By fractionating therapy, normal tissue should recover while pathologic tissue is destroyed. Although fractionation regimens differ depending on the specific pathology, current regimens often involve up to 30 treatments.[35]

Before the 1950s, radiotherapy machines were capable of delivering only relatively low-energy x-rays characterized by rapid energy loss and shallow depth penetration.[35] However, newer machines capable of delivering megaelectron volts (MeV) of x-rays were developed that allowed greater depth penetration and thereby facilitated the treatment of more deep-seated lesions. Today, radiotherapy is primarily delivered with linear accelerators, or linacs, which use electromagnetic waves to accelerate charged particles through a linear tube. These particles emerge from the linac to strike a metal foil and produce x-rays. This process is termed *bremsstrahlung*.[35] Less commonly, cobalt 60 units, which use radioactive isotopes as a high-energy radiation source, are used to deliver radiotherapy.[35] These units have a relatively shallow maximal dose depth of approximately 0.5 cm, thus making them less useful for deeper lesions. Radiotherapy is a well-established treatment of intracranial and extracranial pathologies.[4,9,34,116,119] The medical literature regarding its use is extensive and therefore beyond the scope of this review.

Stereotactic Radiosurgery

Stereotactic radiosurgery refers to the method and corresponding technology for delivering a single high dose of radiation to a well-defined target. It has the potential advantage of delivering a much larger radiation dose to a pathologic lesion without exceeding the radiation tolerance of the surrounding normal tissue. This single, or limited, dose treatment of a small volume of tissue is achieved by targeting the tissue with large numbers of intersecting beams of radiation. "Stereotactic" refers to the fact that radiosurgery uses computer algorithms to coordinate the patient's real-time anatomy in the treatment suite with a preoperative image to allow precise targeting. To achieve this goal, the patient's anatomy is fixed with a stereotactic frame.[34,35] The preoperative images are then taken with the frame in place, and the patient's anatomy is mapped in relation to the frame. This stereotactic frame is rigidly fixed to the patient's skull, thereby limiting movement of the target anatomy. In addition, the frame serves as an external fiducial system that correlates the coordinates of the target tissues determined during preoperative imaging and planning. Leksell first described this technique in 1951 and showed that there was an exponential relationship between dose and the time over which necrosis developed. By using multiple beams at different angles, one can achieve a steep falloff in dose at the periphery of the target volume. For this reason, appropriate definition of the target volume in radiosurgery is of utmost importance. Limited fractionation can now be used in conjunction with stereotactic radiosurgery in a procedure that has recently been termed fractionated or staged radiosurgery.[35] The concept of staging capitalizes on one of the "four R's" by giving surrounding normal tissue time to repair. Because of the cellular makeup, single large fractions tend to be effective on slowly proliferating tissue, such as benign tumors and arteriovenous malformations (AVMs).[35] In contrast, techniques involving staged radiosurgery allow for some normal tissue repair and may be advantageous when ablating larger-volume tumors or lesions that are adjacent to critical normal anatomy.

Currently, several classes of stereotactic radiosurgery systems are in use, including heavy-particle radiosurgery systems, gamma knife radiosurgery, linear accelerator radiosurgery, and frameless image-guided radiosurgery.

Stereotactic Radiosurgery Systems: Current Technology

Heavy-Particle Radiosurgery: Proton-based radiosurgery systems are some of the earliest stereotactic radiosurgery systems used.[55,56,134,135] Charged particles (proton or helium ions) have a unique advantage over photons with respect to radiosurgery.[136] Radiosurgery using photons relies on systems of crossfiring beams from multiple directions to achieve high target tissue radiation delivery while minimizing the radiation exposure of surrounding normal tissue as photons deposit energy along the entire path of the beam. In contrast, charged particles deliver energy in a nonuniform pattern along their beam length. Specifically, they produce a region of intermediate energy dose at the entry site, followed by a zone of high-dose

energy termed the Bragg ionization peak, and then followed by an exit dose of minimal energy.[35] The Bragg ionization peak can be adjusted to precisely deliver peak energy levels to a targeted tissue area.[136] Although this phenomenon is advantageous, heavy-particle radiosurgery systems have several disadvantages that have limited their widespread use. Specifically, the systems are very expensive to construct and maintain and require a working cyclotron. Furthermore, such systems require beam-modifying devices that must be custom made for each patient and require the patient to wear an immobilizing plastic mask or bite block to achieve fixation. Because of these limitations, heavy-particle radiosurgery is currently limited to two active sites in the United States and is used solely for intracranial lesions.[35]

Gamma Knife Radiosurgery: In contrast to heavy-particle radiosurgery systems, gamma knife radiosurgery is significantly less expensive and easier to use. First developed by Leksell in 1967, the Leksell Gamma Knife (Elekta Instruments, Inc., Norcross, GA) uses cobalt 60 as a radiation source.[35] The original gamma knife was used for pallidotomy in the treatment of Parkinson's disease and to treat intracranial tumors and vascular malformations.[34,35,67,90,101] Because the Gamma Knife uses a stereotactic frame, radiosurgical treatments with this system are not fractionated and primarily consist of a one-time therapeutic session.[113] Figure 4-8A and B depicts the Leksell Gamma Knife.

Linear Accelerator Radiosurgery: Linear accelerators, or linacs, have long been the mainstay of standard fractionated

Figure 4–8 *A,* Leksell Gamma Knife. (Courtesy of Elekta Instruments, Inc., Norcross, GA.) *B,* Leksell Gamma Knife layout (*http://www.sh.lsuhsc.edu/ neurosurgery/gammaknife/gamma-knife/*).

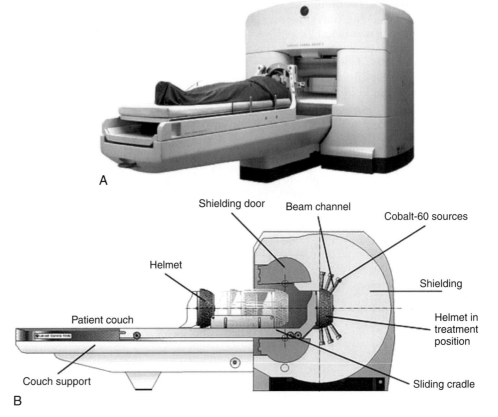

A

B

Shielding door

Beam channel

Cobalt-60 sources

Helmet

Shielding

Patient couch

Helmet in treatment position

Couch support

Sliding cradle

radiotherapy[5,18,39,116] and were modified for radiosurgery in 1982.[35] Linac radiosurgery has subsequently become a cost-effective and widely used alternative to gamma knife radiosurgery. When used for radiosurgery, linacs crossfire a photon beam by moving in multiple arc-shaped paths around the patient's head. The area of crossfire where the multiple fired beams intersect receives a high amount of radiation, with minimal exposure to surrounding normal tissue.[35] Patients treated with linac radiosurgery must also wear a stereotactic frame fixed to the skull for preoperative imaging and therapy. Currently, linac radiosurgery is the predominant modality in the United States, with approximately six times more active centers than gamma knife facilities.[35]

Frameless Image-Guided Radiosurgery: Recently, a novel modified version of linac radiosurgery has been developed that enables frameless image-guided radiosurgery. The system, commercially available as the CyberKnife (Accuray, Inc., Sunnyvale, CA), uses a lightweight linac unit designed for radiosurgery mounted on a highly maneuverable robotic arm.[33] The robotic arm can position and point the linac with 6 degrees of freedom and 0.3-mm precision. In addition, the CyberKnife system features image guidance, which eliminates the need for skeletal fixation.[34,36] The CyberKnife acquires a series of stereoscopic radiographs that identify a preoperatively placed gold fiducial. This fiducial is placed under local anesthesia during the preoperative imaging and planning sessions to allow the system to correlate the patient's target anatomy with the preoperative image for treatment. By actively acquiring radiographs during the treatment session, the system is able to track and follow the target anatomy in nearly real time during treatment.[33,34] With an image guidance system, the CyberKnife functions without a fixed stereotactic frame, thereby enabling fractionation (hypofractionated radiosurgery) of treatment, as well as extracorporeal stereotactic use. In pediatric surgery, this may be a significant technical advantage because it may enable the use of radiosurgery for the treatment of intrathoracic and intra-abdominal pathology (Fig. 4-9).

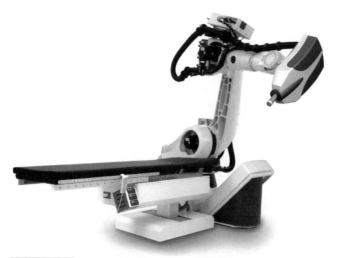

Figure 4–9 CyberKnife System *(http://www.sky.sannet.ne.jp/ybaba/main.html).*

Stereotactic Radiosurgery in Children

Stereotactic radiosurgery of intracranial lesions has been a well-established treatment modality for many years. From the viewpoint of radiosurgery, the fact that the intracranial contents are relatively static results in essentially nonmobile target tissues, thus enabling the delivery of high radiation doses in one or few treatment fractions with minimal risk to adjacent normal tissue. Accuracy is maximized by the use of stereotactic head frames that fix the skull in a given position to allow precise targeting of the desired tissue. This has led to the widespread use of stereotactic radiosurgical techniques in adults for the treatment of benign and malignant otolaryngologic[4,39,41,131,132] and neurosurgical[67,68,80,129,168,201] lesions that are contained within the rigid confines of the skull. Multiple groups have reported the safe and effective use of stereotactic radiosurgery for the treatment of malignant lesions of the brain and neck in children.* In addition to pediatric brain tumors, stereotactic radiosurgery has also been described for the treatment of nonmalignant intracranial lesions in children. The use of radiosurgery for the treatment of cerebral AVMs has been well documented.[102,133,138,156,200] In a series of 30 children with intracranial AVMs (mean age, 11.2 years), the overall obliteration rate after radiosurgery was 35%. The authors concluded that stereotactic radiosurgery was an effective treatment option with acceptably low complication rates for children with cerebral AVMs.[200]

When compared with the adult population, the experience with stereotactic radiosurgery in children is still somewhat limited. Early reports highlight the safety and efficacy of radiosurgery as a treatment modality, but clinical follow-up is still early, with many of the studies limiting the use of radiosurgery to surgically unresectable disease. Despite the relatively limited experience, the use of stereotactic radiosurgery in children may offer several theoretical advantages specific to the pediatric population. In comparison to standard, fractionated radiotherapy, stereotactic radiosurgical techniques deliver conformal radiation treatment with millimeter versus centimeter accuracy. In pediatric patients, the distance between normal and pathologic tissue may be very small. In addition, the developing brain in a child may be more sensitive to the effects of ionizing radiation than adult brains are. Potential cognitive and endocrine disabilities have been described in children after delivery of radiotherapy to the brain.[69,70,201] These concerns have largely limited the use of radiation for the treatment of intracranial tumors in infants. Therefore, the improved accuracy provided by stereotactic radiosurgery may be particularly important in the pediatric population.

In addition to accuracy, stereotactic radiosurgical techniques differ from radiotherapy in that they involve only one to very few treatment sessions. Standard, fractionated radiotherapy often requires tens of treatment sessions to maximize the beneficial effects of the treatment while minimizing the harmful effects to normal tissue. In children, multiple treatment sessions may be a significant challenge.

---

*See references 14, 20, 43, 51, 59, 93, 95, 184, 205, 231, 234, 244.

In smaller children, sedation or anesthesia may be necessary to avoid movement. Such interventions are not without risk, and limiting the number of treatment sessions may serve to minimize the overall risk to pediatric patients.

Although the advantages of stereotactic radiosurgery in children appear promising, there are also specific disadvantages and limitations that must be overcome. Radiosurgical techniques generally use a stereotactic frame to coordinate preoperative imaging with actual radiation delivery. However, these frames must be secured to the skull with pins and screws. In adults, this can often be performed under local anesthesia, but children probably need significant sedation and possibly general anesthesia. Furthermore, an infant's skull is soft and less rigid because the cranial sutures have not yet fused, and standard stereotactic frames often cannot be applied. Similarly, radiosurgery treatment sessions require the patient to remain still for the system to accurately deliver the radiation treatment. Adults are able to cooperate and do not need sedation; however, younger children and infants may require conscious sedation or general anesthesia. Although this drawback is limited by the relatively few sessions needed with radiosurgery, it still diminishes the minimally invasive nature of the therapy in comparison to its application in adults.

Recently, frameless, image-guided stereotactic radiosurgery has been performed with the CyberKnife system using a linac mounted on a robotic arm to deliver radiation energy. In addition, the system uses real-time image guidance to track the movements of a patient's anatomy during the treatment session. Consequently, stereotactic frames are not used with this form of radiosurgery. Recently, Giller et al. described the use of this system in children.[69,70] They used the CyberKnife system in 21 children with brain tumors; their ages ranged from 8 months to 16 years.[69] There were no procedure-related deaths or complications, and local control was achieved in over half the patients. Seventy-one percent of patients received only one treatment session and 38% did not require general anesthesia. None of the patients required rigid skull fixation.[69] In an additional report, the same group highlighted the use of the CyberKnife system to perform radiosurgery in five infants.[70] Although standard stereotactic frames were not required, patient immobilization was aided by general anesthesia, form-fitting head supports, face masks, and body molds. No treatment-related toxicity was encountered, and the authors concluded that "radiosurgery with minimal toxicity can be delivered to infants by use of a robotically controlled system that does not require rigid fixation."[69]

Extracranial Stereotactic Radiosurgery—Implications for General Surgery

Whereas the use of stereotactic radiosurgery for intracranial lesions has been well established, its use for the treatment of extracranial lesions, specifically, intrathoracic and intra-abdominal pathology, is still in its infancy. Although the intracranial contents can easily be immobilized with stereotactic frames, the abdominal and thoracic organs are subject to significant movement because of respiration, peristalsis, and other factors. As a result, only a small body of literature is currently available on the application of stereotactic radiosurgery for extracranial lesions. Recently, several reports have described the efficacy of stereotactic radiosurgery for the treatment of lesions in the liver,[114,216,217,238-241] pancreas,[141,153,154] lung,[236,238,240] and kidney[171,175]—anatomic areas that have traditionally been in the domain of general surgeons. Novel image guidance technologies, as well as soft tissue immobilization devices, have been used to make these therapies possible.[35,152,216,235]

At this time, the majority of the clinical literature is represented by case reports and series detailing the safety and feasibility of extracranial radiosurgery. In addition, many of the reports focus on the technical and engineering aspects of applying radiosurgical techniques to extracranial targets with little data on patient outcomes. All the reports have focused on the adult patient population. However, despite this inexperience, the technology surrounding stereotactic radiosurgery is rapidly developing and shows significant promise for minimally invasive treatment of potentially poorly accessible lesions. Newer systems such as the frameless image-guided CyberKnife system may someday enable the minimally invasive treatment of a variety of pediatric malignancies.

Radioimmunoguided Surgery

Antibodies labeled with radionuclides, when injected systemically, may bind specifically to tumors and thereby allow gamma probe detection.[125,190,204] For the most part, nonspecific binding and systemic persistence have minimized the signal-to-noise ratio, thus limiting this approach. Recently, the Food and Drug Administration (FDA) has approved several new promising radiolabeled antibodies to aid in the identification of occult metastases in patients with functioning endocrine tumors and in the evaluation of lymph node involvement in breast cancer and melanoma.

Surgical Robotics

Innovations in endoscopic technique and equipment continue to broaden the range of applications in MAS. However, many MAS procedures have yet to replace the traditional open approach. Difficulties remain in achieving dexterity and precision of instrument control within the confines of a limited operating space. This problem is further compounded by operating from a 2-D video image. Robotic surgical systems have now evolved that may address these limitations.

Since their introduction in the late 1990s, the use of computer-enhanced robotic surgical systems has grown rapidly. Originally conceived to facilitate battlefield surgery, these systems are now used to enable the performance of complex MAS procedures.* In children, early reports indicate that surgical robots can complete common and

---

*See references 7, 10, 54, 57, 61, 86, 103, 121, 147, 148, 183, 208.

relatively simple pediatric surgical procedures.[79,88] More recently, the use of robotic surgical systems has been described in multiple surgical disciplines, including pediatric surgery, pediatric urology, and pediatric cardiothoracic surgery.[128,140] In addition, complex, technically challenging procedures, such as robot-assisted fetal surgery, have been reported in animal models.[1,96,97,139,143]

Limitations of Standard Minimal Access Surgery Techniques and Technology

Although MAS techniques have revolutionized many operations, they have certain unique complexities not present with conventional open surgery. It is useful to highlight the specific technical challenges that surgical robots can address.

Movement Limitation

MAS instruments work through the body wall. Ports act as pivot points that reverse the direction of motion of the instrument tip in relation to the motion of the instrument handle. To move the instrument tip to the left within the body cavity, the hand of the surgeon must move to the right outside the body. This reversal of movement requires nonintuitive instrument control that is mentally taxing, especially as the complexity of the surgical task increases.

The majority of MAS instruments consist of an endeffector mounted to the tip of a long rigid shaft. The endoscopic cannula allows these instruments to pivot around the fixed point within the body wall, but motion is restricted laterally. The 6 degrees of freedom of position and orientation (defined as motion along the x-, y-, and z-axes and rotation about each of these axes) of open instruments are therefore reduced to 4 degrees of motion (pitch, yaw, roll, and insertion) for MAS procedures (Fig. 4-10A). An additional 2 degrees of freedom could be restored to MAS instruments by constructing articulations at the distal end, past the location of the cannula pivot point (Fig. 4-10B). However, precise and dynamic control of these distal articulations during an operative procedure would be difficult to coordinate without computer-assisted control.

Haptic Limitations

The long shafts of MAS instruments force the surgeon's hands to be separated from the operative anatomy, which significantly decreases tactile sensation and force reflection. The extended instrument length also magnifies any existing hand tremor. Furthermore, the excursion of an instrument tip is highly dependent on its depth of insertion. For instance, an instrument that is shallowly inserted requires comparatively large hand movements to accomplish a given instrument movement inside the body, whereas a deeply inserted instrument requires much less hand movement to sweep the instrument tip around. Consequently, the dynamics of the instrument change constantly throughout a procedure. These factors can lead to less precise and predictable movements than is the case with standard, open surgical techniques.

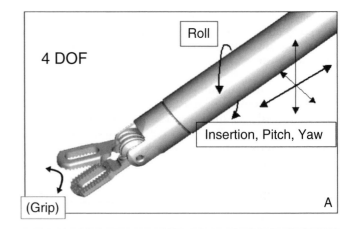

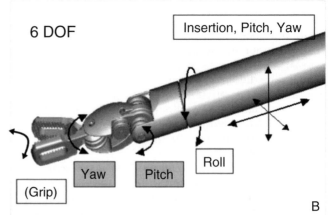

Figure 4–10 *A*, Traditional 4-degree-of-freedom (DOF) endoscopic instrument. *B*, Fully articulated 6-DOF robotic instrument. (Courtesy of Intuitive Surgical, Sunnyvale, CA.)

Visual Limitations

The introduction of an endoscope requires the surgeon to be guided by a video image instead of direct vision. The video monitor is often located on the far side of the patient, and the difference in orientation between the endoscope, instruments, and monitor requires the surgeon to perform a difficult mental transformation between the visual and motor coordinate frame.[214] This problem is further exacerbated when an angled endoscope is used.

Conventional endoscopes are built around a single lens train that displays images in a flat 2-D format. This removes many of the depth cues of normal binocular vision, thereby complicating tasks such as dissection between tissue planes. Some stereoscopic vision systems exist, but their performance is limited by the resolution and contrast characteristics of the endoscopes themselves, as well as display technologies. In addition, conventional endoscopes often require a dedicated assistant to hold and manipulate them. The natural tremors and movements of the assistant are exacerbated by the magnified image.

Robotic Technology in Surgery

For several decades, robots have served in a variety of applications such as manufacturing, deep-sea exploration, munitions detonation, military surveillance, and entertainment. In contrast, the use of robotic technology in surgery is still a relatively young field. Improvements in mechanical design, kinematics, and control algorithms originally created for industrial robots are directly applicable to surgical robotics.

The first recorded application of surgical robotics was for CT-guided stereotactic brain biopsy in 1987.[242] Since then, technologic advancements have led to the development of several different robotic systems. These systems vary significantly in complexity and function.

Classification of Robotic Surgical Systems

One method of classifying robots is by their level of autonomy. Three types of robots are currently used in surgery: autonomous robots, surgical assist devices, and teleoperators (Table 4-2).

An autonomously operating robot carries out a preoperative plan without any immediate control from the surgeon. The tasks performed are typically focused or repetitive but require a degree of precision not attainable by human hands. An example is the Robodoc system used in orthopedic surgery to accurately mill out the femoral canal for hip implants.[11] Another example is the CyberKnife system, which consists of a linac mounted on a robotic arm to precisely deliver radiotherapy to intracranial and spinal tumors.[2,120]

The second class of robots is surgical assist devices, where the surgeon and robot share control. The most well-known example of this group is the AESOP unit (Automatic Endoscopic System for Optimal Positioning; Computer Motion, Inc., Goleta, CA). This system permits the surgeon to attach an endoscope to a robotic arm, which provides a steady image by eliminating the natural movements inherent in a live camera holder. The surgeon is then able to reposition the camera by voice commands. Today, the AESOP has been used by many different surgical disciplines, including general surgery,[6,108] gynecologic surgery,[149] cardiothoracic surgery,[160] and urology.[130]

The final class consists of teleoperator robots, whose every function is explicitly controlled by the surgeon. The hand motions of the surgeon at a control console are tracked by an electronic controller and then relayed to a slave robot so that the instrument tips perfectly mirror every movement of the surgeon. Because the control console is physically separated from the slave robot, these systems are referred to as teleoperators. All the recent advances in robot-assisted surgery have involved this latter class of machines.

History of Teleoperators

The foundation of teleoperator surgical systems can be traced back to the 1970s, when the U.S. National Aeronautics and Space Administration (NASA) began the development of telepresence surgical systems for use in space to accommodate emergency surgery for individuals living in a space station. In the late 1980s and early 1990s the goal was to develop systems capable of battlefield surgery, where surgeons well behind the front lines could operate on injured troops via robots installed on armored vehicles. These projects attempted to develop a form of telemanipulator robot in which the motions of a human operator are translated into movements of mechanical arms some distance away. Although the application of such "master-slave" systems to surgical operations was a revolutionary idea, examples of this technology were already being used in a variety of other industries. The first mechanical master-slave system was developed in 1948 by Raymond Goertz at Argonne National Laboratories. This robot, named the M1, used a series of steel cables and mechanical linkages to connect a master manipulator controlled by a human operator to an identical slave manipulator on the other side of a lead glass barrier for protection from radioactive exposure.

The Stanford Research Institute[72] (now SRI International, Stanford, CA) developed the first master-slave telepresence surgery system capable of performing operations. Consisting of a surgeon's workstation and a remote surgical unit, this system was designed to perform remote, open battlefield surgery. It featured remote articulating robotic arms, stereoscopic imaging, basic force feedback, and an ergonomic design. Although this system was never fully developed, it formed the foundation for the commercial systems in use today.

Current Status of Robotic Technology in Pediatric Surgery

Currently, the use of two robotic surgical systems has been reported in the pediatric surgical literature; the Zeus System (formerly Computer Motion, Goleta, CA; now operated by Intuitive Surgical, Sunnyvale, CA) and the da Vinci Surgical System (Intuitive Surgical). Both systems are classified as teleoperators. The two companies recently merged, and it is predicted that the da Vinci system will become the predominant robotic operative platform. However, at the current time, both systems remain in active clinical use.

Even though these systems are popularly referred to as surgical robots, this is a misnomer because "robot" implies autonomous movement. Neither the da Vinci nor the Zeus system operates without the immediate control of a surgeon. A better term may be "computer-enhanced telemanipulators." However, for the sake of consistency

TABLE 4–2 Classification of Robotic Surgical Systems		
Type of System	**Definition**	**Example**
Autonomous	System carries out treatment without immediate input from the surgeon	CyberKnife Robodoc
Surgical assist	Surgeon and robot share control	Aesop
Teleoperators	Input from the surgeon directs movement of instruments	Intuitive Surgical da Vinci System Computer Motion Zeus System

with the published literature, this chapter will continue to refer to such systems as robots.

The Zeus System

The Zeus system consists of a surgeon's console and three robotic arms (Fig. 4-11A and B). The surgeon operates from a console several feet away from the operating table and uses hand-held manipulators to control the two robotic arms and surgical instruments, a foot pedal to activate the computer-driven system, and voice commands to direct a camera controlled by an AESOP arm.[96] Like the da Vinci system, the Zeus system offers tremor reduction and motion scaling.

The Zeus system consists of three modular, freestanding robotic arms that are attached to the operating table. This design allows the system to be oriented to many different configurations. The Zeus system also features 5-mm instruments capable of increased articulation through the Zeus Microwrist. This joint provides the instrument with an additional degree of freedom at the wrist, for a total of 6 degrees of freedom. More recently, 3.5-mm instruments have been developed. These instruments feature a small diameter and tip size, thus making them particularly useful in pediatric surgery. The Zeus system accommodates a variety of visualization options (3-D and 2-D) and telescope sizes.

The Zeus system has received generalized clearance for surgery under Conformité Européenne (CE) guidelines. In the United States, the Zeus system received FDA clearance for general laparoscopy and has been used for thoracic and cardiac procedures.

The da Vinci Surgical System

The da Vinci system consists of two major components[140] (Fig. 4-12A and B). The first component is the surgeon's console, which houses the visual display system, the surgeon's control handles, and the user interface panels. The second component is the patient side cart, which consists of two to three arms that control the operative instruments and another arm that controls the video endoscope.[50]

The operating surgeon is seated at the surgeon's console, which can be located up to 10 m away from the operating table. Within the console are located the surgeon's control handles, or masters, which act as high-resolution input devices that read the position, orientation, and grip commands from the surgeon's fingertips. This control system also allows for computer enhancement of functions such as motion scaling and tremor reduction.

The image of the operative site is projected to the surgeon through a high-resolution stereo display system that uses two medical-grade cathode ray tube (CRT) monitors to display a separate image to each of the surgeon's eyes. The surgeon's brain then fuses the two separate images into a virtual 3-D construct. The image plane of the stereo viewer is superimposed over the range of motion of the masters, which restores visual alignment and hand-eye coordination. In addition, because the image of the endoscopic instrument tips is overlaid on top of where surgeons sense their hands, the end effect is that surgeons feel that their hands are virtually inside the patient's body. For pediatric surgical applications, a new 2-D, 5-mm endoscope has been developed.

The standard da Vinci instrument platform consists of an array of 8.5-mm-diameter instruments. These instruments provide 7 degrees of freedom via a cable-driven system. Recently, a set of 5-mm instruments has become available. These instruments use a new "snake wrist" design and also provide 7 degrees of freedom (Fig. 4-12C).

Since its inception in 1995, the da Vinci system has received generalized clearance under European CE

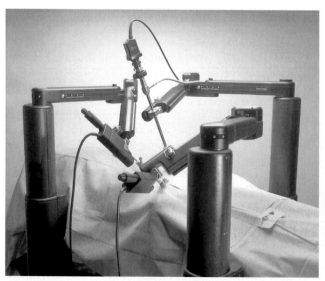

A

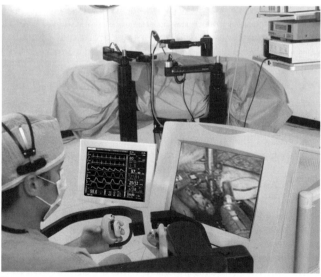

B

Figure 4–11 *A*, The Computer Motion Zeus robotic surgical system. *B*, The Zeus surgeon's console with its video display and master controls. (Courtesy of Intuitive Surgical, Sunnyvale, CA.)

Figure 4–12 The Intuitive Surgical da Vinci robotic surgical system composed of a surgeon's console (*A*) and a patient-side cart (*B*). *C,* Articulated 5-mm robotic instrument. (Courtesy of Intuitive Surgical, Sunnyvale, CA.)

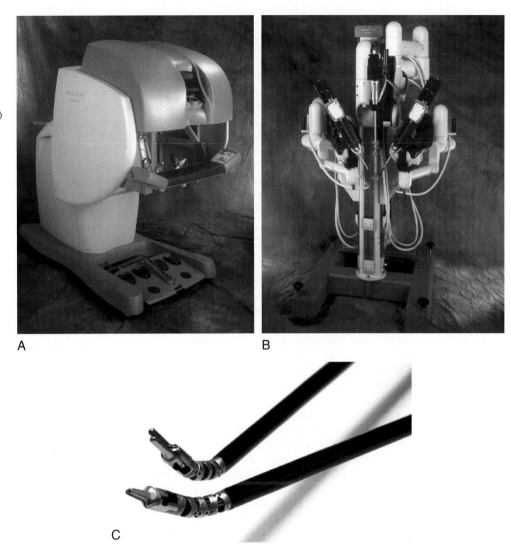

A

B

C

guidelines for all surgical procedures; in the United States it has received clearance for general surgery, thoracic surgery, and urologic procedures. In addition, the da Vinci system recently received FDA clearance for cardiac procedures involving a cardiotomy.

Current Advantages and Limitations of Robotic Pediatric Surgery

The utility of the different robotic surgical systems is highly influenced by the smaller size of pediatric patients and the reconstructive nature of many pediatric surgical procedures. Overall, the advantages of robotic systems stem from technical features and capabilities that directly address many of the limitations of standard endoscopic techniques and equipment. Unlike conventional laparoscopic instrumentation, which requires manipulation in reverse, movement of the robotic device allows the instruments to directly track the movement of the surgeon's hands. Intuitive nonreversed instrument control is therefore restored while preserving the minimal access nature of the approach. The intuitive control of the instruments is particularly advantageous for novice laparoscopists.

In infants and neonates, the use of a magnified image via operating loupes or endoscopes is often necessary to provide more accurate visualization of tiny structures.[207] This enhanced visualization is taken a step further with robotic systems because they are capable of providing a highly magnified 3-D image. The 3-D vision system adds an additional measure of safety and surgical control beyond what is available with the traditional endoscope. The 3-D display improves depth perception, and the ability to magnify images by a factor of 10 allows extremely sensitive and accurate surgical manipulation. The alignment of the visual axis with the surgeon's hands in the console further enhances hand-eye coordination to a degree uncommon in traditional laparoscopic surgery.

Similarly, the presence of a computer control system enables electronic tremor filtration, which makes the motion of the endoscope and the instrument tips steadier than with the unassisted hand. In addition, the systems allow for variable motion scaling from the surgeon's hand to the instrument tips. For instance, a 3:1 scale factor converts 3 cm of movement of the surgeon's hand into 1 cm of motion at the instrument tip. In combination with image magnification from the video endoscope, motion scaling makes delicate motions in smaller anatomic areas easier to perform and more precise.[88]

Both systems use instruments that are engineered with articulations at the distal end, or "wrist," which increases their dexterity in comparison to traditional MAS tools. This technology permits a larger range of motion and rotation, similar to the natural range of articulation of the human wrist, and may be particularly helpful when working space is limited. Specifically, the da Vinci system offers instruments with 7 degrees of freedom, including grip, whereas the Zeus system features instruments capable of 6 degrees of freedom, including grip. Standard laparoscopic instruments are capable of only 5 degrees of freedom, including grip. This increased dexterity may be particularly advantageous during complex, reconstructive operations that require fine dissection and intracorporeal suturing.

Finally, by separating the surgeon from the patient, teleoperator systems feature ergonomically designed consoles that may decrease the fatigue often associated with long MAS procedures. This may become a more significant issue as the field of pediatric bariatric surgery develops because of the larger size and thicker body walls of adolescent bariatric patients. Table 4-3 details the potential advantages of robotic surgical systems in relation to the technical challenges of standard laparoscopic techniques.

Although robotic surgical systems provide several key advantages over standard MAS, a number of technologic limitations are specific to pediatric surgery. First and foremost is the size of the robotic systems. When compared with many pediatric surgical patients, the size of the da Vinci surgical cart or the Zeus modular robotic arms may be overwhelming. This size discrepancy may restrict a bedside surgical assistant's access to the patient while the arms are in use and may require the anesthesiology team to make special preparations to ensure prompt access to the patient's airway.[207]

The size and variety of available robotic instruments are limited in comparison to those offered for standard laparoscopy. Currently, the da Vinci surgical system is the only platform undergoing further development at the industry level. Recently, a new suite of 5-mm instruments with 7 degrees of freedom has been introduced for use with this system. Although these instruments represent a significant improvement over the original 8.5-mm instruments with respect to diameter, the number of instruments offered is still somewhat limited. Furthermore, these instruments use a new "snake wrist" architecture that requires slightly more intracorporeal working room to take full advantage of their enhanced dexterity. Specifically, the instruments are limited by a greater than 10-mm distance from the distal articulating joint, or wrist, and the instrument tip. Similarly, the Zeus system offers several 5-mm instruments capable of 6 degrees of freedom and features a shorter distance between the distal articulating joint and the instrument tip, thus allowing them to function at full capacity in a smaller working area. However, this is accomplished by giving up 1 degree of freedom. Unfortunately, no new resources will be applied to further develop the Zeus system since the corporate merger.

Finally, a number of general limitations currently inherent in the available robotic surgical systems must be overcome before they are universally accepted in pediatric surgery, including the high initial cost of the robotic systems and the relatively high recurring cost of the instruments and maintenance.[140] In addition, neither system offers true haptic feedback.[207] Even though such feedback is reduced in standard MAS in comparison to open procedures, it is further reduced with the robotic interface. This disadvantage is partially compensated for by the improved visualization offered by the robotic systems, but it remains a significant drawback when precise surgical dissection is required.

Finally, the robotic systems require additional, specialized training for the entire operating room team. This translates into robotic procedure times that are predictably longer than those of the conventional laparoscopic approach, at least until the surgical team becomes facile with use of the new technology. Even with an experienced team, setup times have been reported to require an additional 10 to 35 minutes at the beginning of each robot-assisted case.[207] Undoubtedly, many of these issues will be

TABLE 4-3 Potential Advantages of Current Teleoperator Systems

System	Potential Advantage	Standard MAS Limitation Addressed
Da Vinci	3-D visualization	2-D visualization with loss of depth perception
	Instruments with 6 degrees of freedom	Rigid laparoscopic instruments resulting in a high learning curve for complicated tasks such as intracorporeal suturing
	Motion scaling	Magnified tremor because of long length of laparoscopic instruments
	Tremor reduction	Magnified tremor because of long length of laparoscopic instruments
	Intuitive instrument control	Counterintuitive instrument tip control because of fulcrum effect of the laparoscopic cannula
Zeus	3-D visualization	2-D visualization with loss of depth perception
	Instruments with 5 degrees of freedom	Rigid laparoscopic instruments resulting in a high learning curve for complicated tasks such as intracorporeal suturing
	Motion scaling	Magnified tremor because of long length of laparoscopic instruments
	Tremor reduction	Magnified tremor because of long length of laparoscopic instruments
	Intuitive instrument control	Counterintuitive instrument tip control because of fulcrum effect of the laparoscopic cannula

MAS, minimal access surgery.

remedied in the next generation of equipment as the technology continues to improve.

Applications of Robotic Technology in Pediatric Surgery

To date, only a small body of literature regarding the application of robotic technology for pediatric surgical procedures has shown the feasibility of robot-assisted surgery. These reports detailed the completion of relatively routine laparoscopic operations in school-age children. More recently, procedures have been described in much younger patients in multiple fields, including pediatric general surgery, pediatric urology, and pediatric cardiothoracic surgery (Table 4-4). At this time the bulk of the literature represents class IV evidence consisting of case reports and case series, with no class I evidence. However, more recent reports call for a more critical analysis of the technology. The following sections detail the published literature to date, with a focus on current and future applications of robotic surgical systems in pediatric surgery.

Pediatric General Surgery

The first reports describing the use of robotic surgical systems for abdominal procedures in children were published by Gutt et al. and Heller et al. in 2002.[79,88] They described 11 children (mean age, 12 years; range, 7 to 16 years) who underwent either robot-assisted Thal or Nissen fundoplication for gastroesophageal reflux disease. In addition, two children underwent robot-assisted cholecystectomy for symptomatic cholelithiasis, and bilateral oophorectomy for gonadoblastoma was performed in one child. The da Vinci system with 8.5-mm instruments and a 12-mm endoscope was used. The mean operating time for fundoplication was 146 minutes (range, 105 to 180 minutes), with no significant intraoperative or postoperative complications.

In 2003, several authors reported additional case series describing the safety and feasibility of robot-assisted pediatric general surgery. Luebbe et al. described a series of 20 cases treated with the da Vinci system,[140] including 10 Nissen fundoplications (3 with gastrostomy and 1 with pyloroplasty), 3 cholecystectomies, 2 splenectomies, 1 urachus resection, 1 unilateral iliac and retroperitoneal lymphadenectomy, 1 biopsy of a presacral mass, 1 biopsy of a hepatic mass, 1 Gore-Tex patch repair of a Morgagni diaphragmatic hernia, and 1 biopsy of a benign mediastinal mass.[1,140] The mean age of the patients was 8.4 years, although the youngest patient was 4 months old and the smallest was 6.8 kg. The mean console operating time was 93 minutes and the mean operating room setup time was 45 minutes. The intraoperative complication rate was 15%, including conversion to laparotomy during attempted splenectomy to control bleeding at the splenic hilum in two and intraoperative percutaneous evacuation of a pneumothorax during Morgagni hernia repair in one. The conversions to laparotomy were reported to have occurred quickly.

The authors concluded that the 3-D visualization, articulating instruments, and motion scaling were the primary advantages of the robotic system. The primary

disadvantages were the cost, training requirement, loss of tactile sensation, and additional operating room time required for system setup and docking. The authors detailed their technique with regard to patient positioning, port placement, and robotic cart positioning and docking and described their technique of elevating patients lighter than 20 kg off the operating table with foam padding. This enabled more lateral placement of the robotic instrument ports, thereby allowing the robotic arms and assistant surgeon greater mobility to pitch downward without encountering the operating table. We have used this technique and found it to be essential in smaller patients.

Lorincz et al. described seven patients who underwent robot-assisted procedures with the Zeus system.[139] They performed Nissen fundoplications in five children (three with gastrostomy), one cholecystectomy, and one Heller myotomy with partial fundoplication. Specifics regarding patient age and weight, as well as complications, were not included. However, the authors noted that their total procedure times and setup times decreased rapidly as their team gained experience with the robotic system. The first Nissen fundoplication took 4.5 hours, whereas their last took only 1.5 hours. They commented that tissue dissection and suture placement were accurate and knot tying secure.

Most recently, Knight et al. described 15 fundoplications with the Zeus system.[115] They performed 1 Heller myotomy with Dor fundoplication and 14 Nissen fundoplications and collected data regarding setup time, operating time, and outcomes. The mean patient age was 4.3 years (range, 2 months to 18 years) and the mean weight was 13 kg (range, 3.4 to 37.7 kg). Their mean operating time was 195 minutes, 323 minutes for the first case decreasing to 180 minutes for the last case. There were no postoperative complications.

Pediatric Urology

The use of robotic surgical systems in pediatric urology is gaining interest, with recent reports describing their use to perform complex reconstructive operations (see Table 4-4). Pedraza et al. reported the completion of a laparoscopic appendicovesicostomy (Mitrofanoff procedure) in a 7-year-old boy with the use of a four-port transperitoneal approach and the da Vinci system.[165] The total operative time was 6 hours, with no intraoperative or postoperative complications. The authors found the robotic system to be advantageous during the appendicovesical anastomosis. Similarly, the same group performed a robot-assisted laparoscopic bilateral heminephroureterectomy in a 4-year-old girl.[164] The total surgical time for this procedure was 7 hours and 20 minutes, and no complications occurred. The authors suggested that the robotic interface facilitated dissection of the renal hilum and vessels and enabled the completion of a complex MAS operation.

In a review of robotics in pediatric urology, Peters describes the use of robot assistance (da Vinci system) to facilitate complex urologic procedures.[167] Although no case details are provided, the author describes the use of robotic assistance to perform a variety of cases, including

TABLE 4–4 Clinical Experience with Robotic Surgical Systems in Pediatric General Surgery

Author	Robotic System	Type of Study	Patient (N)	Operative Procedure	Results	Comments
Gutt et al.[79] and Heller et al.[88]	Da Vinci	Case series	14	11 fundoplication, 2 cholecystectomy, 1 bilateral salpingo-oophorectomy	Operative times: fundoplication, 146 min (mean); cholecystectomy, 105, 150 min; salpingo-oophorectomy, 95 min	No complications or conversion to laparotomy
Luebbe et al.[140]	Da Vinci	Case series	20	10 fundoplication, 3 cholecystectomy, 2 splenectomy, 1 urachus resection, 1 Morgagni diaphragmatic hernia, 3 biopsies, 1 lymphadenectomy	Mean times: OR setup, 45 min; patient preparation, 17 min; console operating time, 93 min (range, 10-299 min)	15% complications (2 conversions to laparotomy for bleeding, 1 pneumothorax)
Lorincz et al.[139]	Zeus	Case series	7	5 Nissen fundoplication, 1 cholecystectomy, 1 Hellermyotomy	Operative time for fundoplication reduced from 4.5 hr to 1.5 hr	Rapid improvement in case times as team progressed along learning curve
Knight et al.[115]	Zeus	Retrospective case review	15	14 Nissen fundoplication, 1 Heller myotomy with Dor fundoplication	Mean operating time, 195 min; 2 complications within first 30 days after surgery	Rapid improvement with learning; perceived benefit of greater ease and confidence in knot tying and suture placement
Pedraza et al.[165]	Da Vinci	Case report	1	Appendicovesicostomy (Mitrofanoff procedure)	Operative time, 6 hr; no complications	Robotic procedure useful during the appendicovesical anastomosis
Pedraza et al.[164]	Da Vinci	Case report	1	Bilateral heminephroureterectomy	Operative time, 7 hr, 20 min; no complications	Robotic interface facilitated dissection of the renal hilum and vessels
Peters[167]	Da Vinci	Review article	Not provided	Nephrectomies, pyeloplasties (both transperitoneal and retroperitoneal), antireflux procedures (transperitoneal and transvesical), appendicovesicostomy, redo megaureter, pyelolithotomy, and excision of a large müllerian remnant	Not provided	Transperitoneal approach more readily suited for current robotic systems
Le Bret et al.[128]	Zeus	Prospective clinical trial	56	Patent ductus arteriosus ligation (28 thoracoscopic, 28 robotic)	Operating room time: thoracoscopic, 83 min; robotic, 162 min Surgical procedure time: thoracoscopic, 24 min; robotic, 50 min	Longer operative time for robotic group; 1 conversion to videothoracoscopic; no significant difference in complications or outcome
Mihaljevic et al.[150]	Da Vinci	Case series	2	Vascular ring dissection	Total operative times: 172.5 min (mean) Robotic procedure times: 106.5 min (mean)	Total operative time longer than usually required for standard thoracoscopic procedure because of setup; dissection time slightly shorter in robotic cases

nephrectomy, pyeloplasty (both transperitoneal and retroperitoneal), procedures for vesicoureteral reflux (transperitoneal and transvesical), appendicovesicostomy, redo megaureter, pyelolithotomy, and excision of a large müllerian remnant. The author stated that although the robotic system can be used to perform retroperitoneal procedures, the transperitoneal approach is most readily used because of the size of the robotic instruments and arms and stressed the development of a dedicated team approach for efficient use of the robotic system.

Pediatric Cardiothoracic Surgery

At this time, only two reports have been published describing the use of robotic surgical systems in pediatric cardiothoracic surgery (see Table 4-4). Le Bret et al. reported a relatively large series of 56 children who underwent surgical closure of a patent ductus arteriosus.[128] The children were distributed into two groups, one group undergoing standard thoracoscopic repair and the other undergoing robot-assisted repair with the Zeus system. The authors did not detail their method of group assignment. Although the patient characteristics were generally similar, the robot-assisted group tended to consist of smaller and younger patients (mean age, 20 months; mean weight, 10.7 kg) than the standard thoracoscopy group did (mean age, 33 months; mean weight, 13.3 kg). No intraoperative complications occurred in either group. Twenty-seven of twenty-eight procedures allocated to the robot-assisted group were completed, with one patient requiring conversion to standard thoracoscopy because of failure to achieve adequate exposure. The total operating room and surgical procedure time was significantly longer for the robot-assisted group (mean total operating room time, 162 minutes; mean surgical procedure time, 50 minutes) than for the standard thoracoscopy group (mean total operating room time, 83 minutes; mean surgical procedure time, 24 minutes). These differences were statistically significant.

There were no significant differences in postoperative complications, intensive care unit stay, or hospital length of stay between the two groups. The authors concluded that although robot-assisted patent ductus arteriosus closure in small children was safe and feasible, it offered no advantages over standard thoracoscopy. Furthermore, they commented that the additional procedure time required for the robotic approach did not decline with experience and was therefore due to the complexity of the robot and not a learning curve.

In a more recent report, Mihaljevic et al. described use of the da Vinci system for the division of a vascular ring in two patients (ages 10 and 8 years, weighing 48 and 27 kg, respectively).[150] Total operating room times were 180 and 165 minutes with surgical procedure times of 115 and 98 minutes, respectively. The authors concluded that the enhanced visualization and increased dexterity provided by the robotic system represented significant advantages over standard thoracoscopy and highlighted the improved intracorporeal dexterity as an important feature that aided in the division of all fibrous bands around the trachea and esophagus. The authors stated that although the dissection time was slightly shorter in the robot-assisted

cases than in standard thoracoscopy, the total operating room times were generally longer because of setup time.

Experimental Procedures

Although the published human experience has largely focused on relatively routine MAS procedures, several authors have reported the feasibility of performing more complex reconstructive operations in animal models. Hollands et al.,[96-98] Knight et al.,[115] and Lorincz et al.[139] have all described application of the Zeus system in a porcine model. Technically challenging procedures such as enteroenterostomy, hepaticojejunostomy, portoenterostomy, and esophagoesophagostomy were all demonstrated to be technically feasible (Table 4-5). Robot-assisted procedures and standard laparoscopic procedures had reasonably similar operating times and complication rates. In addition, survival studies indicate that the procedures are durable with reasonable long-term outcomes.

Similarly, Aaronson, Malhotra, Olsen, and their colleagues have described application of the da Vinci system in animal models to perform complex pediatric cardiovascular, neurosurgical, and urologic procedures,[1,143,161] including aortic anastomosis in juvenile lambs,[143] transvesical surgery,[161] and simulated myelomeningocele repair in a fetal lamb model.[1] In the latter study, the robotic system enabled the completion of laparoscopic, intrauterine repair of full-thickness skin lesions through small hysterostomies.[1]

Conclusion

At present, robotic surgical systems have been used in pediatric surgery primarily as a tool to facilitate MAS. The current published clinical experience with robotic pediatric surgery has been limited and consists largely of retrospective case reports and case series documenting feasibility and safety. On average, setup and operative times are longer with robotic cases than with standard laparoscopy. However, the rate of complications or conversion to open procedures has been low. At this time, significant long-term follow-up for any differences in clinical outcome has yet to be reported. Because the bulk of the published human experience represents relatively simple and routine MAS procedures, it may be some time before any significant clinical benefits are demonstrated.

In contrast to the human literature, published experimental series have demonstrated the feasibility and occasionally the efficacy of complex, reconstructive robot-assisted procedures in animal models. These applications represent the necessary future for robotic pediatric surgery inasmuch as the benefits of the robotic interface lie in their ability to facilitate fine dissection and intracorporeal suturing. Procedures such as repair of esophageal atresia, portoenterostomy, and ureteral reimplantation can all be performed today with existing laparoscopic equipment. However, mastery of these complex techniques in a MAS environment is extremely challenging. Robotic surgical systems have the potential to enable the completion of these technically challenging operations in a minimally invasive manner that retains the benefits of improved cosmesis, decreased postoperative pain, and potentially shorter hospital stay.

TABLE 4-5 Experimental Pediatric Robotic Procedures in Animal Models

Author	Operative Procedure	Robotic System	Type of Study	Procedure Times, Laparoscopic (mean)	Procedure Times, Robotic (mean)	Additional Results
Hollands et al.[96-98]	Porcine enteroenterostomy (5 laparoscopic, 5 robotic)	Zeus	Acute	Anesthesia, 176 min Operative time, 143 min Anastomotic time, 109 min	Anesthesia, 154 min Operative time, 139 min Anastomotic time, 93 min	All anastomoses were patent without narrowing; 1 small leak occurred in each group; no statistical differences
	Porcine hepaticojejunostomy (5 laparoscopic, 5 robotic)	Zeus	Acute	Anastomotic time, 66 min	Anastomotic time, 93 min	5 complications in the control group (3 leaks and 2 conversions); 1 complication in the robotic group (conversion)
	Porcine esophagoesophagostomy (5 laparoscopic, 5 robotic)	Zeus	Acute	Anesthesia time, 124 min Operative time, 97 min Anastomotic time, 89 min	Anesthesia time, 151 min Operative time, 131 min Anastomotic time, 125 min	All anastomoses were patent with no stricture; 1 anastomosis had a small leak; no statistically significant differences
	Porcine portoenterostomy (10 laparoscopic, 10 robotic)	Zeus	Acute	Anesthesia time, 125 min Operative time, 98 min Anastomotic time, 60 min	Anesthesia time, 164 min Operative time, 137 min Anastomotic time, 94 min	3 complications in the control group (1 narrowed anastomosis and 3 disrupted anastomoses); 4 complications in the robotic group (1 leak, 1 narrowed anastomosis, 2 disrupted anastomoses)
Lorincz et al.[139]	Porcine portoenterostomy (8 robotic)	Zeus	Survival (1 mo)	N/A	Total operative time, 380 min Setup time, 20 min End-to-side anastomosis, 129 min Biliary tract dissection, 36 min Portoenterostomy, 96 min	5/8 animals survived >1 mo postop; all lab values normal; no anastomotic stenoses and the anastomoses were well healed
	Porcine esophagoesophagostomy (7 robotic)	Zeus	Survival (1 mo)	N/A	Mean operative time, 120 min	5/8 animals survived to 1 mo postop; all required 1-2 postop dilatations; postmortem showed well-healed anastomoses
Malhotra et al.[143]	Juvenile ovine thoracic aortic anastomosis (5 robotic)	Da Vinci	Survival (6-12 hr)	N/A	Aortic clamp time, 47 min Anastomotic time, 26 min	All 5 lambs survived the procedure; mean anastomotic burst pressure, 163 ± 9 mm Hg
Aaronson et al.[1]	Intrauterine fetal ovine simulated myelomeningocele repair (6 robotic)	Da Vinci	Survival (7-11 days)	N/A	In utero procedure time, steep learning curve from just under 120 min to just over 30 min within 6 cases	4/6 lambs survived until sacrifice; intrauterine endoscopic surgery is feasible
Olsen et al.[161]	Porcine Cohen cross-trigonal ureter reimplantations (14 robotic reimplantations)	Da Vinci	Survival	N/A	Mean operative time, 68 min	Postop evaluation showed resolution of vesicoureteral reflux

The two systems currently in use offer many of the same advantages over standard MAS techniques: 3-D visualization, articulated instrumentation, intuitive movement, tremor reduction, and motion scaling., In addition, they share many of the same limitations that restrict their widespread adoption in pediatric surgery: high initial and recurring cost, relatively limited instrument selection, necessity for dedicated training, significant setup time, and lack of haptic feedback. In particular, the large system size and instrument dimensions relative to pediatric patients are main issues that must be resolved for robotic pediatric surgery to further develop. However, authors have generally applauded the technologic features of the robotic systems.[50,128,140] Although quantitative clinical value has not yet been demonstrated, most authors have subjectively concluded that the robotic systems appear to enhance surgical precision and make complex MAS procedures easier to perform. Further studies are therefore warranted to fully evaluate the potential benefits and application of robotic surgery to the pediatric population.

The advent of MAS has brought with it a wealth of potential benefits for the patient. However, the inherent limitations of operating in a laparoscopic setting pose significant challenges for the surgeon, and this is only magnified as procedures become more complex, such as those encountered in pediatric surgery. The incorporation of robotic and computer technology has the potential to contribute significantly to the advancement of this area. As the technology continues to be refined, its ultimate acceptance will demand that the issues of cost, training, size, safety, efficacy, and clinical utility all be addressed.

MICROTECHNOLOGIES AND NANOTECHNOLOGIES—SIZE MATTERS

An arsenal of technology will emerge from material science and its application principles to microelectromechanical (MEMS)[211] and nanoelectromechanical (NEMS) systems. Just as the electronics industry was transformed by the ability to manipulate the electronic properties of silicon, manipulation of biomaterials on a similar scale is now possible. For the last 40 years the common materials of stainless steel, polypropylene, polyester, and polytetrafluoroethylene have been unchanged. A recent example of this potential is the use of nitinol (equiatomic nickel-titanium), a metal alloy with the property of shape memory.

An important concept as well as distinction in device manufacturing is that of "top down" versus "bottom up" assembly. Top down refers to the concept of starting with a raw material and shaping it into a device. In a typical MEMS device, silicon is etched, heated, and manipulated to its final form. In the nascent field of nanotechnology, the underlying conceptual principle is that of self-assembly. Here, component ingredients are placed together under optimal conditions and self-assemble into materials. This process is much more one of biologic assembly.

Microelectromechanical Systems

The evolution of surgical technology has followed the trends that are set by most industries—the use of technology that is smaller, more efficient, and more powerful. This trend, which has application in the medical and surgical world, is embodied in MEMS devices.[179]

Most MEMS devices are less than the size of a human hair, and although they are scaled on the micron level, they may be used singly or in groups. MEMS devices have been used for years in automobile airbag systems and in inkjet printers.

Because the medical community relies increasingly on computers to enhance treatment plans, it requires instruments that are functional and diagnostic. Such a level of efficiency lies at the heart of MEMS design technology, which is based on creating devices that can actuate, sense, and modify the outside world on the micron scale. The basic design and fabrication of most MEMS devices resemble the fabrication of a standard integrated circuit, which includes crystal growth, patterning, and etching.[188]

Devices and Examples

MEMS devices have particular usefulness in biologic applications because of their small volume, low energy, and nominal force.[65] Increased efficacy of instrumentation and new areas of application are also emerging from biomedical applications of MEMS systems. There are two basic types of MEMS devices: sensors and actuators. Sensors transduce one type of energy (such as mechanical, optical, thermal, or otherwise) into electrical energy or signals. Actuators take energy and transform it into an action.

Sensors

Sensors transduce or transform energy into an electrical signal. The incoming energy may be mechanical, thermal, optical, or magnetic. Sensors may be active or passive systems. Active sensors derive their own energy from an input signal, whereas passive sensors require an outside energy source to function. Almost all these devices are in their developmental stage, but give form to the concept.

Data Knife and H-Probe Surgical Instruments: MEMS devices are particularly suited to surgical applications because their small dimensions naturally integrate onto the tips of surgical tools. One example is the "Data Knife" (Verimetra, Inc., Pittsburgh), which uses microfabricated pressure sensors attached to the blade of a scalpel (Fig. 4-13). While cutting, the Data Knife pressure sensors cross-reference with previously gathered ex vivo data to inform the surgeon about the type of tissue that is

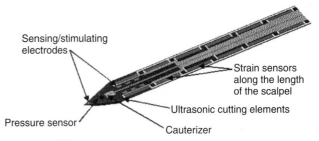

Figure 4-13 Data Knife microelectromechanical-based scalpel. (Courtesy of Verimetra, Inc., Pittsburgh.)

being divided. This information becomes particularly useful during endoscopic cases in which a sense of tactile feedback is reduced or lost entirely.

Verimetra's H-probe uses similar sensors to "palpate" calcified plaque transmurally during coronary bypass surgery. The intention is to eliminate poor positioning of the bypass graft conduit by more precisely targeting an ideal anastomotic site before arteriotomy.

Arterial Blood Gas Analyzer: MEMS technology can be applied to the analysis of arterial blood gas. This MEMS-based analyzer was founded on established methods in infrared spectroscopy. It consists of an infrared light source, an infrared sensor, and an optical filter. The infrared light is passed through the filter, which is designed to monitor the infrared spectra of oxygen, carbon dioxide, and other associated blood gases. Because most gases have a known infrared absorption, the sensor can be designed with specific values for infrared signatures.

Once again, because of microscaling techniques and the relatively small sample size, the test can be performed in less time than needed for conventional arterial blood gas analysis. One specific example is an arterial blood gas catheter for monitoring blood in preterm infants, in which real-time data can be gathered by way of oxygen- and carbon dioxide–specific sensors.

Blood Pressure Sensor: The biggest success story in medical MEMS technology is the disposable blood pressure sensor. Disposable blood pressure sensors replace reusable silicon beam or quartz capacitive pressure transducers, which can cost as much as $600 and have to be sterilized and recalibrated for reuse. These expensive devices measure blood pressure with a saline solution–filled tube-and-diaphragm arrangement that must be connected directly to the arterial lumen. In the silicon MEMS blood pressure transducer, pressure corresponds to deflection of a micromachined diaphragm. A resistive element, a strain gauge, is ion-implanted on the thin silicon diaphragm. The piezoresistor changes output voltage with variations in pressure. Temperature compensation and calibration can be integrated in one sensor.

Other Microelectromechanical Sensors in Medicine: The Wheatstone bridge piezoresistive silicon pressure sensor is a prime example of a MEMS device that is used commonly in medical applications. Able to measure pressures that range from less than 0.1 to more than 10,000 psi, this sensor combines resistors and an etched diaphragm structure to provide an electrical signal that changes with pressure. Primarily, these types of sensors are used in blood pressure monitoring equipment, but their use in the medical field extends far beyond that. These types of sensors can be found in respiratory monitors, dialysis machines, infusion pumps, and medical drilling equipment. They are also used in inflatable hospital bed mattresses or to signal an alarm on detection of lack of motion over a significant time frame in apnea monitors.

Actuators

An actuator is a fluid-powered or electrically powered device that supplies force and motion. Several kinds of actuators are used in MEMS devices, including electrostatic, piezoelectric, thermal, magnetic, and phase recovery. Actuators in medicine are used in valves, accelerometers, and drug delivery systems. Future use to produce muscle activation or "artificial muscles" is predicted.

Drug Delivery Systems: MEMS devices are used in drug delivery systems in the form of micropumps.[126] A typical drug pump consists of a pump chamber, an inlet valve, an outlet valve, a deformable diaphragm, and an electrode. When a charge is applied to the electrode, the diaphragm deforms, which increases the volume in the pump chamber. The change in volume induces a decrease in pressure in the pump chamber. This decreased pressure opens the inlet valve. When the charge is terminated, the pressure returns to normal by closing the inlet valve, opening the outlet valve, and allowing the fluid to exit.

Other micropumps incorporate pistons or pressurized gas to open the outlet valves. One of the more attractive applications for implantable pumps is insulin delivery.

Current insulin micropumps have disadvantages, most notably their expense. The drug supply must be refilled once every 3 months, and each pump costs between $10,000 and $12,000. Furthermore, insulin is unstable at core body temperature. Therefore, an insulin analogue must be synthesized that would be stable at physiologic temperatures. Thinking forward, a biomechanical pancreas that senses glucose and insulin levels and titrates insulin delivery would be an interesting MEMS combination of a sensor and an actuator.

Next Steps

MEMS devices are in the same state today as the semiconductor industry was in the 1960s. Like the first semiconductors, MEMS devices are now largely funded by government agencies such as the Defense Advance Research Projects Agency. Relatively few commercial companies have taken on MEMS devices as a principal product. However, no one could have predicted in 1960 that 40 years later, a semiconductor would be on virtually every desktop in the United States. It is then not unreasonable to predict potential value, including surgical applications, for MEMS devices. Indwelling microsensors for hormone and peptide growth factors might replace episodic examinations, laboratory determinations, or CT scans to monitor tumor recurrence. As more devices are fabricated, the design process becomes easier, and the next technology can be based on what was learned from the last. At some point in the future when more affordable technology becomes available,[179] we will "see" MEMS devices as common surgical modalities, smart instruments, in-line laboratories, surveillance devices, and perhaps, cellular or even DNA insertion.

Nanoelectromechanical Systems

Applications of nanotechnology and NEMS systems in medicine and surgery have recently been reviewed.[68] Size does matter. In medicine and biology the major advantage of decreasing the size scale is the ability to enable materials or particles to find places in body compartments to which they could otherwise not be delivered. Current and future applications of surgical interest include coating and surface manipulation, the self-assembly or biomimicry of existing biologic systems, and targeted therapy in oncology.

Coating and Surface Manipulation

Although most medical devices are composed of a bulk material, biologic incorporation or interaction occurs only at the thinnest of surfaces. To optimize this surface interaction, sintered orthopedic biomaterials have been developed. A thin layer of beads is welded or "sintered" via heat treatment on top of the bulk material.[169] This bead layer optimizes bone ingrowth, whereas the bulk material is responsible for mechanical stability of the device. Hydroxyapatite-coated implants represent a biologic advance in which the device is coated with ceramic hydroxyapatite,[13] thereby inducing bony ingrowth by mimicking (biomimicry) the crystalline nature of bone. Future attempts involve coating with the RGD peptide, the major cell attachment site in many structural proteins.

Cardiovascular stents, and now drug-eluting stents, provide a similar example. The current generation of drug-eluting stents has a micron-thick coating made of a single polymer that releases a drug beginning at the time of implantation.[99] The drug coating of rapamycin or paclitaxel diffuses slowly into the tissue microenvironment to prevent a fibrotic reaction. The future ideal stent will probably be engineered to optimize the bulk material and the coating. Indeed, the perfectly biocompatible material may be one in which the bulk material is artificial and the surface is seeded with the patient's own cells, for example, an endothelialized Gore-Tex vascular stent.[159]

Self-Assembly

NEMS materials are produced from a self-directed or self-assembly process in which mixtures of materials are allowed to condense into particles, materials, or composites.[126] Thus, NEMS processing starts with a nonsolid phase, typically a solution, and by manipulating the environment, materials are created.

Recently, biologic molecules, including proteins and DNA, have been used to stabilize nanoparticle crystals and create materials with unique properties, thus opening the door to unlimited diversity in the next generation of nanoparticles and materials.[144,194] Such processes mimic nature's ability to produce materials such as pearls, coral, and collagen.

Oncology

More than in any other field, microscale and nanoscale technologies will provide the field of oncology with critical therapeutic advances. In considering the perverse biologic process of malignant transformation and spread, our current therapies are gross and nontargeted. Figure 4-14 depicts a complex nanoparticle[84] composed of an iron oxide core surrounded by silicon oxide shells. Ligands may be attached to the silicon oxide coating,

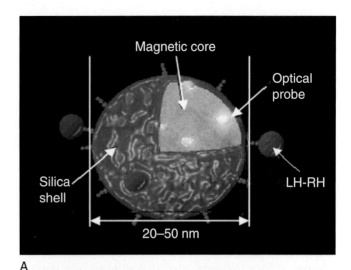

A

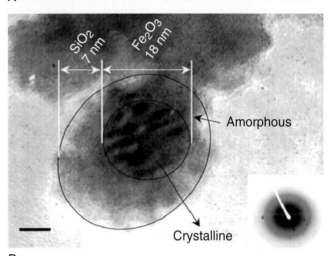

B

Figure 4–14   Schematic of a nanoparticle. An iron oxide core is surrounded by a silicon oxide shelf. Ligands attached to the silicon oxide can target the iron oxide to a specific site or potentially a tumor. The iron oxide can be heated in a magnetic field. Alternatively, the iron oxide may carry a toxin, a gene, or a pharmaceutical.

which may then target the iron oxide to a specific site. Such technology can be used for diagnostic purposes based on tumor permeability or for therapeutic options, or for both.

Harisinghani et al.[84] used iron oxide nanoparticles to identify tumor metastases in lymph nodes in patients with prostate cancer. The authors demonstrated increased sensitivity and specificity in identifying lymph nodes that ultimately contained tumor. Further work with magnetic nanoparticles functionalized with tumor-specific antibodies will enhance specific uptake by tumors.

SURGICAL SIMULATION AND VIRTUAL REALITY

Simulation and virtual reality (VR)[71,146] are two concepts that may reshape the way we think about surgical education, rehearsal, and practice. The practice of surgery is a visual, cognitive, and manual art and science that requires the physician to process increasingly large amounts of information. Techniques are becoming more specific and complex, and decisions are often made with great speed and under urgent circumstances, even when rare problems are being dealt with.

Surgical Simulation

Simulation is a device or exercise that enables the participant to reproduce or represent, under test conditions, phenomena that are likely to occur in actual performance. There must be sufficient realism to suspend the disbelief of the participant. Simulation is firmly established in the commercial airline business as the most cost-effective method of training pilots. Pilots must achieve a certain level of proficiency in the simulator before they are allowed to fly a particular aircraft and must pass regular proficiency testing in the simulator to keep their license. Military organizations use a similar method for training in basic flying skills and find simulation useful in teaching combat skills in complex tactical situations. Surgical simulation therefore has roots in the techniques and experiences that have been validated in other high-performance, high-risk organizations.

The expense and risk of learning to fly motivated Edward Link to construct a mechanical device that he called "the pilot maker" (Link, *http://www.link.com/history.html*). The addition of instrument sophistication enables the training of individuals to fly in bad weather. At the onset of World War II, with an unprecedented demand for pilot trainees, tens of thousands were trained in Link simulators.[89]

The medical community is beginning to use simulation in several areas for training medical personnel, notably surgeons, anesthesiologists, phlebotomists, paramedics, and nurses. The ability of the simulator to drill rehearsed pattern recognition repetitively in clinical practice makes just as much sense for the surgical disciplines as it does for aviators.

Surgical care entails a human risk factor that is related to both the underlying disease and the therapeutic modality. Risk can be reduced through training. One of the ways to accomplish both these goals is through simulation.

Simulation is loosely defined as the act of assuming the outward qualities or appearances of a given object or series of processes.[181] It is commonly assumed that simulation will be coupled with a computer, but this is not requisite. Simulation is a technique (not a technology) used to replace or amplify real experiences with guided experience that involves substantial aspects of the real world in a fully interactive manner.[64] To perform a simulation, it is only necessary to involve the user in a task or environment that is sufficiently "immersive" that the user is able to suspend reality to learn or visualize a surgical teaching point. The knowledge that is gained is then put to use in education or in the live performance of a similar task. Surgeons can learn to tie knots with a Linux-based computer or simulate the actions of a laparoscopic appendectomy with the use of a cardboard box painted to resemble a draped abdomen.

Visual Display Systems in Simulation

Simulator technology involves the design of training systems that are safe, efficient, and effective for orienting new trainees or providing advanced training to established clinicians. This involves teaching specific skills and generating scenarios for the simulation of critical or emergency situations. The entertainment industry is by far the main user and developer of visual displays. So much headway has been made in the advancement of visual technologies by the entertainment industry that many visual devices used in simulation are borrowed from these foundations. Considering that the graphic computing power of a $100,000 supercomputer in 1990 was essentially matched by the graphic capability of a $150.00 video game system in 1998, the available technology today is more than capable of representing a useful surgical simulation faithfully.[232]

Props are a key component of the visual act of simulation. Although laparoscopic surgical procedures can be represented on a desktop computer, a much more immersive experience can be carried out by involving monitors and the equipment used in an actual operating room. As an example, mannequin simulators, though internally complex, can serve to complement the simulation environment. Simulation of procedures such as laparoscopic surgical procedures should use displays similar to those present in the actual operating room.

Simulation of open procedures, on the other hand, requires systems that are presently in the developmental stage. The level of interaction between the surgeon and the simulated patient requires an immersive display system such as a head-mounted display (HMD). The best approach for a developer of a simulator for open procedures would be to choose a system with good optical qualities and concentrate on developing a clear, stable image. Designs for this type of visualization include "see-through displays" in which a synthetic image is superimposed on an actual model.[186] These systems use a high-resolution monitor screen at the level of the operating table because the characteristics of the displayed image must be defined in great detail.

Human/Simulator Interface and Tactile Feedback

Force feedback is the simulation of weight or resistance in a virtual world.[106] Tactile feedback is the perception of a sensation applied to the skin, typically in response to contact. Both tactile feedback and force feedback were necessary developments because the user needs the sensation of touching the involved virtual objects. This so-called *haptic loop*, or human-device interface, was originally developed with remote surgical procedures in mind and has much to offer the evolution of surgical simulation.

Technologies that address haptic feedback are maturing, nurtured by the rapid development of haptic design industries in the United States, Europe, and Japan and in many university-based centers.[106] Haptic technologies have been used in simulations of laparoscopic surgical procedures; however, extending this technology to open procedures in which a surgeon can, at will, select various instruments will require a critical innovation.

Image Generation

The generation of 3-D, interactive graphic images of a surgical field is the next level in surgical simulation. Seeing and manipulating an object in the real world are different from manipulating the same object in virtual space. Most objects that are modeled for simulations are assumed to be solids. In human tissue, with the possible exception of bone, such is not the case. Many organs are deformable semisolids, with potential spaces. Virtual objects must mirror the characteristics of objects in the real world. Even with today's computing power, the task of creating a workable surgical surface (whether skin, organ, or vessel) is extremely difficult.

A major challenge in the creation of interactive surgical objects is the reality that surgeons change the structural aspects of the field through dissection. On a simulator, performing an incision or excising a lesion produces such drastic changes that the computer program supporting the simulation is frequently incapable of handling such complexity. This still does not include the issue of blood flow, which would cause additional changes in the appearance of the simulated organ. Furthermore, the simulation would have to be represented in real time, which means that changes must appear instantaneously.

To be physically realistic, simulated surgical surfaces and internal organs must be compressible in response to pressure applied on the surface, either bluntly or by incision. Several methods of creating deformable, compressible objects exist in computer graphic design.

Frequently, simulator graphic design is based on voxel graphics. A voxel is an approximation of volume, much in the same way a pixel is an approximation of area. Imagine a voxel as a cube in space, with length, width, and depth. Just as pixels have a fixed length and width, voxels have a fixed length, width, and depth. The use of volume as the sole modality to define a "deformable object," however, does not incorporate the physics of pressure, stress, or strain. Therefore, the graphic image will not reflect an accurate response to manipulation. The voxel method does not provide a realistic representation of the real-time changes in an organ's architecture that would occur after a simulated incision.

A more distinct approach to the solution of this problem is provided by the use of finite elements. Finite elements allow the programmer to use volume, pressure, stress, strain, and density as bulk variables. This creates a more detailed image that can be manipulated through blunt pressure or incision. Real-time topologic changes are also supported.

For the moment, a good alternative solution to the problem is to avoid computational models. Some groups have used hollow mannequins with instruments linked to tracking devices that record position. Task trainers allow one to practice laparoscopic skills directly by use of the equivalent of a cardboard box with ports to insert endoscopic tools. These tools are used to complete certain tasks, such as knot tying or object manipulation.

Simulation in Education, Training, and Practice

Historically, surgical training has been likened to an apprenticeship. Residents learn by participating and taking more active roles in patient care or the operative procedure as their experience increases. Despite potential flaws, this model has successfully trained generations of surgeons throughout the world. Error and risk to patients are inherent in this traditional method of education despite honest attempts at mitigation and will always be a factor in the field of surgery, no matter how it is taught. There are new methods of surgical training, however, that can help reduce error and risk to the patient.[155,189]

Training in simulated environments has many advantages. The first advantage is truly the crux of simulation: it provides an environment for consequence-free error, or freedom to fail. Simulator-based training incurs no real harm, injury, or death to the virtual patient. If a student transects the common duct during a simulated cholecystectomy, the student simply notes the technical error and learns from the mistake. Furthermore, simulations can be self-directed and led by a computer instructor or can be monitored and proctored by a real instructor, which means that students can learn on their own time, outside the operating room.[187]

Simulators are pliable tools. Depending on the assessment goals of a particular simulator, tasks can be modified to suit the educational target. For example, self-contained "box trainers" that are used to teach a particular dexterous skill can be modified to be less or more difficult or to teach grasping skills versus tying skills. In more complex computer-based simulations, variables can be changed automatically by the computer or manually by the instructor, even during the simulation. These variables range from changes in the graphic overlay to the introduction of an unexpected medical emergency. Approaches to learning laparoscopic navigational skills within the human body have benefited considerably from such techniques. A prime objective of surgical education is to learn how to function mentally and dexterously in a 3-D environment. Surgical "fly-through" programs can be invaluable resources to learn this kind of special orientation inside the human body.[37]

Perhaps one of the greatest benefits of surgical simulation is the ability of early learners to become skilled in basic tasks that have not previously been presented in formal training. The orientation of medical students, now frequently excluded from patient care tasks, may aid in their engagement, education, and recruitment to surgical careers. Therefore, the most consistent success has been the discovery that simulators are most beneficial to individuals with little or no previous experience in the simulated task.[170]

Looking Forward

Simulation success, particularly in the aviation industry, strongly suggests utility to medical and surgical applications. As with any form of new technology, advances depend on many factors. A product made solely for the sake of technology is doomed to fail; therefore, the simulation market must be driven by clinical and educational need. In these early stages of surgical simulation, simpler, mannequin-based trainers have proved to be more useful. However, as graphic design and human interface technology evolve, simulations become more realistic, and equipment prices fall, more immersive computer-generated models will lead the way for this unique form of continuing medical education.

Virtual Reality

VR, though closely related to simulation, has many unique aspects. Simulation is the method for education and training; VR is the modality for making simulation look more real. VR, simply stated, is the creation of a 3-D artificial environment with which a user in the real world may interact. VR, in contrast to simulation, almost always relies on computers and computer software to generate a virtual environment. Furthermore, an interface device is required to immerse the user.[195] This device could be as simple as a computer mouse or keyboard or as complex as VR-based goggles or headsets. The basic intention of VR is to divert the user's attention from the outside world to a manufactured, virtual world with detailed, interactive content based on visuals, sound, and touch. When optimized, such an experience would immerse the participants such that reality becomes this virtual environment.

The Beginnings

Although the term *virtual reality* was introduced by Jaron Lanier in 1989, the concept of VR as we currently know it emerged long before that time. In 1963, Ivan Sutherland created Sketchpad, one of the first graphics design tools. By this time Sutherland was developing the HMD, which heralded the theories and themes of modern immersive science (Fig. 4-15A) and led to the creation of scene generators for Bell Helicopter Laboratories. With scene generation (Fig. 4-15B), computer graphics would replace the standard video camera–generated display used in flight simulators. Sutherland and Evans designed several VR-based products, and Sutherland developed the first arterial anastomosis simulation in 1971.

With the simultaneous development of computer interface tools, such as the mouse, VR immersion becomes possible because the ordinary user can interact easily with the computer in a manner more intuitive than possible with a keyboard. During the 1970s, major advances in technology meant that computers were becoming more powerful, smaller, and cheaper, and the personal computer, mouse, laser printer, and desktop architecture all were developed.[92]

Science and, even more so, the entertainment industry began to look at VR as a way to enhance their respective businesses. VR has had obvious application in making blockbuster films with dazzling special effects (e.g., *Star Wars, The Terminator,* and *The Perfect Storm*). 3-D mapping of genomes in DNA research led VR into medicine. For the first time, real-time modification of computer-aided design models became available. Thomas Zimmerman designed a "data glove," a type of human interface device, out of the desire to convert gestures into music by feeding these gestures directly into a computer that could interpret the movements as sound. He patented the glove in 1982. The glove could interpret the wearer's hand movements and finger flexion and allow them to interact with a 3-D environment.

Jaron Lanier first combined the HMD and data glove in 1986, thus giving the world a more realistic version of immersive VR. Users could not only see the 3-D environment but also interact with it by feeling the objects and see themselves interacting in VR at the same time. Since then there have been many groups, organizations, and individuals who have been interested in exploring and adding to the general knowledge of this field.

The evolution of VR for surgery began in the 1980s. It was quickly realized that simulation and VR for surgical procedures did not have to rely on an especially detailed

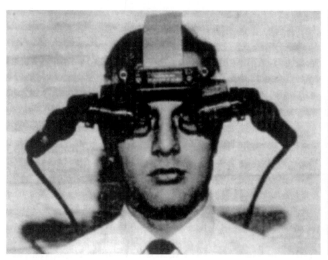
A

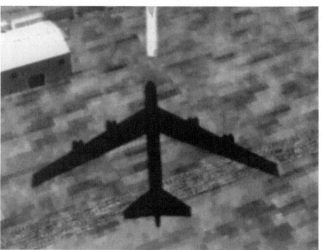
B

Figure 4–15 *A,* Sutherland's head-mounted display. *B,* Scene Generation Software, Evans & Sutherland. (From National Systems Contractors Association Multimedia Online Expo, "Science for the New Millennium.")

graphic terrain, which was the case for complex professional flight simulators. In fact, even moderately detailed surgical VR systems could accomplish the purpose of "task training." This reinforced the fact that for surgeons, one of the primary goals of training was to establish technical skills. Therefore, simple graphic representations of two hollow tubes with an interface for needle holders and forceps would be enough to teach someone about the principles of bowel anastomosis. In the late 1980s, Delp of Stanford University developed one of the first surgical VR-based simulators for lower extremity tendon transfer. In 1991, Satava and Lanier designed the world's first intraabdominal interactive simulation. These seminal events in surgical VR were followed by more improved versions based on similar computer-assisted digitizing and rendering techniques. Although these early iterations lacked the computing power to combine maximum detail with surgical flexibility and dynamic change, they certainly established the concept.

Components

Construction of a virtual environment requires a computer system, a display monitor, an interface device, and compiler software. Surgical simulations and artificial environments are based on the same types of programming methods. Computational speed must be sufficient to power the graphics to deliver a minimum frame rate so that the user does not experience flicker or the perception of frames changing on the monitor. To accomplish this objective, the simulation should be delivered to the user's eye at no less than 30 Hz, or 30 frames per second, equivalent to most television sets. Five years ago, this kind of graphic generation required high-end graphics (Silicon Graphics, Mountain View, CA) or a workstation (SUN, Mountain View, CA). Now, dual- or single-processor personal computers can render graphics at this speed.

The software required to produce virtual worlds has specific requirements. First, the programmer must design the software to match the physical constraints of the real world. The heart, for example, cannot be allowed to float in thin air during a coronary bypass graft simulation. It must have some representation of gravity, compressibility, volume, and mass. These constraints, and more, must be considered for the virtual world to approach reality. Second, the software must be designed so that user interaction will be compiled and processed efficiently and accurately and not become unstable to a user who is dynamically changing the simulation. A forceps pulling on tissue must appropriately deform the graphic representation of that tissue, for example. The software must also be able to communicate force feedback, through external devices, to the user in real time.

Generation of Virtual Bodies from Patient Data

Surgical dissection, though second nature to surgeons, is quite difficult to program into a computer system. The thousands of anatomic interactions can easily exceed processor power, so digital rendering of patient data must be performed as efficiently as possible.

Patient-specific data for VR can come from several sources. MRI, magnetic resonance angiography, CT imaging, PET scanning, US scanning, and SPECT imaging are among the common modalities. Traditionally, a physician mentally organizes these 2-D stacks of data, compiles it in the brain, and visualizes a 3-D representation of the patient, not unlike the visible human data set (Fig. 4-16). With VR, these image stacks are meshed by the computer to realize the data in 3-D automatically; this was previously a mental task performed by the surgeon before an operation.[26]

Using different types of data sources, such as MRI or CT scanning, allows VR programmers to take advantage of the unique properties of each scanning method. CT scanning, for example, is particularly useful for scanning bones. MRI is more useful for soft tissue scanning. These properties can be combined to create a realistic VR image.

The manner in which 3-D images are represented within the system has a profound impact on the overall performance of the simulation. Patient data sets from CT scans, MRI, and other methods originate as voxels.[3,210] Voxel graphics are based on volume and result in an image that contains an infinite number of data points. To compute changes in each point would put a tremendous strain on any computer. Other forms of VR rendering, however, can ease the strain on the system and speed up the simulation.

Surface Rendering

Rendering is the process of digitizing data into a computerized image by applying parameters to the data. To reduce the number of data points that require computation, surface rendering converts volume-based images into geometric primitives that have far fewer data points.[26] This could be a patchwork of polygons that are based on the boundaries of different regions in the image. Boundary regions could be between fascia and fat or gray matter and white matter. Such separation requires knowledge of the properties of each region because some blurring occurs in voxel images, such as CT scans. Shading algorithms can blend layers or regions so that the final product has a smooth appearance (Fig. 4-17). The number of geometric elements is extremely important in the surface method of VR. One must remember that each movement of the simulation by the user in virtual space requires a recalculation of each geometric object by the computer in real time. If there are too many polygons to reproduce quickly, the simulation will "jerk" and thus make it less real and perhaps unusable. When compared with voxel-based imagery, surface-rendered objects run unequivocally faster.

Volume Rendering

Volume rendering requires special equipment to handle the immense amount of data that must be complied. This method works explicitly with volumetric data and renders them each time the data set is manipulated by the user. This differs from surface rendering in that surface rendering splits the volume into groups

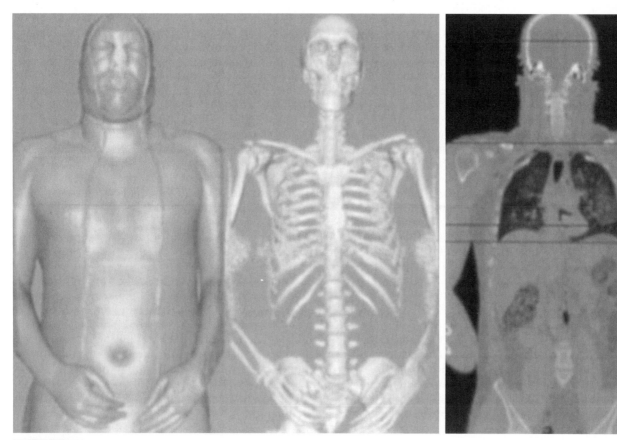

of polygonal surfaces. Surface-rendered objects are fine when the surgeon wants to limit inspection to the surface of an object, but as its name implies, surface rendering displays only the surface part of the data set. Currently, higher-end computer equipment, such as a graphics workstation, is necessary to render volume-based graphics.

Finite Elements

Finite elements are based on geometric networks that are placed under the constraints of physics. Forces of

pressure, elasticity, stress, and strain affect the shape and nature of the object being manipulated. Such manipulation will affect not only the surface of the model but also the volume. When combined with a detailed graphic overlay, finite element models can provide the most accurate simulation to date.[210]

Visual Displays

In a perfect world, VR can incorporate any or all of our five senses, but it usually relies most heavily on our most critical visual sense. The basics of our visual system can

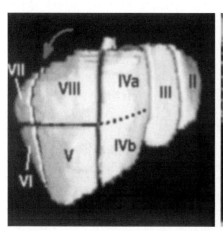

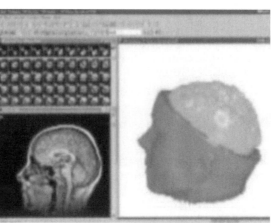

Figure 4–17 Surface-rendered view of the liver. (Courtesy of 3-D Doctor: 3-D Imaging, Rendering, and Measurement Software for Medical Images, Lexington, MA.)

be categorized into three groups: depth perception, field of view, and critical fusion frequency.

Depth perception in humans is limited to approximately 30 m because the eyes are close together in relation to the distance observed. VR systems must allow the user to reproduce these mechanisms, or proper depth cannot be achieved. The eye needs only a limited field of view to feel as though it were part of a virtual environment. Critical fusion frequency is the frequency at which static images, in rapid succession, appear to be a seamless stream of moving data. This is much like the old methods of animation in which shuffled flash cards gave the appearance of an animated cartoon. The approximate frequency for smooth video is around 30 to 40 Hz. Such displays must be capable of delivering a 3-D image. The most dynamic form of VR visual display is the HMD. Although VR can be and often is represented on desktop monitors, the sense of immersion is not as complete when the participant is not in a closed system such as an HMD. On a desktop monitor, a 3-D environment is being projected onto a 2-D screen.

There are two basic methods of 3-D visualization. The first method uses two separate displays, one for each eye, to give a stereoscopic effect. The second method uses a head-mounted tracking system that changes the perspective of the system to match the direction in which the user is looking. This tracking method must coordinate the movement of the user's head and hands.

Many different types of HMDs are available. The capabilities of a particular HMD depend on its final purpose. HMDs exist for personal video gaming, architecture, and missile guidance alike. There are also many modes of

HMD instrumentation. Opaque displays, for example, completely occlude any visual contact with the outside world. Any visual input comes solely from the head-mounted video display.

Fakespace, Inc. (Menlo Park, CA) offers a binocular omni-orientation monitor (BOOM). This head-coupled display is externally supported by a counterbalanced stand. Because it is not worn by the user and is supported by an external platform, the BOOM system can allow for additional hardware technology to be added to the system, thereby creating very high-fidelity visual capability. Resolutions of 1280 × 1024, which are better than most computer monitors, are standard on the Fakespace system. The BOOM device is, of course, weightless to the user and relies on a motion-tracking system to keep face-forward perspective. The swivel stand allows for a superior degree of freedom and field of view.

One of the more novel and immersive visual display systems is the Cave Automatic Virtual Environment (CAVE; Fakespace/Electronic Visualization Laboratories), which is a room-sized multiuser system. Graphics are projected stereoscopically onto the walls and floor and viewed with shutter glasses. Users wear position trackers that monitor the user's position within the CAVE by way of a supercomputer. Changes in perspective are constantly updated as the user moves around this "confined" space. Monocular head-mounted systems allow the wearer to have contact with the outside environment while data are delivered (Fig. 4-18A). Surgical applications include the ability to perform an operation while simultaneously processing data about the patient's vital signs and imaging studies.

Figure 4–18 *A,* eGlass II, with Eye Blocker (Virtual Vision, Redmond, WA). *B,* Retinal display theory (Human Interface Technology Lab, University of Washington). Drive electronics gather an image from a source, such as a computer. The pixels gathered from the computer or other source are beamed 1 pixel at a time through the lens, directly onto the retina. A scanner "paints" an image onto the retina horizontally and vertically at a rate of 18 million pixels per second. Optics refract the image for the viewer's eye.

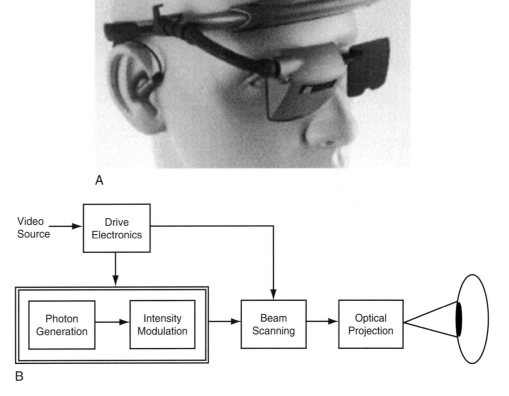

Virtual retinal displays scan light directly onto the viewer's retina (Fig. 4-18B). Because of this feature, the viewer perceives an especially wide field of view. Though still in development, retinal displays have thus far been able to deliver resolutions close to human vision while encased in a lightweight, portable system.[229] Virtual retinal displays have been developed at the University of Washington's Human Interface Technology laboratory.

Input Devices

The best way to interact with the virtual world is with one's hands. It is both natural and intuitive. The DataGlove system (VPL Research, Redwood City, CA [Fig. 4-19]) is the archetypic system.

The DataGlove System frees up the user's hands from a keyboard. Commands are simplified, and tasks are carried out by rudimentary pointing or grasping in the virtual environment. Since conception of the DataGlove, many manufacturers have developed similar interface products. Data gloves process information by many different methods. Some gloves use mechanical sensors or strain gauges over the joints of the hand to determine position. Other gloves use fiber-optic circuits to measure the change in light intensity and angle of the fiber-optic band as the hand flexes and extends. Trackers are also positioned on some gloves to monitor its position in free space. In any configuration, the data glove remains an intuitive solution to a complex problem.

Force and Tactile Feedback

Force (resistance) and tactile (contact or touch) feedback could be the two most important goals of surgical VR, yet they are also among the most difficult to achieve. Surgeons rely on a keen sense of touch and resistance with the human environment, and without these senses, fidelity suffers. LaparQscopy is one example of how touch sense is displaced from the surgeon's hands.[182]

The tangible senses are very hard to generate artificially.[178] Humans can easily judge the force with which to pick up a glass of water to bring it smoothly to the mouth. A computer, if incorrectly programmed, may mistake picking up a glass for hoisting a cinderblock, which would cause the virtual glass of water to be thrown completely across the room. Until recently, the one major component that was lacking in VR simulations has been the sense of touch, or haptics.

Haptic feedback requires two basic features to render the sense of touch back to the user. First, the system needs a computer that is capable of calculating the interaction between the 3-D graphics of the simulation and the user's hand, all in real time. Second, the loop requires some form of interface device (whether a joystick, glove, or other device) for the user to be able to interact with the computer. The computer systems that support haptics are typically 3-D graphics workstations with hardware video acceleration.[46,106] These systems are connected to an interface device, such as the popular PhanToM joystick (SenseAble Technologies, Woburn, MA [Fig. 4-20]). Such joystick-based devices can function to provide up to 6 degrees of freedom. Again, the computer's visuals must refresh at a rate approximately 30 times per second to create a smooth simulation.

Like muscle linkages to bone, because all force must be generated in relation to a point of fixation and an axis of motion, current force feedback systems require an exoskeleton of mechanical linkages. Force feedback systems presently use one of two approaches to this exoskeleton. The first approach consists of an exoskeleton that is mounted on the outside of the hand, similar to the ones used for electromechanical tracking. The linkages consist of several pulleys attached to small motors with long cables. The motors are mounted away from the hand to reduce weight but can exert force on various points of the fingers by pulling the appropriate cable. The second approach consists of a set of small pneumatic pistons between the fingertips and a base plate on the palm of the hand. Force can be applied only to the fingertips by applying pressure to the pistons.

Because these systems reflect all their force back to some point on the hand or wrist, they can allow you to grasp a virtual object and feel its shape but cannot stop you

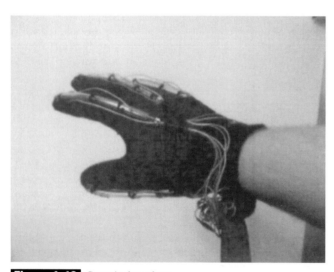

Figure 4-19 Generic data glove.

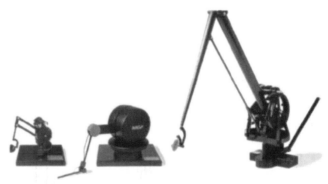

Figure 4-20 PhanToM interfaces (SenseAble Technologies, Woburn, MA).

from passing your hand through that object. To prevent this, the exoskeleton must be extended to a base that is mounted on the floor through more linkages along the arm and body or an external system similar to a robot arm.

Multiple methods of generating force or tactile feedback have been developed.[178] Piezoelectric vibration systems generate slight vibrations onto the user's fingertips when simulated contact is made. Electrotactile feedback works on the same principle of fingertip sensation, although there are no moving parts. A small current is passed over the skin surface in the case of virtual contact. Micropin arrays consist of a bed of fine pins that extend onto a fingertip to produce extremely fine detail. Micropins can re-create the feeling of edges. Pneumatic feedback uses gloves with air pockets placed within the glove. These pockets inflate at the desired time to represent the sense of touching a surface. Temperature feedback uses heating coils on the hand to represent temperature change.

Tracking in Virtual Reality

VR is based on spatial relationships. Even though the user is presented with a virtual representation of certain objects, the computer must know where the user is in relation to such objects. Otherwise, the user's hand, for example, would pass through a virtual glass rather than grasping it. Some VR systems solve this problem by following, or tracking, the critical interface points between the user and the computer. Tracking systems are placed on helmets and gloves so that the computer knows when to react. Several tracking methods exist.[178]

Mechanical tracking systems are physically in connection with the user's interface. The user's helmet is tethered at one end and interfaced with the computer at the other. This direct connection is fast, but the subject is always attached to the system, which limits movement.

Cameras in conjunction with small flashing beacons placed on the body can be used as a method for optical tracking. Multiple cameras taking pictures from different perspectives can analyze the configuration of the flashing light-emitting diodes on the body. These pieces of 2-D data are compiled into a single 3-D image. Such processing takes time, a critical drawback of optical tracking. Magnetic field signals can be used; source elements placed on the hand can be tracked with a sensor. Disadvantages include interference from nearby magnetic sources and a maximum usable distance.

Acoustic trackers use high-frequency sound to triangulate to a source within the work area. These systems rely on line of sight between the source and the microphones and can suffer from acoustic reflections if they are surrounded by hard walls or other acoustically reflective surfaces. If multiple acoustic trackers are used together, they must operate at nonconflicting frequencies, a strategy also used in magnetic tracking.

Challenges of Virtual Reality

As with any emerging technology, there is an ebb and flow of hype and hope.[46] VR is no exception. Areas that have the greatest room for improvement are graphics and haptic feedback. Because of the massive processing power required to create a full VR production, one must currently trade off graphic detail for performance. Consequently, this means that at present VR is defined by the phrase, "it can be good, fast, and cheap; pick two." Such tradeoff results in simulations that have a cartoon quality so that they may have a reasonable run time. Even with a forced reduction in graphic detail, there is still a slight perception of delay, or lag, in the time between user interface and VR reaction. The visual representation of an incision is still very difficult to achieve accurately.

Haptic feedback requires equal computing power (if not more) and can cause instabilities or inaccuracies in the system. Many VR force feedback systems can be compelled to fail by "pushing through" the force feedback and ruining the illusion.

Virtual Reality Preoperative Planning

Beyond simple task training, one of the great advantages and goals of VR is the ability to plan and perform an operation on patient-specific data before actually performing the operation on the same human being. This goes far beyond early learning on a generic task or human. Surgeons, when planning an operation, traditionally compile data such as CT or MRI scans, along with patient examinations and charts, into a solution envisioned in their head. It takes years of experience and training to master such visualization, especially when it comes to translating multiple 2-D images into a 3-D paradigm.

For many surgical specialties, VR techniques can assemble patient-specific data into graphic "before and after" images, which can be manipulated by the surgeon before the operation so that the outcome of the case may be predicted. These outcomes would be based on decisions that the surgeon would make during the operation. Furthermore, as more procedures are developed, VR preplanning can be used as a research model based on actual patient data that would be used to predict the outcome of a novel surgical application. VR enhancement also preemptively speeds up decision processes for complicated cases by providing the surgeon with a preplanned outline of the procedure, thereby making the hospital system more efficient. VR preoperative planning is available for general surgery, vascular surgery, plastic surgery, neurosurgery, and orthopedic surgery.

Craniofacial reconstructive surgery is a difficult task. A surgeon who is asked to handle a difficult or even routine reconstruction reconstructs 3-D data from 2-D CT or MRI scans. No matter how experienced the surgeon, predictions of outcomes in plastic reconstructions are limited, at best, with the use of this traditional method. As a result, the preoperative plan is often modified in the operating room during the procedure. For these reasons, rehearsal and preparation with VR have been applied with increasing frequency in this area.[110,111]

There are many methods of computer-assisted planning for craniofacial surgery, but most of them produce a 3-D interactive image that can predict the outcome of the case on the basis of what the surgeon does on a workstation ahead of time. This process starts with a patient-specific CT or MRI scan that is cut in transverse sections, as is the case in facial reconstruction for trauma or malformation.[151] Once the images are scanned from the patient, they are segmented and specified into bone and soft tissue windows. This process results in a mass of 2-D cuts that must be rendered into a 3-D environment. Patient-specific CT images are typically processed on a graphics workstation.

The University of Erlangen in Germany has demonstrated a method involving "marching cubes" for 2-D to 3-D reconstruction from CT scans.[227] In this process, a Cyberware (Cyberware, Monterey, CA) scanner is used to scan the patient's skin surface features, which are then compressed to reduce the volume of data. The skin and bone windows are compiled similarly into a 3-D image. This image may be cut at any plane to focus on a particular area of interest. Keeve and colleagues[110] simulated a Dal-Pont osteotomy of the mandible with this technique. After the 3-D image is rendered, any number of cutting, moving, and manipulating steps may be performed, which will predict the reconstructive outcome in the operating room (Fig. 4-21). "Before and after" pictures of actual patients with this type of computer-aided design models for facial reconstruction yield positive results.

The National Biocomputational Center at Stanford University uses a slightly different rendering paradigm that is based on CT images; it is called the virtual environment for surgical planning and analysis (VESPA). Montgomery and colleagues[151] developed VESPA for use in craniofacial reconstruction, as well as breast surgery, soft tissue reconstruction, and repair of congenital defects. Once CT images are acquired, voxel, or volume-based, images are focused down the area of interest, which results in very specific, segmented data. 3-D images are broadcast onto a high-definition CRT monitor, and the user, who is wearing tracked CrystalEyes (StereoGraphics, San Rafael, CA) shutter glasses and holding a FasTrak (Polhemus, Colchester, VT) stylus for input, can view and manipulate the virtual object.

The complexity of facial reconstructive surgery almost demands this kind of preoperative power because conventionally, there is only so much planning and prediction that can be performed by a surgeon who uses 2-D conventions. Preplanning will allow the physician and the patient to view almost ensured outcomes; this not only reassures both parties but also allows for reduced anesthesia times.

Virtual Reality–Based Three-Dimensional Surgical Simulators

The actual practice of surgical procedures is a highly visual and, subsequently, manual task with constant visual and haptic feedback and modification.[166] This represents a formidable challenge. To create a VR surgical simulator for education or practice, programmers must develop a system that adequately represents the surgical environment; it must react to the surgical changes (e.g., incision, dissection, resection) that the surgeon imparts to the operative field and must give appropriate force feedback. These prerequisites must be accomplished in a manner that is transparent to the surgeon (i.e., the virtual operating room should mimic a real operating room). Depending on the target audience and application, many surgical simulators have been developed. VR surgical simulators have been applied to open surgical procedures, laparoscopic surgery, and remote telepresence surgery.

The Karlsruhe "VEST" Endoscopic Surgery Trainer (IT VEST Systems AG, Bremen, Germany) is probably the most developed surgical endoscopic simulator (Fig. 4-22). This device mimics the surgically draped human abdomen and allows for the insertion of multiple laparoscopic instruments and an endoscopic camera. Force feedback is provided and applied to the laparoscopic instruments. Visual displays are generated with proprietary KISMET (Kinematic Simulation, Monitoring, and Off-Line Programming Environment for Telerobotics) 3-D generation surgical environments.[77] This software affords the user high-fidelity immersion into a virtual laparoscopic scenario of a minimally invasive cholecystectomy, complete with real-time tissue dynamics and kinematic tissue response to user interaction. The laparoscopic instruments are tracked with sensors to mimic the same degree of freedom of actual endoscopic tools that are placed in a human abdominal cavity. This system is processed by a graphics workstation and has the ability to support total immersion goggles and telepresence training. As computing and graphic power become more developed, the

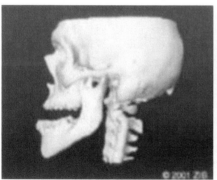
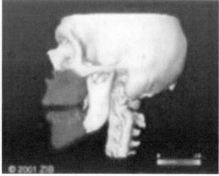
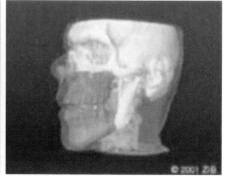

Figure 4–21 Three-dimensional planning of a high Le Fort I osteotomy (Konrad-Zue-Zentrum for Informationstechnik, Berlin, Germany). (Courtesy of SenseAble Technologies, Woburn, MA.)

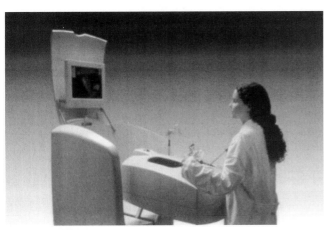

Figure 4–22 VEST/LapSim One endoscopic surgical trainer (IT VEST Systems AG, Bremen, Germany). (Courtesy of IT VEST Systems AG.)

graphic representations will become more detailed and hopefully approach that of the video monitors in an actual operating room.

Other surgical simulation systems are also available. Boston Dynamics (Cambridge, MA) has developed an anastomosis simulation with Pennsylvania State University that is based on force feedback surgical instruments and 3-D vision with shutter goggles. This system allows the user to place sutures in bowel or vessels to simulate the delicate nature of an anastomosis. A "surgical report card" that analyzes the surgeon's performance in real time is a unique implementation in this system. Comments on performance include time, accuracy, angle of needle insertion, and tissue damage.[162]

VR simulators for bronchoscopy, catheter insertion, and endoscopy are so real that residents and fellows use such simulators to get exposure to procedures not already in their arsenal of experience. Stanford University has used the BronchSim and CathSim devices (Immersion Medical Technologies, Gaithersburg, MD) and the VR Med Upper GI Simulator (Fifth Dimension Technologies, Pretoria, South Africa) to evaluate surgical procedure training. A study that involved the BronchSim device consisted of three sections: practice, navigation and visualization, and diagnosis and therapy. The subject was introduced to the bronchoscope and the simulation by a narrative from the training staff, which was supplemented by four videos on basic bronchoscopy that were supplied with the Immersion Medical Technologies software. One of the tasks involved diagnosing an intraluminal bronchial wall tumor from CT scans and plain radiographs of the chest and subsequently using the provided biopsy tool to take a sample of the tumor safely and control hemorrhage.

The BronchSim device was able to distinguish between experts and novices, and subjective data from Likert questionnaires suggest an increase in procedural ability and familiarity with bronchoscopy. Similar educational studies were completed with the same internal structure for evaluation. These studies returned equally encouraging results.

With the advent of computer-assisted medicine, VR training tools have never been so accessible to medical educational programs as they are today. Our results, and the results of many others, suggest that surgical education that incorporates VR systems can be used in a training program for both medical students and residents. Experience suggests that many VR simulator interfaces are realistic enough to serve not only as a teaching tool but also as a method of honing present skills.

Simulation in Surgical Education

Current training in surgery is focused on core knowledge, patient care, team training, and procedural skills. Surgical simulators can be used to enhance each of these components. Simulation can be used for skills training, patient treatment, and crisis training in primary and continuing education for both residents and practicing surgeons.

Surgical simulation has been adopted by several surgical centers and residency programs through the formation of "simulation centers." Mannequin simulators are being used to train surgical interns and residents in crisis treatment and aspects of Advanced Cardiac Life Support (ACLS) and Advanced Trauma Life Support (ATLS) as a formal credentialing method.

As an example of mannequin-based core knowledge training, a simulation of initial burn surgical treatment has been developed. Treatment of acute burn injury is a core surgical skill, and proper treatment ranks in urgency with the care of myocardial infarction. Despite the expertise needed to treat burns, only 20% of surgical residencies have a formal burn rotation.

The MediSim human patient simulator (HPS), a life-sized male mannequin model that is linked to a customizable computer system, was used. The HPS simulates normal and pathologic states reliably and is certified for ATLS and ACLS credentialing. Simulated output is through standard bedside monitoring equipment, spontaneous respiration, eye opening, pulses, voice response, and robotic limb motion. The test scenario demonstrated a 40%, third-degree burn.

Initially, expert intensive care and burn surgeons were asked to validate the scenario for accuracy and relevancy. Next, senior surgery residents were exposed to the 30-minute simulation. Lichert (scale of 1 to 5) questionnaires and expert debriefings were provided to each of the subjects. Each resident's performance was filmed for expert review by an attending physician. The computer-driven response of the HPS was based on the residents' ability to perform ATLS while simultaneously treating the burned patient with fluids, intubation, and escharotomy.

Attending physicians responded that the proposed scenario accurately reflected the key treatment points for ATLS protocols and burn treatment. These experts also perceived that residents who were exposed to the simulation could function as a physician responder in a similar situation. After being debriefed, each subject was more confident with burn treatment, fluid calculation, intubation and ventilator management, and thoracic and extremity escharotomies. Burn treatment simulation can teach residents to process situations that are not experienced in training and can function as a credentialing platform for new faculty. This first validation of simulated burn training with the HPS suggests a feasible solution to a serious educational dilemma.

Also popular are surgical "fly-through" VR-based tools that are designed to provide a medical student or resident with a first exposure to surgical anatomic 3-D relationships. Projects that involve the virtual human male have taken advantage of data sets acquired from this model to create a virtual human anatomy resource that allows students to approach any anatomic structure from any angle or route. The Visible Human Project data sets can be rendered in a 3-D format to create virtual detailed fly-through movies. These fly-throughs can be modified to demonstrate the before and after effects of many common surgical procedures and provide an "endoscopic" view of the abdominal cavity. As more surgical procedures are developed that require more detailed and specific knowledge of surgical relationships and as the time for surgical education continues to decrease, VR fly-throughs may provide an educational solution.

SURGICAL INNOVATION

Technology continues to advance rapidly and has become more complex and interdisciplinary; at the same time clinical surgery has become increasingly demanding, with intense focus required. As a result, the gap between technical advances and creative surgeons is growing. This chapter is an attempt to narrow that gap.

If, indeed, change is constant and constant cycling has advanced our field, it is incumbent on us as a specialty to understand, thoughtfully incorporate, and even direct the useful change of surgical innovation. Surgeons are undeniably uniquely positioned and privileged to contribute to this cycle, but the growing gap has created a special field of knowledge requiring a specialized education program.

A formal education program that teaches the process of innovation to young surgeons has been established as a 2-year fellowship in surgical innovation (*http://surgery.stanford.edu/innovation*). In the first year, fellows participate in didactic courses that address practical issues in needs assessment, technology solutions, intellectual property, ownership, the FDA approval process, and the underpinning economics of this process. A team-based project course is a large component of the first year.

A second year is spent further developing an identified project. At the completion of the program the fellow will possess the requisite skills to become a significant contributor to the next cycle of surgical innovation in children and adults. Depending on the background of the fellow, a master's degree in bioengineering is also achievable.

The surgical innovation program at Lucile Packard Children's Hospital leverages heavily on the well-established biodesign program led by Drs. Paul Yock and Joshua Makower (*http://inovation.stanford.edu/isp/home.isp*). This network focuses explicitly on technology transfer that brings innovations bidirectionally to the bedside-to-bench cycle. This unique academic program is focused on invention and implementation of new health care technologies through interdisciplinary research and education at the emerging frontiers of biomedical engineering.

The Surgical Innovation Program and Biodesign are part of a campus-wide interdisciplinary program titled "Stanford's Bio-X Initiative"; it involves over 500 scientists from the life sciences, engineering, chemistry, and physics with broad research themes in biocomputation, biophysics, genomics and proteomics, regenerative medicine, and chemical biology.

CONCLUSION

If pediatric surgery is to remain an active participant in the endless cycle of change, acknowledgment of the role of technology in advancing our care and a desire to actively embrace and drive the process forward in an ethical fashion are essential. To sit on the sideline is to invite a slow and agonizing demise of us as individuals and, more critically, our field and our responsibility to its future. This two-volume text is a tribute to those who came before us and in the space of less than 50 years defined our specialty. We as stewards of this generation must be architects of the next 50 years.

REFERENCES

1. Aaronson OS, Tulipan NB, Cywes R, et al: Robot-assisted endoscopic intrauterine myelomeningocele repair: A feasibility study. Pediatr Neurosurg 2002;36:85.
2. Adler JR Jr, Chang SD, Murphy MD, et al: The CyberKnife: A frameless robotic system for radiosurgery. Stereotact Funct Neurosurg 1997;69:124-128.
3. Aharon S, Robb RA: 3-D surface reconstruction of patient-specific anatomic data using a pre-specified number of polygons. Stud Health Technol Inform 1997;39:430.
4. Ahn YC, Lee KC, Kim DY, et al: Fractionated stereotactic radiation therapy for extracranial head and neck tumors. Int J Radiat Oncol Biol Phys 2000;48:501.
5. Alexander E 3rd, Loeffler JS: Radiosurgery using a modified linear accelerator. Neurosurg Clin North Am 1992;3:167.
6. Arezzo A, Testa T, Ulmer F, et al: Positioning systems for endoscopic solo surgery. Minerva Chir 2000;55:635.
7. Argenziano M, Oz MC, Kohmoto T, et al: Totally endoscopic atrial septal defect repair with robotic assistance. Circulation 2003;108(Suppl 1):II191.
8. Arjomand H, Turi ZG, McCormick D, et al: Percutaneous coronary intervention: Historical perspectives, current status, and future directions. Am Heart J 2003;146:787.
9. Bajada C, Selch M, De Salles A, et al: Application of stereotactic radiosurgery to the head and neck region. Acta Neurochir Suppl (Wien) 1994;62:114.
10. Ballantyne GH, Moll F: The da Vinci telerobotic surgical system: The virtual operative field and telepresence surgery. Surg Clin North Am 2003;83:1203.
11. Bargar WL, Bauer A, Borner M: Primary and revision total hip replacement using the Robodoc system. Clin Orthop 1998;354:82.
12. Bergonié J: De quelques resultats de la radiotherapie et essai de fixation d'une technique rationelle. C R Acad Sci (Paris) 1906;143:983.
13. Billotte W: Ceramic biomaterials. In Bronzino JD (ed): Biomedical Engineering Handbook, 2nd ed. Boca Raton, Florida, CRC Press, 1999.

14. Black PM, Tarbell NJ, Alexander E 3rd, et al: Stereotactic techniques in managing pediatric brain tumors. Childs Nerv Syst 1993;9:343.

15. Blasberg RG, Gelovani J: Molecular-genetic imaging: A nuclear medicine–based perspective. Mol Imaging 2002;1:280.

16. Blomgren H, Lax I, Naslund I, et al: Stereotactic high dose fraction radiation therapy of extracranial tumors using an accelerator. Clinical experience of the first thirty-one patients. Acta Oncol 1995;34:861.

17. Brown PO, Botstein D: Exploring the new world of the genome with DNA microarrays. Nat Genet 1999; 21(Suppl 1):S33.

18. Buatti JM, Friedman WA, Bova FJ, et al: Linac radiosurgery for locally recurrent nasopharyngeal carcinoma: Rationale and technique. Head Neck 1995;17:149.

19. Buatti JM, Friedman WA, Meeks SL, et al: The radiobiology of radiosurgery and stereotactic radiotherapy. Med Dosim 1998;23:201.

20. Buatti JM, Meeks SL, Marcus RB Jr, et al: Radiotherapy for pediatric brain tumors. Semin Pediatr Neurol 1997;4:3049.

21. Burns PN: Harmonic imaging with ultrasound contrast agents. Clin Radiol 1996;51(Suppl 1):S50.

22. Bush RL, Lin PH, Lumsden AB: Endovascular treatment of the thoracic aorta. Vasc Endovasc Surg 2003;37:399.

23. Bush RL, Lin PH, Lumsden AB: Endovascular management of abdominal aortic aneurysms. J Cardiovasc Surg (Torino) 2003;44:527.

24. Callahan MJ, Rodriguez DP, Taylor GA: CT of appendicitis in children. Radiology 2002;224:325.

25. Cannon JW, Stoll JA, Salgo IS, et al: Real-time three-dimensional ultrasound for guiding surgical tasks. Comput Aided Surg 2003;8:82.

26. Carmine J, Allen P, Ardrey P, et al: Medical Applications of Virtual Reality. Raleigh, NC, Department of Biological and Agricultural Engineering, North Carolina State University, 1999.

27. Chang CH, Chang FM, Yu CH, et al: Three-dimensional ultrasound in the assessment of fetal cerebellar transverse and antero-posterior diameters. Ultrasound Med Biol 2000;26:175.

28. Chang CH, Chang FM, Yu CH, et al: Assessment of fetal cerebellar volume using three-dimensional ultrasound. Ultrasound Med Biol 2000;26:981.

29. Chang CH, Yu CH, Chang FM, et al: Assessment of fetal adrenal gland volume using three-dimensional ultrasound. Ultrasound Med Biol 2002;28:1383.

30. Chang CH, Yu CH, Chang FM, et al: Volumetric assessment of normal fetal lungs using three-dimensional ultrasound. Ultrasound Med Biol 2003;29:935.

31. Chang FM, Hsu KF, Ko HC, et al: Fetal heart volume assessment by three-dimensional ultrasound. Ultrasound Obstet Gynecol 1997;9:42.

32. Chang FM, Hsu KF, Ko HC, et al: Three-dimensional ultrasound assessment of fetal liver volume in normal pregnancy: A comparison of reproducibility with two-dimensional ultrasound and a search for a volume constant. Ultrasound Med Biol 1997;23:381.

33. Chang SD, Adler JR: Robotics and radiosurgery—the cyberknife. Stereotact Funct Neurosurg 2001;76:204.

34. Chang SD, Adler JR Jr: Current status and optimal use of radiosurgery. Oncology (Huntingt) 2001;15:209.

35. Chang SD, Adler JR, Steinberg GK: General and Historical Considerations of Radiotherapy and Radiosurgery, vol 3. Philadelphia, WB Saunders, 2003.

36. Chang SD, Main W, Martin DP, et al: An analysis of the accuracy of the CyberKnife: A robotic frameless stereotactic radiosurgical system. Neurosurgery 2003;52:140.

37. Chopra V, Gesink BJ, de Jong J, et al: Does training on an anesthesia simulator lead to improvement in performance? Br J Anaesth 1994;73:293.

38. Choy G, Choyke P, Libutti SK: Current advances in molecular imaging: Noninvasive in vivo bioluminescent and fluorescent optical imaging in cancer research. Mol Imaging 2003;2:303.

39. Chua DT, Sham JS, Kwong PW, et al: Linear accelerator–based stereotactic radiosurgery for limited, locally persistent, and recurrent nasopharyngeal carcinoma: Efficacy and complications. Int J Radiat Oncol Biol Phys 2003;56:177.

40. Cleary K, Anderson J, Brazaitis M, et al: Final report of the technical requirements for image guided spine procedures workshop, April 17-20, 1999, Ellicott City, Maryland, USA. Comput Aided Surg 2000;5:180.

41. Cmelak AJ, Cox RS, Adler JR, et al: Radiosurgery for skull base malignancies and nasopharyngeal carcinoma. Int J Radiat Oncol Biol Phys 1997;37:997.

42. Coleman BG, Adzick NS, Crombleholme TM, et al: Fetal therapy: State of the art. J Ultrasound Med 2002;21:1257.

43. Colombo F, Benedetti A, Casentini L, et al: Stereotactic radiosurgery of intracranial tumors in childhood. J Neurosurg Sci 1985;29:233.

44. Costa GL, Sandora MR, Nakajima A, et al: Adoptive immunotherapy of experimental autoimmune encephalomyelitis via T-cell delivery of the IL-12 p40 subunit. J Immunol 2001;167:2379.

45. Crisera CA, Marosky JK, Longaker MT, et al: Organogenesis particularly relevant to fetal surgery. World J Surg 2003; 27:38.

46. Delany B, Abouaf J: The Market for Visual Simulation/Virtual Reality Systems, 4th ed. New York, CyberEdge Information Services, 2001.

47. Denecke T, Frush DP, Li J: Eight-channel multidetector computed tomography: Unique potential for pediatric chest computed tomography angiography. J Thorac Imaging 2002;17:306.

48. Detre JA, Wang J: Technical aspects and utility of fMRI using BOLD and ASL. Clin Neurophysiol 2002;113:621.

49. Donnelly LF, Frush DP: Pediatric multidetector body CT. Radiol Clin North Am 2003;41:637.

50. Drasin T, Gracia C, Atkinson J: Pediatric applications of robotic surgery. Pediatr Endosurg Innovative Tech 2003;7:377.

51. Dunbar SF, Tarbell NJ, Kooy HM, et al: Stereotactic radiotherapy for pediatric and adult brain tumors: Preliminary report. Int J Radiat Oncol Biol Phys 1994;30:531.

52. Dyson RL, Pretorius DH, Budorick NE, et al: Three-dimensional ultrasound in the evaluation of fetal anomalies. Ultrasound Obstet Gynecol 2000;16:321.

53. Edelman RR, Hahn PF, Buxton R, et al: Rapid MR imaging with suspended respiration: Clinical application in the liver. Radiology 1986;161:125.

54. Even-Bendahan G, Lazar I, Erez I, et al: Role of imaging in the diagnosis of acute appendicitis in children. Clin Pediatr (Phila) 2003;42:23.

55. Fabrikant JI, Levy RP, Steinberg GK, et al: Heavy-charged-particle radiosurgery for intracranial arteriovenous malformations. Stereotact Funct Neurosurg 1991;57:50.

56. Fabrikant JI, Lyman JT, Frankel KA: Heavy charged-particle Bragg peak radiosurgery for intracranial vascular disorders. Radiat Res Suppl 1985;8:S244.

57. Falk V, Jacobs S, Gummert J, et al: Robotic coronary artery bypass grafting (CABG)—the Leipzig experience. Surg Clin North Am 2003;83:1391.

58. Fox LA: Images in clinical medicine. Three-dimensional CT diagnosis of maxillofacial trauma. N Engl J Med 1993;329:102.

59. Freeman CR, Souhami L, Caron JL, et al: Stereotactic external beam irradiation in previously untreated brain tumors in children and adolescents. Med Pediatr Oncol 1994;22:173.

60. Freiherr G: Harmonic imaging: What is it, how it works. Diagnostic Imaging Europe 1998;HU6.

61. Frinking PJ, Bouakaz A, Kirkhorn J, et al: Ultrasound contrast imaging: Current and new potential methods. Ultrasound Med Biol 2000;26:965.

62. Frush DP, Donnelly LF: Pulmonary sequestration spectrum: A new spin with helical CT. AJR Am J Roentgenol 1997;169:679.

63. Frush DP, Donnelly LF: Helical CT in children: Technical considerations and body applications. Radiology 1998;209:37.

64. Gaba DM: The future vision of simulation in health care. Qual Saf Health Care 2004;12(Suppl 1):i2.

65. Garcia-Ruiz A, Gagner M, Miller JH, et al: Manual vs robotically assisted laparoscopic surgery in the performance of basic manipulation and suturing tasks. Arch Surg 1998;133:957.

66. Gardner E, Linskey ME, Penagaricano JA, et al: Stereotactic radiosurgery for patients with cancer of the head and neck. Curr Oncol Rep 2003;5:164.

67. Gerosa M, Nicolato A, Foroni R: The role of gamma knife radiosurgery in the treatment of primary and metastatic brain tumors. Curr Opin Oncol 2003;15:188.

68. Gertner ME, Krummel TM: Micro- and nanoelectromechanical systems in medicine and surgery. In Greco R (ed): Nanobiology: Nano Scale Fabrication of New Generation of Biomedical Devices. Boca Raton, FL, CRC Press, 2005, pp 25-38.

69. Giller CA, Berger BD, Gilio JP, et al: Feasibility of radiosurgery for malignant brain tumors in infants by use of image-guided robotic radiosurgery: Preliminary report. Neurosurgery 2004;55:916.

70. Giller CA, Berger BD, Pistenmaa DA, et al: Robotically guided radiosurgery for children. Pediatr Blood Cancer 2005;45:304.

71. Gorman P, Krummel T: Simulation and virtual reality in surgical education: Real or unreal? Arch Surg 1999;134:1203.

72. Greco R (ed): Nanobiology: Nano Scale Fabrication of New Generation of Biomedical Devices. Boca Raton, FL, CRC Press 2005, pp 1-24.

73. Gressens P, Luton D: Fetal MRI: Obstetrical and neurological perspectives. Pediatr Radiol 2004;34:682.

74. Gritzmann N, Hollerweger A, Macheiner P, et al: Transabdominal sonography of the gastrointestinal tract. Eur Radiol 2002;12:1748.

75. Gropler RJ: Methodology governing the assessment of myocardial glucose metabolism by positron emission tomography and fluorine 18–labeled fluorodeoxyglucose. J Nucl Cardiol 1994;1(2 Pt 2) (Suppl):S4.

76. Gropler RJ, Soto P: Recent advances in cardiac positron emission tomography in the clinical management of the cardiac patient. Curr Cardiol Rep 2004;6:2026.

77. Gruener G: Telementoring using tactile cues. In Mechanical Engineering. Boulder, CO, University of Colorado, 1998.

78. Gunven P, Blomgren H, Lax I: Radiosurgery for recurring liver metastases after hepatectomy. Hepatogastroenterology 2003;50:1201.

79. Gutt CN, Markus B, Kim ZG, et al: Early experiences of robotic surgery in children. Surg Endosc 2002;16:1083.

80. Hadjipanayis CG, Kondziolka D, Gardner P, et al: Stereotactic radiosurgery for pilocytic astrocytomas when multimodal therapy is necessary. J Neurosurg 2002;97:56.

81. Hahn PF, Saini S, Cohen MS, et al: An aqueous gastrointestinal contrast agent for use in echo-planar MR imaging. Magn Reson Med 1992;25:380.

82. Hall E: Radiobiology for the Radiologist, vol 5. Philadelphia, JB Lippincott, 2000.

83. Hall EJ, Brenner DJ: The radiobiology of radiosurgery: Rationale for different treatment regimes for AVMs and malignancies. Int J Radiat Oncol Biol Phys 1993;25:381.

84. Harisinghani M, Barentsz J, Hahn PF, et al: Noninvasive detection of clinically occult lymph-node metastases in prostate cancer. N Engl J Med 2003;348:2491.

85. Harrison MR, Evans MI, Adzick NS, et al (eds): The Unborn Patient: The Art and Science of Fetal Therapy, 3rd ed. Philadelphia, WB Saunders, 2001.

86. Hashizume M, Shimada M, Tomikawa M, et al: Early experiences of endoscopic procedures in general surgery assisted by a computer-enhanced surgical system. Surg Endosc 2002;16:1187.

87. Hedequist DJ, Hall JE, Emans JB: The safety and efficacy of spinal instrumentation in children with congenital spine deformities. Spine 2004;29:2081.

88. Heller K, Gutt C, Schaeff G, et al: Use of the robot system da Vinci for laparoscopic repair of gastro-oesophageal reflux in children. Eur J Pediatr Surg 2002;12:239.

89. Henriksen K, Moss F: From the runway to the airway and beyond. Qual Saf Health Care 2004;13(Suppl 1):S11.

90. Hernandez L, Zamorano L, Sloan A, et al: Gamma knife radiosurgery for renal cell carcinoma brain metastases. J Neurosurg 2002;97(5 Suppl):S489.

91. Herschman HR: Molecular imaging: Looking at problems, seeing solutions. Science 2003;302:605.

92. Hiltzik M (ed): Dealers of Lightning: Xerox PARC and the Dawn of the Computer Age. New York, HarperBusiness, 1999.

93. Hirth A, Pedersen PH, Baardsen R, et al: Gamma-knife radiosurgery in pediatric cerebral and skull base tumors. Med Pediatr Oncol 2003;40:99.

94. History of PET and MRI. Advanced Biomedical Technology Research [website] 11/17/03; accessed 12/9/04.

95. Hodgson DC, Goumnerova LC, Loeffler JS, et al: Radiosurgery in the management of pediatric brain tumors. Int J Radiat Oncol Biol Phys 2001;50:929.

96. Hollands CM, Dixey LN: Applications of robotic surgery in pediatric patients. Surg Laparosc Endosc Percutan Tech 2002;12:71.

97. Hollands CM, Dixey LN: Robotic-assisted esophago-esophagostomy. J Pediatr Surg 2002;37:983.

98. Hollands CM, Dixey LN, Torma MJ: Technical assessment of porcine enteroenterostomy performed with ZEUS robotic technology. J Pediatr Surg 2001;36:1231.

99. Honda Y, Fitzgerald P: Stent thrombosis: An issue revisited in a changing world. Circulation 2003;108:2.

100. Horton KM, Fishman EK: Multidetector-row computed tomography and 3-dimensional computed tomography imaging of small bowel neoplasms: Current concept in diagnosis. J Comput Assist Tomogr 2004;28:106.

101. Hoshi S, Jokura H, Nakamura H, et al: Gamma-knife radiosurgery for brain metastasis of renal cell carcinoma: Results in 42 patients. Int J Urol 2002;9:618.

102. Humphreys RP, Hoffman HJ, Drake JM, et al: Choices in the 1990s for the management of pediatric cerebral arteriovenous malformations. Pediatr Neurosurg 1996;25:2775.

103. Jacob BP, Gagner M: Robotics and general surgery. Surg Clin North Am 2003;83:1405.

104. Jodicke A, Berthold LID, Scharbrodt W, et al: Endoscopic surgical anatomy of the paediatric third ventricle studied using virtual neuroendoscopy based on 3-D ultrasonography. Childs Nerv Syst 2003;19:325.

105. Jodicke A, Daentzer D, Kastner S, et al: Risk factors for outcome and complications of dorsal foraminotomy in cervical disc herniation. Surg Neurol 2003;60:124.

106. John N: Surgical Simulators on the World Wide Web—This Must Be the Way Forward? Manchester, England, Manchester Visualisation Centre, University of Manchester, 1999.

107. Kapoor V, McCook BM, Torok FS: An introduction to PET-CT imaging. Radiographics 2004;24:523.

108. Kasalicky MA, Svah J, Fried M, et al: AESOP 3000—computer-assisted surgery, personal experience. Rozhl Chir 2002;81:346.

109. Kaste SC: Issues specific to implementing PET-CT for pediatric oncology: What we have learned along the way. Pediatr Radiol 2004;34:205.

110. Keeve E, Girod S, Girod B: Computer aided craniofacial surgery. In Computer Assisted Radiology. Paris, Telecommunications Institute, University of Erlangen, 1996.

111. Keeve E, Girod S, Kikinis R, Girod B: Deformable modeling of facial tissue for craniofacial surgery simulation. Comput Aided Surg 1999;3:228.

112. Kelly PJ: State of the art and future directions of minimally invasive stereotactic neurosurgery. Cancer Control 1995;2:287.

113. Kelly PJ: Stereotactic surgery: What is past is prologue. Neurosurgery 2000;46:16.

114. Kitamura K, Shirato H, Seppenwoolde Y, et al: Tumor location, cirrhosis, and surgical history contribute to tumor movement in the liver, as measured during stereotactic irradiation using a real-time tumor-tracking radiotherapy system. Int J Radiat Oncol Biol Phys 2003;56:221.

115. Knight CG, Lorincz A, Gioell KM, et al: Computer-assisted robot-enhanced laparoscopic fundoplication in children. J Pediatr Surg 2004;39:864.

116. Kocher M, Voges J, Staar S, et al: Linear accelerator radiosurgery for recurrent malignant tumors of the skull base. Am J Clin Oncol 1998;21:18.

117. Kondziolka D, Lunsford LID, Flickinger JC: The radiobiology of radiosurgery. Neurosurg Clin North Am 1999;10:157.

118. Kondziolka D, Lunsford LID, Loeffler JS, et al: Radiosurgery and radiotherapy: Observations and clarifications. J Neurosurg 2004;101:585.

119. Kondziolka D, Lunsford LID, Witt TC, et al: The future of radiosurgery: Radiobiology, technology, and applications. Surg Neurol 2000;54:406.

120. Kuo JS, Yu C, Petrovich A, et al: The CyberKnife stereotactic radiosurgery system: Description, installation, and an initial evaluation of use and functionality. Neurosurgery 2003;53:1235.

121. Lanfranco AR, Castellanos AE, Desai JP, et al: Robotic surgery: A current perspective. Ann Surg 2004;239:14.

122. Lange A, Mankad P, Walayat M, et al: Transthoracic three-dimensional echocardiography in the preoperative assessment of atrioventricular septal defect morphology. Am J Cardiol 2000;85:630.

123. Langer SG, Carter SJ, Haynor DR, et al: Image acquisition: Ultrasound, computed tomography, and magnetic resonance imaging. World J Surg 2001;25:1428.

124. Larson DA, Flickinger JC, Loeffler JS: The radiobiology of radiosurgery. Int J Radiat Oncol Biol Phys 1993; 25:557.

125. LaValle GJ, Martinez DA, Sobel D, et al: Assessment of disseminated pancreatic cancer: A comparison of traditional exploratory laparotomy and radioimmunoguided surgery. Surgery 1997;122:867.

126. Lavan D, McQuire T, Langer R: Small-scale systems for in vivo drug delivery. Nat Biotechnol 2003;21:1184.

127. Lawler LP, Fishman EK: Multidetector row computed tomography of the aorta and peripheral arteries. Cardiol Clin 2003;21:607.

128. Le Bret E, Papadatos S, Folliguet T, et al: Interruption of patent arteriosus in children: Robotically assisted versus videothoracoscopic surgery. J Thorac Cardiovasc Surg 2002;123:973.

129. Lederman G, Wronski M, Fine M: Fractionated radiosurgery for brain metastases in 43 patients with breast carcinoma. Breast Cancer Res Treat 2001;65:145.

130. Lee BR, Chow GK, Ratner LE, et al: Laparoscopic live donor nephrectomy: Outcomes equivalent to open surgery. J Endourol 2000;14:811.

131. Lee N, Millender LE, Larson DA, et al: Gamma knife radiosurgery for recurrent salivary gland malignancies involving the base of skull. Head Neck 2003;25:210.

132. Lee N, Xia P, Quivey JM, et al: Intensity-modulated radiotherapy in the treatment of nasopharyngeal carcinoma: An update of the UCSF experience. Int J Radiat Oncol Biol Phys 2002;53:12.

133. Levy EL, Niranjan A, Thompson TP, et al: Radiosurgery for childhood intracranial arteriovenous malformations. Neurosurgery 2000;47:834.

134. Levy RP, Fabrikant JI, Frankel KA, et al: Stereotactic heavy-charged-particle Bragg peak radiosurgery for the treatment of intracranial arteriovenous malformations in childhood and adolescence. Neurosurgery 1989; 24:841.

135. Levy RP, Fabrikant JI, Frankel KA, et al: Heavy-charged-particle radiosurgery of the pituitary gland: Clinical results of 840 patients. Stereotact Funct Neurosurg 1991;57:22.

136. Levy RP, Schulte RW, Slater JD, et al: Stereotactic radiosurgery—the role of charged particles. Acta Oncol 1999;38:165.

137. Light ED, Idriss SF, Wolf PD, et al: Real-time three-dimensional intracardiac echocardiography. Ultrasound Med Biol 2001;27:1177.

138. Loeffler JS, Rossitch E Jr, Siddon R, et al: Role of stereotactic radiosurgery with a linear accelerator in treatment of intracranial arteriovenous malformations and tumors in children. Pediatrics 1990;85:774.

139. Lorincz A, Langenburg S, Klein M: Robotics and the pediatric surgeon. Curr Opin Pediatr 2003;15:262.

140. Luebbe B, Woo R, Wolf S, et al: Robotically assisted minimally invasive surgery in a pediatric population: Initial experience, technical considerations, and description of the da Vinci Surgical System. Pediatr Endosurg Innovative Tech 2003;7:385.

141. Machado LG, Savi MA: Medical applications of shape memory alloys. Braz J Med Biol Res 2003;36:683.

142. Mack M: Minimally invasive and robotics surgery. JAMA 2001;285:568.

143. Malhotra SP, Le D, Thelitz S, et al: Robotic-assisted endoscopic thoracic aortic anastomosis in juvenile lambs. Heart Surg Forum 2002;6:38.

144. Mao C, Flynn CE, Hayhurst A, et al: Viral assembly of oriented quantum dot nanowires. Proc Natl Acad Sci U S A 2003;100:6946.

145. McCaffrey A, Kay MA, Contag CH: Advancing molecular therapies through in vivo bioluminescent imaging. Mol Imaging 2003;2:75.

146. Meier AH, Rawn RI, Krummel TM: Virtual reality: Surgical application, a challenge for the new millennium. J Am Coll Surg 2000;192:372.

147. Menkis AH, Kodera K, Kiaii B, et al: Robotic surgery, the first 100 cases: Where do we go from here? Heart Surg Forum 2004;7:1.

148. Menon M, Srivastava A, Tewari A, et al: Laparoscopic and robot assisted radical prostatectomy: Establishment of a structured program and preliminary analysis of outcomes. J Urol 2002;168:945.

149. Mettler L, Ibrahim M, Ionat W: One year of experience working with the aid of a robotic assistant (the voice-controlled optic holder AESOP) in gynaecological endoscopic surgery. Hum Reprod 1998;13:2748.

150. Mihaljevic T, Cannon JW, del Nido PJ: Robotically assisted division of a vascular ring in children. J Thorac Cardiovasc Surg 2003;125:1163.

151. Montgomery K, Stephanides M, Schendel S: User Interface Paradigms for VR-Surgical Based Planning, Lessons Learned over a Decade of Research. Stanford, CA, Stanford University, 1996-2000.

152. Murphy MJ, Adler JR Jr, Bodduluri M, et al: Image-guided radiosurgery for the spine and pancreas. Comput Aided Surg 2000;5:278.

153. Murphy MJ, Chang SD, Gibbs IC, et al: Patterns of patient movement during frameless image-guided radiosurgery. Int J Radiat Oncol Biol Phys 2003;55:1400.

154. Murphy MJ, Martin D, Whyte R, et al: The effectiveness of breath-holding to stabilize lung and pancreas tumors during radiosurgery. Int J Radiat Oncol Biol Phys 2002;53:4752.

155. Murray W, Schneider A: Using simulators for education and training in anesthesiology. Anesthesia Patient Safety Foundation Newsletter, 1996.

156. Nicolato A, Gerosa M, Ferraresi P, et al: Stereotactic radiosurgery for the treatment of arteriovenous malformations in childhood. J Neurosurg Sci 1997;41:359.

157. Nordberg A: Application of PET in dementia disorders. Acta Neurol Scand Suppl 1996;168:71.

158. Nordberg A: PET imaging of amyloid in Alzheimer's disease. Lancet Neurol 2004;3:519.

159. Nugent H, Edelman E: Tissue engineering therapy for cardiovascular disease. Circ Res 2003;92:1068.

160. Okada S, Tanaba Y, Yaegashi S, et al: Initial use of the newly developed voice-controlled robot system for a solitary pulmonary arterio-venous malformation. Kyobu Geka 2002;55:871.

161. Olsen LH, Deding D, Yeung CK, Jorgensen TM: Computer assisted laparoscopic pneumovesical ureter reimplantation. In Cohen: Initial experience in a pig model. APMIS Suppl 2003;109:23.

162. O'Toole RV, Playter RR, Krummel TM, et al: Measuring and developing suturing technique with a virtual reality surgical simulator. J Am Coll Surg 1999;189:127.

163. Paek B, Goldberg JD, Albanese CT: Prenatal diagnosis. World J Surg 2003;27:27.

164. Pedraza R, Palmer I, Moss V, et al: Bilateral robotic assisted laparoscopic heminephroureterectomy. J Urol 2004;171:2394.

165. Pedraza R, Weiser A, Franco I: Laparoscopic appendicovesicostomy (Mitrofanoff procedure) in a child using the da Vinci robotic system. J Urol 2004;171:1652.

166. Peitgen H, Preim B, Selle D, et al: Risk Analysis for Liver Surgery. Center for Medical Diagnostic Systems and Visualization. Bremen, Germany, 1999.

167. Peters C: Robot assisted surgery in pediatric urology. Pediatr Endosurg Innovative Tech 2003;7:403.

168. Petrovich Z, Jozsef G, Yu C, et al: Radiotherapy and stereotactic radiosurgery for pituitary tumors. Neurosurg Clin North Am 2003;14:147.

169. Pilliar RM: Powder metal-made orthopedic implants with porous surface for fixation by tissue ingrowth. Clin Orthop 1983;176:242.

170. Pimentel K, Teixeira K: Virtual Reality: Through the New Looking Glass. Windcrest, New York, McGraw-Hill, 1993.

171. Ponsky LE, Crownover RL, Rosen MJ, et al: Initial evaluation of Cyberknife technology for extracorporeal renal tissue ablation. Urology 2003;61:498.

172. Powers JE, Burns PN, Souquet J: Imaging instrumentation for ultrasound contrast agents. In Nanda N, Schlief R, Goldberg B (eds): Advances in Echo Imaging Using Contrast Enhancement. Dordrecht, The Netherlands, Kluwer Academic, 1997, p 139.

173. Powers WJ, Zazulia AR: The use of positron emission tomography in cerebrovascular disease. Neuroimaging Clin North Am 2003;13:741.

174. Prayer D, Brugger PC, Prayer L: Fetal MRI: Techniques and protocols. Pediatr Radiol 2004;34:685.

175. Qian G, Lowry J, Silverman P, et al: Stereotactic extracranial radiosurgery for renal cell carcinoma. Int J Radiat Oncol Biol Phys 2003;57(2 Suppl):S283.

176. Radford IR: Evidence for a general relationship between the induced level of DNA double-strand breakage and cell-killing after X-irradiation of mammalian cells. Int J Radiat Biol Relat Stud Phys Chem Med 1986;49:611.

177. Rickers C, Sasse K, Buchert R, et al: Myocardial viability assessed by positron emission tomography in infants and children after the arterial switch operation and suspected infarction. J Am Coll Cardiol 2000;36:1676.

178. Riva G, Bolzoni M, Melis L: Sensing in VR. Milan, Applied Technology for Psychology Laboratory, 1996.

179. Roberts B: Is there money in MEMS? Electronic Business Magazine, May 1999.

180. Roberts EG, Shulkin BL: Technical issues in performing PET studies in pediatric patients. J Nucl Med Technol 2004;32:5.

181. Rosen J, Lasko-Harvill A, Satava R: Virtual reality and surgery. In Taylor R (ed): Computer Integrated Surgery. Cambridge, MA, MIT Press, 1996.

182. Rosenberg LB, Stredney D: A haptic interface for virtual simulation of endoscopic surgery. Stud Health Technol Inform 1996;29:371.

183. Rubin GD: 3-D imaging with MDCT. Eur J Radiol 2003; 45(Suppl 1):S37.

184. Rutten I, Deneufbourg JM: Radiotherapy in pediatric head and neck tumours. Acta Otorhinolaryngol Belg 2000;54:1.

185. Salo JA, Salminen JT, Kiviluoto TA, et al: Treatment of Barrett's esophagus by endoscopic laser ablation and antireflux surgery. Ann Surg 1998;227:40.

186. Salzberg A, Krummel TM (eds): Patient Safety: The Surgeon's Role. Patient Safety Manual. Chicago, American College of Surgeons, 2001.

187. Salzberg A, Krummel TM: Use of a virtual reality flexible bronchoscopy simulator for use in medical and surgical training. Paper presented at a meeting of the Society of Critical Care Medicine, 2001, San Diego, CA.

188. Salzberg D, Bloom M, Krummel TM: Current problems in surgery. Curr Probl Surg Adv Technol 2003;39:733.

189. Satava RM: Virtual endoscopy: Diagnosis using 3-D visualization and virtual representation. Surg Endosc 1996;19:173.

190. Schneebaum S, Papo J, Graif M, et al: Radioimmunoguided surgery benefits for recurrent colorectal cancer. Ann Surg Oncol 1997;4:371.

191. Schnepp R, Hua X: A tumor-suppressing duo: TGFbeta and activin modulate a similar transcriptome. Cancer Biol Ther 2003;2:171.

192. Schoder H, Erdi YE, Larson SM, et al: PET/CT: A new imaging technology in nuclear medicine. Eur J Nucl Med Mol Imaging 2003;30:1419.

193. Schoder H, Larson SM, Yeung HW: PET/CT in oncology: Integration into clinical management of lymphoma,

melanoma, and gastrointestinal malignancies. J Nucl Med 2004;45(Suppl 1):72S.

194. Seeman N, Belcher A: Emulating biology: Building nanostructures from the bottom up. Proc Natl Acad Sci U S A 2002;99(Suppl 2):S6451.

195. Semwal SK, Barnhart BK: Ray casting and the enclosing-net algorithm for extracting shapes from volume data. Comput Biol Med 1995;25:261.

196. Seymour CB, Mothersill C, Alper T: High yields of lethal mutations in somatic mammalian cells that survive ionizing radiation. Int J Radiat Biol Relat Stud Phys Chem Med 1986;50:167.

197. Shahidi R, Clarke L, Bucholz RD, et al: White paper: Challenges and opportunities in computer-assisted interventions, January 2001. Comput Aided Surg 2001; 6:176.

198. Shrieve DC, Klish M, Wendland MM, et al: Basic principles of radiobiology, radiotherapy, and radiosurgery. Neurosurg Clin North Am 2004;15:467.

199. Singh RK, Smith JT, Wilkinson ID, et al: Ultrafast MR imaging in pediatric neuroradiology. Acta Radiol 2003;44:550.

200. Smyth MD, Sneed PK, Ciricillo SF, et al: Stereotactic radiosurgery for pediatric intracranial arteriovenous malformations: The University of California at San Francisco experience. J Neurosurg 2002;97:48.

201. Somaza SC, Kondziolka D, Lunsford LID, et al: Early outcomes after stereotactic radiosurgery for growing pilocytic astrocytomas in children. Pediatr Neurosurg 1996;25:109.

202. Stahl A, Wieder H, Wester JH, et al: PET/CT molecular imaging in abdominal oncology. Abdom Imaging 2004;29:388.

203. Steichen FM, Ravitch MM (eds): Stapling in Surgery. Chicago, Year Book, 1984.

204. Stigbrand T, Ullen A, Sandstrom P, et al: Twenty years with monoclonal antibodies: State of the art—where do we go? Acta Oncol 1996;35:259.

205. Suh JH, Barnett GH: Stereotactic radiosurgery for brain tumors in pediatric patients. Technol Cancer Res Treat 2003;2:141.

206. Takacs I, Hamilton AJ: Extracranial stereotactic radiosurgery: Applications for the spine and beyond. Neurosurg Clin North Am 1999;10:257.

207. Talamini MA: Robotic surgery: Is it for you? Adv Surg 2002;36:1.

208. Talamini MA, Chapman S, Horgan S, et al: A prospective analysis of 211 robotic-assisted surgical procedures. Surg Endosc 2003;17:1521.

209. Tanaka H, Hashimoto K, Yamada I, et al: Interstitial photodynamic therapy with rotating and reciprocating optical fibers. Cancer 2001;91:1791.

210. Taylor CA, Hughes TJ, Zarins CK: Finite element modeling of three-dimensional pulsatile flow in the abdominal aorta: Relevance to atherosclerosis. Ann Biomed Eng 1998;26:975.

211. Taylor R, Stulberg D: Excerpts from the final report for the second international workshop on robotics and computer assisted medical interventions, June 23-26, 1996, Bristol, England. Comput Aided Surg 1997;2:78.

212. Tempany C, McNeil B: Advances in biomedical imaging. JAMA 2001;285:5627.

213. Temple MJ, Langer JC: Image-guided surgery for the pediatric patient: Ultrasound, computerized tomography, and magnetic resonance imaging. Curr Opin Pediatr 2003;15:256.

214. Tendick F Jr, Tharp G, Stark L: Sensing and manipulation problems in endoscopic surgery: Experiment, analysis and observation. Presence 1993;2:66.

215. Timmerman R, Papiez L, McGarry R, et al: Extracranial stereotactic radioablation: Results of a phase I study in medically inoperable stage I non–small cell lung cancer. Chest 2003;124:1946.

216. Timmerman R, Papiez L, Suntharalingam M: Extracranial stereotactic radiation delivery: Expansion of technology beyond the brain. Technol Cancer Res Treat 2003; 2:153.

217. Tokuuye K, Sumi M, Ikeda H, et al: Technical considerations for fractionated stereotactic radiotherapy of hepatocellular carcinoma. Jpn J Clin Oncol 1997;27:170.

218. Tome WA, Mehta MP, Meeks SL, et al: Fractionated stereotactic radiotherapy: A short review. Technol Cancer Res Treat 2002;1:153.

219. Townsend DW: Physical principles and technology of clinical PET imaging. Ann Acad Med Singapore 2004;33:133.

220. Townsend DW, Carney JP, Yap JT, et al: PET/CT today and tomorrow. J Nucl Med 2004;45(Suppl 1):4S.

221. Tranquart F, Grenier N, Eder V, et al: Clinical use of ultrasound tissue harmonic imaging. Ultrasound Med Biol 1999;25:889.

222. Treece GM, Prager RW, Gee AH, et al: Correction of probe pressure artifacts in freehand 3D ultrasound. Med Image Anal 2002;6:199.

223. Triadafilopoulos G, DiBaise JK, Nostrant TT, et al: The Stretta procedure for the treatment of GERD: 6 and 12 month follow-up of the U.S. open label trial. Gastrointest Endosc 2002;55:149.

224. Uematsu M: [Stereotactic radiation therapy for non small cell lung cancer.] Nippon Geka Gakkai Zasshi 2002; 103:256.

225. Uhlendorf V: Physics of ultrasound contrast imaging: Scattering in the linear range. IEEE Trans Ultrasonics Ferroelectrics Frequency Control 1994;41:70.

226. Unger EC, Cohen MS, Gatenby RA, et al: Single breath-holding scans of the abdomen using FISP and FLASH at 1.5 T. J Comput Assist Tomogr 1988;12:575.

227. van Leeuwen MS, Obertop H, Hennipman AH, Fernandez MA: 3-D reconstruction of hepatic neoplasms: A preoperative planning procedure. Baillieres Clin Gastroenterol 1995;9:121.

228. Verheij M, Bartelink H: Radiation-induced apoptosis. Cell Tissue Res 2000;301:133.

229. Viirre E, Pryor H, Nagata S, Furness TA 3rd: The virtual retinal display: A new technology for virtual reality and augmented vision in medicine. Stud Health Technol Inform 1998;50:252.

230. Vooijs M, Jonkers J, Lyons S, et al: Noninvasive imaging of spontaneous retinoblastoma pathway–dependent tumors in mice. Cancer Res 2002;62:1892.

231. Wara W, Bauman G, Gutin P, et al: Stereotactic radiosurgery in children. Stereotact Funct Neurosurg 1995; 64(Suppl 1):118.

232. Waterworth JA: Virtual Reality in Medicine: A Survey of the State of the Art. Umea, Sweden, Umea University, 1998, p 1.

233. Weissleder R, Mahmood U: Molecular imaging. Radiology 2001;219:316.

234. Weprin BE, Hall WA, Cho KH, et al: Stereotactic radiosurgery in pediatric patients. Pediatr Neurol 1996;15:193.

235. Whyte RI, Crownover R, Murphy MJ, et al: Stereotactic radiosurgery for lung tumors: Preliminary report of a phase I trial. Ann Thorac Surg 2003;75:1097.

236. Wilke M, Holland SK, Myseros JS, et al: Functional magnetic resonance imaging in pediatrics. Neuropediatrics 2003;34:225.

237. Wilson RD: Prenatal evaluation for fetal surgery. Curr Opin Obstet Gynecol 2002;14:187.

238. Wulf J, Hadinger U, Oppitz U, et al: Stereotactic radiotherapy of extracranial targets: CT-simulation and accuracy of treatment in the stereotactic body frame. Radiother Oncol 2000;57:225.

239. Wulf J, Hadinger U, Oppitz U, et al: Stereotactic radiotherapy of targets in the lung and liver. Strahlenther Onkol 2001;177:645.

240. Wulf J, Hadinger U, Oppitz U, et al: Impact of target reproducibility on tumor dose in stereotactic radiotherapy of targets in the lung and liver. Radiother Oncol 2003;66:141.

241. Yin F, Kim JG, Haughton C, et al: Extracranial radiosurgery: Immobilizing liver motion in dogs using high-frequency jet ventilation and total intravenous anesthesia. Int J Radiat Oncol Biol Phys 2001;49:211.

242. Young RF: Application of robotics to stereotactic neurosurgery. Neurol Res 1987;9:123.

243. Zimmerman RA, Haselgrove JC, Wang Z, et al: Advances in pediatric neuroimaging. Brain Dev 1998;20:275.

244. Zissiadis Y, Dutton S, Kieran M, et al: Stereotactic radiotherapy for pediatric intracranial germ cell tumors. Int J Radiat Oncol Biol Phys 2001;51:108.

Chapter 5

The Fetus as a Patient

Michael R. Harrison

Many congenital defects of interest to pediatric surgeons can now be detected before birth. Although some inherited anatomic malformations may be sought specifically, most are identified serendipitously during sonography performed for obstetric indications. Sometimes the conditions that lead to prenatal diagnosis are associated with underlying fetal malformations, such as oligohydramnios associated with fetal urinary tract obstruction, or polyhydramnios associated with fetal intestinal obstruction.

Prenatal diagnosis improves perinatal care. Severe lesions detected early enough may lead to counseling and termination of pregnancy. Most correctable defects are best managed by maternal transport to an appropriate center and delivery near term; some may benefit from a change in the timing or mode of delivery (Table 5-1). Finally, serial study of affected fetuses may help unravel the developmental pathophysiology of some surgically correctable lesions and thus lead to improved treatment before or after birth. It is important that surgeons familiar with the management of these lesions after birth be involved in management decisions and family counseling.[28]

FETAL IMAGING

Direct imaging of the fetus has advanced rapidly in the past 3 decades. Fetal anatomy, normal and abnormal, can be accurately delineated by ultrasonography (US). This noninvasive technique appears to be safe for both the fetus and the mother and is now routinely applied in most pregnancies. The details of ultrasonographic diagnosis are covered elsewhere,[28] but it is important to remember that sonography is operator dependent. The scope and reliability of the information obtained are directly proportional to the skill and experience of the sonographer, and that information can be crucial to management. For example, management of a fetal defect requires a thorough evaluation of the fetus for other abnormalities, because malformations often occur as part of a syndrome. Three-dimensional US has not added much to the accuracy or sensitivity of diagnosis but may prove advantageous for US-guided interventions.

Real-time US may yield important information on fetal movement and fetal vital functions (heart rate variability, breathing movements) that reflect fetal well-being. Serial US evaluation is particularly useful in defining the natural history and progression of fetal disease. Increased nuchal translucency is a finding that correlates with chromosomal and some structural abnormalities; thus US can be used as a noninvasive screening technique at 11 to 14 weeks' gestation. Finally, fetal fluids (urine, ascites, pleural fluid, blood, cerebrospinal fluid) can be aspirated under real-time US guidance for both diagnosis and therapy.[28] In my experience with more than 500 cases, this technique has proved safe and relatively easy.

Although US has supplanted most conventional radiographic studies, very fast computed tomography and magnetic resonance imaging scanners allow imaging of the fetus without the need for anesthesia or paralysis in most cases. Volume measurement of organs (e.g., hypoplastic lungs) is possible, but this has not proved significantly better than earlier US measurements (e.g., lung-to-head ratio) in determining prognosis. Magnetic resonance imaging is far superior for central nervous system malformations and acquired lesions and thus may be crucial in determining neurologic prognosis.[28]

BIOCHEMICAL SCREENING

An elevated alpha fetoprotein (AFP) level in maternal serum and amniotic fluid is a reliable indicator of a fetal abnormality. Although used to screen for neural tube defects, AFP is also elevated in such defects as omphalocele, gastroschisis, and sacrococcygeal teratoma, in which transudation of fetal serum is increased. AFP is the major glycoprotein of fetal serum and resembles albumin in molecular weight, amino acid sequence, and immunologic characteristics. The AFP level in fetal serum reaches a peak of 3 mg/mL at 13 to 15 menstrual weeks. AFP concentration in amniotic fluid follows a curve similar to that of fetal serum, but at a 150-fold dilution. Measuring other markers (e.g., estriol and chorionic gonadotropins) enhances aneuploidy screening.

TABLE 5-1 Management of Prenatally Diagnosed Defects

Defects Usually Managed by Pregnancy Termination
Anencephaly, hydranencephaly, alobar holoprosencephaly
Severe anomalies associated with chromosomal abnormalities
   (e.g., trisomy 13)
Bilateral renal agenesis, infantile polycystic kidney disease
Severe, untreatable, inherited metabolic disorders
   (e.g., Tay-Sachs disease)
Lethal bone dysplasias (e.g., thanatophoric dysplasia, recessive
   osteogenesis imperfecta)

Defects Detectable in Utero but Best Corrected after Delivery Near Term
Esophageal, duodenal, jejunoileal, and anorectal atresias
Meconium ileus (cystic fibrosis)
Enteric cysts and duplications
Small, intact omphalocele and gastroschisis
Unilateral multicystic dysplastic kidney, hydronephrosis
Craniofacial, limb, and chest wall deformities
Simple cystic hygroma
Small sacrococcygeal teratoma, mesoblastic nephroma,
   neuroblastoma
Benign cysts (e.g., ovarian, mesenteric, choledochal)

Defects That May Lead to Cesarean Delivery
Conjoined twins
Giant or ruptured omphalocele, gastroschisis
Severe hydrocephalus, large or ruptured meningomyelocele
Large sacrococcygeal teratoma or cervical cystic hygroma
Malformations requiring preterm delivery in the presence of
   inadequate labor or fetal distress

Defects That May Lead to Induced Preterm Delivery
Progressively enlarging hydrocephalus, hydrothorax
Gastroschisis or ruptured omphalocele with damaged bowel
Intestinal ischemia and necrosis secondary to volvulus or
   meconium ileus
Progressive hydrops fetalis
Intrauterine growth retardation
Arrhythmias (e.g., supraventricular tachycardia with failure)

Defects That May Require EXIT Procedure
Congenital high airway obstruction syndrome (CHAOS)
Large cervical tumor (e.g., teratoma)
Mass obstructing trachea or mouth (e.g., cystic hygroma)
Conditions requiring immediate ECMO cannulation
Chest mass preventing lung expansion

ECMO, extracorporeal membrane oxygenation; EXIT, ex utero intrapartum treatment.

FETAL SAMPLING

Cells can be obtained for karyotyping and for DNA-based diagnosis of many genetic defects and inherited metabolic abnormalities. Chorionic villus sampling (transvaginal or transabdominal) allows diagnosis in the first trimester, whereas amniocentesis is usually performed in the second trimester. The most common indication is advanced maternal age, known carrier state, or previous child with a genetic disorder. Fetal blood can be obtained by US-guided percutaneous umbilical cord sampling as early as 14 weeks' gestation. Culture of blood cells allows more

rapid karyotyping (2 days versus 7 days for amniocentesis). Biopsies of fetal skin and liver can be performed using sonography or fetoscopy. The risk of fetal loss from sampling techniques ranges from 1% to 5%.

Powerful new sorting techniques now allow isolation of fetal cells in the maternal circulation, allowing genetic testing for some diseases from a maternal blood sample alone. Rapid advances in molecular analysis combined with mapping of the human genome will allow genetic diagnosis of an ever-increasing number of diseases.[28]

FETAL ACCESS

Although most anatomic malformations diagnosed by prenatal US are best managed by appropriate medical and surgical therapy after delivery, a few simple anatomic abnormalities that have predictable devastating developmental consequences may require correction before birth.[18,19,29] In the 1980s the developmental pathophysiology of several potentially correctable lesions was studied in animal models; the natural history was determined by serial observation of human fetuses; selection criteria for intervention were developed; and anesthetic, tocolytic, and surgical techniques for hysterotomy and fetal surgery were refined.[2,19,21,23,28,29]

This investment in basic and clinical research has already benefited some fetal patients with a few relatively rare defects and will benefit many more as new forms of therapy, including stem cell transplantation, tissue engineering, and gene therapy, are applied to a wide variety of anatomic and biochemical defects. Some milestones in the development of fetal therapy are listed in Table 5-2.

The technical aspects of hysterotomy for open fetal surgery, which evolved over 30 years of experimental and clinical work, are presented in Figure 5-1.[28] Because the morbidity of hysterotomy (particularly preterm labor) is significant, videoendoscopic fetal surgery (FETENDO) techniques that obviate the need for a uterine incision were developed (Fig. 5-2).[17] Complex fetoscopic surgery with multiple ports may require maternal mini-laparotomy (e.g., FETENDO clip or FETENDO balloon for tracheal occlusion). Percutaneous fetoscopic intervention has been applied clinically for diagnostic biopsies, laser ablation of placental vessels in twin-twin transfusion syndrome,[53] fetal cystoscopy and urinary tract decompression,[40] cord ligature or division for anomalous twins,[12,45] and division of amniotic bands. Percutaneous US-guided intervention has been applied to the placement of catheter-shunts (bladder, chest),[40,47] vascular access (heart, umbilical vessels), radiofrequency ablation of large tumors or anomalous twins,[55] aspiration of fluid from fetal body cavities,[50] and administration of drugs or cells directly to the fetus.[16]

MANAGEMENT OF MOTHER AND FETUS

Breaching the uterus, whether by puncture or incision, incites uterine contractions. Despite technical advances,

TABLE 5–2 Milestones in Fetal Therapy

Event	Place	Year
IUT for Rh disease	Women's National Hospital, Auckland, NZ	1961
Hysterotomy for fetal vascular access—IUT	University of Puerto Rico	1964
Fetoscopy—diagnostic	Yale	1974
Experimental pathophysiology (sheep model)	UCSF	1980
Hysterotomy and maternal safety (monkey model)	UCSF	1981
Vesicoamniotic shunt for uropathy	UCSF	1982
Vesicoamniotic shunt for hydrocephalus	Denver	1982
International Fetal Medicine and Surgery Society founded	Santa Barbara, Calif	1982
Open fetal surgery for uropathy	UCSF	1983
CCAM resection	UCSF	1984
First edition, *Unborn Patient: Prenatal Diagnosis and Treatment*	UCSF	1984
Intravascular transfusion	King's College, London University	1985
CDH open repair	UCSF	1989
Anomalous twin-cord ligation, RFA	King's College, London University	1990
NIH trial: open repair CDH	UCSF	1990
Aortic balloon valvuloplasty	King's College, London University	1991
SCT resection	UCSF	1992
Laser ablation of placental vessels	St. Joseph's Hospital, Milwaukee; King's College, London University	1995
EXIT procedure for airway obstruction	UCSF	1995
Fetoscopic surgery (FETENDO)	UCSF	1996
Stem cell treatment for SCIDS	Detroit	1996
CDH—FETENDO clip, balloon	UCSF	1997
Myelomeningocele—open repair	Vanderbilt	1997
NIH trial: FETENDO balloon in CDH	UCSF	1998
Resection of pericardial teratoma	UCSF	2000
EuroFetus trial for twin-twin transfusion syndrome	University Hospital, Gasthuisberg, Belgium; Université Paris-Ouest, Versailles, France	2001
Resection of cervical teratoma	UCSF	2001
NIH trial: open repair myelomeningocele	UCSF, CHOP, Vanderbilt	2002
NIH trial: twin-twin transfusion syndrome	CHOP, UCSF, Perinatal Network	2002
Balloon dilatation for hypoplastic heart	Harvard	2003

CCAM, congenital cystic adenomatoid malformation; CDH, congenital diaphragmatic hernia; CHOP, Children's Hospital of Philadelphia; EXIT, ex utero intrapartum treatment; IUT, intrauterine transfusion; NIH, National Institutes of Health; RFA, radiofrequency ablation; SCIDS, severe combined immunodeficiency syndrome; SCT, sacrococcygeal teratoma; UCSF, University of California–San Francisco.

disruption of membranes and preterm labor are the Achilles' heel of fetal therapy. Although halogenated inhalation agents provide satisfactory anesthesia for mother and fetus, the depth of anesthesia necessary to achieve intraoperative uterine relaxation can produce fetal and maternal myocardial depression and affect placental perfusion.[52] Indomethacin can constrict the fetal ductus arteriosus, and the combination of magnesium sulfate and betamimetics can produce maternal pulmonary edema. The search for a more effective and less toxic tocolytic regimen led to the demonstration in monkeys that exogenous nitric oxide ablates preterm labor induced by hysterotomy.[39] Intravenous nitroglycerin is a potent tocolytic but requires careful control to avoid serious complications.[28]

Postoperative management takes place in the fetal intensive care unit. Maternal arterial pressure, central venous pressure, urine output, and oxygen saturation are continuously monitored. Fetal well-being and uterine activity are recorded externally by tocodynamometer. Patient-controlled analgesia, continuous epidural analgesics, or both ease maternal stress and aid tocolysis.

When labor is controlled and the fetus is stable, the patient is transferred to the obstetric ward. Outpatient monitoring and tocolysis continue, and fetal sonograms are performed at least weekly. Open hysterotomy requires cesarean delivery in this and future pregnancies.[11,43]

RISKS OF MATERNAL-FETAL SURGERY

For the fetus, the risk of the procedure is balanced against the benefit of correction of a fatal or debilitating defect. The risks and benefits for the mother are more difficult to assess. Most fetal malformations do not directly threaten the mother's health, yet she is subject to significant risk and discomfort from the procedure. She may choose to accept the risk for the sake of the unborn fetus and to alleviate the burden of raising a child with a severe malformation.

There is a paucity of published data on the maternal impact of fetal surgical interventions.[43] My colleagues and I analyzed maternal morbidity and mortality associated with different types of fetal intervention (open hysterotomy, various endoscopic procedures, and percutaneous

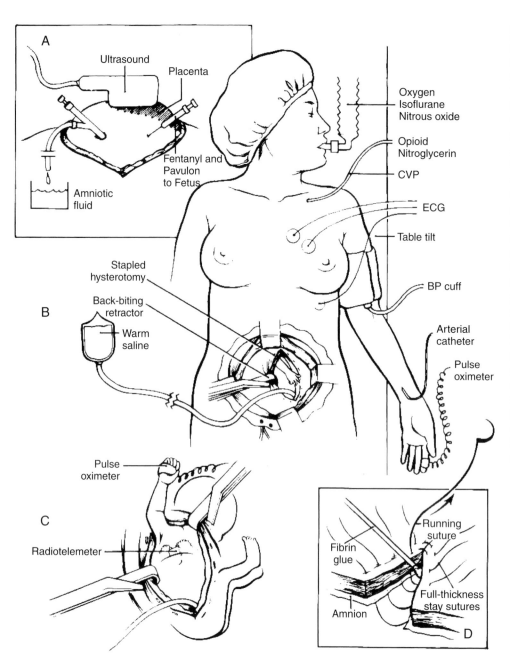

Figure 5-1 Summary of open fetal surgery techniques. *A,* The uterus is exposed through a low, transverse abdominal incision. Ultrasonography is used to localize the placenta, inject the fetus with narcotic and muscle relaxant, and aspirate amniotic fluid. *B,* The uterus is opened with staples that provide hemostasis and seal the membranes. Warm saline solution is continuously infused around the fetus. Maternal anesthesia, tocolysis, and monitoring are shown. Absorbable staples and back-biting clamps facilitate hysterotomy exposure of the pertinent fetal part. *C,* A miniaturized pulse oximeter records pulse rate and oxygen saturation intraoperatively. A radiotelemeter monitors fetal electrocardiogram (ECG) and amniotic pressure during and after the operation. *D,* After fetal repair, the uterine incision is closed with absorbable sutures and fibrin glue. Amniotic fluid is restored with warm lactated Ringer's solution. BP, blood pressure; CVP, central venous pressure.

techniques) to quantify this risk. We performed a retrospective evaluation of a continuous series of 187 cases performed between July 1989 and May 2003 at the University of California at San Francisco Fetal Treatment Center. Fetal surgery was performed by open hysterotomy in 87 cases, endoscopic techniques in 69, and percutaneous techniques in 31. There was no maternal mortality. Endoscopic procedures, even with a laparotomy, showed statistically significantly less morbidity compared with the open hysterotomy group in terms of cesarean section as delivery mode (94.8% versus 58.8%, $P < 0.001$), requirement for intensive care unit stay (1.4% versus 26.4%, $P < 0.001$), length of hospital stay (7.9 versus 11.9 days, $P = 0.001$), and requirement for blood transfusions (2.9% versus 12.6%, $P = 0.022$). It was not significant for premature rupture of membranes, pulmonary edema, abruptio placentae, postoperative vaginal bleeding,

uncontrollable preterm labor leading to preterm delivery, or interval from fetal surgery to delivery. Chorion-amnion membrane separation occurred more often in the endoscopy group (64.7% versus 20.3%, $P < 0.001$). The percutaneous procedure group had the least morbidity.[11] This study confirmed that fetal surgery can be performed without maternal mortality. Short-term morbidity can be serious, however, impacting maternal health, length of the pregnancy, and survival of the fetus.

Because midgestation hysterotomy is not done in the lower uterine segment, delivery after fetal surgery and all future deliveries should be by cesarean section. In our series, two uterine disruptions occurred in subsequent pregnancies; uterine closure and neonatal outcome were excellent in both cases. Finally, the ability to carry and deliver subsequent infants does not appear to be jeopardized by fetal surgery.

Figure 5-2 Operating room setup. Note that there are two monitors at the head of the table: one for the fetoscopic picture, and the other for the real-time ultrasound image.

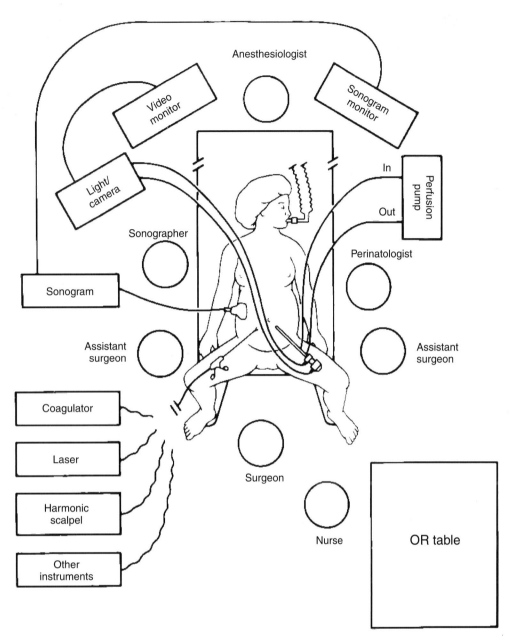

PRENATAL DIAGNOSIS DICTATES PERINATAL MANAGEMENT

The nature of the defect determines perinatal management (see Table 5-1).[28] When serious malformations that are incompatible with postnatal life are diagnosed early enough, the family has the option of terminating the pregnancy. Most correctable malformations that can be diagnosed in utero are best managed by appropriate medical and surgical therapy after delivery near term; prenatal diagnosis allows delivery at a center where a neonatal surgical team is prepared to act. Elective cesarean delivery rather than a trial at vaginal delivery may be indicated for fetal malformations that cause dystocia or that will benefit from immediate surgical repair in a sterile environment.

Early delivery may be indicated for fetal conditions that require treatment as soon as possible after diagnosis,

but the risk of prematurity must be carefully considered. The rationale for early delivery is unique to each anomaly, but the principle remains the same: continued gestation will have progressive ill effects on the fetus. In some cases, the function of a specific organ system is compromised by the lesion (e.g., hydronephrosis) and will continue to deteriorate until the lesion is corrected. In some malformations, the progressive ill effects on the fetus result directly from being in utero (e.g., the bowel damage in gastroschisis from exposure to amniotic fluid).

Some fetal deficiency states may be alleviated by treatment before birth (Table 5-3). For example, blood can be transfused into the fetal peritoneal cavity or directly into the umbilical artery, and antiarrhythmic drugs can be given transplacentally to convert fetal supraventricular tachycardia. When the necessary substrate, medication, or nutrient cannot be delivered across the placenta,

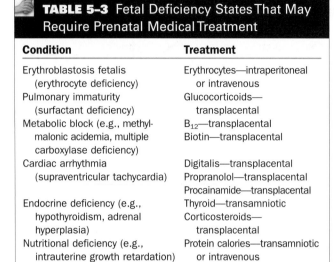

TABLE 5-3 Fetal Deficiency States That May Require Prenatal Medical Treatment

Condition	Treatment
Erythroblastosis fetalis (erythrocyte deficiency)	Erythrocytes—intraperitoneal or intravenous
Pulmonary immaturity (surfactant deficiency)	Glucocorticoids—transplacental
Metabolic block (e.g., methyl-malonic acidemia, multiple carboxylase deficiency)	B$_{12}$—transplacental Biotin—transplacental
Cardiac arrhythmia (supraventricular tachycardia)	Digitalis—transplacental Propranolol—transplacental Procainamide—transplacental
Endocrine deficiency (e.g., hypothyroidism, adrenal hyperplasia)	Thyroid—transamniotic Corticosteroids—transplacental
Nutritional deficiency (e.g., intrauterine growth retardation)	Protein calories—transamniotic or intravenous

it may be injected into the amniotic fluid, where it can be swallowed and absorbed by the fetus. In the future, it is possible that deficiencies in cellular function will be corrected by providing the appropriate stem cell graft or the appropriately engineered gene.[14,16]

FETAL PROBLEMS AMENABLE TO SURGICAL CORRECTION BEFORE BIRTH

The only anatomic malformations that warrant consideration are those that interfere with fetal organ development and that, if alleviated, would allow normal development to proceed (Table 5-4). Initially, a few life-threatening malformations were intensively studied and successfully corrected. Over the last decade, an increasing number of fetal defects have been defined and new treatments devised.[21,28] As less invasive interventional techniques have been developed and proved safe, a few nonlethal anomalies (e.g., myelomeningocele) are now candidates for fetal surgical correction.[10,38,58] Finally, stem cell transplantation, gene therapy, and tissue engineering should allow the treatment of a variety of inherited disorders.[14,16,32,51]

TABLE 5-4 Fetal Conditions Amenable to Treatment before Birth

	Effect on Development (Rationale for Treatment)	Result without Treatment	Recommended Treatment
Life-Threatening Defects			
Urinary obstruction (urethral valves)	Hydronephrosis Lung hypoplasia	Renal failure Pulmonary failure	Percutaneous vesicoamniotic shunt Fetoscopic ablation of valves Open vesicostomy
Cystic adenomatoid malformation	Lung hypoplasia, hydrops	Hydrops, death	Open pulmonary lobectomy Ablation (laser, RFA) Steroids Open complete repair
Congenital diaphragmatic hernia	Lung hypoplasia	Pulmonary failure	Temporary tracheal occlusion: tracheal clip (open and fetoscopic), fetoscopic balloon (percutaneous, reversible)
Sacrococcygeal teratoma	High-output failure	Hydrops, death	Open resection of tumor Vascular occlusion: RFA, alcohol RFA
Twin-twin transfusion syndrome	Donor-recipient steal through placenta	Fetal hydrops, death; neurologic damage to survivor	Fetoscopic laser ablation of placental vessels (NIH trial) Amnioreduction (NIH trial) Selective reduction
Acardiac or anomalous twin (TRAP)	Vascular steal Embolization	Death or damage to surviving twin	Selective reduction Cord occlusion or division RFA
Aqueductal stenosis	Hydrocephalus	Brain damage	Ventriculoamniotic shunt
Valvular obstruction	Hypoplastic heart	Heart failure	Balloon valvuloplasty
Congenital high airway obstruction syndrome (CHAOS)	Overdistention by lung fluid	Hydrops, death	Fetoscopic tracheostomy EXIT
Cervical teratoma	Airway obstruction High-output failure	Hydrops, death	Open resection EXIT Vascular occlusion: alcohol, RFA RFA

Continued

TABLE 5–4 Fetal Conditions Amenable to Treatment before Birth—Cont'd			
	Effect on Development (Rationale for Treatment)	**Result without Treatment**	**Recommended Treatment**
Non-Life-Threatening Defects			
Myelomeningocele	Spinal cord damage	Paralysis, neurogenic bladder or bowel, hydrocephalus	Open repair (NIH trial) Fetoscopic coverage
Gastroschisis	Bowel damage	Malnutrition, short bowel	Serial amnio-exchange
Cleft lip and palate	Facial defect and deformity	Persistent	Fetoscopic repair* Open repair
Metabolic and Cellular Defects			
Stem cell or enzyme defects	Hemoglobinopathy Immunodeficiency Storage diseases	Anemia, hydrops Infection, death Retardation, death	Fetal stem cell transplant Fetal gene therapy*
Predictable organ defect	Agenesis or hypoplasia of heart, lung, kidney	Neonatal heart, lung, kidney failure	Induce tolerance for postnatal organ transplant* Tissue engineering*

*Not yet attempted in human fetuses.
EXIT, ex utero intrapartum treatment; NIH, National Institutes of Health; RFA, radiofrequency ablation; TRAP, twin reversed arterial perfusion.

Urinary Tract Obstruction

Fetal urethral obstruction results in pulmonary hypoplasia and renal dysplasia, but these often fatal consequences can be ameliorated by urinary tract decompression before birth.[1] The natural history of untreated fetal urinary tract obstruction is well documented, and selection criteria based on fetal urine electrolyte and β_2-microglobulin levels and the ultrasonographic appearance of fetal kidneys have proved reliable.[40] Of all fetuses with urinary tract dilatation, as many as 90% do not require intervention. However, fetuses with bilateral hydronephrosis due to urethral obstruction who subsequently develop oligohydramnios require treatment. If the lungs are mature, the fetus can be delivered early for postnatal decompression. If the lungs are immature, the bladder can be decompressed in utero by a Harrison vesicoamniotic shunt placed percutaneously under ultrasound guidance, by fetoscopic vesicostomy, or by fetocystoscopic ablation of urethral valves.[40,47] Experience treating several hundred fetuses in many institutions suggests that selection is good enough to avoid inappropriate intervention, and that restoration of amniotic fluid can prevent the development of fatal pulmonary hypoplasia. It is not yet clear how much renal functional damage can be reversed by decompression.

Cystic Adenomatoid Malformation

Although congenital cystic adenomatoid malformation often presents as a benign pulmonary mass in infants and children, some fetuses with large lesions die in utero or at birth from hydrops and pulmonary hypoplasia. The pathophysiology of hydrops and the feasibility of resecting the fetal lung have been studied in animals. Experience managing more than 200 cases suggests that most lesions can be successfully treated after birth and that some lesions resolve before birth. Although only a few fetuses with very large lesions develop hydrops before 26 weeks' gestation, these lesions may progress rapidly, leading to the fetuses' death in utero. Careful US surveillance of large lesions is necessary to detect the first signs of hydrops, because fetuses who develop this condition can be successfully treated by emergency resection of the cystic lobe in utero.[25] Fetal pulmonary lobectomy has proved to be surprisingly simple and quite successful at two large fetal surgery centers.[1] For lesions consisting of single large cysts, thoracoamniotic shunting has also been successful.[59] Percutaneous ablation techniques are being investigated. Regression of very large lesions and hydrops has been observed after maternal steroid treatment.[56]

Congenital Diaphragmatic Hernia

Congenital diaphragmatic hernia (CDH) can now be accurately diagnosed by midgestation, and the outcome for individual cases can be predicted by ultrasonographic measurement of the lung-to-head ratio (LHR) and the presence or absence of liver herniation into the thorax. Fetuses without liver herniation and a favorable LHR (>1.4) have low mortality after term delivery at tertiary centers. However, fetuses with liver herniation and a low LHR have a high mortality and morbidity despite recent advances in intensive neonatal care, including extracorporeal membrane oxygenation (ECMO), nitric oxide inhalation, high-frequency ventilation, and delayed operative repair of the hernia.[4-6,8,23,41,50]

The fundamental problem in babies born with CDH is pulmonary hypoplasia. The aim of research in experimental animal models and later in human subjects over 2 decades has been to improve growth of the hypoplastic lungs before they are needed for gas exchange at birth. Anatomic repair of the hernia by open hysterotomy proved feasible but did not decrease mortality and was abandoned.[22,26] Fetal tracheal occlusion was developed as an alternative strategy to promote fetal lung growth by preventing normal egress of lung fluid. Occlusion of the fetal trachea was shown to stimulate fetal lung growth in a variety of animal models.[9,13,46] Techniques to achieve reversible fetal tracheal occlusion were explored in animal models and then applied clinically, evolving from external metal clips placed on the trachea by open hysterotomy or fetoscopic neck dissection to internal tracheal occlusion with a detachable silicone balloon placed by fetal bronchoscopy through a single 5-mm uterine port.[3,7,27]

The initial experience suggested that fetal endoscopic tracheal occlusion improved survival in human fetuses with severe CDH.[27,31,33] To evaluate this novel therapy, my colleagues and I conducted a randomized, controlled trial comparing tracheal occlusion with standard care.[30] Survival with fetal endoscopic tracheal occlusion met expectations (73% actual; 75% predicted) and was better than that of historical controls (37%), but it was no better than that of concurrent randomized controls. The higher-than-expected survival in the standard-care group may be because the study design mandated that patients in both treatment groups be delivered, resuscitated, and intensively managed in a unit experienced in caring for critically ill newborns with pulmonary hypoplasia.[30]

Attempts to improve the outcome of severe CDH by treatment either before or after birth have been double-edged swords. Intensive care after birth has improved survival but increased long-term sequelae in survivors, and it is expensive.[5,6,8,23,50] Intervention before birth may increase lung size, but prematurity caused by the intervention itself can be detrimental.[15,20,22,24,31] In our study, babies with severe CDH who had tracheal occlusion before birth were born, on average, at 31 weeks as a consequence of the intervention. Their survival rates and respiratory outcomes (including duration of oxygen requirement) were comparable to those of infants without tracheal occlusion who were born at 37 weeks, suggesting that tracheal occlusion improves pulmonary hypoplasia, but the improvement in lung growth is affected by pulmonary immaturity related to earlier delivery.[30]

These results underscore the important role of randomized trials in evaluating promising new therapies. This was the second National Institutes of Health–sponsored trial evaluating a new prenatal intervention for severe fetal CDH. The first trial showed that complete surgical repair of the anatomic defect (which required hysterotomy), though feasible, was no better than postnatal repair in improving survival and was ineffective when the liver as well as the bowel was herniated.[22] That trial led to the abandonment of open complete repair at our institution and subsequently around the world. Information derived from that trial regarding measures of the severity of pulmonary hypoplasia (including liver herniation and development of the LHR) led to an alternative physiologic strategy to enlarge the hypoplastic fetal lung by temporary tracheal occlusion[20,24,33] and to the development of less invasive fetal endoscopic techniques that did not require hysterotomy to achieve temporary, reversible tracheal occlusion.[3,17,27]

Our ability to accurately diagnose and assess the severity of CDH before birth has improved dramatically.

Fetuses with CDH who have associated anomalies do poorly, whereas fetuses with isolated CDH, no liver herniation, and LHRs above 1.4 have an excellent prognosis (100% in our experience). In our study, fetuses with LHRs between 0.9 and 1.4 had a better than 80% chance of survival when delivered at a tertiary care center. The small number of fetuses with LHRs below 0.9 had a poor prognosis in both treatment groups and should be the focus of further studies.[30]

Because tracheal occlusion is effective in enlarging hypoplastic lungs, other approaches to tracheal occlusion might be beneficial. Although the duration of occlusion in this study (36.2 ± 14.7 days) is comparable to that studied in animal models, the optimal timing and duration of occlusion are not known in humans. Short-term occlusion later in gestation and earlier occlusion (with possible reversal in utero) have been studied in animal models[13,46] and applied in humans.[7] It is also possible that the risk of premature rupture of membranes leading to preterm labor and delivery might be reduced by using smaller 2-mm fetoscopes percutaneously and newly developed techniques to seal membranes.

Myelomeningocele

Myelomeningocele is a devastating birth defect with sequelae that affect both the central and peripheral nervous systems. Altered cerebrospinal fluid dynamics results in the Chiari II malformation and hydrocephalus. Damage to the exposed spinal cord results in lifelong lower extremity neurologic deficiency, urinary incontinence, sexual dysfunction, and skeletal deformities. This defect carries enormous personal, familial, and societal costs, because the near-normal life span of affected children is characterized by hospitalization, multiple operations, disability, and institutionalization. Although it has been assumed that the spinal cord itself is intrinsically malformed in children with this defect, recent work suggests that the neurologic impairment after birth may be due to exposure of and trauma to the spinal cord in utero, and that covering the exposed cord may prevent the development of the Chiari malformation.[10,49,58]

Since 1997, more than 200 fetuses have had in utero closure of myelomeningocele by open fetal surgery. Preliminary clinical evidence suggests that this procedure reduces the incidence of shunt-dependent hydrocephalus and restores the cerebellum and brainstem to a more normal configuration.[58] However, clinical results of fetal surgery for myelomeningocele are based on comparisons with historical controls; examine only efficacy, not safety; and lack long-term follow-up.

The National Institutes of Health has funded a multicenter, randomized clinical trial (the Management of Myelomeningocele Study [MOMS]) of 200 patients that will be conducted at three fetal surgery units—University of California–San Francisco, Children's Hospital of Philadelphia, and Vanderbilt University Medical Center; the George Washington University Biostatistics Center will be the independent data and study coordinating center. The primary objectives of this randomized trial are to determine (1) whether intrauterine repair of fetal myelomeningocele at 19 to 26 weeks' gestation using a standard multilayer closure improves outcome, as measured by death or the need for ventricular decompressive shunting by 1 year of life, compared with standard postnatal care; and (2) whether intrauterine repair of myelomeningocele can improve cognitive function as measured by the Bayley Scales of Infant Development mental development index at 30 months' corrected age. There is a moratorium on performing this surgery outside the trial until the results are reported.

Airway Obstruction

The tracheal occlusion strategy for fetal CDH required the development of techniques to safely reverse the obstruction at birth. The ex utero intrapartum treatment (EXIT) procedure is a technique in which the principles of fetal surgery (anesthesia for mother and fetus, complete uterine relaxation, and maintenance of umbilical circulation to support the fetus) are used during cesarean delivery to allow the airway to be secured while the fetus remains on maternal bypass. The EXIT procedure has been used successfully to reverse tracheal occlusion, repair the trachea, secure the airway by tracheotomy, resect large cervical tumors, place vascular cannulas for immediate extracorporeal life support using ECMO, and manage laryngeal obstruction in congenital high airway obstruction syndrome.[1,35,36]

The EXIT procedure provides a wonderful opportunity for surgeons, perinatologists, neonatologists, and anesthesiologists to learn to work together and should be one of the first procedures performed in new fetal treatment centers.

Sacrococcygeal Teratoma

Most neonates with sacrococcygeal teratoma survive, and malignant invasion is unusual. However, the prognosis of patients with sacrococcygeal teratoma diagnosed prenatally (by US or elevated AFP) is less favorable. There is a subset of fetuses (<20%) with large tumors who develop hydrops from high output failure secondary to extremely high blood flow through the tumor. Because hydrops progresses rapidly to fetal death, frequent US follow-up is mandatory. Excision of the tumor reverses the pathophysiology if it is performed before the mirror syndrome (maternal eclampsia) develops in the mother.[28,34] Attempts to interrupt the vascular steal by ablating blood flow to the tumor by alcohol injection or embolization have not been successful. US-guided radiofrequency ablation of the vascular pedicle has worked, but with unacceptable damage to adjacent structures.

Twin-Twin Transfusion Syndrome

Twin-twin transfusion syndrome (TTTS) is a complication of monochorionic multiple gestations resulting from an imbalance in blood flow through vascular communications, or chorioangiopagus, such that one twin is compromised and the other is favored. It is the most common serious complication of monochorionic twin gestations, affecting between 4% and 35% of such pregnancies, or approximately 0.1 to 0.9 births per 1000 in the United States each year. Despite the relatively low incidence, TTTS disproportionately accounts for 17% of all perinatal mortality associated with twin gestations. Standard therapy has been limited to serial amnioreduction, which improves the overall outcome but has little impact on the more severe end of the spectrum in TTTS. In addition, survivors of TTTS treated by serial amnioreduction have an 18% to 26% incidence of significant neurologic and cardiac morbidity. Selective fetoscopic laser photocoagulation of chorioangiopagus has emerged as an alternative treatment strategy with at least comparable, if not superior, survival to serial amnioreduction, as demonstrated in a randomized trial in Europe.[12,53]

Twin Reversed Arterial Perfusion Syndrome

Acardiac twinning is a rare anomaly in which a normal "pump" twin perfuses an acardiac twin, resulting in twin reversed arterial perfusion (TRAP) syndrome. In acardiac monochorionic twin gestations, this compromises the viability of the morphologically normal pump twin. Selective reduction and obliteration of blood flow in the acardiac twin have been accomplished by a variety of techniques, including fetectomy; ligation, division, and cauterization of the umbilical cord; and obliteration of the circulation in the anomalous twin by alcohol injection, electrocautery, or radiofrequency ablation.[12,45] My colleagues and I have used a 14- or 17-gauge radiofrequency ablation probe and real-time US guidance in a minimally invasive, percutaneous technique that effectively obliterates the blood supply of the acardiac fetus and protects the pump twin.[55] Our experience with more than 30 cases has been excellent.

Aqueductal Stenosis

Obstruction to the flow of cerebrospinal fluid dilates the ventricles, compresses the developing brain, and eventually compromises neurologic function. For severe cases with progression in utero, decompressing the ventricles may ameliorate the adverse effects on the developing brain; however, percutaneously placed ventriculoamniotic shunts have not improved outcome.[47] As a result, a moratorium is being observed until the natural history is clarified and selection criteria and better fetal shunting techniques are developed.[37]

Aortic Obstruction and Hypoplastic Heart

A few simple structural cardiac defects that interfere with development may benefit from prenatal correction. If obstruction of blood flow across the pulmonary or aortic valve interferes with development of the ventricles or pulmonary or systemic vasculature, relief of the anatomic obstruction may allow normal development with an improved outcome.[48] For example, congenital aortic stenosis may lead to hypoplastic left heart syndrome. Stenotic aortic valves have been dilated by a balloon catheter placed percutaneously or in a transuterine procedure with maternal laparotomy, with promising results.[42,57] The procedure is technically difficult, however. Several centers are developing experimental techniques to correct fetal heart defects.

Gastroschisis

Patients born with gastroschisis require immediate surgical intervention after birth with either primary or staged closure of the abdominal wall. Despite closure of the abdominal wall defect, many babies face prolonged difficulty with nutrient absorption and intestinal motility. At birth, the intestines of these patients are frequently thickened and covered by a fibrinous "peel." Mesenteric shortening and intestinal atresia may also be present. The bowel damage may be due to constriction of the mesentery (like a napkin ring), causing poor lymphatic and venous drainage from the bowel, or to an inflammatory reaction to various substances in the amniotic fluid bathing the bowel.[54]

Serial amniotic fluid exchange has been used to dilute putative inflammatory mediators in an attempt to prevent bowel damage.[60] However, the ability to select those fetuses with damaged bowel is limited, and the volume of exchange may be inadequate to alter the outcome.

Cleft Lip and Palate

The observation that fetal wounds heal without scar formation has stimulated interest in the possibility of correcting cleft lip and palate in utero to avoid scarring, midfacial growth restriction, and secondary nasal deformity. However, the theoretical benefits of such repair are unproved and do not yet justify the risks of intervention.[44]

Inherited Defects Correctable by Fetal Stem Cell Transplantation

Various inherited defects that are potentially curable by hematopoietic stem cell (HSC) transplantation (e.g., immunodeficiencies, hemoglobinopathies, storage diseases) can now be detected early in gestation. Postnatal bone marrow transplantation is limited by donor availability, graft rejection, graft-versus-host disease, and patient deterioration before transplantation, which often begins in utero. Transplantation of fetal HCSs early in gestation may circumvent these difficulties.[14,32,51]

The rationale for in utero rather than postnatal transplantation is that the preimmune fetus (<15 weeks) should not reject the transplanted cells, and the fetal bone marrow is primed to receive HSCs that migrate from the fetal liver. Thus, myeloablation and immunosuppression may not be necessary. In addition, in utero transplantation allows treatment before fetal health is compromised by the underlying disease. The disadvantage of treatment in utero is that the fetus is difficult to access for diagnosis and treatment. Definitive diagnosis using molecular genetic techniques requires fetal tissue obtained by transvaginal or transabdominal chorionic villus sampling, amniocentesis, or fetal blood sampling. Delivering even a small volume (<1 mL) of cells to an early-gestation fetus by intra-abdominal or intravenous injection requires skill and carries significant risks. The greatest potential problem with in utero transplantation of HSCs is that the degree of engraftment or chimerism may not be sufficient to cure or palliate some diseases. In chronic granulomatous disease and severe combined immunodeficiency, relatively few normal donor cells can provide sufficient enzyme activity to alleviate symptoms. However, a significantly higher degree of donor cell engraftment and expression in the periphery might be necessary to change the course of such diseases as β-thalassemia or sickle cell disease. For diseases that require a high percentage of donor cells, a promising strategy is to induce tolerance in utero for subsequent postnatal booster injections from a living relative. The optimal source of donor HSCs for in utero transplantation is not known. Donor cells can be obtained from adult bone marrow or peripheral blood, from neonatal umbilical cord blood, or from the liver of aborted fetuses.

Clinical experience with fetal HSC transplantation is limited. Although engraftment has been successful in cases of severe combined immunodeficiency syndrome, for most other diseases, low levels of engraftment after injection have limited clinical efficacy.[14,16,32,51]

THE PAST AND FUTURE OF FETAL INTERVENTION

Although only a few fetal defects are currently amenable to surgical treatment, the enterprise of fetal surgery has produced some unexpected spin-offs that are of interest beyond this narrow therapeutic field. For pediatricians, neonatologists, and dysmorphologists, the natural history and pathophysiology of many previously mysterious conditions of newborns have been clarified by following the development of the disease in utero. For obstetricians, perinatologists, and fetologists, techniques developed during experiments in lambs and monkeys will prove to be useful in managing high-risk pregnancies. For example, an absorbable stapling device developed for fetal surgery has been applied to cesarean sections, radiotelemetric monitoring has applications outside fetal surgery, and videoendoscopic techniques have allowed fetal manipulation without hysterotomy. These techniques will greatly expand the indications for fetal intervention. Finally, the intensive effort to solve the vexing problem of preterm labor after hysterotomy for fetal surgery has yielded new insight into the role of nitric oxide in myometrial contractions and has spawned interest in treating spontaneous preterm labor with nitric oxide donors.

Fetal surgical research has yielded advances in fetal biology with implications beyond fetal therapy. The serendipitous observation that fetal incisions heal without scarring has provided new insights into the biology of wound healing and has stimulated efforts to mimic the fetal process postnatally. Fetal tissue seems to be biologically and immunologically superior for transplantation and for gene therapy, and fetal immunologic tolerance may allow a wide variety of inherited nonsurgical diseases to be cured by fetal HSC transplantation.

The great promise of fetal therapy is that, for some diseases, the earliest possible intervention (before birth) produces the best possible outcome (the best quality of life for the resources expended). However, the promise of cost-effective, preventive fetal therapy can be subverted by misguided clinical applications, such as a complex in utero procedure that only half saves an otherwise doomed fetus for a life of intensive (and expensive) care. Enthusiasm for fetal interventions must be tempered by reverence for the interests of the mother and her family, careful study of the disease in experimental fetal animals and untreated human fetuses, and a willingness to abandon therapy that does not prove to be effective and cost-effective in properly controlled trials.

REFERENCES

1. Adzick NS: Management of fetal lung lesions. Clin Perinatol 2003;30:481-492.
2. Adzick NS, Harrison MR, Glick PL, et al: Fetal surgery in the primate. III. Maternal outcome after fetal surgery. J Pediatr Surg 1986;21:477-480.
3. Albanese CT, Jennings RW, Filly RA, et al: Endoscopic fetal tracheal occlusion: Evolution of techniques. Pediatr Endosurg Innov Techn 1998;2:47-53.
4. Albanese CT, Lopoo J, Goldstein RB, et al: Fetal liver position and perinatal outcome for congenital diaphragmatic hernia. Prenat Diagn 1998;18:1138-1142.
5. Boloker J, Bateman DA, Wung JT, Stolar CJ: Congenital diaphragmatic hernia in 120 infants treated consecutively with permissive hypercapnea/spontaneous respiration/elective repair. J Pediatr Surg 2002;37:357-366.
6. Congenital Diaphragmatic Hernia Study Group: Does extracorporeal membrane oxygenation improve survival in neonates with congenital diaphragmatic hernia? J Pediatr Surg 1999;34:720-724.
7. Deprest J, Gratacos E, Nicolaides KH, FETO Task Group: Fetoscopic tracheal occlusion (FETO) for severe congenital diaphragmatic hernia: Evolution of a technique and preliminary results. Ultrasound Obstet Gynecol 2004;24:121-126.
8. Desfrere L, Jarreau PH, Dommergues M, et al: Impact of delayed repair and elective high-frequency oscillatory ventilation on survival of antenatally diagnosed congenital diaphragmatic hernia: First application of these strategies in the more "severe" subgroup of antenatally diagnosed newborns. Intensive Care Med 2000;26:934-941.
9. DiFiore JW, Fauza DO, Slavin R, et al: Experimental fetal tracheal ligation reverses the structural and physiologic effects of pulmonary hypoplasia in congenital diaphragmatic hernia. J Pediatr Surg 1994;29:248-256.
10. Farmer DL, von Koch CS, Peacock WJ, et al: In utero repair of myelomeningocele: Experimental pathophysiology, initial clinical experience, and outcomes. Arch Surg 2003;138:872-878.
11. Farrell JA, Albanese CT, Jennings RW, et al: Maternal fertility is not affected by fetal surgery. Fetal Diagn Ther 1999;14:190-192.
12. Feldstein VA, Machin GA, Albanese CT, et al: Twin-twin transfusion syndrome: The "select" procedure. Fetal Diagn Ther 2000;15:257-261.
13. Flageole H, Evrard VA, Piedboeuf B, et al: The plug-unplug sequence: An important step to achieve type II pneumocyte maturation in the fetal lamb model. J Pediatr Surg 1998;33:299-303.
14. Flake AW: Stem cell and genetic therapies for the fetus. Semin Pediatr Surg 2003;12:202-208.
15. Flake AW, Crombleholme TM, Johnson MP, et al: Treatment of severe congenital diaphragmatic hernia by fetal tracheal occlusion: Clinical experience with fifteen cases. Am J Obstet Gynecol 2000;183:1059-1066.
16. Flake AW, Harrison MR, Adzick NS, Zanjani ED: Transplantation of fetal hematopoietic stem cells in utero: The creation of hematopoietic chimeras. Science 1986;233:776-778.
17. Fowler SF, Sydorak RM, Albanese CT, et al: Fetal endoscopic surgery: Lessons learned and trends reviewed. J Pediatr Surg 2002;37:1700-1702.
18. Harrison MR: Unborn: Historical perspective of the fetus as a patient. Pharos 1982;45:19-24.
19. Harrison MR: Fetal surgery. Am J Obstet Gynecol 1996;174:1255-1264.
20. Harrison MR: Fetal surgery: Trials, tribulations, and turf. J Pediatr Surg 2003;38:275-282.
21. Harrison MR: The University of California at San Francisco Fetal Treatment Center: A personal perspective. Fetal Diagn Ther 2004;19:513-524.
22. Harrison MR, Adzick NS, Bullard KM, et al: Correction of congenital diaphragmatic hernia in utero. VII. A prospective trial. J Pediatr Surg 1997;32:1637-1642.
23. Harrison MR, Adzick NS, Estes JM, Howell LJ: A prospective study of the outcome of fetuses with congenital diaphragmatic hernia. JAMA 1994;271:382-384.
24. Harrison MR, Adzick NS, Flake AW, et al: Correction of congenital diaphragmatic hernia in utero. VIII. Response of the hypoplastic lung to tracheal occlusion. J Pediatr Surg 1996;31:1339-1348.
25. Harrison MR, Adzick NS, Jennings RW, et al: Antenatal intervention for congenital cystic adenomatoid malformation. Lancet 1990;336:965-967.
26. Harrison MR, Adzick NS, Longaker MT, et al: Successful repair in utero of a fetal diaphragmatic hernia after removal of herniated viscera from the left thorax. N Engl J Med 1990;322:1582-1584.
27. Harrison MR, Albanese CT, Hawgood S, et al: Fetoscopic temporary tracheal occlusion by means of detachable balloon for congenital diaphragmatic hernia. Am J Obstet Gynecol 2000;185:730-733.
28. Harrison MR, Evans MI, Adzick NS, Holzgreve W (eds): The Unborn Patient: The Art and Science of Fetal Therapy, 3rd ed. Philadelphia, WB Saunders, 2001, pp 297-314.
29. Harrison MR, Golbus MS, Filly RA: Management of the fetus with a correctable congenital defect. JAMA 1981;246:774-777.
30. Harrison MR, Keller RL, Hawgood SB, et al: A randomized trial of fetal endoscopic tracheal occlusion for severe fetal congenital diaphragmatic hernia. N Engl J Med 2003;349:1916-1924.
31. Harrison MR, Mychaliska GB, Albanese CT, et al: Correction of congenital diaphragmatic hernia in utero. IX. Fetuses with poor prognosis (liver herniation and low lung-to-head ratio) can be saved by fetoscopic temporary tracheal occlusion. J Pediatr Surg 1998;33:1017-1022.
32. Harrison MR, Slotnick RN, Crombleholme TM, et al: In utero transplantation of fetal liver haematopoietic stem cells in monkeys. Lancet 1989;2:1425-1427.
33. Harrison MR, Sydorak RM, Farrell JA, et al: Fetoscopic temporary tracheal occlusion for congenital diaphragmatic hernia: Prelude to a randomized controlled trial. J Pediatr Surg 2003;38:1012-1026.
34. Hedrick HL, Flake AW, Crombleholme TM, et al: Sacrococcygeal teratoma: Prenatal assessment, fetal intervention, and outcome. J Pediatr Surg 2004;39:430-438.

35. Hedrick MH, Ferro MM, Filly RA, et al: Congenital high airway obstruction (CHAOS): A potential for perinatal intervention. J Pediatr Surg 1994;29:271-274.

36. Hirose S, Farmer DL, Lee H, et al: The ex utero intrapartum treatment procedure: Looking back at the EXIT. J Pediatr Surg 2004;39:375-380.

37. Hudgins RJ, Edwards MS, Goldstein R, et al: Natural history of fetal ventriculomegaly. Pediatrics 1988;82:692-697.

38. Jennings RW, MacGillivray TE, Harrison MR: Nitric oxide inhibits preterm labor in the rhesus monkey. J Matern Fetal Med 1993;2:170.

39. Johnson MP, Bukowski TP, Reitleman C, et al: In utero surgical treatment of fetal obstructive uropathy: A new comprehensive approach to identify appropriate candidates for vesicoamniotic shunt therapy. Am J Obstet Gynecol 1994;170:1770-1776.

40. Johnson MP, Sutton LN, Rintoul N, et al: Fetal myelomeningocele repair: Short-term clinical outcomes. Am J Obstet Gynecol 2003;189:482-487.

41. Keller RL, Glidden DV, Paek BW, et al: Lung-to-head ratio and fetoscopic temporary tracheal occlusion: Prediction of survival in severe left congenital diaphragmatic hernia. Am J Obstet Gynecol 2003;21:244-249.

42. Kohl T, Sharland G, Allan LD, et al: World experience of percutaneous ultrasound-guided balloon valvuloplasty in human fetuses with severe aortic valve obstruction. Am J Cardiol 2000;85:1230-1233.

43. Longaker MT, Golbus MS, Filly RA, et al: Maternal outcome after open fetal surgery: A review of the first 17 human cases. JAMA 1991;265:737-741.

44. Longaker MT, Whitby DJ, Adzick NS, et al: Fetal surgery for cleft lip: A plea for caution. Plast Reconstr Surg 1991;88:1087-1092.

45. Lopoo JB, Paek BW, Machin GA, et al: Cord ultrasonic transection procedure for selective termination of a monochorionic twin. Fetal Diagn Ther 2000;15:177-179.

46. Luks FI, Wild YK, Piasecki GJ, De Paepe ME: Short-term tracheal occlusion corrects pulmonary vascular anomalies in the fetal lamb with diaphragmatic hernia. Surgery 2000;128:266-272.

47. Manning FA, Harrison MR, Rodeck C: Catheter shunts for fetal hydronephrosis and hydrocephalus: Report of the International Fetal Surgery Registry. N Engl J Med 1986;315:336-346.

48. Marshall AC, van der Velde ME, Tworetzky W, et al: Creation of an atrial septal defect in utero for fetuses with hypoplastic left heart syndrome and intact or highly restrictive atrial septum. Circulation (online), June 28, 2004.

49. Meuli M, Meuli-Simmen C, Hutchins GM, et al: In utero surgery rescues neurologic function at birth in sheep with spina bifida. Nat Med 1995;1:342-347.

50. Muratore CS, Kharasch V, Lund DP, et al: Pulmonary morbidity in 100 survivors of congenital diaphragmatic hernia monitored in a multidisciplinary clinic. J Pediatr Surg 2001;36:133-140.

51. Peranteau WH, Hayashi S, Kim HB, et al: In utero hematopoietic cell transplantation: What are the important questions? Fetal Diagn Ther 2004;19:9-12.

52. Rychik J, Tian Z, Cohen MS, et al: Acute cardiovascular effects of fetal surgery in the human. Circulation 2004;110:1549-1556.

53. Senat MV, Deprest J, Boulvain M, et al: Endoscopic laser surgery versus serial amnioreduction for severe twin-to-twin transfusion syndrome. N Engl J Med 2004;351:136-144.

54. Sydorak RM, Nijagal A, Sbragia L, et al: Gastroschisis: Small hole, big cost. J Pediatr Surg 2002;37:1669-1672.

55. Tsao K, Feldstein VA, Albanese CT, et al: Selective reduction of acardiac twin by radiofrequency ablation. Am J Obstet Gynecol 2002;187:635-640.

56. Tsao K, Hawgood S, Vu L, et al: Resolution of hydrops fetalis in congenital cystic adenomatoid malformation after prenatal steroid therapy. J Pediatr Surg 2003;38:508-510.

57. Tworetzky W, Marshall AC: Balloon valvuloplasty for congenital heart disease in the fetus. Clin Perinatol 2003;30:541-550.

58. Walsh DS, Adzick NS: Foetal surgery for spina bifida. Semin Neonatol 2003;8:197-205.

59. Wilson RD, Baxter JK, Johnson MP, et al: Thoracoamniotic shunts: Fetal treatment of pleural effusions and congenital cystic adenomatoid malformations. Fetal Diagn Ther 2004;19:4113-4120.

60. Wilson RD, Johnson MP: Congenital abdominal wall defects: An update. Fetal Diagn Ther 2004;19:385-398.

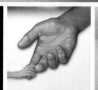

Chapter 6

Neonatal Physiology and Metabolic Considerations

Agostino Pierro, Simon Eaton, and Evelyn Ong

Advances in neonatal intensive care and surgery have significantly improved the survival of neonates with congenital or acquired abnormalities. This has been matched by an improvement in our understanding of the physiology of infants and their metabolic response to starvation, anesthesia, operative stress, and systemic inflammation. Newborn infants are not just small adults; their physiology in terms of thermoregulation and fluid and caloric needs can be very different, particularly if the neonate is premature or growth retarded. This chapter focuses on the physiology and metabolism of newborn infants undergoing surgery, with particular emphasis on the characteristics of preterm neonates. We discuss fluid and electrolyte balance, neonatal energy metabolism and thermoregulation, and the metabolism of carbohydrate, fat, and protein. In addition, we present the current knowledge on the neonatal response to operative trauma and sepsis—two of the major factors that alter neonatal physiology.

PREMATURE, SMALL-FOR-GESTATIONAL-AGE, AND INTRAUTERINE GROWTH-RETARDED NEONATES

The greatest growth rate occurs during fetal life. In fact, the evolution from one fertilized cell to a 3.5-kg neonate encompasses a 5000-fold increase in length, a 61×10^6 increase in surface area, and a 6×10^{12} increase in weight. The greatest postnatal growth rate occurs just after birth. It is not unusual to notice a period of slow or arrested neonatal growth during critical illness or soon after surgery.

Neonates can be classified as premature, term, or postmature according to gestational age. Any infant born before 37 weeks' gestation is considered premature, term infants are those born between 37 and 42 weeks' gestation, and post-term neonates are born after 42 weeks' gestation. Previously, any infant weighing less than 2500 g was termed premature. This definition is inappropriate, because many neonates weighing less than 2500 g are mature or postmature but small for their gestational age; they have a different appearance and different problems than do premature infants. The gestational age can be estimated antenatally or in the first days after birth using the Ballard score (Fig. 6-1).[15] By plotting body weight versus gestational age (Fig. 6-2),[49] newborn infants can be classified as small, appropriate, or large for gestational age. Head circumference and length are also plotted against gestational age to estimate intrauterine growth (Fig. 6-3).[49] Any infant whose weight is below the 10th percentile for gestational age is defined as small for gestational age. Large-for-gestational-age infants are those whose weights are above the 90th percentile for gestational age (see Fig. 6-2).[49] In general, preterm infants weigh less than 2500 g and have a crown-heel length less than 47 cm, a head circumference less than 33 cm, and a thoracic circumference less than 30 cm. Preterm infants have physiologic handicaps due to functional and anatomic immaturity of various organs. Body temperature is difficult to maintain, respiratory problems are common, renal function is immature, the ability to combat infection is inadequate, the conjugation and excretion of bilirubin is impaired, and hemorrhagic diathesis is more common.

Premature infants are usually assigned to subgroups on the basis of birth weight, as follows:

1. Moderately low birth weight (1501 to 2500 g). This group represents 82% of all premature infants. The mortality rate in this group is 40 times that in term infants.
2. Very low birth weight (1001 to 1500 g). This group represents 12% of premature infants. The mortality rate in this group is 200 times that in full-term babies.
3. Extremely low birth weight ($\leq$1000 g). These babies represent 6% of premature births but account for a disproportionate number of newborn deaths. The mortality rate is 600 times that in term infants.

The definition of intrauterine growth retardation (IUGR) is often confused and unclear in the medical literature. IUGR is usually defined as a documented decrease in intrauterine growth noted by fetal ultrasonography. IUGR can be temporary, leading to a normal-size neonate at birth. There are two types of IUGR: symmetrical and asymmetrical. Symmetrical IUGR denotes normal body proportions (small head and small body) and is considered a more severe form of IUGR.[165]

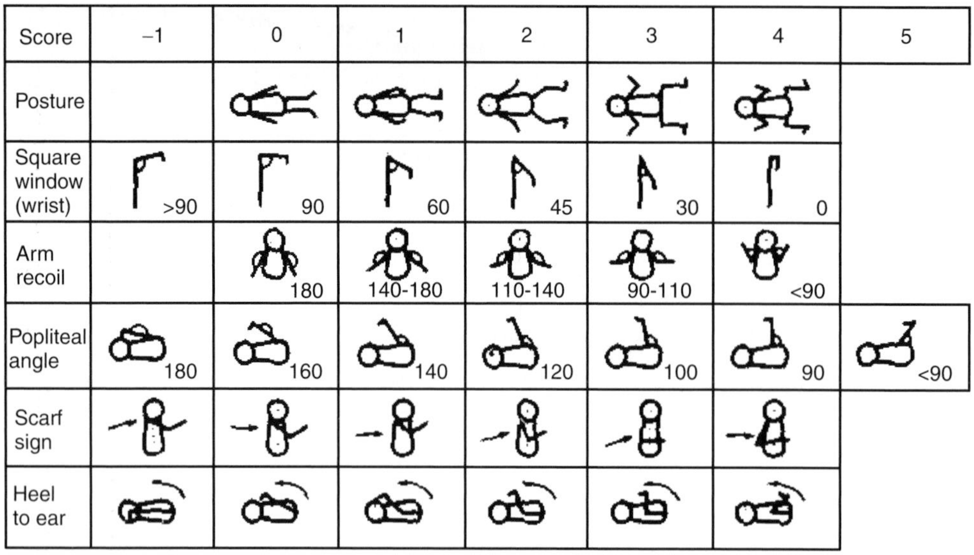

Score	−1	0	1	2	3	4	5
Posture							
Square window (wrist)	>90	90	60	45	30	0	
Arm recoil		180	140-180	110-140	90-110	<90	
Popliteal angle	180	160	140	120	100	90	<90
Scarf sign							
Heel to ear							

Physical Maturity

Skin	Sticky friable, transparent	Gelatinous, red, translucent	Smooth, pink, visible veins	Superficial peeling and/or rash; few veins	Cracking, pale areas; rare veins	Parchment, deep cracking; no vessels	Leathery, cracked, wrinkled
Lanugo	None	Sparse	Abundant	Thinning	Bald areas	Mostly bald	Maturity Rating
Plantar surface	Heel-toe 40-50 mm: −1 <40 mm: −2	>50 mm, no crease	Faint red marks	Anterior transverse crease only	Creases anterior ⅔	Creases over entire sole	
Breast	Imperceptible	Barely perceptible	Flat areola, no bud	Stippled areola, 1–2 mm bud	Raised areola, 3–4 mm bud	Full areola, 5–10 mm bud	
Eye/ear	Lids fused loosely: −1 lightly: −2	Lids open; pinna flat; stays folded	Slightly curved pinna; soft; slow recoil	Well-curved pinna; soft but ready recoil	Formed and firm, instant recoil	Thick cartilage, ear stiff	
Genitals (male)	Scrotum flat, smooth	Scrotum empty, faint rugae	Testes in upper canal, rare rugae	Testes descending, few rugae	Testes down, good rugae	Testes pendulous, deep rugae	
Genitals (female)	Clitoris prominent, labia flat	Clitoris prominent, small labia minora	Clitoris prominent, enlarging minora	Majora and minora equally prominent	Majora large, minora small	Majora cover clitoris and minora	

Maturity Rating

Score	Weeks
−10	20
−5	22
0	24
5	26
10	28
15	30
20	32
25	34
30	36
35	38
40	40
45	42
50	44

Figure 6–1 Ballard score for gestational age. (From Ballard JL, Khoury JC, Wedig K, et al: New Ballard score, expanded to include extremely premature infants. J Pediatr 1991;119:417-423.)

Asymmetrical IUGR denotes a small abdominal circumference, decreased subcutaneous and abdominal fat, reduced skeletal muscle mass, and head circumference in the normal range. Infants with asymmetrical IUGR exhibit catch-up growth more frequently than do those with symmetrical IUGR, although 10% to 30% of all infants with IUGR remain short as children and adults. Premature infants are expected to have catch-up growth by 2 years of age. Those born after 29 weeks' gestation usually exhibit catch-up growth, whereas those born before 29 weeks are more likely to have a decreased rate of height and weight gain, which may be noted in the first week after birth and last up to 2 years.[32,66,68]

PREDICTING NEONATAL MORTALITY

Various factors contribute to the mortality of neonates. The most common factors are listed in Table 6-1. Overall, there has been an improvement in neonatal mortality during the past decade (Fig. 6-4).[48] Birth weight and gestational age are strong indicators of mortality. The survival of neonates born weighing 500 g at 22 weeks' gestational age is close to 0%. With increasing gestational age, survival rates increase to approximately 15% at 23 weeks, 56% at 24 weeks, and 79% at 25 weeks. Scoring systems to predict mortality would be particularly useful to neonatal surgeons in planning treatment, counseling parents, and comparing outcomes among different centers. However, these scoring systems have not been developed and validated in patients requiring neonatal surgery. Generic scoring systems for neonates are available, but these do not take into consideration the anatomic abnormality requiring surgery. They are based on physiologic abnormalities such as hypotension or hypertension, acidosis, hypoxia, hypercapnia, anemia, and neutropenia (Score for Neonatal Acute Physiology [SNAP]) or clinical parameters such as gestational age, birth weight, anomalies, acidosis, and FiO_2

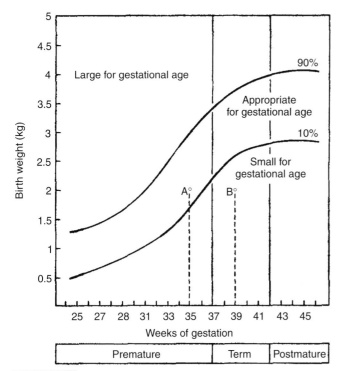

Figure 6–2 Level of intrauterine growth based on birth weight and gestational age of live-born, single white infants. (From Disturbances in newborns and infants. In Beers MF, Berkow R [eds]: The Merck Manual of Diagnosis and Therapy, 17th ed. White House Station, NJ, Merck Research Laboratories, 1999, pp 2127-2145.)

TABLE 6–1 Major Causes of Mortality in Surgical Neonates	
Preterm Neonates	**Term Neonates**
Necrotizing enterocolitis	Congenital anomalies
Congenital anomalies	Infection
Severe immaturity	Persistent pulmonary hypertension
Respiratory distress syndrome	Meconium aspiration
Intraventricular hemorrhage	Birth asphyxia, trauma
Infection	
Bronchopulmonary dysplasia	

children,[12,118,179,180] to monitor the clinical status of neonates with acute abdominal emergencies requiring surgery. Combining the surgeon's judgment and an objective score may produce an accurate assessment of the clinical progress of critically ill neonates and estimate their risk of mortality.

FLUID AND ELECTROLYTE BALANCE

Body Water Composition

Total body water (TBW) is divided into two compartments: intracellular and extracellular. During the first trimester, about 90% of body mass is TBW; 65% of body mass is extracellular fluid, and 25% is intracellular fluid.[61] Only 1% of body mass is fat. However, these percentages change throughout gestation as the amount of body protein and fat increases. TBW declines to 80% by 32 weeks' gestation and is approximately 68% to 75% by term.[60] By the age of 3 months, TBW constitutes 60% of total body mass. This is accompanied by a decrease in the ratio of extracellular compartment fluid (ECF) to intracellular compartment fluid (ICF). ECF is 60% of total

(Clinical Risk Index for Babies [CRIB]).[4,141] CRIB includes 6 parameters collected in the first 12 hours after birth, and SNAP has 26 variables collected during the first 24 hours; there have been various modifications to each of these scoring systems.[63] We recently used a modified organ failure score (Table 6-2), based on the Sepsis-Related Organ Failure Assessment (SOFA) used in adults and

Figure 6–3 Level of intrauterine growth based on gestational age, body length (A), and head circumference (B) at birth.

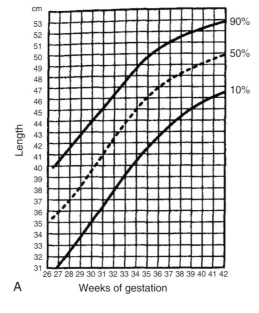

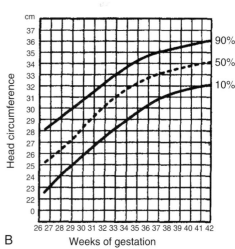

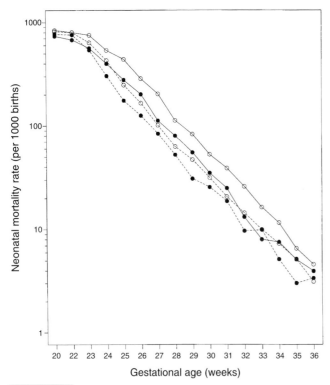

Figure 6–4 Neonatal mortality, by gestational age, for black (●) and white (○) infants in the United States. Solid lines denote data for 1989; dashed lines are for 1997. Data shown are for less than 37 weeks' gestation only. (From Demissie K, Rhoads GG, Ananth CV, et al: Trends in preterm birth and neonatal mortality among blacks and whites in the United States from 1989 to 1997. Am J Epidemiol 2001;154:307-315.)

body mass at 20 weeks' gestation and declines to 40% at term, whereas ICF increases from 25% at 20 weeks' gestation to 35% at term and then to 43% at 2 months of age. Thereafter, both ECF and ICF decrease with time relative to body weight. Among preterm infants, those who are small for gestational age have a significantly higher body

water content (approximately 90%) than do appropriate-for-gestational-age infants (approximately 84%).[78]

In addition to the fluid compartments seen in adults, significant volumes of fluid are contained in the fetus's lungs. This pulmonary fluid is formed by the secretion of chloride into the alveolar spaces. The fluid accumulates and flows out of the trachea to communicate with the amniotic fluid sac, where it contributes up to one third of its total volume[108] or is swallowed. The production of pulmonary fluid appears to increase until 36 weeks' gestation and then plateaus until term.[67,92,99] It is not clear how much fluid exchange can occur between the alveolar fluid and the blood circulation. The stomach may also act as a large fluid reservoir in the fetus. Previously, it was estimated that 200 to 1500 mL of amniotic fluid was swallowed a day; it is now thought to be equivalent to 20% to 25% of total body mass per day.[24,155] These pathways within the amniotic sac are shown in Figure 6-5.

Neonatal Fluid Shifts

Fluid balance in the neonate represents adaptation of homeostatic mechanisms to the dramatic change in environment and circulation of the neonate peripartum (Fig. 6-5).

Peripartum

Before labor, pulmonary fluid production decreases, and existing fluid is reabsorbed. During labor, efflux through the trachea increases and accelerates, thereby drying out the lungs; arterial pressure increases and causes shifts in plasma from the vascular compartment and a slight rise in hematocrit. Placental transfusion can occur if there is delayed clamping of the cord and the neonate is placed at or below the level of the placenta, resulting in up to a 50% increase in red blood cells and blood volume. This polycythemia may have severe consequences such as neurologic impairment, thrombus formation, and tissue ischemia.[146]

TABLE 6–2 Modified Organ Failure Score

Organ System	Score*				
	0	1	2	3	4
Respiratory (Pao_2/Fio_2)	>400	≤400	≤300	≤200 with respiratory support	≤100 with respiratory support
Renal (urine output)			<1 mL/kg/hr for 6 hr	<0.5 mL/kg/hr for 6 hr	Anuria
Hepatic (serum bilirubin in μmol/L [mg/dL])		20-32 [1.17-1.9]	33-101 [2.0-5.9]	102-204 [6.0-12.0]	>204 [>12.0]
Cardiovascular (hypotension)	No hypotension	MAP (mm Hg) < gestational age + age (wk)	Dopamine <5.0 μg/kg/min, or dobutamine any dose	Dopamine >5.0 μg/kg/min, epinephrine <0.1 μg/kg/min, or norepinephrine <0.1 μg/kg/min	Dopamine >15.0, μg/kg/min, epinephrine >0.1 μg/kg/min, or norepinephrine >0.1 μg/kg/min
Coagulation (platelet count)	>150	≤150	≤100	≤50	≤20 or platelet transfusion

*To calculate the aggregate score, the worst value of each parameter in each time interval is recorded.
MAP, mean arterial pressure.
From references 12, 118, 179, 180.

Figure 6–5 Major routes of fluid movement in *A*, adult, and *B*, late-gestation fetus. (From Brace RA: Fetal and amniotic fluid balance. In Gluckman PD, Heymann MA (eds): Pediatrics and Perinatology: The Scientific Basis, 2nd ed. London, Arnold, 1996, pp 233-241.

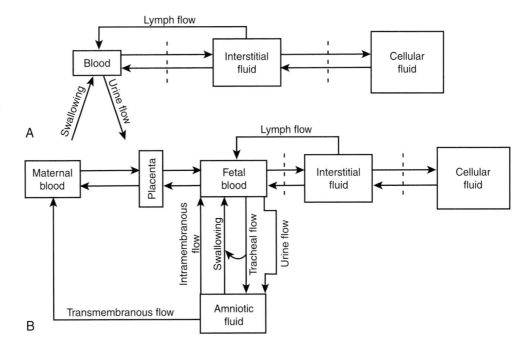

Postpartum

On postpartum day 1, the neonate is oliguric. Over the next 1 to 2 days, dramatic shifts in fluid from the intracellular to extracellular compartment result in a diuresis and natriuresis; this contributes to weight loss during the first week of life—approximately 5% to 10% in term neonates and 10% to 20% in premature infants. The proportion of fluid loss from ECF and ICF is controversial, and the mechanism has yet to be determined. This diuresis occurs regardless of fluid intake or insensible losses and may be related to a postnatal surge in atrial natriuretic peptide.[116] Limitations in the methodology of measuring ECF and ICF have limited our understanding of the processes. It has been demonstrated, however, that large increases in water and calorie intake are required to reduce the weight loss. Higher calorie intake alone reduces weight loss, but the ECF still decreases. Subsequent weight gain appears to be the result of increases in tissue mass and ICF per kilogram body weight, but not ECF per kilogram body weight. By the fifth postpartum day, urinary excretion begins to reflect the fluid status of the infant.

Renal Function

The first functional nephrons appear at 8 weeks' gestation, and the full number of glomeruli is reached by 34 weeks. Glomerular filtration starts at between 9 and 12 weeks. The renal arteries derived from the aorta at the T12 to L2 levels divide into segmental end arteries and are vulnerable to ischemia in the peripartum period. In utero, renal blood flow and glomerular filtration rate (GFR) gradually increase owing to the development of new nephrons. Renovascular resistance is initially high; therefore, renal blood flow is limited in utero despite the gradual increase in the proportion of cardiac output distributed to the kidneys during gestation.

During the first day of life, the distribution of cortical perfusion alters, with increased perfusion of the outer cortex. GFR rises rapidly during this time, despite total renal blood flow being unchanged. In subsequent days, inner cortex perfusion is maintained while outer cortex perfusion increases. Eventually, renovascular resistance decreases, resulting in a rapid rise in GFR over the first 3 months of life followed by a slower rise to adult levels by 12 to 24 months of age. Premature and low-birth-weight infants may have a lower GFR than term infants, and the initial rapid rise in GFR is absent. However, GFR increases gradually until it reaches that of a term infant at 40 weeks' gestation. Because of these rapid changes in GFR, interpretation of plasma creatinine to determine renal function status is difficult immediately post partum.

Urine osmolality is controlled by two mechanisms. Urine is concentrated in the loop of Henle using a countercurrent system dependent on the osmolality of the medullary interstitium. In neonates, the low osmolality in the renal medulla means that the countercurrent system is less effective; urine concentration capacity is between 500 and 700 mOsm/kg, compared with 1200 mOsm/kg in the adult kidney, resulting in less tolerance for fluid overload.

As in adults, neonates respond to fluctuations in serum osmolality. Antidiuretic hormone (ADH) regulates serum osmolality by increasing reabsorption of water from the renal collecting tubules and is produced by the fetal pituitary from 12 weeks' gestation. There is a peripartum increase in ADH secretion, and both preterm and term infants are capable of producing ADH in response to appropriate stimuli. In term infants, ADH levels measure between 275 and 280 mOsm/kg, and it is secreted at almost adult levels. However, in comparison with those of adults, neonatal renal tubules are relatively insensitive to ADH, possibly because there are fewer ADH receptors present or because the lower concentration gradient in the renal medulla reduces its effect.

The syndrome of inappropriate (excess) ADH secretion (SIADH) may occur following cerebral or pulmonary injury, painful surgery, or hypoxia. It manifests as an increase in weight, hyponatremia, oliguria with high urine osmolality, and high urinary sodium in disproportion to plasma sodium. It is treated by fluid restriction and administration of nasal synthetic desmopressin (DDAVP).

Sodium

Normal neonatal serum sodium levels are 135 to 140 mmol/L, controlled by moderating renal excretion. Serum sodium is the major determinant of serum osmolality and therefore extracellular fluid volume. Urinary sodium excretion is dependent on the GFR and is therefore low in neonates compared with adults. In addition, neonates have a limited tubular capacity to reabsorb sodium and thus have greater urinary sodium losses, more so in preterm than term infants. During the period of oliguria on day 1 of life, sodium supplementation is not normally required. The normal maintenance sodium requirement following normal diuresis is 2 to 4 mmol/kg per day.

Hyponatremia

Serum sodium concentrations of less than 135 mmol/L can occur in a state of hypovolemia, euvolemia, or hypervolemia (Table 6-3). Symptoms are often not apparent until serum sodium falls below 120 mmol/L and manifest as the effects of cerebral edema: apathy, nausea, vomiting, headache, seizure, and coma. The severity of symptoms is directly related to the rapidity of onset and magnitude of hyponatremia.

The kidneys respond to a fall in serum sodium by excreting more dilute urine, but the secretion of ADH in response to hypovolemia affects this. Therefore, measurements of urinary sodium can be used to help determine the underlying cause of hyponatremia. Urine sodium concentrations less than 10 mmol/L indicate an appropriate renal response to euvolemic hyponatremia. However, if the urinary sodium is greater than 20 mmol/L, this can indicate either sodium leak from damaged renal tubules or hypervolemia.

Hypernatremia

Hypernatremia (serum sodium >145 mmol/L) can occur in varying states of hydration (see Table 6-3). This most commonly occurs in children secondary to hypotonic fluid loss, such as occurs with diarrhea. Clinical signs include dry mucous membranes, loss of skin turgidity, drowsiness, irritability, hypertonicity, seizure, and coma. Fluid loss from the cerebral tissues can result in tearing blood vessels and cerebral hemorrhage. Cerebral tissues respond by retaining intracellular taurine to increase the return of water from the extracellular compartment. Hypocalcemia can often accompany hypernatremia.

Potassium

Potassium is the most abundant intracellular cation and is essential for maintaining the cellular transmural ion gradient. The normal serum concentration is 3.5 to 5.8 mmol/L. In the first 24 to 72 hours post partum, a large shift of potassium from intracellular to extracellular compartments occurs, resulting in a rise in plasma potassium. This is compounded by the diuresis phase, which limits the amount of tubular excretion of potassium by limiting the availability of water and sodium. This effect is directly related to the degree of prematurity and can cause significant morbidity. However, potassium eventually falls as the diuresis phase ends and potassium excretion rises. Potassium supplementation is therefore not required in the first day of life, but after diuresis, a maintenance intake of 1 to 3 mmol/kg per day is required.

Hypokalemia

Hypokalemia is most commonly iatrogenic, due to either inadequate potassium intake or use of diuretics, but it can also be caused by vomiting, diarrhea, alkalosis (which drives potassium intracellularly), or polyuric renal failure. Insulin and sympathetic system stimulation also drive potassium into cells and can exaggerate preexisting hypokalemia. The normal ion gradient is disrupted and predisposes to muscle current conduction abnormalities, such as cardiac arrhythmias, paralytic ileus, urinary retention, and respiratory muscle paralysis.

TABLE 6-3 Sodium Abnormalities and Hydration Status

	Hypovolemic	Euvolemic	Hypervolemic
Hyponatremia	Gastrointestinal losses: vomiting, diarrhea, small bowel fistula, ileostomy Intake of hypotonic solutions Renal disease Cerebral salt-wasting disease Perspiration: cystic fibrosis, adrenal insufficiency	Syndrome of inappropriate secretion of antidiuretic hormone Diuretics	Congestive cardiac failure Liver cirrhosis Nephrotic syndrome Renal failure
Hypernatremia	Diabetes insipidus Excessive sweating Increased insensible losses	Antidiuretic hormone insufficiency	Excess sodium intake

Hyperkalemia

Causes of hyperkalemia include severe metabolic acidosis, cell necrosis with release of intracellular potassium (e.g., severe crush injuries), acute renal failure, iatrogenic excessive intake, adrenal insufficiency, insulin-dependent diabetes mellitus, or severe hemolysis. Hyperkalemia can be exacerbated in the presence of hypoxia, metabolic acidosis, catabolic stress, and oliguria. Preterm infants may also suffer from hyperkalemia with high insensible fluid losses. As in hypokalemia, hyperkalemia alters the electrical gradient of cell membranes, and patients are vulnerable to cardiac arrhythmias, including asystole.

Calcium

Calcium plays an important role in enzyme activity, muscle contraction and relaxation, the blood coagulation cascade, bone metabolism, and nerve conduction. Calcium is maintained at a total serum concentration of 1.8 to 2.1 mmol/L in neonates and 2.0 to 2.5 mmol/L in term infants and is divided into three fractions. Thirty percent to 50% is protein bound, and 5% to 15% is complexed with citrate, lactate, bicarbonate, and inorganic ions. The remaining free calcium ions are metabolically active, and concentrations fluctuate with serum albumin levels. Hydrogen ions compete reversibly with calcium for albumin binding sites; therefore, free calcium concentrations increase in acidosis.

Calcium metabolism is under the control of many hormones, but primarily 1,25-dihydroxycholecalciferol (gastrointestinal absorption of calcium, bone resorption, increased renal calcium reabsorption), parathyroid hormone (bone resorption, decreased urinary excretion), and calcitonin (bone formation and increased urinary excretion). Calcium is actively transported from maternal to fetal circulation against the concentration gradient, resulting in peripartum hypercalcemia. There is a transient fall in calcium post partum to 1.8 to 2.1 mmol/L and a gradual rise to normal infant levels over 24 to 48 hours.

Hypocalcemia

In addition to the physiologic hypocalcemia of neonates, which is usually asymptomatic, other causes of hypocalcemia are hypoparathyroidism, including DiGeorge syndrome, and parathryoid hormone insensitivity in infants of diabetic mothers, which may also be related to hypomagnesemia. Clinical manifestations are tremor, seizures, and a prolonged QT interval on the electrocardiogram.

Hypercalcemia

Hypercalcemia is less common than hypocalcemia but can result from inborn errors of metabolism, such as familial hypercalcemic hypocalciuria or primary hyperparathyroidism. Iatrogenic causes are vitamin A overdose or deficient dietary phosphate intake. Less common causes in children are tertiary hyperparathyroidism, paraneoplastic syndromes, and metastatic bone disease.

Magnesium

As an important enzyme cofactor, magnesium affects adenosine triphosphate (ATP) metabolism and glycolysis. Only 20% of total body magnesium is exchangeable with the biologically active free ion form. The remainder is bound in bone or to intracellular protein, RNA, or ATP, mostly in muscle and liver. Gastrointestinal absorption of magnesium is controlled by vitamin D, parathyroid hormone, and sodium reabsorption. As previously stated, hypomagnesemia is often related to hypocalcemia.

Acid-Base Balance

Acid-base balance is achieved by intracellular and extracellular buffer systems, respiration, and renal function. Intracellular systems consist of conjugate acid-base pairs in equilibrium, as shown by the following equation:

$$HA \leftrightarrow H^+ + A^-$$

where H is proton and A is acid. The pH can be derived from the Henderson-Hasselbalch equation:

$$pH = \frac{pK + \log [A^-]}{[HA]}$$

where pK is the dissociation constant of the weak acid, $[A^-]$ is the concentration of the dissociated acid, and $[HA]$ is the concentration of the acid. The most important of these intracellular buffer systems is the carbonic anhydrase system:

$$CO_2 + H_2O \leftrightarrow H^+ + HCO_3^-$$

Extracellular buffer systems are similar, but the proton is loosely associated with proteins, hemoglobin, or phosphates and takes several hours to equilibrate.

Respiratory compensation uses the carbonic anhydrase system, ridding the body of carbon dioxide (CO_2) and thereby shifting equilibrium to the left of the reaction and reducing the number of protons. The extent of the shift is influenced by the active transport of bicarbonate across the blood-brain barrier, thereby triggering central respiratory drive.

Normal extracellular pH is maintained at 7.35 to 7.45. Normal metabolic processes produce carbonic acid, lactic acid, ketoacids, phosphoric acid, and sulfuric acid, all of which are either excreted or controlled by a number of buffer systems.

Fetal Acid-Base Balance

The carbonic anhydrase–bicarbonate buffer system is particularly important to the fetus because CO_2 can be readily excreted via the placental circulation. The intracellular buffering system in the developing fetus is considerably smaller than that of a child or adult but still has a greater capacity than the extracellular buffering system.

Respiratory compensation is limited by the placental function, fetomaternal circulation, and maternal respiratory compensation. However, renal compensation contributes more to acid-base balance.

Neonatal Acid-Base Balance

Loss of the contribution of the fetomaternal circulation and maternal respiratory and renal compensation mechanisms forces the neonate to adapt and the systems to mature. There is a suggestion that increased sensitivity of the respiratory centers to fluctuations in pH changes allows the neonate to better control acid-base balance. Increases in the intracellular protein mass allow greater intracellular buffering. The extracellular buffer systems are already functional.

Respiratory compensation becomes active as respiration is established. Because it relies on pulmonary function and lung maturity, neonates with lung disease may have impaired respiratory compensation. CO_2 passes freely across the blood-brain barrier, allowing almost immediate response from respiratory drive centers to respiratory acidosis. The response to metabolic acidosis is delayed because interstitial bicarbonate requires a few hours to equilibrate with the cerebral bicarbonate.

Renal compensation is the most important mechanism available to neonates for acid-base balance. Adjustments in urine acidity have been seen as soon as a few hours post partum, but 2 to 3 days are required for renal compensation to fully mature. Consequent to the changes in renal function and perfusion described previously, the neonate's ability to handle acid-base balance is limited in the first few days of life. Proximal tubules are responsible for the reabsorption of 85% to 90% of filtered bicarbonate, but they function less efficiently in premature neonates. Reabsorption can also be affected by some drugs used in neonates. Dopamine inhibits sodium-proton pump activity in the proximal tubules and therefore decreases the amount of bicarbonate that is reabsorbed. The remaining bicarbonate reabsorption takes place in the distal tubules, but they differ from the proximal tubules in that they lack carbonic anhydrase. Aldosterone is the most important hormone affecting distal tubular function and stimulates proton excretion in the distal tubules. However, the distal nephrons of premature infants are developmentally insensitive to aldosterone. Protons are excreted in the urine as phosphate, sulfate, and ammonium salts. This increases with age and gestation. However, the introduction of phosphate-containing drugs increases phosphate delivery to the distal tubules and therefore can increase the capacity to excrete H^+. Dopamine decreases the reabsorption of protons in the distal tubules, thereby increasing proton excretion.

Causes of Acid-Base Imbalance

Arterial blood gases are used to help identify the cause of an acid-base imbalance (Table 6-4). Acid-base state is indicated by the pH, whereas high or low bicarbonate and CO_2 partial pressures indicate whether the source is metabolic or respiratory. The priority is to treat any underlying cause, such as metabolic acidosis caused by dehydration or sepsis. The slow infusion of buffers such as sodium bicarbonate or tris(hydroxymethyl)aminomethane (a sodium-free buffer) should be used as therapeutic adjuncts. The amount of sodium bicarbonate required can be calculated using the following equation:

$$NaHCO_2 \text{ (mmol)} = \frac{\text{Base excess} \times \text{Body weight (kg)}}{3}$$

ENERGY METABOLISM

Energy is the ability to do work and is essential to all life processes. The unit of energy is the calorie or joule. One calorie equals 4.184 joules; it is the energy required to raise 1 g of water from 15°C to 16°C. The most widely used medical unit of energy is the kilocalorie (kcal), which is equal to 1000 calories. One joule equals the energy required to move 1 kg the distance of 1 m with 1 newton of force. The first law of thermodynamics states that energy cannot be created or destroyed. Thus:

$$\text{Energy in} = \text{Energy out} + \text{Energy stored}$$

In the case of neonates, this can be expressed as follows[143]:

$$\text{Energy intake} = \text{Energy losses in excreta} + \text{Energy stored} \\ + \text{Energy of tissue synthesis} \\ + \text{Energy expended on activity} \\ + \text{Basal metabolic rate}$$

TABLE 6-4 Causes of Acid-Base Imbalance in the Fetus and Neonate

	Fetus	Neonate
Metabolic acidosis	Hypoxia secondary to placental dysfunction Maternal hypoxia Maternal diabetes mellitus Sepsis Renal tubular abnormalities	Hypoxia Perinatal asphyxia Severe pulmonary disease Hypovolema Myocardial dysfunction of prematurity Vasoregulation abnormalities Sepsis Metabolic disorder Prematurity (renal immaturity)
Metabolic alkalosis	Hyperemesis gravidarum	Prolonged diuretic use
Respiratory acidosis	Maternal hypoventilation: Asthma Airway obstruction Narcotic overdose Anesthesia Magnesium sulfate toxicity	Respiratory distress syndrome
Respiratory alkalosis	Maternal hyperventilation	Pyrexia Iatrogenic hyperventilation Urea cycle disorder

Energy Intake

The principal foodstuffs are carbohydrates, fats, and proteins (see later). The potential energy that can be derived from these foods is the energy released when the food is completely absorbed and oxidized. The metabolizable energy is somewhat less than the energy intake, because energy is lost in the feces, in the form of indigestible elements, and in the urine, in the form of incompletely metabolized compounds such as urea from amino acids or ketone bodies from fats. Thus, metabolizable energy can be calculated as follows:

$$\text{Metabolizable energy} = \text{Energy intake} - \text{Energy losses in urine and stool}$$

Food is metabolized through a variety of complex metabolic pathways. Complete metabolism of a food requires that it be oxidized to CO_2, water, and, in the case of proteins, urea and ammonia. This metabolism takes place according to predictable stoichiometric equations.[109] The energy liberated by oxidation is not used directly but is used to create high-energy intermediates from which energy can be released where and when it is required. Such intermediates include ATP, guanosine triphosphate, cytidine triphosphate, uridine triphosphate, inosine triphosphate, and creatine phosphate. These intermediates store energy in the form of a high-energy phosphate bond. The energy is released when the bond is hydrolyzed. Creation of these high-energy intermediates may result directly from a step in the metabolic pathway. More often, however, they are created indirectly, as the result of oxidative phosphorylation, the process by which a compound is oxidized by the sequential removal of hydrogen ions, which are then transferred through a variety of flavoproteins and cytochromes until they are combined with oxygen to produce water. This process releases large amounts of energy, which is used to create the high-energy phosphate bonds in the intermediates. Thus, the energy in food is used to produce high-energy intermediates, in which form energy is available for all the processes of life.

The respiratory quotient is calculated as CO_2 production divided by oxygen consumption, and it varies with the substrate being oxidized. It has a numerical value of 1.0 for glucose oxidation and 0.70 to 0.72 for fat oxidation, depending on the chain length of the fat oxidized. Thus the respiratory quotient, measured by indirect calorimetry, reflects the balance of substrate use. This situation is complicated, however, by the partial oxidation of, for example, fats to ketone bodies or carbohydrate conversion to lipids, which results in a respiratory quotient of greater than 1.0. Tables of precise respiratory quotients for individual carbohydrates, fats, and amino acids are available.[109]

Birth represents a transition from the fetal state, in which carbohydrate is the principal energy substrate (approximately 80% of energy expended), to the infant state, in which both carbohydrate and fat are used to provide energy.[69] This transition is evidenced by the change in respiratory quotient, which declines from 0.97 at birth to 0.80 by 3 hours of age,[74,153] such that fat provides 60% to 70% of energy. This is probably due to the fact that newborn infants have some initial difficulty obtaining enough exogenous energy to meet their energy needs and are thus more dependent on endogenous energy stores. Thereafter, the respiratory quotient has been shown to increase slightly during the first week of life,[28,29,153] which suggests that newborn infants may preferentially metabolize fat in the first instance. Low-birth-weight infants have a respiratory quotient higher than 0.90.[138]

Energy Storage

Energy is stored mainly as fat. A normal 70-kg man has about 17 kg of fat, which is capable of yielding 150,000 kcal of energy upon oxidation—enough energy for a 2-month fast. Energy is also stored as glycogen in the liver, kidneys, and muscles. Muscle glycogen can be used only in situ, but liver and kidney glycogen can be used to produce glucose for metabolism in other sites. Glycogen stores contain between 1000 and 3000 kcal worth of glycogen, enough for about 6 to 24 hours of fasting. Protein performs functions other than energy storage, and of the 11 kg of protein (7 kg intracellular, 4 kg extracellular) in a 70-kg man, about half (equivalent to about 22,000 kcal) can be used as a source of energy during severe fasting. The serious consequences of mobilizing protein include wasting, reduced wound healing, edema, failure of growth and neurologic development, and reduced resistance to infection. Studies of growing infants have shown that each gram of weight gain (i.e., each gram of energy stored) requires an average of 5 kcal of energy.[74,143] The energy required to lay down tissue stores includes (1) the energy stored within the tissue itself (e.g., 9 kcal/g of fat) and (2) the energy investment needed to convert the food into storable and usable substrates. Studies have shown this additional investment to be on the order of 5% to 30% of the energy value of the tissue.[94]

Energy of Growth and Tissue Synthesis

In stable, mature adults, little energy is needed for growth. However, in neonates, the energy requirements for growth are considerable. In infants, up to 50% of the energy intake can be used for growth.[35,143] The energy needed for growth includes the energy stored in tissues and the energy investment needed for tissue synthesis. The energy stored can be measured by recording the difference between the metabolizable energy intake and the energy expenditure.[143] The energy needed for tissue synthesis is believed to be the same as the diet-induced thermogenesis (i.e., the energy cost of interconversion of nutrients for metabolism, organization, and deposition).[13,27,143] By recording the difference in resting energy expenditure (REE) before and after feeding, Reichman et al.[143] estimated the cost of tissue synthesis as 3 to 6 kcal/kg per day. From longitudinal studies of energy expenditure over a period of weeks in growing infants, the cost of tissue synthesis has been found to be 9.3 kcal/kg per day, or 7.6% of total energy intake.[35] The rate of growth of premature infants is on the order of 17 to 19 g/kg per day,[36] compared with 4 to 8 g/kg per day for full-term infants.[185] Thus, the energy cost of growth is much greater in premature infants.[130] Studies of premature infants have shown that the metabolic cost of growth is related to the rate of protein accretion.[33,59,115,130] This is because protein has a lower energy value per unit weight than fat but requires a greater energy investment. In rapidly growing premature infants, the metabolic cost of growth is mainly due to protein anabolism and has been estimated to be 1.2 kcal/g of weight gained, which represents about 30% of total energy expenditure.[33,115]

Energy Losses

Infants may lose energy in the excreta. Because of the immaturity of the gut and kidney and the potentially inadequate supply of bile acids, stool and urine losses may be proportionally higher than in adults.

Energy of Activity

Studies have shown that energy expenditure varies considerably with changes in an infant's activity. Vigorous activity such as crying may double the energy expenditure,[130] but because most of the time is spent sleeping,[130] the energy expended on activity is less than 5% of the total daily energy expenditure.[143] Studies have shown that daily energy expenditure is related to both the duration and the level of activity.[29,59]

Basal Metabolic Rate and Resting Energy Expenditure

Because of ethical considerations, it is not possible to completely starve a newborn infant for the 14 hours required to measure basal metabolic rate. As a result, REE is much more commonly used as the basis of metabolic studies. REE is influenced by a number of factors, including age, body composition, size of vital organs, and energy intake.

Age: The REE of a full-term, appropriate-for-gestational-age infant increases from 33 kcal/kg per day at birth to 48 kcal/kg per day by the end of the first week of life.[85,149] It then remains constant for 1 month before declining. REE is higher in premature and small-for-gestational-age infants.[117] These age-related differences probably reflect changes in body composition,[85] although it has been suggested that the increase in basal metabolism during the first week of life may represent increased enzyme activity in functioning organs.[93]

Body Composition: During the first weeks of life, infants lose body water. This is accompanied by a well-recognized loss of body weight.[74] Before birth, a fetus is approximately 75% water, but by 1 month of age, water content has declined to 45%.[56,57] Thus, the increase in REE observed during the first weeks of life may reflect the relative increase in body tissue and the relative decrease in body water.

Size of Vital Organs: The brain, liver, heart, and kidneys account for up to 66% of the basal metabolic rate in adults yet constitute only 7% of total body weight. In infants, these organs (particularly the brain) account for a greater proportion of body weight. It is believed that the brain alone may account for 60% to 65% of the basal metabolic rate during the first month of life. In premature and small-for-gestational-age infants, the vital organs are less affected by intra- and extrauterine malnutrition than are other organs.[85,117] Thus, their contribution to basal metabolism is even greater[36]; the brain alone may account for up to 70% of basal metabolism.[88] Premature and small-for-gestational-age infants also tend to have a greater proportion of metabolically active brown adipose tissue relative to inactive white adipose tissue.[130] By contrast, full-term, appropriate-for-gestational-age infants may have only 40 g of brown adipose tissue versus 520 g of white adipose tissue.[85]

Dietary Intake: The REE of infants is related to caloric intake and weight gain. A significant linear correlation between increasing REE and increasing energy intake has been demonstrated.[35] In one study, REE increased by 8.5 kcal/kg per day following a meal, which was equivalent to 5.7% of the gross energy intake; this correlates well with the energy cost of growth.[35] Salomon et al.[150] measured the diet-induced thermogenesis of each dietary constituent in infants. They found that amino acids increased REE by 11% (4.4% of caloric intake), fat increased it by 8% (3% of caloric intake), and glucose did not increase REE at all. This study is somewhat at odds with the results of other studies, which have shown that REE increases considerably after a glucose load, particularly at high doses.[1,134]

The energy metabolism of neonates is different from that of adults and children, and this reflects their special physiologic status. Newborn infants have a significantly higher metabolic rate and energy requirement per unit body weight than do children and adults (Fig. 6-6).[170] They require approximately 40 to 70 kcal/kg per day for maintenance metabolism, 50 to 70 kcal/kg per day for growth (tissue synthesis and energy stored), and up to 20 kcal/kg per day to cover energy losses in excreta (see Fig. 6-6).[59,130]

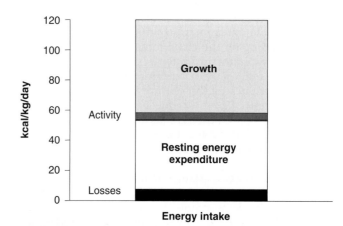

Figure 6-6 Partition of energy intake in newborn infants undergoing surgery. (Adapted from Pierro A, Carnielli V, Filler RM, et al: Partition of energy metabolism in the surgical newborn. J Pediatr Surg 1991;26:581-586.)

Computerization and miniaturization of indirect calorimeters have allowed the noninvasive investigation of energy metabolism in neonates.[130,132,137,170] The total energy requirements for a newborn infant fed enterally is 100 to 120 kcal/kg per day, compared with 60 to 80 kcal/kg per day for a 10-year-old and 30 to 40 kcal/kg per day for a 20-year-old individual. Newborn infants receiving total parenteral nutrition require fewer calories (80 to 100 kcal/kg per day). This is due to the absence of energy losses in excreta and to the fact that energy is not required for thermoregulation when the infant is nursed in a thermoneutral environment using a double-insulated incubator.

Several equations have been published to predict energy expenditure in adults.[46] In stable neonates, REE can be predicted from parameters such as weight, heart rate, and age using the following equation[132]:

$$REE \text{ (cal/min)} = -74.436 + (34.661 \times \text{Body weight in kg}) \\ + (0.496 \times \text{Heart rate in beats/min}) \\ + (0.178 \times \text{Age in days})$$

The major predictor of REE in this equation is body weight, which is also the strongest individual predictor of REE and represents the total mass of living tissue. Heart rate provides an indirect measure of the hemodynamic and metabolic status of the infant, and postnatal age has been shown to influence REE in the first few weeks of life.

THERMOREGULATION

After delivery, the relatively low ambient temperature and evaporation of the residual amniotic fluid from the skin increase the heat loss from the newborn infant. Neonates are homeotherms. They are far more susceptible to changes in environmental temperature than adults are because they have a small mass and a relatively large surface area, they possess relatively little insulating tissue such as fat and hair, they are unable to make significant behavioral alterations such as turning up the thermostat or putting on extra clothing, and they have limited energy reserves.[28] The thermoneutral zone is critical to infants[85] and is higher than it is for adults (32°C to 34°C for full-term, appropriate-for-gestational-age infants).[86] There are a number of published tables giving the optimal environmental temperature for infants of different weights and ages.[86] Numerous studies have shown that the morbidity and mortality of infants nursed outside the thermoneutral zone are significantly increased.

Heat is lost through radiation, conduction, and convection (70%) and evaporation (25%); by raising the temperature of feedings (3%); and with the excreta (2%).[85] The infant's response to cooling depends on the maturation of hypothalamic regulatory centers and the availability of substrates for thermogenesis.[85] The initial response, which is mediated by the sympathetic nervous system, is to reduce heat losses by vasoconstriction[28] and to increase heat production by shivering and nonshivering thermogenesis. Newborn infants are unable to respond to cold exposure by shivering but have a highly specialized tissue—brown adipose tissue—that is capable of generating heat

without shivering. The brown adipose tissue is well established by 22 weeks' gestation and makes up 90% of the total body fat by 29 weeks' gestation.[114] It is the most important site of nonshivering thermogenesis; other sites include the brain, liver, and kidneys. Studies have shown that the preferred fuels for nonshivering thermogenesis are free fatty acids.[31] The energy cost of thermoregulation in a cold environment is considerable. Even within the thermoneutral zone, thermoregulation can account for up to 8% of total energy expenditure.[157] REE can double when full nonshivering thermogenesis is taking place.

Neonates undergoing major operations under general anesthesia frequently become hypothermic.[122,152] Compared with adults, newborn infants experience greater difficulty maintaining their physiologic body temperature in the presence of a cold environmental challenge.[2] Hypothermia may increase the incidence of postoperative complications such as acidosis, impaired immune function, and delayed wound healing.[105] As the environmental temperature decreases, an increased blood flow to brown fat stores is observed, and heat is produced in brown fat mitochondria. During an operation, a neonate is exposed not only to a cool environment but also to a wide variety of anesthetic and paralytic agents that may have detrimental effects on heat production (energy expenditure) and core temperature.[95,97] Nonshivering thermogenesis is inhibited by anesthetic agents in experimental animals.[2,121] Albanese et al.[2] showed that termination of general anesthesia during cold exposure causes a rapid and profound increase in nonshivering thermogenesis in rabbits. This may explain the sudden and rapid increase in energy expenditure observed in young infants at the end of an operation.[41,97]

It has long been known that brown adipose tissue contains a protein, uncoupling protein 1, that dissipates the proton gradient formed across the mitochondrial inner membrane during substrate oxidation.[31] However, only recently has it been postulated that a proton leak contributes to thermogenesis in the liver.[144] The magnitude of the proton leak may be a major determinant of metabolic rate.[135] The oxidative breakdown of nutrients releases energy, which is converted to usable chemical fuel (ATP) in the mitochondria of cells by oxidative phosphorylation. This is used to drive energy-consuming processes in the body. During oxidative phosphorylation, protons are pumped from the mitochondrial matrix to the intermembrane space. Proton pumping is directly proportional to the rate of oxygen consumption ($\dot{V}O_2$) and generates and maintains a difference in the electrochemical potential of protons across the inner membrane. Protons return to the matrix by one of two routes: the phosphorylation pathway, which generates ATP, or the leak pathway, which is nonproductive and releases energy as heat. A significant proportion (20% to 30%) of oxygen consumed by resting hepatocytes from adult rats is used to drive the heat-producing proton leak.[25] This leak pathway in the liver and other organs is a significant contributor to the reactions that constitute the standard REE, resulting in significant resting heat production.[26,145] The proton permeability of the inner mitochondrial membrane in rat liver mitochondria is high in fetuses, is significantly reduced during early neonatal life, and reaches the lowest maintained level in adults.[175] Valcarce et al.[175] suggest that this could provide a protective mechanism for thermal adaptation of newborn rats during the perinatal period, before the establishment of brown adipose tissue thermogenesis. It is conceivable that newborn infants are "preprogrammed" with similar protective mechanisms that allow them to survive the stresses of birth (cold adaptation), surgery (cord division), and starvation (transient hypoglycemia).

CARBOHYDRATE, FAT, AND PROTEIN METABOLISM

The profound physiologic changes that take place in the perinatal period are reflected by equally dramatic changes in nutrition and metabolism. The fetus exists within a thermostable environment in which nutrition is continually supplied intravenously and waste products are efficiently removed. At birth, this continual nutrient supply ceases abruptly, resulting in a brief period of starvation. At the end of this period of starvation, nutrition also changes from the placental supply of glucose to milk, which is high in fat and low in carbohydrate. In addition, the kidneys and lungs of the neonate have to become much more metabolically active, and the neonate must maintain its own body temperature by activating both metabolic and physiologic mechanisms of thermogenesis and heat conservation. The neonate's successful adaptation to extrauterine life requires carefully regulated changes in glucose and fat metabolism, together with the use of stored protein reserves until an adequate nutritional supply of protein or amino acids is established. Toward the end of the neonatal period, nutrition again changes as the baby is started on a diet that is higher in carbohydrate and lower in fat than the milk diet of the neonatal period. Hence, a healthy neonate is in a state of metabolic flux, and these changes must be carefully regulated to maintain growth and brain development in this critical period. It is now known that nutrition and growth during the neonatal period are important later determinants of cardiovascular disease[158] and neurodevelopment.[107] Additional physiologic stresses caused by prematurity, infection, gastrointestinal dysfunction, anesthesia, and surgical stress present a considerable challenge to the neonate's maintenance of metabolic homeostasis. Careful management of nutrition and metabolism by surgeons and physicians is necessary to avoid additional morbidity and mortality caused by malnutrition and the neurologic sequelae of hypo- or hyperglycemia.[40] The long-term metabolic, neurologic, and cardiovascular sequelae of surgery, parenteral nutrition, or sepsis during the neonatal period are unknown, but given the importance of this period for subsequent development, nutritional management of the neonatal surgical patient likely plays a role in adult health.

Neonatal Glucose Metabolism

Most of the energy supply (approximately 70% of total calories as carbohydrate, <10% as fat)[69] of the fetus comes from maternally supplied glucose. At birth, the switch from a high-carbohydrate diet to one that is higher in lipids and lower in carbohydrates (approximately 40% of calories as carbohydrate, 50% as fat)[69] means that the neonate must not only adapt to a difference in timing and magnitude of carbohydrate supply but also regulate its own level of glycemia by insulin and glucagons, gluconeogenesis, and the other mechanisms of glucose homeostasis. The brain can use only glucose or ketone bodies; it is unable to directly oxidize lipids. Thus, maintenance of euglycemia during the neonatal period is particularly important for a favorable neurologic outcome. Despite the greater supply of fats as a fuel source in neonates than in adults, glucose turnover is greater in neonates (3 to 5 mg/kg per minute) than in adults (2 to 3 mg/kg per minute), partly due to the relatively increased brain–body mass ratio. Premature infants have an even greater glucose turnover rate (5 to 6 mg/kg per minute).[120] In premature and term infants, 90% of glucose is used by the brain; this decreases to about 40% in adults.[5] Term infants have two important means of glucose production to maintain euglycemia: glycogenolysis and gluconeogenesis. Glucose production in term neonates originates from glycogenolysis (approximately 40%) and gluconeogenesis from glycerol (20%), alanine and other amino acids (10%), and lactate (30%).[100]

The Glucagon-Insulin Axis in the Perinatal Period

Although the fetus is capable of synthesizing and releasing glucagon and insulin, the function of insulin during pregnancy is probably to promote anabolism and enhance growth rather than to regulate circulating glucose.[120] Glucagon is important for the induction of gluconeogenic enzymes during pregnancy, and the surge in glucagon at birth, due to cord clamping, is probably responsible for the rapid postnatal increase in gluconeogenic capacity.[160] Islet cell function is relatively unresponsive for the first 2 weeks of neonatal life, so that increases in insulin secretion and decreases in glucagon secretion are relatively slow in response to increased glucose concentration.[120] There is a similarly slow response to hypoglycemia in the neonate, so that if a neonate starts to become hypoglycemic, it may be some time before insulin secretion is decreased and glucagon secretion is increased to stimulate gluconeogenesis. In addition, insulin sensitivity is lower in the end-organs of neonates than in adults; thus, plasma insulin is less closely linked to blood glucose, and plasma glucagon is more closely linked to glycemia.[81,82] The maturation of the response to glucose is even slower in preterm infants than in term neonates.[43]

Glycogen and Glycogenolysis in the Perinatal Period

During the third trimester of pregnancy, maternal glucose is stored as glycogen. Most fetal storage is in the liver; some glycogen is also stored in fetal skeletal muscle, kidney, and intestine, but only a small amount in the brain. Hepatic and renal glycogen is mobilized at and immediately after birth to maintain a circulating glucose concentration; however, the hepatic glycogen stores are exhausted within 24 hours of birth or even sooner in premature babies (who had an abbreviated or no third trimester), small-for-gestational-age babies, or babies that experienced extensive perinatal stress and therefore had early catecholamine-stimulated mobilization of hepatic glycogen. Other tissues, such as heart, skeletal muscle, and lung, can metabolize stored glycogen intracellularly but cannot mobilize it to the circulation, due to a lack of the enzyme glucose-6-phosphatase. Mobilization and use of glycogen stores take place in response to the perinatal surge in glucagon or catecholamine.

Neonatal Gluconeogenesis

Key enzymes of gluconeogenesis are present in the fetus from early in gestation and increase throughout gestation and during the neonatal period. However, gluconeogenesis in vivo in the fetus has not been demonstrated, and it is not known whether cytosolic phospho*enol*pyruvate carboxykinase (necessary for gluconeogenesis from amino acids or lactate) or glucose-6-phosphatase (necessary for gluconeogenesis from all substrates and for glucose export following glycogenolysis) is expressed adequately to support gluconeogenesis by the fetal liver. Glucose-6-phosphatase expression is low in the fetus but increases within a few days of birth in term neonates.[30] Studies measuring gluconeogenesis from glycerol in preterm infants suggest that some gluconeogenesis from glycerol can occur,[169] but in preterm infants, this can only partly compensate for a decrease in exogenous glucose supply, probably owing to limited levels of glucose-6-phosphatase.[177] Parenteral glycerol supports enhanced rates of gluconeogenesis in preterm infants,[166] whereas no increase in gluconeogenesis was observed with the provision of mixed amino acids[167] or alanine[178] to preterm neonates, supporting the hypothesis that gluconeogenesis from amino acids or lactate is limited by a lack of phospho*enol*pyruvate carboxykinase activity in preterm infants. Parenteral lipids stimulate gluconeogenesis in preterm infants,[167] probably by providing carbon substrate (glycerol) and fatty acids. Fatty acid oxidation is indispensable for gluconeogenesis, providing both an energy source (ATP) to support gluconeogenesis and acetyl coenzyme A to activate pyruvate carboxylase. In experimental animals, the increase in the glucagon-insulin ratio at birth stimulates maturation of the enzymes of gluconeogenesis, particularly phospho*enol*pyruvate carboxykinase, although little is known about the induction of gluconeogenesis in human neonates. Gluconeogenesis is evident within 4 to 6 hours after birth in term neonates.[58,101]

Neonatal Hypoglycemia

Blood glucose levels fall immediately after birth but rise either spontaneously due to glycogenolysis or gluconeogenesis or as a result of feeding. This period of hypoglycemia is not considered clinically significant, but subsequent hypoglycemia should be avoided. There is considerable controversy over the blood glucose level below which infants should be considered hypoglycemic and the duration of hypoglycemia before preventive or investigational measures should be instigated,[80] particularly because glucose concentrations fluctuate significantly during this period of massive metabolic, physiologic, and nutritional change. In addition, the symptoms of neonatal

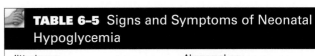

TABLE 6-5 Signs and Symptoms of Neonatal Hypoglycemia

Jitteriness	Abnormal cry
Tremors	Cardiac arrest
Apnea	Hypothermia
Cyanosis	Tachypnea
Limpness, apathy, lethargy	Seizures

hypoglycemia are nonspecific and may include those listed in Table 6-5, many of which are subjective. Recent operational thresholds for circulating glucose levels are less than 45 mg/dL (2.5 mmol/L) for term neonates with abnormal clinical signs, persistently below 36 mg/dL (2.0 mmol/L) for term neonates with risk factors for compromised metabolic adaptation, 47 mg/dL (2.6 mmol/L) for preterm infants (although data are limited), and greater than 45 mg/dL (2.5 mmol/L) at all times in parenterally fed infants because of the likelihood of increased insulin (and therefore suppressed lipolysis and ketogenesis) in these infants.[42]

Causes of hypoglycemia in the neonatal period are shown in Table 6-6. Glucose metabolism is particularly important for the brain during this critical growth period, and hypoglycemia below 2.6 mmol/L is associated

TABLE 6-6 Causes of Hypoglycemia in the Neonate

Associated with Changes in Maternal Metabolism
Intrapartum administration of glucose
Drug treatment
    Terbutaline, ritodrine, propranolol
    Oral hypoglycemic agents
Diabetes in pregnancy; infant of diabetic mother
Severe Rh incompatibility

Associated with Neonatal Problems
Idiopathic condition or failure to adapt
Perinatal hypoxia-ischemia
Infection, sepsis
Hypothermia
Hyperviscosity
Erythroblastosis fetalis, fetal hydrops
Exchange transfusion
Other
    Iatrogenic causes
    Congenital cardiac malformations

Intrauterine Growth Restriction
Endocrine and Metabolic Disorders
Hyperinsulinism (e.g., congenital hyperinsulinism, Beckwith-
    Wiedemann syndrome)
Other endocrine disorders
    Panhypopituitarism
    Isolated growth hormone deficiency
    Cortisol deficiency
Inborn errors of metabolism
    Glycogen storage diseases 1a and 1b
    Fructose 1,6-diphosphatase deficiency
    Pyruvate carboxylase deficiency
    Fatty acid oxidation disorders

with short-term neurophysiologic changes[103] and poor neurodevelopmental outcome.[51,111] However, it is difficult in these studies to reliably delineate hypoglycemia as a risk factor independent from the comorbidities and causes of hypoglycemia, such as prematurity, congenital hyperinsulinism,[113] being small for gestational age,[51] or having a diabetic mother,[164] and there is uncertainty concerning the frequency, degree, and duration of hypoglycemia that may cause neurologic problems.[79] Recent advances in neonatal cerebral imaging modalities have suggested characteristic features that may result from neonatal hypoglycemia, although the number of patients studied is small, and it is still difficult to distinguish these features from those due to comorbidities.[187]

Treatment of hypoglycemia in neonates depends on the feeding route and whether risk factors have been identified. Frequent monitoring of blood glucose is necessary, and treatment or investigational algorithms suggest increased enteral feeds along with intravenous administration of glucose if clinical signs of hypoglycemia are present.[80]

Neonatal Hyperglycemia

Neonatal hyperglycemia can also occur and has been recognized as representing several distinct clinical entities. Diabetes mellitus can present in the neonatal period, although the condition is rare, occurring in approximately 1 in 400,000 to 500,000 live births.[156,181] Both permanent and transient neonatal diabetes can occur. Transient neonatal diabetes mellitus accounts for about 50% of cases and usually resolves within 3 to 6 months; however, it may lead to the development of permanent diabetes in childhood or adolescence. Permanent neonatal diabetes mellitus accounts for the other 50% of cases. The transient type is due to paternal imprinting,[64,112] and one of the molecular causes of the permanent type has been elucidated.[70]

Most hyperglycemia in neonates is self-limited, resolves spontaneously, and has few features in common with diabetes. Its frequency appears to be increasing in parallel with increased survival of extremely low-birth-weight infants who are fed parenterally and receive corticosteroids. The etiology of neonatal hyperglycemia is not well understood, but possible causes are inability to suppress gluconeogenesis in response to glucose infusion, excessive glucose infusion rates, end-organ insulin resistance, or low plasma insulin in combination with high catecholamine levels (e.g., due to corticosteroid administration); as a result of infection; or in response to pain or surgery (see later).[80] The management of hyperglycemia in neonates is to treat its cause (e.g., treat infection or pain, decrease excessive glucose infusion rates). There is still controversy regarding insulin administration[168]: on the one hand, insulin infusion allows the maintenance of high glucose infusion rates; on the other hand, there are reports of adverse effects. Neither the acute nor the long-term sequelae of hyperglycemia in neonates are well understood; ketosis or metabolic acidosis does not occur as a result of hyperglycemia, but osmotic diuresis and glycosuria may lead to dehydration. Although the evidence for cerebral pathology and adverse neurodevelopmental outcome as a result of neonatal hyperglycemia is scant, there is a risk of increased cerebral bleeds due to osmotic shifts. There has recently been a great deal of interest in the tight control of blood glucose in adult intensive care unit patients following the study of Van den Berghe et al.[176] Although it remains to be demonstrated whether tight control of blood glucose concentration is beneficial in neonates or in specific subgroups of neonates, it has been demonstrated that peak blood glucose and duration of hyperglycemia correlate with mortality in children[162] and that hyperglycemia is associated with increased morbidity and mortality in neonates with necrotizing enterocolitis.[76]

Neonatal Lipid and Fat Metabolism

Fat is the main energy source of neonates, providing 40% to 50% of calories in milk or formula. As discussed earlier, fat oxidation becomes a major fuel used within 3 hours of birth.[74,153] In addition, fat is the main store of energy within the body. Although most chain lengths of fatty acids can be used for energy, fatty acids in the form of phospholipids and other fat-derived lipids are extremely important structural components of cell membranes, and the function of these membranes is dependent on the availability of the correct chain length and degree of unsaturation of fatty acids. Thus, throughout the period of neonatal growth, an array of different fatty acids, either supplied by the diet or metabolized by the body, is essential to support growth, particularly that of the brain, which is rich in complex lipids.

Neonatal Fatty Acid Oxidation and Ketogenesis

Fatty acid beta oxidation is the major process by which fatty acids are oxidized. The sequential removal of two-carbon units from the acyl chain provides a major source of ATP for heart and skeletal muscle. Hepatic beta oxidation serves a different role by providing ketone bodies (acetoacetate and β-hydroxybutyrate) to the peripheral circulation and supporting hepatic gluconeogenesis by providing ATP and acetyl coenzyme A to instigate pyruvate carboxylase activity. In addition, kidney,[172] small intestine,[19] white adipose tissue,[173] and brain astrocytes[45] may be ketogenic under some conditions. Ketone bodies are another significant fuel for extrahepatic organs, especially the brain, when blood glucose levels are low. Consequently, ketogenesis is extremely important to provide an alternative fuel for the brain when glucose levels may be fluctuating because of alterations in the feeding pattern and adaptation of physiologic and metabolic homeostasis. For oxidation of the acyl groups of stored, ingested, or infused triacylglycerol to take place, nonesterified fatty acids must be released. This can occur distant from the site of use by the action of hormone-sensitive lipase in the adipocyte, or locally by the action of endothelial lipoprotein lipase.[55,71] Nonesterified fatty acids bound to albumin provide the main substrate that is taken up and oxidized by tissues. In addition, intracellular triacylglycerol stores can provide a significant source of acyl moieties for beta oxidation in the heart and skeletal muscle, again through the action of hormone-sensitive lipase. Hormone-sensitive lipase and lipoprotein lipase are under the control of the hormonal and nutritional milieu, so that fatty acid oxidation is partly controlled by the supply of nonesterified fatty acids to the tissue (Fig. 6-7).[52] The pathway of hepatic fatty acid oxidation and ketogenesis is shown in Figure 6-8. In the immediate postnatal period, the plasma levels of nonesterified fatty acids increase rapidly, in response to the glucagon-catecholamine surge that stimulates lipolysis and the fall in insulin that occurs as a result of birth and cord division.[119,127] This lipolysis also results in the release of glycerol, which can be used as a gluconeogenic precursor (see earlier).[119,127] Ketone bodies are formed fairly soon after birth,[22,47,69,84,126,183] reaching 0.2 to 0.5 mM in the first 2 postnatal days and 0.7 to 1.0 mM between 5 and 10 days,[183] although this may be impaired in premature or small-for-gestational-age babies.[47,83,84] During hypoglycemia, ketone body concentrations can rise to 1.5 to 5.0 mM.[183] The enzymes of fatty acid oxidation and ketogenesis all increase in activity postnatally in experimental animals, accounting for this increased capacity for fatty acid oxidation and ketogenesis,[69] although little is known about the induction of fatty acid oxidation enzymes in humans. Hydroxymethylglutaryl-coenzyme A synthase is thought to be particularly important in the control of ketogenesis and is subject to short-term activation by glucagon, which may account for the rapid surge in ketogenesis at birth.[139]

Ketone Body Utilization

Little is known about the ontogeny of the enzymes of ketone body use in human tissues. Heart, muscle, kidney, and brain are all capable of ketone body use, and the

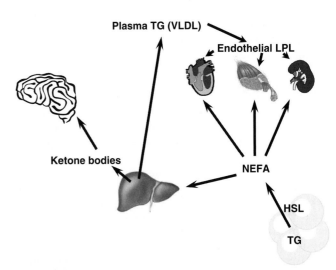

Figure 6–7 Physiology of fatty acid metabolism. Fatty acids (nonesterified fatty acids [NEFAs]) are released from adipose tissue triacylglycerol (TG) stores by the action of hormone-sensitive lipase (HSL). NEFAs can be taken up and oxidized to carbon dioxide, yielding adenosine triphosphate (ATP), by heart, muscle, and kidney; they can be oxidized to ketone bodies or re-esterified to circulating TG very-low density lipoprotein (VLDL) by the liver. Ketone bodies are oxidized by the brain, which cannot oxidize fatty acids directly. Endothelial lipoprotein lipase (LPL) releases NEFAs from circulating TG, which are then taken up and oxidized.

enzymes required have been found in human tissue.[62,123,124] In rats, the activities of the ketone body enzymes are very high in neonatal brain and decrease at weaning, whereas they are lower than adult levels in

Figure 6–8 Hepatic fatty acid oxidation. Circulating nonesterified fatty acids (NEFAs), bound to albumin, are taken up by hepatocytes. Fatty acids can be oxidized in the mitochondria or esterified to triacylglycerol and re-exported. Acetyl coenzyme A from fatty acid oxidation can be used to generate adenosine triphosphate (ATP) via the Krebs cycle or used to generate ketone bodies for peripheral utilization.

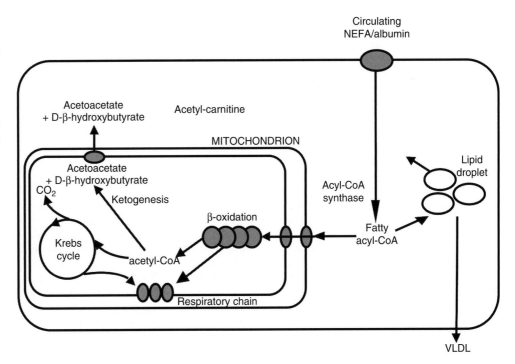

neonatal muscle and kidney, suggesting preferential use by the brain.[69]

Neonatal Protein and Amino Acid Metabolism

In contrast to healthy adults who exist in a state of neutral nitrogen balance, infants need to be in positive nitrogen balance to achieve satisfactory growth and development. Infants are efficient at retaining nitrogen and can retain up to 80% of the metabolizable protein intake on both oral and intravenous diets.[33,159,190] Protein metabolism is dependent on both protein and energy intake. The influence of dietary protein is well established. An increased protein intake has been shown to enhance protein synthesis,[65,72] reduce endogenous protein breakdown,[125] and thus enhance net protein retention.[125,191] The influence of nonprotein energy intake on protein metabolism is more controversial. Protein retention can be enhanced by the intake of carbohydrate and fat,[16,34,110,128,147,174] which are thus said to be protein sparing. Although some studies have suggested that the protein-sparing effect of carbohydrate is greater than that of fat,[34,110,174] others have suggested that the protein-sparing effect of fat may be equivalent to or greater than that of carbohydrate.[16,128,147] The addition of fat calories to the intravenous diets of newborn surgical patients reduces protein oxidation and protein contribution to energy expenditure and increases protein retention.[128] To further investigate this positive effect on protein metabolism, we studied the various components of whole protein metabolism by the combined technique of indirect calorimetry and use of a stable isotope (^{13}C-leucine) tracer. Two groups of neonates receiving isonitrogenous and isocaloric total parenteral nutrition were studied: one group received a high-fat diet, and the other a high-carbohydrate diet.[95] There was no significant difference between the two groups with regard to any of the components of whole-body protein metabolism: protein synthesis, protein breakdown, protein oxidation and excretion, and total protein flux. This study confirms previous observations that infants have high rates of protein turnover, synthesis, and breakdown, which may be up to eight times greater than those reported in adults. In newborn infants receiving parenteral nutrition, synthesis and breakdown of endogenous body protein far exceed intake and oxidation of exogenous protein. Infants are avid retainers of nitrogen, and carbohydrate and fat have an equivalent effect on protein metabolism. This supports the use of fat in the intravenous diets of newborn surgical patients.

The protein requirements of newborn infants are between 2.5 and 3.0 g/kg per day. Amino acids, the building blocks of protein, can be widely interconverted, so that several are described as dispensable (or nonessential): alanine, aspartate, asparagine, glutamate, and serine. Others are described as indispensable (or essential): histidine, isoleucine, leucine, lysine, methionine, phenylalanine, threonine, tryptophan, and valine. Still other amino acids (arginine, cysteine, glycine, glutamine, proline, and tyrosine) are not usually essential but can become important during metabolic stress, such as sepsis. Sulfur amino acids (cysteine, methionine) and tyrosine, in particular, are abundant in acute phase proteins, so their supply becomes particularly important during acute phase responses. Human milk provides amino acids in the form of protein and as free amino acids. Milk proteins are important not only for their nutritive value; they possess other important properties such as anti-infective activity (IgA, IgM, IgG, lactoferrin, lysozyme).[77] It has been suggested that the platelet-activating factor acetylhydrolase, a minor component of human milk, is responsible for some of breast milk's protective effect against necrotizing enterocolitis.[142] The amino acid glutamine is of particular interest in premature infants and neonates undergoing surgery.

The nitrogen source of total parenteral nutrition is usually provided as a mixture of crystalline amino acids. Commercially available solutions contain the eight known essential amino acids plus histidine, which is essential in children.[191] Complications such as azotemia, hyperammonemia, and metabolic acidosis have been described in patients receiving high levels of intravenous amino acids,[102] but these complications are rarely seen with an amino acid intake of 2 to 3 g/kg per day.[4] In patients with severe malnutrition or with additional losses (e.g., jejunostomy, ileostomy), the protein requirements are higher.[191] The ideal quantitative composition of amino acid solutions is still controversial. In newborn infants, cysteine, taurine, and tyrosine seem to be essential amino acids. However, the addition of cysteine in the parenteral nutrition of neonates does not cause any difference in growth rate or nitrogen retention.[190] The essentiality of these amino acids could be related to the synthesis of neurotransmitter, bile salts, and hormones. Failure to supply these amino acids may result in poor long-term neurologic or gastrointestinal function.[140] The incidence of abnormal plasma aminograms during parenteral nutrition is low. There are no convincing data to support the selection of one crystalline amino acid solution over another in newborn infants. Glutamine is a nonessential amino acid that has many important biologic functions, such as being a preferential fuel for the immune system and the gut. Various authors have postulated that glutamine may become "conditionally essential" during sepsis and that addition of glutamine to parenteral feeds of premature or surgical neonates may help preserve mucosal structure, prevent bacterial location, and hence reduce the number of infections and the time before full enteral feeding can be established.

METABOLIC RESPONSE TO STRESS

The body has developed a system of responses to deal with various noxious stimuli that threaten survival. In some respects, these responses are stereotypical and lead to the so-called stress response. Stress can be defined as "factors that cause disequilibrium to an organism and therefore threaten homeostasis."[184] Initiators of the stress response in newborn infants include operative trauma and sepsis. In this chapter we discuss the response to operative trauma; the physiologic changes due to sepsis are discussed in Chapter 10.

The stress response is initiated and coordinated by several messengers and affects whole-body systems. The insult of operative trauma can be considered a form of "controlled" injury that results in alterations in the metabolic, inflammatory, endocrine, and immune responses. These responses have evolved to enhance the survival of trauma and infection in the absence of iatrogenic intervention. They limit patient activity in the area of injury to prevent secondary damage and start the healing process through the inflammatory signals produced. Changes in metabolism increase the availability of substrates needed by regenerating and healing tissue. Immune stimulation leads to the swift eradication of any causal or secondary opportunistic microbial invasion, and the subsequent immunoparesis dampens this stimulation to allow healing to ensue.

In contrast with adults, the energy requirements of infants and children undergoing major operations seem to be minimally modified by the operative trauma per se. In adults, trauma or surgery causes a brief "ebb" period with a depressed metabolic rate, followed by a "flow" phase characterized by an increase in oxygen consumption to support the massive exchanges of substrate between organs (Fig. 6-9).[87] In newborn infants, major abdominal surgery causes a moderate (15%) and immediate (peak at 4 hours) elevation of oxygen consumption and REE and a rapid return to baseline 12 to 24 hours postoperatively (see Fig. 6-9).[97] There is no further increase in

energy expenditure in the first 5 to 7 days following an operation.[97,154] The timing of these changes corresponds with the postoperative increase in catecholamine levels described by Anand et al.[10] Maximal endocrine and biochemical changes are observed immediately after the operation and gradually return to normal over the next 24 hours. Interestingly, infants having a major operation after the second day of life have a significantly greater increase in REE than do infants undergoing surgery within the first 48 hours of life. A possible explanation may be the secretion of endogenous opioids by newborn infants. It has been suggested that nociceptive stimuli during the operation are responsible for the endocrine and metabolic stress response, and that these stimuli may be inhibited by opioids.[9,10] This is supported by studies showing that moderate doses of opioids blunt the endocrine and metabolic responses to operative stress in infancy.[9,10] The levels of endogenous opioids in the cord blood of newborn infants are five times higher than the plasma levels in resting adults.[54] Thus, it is possible that the reduced metabolic stress response observed in infants younger than 48 hours old is related to higher circulating levels of endogenous opioids. This may constitute a protective mechanism, blunting the response to stress in the perinatal period.

Chwals et al.[38] demonstrated that the postoperative increase in energy expenditure can result from severe underlying acute illness (e.g., sepsis, intense inflammation). REE is directly proportional to growth rate in healthy infants, and growth is retarded during acute metabolic stress. These authors suggest that energy is used for growth recovery after resolution of the acute injury response in infants undergoing surgery. They indicate that serial measurement of postoperative REE can be used to stratify injury severity and may be an effective parameter to monitor the return of normal growth metabolism in infants after surgery.

Operative trauma initiates a constellation of inflammatory pathways that regulate a whole-body response to operative stress, which is similar to that seen after injury. The responses can be initiated and controlled by both chemical or hormonal signals and afferent nervous signals. Some of the chemical signals responsible for these responses originate in the operative wound in response to cellular injury.

ADULTS

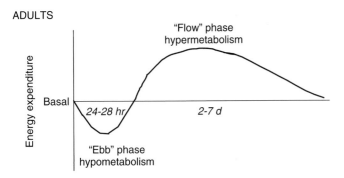

INFANTS

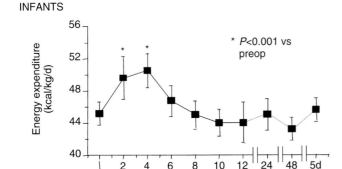

Figure 6–9 Postoperative variations in energy expenditure in adults and neonates undergoing major operations. Data for infants are expressed as mean ± SEM. (Adapted from Jones MO, Pierro A, Hammond P, et al: The metabolic response to operative stress in infants. J Pediatr Surg 1993;28:1258-1262; and Pierro A: J Pediatr Surg 2002; 37: 811–822.)

Cytokines

Cytokines constitute one of the key chemical messenger systems in the control and coordination of the response to injury. They are a group of low-molecular-weight polypeptides or glycoproteins that act to regulate the local and systemic immune function and modulate the inflammatory response. Cytokines are active at very low concentrations, usually at the picogram level, and their production is normally transient. They act by altering gene expression in target cells. Cytokines act in a paracrine and autocrine manner at concentrations in the picomolar to nanomolar range, but they can have systemic effects if there is spillover into the circulation.

Cytokines generally have a wide range of actions in the body. Because they are not usually stored intracellularly, they must be synthesized de novo and released into the tissues upon appropriate stimulation and gene transcription. One of the crucial controllers of cytokine gene regulation is nuclear factor kappa B,[21,89] a protein transcription factor that enhances the transaction of a variety of cytokine genes. Lymphocytes are activated at the site of injury. The first cells to be recruited to the site of inflammation are monocytes and neutrophils, which produce cytokines in the first few hours after the onset of a surgical or traumatic wound.[104] These cytokines are chemoattractant to other white cells.

Cytokines are divided into pro- and anti-inflammatory types on the basis of whether they stimulate the immune system or dampen the immune response. Although most cytokines have a clear pro- or anti-inflammatory response, a few have dual properties. Some cytokines may exhibit a proinflammatory action in a particular cell or under certain conditions but an anti-inflammatory response in a different cell or under different conditions.[188] The presence of anti-inflammatory cytokines is important in inhibiting the immune response to prevent excessive tissue destruction and death. The presence of naturally occurring inhibitors helps abate the otherwise catastrophic positive feedback loop that could lead to widespread tissue destruction from excessive inflammation. The cytokines that are commonly released following trauma include the proinflammatory interleukin (IL)-1, IL-6, and tumor necrosis factor (TNF)-α and the anti-inflammatory IL-1ra and IL-10.

Both pro- and anti-inflammatory cytokines are produced in response to operative stress. The actual cytokine cascade is heterogeneous and is determined by various factors, including the type and magnitude of the operation. The cytokine cascade in response to operations in adults has been well characterized,[44] but there have been limited studies in neonates. Cytokines bond to specific membrane receptors of target organs. Their actions in the acute stress response include (1) changes in gene expression and proliferation, thereby affecting wound healing and immunocompetence; (2) release of counterregulatory hormones; and (3) facilitation of cell-to-cell communication.[37] Substrate utilization is also affected by cytokine release. Glucose transport is increased by TNF, hepatic gluconeogenesis is stimulated by IL-1, and hepatic lipogenesis is stimulated by IL-1, IL-6, and TNF. IL-1 and TNF also appear to promote muscle proteolysis. In neonates, IL-6 increases maximally 12 hours after major surgery; this increase is proportional to the degree of operative trauma,[98] indicating that this cytokine is a marker of the stress response in neonates. IL-1 and TNF may have a synergistic effect in producing the metabolic manifestations seen after injury and infection.[87] However, systemic cytokine release cannot account for all the metabolic changes seen after injury, because cytokines are not consistently found in the bloodstream of injured patients, and systemic cytokine administration does not produce all the metabolic effects observed in injured adults.

Other mediators of the response to tissue injury include histamine, a well-known chemical mediator in acute inflammation that causes vascular dilatation and the immediate transient phase of increased vascular permeability; 5-hydroxytryptamine (serotonin), a potent vasoconstrictor; lysosomal compounds released from activated neutrophils, monocytes, and macrophages; lymphokines, chemicals involved in the inflammatory cascade with vasoactive or chemotactic properties; the complement system; and the kinin system. These mediators cause vasodilatation, increased vascular permeability, and emigration and stimulation of white blood cells. The postoperative changes that occur also affect the immune system. There is a period of immune stimulation that is often followed by period of immunoparesis. There is a proinflammatory response that is balanced by an anti-inflammatory response. The balance often determines and predicts the development of complications and the outcome in terms of morbidity and mortality.

Other responses may be initiated by peripheral and central nervous system stimulation. Peripheral efferents from pain receptors, for instance, can feed back to the central nervous system and produce some of the clinical signs of inflammation and the responses seen after operative stress. Indeed, blockage of this afferent stimulus is associated with dampening of the stress response.[10] Fentanyl and morphine are commonly used in pediatric anesthesia for pain relief. Studies in preterm infants and neonates have shown that fentanyl blunts the metabolic response to operative stress.[9-11]

Endocrine Response

Various studies have characterized the endocrine response to surgery in infants and children.[7,8,73] These studies reveal that the response lasts between 24 and 48 hours postoperatively; in adults, it usually lasts longer.[20,171] Compared with values seen after an overnight fast, there is an increase in insulin levels in the early postoperative period; however, this increase in insulin is not proportional to the increase in glucose. There is a change in the insulin-glucose ratio in the postoperative period that lasts more than 24 hours.[8,182] Anand et al.[8] found that neonates exhibited an initial decrease in the insulin-glucose ratio in the immediate postoperative period that was restored by 6 hours. Ward-Platt et al.[182] found an instantaneous and continuous rise in the ratio in older infants and children.

Cortisol is significantly elevated postoperatively and remains elevated for 24 hours, accompanied by a rise in catecholamines.[75,148] Both hormones have anti-insulin effects. The rise in cortisol and catecholamines partially drives the postoperative hyperglycemic response and may be responsible for the relative insulin insensitivity in the postoperative period. Anand et al.[8] found a very significant correlation between glucose and adrenaline levels in neonates at the end of abdominal surgery. There is an increase in lactate levels in the postoperative period both in adults and in infants and children.[6,9,91] This increase in lactate is related to the alteration in glucose metabolism[8] and, more acutely, the presence of tissue hypoperfusion related to surgery.[91] The degree of lactate increase may represent a means of determining the magnitude of operative stress. Changes in hormone levels are related to the magnitude of operative stress and have been shown in some, but not all, procedures to be lessened by laparoscopic surgery.

Effect of Surgery on Glucose Metabolism in Neonates

Surgery in adults is well known to cause hyperglycemia, and a hyperglycemic response to surgery has also been well documented in neonates,[8-11,23,53,106,133,161] with the degree of hyperglycemia being negatively correlated with age.[161] In contrast to adults, however, in whom blood glucose concentrations may remain high for several days postoperatively, the rise in glucose levels in neonates is short-lived, lasting only up to 12 hours. In an elegant study, Anand and Aynsley-Green[7] showed a strong correlation between the degree of surgical stress and the increase in glucose levels. In the same study, stress scores were also strongly positively correlated with plasma adrenaline, noradrenaline, glucagon, and insulin and less strongly

with cortisol.[7] The hyperglycemic response to surgery is probably multifactorial, including increased glycogenolysis and gluconeogenesis in response to increases in plasma catecholamines and, subsequently, glucagon. In addition, the insulin response to hyperglycemia may be inappropriately low, especially in preterm neonates undergoing surgery,[8] and tissues may become relatively refractory to insulin. Support for the hypothesis that these effects are driven by catecholamine release is provided by the studies of Anand's group, who showed that blunting the catecholamine response to surgery by modulating the anesthetic regimen led to a blunting of the hyperglycemic and endocrine response to surgery.[9-11] The timing of the adrenaline, noradrenaline, and glucose response to neonatal surgery is shown in Figure 6-10.

Carbohydrate conversion to fat (lipogenesis) occurs when glucose intake exceeds metabolic needs. The risks associated with this process are twofold: accumulation of the newly synthesized fat in the liver,[163] and aggravation of respiratory acidosis resulting from increased CO_2 production, particularly in patients with compromised pulmonary function.[14] Jones et al.[96] showed that in infants receiving parenteral nutrition after surgery, there is a negative linear relationship between glucose intake and fat utilization (oxidation and conversion to fat) expressed in grams/kilograms per day ($y = 4.547 - 0.254x$; $r = -0.937$; $P = <0.0001$). From this it was calculated that net fat synthesis from glucose exceeds net fat oxidation when the glucose intake is greater than 18 g/kg per day. Jones et al.[96] also found a significant relationship between glucose intake and CO_2 production ($y = 3.849 + 0.183x$; $r = 0.825$; $P = <0.0001$). The slope of this relationship was steeper when glucose intake exceeded 18 g/kg per day ($y = 2.62 + 0.244x$; $r = 0.746$; $P = <0.05$) than when it was less than 18 g/kg per day ($y = 5.30 + 0.069x$; $r = 0.264$; $P = 0.461$). Thus, the conversion of glucose to fat results in a significantly increased production of CO_2. Glucose intake exceeding 18 g/kg per day is also associated with a significant increase in respiratory rate and plasma triglyceride levels. In summary:

1. Glucose intake is the principal determinant of carbohydrate and fat utilization.
2. The maximal oxidative capacity for glucose in infants undergoing surgery is 18 g/kg per day, which is equivalent to the energy expenditure of the infant.
3. If glucose is given in excess of the maximal oxidative capacity, (a) net fat oxidation ceases; (b) net fat synthesis begins; (c) the thermogenic effect of glucose increases, and the efficiency with which glucose is metabolized decreases; (d) carbon dioxide production and respiratory rate increase; and (e) plasma triglyceride levels increase.

It is therefore advisable in stable surgical newborn infants requiring parenteral nutrition not to exceed 18 g/kg per day of intravenous glucose intake.[96,129]

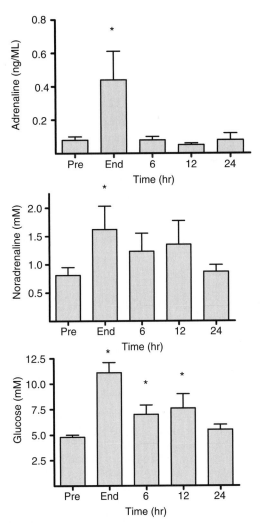

Figure 6–10 Response of adrenaline, noradrenaline, and glucose to surgery in neonates. (Data from Anand KJS, Brown MJ, Causon RC, et al: Can the human neonate mount an endocrine and metabolic response to surgery? J Pediatr Surg 1985;20:41–48.)*p < 0.05 *vs.* preoperative sample.

Effect of Surgery on Fat Metabolism in Neonates

Surgery in neonates causes an increase in nonesterified fatty acid and ketone body levels[8,9,11,133] that can be decreased by modulating the catecholamine release,[9,11] suggesting that catecholamine stimulation of lipolysis is responsible for this increase. Pierro et al.[129] studied intravenous fat utilization by infusing for 4 hours Intralipid 10% in isocaloric and isovolemic amounts into the previously given mixture of glucose and amino acids. Gas exchange was measured by indirect calorimetry to calculate the patient's oxygen consumption and CO_2 production and net fat utilization. The study showed that (1) surgical infants adapt rapidly (within 2 hours) to the intravenous infusion of fat, (2) more than 80% of the exogenous fat can be oxidized, and (3) CO_2 production is reduced during fat infusion as a consequence of the cessation of carbohydrate conversion to fat.[129] This study did not measure the rate of fat utilization during a mixed intravenous diet including carbohydrate, amino acids, and fat. More recent studies on stable surgical newborn infants receiving fixed amounts of carbohydrate and amino acids and variable amounts of intravenous long-chain triglyceride fat emulsion have shown that at a carbohydrate intake of 15 g/kg per day (56.3 kcal/kg per day), the proportion of energy metabolism derived from fat oxidation does not exceed 20%, even with a fat intake as high as 6 g/kg per day. At a carbohydrate intake of 10 g/kg per day, this proportion can be as high as 50%.[131] This study seems to indicate that during postoperative parenteral nutrition in infants, the majority of the intravenous fat infused is not oxidized but deposited. Net fat oxidation seems to be significantly influenced by the carbohydrate intake and by the REE of the neonate. When the intake of glucose calories exceeds the REE of the infant, net fat oxidation is minimal regardless of fat intake.[131] Therefore, to use intravenous fat as an energy source (i.e., oxidation to CO_2 and H_2O), carbohydrate intake must be maintained below basal energy requirements.

Commonly used fat emulsions for parenteral nutrition in pediatrics are based on long-chain triglycerides (LCTs). The rate of intravenous fat oxidation during total parenteral nutrition can theoretically be enhanced by adding L-carnitine or medium-chain triglycerides (MCTs) to the intravenous diet. Important differences between MCTs and LCTs have been observed with respect to physical and metabolic properties. MCTs are cleared from the bloodstream at a faster rate and are oxidized more completely for energy production than are LCTs. Therefore, they seem to serve as a preferential energy source for the body. We investigated the effects of MCTs on intravenous fat utilization during total parenteral nutrition in two groups of stable surgical newborn infants.[50] One group received LCT-based (100% LCTs) fat emulsion, and the other group received an isocaloric amount of MCT-based (50% MCTs + 50% LCTs) fat emulsion. In infants receiving carbohydrate calories in excess of the measured REE (56 kcal/kg per day), net fat oxidation was not enhanced by the administration of MCT-based fat emulsion. Conversely, in infants receiving carbohydrate calories below the REE (41 kcal/kg per day), the administration of MCT fat emulsion increased net fat oxidation from 0.6 ± 0.2 to 1.7 ± 0.2 g/kg per day. The administration of MCT-based fat emulsion did not increase the metabolic rate of the infants. Fats that are not used can become the substrates for free lipid peroxidation and free radical production. Peroxidation has specifically been linked with lipids in parenteral nutrition[18,186] and has been shown to be dependent on the amount of carbohydrate given: if net fat oxidation is not taking place because carbohydrate intake is high, more lipid is present to be peroxidized.[17]

Effect of Surgery on Protein and Amino Acid Metabolism in Neonates

Major operative stress in adults results in a negative nitrogen balance due to muscle protein catabolism. Neonates are already in a more precarious position regarding nitrogen balance, so if major protein catabolism were to take place, growth and other important functions would be impaired. Nitrogen losses are increased after surgery in neonates,[39,90,151,189] and muscle protein breakdown has also been demonstrated by increased 3-methylhistidine excretion.[10,11] However, these changes are relatively short-lived and can be overcome by providing additional dietary nitrogen or calories. Powis et al.[136] investigated protein metabolism kinetics in infants and young children who had undergone major operations. Patients were studied for 4 hours preoperatively and for the first 6 hours following surgery. There were no significant differences in the rates of whole-body protein flux, protein synthesis, amino acid oxidation, and protein degradation preoperatively and postoperatively, indicating that infants and children do not increase their whole-body protein turnover after major operations. It is possible that infants and children are able to convert energy expended on growth to energy directed toward wound repair and healing, thereby avoiding the overall increase in energy expenditure and catabolism seen in adults.[136] However, little is known about the components of protein turnover in neonates. The only available study, on six neonates with necrotizing enterocolitis, showed no differences in protein turnover between acute and recovery phases of the disease.[137]

REFERENCES

1. Acheson KJ, Schutz Y, Bessard T, et al: Nutritional influences on lipogenesis and thermogenesis after a carbohydrate meal. Am J Physiol 1984;246:E62-E70.
2. Albanese CT, Nour BM, Rowe MI: Anesthesia blocks non-shivering thermogenesis in the neonatal rabbit. J Pediatr Surg 1994;29:983-986.
3. Alroomi L, Barclay S, Beattie J, et al: CRIB (Clinical Risk Index for Babies), mortality, and impairment after neonatal intensive-care. Lancet 1995;345:1020-1022.
4. American Academy of Pediatrics Committee on Nutrition: Commentary on parenteral nutrition. Pediatrics 1983;71:547-552.
5. American Academy of Pediatrics Committee on Nutrition: Hypoglycemia in infants and children. In Kleinman RE (ed): Pediatric Nutrition Handbook, 5th ed. Elk Grove, IL, American Academy of Pediatrics, 2004, pp 515-535.
6. Anand KJS: Neonatal stress responses to anesthesia and surgery. Clin Perinatol 1990;17:207-214.
7. Anand KJS, Aynsley-Green A: Measuring the severity of surgical stress in newborn infants. J Pediatr Surg 1988;23:297-305.

8. Anand KJS, Brown MJ, Causon RC, et al: Can the human neonate mount an endocrine and metabolic response to surgery? J Pediatr Surg 1985;20:41-48.

9. Anand KJS, Hickey PR: Halothane-morphine compared with high-dose sufentanil for anesthesia and postoperative analgesia in neonatal cardiac surgery. N Engl J Med 1992;326:1-9.

10. Anand KJS, Sippell WG, Aynsley-Green A: Randomised trial of fentanyl anaesthesia in preterm babies undergoing surgery: Effects on the stress response. Lancet 1987;1:62-66.

11. Anand KJS, Sippell WG, Schofield NM, et al: Does halothane anaesthesia decrease the metabolic and endocrine stress responses of newborn infants undergoing operation? BMJ 1988;296:668-672.

12. Antonelli M, Moreno R, Vincent JL, et al: Application of SOFA score to trauma patients: Sequential Organ Failure Assessment. Intensive Care Med 1999;25:389-394.

13. Ashworth A, Bell R, James WP, et al: Calorie requirements of children recovering from protein-calorie malnutrition. Lancet 1968;2:600-603.

14. Askanazi J, Nordenstrom J, Rosenbaum SH, et al: Nutrition for the patient with respiratory failure: Glucose vs fat. Anesthesiology 1981;54:373-377.

15. Ballard JL, Khoury JC, Wedig K, et al: New Ballard score, expanded to include extremely premature infants. J Pediatr 1991;119:417-423.

16. Bark S, Holm I, Hakansson I, et al: Nitrogen-sparing effect of fat emulsion compared with glucose in the postoperative period. Acta Chir Scand 1976;142:423-427.

17. Basu R, Muller DPR, Eaton S, et al: Lipid peroxidation can be reduced in infants on total parenteral nutrition by promoting fat utilisation. J Pediatr Surg 1999;34:255-259.

18. Basu R, Muller DPR, Papp E, et al: Free radical formation in infants: The effect of critical illness, parenteral nutrition, and enteral feeding. J Pediatr Surg 1999;34:1091-1095.

19. Bekesi A, Williamson DH: An explanation for ketogenesis by the intestine of the suckling rat—the presence of an active hydroxymethylglutaryl-coenzyme-A pathway. Biol Neonate 1990;58:160-165.

20. Bellon JM, Manzano L, Larrad A, et al: Endocrine and immune response to injury after open and laparoscopic cholecystectomy. Int Surg 1998;83:24-27.

21. Blackwell TS, Christman JW: The role of nuclear factor-kappa B in cytokine gene regulation. Am J Respir Cell Mol Biol 1997;17:3-9.

22. Bougneres PF, Lemmel C, Ferre P, et al: Ketone-body transport in the human neonate and infant. J Clin Invest 1986;77:42-48.

23. Bouwmeester NJ, Anand KJS, van Dijk M, et al: Hormonal and metabolic stress responses after major surgery in children aged 0-3 years: A double-blind, randomized trial comparing the effects of continuous versus intermittent morphine. Br J Anaesth 2001;87:390-399.

24. Brace RA: Physiology of amniotic fluid volume regulation. Clin Obstet Gynecol 1997;40:280-289.

25. Brand MD: The proton leak across the mitochondrial inner membrane. Biochim Biophys Acta 1990;1018:128-133.

26. Brand MD, Chien LF, Ainscow EK, et al: The causes and functions of mitochondrial proton leak. Biochim Biophys Acta 1994;1187:132-139.

27. Brooke OG, Ashworth A: The influence of malnutrition on the postprandial metabolic rate and respiratory quotient. Br J Nutr 1972;27:407-415.

28. Bruck K: Temperature regulation in the newborn infant. Biol Neonate 1961;3:65-119.

29. Bruck K, Parmlee AH, Bruck M: Neutral temperature range and range of "thermal comfort" in premature infants. Biol Neonate 1962;4:32-51.

30. Burchell A, Gibb L, Waddell ID, et al: The ontogeny of human hepatic microsomal glucose-6-phosphatase proteins. Clin Chem 1990;36:1633-1637.

31. Cannon B, Nedergaard J: Brown adipose tissue: Function and physiological significance. Physiol Rev 2004;84:277-359.

32. Casey PH, Kraemer HC, Bernbaum J, et al: Growth patterns of low birth weight preterm infants: A longitudinal analysis of a large, varied sample. J Pediatr 1990;117:298-307.

33. Catzeflis C, Schutz Y, Micheli JL, et al: Whole-body protein-synthesis and energy-expenditure in very low birth-weight infants. Pediatr Res 1985;19:679-687.

34. Chessex P, Gagne G, Pineault M, et al: Metabolic and clinical consequences of changing from high-glucose to high-fat regimens in parenterally fed newborn-infants. J Pediatr 1989;115:992-997.

35. Chessex P, Reichman BL, Verellen GJ, et al: Influence of postnatal age, energy intake, and weight gain on energy metabolism in the very low-birth-weight infant. J Pediatr 1981;99:761-766.

36. Chessex P, Reichman B, Verellen G, et al: Metabolic consequences of intrauterine growth retardation in very low birthweight infants. Pediatr Res 1984;18:709-713.

37. Chwals WJ: The newborn as a surgical patient: Metabolic considerations. In O'Neill JA Jr, Rowe MI, Grosfeld JL, et al (eds): Pediatric Surgery, 5th ed. St Louis, Mosby-Year Book, 1998, pp 57-70.

38. Chwals WJ, Letton RW, Jamie A, et al: Stratification of injury severity using energy-expenditure response in surgical infants. J Pediatr Surg 1995;30:1161-1164.

39. Colle E, Paulsen EP: Response of the newborn infant to major surgery. 1. Effects on water, electrolyte, and nitrogen balances. Pediatrics 1959;23:1063-1084.

40. Coran AG: Nutrition of the surgical patient. In Welch KJ, Randolph JG, Reed DJ (eds): Pediatric Surgery. Chicago, Year Book, 1986, pp 96-108.

41. Coran AG, Pierro A, Schmeling DJ: Metabolism of the neonate requiring surgery. In Cowett RM (ed): Principles of Perinatal-Neonatal Metabolism, 2nd ed. New York, Springer, 1998, pp 1131-1151.

42. Cornblath M, Hawdon JM, Williams AF, et al: Controversies regarding definition of neonatal hypoglycemia: Suggested operational thresholds. Pediatrics 2000;105:1141-1145.

43. Cowett RM, Farrag HM: Neonatal glucose metabolism. In Cowett RM (ed): Principles of Perinatal-Neonatal Metabolism, 2nd ed. New York, Springer, 1998, pp 683-722.

44. Cruickshank AM, Fraser WD, Burns HJ, et al: Response of serum interleukin-6 in patients undergoing elective surgery of varying severity. Clin Sci (Colch) 1990;79:161-165.

45. Cullingford TE, Dolphin CT, Bhakoo KK, et al: Molecular cloning of rat mitochondrial 3-hydroxy-3-methylglutaryl-CoA lyase and detection of the corresponding mRNA and of those encoding the remaining enzymes comprising the ketogenic 3-hydroxy-3-methylglutaryl-CoA cycle in central nervous system of suckling rat. Biochem J 1998;329:373-381.

46. Cunningham JJ: Body composition as a determinant of energy expenditure: A synthetic review and a proposed general prediction equation. Am J Clin Nutr 1991;54:963-969.

47. Deboissieu D, Rocchiccioli F, Kalach N, et al: Ketone-body turnover at term and in premature newborns in the first 2 weeks after birth. Biol Neonate 1995;67:84-93.

48. Demissie K, Rhoads GG, Ananth CV, et al: Trends in preterm birth and neonatal mortality among blacks and whites in the United States from 1989 to 1997. Am J Epidemiol 2001;154:307-315.

49. Disturbances in newborns and infants. In Beers MF, Berkow R (eds): The Merck Manual of Diagnosis and Therapy, 17th ed. White House Station, NJ, Merck Research Laboratories, 1999, pp 2127-2145.

50. Donnell SC, Lloyd DA, Eaton S, et al: The metabolic response to intravenous medium-chain triglycerides in infants after surgery. J Pediatr 2002;141:689-694.

51. Duvanel CB, Fawer CL, Cotting J, et al: Long-term effects of neonatal hypoglycemia on brain growth and psychomotor development in small-for-gestational-age preterm infants. J Pediatr 1999;134:492-498.

52. Eaton S: Control of mitochondrial β-oxidation flux. Prog Lipid Res 2002;41:197-239.

53. Elphick MC, Wilkinson AW: The effects of starvation and surgical injury on the plasma levels of glucose, free fatty acids, and neutral lipids in newborn babies suffering from various congenital anomalies. Pediatr Res 1981;15:313-318.

54. Facchinetti F, Bagnoli F, Bracci R, et al: Plasma opioids in the first hours of life. Pediatr Res 1982;16:95-98.

55. Fielding BA, Frayn KN: Lipoprotein lipase and the disposition of dietary fatty acids. Br J Nutr 1998;80:495-502.

56. Fomon SJ: Body composition of male reference infant during first year of life—Borden Award address, October 1966. Pediatrics 1967;40:863-870.

57. Fomon SJ, Nelson SE: Body composition of the male and female reference infants. Annu Rev Nutr 2002;22:1-17.

58. Frazer TE, Karl IE, Hillman LS, et al: Direct measurement of gluconeogenesis from [2,3-C-13(2)]alanine in the human neonate. Am J Physiol 1981;240:E615-E621.

59. Freymond D, Schutz Y, Decombaz J, et al: Energy-balance, physical-activity, and thermogenic effect of feeding in premature-infants. Pediatr Res 1986;20:638-645.

60. Friis-Hansen B: Body water compartments in children: Changes during growth and related changes in body composition. Pediatrics 1961;28:169-181.

61. Friis-Hansen B: Water distribution in the foetus and newborn infant. Acta Paediatr Scand Suppl 1983;305:7-11.

62. Fukao T, Song XQ, Mitchell GA, et al: Enzymes of ketone body utilization in human tissues: Protein and messenger RNA levels of succinyl-coenzyme A (CoA), 3-ketoacid CoA transferase and mitochondrial and cytosolic acetoacetyl-CoA thiolases. Pediatr Res 1997;42:498-502.

63. Gagliardi L, Cavazza A, Brunelli A, et al: Assessing mortality risk in very low birthweight infants: A comparison of CRIB, CRIB-II, and SNAPPE-II. Arch Dis Child 2004;89:F419-F422.

64. Gardner RJ, Mungall AJ, Dunham I, et al: Localisation of a gene for transient neonatal diabetes mellitus to an 18.72 cR(3000) (similar to 5.4 Mb) interval on chromosome 6q. J Med Genet 1999;36:192-196.

65. Garlick PJ, Clugston GA, Swick RW, et al: Diurnal pattern of protein and energy metabolism in man. Am J Clin Nutr 1980;33:1983-1986.

66. Gibson AT, Carney S, Cavazzoni E, et al: Neonatal and postnatal growth. Horm Res 2000;53(Suppl 1):S42-S49.

67. Gilbert WM, Brace RA: Amniotic fluid volume and normal flows to and from the amniotic cavity. Semin Perinatol 1993;17:150-157.

68. Gill A, Yu VY, Bajuk B, et al: Postnatal growth in infants born before 30 weeks' gestation. Arch Dis Child 1986;61:549-553.

69. Girard J, Ferré P, Pégorier J-P, et al: Adaptations of glucose and fatty-acid metabolism during perinatal-period and suckling-weaning transition. Physiol Rev 1992;72:507-562.

70. Gloyn AL, Pearson ER, Antcliff JF, et al: Activating mutations in the gene encoding the ATP-sensitive potassium-channel subunit Kir6.2 and permanent neonatal diabetes. N Engl J Med 2004;350:1838-1849.

71. Goldberg IJ: Lipoprotein lipase and lipolysis: Central roles in lipoprotein metabolism and atherogenesis. J Lipid Res 1996;37:693-707.

72. Golden M, Waterlow JC, Picou D: The relationship between dietary intake, weight change, nitrogen balance, and protein turnover in man. Am J Clin Nutr 1977;30:1345-1348.

73. Gruber EM, Laussen PC, Casta A, et al: Stress response in infants undergoing cardiac surgery: A randomized study of fentanyl bolus, fentanyl infusion, and fentanyl-midazolam infusion. Anesth Analg 2001;92:882-890.

74. Gudinchet F, Schutz Y, Micheli J-L, et al: Metabolic cost of growth in very-low birthweight infants. Pediatr Res 1992;16:1025-1030.

75. Hakanson E, Rutberg H, Jorfeldt L, et al: Endocrine and metabolic responses after standardized moderate surgical trauma: Influence of age and sex. Clin Physiol 1984;4:461-473.

76. Hall NJ, Peters M, Eaton S, et al: Hyperglycemia is associated with increased morbidity and mortality rates in neonates with necrotizing enterocolitis. J Pediatr Surg 2004;39:898-901.

77. Hamosh M: Human milk composition and function in the infant. In Polin RA, Fox WW, Abman SH (eds): Fetal and Neonatal Physiology, 3rd ed. Philadelphia, WB Saunders, 2004, pp 275-284.

78. Hartnoll G, Betremieux P, Modi N: Body water content of extremely preterm infants at birth. Arch Dis Child Fetal Neonatal Ed 2000;83:F56-F59.

79. Hawdon JM: Hypoglycaemia and the neonatal brain. Eur J Pediatr 1999;158:S9-S12.

80. Hawdon JM, Aynsley-Green A: Disorders of blood glucose homoeostasis in the neonate. In Rennie JM, Roberton NRC (eds): Textbook of Neonatology. Edinburgh, Churchill Livingstone, 1999, pp 939-956.

81. Hawdon JM, Aynsley-Green A, Alberti K, et al: The role of pancreatic insulin-secretion in neonatal glucoregulation. 1. Healthy term and preterm infants. Arch Dis Child 1993;68:274-279.

82. Hawdon JM, Aynsley-Green A, Bartlett K, et al: The role of pancreatic insulin-secretion in neonatal glucoregulation. 2. Infants with disordered blood-glucose homeostasis. Arch Dis Child 1993;68:280-285.

83. Hawdon JM, Ward-Platt MP: Metabolic adaptation in small-for-gestational-age infants. Arch Dis Child 1993;68:262-268.

84. Hawdon JM, Ward-Platt MP, Aynsley-Green A: Patterns of metabolic adaptation for preterm and term infants in the 1st neonatal week. Arch Dis Child 1992;67:357-365.

85. Heim T: Homeothermy and its metabolic cost. In Davis JA, Dobbing J (eds): Scientific Foundations of Paediatrics. London, Heinemann, 1981, pp 91-128.

86. Hey EN, Katz G: The optimum thermal environment for naked babies. Arch Dis Child 1970;45:328-334.

87. Hill AG, Hill GL: Metabolic response to severe injury. Br J Surg 1998;85:884-890.

88. Hofman MA: Energy metabolism and relative brain size in human neonates from single and multiple gestations: An allometric study. Biol Neonate 1984;45:157-164.

89. Holmes-McNary M: Nuclear factor kappa B signaling in catabolic disorders. Curr Opin Clin Nutr Metab Care 2002;5:255-263.

90. Hughes EA, Stevens LH, Toms DA, Wilkinson AW: Oesophageal atresia: Metabolic effects of operation. Br J Surg 1965;52:403-410.

91. Ishida H, Murata N, Yamada H, et al: Effect of CO_2 pneumoperitoneum on growth of liver micrometastases in a rabbit model. World J Surg 2000;24:1004-1008.

92. Jain L: Alveolar fluid clearance in developing lungs and its role in neonatal transition. Clin Perinatol 1999;26:585-599.

93. Jansky L: Non-shivering thermogenesis and its thermoregulatory significance. Biol Rev Camb Philos Soc 1973;48: 85-132.

94. Jequier E: The influence of nutrient administration on energy-expenditure in man. Clin Nutr 1986;5:181-186.

95. Jones MO, Pierro A, Garlick PJ, et al: Protein metabolism kinetics in neonates: Effect of intravenous carbohydrate and fat. J Pediatr Surg 1995;30:458-462.

96. Jones MO, Pierro A, Hammond P, et al: Glucose utilization in the surgical newborn infant receiving total parenteral nutrition. J Pediatr Surg 1993;28:1121-1125.

97. Jones MO, Pierro A, Hammond P, et al: The metabolic response to operative stress in infants. J Pediatr Surg 1993;28:1258-1262.

98. Jones MO, Pierro A, Hashim IA, et al: Postoperative changes in resting energy-expenditure and interleukin-6 level in infants. Br J Surg 1994;81:536-538.

99. Kalache KD, Chaoui R, Marks B, et al: Does fetal tracheal fluid flow during fetal breathing movements change before the onset of labour? Br J Obstet Gynaecol 2002;109:514-519.

100. Kalhan SC: Metabolism of glucose and methods of investigation in the fetus and newborn. In Polin RA, Fox WW, Abman SH (eds): Fetal and Neonatal Physiology, 3rd ed. Philadelphia, WB Saunders, 2004, pp 449-464.

101. Kalhan SC, Parimi P, Van Beek R, et al: Estimation of gluconeogenesis in newborn infants. Am J Physiol Endocrinol Metab 2001;281:E991-E997.

102. Kerner JA: Carbohydrate requirements. In Kerner JA (ed): Manual of Pediatric Parenteral Nutrition. New York, Wiley, 1983, pp 79-88.

103. Koh THHG, Aynsley-Green A, Tarbit M, et al: Neural dysfunction during hypoglycaemia. Arch Dis Child 1988; 63:1353-1358.

104. Kondo T, Ohshima T, Mori R, et al: Immunohistochemical detection of chemokines in human skin wounds and its application to wound age determination. Int J Legal Med 2002;116:87-91.

105. Kurz A, Sessler DI, Lenhardt R: Perioperative normothermia to reduce the incidence of surgical-wound infection and shorten hospitalization: Study of Wound Infection and Temperature Group. N Engl J Med 1996;334: 1209-1215.

106. Larsson LE, Nilsson K, Niklasson A, et al: Influence of fluid regimens on perioperative blood-glucose concentrations in neonates. Br J Anaesth 1990;64:419-424.

107. Latal-Hajnal B, von Siebenthal K, Kovari H, et al: Postnatal growth in VLBW infants: Significant association with neurodevelopmental outcome. J Pediatr 2003;143: 163-170.

108. Laudy JA, Wladimiroff JW: The fetal lung. 1. Developmental aspects. Ultrasound Obstet Gynecol 2000;16:284-290.

109. Livesey G, Elia M: Estimation of energy expenditure, net carbohydrate utilization, and net fat oxidation and synthesis by indirect calorimetry: Evaluation of errors with special reference to the detailed composition of fuels. Am J Clin Nutr 1988;47:608-628.

110. Long JM, Wilmore DW, Mason AD, et al: Effect of carbohydrate and fat intake on nitrogen excretion during total intravenous feeding. Ann Surg 1977;185:417-422.

111. Lucas A, Morley R, Cole TJ: Adverse neurodevelopmental outcome of moderate neonatal hypoglycaemia. BMJ 1988;297:1304-1308.

112. Ma D, Shield JPH, Dean W, et al: Impaired glucose homeostasis in transgenic mice expressing the human transient neonatal diabetes mellitus locus, TNDM. J Clin Invest 2004;114:339-348.

113. Menni F, de Lonlay P, Sevin C, et al: Neurologic outcomes of 90 neonates and infants with persistent hyperinsulinemic hypoglycemia. Pediatrics 2001;107:476-479.

114. Merklin RJ: Growth and distribution of human fetal brown fat. Anat Rec 1974;178:637-645.

115. Micheli JL, Schutz Y: Protein metabolism and postnatal growth in very low birthweight infants. Biol Neonate 1987;52(Suppl 1):S25-S40.

116. Modi N, Betremieux P, Midgley J, et al: Postnatal weight loss and contraction of the extracellular compartment is triggered by atrial natriuretic peptide. Early Hum Dev 2000;59:201-208.

117. Montgomery RD: Changes in the basal metabolic rate of the malnourished infant and their relation to body composition. J Clin Invest 1962;41:1653-1663.

118. Moreno R, Vincent JL, Matos R, et al: The use of maximum SOFA score to quantify organ dysfunction/failure in intensive care: Results of a prospective, multicentre study. Working Group on Sepsis Related Problems of the ESICM. Intensive Care Med 1999;25:686-696.

119. Novak M, Melichar V, Hahn P: Postnatal changes in blood serum content of glycerol and fatty acids in human infants. Biologia Neonatorum 1964;7:179-184.

120. Ogata ES: Carbohydrate homeostasis. In Avery GB, Fletcher MA, MacDonald MG (eds): Neonatology: Pathophysiology and Management of the Newborn, 5th ed. Philadelphia, Lippincott Williams & Wilkins, 1999, pp 699-714.

121. Ohlson KB, Mohell N, Cannon B, et al: Thermogenesis in brown adipocytes is inhibited by volatile anesthetic agents: A factor contributing to hypothermia in infants? Anesthesiology 1994;81:176-183.

122. Okada Y, Powis M, Mcewan A, et al: Fentanyl analgesia increases the incidence of postoperative hypothermia in neonates. Pediatr Surg Int 1998;13:508-511.

123. Page MA, Williams DH: Enzymes of ketone-body utilisation in human brain. Lancet 1971;2:66-68.

124. Patel MS, Johnson CA, Rajan R, et al: Metabolism of ketone-bodies in developing human brain—development of ketone-body-utilizing enzymes and ketone-bodies as precursors for lipid-synthesis. J Neurochem 1975;25:905-908.

125. Pencharz PB, Masson M, Desgranges F, et al: Total-body protein-turnover in human premature neonates—effects of birth-weight, intrauterine nutritional-status and diet. Clin Sci 1981;61:207-215.

126. Persson B: Determination of plasma acetoacetate and D-beta-hydroxybutyrate in new-born infants by an enzymatic fluorometric micro-method. Scand J Clin Lab Invest 1970;25:9-18.

127. Persson B, Gentz J: Pattern of blood lipids, glycerol and ketone bodies during neonatal period, infancy and childhood. Acta Paediatr Scand 1966;55:353-362.

128. Pierro A, Carnielli V, Filler RM, et al: Characteristics of protein sparing effect of total parenteral nutrition in the surgical infant. J Pediatr Surg 1988;23:538-542.

129. Pierro A, Carnielli V, Filler RM, et al: Metabolism of intravenous fat emulsion in the surgical newborn. J Pediatr Surg 1989;24:95-101.

130. Pierro A, Carnielli V, Filler RM, et al: Partition of energy metabolism in the surgical newborn. J Pediatr Surg 1991; 26:581-586.

131. Pierro A, Jones MO, Hammond P, et al: Utilisation of intravenous fat in the surgical newborn infant. Proc Nutr Soc 1993;52:237A.

132. Pierro A, Jones MO, Hammond P, et al: A new equation to predict the resting energy expenditure of surgical infants. J Pediatr Surg 1994;29:1103-1108.

133. Pinter A: Metabolic effects of anesthesia and surgery in newborn infant—changes in blood levels of glucose, plasma free fatty-acids, alpha-amino-nitrogen, plasma amino-acid ratio and lactate in neonate. Z Kinder Grenzgebiete 1973; 12:149-162.

134. Pittet P, Gygax PH, Jequier E: Thermic effect of glucose and amino acids in man studied by direct and indirect calorimetry Br J Nutr 1974;31:343-349.

135. Porter RK, Brand MD: Body-mass dependence of H+ leak in mitochondria and its relevance to metabolic-rate. Nature 1993;362:628-630.

136. Powis MR, Smith K, Rennie M, et al: Effect of major abdominal operations on energy and protein metabolism in infants and children. J Pediatr Surg 1998;33:49-53.

137. Powis MR, Smith K, Rennie M, et al: Characteristics of protein and energy metabolism in neonates with necrotizing enterocolitis—a pilot study. J Pediatr Surg 1999;34:5-10.

138. Putet G: Lipids as an energy source for the premature and full-term neonate. In Polin RA, Fox WW, Abman SH (eds): Fetal and Neonatal Physiology, 3rd ed. Philadelphia, WB Saunders, 2004, pp 415-418.

139. Quant PA, Robin D, Robin P, et al: Control of hepatic mitochondrial 3-hydroxy-3-methylglutaryl-CoA synthase during the fetal neonatal transition, suckling and weaning in the rat. Eur J Biochem 1991;195:449-454.

140. Rassin DK: Amino acid requirements and profiles in total parenteral nutrition. In Lebenthal E (ed): Total Parenteral Nutrition: Indications, Utilization, Complications, and Pathophysiological Considerations. New York, Raven Press, 1986, pp 5-15.

141. Rautonen J, Makela A, Boyd H, et al: CRIB and SNAP: Assessing the risk of death for preterm neonates. Lancet 1994;343:1272-1273.

142. Reber KM, Nankervis CA: Necrotizing enterocolitis: Preventative strategies. Clin Perinatol 2004;31:157-167.

143. Reichman BL, Chessex P, Putet G, et al: Partition of energy metabolism and energy cost of growth in the very low-birth-weight infant. Pediatrics 1982;69:446-451.

144. Rolfe DF, Brand MD: The physiological significance of mitochondrial proton leak in animal cells and tissues. Biosci Rep 1997;17:9-16.

145. Rolfe DF, Hulbert AJ, Brand MD: Characteristics of mitochondrial proton leak and control of oxidative phosphorylation in the major oxygen-consuming tissues of the rat. Biochim Biophys Acta 1994;1188:405-416.

146. Rosenkrantz TS: Polycythemia and hyperviscosity in the newborn. Semin Thromb Hemost 2003;29:515-527.

147. Rubecz I, Mestyan J, Varga P, et al: Energy metabolism, substrate utilization, and nitrogen balance in parenterally fed postoperative neonates and infants: The effect of glucose, glucose + amino acids, lipid + amino acids infused in isocaloric amounts. J Pediatr 1981;98:42-46.

148. Rutberg H, Hakanson E, Anderberg B, et al: Effects of the extradural administration of morphine, or bupivacaine, on the endocrine response to upper abdominal surgery. Br J Anaesth 1984;56:233-238.

149. Rutter N, Brown SM, Hull D: Variations in the resting oxygen consumption of small babies. Arch Dis Child 1978; 53:850-854.

150. Salomon JW, Swyer PR, Jequier E: Thermic effects of glucose, amino acid and lipid in the term newborn. Biol Neonate 1979;35:8-16.

151. Schmeling DJ, Coran AG: The hormonal and metabolic response to stress in the neonate. Pediatr Surg Int 1990;5:307-321.

152. Sellden E, Brundin T, Wahren J: Augmented thermal effect of amino-acids under general-anesthesia—a mechanism useful for prevention of anesthesia-induced hypothermia. Clin Sci 1994;86:611-618.

153. Senterre J, Karlberg P: Respiratory quotient and metabolic rate in normal full-term and small-for-date newborn infants. Acta Paediatr Scand 1970;59:653-658.

154. Shanbhogue RLK, Lloyd DA: Absence of hypermetabolism after operation in the newborn- infant. JPEN J Parenter Enteral Nutr 1992;16:333-336.

155. Sherer DM: A review of amniotic fluid dynamics and the enigma of isolated oligohydramnios. Am J Perinatol 2002;19:253-266.

156. Shield JP, Gardner RJ, Wadsworth EJ, et al: Aetiopathology and genetic basis of neonatal diabetes. Arch Dis Child Fetal Neonatal Ed 1997;76:F39-F42.

157. Sinclair JC: Heat production and thermoregulation in the small-for-date infant. Pediatr Clin North Am 1970;17: 147-158.

158. Singhal A, Lucas A: Early origins of cardiovascular disease: Is there a unifying hypothesis? Lancet 2004;363:1642-1645.

159. Snyderman SE, Boyer A, Kogut MD, et al: The protein requirement of the premature infant. I. The effect of protein intake on the retention of nitrogen. J Pediatr 1969;74:872-880.

160. Sperling MA, DeLamater PV, Phelps D, et al: Spontaneous and amino acid-stimulated glucagon secretion in the immediate postnatal period: Relation to glucose and insulin. J Clin Invest 1974;53:1159-1166.

161. Srinivasan G, Jain R, Pildes RS, et al: Glucose-homeostasis during anesthesia and surgery in infants. J Pediatr Surg 1986;21:718-721.

162. Srinivasan V, Spinella PC, Drott HR, et al: Association of timing, duration, and intensity of hyperglycemia with intensive care unit mortality in critically ill children. Pediatr Crit Care Med 2004;5:329-336.

163. Stein TP: Why measure the respiratory quotient of patients on total parenteral nutrition? J Am Coll Nutr 1985;4:501-513.

164. Stenninger E, Flink R, Eriksson B, et al: Long term, neurological dysfunction and neonatal hypoglycaemia after diabetic pregnancy. Arch Dis Child 1998;79:F174-F179.

165. Styne DM: Endocrine factors affecting neonatal growth. In Polin RA, Fox WW, Abman SH (eds): Fetal and Neonatal Physiology, 3rd ed. Philadelphia, WB Saunders, 2004, pp 266-275.

166. Sunehag AL: Parenteral glycerol enhances gluconeogenesis in very premature infants. Pediatr Res 2003;53:635-641.

167. Sunehag AL: The role of parenteral lipids in supporting gluconeogenesis in very premature infants. Pediatr Res 2003;54:480-486.

168. Sunehag AL, Haymond MW: Glucose extremes in newborn infants. Clin Perinatol 2002;29:245-260.

169. Sunehag AL, Haymond MW, Schanler RJ, et al: Gluconeogenesis in very low birth weight infants receiving total parenteral nutrition. Diabetes 1999;48:791-800.

170. Teitelbaum DH, Coran AG: Perioperative nutritional support in pediatrics. Nutrition 1998;14:130-142.

171. Thorell A, Efendic S, Gutniak M, et al: Insulin resistance after abdominal surgery. Br J Surg 1994;81:59-63.

172. Thumelin S, Forestier M, Girard J, et al: Developmental-changes in mitochondrial 3-hydroxy-3-methylglutaryl-CoA synthase gene-expression in rat-liver, intestine and kidney. Biochem J 1993;292:493-496.

173. Thumelin S, Kohl C, Girard J, et al: Atypical expression of mitochondrial 3-hydroxy-3-methylglutaryl-CoA synthase in subcutaneous adipose tissue of male rats. J Lipid Res 1999;40:1071-1077.

174. Tulikoura I, Huikuri K: Changes in nitrogen metabolism in catabolic patients given three different parenteral nutrition regimens. Acta Chir Scand 1981;147:519-524.

175. Valcarce C, Vitorica J, Satrustegui J, et al: Rapid postnatal developmental changes in the passive proton permeability

of the inner membrane in rat-liver mitochondria. J Biochem 1990;108:642-645.

176. Van den Berghe G, Wouters P, Weekers F, et al: Intensive insulin therapy in critically ill patients. N Engl J Med 2001;345:1359-1367.

177. van Kempen AA, Romijn JA, Ruiter AF, et al: Adaptation of glucose production and gluconeogenesis to diminishing glucose infusion in preterm infants at varying gestational ages. Pediatr Res 2003;53:628-634.

178. van Kempen AA, Romijn JA, Ruiter AF, et al: Alanine administration does not stimulate gluconeogenesis in preterm infants. Metabolism 2003;52:945-949.

179. Vincent JL, De Mendonca A, Cantraine F, et al: Use of the SOFA score to assess the incidence of organ dysfunction/failure in intensive care units: Results of a multicenter, prospective study. Working Group on Sepsis-Related Problems of the European Society of Intensive Care Medicine. Crit Care Med 1998;26:1793-1800.

180. Vincent JL, Moreno R, Takala J et al: The SOFA (Sepsis-Related Organ Failure Assessment) score to describe organ dysfunction/failure. On behalf of the Working Group on Sepsis-Related Problems of the European Society of Intensive Care Medicine. Intensive Care Med 1996;22:707-710.

181. Vonmuhlendahl E, Herkenhoff H: Long-term course of neonatal diabetes. N Engl J Med 1995;333:704-708.

182. Ward-Platt MP, Tarbit MJ, Aynsley-Green A: The effects of anesthesia and surgery on metabolic homeostasis in infancy and childhood. J Pediatr Surg 1990;25:472-478.

183. Williamson DH, Thornton PS: Ketone body production and metabolism in the fetus and neonate. In Polin RA, Fox WW, Abman SH (eds): Fetal and Neonatal Physiology, 3rd ed. Philadelphia, WB Saunders, 2004, pp 419-428.

184. Wilmore DW: From Cuthbertson to fast-track surgery: 70 years of progress in reducing stress in surgical patients. Ann Surg 2002;236:643-648.

185. Winthrop AL, Jones PJ, Schoeller DA, et al: Changes in the body composition of the surgical infant in the early postoperative period. J Pediatr Surg 1987;22:546-549.

186. Wispe JR, Bell EF, Roberts RJ: Assessment of lipid peroxidation in newborn infants and rabbits by measurements of expired ethane and pentane: Influence of parenteral lipid infusion. Pediatr Res 1985;19:374-379.

187. Yager JY: Hypoglycemic injury to the immature brain. Clin Perinatol 2002;29:651-674.

188. Yasukawa H, Ohishi M, Mori H, et al: IL-6 induces an anti-inflammatory response in the absence of SOCS3 in macrophages. Nat Immunol 2003;4:551-556.

189. Zlotkin SH: Intravenous nitrogen intake requirements in full-term newborns undergoing surgery. Pediatrics 1984;73:493-496.

190. Zlotkin SH, Bryan MH, Anderson GH: Intravenous nitrogen and energy intakes required to duplicate in utero nitrogen accretion in prematurely born human infants. J Pediatr 1981;99:115-120.

191. Zlotkin SH, Stallings VA, Pencharz PB: Total parenteral nutrition in children. Pediatr Clin North Am 1985;32: 381-400.

Chapter 7

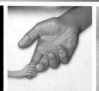

Respiratory Physiology and Care

Jay M. Wilson and John W. DiFiore

"The body is but a pair of pincers set over a bellows and a stewpan and the whole fixed upon stilts."[35] This chapter discusses the bellows. In doing so, we examine normal lung development, pulmonary physiology, devices (invasive and noninvasive) for patient monitoring, and devices designed to provide ventilatory support. Finally, we discuss how to apply this information to the management of patients with respiratory failure in the modern intensive care unit.

LUNG DEVELOPMENT

Although the structural development of the lung is complex, the following three "laws of lung development" put forth by Reid offer a useful summary.[157,158]

Airway: The bronchial tree is fully developed by the 16th week of gestation.

Alveoli: Alveoli develop after birth and increase in number until 8 years of age. The size of the alveoli increases until the growth of the chest wall finishes during adulthood.

Blood Vessels: The preacinar vessels (arteries and veins) follow the development of the airways, and the intra-acinar vessels follow that of the alveoli. Muscularization of the intra-acinar arteries does not keep pace with the appearance of new arteries.

Lung development is divided into five phases: embryonic, pseudoglandular, canalicular, saccular, and alveolar. The boundaries between these phases are not sharp; they blend into one another, with considerable overlap between areas within the lung. There is also some variation from individual to individual.[148]

Embryonic Phase

The human fetal lung originates in the 3-week-old embryo as a ventral diverticulum that arises from the caudal end of the laryngotracheal groove of the foregut.[28] This diverticulum grows caudally to form the primitive trachea. By 4 weeks, the end of the diverticulum divides, forming the two primary lung buds. These lung buds develop lobar buds, which correspond to the mature lung lobes (three on the right side and two on the left side). By the sixth week of gestation, the lobar buds have further subdivided to form the bronchopulmonary segments.

The primitive lung bud is lined by an epithelium derived from endoderm; it differentiates into both the respiratory epithelium that lines the airways[30] and the specialized epithelium that lines the alveoli and permits gas exchange.[198] The lung bud grows into a rounded mass of mesodermal cells from which the blood vessels, smooth muscle, cartilage, and other connective tissues that form the framework of lung differentiate.[107] Ectoderm contributes to the innervation of the lung (Fig. 7-1A).[160]

Pseudoglandular Phase

From the 7th to 16th weeks of gestation, conducting airways are formed by repeated dichotomous branching, resulting in 16 to 25 generations of primitive airways.[28] During this phase, the lung has a distinctly glandular appearance (hence the term *pseudoglandular*), created by small epithelium-lined tubules surrounded by abundant mesenchyma (Fig. 7-1B).[107] By the 16th week of gestation, all the bronchial airways have been formed.[155,157,158] After this time, further growth occurs only by elongation and widening of existing airways and not by further branching. During this period, the respiratory epithelium begins to differentiate, cilia appear in proximal airways, and cartilage begins to form.

During the pseudoglandular phase, mesenchymal-epithelial interactions are necessary for normal lung airway morphogenesis.[116] In vitro, endodermal lung buds undergo normal bronchiolar branching only if they are exposed to bronchial mesoderm. No other mesoderm, including tracheal, induces bronchial branching.[175] Moreover, the rate and extent of bronchial branching are directly proportional to the amount of mesenchyma present.[116]

In addition to bronchial branching, mesenchyma is necessary for bronchial cytodifferentiation. With increasing amounts of mesenchyma, epithelial differentiation is shifted from bronchial (ciliated columnar cells and goblet

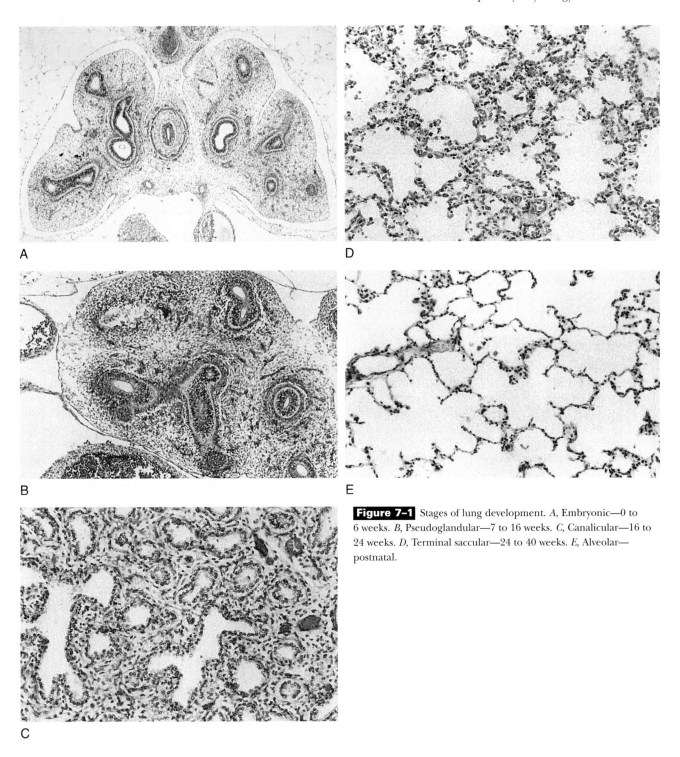

Figure 7-1 Stages of lung development. *A,* Embryonic—0 to 6 weeks. *B,* Pseudoglandular—7 to 16 weeks. *C,* Canalicular—16 to 24 weeks. *D,* Terminal saccular—24 to 40 weeks. *E,* Alveolar—postnatal.

cells) to alveolar (primarily type II pneumocytes).[116] Similarly, differentiation of lung mesenchyma into smooth muscle, blood vessels, and cartilage occurs only when lung epithelium and lung mesenchyma are co-cultivated.[183]

Canalicular Phase

The canalicular phase takes place from the 16th to 24th weeks of gestation. During this time, the basic structure

of the gas-exchanging portion of the lung is formed and vascularized.

Early in the canalicular period, the lungs have a simple airspace configuration. Potential gas-exchanging structures are smooth-walled, blind-ending channels that are lined by cuboidal epithelium and supported by abundant loose interstitium and scattered small blood v essels. As the canalicular period progresses, interstitial tissue decreases, capillary growth increases, and these "channels" assume a more complex, irregular pattern (Fig. 7-1C).

At approximately 20 weeks' gestation, differentiation of the primitive epithelial cells begins. The first morphologic evidence of this phase of differentiation is the growth of capillaries beneath the epithelial cells that line the primitive gas-exchanging channels. In one population of overlying epithelial cells, capillary ingrowth results in thinning of the cytoplasm, narrowing of the air-blood interface, and differentiation into type I pneumocytes—the cells ultimately responsible for gas exchange. In other overlying epithelial cells, the lamellar bodies that are associated with surfactant synthesis begin to appear; these bodies identify the type II cells that will ultimately produce surfactant. Although some investigators have concluded that the progenitor of type I cells is an undifferentiated epithelial cell, a more convincing body of evidence suggests that type I cells develop from differentiated type II cells.[3,4,64,173,177] By the end of the canalicular period, structural development of the lung has progressed to the point where gas exchange is possible.

Terminal Saccular Phase

The terminal saccular phase of lung development takes place from 24 weeks' gestation until term and is associated with remarkable changes in the appearance of the lung. Interstitial tissue becomes less prominent, and airspace walls demonstrate marked thinning. Tissue projections into the distal airspace regions divide the distal airspaces into saccules, where capillaries are generally exposed to only one respiratory surface (Fig. 7-1D). Later, in the mature alveolus, each capillary is simultaneously exposed to at least two alveoli.[34]

The cells that line the saccules of the human fetal lung at this stage of development are recognizable type I and type II pneumocytes. Morphologically, they are indistinguishable from the corresponding cells described in neonatal or adult human lung tissue. However, the surfactant produced by the early fetal lung differs biochemically from that produced later in gestation. Although no apparent morphologic differences in the lamellar bodies exists, immature lungs produce surfactant that is rich in phosphatidylinositol, whereas the surfactant produced by lungs late in gestation is rich in phosphatidylglycerol.[80]

Postnatal or Alveolar Phase

An alveolus is defined as an open outpouching of an alveolar duct, lined almost exclusively by the thin processes of type I pneumocytes. Its interstitial capillaries are simultaneously exposed to at least two alveoli, and because the nuclei of all cells are located away from the gas-exchange surface, the barrier to gas exchange is usually only a few nanometers thick.[148] The barrier between the gas in the alveoli and the blood in the capillaries is composed of three layers: the thin processes of the type I cells, a basement membrane that appears to be common to the endothelial and alveolar cells, and the thin extensions of the endothelial cells (Fig. 7-2A). The type I cell is responsible for gas exchange, and the type II cell synthesizes and secretes surfactant.

At birth, the lung has no mature alveoli but instead contains approximately 20 million primitive terminal sacs.[26,27,51,60] These sacs are lined by mature alveolar epithelium; in shape they resemble large, shallow cups.[26,27,51,60,157] At approximately 5 weeks after birth, these 20 million primitive terminal sacs begin to develop into the 300 million alveoli that will be present by 8 years of age, with the fastest multiplication occurring before 4 years of age (Fig. 7-1E).[51,60,199] After age 8 years, increases in lung volume result from increases in alveolar size but not number.[51]

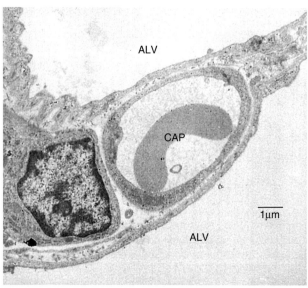

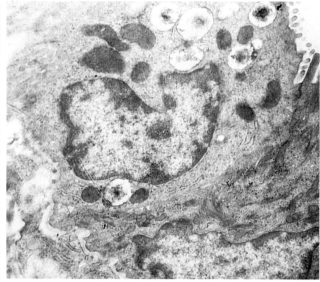

A   B

Figure 7–2 *A,* Electrophotomicrograph of a type I pneumocyte. Note the thin alveolar-arterial interface. *B,* Electrophotomicrograph of a type II pneumocyte. Note the lamellar bodies filled with surfactant. ALV, alveolar; CAP, cappillary.

Arterial Growth

The pattern of growth of pulmonary arteries differs, depending on the location of the artery relative to the acinus. The preacinar region refers to the conducting airways and includes the trachea, major bronchi, and bronchial branches to the level of the terminal bronchiolus. The acinus refers to the functional respiratory unit of the lung and includes structures that are distal to the terminal bronchiolus (specifically the respiratory bronchioli, alveolar ducts, and alveoli). In the preacinar region, the pulmonary artery gives off a branch to accompany each airway branch—a "conventional" artery that ultimately provides terminal branches to the acini. Many additional branches arise from the conventional arteries and pass directly into adjacent respiratory tissue to supply the peribronchial parenchyma; these are called "supernumerary" arteries.[89,156]

Mirroring the branching of bronchial airways, the development of all preacinar conventional and supernumerary arteries is complete by 16 weeks' gestation.[88,89] Subsequent changes in the preacinar arteries involve only size, not number. In the intra-acinar region, terminal branches of the conventional pulmonary arterioles supply the capillary bed. Concurrent with alveolar development, these small vessels of the lung multiply rapidly after birth to keep pace with alveolar multiplication.

In adults, complete muscularization of pulmonary arteries is found throughout the acinus, even in the walls of alveoli immediately under the pleura. In the fetus, however, complete muscularization of the arteries occurs proximal to or at the level of the terminal bronchioli. Consequently, only partially muscular or nonmuscular arteries are found within the acinus itself. New alveoli appear during early childhood simultaneously with the accompanying intra-acinar arteries. However, muscularization of these arteries is a slow process.[157]

Mediators of Fetal Lung Development

There is a large body of evidence supporting the role of lung liquid in normal and experimental fetal lung growth. Naturally occurring airway occlusions in humans have resulted in large, fluid-filled lungs that histologically have either normal or slightly distended alveoli.[2,74,77,110,125] In other instances, intrauterine airway occlusion results in large lungs despite the presence of other anatomic abnormalities, such as Potter's syndrome or congenital diaphragmatic hernia, that would normally lead to pulmonary hypoplasia.[145,146,202]

The clue that lung liquid dynamics may play a pivotal role in lung development stems from investigations in fetal lambs. In the final stages of gestation, lambs' rate of production of liquid in the lungs increases substantially, as does the intratracheal-intrapulmonary pressure. More significantly, these changes coincide with the most rapid period of lung growth, with dramatic increases in lung volume and total alveolar number in the 12 to 14 days following these changes in lung liquid dynamics.[6,58] Experimental studies of normal fetal lambs have confirmed that retention of lung liquid leads to pulmonary hyperplasia, whereas drainage of liquid leads to hypoplasia.

Fetal tracheal occlusion prevents the alveolar and vascular components of pulmonary hypoplasia associated with bilateral fetal nephrectomy and experimental fetal diaphragmatic hernia.[56,57,161,203] Since these initial studies, multiple experimental animal models of fetal tracheal occlusion have shown dramatic increases in lung growth. Prolonged tracheal occlusion, although inducing pulmonary hyperplasia, significantly decreases surfactant production and the number of type II pneumocytes.[32,67,108,138,143] This effect can be alleviated by temporary tracheal occlusion, which does not cause the dramatic decrease in type II pneumocytes seen after prolonged tracheal occlusion.[52,53,140] Postnatal intrapulmonary distention accelerates neonatal lung growth but not adult lung growth, underscoring the malleable nature of the immature lung.[135]

Although increased intrapulmonary pressure has been cited as the primary stimulus for lung growth in tracheal occlusion models, it is likely only a trigger for more complex downstream regulatory changes. Alteration in the chemical composition of lung liquid in tracheal occlusion models has been implicated.[141] Tracheal occlusion has been associated with increased expression or production of multiple growth factors, including keratinocyte growth factor, vascular endothelial growth factor, transforming growth factor-β2, insulin-like growth factor I, hepatoma-derived growth factor, ribosomal protein S24, and stathmin, all of which may participate in a complex regulatory pathway for lung development enhanced by tracheal occlusion.[43,119,130,134,150]

Detailed signals and pathways mediating control and regulation of lung development have recently been uncovered in other animal models of lung growth and pulmonary hypoplasia.[164] Studies of hormonal influences on lung development are scarce, but those that are available suggest that hormones do not play a major role in lung growth,[31,37,62,101,105] although they may have more influence on development of the surfactant system. Epidermal growth factor, hepatoma-derived growth factor, and keratinocyte growth factor are also believed to be involved in lung development.[38,115,124,139,181] Maternal corticosteroid treatment causes structural changes in fetal lungs that are independent of surfactant secretion.[18,33,99,179]

PULMONARY PHYSIOLOGY

The process of breathing is complex and involves contraction of the inspiratory muscles to generate negative pressure in the trachea to bring fresh air into the lungs. In the lungs, the process of oxygen uptake and carbon dioxide elimination occurs by means of diffusion across the ultrathin alveolar capillary membrane. This process is critical not only to fuel the cells of the body with oxygen for metabolism but also to maintain appropriate acid-base status by careful regulation of carbon dixoide. Dysfunction in any part of this process can lead to respiratory failure and the need for mechanical ventilatory support.

To understand the process of respiration, it is necessary to understand the terminology associated with the assessment of pulmonary function.

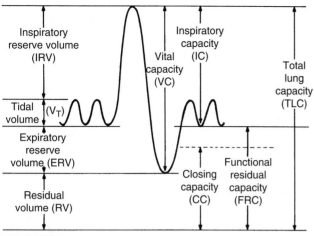

Figure 7-3 Functional components of lung volume.

Lung Volumes

The total volume of the lung is divided into subcomponents, defined as follows (Fig. 7-3).

Functional Residual Capacity (FRC): The volume of gas in the lung that is present at the end of a normal expiration when airflow is zero and alveolar pressure equals ambient pressure.

Expiratory Reserve Volume: The additional gas that can be exhaled beyond FRC to reach residual volume.

Residual Volume: The minimum lung volume possible. This is the gas that remains in the lung after all exhalable gas has been removed.

Total Lung Capacity: The total volume present in the lung.

Inspiratory Capacity: The difference in inhaled volume between FRC and total lung capacity.

Vital Capacity: The amount of gas inhaled from FRC to total lung capacity.

Inspiratory Reserve Volume: The amount of gas inhaled from peak normal inspiratory volume to total lung capacity.

Tidal Volume: The volume of a normal inspiration.
Refer to Table 7-1 for a list of abbreviations and symbols and Table 7-2 for related formulas.

Tidal volume, vital capacity, inspiratory capacity, inspiratory reserve volume, and expiratory reserve volume can be directly measured by spirometry. Conversely, total lung volume, FRC, and residual volume cannot be measured by spirometry, and one of the following techniques must be used: (1) the nitrogen washout test, in which the nitrogen eliminated from the lungs while breathing pure oxygen is measured, (2) the helium dilution test, which measures the equilibration of helium into the lung; or (3) total-body plethysmography, which measures changes in body volume and pressure to calculate FRC using Boyle's law.[127]

TABLE 7-1 Abbreviations and Symbols

Cao_2	Concentration of oxygen in arterial blood
Cco_2	Concentration of oxygen in end-capillary blood
$C\bar{v}o_2$	Concentration of oxygen in mixed venous blood
DL_{CO}	Diffusing capacity of the lung for carbon monoxide
DL_{O_2}	Diffusing capacity of the lung for oxygen
ERV	Expiratory reserve volume
Fio_2	Fraction of oxygen in inspired air
FRC	Functional residual capacity
IC	Inspiratory capacity
IRV	Inspiratory reserve volume
$P\bar{A}_{CO}$	Mean partial pressure of carbon monoxide in alveolar gas
$Paco_2$	Partial pressure of carbon dioxide in arterial blood
$PACO_2$	Partial pressure of carbon dioxide in alveolar gas
$P\bar{A}CO_2$	Mean partial pressure of carbon dioxide in alveolar gas
Pao_2	Partial pressure of oxygen in arterial blood
PAO_2	Partial pressure of oxygen in alveolar gas
$P\bar{A}O_2$	Mean partial pressure of oxygen in alveolar gas
Pco_2	Partial pressure of carbon dioxide
$P\bar{C}O_2$	Mean partial pressure of oxygen in capillary blood
$P\bar{E}CO_2$	Mean partial pressure of carbon dioxide in mixed expired air
Po_2	Partial pressure of oxygen
$\dot{Q}s$	Shunt flow
$\dot{Q}t$	Total cardiac output
R	Respiratory exchange ratio
RQ	Respiratory quotient
RV	Residual volume
Sao_2	Percentage saturation of hemoglobin with oxygen in arterial blood
Svo_2	Percentage saturation of hemoglobin with oxygen in mixed venous blood
TLC	Total lung capacity
V_A	Volume of alveolar gas
VC	Vital capacity
V_D	Volume of dead space gas
V_T	Tidal volume
$\dot{V}_A/\dot{Q}_C$	Ratio of alveolar ventilation to pulmonary capillary blood flow
$\dot{V}co_2$	Amount of carbon dioxide eliminated per minute
$\dot{V}_E$	Expired volume of ventilation per minute
$\dot{V}_I$	Inspired volume of ventilation per minute
$\dot{V}o_2$	Rate of oxygen uptake per minute

TABLE 7-2 Formulas

Diffusion capacity	$DL_{CO} = \dot{V}_{CO}/P\bar{A}_{CO}$
Dead space	$V_D = V_T (P\bar{A}CO_2 - P\bar{E}CO_2/P\bar{A}CO_2)$
Shunt fraction	$\dot{Q}s/\dot{Q}t = Cco_2 - Cao_2/Cco_2 - C\bar{v}o_2$
Respiratory quotient	R = Rate of CO_2 output/Rate of O_2 uptake
Mixed venous oxygen saturation	$S\bar{v}o_2 = Sao_2 - \dot{V}o_2/13.9 \times \dot{Q} \times (Hb)$
Pulmonary blood flow	$\dfrac{\text{Oxygen uptake}}{\text{Arterial} - \text{venous oxygen content difference}}$
Henderson-Hasselbalch equation	$pH = \dfrac{pK + \log [HCO_3]}{0.03\, Pco_2}$

Closing Capacity

Inspiratory pressure within the airway decreases as gas travels in a distal direction. Eventually, the intraluminal pressure stenting the airway open equals the surrounding parenchymal pressure; this is called the equal pressure point.[122] Downstream of the equal pressure point, intraluminal pressure drops below surrounding parenchymal pressure, and airway closure occurs, leading to unventilated alveoli and a physiologic shunt. In normal lungs, little or no unventilated area exists at FRC. However, any reduction in FRC (which frequently occurs in diseased lungs) will cause more areas of the lung to reach closing volume and become atelectatic and increase the shunt.[120] Conversely, an increase in FRC (achieved by positive-pressure ventilation) may open some areas that were closed, thereby reducing the physiologic shunt.

Pulmonary Compliance

Pulmonary compliance is defined as the change in lung volume per unit change in pressure.[114] Dynamic compliance is the volume change divided by the peak inspiratory transthoracic pressure. Static compliance is the volume change divided by the plateau inspiratory pressure.[71] With the initiation of an inspiratory breath, the transthoracic pressure gradient increases to a peak value. This increase is a function of elastic resistance of the lung and chest wall, as well as airway resistance. The pressure then falls to a plateau level as the gas redistributes in alveoli. Consequently, dynamic compliance is always lower than static compliance. Figure 7-4 demonstrates a standard static compliance curve.[151] Ventilation normally occurs in the steep portion of the curve, whereas large changes in volume occur in response to small changes in pressure. However, at low and high volumes, large changes in pressure result in minimal changes in volume. In diseased lungs in which compliance has dropped into the flat portion of the curve, the goal of mechanical ventilation is to return it to the steep portion. Excessive pressure applied by the ventilator

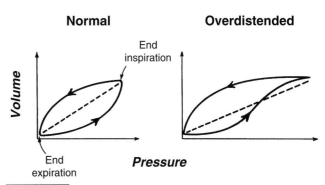

Normal   **Overdistended**

End inspiration

Volume

Pressure

End expiration

Figure 7-5 Dynamic pressure-volume loop demonstrating an idealized ventilatory cycle and overdistention during positive-pressure ventilation.

results in ventilation at the top of the curve, where the process once again becomes inefficient.[91]

Changes in lung volume and pleural pressure during a normal breathing cycle, which reflect the elastic and flow-resistant properties of the lung, are displayed as a pressure-volume loop (Fig. 7-5). The slope of the line that connects the end-expiratory and end-inspiratory points provides a measure of the dynamic compliance of the lung. The area that falls between this line and the curved lines to the right and left represents the additional work required to overcome flow resistance during inspiration and expiration, respectively.

Airway Resistance

Resistance to gas flow is a function of the physical property of the gas (molecules interact with one another and with airway walls), as well as the length of the tube through which the gas travels. Most important, resistance is a function of the internal diameter of the tube. Because the airways in small children are narrow, a slight change in diameter secondary to airway swelling can result in a dramatic increase in resistance. Because airways are smaller at the base of the lung, resistance is greater there than in the apical region.[121] In addition, the velocity of flow affects resistance because, below critical velocity, gas flow is laminar. However, above critical velocity, there is turbulent flow, and resistance increases.

Time Constants

The time constant is a product of the compliance and resistance of the lung and calculates how quickly exhalation can occur. Consequently, increases in compliance or resistance of individual alveolar units or areas of the lung increase the time constant. One time constant is defined as the time required to complete 63% of tidal volume expiration (two, three, and four time constants = 87%, 95%, and 99%, respectively).[137] Because the resistance of the airways leading to individual alveoli varies, depending on alveolar location, and because the compliance of individual alveoli also varies, the measured time constant is actually an average of many different time constants

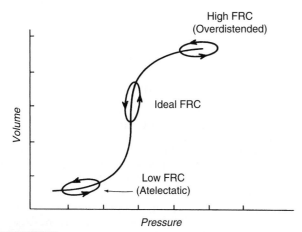

High FRC (Overdistended)

Ideal FRC

Volume

Low FRC (Atelectatic)

Pressure

Figure 7-4 Static compliance curve with superimposed dynamic flow-volume loops for high, low, and ideal functional residual capacities (FRCs).

throughout the lung. The importance of understanding time constants becomes apparent when assisted mechanical ventilation is contemplated. In a lung with high compliance or high resistance, the time constant is prolonged. Mechanical ventilator settings would consequently need to be adjusted to allow for near-complete expiration (three time constants, or 95% expiration) to avoid breath stacking and overdistention. Conversely, in lungs with low compliance or low resistance, the time constant is less; under these circumstances, an increase in minute ventilation should be accomplished with increases in respiratory rate rather than increases in tidal volume. Because of low compliance, tidal volume would be more likely to lead to high pressure and barotrauma.

Pulmonary Circulation

Mixed venous blood from the systemic circulation collects in the right atrium, passes into the right ventricle, and then travels into the pulmonary capillary bed, where gas exchange occurs. Blood subsequently drains into the left atrium, where it is pumped into the left ventricle and ultimately into the systemic circulation. Desaturated blood that originates from systemic sources through the bronchial and pleural circulation represents 1% to 3% of the total volume of blood that exits the left atrium. In pathologic situations, this anatomic right-to-left shunting can approach 10%.[65] In addition, under any circumstance in which pressure in the right atrium exceeds that of the left atrium, the foramen ovale (which is anatomically patent in all neonates and in 20% to 30% of older children) becomes another major area for extrapulmonary right-to-left shunting.

Because blood is a fluid and is affected by gravity, in an upright individual, blood pressure and thus blood flow in the pulmonary capillary bed are lowest at the apex of the lung and greatest at the base. Under normal circumstances, pulmonary artery pressure is adequate to deliver some blood to the apex of the lung; however, in pathologic situations such as hemorrhage or shock, blood flow to the apex can fall to zero, resulting in an area that is ventilated but not perfused; such areas are referred to as dead space. The lung can be divided into four regions, designated progressively in a caudal direction from apex to base. In zone 1 (the apex), the alveolar pressure exceeds pulmonary artery pressure, and little or no flow occurs. In zone 2, the arterial pressure exceeds alveolar pressure, but alveolar pressure exceeds venous pressure. In this region, flow is determined by arterial-alveolar pressure differences. In zone 3, the pulmonary venous pressure exceeds alveolar pressure, and flow is determined by the arterial-venous pressure differences. In zone 4 (the base), pulmonary interstitial pressure exceeds both pulmonary venous and alveolar pressure, and flow in this region is determined by arterial interstitial pressure differences.[106]

Because oxygen is a pulmonary vasodilator, hypoxemia is a potent stimulus for vasoconstriction in the pulmonary vascular bed. In addition, because acidosis is a pulmonary vasoconstrictor and alkalosis is a vasodilator, the partial pressure of carbon dioxide (PCO_2) indirectly affects the capillary bed because of its effect on pH.

Pulmonary Gas Exchange

Diffusion

Oxygen and carbon dioxide pass between the alveolus and the pulmonary capillary bed by passive diffusion.[192] Because diffusion in a gaseous environment is a function of molecular weight, oxygen diffuses more rapidly through air than through carbon dioxide. However, because diffusion across the capillary alveolar membrane involves a shift from the gaseous phase to the liquid phase, solubility of the gas in liquid becomes rate limiting, and carbon dioxide (because it is more soluble than oxygen) diffuses 20 times more rapidly.[162]

Diffusion is driven not only by differences in solubility but also by differences in partial pressure of the gases across the capillary alveolar membrane. Gas exchange is consequently most rapid at the beginning of the capillary, where the differences in the partial pressure of oxygen (PO_2) and PCO_2 between the alveoli and the capillaries are greatest; gas exchange is virtually complete one third of the way across the pulmonary capillary bed.[194] Consequently, in normal individuals, the principal limiting factor for oxygen uptake at rest or during exercise is pulmonary blood flow.[201] Although the rate of diffusion is not rate limiting in the healthy state, in circumstances in which the alveolar capillary membrane is thickened, diffusion may become sufficiently impaired to prevent complete saturation of available hemoglobin. Carbon monoxide, which has diffusion characteristics similar to those of oxygen, is used to measure diffusion capacity.

Dead Space

Minute ventilation, which is defined as the total volume of air inspired each minute, is calculated as the product of the tidal volume and the respiratory rate. However, the entire volume of gas does not participate in gas exchange; the portion of each tidal breath that ventilates only the oropharynx, larynx, trachea, and major conducting bronchi (the anatomic dead space) does not participate in gas exchange.[196] In addition to the anatomic dead space, a certain volume of gas ventilates unperfused alveoli and consequently does not participate in gas exchange. This is known as alveolar dead space and is minimal in the absence of disease. The combination of anatomic and alveolar dead space, known as physiologic dead space, is equal to approximately one third of the normal tidal volume; dead space that exceeds this amount is considered pathologic.[152]

Ventilation-Perfusion Matching

For optimal gas exchange, the ventilation (V) and perfusion (Q) to a given segment of the lung should be matched.[200] The V/Q ratios of different lung units are not identical,[193] but the averaged ratio of alveolar ventilation to blood flow in the lung is approximately 0.8. At the apex of the lung, the V/Q ratio is higher; at the base of the lung, the ratio is lower. Under normal circumstances, V/Q mismatching is minimal and inconsequential. However, in disease states, mismatching can contribute significantly to the impairment of gas exchange. In circumstances in which blood is flowing through regions of the lung with no ventilation, a right-to-left shunt that can significantly decrease the arterial oxygen saturation is created.

Oxygen Transport

Oxygen is transported through the bloodstream in one of two ways. It may be transported in aqueous solution in the plasma or in chemical combination within hemoglobin in erythrocytes. The amount of oxygen transported in solution is negligible. Thus, most oxygen is carried bound to hemoglobin in erythrocytes. At full saturation, 1 g of hemoglobin is capable of carrying 1.34 mL of oxygen. However, the actual amount of oxygen carried by hemoglobin varies and is defined by a sigmoid-shaped curve referred to as the oxyhemoglobin dissociation curve (Fig. 7-6). Under normal circumstances, hemoglobin is 100% saturated with oxygen; however, the sigmoid shape of this curve ensures that the oxygen carrying capacity of hemoglobin remains relatively high, even at a PO_2 as low as 60. As a result, mild pulmonary disorders do not interfere with oxygen delivery. At the same time, the steep area of the dissociation curve ensures that a large quantity of oxygen can be unloaded into the peripheral tissues as PO_2 drops. The oxyhemoglobin dissociation curve can be shifted to the left or right by changes in the affinity of hemoglobin for oxygen. A shift to the left results in a higher affinity of hemoglobin for oxygen and is caused by alkalosis,[90] hypothermia, decreased erythrocyte 2,3-diphosphoglycerate (2,3-DPG)[21] (which often occurs in old banked blood),[17] or fetal hemoglobin.[81] In this situation, at a given PO_2, the hemoglobin is more saturated than normal, and tissue perfusion should therefore be increased to deliver the same amount of oxygen for metabolic needs. A shift to the right is the result of a lowered affinity of hemoglobin for oxygen and is caused by acidosis,[90] hyperthermia, and an increased red blood cell 2,3-DPG content.[21] This rightward shift results in hemoglobin that is less saturated at a given PO_2, thereby allowing the unloading of more oxygen at lower rates of flow to the peripheral tissues.

Carbon Dioxide Equilibrium and Acid-Base Regulation

Because carbon dioxide is produced as an end product of metabolism, its rate of production is a function of metabolic rate. Under normal circumstances, the amount of carbon dioxide produced is slightly less than the amount of oxygen consumed. This is defined by the respiratory quotient (R):

$$R = \frac{\text{Rate of } CO_2 \text{ output}}{\text{Rate of } O_2 \text{ uptake}}$$

Under normal circumstances, the respiratory quotient is 0.8, but it can vary from 1.0 to 0.7, depending on whether carbohydrate or fat is used as the principal source of nutrition. The lungs are primarily responsible for the elimination of carbon dioxide, and the rate of elimination depends on pulmonary blood flow and alveolar ventilation. Carbon dioxide is carried in the bloodstream in several forms. In aqueous solution, it exists in a state of equilibrium as dissolved carbon dioxide and as carbonic acid ($CO_2 + H_2O \rightleftharpoons H_2CO_3$). This equation normally is shifted markedly to the left. In erythrocytes, however, the enzyme carbonic anhydrase catalyzes the reaction, which shifts the equation to the right.[102,113] The ability of carbonic acid to dissociate and reassociate ($H_2C_3 \rightleftharpoons H^+ + HCO_5$) is an important factor in buffering plasma to maintain a physiologic pH. The relationship is defined using the Henderson-Hasselbalch equation. A small amount of carbon dioxide is also carried combined with hemoglobin in the form of carbaminohemoglobins.[102]

MONITORING

Because the condition of acutely ill infants and children can deteriorate rapidly, continuous surveillance of their physiologic status is necessary to provide ideal care. Many options for physiologic monitoring are available to the clinician in the modern intensive care unit; the most useful are discussed in this section.

Noninvasive Monitoring

Pulse Oximetry

Pulse oximetry provides continuous noninvasive monitoring of hemoglobin saturation. The principle of pulse oximetry is based on spectrophotometry and relies on the fact that oxygenated and deoxygenated hemoglobin transmit light at different frequencies. Oxygenated hemoglobin

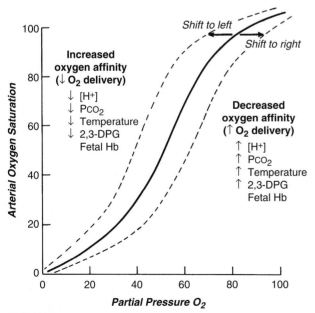

Figure 7-6 Oxyhemoglobin dissociation curve. DPG, diphosphoglycerate; Hb, hemoglobin.

selectively absorbs infrared light (940 nm) and transmits red light (660 nm), whereas deoxyhemoglobin absorbs red light and transmits infrared light. The pulse oximeter probe contains two light-emitting diodes that pass light at the wavelengths noted earlier through a perfused area of tissue to a photodetector on the other side. The photodiode compares the amounts of infrared, red, and ambient light that reach it to calculate the oxygen saturation in arterial blood (SaO_2).[7,185]

The advantages of pulse oximetry are that it is noninvasive and has a rapid response time, making changes in clinical status immediately apparent. Disadvantages of oximetry are that it is insensitive to large changes in arterial PO_2 at the upper end of the oxygenated hemoglobin dissociation curve. In addition, at an oxygen saturation below 70%, the true SaO_2 is significantly underestimated by most oximeters. When SaO_2 measurements are routinely below 85%, determination of its correlation with actual partial pressure of oxygen in arterial blood (PaO_2) through the use of indwelling arterial catheters is necessary. Errors can also occur when other forms of hemoglobin exist.[165] The presence of carboxyhemoglobin and methemoglobin results in falsely elevated SaO_2 readings.[17] Conversely, certain dyes such as methylene blue result in a marked decrease in measured SaO_2.[197] The presence of fetal hemoglobin, which has an absorption spectrum similar to that of adult hemoglobin, has no impact on the accuracy of SaO_2 measurements. Physical factors, including poor peripheral perfusion, abnormally thick or edematous tissue at the site of sensor placement, the presence of nail polish, and excessive ambient light, also lead to inaccurate readings.[36,144,166]

Capnometry

Capnometry is a noninvasive method that measures the end-tidal partial pressure of carbon dioxide in the expired gas.[172] As with pulse oximetry, capnometry is based on the principle that carbon dioxide absorbs infrared light. Exhaled gas passes through a sampling chamber that has an infrared light source on one side and a photodetector on the other side. Based on the amount of infrared light that reaches the photodetector, the amount of carbon dioxide present in the gas can be calculated. Depending on the equipment, data can be reported as the maximum concentration of carbon dioxide (end-tidal carbon dioxide), or it can provide a display of the entire exhaled carbon dioxide waveform; this display is known as a capnogram.[178]

Two categories of carbon dioxide monitors exist: mainstream monitors and sidestream monitors.[83] Mainstream monitors, in which the sampling cell is connected to the airway between the ventilator and the endotracheal tube, respond faster to changes in carbon dioxide but must be heated to prevent water condensation. These chambers are consequently heavy and hot and must be supported to avoid contact with the patient. Sidestream monitors draw a continuous sample of gas from the respiratory circuit into the measuring cell. This system is lightweight and can theoretically be used in nonintubated patients[25]; however, because of the longer transit time to the sampling chamber, this unit is slow in responding to changes in carbon dioxide.

Because the carbon dioxide that is measured in expired gases is a product of metabolic rate, pulmonary circulation, and alveolar ventilation, these variables must all be considered when interpreting changes in end-tidal carbon dioxide measurements.

Transcutaneous Measurement of Gas Tension

Measurement of PO_2 and PCO_2 at the skin surface is possible by means of transcutaneous monitoring.[126] The principle of this device is based on the fact that PO_2 and PCO_2 approximate arterial values in areas where blood flow exceeds the metabolic requirements of the tissue. To increase blood flow, the devices used to measure transcutaneous PO_2 and PCO_2 contain a sampling electrode and a warming device to increase local blood flow.[186] The advantage of transcutaneous monitoring is that it may reduce the number of (but not eliminate the need for) arterial blood gas determinations required in a sick individual. One limitation of the device is that the measured transcutaneous PO_2 and PCO_2 are not equal to arterial blood gas tensions and can frequently be 5 to 10 mm Hg higher or lower than the arterial counterpart. Changes in peripheral perfusion caused by shock or vasopressors can make these values even more inaccurate.[187] Another disadvantage is that burns or blisters may occur at the electrode site because of the warming component. This requires frequent changing of the monitoring site, at which time recalibration is necessary.

Impedance Pneumography

Impedance pneumography is a noninvasive method of measuring changes in respiratory rate and breathing patterns.[15] It is based on the principle that impedance (resistance) to an electrical current passing through the thorax changes between inspiration and expiration because of the difference in the amount of gas in the lungs.[94] The technique is relatively easy to perform. The disadvantage of the system is that it is quite sensitive to body movement, which can lead to artifacts. In addition, because the device measures only impedance, it is not reliable to assess the quality of the respiratory effort or significant changes in tidal volume.[133]

Invasive Monitoring

Mixed Venous Oxygen Monitoring

Measurement of mixed venous oxygen saturation (SvO_2) may be the single most useful measurement in determining critical impairment in oxygen delivery to the tissues (usually interpreted as an SvO_2 <60%). Because the SvO_2 is a function of arterial saturation, cardiac output, and hemoglobin concentration, any deviation in these values is detected in the SvO_2.

Although a lowered SvO_2 does not identify the cause of the impairment, it provides several hints to solving the problem. Increasing the fractional concentration of oxygen in inspired gas (FiO_2) to elevate SaO_2, using pressors or volume expansion to increase the cardiac output, or increasing the hemoglobin concentration with transfusions can all be used to correct a critically low SvO_2. The SvO_2 can be monitored by intermittent measurement of blood withdrawn from a pulmonary artery catheter or by continuous monitoring using a pulmonary artery catheter equipped with a fiber-optic bundle.[174]

Arterial Catheterization

Indwelling arterial catheterization provides access for continuous monitoring of arterial blood pressure and intermittent arterial blood gas sampling. This method is indicated for patients who require frequent blood gas sampling or who are hemodynamically unstable.

In children, the most common locations for arterial catheter placement are the radial, posterior tibial, or dorsalis pedis arteries. When placing a radial artery catheter, it is imperative to ascertain the patency of the ulnar artery by assessing blood flow to the hand and fingers while the radial artery is compressed (Allen's test).[93] Otherwise, ischemic necrosis of the hand may occur.[20] In newborn infants, the umbilicus provides two additional arteries for access. The catheter tip is generally placed at one of two positions. The high position (T6 through T8) places the tip below the ductus arteriosus but above the major abdominal tributaries. The low position (L3 through L4) places the catheter tip between the renal arteries and inferior mesenteric arteries. These positions have the advantage of minimizing the potential complications of thrombus or embolus into the tributary vessels.

The advantage of direct arterial catheterization is that it provides the most accurate continuous measurement of blood pressure, as well as the most accurate assessment of PaO_2 and $PaCO_2$. The disadvantage is that the technique is invasive and therefore involves a risk of infection,[149,170] embolization,[118] and thrombosis[19]; this risk increases with time.[72] Another complication is the potential for anemia, because the presence of indwelling arterial lines has been associated with excessive blood testing.[128] Consequently, daily assessment of the necessity of direct arterial monitoring is essential, and catheters should be removed as soon as the patient can be managed without them.

In infants, the right radial artery is unique, in that it provides peripheral arterial access to preductal blood (i.e., blood ejected from the left ventricle before being mixed in the aorta with blood from a patent ductus arteriosus). When pulmonary hypertension exists (e.g., congenita diaphragmatic hernia), significant differences in preductal and postductal arterial saturation may occur, and monitoring of both sites is often useful in guiding therapy.

Pulmonary Artery Catheterization

The pulmonary artery catheter (PAC) enables the direct measurement of right atrial pressure, right ventricular end-diastolic pressure, pulmonary artery pressure, and SvO_2.[13,44,48,49,169,190] In addition, calculation of cardiac output and left heart filling pressures can be calculated indirectly. Measurement of cardiac output is based on the technique of thermodilution,[69] in which a bolus of cold fluid is injected through the port of the PAC in the right atrium. By measuring the temperature drop in the pulmonary artery, the cardiac output can be calculated using the Stuart Hamilton equation.[131]

Left atrial pressure can be approximated by measuring the pulmonary artery occlusion pressure, which is accomplished by inflating the balloon on the PAC until the forward flow of blood is impeded. Complications include cardiac arrhythmias in up to 50% of critically ill patients, conduction defects (6%), pulmonary infarction (<1%), pulmonary artery rupture (0.2%), catheter knotting, balloon rupture (5%), and infection.[16,61,68,142,171,176,184] Recently the efficacy of PACs has been called into question because several large series in adults suggested that pulmonary artery catheterization did not improve outcome and was associated with increased morbidity and resource use.[49] Because of these concerns and the evolution of less invasive methods, such as echocardiography, use of PACs in noncardiac pediatric patients is now rare.

MECHANICAL VENTILATORS

A basic knowledge of mechanical ventilators is important for pediatric surgeons because respiratory failure is the most frequent diagnosis requiring admission to the pediatric intensive care unit.[63] The goals of mechanical ventilation are to achieve adequate excretion of carbon dioxide by maintaining alveolar ventilation, maintain adequate arterial oxygenation, expand areas of atelectasis by increasing lung volume, and reduce the mechanical work of breathing. While achieving these goals, mechanical ventilation must also avoid inflicting further injury from barotrauma, oxygen toxicity, or both.[41]

The first-generation ventilator developed by O'Dwyer in 1968 was powered by a foot pump and was not significantly improved upon until 1970, when Siemens introduced the 900A. Since then, ventilators have evolved from simple devices delivering bulk volumes of air based on cycling pressure and time to more advanced models with intermittent mandatory ventilation (IMV), synchronized IMV, and positive end-expiratory pressure (PEEP). In the 1980s, the addition of microprocessors to ventilators provided new functions, such as pressure support ventilation (PSV), mandatory minute ventilation, airway pressure release ventilation, and, more recently, proportional assist ventilation and volume-assured PSV.

Cycling Mechanisms

Mechanical Breath Phases

All mechanical breaths cycle through four distinct phases: inspiration, cycling, expiration, and triggering. Inspiration is the point where expiratory valves close and fresh gas is introduced under pressure into the lungs. Cycling is the point where inspiration changes to expiration and can occur in response to elapsed time, delivered volume, or pressure met. At this point, inflow of gas stops and expiratory valves open to allow passive release of gas from the lungs. Triggering is the changeover from expiration to inspiration and can occur in response to elapsed time (control mode) or in response to a patient-initiated event (assist mode), such as changes in airway pressure or gas flow. Most of the recent refinements in ventilator design are aimed at decreasing the mechanical lag time between patient effort and ventilator response, thereby increasing patient comfort and reducing the work of breathing.[29,188]

Ventilators are broadly classified into two groups—volume and pressure controlled—based on the specific parameter by which the ventilator cycles are controlled.

Pressure Ventilation

Pressure ventilation uses pressure as the main parameter to define inspiration; this method is currently the most common form of ventilation used in infants. In these ventilators, the inspiratory phase ceases when a preset peak inspiratory pressure (PIP) is reached. Some ventilators, known as time-cycled ventilators, use a preset inspiratory time to determine inspiration but are pressure limited and thus classified as pressure ventilators. The major advantage of pressure ventilation is that it allows careful control of PIP and mean airway pressure, thereby avoiding barotrauma. The disadvantage is that tidal volume is a function of not only the difference between PIP and PEEP but also the inspiratory time and compliance. Consequently, as lung compliance changes during the course of an illness, tidal volumes may change dramatically. Therefore, use of pressure-cycled ventilators requires careful attention to the tidal volume being delivered at a given setting to avoid underventilation as compliance worsens or overdistention and barotrauma as compliance improves (see Fig. 7-5).

Volume-Cycled Ventilation

Volume ventilation uses a preset tidal volume to define inspiration. The major advantage of this type of ventilator is that a consistent tidal volume is delivered. The disadvantage is that PIP and mean airway pressure vary with changes in compliance. Frequently, as the pathologic process progresses, adjustments in tidal volume and rate are necessary to maintain the desired minute ventilation and avoid high pressures and barotrauma. To avoid dangerously high PIPs, most volume-cycled ventilators have a pressure-limit valve that prematurely interrupts inspiration when the preset limit is reached. Because this can lead to significant alveolar hyperventilation, a pressure-limit alarm sounds to alert the clinician that this is occurring. Volume-cycled ventilation is more commonly used in older children but can be used in infants.[41]

Modes of Ventilation

The mode of ventilation indicates how the ventilator interfaces with the patient's own breathing efforts. Most ventilators are capable of providing several modes, which vary from total control of ventilation to simple maintenance of PEEP without ventilatory assistance.

Control Mode

Total control is used when it is necessary to maintain complete control of the patient's ventilation.[25] Because the mechanisms for patient-triggered assist modes are disabled, it is generally necessary to paralyze and sedate the patient to eliminate asynchrony with the ventilator. The control mode is generally used when extremes of ventilation are necessary, such as very high minute ventilation requiring rapid respiratory rates.

Assist-Control Mode

Assist-control is similar to the control mode in that the variables of volume pressure and inspiratory time are preset. However, the patient is allowed to override the preset respiratory rate with patient-triggered breaths, which are then completely supported by the ventilator. In the assist-control mode, each breath, whether the patient or the ventilator triggers it, is fully supported by the ventilator. This method may be advantageous if the goal is to reduce the work of breathing or disadvantageous in situations such as weaning, when exercise of the patient's respiratory muscles is desirable.[9] Another disadvantage is that in small infants with high respiratory rates, hyperventilation and asynchrony with the ventilator are common.

Intermittent Mandatory Ventilation

IMV differs from the control and assist-control methods in that the ventilator controls are preset for mandatory inflations, but spontaneous unsupported ventilation is also allowed. The advantage of this method is that it allows exercise of the respiratory muscles. IMV is also an excellent weaning technique, and in infants with high respiratory rates, it can avoid the hyperventilation seen with control modes. One disadvantage is the potential for asynchrony with the ventilator because a machine-driven inspiration may be stacked on top of a patient's spontaneous exhalation. This increases the work of breathing and may result in hypoventilation or even pneumothorax.[75]

Synchronized Intermittent Mandatory Ventilation

Synchronized IMV allows the mandatory ventilator-delivered breaths to be synchronized with the patient's spontaneous efforts. The obvious advantage of this mode is synchronization of breaths, which should reduce the work of breathing.[47] Disadvantages relate to the sensitivity of the synchronizing mechanisms, because a spontaneous inspiratory effort (usually identified by a change in airway pressure) that is not immediately responded to with a synchronous breath can actually increase the work of breathing.[9]

Pressure Support Ventilation

PSV is a spontaneous mode of ventilation in which each breath is initiated by the patient but is supported by constant pressure inflation. This method has been shown to increase the efficiency of inspiration and decrease the work of breathing.[98,111] Like IMV, PSV is useful for weaning patients from mechanical ventilation. Unlike IMV, in which weaning involves decreasing the number of mandatory breaths with maintenance of inspiratory pressures, PSV involves steady decreases in the level of pressure support because the rate is controlled by the patient.

Continuous Positive Airway Pressure and Positive End-Expiratory Pressure

With continuous positive airway pressure (CPAP), a predetermined positive airway pressure is applied to the patient throughout the respiratory cycle.[10] The patient, however, is responsible for generating the tidal volume. This method increases the FRC and usually improves oxygenation by preventing atelectasis.[195] However, this technique can increase the work of breathing.

PEEP provides continuous positive pressure throughout the ventilatory cycle, which can prevent atelectasis, increase FRC, and improve oxygenation. PEEP is commonly employed in the range of 2 to 10 cm/H_2O in neonates and 5 to 20 cm/H_2O in older children, although most ventilators can provide PEEP at significantly higher levels.

Airway Pressure Release Ventilation

Airway pressure release ventilation allows brief expiration to ambient pressure followed by rapid reinflation to regenerate baseline CPAP. Theoretically, this allows the maintenance of pressure to minimize atelectasis while allowing for increased carbon dioxide elimination. Animal trials and preliminary human trials appear to support this claim.[42,182]

Mandatory Minute Ventilation

Mandatory minute ventilation is a relatively new mode in which the ventilator adjusts the rate or pressure to maintain a predetermined expired volume. This may be useful as a weaning mode because the ventilator reduces its support in response to increased activity by the patient.

Proportional Assist Ventilation

Proportional assist ventilation varies support with each breath, depending on patient effort. It is based on amplification of parameters derived from the patient's compliance and inspiratory resistance.[205] The objective is to improve patient synchrony and comfort with the ventilator. To date, there have been no published trials in children to support or refute these proposed benefits.

Volume-Assisted Pressure Support Ventilation

Volume-assisted PSV was designed to ensure that an adequate expired volume is maintained in patients receiving PSV when inspiratory demand falls below a preset level.[8] Preliminary studies in adults have been promising.[78]

Inverse Ratio Ventilation

With inverse ratio ventilation, the inspiratory-expiratory time ratio is greater than 1, as opposed to the typical ratio of 1:2 to 1:5. It has been advocated for use in severe acute respiratory distress syndrome (ARDS) or acute lung injury to improve oxygenation while minimizing volutrauma or barotrauma.[1] This is because inverse ratio ventilation allows for increases in mean airway pressure without increases in tidal volume or PIP. Its use remains controversial; several small studies support its use, but others report higher complication rates than with more conventional modes of ventilation.[1,123,129,154,163] However, it should be considered when traditional modes of ventilation have failed to reverse hypoxemia despite high airway pressures.[168]

High-Frequency Ventilation

High-frequency ventilation (HFV) is defined as mechanical ventilation that uses a tidal volume less than or equal to dead space delivered at superphysiologic rates (>150 breaths per minute).[22] The potential advantages of HFV include smaller volume and pressure changes during the respiratory cycle, gas exchange at significantly lower pressures, and less depression of endogenous surfactant production. A large body of animal data suggests that ventilator-induced lung injury results from changes in pulmonary volume rather than from changes in pressure.[82] Large cyclic volume changes during conventional ventilation have been shown to disrupt the alveolar capillary interface, resulting in increased microvascular permeability and pulmonary interstitial edema.[117] This combination of fluid and protein in the interstitial and alveolar space results in surfactant inhibition, further reducing lung compliance. Conversely, it has been shown that maintaining high lung volume with minimal changes in alveolar pressure or volume does not result in significant pulmonary injury.[180]

Several techniques of HFV exist. High-frequency positive-pressure ventilation is a modification of conventional pressure-limited ventilators, providing rates up to 150 breaths per minute.[23] High-frequency flow interrupters deliver high-pressure, short-duration breaths, with passive expiration.[39] High-frequency jet ventilators deliver short jet breaths at the distal end of the endotracheal tube; expiration is passive.[24] High-frequency oscillatory ventilation (HFOV) uses extremely small tidal volumes delivered at very high rates.[46,153] Unlike the other forms of HFV, the expiratory phase of oscillating ventilators is active.

The mechanism of gas exchange is poorly understood in HFV. With a tidal volume below dead space volume, alveolar ventilation should equal zero, and the technique should not work. However, the probable mechanisms are bulk axial flow, interregional gas mixing (pendelluft), and molecular diffusion.

Oxygenation is improved by recruiting or maintaining lung volume. Unlike conventional ventilation, which requires elevated peak pressure, mean lung volumes can be maintained with ventilation occurring around a relatively fixed intrapulmonary pressure.[40] Elimination of carbon dioxide is much more sensitive to changes in tidal volume than changes in rate.[70] Consequently, when a lower PCO_2 is desired, this can be accomplished by reducing breathing frequency, because the benefit of the increased volume output per stroke exceeds the detriment of decreasing the rate.

Currently, there are two strategies for applying HFV. The high-volume strategy is designed for patients with atelectasis-prone lungs. The mean airway pressure is steadily increased in small increments while monitoring oxygenation. Risks of this approach include using inadequate pressure, thereby worsening atelectasis, or using excessive pressure, leading to injury and air leak.[100] The low-volume strategy is for patients with pneumothorax or air trapping.[45] A higher FiO_2 is frequently necessary with this strategy, and a higher $PaCO_2$ (50 to 60 mm Hg) is frequently tolerated.

The initial clinical experience with HFOV (the most widely used HFV at present) was in premature infants with hyaline membrane disease.[84] That initial study did not show a particular benefit of HFV over conventional ventilation, but its methods have been criticized and its conclusions have not been corroborated by subsequent studies. Later studies of HFOV in neonates demonstrated a significant reduction in the incidence of chronic lung disease,[46] improvement in oxygenation, and reduction in the incidence of air-leak syndrome.[153] Several other studies have shown HFOV to be a reasonable alternative to extracorporeal membrane oxygenation (ECMO) for infants who meet ECMO criteria.[50,189]

Clinical data in older children are sparse; however, a series from Children's Hospital in Boston demonstrated that HFOV has some efficacy as a rescue therapy for pediatric patients who meet ECMO criteria.[12] In this study, the high-volume strategy was used to rapidly attain and maintain optimal lung volume. A multicenter prospective, randomized trial has since been completed, comparing HFOV with conventional mechanical ventilation in pediatric patients with diffuse alveolar disease or air-leak syndrome.[11] Those data showed that HFOV offered rapid and sustained improvements in oxygenation, and despite the use of higher mean airway pressures, a lower incidence of barotrauma was seen with HFOV than with conventional mechanical ventilation.

Extreme Modes of Gas Exchange

Extracorporeal Life Support

Extracorporeal life support (ECLS) sits at the extreme end of the gas-exchange spectrum. It supports or temporarily replaces the function of the heart, the lungs, or both with an extracorporeal mechanical device. Further details and indications for its use are discussed in Chapter 8.

Intravascular Oxygenation

Intravascular oxygenation involves an intracorporeal gas-exchange device inserted into the inferior vena cava that functions similarly to the ECLS circuit. Space constraints

in the inferior vena cava limit its use to a supportive role. This is discussed in greater detail in Chapter 8.

Extracorporeal Carbon Dioxide Removal

Extracorporeal removal of carbon dioxide is similar to ECLS, but it is used when carbon dioxide elimination is the principal problem. This is discussed further in Chapter 8.

Liquid Ventilation

Although the ability to provide gas exchange by means of a liquid medium was first demonstrated in the laboratory almost 30 years ago, liquid ventilation did not become a reality until 1990, when the first clinical evaluations were performed in moribund premature newborn infants with respiratory distress syndrome.[76] That study was the first to demonstrate that gas exchange could be supported clinically using a liquid medium. Since then, additional clinical studies have been performed to assess the safety and efficacy of liquid ventilation in adults and children.[73,86,87,104]

To date, the clinical trials of liquid ventilation have used perfluorocarbons as the liquid vehicle. Perfluorocarbons are clear, colorless, odorless fluids that have low surface tension and carry a large amount of oxygen and carbon dioxide. There are currently two methods of liquid ventilation: total liquid ventilation (TLV) and partial liquid ventilation (PLV). In TLV, the lungs are completely filled with perfluorocarbon to FRC. Subsequently, tidal volumes of additional perfluorocarbon are administered using a device similar to the ECMO circuit. The tidal volume of perfluorocarbon must pass through an external membrane oxygenator (where gas exchange occurs) before being reinstalled into the lungs. Because of the complexity of this process, to date, TLV has been done only in laboratory investigations. PLV, in contrast, is quite easy to perform and very similar to standard mechanical ventilation. In PLV, the lungs are filled with the perfluorocarbon liquid to FRC. Tidal volume, however, is provided by a standard ventilator that uses gas.[85,167] The mixing of the liquid and the gas in the conducting airways of the lung allows the transfer of gases between the two mediums. Because of its ease of use, PLV has been employed exclusively for all clinical trials to date.

The mechanism by which liquid ventilation improves gas exchange is probably a combination of a direct surfactant effect of the perfluorocarbon resulting from its low surface tension and a lavage effect that removes exudates in the peripheral airways. These two effects result in recruitment of atelectatic lung regions and better ventilation-perfusion matching.

After the initial clinical evaluation of perfluorocarbon liquid in newborns with respiratory distress, several other noncontrolled clinical studies were done in adults and children; these studies generally demonstrated improvement in pulmonary function with liquid ventilation.[73,86,87,104] Laboratory studies evaluating the effect of PLV on newborn lambs with congenital diaphragmatic hernia also demonstrated improvements in gas exchange and pulmonary compliance in the liquid ventilation group.[112]

At present, nine human infants with congenital diaphragmatic hernia have received PLV while being supported by ECMO (J. Wilson, unpublished data).[147]

Investigational Adjuncts to Mechanical Ventilation

Prone Positioning

Placing patients with ARDS in the prone position is purported to improve oxygenation by redistributing gravity-dependent blood flow into nonatelectatic areas of nondependent lung by placing them in a dependent position. Several small series have demonstrated at least transient improvements in oxygenation,[132,191] but a recently completed study evaluating prone positioning in pediatric patients failed to show significant improvements in ventilator-free days or survival. In addition, this study noted significant complications with this technique.[136] The value of this adjunct continues to be investigated.

Inhaled Nitric Oxide

Nitric oxide is a potent, short-acting pulmonary vasodilator that has been in clinical trial for more than a decade. In neonates with primary pulmonary hypertension, it has been shown to improve oxygenation and decrease the use of ECLS. However, despite a transient improvement in oxygenation, it has failed to improve ventilator weaning or survival in three large trials of patients with ARDS.[54,79,109]

Pharmacologic Adjuncts in Acute Respiratory Distress Syndrome

Several pharmacologic adjuncts have been proposed for patients with ARDS, including prostaglandin E, acetylcysteine, high-dose corticosteroids, surfactant, and a variety of antioxidants. Unfortunately, despite encouraging results from several small series, a recent meta-analysis of all published trials demonstrated no effect on early mortality and a greater number of adverse events in the active therapy arm in the prostaglandin, surfactant, and steroid trials.[5] Consequently, none of these agents can be routinely recommended as adjunctive measures in the treatment of respiratory failure or ARDS at this time. Investigation continues.

MANAGEMENT OF RESPIRATORY FAILURE

Respiratory failure is defined as inadequate oxygenation leading to hypoxemia or inadequate ventilation leading to hypercarbia. The first step in treating respiratory failure is to establish an adequate airway. Usually this is accomplished using an endotracheal tube, which can be placed either orally or nasally. The approximate internal diameter of the endotracheal tube can be estimated in children older than 2 years using the following formula:

$$\frac{16 + \text{age of child}}{4}$$

In children older than 8 years, uncuffed tubes are often used, and there should be an air leak present when positive pressure between 20 and 30 cm H_2O is achieved. If properly cared for, these tubes can be left in place for several weeks.

The goal of mechanical ventilation is to restore alveolar ventilation and oxygenation toward normal without causing injury from barotrauma or oxygen toxicity. In general, this correlates to maintaining PaO_2 between 50 and 80 mm Hg, $PaCO_2$ between 40 and 60 mm Hg, pH between 7.35 and 7.45, and mixed venous oxygen saturation less than 70.

Initial ventilator settings on pressure-cycled ventilators should be $FiO_2 = 100\%$, rate = 20 to 30 breaths per minute, PIP = 20 to 30 torr, PEEP = 3 to 5 torr, and inspiratory-expiratory ratio = 1:2. The aim is to provide an initial tidal volume of 6 to 8 mL/kg. PEEP should be employed in cases of diffuse lung injury to support oxygenation. Support should be started at 2.0 cm H_2O and adjusted in increments of 1 to 2 cm H_2O. PEEP greater than 10.0 cm H_2O in infants and 15.0 cm H_2O in older children is rarely indicated. Sedation often enhances the response to mechanical support by allowing better synchrony between patient and machine. After the patient has been stabilized for a brief period, the ventilatory management must be individualized, depending on the underlying physiologic condition.

Manipulating the Ventilator Settings

Various parameters can be preset on most ventilators, including the respiratory rate, PIP, PEEP, inspiratory time, and gas flow rate. When adjusting these parameters, it is necessary to consider the pathologic condition present in the lung. Infants with primary pulmonary hypertension have very compliant lungs that are easily overdistended. In these patients, adequate minute ventilation may be achieved with low PIP and PEEP, a short inspiratory time, and a moderate respiratory rate. Conversely, a child with ARDS has noncompliant lungs and may require a relatively high PIP and PEEP, a short inspiratory time, and a high respiratory rate to achieve adequate alveolar ventilation. Obstructive disorders, such as meconium aspiration syndrome or asthma, have a longer time constant and require ventilation at a slower rate. After determining the initial settings, however, the patient's response must be evaluated, and adjustments must be made to stay abreast of dynamic changes in pulmonary compliance and resistance that occur over time.

Adjusting the Partial Pressure of Carbon Dioxide

The $PaCO_2$ is directly related to alveolar ventilation and, consequently, to minute ventilation (tidal volume × respiratory rate). An increase in minute ventilation can be achieved by adjusting either tidal volume or, more frequently, respiratory rate. However, at high rates or in lungs with prolonged time constants, increases in respiratory rate can lead to breath stacking, overdistention, reduced alveolar ventilation, and a subsequent rise in PCO_2.

Adjusting the Partial Pressure of Oxygen

In most conditions requiring mechanical ventilation, patchy atelectasis, caused by a drop in FRC toward closing capacity, results in a significant intrapulmonary shunt that is relatively insensitive to increases in FiO_2. Recruitment of the atelectatic areas by increasing the mean airway pressure is far more likely to be effective in increasing PaO_2. This can be achieved by increasing PIP, PEEP, or the inspiratory-expiratory ratio. High PIP has been shown to cause barotrauma, most likely as a result of overdistention of the more compliant (i.e., healthier) portions of the lung.[151] Consequently, increases in PIP should be used sparingly. An increased PEEP is generally preferable to an increased PIP because the PEEP can recruit collapsed alveoli (by increasing FRC), thereby decreasing the intrapulmonary shunt without significant risk of barotrauma. However, if a pressure-cycled ventilator is used, increases in PEEP without changes in PIP will result in a lower tidal volume and require adjustments in respiratory rate to maintain minute ventilation. Monitoring compliance also ensures that breaths are provided at the most compliant part of the ventilation curve.

Weaning

Weaning is the process during which mechanical ventilation is slowly withdrawn, allowing the patient to assume an increasing amount of the work of breathing. The specific technique of weaning depends on which form of ventilation is being used. Weaning from mechanical ventilation should be attempted only when the patient is hemodynamically stable on acceptable ventilator settings and is able to spontaneously maintain an acceptable $PaCO_2$. In general, this translates into an FiO_2 less than 0.4, PIP less than 30, PEEP less than 5, and ventilator-assisted breaths less than 15 per minute. The child should also have adequate nutrition and a ratio of dead space gas to tidal volume of less than 0.6 (normal = 0.3).

Weaning from IMV support involves a gradual decrease in the frequency of ventilator-delivered breaths. The rate of weaning depends on the patient's clinical condition and response. Monitoring the patient's spontaneous respiratory efforts and blood gas parameters can assist in this process. In older patients, the IMV rate can be reduced to as low as 2 to 4 breaths per minute before the patient is extubated. Because of higher airway resistance in the smaller endotracheal tubes used in younger patients, extubation is generally attempted when the rate is reduced to 8 to 10 breaths per minute.

Weaning from PSV involves a slow decrease in the level of pressure support while monitoring the quality and quantity of the patient's spontaneous respiratory effort. In general, this type of ventilation is withdrawn by reducing the pressure in increments of 1 to 2 cm H_2O.

Weaning Failure

Despite multiple indicators that predict successful weaning, 10% of patients will fail extubation. In most cases, this failure is due to excessive respiratory load. This is manifested clinically as the development of rapid shallow breathing, worsening of lung mechanics, and increase in respiratory muscle load.[96,97] Factors that contribute to this are increased ratio of dead space gas to tidal volume, which accompanies the onset of rapid, shallow breathing; excessive carbon dioxide production due to increased work of breathing; and, sometimes, excessive carbohydrate calories. Respiratory muscle fatigue due to increased respiratory load can cause prolonged (>24 hours) impairment in diaphragmatic and respiratory muscle function.[159] Consequently, time must be allowed for recovery before attempting to wean again. Metabolic abnormalities, such as acute respiratory acidosis, decrease the contractility and endurance of the diaphragm.[95] Imbalances in phosphate, calcium, potassium, and magnesium also impair respiratory muscle function,[14,55,66] as does hypothyroidism.[103] Correction of these variables toward normal ensures that the patient's best effort is being evaluated.

Complications of Mechanical Ventilation

Barotrauma is the principal complication of mechanical ventilation. It is caused by overdistention of alveoli by inappropriately high PIP or PEEP or excessive tidal volumes. The consequences of barotrauma include pneumothorax, pneumomediastinum, and pulmonary interstitial emphysema.[59] In addition, because barotrauma seems to be more closely related to volume changes than to pressure changes, the incidence and severity of barotrauma can potentially be lowered by the use of lower tidal volumes (5 to 7 mL/kg) and by accepting a lower pH and a higher PCO_2—a ventilatory technique known as permissive hypercapnea.[204]

Oxygen toxicity is another complication of mechanical ventilation. The mechanism of injury is purported to be damage to the capillary endothelium, as well as type I and II pneumocytes, from oxygen free radicals.[92] Every attempt should be made to maintain the FiO_2 below 0.6 by adjusting mean airway pressure to improve intrapulmonary shunt and by accepting marginal levels of PO_2 (50 to 60 mm Hg) as long as SvO_2 remains adequate.

Bronchopulmonary dysplasia is a progressive chronic condition that may occur in 15% of infants that require mechanical ventilation. It is unclear whether the cause of this dysplasia is related to barotrauma, oxygen toxicity, or both. Consequently, bronchopulmonary dysplasia can best be avoided by paying careful attention to providing adequate ventilatory support at the lowest possible pressures and oxygen concentration.

These complications are all a direct consequence of positive-pressure inflation of an organ designed to function in a negative-pressure environment. Consequently, it is unlikely that any current or future variation of positive-pressure ventilation will ever be completely safe.

Other common complications not directly related to the mechanics of ventilation itself include nosocomial pneumonia acquired due to the ubiquitous nature of pathogens in the intensive care unit and breach of upper airway defenses by the endotracheal tube. Deep vein thrombosis and pulmonary emboli are not uncommon in older pediatric patients, who should receive prophylaxis. Laryngeal trauma during intubation, tracheal stenosis caused by ill-fitting tubes and prolonged intubation, and sinusitis principally associated with nasal intubation round out the list of the more common complications. Most can be avoided or treated by careful attention to detail.

REFERENCES

1. Abraham E, Yoshihara G: Cardiorespiratory effects of pressure controlled inverse ratio ventilation in severe respiratory failure. Chest 1989;96:1356.
2. Adams FH, Fujiwara T, Rowshan G: The nature and origin of the fluid in the fetal lamb lung. J Pediatr 1963;63:881.
3. Adamson IY, Bowden DH: The type 2 cell as progenitor of alveolar epithelial regeneration: A cytodynamic study in mice after exposure to oxygen. Lab Invest 1974;30:35.
4. Adamson IY, Bowden DH: Derivation of type 1 epithelium from type 2 cells in the developing rat lung. Lab Invest 1975;32:736.
5. Adhikari N, Burns KE, Meade MO: Pharmacologic treatments for acute respiratory distress syndrome and acute lung injury: Systematic review and meta-analysis. Treat Respir Med 2004;3:307.
6. Alcorn DG, Adamson TM, Maloney JE, et al: A morphologic and morphometric analysis of fetal lung development in the sheep. Anat Rec 1981;201:655.
7. Alexander CM, Teller LE, Gross JB: Principles of pulse oximetry: Theoretical and practical considerations. Anesth Analg 1989;68:368.
8. Amato MB, Barbas CS, Bonassa J, et al: Volume-assured pressure support ventilation (VAPSV): A new approach for reducing muscle workload during acute respiratory failure. Chest 1992;102:1225.
9. American College of Chest Physicians: Consensus conference: Mechanical ventilation. Chest 1993;104:1835.
10. American College of Chest Physicians–American Thoracic Society Joint Committee on Pulmonary Nomenclature: Pulmonary terms and symbols. Chest 1975;67:583.
11. Arnold JH, Hanson JH, Toro-Figuero LO, et al: Prospective, randomized comparison of high-frequency oscillatory ventilation and conventional mechanical ventilation in pediatric respiratory failure. Crit Care Med 1994;22:1530.
12. Arnold JH, Truog RD, Thompson JE, et al: High-frequency oscillatory ventilation in pediatric respiratory failure. Crit Care Med 1993;21:272.
13. Artery Catheter Consensus Conference: Consensus statement. Crit Care Med 1997;25:910.
14. Aubier M, Viires N, Piquet J, et al: Effects of hypocalcemia on diaphragmatic strength generation. J Appl Physiol 1985;58:2054.
15. Baird TM, Goydos JM, Neuman MR: Optimal electrode location for monitoring the ECG and breathing in neonates. Pediatr Pulmonol 1992;12:247.
16. Barash PG, Nardi D, Hammond G, et al: Catheter-induced pulmonary artery perforation: Mechanisms, management, and modifications. J Thorac Cardiovasc Surg 1981;82:5.
17. Barker SJ, Tremper KK: The effect of carbon monoxide inhalation on pulse oximetry and transcutaneous Po_2. Anesthesiology 1987;66:677.
18. Beck JC, Mitzner W, Johnson JW, et al: Betamethasone and the rhesus fetus: Effect on lung morphometry and connective tissue. Pediatr Res 1981;15:235.
19. Bedford RF: Long-term radial artery cannulation: Effects on subsequent vessel function. Crit Care Med 1978;6:64.
20. Bedford RF, Wollman H: Complications of percutaneous radial-artery cannulation: An objective prospective study in man. Anesthesiology 1973;38:228.
21. Benesch R, Benesch RE, Yu CI: Reciprocal binding of oxygen and diphosphoglycerate by human hemoglobin. Proc Natl Acad Sci U S A 1968;59:526.
22. Bland RD, Kim MH, Light MJ, et al: High frequency mechanical ventilation in severe hyaline membrane disease an alternative treatment? Crit Care Med 1980;8:275.
23. Borg U, Eriksson I, Sjostrand U: High-frequency positive-pressure ventilation (HFPPV): A review based upon its use during bronchoscopy and for laryngoscopy and microlaryngeal surgery under general anesthesia. Anesth Analg 1980;59:594.
24. Boros SJ, Mammel MC, Coleman JM, et al: Neonatal high-frequency jet ventilation: Four years' experience. Pediatrics 1985;75:657.
25. Bowe EA, Boysen PG, Broome JA, et al: Accurate determination of end-tidal carbon dioxide during administration of oxygen by nasal cannulae. J Clin Monit 1989;5:105.
26. Boyden EA: The terminal air sacs and their blood supply in a 37-day infant lung. Am J Anat 1965;116:413.
27. Boyden EA: The pattern of the terminal air spaces in a premature infant of 30-32 weeks that lived nineteen and a quarter hours. Am J Anat 1969;126:31.
28. Boyden EA: Development and growth of the airways. In Hodson WA (ed): Development of the Lung. Philadelphia, Marcel Dekker, 1977, p 121.
29. Branson RD, Campbell RS, Davis K Jr, et al: Comparison of pressure and flow triggering systems during continuous positive airway pressure. Chest 1994;106:540.
30. Breeze RG, Wheeldon EB: The cells of the pulmonary airways. Am Rev Respir Dis 1977;116:705.
31. Brumley GW, Chernick V, Hodson WA, et al: Correlations of mechanical stability, morphology, pulmonary surfactant, and phospholipid content in the developing lamb lung. J Clin Invest 1967;46:863.
32. Bullard KM, Sonne J, Hawgood S, et al: Tracheal ligation increases cell proliferation but decreases surfactant protein in fetal murine lungs in vitro. J Pediatr Surg 1997;32:207.
33. Bunton TE, Plopper CG: Triamcinolone-induced structural alterations in the development of the lung of the fetal rhesus macaque. Am J Obstet Gynecol 1984;148:203.
34. Burri PH: Fetal and postnatal development of the lung. Annu Rev Physiol 1984;46:617.
35. Butler S: In Wilkins R (ed): The Doctor's Quotation Book. New York, Barnes & Noble Books, 1992, p 81.
36. Cahan C, Decker MJ, Hoekje PL, et al: Agreement between noninvasive oximetric values for oxygen saturation. Chest 1990;97:814.
37. Carpenter G, Cohen S: Epidermal growth factor. Annu Rev Biochem 1979;48:193.
38. Catterton WZ, Escobedo MB, Sexson WR, et al: Effect of epidermal growth factor on lung maturation in fetal rabbits. Pediatr Res 1979;13:104.
39. Cavanaugh K, Bloom B: Combined HFV and CMV for neonatal air leak. Respir Manage 1990;20:43.
40. Chang HK: Mechanisms of gas transport during ventilation by high-frequency oscillation. J Appl Physiol 1984;56:553.
41. Chatburn RL: Principles and practice of neonatal and pediatric mechanical ventilation. Respir Care 1991;36:569.
42. Chiang AA, Steinfeld A, Gropper C, et al: Demand-flow airway pressure release ventilation as a partial ventilatory support mode: Comparison with synchronized intermittent mandatory ventilation and pressure support ventilation. Crit Care Med 1994;22:1431.

43. Cilley RE, Zgleszewski SE, Chinoy MR: Fetal lung development: Airway pressure enhances the expression of developmental genes. J Pediatr Surg 2000;35:113.

44. Clark C, Harman E: Hemodynamic monitorying: Pulmonary artery catheters. In Civetta J, Taylor R, Kirby R (eds): Critical Care. Philadelphia, JB Lippincott, 1988, p 319.

45. Clark RH, Gerstmann DR, Null DM, et al: Pulmonary interstitial emphysema treated by high-frequency oscillatory ventilation. Crit Care Med 1986;14:926.

46. Clark RH, Gerstmann DR, Null DM Jr, et al: Prospective randomized comparison of high-frequency oscillatory and conventional ventilation in respiratory distress syndrome. Pediatrics 1992;89:5.

47. Clear J: Improved oxygenation during synchronized vs intermittent mandatory ventilation in VLBW infants with respiratory distress: A randomized crossover design. Pediatr Res 1993;33:1226A.

48. Coleman SS, Anson BJ: Arterial patterns in the hand based upon a study of 650 specimens. Suvr Med (Sofiia) 1961; 113:409.

49. Connors AF Jr, Speroff T, Dawson NV, et al: The effectiveness of right heart catheterization in the initial care of critically ill patients. SUPPORT investigators. JAMA 1996;276:889.

50. Cornish JD, Gerstmann DR, Clark RH, et al: Extracorporeal membrane oxygenation and high-frequency oscillatory ventilation: Potential therapeutic relationships. Crit Care Med 1987;15:831.

51. Davies G, Reid L: Growth of the alveoli and pulmonary arteries in childhood. Thorax 1970;25:669.

52. De Paepe ME, Johnson BD, Papadakis K, et al: Temporal pattern of accelerated lung growth after tracheal occlusion in the fetal rabbit. Am J Pathol 1998;152:179.

53. De Paepe ME, Papadakis K, Johnson BD, et al: Fate of the type II pneumocyte following tracheal occlusion in utero: A time-course study in fetal sheep. Virchows Arch 1998;432:7.

54. Dellinger RP, Zimmerman JL, Taylor RW, et al: Effects of inhaled nitric oxide in patients with acute respiratory distress syndrome: Results of a randomized phase II trial. Inhaled Nitric Oxide in ARDS Study Group. Crit Care Med 1998;26:15.

55. Dhingra S, Solven F, Wilson A, et al: Hypomagnesemia and respiratory muscle power. Am Rev Respir Dis 1984; 129:497.

56. DiFiore JW, Fauza DO, Slavin R, et al: Experimental fetal tracheal ligation reverses the structural and physiological effects of pulmonary hypoplasia in congenital diaphragmatic hernia. J Pediatr Surg 1994;29:248.

57. DiFiore JW, Fauza DO, Slavin R, et al: Experimental fetal tracheal ligation and congenital diaphragmatic hernia: A pulmonary vascular morphometric analysis. J Pediatr Surg 1995;30:917.

58. Docimo SG, Crone RK, Davies P, et al: Pulmonary development in the fetal lamb: Morphometric study of the alveolar phase. Anat Rec 1991;229:495.

59. Dreyfuss D, Soler P, Basset G, et al: High inflation pressure pulmonary edema: Respective effects of high airway pressure, high tidal volume, and positive end-expiratory pressure. Am Rev Respir Dis 1988;137:1159.

60. Dunnill M: Postnatal growth of the lung. Thorax 1962;17:329.

61. Elliott CG, Zimmerman GA, Clemmer TP: Complications of pulmonary artery catheterization in the care of critically ill patients: A prospective study. Chest 1979;76:647.

62. Erenberg A, Rhodes ML, Weinstein MM, et al: The effect of fetal thyroidectomy on ovine fetal lung maturation. Pediatr Res 1979;13:230.

63. Esteban A, Anzueto A, Alia I, et al: How is mechanical ventilation employed in the intensive care unit? An international utilization review. Am J Respir Crit Care Med 2000; 161:1450.

64. Evans MJ, Cabral LJ, Stephens RJ, et al: Renewal of alveolar epithelium in the rat following exposure to NO_2. Am J Pathol 1973;70:175.

65. Finch CA, Lenfant C: Oxygen transport in man. N Engl J Med 1972;286:407.

66. Fisher J, Magid N, Kallman C, et al: Respiratory illness and hypophosphatemia. Chest 1983;83:504.

67. Flageole H, Evrard VA, Piedboeuf B, et al: The plug-unplug sequence: An important step to achieve type II pneumocyte maturation in the fetal lamb model. J Pediatr Surg 1998;33:299.

68. Foote GA, Schabel SI, Hodges M: Pulmonary complications of the flow-directed balloon-tipped catheter. N Engl J Med 1974;290:927.

69. Forrester JS, Ganz W, Diamond G, et al: Thermodilution cardiac output determination with a single flow-directed catheter. Am Heart J 1972;83:306.

70. Fredberg JJ, Glass GM, Boynton BR, et al: Factors influencing mechanical performance of neonatal high-frequency ventilators. J Appl Physiol 1987;62:2485.

71. Fry DL, Hyatt RE: Pulmonary mechanics: A unified analysis of the relationship between pressure, volume and gas flow in the lungs of normal and diseased human subjects. Am J Med 1960;29:672.

72. Gardner RM, Schwartz R, Wong HC, et al: Percutaneous indwelling radial-artery catheters for monitoring cardiovascular function: Prospective study of the risk of thrombosis and infection. N Engl J Med 1974;290:1227.

73. Gauger P: Initial experience with partial liquid ventilation in pediatric patients with the acute respiratory distress syndrome. Crit Care Med 1996;24:4.

74. Goodlin R, Lloyd D: Fetal tracheal excretion of bilirubin. Biol Neonate 1968;12:1.

75. Greenough A, Morley C, Davis J: Interaction of spontaneous respiration with artificial ventilation in preterm babies. J Pediatr 1983;103:769.

76. Greenspan JS, Wolfson MR, Rubenstein SD, et al: Liquid ventilation of human preterm neonates. J Pediatr 1990; 117:106.

77. Griscom NT, Harris GB, Wohl ME, et al: Fluid-filled lung due to airway obstruction in the newborn. Pediatrics 1969;43:383.

78. Groeger JS, Levinson MR, Carlon GC: Assist control versus synchronized intermittent mandatory ventilation during acute respiratory failure. Crit Care Med 1989;17:607.

79. Groupe d'Etude sur le NO inhale au cours de lards (GENOA): Inhaled NO in ARDS: Presentation of a double blind randomized multicentric study [abstract]. Am J Respir Crit Care Med 1996;275:383.

80. Hallman M, Kulovich M, Kirkpatrick E, et al: Phosphatidylinositol and phosphatidylglycerol in amniotic fluid: Indices of lung maturity. Am J Obstet Gynecol 1976; 125:613.

81. Hellegers AE, Schruefer JJ: Nomograms and empirical equations relating oxygen tension, percentage saturation, and pH in maternal and fetal blood. Am J Obstet Gynecol 1961;81:377.

82. Hernandez LA, Peevy KJ, Moise AA, et al: Chest wall restriction limits high airway pressure-induced lung injury in young rabbits. J Appl Physiol 1989;66:2364.

83. Hess D: Capnometry and capnography: Technical aspects, physiologic aspects and clinical applications. Respir Care 1990;35:557.

84. High-frequency oscillatory ventilation compared with conventional mechanical ventilation in the treatment of respiratory failure in preterm infants. The HIFI Study Group. N Engl J Med 1989;320:88.

85. Hirschl RB, Merz SI, Montoya JP, et al: Development and application of a simplified liquid ventilator. Crit Care Med 1995;23:157.

86. Hirschl RB, Pranikoff T, Gauger P, et al: Liquid ventilation in adults, children, and full-term neonates. Lancet 1995;346:1201.

87. Hirschl RB, Pranikoff T, Wise C, et al: Initial experience with partial liquid ventilation in adult patients with the acute respiratory distress syndrome. JAMA 1996;275:383.

88. Hislop A, Reid L: Intra-pulmonary arterial development during fetal life: Branching pattern and structure. J Anat 1972;113:35.

89. Hislop A, Reid L: Pulmonary arterial development during childhood: Branching pattern and structure. Thorax 1973;28:129.

90. Hlastala MP, Woodson RD: Saturation dependency of the Bohr effect: Interactions among H^+, CO_2, and DPG. J Appl Physiol 1975;38:1126.

91. Hoppin F, Hildebrandt J: Mechanical properties of the lung. In West J (ed): Lung Biology in Health and Disease: Bioengineering Aspects of the Lung. New York, Dekker, 1978, p 263.

92. Jenkinson S: Oxygen toxicity in acute respiratory monitoring. Respir Care 1983;28:614.

93. Jordan W: Arterial catheters. In Blumer J (ed): A Practical Guide to Pediatric Intensive Care, 3rd ed. St Louis, Mosby-Year Book, 1990, p 263.

94. Jordan W: Electrographic and respiratory monitoring. In Blumer J (ed): A Practical Guide to Pediatric Intensive Care, 3rd ed. St Louis, Mosby-Year Book, 1990, p .

95. Juan G, Calverley P, Talamo C, et al: Effect of carbon dioxide on diaphragmatic function in human beings. N Engl J Med 1984;310:874.

96. Jubran A, Tobin MJ: Pathophysiologic basis of acute respiratory distress in patients who fail a trial of weaning from mechanical ventilation. Am J Respir Crit Care Med 1997;155:906.

97. Jubran A, Tobin MJ: Passive mechanics of lung and chest wall in patients who failed or succeeded in trials of weaning. Am J Respir Crit Care Med 1997;155:916.

98. Kacmarek R: The role of pressure support ventilation in reducing work of breathing. Respir Care 1988;33:99.

99. Kauffman SL: Acceleration of canalicular development in lungs of fetal mice exposed transplacentally to dexamethasone. Lab Invest 1977;36:395.

100. Kinsella JP, Gerstmann DR, Clark RH, et al: High-frequency oscillatory ventilation versus intermittent mandatory ventilation: Early hemodynamic effects in the premature baboon with hyaline membrane disease. Pediatr Res 1991;29:160.

101. Kitterman JA, Liggins GC, Campos GA, et al: Prepartum maturation of the lung in fetal sheep: Relation to cortisol. J Appl Physiol 1981;51:384.

102. Klocke R: Carbon dioxide transport. In Farhi L, Tenney S (eds): Handbook of Physiology. Washington, DC, American Physiological Society, 1987, p 88.

103. Laroche CM, Cairns T, Moxham J, et al: Hypothyroidism presenting with respiratory muscle weakness. Am Rev Respir Dis 1988;138:472.

104. Leach D: Partial liquid ventilation with perflubron (LiquiVent): A pilot safety and efficacy study in premature newborns with severe RDS who have failed conventional therapy and exogenous surfactant. Paper presented at the American Academy of Pediatrics meeting, 1994, Dallas.

105. Liggins GC, Kitterman JA, Campos GA, et al: Pulmonary maturation in the hypophysectomised ovine fetus: Differential responses to adrenocorticotrophin and cortisol. J Dev Physiol 1981;3:1.

106. Lloyd TC Jr, Wright GW: Pulmonary vascular resistance and vascular transmural gradient. J Appl Physiol 1960; 15:241.

107. Loosli CG, Potter EL: Pre- and postnatal development of the respiratory portion of the human lung with special reference to the elastic fibers. Am Rev Respir Dis 1959;80:5.

108. Luks FI, Roggin KK, Wild YK, et al: Effect of lung fluid composition on type II cellular activity after tracheal occlusion in the fetal lamb. J Pediatr Surg 2001;36:196.

109. Lundin S, Mang H, Smithies M, et al: Inhalation of nitric oxide in acute lung injury: Results of a European multicentre study. The European Study Group of Inhaled Nitric Oxide. Intensive Care Med 1999;25:911.

110. MacGregor A: Pathology of Infancy and Childhood. London, Livingston, 1960.

111. MacIntyre N: Weaning from mechanical ventilatory support: Volume-assisting intermittent breaths versus pressure-assisting every breath. Respir Care 1988;33:121.

112. Major D, Cadenas M, Cloutier R, et al: Combined gas ventilation and perfluorochemical tracheal instillation as an alternative treatment for lethal congenital diaphragmatic hernia in lambs. J Pediatr Surg 1995;30:1178.

113. Maren TH: Carbonic anhydrase: Chemistry, physiology, and inhibition. Physiol Rev 1967;47:595.

114. Marshall R: The physical properties of the lungs in relation to the subdivisions of lung volume. Clin Sci (Colch) 1957;16:507.

115. Mason RJ, Leslie CC, McCormick-Shannon K, et al: Hepatocyte growth factor is a growth factor for rat alveolar type II cells. Am J Respir Cell Mol Biol 1994;11:561.

116. Masters JR: Epithelial-mesenchymal interaction during lung development: The effect of mesenchymal mass. Dev Biol 1976;51:98.

117. Mathieu-Costello OA, West JB: Are pulmonary capillaries susceptible to mechanical stress? Chest 1994;105(Suppl): 102S.

118. Matthews JI, Gibbons RB: Embolization complicating radial artery puncture. Ann Intern Med 1971;75:87.

119. McCabe AJ, Carlino U, Holm BA, et al: Upregulation of keratinocyte growth factor in the tracheal ligation lamb model of congenital diaphragmatic hernia. J Pediatr Surg 2001;36:128.

120. McCarthy DS, Spencer R, Greene R, et al: Measurement of "closing volume" as a simple and sensitive test for early detection of small airway disease. Am J Med 1972;52:747.

121. Mead J, Takishima T, Leith D: Stress distribution in lungs: A model of pulmonary elasticity. J Appl Physiol 1970;28:596.

122. Mead J, Turner JM, Macklem PT, et al: Significance of the relationship between lung recoil and maximum expiratory flow. J Appl Physiol 1967;22:95.

123. Mercat A, Graini L, Teboul JL, et al: Cardiorespiratory effects of pressure-controlled ventilation with and without inverse ratio in the adult respiratory distress syndrome. Chest 1993;104:871.

124. Messmer TO, Armour R, Holley RW: Factors influencing the growth of alveolar type II epithelial cells isolated from rat lungs. Exp Cell Res 1982;142:417.

125. Milles G, Dorsey DB: Intra-uterine respiration-like movements in relation to development of the fetal vascular system: A discussion of intra-uterine physiology based upon cases of congenital absence of the trachea, abnormal vascular development, and other anomalies. Am J Pathol 1950;26:411.

126. Monaco F, McQuitty JC: Transcutaneous measurements of carbon dioxide partial pressure in sick neonates. Crit Care Med 1981;9:756.

127. Morris A: Clinical Pulmonary Function Testing: A Manual of Uniform Laboratory Procedures. Salt Lake City, Intermountain Thoracic Society, 1984.

128. Muakkassa FF, Rutledge R, Fakhry SM, et al: ABGs and arterial lines: The relationship to unnecessarily drawn arterial blood gas samples. J Trauma 1900;30:1087.

129. Munoz J, Guerrero JE, Escalante JL, et al: Pressure-controlled ventilation versus controlled mechanical ventilation with decelerating inspiratory flow. Crit Care Med 1993;21:1143.

130. Muratore CS, Nguyen HT, Ziegler MM, et al: Stretch-induced upregulation of VEGF gene expression in murine pulmonary culture: A role for angiogenesis in lung development. J Pediatr Surg 2000;35:906.

131. Nadeau S, Noble WH: Limitations of cardiac output measurements by thermodilution. Can Anaesth Soc J 1986;33:780.

132. Nakos G, Tsangaris I, Kostanti E, et al: Effect of the prone position on patients with hydrostatic pulmonary edema compared with patients with acute respiratory distress syndrome and pulmonary fibrosis. Am J Respir Crit Care Med 2000;161:360.

133. Neuman M: The biophysical and bioengineering bases of perinatal monitoring. Part V. Neonatal cardiac and respiratory monitoring. Perinatal Neonatal 1979;3:17.

134. Nobuhara KK, DiFiore JW, Ibla JC, et al: Insulin-like growth factor-I gene expression in three models of accelerated lung growth. J Pediatr Surg 1998;33:1057.

135. Nobuhara KK, Fauza DO, DiFiore JW, et al: Continuous intrapulmonary distension with perfluorocarbon accelerates neonatal (but not adult) lung growth. J Pediatr Surg 1998;33:292.

136. Offner PJ, Haenel JB, Moore EE, et al: Complications of prone ventilation in patients with multisystem trauma with fulminant acute respiratory distress syndrome. J Trauma 2000;48:224.

137. Otis AB, McKerrow CB, Bartlett RA, et al: Mechanical factors in distribution of pulmonary ventilation. J Appl Physiol 1956;8:427.

138. O'Toole SJ, Sharma A, Karamanoukian HL, et al: Tracheal ligation does not correct the surfactant deficiency associated with congenital diaphragmatic hernia. J Pediatr Surg 1996;31:546.

139. Panos RJ, Rubin JS, Csaky KG, et al: Keratinocyte growth factor and hepatocyte growth factor/scatter factor are heparin-binding growth factors for alveolar type II cells in fibroblast-conditioned medium. J Clin Invest 1993;92:969.

140. Papadakis K, De Paepe ME, Tackett LD, et al: Temporary tracheal occlusion causes catch-up lung maturation in a fetal model of diaphragmatic hernia. J Pediatr Surg 1998;33:1030.

141. Papadakis K, Luks FI, De Paepe ME, et al: Fetal lung growth after tracheal ligation is not solely a pressure phenomenon. J Pediatr Surg 1997;32:347.

142. Patel C, Laboy V, Venus B, et al: Acute complications of pulmonary artery catheter insertion in critically ill patients. Crit Care Med 1986;14:195.

143. Piedboeuf B, Laberge JM, Ghitulescu G, et al: Deleterious effect of tracheal obstruction on type II pneumocytes in fetal sheep. Pediatr Res 1997;41:473.

144. Poets CF, Samuels MP, Noyes JP, et al: Home monitoring of transcutaneous oxygen tension in the early detection of hypoxaemia in infants and young children. Arch Dis Child 1991;66:676.

145. Potter E: Bilateral renal agenesis. J Pediatr 1946;29:68.

146. Potter E, Bohlender G: Intrauterine respiration in relation to development of the fetal lung. Am J Obstet Gynecol 1941;42:14.

147. Pranikoff T, Gauger PG, Hirschl RB: Partial liquid ventilation in newborn patients with congenital diaphragmatic hernia. J Pediatr Surg 1996;31:613.

148. Pringle K: Lung development in congenital diaphragmatic hernia. In Puri P (ed): Congenital Diaphragmatic Hernia. New York, Karger, 1989, p 62.

149. Puri VK, Carlson RW, Bander JJ, et al: Complications of vascular catheterization in the critically ill: A prospective study. Crit Care Med 1980;8:495.

150. Quinn TM, Sylvester KG, Kitano Y, et al: TGF-beta2 is increased after fetal tracheal occlusion. J Pediatr Surg 1999;34:701.

151. Rahn H: The pressure-volume diagram of the thorax and lung. Am J Physiol 1946;146:161.

152. Raine JM, Bishop JM: A-a difference in O_2 tension and physiological dead space in normal man. J Appl Physiol 1963;18:284.

153. Randomized study of high-frequency oscillatory ventilation in infants with severe respiratory distress syndrome. HiFO Study Group. J Pediatr 1993;122:609.

154. Rappaport SH, Shpiner R, Yoshihara G, et al: Randomized, prospective trial of pressure-limited versus volume-controlled ventilation in severe respiratory failure. Crit Care Med 1994;22:22.

155. Reid L: The embryology of the lung. In Ciba Foundation Symposium: Development of the Lung. London, Churchill, 1967, p 109.

156. Reid L: Structural and functional reappraisal of the pulmonary artery system. In British Postgraduate Medical Federation: Scientific Basis of Medicine, Annual Reviews. London, Athlone Press, 1968, p 235.

157. Reid L: 1976 Edward B. D. Neuhauser lecture: The lung: growth and remodeling in health and disease. AJR Am J Roentgenol 1977;129:777.

158. Reid LM: Lung growth in health and disease. Br J Dis Chest 1984;78:113.

159. Reid WD, Huang J, Bryson S, et al: Diaphragm injury and myofibrillar structure induced by resistive loading. J Appl Physiol 1994;76:176.

160. Richardson JB: Nerve supply to the lungs. Am Rev Respir Dis 1979;119:785.

161. Roubliova XI, Verbeken EK, Wu J, et al: Effect of tracheal occlusion on peripheral pulmonary vessel muscularization in a fetal rabbit model for congenital diaphragmatic hernia. Am J Obstet Gynecol 2004;191:830.

162. Roughton FJ, Forster RE: Relative importance of diffusion and chemical reaction rates in determining rate of exchange of gases in the human lung, with special reference to true diffusing capacity of pulmonary membrane and volume of blood in the lung capillaries. J Appl Physiol 1957;11:290.

163. Sassoon CS, Mahutte CK, Light RW: Ventilator modes: Old and new. Crit Care Clin 1990;6:605.

164. Schnitzer JJ: Control and regulation of pulmonary hypoplasia associated with congenital diaphragmatic hernia. Semin Pediatr Surg 2004;13:37.

165. Severinghaus JW, Kelleher JF: Recent developments in pulse oximetry. Anesthesiology 1992;76:1018.

166. Severinghaus JW, Spellman MJ Jr: Pulse oximeter failure thresholds in hypotension and vasoconstriction. Anesthesiology 1990;73:532.

167. Shaffer TH, Moskowitz GD: Demand-controlled liquid ventilation of the lungs. J Appl Physiol 1974;36:208.

168. Shanholtz C, Brower R: Should inverse ratio ventilation be used in adult respiratory distress syndrome? Am J Respir Crit Care Med 1994;149:1354.

169. Shaw TJ: The Swan-Ganz pulmonary artery catheter: Incidence of complications, with particular reference to ventricular dysrhythmias, and their prevention. Anaesthesia 1979;34:651.

170. Shinozaki T, Deane RS, Mazuzan JE Jr, et al: Bacterial contamination of arterial lines: A prospective study. JAMA 1983;249:223.

171. Sise MJ, Hollingsworth P, Brimm JE, et al: Complications of the flow-directed pulmonary artery catheter: A prospective analysis in 219 patients. Crit Care Med 1981;9:315.

172. Sivan Y, Eldadah MK, Cheah TE, et al: Estimation of arterial carbon dioxide by end-tidal and transcutaneous P_{CO_2} measurements in ventilated children. Pediatr Pulmonol 1992;12:153.

173. Snyder JM, Johnston JM, Mendelson CR: Differentiation of type II cells of human fetal lung in vitro. Cell Tissue Res 1981;220:17.

174. Spinale FG, Smith AC, Crawford FA: Relationship of bioimpedance to thermodilution and echocardiographic measurements of cardiac function. Crit Care Med 1900;18:414.

175. Spooner BS, Wessells NK: Mammalian lung development: Interactions in primordium formation and bronchial morphogenesis. J Exp Zool 1970;175:445.

176. Sprung CL, Jacobs LJ, Caralis PV, et al: Ventricular arrhythmias during Swan-Ganz catheterization of the critically ill. Chest 1981;79:413.

177. Stahlman MT, Gray ME: Anatomical development and maturation of the lungs. Clin Perinatol 1978;5:181.

178. Stock MC: Noninvasive carbon dioxide monitoring. Crit Care Clin 1988;4:511.

179. Suen H, Bloch K, Donahoe P: Antenatal glucocorticoid treatment corrects the pulmonary immaturity of CDH. Program of the 24th annual meeting of the American Pediatric Surgical Association, 1993, Hilton Head, SC.

180. Sugiura M, McCulloch PR, Wren S, et al: Ventilator pattern influences neutrophil influx and activation in atelectasis-prone rabbit lung. J Appl Physiol 1994;77:1355.

181. Sundell HW, Gray ME, Serenius FS, et al: Effects of epidermal growth factor on lung maturation in fetal lambs. Am J Pathol 1980;100:707.

182. Sydow M, Burchardi H, Ephraim E, et al: Long-term effects of two different ventilatory modes on oxygenation in acute lung injury: Comparison of airway pressure release ventilation and volume-controlled inverse ratio ventilation. Am J Respir Crit Care Med 1994;149:1550.

183. Taderera JV: Control of lung differentiation in vitro. Dev Biol 1967;16:489.

184. Thomson IR, Dalton BC, Lappas DG, et al: Right bundle-branch block and complete heart block caused by the Swan-Ganz catheter. Anesthesiology 1979;51:359.

185. Tremper KK, Barker SJ: Pulse oximetry. Anesthesiology 1989;70:98.

186. Tremper KK, Mentelos RA, Shoemaker WC: Effect of hypercarbia and shock on transcutaneous carbon dioxide at different electrode temperatures. Crit Care Med 1980; 8:608.

187. Tremper KK, Shoemaker WC: Transcutaneous oxygen monitoring of critically ill adults, with and without low flow shock. Crit Care Med 1981;9:706.

188. Tutuncu AS, Cakar N, Camci E, et al: Comparison of pressure- and flow-triggered pressure-support ventilation on weaning parameters in patients recovering from acute respiratory failure. Crit Care Med 1997;25:756.

189. Varnholt V, Lasch P, Suske G, et al: High frequency oscillatory ventilation and extracorporeal membrane oxygenation in severe persistent pulmonary hypertension of the newborn. Eur J Pediatr 1992;151:769.

190. Varon A: Hemodynamic monitoring: Arterial and pulmonary artery catheters. In Civetta J, Taylor R, Kirby R (eds): Critical Care, 2nd ed. Philadelphia, JB Lippincott, 1992, p 321.

191. Voggenreiter G, Neudeck F, Aufmkolk M, et al: Intermittent prone positioning in the treatment of severe and moderate posttraumatic lung injury. Crit Care Med 1999;27:2375.

192. Wagner PD: Diffusion and chemical reaction in pulmonary gas exchange. Physiol Rev 1977;57:257.

193. Wagner PD, Laravuso RB, Uhl RR, et al: Continuous distributions of ventilation-perfusion ratios in normal subjects breathing air and 100 per cent O_2. J Clin Invest 1974;54:54.

194. Wagner PD, West JB: Effects of diffusion impairment on O_2 and CO_2 time courses in pulmonary capillaries. J Appl Physiol 1972;33:62.

195. Waldhorn RE, Herrick TW, Nguyen MC, et al: Long-term compliance with nasal continuous positive airway pressure therapy of obstructive sleep apnea. Chest 1990;97:33.

196. Wasserman K, Whipp BJ: Exercise physiology in health and disease. Am Rev Respir Dis 1975;112:219.

197. Watcha MF, Connor MT, Hing AV: Pulse oximetry in methemoglobinemia. Am J Dis Child 1989;143:845.

198. Weibel ER: Morphological basis of alveolar-capillary gas exchange. Physiol Rev 1973;53:419.

199. Weibel ER, Gomez DM: A principle for counting tissue structures on random sections. J Appl Physiol 1962;17:343.

200. West JB, Wagner PD, Derks CM: Gas exchange in distributions of VA-Q ratios: Partial pressure-solubility diagram. J Appl Physiol 1974;37:533.

201. Whipp BJ, Wasserman K: Alveolar-arterial gas tension differences during graded exercise. J Appl Physiol 1969; 27:361.

202. Wigglesworth JS, Desai R, Hislop AA: Fetal lung growth in congenital laryngeal atresia. Pediatr Pathol 1987;7:515.

203. Wilson JM, DiFiore JW, Peters CA: Experimental fetal tracheal ligation prevents the pulmonary hypoplasia associated with fetal nephrectomy: Possible application for congenital diaphragmatic hernia. J Pediatr Surg 1993; 28:1433.

204. Wung JT, James LS, Kilchevsky E, et al: Management of infants with severe respiratory failure and persistence of the fetal circulation, without hyperventilation. Pediatrics 1985;76:488.

205. Younces M, Roberts D, Light R, et al: Proportional assist ventilation: A new approach to ventilatory support [abstract]. Am Rev Respir Dis 1989;139:A363.

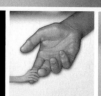

Chapter 8

Extracorporeal Life Support for Cardiopulmonary Failure

Ronald B. Hirschl and Robert H. Bartlett

Extracorporeal life support (ECLS) or extracorporeal membrane oxygenation (ECMO) denotes the use of prolonged extracorporeal cardiopulmonary bypass, usually via extrathoracic cannulation, in patients with acute, reversible cardiac or respiratory failure who are unresponsive to conventional medical or pharmacologic management.[7,42] It is important to recognize that ECLS is not a therapeutic intervention; it simply provides cardiopulmonary support so that the patient is spared the deleterious effects of high airway pressure, high oxygen fraction in inspired air (FiO_2), vasoactive drugs, and perfusion impairment while reversible pathophysiologic processes are allowed to resolve either spontaneously or by medical or surgical intervention. The technology of ECLS is similar for all applications, but the indications, management, and results are best considered separately for adults, children, and neonates with either respiratory or cardiac failure. This chapter is limited to neonates and children with respiratory or cardiac failure.

In 1989 the active ECLS centers formed the Extracorporeal Life Support Organization (ELSO), which standardized many aspects of ECLS. ELSO maintains a registry of all cases treated by the member centers. Much of the information provided here is based on reports from the ELSO Registry.[28]

BACKGROUND

ECLS was first successfully applied in a newborn with respiratory failure in 1975.[9] By 1982 ECLS had been used in 45 newborns with respiratory failure, both premature and full term, demonstrating a survival of 55% and short-term normal growth and development in 80% of the survivors.[8-10] Three prospective, randomized trials compared the effectiveness of ECLS with that of conventional mechanical ventilation in full-term newborns with severe respiratory insufficiency. In 1985 our group used an adaptive design known as "play-the-winner," which weighted randomization toward the successful and away from the unsuccessful intervention.[12] The randomization scheme resulted in 11 ECLS patients who survived and 1 control patient who died. Although statistically significant in

view of the 80% to 90% predicted mortality among the enrolled patients, this study was highly controversial and was not well accepted by the medical community. In 1989 O'Rourke et al.[68] conducted a randomized trial using a similar adaptive design. Survival in the control group was 6 of 10 patients (60%) and in the ECLS group 28 of 29 (97%). A traditional randomized, prospective study was performed in the United Kingdom that demonstrated a significant difference in survival between full-term newborns managed with ECLS (72%) and those managed by conventional means (41%).[30] Based on these studies, ECLS is considered to be indicated in neonatal respiratory failure whenever the risk of mortality is high. As of July 2004, the ELSO Registry database reported 27,407 adult, pediatric, and newborn patients with cardiorespiratory failure who were supported with ECLS, with an overall 73% survival rate.[28]

Timmons et al.[94] conducted a multicenter data-collection study of pediatric respiratory failure in 1991. The only treatment variable that correlated with improved outcome was ECLS. This large database was further evaluated by Green et al.[39] They did a matched-pair study of patients who were managed with ECLS (74% survival) compared with those managed by conventional means (53% survival). As of July 2004, there were 2762 cases of respiratory failure in children more than 30 days old in the registry, with an overall survival of 56%.

ECLS has been used successfully for pediatric cardiac failure since 1972. Intra- or postoperative cardiac failure is the most common indication. ECLS is the only mechanical support system for children, unlike adults, for whom balloon pumps and ventricular assist devices are available. As of July 2004, 5584 cases of cardiac failure in children had been recorded in the registry, with an overall survival of 41%.

INDICATIONS

ECLS is indicated for acute severe respiratory or cardiac failure when recovery can be expected within 2 to 4 weeks. Severe cardiac or respiratory failure can be defined as any acute failure in which the mortality risk is greater than 50%; survival ranges from 50% to 90% in different categories of patients. In some cases the risk is easy to identify (e.g., cardiac arrest or inability to come off cardiopulmonary bypass in the operating room). In other cases it is more difficult to quantitate (e.g., a neonate with borderline oxygenation on 80% oxygen on moderate ventilatory settings with nitric oxide). Some scoring systems have been devised in these categories of patients to try to define high mortality risk.

Mortality risk in neonatal respiratory failure can be measured by an oxygen index (OI) that is based on arterial oxygenation (PaO_2) and mean airway pressure (MAP) despite and after all appropriate treatment. It is computed according to the following formula:

$$OI = (MAP \times FiO_2 \times 100)/PaO_2$$

In the early ECLS studies, an OI greater than 40 in three of five postductal arterial blood gases, each drawn 30 to 60 minutes apart, was predictive of a mortality greater than 80%.[11,69] A randomized, controlled study performed by our group suggested that "early" initiation of ECLS based on an OI greater than 25, which is predictive of a 50% mortality rate, is associated with a trend toward higher mental developmental scores and a lower incidence of morbidity at 1 year of age when compared with a control group of patients in whom ECLS was initiated at an OI greater than 40.[79] We currently consider institution of ECLS when a series of postductal arterial blood gases demonstrates an OI greater than 25, with mandatory application of ECLS when the OI is greater than 40.

Criteria for high mortality risk among older children with respiratory failure are based on the OI or alveolo-arterial oxygen (AaO_2) gradient. Rivera et al.[75] suggest that a ventilation index (respiratory rate × $PaCO_2$ × peak inspiratory pressure/1000) greater than 40 and an OI greater than 40 are associated with a mortality of 77%, and a combination of peak inspiratory pressure of 40 cm H_2O or greater and an $AaDO_2$ greater than 580 mm Hg are associated with a mortality of 81%. We consider $AaDO_2$ greater than 600 on FiO_2 1.0—despite and after optimal treatment—an indication of high mortality risk in children.

Criteria for the initiation of ECLS in pediatric patients with cardiac failure are clinical signs of decreased peripheral perfusion, including oliguria (urine output <0.5 mL/kg per hour), metabolic acidosis, and hypotension, despite the administration of inotropic agents and volume resuscitation.[22,60] ECLS is applied in pediatric cardiac patients in the setting of cardiogenic shock (20%), cardiac arrest (20%), and acute deterioration (10%); an additional 20% of patients are placed on ECLS directly in the operating room due to inability to wean from heart-lung bypass.

Current relative contraindications are as follows:

1. Prematurity. The lower limit for newborns is 1 kg and 30 weeks' gestational age because of a higher incidence of intracranial bleeding in smaller, younger infants.[18,44]
2. Pre-ECMO intracranial hemorrhage higher than grade 2.[73]
3. Prolonged mechanical ventilation. Mechanical ventilation for longer than 7 days in newborn and pediatric patients has been considered a contraindication to ECLS because of the high incidence of bronchopulmonary dysplasia and irreversible fibroproliferative lung disease. However, reviews of the ELSO Registry data suggest that the survival rate remains at approximately 50% to 60% after 14 days of pre-ECLS mechanical ventilation in neonatal and pediatric patients with respiratory failure.[72] We currently consider ECLS in any patient who has been mechanically ventilated for up to 14 days, keeping in mind that morbidity and mortality increase with time on the ventilator.
4. Cardiac arrest. Cardiac arrest that requires cardiopulmonary resuscitation in the pre-ECLS period has been considered a contraindication to the institution of extracorporeal support. However, survival rates of up to 60% have been observed among neonates who suffer cardiac arrest before or during cannulation.[25,99] Of those who survive, at least 60% have a reasonable neurologic outcome. Similar survival rates (64%), without long-term sequelae, were noted among pediatric cardiac failure patients who endured cardiac arrest for 65 ± 9 minutes before the institution of ECLS.[23] Based on these data, many centers now consider patients who sustain pre-ECLS cardiac arrest to be candidates for extracorporeal support.
5. Congenital diaphragmatic hernia (CDH) with bilateral hypoplasia. Although CDH was originally a contraindication,[40] it was subsequently demonstrated that a number of patients who met this exclusion criteria survived. Thus, most centers now consider any patient with CDH a candidate for ECLS.[66,87] Stolar et al.[90] suggest that failure to generate a best preductal PaO_2 greater than 100 mm Hg and $PaCO_2$ less than 50 mm Hg accurately identifies nonsalvageable newborns with CDH who should be excluded from ECLS.
6. Profound neurologic impairment, multiple congenital anomalies, or other conditions not compatible with meaningful life.

Additional relative contraindications for older children are multiorgan system failure, major burns, immunodeficiency, active bleeding, and the presence of an incurable disease process.

METHODS OF EXTRACORPOREAL SUPPORT

The goal of ECLS is to perfuse warmed, arterialized blood into the patient.[7] To achieve this goal, the extracorporeal blood flow is used in venoarterial (VA) mode for cardiac support and venovenous (VV) mode for respiratory support. VA mode provides complete support, but there are significant disadvantages: (1) a major artery must be cannulated and at least temporarily sacrificed, (2) the risk of dissemination of particulate or gaseous emboli into the systemic circulation is substantial, (3) pulmonary perfusion may be markedly reduced, (4) left ventricular output may be compromised owing to the presence of increased ECLS circuit-induced afterload resistance, and (5) the coronary arteries are perfused predominantly by the relatively hypoxic left ventricular blood.[80] VV access, either by two vessels or by a single vessel via a double-lumen catheter, supports gas exchange without the disadvantages of VA support. VV or double-lumen VV ECLS is now the preferred method for patients of all age groups who do not require cardiac support (Fig. 8-1).[20] Data from the ELSO

Registry and a nonrandomized multicenter study suggest that bypass performed with the double-lumen VV configuration may increase the survival rate and reduce the incidence of intracranial hemorrhage in neonates.[3] However, a matched-pairs analysis that corrected for pre-ECLS severity of cardiopulmonary dysfunction revealed no difference in either parameter between patients undergoing bypass with a double-lumen VV or VA configuration.[32] There are no double-lumen catheters available for children weighing more than 10 kg. Femoral and jugular cannulation is used for older children.

THE EXTRACORPOREAL LIFE SUPPORT CIRCUIT

The ECLS circuit comprises a pump, a membrane lung, and a heat exchanger (Fig. 8-2), as well as other devices associated with safety and monitoring functions. A full description of the technology, including device function and malfunction, is published in the ELSO's textbook.[27] Right atrial blood is drained by gravity siphon via a cannula placed through the right internal jugular or right femoral vein. Roller pumps are the most common perfusion devices used and require continuous servoregulation and monitoring to prevent the application of high levels of negative pressure to the drainage circuit and high levels of positive pressure, with a risk of circuit disruption, to the infusion limb of the circuit should occlusion occur. Application of high negative pressures to the drainage circuit (with a centrifugal pump, for example) results in hemolysis, damage to the endothelium of the

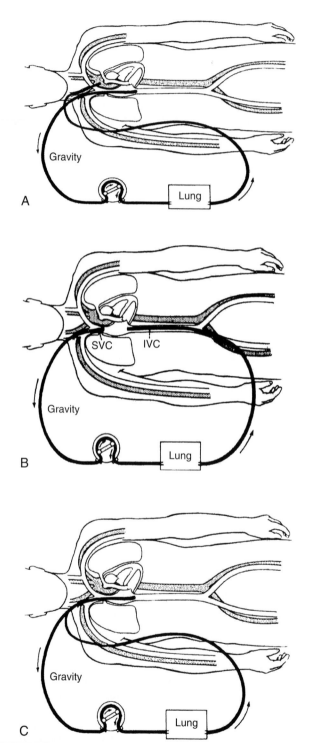

Figure 8-1 Three most common extracorporeal bypass configurations. *A,* Venoarterial with drainage from the internal jugular vein and reinfusion into the carotid artery. *B,* Venovenous via drainage from the internal jugular vein and reinfusion into the femoral vein. *C,* Venovenous via a double-lumen cannula placed into the internal jugular vein. IVC, inferior vena cava; SVC, superior vena cava.

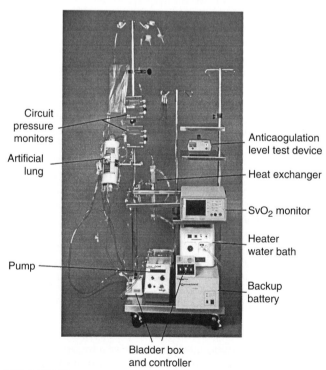

Figure 8-2 Extracorporeal life support circuit. The essential components include the roller pump, the membrane lung, and the heat exchanger. The remainder of the devices shown perform monitoring and safety functions.

TABLE 8-1 Circuit Components and Prime for Patients of Different Sizes Receiving Venovenous Support

	Weight (kg)					
	2-4	**4-15***	**15-20**	**20-30**	**30-50**	**50+**
Drainage tubing (inches)	$\frac{1}{4}$	NA	$\frac{3}{8}$	$\frac{3}{8}$	$\frac{1}{2}$	$\frac{1}{2}$
Raceway (inches)	$\frac{1}{4}$	NA	$\frac{3}{8}$-$\frac{1}{2}$	$\frac{1}{2}$	$\frac{1}{2}$	$\frac{1}{2}$
Oxygenator (m²)	0.8-1.5	NA	2.5-3.5	3.5-4.5	4.5	4.5 × 2
Cannulas† (French)	12-15	NA	Inf: 16-19	Inf: 17-21	Inf: 21	Inf: 21
	DLVV‡	NA	Dr: 14-19	Dr: 17-21	Dr: 19-23§	Dr: 21-23§
Prime	RBC: 1-2 U	NA	RBC: 3 U	RBC: 4 U	RBC: 4 U¶	RBC: 5 U¶
	FFP: 50-100 mL	NA	FFP: $\frac{1}{2}$ U	FFP: 1 U	FFP:1 U	FFP: 1 U

*Venovenous ECLS is not currently recommended in patients weighing 4 to 15 kg (younger than 3 years).
†All cannulas are the shortest Biomedicus cannula available in the specified size. These are only guidelines, and individual patient variables must be considered.
‡12 and 15 French DLVV cannulas are manufactured by Jostra. The 14 French DLVV cannula is manufactured by Kendall.
§The M-number (2.4) of the 23 French Biomedicus (38 cm) custom cannula is nearly the same as that of the 29 French Biomedicus (50 cm) cannula.
¶Normosol (3 L) with 12.5 g albumin and 1 g CaCl is usually used.
DLVV, double-lumen venovenous; Dr, drainage; ECLS, extracorporeal life support; FFP, fresh frozen plasma; Inf, infusion; NA, not applicable; RBC, red blood cells; U, units.

right atrium or vena cava, and cavitation as air is drawn out of solution.

The artificial lung most commonly used is the Kolobow spiral coil, solid silicone rubber membrane lung.[52] The size of the various ECLS components required as a function of patient weight is demonstrated in Table 8-1. Hollow-fiber artificial lungs made of microporous materials are highly efficient with regard to gas exchange, have low resistance to blood flow, and are easy to prime. The disadvantage of the microporous membrane is the increased rate of condensation of water in the gas phase and the frequent need for replacement owing to the development of plasma leak.[62] Phospholipid adsorption onto the blood surface of the hollow fiber at the site of 5-μm pores is the mechanism by which the plasma leak occurs.[62] Artificial lungs with hollow fibers that do not have pores resolve this problem and are preferred for ECLS. These devices have been used in Europe and Japan but are not available in the United States.

The volume of the neonatal circuit is approximately 400 to 500 mL, which is one to two times the newborn blood volume. The circuit must therefore be primed carefully to perfuse the neonate at the onset of bypass with blood containing the appropriate pH, hematocrit, calcium, clotting factors, and electrolytes and at the appropriate temperature. However, as shown in Table 8-1, ECLS may be instituted in patients weighing more than 35 kg without the addition of blood to the prime.

PATIENT MANAGEMENT

Patient management is described in detail in the ELSO's textbook.[27] The size of the venous cannula is the factor that determines the blood flow rate and, therefore, the level of extracorporeal support. The largest possible venous access cannula should be placed; it should be of sufficient size to provide adequate blood flow (100 mL/kg per minute) with the assistance of a 100 cm H_2O gravity siphon pressure. The flow-pressure characteristics of a given cannula are determined by a number of geometric factors, including length, internal diameter, and side-hole placement. The M-number provides a standardized means for describing the flow-pressure relationships in a variety of vascular access devices.[63,83]

The first choice for venous access is the internal jugular vein because it is large and provides easy access to the right atrium via a short cannula. The femoral vein is the second choice for venous drainage access during ECLS and the first choice for drainage during VV support. In children younger than 5 years, the femoral vein is too small to function as the primary drainage site, and VV access is used in a jugular to femoral fashion in young children. A proximal venous drainage cannula can be placed in the proximal internal jugular vein to enhance venous drainage to the extracorporeal circuit.[85] One study demonstrated a reduction in intracranial hemorrhage following initiation of the use of such a cannula when compared with historical controls.[67] An ELSO Registry study, however, failed to demonstrate an effect on intracranial hemorrhage or survival during routine use of a proximal venous drainage cannula.[29]

The size of the reinfusion cannula is less critical than that of the venous cannula, although it must be large enough to tolerate the predicted blood flow rate at levels of total support without generating a pressure greater than 350 mm Hg proximal to the membrane lung. The first choice for placement of a cannula into the arterial circulation is the carotid artery in all age groups because it provides easy access to the aortic arch. Few complications have been associated with carotid artery cannulation and ligation in newborns and children.[58,77] The second choice for arterial access is the femoral artery. Distal perfusion of the lower extremity arterial circulation is required when the femoral artery is cannulated.

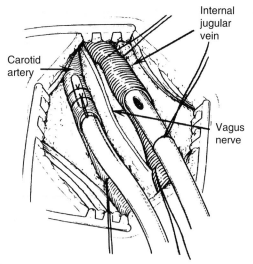

Figure 8-3 Cannulation for venoarterial extracorporeal support. The transverse right supraclavicular incision is shown. In neonates, the cannulas are placed 2.5 cm into the artery and 6.0 cm into the vein. They are secured using two circumferential 2-0 silk ligatures with a small piece of plastic vessel loop placed underneath to protect the vessels from injury during decannulation. One of the ends of the marking ligature is tied to the most distal circumferential suture for extra security.

The cannulation procedure is usually performed by direct cutdown using local anesthesia (Fig. 8-3). The tips of the arterial and venous cannulas (see Table 8-1 for sizes) are optimally located at the opening of the right brachiocephalic artery and the inferior aspect of the right atrium, respectively. The double-lumen VV cannula must be placed such that the tip is in the mid–right atrium, with the reinfusion ports oriented toward the tricuspid valve to minimize recirculation of reinfused blood. Percutaneous access to the internal jugular and femoral veins is the preferred approach to cannulation in adults and children older than 3 years. Sequentially larger dilators are placed over a wire, and a Seldinger technique allows final access of the cannula itself into these large veins. A 12 or 15 French double-lumen VV cannula is amenable to percutaneous introduction into the internal jugular vein in neonates.

The cannulas are connected to the ECLS circuit, and cardiopulmonary bypass is initiated. Flow is increased over the ensuing 10 to 15 minutes to levels of 100 mL/kg. Once a patient is on extracorporeal support, there is typically rapid cardiopulmonary stabilization. All paralyzing agents, vasoactive drugs, and other infusions are discontinued during VA support; some pressor or inotropic support may be necessary when VV bypass is used.[20] Ventilator settings are adjusted to minimal levels (peak inspiratory pressure <25 and FiO_2 <0.4) to allow the lung to rest and any air leaks secondary to barotrauma to seal.[7] Application of positive end-expiratory pressure in the range of 12 to 14 cm H_2O during the course on extracorporeal support has been demonstrated to decrease the duration of ECLS from 132 ± 55 hours to 97 ± 36 hours.[48] Because only partial bypass is used, oxygenation and carbon dioxide elimination are

determined by a combination of native lung function and extracorporeal flow. The mixed venous oxygen saturation (SvO_2) is conveniently monitored by a fiber-optic Oximetrix catheter placed in the venous limb of the circuit, which allows one to determine the adequacy of oxygen delivery in relation to oxygen consumption. Pump flow is adjusted to maintain oxygen delivery such that the SvO_2 is above 70% during VA support and above 85% during VV support. The $PaCO_2$ is inversely proportional to the flow rate of gas ventilating the membrane lung.

CANNULATION FOR CARDIAC SUPPORT

Deterioration in myocardial function is observed in approximately 7% of neonates after initiation of ECLS.[26,43,57] This "myocardial stun" usually occurs in those patients with exaggerated levels of hypoxia, with more frequent episodes of cardiac arrest, and who required more frequent epinephrine pressor support before ECLS. It typically resolves over the first 24 to 48 hours after initiation of ECLS.

If the left ventricle does not eject (no arterial pulse contour), the left ventricle and atrium will distend and cause pulmonary edema. If this occurs, balloon or blade atrial septostomy may be required to decompress the left heart and allow the resolution of pulmonary edema and eventual improvement in cardiac function.[51]

Heparin is titrated to prevent thrombus formation throughout the course of ECLS. The level of anticoagulation is monitored hourly by the whole-blood activated clotting time (ACT).[7,42] The ACT is maintained 50% to 60% above normal (180 seconds for the Hemochron device). Transfusion of red blood cells to maintain the hematocrit greater than 45% and fresh frozen plasma to maintain the fibrinogen levels greater than 200 mg/dL are frequently required. Platelets are transfused to maintain the platelet count greater than 100,000/mm^3, although the decrease in platelet function and count associated with extracorporeal support appears to be only transiently corrected by platelet administration.[76] Stallion et al.[86] suggested that maintaining the platelet count greater than 200,000/mm^3 appears to be associated with a decrease in bleeding complications. We continue to maintain the platelet count greater than 100,000/mm^3, except in a patient who is at high risk for or has ongoing hemorrhage, in which case the platelet count is maintained greater than 150,000/mm^3.

Diuresis or hemofiltration is titrated to normal "dry" weight. Renal function may be transiently impaired during ECLS; therefore, use of a hemofilter placed in the circuit to supplement urine output may be necessary in some patients.[41] Renal insufficiency that develops before or during ECLS can also be easily managed via a hemofilter placed in the extracorporeal circuit as necessary.[81] Nutrition remains a high priority in a critically ill patient requiring ECLS.

Most operative procedures performed during ECLS are carried out in the intensive care unit.[6] Either isoflurane gas anesthesia administered via the oxygenator of the ECLS circuit or intravenous anesthesia with fentanyl or sufentanil and vecuronium may be employed. Nagaraj et al.[65] described 44 procedures performed in 37 neonates on ECLS. These procedures consisted of recannulation or repositioning of cannulas (14), tube thoracostomy (11), cardiac surgery (6), cardiac catheterization (4), repair of CDH (5), and thoracotomy (4). Hemorrhagic complications, which occurred in 46% to 55% of patients, were associated with a higher mortality. Therefore, one should strongly consider whether the procedure is necessary, such as placement of thoracostomy tubes for small pneumothoraces, or whether the operation can be delayed until ECLS is discontinued. During procedures performed while the patient is on ECLS, electrocautery should be used generously, the ACT reduced to a maximum of 160 to 180 seconds, and the platelet count maintained at greater than 150,000/mm³. One should also consider perioperative administration of aminocaproic acid.[106]

Repair of CDH can be done before, during, or after ECLS. Practice changed when we realized that lung dysfunction is caused by hypoplasia and vasospasm, not the hernia. Connors et al.[19] first described the repair of CDH in six newborns at a mean of 25 hours following initiation of ECLS, with four survivors. Lally et al.[54] reported a 43% survival rate among 42 newborns undergoing diaphragmatic hernia repair while on extracorporeal support. Vazquez and Cheu[98] reported that up to 48% of patients with CDH who require ECLS undergo repair while on extracorporeal support. Other studies suggest that operative repair in a newborn with CDH can be performed following discontinuation of ECLS and after continued resolution of pulmonary hypertension and ventilator weaning. Based on data from the ELSO Registry, Vazquez and Cheu[98] demonstrated that surgical hemorrhage requiring transfusion occurred in 38% of those repaired while on ECLS, versus 18% and 6% of those repaired before and after, respectively. Wilson et al.[106] observed a reduction in blood loss and transfusion requirement in a group of 22 patients in whom repair was performed on ECLS electively before decannulation. In these patients, the ACT was maintained at the 180- to 200-second level, and aminocaproic acid was administered continuously for 72 hours postoperatively or until decannulation in all patients. Re-exploration for hemorrhage was not required. Our current practice is to repair the hernia after weaning from ECLS.

When lung function improves, ECLS flow is decreased, leading to a "trial off" (without ECLS). During VV bypass, the gas phase of the membrane lung can simply be capped indefinitely, so that the patient remains on extracorporeal blood flow but without the artificial lung's contribution to gas exchange. Patients on VA bypass are tested by clamping the lines (no flow). Such trials are performed on a daily basis with optimal pressor support and are frequently accompanied by echocardiographic evaluation.

Once it has been determined that ECLS can be discontinued, the cannulation site incisions are opened and the right carotid artery, internal jugular vein, or both are ligated. The carotid artery can be repaired following a course of VA extracorporeal support, although there is no proven benefit and there is the potential risk of distal embolism, late stenosis, and development of atherosclerosis.[13,85] Percutaneously placed cannulas can simply be removed and pressure applied, without concern about the patient's anticoagulation status.

The duration of ECLS (mean ± standard deviation) is 149 ± 162 hours for neonates with respiratory failure, 280 ± 204 hours for children with respiratory failure, and 140 ± 113 hours for patients with congenital heart disease. Reasons to discontinue extracorporeal support other than when indicated by improvement of cardiopulmonary function include the presence of irreversible brain damage, other lethal organ failure, and uncontrollable bleeding. Those neonates with CDH or pneumonia and pediatric patients with cardiac or pulmonary failure may require substantially longer periods on ECLS before resolution of the cardiopulmonary process is observed.

COMPLICATIONS

In general, the complications associated with ECLS fall into one of three major categories: (1) bleeding associated with heparinization, (2) technical failure, and (3) neurologic sequelae, a majority of which are secondary to the hypoxia and hemodynamic instability that occur before the onset of extracorporeal support.

The average number of patient complications per ECLS case is 2.1.[108] Because of systemic heparinization, bleeding complications are the most common and devastating.[96] Intracranial hemorrhage occurs in approximately 13% of neonates, 5% of pediatric patients, and 4% of cardiac patients. It is the most frequent cause of death in newborns managed with ECLS.[46] Because of the associated heparinization, intracranial hemorrhage may be unusual in terms of both extent and location.[15,16] The mechanism by which it occurs in newborns on ECLS is multifactorial. In addition to heparin administration, platelet function and number are decreased for up to 48 hours after discontinuation of ECLS, as are coagulation factor levels.[2] Wilson et al.[105] noted a reduction in the incidence of intracranial hemorrhage, compared with historical controls, among a cohort of 42 newborns considered to be at high risk for bleeding complications who received 100 mg/kg of aminocaproic acid (Amicar) just before or after cannulation, followed by a continuous infusion of 30 mg/kg per hour until decannulation. The incidence of intracranial hemorrhage is clearly increased in patients who are premature, especially those less than 37 weeks' gestational age. Although carotid ligation and institution of ECLS in normal animals do not affect carotid artery or cerebral blood flow, initiation of ECLS in the setting of hypoxia results in augmentation of carotid artery and cerebral blood flow and loss of cerebral autoregulation.[82] In addition, decreases in $PaCO_2$ result in marked decreases in cerebral blood flow.[100] Therefore, carotid artery and internal jugular vein ligation, along with rapid institution of ECLS, in the setting of hypoxia or hypercarbia may result in alterations in cerebral blood flow and cerebral autoregulation, with the potential induction of intracranial hemorrhage in an anticoagulated patient.

Bleeding at extracranial sites is observed in 21% of neonatal cases, 44% of pediatric respiratory cases, and 40% of neonatal and pediatric cardiac cases. These sites include gastrointestinal hemorrhage (2% to 5%); cannulation site bleeding (up to 6%); bleeding at another surgical site (neonatal respiratory cases, 6%; pediatric respiratory cases, 24%; neonatal and pediatric cardiac cases, 28%); and a miscellaneous group of bleeding sites, including pericardial, intrathoracic, and retroperitoneal (7% to 15%). Bleeding during ECLS is managed by maintaining the platelet count greater than 150,000/mm[3] and decreasing the ACT to a maximum of 160 to 180 seconds. Occasionally, discontinuation of heparin or, if tolerated, temporary discontinuation of bypass with normalization of the coagulation status may be necessary to achieve resolution of the bleeding.[104] If hemorrhage persists, aggressive surgical intervention is indicated. We have found that intra-abdominal or intrathoracic packing with planned daily re-exploration allows control of hemorrhage in most situations. Only in extreme circumstances should permanent discontinuation of bypass be considered in a patient with persistent cardiopulmonary failure.

Neurologic injury induced either before or after the onset of ECLS is a constant concern. Many neonates must endure the insult of hypoxia or ischemia before the institution of bypass. Streletz et al.[92] noted no increase in the electroencephalographic abnormalities present before and during ECLS among 145 neonates. In addition, Walsh-Sukys et al.,[102] in a prospective evaluation of 26 neonates managed with conventional mechanical ventilation and 43 neonates managed with ECLS, noted a similar 25% rate of neurodevelopmental impairment in both groups at 8 to 20 months of age. The incidence of any neurodevelopmental impairment at age 1 year was 28% among survivors of both groups in the United Kingdom neonatal randomized study.[30] It has been suggested that ligation of the carotid artery in the minutes before the onset of ECLS, at a time when hypoxemia and hemodynamic instability are maximized, results in a further decrease in cerebral tissue oxygenation, which in turn might exacerbate the neurologic injury.[55]

Seizures have been noted in 10% to 13% of patients undergoing ECLS.[17] The presence of seizures in newborns during ECLS portends a poor prognosis: 50% to 65% with electrographic seizures during ECLS either died or were developmentally handicapped at 1 to 2 years of age.

Hemolysis (serum hemoglobin >100 mg/dL) occurs in 6% to 12% of patients. This complication is likely due to red blood cell trauma during extracorporeal support, which is often related to clot formation within the circuit, overocclusion of the roller pump, or use of a centrifugal pump. Hyperbilirubinemia is noted in 8% of patients, and renal insufficiency in 10%. Pneumothorax (occurring in 4% to 14%) and pericardial tamponade are life-threatening intrathoracic complications that manifest with increasing PaO_2 and decreasing peripheral perfusion and SvO_2, followed by decreasing ECLS flow and progressive deterioration. Initial emergent placement of a pleural or pericardial drainage catheter, followed by thoracotomy for definitive treatment of a pericardial tamponade, may be lifesaving.

Technical complications occurred in 27% of the cases reported to the ELSO Registry.[91] The average number of mechanical complications per ECLS case was 0.75. The most notable technical complications included the presence of thrombus in the circuit (26%), incorrect cannula positioning (6% to 15%), oxygenator failure (5% to 17%), pump malfunction (1% to 4%), and presence of air in the circuit (6%). The effect of technical complications on survival was not substantial, although there was a significant decrease among neonatal patients—from 84% in those without technical complications to 80% in those with them.

RESULTS AND FOLLOW-UP

A total of 27,520 cases have been reported to the ELSO Registry since 1975.[28,91,95] Of these, there have been 19,296 cases of neonatal respiratory failure, 2762 cases of pediatric respiratory failure, and 5157 of pediatric cardiac failure. The number and diagnosis of neonatal respiratory failure survivors are given in Table 8-2. Overall survival is 77%, with the best survival noted among neonatal patients with the diagnoses of meconium aspiration syndrome (94% survival), respiratory distress syndrome (84%), and persistent pulmonary hypertension of the newborn (78%). CDH patients continue to have the poorest survival among those who receive ECLS, likely because of the "irreversible" pulmonary hypoplasia associated with that condition. In fact, the survival in patients with CDH requiring ECLS has fallen from a high of 71% in 1987 to the current rate of 53%. The total number of neonatal respiratory ECLS cases peaked in 1992, with 1488 cases. There was a trend downward in the total number of neonatal cases in 1993 (1306) and

TABLE 8–2 Extracorporeal Life Support Organization Registry: Summary Data on Neonatal Respiratory Failure Cases Managed with Extracorporeal Life Support (as of July 2004)

Primary Diagnosis	Total Number of Patients	Number Survived	Percent Survived
Congenital diaphragmatic hernia	4491	2367	53
Meconium aspiration syndrome	6560	6160	94
Persistent pulmonary hypertension of the newborn/persistent fetal circulation	2914	2287	78
Respiratory distress syndrome/hyaline membrane disease	1380	1161	84
Pneumonia/sepsis	2650	1857	70
Air-leak syndrome	96	69	72
Other	1205	777	64
Total	19,296	14,678	76

TABLE 8-3 Pediatric Respiratory Failure Cases Managed with Extracorporeal Life Support at the University of Michigan between Novemer 1982 and July 2004

Primary Diagnosis	Total Number of Patients	Number Survived	Percent Survived
Viral pneumonia	53	44	83
Bacterial pneumonia or sepsis	17	10	59
Aspiration	13	10	77
Trauma	7	7	100
Acute respiratory distress syndrome	67	42	63
Other	40	34	85
Total	197	147	75

1994 (1151) owing to improved results with neonatal respiratory management, including the use of nitric oxide and high-frequency oscillatory ventilation.[28]

The experience with pediatric patients with respiratory failure who were managed with ECLS at the University of Michigan is demonstrated in Table 8-3. Although the overall survival rate since 1982 is 75%, the survival rate in the most recent 2 years is 88%.[93] In addition, patients in the younger age groups demonstrate greater survival rates, including 100% survival in infants younger than 1 year of age. The ELSO Registry demonstrates that pediatric respiratory cases are accumulating at a rate of 150 to 200 per year, with an overall survival rate of 56% (Table 8-4).[28] One of the most frequent diagnoses is viral pneumonia, which is predominated by respiratory syncytial virus, an entity associated with 49% to 58% survival.[61,89] Other studies from individual centers also suggest that the survival rate of pediatric patients with

respiratory failure managed with ECLS is 41% to 53%.[64,103] An approximately 50% survival rate is noted in pediatric patients with multiorgan system failure and in those with overwhelming septic shock who are managed with ECLS.[14] Green et al.,[38] analyzing data from the ELSO Registry, demonstrated that the survival rate in pediatric respiratory failure patients on ECLS for longer than 2 weeks was similar to the survival rate of patients supported for shorter periods. However, judgment must be used regarding the reversible nature of the respiratory dysfunction, the presence of associated organ system failure, and the development of complications associated with ECLS in determining whether continuation is warranted after prolonged periods on ECLS.

The ELSO Registry results for cardiac support cases are summarized in Table 8-5.[28] Between 200 and 300 cardiac cases are reported to the registry each year, the vast majority of which are pediatric cardiac surgical cases. The overall survival is 41%. Almost all patients are managed with VA bypass. The survival rate is especially poor (0 to 25%) in those patients with an anomaly that consists of a single ventricle.[53] Although Ziomek et al.[107] demonstrated a 47% survival among 17 patients in whom ECLS was initiated in the operating room, other studies suggest a poor outcome when ECLS is initiated in the operating room or at a point more than 50 hours following operation or among those who are on ECLS for more than 6 to 9 days.[107] Data from numerous centers demonstrate a survival rate ranging from 46% to 53%,[47,74] with Klein et al.[50] observing a survival rate of 61% among 39 infants and children. The cause of death was lack of improvement in cardiovascular function in 37% of patients and major central nervous system damage in 15%, suggesting that earlier intervention with ECLS could improve outcome.[74] In a large series from Children's Hospital of Philadelphia, ECLS was used for 3.4% of children having cardiac operations; the overall survival was 39%.[59] Survival among patients who were bridged with ECLS to heart transplantation was 40% to 60%.[31] Application of ECLS to patients with cardiac failure following pediatric cardiac transplantation is associated with a long-term survival of 35% to 41%.

TABLE 8-4 Extracorporeal Life Support Organization Registry: Summary Data on Pediatric Respiratory Failure Cases Managed with Extracorporeal Life Support (as of July 2004)

Primary Diagnosis	Total Number of Patients	Number Survived	Percent Survived
Bacterial pneumonia	290	157	54
Viral pneumonia	728	457	63
Trauma	70	44	63
Aspiration	168	110	65
Pneumocystis	22	9	41
Acute respiratory distress syndrome	278	144	52
Other	1206	615	51
Total	2762	1536	56

TABLE 8-5 Extracorporeal Life Support Organization Registry: Summary Data on Cardiac Failure Cases (Children Aged 1 Day to 16 Years) Managed with Extracorporeal Life Support (as of July 2004)

Primary Diagnosis	Total Number of Patients	Number Survived	Percent Survived
Cardiac surgery	4064	1564	38
Cardiac arrest	98	30	31
Myocarditis	156	89	57
Myocardiopathy	333	181	54
Other	933	409	44
Total	5584	2273	41

ECLS has been effective in other clinical situations, such as blunt trauma in children and adults, with survival rates of approximately 65%.[4,88] Although thermal injury was previously considered a contraindication, ECLS has been applied in pediatric burn patients (mean of 46% of total body surface area burned), with survival in three of five patients.[37] ECLS has also been successfully applied to patients undergoing tracheal repair, those with alveolar proteinosis who require lung lavage, and those with lung hypoplasia due to in utero renal insufficiency, asthma, sickle cell disease, and lung failure following lung transplantation.[33-35,45,49,84,101] Another application of ECLS has been in the form of extracorporeal cardiopulmonary resuscitation in adult or pediatric patients with cardiogenic shock, post-traumatic hypotension, hypothermia, arrhythmias, and cardiac arrest.[24]

Multiple studies have involved the long-term follow-up of newborn and pediatric patients after a course of ECLS. Most documented normal neurologic function in 70% to 80% of patients.[1,5,36,78] Such studies demonstrate that neurologic morbidity is no different in ECLS-managed newborns than in those managed by conventional mechanical ventilation.

Patients with CDH who are managed with ECLS demonstrate a high incidence of morbidity, including gastroesophageal reflux in up to 81%, the need for tube feeding in up to 69%, the development of chronic lung disease in up to 62%, the development of extra-axial fluid collections or enlarged ventricles in 30%, and growth delay in 40% to 50%.[21,56,97] These problems tend to resolve with time. The neurodevelopmental outcome among newborns with CDH was not dissimilar to that of other ECLS-treated children. Although most cardiac and pediatric respiratory failure patients demonstrate few sequelae at follow-up, long-term studies in these groups have been less complete.

Three studies have evaluated the relative cost of treating newborn patients with ECLS compared with more conventional means. All demonstrated that the hospital charges were not significantly different: $49,500 for ECLS patients versus $53,700 for those managed with conventional mechanical ventilation.[79] Pearson and Short[70] found that the average daily charge for neonates receiving ECLS was twice that for patients receiving conventional mechanical ventilation, but the mean hospital stay was decreased by 50% in the ECLS group. Hospital charges were 43% lower in the ECLS group compared with the conventionally treated group when only the survivors were considered.

Maintaining a patient on extracorporeal support for days or weeks requires a prepared, organized, well-trained, and highly skilled team of physicians, respiratory therapists, nurses, and ECLS technicians. It is not a technique to be undertaken in a haphazard fashion on the spur of the moment without prior preparation and organization. The current recommendations by the American Academy of Pediatrics Committee on the Fetus and Newborn suggest that neonatal ECLS centers be established only at recognized level III regional centers with appropriate educational programs, ongoing research activity, and infant follow-up programs.[71]

THE FUTURE OF EXTRACORPOREAL LIFE SUPPORT

Although current devices allow safe and effective prolonged extracorporeal support, the future of ECLS depends on improvements in component technology, accompanied by circuit simplification and autoregulation. VV support may be performed via a tidal-flow single-cannula system in which a nonocclusive roller pump and alternating clamps generate cyclic drainage and reinfusion of blood through a percutaneously placed venous cannula. Once a compact, servoregulated device is developed with the ability to provide extracorporeal support without anticoagulation, ECLS will be a simple technique rather than a complex, labor-intensive intervention. At that point, the indications for extracorporeal support will broaden as the technique is applied to a wider population of patients with less severe cardiopulmonary insufficiency.

One of the major benefits of the ECLS experience may be the ability to explore the pathophysiology of cardiac and respiratory failure. Improved understanding of pulmonary and cardiac organ failure may lead to new preventive measures and improved treatment modalities that eventually eliminate the need for ECLS in patients with cardiorespiratory failure.

REFERENCES

1. Adolph V, Ekelund C, Smith C, et al: Developmental outcome of neonates treated with extracorporeal membrane oxygenation. J Pediatr Surg 1990;25:43.
2. Anderson H, Cilley RE, Zwischenberger JB, et al: Thrombocytopenia in neonates after extracorporeal membrane oxygenation. ASAIO Trans 1986;32:534.
3. Anderson H, Snedecor SM, Otsu T, et al: Multicenter comparison of conventional venoarterial access versus venovenous double-lumen catheter access in newborn infants undergoing extracorporeal membrane oxygenation. J Pediatr Surg 1983;28:530.
4. Anderson HL, Shapiro MB, Delius RE, et al: Extracorporeal life support for respiratory failure after multiple trauma. J Trauma 1994;37:266.
5. Andrews AF, Nixon CA, Cilley RE, et al: One- to three-year outcome for 14 neonatal survivors of extracorporeal membrane oxygenation. Pediatrics 1986;78:692.
6. Atkinson JB, Kitagawa H, Humphries B: Major surgical intervention during extracorporeal membrane oxygenation. J Pediatr Surg 1992;27:1197.
7. Bartlett R: Extracorporeal life support for cardiopulmonary failure. Curr Probl Surg 1990;27:621.
8. Bartlett RH, Andrews AF, Toomasian JM, et al: Extracorporeal membrane oxygenation for newborn respiratory failure: Forty-five cases. Surgery 1982;92:425.
9. Bartlett RH, Gazzaniga AB, Huxtable RF, et al: Extracorporeal circulation (ECMO) in neonatal respiratory failure. J Thorac Cardiovasc Surg 1977;74:826.
10. Bartlett RH, Gazzaniga AB, Huxtable RH, et al: Extracorporeal membrane oxygenation (ECMO) in newborn respiratory failure: Technical consideration. Trans Am Soc Artif Intern Organs 1979;25:473.
11. Bartlett RH, Gazzaniga AB, Toomasian J, et al: Extracorporeal membrane oxygenation (ECMO) in neonatal respiratory failure: 100 cases. Ann Surg 1986;204:236.

12. Bartlett RH, Roloff DW, Cornell RG, et al: Extracorporeal circulation in neonatal respiratory failure: A prospective randomized study. Pediatrics 1985;76:479.

13. Baumgart S, Streletz LJ, Needleman L, et al: Right common carotid artery reconstruction after extracorporeal membrane oxygenation: Vascular imaging, cerebral circulation, electroencephalographic, and neurodevelopmental correlates to recovery. J Pediatr 1994;125:295.

14. Beca J, Butt W: Extracorporeal membrane oxygenation for refractory septic shock in children. Pediatrics 1994;93:726.

15. Bowerman RA, Zwischenberger JB, Andrews AF, et al: Cranial sonography of the infant treated with extracorporeal membrane oxygenation. AJR Am J Roentgenol 1985; 145:161.

16. Bulas DI, Taylor GA, Fitz CR, et al: Posterior fossa intracranial hemorrhage in infants treated with extracorporeal membrane oxygenation: Sonographic findings. AJR Am J Roentgenol 1991;156:571.

17. Campbell LR, Bunyapen C, Gangarosa ME, et al: Significance of seizures associated with extracorporeal membrane oxygenation. J Pediatr 1991;119:789.

18. Cilley RE, Zwischenberger JB, Andrews AF, et al: Intracranial hemorrhage during extracorporeal membrane oxygenation in neonates. Pediatrics 1986;78:699.

19. Connors RH, Tracy T Jr, Bailey PV, et al: Congenital diaphragmatic hernia repair on ECMO. J Pediatr Surg 1990;25:1043.

20. Cornish JD, Heiss KF, Clark RH, et al: Efficacy of venovenous extracorporeal membrane oxygenation for neonates with respiratory and circulatory compromise. J Pediatr 1993; 122:105.

21. D'Agostino J, Bernbaum J, Gerdes M, et al: Outcome for infants with congenital diaphragmatic hernia requiring extracorporeal membrane oxygenation: The first year. J Pediatr Surg 1995;30:10.

22. Dalton HJ, Siewers RD, Fuhrman BP, et al: Extracorporeal membrane oxygenation for cardiac rescue in children with severe myocardial dysfunction. Crit Care Med 1993;21:1020.

23. del Nido PJ, Dalton HJ, Thompson AE, et al: Extracorporeal membrane oxygenator rescue in children during cardiac arrest after cardiac surgery. Circulation 1992;86 (Suppl II):II-300.

24. Dembitsky WP, Moreno-Cabral RJ, Adamson RM, et al: Emergency resuscitation using portable extracorporeal membrane oxygenation. Ann Thorac Surg 1993;55:304.

25. Dickey LA, Cheu HW: Neonates requiring cardiopulmonary resuscitation before extracorporeal membrane oxygenation: Prognostic factors for survival and neurologic outcome. Paper presented at the 9th Annual Children's National Medical Center ECMO Symposium, Feb 28, 1993, Keystone, Colo.

26. Dickson ME, Hirthler MA, Simoni J, et al: Stunned myocardium during extracorporeal membrane oxygenation. Am J Surg 1990;160:644.

27. ECMO Extracorporeal Cardiopulmonary Support in Critical Care. Ann Arbor, Mich, ELSO, 1995.

28. ELSO: The Registry of the Extracorporeal Life Support Organization. (updated annually). Available at elso@med.umich.edu.

29. Fazzalari FL, Hirschl RB, Delosh T, et al: The routine use of a proximal venous cannula in neonatal ECLS does not reduce the incidence of intracranial hemorrhage. Paper presented at the American Academy of Pediatrics, 1994.

30. Firmin R: United Kingdom neonatal ECMO study. Paper presented at the 7th International ELSO Conference, Sep 30, 1995, Dearborn, Mich.

31. Galantowicz ME, Stolar CJ: Extracorporeal membrane oxygenation for perioperative support in pediatric heart transplantation. J Thorac Cardiovasc Surg 1991;102:148.

32. Gauger PG, Hirschl RB, Delosh TN, et al: A matched pairs analysis of venoarterial and venovenous extracorporeal life support in neonatal respiratory failure. ASAIO J 1995; 41:M573.

33. Geiduschek JM, Inglis A Jr, O'Rourke PP, et al: Repair of a laryngotracheoesophageal cleft in an infant by means of extracorporeal membrane oxygenation. Ann Otol Rhinol Laryngol 1993;102:827.

34. Gibbons MD, Horan JJ, Dejter S Jr, et al: Extracorporeal membrane oxygenation: An adjunct in the management of the neonate with severe respiratory distress and congenital urinary tract anomalies. J Urol 1993;150:434.

35. Gillett DS, Gunning KE, Sawicka EH, et al: Life threatening sickle chest syndrome treated with extracorporeal membrane oxygenation. BMJ 1987;294:81.

36. Glass P, Miller M, Short B: Morbidity for survivors of extracorporeal membrane oxygenation: Neurodevelopmental outcome at 1 year of age. Pediatrics 1989;83:72.

37. Goretsky MJ, Greenhalgh DG, Warden GD, et al: The use of extracorporeal life support in pediatric burn patients with respiratory failure. J Pediatr Surg 1995;30:620.

38. Green TP, Moler FW, Goodman DM: Probability of survival after prolonged extracorporeal membrane oxygenation in pediatric patients with acute respiratory failure: Extracorporeal Life Support Organization. Crit Care Med 1995;23:1132.

39. Green TP, Timmons OD, Fackler JC, et al: The impact of extracorporeal membrane oxygenation on survival in pediatric patients with acute respiratory failure. Paper presented at the Society of Critical Care Medicine, 1994.

40. Heiss K, Manning P, Oldham KT, et al: Reversal of mortality for congenital diaphragmatic hernia with ECMO. Ann Surg 1989;209:225.

41. Heiss KF, Pettit B, Hirschl RB, et al: Renal insufficiency and volume overload in neonatal ECMO managed by continuous ultrafiltration. ASAIO Trans 1987;33:557.

42. Hirschl RB, Bartlett RH: Extracorporeal membrane oxygenation support in cardiorespiratory failure. Adv Surg 1987;21:189.

43. Hirschl RB, Heiss KF, Bartlett RH: Severe myocardial dysfunction during extracorporeal membrane oxygenation. J Pediatr Surg 1992;27:48.

44. Hirschl RB, Schumacher RE, Snedecor SN, et al: The efficacy of extracorporeal life support in premature and low birth weight newborns. J Pediatr Surg 1993;28:1336.

45. Hurrion EM, Pearson GA, Firmin RK: Childhood pulmonary alveolar proteinosis: Extracorporeal membrane oxygenation with total cardiopulmonary support during bronchopulmonary lavage. Chest 1994;106:638.

46. Jarjour IT, Ahdab-Barmada M: Cerebrovascular lesions in infants and children dying after extracorporeal membrane oxygenation. Pediatr Neurol 1994;10:13.

47. Kanter KR, Pennington G, Weber TR, et al: Extracorporeal membrane oxygenation for postoperative cardiac support in children. J Thorac Cardiovasc Surg 1987;93:27.

48. Keszler M, Ryckman FC, McDonald J Jr, et al: A prospective, multicenter, randomized study of high versus low positive end-expiratory pressure during extracorporeal membrane oxygenation. J Pediatr 1992;120:107.

49. King D, Smales C, Arnold AG, et al: Extracorporeal membrane oxygenation as emergency treatment for life-threatening acute severe asthma. Postgrad Med J 1986; 62:855.

50. Klein MD, Shaheen KW, Whittlesey GC, et al: Extracorporeal membrane oxygenation for the circulatory support of children after repair of congenital heart disease. J Thorac Cardiovasc Surg 1990;100:498.

51. Koenig PR, Ralston MA, Kimball TR, et al: Balloon atrial septostomy for left ventricular decompression in patients receiving extracorporeal membrane oxygenation for myocardial failure. J Pediatr 1993;122 (Suppl):S95.

52. Kolobow T, Boman RL: Construction and evaluation of an alveolar membrane artificial heart lung. ASAIO Trans 1963;9:238.

53. Kulick TJ, Moler FW, Palmisano JM, et al: Outcome-associated factors in pediatric patients treated with ECMO following cardiac surgery. Circulation (in press).

54. Lally KP, Paranka MS, Roden J, et al: Congenital diaphragmatic hernia: Stabilization and repair on ECMO. Ann Surg 1992;216:569.

55. Liem KD, Hopman JC, Oeseburg B, et al: Cerebral oxygenation and hemodynamics during induction of extracorporeal membrane oxygenation as investigated by near infrared spectrophotometry. Pediatrics 1995;95:555.

56. Lund DP, Mitchell J, Kharasch V, et al: Congenital diaphragmatic hernia: The hidden morbidity. J Pediatr Surg 1994;29:258.

57. Martin GR, Short BL, Abbott C, et al: Cardiac stun in infants undergoing extracorporeal membrane oxygenation. J Thorac Cardiovasc Surg 1991;101:607.

58. Matsumoto JS, Babcock DS, Brody AS, et al: Right common carotid artery ligation for extracorporeal membrane oxygenation: Cerebral blood flow velocity measurement with Doppler duplex US. Radiology 1990;175:757.

59. Meliones JN, Custer JR, Snedecor S, et al: Extracorporeal life support for cardiac assist in pediatric patients: Review of ELSO Registry data. Circulation 1991;84:168.

60. Moler FW, Custer JR, Bartlett RH, et al: Extracorporeal life support for severe pediatric respiratory failure: An updated experience, 1991-1993. J Pediatr 1994;124:875.

61. Moler FW, Palmisano JM, Green TP, et al: Predictors of outcome of severe respiratory syncytial virus-associated respiratory failure treated with extracorporeal membrane oxygenation. J Pediatr 1993;123:46.

62. Montoya J, Shanley C, Merz S, et al: Plasma leakage through microporous membranes: Role of phospholipids. ASAIO J 1992;38:M399.

63. Montoya JP, Merz SI, Bartlett RH: A standardized system for describing flow/pressure relationships in vascular access devices. ASAIO Trans 1991;37:4.

64. Morton A, Dalton H, Kochanek P, et al: Extracorporeal membrane oxygenation for pediatric respiratory failure: Five-year experience at the University of Pittsburgh. Crit Care Med 1994;22:1659.

65. Nagaraj HS, Mitchell KA, Fallat ME, et al: Surgical complications and procedures in neonates on extracorporeal membrane oxygenation. J Pediatr Surg 1992;27:1106.

66. Newman KD, Anderson KD, Van Meurs K, et al: Extracorporeal membrane oxygenation and congenital diaphragmatic hernia: Should any infant be excluded? J Pediatr Surg 1990;25:1048.

67. O'Connor TA, Haney BM, Grist GE, et al: Decreased incidence of intracranial hemorrhage using cephalic jugular venous drainage during neonatal extracorporeal membrane oxygenation. J Pediatr Surg 1993;28:1332.

68. O'Rourke PP, Crone RK, Vacanti JP, et al: Extracorporeal membrane oxygenation and conventional medical therapy in neonates with persistent pulmonary hypertension of the newborn: A prospective randomized study. Pediatrics 1989;84:957.

69. Ortega M, Ramos AD, Platzker AC, et al: Early prediction of ultimate outcome in newborn infants with severe respiratory failure. J Pediatr 1988;113:744.

70. Pearson GD, Short BL: An economic analysis of extracorporeal membrane oxygenation. J Intensive Care Med 1987;2:116.

71. Poland RL, Cassady G, Erenbery A, et al: Recommendations on extracorporeal membrane oxygenation. Pediatrics 1990;85:618.

72. Pranikoff T, Hirschl RH, Custer JR, et al: Survival is inversely proportional to the duration of mechanical ventilation prior to pediatric extracorporeal life support. Paper presented at the American Academy of Pediatrics Section on Surgery, Oct 22, 1994, Dallas, Tex.

73. Radack DM, Baumgart S, Gross GW: Subependymal (grade 1) intracranial hemorrhage in neonates on extracorporeal membrane oxygenation: Frequency and patterns of evolution. Clin Pediatr 1994;33:583.

74. Raithel SC, Pennington DG, Boegner E, et al: Extracorporeal membrane oxygenation in children after cardiac surgery. Circulation 1992;86:305.

75. Rivera RA, Butt W, Shann F: Predictors of mortality in children with respiratory failure: Possible indications for ECMO. Anesth Intensive Care 1990;18:385.

76. Robinson TM, Kickler TS, Walker LK, et al: Effect of extracorporeal membrane oxygenation on platelets in newborns. Crit Care Med 1993;21:1029.

77. Schumacher RE, Barks JD, Johnston MV, et al: Right-sided brain lesions in infants following extracorporeal membrane oxygenation. Pediatrics 1988;82:155.

78. Schumacher RE, Palmer TW, Roloff DW, et al: Follow-up of infants treated with extracorporeal membrane oxygenation for newborn respiratory failure. Pediatrics 1991;87:451.

79. Schumacher RE, Roloff DW, Chapman R, et al: Extracorporeal membrane oxygenation in term newborns: A prospective cost-benefit analysis. ASAIO J 1993;39:873.

80. Secker-Walker JS, Edmonds JF, Spratt EH, et al: The source of coronary perfusion during partial bypass for extracorporeal membrane oxygenation (ECMO). Ann Thorac Surg 1976;21:138.

81. Sell LL, Cullen ML, Whittlesey GC, et al: Experience with renal failure during extracorporeal membrane oxygenation: Treatment with continuous hemofiltration. J Pediatr Surg 1987;22:600.

82. Short BL, Walker LK, Traystman RJ: Impaired cerebral autoregulation in the newborn lamb during recovery from severe, prolonged hypoxia, combined with carotid artery and jugular vein ligation. Crit Care Med 1994;22:1262.

83. Sinard JM, Merz SI, Hatcher MD, et al: Evaluation of extracorporeal perfusion catheters using a standardized measurement technique—the M-number. ASAIO Trans 1991;37:60.

84. Slaughter MS, Nielsen K, Bolman RD: Extracorporeal membrane oxygenation after lung or heart-lung transplantation. ASAIO J 1993;39:M453.

85. Spector ML, Wiznitzer M, Walsh-Sukys MC, et al: Carotid reconstruction in the neonate following ECMO. J Pediatr Surg 1991;26:357.

86. Stallion A, Cofer BR, Rafferty JA, et al: The significant relationship between platelet count and hemorrhagic complications on ECMO. Perfusion 1994;9:265.

87. Steimle CN, Meric F, Hirschl RB, et al: Effect of extracorporeal life support on survival when applied to all patients with congenital diaphragmatic hernia. J Pediatr Surg 1994;29:997.

88. Steiner RB, Adolph VR, Heaton JF, et al: Pediatric extracorporeal membrane oxygenation in posttraumatic respiratory failure. J Pediatr Surg 1991;26:1011.

89. Steinhorn RH, Green TP: Use of extracorporeal membrane oxygenation in the treatment of respiratory syncytial virus bronchiolitis: The national experience, 1983 to 1988. J Pediatr 1990;116:338.

90. Stolar C, Dillon P, Reyes C: Selective use of extracorporeal membrane oxygenation in the management of

congenital diaphragmatic hernia. J Pediatr Surg 1988; 23:207.

91. Stolar CJ, Snedecor SM, Bartlett RH: Extracorporeal membrane oxygenation and neonatal respiratory failure: Experience from the extracorporeal life support organization. J Pediatr Surg 1991;26:563.

92. Streletz LJ, Bej MD, Graziani LJ, et al: Utility of serial EEGs in neonates during extracorporeal membrane oxygenation. Pediatr Neurol 1992;8:190.

93. Swaniker F, Kolla S, Moler F, et al: Extracorporeal life support outcome for 128 pediatric patients with respiratory failure. J Pediatr Surg 2000;35:197.

94. Timmons OD, Dean JM, Vernon DD: Mortality rates and prognostic variables in children with ARDS. J Pediatr 1991;119:896.

95. Toomasian JM, Snedecor SM, Cornell RG, et al: National experience with extracorporeal membrane oxygenation for newborn respiratory failure: Data from 715 cases. ASAIO Trans 1988;34:140.

96. Upp J Jr, Bush PE, Zwischenberger JB: Complications of neonatal extracorporeal membrane oxygenation. Perfusion 1994;9:241.

97. Van Meurs KP, Robbins ST, Reed VL, et al: Congenital diaphragmatic hernia: Long-term outcome in neonates treated with extracorporeal membrane oxygenation. J Pediatr 1993;122:893.

98. Vazquez WD, Cheu HW: Hemorrhagic complications and repair of congenital diaphragmatic hernias: Does timing of the repair make a difference? Data from the Extracorporeal Life Support Organization. J Pediatr Surg 1994;29:1002.

99. von Allmen D, Ryckman FC: Cardiac arrest in the ECMO candidate. J Pediatr Surg 1991;26:143.

100. Walker LK, Short BL, Gleason CA, et al: Cerebrovascular response to carbon dioxide in lambs receiving extracorporeal membrane oxygenation. Crit Care Med 1994;22:291.

101. Walker LK, Wetzel RC, Haller J Jr: Extracorporeal membrane oxygenation for perioperative support during congenital tracheal stenosis repair. Anesth Analg 1992; 75:825.

102. Walsh-Sukys MC, Bauer RE, Cornell DJ, et al: Severe respiratory failure in neonates: Mortality and morbidity rates and neurodevelopmental outcomes. J Pediatr 1994; 125:104.

103. Weber TR, Tracy T Jr, Connors R, et al: Prolonged extracorporeal support for non neonatal respiratory failure. J Pediatr Surg 1992;27:1100.

104. Whittlesey GC, Drucker DE, Salley SO, et al: ECMO without heparin: Laboratory and clinical experience. J Pediatr Surg 1991;26:320.

105. Wilson JM, Bower LK, Fackler JC, et al: Aminocaproic acid decreases the incidence of intracranial hemorrhage and other hemorrhagic complications of ECMO. J Pediatr Surg 1993;28:536.

106. Wilson JM, Bower LK, Lund DP: Evolution of the technique of congenital diaphragmatic hernia repair on ECMO. J Pediatr Surg 1994;29:1109.

107. Ziomek S, Harrell J Jr, Fasules JW, et al: Extracorporeal membrane oxygenation for cardiac failure after congenital heart operation. Ann Thorac Surg 1992;54:861.

108. Zwischenberger JB, Nguyen TT, Upp J Jr, et al: Complications of neonatal extracorporeal membrane oxygenation: Collective experience from the Extracorporeal Life Support Organization. J Thorac Cardiovasc Surg 1994; 107:838.

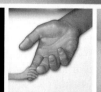

Chapter 9

Neonatal Cardiovascular Physiology and Care

Albert P. Rocchini

To appropriately meet the cardiovascular needs of patients, it is important to understand the normal cardiovascular physiology. This chapter summarizes normal fetal and neonatal cardiovascular physiology and describes principles for the medical management of common cardiovascular problems in neonates.

CARDIOVASCULAR PHYSIOLOGY

Regardless of age, the major variables that affect cardiovascular function are preload (end-diastolic volume), heart rate, arterial pressure (afterload), and contractility (inotropic state of the heart).[5,6,58] At all ages, increasing the myocardial muscle length, heart rate, and other factors that alter the inotropic state of the heart has a positive effect on cardiac function, whereas increasing afterload has a negative effect. However, in an intact animal or human, it is almost impossible to change one of these factors without also affecting another. The net physiologic response is the combined effect of the intervention. For example, in an isolated muscle preparation, increasing the rate of stimulation of the muscle always results in an increase in the force of contraction.[6] However, in animals and children, pacing the heart at a faster rate causes a decrease in stroke volume and no change or a slight decrease in cardiac output. These opposite effects result from the difficulty of controlling the interaction of venous return, end-diastolic volume, inotropic state, heart rate, and afterload.

In addition, the subject's age can affect cardiovascular function. For example, in the fetus, increases in systemic afterload have a much greater effect on fetal right ventricular function (decreasing it) than on left ventricular function, whereas in the infant, increases in systemic afterload have a much greater effect on left ventricular function (decreasing it) than on right ventricular function.[50] The following sections focus individually on heart rate, preload, afterload, and contractility in the fetus and neonate.

Heart Rate

Changes in heart rate have the same effect on ventricular output in both the immature and the adult heart.[4] Increases in heart rate induced by atrial pacing can also result in a decrease in ventricular performance. Stroke volume falls with an increase in heart rate, a consequence of decreasing end-diastolic filling time and end-diastolic volume; however, because the decrease in stroke volume is usually proportional to the increase in heart rate, the net effect is either no change or a slight fall in cardiac output. In comparison to the adult, the fetus and neonatal infant have a relatively high resting heart rate. Because of the high basal heart rate, a neonate's cardiac output can rarely be increased by increasing the heart rate. Similarly, in the neonate or fetus, decreases in heart rate to near adult levels, around 60 beats per minute, are usually associated with marked decreases in cardiac output. Unlike pacing, a spontaneous increase in heart rate is usually associated with an increase in cardiac output. A spontaneous heart rate change differs from a similar change induced by atrial pacing because the underlying stimuli that cause the spontaneous change also affect inotropy, venous return, or afterload. For example, an increase in venous return that maintains end-diastolic volume despite a rate-induced shortening of diastolic filling can result in an increase in stroke volume. Similarly, if the stimulus to increase the heart rate is associated with an increase in contractility, even though venous return may not increase, the increase in heart rate will result in an increase in cardiac output. Exceptions to the positive effect of a spontaneous increase in heart rate on cardiac output can usually be explained by an increase in arterial pressure.[58] The negative effect of afterload on ventricular function results in a fall in stroke volume and cardiac output.

Preload

At all ages, ventricular output depends on end-diastolic volume. An increase in stroke volume or cardiac output occurs when end-diastolic volume is increased (the Frank-Starling relation).[5,14] This relation depends on the number of cross-bridges that can be made at a given sarcomere length, and the sarcomere length depends on myofilament sensitivity to calcium.[60] Although this relationship exists in both the newborn and the adult, the magnitude of the relationship is frequently diminished in the newborn. It is well known that when left ventricular end-diastolic pressure is high, only small increments in end-diastolic volume and stroke volume follow from a further increase in filling pressure. As can be seen in Figure 9-1, the end-diastolic pressure at which further increases result in little change in cardiac output is called preload reserve. In the newborn, because the myocardium is immature and has greater stiffness (reduced compliance), the preload reserve occurs at a lower pressure than in the adult.[28]

Afterload

The cardiovascular function of both the immature and the adult heart is negatively affected by an increase in afterload.[32,46,58] There is a maturational difference in the effect of afterload on myocardial function. The immature ventricle cannot eject against arterial pressures that are well tolerated by the adult heart. This quantitative difference in response to afterload is due to the weaker contraction of the immature myocardium (corrected for muscle cross-sectional area) and the thinner ventricular wall of the immature heart. Afterload also has a quantitatively different effect on right and left ventricular function. In both the neonate and the adult, increases in arterial pressure have a much greater negative effect on the stroke volume of the right ventricle than that of the left. In the fetus and the neonate with a widely patent ductus arteriosus, this difference is a consequence of the relatively larger right ventricular stroke volume, end-diastolic volume, and free-wall curvature

in the presence of similar right and left ventricular free-wall thicknesses.[46] Because of Laplace's law, the systolic wall stress of the right ventricle is greater than that of the left ventricle in the face of similar arterial pressures. This increase in right ventricular systolic wall stress causes the right ventricular ejection to be more negatively affected by an increase in arterial pressure.

Contractility

An intervention that does not alter preload or afterload yet increases the force of contraction or increases cardiac output is said to have a positive inotropic effect. This positive effect usually arises from either an increase in the sensitivity of the myofilaments to calcium or an increase in the cytosolic calcium transient. The immature heart responds to positive inotropic agents with an increase in left ventricular output; however, in comparison to the adult heart, this response is reduced. In cardiac muscle, the movement of calcium through the dihydropyridine-sensitive calcium channel is essential for calcium-induced calcium release from the sarcoplasmic reticulum.[24,27,35,43,59] Calcium-induced calcium release amplifies the effect of the calcium current on cytosolic calcium concentration.[54,59] In the absence of calcium-induced calcium release, trans-sarcolemmal calcium flow results in a contraction whose peak force is only a fraction of that achieved in the presence of the amplification system. Both the dihydropyridine-sensitive calcium channels and the sarcoplasmic reticulum calcium-release channels (ryanodine receptors) are necessary for calcium-induced calcium release. Compared with the adult heart, the immature heart has a greater dependence on extracellular calcium because it has reduced calcium-induced calcium release. The reduced dependence of the adult myocardium on extracellular calcium is due to maturation of the sarcoplasmic reticulum. Both absolute and relative sarcoplasmic reticulum volumes increase with age, as does sarcoplasmic reticulum calcium release. For example, ryanodine has little effect on the force of contraction of the newborn myocardium. The immaturity of the sarcoplasmic reticulum and the greater dependence on extracellular calcium concentrations are two explanations for why calcium channel blockers, such as verapamil, are poorly tolerated in the newborn.

FETAL CIRCULATION

In addition to understanding how preload, afterload, heart rate, and contractility affect neonatal cardiovascular function, it is important to understand how birth affects the cardiovascular system. The fetal circulation differs from the adult circulation in a number of ways. The adult circulation is characterized by blood flow in series. That is, blood returns to the heart from the venous system to the right atrium and ventricle and is then injected into the lungs for oxygenation. Oxygenated blood then returns through the pulmonary veins to the left atrium and ventricle and is ejected into the arterial system. The right ventricle works against the low afterload of

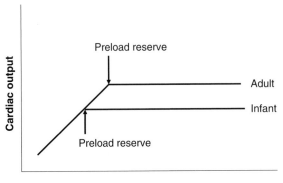

Figure 9–1 Frank-Starling relation between cardiac output and left ventricular end-diastolic pressure. The point at which further increases in end-diastolic volume result in no further increase in cardiac output is referred to as the preload reserve *(arrow)*. Because the neonatal myocardium is stiffer and less compliant, the preload reserve occurs at a lower pressure than in the mature adult heart.

the pulmonary circulation, whereas the left ventricle works against the high afterload of the systemic circulation. In the fetus, oxygenation and carbon dioxide elimination take place in the placenta. Oxygenated blood flows to the fetus through the umbilical veins, which connect to the inferior vena cava through the ductus venosus.[16,47,52] The oxygenated umbilical blood flow mixes with the poorly oxygenated portal blood from the gastrointestinal tract. Because of the eustachian valve in the right atrium, the higher-saturated umbilical venous blood preferentially streams across the foramen ovale into the left atrium,[21,36] whereas the lower-saturated blood from the distal inferior vena cava and superior vena cava enters the tricuspid valve and is directed to the right ventricle. Although these are the preferential patterns of flow, some blood from the placenta does enter the tricuspid valve, and some blood from the distal inferior vena cava and superior vena cava enters the foramen ovale. Both the right and left ventricles pump to the systemic circulation. The right ventricular output is directed through the ductus arteriosus to the descending thoracic aorta, and the left ventricular output is directed although the aortic valve to the ascending aorta. Because of the preferential streaming of umbilical venous return, the most oxygenated blood goes to the left ventricle and is distributed to the heart and cerebral circulation, whereas the less oxygenated blood goes to the right ventricle and is distributed to the pulmonary arteries, abdominal organs, and placental arteries.[52]

Because of this unique fetal circulation, many types of congenital heart disease that are not compatible with life after birth are well tolerated in utero. For example, infants with hypoplastic or atretic left or right ventricular outflow tracts develop normally in utero, whereas after birth these lesions are fatal unless surgery is performed. With birth, there is a rapid transformation from the fetal circulation to the adult circulation. This transformation involves elimination of the umbilical-placental circulation, establishment of an adequate pulmonary circulation, and separation of the left and right sides of the heart by closure of the ductus arteriosus and foramen ovale. Figure 9-2 depicts the fetal, immediate postbirth, and a few days postbirth hemodynamics.[51] Persistence of the fetal circulation after birth usually means that adequate pulmonary circulation is not achieved and fetal channels have not closed. For example, infants with congenital diaphragmatic hernia have persistence of the fetal circulation because of high pulmonary resistance due to poor oxygenation and persistent patency of the foramen ovale and ductus arteriosus.

MANAGEMENT OF COMMON CARDIOVASCULAR PROBLEMS IN THE NEONATE

Congestive Heart Failure

The common causes of heart failure in the neonate include rhythm disturbances and congenital cardiovascular malformations. Table 9-1 lists common congenital heart lesions and the age at which congestive heart failure

is likely to occur. In an infant with cyanotic congenital heart disease, congestive heart failure usually occurs with lesions that have large amounts of pulmonary blood flow or regurgitant atrioventricular valves. The ultimate management of heart failure is to treat the underlying congenital malformation; however, medical management is essential to stabilize the infant and enable surgical correction to be performed with reduced risk. Standard medical management includes the principles of rate control, preload control, afterload control, and improvement in contractility. Because of the high resting heart rate of the neonate, one cannot use increasing heart rate to increase cardiac output. In fact, chronic supraventricular tachycardia, frequently the result of an atrial ectopic focus, is a cause of congestive cardiomyopathy.

Preload control is the mainstay of symptomatic therapy for heart failure. This is accomplished with the use of diuretics. The most common diuretic used to treat heart failure in the infant is furosemide (Lasix). Table 9-2 lists some commonly used diuretics and current dose recommendations. One diuretic that may have benefits beyond symptomatic therapy is spironolactone (Aldactone).[13,33] Recent evidence suggests that in addition to causing fluid retention, aldosterone can cause myocardial fibrosis. There are now a number of clinical trials in adults that suggest that chronic blockade of mineralocorticoid receptors results in improved cardiac remodeling.[33] It is important when considering the use of diuretics to avoid too much diuresis. If the child's preload is reduced below the preload reserve, cardiac output will decrease (see Fig. 9-1).

Afterload agents work by decreasing ventricular loading, predominantly by reducing systemic vascular resistance. The pharmacologic agents that are most useful in altering afterload are vasodilators (see Table 9-2). These drugs are important therapeutic agents in the treatment of infants with heart failure secondary to a large left-to-right shunt, severe atrioventricular and semilunar valve regurgitation, dilated cardiomyopathy, and postoperative low-output states.[7-10,29] Angiotensin-converting enzyme inhibitors are the most commonly used class of afterload-reducing agents.[38,42,55,61] In addition to reducing ventricular afterload, they have been shown to improve cardiovascular remodeling in adults with congestive cardiomyopathy.[33] Another means of afterload control is beta-receptor blockade. Low-dose beta blockers have been used successfully in the treatment of congestive cardiomyopathy. They work by interfering with the deleterious effects of increased sympathetic activity.[3,22]

The final group of agents used to treat congestive heart failure in infants and young children increases the inotropy of the heart (see Table 9-2). The oldest agent in this class is digitalis. Digoxin is still the most commonly used chronic inotropic agent. It increases contractility by inhibiting the sodium–potassium–adenosine triphosphatase pump, resulting in an increase in intracellular sodium, which in turn stimulates calcium entry into the cell by the sodium-calcium exchanger; the increased intracellular calcium leads to increased contractility. Recent studies suggest that digitalis also

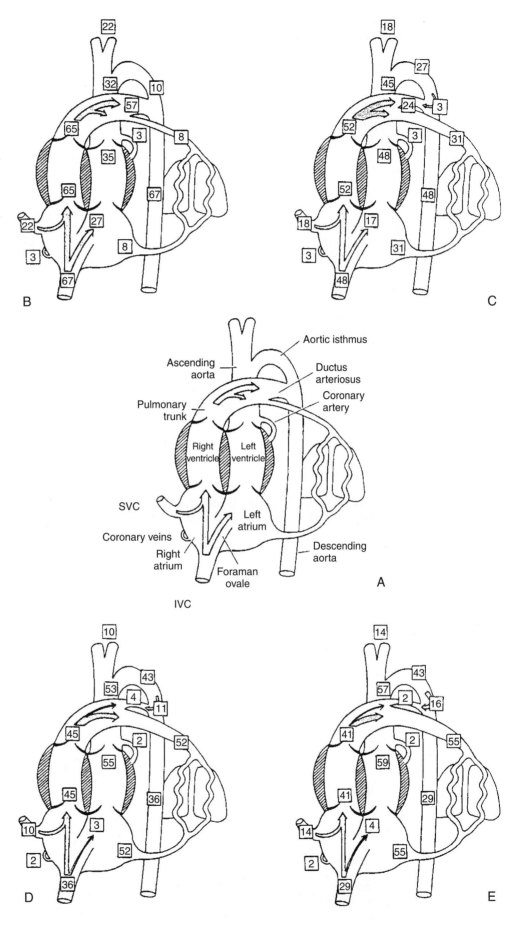

Figure 9–2 Distribution of the circulation in the fetal lamb. Percentages of combined ventricular output are shown in boxes. *A,* Anatomy of the fetal circulation. *B,* Undisturbed state. *C,* After ventilation with 3% oxygen, so as not to alter fetal blood gases. *D,* After ventilation with oxygen. *E,* After ventilation with oxygen and umbilical cord occlusion. IVC, inferior vena cava; SVC, superior vena cava. (From Rudolph AM: The fetal circulation and its adjustments after birth. In Moller JH, Hoffman JIE [eds]: Pediatric Cardiovascular Medicine. Philadelphia, Churchill Livingstone, 2000, p 62.)

TABLE 9-1 Causes of Congestive Heart Failure at Various Ages

Fetus to 1 Day of Life	First Week to 6 Weeks of Life	6 Weeks to 3 Months of Life	After 6 Months of Life
Tachyarrhythmias	Critical aortic stenosis	Ventricular septal defects	Myopericarditis
Anemia or hemolytic disease	Coarctation of aorta (simple or complex)	Patent ductus arteriosus	Endocarditis
Atrioventricular valve regurgitation	Hypoplastic left heart syndrome	Atrioventricular septal defects	Primary pulmonary hypertension*
Heart block	Interrupted aortic arch	Atrial septal defects*	Rheumatic heart disease
Cardiac or pericardial tumors*	Critical pulmonary stenosis	Tachyarrhythmias	Kawasaki disease
Arteriovenous malformations (usually brain or liver)*	Common mixing lesions (e.g., truncus, single ventricle)	Anomalous left coronary artery from pulmonary artery	Postoperative congenital heart disease
Birth asphyxia	Tachyarrhythmias	Myocarditis or cardiomyopathy	Neuromuscular disease
Fetal-maternal or fetal-fetal transfusions	Obstructed or nonobstructed total anomalous pulmonary venous return	Nonobstructive total anomalous pulmonary venous return	Cardiomyopathies (restrictive, hypertrophic, dilated)
Myocarditis	Myocarditis or cardiomyopathy		Systemic hypertension
Hyperviscosity	Systemic hypertension*		Collagen vascular disease*
Premature closure of foramen ovale or patent ductus*	Endocrine disorders: thyroid disease, adrenal insufficiency, parathyroid disease*		Drugs: anthracycline, ipecac, cocaine, heavy metal
Semilunar valve insufficiency (e.g., absent pulmonary valve, aortic to left ventricular tunnel)*	Persistent pulmonary hypertension		Anemia: sickle cell, thalassemia, hemolytic*
	Patent ductus arteriosus (especially premature infants)		
	Infant of diabetic mother		

*Rare cause of heart failure.

TABLE 9-2 Medications Used to Treat Congestive Heart Failure

Class	Drug	Dose	Dosing Interval	Comments
Diuretic	Hydrochlorothiazide	2.0-3.0 mg/kg up to 50 mg/day	bid	Increases uric acid level.
	Furosemide	0.5-2.0 mg/kg up to 6.0 mg/kg/day	qd or bid	
	Spironolactone	1.0-3.3 mg/kg	bid	Potassium-sparing; used with causing with CEI
	Metolazone	0.2-0.4 mg/kg	qd	
ACE inhibitor	Benazepril	0.2 mg/kg up to 10 mg/day	qd	Contraindicated in pregnancy; check serum potassium, creatinine; cough and angioedema are side effects
	Captopril	0.3-0.5 mg/kg up to 6.0 mg/kg	tid	
	Enalapril	0.08 mg/kg up to 5.0 mg/day	qd-bid	
	Lisinopril	0.07 mg/kg up to 40 mg/day	qd	
Angiotensin receptor blocker	Irbesartan	6-12 yr: 75-150 mg/day	qd	Contraindicated in pregnancy; check serum potassium, creatinine
	Losartan	0.7 mg/kg/day up to 50 mg/day	qd	
Beta blocker	Metoprolol	1.0-2.0 mg/day up to 6.0 mg/kg/day	qd	
Vasodilator	Hydralazine	0.75 mg/kg up to 7.5 mg/kg	qid	May cause tachycardia, fluid retention, lupus-like syndrome
	Prazosin	0.05-0.1 mg/kg up to 0.5 mg/kg	tid	
Inotrope	Digoxin	Digitalizing dose: 20-40 µg/kg, depending on age Maintenance dose: 5-10 µg/kg	bid	
	Dobutamine	2-20 µg/kg/min IV		
	Dopamine	2-20 µg/kg/min IV		
	Milrinone	Loading dose 0.05-1.0 mg/kg, then 0.5-0.75 µg/kg/min		
	Epinephrine	0.05-2.0 µg/kg/min IV		

ACE, angiotensin-converting enzyme.

helps heart failure by inhibiting sympathetic nerve traffic and thus decreasing cardiac metabolic demands.[25] In addition to digoxin, there are other intravenous inotropic agents, the majority of which stimulate the β-adrenergic receptor in the heart, which in turn increases adenyl cyclase activity and ultimately contractility. These agents are especially useful in managing severe acute congestive heart failure and cardiogenic shock. Depending on the individual agent, blood pressure can be either increased or slightly decreased. For example, dopamine can cause alpha-receptor stimulation with some degree of vasoconstriction,[11] whereas dobutamine tends to produce more systemic vasodilatation and either slightly decreases or has no effect on systemic pressure.[20,44] Milrinone is another intravenous inotrope that is frequently used in infants. It is a phosphodiesterase inhibitor and increases contractility by inhibiting the breakdown of cyclic adenosine monophosphate. Besides being a positive inotropic agent, it reduces afterload as well. Thus milrinone is likely to lower blood pressure slightly. It is also useful in producing some degree of pulmonary artery vasodilatation and is therefore an ideal agent for an infant with severe congestive heart failure and pulmonary artery hypertension.[19]

If pharmacologic therapy is not enough to maintain adequate cardiac output, mechanical devices can be used to support the circulation. The most commonly used mechanical support device is extracorporeal membrane oxygenation. More recently, ventricular assist devices have been used in infants with end-stage cardiomyopathy as a bridge to cardiac transplantation.[17,30,56]

Abnormalities in Cardiac Rhythm

Heart Block

Both slow and fast heart rates can severely compromise the cardiovascular circulation of an infant. Complete heart block may be either congenital or acquired and occurs in 1 per 20,000 live births.[12,41,53] There is a strong association between maternal connective tissue disease and congenital complete heart block. For example, a woman with systemic lupus erythematosus has a 1 in 20 risk of having a child with complete heart block if she is anti-Ro positive.[48] Maternal immunoglobulin G antibodies to soluble ribonucleoprotein antigens (anti-Ro and anti-La) cross the placenta after the 12th to 16th week of gestation. This transfer of antibodies results in an inflammatory response in the fetal heart, particularly in the conduction system, with destruction of the atrioventricular node.[34,37,40,48,49,53,57] Complete heart block in the neonate may or may not need treatment. The decision whether to place a pacemaker in an infant with heart block depends on the presence of in utero heart failure (hydrops) or the development of postnatal congestive heart failure. Heart rate alone is usually not an indication for pacemaker placement; however, if the infant's heart rate remains below 50 beats per minute, a pacemaker is frequently required. Some forms of congenital heart disease also have a high incidence of heart block. These lesions include Ebstein's anomaly

of the tricuspid valve and corrected transposition of the great arteries.

Tachyarrhythmias

Tachyarrhythmias can occur in infants and young children and cause heart failure. The most common type of tachyarrhythmia is supraventricular tachycardia. The incidence of paroxysmal supraventricular tachycardia is 1 in 250 to 1000 children.[31] It occurs most commonly in males younger than 4 months old and is frequently present in the fetus. The pathologic mechanism underlying the tachycardia is usually either Wolff-Parkinson-White syndrome (an accessory pathway between the atria and ventricles) or atrioventricular nodal reentry (dual conduction pathways within the atrioventricular node). If the supraventricular tachycardia is sustained, heart failure will likely occur within 24 to 48 hours. The treatment of supraventricular tachycardia, regardless of the cause, is similar. If the infant becomes acidotic or hypotensive, immediate synchronized direct-current cardioversion should be performed, at a dosage of 1 to 2 watt-sec/kg.[2] If the infant is stable and relatively asymptomatic, any intervention that increases atrioventricular node refractoriness is likely to work. Application of ice or an ice-water bag directly to the center of the infant's face recruits the diving reflex and stops the tachycardia. A rapid intravenous infusion of adenosine is also very effective in terminating supraventricular tachycardia.[15] The usual dose is a 100 μg/kg bolus, increasing by 100-μg increments to a maximum of 400 μg/kg. A few serious side effects have been associated with adenosine administration, including atrial fibrillation, ventricular tachycardia, asystole, apnea, and bronchospasm. Therefore, adenosine should be administered in an area where cardioversion and cardiopulmonary resuscitation can be performed.

Children with supraventricular tachycardia and mild to moderate congestive heart failure can be treated initially with adenosine; other pharmacologic agents such as digoxin, amiodarone, and procainamide may be helpful if adenosine fails to convert the tachycardia. Table 9-3 lists some commonly used antiarrhythmic agents and current dose recommendations. In infants, the intravenous route is preferred for the administration of digoxin. The digitalizing dose may be given as often as every 2 to 4 hours. If tachycardia persists after three doses, one more dose equivalent to one fourth of the total digitalizing dose may be given. If the tachycardia still has not converted, vagal stimulation or adenosine may be effective in terminating the tachycardia after digitalization. The maintenance dose of digoxin depends on the total digitalizing dose required to terminate the tachycardia; it is one eighth of the total digitalizing dose twice daily. Digoxin should be avoided in patients with wide QRS tachycardia and when Wolff-Parkinson-White syndrome is a possible cause. Digoxin in the presence of Wolff-Parkinson-White with atrial fibrillation can result in acceleration of the ventricular response and resultant ventricular fibrillation.

Esmolol or propranolol, which may further depress cardiac function, should be used with caution in critically

TABLE 9–3 Pharmacologic Agents Used to Treat Tachyarrhythmias

Drug	Dosage	Onset of Action	Potential Adverse Effects	Drug Interactions	Cardiovascular Contraindications	Comments
Adenosine	100-150 µg/kg given rapid IV; double dose sequentially up to max of 300 µg/kg	<5 sec	Dyspnea, bronchospasm, headache, chest pains, AV block/asystole, PVCs, atrial fibrillation, torsades de pointes, hypotension	Theophylline: adenosine less effective Digoxin: increased risk of VT Diazepam: potentiates effects of adenosine	Prolonged QT Second- or third-degree AV block, except in presence of pacemaker Sick sinus syndrome	Have defibrillator available when administering, in case of ventricular rate acceleration, torsades de pointes, VF
Amiodarone	Bolus: 5 mg/kg over 10 min Infusion: 10-15 µg/kg/day	Within 5 min of initial bolus	Hypotension, sinus arrest or bradycardia, AV block	Digoxin: increases digoxin levels Procainamide: causes increased levels Warfarin: increases INR	Sick sinus syndrome or AV block, except if pacemaker present Cardiogenic shock.	Closely monitor BP, heart rate and rhythm Hypotension can be treated with volume and calcium
Esmolol	Load: 500 µg/kg over 1-2 min Maintenance: 50-200 µg/kg/min	Within 1-2 min	Hypotension, dizziness, headache, nausea, bronchospasm, decreased cardiac output	Digoxin: increase level Morphine: causes increased esmolol level	Sinus bradycardia, second- or third-degree heart block, cardiogenic shock, overt heart failure	Use with caution in patients with decreased renal function, diabetes, or asthma
Procainamide	Load: infants 7-10 mg/kg over 45 min; older children 12 mg/kg Infusion: 40-50 µg/kg/min; occasionally may need up to 100 µg/kg/min	Within 30 min	Hypotension, increased ventricular response with atrial flutter, bradycardia, asystole, depressed ventricular function, fever, myalgia, AV block, confusion, dizziness, headache	Amiodarone: causes increased concentration of procainamide Digoxin: causes increase in digoxin levels	Second- and third-degree AV block without pacemaker Congestive heart failure Prolonged QT interval	Continuously monitor ECG and BP Monitor potassium levels—if potassium decreases, arrhythmias may increase

AV, atrioventricular; BP, blood pressure; ECG, electrocardiogram; INR, international normalized ratio; PVC, premature ventricular contraction; VF, ventricular fibrillation; VT, ventricular tachycardia.

ill infants with congestive heart failure. Once the tachycardia has been terminated and the congestive heart failure is controlled, beta blockers can be used as effective long-term antiarrhythmic therapy in infants with supraventricular tachycardia.

Amiodarone is now being used with increasing frequency for the emergency treatment of supraventricular tachycardia, especially in postoperative patients. Intravenous administration of amiodarone has been reported to terminate tachycardia within 2 hours of the initial bolus in more than 40% of patients.[26,45] The major side effects of amiodarone include hypotension, decreased ventricular function, and bradycardia.

Intravenous procainamide can be very effective in patients with refractory supraventricular tachycardia. The combination of procainamide and a beta blocker is especially effective in treating refractory atrial flutter in the neonate.

Verapamil, though an effective agent to treat supraventricular tachycardia in adults, is contraindicated in infants with congestive heart failure. Use of verapamil in infants has resulted in cardiovascular collapse and death.[1,23]

In my institution, we frequently use esophageal overdrive pacing to convert supraventricular tachycardia in infants. Esophageal pacing has the advantage of not only treating the arrhythmia but also helping to arrive at a definitive diagnosis of the tachycardia. Overdrive pacing involves pacing the atrium via the esophagus at a rate slightly higher than the rate of the tachycardia. With cessation of pacing, sinus rhythm usually returns. Esophageal pacing is effective in most forms of supraventricular tachycardia, including atrial flutter.[18,39]

Ventricular tachycardia is extremely unusual in the newborn. It is most often seen in infants with intracardiac tumors, such as rhabdomyomas, and in infants with long QT syndrome.

Congenital Heart Disease

Certain types of congenital heart disease are frequently associated with other congenital lesions that require general surgical procedures in the newborn period. For example, tetralogy of Fallot and ventricular septal defects are common in infants with tracheoesophageal fistulas, anal atresia, and other lesions common to the VATER complex. Interrupted aortic arch, truncus arteriosus, and tetralogy of Fallot are frequently present in infants with DiGeorge syndrome. Hypoplastic left heart syndrome has been reported to occur in infants with congenital diaphragmatic hernia. More than 60% of infants with Down syndrome have congenital heart disease (patent ductus arteriosus, ventricular septal defects, atrioventricular septal defects, and tetralogy of Fallot). Because of the strong association between congenital heart disease and other congenital anomalies that require general surgery in the newborn period, a cardiology consultation and echocardiogram are often necessary before the surgical procedure. The exact management depends on the type of congenital heart disease.

In infants with restricted pulmonary blood flow, such as seen with tetralogy of Fallot or pulmonary atresia, ductal patency is necessary to maintain adequate oxygenation. If a ductus was present in fetal life, it can usually be maintained patent with the administration of prostaglandin E_1, at a usual starting dose of 0.1 to 0.05 µg/kg per minute. If the ductus is patent, I use low-dose prostaglandin (0.02 to 0.03 µg/kg per minute) to maintain its patency; if the ductus is virtually closed, I start with a higher dose of prostaglandin until patency is achieved and then cut back to low-dose therapy. Side effects associated with prostaglandin administration include apnea, seizures, fever, hypotension, and flushing. Once the infant has been stabilized, more definitive therapy can be contemplated. At my institution, whenever possible, we choose complete repair of these lesions over palliation with a systemic–to–pulmonary artery shunt.

In infants with hypoplastic left heart syndrome, initial management requires that an atrial septal defect be present and that ductal patency be maintained. In these infants, systemic blood flow is directly related to pulmonary artery resistance, and oxygen saturation is inversely related to pulmonary vascular resistance (i.e., as pulmonary resistance decreases, pulmonary blood flow increases, resulting in a higher oxygen saturation and a lower systemic blood flow). The ideal systemic oxygen saturation in an infant with hypoplastic left heart syndrome is around 80%. When the oxygen saturation is in the high 80s to low 90s, the ratio of pulmonary to systemic blood flow is usually greater than 4:1, and systemic hypoperfusion is usually present; when the oxygen saturation is in the high 70s to low 80s, the pulmonary-to-systemic flow ratio is nearly balanced. Ideally, I like to let these infants maintain spontaneous respirations and withhold supplemental oxygen. In some cases, it may be necessary to cause pulmonary vasoconstriction, which can be accomplished by placing the infant in a mixture of room air and nitrogen. The lower inspired oxygen concentration causes pulmonary artery vasoconstriction, which results in a reduction in pulmonary blood flow and maintenance of adequate systemic perfusion. Once the infant has been stabilized, it is my policy to perform Norwood palliation. In some selected cases, cardiac transplantation may be the best surgical option for the infant.

Infants with ventricular septal defects or atrioventricular septal defects usually have no symptoms during the first month of life. Congestive heart failure from a ventricular septal defect is usually the result of excess pulmonary blood flow. The two major determinants of left-to-right shunt flow across a ventricular septal defect are the size of the defect and the ratio of pulmonary arteriolar to systemic arteriolar resistance. In a full-term infant, it usually takes 4 to 6 weeks for the pulmonary resistance to drop to normal levels; thus, infants with large septal defects do not usually develop heart failure until the second month of life. Causes of early heart failure in an infant with a ventricular septal defect include prematurity and other associated cardiac lesions. The two lesions most often associated with the early development of congestive heart failure are coarctation of the aorta and, in the case of an atrioventricular septal defect, significant atrioventricular valvular regurgitation.

REFERENCES

1. Abinader E, Borochowitz Z, Berger A: A hemodynamic complication of verapamil therapy in a neonate. Helv Paediatr Acta 1981;36:451.

2. Adkins DL, Kerger RE: Pediatric defibrillation: Current flow is improved by using "adult" electrode paddles. Pediatrics 1994;94:90.

3. Anderson JL, Bilbert EM, O'Connell JB, et al: Long term (2 year) beneficial effects of beta receptor blockade with bucindolol in patients with dilated cardiomyopathy. J Am Coll Cardiol 1991;17:1373.

4. Anderson PAW, Glick KL, Killman AP, et al: The effect of heart rate on in utero left ventricular output in the fetal sheep. J Physiol (Lond) 1986;372:557.

5. Anderson PAW, Glick K, Manring A, et al: Developmental changes in cardiac contractility in fetal and postnatal sheep: In vitro and in vivo. Am J Physiol 1984;247:H371.

6. Anderson PAW, Manring A, Glick K, et al: Biophysics of the developing heart. III. A comparison of the left ventricular dynamics of the fetal and neonatal lamb heart. Am J Obstet Gynecol 1982;143:195.

7. Artman M, Graham TP: Guidelines for vasodilator therapy of congestive heart failure in infants and children. Am Heart J 1987;113:994.

8. Beekman RH, Rocchini AP, Dick M, et al: Vasodilator therapy in children: Acute and chronic effects in children with left ventricular dysfunction or mitral regurgitation. Pediatrics 1983;52:112.

9. Beekman RH, Rocchini AP, Rosenthal A: Hemodynamic effects of hydralazine in infants with a large ventricular septal defect. Circulation 1982;65:523.

10. Bengur AR, Beekman RH, Rocchini AP, et al: Acute hemodynamic effects of captopril in children with a congestive or restrictive cardiomyopathy. Circulation 1991;83:523.

11. Bhatt-Mehta V, Nahata MC: Dopamine and dobutamine in pediatric therapy. Pharmacology 1989;9:303.

12. Chameides LM, Truex RC, Vetter VL, et al: Association of maternal systemic lupus erythematosus with congenital complete heart block. N Engl J Med 1977;297:1204.

13. Chatterje K: Congestive heart failure: What should be the initial therapy and why? Am J Cardiovasc Drugs 2002;2:1.

14. Clyman RI, Teitel D, Padbury C, et al: The role of β-adrenergic receptor stimulation and contractile state in the preterm lamb's response to altered ductus arteriosus patency. Pediatr Res 1988;23:316.

15. Crosson JE, Etheridge SP, Milstein S, et al: Therapeutic and diagnostic utility of adenosine during tachycardia evaluation in children. Am J Cardiol 1994;74:155.

16. Dawes GS, Mott JC, Widdicombe JG: The foetal circulation in the lamb. J Physiol 1952;126:563.

17. delNido PJ, Armitage JM, Fricker FJ, et al: Extracorporeal membrane oxygenation support as a bridge to pediatric heart transplantation. Circulation 1994;90:66.

18. Dick M II, Scott WA, Serwer GS, et al: Acute termination of supraventricular tachyarrhythmias in children by transesophageal pacing. Am J Cardiol 1988;61:925.

19. DiDomenico RJ, Park HY, Southworth MR, et al: Guidelines for acute decompensated heart failure treatment. Ann Pharmacother 2004;38:649.

20. Driscoll DJ, Gillete PC, Duff DF, et al: Hemodynamic effects of dobutamine in children. Am J Cardiol 1979;43:581.

21. Edelstone DI, Rudolph AM, Heymann MA: Liver and ductus venosus blood flows in fetal lambs in utero. Cir Res 1978; 42:426.

22. Eichhorn EJ: Paradox of beta-adrenergic blockade for the management of congestive heart failure. Am J Med 1992; 92:527.

23. Epstein MC, Kiel EA, Victoria BE: Cardiac decompensation following verapamil therapy in infants with supraventricular tachycardia. Pediatrics 1985;75:737.

24. Fabiato A: Appraisal of the physiological relevance of two hypotheses for the mechanisms of calcium release from the mammalian cardiac sarcoplasmic reticulum: Calcium-induced release versus charge-coupled release. Mol Cell Biochem 1989;89:135.

25. Ferguson DW, Berg WJ, Sanders SJ, et al: Somatoinhibitory responses in digitalis glycosides in heart failure patients: Direct evidence from sympathetic neural recordings. Circulation 1989;80:65.

26. Figa FH, Bow RM, Hamilton BF, et al: Clinical efficacy and safety of intravenous amiodarone in infants and children. Am J Cardiol 1994;74:573.

27. Fisher DJ, Tate CA, Phillips S: Development regulation of the sarcoplasmic reticulum calcium pump in the rabbit heart. Pediatr Res 1992;31:474.

28. Friedman WF: The intrinsic physiologic properties of the developing heart. Prog Cardiovasc Dis 1972;15:87.

29. Friedman WF, George BL: Medical progress—treatment of congestive heart failure by altering loading conditions of the heart. J Pediatr 1985;106:697.

30. Gajarski RJ, Mosca RS, Ohye RG, et al: Use of extracorporeal life support as a bridge to pediatric cardiac transplantation. J Heart Lung Transplant 2003;22:28.

31. Garson A Jr, Ludomirsky A: Supraventricular tachycardia. In Garson A Jr, Bricker JT, McNamara DG (eds): The Science and Practice of Pediatric Cardiology. Philadelphia, Lea & Febiger, 1990, p 1809.

32. Gilbert RD: Control of fetal cardiac output during changes in blood volume. Am J Physiol 1980;238:H80.

33. Gonzalez A, Lopez B, Diez J: Fibrosis in hypertensive heart disease: Role of the renin-angiotensin-aldosterone system. Med Clin North Am 2004;88:83.

34. Hartley JB, Kaine JL, Fox OF, et al: Ro(SS-A) antibody antigen in a patient with congenital complete heart block. Arthritis Rheum 1985;28:1321.

35. Hille B: Calcium channels. In Ionic Channels of Excitable Membranes, 2nd ed. Sunderland, Mass, Sinauer Associates, 1991, p 83.

36. Kiserud T, Eik-Nes SH, Blaas HG, et al: Foramen ovale: An ultrasonographic study of its relation to the inferior vena cava, ductus venosus and hepatic veins. Ultrasound Obstet Gynecol 1992;2:389.

37. Lee LA, Coutler S, Erner S, et al: Cardiac immunoglobulin deposition and congenital heart block associated with maternal anti-Ro autoantibodies. Am J Med 1987; 83:793.

38. Lewis AB, Chabot M: The effect of treatment with angiotensin converting enzyme inhibitors on survival of pediatric patients with dilated cardiomyopathy. Pediatr Cardiol 1993;14:9.

39. Lister JW, Cohen LS, Bernstein WH, et al: Treatment of supraventricular tachycardia by rapid atrial stimulation. Circulation 1968;38:1044.

40. Litsey SE, Noonan JA, O'Connor WN, et al: Maternal connective tissue disease and congenital heart block: Demonstration of immunoglobulin in cardiac tissue. N Engl J Med 1985;312:98.

41. McCue CM, Mantakas ME, Tingelstad JB, et al: Congenital heart block in newborns of mothers with connective tissue disease. Circulation 1977;56:82.

42. Montigny M, Davignon A, Fouron JC, et al: Captopril in infants in congestive heart failure secondary to a large ventricular left-to-right shunt. Am J Cardiol 1989; 63:631.

43. Ogawa Y: Role of ryanodine receptors. Crit Rev Biochem Mol Biol 1994;29:229.

44. Opie LH: Drugs for the Heart, 3rd ed. Philadelphia, WB Saunders, 1991, p 142.

45. Perry JC, Fenrich AL, Hulse JE, et al: Pediatric use of intravenous amiodarone: Efficacy and safety in critically ill patients from multicenter protocol. J Am Coll Cardiol 1996;27:1246.

46. Pinson CW, Morton MJ, Thornburg KL, et al: An anatomic basis for fetal right ventricular dominance and arterial pressure sensitivity. J Dev Physiol 1987;9:253.

47. Pohlman AG: The fetal circulation through the heart. Bull Johns Hopkins Hosp 1907;18:409.

48. Ramsey-Goldman R, Hom D, Deng J, et al: Anti-SS-A antibodies and fetal outcome in maternal systemic lupus erythematosus. Arthritis Rheum 1986;28:1321.

49. Reed BR, Lee LA, Harmon C, et al: Autoantibodies to SS-A/Ro in infants with congenital heart block. J Pediatr 1983;6:889.

50. Reller MD, Morton MJ, Reid DL, et al: Fetal lamb ventricles respond differently to filling and arterial pressures and to in utero ventilation. Pediatr Res 1987;22:621.

51. Rudolph AM: The fetal circulation and its adjustments after birth. In Moller JH, Hoffman JIE (eds): Pediatric Cardiovascular Medicine. Philadelphia, Churchill Livingstone, 2000, p 62.

52. Rudolph AM, Heymann MA: The circulation of the fetus in utero: Methods for studying distribution of blood flow, cardiac output and organ blood flow. Circ Res 1966; 21:163.

53. Scott JS, Maddison PJ, Taylor PV, et al: Connective-tissue disease, antibodies to ribonucleoprotein, and congenital heart block. N Engl J Med 1983;309:209.

54. Sham JSK, Cleemann L, Morad M: Gating of the cardiac Ca^{2+} release channel: The role of Na^+ current and Na^+-Ca^{2+} exchange. Science 1992;255:850.

55. Stern H, Weil J, Genz T, et al: Captopril in children with dilated cardiomyopathy: Acute and long-term effects in a prospective study of hemodynamic and hormonal effects. Pediatr Cardiol 1990;11:22.

56. Takano H, Nakatani T, Tanaka Y, et al: Clinical experience with ventricular assist systems in Japan. Ann Thorac Surg 1993;55:250.

57. Taylor PV, Scott JS, Gerlis LM, et al: Maternal antibodies against fetal cardiac antigens in congenital complete heart block. N Engl J Med 1986;315:667.

58. Thornburg KL, Morton MJ: Filling and arterial pressures as determinants of left ventricular stroke volume in fetal lambs. Am J Physiol 1986;251:H961.

59. Valdivia HH, Kaplan JH, Ellis-Davies GC, et al: Rapid adaptation of cardiac ryanodine receptors: Modulation by Mg^{2+} and phosphorylation. Science 1997;267:1997.

60. Wang Y-P, Fuchs F: Osmotic compression of skinned cardiac and skeletal muscle bundles: Effects on force generation, Ca^{2+} sensitivity and Ca^{2+} binding. J Mol Cell Cardiol 1995;27:1235.

61. Webster MW, Neutze JM, Calder AL: Acute hemodynamic effects of converting enzyme inhibition in children with intracardiac shunts. Pediatr Cardiol 1992;13:129.

Chapter 10

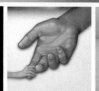

Sepsis and Related Considerations

Jeffrey S. Upperman and Henri R. Ford

Despite recent advances in neonatology and pediatric critical care and the widespread use of broad-spectrum antimicrobial agents, infection remains a leading cause of morbidity and mortality in infants and children. Microbial infections usually result from failure of the intrinsic host defense mechanisms to combat putative virulence factors of invading microorganisms. Immunocompromised infants and children, along with preterm and term neonates, who characteristically have significant impairment of their host defense systems, are particularly vulnerable to bacterial infections. Such infections initially elicit a localized inflammatory response aimed at destroying the bacteria. Failure to control either the infection itself or the inflammatory response to infection may evoke a constellation of clinical symptoms that have been variably defined as the sepsis syndrome.

Traditionally, the term *sepsis* was used to denote the profound clinical alterations in vital signs, homeostasis, and metabolism that occur in response to the presence of gram-negative or gram-positive microbial pathogens in the bloodstream of affected individuals. However, a growing body of evidence suggests that neither bacteremia nor an active infection is required for the development of the sepsis syndrome; a number of critically injured patients die of apparent overwhelming sepsis without any identifiable source of infection.[54] In these patients, the large amount of necrotic or injured tissue is sufficient to activate the inflammatory cascade and culminate in serious hemodynamic compromise, characterized by fever, shock or cardiovascular collapse, hypoperfusion with attendant organ dysfunction, and generalized edema. This cluster of events is now defined as the systemic inflammatory response syndrome (SIRS). Thus, the concept of SIRS may be invoked in the absence of identifiable systemic infection. It may represent the final common pathway through which overwhelming infection results in the death of the host.

Sepsis, which is the term used when SIRS is derived from an infectious cause, remains a major cause of morbidity and mortality in the United States. In fact, in a review of discharge data on approximately 750 million hospitalizations from 1979 to 2000, Martin et al.[90] found 10,319,418 cases of sepsis. During the study period, there was an 8.7% annual increase in the incidence of sepsis, from about 164,000 cases to nearly 660,000 cases. Watson et al.[141] reported results from a national survey that demonstrated

that for nearly 1.6 million hospitalizations in children aged 19 years or younger, there were 42,364 pediatric cases of severe sepsis per year. The incidence was greatest in infants (5.16 per 1000), fell markedly in older children (0.20 per 1000 in 10- to 14-year-olds), and was higher in boys than in girls. They also reported that hospital mortality for patients who met severe sepsis criteria was approximately 10%, or 4383 deaths nationally (6.2 per 100,000 population). In patients with altered host defense mechanisms, as seen with diabetes mellitus, hepatic failure, burns, trauma, malignant neoplasms, or drug-induced immunosuppression, sepsis is the most common cause of death.[148] Approximately 30% of patients with sepsis have gram-negative bacteria in their blood. The most common organisms identified in adults and older children include *Escherichia coli, Pseudomonas aeruginosa, Klebsiella,* and *Bacteroides* species.[28,156] In the neonatal population, the most common microbial pathogens are group B streptococci and gram-negative enteric bacilli (predominantly *E. coli*). Although the specific clinical symptoms elicited by these microbes may vary based on the developmental maturity of the host, the ultimate consequence of such infections (if uncontrolled) may be SIRS or death.

A detailed examination of specific infections encountered in surgical neonates and children is beyond the scope of this chapter. Rather, this chapter examines the mechanisms by which infections in neonates and children result in full-blown SIRS. To fully comprehend the pathogenesis of SIRS, we must first examine the mechanisms by which microbial pathogens gain access to the tissues or systemic circulation to cause infection and incite the inflammatory cascade. Similarly, we need to study how the intrinsic host defense mechanisms permit bacterial invasion or allow the amplification of potentially harmful soluble inflammatory mediators responsible for the development of SIRS.

The first part of this chapter focuses on the determinants of infection, such as bacterial virulence and host defense mechanisms. The cellular and humoral (including antibody, complement, and cytokine) responses to infection and tissue injury are closely examined because they represent the final common pathway for the development of SIRS. Alterations in neonatal host defense mechanisms are considered separately. The second part examines the pathogenesis as well as the hemodynamic and metabolic consequences of SIRS in older children and neonates. The third part stresses the diagnostic approach to neonatal sepsis, and the last part focuses on new treatment modalities, especially the biologic response modifiers.

DETERMINANTS OF INFECTION

Barriers to Infection

The human body is normally colonized by a wide array of microbes. Bacteria are ubiquitous on the skin, in the oropharynx, and in the respiratory, gastrointestinal, and genitourinary tracts. However, clinical infections do not develop unless the intrinsic equilibrium that exists between the indigenous microbial flora and the local host defense mechanisms is altered. The indigenous microflora help prevent colonization by pathogenic microbes by blocking their adherence to the epithelial barrier or by competing for available nutrients. Other protective mechanisms specific for each organ system help minimize colonization by microbial pathogens. For instance, the skin not only maintains a relatively acidic environment that limits bacterial replication but also

undergoes desquamation at regular intervals, a phenomenon that severely hinders bacterial adherence. Intestinal mucus and peristalsis prevent bacterial attachment to the enterocyte, and the cilia of the respiratory epithelium prevent attachment to the respiratory tract. Gastric acidity impedes bacterial replication and colonization. Oropharyngeal, nasopharyngeal, and tracheobronchial secretions are rich in immunoglobin A (IgA), which impairs the ability of bacteria to adhere to mucosal cells. Thus, for infection to occur, typically there must be a breach of the integrity of the normal protective barrier to permit bacterial adherence and subsequent penetration or internalization (Fig. 10-1). Alternatively, the microbial pathogen must be sufficiently virulent to penetrate this barrier. Finally, the internalized bacteria must be able to evade both the local cellular and humoral host defense mechanisms to survive and replicate within the host.

Barrier failure plays an important role in the development of local or systemic infection. Diverse insults may lead to barrier failure. These include trauma or direct tissue injury; surgery, malnutrition, burns, immunosuppression, shock, and reperfusion injury following ischemia.[142] For instance, during ischemia, utilization of adenosine triphosphate results in the accumulation of adenosine

Figure 10–1   The gut barrier is envisioned as a series of "hurdles" that bacteria must overcome to penetrate the epithelial layer and disseminate systemically. *First hurdle:* Gastric acid lowers intragastric pH, promoting a hostile environment for bacterial growth. *Second hurdle:* Coordinated peristalsis continually sweeps bacteria downstream, thus limiting their attachment to the mucosal surface. *Third hurdle:* Indigenous microbial flora (aerobes and anaerobes) prevent the overgrowth of pathogenic gram-negative aerobic bacteria. *Fourth hurdle:* IgA, a nonbactericidal immunoglobulin, coats and aggregates bacteria, preventing their attachment to the mucosal surface. *Fifth hurdle:* Intestinal mucus forms a weblike barrier to prevent bacterial attachment to the enterocyte.

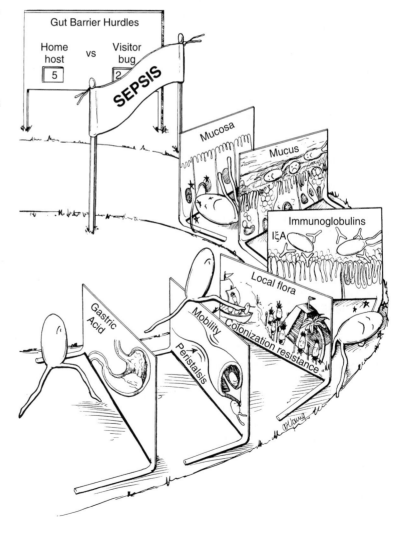

diphosphate, adenosine monophosphate, inosine, and hypoxanthine. Xanthine oxidase activity is also increased, but its effect is initially blunted because oxygen is required to oxidize hypoxanthine to xanthine. However, during reperfusion, oxygen is supplied, hypoxanthine is oxidized, and toxic reactive oxygen intermediates (ROIs), or species, such as superoxide (O_2^-) and hydrogen peroxide (H_2O_2) are formed. These ROIs can mediate direct tissue injury and thus result in gut barrier failure.[7,32,33,143] As a result, bacteria can attach to the injured epithelial surface and undergo internalization, or they can gain direct access to the bloodstream through the damaged mucosa. As discussed later, once the organism has become internalized, the development of clinical infection is dependent on the interplay between microbial virulence and local host defense mechanisms beyond the barrier that has been violated.

Bacterial Virulence

Microbial pathogens possess unique biochemical properties known as virulence factors that permit the successful establishment of infection within the host. If these virulence factors escape the host immune system, the net result will be sufficient multiplication or persistence of the microorganism within the host to cause significant damage to local tissue or allow transmission of the microorganism to other susceptible hosts.

The first and perhaps the most critical step in the process of microbial infection is attachment of the pathogenic microorganism to the cell surface. Some organisms multiply at the site of attachment, while others use this attachment as a prerequisite for microbial invasion. Elimination of this first step may completely abrogate colonization and invasion by microbial pathogens.

The process of microbial adherence or attachment requires intricate interaction between specific molecules on the surface of the bacteria, known as adhesins, and specialized receptors on the host cell. Bacterial fimbriae or pili are perhaps the best studied adhesins that have been shown to promote bacterial adherence to mucosal surfaces. Members of the Enterobacteriaceae family exhibit prominent, morphologically similar pili—type I fimbriae—that permit their attachment to the D-mannose receptor sites on epithelial cells.[26,28] Further, certain bacteria, such as *E. coli*, can simultaneously express different types of adhesins—type I, X, and P fimbriae—a property that clearly enhances the microbe's ability to attach to host surfaces.[48] Other adhesins include invasins, proteins that not only mediate bacterial attachment but also facilitate entry into the host, and hemaglutinin, which is expressed on pathogens such as *Bordetella pertussis, Salmonella typhimurium,* and influenza virus.[48] The host also secretes proteins that indirectly facilitate bacterial adherence; these include proteins of the extracellular matrix—namely, fibronectin, laminin, collagen, and vitronectin. These proteins share a common peptide sequence Arg-Gly-Asp (RGD), which is also found on many microbial pathogens that bind to mammalian cells.[69] For instance, *Staphylococcus aureus* and *Streptococcus pyogenes* are known to bind fibronectin on epithelial surfaces.[48]

Fortunately, bacterial binding to extracellular matrix proteins is usually of low affinity and rarely leads to microbial invasion.

Bacterial adherence allows microorganisms to penetrate the intact epithelial barrier of the host and eventually replicate. However, the mere adherence of the bacteria may not be sufficient for subsequent entry into the host cell. Bacterial internalization requires a high-affinity interaction between adhesins and specific receptors on the cell surface. The integrin receptors appear to be the primary targets on the cell surface for these interactions because they can bind bacterial adhesins as well as extracellular matrix proteins such as fibronectin, laminin, collagen, and vitronectin. In fact, numerous microbial pathogens have been reported to bind host cell integrin receptors. It is the affinity of this interaction that determines whether the microbe becomes internalized or remains adherent to the host cell surface.[69]

Other bacterial virulence factors may also facilitate internalization. For instance, the cell surface protein invasin, found on *Yersinia* species, serves a dual purpose as an adhesin and an enhancer of bacterial invasion. It binds to β_1 integrins on the cell surface, resulting in internalization of *Yersinia*. Transfer of the invasin gene to nonpathogenic *E. coli* renders the organism capable of internalization and host tissue invasion.[69,97] Another variant of the invasin gene, termed the attachment invasion locus, has been identified in *Yersinia* species that cause clinical disease but not in those species that do not cause clinical infection. This molecule may serve as a potential marker of bacterial virulence.

Once bacterial internalization has occurred, the microbe is now located in an endosomal compartment, known as a phagosome, and must escape the intracellular host defense mechanisms (discussed in the next section) to multiply. For internalized bacteria to survive, (1) fusion of the host cell lysosome with the phagosome to form a phagolysosome must be avoided, (2) acidification of the phagolysosome must be prevented, or (3) the antibacterial activity of the phagolysosome must be neutralized. Successful avoidance of these host defense mechanisms permits the establishment and multiplication of the organisms within the host. Bacterial toxins may play an important role in this process, either by causing direct damage to host cells or by interfering with host defense mechanisms. For instance, diphtheria toxin creates a layer of dead cells that serves as a medium for bacterial growth. *Clostridium difficile* secretes both an enterotoxin (toxin A) and a cytotoxin (toxin B) that can damage the mucosal epithelium. *Clostridium perfringens* secretes numerous exotoxins with well-defined roles in the microbe's virulence. These toxins are enzymes with specific targets; they include hyaluronidase, collagenase, proteinase, deoxyribonuclease, and lecithinase. Several organisms such as *Haemophilus influenzae, Streptococcus pneumoniae, Neisseria meningitidis,* and other bacteria that infect the oral cavity produce proteases that are capable of neutralizing local host defense mechanisms.[47] *S. aureus* is able to neutralize ROIs such as hydrogen peroxide through the production of catalase. Likewise, bacterial endotoxins have potent biologic properties. Lipopolysaccharide (LPS) consists of three regions: an O-specific side chain, a core polysaccharide, and an inner lipid A region. Most of the biologic properties of LPS (also known as endotoxin) are attributed to the lipid A region. In fact, lipid A is believed to be the principal mediator of septic shock. LPS (lipid A) triggers an inflammatory cascade, leading to the release of various inflammatory mediators, including arachidonic acid derivatives, leukotrienes, and proinflammatory cytokines, and complement activation. Endotoxin interacts with inflammatory cells by binding to a complex consisting of soluble and membrane-bound receptors; this leads to a cascade of signaling events that result in increased expression of proinflammatory cytokines. These inflammatory mediators are responsible for the hemodynamic and metabolic events that characterize SIRS. We detail the LPS binding mechanism in the next section.

Another method of evading the host defense mechanisms is for the bacteria to avoid phagocytosis or engulfment by the professional phagocytes, such as the neutrophils and macrophages. Streptococci secrete a streptolysin that inhibits neutrophil migration or chemotaxis and impairs phagocyte cytotoxicity. Encapsulated organisms cannot be eliminated unless specific opsonizing antibodies that bind to the surface of the bacteria and facilitate their attachment to the Fc receptors on the neutrophil are present. These organisms are virulent pathogens in splenectomized patients, especially those younger than 4 years. Last, certain microbial pathogens may avoid phagocytosis by binding the Fc receptor of IgG with the bacterial cell wall protein A, which is found in many bacteria, including virulent strains of staphylococci. This interaction prevents binding of the Fc receptor of the IgG antibody to the Fc receptor of the neutrophil.

Host Defense

Successful establishment of infection requires bacterial adhesion and internalization, as well as the ability to avoid intracellular and extracellular host defense mechanisms. Phagocytes, including neutrophils, monocytes-macrophages, lymphocytes, and humoral elements, constitute the host's principal armamentarium against invading microbial pathogens. The immune system typically mounts a well-orchestrated response aimed at destroying the invading microbe. However, as we show later, this response may be exaggerated at times and result in significant host tissue destruction.

Neutrophils

Neutrophils are terminally differentiated effector cells that constitute the first line of defense in response to infection, tissue injury, or other events that stimulate the release of inflammatory mediators or cytokines. Normally, neutrophils circulate in the bloodstream for 6 to 7 hours. Nearly 50% of circulating neutrophils adhere to the vascular endothelium after release from the bone marrow. Functionally they represent the "foot soldiers" of the immune system. As such, they must leave the circulation via a process known as diapedesis to reside in the tissues,

where they survive an additional 48 hours, effecting phagocytosis and microbial killing. Egress into the tissues is a highly regulated process that involves complex interactions between receptors on the phagocytes and the vascular endothelial cells. These interactions are governed at least in part by cytokines or other inflammatory mediators. Three specific events must occur: (1) neutrophil adherence to the endothelium, (2) migration of the neutrophil through the endothelium to the site of injury or inflammation (diapedesis), followed by (3) stimulation or priming of the neutrophil for killing. Neutrophil adherence is governed by adhesion molecules on the neutrophil and endothelial cell. There are three important classes of adhesion molecules involved in neutrophil–endothelial cell interactions: selectins, integrins, and the immunoglobulin superfamily. The first step in the adhesion cascade involves rolling of the neutrophil along the vascular endothelium, a process regulated by the selectins—specifically, leukocyte (L)-selectin, which binds to endothelial (E)-selectin and platelet (P)-selectin, which are both present on activated endothelial cells.[13] Injury or infectious or inflammatory stimuli up-regulate P-selectin expression on the surface of endothelial cells within minutes. This process permits low-avidity adhesion between L-selectin on the neutrophil and P-selectin on the endothelium, which in turn facilitates leukocyte rolling. Migration of the neutrophil to the site of inflammation requires the formation of a firm adhesion between the neutrophil and the endothelial cell. This interaction is governed by the β_2 integrin CD11b/CD18 on the neutrophil and the intercellular adhesion molecule 1 (ICAM-1), a member of the immunoglobulin superfamily, on the endothelial cell.[138]

LPS release by bacteria may play an important role in neutrophil adhesion and migration by stimulating the release of inflammatory mediators such as tumor necrosis factor-α (TNF-α), interleukin-1 (IL-1), and interferon-γ (IFN-γ), which are known to up-regulate ICAM-1 and E-selectin expression on endothelial cells.[13,150] Up-regulation of E-selectin permits enhanced neutrophil rolling, and up-regulation of ICAM-1 promotes high-affinity adhesion between neutrophil and endothelial cell, which facilitates neutrophil migration to the site of inflammation. In addition, LPS forms a complex with lipopolysaccharide binding protein (LBP), which in turn binds to the CD14 molecule and the Toll-like receptor 4 (TLR-4) on the neutrophil (and monocyte) and leads to up-regulation of the β_2 integrin CD11b/ CD18. Thus bacterial LPS can enhance neutrophil-endothelial interactions both directly and indirectly.[68,118]

The net result of the adhesive interactions between neutrophils and endothelial cells is stationary adherence of the neutrophil. Neutrophil egress or migration through the endothelial cell is regulated by platelet–endothelial cell adhesion molecule 1 (PECAM-1).[98-100,106] PECAM-1 is highly expressed in blood vessels, especially on the surface of endothelial cells and on neutrophils. It has been implicated in maintenance of the vascular permeability barrier, modulation of cell migration, and transendothelial migration of monocytes and neutrophils. Antibodies to PECAM-1 lead to leaky barriers and inhibit neutrophil transmigration.[71] In addition to PECAM-1, neutrophil egress requires the presence of a chemotactic gradient through the extracellular matrix. A wide variety of chemotaxins have been described. These include small bacterial peptides, monocyte chemotactic protein 1 (MCP-1), platelet-activating factor (PAF), and leukotriene B_4. Chemotaxins abound at sites of inflammation. Perhaps the two most important chemotaxins for neutrophil migration are IL-8 and C5a, the latter a product of the classic and alternative pathways of complement activation (discussed later). Neutrophils are extremely responsive or sensitive to these chemotaxins; even a concentration as low as 0.1% can be detected.[87,126,127] Interaction between specific receptors on the neutrophils and the chemotaxin evokes a series of secondary intracellular signaling events, leading to translocation of protein kinase C from the cytoplasm to the cell membrane, protein kinase C–dependent phosphorylation, and an increase in free cytosolic calcium. These events lead to conformational changes in the cytoskeleton of the neutrophil that permit its transendothelial egress and rapid movement toward the chemotactic gradient.[37]

The well-orchestrated series of adhesive interactions between the neutrophil and the endothelial cell permit its margination, diapedesis, and extravasation at sites of inflammation. Neutrophils are the first inflammatory cells to accumulate at sites of injury, where they serve to limit or restrict infections through their potent phagocytic and cytotoxic properties. Evidence suggests that early release of certain inflammatory mediators or chemotaxins following injury or infection may enhance adhesive interactions between the neutrophil and the endothelial cell and prime the neutrophil for a more potent cytotoxic response.[3] Disruption of neutrophil–endothelial cell interaction with specific monoclonal antibodies against adhesion molecules inhibits neutrophil chemotaxis at sites of injury, thus potentially impairing the ability to combat bacterial infection.[95] In fact, patients with leukocyte adhesion deficiency are susceptible to recurrent bacterial infections because they lack the β_2 integrin receptor CD11b/CD18. As a result, their neutrophils cannot adhere to the endothelium, and diapedesis into the tissues fails to occur.[8] Patients who are unable to synthesize selectin ligands (leukocyte adhesion deficiency II) also experience recurrent bacterial infections owing to their inability to recruit neutrophils to areas of inflammation.[43,63]

In the tissues, efficient disposal of the microorganism by the neutrophil requires phagocytosis of the microbe, followed by intracellular killing (Fig. 10-2). Phagocytosis is greatly enhanced by prior opsonization of the microbe with specific immunoglobulins. This process results in complement activation, which leads to the deposition of additional ligands or receptors on the bacterial surface. These ligands in turn facilitate neutrophil adherence to the microbe. Signal transduction as a result of the interaction between neutrophil and bacteria elicits secondary changes in membrane fluidity, resulting in pseudopod formation and complete internalization of the microbe into endosomal compartments known as phagosomes. Prior stimulation or priming of the neutrophil by inflammatory cytokines or chemotaxins activates it for more efficient killing. Bacterial killing is then effected through the fusion of lysosomes containing potent microbicidal

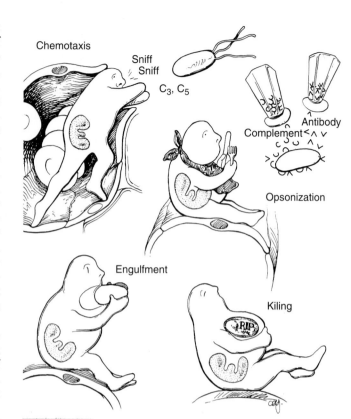

Figure 10–2 Summary of the steps involved in bacterial killing by the neutrophil. *A*, Neutrophil chemotaxis is governed by adhesion molecules on the neutrophils and endothelial cells, inflammatory cytokines, and chemotaxins such as C5a and interleukin-8. *B*, Bacteria are "prepared" or opsonized before engulfment (phagocytosis) occurs. *C*, The opsonized bacteria are engulfed by the neutrophil into endosomal compartments known as phagosomes. *D*, The neutrophil destroys the ingested bacteria by fusing its lysosome, containing potent microbicidal agents, with the phagosome. Both oxygen-dependent and oxygen-independent killing occurs in the phagolysosome.

agents with the phagosome. In the phagolysosome, bacterial killing occurs through both oxygen-dependent and oxygen-independent pathways.

The principal oxygen-dependent mechanisms involve the formation of ROIs by the enzyme NADPH oxidase. The active form of the enzyme is assembled in the cell membrane and catalyzes the reduction of molecular oxygen (O_2) to superoxide (O_2^-)—the so-called respiratory burst. Superoxide is converted to hydrogen peroxide (H_2O_2) by superoxide dismutase. H_2O_2 in turn can react with superoxide in the presence of iron or other metal to give the potent ROI hydroxyl radical (°OH). Alternatively, H_2O_2 can react with chloride (Cl^-) in the presence of myeloperoxidase, an enzyme found in the cytoplasmic granules, to give the highly reactive hypochlorous acid (HOCl). HOCl in turn reacts with endogenous nitrogen-containing compounds to form the powerful oxidizing agents chloramines, which account for much of the neutrophil's cytotoxicity.[110,144]

The oxygen-independent microbicidal pathway of the neutrophil is effected principally by a number of peptides contained in specific cytoplasmic granules. Among these are lysozyme, elastase, lactoferrin, cathepsin, and defensins. Many of these peptides act synergistically to promote microbial killing. For instance, defensins and elastase increase bacterial membrane permeability, allowing penetration by other microbicidal peptides or ROIs. However, as we show later, under certain circumstances, such as prior priming of the neutrophil by cytokines or the presence of a potent stimulus, the cytotoxic arsenal of the neutrophil may induce severe tissue injury through intense degranulation and indiscriminate fusion of specific granules (lysosomes) with the cell membrane (in addition to the phagosome), leading to the release of ROIs and other microbicidal agents into the surrounding microenvironment.

Monocytes-Macrophages

The monocyte-macrophage represents a complex, heterogeneous group of phenotypically related cells that arise from the same stem cell as the granulocyte. As such, the monocyte-macrophage exhibits many similarities with the neutrophil in host defense against microbes. The primordial stem cell gives rise to the monoblast, which differentiates into a promonocyte as it acquires specific granules in the bone marrow. Further maturation leads to the formation of the monocyte, which possesses enhanced phagocytic and immunologic abilities. Following their release into the bloodstream, the monocytes migrate to various tissues and organs, where they differentiate into mature macrophages, characterized by the acquisition of specific granules (enzymes) as well as receptors for growth factors and complement.[70,80,136] Although there are regional differences in their functional and metabolic properties, in general, tissue macrophages are able to recognize a wide variety of inflammatory and immunologic stimuli, including bacteria and their by-products, complement fragment, and cytokines. These stimuli are then processed and transduced into specific immunologic responses, resulting in the release of diverse cytokines as part of a coordinated attempt to promote tissue repair or effect cytotoxicity against microbes.

Macrophages are the principal effectors in the armamentarium against intracellular pathogens, including certain bacteria, mycobacteria, and plasmodia. In addition, they can phagocytose and kill many common bacteria, although with less efficiency than the neutrophil. Like neutrophils, they express adhesion molecules such as L-selectin as well as β_2 and β_1 integrins. The latter is an important distinction from the neutrophil because it permits the macrophage to migrate to sites of injury or inflammation in patients with β_2 integrin deficiency (leukocyte adhesion deficiency). Macrophages migrate to sites of inflammation or tissue injury in response to various chemotaxins, including complement (C5a), bacterial peptides, foreign antigens, and cytokines such as IL-1, TNF-α, and MCP-1. These cytokines can act in an autocrine (cell of origin) or paracrine (distant cell) fashion to recruit additional macrophages and other inflammatory cells to the sites of injury or infection. Ligand-receptor interactions (specific and nonspecific) lead to phagocytosis of bacteria, followed by intracellular killing. Antigenic fragments derived from these bacteria are processed by the macrophage and then presented to T lymphocytes in the context of major histocompatibility complex (MHC) class II molecules. This cognate interaction between macrophage and T cell elicits specific immune responses that amplify the cytokine (and cellular) response to further enhance microbicidal activity. This highly specialized function is one of the key distinguishing features of the macrophage in host defense against microbes.

The mechanisms of microbial killing used by the macrophage closely resemble those employed by the neutrophil. Bacteria are internalized in phagosomes and then killed by virtue of fusion of the phagosomes with lysosomes, with the release of cytotoxic substances (granules). Both oxygen-dependent and oxygen-independent mechanisms are used by the macrophage. Like the neutrophil, the macrophage produces ROIs, but in addition, it produces a substantial amount of the potent molecule nitric oxide (NO), which has been shown to have diverse biologic properties, including antimicrobial activity. Prior priming of the macrophage by LPS or IFN-γ, for instance, leads to increased production of both ROIs and NO—a phenomenon that may be beneficial for eliminating microbes but harmful if it is uncontrolled or directed at host tissues.

NO is the product of the conversion of arginine to citrulline by nitric oxide synthase (NOS). There are three isoforms of NOS: NOS-1 (neuronal NOS) and NOS-3 (endothelial NOS) are calcium dependent and are expressed constitutively at low levels; they produce picomolar amounts of NO. NOS-2 (also known as inducible NOS or iNOS) is usually absent except when induced in response to inflammatory mediators (e.g., LPS, cytokines); it is the principal isoform found in macrophages.[4,121] NO has been shown to have both cytotoxic and cytostatic activity against a wide range of microorganisms in vitro and in vivo; these include parasites, mycobacteria, fungi, viruses, bacteria, and chlamydia.[30] However, there is no clear evidence that human phagocytes produce sufficient amounts of NO to account for its antimicrobial activity.[121] In fact, evidence suggests that NO must react with ROIs to exert its cytotoxicity.[84] However, the precise nature of this reaction is not completely understood; under certain conditions NO may be cytostatic or cytotoxic, while under others it may be cytoprotective.[31,75,121]

Diverse molecular targets of NO have been identified. NO directly inhibits heme proteins such as myoglobin, hemoglobin, catalase, peroxidase, and cytochrome c, as well as nonheme iron proteins such as ferritin and ribonucleotide reductase, the rate-limiting enzyme in DNA synthesis.[103] Alternatively, NO may induce conformational changes in iron-sulfur linkages within the catalytic domain of enzymes involved in the mitochondrial electron transport chain, such as NADH–ubiquinone oxidoreductase, NADH–succinate oxidoreductase, and aconitase of the Krebs cycle.[103] In addition, NO may cause direct DNA damage through deamination reactions,[105] increased oxidative stress caused by the depletion of antioxidants such as thiols, or reactions with ROIs to form even more toxic metabolites such as peroxynitrite.[31] A potential consequence of NO-induced DNA strand break is the activation of the DNA repair enzyme poly(ADP) ribosyl transferase, which leads to a futile repair cycle resulting in depletion of reducing equivalents (NAD+)

and bioenergetic deprivation.[157] Stimuli that promote NO production in activated macrophages may also induce ROI generation.[67] NO, with its unpaired electron, preferentially reacts with other species possessing unpaired electrons, such as heme iron and nonheme iron proteins and superoxide. The more biologically relevant reactions of NO are listed in Table10-1.[67]

The biologic effects of NO can be classified as direct or indirect. The direct effects are those reactions whereby NO reacts specifically with the biologic target, such as metals or other radicals; the indirect effects are those whereby NO reacts first with oxygen or superoxide to form redox species, which then mediate alterations of macromolecules. The fastest and most biologically relevant reaction of NO is with O_2^- to produce the potent oxidant peroxynitrite ($ONOO^-$) (Table 10-1, Equation 1). At physiologic pH, $ONOO^-$ undergoes protonation to form the highly reactive peroxynitrous acid (ONOOH, not shown), which can (theoretically) undergo homolytic fission to form OH and NO_2. However, this latter reaction is thermodynamically unfavorable because these two free radicals react so rapidly together that the equilibrium lies almost exclusively to the left.[27] Evidence suggests that peroxynitrite is a key reactive nitrogen intermediate that is generated in inflammatory lesions in vivo and is responsible for some of the pathologic or cytopathic effects of NO.[27] NO may react with hemoglobin to form methemoglobin and nitrate, which is fairly innocuous. Alternatively, NO or $ONOO^-$ may react with metalloproteins to produce a nitrosonium cation (NO^+) intermediate, which may in turn oxidize reduced thiol (R—SH) to form S-nitrosothiol (R—SN≡O) (Equation 2). S-nitrosothiols are biologically active compounds that have been shown to be cytostatic for *S. typhimurium*[31] and can serve as NO donors (Equations 3a and 3b) or as NO^+ donors.[27,130] Release of bound iron from the reaction of NO or $ONOO^-$ with metalloproteins or Fe^{3+} (see Equation 2) may lead to further oxidative injury by providing the necessary catalyst for °OH formation in the Haber-Weiss reaction (Equation 4).

NO chemistry is quite complex in vitro. Under certain conditions, the reaction of NO with O_2^- to form $ONOO^-$ may result in a reduction of oxidant-mediated injury if

peroxynitrite decomposes to nitrate (see Equation 1). In fact, the interaction of NO and O_2^- results in decreased O_2^--mediated staphylococcal killing at early time points, whereas NO enhances killing during prolonged incubation periods.[75] Pacelli et al.[108] reported similar findings for *E. coli*. However, other mechanisms may augment the cytotoxic effect of NO. For instance, the normally innocuous end product of NO metabolism, nitrite (NO_2^-), can be converted to nitrous acid at pH 5.0, which is commonly attained in the phagolysosome.[21] Nitrous acid, in turn, can give rise to NO. In fact, this reaction is associated with natural resistance-associated macrophage protein 1, a gene that confers resistance to certain microbes.[104] The gene permits cells that normally do not produce NO to make the molecule by transporting NO_2^- generated by other cells in the vicinity into their own acidic lysosome or phagolysosome, where it can undergo protonation to give rise to nitrous acid. Nitrous acid can then dismutate to give rise to NO. Thus microbes can be killed in phagosomes of cells that do not make NO.

From the foregoing discussion it is apparent that the antimicrobial properties of NO are mediated principally by $ONOO^-$, NO^+, OH, and R—SN≡O. However, sustained overproduction of these compounds by the activated macrophage may also lead to cellular injury and multisystem organ dysfunction or SIRS.

Lymphocytes

Although neutrophils and monocytes-macrophages represent the major effectors of the host defense against microbes, certain microorganisms, especially the intracellular pathogens, are able to evade their cytotoxic arsenal. Therefore, these organisms must be eliminated through different means. The lymphocytes and, to a lesser extent, the natural killer (NK) cells form the secondary line of defense against such microbes.

Lymphocytes arise from a hematopoietic stem cell in the bone marrow. Early in the differentiation pathway, the lymphoid progenitor cell undergoes maturation in one of two distinct compartments, where it acquires its phenotypic and functional characteristics. Certain cells leave the bone marrow to undergo a process of "education" or

---

TABLE 10–1 Nitric Oxide Reactions

1. °NO + °O_2^- (Superoxide) $\longrightarrow$ $ONOO^-$ (Peroxynitrite) $\xleftarrow{\ \ }$ $\xrightarrow{H^4}$ °OH (Hydroxyl Radical) + °NO_2 (Nitrogen Dioxide)

    $\downarrow$

    NO_3^- (Nitrate)

2. °NO or ONNO$^-$ + Fe^{+3} $\longrightarrow$ Fe^{+2} NO^+ $\xrightarrow{R—SN}$ RS—N≡O

3. a. RS—N≡O + °O_2^- H^+ $\longrightarrow$ R—SH + °O_2 + °NO

    b. °NO + °O_2^- $\longrightarrow$ ONNO$^-$

4. °O_2^- + H_2O_2 $\xrightarrow{Fc}$ O_2 + OH^- + OH

maturation in the thymus. These mature T cells migrate from the thymus to reside in peripheral lymphoid organs such as the spleen, lymph nodes, and intestinal Peyer's patches. Other lymphoid progenitor cells undergo maturation either in the bone marrow or in the fetal liver, where they become committed to immunoglobulin synthesis (B cells).

Both B cells and T cells play an important role in the elimination of microbes. B cells in particular produce opsonizing antibodies that facilitate phagocytosis of encapsulated organisms. They also secrete other immunoglobulins, such as IgA, that play a central role in mucosal immunity by preventing bacterial adherence and invasion. In addition, B cells participate in antibody-dependent cell-mediated cytotoxicity. T lymphocytes, in contrast, are the principal effectors of cell-mediated immunity against intracellular pathogens. T-cell-mediated killing requires (1) recognition of the inciting antigen or microbe, (2) cellular activation, (3) clonal expansion, and (4) targeted killing. Antigen presentation and recognition are governed in part by a family of normally occurring cell surface proteins known as MHC proteins. There are two classes of MHC proteins: class I, which is expressed in virtually all nucleated cells, and class II, which is expressed primarily in antigen-presenting cells such as macrophages, dendritic cells, and B lymphocytes. These cells phagocytose bacteria, processing or breaking down the organism into smaller fragments or peptides that are then bound to MHC class II proteins and inserted into the cell membrane of the antigen-presenting cells. T cells bearing the same MHC molecules are able to recognize this MHC-plus-peptide complex on the antigen-presenting cell. Interaction between this complex and specific ligands on T helper (TH) cells (CD4+) leads to cytokine production, recruitment of additional phagocytic (inflammatory) cells, and proliferation of different classes of lymphocytes: B cells, CD8+ cytotoxic T lymphocytes (CTLs), and TH cells. Ultimately, microbial killing is effected primarily by the CTLs. Infected cells that cannot process antigen in the context of an MHC class II protein form a complex between MHC class I molecules in the cell and antigenic peptides derived from the invading pathogen. This complex is readily recognized and targeted for destruction by the CTLs. Thus, although only antigen-presenting cells can process antigen in the context of MHC class II molecules and elicit a TH response, all cells infected by an intracellular pathogen can present foreign antigen in association with MHC class I molecules, which serve as the target for the CTLs.

Two important events are required for T-cell activation: stimulation via the T-cell receptor signal-transducing protein complex CD3, and simultaneous cross-linking of the CD4 or CD8 ligand to the appropriate MHC-plus-peptide complex on an antigen-presenting cell or infected cell. Signal transduction initiates a cascade of events leading to calcium mobilization, activation of protein kinases, and transcription and translation of specific genes encoding proteins that can help eliminate the pathogen. Such proteins include perforins and serine proteases in CTLs and various cytokines in TH cells. Two classes of TH cells have been described based on their cytokine profile: TH1 cells produce IL-2 and IFN-γ, while TH2 cells produce IL-4, IL-5, IL-10, and IL-13. Other cytokines, such as IL-3 and granulocyte-macrophage colony-stimulating factor, are produced by both TH1 and TH2 cells. Secreted cytokines bind specific receptors on target cells and activate signal transduction pathways, resulting in the elaboration of new proteins and cellular proliferation or differentiation, with acquisition of a distinct effector phenotype based on the class of cytokine released. For instance, TH1 cytokines evoke primarily a T-cell-mediated response characterized in part by recruitment of macrophages to the site of infection, followed by macrophage activation by IFN-γ.[22,101] In contrast, TH2 cytokines shift the balance toward a humoral (B-cell) response. Activated CTLs bind to cells expressing MHC-plus-peptide complex and release cytotoxic granules such as perforin, which can create a "hole" in the cell membrane and lead to osmotic lysis. Alternatively, such CTLs may release serine proteases that induce apoptosis (programmed cell death) in the infected cell without affecting the effector cell (CTL).[65,91,113]

Similar to the CTL, NK cells, which represent a variant of the lymphocyte family, can also employ granule exocytosis to kill infected target cells. In addition, these cells possess Fc receptors for immunoglobulin and therefore can participate in antibody-dependent, cell-mediated cytotoxicity.

Humoral Factors

The previous sections emphasized the importance of cell-mediated immunity in the host defense against microbes. However, it should be apparent that the cellular response is a highly complex phenomenon that is often initiated and optimized by diverse humoral factors, including immunoglobulins, complement activation, and cytokines.

Immunoglobulins

Immunoglobulins or antibodies represent a class of proteins that are synthesized by mature B lymphocytes or plasma cells, mainly as a result of cognate interaction between a TH cell and an antigen-presenting cell bearing an MHC-plus-peptide complex. This interaction may lead to cytokine synthesis and B-cell proliferation and maturation, with production of distinct classes of immunoglobulin. The primary role of antibodies in the host defense against microbes is to prevent bacterial adherence to, and subsequent invasion of, susceptible host cells. The mechanisms involved in this process include opsonization of the microbe to facilitate phagocytosis, complement activation with deposition of complement fragments on bacterial membranes to further enhance phagocytosis and subsequent bacterial killing, and neutralization of intrinsic microbial toxins or virulence factors to impede bacterial attachment to cell surfaces. There are five major classes of immunoglobulins: IgA, IgG, IgM, IgD, and IgE. Among these groups, IgG, IgM, and IgA are the predominant antibodies that mediate the host defense against microbes.

IgM is the largest of the immunoglobulins. It is the main component of the initial response to infection or antigenic stimulus. As such, it has a half-life of only 5 to 6 days, and its level declines steadily as IgG levels increase. Because of its size, IgM is found exclusively in the intravascular space, serving as an efficient bacterial agglutinin and as a potent activator of the complement system.

IgG is perhaps the most abundant antibody, constituting nearly 85% of serum immunoglobulins. It is found in both intravascular and extravascular (tissue) spaces. It is the only immunoglobulin that crosses the placenta from the mother to the fetus. IgG is the predominant class of antibody directed against bacteria and viruses. The biologic potency of the molecule resides in its ability to opsonize bacteria by binding the antigen with its Fab component, while simultaneously binding the Fc receptor on the neutrophil, monocyte, or macrophage with its own Fc component. Moreover, IgG aggregates can activate the complement system.

Antibodies of the IgA isotype play a critical role in local mucosal immunity. They are synthesized by plasma cells within lymphoid tissue situated subjacent to the epithelial surfaces where they are secreted. IgA is released as a dimer and acquires a secretory component as it passes through the epithelial cell to exit at the mucosal surface in the form of secretory IgA. The latter serves as an antiseptic paint that binds pathogenic microbes and thus prevents their attachment, colonization, and subsequent invasion of tissue. Note, however, that IgG, IgM, and, to a lesser extent, IgE can also play a role in local mucosal immunity, especially in patients with congenital IgA deficiency.

Complement System

Although antibodies are effective at recognizing antigenic determinants on microbial pathogens, they are unable to independently kill the microorganisms. Following opsonization, they must rely on phagocytes to ingest the microbe and on complement activation to further enhance or augment their opsonic ability to neutralize and ultimately kill the ingested pathogen. There are two distinct pathways for complement activation: classic and alternative (Fig. 10-3). Antigen-antibody complexes are the predominant initiators of the classic pathway. In contrast, bacterial cell wall fragments, endotoxin (or LPS), cell surfaces, burned and injured tissue, and complex polysaccharides are capable of activating the

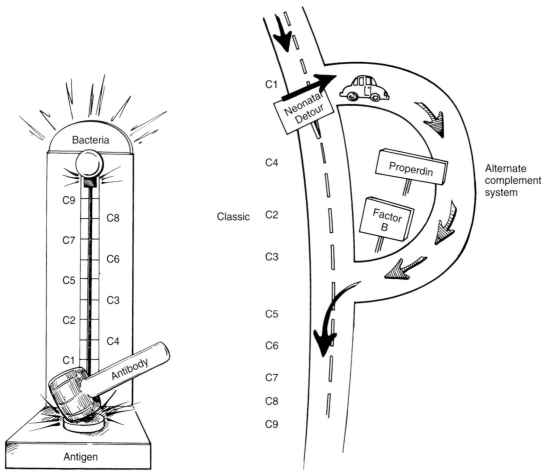

Figure 10–3 The classic and alternative pathways of complement activation. The classic pathway is activated by antigen-antibody complexes. The alternative (properdin) pathway is activated by numerous factors, including bacterial cell wall fragments and lipopolysaccharide. The most critical point in the complement cascade occurs at C3, where both pathways converge to form C3a and C3b. C3b can lead to dramatic amplification of the complement system. Further, C3b is a potent opsonin and activates the distal components of the cascade.

alternative (properdin) pathway. Stimulation through either pathway initiates a cascade of events that can lead to marked complement activation as a result of an elaborate amplification process. The most critical point in this cascade occurs at C3, where both pathways converge to form C3a and C3b. C3a is both a vasodilator and a chemotaxin for phagocytes. The C3b molecule, in contrast, is the most critical component of the complement cascade because this enzyme permits dramatic amplification of the system by facilitating further cleavage of C3 to C3a and C3b, as well as enhanced C3b production via the alternative pathway. Moreover, C3b is the most potent biologic opsonin, with cell surface receptors present on most phagocytes. Deposition of C3b on the surface of bacteria can promote its lysis by activating the distal components of the complement cascade (C8 and C9), which insert into and damage the cell membrane, resulting in osmotic lysis. In the process, another even more potent chemotaxin, C5a, is released that is also capable of inducing a respiratory burst in the phagocyte and thus facilitate bacterial killing.

Cytokines

The mediators that orchestrate or regulate the complex interactions among the various cellular effectors in the cytotoxic arsenal against microbes are generally known as cytokines. They represent a heterogeneous class of glycoproteins that are secreted by a variety of cells, including neutrophils, monocytes-macrophages, B and T lymphocytes, NK cells, endothelial cells, and fibroblasts. These cells synthesize and release cytokines de novo in response to inflammatory and antigenic stimuli such as LPS. Because of their potent biologic activity, their production, secretion, and duration of activity are closely regulated, especially at the messenger RNA (mRNA) level. Cytokines typically exert their functions in a paracrine, autocrine, or endocrine fashion by binding specific receptors on the surface of adjacent, originating, or distant target cells, respectively. Interaction between a cytokine and its receptor leads to signal transduction, resulting in new gene transcription, mRNA translation, and protein synthesis. The last may evoke phenotypic changes in the target cell, priming it for a cytotoxic effector function, for instance; alternatively, it may down-regulate or up-regulate the production of other cytokines. In general, there is extensive pleiotropy and redundancy in cytokine function. Some cytokines serve to amplify the inflammatory response, while others function to limit its extent. Proinflammatory cytokines such as TNF-α, IL-1, IL-6, IL-8, IL-11, and IL-18 share a number of similar properties; other cytokines that confer more specific immunity against certain pathogens, such as IL-2, IL-4, IL-12, and IL-13, also exhibit a number of similarities. Anti-inflammatory cytokines such as IL-10 and transforming growth factor-β neutralize the biologic activities of the proximal mediators of inflammation—the monocytes-macrophages and their secretory products.

TNF-α is one of the earliest inflammatory mediators released in response to infection. The predominant source of TNF-α is the monocyte-macrophage, although NK cells, mast cells, and some activated T cells also produce it, but to a lesser extent. TNF-α exerts a number of important functions in the inflammatory response. At low levels, it may (1) enhance endothelial cell adhesiveness for leukocytes; (2) promote neutrophil chemotaxis or recruitment to sites of inflammation; (3) stimulate the production of other proinflammatory cytokines that mimic TNF function, such as IL-1, IL-6, and IL-8; (4) prime neutrophils and monocytes-macrophages for microbial killing; and (5) up-regulate the expression of MHC class I molecules on target cells to facilitate killing. However, excess or uncontrolled TNF production, as occurs in overwhelming sepsis, may contribute to profound hemodynamic instability due to cardiovascular collapse, depressed myocardial contractility, and disseminated intravascular coagulation. It should be noted, however, that soluble TNF-α receptors are readily detected in the serum of trauma patients with markedly elevated TNF-α levels and thus may help limit the deleterious effects of excess TNF-α.[64]

IL-1 is released relatively early during the inflammatory response to infection or injury. It is produced by monocytes-macrophages and by epithelial, endothelial, and dendritic cells in response to endotoxin challenge or TNF stimulation. There are two biologically active forms of the molecule: IL-1α, which may be membrane associated, and IL-1β, which is active in soluble form. They share similar properties with TNF-α, including induction of other cytokines such as IL-2, IL-6, and IL-8. However, unlike TNF-α, they exert little or no effect on MHC class I expression. Nor do they play a role in hemodynamic collapse, perhaps due to concomitant release of IL-1 receptor antagonist, which shares structural homology with IL-1α and IL-1β.

IL-6 is the most important regulator of hepatic production of acute phase proteins. It is produced by a variety of cells, including mononuclear phagocytes, TH2 cells, and fibroblasts, in response to tissue injury, infection, TNF, and IL-1. It stimulates B-cell differentiation and enhances CTL maturation. IL-6 acts through a membrane-bound receptor that can shed and continue to regulate IL-6 activity away from the site of production.[72]

IL-8 is secreted by monocytes-macrophages, T cells, endothelial cells, and platelets in response to inflammation, IL-1, and TNF. It is one of the most potent chemotactic and activating factors for neutrophils. IL-8 belongs to a family of chemoattractants that includes other chemokines such as MCP-1, -2, and –3; macrophage inflammatory protein (MIP-1a, MIP-1b); and RANTES (regulated on activation, normal T expressed and secreted). These mediators are released early in inflammation, mainly by monocytes-macrophages but also by neutrophils and platelets. MIP-1a and MCP-1 may act in an autocrine fashion to recruit additional mononuclear phagocytes to sites of inflammation, thus potentially amplifying the inflammatory response. Another proinflammatory macrophage product, migration inhibitory factor, appears to be induced by TNF at sites of inflammation and serves to "trap" macrophages at those sites and elicit further TNF-α production by them.[64] RANTES is a lymphocyte-derived chemoattractant that promotes macrophage chemotaxis, up-regulates adhesion molecules, and enhances the release of inflammatory mediators.[64] Other chemoattractants include PAF, which is secreted by endothelial cells and macrophages, and leukotriene B$_4$. In addition to serving as a chemoattractant for neutrophils, PAF up-regulates CD11b/CD18 (ß$_2$ integrin) on the neutrophil.[87] In general, the chemoattractants not only recruit phagocytes to sites of inflammation but also appear to prime these cells for subsequent cytotoxic effector function.[77,117,153]

Other cytokines that play an important role in the elimination of invading microbial pathogens include products of TH1 cells, such as IL-2 and IFN-γ, as well as products of TH2 cells, such as IL-4 and IL-13. In general, TH1 cytokines are produced in response to bacterial, viral, or protozoan infections, and TH2 cytokines are secreted mostly in response to metazoa or allergens.[122,123] IL-2, the prototypical T-cell growth factor, directly amplifies the immune response by inducing cellular proliferation. It also augments killing by activating NK cells. IFN-γ is perhaps one of the most important macrophage activating factors. It stimulates the macrophage to express MHC class II molecules, which is necessary for antigen processing and for amplification of the immune response. In addition, it induces NOS activity (NOS-2), which is critical for intracellular killing of invading pathogens.[30,36] IFN-γ may enhance microbial killing by inducing TNF-α production and TNF-α receptor expression by macrophages and by activating NK cells. IFN-γ is also produced by activated CTLs in response to IL-2 and antigen expressed in the context of MHC class I molecules and by NK cells in response to IL-12.

IL-12, primarily a macrophage product, is the most potent inducer of IFN-γ production by NK cells. In addition, it influences the uncommitted TH cell to differentiate into the TH1 phenotype, secreting IL-2 and IFN-γ.[51] IL-12 can support most of the functions performed by IL-2, except perhaps its proliferative effect. Therefore, IL-12 plays an important role in the elimination of intracellular organisms.

The role of TH2 cytokines such as IL-4 and IL-13 is less clear. Although they partly promote monocyte differentiation and may induce the expression of adhesion molecules in the endothelium, they are mostly responsible for immunoglobulin isotype switching in B cells, leading predominantly to IgG4 and IgE production.

Often there is no direct correlation between plasma cytokine levels and local tissue events. This finding may be due to the presence of anti-inflammatory or regulatory cytokines that target the initiators of the inflammatory cascade. For instance, the IL-1 receptor antagonist and soluble receptor to TNF-α neutralize the biologic activity of IL-1β and TNF-α, respectively.[25,42,64] The TH2 cytokine, IL-10, down-regulates macrophage function by suppressing TNF-α and IL-1 receptor antagonist production.[25,137] It also impedes the macrophage's ability to amplify the immune response as an antigen-presenting cell by down-regulating class II MHC molecule expression.[64] Transforming growth factor-β released by degranulating platelets and activated macrophages may serve as an autocrine down-regulator of macrophage function. Similarly, prostaglandin E$_2$, catecholamines, and glucocorticoids, which are released in significant quantities in response to injury and inflammation, have been shown to suppress macrophage function.[64] The exact mechanisms of this suppression are still undefined, although in the case of catecholamines, it may involve increased IL-10 production[155]; in the case of glucocorticoids, it may involve decreased IFN-γ, TNF-α, and IL-1β production.[60,76,140]

In addition to the foregoing regulatory cytokines, recent evidence suggests the existence of another class of proteins that suppress cytokine signal transduction.[79] Known as suppressors of cytokine signaling (SOCS), they belong to a family of proteins that negatively regulate cytokine signal transduction. They signal through Janus tyrosine kinases and signal transducer and activators of transcription. The biologic result is attenuation of the cytokine response. Little is known about the downstream targets of SOCS, but clearly, elucidation of this pathway will offer potential therapeutic targets.

Cytokine production and signaling are central to the sepsis response. Yet, under similar clinical and demographic circumstances, individuals may exhibit distinct responses to an identical stimulus. Although it may be simplistic to say that all individuals are intrinsically different, in reality, it appears that the uniqueness of the genetic machinery from one individual to the next may explain the distinct variations in cytokine responses between two similar patients. One possible explanation is differential protein expression between the two patients. For example, whereas a traumatic insult in one patient may lead to overwhelming sepsis and result in admission to the intensive care unit, another individual may exhibit a more attenuated response characterized by fever and tachycardia for a couple of hours, followed by resolution of the symptoms. Proteins may be expressed differently for a number of reasons, but one significant factor may be the gene structure of the individual. Gene polymorphisms or single nucleotide polymorphisms are differences in nucleic acid base pairs that occur every 100 bases. The change in base pairs that occurs in the promoter region of the gene may lead to over- or underproduction of a gene product. For instance, a patient with sickle cell disease, which is associated with a gene polymorphism, may have a devastating hematologic disease, but when this same individual is exposed to the agent that causes malaria (*Plasmodium falciparum*), the deviation in genetic programming protects the patient from developing malaria. Recent evidence suggests that the presence of one gene polymorphism may serve as a marker for additional protective gene polymorphisms.[134] Cytokine gene polymorphisms may explain differences in the inflammatory response among individuals.[151] There are ongoing studies in this area, and although the complexity continues to mount, it is hoped that supercomputers will simplify the massive amount of data and provide a concise and simple readout for estimating the cytokine variability of an individual. Such advances are likely to provide clinicians with data that increase their vigilance or assist them in making rational therapeutic decisions to combat pathogenic insults, similar to the way one now uses coagulation parameters before performing an operation.

Neonatal Host Defense

In general, neonates, especially premature infants, show increased susceptibility to bacterial infections and sepsis.

This predisposition is closely linked to intrinsic deficiencies in the neonatal host defense apparatus. In this section we review some of the salient features that may account for the neonate's vulnerability to infection.

At term, production of neutrophils is near the maximal level in human neonates. Neutrophils constitute approximately 60% of circulating leukocytes; 15% of these neutrophils are immature (bands). These percentages are substantially lower in premature infants. Perhaps one of the most important factors in neonates' increased propensity for bacterial infections is their relative inability to significantly increase the levels of circulating neutrophils in response to stress or infection, owing primarily to a limited neutrophil storage pool and, to a lesser extent, to increased margination of neutrophils.[24,139] In fact, experimental data from neonatal rats suggest that their neutrophil storage pool is only 20% to 30% of that in adults.[24] Increased production of neutrophils in response to infection is dependent on increased formation of myeloid progenitor stem cells, a process that takes at least 5 to 7 days before it can lead to de novo neutrophil production. As a result, systemic infections often lead to severe neutropenia because neonates cannot sufficiently augment the numbers of circulating neutrophils. In fact, the relative degree of depletion of the neutrophil storage pool is a predictor of fatal outcome in neonatal sepsis.[24]

In addition to an already diminished storage pool, neonatal neutrophils show decreased adhesion to activated endothelium.[6,125] This process may be due to decreased L-selectin expression on the surface of neonatal neutrophils and an inability to up-regulate cell surface β_2 integrin.[6,125] Consequently, the neutrophils are unable to form the high-affinity adhesion to the endothelium that is necessary to effectively respond to a chemotactic gradient and migrate into tissues at sites of inflammation. In fact, several studies have shown that chemotaxis of neonatal neutrophils is substantially less than that of adult neutrophils.[66,114] Further, accumulating evidence suggests that abnormal signal transduction following the binding of chemotactic receptors to membrane receptors on neonatal neutrophils may also contribute to impaired chemotaxis.

Under normal conditions, neonatal neutrophils bind, ingest, and kill bacteria as effectively as adult neutrophils do. However, in the presence of a suboptimal concentration of opsonins, neonatal neutrophils are less efficient at phagocytosis[96]—an important consideration, because neonatal serum is deficient in opsonins.

Neonatal neutrophils show normal production of superoxide but a relative decrease in the amount of hydroxyl radical and in the number of specific granules (defensins).[5] Therefore, they may exhibit decreased oxygen-dependent and oxygen-independent microbial killing.[5] However, the deficiencies in microbicidal activity appear to be less critical than the substantial reduction in the neonatal neutrophil storage pool and the impairment in neutrophil chemotaxis, except perhaps in the presence of a high bacterial load, when efficient microbial killing becomes crucial.

Although the neonatal neutrophil storage pool may be diminished, the number of monocytes per blood volume in term infants appears to be equal to or greater than that of adults.[23] However, migration of these monocytes to sites of inflammation is significantly delayed compared with adults. Possible explanations for this relative delay in migration include decreased generation of chemoattractant factors for monocytes, impaired monocyte chemotaxis (as has been shown for neutrophils), and inability to up-regulate adhesion molecules on the surface of neonatal monocytes. Yet numerous studies have shown that neonatal monocytes have normal chemotaxis; others suggest that they may have normal migratory capacity but fail to properly orient toward the chemotactic gradient. Similarly, there are several conflicting reports regarding the expression of adhesion molecules on the surface of neonatal monocytes. Some studies show increased expression of β_2 integrins, while others suggest that these molecules are down-regulated in activated and resting neonatal monocytes. Nevertheless, once they reach the site of active inflammation, neonatal monocytes phagocytose and kill bacteria as effectively as adult monocytes do. They probably use similar microbicidal mechanisms as adult monocytes, as they can generate comparable levels of ROIs. However, data on NO production by neonatal monocytes relative to adult monocytes are scant. Activated neonatal monocytes and macrophages produce substantially less IL-6 and TNF-α than their adult counterparts. IL-1 production, in contrast, is equivalent.

Term neonates have a substantially greater number of circulating T lymphocytes than adults do. They also have a greater proportion of CD4+ versus CD8+ T cells compared with adults. These T cells express predominantly a virgin phenotype secondary to their relative lack of exposure to foreign antigens. However, they proliferate effectively in response to mitogenic stimuli. Stimulated neonatal T cells produce large quantities of IL-2. In contrast, production of other cytokines such as TNF-α, IFN-γ, IL-3, IL-4, IL-5, and IL-10 is either moderately or significantly suppressed.[40,41,83] Neonates show decreased T-cell-mediated (CTL) cytotoxicity; this phenomenon may be due in part to the relative lack of prior antigenic exposure and the deficiency in cytokine production. Alternatively, the relative decrease in T-cell function may be the result of impaired monocyte-macrophage chemotaxis, resulting in diminished MHC-restricted cognate interactions between antigen-presenting cells and TH cells. Thus cytokine production is significantly reduced, and the inflammatory response is not amplified.

Term neonates also show relative immaturity of B-cell function and development. Although neonatal B cells can differentiate into IgM-secreting plasma cells, they do not differentiate into IgG- or IgA-secreting plasma cells until much later. IgM is more abundant in neonatal than in adult secretions. In contrast, virtually all circulating neonatal serum IgG is derived from maternal placental transfer. In fact, it is not until the third or fourth month of life that neonatal IgG production begins to account for a greater proportion of circulating IgG. As a result, the fetus is protected against most infectious agents for which the mother has adequate levels of circulating IgG antibodies, but not against those microbes that elicit a different immunoglobulin isotype, such as *E. coli* and *Salmonella*. Premature neonates are particularly vulnerable to such infections because they do not receive sufficient maternal IgG. IgM and secretory IgA, which is detected in neonatal secretions within the first week of life and is abundant in breast milk, may provide compensatory protection against bacterial infection.

In term neonates, the percentage of NK cells, which play an important role against intracellular pathogens by promoting target cell lysis in a non-MHC-restricted fashion, is similar to that of the adult. However, they are functionally and phenotypically immature (CD56-).[74,93] At birth, their lytic potential is only 50% of that of adult NK cells, and it does not reach mature levels until late in infancy. This phenomenon may be partly due to decreased cytokine production (especially IFN-γ) in neonates, as previously discussed.

In general, because of their reduced levels of immunoglobulins, neonates rely primarily on the alternative (antibody-independent) pathway of complement activation (see Fig. 10-3). However, a substantial proportion of term and preterm neonates exhibits a significant reduction in components of both the classic and the alternative pathways of complement activation. The level of C9, a terminal component of the complement system that is critical for killing gram-negative organisms, is diminished, especially in preterm infants. The relative opsonic capacity of both term and preterm neonates is also impaired. This observation may be the result of inefficient cross-linking of the opsonin C3b after it has been deposited on the microorganism. Alternatively, it may reflect diminished levels of fibronectin, which plays an important role in cell adhesion and facilitates the binding of certain bacteria to phagocytes. Neonates also show decreased production of the potent chemotactic factor C5a. These defects further predispose term and preterm neonates to bacterial infections, because in addition to their already reduced neutrophil storage pool and their depressed levels of immunoglobulin, they cannot effectively use the most potent biologic opsonin, C3b, which is also responsible for amplification of the complement pathway; in addition, they have a decreased influx of phagocytes and impaired killing at the sites of infection owing to the decrease in C5a and in C9.

PATHOGENESIS OF SYSTEMIC INFLAMMATORY RESPONSE SYNDROME

The development of clinical infection is largely governed by complex, intricate interactions between the intrinsic host defense mechanisms and the virulence factors of the microbial pathogen. Failure of the immune system to prevent bacterial invasion results in proliferation of the microorganism at the portal of entry or nidus of infection. Such infections initially evoke a localized, well-orchestrated inflammatory response aimed at destroying the microbe. It consists primarily of the local release of inflammatory cytokines such as TNF-α and IL-1β by macrophages activated at least in part by bacteria and their by-products, such as endotoxin (LPS). The lipid A moiety of LPS binds LBP, a 60-kD protein normally present in human serum. This complex, in turn, binds the CD14 molecule, a receptor found on macrophages, neutrophils,

and endothelial cells, and then interacts with the TLR on these cells to induce the release of cytokines such as TNF-α, IL-6, and PAF (Fig.10-4). LPS-LBP binds with TLR and signals through mitogen-activated kinases.[14] Interestingly, there may be an age-dependent decrease in LPS-induced cytokine production in macrophages, suggesting that younger individuals may mount a more exuberant proinflammatory response.[14] These molecules up-regulate the expression of adhesion molecules on endothelial cells and neutrophils. Subsequent release of IL-8 helps recruit and activate additional inflammatory cells, especially neutrophils, at the site of infection. Neutrophil migration results from rolling, adhesion, and diapedesis through the endothelium toward the chemotactic gradient. The activated neutrophil phagocytoses the microorganism at the site of infection and kills it within its phagolysosomes. Other exogenous factors, such as antibiotics, may help control or eradicate infections. However, failure to control infections or a significant delay in treating them may result in bacterial proliferation, with systemic (bloodstream) invasion and further activation and amplification of the inflammatory cascade. Occasionally, this latter phenomenon occurs even after successful treatment of the infectious process. The hallmark of this uncontrolled stimulation of the inflammatory cascade is SIRS, characterized by profound clinical alterations in vital signs, homeostasis, and metabolism, with attendant organ dysfunction.

The diagnosis of SIRS in older children and adults requires the presence of at least two of the following clinical criteria: (1) body temperature greater than 38°C or less than 36°C; (2) heart rate greater than 90 beats per minute; (3) respiratory rate greater than 20 breaths per minute or a PaCO$_2$ less than 32 mm Hg; and (4) white blood cell count greater than 12,000 cells/mm^3 or less than 4000 cells/mm^3, or the presence of greater than 10% bands. Many noninfectious entities, such as trauma, burns, and acute pancreatitis, can stimulate SIRS. As a result, the term *sepsis* is used when SIRS has an infectious cause. Risk factors for the development of progressive organ dysfunction in patients with SIRS include the presence of a persistent focus of infection or inflammation, as in an undrained abscess; persistent hypoperfusion; and persistence of the inflammatory response itself.

An uncontrolled inflammatory response leads to sustained cytokine release (TNF-α and IL-1β) by activated macrophages. Systemic release of cytokines up-regulates adhesion molecules in endothelial cells of distant organs, such as the lung, and thus may potentiate neutrophil-mediated acute lung injury. IL-8 recruits and activates neutrophils; the latter may cause direct cytotoxicity to the endothelial cells through premature degranulation and release of cytotoxic granules or ROIs. This phenomenon results in pulmonary interstitial injury, capillary leak, and respiratory failure. In addition, neutrophils may persist in the circulation of patients with SIRS by virtue of increased shedding of L-selectin,[94] as well as a reduced rate of spontaneous apoptosis, which may be related to IL-6 or PAF release.[15] As a result of their increased half-life, these activated neutrophils can mediate injury in a variety of organs, resulting in capillary leak syndrome, decreased perfusion, and end-organ damage.

Figure 10–4 Pathogenesis of systemic inflammatory response syndrome (SIRS). Bacterial invasion secondary to barrier failure leads to the local release of lipopolysaccharide (LPS), with consequent formation of an LPS–lipopolysaccharide binding protein (LBP)–CD14–Toll-like receptor 4 (TLR-4) complex on neutrophils, macrophages, and endothelial cells, resulting in cellular activation. Inflammatory cytokines are released, up-regulate adhesion molecules, and promote chemotaxis of neutrophils and macrophages. (The complement system, clotting cascade, and lymphocyte population may also be activated, but this is not shown in the diagram.) The activated cells release microbicidal agents typically designed for bacterial killing, but they may be injurious and promote distant organ injury and SIRS if the inflammatory process is "uncontrolled." ICAM, intercellular adhesion molecule; IL, interleukin; MCP, monocyte chemotactic protein; MIP, macrophage inflammatory protein; NO, nitric oxide; PAF, platelet-activating factor; PECAM, platelet–endothelial cell adhesion molecule; ROI, reactive oxygen intermediate (or species); TNF, tumor necrosis factor.

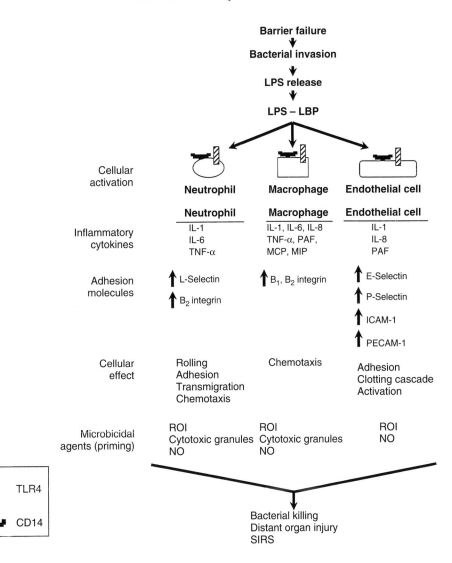

Tissue hypoxia further amplifies this inflammatory cascade by stimulating additional release of TNF-α, IL-1, and IL-8 by macrophages and by up-regulating adhesion molecules on both neutrophils and endothelial cells.[9,119,145]

Numerous other mechanisms may help perpetuate the inflammatory response. For instance, both TNF-α and IL-1β can activate a transcriptional regulatory factor, nuclear factor kappa B, which binds to the promoter region of each gene. Such activation results in increased gene transcription and additional production of these proinflammatory cytokines.[1,78,86,152] Further, TNF-α and IL-1 can activate macrophages in an autocrine fashion to produce additional proinflammatory cytokines. Interaction between macrophages and CD4+ TH lymphocytes results in production of IFN-γ, which is one of the most potent macrophage activators. Thus, through these varied interactions, the macrophage is able to achieve a self-sustaining inflammatory phenotype that can perpetuate the inflammatory cascade. In fact, a retrospective analysis of the cytokine profile of 97 septic patients revealed that the magnitude of the systemic inflammatory response (defined as the plasma concentrations of inflammatory mediators) clearly affected the mortality rate.[15,20] Last,

genetic polymorphism within the TNF locus may influence plasma TNF-α levels during infection and therefore may affect outcome. Patients who are homozygotes for the *TNFB1* allele have reduced levels of TNF-α in their plasma and a lower mortality rate after infection than do patients who are homozygotes for the *TNFB2* allele or heterozygotes for *TNFB1* and *TNFB2*.[131]

Physiologic and Metabolic Consequences

The most prominent clinical and hemodynamic alterations in patients with SIRS or sepsis are reduced systemic vascular resistance and decreased peripheral extraction of oxygen.[109] Therefore, a consistent increase in oxygen delivery or supply is required to maintain adequate tissue oxygenation. The decrease in systemic vascular resistance may be initiated in part by NO as well as by prostacyclin or complement activation. However, one report failed to demonstrate a role for inducible NOS in the hemodynamic decompensation seen after untreated hemorrhagic shock.[76] The increase in oxygen delivery is achieved by increasing cardiac output and by increasing minute ventilation. Patients who are unable to balance the need for increased oxygen delivery and increased demand, owing to depressed myocardial function, pulmonary failure, or reduced cellular metabolism secondary to underlying organ dysfunction, have an increased risk of mortality. These patients may exhibit marked anaerobic metabolism with excess lactate production.[12]

A significant loss of lean body mass typifies the patient with SIRS or sepsis. Activation of the neurohumoral axis by proinflammatory cytokines results in the release of adrenocorticotropic hormone, cortisol, catecholamines, and other gluconeogenic hormones, such as glucagon, to increase energy substrate. Skeletal muscle breakdown occurs as the body attempts to generate the substrate necessary for energy production, hepatic gluconeogenesis, and protein synthesis. The febrile response, which is most likely mediated by TNF-α, IL-1, and IL-6, further augments the catabolic rate. This increased catabolic rate is relatively unresponsive to exogenous amino acids, although protein synthesis in the liver does respond to an exogenous supply of amino acids. TNF-α and IL-1 are also known to reduce lipoprotein lipase activity,[85,133] which leads to total-body lipogenesis, as well as decreased peripheral clearance of triglycerides.

Neonatal Sepsis

Neonates are particularly vulnerable to bacterial infections during the first 4 weeks of life as a result of intrinsic deficiencies in their host defense systems. These "compromised" hosts are unable to efficiently localize bacterial infections. As a result, they are at risk of developing bacteremia or meningitis, which may lead to full-blown neonatal sepsis. Bone's criteria have been modified to more accurately define the sepsis syndrome in the pediatric population. They include (1) clinical evidence of sepsis, with fever (rectal temperature >38.0°C) or hypothermia (<35.6°C); (2) tachycardia (heart rate >95th percentile for age); (3) tachypnea (respiratory rate >95th percentile for age); (4) hypotension (mean arterial blood pressure <5th percentile for age); and (5) altered mental status, metabolic acidosis (arterial pH <7.35 or base deficit >–5), oliguria (urine output <1 mL/kg per hour), or signs of poor peripheral perfusion, such as delayed capillary refill.[38] Although the incidence of clinically proven sepsis in neonates is only 1 to 5 cases per 1000 live births, the fatality rate is high—30% to 50%.[129] Moreover, surviving patients experience significant morbidity. Risk factors for the development of neonatal sepsis can be classified into two broad categories: maternal and neonatal.

Maternal Factors

Premature onset of labor, prolonged (>24 hours) rupture of the membrane, clinically proven chorioamnionitis, colonization of the genital tract with pathogenic bacteria (e.g., group B streptococcus or E. coli), urinary tract infection, and sexual intercourse near the time of delivery are all independent risk factors for the development of neonatal infection. They increase the risk of infection by exposing the neonate to pathogens in utero as well as during vaginal delivery. In fact, these risk factors increase the rate of systemic infection more than 10-fold.[129]

Neonatal Factors

As previously discussed, the neonate's host defense mechanism is markedly impaired. This impairment results from a diminished neutrophil storage pool, abnormal neutrophil and monocyte chemotaxis, decreased cytokine and complement production, and diminished levels of type-specific IgG, secretory IgA, and IgM, which, along with indwelling catheters, may result in compromised anatomic barriers. These deficiencies are even more accentuated in the preterm neonate. Low birth weight may also be an independent risk factor, because infants weighing less than 2500 g have a nearly eightfold increased risk of infection compared with those who weigh more.[35,129]

The organisms that are most commonly involved in neonatal sepsis are group B streptococcus and E. coli K-1. These organisms typically colonize the gastrointestinal tract of the mother and can be detected in rectal or vaginal cultures. Other organisms implicated in neonatal sepsis include Staphylococcus epidermidis and the intracellular pathogen Listeria monocytogenes. In addition to the intrinsic deficiencies in the neonatal host defense mechanisms, the virulence factors of these organisms influence the likelihood of developing systemic infection. Group B streptococcus possesses a capsular polysaccharide that prevents its phagocytosis by the neutrophil in the absence of adequate opsonins, which, as discussed earlier, are deficient in the neonate.[45,147] Similarly, the capsular polysaccharide of E. coli K-1 serves as one of its most important structural virulence factors. Other potential virulence factors include the presence of pili, specific O antigens, and α-hemolysins in E. coli K-1 and neuraminidase and toxin in group B streptococcus.[45,147] The intrinsic pathogenicity of S. epidermidis is derived from its ability to elaborate lectins that promote adherence to the epithelium, along with a surface slime that protects the organism from phagocytosis as well as from the toxic effects of antibiotics.[55,111] In contrast to bacterial infections, neonatal infections with L. monocytogenes and certain viruses, such as herpes simplex virus, reflect a deficiency in T-cell-mediated immunity.

The hallmark of neonatal sepsis is temperature instability, apnea, respiratory distress, cardiovascular instability, lethargy, feeding intolerance, and other gastrointestinal disturbances. In term as well as preterm neonates, group B streptococcus infection may follow a fulminant course within the first 96 hours of life. Respiratory distress, hypotension, and disseminated intravascular coagulation can be seen within the first 24 hours and may lead to death if aggressive supportive therapy and antibiotics are not initiated. Hypoglycemia is also a common feature of neonatal sepsis. It is mainly the result of glycogenolysis, decreased gluconeogenesis despite increased production of gluconeogenic hormones such as glucagon, and increased glucose utilization by tissues.

Evidence suggests that, as in adults and older children, proinflammatory cytokines such as TNF-α, IL-1, IL-6, IL-8, and PAF may play an important role in the hemodynamic instability that characterizes neonatal sepsis. Sullivan et al.[132] reported elevated levels of IL-1, IL-6, and TNF-α in children with both gram-positive and gram-negative infections. Similarly, IL-6 (especially combined with C-reactive protein levels) was found to be a sensitive marker for the diagnosis of neonatal bacterial infection.[18] Administration of pentoxifylline (an inhibitor of TNF-α) to neonatal piglets with group B streptococcal sepsis attenuated TNF production and improved the piglets' pulmonary hemodynamics.[52] Wong et al.[149] found elevated levels of nitrite and nitrate, the stable end products of NO metabolism in the plasma of infants and children with sepsis, suggesting that NO may also be an important mediator of the hemodynamic instability that characterizes neonatal sepsis.

DIAGNOSIS

The various clinical signs of SIRS and sepsis have already been reviewed, but these signs are nonspecific. For instance, one group of investigators reported that among febrile full-term neonates, only 10% had documented bacterial infection; in premature infants, this number decreased to 3%.[129] Prompt and accurate diagnosis of infection remains the primary objective of the clinician, especially in term and preterm neonates, so that proper antibiotic therapy can be initiated to minimize both the mortality and the morbidity of neonatal sepsis. Although isolating the microorganism from the blood, cerebrospinal fluid, urine, body fluids, or tissues remains the gold standard for the diagnosis of bacterial infection, such cultures may be negative. Sensitivity of blood cultures can be enhanced if a minimum of 0.5 mL of blood is withdrawn. Cultures should be obtained from peripheral blood as well as from indwelling catheters. Urine culture should be obtained by suprapubic aspiration or direct bladder catheterization, and the urine should be concentrated 25- to 50-fold. Positive urine cultures within the first 7 days of life (especially the first 72 hours) presuppose an antecedent bacteremia. Because up to one third of neonates with sepsis have meningitis, lumbar puncture should also be performed. The presence of meningeal infection should be suspected if (1) the white blood cell count in the cerebrospinal fluid is greater than 32 cells/mm³ with more than 60% neutrophils, (2) the glucose concentration in the cerebrospinal fluid is less than 50% of a simultaneously drawn serum glucose, (3) the cerebrospinal fluid protein is greater than 150 mg/dL, or (4) bacteria are detected by Gram stain or by counterimmunoelectrophoresis.

Numerous laboratory studies have been used to provide direct or indirect evidence of bacterial infection. Unfortunately, no single test has proved to be sufficiently reliable in establishing or excluding the diagnosis of bacterial sepsis.

Total Leukocyte Count: By itself, the total leukocyte count is of limited value in the diagnosis of neonatal sepsis. Less than 50% of neonates with a white blood cell count less than 5000/mm³ or greater than 20,000/mm³ are ultimately identified as being infected.[112,128] Because of the low predictive accuracy of the total leukocyte count,

various investigators have sought other neutrophil indices of neonatal infection. The total neutrophil count, which takes into account both mature and immature forms, has not been reliable because only two thirds of infants with sepsis have abnormal neutrophil counts. Similarly, the immature neutrophil count is of little diagnostic value because the number of bands and metamyelocytes entering the bloodstream in response to infection is inconsistent or unpredictable and reflects the fact that the neonatal neutrophil storage pool may be limited. One of the most useful but still unreliable indices is the ratio of immature to total neutrophils; normally, this ratio is approximately 0.2. A normal ratio usually suggests that infection is highly unlikely. A ratio greater than 0.2 is a sensitive indicator of infection in the absence of perinatal asphyxia or pregnancy-induced hypertension. Severe neutropenia (ratio >0.8) usually signifies severe bone marrow depletion and a poor prognosis.

Platelet Count: Thrombocytopenia has been shown to be a nonspecific, late predictor of neonatal sepsis. It may be seen in viral, fungal, and bacterial infections. Moreover, it is often not detected until hemodynamic changes have already occurred.

Acute Phase Reactants: In response to infection, the liver synthesizes large quantities of certain proteins known as acute phase reactants. These proteins are stimulated mostly in response to IL-6 and include C-reactive protein, albumin, fibrinogen, and haptoglobin. C-reactive protein is the most extensively studied. Its primary role is to serve as a carrier protein to bind and promote the clearance of potentially toxic microbial by-products. However, levels up to 10 times normal have been associated with other noninfectious causes, including perinatal asphyxia, meconium aspiration, and respiratory distress syndrome. Measuring C-reactive protein levels may be useful in monitoring the response to therapy. The concentration of C-reactive protein increases within the first 8 hours of infection and peaks within 2 to 3 days; levels fall promptly as the inflammatory process subsides. Haptoglobin and fibrinogen, as well as the erythrocyte sedimentation rate, are of little or limited value in diagnosing bacterial infection.

Investigators have tried to combine data from various screening tests in an effort to improve predictive accuracy. These screening panels have not shown an enhanced ability to diagnose infection compared with the individual tests. However, the negative predictive value of these tests—that is, the likelihood that a normal test excludes the presence of bacterial sepsis—approaches 100%. To date, measuring the levels of various cytokines in plasma has not proved to be useful in the diagnosis of bacterial infection.

An emerging concept in sepsis research is the PIRO system. This is an approach to stratify patients on the basis of their predisposing conditions (P), the nature and extent of the infection (I), the nature and magnitude of the host response (R), and the degree of concomitant organ dysfunction (O).[81,82] The proposed PIRO model discriminates between morbidity arising from infection and sickness secondary to the host response to infection. In addition, the PIRO system accounts for premorbid ailments that may enhance the risk of an adverse outcome independent of the infectious process.

THERAPY

Successful treatment of sepsis and SIRS is contingent on prompt recognition of the signs and symptoms of the syndrome and aggressive early intervention. In particular, adequate cardiovascular and pulmonary support is essential, especially in the early stages of SIRS, when the capillary leak syndrome and decreased systemic vascular resistance may compromise blood pressure as well as tissue oxygenation. The principal objective is to restore oxygen delivery to the tissues in view of the decreased peripheral oxygen utilization and the increased oxygen demand. This goal can be achieved by ensuring that the patient is adequately resuscitated. Evidence suggests that children who present with sepsis are often grossly underresuscitated.[19,61] Inadequate volume replenishment in a patient with SIRS results in hypotension, decreased tissue perfusion, and exacerbation of the oxygen debt. These patients should undergo aggressive early resuscitation to improve outcome.[19,61] Vasopressors should not be initiated until the volume deficit has been corrected. Mechanical ventilation may be an important adjunct in patients with obvious pulmonary dysfunction or failure. Urine output and hemodynamic parameters should be monitored closely, and appropriate adjustments made. Nutritional support should be initiated early (preferably enterally) to minimize the catabolic state and provide nutrients for the gut. This is particularly true for term and premature infants who have reduced glycogen stores and often exhibit significant hypoglycemia.

Besides fluid resuscitation and respiratory support, antibiotic therapy is the cornerstone of treatment for sepsis. Empirical broad-spectrum antibiotic therapy should be started without delay. Sepsis or SIRS is often the result of systemic gram-negative infection, even though less than 50% of patients with SIRS have positive blood cultures. The most common offending organisms include *E. coli*, *P. aeruginosa*, *Klebsiella*, and *Bacteroides* species. In term and preterm neonates, group B streptococcus, *E. coli*, and *L. monocytogenes* account for the majority of the bacterial isolates. In this population, ampicillin and gentamicin should provide more than adequate initial coverage, because *S. epidermidis* and other organisms (e.g., *Candida* species) are not encountered until later. Blood cultures should be obtained within 24 to 48 hours following initiation of antibiotic therapy to determine whether the patient is responding to treatment. Persistent positive cultures on optimal therapy suggest antibiotic resistance, the presence of an undrained infectious collection, or a colonized indwelling catheter.

Antibiotic therapy may initially be associated with acute or subacute deterioration in a patient with sepsis. This phenomenon results from the release of large quantities of endotoxin in the bloodstream by killed bacteria. In fact, intravenous antibiotics have been shown to increase free endotoxin levels by 50-fold in humans.[124] Binding of LPS with LBP results in the formation of a complex that is 1000-fold more potent than LPS alone. Binding of this LPS-LBP complex to the CD14 molecule and TLR-4 on macrophages, neutrophils, or endothelial cells induces the synthesis and release of numerous proinflammatory cytokines capable of further activating or amplifying the inflammatory cascade that characterizes SIRS. Therefore, in recent years, there have been numerous attempts to block the inflammatory response in septic patients with the use of monoclonal antibodies to the lipid A moiety of LPS.

The first large trial of the human monoclonal (IgM) anti–lipid A antibody (HA-1A) in patients with SIRS suggested that those with documented, culture-positive, gram-negative bacteremia were most likely to benefit from this treatment.[156] However, a subsequent clinical trial involving patients with gram-negative bacteremia and septic shock failed to support this theory, finding no difference in mortality rate among patients receiving HA-1A and those receiving placebo.[92] Similar observations were made by Rogy et al.,[116] who compared HA-1A with bactericidal permeability-increasing protein (BPI), an endogenously produced human LPS-neutralizing protein, in baboons receiving *E. coli* infusions. Another clinical trial using a different anti-LPS monoclonal antibody, E5, failed to show any improvement in mortality in nonshock patients with gram-negative sepsis; however, E5 treatment resulted in greater resolution of organ failure and prevented the development of adult respiratory distress syndrome.[16] Possible explanations for the failure of anti-LPS therapy to affect mortality in sepsis include persistent endotoxemia, owing to either uncontrolled infection or inadequate neutralization of LPS by the antibody.[28] Alternatively, it is possible that once LPS has initiated the inflammatory cascade, neutralization with HA-1A or another anti-LPS antibody will be ineffective. In addition, because SIRS can result from other causes, including gram-positive infections, severe trauma, or burns, it may be more practical to attempt to block the proximal soluble mediators of the inflammatory response rather than targeting LPS. Such a strategy has been employed by other investigators using CDP57, a fully humanized anti–TNF-α antibody. The administration of CDP57 to patients with rapidly evolving septic shock resulted in a prompt (within 30 minutes) decrease in circulating TNF-α levels and a slower decrease in circulating IL-1β and IL-6 levels; however, the survival rate was not affected.[34] A phase III trial evaluating an interleukin-1 receptor antagonist in patients with SIRS did not show any survival advantage, except in patients with end-organ dysfunction or a predicted mortality risk greater than 242 using the Acute Physiology and Chronic Health Evaluation (APACHE) III score.[49,50]

Activation of the cytokine cascade triggers a diverse set of reactions, including activation of the coagulation cascade and inhibition of the fibrinolytic pathway.[59] Coagulation activation leads to thrombin production and fibrin deposition in the microvasculature, thus leading to micro- and macrovascular thromboses. This process makes evolutionary sense because its purpose is to limit microbial dissemination throughout the host; unchecked, however, it can lead to organ dysfunction and ultimately death. Activated protein C is an endogenous regulator of coagulation and inflammation. Once protein C is activated by the thrombin-thrombomodulin complex, it exerts antithrombotic[58,88] and profibrinolytic effects.[11,29,135] The anti-inflammatory effects of activated protein C are direct, by means of inhibition of nuclear factor kappa B translocation,[73] cytokine formation,[56,62] and selectin activity.[57] Activated protein C is a promising therapeutic target because many patients with severe sepsis have an acquired deficiency of activated protein C and an increased risk of mortality.[46] Recent adult and pediatric studies examining drotrecogin alfa (activated), a recombinant form of human activated protein C, suggest that the drug is safe and beneficial. The PROWESS study[12a] was a large multicenter, randomized, double-blind, placebo-controlled trial in adults with severe sepsis. The results of this trial demonstrated a substantial decrease in the 28-day mortality from all causes in adults with sepsis receiving drotrecogin alfa (activated) compared with patients receiving placebo. The pediatric trial, which started during the interim analysis of the adult trial, was an open-label, nonrandomized, sequential international multicenter study (conducted in the United States and United Kingdom). The investigators found a significant increase in baseline levels of protein C and antithrombin over the study period; they also found about a 5% incidence of serious bleeding. These results were comparable to those of the adult trial and provide reason to conduct a large phase III randomized, placebo-controlled study.

Among potential anticytokine therapeutic agents, the administration of soluble TNF receptors or BPI may prove to be quite useful. In particular, BPI, which is normally produced by the neutrophil, has a high affinity for LPS and has been shown to be protective in an endotoxin-challenge model of sepsis.[50,89] Numerous other potential immunomodulators have been used, including taurolidine, an antiendotoxic drug,[146] and monophosphoryl lipid A, a hydrolyzed derivative of endotoxin derived from *Salmonella minnesota* R595. However, no benefit has been documented to date.[10] Other strategic approaches to the biologic therapy of sepsis have targeted the endothelial cell and its products. Antioxidant therapy and PAF receptor antagonists can attenuate damage due to the deleterious effects of ROIs and PAF. However, clinical trials have not yet been carried out. Antibodies to P-selectin, E-selectin, ICAM-1, CD11/CD18 integrins, and PECAM-1 have shown promising results in experimental models of reperfusion injury.[87]

Phosphodiesterase inhibitors represent another important class of immunomodulators. These agents increase intracellular levels of cyclic adenosine monophosphate (cAMP), which leads to a decrease in the accumulation of mRNA for TNF-α following LPS stimulation. Pentoxifylline is one of the best known drugs in this class. It has been shown to decrease the production of TNF-α in experimental models of endotoxic shock and in human volunteers.[115,120,154] Both beta and alpha agonists, which may play an important role in the cardiovascular stabilization of septic patients, have also been shown to diminish TNF-α production, presumably by increasing intracellular levels of cAMP.[76] Corticosteroids have been shown to play a protective role in various models of septic shock. The mechanism may involve inhibition of translational activation of TNF-α.[53] Administration of low-dose dexamethasone to pediatric patients with meningitis decreases cytokine levels in the cerebrospinal fluid and improves inflammation as well as overall neurologic outcome.[102,107] In contrast, high-dose corticosteroids may be detrimental in septic shock because only a small dose is required to block the translation of TNF-α mRNA; a high dose may cause unnecessary prolonged immunosuppression that obviates the salutary effects of TNF blockade.[17,39] Steroids probably exert the greatest anti-inflammatory effect when administered before initiating antibiotic therapy because they can block the increase in TNF-α that would normally result from the endotoxemia caused by the antibiotic-induced bacterial lysis. The same argument regarding optimal time for administration also applies to the other biologic response modifiers.

Both intravenous gamma globulin and fresh frozen plasma have been advocated as adjunctive therapy for septic neonates, especially premature neonates who are deficient in IgG, IgM, IgA, and complement. A controlled clinical trial failed to demonstrate any advantage to prophylactic use of intravenous gamma globulin in very-low-birth-weight infants.[44] Similarly, no benefit was found when fresh frozen plasma was administered prophylactically to infants with suspected infection.[2] Nevertheless, the data suggest that intravenous gamma globulin (700 mg/kg) may be useful in preterm neonates with overwhelming gram-negative sepsis, which often follows intestinal perforation secondary to necrotizing enterocolitis.

REFERENCES

1. Abraham E: Alterations in transcriptional regulation of proinflammatory and immunoregulatory cytokine expression by hemorrhage, injury, and critical illness. New Horiz 1996;4:184-193.

2. Acunas BA, Peakman M, Liossis G, et al: Effect of fresh frozen plasma and gammaglobulin on humoral immunity in neonatal sepsis. Arch Dis Child Fetal Neonatal Ed 1994;70: F182-F187.

3. Albelda SM, Smith CW, Ward PA: Adhesion molecules and inflammatory injury. FASEB J 1994;8:504-512.

4. Albina JE, Cui S, Mateo RB, Reichner JS: Nitric oxide-mediated apoptosis in murine peritoneal macrophages. J Immunol 1993;150:5080-5085.

5. Ambruso DR, Altenburger KM, Johnston RB Jr: Defective oxidative metabolism in newborn neutrophils: Discrepancy between superoxide anion and hydroxyl radical generation. Pediatrics 1979;64(Suppl):722-725.

6. Anderson DC, Abbassi O, Kishimoto TK, et al: Diminished lectin-, epidermal growth factor-, complement binding domain-cell adhesion molecule-1 on neonatal neutrophils underlies their impaired CD18-independent adhesion to endothelial cells in vitro. J Immunol 1991;146:3372-3379.

7. Ar'Rajab A, Dawidson I, Fabia R: Reperfusion injury. New Horiz 1996;4:224-234.

8. Arnaout MA: Leukocyte adhesion molecules deficiency: Its structural basis, pathophysiology and implications for modulating the inflammatory response. Immunol Rev 1990;114:145-180.

9. Arnould T, Michiels C, Remacle J: Increased PMN adherence on endothelial cells after hypoxia: Involvement of PAF, CD18/CD11b, and ICAM-1. Am J Physiol 1993;264:C1102-C1110.

10. Astiz ME, Rackow EC, Still JG, et al: Pretreatment of normal humans with monophosphoryl lipid A induces tolerance to

endotoxin: A prospective, double-blind, randomized, controlled trial. Crit Care Med 1995;23:9-17.

11. Bajzar L, Kalafatis M, Simioni P, Tracy PB: An antifibrinolytic mechanism describing the prothrombotic effect associated with factor V Leiden. J Biol Chem 1996;271: 22949-22952.

12. Beal AL, Cerra FB: Multiple organ failure syndrome in the 1990s: Systemic inflammatory response and organ dysfunction. JAMA 1994;271:226-233.

12a. Bernard GR, Vincent JL, Laterre PF, et al: Recombinant human protein C Worldwide Evaluation in Severe Sepsis (PROWESS) Study group. Efficacy and safety of recombinant human activated protein C for severe sepsis. N Engl J Med 2001;344:699-709.

13. Bevilacqua MP, Nelson RM: Selectins. J Clin Invest 1993; 91:379-387.

14. Boehmer ED, Goral J, Faunce DE, Kovacs EJ: Age-dependent decrease in Toll-like receptor 4-mediated proinflammatory cytokine production and mitogen-activated protein kinase expression. J Leukoc Biol 2004;75:342-349.

15. Bone RC: Sepsis and its complications: The clinical problem. Crit Care Med 1994;22(Suppl):S8-S11.

16. Bone RC, Balk RA, Fein AM, et al: A second large controlled clinical study of E5, a monoclonal antibody to endotoxin: Results of a prospective, multicenter, randomized, controlled trial. The E5 Sepsis Study Group. Crit Care Med 1995;23:994-1006.

17. Bone RC, Fisher CJ Jr, Clemmer TP, et al: A controlled clinical trial of high-dose methylprednisolone in the treatment of severe sepsis and septic shock. N Engl J Med 1987;317: 653-658.

18. Buck C, Bundschu J, Gallati H, et al: Interleukin-6: A sensitive parameter for the early diagnosis of neonatal bacterial infection. Pediatrics 1994;93:54-58.

19. Carcillo JA, Davis AL, Zaritsky A: Role of early fluid resuscitation in pediatric septic shock. JAMA 1991;266:1242-1245.

20. Casey LC, Balk RA, Bone RC: Plasma cytokine and endotoxin levels correlate with survival in patients with the sepsis syndrome. Ann Intern Med 1993;119:771-778.

21. Chan J, Xing Y, Magliozzo RS, Bloom BR: Killing of virulent *Mycobacterium tuberculosis* by reactive nitrogen intermediates produced by activated murine macrophages. J Exp Med 1992;175:1111-1122.

22. Cher DJ, Mosmann TR: Two types of murine helper T cell clone. II. Delayed-type hypersensitivity is mediated by TH1 clones. J Immunol 1987;138:3688-3694.

23. Christensen RD: Hematopoiesis in the fetus and neonate. Pediatr Res 1989;26:531-535.

24. Christensen RD, Rothstein G: Exhaustion of mature marrow neutrophils in neonates with sepsis. J Pediatr 1980;96: 316-318.

25. Cinat M, Waxman K, Vaziri ND, et al: Soluble cytokine receptors and receptor antagonists are sequentially released after trauma. J Trauma 1995;39:112-118.

26. Clegg S, Gerlach GF: Enterobacterial fimbriae. J Bacteriol 1987;169:934-938.

27. Crow JP, Beckman JS: Reactions between nitric oxide, superoxide, and peroxynitrite: Footprints of peroxynitrite in vivo. Adv Pharmacol 1995;34:17-43.

28. Danner RL, Elin RJ, Hosseini JM, et al: Endotoxemia in human septic shock. Chest 1991;99:169-175.

29. de Fouw NJ, van Tilburg NH, Haverkate F, Bertina RM: Activated protein C accelerates clot lysis by virtue of its anticoagulant activity. Blood Coagul Fibrinolysis 1993; 4:201-210.

30. De Groote MA, Fang FC: NO inhibitions: Antimicrobial properties of nitric oxide. Clin Infect Dis 1995;21(Suppl 2): S162-S165.

31. De Groote MA, Granger D, Xu Y, et al: Genetic and redox determinants of nitric oxide cytotoxicity in a *Salmonella typhimurium* model. Proc Natl Acad Sci U S A 1995;92: 6399-6403.

32. Deitch EA, Rutan R, Waymack JP: Trauma, shock, and gut translocation. New Horiz 1996;4:289-299.

33. Deitch EA, Specian RD, Berg RD: Endotoxin-induced bacterial translocation and mucosal permeability: Role of xanthine oxidase, complement activation, and macrophage products. Crit Care Med 1991;19:785-791.

34. Dhainaut JF, Vincent JL, Richard C, et al: CDP571, a humanized antibody to human tumor necrosis factor-alpha: Safety, pharmacokinetics, immune response, and influence of the antibody on cytokine concentrations in patients with septic shock. CPD571 Sepsis Study Group. Crit Care Med 1995;23:1461-1469.

35. Dillon HC Jr, Khare S, Gray BM: Group B streptococcal carriage and disease: A 6-year prospective study. J Pediatr 1987;110:31-36.

36. Ding A, Nathan C, Stuehr D: Release of reactive nitrogen intermediates and reactive oxygen intermediates from mouse peritoneal macrophages: Comparison of activating cytokines and evidence for independent production. J Immunol 1988;141:2407.

37. Ding J, Badwey JA: Neutrophils stimulated with a chemotactic peptide or a phorbol ester exhibit different alterations in the activities of a battery of protein kinases. J Biol Chem 1993;268:5234-5240.

38. Duke T, South M, Stewart A: Activation of the L-arginine nitric oxide pathway in severe sepsis. Arch Dis Child 1997; 76:203-209.

39. Effect of high-dose glucocorticoid therapy on mortality in patients with clinical signs of systemic sepsis. The Veterans Administration Systemic Sepsis Cooperative Study Group. N Engl J Med 1987;317:659-665.

40. Ehlers S, Smith KA: Differentiation of T cell lymphokine gene expression: The in vitro acquisition of T cell memory. J Exp Med 1991;173:25-36.

41. English BK, Burchett SK, English JD, et al: Production of lymphotoxin and tumor necrosis factor by human neonatal mononuclear cells. Pediatr Res 1988;24:717-722.

42. Ertel W, Keel M, Bonaccio M, et al: Release of anti-inflammatory mediators after mechanical trauma correlates with severity of injury and clinical outcome. J Trauma 1995;39: 879-885.

43. Etzioni A, Doerschuk CM, Harlan JM: Of man and mouse: Leukocyte and endothelial adhesion molecule deficiencies. Blood 1999;94:3281-3288.

44. Fanaroff AA, Korones SB, Wright LL, et al: A controlled trial of intravenous immune globulin to reduce nosocomial infections in very-low-birth-weight infants. National Institute of Child Health and Human Development Neonatal Research Network. N Engl J Med 1994;330:1107-1113.

45. Ferrieri P: Neonatal susceptibility and immunity to major bacterial pathogens. Rev Infect Dis 1990;12(Suppl 4): S394-S400.

46. Fijnvandraat K, Derkx B, Peters M, et al: Coagulation activation and tissue necrosis in meningococcal septic shock: Severely reduced protein C levels predict a high mortality. Thromb Haemost 1995;73:15-20.

47. Finlay BB, Falkow S: Common themes in microbial pathogenicity. Microbiol Rev 1989;53:210-230.

48. Finlay BB, Falkow S: Salmonella interactions with polarized human intestinal Caco-2 epithelial cells. J Infect Dis 1990; 162:1096-1106.

49. Fisher CJ Jr, Dhainaut JF, Opal SM, et al: Recombinant human interleukin 1 receptor antagonist in the treatment of patients with sepsis syndrome: Results from a randomized,

double-blind, placebo-controlled trial. Phase III rhIL-1ra Sepsis Syndrome Study Group. JAMA 1994;271:1836-1843.

50. Fisher CJ Jr, Marra MN, Palardy JE, et al: Human neutrophil bactericidal/permeability-increasing protein reduces mortality rate from endotoxin challenge: A placebo-controlled study. Crit Care Med 1994;22:553-558.

51. Gazzinelli RT, Hieny S, Wynn TA, et al: Interleukin 12 is required for the T-lymphocyte-independent induction of interferon gamma by an intracellular parasite and induces resistance in T-cell-deficient hosts. Proc Natl Acad Sci U S A 1993;90:6115-6119.

52. Gibson RL, Redding GJ, Henderson WR, Truog WE: Group B streptococcus induces tumor necrosis factor in neonatal piglets: Effect of the tumor necrosis factor inhibitor pentoxifylline on hemodynamics and gas exchange. Am Rev Respir Dis 1991;143:598-604.

53. Giroir BP: Mediators of septic shock: New approaches for interrupting the endogenous inflammatory cascade. Crit Care Med 1993;21:780-789.

54. Goris RJ, te Boekhorst TP, Nuytinck JK, Gimbrere JS: Multiple-organ failure: Generalized autodestructive inflammation? Arch Surg 1985;120:1109-1115.

55. Gray ED, Peters G, Verstegen M, Regelmann WE: Effect of extracellular slime substance from *Staphylococcus epidermidis* on the human cellular immune response. Lancet 1984;1: 365-367.

56. Grey ST, Tsuchida A, Hau H, et al: Selective inhibitory effects of the anticoagulant activated protein C on the responses of human mononuclear phagocytes to LPS, IFN-gamma, or phorbol ester. J Immunol 1994;153: 3664-3672.

57. Grinnell BW, Hermann RB, Yan SB: Human protein C inhibits selectin-mediated cell adhesion: Role of unique fucosylated oligosaccharide. Glycobiology 1994;4:221-225.

58. Gruber A, Hanson SR, Kelly AB, et al: Inhibition of thrombus formation by activated recombinant protein C in a primate model of arterial thrombosis. Circulation 1990;82: 578-585.

59. Hack CE, Zeerleder S: The endothelium in sepsis: Source of and a target for inflammation. Crit Care Med 2001; 29(Suppl):S21-S27.

60. Han J, Thompson P, Beutler B: Dexamethasone and pentoxifylline inhibit endotoxin-induced cachectin/tumor necrosis factor synthesis at separate points in the signaling pathway. J Exp Med 1990;172:391-394.

61. Han YY, Carcillo JA, Dragotta MA, et al: Early reversal of pediatric-neonatal septic shock by community physicians is associated with improved outcome. Pediatrics 2003;112: 793-799.

62. Hancock WW, Grey ST, Hau L, et al: Binding of activated protein C to a specific receptor on human mononuclear phagocytes inhibits intracellular calcium signaling and monocyte-dependent proliferative responses. Transplantation 1995;60:1525-1532.

63. Harlan JM: Leukocyte adhesion deficiency syndrome: Insights into the molecular basis of leukocyte emigration. Clin Immunol Immunopathol 1993;67(Suppl):S16-S24.

64. Hauser CJ: Regional macrophage activation after injury and the compartmentalization of inflammation in trauma. New Horiz 1996;4:235-251.

65. Hayes MP, Berrebi GA, Henkart PA: Induction of target cell DNA release by the cytotoxic T lymphocyte granule protease granzyme A. J Exp Med 1989;170:933-946.

66. Hill HR: Biochemical, structural, and functional abnormalities of polymorphonuclear leukocytes in the neonate. Pediatr Res 1987;22:375-382.

67. Hogg N, Darley-Usmar VM, Wilson MT, Moncada S: Production of hydroxyl radicals from the simultaneous generation of superoxide and nitric oxide. Biochem J 1992;281:419-424.

68. Huber AR, Kunkel SL, Todd RF 3rd, Weiss SJ: Regulation of transendothelial neutrophil migration by endogenous interleukin-8. Science 1991;254:99-102.

69. Isberg RR, Tran Van Nhieu G: Binding and internalization of microorganisms by integrin receptors. Trends Microbiol 1994;2:10-14.

70. Iwama A, Wang MH, Yamaguchi N, et al: Terminal differentiation of murine resident peritoneal macrophages is characterized by expression of the STK protein tyrosine kinase, a receptor for macrophage-stimulating protein. Blood 1995;86:3394-3403.

71. Jackson DE: The unfolding tale of PECAM-1. FEBS Lett 2003;540:7-14.

72. Jones SA, Horiuchi S, Topley N, et al: The soluble interleukin 6 receptor: Mechanisms of production and implications in disease. FASEB J 2001;15:43-58.

73. Joyce DE, Gelbert L, Ciaccia A, et al: Gene expression profile of antithrombotic protein C defines new mechanisms modulating inflammation and apoptosis. J Biol Chem 2001;276:11199-11203.

74. Kaplan J, Shope TC, Bollinger RO, Smith J: Human newborns are deficient in natural killer activity. J Clin Immunol 1982;2:350-355.

75. Kaplan SS, Lancaster JR Jr, Basford RE, Simmons RL: Effect of nitric oxide on staphylococcal killing and interactive effect with superoxide. Infect Immun 1996;64:69-76.

76. Kern J, Lamb R, Reed J, et al: Dexamethasone inhibition of interleukin-1 beta production by human monocytes: Posttranscriptional mechanisms. J Clin Invest 1988;81:237.

77. Koefoed-Johnsen V, Ussing HH: The nature of the frog skin potential. Acta Physiol Scand 1958;42:298-308.

78. Kolesnick R, Golde DW: The sphingomyelin pathway in tumor necrosis factor and interleukin-1 signaling. Cell 1994;77:325-328.

79. Krebs DL, Hilton DJ: SOCS: Physiological suppressors of cytokine signaling. J Cell Sci 2000;113:2813-2819.

80. Leonard EJ, Skeel A: A serum protein that stimulates macrophage movement, chemotaxis and spreading. Exp Cell Res 1976;102:434-438.

81. Levy MM, Fink MP, Marshall JC, et al: 2001 SCCM/ ESICM/ACCP/ATS/SIS International Sepsis Definitions Conference. Crit Care Med 2003;31:1250-1256.

82. Levy MM, Fink MP, Marshall JC, et al: 2001 SCCM/ ESICM/ACCP/ATS/SIS International Sepsis Definitions Conference. Intensive Care Med 2003;29:530-538.

83. Lewis DB, Yu CC, Meyer J, et al: Cellular and molecular mechanisms for reduced interleukin 4 and interferon-gamma production by neonatal T cells. J Clin Invest 1991;87:194-202.

84. Lipton SA, Choi YB, Pan ZH, et al: A redox-based mechanism for the neuroprotective and neurodestructive effects of nitric oxide and related nitroso-compounds. Nature 1993;364:626-632.

85. Lowry SF: Anticytokine therapies in sepsis. New Horiz 1993;1:120-126.

86. Machleidt T, Wiegmann K, Henkel T, et al: Sphingomyelinase activates proteolytic I kappa B-alpha degradation in a cell-free system. J Biol Chem 1994;269: 13760-13765.

87. Maier RV, Bulger EM: Endothelial changes after shock and injury. New Horiz 1996;4:211-223.

88. Marlar RA, Kleiss AJ, Griffin JH: Human protein C: Inactivation of factors V and VIII in plasma by the activated molecule. Ann N Y Acad Sci 1981;370:303-310.

89. Marra MN, Thornton MB, Snable JL, et al: Endotoxin-binding and -neutralizing properties of recombinant

bactericidal/permeability-increasing protein and monoclonal antibodies HA-1A and E5. Crit Care Med 1994;22:559-565.

90. Martin GS, Mannino DM, Eaton S, Moss M: The epidemiology of sepsis in the United States from 1979 through 2000. N Engl J Med 2003;348:1546-1554.

91. Masson D, Tschopp J: A family of serine esterases in lytic granules of cytolytic T lymphocytes. Cell 1987;49:679-685.

92. McCloskey RV, Straube RC, Sanders C, et al: Treatment of septic shock with human monoclonal antibody HA-1A: A randomized, double-blind, placebo-controlled trial. CHESS Trial Study Group. Ann Intern Med 1994;121:1-5.

93. McDonald T, Sneed J, Valenski WR, et al: Natural killer cell activity in very low birth weight infants. Pediatr Res 1992;31:376-380.

94. McGill SN, Ahmed NA, Hu F, et al: Shedding of L-selectin as a mechanism for reduced polymorphonuclear neutrophil exudation in patients with the systemic inflammatory response syndrome. Arch Surg 1996;131:1141-1146.

95. Mileski W, Borgstrom D, Lightfoot E, et al: Inhibition of leukocyte-endothelial adherence following thermal injury. J Surg Res 1992;52:334-339.

96. Miller ME: Phagocyte function in the neonate: Selected aspects. Pediatrics 1979;64(Suppl):S709-S712.

97. Miller VL, Falkow S: Evidence for two genetic loci in *Yersinia enterocolitica* that can promote invasion of epithelial cells. Infect Immun 1988;56:1242-1248.

98. Muller W, Weigl S, Deng X, Phillips DM: PECAM-1 is required for transendothelial migration of leukocytes. J Exp Med 1993;178:449-460.

99. Muller WA: The role of PECAM-1 (CD31) in leukocyte emigration: Studies in vitro and in vivo. J Leukoc Biol 1995;57:523-528.

100. Muller WA: Migration of leukocytes across endothelial junctions: Some concepts and controversies. Microcirculation 2001;8:181-193.

101. Murray HW, Spitalny GL, Nathan CF: Activation of mouse peritoneal macrophages in vitro and in vivo by interferon-gamma. J Immunol 1985;134:1619-1622.

102. Mustafa MM, Ramilo O, Saez-Llorens X, et al: Cerebrospinal fluid prostaglandins, interleukin 1 beta, and tumor necrosis factor in bacterial meningitis: Clinical and laboratory correlations in placebo-treated and dexamethasone-treated patients. Am J Dis Child 1990;144:883-887.

103. Nathan C: Nitric oxide as secretory product of mammalian cells. FASEB J 1992;6:3051-3064.

104. Nathan C: Natural resistance and nitric oxide. Cell 1995;82:873-876.

105. Nguyen T, Brunson D, Crespi CL, et al: DNA damage and mutation in human cells exposed to nitric oxide in vitro. Proc Natl Acad Sci U S A 1992;89:3030-3034.

106. O'Brien CD, Lim P, Sun J, Albelda SM: PECAM-1-dependent neutrophil transmigration is independent of monolayer PECAM-1 signaling or localization. Blood 2003;101:2816-2825.

107. Odio CM, Faingezicht I, Paris M, et al: The beneficial effects of early dexamethasone administration in infants and children with bacterial meningitis. N Engl J Med 1991;324:1525-1531.

108. Pacelli R, Wink DA, Cook JA, et al: Nitric oxide potentiates hydrogen peroxide-induced killing of *Escherichia coli*. J Exp Med 1995;182:1469-1479.

109. Parrillo JE, Parker MM, Natanson C, et al: Septic shock in humans: Advances in the understanding of pathogenesis, cardiovascular dysfunction, and therapy. Ann Intern Med 1990;113:227-242.

110. Partrick DA, Moore FA, Moore EE, et al: Neutrophil priming and activation in the pathogenesis of postinjury multiple organ failure. New Horiz 1996;4:194-210.

111. Peters G, Locci R, Pulverer G: Adherence and growth of coagulase-negative staphylococci on surfaces of intravenous catheters. J Infect Dis 1982;146:479-482.

112. Philip AG, Hewitt JR: Early diagnosis of neonatal sepsis. Pediatrics 1980;65:1036-1041.

113. Podack ER, Young JD, Cohn ZA: Isolation and biochemical and functional characterization of perforin 1 from cytolytic T-cell granules. Proc Natl Acad Sci U S A 1985;82:8629-8633.

114. Raghunathan R, Miller ME, Everett S, Leake RD: Phagocyte chemotaxis in the perinatal period. J Clin Immunol 1982;2:242-245.

115. Refsum SE, Halliday MI, Campbell G, et al: Modulation of TNF alpha and IL-6 in a peritonitis model using pentoxifylline. J Pediatr Surg 1996;31:928-930.

116. Rogy MA, Moldawer LL, Oldenburg HS, et al: Anti-endotoxin therapy in primate bacteremia with HA-1A and BPI. Ann Surg 1994;220:77-85.

117. Rollins BJ, Sunday ME: Suppression of tumor formation in vivo by expression of the JE gene in malignant cells. Mol Cell Biol 1991;11:3125-3131.

118. Rosengren S, Olofsson AM, von Andrian UH, et al: Leukotriene B4-induced neutrophil-mediated endothelial leakage in vitro and in vivo. J Appl Physiol 1991;71:1322-1330.

119. Scannell G: Leukocyte responses to hypoxic/ischemic conditions. New Horiz 1996;4:179-183.

120. Schade UF: Pentoxifylline increases survival in murine endotoxin shock and decreases formation of tumor necrosis factor. Circ Shock 1990;31:171-181.

121. Schoedon G, Schneemann M, Walter R, et al: Nitric oxide and infection: Another view. Clin Infect Dis 1995;21(Suppl 2):S152-S157.

122. Scott P: IL-12: Initiation cytokine for cell-mediated immunity. Science 1993;260:496-497.

123. Scott P, Kaufmann SH: The role of T-cell subsets and cytokines in the regulation of infection. Immunol Today 1991;12:346-348.

124. Shenep JL, Flynn PM, Barrett FF, et al: Serial quantitation of endotoxemia and bacteremia during therapy for gram-negative bacterial sepsis. J Infect Dis 1988;157:565-568.

125. Smith JB, Kunjummen RD, Kishimoto TK, Anderson DC: Expression and regulation of L-selectin on eosinophils from human adults and neonates. Pediatr Res 1992;32:465-471.

126. Snyderman R, Goetzl EJ: Molecular and cellular mechanisms of leukocyte chemotaxis. Science 1981;213:830-837.

127. Snyderman R, Pike MC: Chemoattractant receptors on phagocytic cells. Annu Rev Immunol 1984;2:257-281.

128. Squire E, Favara B, Todd J: Diagnosis of neonatal bacterial infection: Hematologic and pathologic findings in fatal and nonfatal cases. Pediatrics 1979;64:60-64.

129. St Gene J, Polin R: Neonatal sepsis: Progress in diagnosis and management. Drugs 1988;36:784-800.

130. Stamler JS: Redox signaling: Nitrosylation and related target interactions of nitric oxide. Cell 1994;78:931-936.

131. Stuber F, Petersen M, Bokelmann F, Schade U: A genomic polymorphism within the tumor necrosis factor locus influences plasma tumor necrosis factor-alpha concentrations and outcome of patients with severe sepsis. Crit Care Med 1996;24:381-384.

132. Sullivan JS, Kilpatrick L, Costarino AT Jr, et al: Correlation of plasma cytokine elevations with mortality rate in children with sepsis. J Pediatr 1992;120:510-515.

133. Tracy K: Tumor necrosis factor (cachectin) in the biology of septic shock syndrome. Circ Shock 1991;35:123.

134. Upperman JS, Pillage G, Siddiqi MQ, et al: Dominance of high-producing IL-6 and low-producing IL-10 and IFN-γ alleles in glucose-6-phosphate dehydrogenase deficient trauma patients. Shock (in press).

135. van Hinsbergh VW, Bertina RM, van Wijngaarden A, et al: Activated protein C decreases plasminogen activator-inhibitor activity in endothelial cell-conditioned medium. Blood 1985;65:444-451.

136. VanFurth R, Hirsh J, Fedurko M: Morphology and peroxidase cytochemistry of mouse promonocytes, monocytes, and macrophages. J Exp Med 1970;132:794.

137. Vannier E, Miller L, Dinarello C: Coordinated anti-inflammatory effects of interleukin 4: Interleukin 4 suppresses interleukin1 but up-regulates gene expression and synthesis of interleukin1 receptor antagonist. Proc Natl Acad Sci U S A 1992;89:4076-4080.

138. VonAndrian U, Hansell P, Chambers J, et al: L-selectin function is required for β$_2$-integrin-mediated neutrophil adhesion at physiologic shear rates in vivo. Am J Physiol 1992;263:H1034-H1044.

139. Walker RI, Willemze R: Neutrophil kinetics and the regulation of granulopoiesis. Rev Infect Dis 1980;2:282-292.

140. Warren MK, Vogel SN: Opposing effects of glucocorticoids on interferon-gamma-induced murine macrophage Fc receptor and Ia antigen expression. J Immunol 1985;134:2462-2469.

141. Watson RS, Carcillo JA, Linde-Zwirble WT, et al: The epidemiology of severe sepsis in children in the United States. Am J Respir Crit Care Med 2003;167:695-701.

142. Waxman K: Shock: Ischemia, reperfusion, and inflammation. New Horiz 1996;4:153-160.

143. Waxman K: What mediates tissue injury after shock? N Horiz 1996;4:151-152.

144. Weiss SJ: Tissue destruction by neutrophils. N Engl J Med 1989;320:365-376.

145. West MA, Wilson C: Hypoxic alterations in cellular signal transduction in shock and sepsis. New Horiz 1996;4:168-178.

146. Willatts SM, Radford S, Leitermann M: Effect of the antiendotoxic agent, taurolidine, in the treatment of sepsis syndrome: A placebo-controlled, double-blind trial. Crit Care Med 1995;23:1033-1039.

147. Wilson CB: Immunologic basis for increased susceptibility of the neonate to infection. J Pediatr 1986;108:1-12.

148. Wilson RF: Special problems in the diagnosis and treatment of surgical sepsis. Surg Clin North Am 1985;65:965-989.

149. Wong HR, Carcillo JA, Burckart G, et al: Increased serum nitrite and nitrate concentrations in children with the sepsis syndrome. Crit Care Med 1995;23:835-842.

150. Wright SD, Ramos RA, Tobias PS, et al: CD14, a receptor for complexes of lipopolysaccharide (LPS) and LPS binding protein. Science 1990;249:1431-1433.

151. Wunderink RG, Waterer GW: Genetics of sepsis and pneumonia. Curr Opin Crit Care 2003;9:384-389.

152. Yang Z, Costanzo M, Golde DW, Kolesnick RN: Tumor necrosis factor activation of the sphingomyelin pathway signals nuclear factor kappa B translocation in intact HL-60 cells. J Biol Chem 1993;268:20520-20523.

153. Yoshimura T, Yuhki N, Moore SK, et al: Human monocyte chemoattractant protein-1 (MCP-1): Full-length cDNA cloning, expression in mitogen-stimulated blood mononuclear leukocytes, and sequence similarity to mouse competence gene JE. FEBS Lett 1989;244:487-493.

154. Zabel P, Wolter DT, Schonharting MM, Schade UF: Oxpentifylline in endotoxaemia. Lancet 1989;2:1474-1477.

155. Zhong W, Chavali S, Utsunomiya T, et al: Cytokine regulation by a β-adrenergic agonist improves mortality in mice with severe endotoxemia. Surg Forum 1995;46:99-101.

156. Ziegler EJ, Fisher CJ Jr, Sprung CL, et al: Treatment of gram-negative bacteremia and septic shock with HA-1A human monoclonal antibody against endotoxin: A randomized, double-blind, placebo-controlled trial. The HA-1A Sepsis Study Group. N Engl J Med 1991;324:429-436.

157. Zingarelli B, O'Connor M, Wong H, et al: Peroxynitrite-mediated DNA strand breakage activates poly-adenosine diphosphate ribosyl synthetase and causes cellular energy depletion in macrophages stimulated with bacterial lipopolysaccharide. J Immunol 1996;156:350-358.

Chapter 11

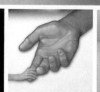

Surgical Implications of Hematologic Disease

Raymond J. Hutchinson

Hematologists and pediatric surgeons frequently interact with each other in the comprehensive management of pediatric surgical patients. The evaluation and management of anemia, thrombocytopenia, platelet dysfunction, clotting factor deficiencies, and thrombosis are the common meeting grounds; in addition, the judicious use of transfusion therapy often raises questions of interest to both groups of physicians. The most important considerations in each of these areas are discussed here.

ANEMIA

An inadequate mass of red blood cells (RBCs), resulting in insufficient delivery of oxygen to the tissues, can occur for three major pathophysiologic reasons: (1) inadequate production or maturation of RBCs in the bone marrow (e.g., Diamond-Blackfan anemia, transient erythroblastopenia of childhood), (2) loss of red cell mass as a result of bleeding (e.g., gastrointestinal blood loss from Meckel's diverticulum) or splenic sequestration (as seen in sickle cell diseases), or (3) RBC destruction (hemolytic disorders).[75] Clearly, a thorough history and physical examination provide invaluable data when planning the workup for a pale child or for the evaluation of a low hematocrit or hemoglobin concentration noted on a complete blood cell count (CBC). In pediatric medicine and surgery, individual and family histories are particularly relevant because of the frequency of congenital and genetic anemias. Of course, the child's age at diagnosis determines, at least in part, the importance of neonatal or genetic factors.

In the history, items of importance include evidence of intrauterine bleeding in the mother or neonatal hemolysis (e.g., from placental abruption or erythroblastosis fetalis, respectively), neonatal jaundice or neonatal bleeding, the rate of development of pallor, the presence of scleral icterus, and a history of rectal bleeding. The family history is relevant for identifying other family members with anemia or treatment for anemia, splenectomy, or cholecystectomy. A complete physical examination includes assessment of jaundice and degree of pallor,

documentation of the size of the spleen and lymph nodes, evaluation for signs of bleeding (including testing the stool for blood), and assessment of cardiovascular stability.

The CBC yields much information regarding the causes of anemia. It provides information regarding two lineages in addition to the red cell lineage: the white cell (myeloid) and the platelet (megakaryocytic). Involvement of more than one hematopoietic lineage often indicates a production problem occurring in the bone marrow; hence, bone marrow aspiration and biopsy are typically done early in the workup of children with multiple cytopenias. The mean corpuscular volume (MCV) allows the classification of anemias into microcytic, normocytic, and macrocytic categories; this can be a useful diagnostic clue and can facilitate a directed workup. Similarly, a mean corpuscular hemoglobin concentration value that exceeds 36 is highly suggestive of the presence of a large number of spherocytes, as seen in hereditary spherocytosis.[66] The RBC distribution width index provides information about the size distribution of circulating red cells, allowing the physician to categorize the red cell population as homogeneously small or large or as heterogeneous with biphasic or multiphasic characteristics. This information, when coupled with the MCV, allows a more cost-effective workup. Figure 11-1 provides an algorithm for the workup of a patient with anemia.

Nonhemolytic Anemias

Underproduction of RBCs because of marrow failure or as a result of deficiency of an essential nutrient, such as iron, is a common mechanism that can lead to severe degrees of anemia. This anemia can interfere with the appropriate management of surgical emergencies.

Marrow Failure

One major clue to the existence of bone marrow failure is the presence of multilineage cytopenias. The concomitant existence of anemia with neutropenia or thrombocytopenia

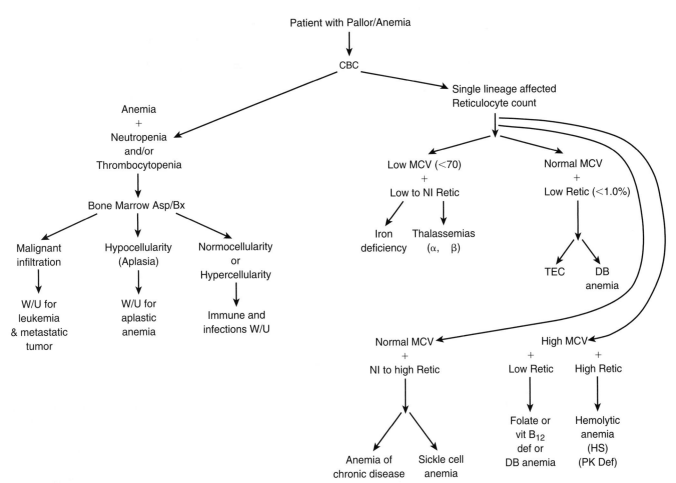

Figure 11–1 Algorithm for the workup of a patient with anemia. Asp/Bx, aspirate/biopsy; CBC, complete blood count; DB, Diamond-Blackfan; Def, deficiency; HS, hereditary spherocytosis, MCV, mean corpuscular volume; Nl, normal; PK def, pyruvate kinase deficiency; Retic, reticulocyte; TEC, transient erythroblastopenia of childhood; W/U, workup.

suggests (1) the existence of primary marrow failure resulting from constitutional (Fanconi's) anemia or acquired aplastic anemia or (2) failure of the bone marrow as a result of infiltrative disease, which occurs in cases of acute leukemia or metastatic neuroblastoma. Bone marrow aspiration and biopsy can often quickly resolve uncertainty regarding the diagnosis.

Fanconi's anemia is transmitted in an autosomal recessive pattern but affects males slightly more often than females (1.3:1).[8] The hematologic presentation is variable, with a single cell lineage often affected early, followed by evolution to multilineage aplastic anemia. The age at presentation ranges from birth to 35 years (mean, 8 years; median, 7 years).[8] Patients affected by Fanconi's anemia often exhibit congenital malformations (e.g., cutaneous hyperpigmentation, anomalies of the thumb and radial side of the forearm, microsomy, mental retardation).[40] They are predisposed to malignancies (e.g., leukemia and liver tumors) as a consequence of the associated chromosomal breakage.[20,86]

Acquired aplastic anemia is idiopathic in at least 50% of cases; commonly observed associations include occurrence after hepatitis B or after the use of such drugs as chloramphenicol, sulfonamides, phenothiazines,

and anticonvulsants.[7] Anabolic steroids provide reasonable, though usually temporary, improvement in the blood counts of patients with Fanconi's anemia[88]; however, they fail to do so for patients with acquired aplasia.[61] Allogeneic bone marrow transplantation from a well-matched donor, preferably a sibling, is potentially curative for Fanconi's and acquired aplastic anemia.[38,79] The use of recombinant human hematopoietic growth factors, such as erythropoietin, granulocyte colony-stimulating factor, granulocyte-macrophage colony-stimulating factor, and interleukin-3, is currently limited because of transient or incomplete responses.[33,58,100]

Single-lineage RBC hypoplasia is characterized by normal white blood cell and platelet counts, a low reticulocyte count (<1.0%), and the absence of erythroid precursors on marrow aspirate smears. Two conditions should come to mind when confronted with this clinical picture: Diamond-Blackfan anemia (congenital hypoplastic anemia) and transient erythroblastopenia of childhood (TEC). The former condition is characterized by elements of persistent fetal erythropoiesis, such as high fetal hemoglobin percentage on hemoglobin electrophoresis, retained expression of fetal red cell antigen i, and high MCV of red cells.[5] Patients with TEC usually do not exhibit these features.[105] TEC resolves within 2 to 8 weeks, which is consistent with suppression due to a presumed viral cause.[34] Corticosteroids are the mainstay of therapy for Diamond-Blackfan anemia; prednisone 2 mg/kg per day is used initially, followed by tapering to alternate-day dosing or less as the patient's condition allows.[6] Patients with Diamond-Blackfan anemia occasionally become transfusion dependent; in rare cases, patients require allogeneic bone marrow transplantation.[57] Although RBC transfusions are occasionally required for patients with TEC, most do not require therapy because recovery is sufficiently rapid.

Blood Loss

Anemia is an important manifestation of acute and chronic hemorrhage. Significant acute hemorrhage is usually accompanied by signs of cardiovascular stress, consisting of peripheral vasoconstriction, hypotension, tachycardia, and oliguria.[69] If the patient loses more than 30% of the total blood volume, hypovolemic shock often occurs. After acute hemorrhage, it may take several hours before the full effect on the hemoglobin and hematocrit levels can be assessed; a precipitous drop in these values within 1 to 2 hours of the hemorrhage usually indicates blood loss in excess of 20% of the total volume.[54]

Conversely, chronic blood loss resulting from low-grade, slow, or intermittent bleeding is usually not associated with the symptoms of cardiovascular stress. Patients with chronic anemia often exhibit a compensated picture that may not require intervention with transfusion. When transfusion is unavoidable, a judicious approach should be taken because multiple transfusions carry notable risks, including transmission of viral infection[55] and transfusional hemosiderosis.[21]

Sequestration of blood in the spleen is another mechanism of significant blood loss that can lead to anemia.[87] Splenomegaly caused by hemolytic anemias, portal vascular anomalies, or primary pathologic conditions of the liver can lead to sequestration of blood in dilated splenic sinusoids.

The therapeutic approach to the management of patients with anemia resulting from blood loss varies according to the rate at which the anemia developed. To restore blood volume and oxygen carrying capacity to a patient who has lost a large amount of blood, it may be necessary to transfuse a unit of blood quickly. This can usually be accomplished safely, even in young children, over a 15- to 30-minute period, as long as the volume and rate of delivery are adjusted to the child's size and estimated blood loss. Excessive volume expansion can usually be prevented through careful monitoring of the heart rate, arterial blood pressure, venous pressure, and core and peripheral temperatures.[69] Patients with chronic anemia that has gradually reached a level that compromises cardiopulmonary status should receive transfusions of RBCs in amounts that are appropriate to restore cardiopulmonary function to a compensated level. Overtransfusion should be avoided; this is particularly relevant for children with chronic anemia that requires repeated transfusions. For such children, frequent transfusions may result in transfusional hemosiderosis; the greater the number of

RBC units transfused, the greater the iron load transfused. After the serum ferritin exceeds 1000 µg/L, transferrin becomes saturated, and patients are at risk for cardiac and hepatic iron deposition[21]; these patients should be considered for chelation therapy with deferoxamine. Patients who develop moderate anemia resulting from blood loss or aggressive hemolysis should be slowly transfused back to the baseline level in aliquots of 5 to 10 mL/kg over 2 hours each, with time allowed between aliquots for re-equilibration and reassessment of the patient's cardiac status.

Nutritional Anemias

Iron-deficiency anemia results from inadequate intake of dietary iron, poor absorption, misutilization as a result of defective transport, loss of iron through bleeding, or sequestration of iron in an atypical location (e.g., the lungs in cases of pulmonary hemosiderosis). The age of the patient influences whether he or she will become iron deficient. In infants, who experience rapid expansion of blood volume during growth, 30% of the iron required for hemoglobin production must come from the diet. In adult men, only 5% is derived from the diet,[25] and the remainder is generated by RBC degradation.

The American Academy of Pediatrics[9-11] recommends dietary iron intake of 1.0 mg/kg per day to a maximum of 15 mg/day for full-term infants, starting no later than 4 months of age and continuing until 3 years of age. Preterm infants weighing between 1500 and 2500 g require 2 mg/kg per day to a maximum of 15 mg/day, starting no later than 2 months of age. Recommendations for very-low-birth-weight infants are even higher: 4 mg/kg per day for those weighing less than 1500 g at birth. In older children and adults, dietary iron requirements vary, depending on growth and gender:

4 to 10 years old	10 mg/day
11 to 16 years old	18 mg/day
Adult men	10 mg/day
Adult women	18 mg/day

The peak age range for developing nutritional iron deficiency is 6 months to 2 years. During this period, children make the transition from being dependent on breast milk or iron-fortified formula to a mixed diet of milk (often cow's milk) and solid foods. Depending on which foods constitute most of the child's diet, dietary iron may be adequate or inadequate. Children who depend heavily on cow's milk, at the expense of solid foods, are especially prone to iron-deficiency anemia. The typical presentation for such children is the gradual development of pallor, a hemoglobin concentration of 3.0 to 6.0 g/dL, and an MCV of 45 to 60 fL. Older individuals are much less likely to develop iron-deficiency anemia, especially from an inadequate diet, unless they participate in fad diets.

Consumption of unprocessed cow's milk by infants, intestinal parasitic infestations, and preexistent iron deficiency may lead to intestinal blood loss. The use of aspirin or aspirin-containing medications may increase intestinal blood loss sufficiently to cause anemia. Other anatomic sources of blood loss and iron deficiency include the following: in the perinatal period—fetal-maternal hemorrhage, placental injury at delivery, and twin-to-twin transfusion through placental communications; in older children—Meckel's diverticulum, intestinal duplication, hemorrhagic telangiectasia, and, rarely, bleeding ulcers or gastroesophageal reflux.

The diagnosis of iron deficiency is made by confirming the existence of microcytic, hypochromic anemia in the context of a clinical situation that suggests a possible cause. The low MCV and mean corpuscular hemoglobin should be corroborated with a careful review of the blood smear. Serum iron studies that measure the serum iron level, total iron-binding capacity, and serum ferritin level finalize the diagnosis. The typical pattern consists of a low serum iron level, high total iron-binding capacity, low serum ferritin, and low total-body iron stores. Finally, a therapeutic trial of iron should result in an increasing reticulocyte count within 1 week, and the hemoglobin and hematocrit levels should rise soon thereafter.

Treatment consists of the administration of oral iron (ferrous sulfate) at a dose of 6 mg/kg per day of elemental iron. Because ferrous sulfate is only 20% elemental iron, this must be taken into consideration when calculating the dose (e.g., a 325-mg tablet of ferrous sulfate contains 65 mg of elemental iron). The iron must be continued for 3 to 4 months. Correction of the anemia, correction of microcytosis, and elevation of the free erythrocyte protoporphyrin level usually occur within that period.[99]

Hemolytic Anemias

The sickle cell diseases, β-thalassemia, hereditary spherocytosis, and pyruvate kinase deficiency all have potential ramifications for pediatric surgeons.

Sickle Cell Diseases

The sickle hemoglobinopathies present early in life with episodes of painful crisis, acute chest syndrome, bacteremia, and splenic sequestration.[36] In a report of the Cooperative Study of Sickle Cell Disease, patients with homozygous sickle cell anemia and those with sickle cell–hemoglobin C disease demonstrated significant incidence rates of painful crisis, acute chest syndrome, and bacteremia; however, all 20 deaths in a cohort of 694 infants followed for 10 years occurred among the patients with homozygous sickle cell anemia.[36] It was also clear from this study that most hand-foot syndromes occurred among the sickle cell anemia patients, in the first 3 years of life.

Several sequelae of the sickle cell disorders are of interest to pediatric surgeons. Painful vaso-occlusive crises occasionally masquerade as acute abdominal events that typically require surgical intervention (e.g., appendicitis). Because painful crises are usually accompanied by an elevated leukocyte count, this parameter is not useful in distinguishing appendicitis from a painful crisis. Serial examinations and collaborative evaluation with a hematologist who is skilled in the evaluation of patients with sickle cell diseases reduce the frequency of unnecessary and potentially harmful surgical interventions during painful crises.

Acute chest syndrome can represent a life-threatening situation. Correction of this process requires rapid transfusion to raise the oxygen carrying capacity of the blood and lower the percentage of hemoglobin S, to reverse the sickling process.

For patients with repeated episodes of splenic sequestration, the surgeon may be called on to remove the spleen to reduce the risk of subsequent sequestration, which is characterized by rapid drops in hemoglobin concentration, hematocrit value, and platelet count. At times, progressive sequestration may lead to hypovolemic shock and have life-threatening implications. Typically, splenectomy is justified after two episodes of sequestration, even in young patients (younger than 4 years old).[87] Similarly, the development of symptomatic cholelithiasis usually dictates that cholecystectomy be performed.[81]

Patients with sickle cell anemia have a high incidence of perioperative morbidity.[29] Complications that occur at an increased rate in patients with sickle cell disease undergoing surgery include painful crises, acute chest syndromes, and transfusion reactions due to erythrocyte alloimmunization.

Another consideration for pediatric surgeons managing patients with sickle cell diseases is related to the percentage of sickle hemoglobin and the safety of general anesthesia. In the past, RBC transfusion to lower the percentage of sickle hemoglobin to less than 30% has been the preferred approach. However, data suggest that patients do just as well with a more conservative approach that aims at achieving a preoperative hemoglobin level of 10 g/dL but does not attempt to lower the hemoglobin S level below an arbitrary cutoff point.[103] Care should be taken to ensure adequate blood oxygenation during a surgical procedure, but excessive transfusion should be avoided.

Further, reducing preoperative transfusions reduces the risk of alloimmunization and of transfusion reactions. The development of non-ABO erythrocyte antibodies occurs in 8% to 50% of patients with sickle cell disease, varying with the number of RBC transfusions administered.[27] Clearly, the development of these antibodies adds complexity to surgical procedures and increases the risk of reactions with subsequent transfusions. RBC phenotyping with matching for E, C, and Kell group antigens is recommended because it reduces the risk of alloimmunization.[19,104] Several published studies have questioned the benefit of aggressive preoperative transfusion, suggesting that young patients undergoing low-risk surgery do not require transfusion.[44,103] For others, a conservative transfusion regimen designed to increase the plasma hemoglobin concentration to 10 g/dL offers as much benefit as an aggressive regimen aimed at decreasing the hemoglobin S concentration, with a lower risk of complications.[103]

Postoperative complications of surgery vary, depending on the type of surgical procedure performed, the age of the patient, the status of disease activity and disease-related organ dysfunction, the presence of infection, evidence of chronic lung disease, the presence of pregnancy in female patients, and the genetic form of sickle cell disease.[29] Preoperative assessment of lung function with a chest radiograph, oxygen saturation determination, and pulmonary function tests, and of renal function with serum blood urea nitrogen and creatinine measurements, blood pressure measurement, and screening for urinary infection and proteinuria, is a useful strategy for decreasing intraoperative risks.

β-Thalassemia

β-Thalassemia is characterized by the inability to synthesize normal amounts of β-chain hemoglobin polypeptide,[101] resulting in ineffective erythropoiesis. Patients with homozygous β-thalassemia become dependent on RBC transfusions early in life. As a consequence of extramedullary hematopoiesis, splenomegaly is a frequent finding. Splenic sequestration of RBCs often leads to an enhanced transfusion requirement. When the RBC transfusion requirement exceeds 250 mL/kg per year, splenectomy should be considered because it often reduces the transfusion requirement.[22]

Hereditary Spherocytosis and Erythrocyte Enzyme Deficiencies

Hereditary spherocytosis and RBC enzyme deficiencies, such as pyruvate kinase deficiency, result in hemolytic anemia, often associated with gallstone formation. When cholelithiasis is symptomatic, cholecystectomy is necessary. In the case of hereditary spherocytosis, when patients maintain a relatively high reticulocyte count (≥10%) in the presence of moderate to severe anemia, splenectomy should be considered when patients reach the age of 5 to 6 years.[93] Splenectomy reduces the risk of developing gallstones, and it minimizes the chance of a precipitous drop in the hemoglobin concentration when a patient with hereditary spherocytosis develops a viral infection. The therapeutic value of splenectomy also needs to be considered in patients with other types of hemolytic anemia, such as pyruvate kinase deficiency and refractory autoimmune hemolytic anemia.

THROMBOCYTOPENIA AND DISORDERS OF PLATELET FUNCTION

Thrombocytopenia

A platelet count below 150,000/μL is usually considered the lower limit of the normal range,[97] and thrombocytopenia exists when the platelet count falls below this value. Thrombocytopenia can have a genetic or an acquired origin.

Genetic Thrombocytopenia

Several genetic conditions should be considered when thrombocytopenia is diagnosed early in life. Thrombocytopenia in a patient with absent radii is noted at birth, is inherited in an autosomal recessive fashion, and often spontaneously improves after the first year of life. However, these children have up to 35% mortality during their first year from central nervous system and gastrointestinal bleeding.[46] Amegakaryocytic thrombocytopenia is present at birth or shortly thereafter, is not associated with physical anomalies, and has a notable incidence of progression to aplastic anemia.[28,45] As its name implies, amegakaryocytic thrombocytopenia is a marrow failure state and is typically inherited as an autosomal recessive trait. As mentioned earlier, Fanconi's anemia may present with isolated thrombocytopenia before full expression of the aplastic state is evident; however, the physical stigmata and chromosomal breakage associated with Fanconi's anemia allow the distinction between this and amegakaryocytic thrombocytopenia. In addition, familial thrombocytopenias occur in autosomal dominant, autosomal recessive, and sex-linked genetic forms. Wiskott-Aldrich syndrome is an example of the sex-linked variety, with thrombocytopenia occurring in association with eczema or frequent infections. This syndrome affects primarily males, as expected based on the genetics. It occurs in the background of underlying T-lymphocyte dysfunction.[76]

Acquired Thrombocytopenia

Exposure to maternal antibodies with antiplatelet surface antigen specificity (arising because of exposure to certain therapeutic drugs or to various viral infections or because of the existence of an autoimmune state) can lead to acquired thrombocytopenia. Certain classes of drugs are more likely to induce thrombocytopenia, including antibacterial drugs (e.g., trimethoprim-sulfamethoxazole), anticonvulsants (e.g., phenytoin and carbamazepine), and the phenothiazines (e.g., chlorpromazine). Two disorders merit special mention: neonatal isoimmune thrombocytopenia and idiopathic thrombocytopenic purpura.

Neonatal isoimmune thrombocytopenia occurs when an infant's mother becomes sensitized to a paternal platelet antigen inherited by the infant and expressed on platelets during gestation. The mother develops an antiplatelet IgG titer when the maternal-fetal blood barrier breaks down, allowing the infant's platelets to enter the maternal circulation. The platelet antigen most frequently responsible for this sensitization is PL[A1], an antigen for which 98% of the population is positive.[32] Random platelet transfusions generally do not raise the infant's platelet count, especially when a common antigen (such as PL[A1]) has led to sensitization; such transfused platelets are rapidly destroyed. Conversely, the use of maternal platelets (PL[A1] negative) typically leads to a sustained rise in the infant's platelet count; when the mother's postpartum condition allows for platelet pheresis, this can be a lifesaving intervention.[4]

Idiopathic thrombocytopenic purpura occurs in children and adolescents of all ages but is most typical in children 2 to 5 years of age.[64] It often occurs after a viral infection and is believed to be caused by a misdirected antiviral immune response, with antibodies cross-reacting with platelets and leading to primary splenic destruction.

Interventions of demonstrated benefit include intravenous administration of immune globulin (IgG), intravenous administration of anti-D immunoglobulin, and oral administration of prednisone.[31] Although all three treatments lead to elevation of the platelet count, the intravenous IgG and prednisone produce a faster response, with measurable improvement in 1 to 2 days. Before prednisone is used, consideration should be given to performing bone marrow aspiration to rule out leukemia, because leukemia may be partially but inadequately treated by prednisone. Response to these treatments may be short-lived, but despite the temporary response, 55% to 75% of patients fully recover within the first month after diagnosis and 80% to 90% by the sixth month after diagnosis.[65,68] As with neonatal isoimmune thrombocytopenia, the administration of random donor platelets is of little therapeutic benefit because of rapid consumption by the reticuloendothelial system. Splenectomy is sometimes undertaken in children refractory to other treatments to reverse the thrombocytopenia; approximately 70% of children achieve complete remission after splenectomy.[80]

Disorders of Platelet Function

Cutaneous or mucous membrane bleeding despite a normal platelet count suggests the presence of a disorder of platelet function. The detrimental effects of aspirin on platelet function have been recognized for many years. Aspirin inhibits platelet cyclooxygenase, resulting in deficiency of thromboxane A_2 and inhibition of platelet aggregation.[47] A prolonged bleeding time characterizes platelet dysfunction due to aspirin ingestion or other functional defects.

Von Willebrand's disease is notable for abnormal platelet adhesion and aggregation. This disorder is associated with subnormal levels of factor VIII procoagulant activity and of von Willebrand's factor.[53,72] A number of variants of this disorder are now known to exist, although most cases are genetic in origin, with autosomal dominant transmission. Correction of the functional defect is usually achieved with administration of cryoprecipitate; each unit of cryoprecipitate contains 60 to 80 units of factor VIII procoagulant activity. A dose of cryoprecipitate providing 10 units of factor VIII activity per kilogram of body weight is sufficient to achieve adequate hemostasis for surgery. Failure to correct von Willebrand's disease before a patient undergoes surgery increases the risk for mucosal bleeding, surface bleeding, or both.

Two other conditions that may be relevant to pediatric surgeons are Glanzmann's thrombasthenia[13] and Bernard-Soulier syndrome.[37] Both disorders are genetically transmitted and associated with severe defects of platelet function. A screening bleeding time longer than 20 minutes is consistent with these disorders. Infusion of platelet concentrate is the appropriate corrective measure for serious bleeding, using either 0.2 unit/kg or 4 units/m². However, patients quickly become resistant to platelet transfusions because of the high risk for alloimmunization.

DISORDERS OF COAGULATION

In evaluating children for bleeding tendencies, the physician should start with a review of items that pertain to a bleeding history. This includes bleeding after surgical procedures, circumcision, or dental extractions; delayed bleeding from the umbilical stump; hematoma formation after intramuscular injections; easy bruising with minor trauma; bleeding into joints; prolonged bleeding from lacerations; menorrhagia; hematuria; and bleeding from the gastrointestinal tract. A history of the use of or exposure to aspirin, aspirin-containing medications, or anticoagulant drugs should be ascertained. The presence of systemic illnesses that predispose to bleeding (e.g., lupus erythematosus, nephrosis, hypothyroidism, sepsis) should also be discussed. Finally, taking a family history of bleeding tendencies is essential and enhances or reduces the probability of diagnosing a bleeding disorder in the patient being evaluated (Fig. 11-2).

The physical examination provides further data that offer a perspective on the likelihood of a bleeding disorder. Bleeding in the skin or mucous membranes (petechiae, ecchymoses), soft tissues (hematomas), or joints or on funduscopic examination should be noted.

A good laboratory screening panel consists of the following tests: platelet count, bleeding time, prothrombin time (PT), and activated partial thromboplastin time (APTT) (Table 11-1). The bleeding time reflects platelet number and function. Template methods are preferred over the older lancet methods because better standardization is achieved. Nevertheless, the bleeding time is subject to considerable variation related to the experience of the person performing the test, the patient's skin temperature, and the length and depth of the incision. The normal range for the bleeding time is 3½ to 11½ minutes. Times in the 12- to 15-minute range must be viewed circumspectly, whereas values in excess of 15 minutes are prolonged and abnormal. When planning to obtain a bleeding time or evaluating a prolonged test result, the physician should ask about the use of aspirin or aspirin-containing medications, which can significantly prolong the bleeding time.

Several screening tests for deficient or defective coagulation factors are available. The whole-blood clotting time is not sensitive enough for screening, and the activated clotting time, though more sensitive, is not adequate. The APTT is the most sensitive of the global screening tests. In this test, plasma is incubated with an inert activating agent (e.g., kaolin) and a partial thromboplastin as a platelet substitute, followed by the addition of calcium. The APTT detects deficient clotting factors in the intrinsic and the common pathways. However, mild deficiencies of factors VIII and IX are not detected by the APTT, and deficiencies of factors VII and XIII are not detected at all. The normal range for the APTT is 25 to 35 seconds; the precise upper limit depends on the reagents and the specific method used.[63] The other major screening test, the PT, is done by adding tissue factor (a complete thromboplastin) to plasma with simultaneous or subsequent recalcification. The normal range for the PT is 11 to 12 seconds[63]; this test detects deficiencies of factor VII and factors in the common pathway.

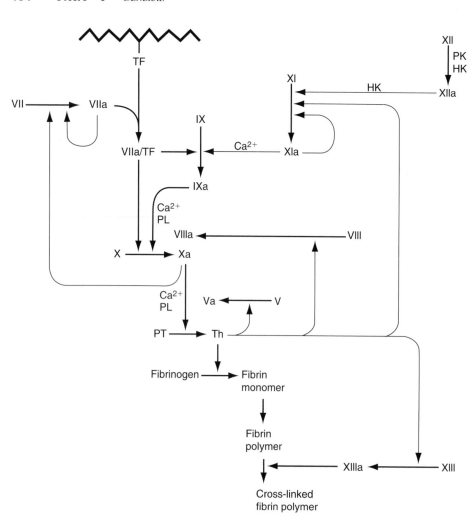

Figure 11–2 Coagulation cascade. HK, high-molecular-weight kininogen; PK, prekallikrein; PL, phospholipid; PT, prothrombin; TF, tissue factor; Th, thrombin. (From Schafer AI: Coagulation cascade: An overview. In Loscalzo J, Schafer AI [eds]: Thrombosis and Hemorrhage. Boston, Blackwell Scientific, 1994.)

TABLE 11–1 Tests to Detect Bleeding Disorders

Test	Parameters Measured
Platelet count	Platelet number
Bleeding time	Systemic primary hemostasis
	Defect of platelet number or function
	Defect in platelet-vessel wall interaction
	Primary vascular disorder
Prothrombin time (PT)	Extrinsic and common pathways: factors VII, X, V; prothrombin; fibrinogen
Activated partial thromboplastin time (APTT)	Intrinsic and common pathways: factors XII, IX, XI, VIII, X, V; prothrombin; fibrinogen; prekallikrein; high-molecular-weight kininogen
Thrombin time	Fibrinogen
Fibrinogen quantitation	Level of fibrinogen in plasma (mg/dL)
Fibrin degradation products	Breakdown products of fibrinogen or fibrin—elevated with increased fibrinolysis or disseminated intravascular coagulation
D-dimer assay	Fibrin-specific degradation product; indicator of both thrombin and plasmin generation
Euglobulin lysis time	Screening test of fibrinolytic activity
Mixing study (using PT or APTT)	Presence of a circulating anticoagulant
Antithrombin III (AT III) activity	Level of the antithrombotic AT III
Protein C, protein S antigen activity	Levels of the antithrombotic proteins C and S
Activated protein C resistance assay	Presence of mutant, functionally deficient factor V Leiden (predisposing to thrombosis)

From Schafer AI: Approach to bleeding. In Loscalzo J, Schafer AI (eds): Thrombosis and Hemorrhage. Boston, Blackwell Scientific, 1994; Comp PC: Approach to thrombosis. In Loscalzo J, Schafer AI (eds): Thrombosis and Hemorrhage. Boston, Blackwell Scientific, 1994; and Santoro SA: Laboratory evaluation of hemostatic disorders. In Hoffman R, et al (eds): Hematology: Basic Principles and Practice. New York, Churchill Livingstone, 1991.

Specific assays to determine the presence of a single factor deficiency are available. If a satisfactory conclusion cannot be achieved despite attempts to identify one or more factor deficiencies, a search for a plasma inhibitor of coagulation should be initiated. This can be accomplished by performing mixing studies with the APTT or PT, depending on which is more abnormal. For these studies, normal plasma is mixed with the deficient (patient) plasma in ranging concentrations (1:3, 1:1, 3:1). Failure to totally correct the test at the 3:1 (normal-patient) mix suggests the presence of an inhibitor, whereas factor deficiencies should be totally corrected at the 1:3 and certainly at the 1:1 mixtures.

Coagulation Factor Deficiencies

The most common inherited factor deficiencies include hemophilia A (factor VIII deficiency) and hemophilia B (factor IX deficiency); both disorders are inherited as X-linked recessive traits and affect males almost exclusively. In hemophilia A, the factor VIII procoagulant activity is deficient or defective, and the severity of bleeding correlates strongly with factor VIII levels; levels of less than 3% are associated with spontaneous hemorrhage into joints and soft tissues. Hemophilia B is characterized by deficient or defective factor IX. Very low levels (<3% of normal) can also be associated with spontaneous bleeding into joints and soft tissues. Different molecular defects account for the various subtypes of hemophilia A and hemophilia B. Hemophilia A is more common than hemophilia B. In the United States, the former occurs in 1 in 10,000 males; the latter occurs in 1 in 40,000 males.[63]

In general, levels of factor VIII or IX in excess of 30% are associated with reasonably normal hemostasis. Individuals with levels of 8% to 20% often lead near-normal lives, with significant bleeding only after surgery or significant trauma.[63]

The diagnosis of factor VIII deficiency can be made at birth. A prolonged APTT characterizes children who will ultimately be diagnosed with hemophilia A. Further workup reveals deficient levels of functioning factor VIII in a specific factor assay. In the evaluation of factor IX deficiency, however, the physician must consider the physiologic delay in achieving normal levels of the vitamin K–dependent factors in infants. Though confounding the interpretation of factor IX levels in infants, this physiologic delay does not lead to misinterpretation of the near-complete deficiency seen in hemophilia B. A prolonged APTT with a subsequent factor IX level of less than 10% is consistent with a diagnosis of hemophilia B. Infants with levels in the 10% to 50% range should be retested at 3 to 6 months of age or sooner if clinically significant bleeding occurs.

Other Factor Deficiencies

Congenital afibrinogenemia is associated with abnormal bleeding (e.g., melena, hematemesis, mucosal bleeding, hematoma, umbilical cord hemorrhage) early in life. In older children, bleeding after minor trauma, menorrhagia, hemarthrosis, and cerebral hemorrhage may occur. The diagnosis is confirmed by quantitative measurement of fibrinogen; immunologic methods may detect small amounts of fibrinogen even when other methods (e.g., precipitation and coagulation) fail to do so. Fibrinogen levels above 50 mg/dL are usually adequate for hemostasis.[3] Whole blood, plasma, or cryoprecipitate can be used to correct fibrinogen levels.

Dysfibrinogenemias are disorders of fibrinogen function caused by structural defects in the protein; more than 300 abnormal fibrinogens have been described.[15,63] Many individuals affected by dysfibrinogenemias do not have clinical histories of bleeding and are diagnosed during routine screening. In patients with bleeding tendencies, menorrhagia, easy bruising, and prolonged bleeding after minor trauma or surgery are observed. Although afibrinogenemia is transmitted as an autosomal recessive trait, dysfibrinogenemias seem to be transmitted in an autosomal dominant fashion. Quantitative immunologic or precipitation techniques usually produce normal results in dysfibrinogenemias, but assays that assess the functional contribution of fibrinogen to coagulation are abnormal. Most patients with dysfibrinogenemia do not require treatment, but plasma or cryoprecipitate can be used for patients with significant bleeding.

Table 11-2 lists the recognized clotting factors and their propensity for associated clinical bleeding. Deficiencies of prothrombin (factor II), factor V, and factor XI predispose to mild bleeding tendencies, whereas deficiencies of factors VII and X predispose to variable bleeding tendencies, with some individuals exhibiting significant hemorrhagic events. Of note is that deficiencies of the contact-activated factors—factor XII (Hageman factor), prekallikrein (Fletcher factor), and high-molecular-weight kininogen—are not associated

TABLE 11-2 Clotting Factor Deficiencies

Deficient Factor	Clinical Relevance
I	Risk of hemorrhage at levels <50 mg/dL
II	Mild bleeding tendency after injuries, dental extractions, surgery
V	Mild bleeding tendency (menorrhagia, significant bleeding after injury or surgery)
VII	Variable bleeding tendency (intracranial hemorrhage in newborns, menorrhagia)
VIII	Moderate to severe bleeding tendency at levels <5%
IX	Moderate to severe bleeding tendency at levels <5%
X	Variable bleeding tendency (neonatal hemorrhage, bleeding after trauma, menorrhagia)
XI	Mild bleeding tendency (menorrhagia, epistaxis, postoperative bleeding)
XII	Generally asymptomatic
Prekallikrein	Asymptomatic
High-molecular-weight kininogen	Asymptomatic

with bleeding, and their presence should not preclude required surgery.

Acquired Defects

Severe liver disease is often associated with significant clotting factor deficiency. The healthy liver is the site of synthesis of most coagulation factors (fibrinogen; prothrombin; factors V, VII, IX, X, XI, XII, and XIII; prekallikrein; and high-molecular-weight kininogen).[63] The liver is also the source of the natural anticoagulants (antithrombin III [AT III], protein C, and protein S), as well as of inhibitors of fibrinolysis (antiplasmin and α_1-antitrypsin). Because the liver is also involved in the clearance of activated clotting factors, liver failure can lead to disseminated intravascular coagulation (DIC) as a consequence of the inability to clear activated factors and the failure to synthesize AT III. However, severe hepatic injury and failure are more typically associated with a hemorrhagic tendency caused by insufficient production of clotting factors. Increased fibrinolysis resulting from decreased hepatic synthesis of inhibitors may contribute to the hemorrhagic tendency.

In infants, vitamin K deficiency, caused by dietary deficiency, failure of absorption, or specific drug antagonism,[63] can result in a severe bleeding diathesis. Deficiency of vitamin K interferes with the development of essential calcium-binding sites on the vitamin K–dependent coagulation factors,[78] including prothrombin and factors VII, IX, and X. Although newborns depend on exogenous sources of vitamin K, older infants absorb vitamin K from the colon, and synthesis by bacteria is the primary source. In older children and adults, vitamin K is absorbed from the ileum. The daily requirement of approximately 1 μg/kg is supplied by leafy green vegetables in the diet.[74] Vitamin K is stored in the liver after absorption.

Vitamin K stores are deficient in most normal newborn infants. However, few develop a bleeding diathesis. Without early supplementation, infants may bruise, have cephalohematomas, and experience gastrointestinal and umbilical hemorrhage and oozing from puncture sites. Platelet and fibrinogen levels are normal in these infants, but marked prolongation of the PT and APTT, which results from deficiencies of factors II, VII, IX, and X, is noted. Administration of parenteral vitamin K leads to quick correction of the clotting tests and cessation of bleeding. Breast-feeding accentuates the vitamin K deficiency because breast milk contains far less vitamin K (2 to 15 μg/L) than cow's milk (60 μg/L).[48] Hemorrhagic disease in newborns can be prevented by intramuscular administration of vitamin K shortly after birth. A dose of 0.5 to 1.0 mg of vitamin K_1 oxide is recommended; this dose far exceeds the requirement of 25 μg.[49]

Outside of the neonatal period, malabsorption can lead to vitamin K deficiency and a hemorrhagic tendency. Cystic fibrosis, biliary atresia, chronic hemolytic anemia with secondary cholelithiasis and obstructive jaundice, and disorders leading to upper small intestinal dysfunction are conditions that can cause vitamin K malabsorption.

Use of coumarin compounds can lead to vitamin K deficiency and resultant hemorrhage. Bleeding as a result of vitamin K deficiency ranges from massive ecchymoses and significant mucous membrane hemorrhage to central nervous system hemorrhage. PT and APTT assays are typically prolonged but normalize after vitamin K therapy. Administration of vitamin K intravenously at a dose of 5 to 10 mg leads to clinical improvement within a few hours and to correction of coagulation studies within 24 hours.[63]

DIC occurs after in vivo activation of the coagulation mechanism, resulting in the transformation of fibrinogen to fibrin. A wide range of pathophysiologic states can cause DIC, including intrauterine infection; maternal toxemia; abrupted placenta; severe respiratory distress syndrome; necrotizing enterocolitis; disseminated bacterial, viral, and rickettsial infections; leukemia and other malignancies; giant cavernous hemangiomas; severe traumatic events; acute anaphylaxis; and snakebite.[63] Diffuse endothelial damage or tissue injury with release of procoagulant materials can lead to activation of factor XII and platelet adherence to damaged endothelium, with subsequent platelet aggregation and release of phospholipids.

The diagnosis of DIC is facilitated by reviewing the peripheral blood smear, searching for erythrocyte fragmentation, and documenting a decreased number of platelets. Studies of coagulation parameters, including a platelet count, PT, APTT, thrombin time, and fibrinogen quantitation, should be undertaken. Tests to document the presence of fibrin monomer resulting from thrombin activity, fibrin degradation products secondary to fibrinolysis, and D-dimer levels are useful to confirm the diagnosis of DIC.

Treatment of DIC consists of correction of the underlying or precipitating process and supportive care. Further therapy should be determined by the patient's general condition and the hemorrhagic or thrombotic manifestations. Heparin may be indicated in children with purpura fulminans and signs of thrombosis; however, use of heparin for less severe forms of DIC is questionable. In the presence of decreased AT III levels, heparin may not be effective. AT III can be supplemented by the infusion of fresh frozen plasma or AT III concentrates. The patient's platelet count and fibrinogen level can be monitored as indices of response to therapy. For patients with primary hemorrhagic manifestations and little if any thrombosis, the administration of platelets and fresh frozen plasma is indicated if bleeding is moderately severe and associated with a decreasing platelet count and prolonged PT and APTT.

Thrombotic Disorders

The naturally occurring anticoagulants AT III, protein C, and protein S work to contain excessive in vivo blood coagulation. Thrombosis often results when the activity of these anticoagulants is deficient. In addition, genetic abnormalities of factor V (G1691A) and prothrombin

(G20210A), as well as abnormal homocysteine and lipoprotein (a) levels, have been associated with thrombosis in children.[67] Finally, the presence of antiphospholipid antibodies (e.g., lupus anticoagulant, anticardiolipin antibody) is associated with an increased risk of venous thrombosis.

AT III is a heparin cofactor that is essential to heparin therapy and is a major inhibitor of blood clotting. AT III is a physiologic inhibitor of thrombin and of activated factor X. This cofactor, which is synthesized in the liver, has a biologic half-life of 2 to 5 days. Congenital AT III deficiency occurs at a frequency of 1 per 2000 to 5000 individuals.[73,89] Thrombotic events are often first noted in the second and third decades of life. Surgery, trauma, infection, and pregnancy predispose to thrombotic events. Large amounts of heparin may be required to effectively anticoagulate the patient because AT III is necessary for full heparin activity. Diagnosis is made by specific assay for AT III; immunologic, enzymatic, and clotting assays are available. Although most patients exhibit quantitative deficiency, some patients have qualitative defects that might be overlooked in an immunologic assay. Oral anticoagulation has been the mainstay of therapy. However, purified concentrates of AT III are now available and can be used at a dose of 50 IU/kg for the short term to prevent thrombosis in high-risk situations, such as in acute thrombosis, during surgery, or during the third trimester of pregnancy.[59,98] A level of 80% or more should be achieved. For long-term prophylaxis, warfarin should be used.

Both protein C and protein S are vitamin K–dependent plasma proteins that act in concert to inactivate procoagulants, thereby reducing the risk for thrombosis. Protein C functions by inactivating factors V and VIII; in its active form, protein C also indirectly facilitates clot lysis.[63] Deficiency of protein C is inherited as an autosomal dominant trait. The homozygous state in infants is characterized by pupura fulminans, retinal thrombotic events with retinal detachment and loss of vision, and other thrombotic events.[43] Heterozygous deficiency of protein C is often asymptomatic during childhood but causes venous thrombosis in adolescents and young adults. Heterozygotes generally have levels of approximately 50%, but these individuals are still at risk for thrombotic events. Protein C assays are functional and immunologic. Although it has a role in preventing thrombosis in homozygous individuals who are essentially deficient of protein C, warfarin should be used cautiously in these individuals because their thrombotic tendency can be exacerbated by a further reduction in vitamin K–dependent protein C. In fact, heterozygotes often develop purpuric, thrombotic cutaneous lesions while receiving warfarin, a contraindication to its use. These side effects are presumably caused by further lowering of the protein C level. Heparin should be used to treat acute venous thrombosis, and protein C concentrates are now available to facilitate the management of acute thrombosis in protein C–deficient patients.

Protein S acts as a cofactor for protein C. Deficiency of protein S is associated with recurrent venous thrombosis. Heterozygotes with 35% to 50% of the normal levels of the protein develop recurrent thromboses in adolescence and early adulthood.[85] The same guidelines for the use of heparin in treating venous thrombosis apply to patients who are deficient in protein S (as well as those deficient in AT III and protein C). Caution should be exercised when warfarin is used in protein S–deficient patients.

Recently, mutations in factor V (e.g., factor V Leiden) have been associated with the failure of activated protein C to inactivate factor V.[14,24] Because protein C typically prevents thrombosis by inactivating factors V and VIII, loss of this effect on factor V should theoretically lead to an increased risk for thrombosis. In fact, studies done on families with a high incidence of thromboembolic events confirm the association among activated protein C resistance, factor V mutations, and thrombosis.[106] Mutation of factor V may be the most common cause of venous thromboembolism.

TRANSFUSION THERAPY

Greater accessibility to improved blood products has increased the survival of critically ill patients who need enhanced oxygen delivery, intravascular volume expansion, and improved coagulability. The estimated blood volume for infants and young children weighing 10 to 30 kg is approximately 75.4 mL/kg.[84] RBC transfusions should be used to correct pathophysiologic events that cause inadequate oxygen delivery and resultant tissue hypoxia. The decision to transfuse RBCs should be based on several factors: signs of tissue hypoxia (tachycardia, tachypnea), extent of blood loss, rate at which anemia has developed, age of the patient, and concomitant or subsequent physiologic stress that the patient may be forced to undergo (e.g., infection, pulmonary compromise, surgery). Transfused RBCs survive for a relatively long time; less than 1% of the number transfused is destroyed daily.[69] Typically, the number of transfused cells in the recipient's circulation decreases steadily over 110 to 120 days.[106]

Historically, whole blood was the preferred product for transfusion in patients with severe acute blood loss. However, with the increased use of blood fractionation to produce several products from each unit of blood, greater emphasis is now placed on the use of packed RBCs in conjunction with a plasma substitute, if necessary. For hemorrhage of moderate severity, packed RBCs are as effective as citrated whole blood.[84] For severe hemorrhage, plasma substitutes are required when packed RBCs are transfused to prevent an unacceptable increase in hematocrit levels.[69]

To restore blood volume and oxygen carrying capacity to a patient who has lost a large amount of blood, it may be necessary to transfuse a unit of blood quickly. This can usually be done in the same way as discussed in the section on blood loss resulting from anemia. When replacement is less urgent, 10 to 15 mL/kg is transfused over 1 to 2 hours. Massive transfusions that involve replacing an amount of blood equal to the patient's blood volume in 24 hours carry the risk of citrate toxicity, electrolyte imbalance, decreased release of oxygen to tissues resulting from diminished RBC 2,3-bisphosphoglycerate content, pulmonary microembolism, decreased core temperature (if massive amounts of cold blood have been transfused), and thrombocytopenia or DIC. Prevention and successful treatment of the side effects of massive transfusion require careful reassessment of the patient during and after transfusion.

Various plasma substitutes, such as dextran, modified fluid gelatin, and hydroxyethyl starch, have been used to expand plasma volume in hypovolemic patients. However, the possibility of allergic reactions and abnormal bleeding has tempered enthusiasm for their use. Perfluorocarbon compounds, in which oxygen is highly soluble, have been shown to act as effective blood substitutes for oxygen delivery in animals.[70] However, side effects, including lowered platelet count,[82] diminished macrophage function,[35] and activation of complement with resultant pulmonary changes,[23] have severely hampered the use of these compounds; they are being evaluated in clinical trials.[95]

Transfusion in Patients with Cancer or Immunodeficiencies

The basic principle of transfusing to correct altered hemodynamics and insufficient delivery of oxygen applies when treating immunodeficient patients and those with cancer. No absolute value of peripheral blood hemoglobin concentration or hematocrit below which transfusion is mandated exists. In fact, absolute threshold criteria for transfusion therapy are being abandoned in many centers as a result of concerns about transfusion risks, the high cost of transfusion therapy, and the growing perception that many patients can tolerate lower hemoglobin values than previously believed without adverse physiologic effects. Clearly, the age of the patient, the rate at which hemoglobin or hematocrit values are falling, and concomitant problems influence the decision to transfuse. Children younger than 10 years tolerate hemoglobin values as low as 6 to 7 g/dL without adverse effects. Nevertheless, a rapid decline to this level usually requires RBC transfusion. Similarly, concomitant infection, space-occupying pulmonary disease, pleural effusion, cardiomyopathy, central nervous system insult, or injury to any major organ may mandate earlier transfusion. The immune state of the patient often warrants special consideration with respect to the type of RBC product chosen and the handling of that product. Many patients with primary immunodeficiency and those with immunodeficiency secondary to therapy should receive blood products that have been irradiated at a level of at least 1500 cGy to prevent graft-versus-host disease. In addition, severely immunocompromised patients, such as bone marrow transplant recipients, who are serologically cytomegalovirus (CMV) negative at the time of transfusion should receive CMV-negative or CMV-safe (leukocyte-reduced) blood products. In fact, many blood banks are releasing only leukocyte-reduced cellular products for all transfusion recipients.

Choice of Red Blood Cell Product

Fresh whole blood is a suitable choice for use in exchange transfusions when the whole blood being removed from the patient is being replaced (milliliter for milliliter) and when patients with massive blood loss resulting from acute hemorrhage are being treated. For patients in whom excessive increases in intravascular volume may cause problems, other RBC products are preferred.

Packed RBCs are the product of choice for patients with moderate acute blood loss or chronic anemia resulting from underproduction or hemolysis. Advantages of packed RBCs include removal of the anticoagulant citrate and 60% to 70% of the plasma.[17] This consideration is particularly important for patients with volume overload, poor cardiac function, or both.

One advantage of washed RBCs is that 85% to 90% of the leukocytes and more than 95% of the plasma have been removed[17]; however, additional expense is incurred for the preparation of this product. Washed RBCs can be used to transfuse patients with a history of nonhemolytic transfusion reactions.

More than 90% of the white blood cells have been removed from frozen deglycerolized RBCs, with retention of minimal plasma (<0.5% of original plasma).[17] This product is often chosen for patients who require chronic transfusions.

Leukocyte-reduced RBCs are relatively free of leukocytes (>70% removed)[102] and may be less likely to transmit CMV and other viruses. This product is advantageous for patients with a history of transfusion reactions and for immunodeficient patients at risk for CMV disease.

Each of the products mentioned has a place in transfusion therapy. However, physicians who use these products should bear in mind the appropriate indications for each and the increased cost associated with additional processing of RBCs (e.g., washing, freezing, thawing).

Transfusion Reactions and Toxicity

Citrate toxicity resulting from transfusion of the plasma anticoagulant citrate, which binds calcium, may manifest as symptomatic hypocalcemia. Development of this toxicity is the major drawback for using whole blood for rapid RBC and volume replacement.

Transfusion reactions take several forms and usually occur because of patient exposure to proteins from plasma, RBCs, white blood cells, or platelets to which the individual has a natural or an acquired sensitivity. Reactions occur in 2% to 3% of transfusions; of these, 41% are febrile and nonhemolytic, 58% are urticarial, and 1% are delayed hemolytic.[12] For patients with repeated urticaria, the use of washed or frozen RBCs in conjunction with pretreatment of the recipient with an antihistamine or corticosteroid may reduce the incidence of recurrence. Febrile nonhemolytic reactions are usually caused by acquired antibodies to plasma protein or leukocyte alloantigens and occur exclusively in patients with a history of previous transfusion or pregnancy. Pretreatment of the patient with antipyretics, antihistamines, or corticosteroids may alleviate symptoms. Because of the sophisticated quality-control measures currently in place in modern blood banks, hemolytic reactions are rare. Fever, chills, pain in the abdomen and lower back, tachycardia, hypotension, renal failure, and shock may be manifestations of a hemolytic reaction caused by major blood group incompatibility. When these symptoms are associated with transfusion, the infusion should be stopped, and a sample of the patient's blood should be sent to the blood bank along with the remainder of the aborted RBC unit. Delayed transfusion reactions occur 3 to 10 days after transfusion, are caused by minor blood group sensitization from previous transfusion, and are usually less severe than reactions due to major blood group incompatibility.

The risk of transfusing infectious agents in blood products has been re-emphasized by the acquired immunodeficiency syndrome (AIDS) epidemic. Although less than 5% of AIDS cases have been caused by blood transfusion, fear of acquiring the human immunodeficiency virus (HIV) from transfused blood products remains high because of the associated high mortality. Preferential collection of blood products from volunteer donors and HIV screening have reduced the risk for HIV transmission to 1 in 153,000 units of blood product transfused. The risk of transmitting certain hepatitis viruses, CMV, and Epstein-Barr virus must also be considered when ordering transfusions. Screening for hepatitis B and hepatitis C has had a positive effect on reducing the risk of acquiring these viruses from transfusions; hepatitis A is not considered to be a risk of transfusion. With the use of volunteer donors and screening for the hepatitis B antigen, the incidence of transfusion-acquired hepatitis B has fallen to 1 in 1000 transfusions.[12] The use of hepatitis B vaccine for patients who are likely to receive multiple transfusions is a recommended practice. The virus that causes hepatitis C has been identified, and a screening test is now used to detect that virus in the blood of potential donors. Use of this test is expected to decrease the 6% incidence of acquiring this infection through transfusion.[52] CMV is carried in transfused lymphocytes, and infusion of such lymphocytes in immunodeficient individuals can cause serious infection. Use of frozen or washed RBCs, blood products from CMV-negative donors, or leukocyte-reduced RBCs reduces the risk of acquiring CMV-related illness for immunodeficient individuals.[30,96]

Graft-versus-host disease is a potential transfusion-related problem for immunodeficient individuals. This disorder, which is well documented to occur after allogeneic bone marrow transplantation, has been recognized in an increasing number of immunodeficient patients receiving transfusions. Transfusion-associated graft-versus-host disease has been reported in 131 patients.[3] High fever, scaly maculopapular erythematous rash, diarrhea, hepatocellular damage with morbid elevation of liver enzymes, and pancytopenia characterize transfusion-associated graft-versus-host disease. The disorder typically occurs 8 to 12 days after transfusion. Overall mortality is 90%, with most deaths occurring within 1 month of onset. Steroids, antithymocyte globulin, cyclophosphamide, and anti-T-cell monoclonal antibodies have been disappointing in the treatment of this disease. Transfusion-associated graft-versus-host disease is readily avoided by irradiation of all cellular blood products to be transfused to immunodeficient patients. Irradiation of cellular products with doses of 1500 to 5000 cGy lethally damages lymphocytes without adversely affecting the function of RBCs, platelets, and neutrophils. The treated blood product is not radioactive and can be handled by hospital personnel in the usual fashion. Transfusion-associated graft-versus-host disease has not been reported to occur after transfusion of fresh frozen plasma or cryoprecipitate.

Platelet Transfusion

The normal platelet count in children and adults ranges from $150,000/\mu L$ to $450,000/\mu L$[51]; levels in newborn infants are occasionally as low as $80,000/\mu L$.[42] Once released into the bloodstream, platelets circulate for approximately 8 to 10 days. Patients with platelet counts below $10,000/\mu L$ are clearly at risk for hemorrhage,[16] whereas individuals with platelet counts below $50,000/\mu L$ carry a risk for bleeding during surgical intervention.[1] Replacing circulating platelets with a transfusion of platelet concentrate reduces the risks for spontaneous bleeding in patients with platelet counts below $10,000/\mu L$ and of intraoperative and postoperative bleeding in individuals with platelet counts below $50,000/\mu L$.

Random donor concentrates are obtained from whole-blood collections through a two-step centrifugation procedure.[39] An initial soft spin brings down the RBCs and leaves the platelets suspended in the supernatant plasma. The platelet-rich plasma is then centrifuged at high speeds to pellet the platelets, resulting in a platelet button than is resuspended in 50 mL of plasma. The platelet concentrate is then stored at 20° C to 24° C for up to 5 days. The pH of the concentrate should be maintained at 6.0 or higher.

Single-donor platelets are collected by apheresis techniques; approximately 3×10^{14} platelets, which is equal to six to eight individual concentrates, are contained in 200 to 400 mL of plasma.[39] These platelets can be stored for up to 5 days. Single-donor collections are useful for transfusion in patients who have become alloimmunized to random donor concentrates. Identification of compatible single donors through trial and error or by HLA-matching prospective donors often results in greater augmentation of the platelet count after transfusion for patients with alloantibodies to platelets.

The use of 1-hour post-transfusion platelet counts in patients who are apparently alloimmunized to random donor platelet concentrates is of value in determining the need for single-donor or HLA-matched platelets.[90] If the patient is not septic or sequestering platelets in the spleen, failure to demonstrate an increase in the circulating platelet count 1 hour after transfusion of random donor concentrates usually indicates the existence of platelet alloantibodies.

Platelet concentrates are usually used for patients with thrombocytopenia and concomitant bleeding or thrombocytopenia of sufficient magnitude to impart a significant threat of bleeding during surgery or other invasive procedures. When surgery or invasive procedures are required, administration of prophylactic transfusions to thrombocytopenic patients is reasonable for platelet counts below 50,000/μL.[39] The same threshold for platelet transfusion is reasonable for head trauma patients with thrombocytopenia. Many oncology centers transfuse cancer patients in a prophylactic manner, with the threshold for transfusion ranging from 10,000 to 30,000/μL.[2,26,77] Data suggest that minimal risk for bleeding exists when the platelet count is above 10,000/μL, provided the patient is afebrile and uninfected.[16] Finally, it is important to consider that platelet concentrates can be used to stop bleeding resulting from impaired platelet function (e.g., Glanzmann's thrombasthenia, Bernard-Soulier syndrome) or in acquired platelet functional defects (e.g., aspirin ingestion).

To stop bleeding in a thrombocytopenic patient, an increase in the platelet count of 40,000/μL is believed to be necessary.[50] For children, 0.1 unit of concentrate per kilogram of body weight usually produces an increment of 40,000/μL; similarly, 4 units/m² of body surface area accomplishes the same result.[56] In clinical practice, a minimum of 2 units of platelet concentrate is administered, even to infants. This algorithm can be applied to meet the needs of thrombocytopenic surgical patients. A platelet count done 1 hour after the platelet transfusion usually provides an accurate assessment of the increment achieved; in bleeding patients, cessation of bleeding is the ultimate index. The half-life of transfused platelets averages approximately 4 days; concomitant fever, infection, or conditions favoring platelet consumption decrease platelet survival.[91] The use of ABO-compatible platelets may lengthen survival, although this is controversial.[18,92] Use of single-donor platelets or HLA-matched platelets often lengthens platelet survival in an allosensitized recipient. When a patient demonstrates increments of less than 10,000/μL on two or three successive administrations of random donor platelets, consideration should be given to using single-donor or HLA-matched platelets. However, if a thrombocytopenic patient is a candidate for bone marrow transplantation from a related donor, use of matched platelets from family members should be avoided to prevent sensitization to minor antigens, because this might increase the potential for graft rejection.

Platelet concentrates are administered through blood filters. The standard 170-μm screen filters remove blood clots and are commonly used to administer platelet concentrates.[39] Contemporary microaggregate blood filters remove lymphocytes while allowing platelets to pass through. These filters may reduce the risk for febrile transfusion reactions and may prevent sensitization to HLA antigens through the removal of lymphocytes.[39] However, filters used to prepare leukocyte-reduced RBCs should not be used to transfuse platelet concentrates because they also remove most of the platelets.[60] Irradiation of platelet units to 1500 cGy is appropriate to lower the risk for graft-versus-host disease in high-risk patients. Platelet function measured by in vitro assays is not altered by this dose of radiation.[62,71,83,94]

Small amounts of Rh-positive RBCs in platelet concentrates may be sufficient to stimulate the production of anti-D in Rh-negative individuals.[41] Administration of Rh-immune globulin may prevent this sensitization in Rh-negative female recipients of platelet concentrates. Transfusion reactions caused by leukoagglutinins that combine with leukocytes and platelets may occur during or shortly after a platelet transfusion.[39] Fever and rigor are often associated with reactions to platelet transfusions. Decreasing the rate of infusion may reduce the risk of a febrile reaction. Acetaminophen, intravenous corticosteroids, and parenteral meperidine can be used to ameliorate this type of reaction. Allergic transfusion reactions are characterized by hives and occasional hypotension or bronchospasm.[39] Antihistamines and occasionally epinephrine are useful to treat allergic reactions.

A small risk for the transmission of viral infection is associated with the transfusion of platelet concentrate. In addition, because platelets are stored at room temperature, the possibility of bacterial contamination must be considered when transfused patients develop fever, chills, hypotension, or DIC.

REFERENCES

1. Aballi AJ, Puapondh Y, Desposito F: Platelet counts in thriving premature infants. Pediatrics 1968;42:685.
2. Aderka D, et al: Bleeding due to thrombocytopenia in acute leukemias and reevaluation of the prophylactic platelet transfusion policy. Am J Med Sci 1986;291:147.
3. Adler SP: Transfusion associated cytomegalovirus infections. Rev Infect Dis 1983;5:977.
4. Adner MM, et al: Use of "compatible" platelet transfusions in treatment of congenital isoimmune thrombocytopenic purpura. N Engl J Med 1969;280:244.
5. Alter BP: Fetal erythropoiesis in stress hematopoiesis. Exp Hematol 1979;7:200.
6. Alter BP: The bone marrow failure syndromes. In Nathan DG, Oski FA (eds): Hematology of Infancy and Childhood, 3rd ed. Philadelphia, WB Saunders, 1987.
7. Alter BP, Potter NU: Long-term outcome in Fanconi's anemia: Description of 26 cases and review of the literature. In German J (ed): Chromosome Mutation and Neoplasia. New York, AR Liss, 1983.
8. Alter BP, et al: Classification and aetiology of the aplastic anemias. Clin Haematol 1978;7:431.
9. American Academy of Pediatrics, Committee on Nutrition: Iron balance and requirements in infancy. Pediatrics 1969; 43:134.

10. American Academy of Pediatrics, Committee on Nutrition: Iron supplementation for infants. Pediatrics 1976;58:765.

11. American Academy of Pediatrics, Committee on Nutrition: Iron fortification of infant formulas. Pediatrics 1999; 104:119.

12. American Medical Association: General Principles of Blood Transfusion, 3rd ed. Chicago, AMA, 1985.

13. Bernard J, Soulier J: Sur une nouvelle variété de dystrophie thrombocytaire hemorragipore congenitale. Sem Hop Paris 1948;24:3217.

14. Bertina RM, et al: Mutation in blood coagulation factor V associated with resistance to activated protein C. Nature 1994;369:64.

15. Bolton PHB, et al. The rare coagulation disorders—review with guidelines for management from the United Kingdom Haemophilia Centre Doctors' Organisation. Haemophilia 2004;10:593.

16. Brecher G, Schneiderman M, Cronkite EP: The reproducibility and constancy of the platelet count. Am J Clin Pathol 1953;23:15.

17. Bucala R, Kawakami M, Cerani A: Cytotoxicity of a perfluorocarbon blood substitute to macrophages in vitro. Science 1983;220:965.

18. Cable R: Platelet transfusion. In Nathan DG, Oski FA (eds): Hematology of Infancy and Childhood. Philadelphia, WB Saunders, 1987.

19. Castro O, et al: Predicting the effects of transfusing only phenotyped-matched RBCs to patients with sickle cell disease: Theoretical and practical implications. Transfusion 2002;42:684.

20. Cattan D, et al: Maladie de Fanconi et cancer du foie. Arch Fr Mal App Dig 1974;63:41.

21. Cohen A: Management of iron overload in the pediatric patient. Hematol Oncol Clin North Am 1987;1:521.

22. Cohen A, Markenson AL, Schwartz E: Transfusion requirements and splenectomy in thalassemia major. J Pediatr 1980;97:100.

23. Colman RW, et al: Effects of a perfluoro erythrocyte substitute on platelets in vitro and in vivo. J Lab Clin Med 1980;95:553.

24. Dahlbäck B, Hildebrand B: Inherited resistance to activated protein C is corrected by anticoagulant cofactor activity found to be a property of factor V. Proc Natl Acad Sci U S A 1994;91:1396.

25. Dallman PR: Iron deficiency and related nutritional anemias. In Nathan DG, Oski FA (eds): Hematology of Infancy and Childhood, 3rd ed. Philadelphia, WB Saunders, 1987.

26. Daly PA, et al: Platelet transfusion therapy: One-hour posttransfusion increments are valuable in predicting the need for HLA-matched preparations. JAMA 1980;243:435.

27. Davies SC: Blood transfusion in sickle cell disease. Curr Opin Hematol 1996;3:485.

28. Eisenstein EM: Congenital amegakaryocytic thrombocytopenic purpura. Clin Pediatr 1966;5:143.

29. Firth PG, Head CA: Sickle cell disease and anesthesia. Anesthesiology 2004;101:766.

30. Fosburg MT, Kevy SV: Red cell transfusion. In Nathan DG, Oski FA (eds): Hematology of Infancy and Childhood, 3rd ed. Philadelphia, WB Saunders, 1987.

31. Gadner H: Management of immune thrombocytopenic purpura in children. Rev Clin Exp Hematol 2001;5:201.

32. Galea P, et al: Isoimmune neonatal thrombocytopenic purpura. Arch Dis Child 1981;56:112.

33. Ganser A, et al: Effects of recombinant human interleukin-3 in aplastic anemia. Blood 1990;76:1287.

34. Gasser C: Akute erythroblastopenie. Schweiz Med Wochenschr 1949;79:838.

35. Geyer RP: "Bloodless" rats through use of artificial blood substitutes. Fed Proc 1975;34:1499.

36. Gill FM, et al: Clinical events in the first decade in a cohort of infants with sickle cell disease. Blood 1995; 86:776.

37. Glanzmann E: Hereditaire haemorrhagische thromboasthenie E in beitrag zur pathologie der blut plattchen. Jahrb Kinderheilk 1918;88:1.

38. Gluckman E, et al: Bone marrow transplantation in Fanconi anaemia. Br J Haematol 1980;45:557.

39. Gmur J, et al: Safety of stringent prophylactic platelet transfusion policy for patients with acute leukemia. Lancet 1991; 338:1223.

40. Gmyrek D, Syllm-Rapoport I: Zur Fanconi-Anämie FA: Analyse von 129 beschriedenen Fällen. Z Kinderheilk 1964; 91:297, 1964.

41. Goldfinger D, McGinniss MH: Rh-incompatible platelet transfusions: Risks and consequences of sensitizing immunosuppressed patients. N Engl J Med 1971; 284:942.

42. Greenbaum BH: Transfusion-associated graft-versus-host disease: Historical perspectives, incidence, and current use of irradiated blood products. J Clin Oncol 1991; 9:1889.

43. Griffin JH: Clinical studies of protein C. Semin Thromb Hemost 1984;10:162.

44. Griffin TC, Buchanan GR: Elective surgery in children with sickle cell disease without preoperative blood transfusion. J Pediatr Surg 1993;28:681.

45. Gross S, Kiwanuka J: Chronic ITP terminating in aplastic anemia. Am J Pediatr Hematol Oncol 1981;3:446.

46. Hall JG, et al: Thrombocytopenia with absent radius (TAR). Medicine 1969;48:411.

47. Hamberg M, et al: Isolation and structure of two prostaglandin endoperoxides that cause platelet aggregation. Proc Natl Acad Sci U S A 1974;71:345.

48. Haroon Y, et al: The content of phylloquinone (vitamin K_1) in human milk, cows' milk and infant formula foods determined by high-performance liquid chromatography. J Nutr 1982;112:1105.

49. Hathaway WE: New insights on vitamin K. Hematol Oncol Clin North Am 1987;1:367.

50. Higby DJ, et al: The prophylactic treatment of thrombocytopenic leukaemic patients with platelets: A double blind study. Transfusion 1974;14:440.

51. Hillyer CD, et al: Methods for the reduction of transfusion-transmitted cytomegalovirus infection: Filtration versus the use of seronegative donor units. Transfusion 1994;34:929.

52. Holland PV, Schmidt PJ (eds): Committee on Standards, American Association of Blood Banks: Standards for Blood Banks and Transfusion Services, 12th ed. Arlington, Va, American Association of Blood Banks, 1987.

53. Howard MA, Firkin B: Ristocetin—a new tool in the investigation of platelet aggregation. Thromb Diath Haemorrhag 1971;26:362.

54. Howarth S, Sharpey-Schafer EP: Low blood pressure phases following hemorrhage. Lancet 1947;1:19.

55. Hutchinson RJ: Blood products. Semin Pediatr Surg 1992;1:231.

56. Ilett SJ, Lilleyman JS: Platelet transfusion requirements of children with newly diagnosed lymphoblastic leukemia. Acta Haematol 1979;62:86.

57. Iriondo A, et al: Complete recovery of hemopoiesis following bone marrow transplant in a patient with

unresponsive congenital hypoplastic anemia (Blackfan-Diamond syndrome). Blood 1984;64:348.

58. Kojima S, et al: Treatment of aplastic anemia in children with recombinant human granulocyte colony-stimulating factor. Blood 1991;77:937.

59. Laharrague P, et al: Antithrombin III: Substitutive treatment of the hereditary deficiency. Thromb Haemost 1980;1:72.

60. Lee EJ, Schiffer CA: ABO compatibility can influence the results of platelet transfusion: Results of a randomized trial. Transfusion 1989;29:384.

61. Li FP, et al: The mortality of acquired aplastic anemia in children. Blood 1972;40:153.

62. Lohrmann HP, et al: Platelet transfusions from HL-a compatible unrelated donors to alloimmunized patients. Ann Intern Med 1974;80:9.

63. Lusher JM: Diseases of coagulation: The fluid phase. In Nathan DG, Oski FA (eds): Hematology of Infancy and Childhood, 3rd ed. Philadelphia, WB Saunders, 1987.

64. Lusher JM, Iyer R: Idiopathic thrombocytopenic purpura in children. Semin Thromb Hemost 1977;3:175.

65. Lusher JM, et al: Idiopathic thrombocytopenic purpura in children. Am J Pediatr Hematol Oncol 1984;6:149.

66. MacKinney AA, et al: Ascertaining genetic carriers of hereditary spherocytosis by statistical analysis of multiple laboratory tests. J Clin Invest 1962;41:554.

67. Manco-Johnson MJ, et al: Recommendations for tPA thrombolysis in children. On behalf of the Scientific Subcommittee on Perinatal and Pediatric Thrombosis of the Scientific and Standardization Committee of the International Society of Thrombosis and Haemostasis. Thromb Haemost 2002;88:157.

68. McClure PD: Idiopathic thrombocytopenic purpura in children: Diagnosis and management. Pediatrics 1975;55:68.

69. Mollison PL, Engelfriet CP, Contreras M: Blood Transfusion in Clinical Medicine, 8th ed. Oxford, Blackwell Scientific, 1987.

70. Mollison PL, Young IM: In vivo survival in the human subject of transfused erythrocytes after storage in various preservative solutions. Q J Exp Physiol 1942;31:359.

71. Moroff G, et al: The influence of irradiation on stored platelets. Transfusion 1986;26:453.

72. Nilsson IM, Blombäck M, Von Francken I: On an inherited autosomal hemorrhagic diathesis with antihaemophilic globulin (AHG) deficiency and prolonged bleeding time. Acta Med Scand 1957;159:35.

73. Odegard OR, Abildgaard U: Antifactor X a activity in thrombophilia: Studies in a family with AT III deficiency. Scand J Haematol 1977;18:86.

74. Olson RE: Vitamin K. In Colman PW, et al (eds): Hemostasis and Thrombosis: Basic Principles and Clinical Practice. Philadelphia, JB Lippincott, 1982.

75. Oski FA: The erythrocyte and its disorders. In Nathan DG, Oski FA (eds): Hematology of Infancy and Childhood, 3rd ed. Philadelphia, WB Saunders, 1987.

76. Perry GS III, et al: The Wiskott-Aldrich syndrome in the United States and Canada (1892-1979). J Pediatr 1980;97:72.

77. Pisciotto PT, Snyder EL: Platelet defects and their therapy. In Luban NLC (ed): Transfusion Therapy in Infants and Children. Baltimore, Johns Hopkins University Press, 1991.

78. Prydz H: Vitamin K-dependent clotting factors. Semin Thromb Hemost 1977;4:1.

79. Ramsay NKC, et al: Total lymphoid irradiation and cyclophosphamide as preparation for bone marrow transplantation in severe aplastic anemia. Blood 1980;55:344.

80. Reid NM: Chronic idiopathic thrombocytopenic purpura: Incidence, treatment, and outcome. Arch Dis Child 1995;72:125.

81. Rennels MB, et al: Cholelithiasis in patients with major sickle hemoglobinopathies. Am J Dis Child 1983;138:66.

82. Robertson HD, Polk HC: Blood transfusions in elective operations: Comparison of whole blood versus packed red cells. Ann Surg 1975;181:778.

83. Rock G, Adams GA, Labow RS: The effects of irradiation on platelet function. Transfusion 1988;28:451.

84. Russell SJM: Blood volume studies in healthy children. Arch Dis Child 1949;24:88.

85. Schafer AI: The hypercoagulable states. Ann Intern Med 1985;102:814.

86. Schaison G, et al: L' anémie de fanconi. fréquence de l' évolution vers la leucémie. Presse Med 1983;12:1269.

87. Seeler RA, Shwiaki MZ: Acute splenic sequestration crises (ASSC) in young children with sickle cell anemia. Clin Pediatr 1972;11:701.

88. Shahidi NT, Diamond LK: Testosterone-induced remission in aplastic anemia of both acquired and congenital types: Further observations in 24 cases. N Engl J Med 1961;264:953.

89. Shapiro SS, Anderson DB: Thrombin inhibition in normal plasma. In Lundblad R, Fenton J, Mann K (eds): Chemistry and Biology of Thrombin. Ann Arbor, Mich, Science Publishers, 1977.

90. Simpson MB: Platelet function and transfusion therapy in the surgical patient. In Schiffer CA (ed): Platelet Physiology and Transfusion. Washington DC, American Association of Blood Banks, 1978.

91. Slichter SJ: Controversies in platelet transfusion therapy. Annu Rev Med 1980;31:509.

92. Slichter SJ, Harker LA: Preparation and storage of platelet concentrates. II. Storage variables influencing platelet viability and function. Br J Haematol 1976;34:403.

93. Smedley JC, Bellingham AJ: Current problems in haematology. 2. Hereditary spherocytosis. J Clin Pathol 1991;44:441.

94. Snyder EL, DePalma L, Napychank P: Use of polyester filters for preparation of leukocyte-poor platelet concentrates. Vox Sang 1988;54:21.

95. Squires JE: Artificial blood. Science 2002;295:1002.

96. Stevens CE, et al: Hepatitis B virus antibody in blood donors and the occurrence of non-A, non-B hepatitis in transfusion recipients: An analysis of the transfusion-transmitted viruses study. Ann Intern Med 1984;101:733.

97. Stuart MJ, Kelton JG: The platelet: Quantitative and qualitative abnormalities. In Nathan DG, Oski FA (eds): Hematology of Infancy and Childhood, 3rd ed. Philadelphia, WB Saunders, 1987.

98. Thaler E, et al: Antithrombin III replacement therapy in patients with congenital and acquired antithrombin III deficiency. Thromb Haemost 1979;42:327.

99. Thomas WJ, et al: Free erythrocyte protoporphyrin: Hemoglobin ratios, serum ferritin and transferrin saturation levels during treatment of infants with iron deficiency anemia. Blood 1977;49:455.

100. Vadhan-Raj S, et al: Stimulation of myelopoiesis in patients with aplastic anemia by recombinant human granulocyte-macrophage colony-stimulating factor. N Engl J Med 1988;319:1268.

101. Valentine WN, Neel JV: Hematologic and genetic study of transmission of thalassemia (Cooley's anemia; Mediterranean anemia). Arch Intern Med 1944;74:185.

102. Vercellotti GM, et al: Activation of plasma complement by perfluorocarbon artificial blood: Probable mechanism of adverse pulmonary reactions in treated patients and rationale for corticosteroid prophylaxis. Blood 1982; 59:1299.

103. Vichinsky EP, et al: A comparison of conservative and aggressive transfusion regimens in the perioperative management of sickle cell disease. N Engl J Med 1995; 333:206.

104. Vichinsky EP, et al: Prospective RBC phenotype matching in a stroke-prevention trial in sickle cell anemia: A multicenter transfusion trial. Transfusion 2001;41:1086.

105. Wang WC, Mentzer WC: Differentiation of transient erythroblastopenia of childhood from congenital hypoplastic anemia. J Pediatr 1976;88:784.

106. Zöller B, Dahlbäck B: Linkage between inherited resistance to activated protein C and factor V gene mutation in venous thrombosis. Lancet 1994;343:1536.

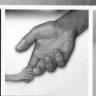

Chapter 12

Nutritional Support

Daniel H. Teitelbaum and Arnold G. Coran

The development of modern nutritional support is the result of numerous investigators' contributions during the past 350 years. The first known person to attempt to deliver intravenous nutrition was Sir Christopher Wren in 1658, the architect of St. Paul's Cathedral in London. Wren used hollow goose quills to infuse wine into dogs. In the 19th century Claude Bernard, the first physiologist, infused numerous substrates into animals. He discovered that intravenously administered sugars could be effectively metabolized only if they were predigested by gastric juices; this constituted the first understanding of the digestion of carbohydrates.[172] In the 1930s Elman[62] delivered the first successful infusion of protein, as hydrolysates of casein, into patients. In 1949 Rhoads et al.[171] developed an apparatus for the continuous infusion of intravenous substances into dogs. It definitively showed that weight gain in puppies could be achieved by means of intravenous nutrition. Critical refinements in the application, and the use of a central venous catheter, allowed Dudrick and colleagues to infuse concentrated solutions of glucose and amino acids into patients.[59,60,228] This technique allowed the use of total parenteral nutrition (TPN) in adult and pediatric patients. One of the most dramatic cases of the use of TPN was in a newborn with jejunoileal atresia; the infant was maintained by this route for more than 22 months and had weight gain and an increased head circumference.[228] Application of this technique in other infants caused a dramatic improvement in survival among those who previously would have died after the surgical correction of congenital anomalies. The past 50 years has led to dramatic developments in both specialized enteral and parenteral products for infants and children. Use of intravenous administration devices and central venous catheterization has allowed the administration of parenteral nutrition (PN) to numerous surgical patients who otherwise would have suffered from the consequences of malnutrition due to prolonged periods of starvation.

NORMAL PEDIATRIC GROWTH

Unique to the pediatric patient is growth and development. The term newborn grows at a rate of 25 to 30 g/day over the first 6 months of life, leading to a doubling of the birth weight by 5 months of age.[125] The average infant triples his or her birth weight by 12 months. By 3 years of age, the weight is four times the birth weight, and by the completion of the first decade, the weight increases by 20-fold. Body length increases 50% by the end of the first year of life and increases threefold by the end of the first decade. The preterm infant's growth pattern is quite distinct from that of a term infant. Most nutrients are accumulated by the fetus in the third trimester of pregnancy. Thus, fat accounts for only 1% to 2% of body weight in a 1-kg infant, compared with 16% in a term (3.5-kg) infant. An anticipated loss of 15% of a preterm infant's birth weight is usual in the first 7 to 10 days of life, compared with a 7% to 10% weight loss for a term infant. After this initial period of weight loss, a preterm infant less than 27 weeks' gestation gains weight at a slower rate of approximately 10 to 20 g/day because he or she has not yet entered the accelerated weight gain of the third trimester.[176]

NUTRITIONAL ASSESSMENT

Nutritional assessment is a critical aspect of the initial evaluation of all surgical patients.[13] The incidence of malnutrition in surgical patients has been well documented in several reviews.[25] Classic work by Cooper et al.[46] showed that 18% to 40% of pediatric surgical patients suffer malnutrition; this rate of malnutrition has also been documented in other pediatric patients.[84] Other patients at risk for malnutrition include those with large, open wounds with concomitant loss of protein and increased metabolic needs; extensive burns; blunt trauma; and sepsis. An important question is how long the gastrointestinal (GI) tract will be dysfunctional after major surgery; this information must be integrated into the nutritional support delivered in the perioperative period. Nutritional assessment can be divided into subjective and objective components.

A subjective global assessment is performed during the history and physical examination. This should include an evaluation of weight loss (5% indicates mild malnutrition; 10%, moderate to severe malnutrition), anorexia, vomiting, as well as physical evidence of muscle wasting (indicative of severe malnutrition); this evaluation has been modified for pediatric patients, but it is not as well validated as that for adults.[184] The subjective global assessment has been shown to be an accurate means of assessing malnutrition in both hospitalized and nonhospitalized patients.

The objective portion of the assessment begins with the basic anthropometric measurements of height, weight, and head circumference. Measurements are placed on a standardized growth curve such as that of the National Center for Health Statistics. From these growth charts, the expected weight-for-height index can be calculated. Because length and head circumference are less affected by excess fat or postoperative fluid fluctuations, length is an excellent indicator of long-term body growth. Acute changes in nutritional status have a more immediate effect on body weight than on length and thus decrease the child's weight-for-height index. Chronic undernutrition, in contrast, results in a lag in both height and weight.

Biochemical Measurements of Nutritional Status

The serum albumin level has been used as an indication of chronic nutritional status. However, albumin turnover is slow (half-life of 18 days). Therefore, other proteins such as prealbumin binding protein (half-life of 2 days) and retinol binding protein (half-life of 12 hours) are indications of more current intake. There are no established norms for prealbumin or retinol binding protein in infants and young children.[132] Ideally, a baseline level is obtained, and then subsequent levels can be used to determine the effects of disease or nutritional supplementation. Other parameters that may be useful for measuring nutritional status include bone age and dental status. Malnutrition is a common cause of delayed bone maturation.[58]

Direct Measurement of Body Composition

Various methods have been created over the past 25 years to more directly measure the body composition of adults and children. Many of these methods are not readily accessible to most clinicians. Some, however, are becoming more common in pediatric centers. Measurement of body water has been done for several years using isotope dilution techniques. This is based on the principle that fat is anhydrous, so most of the isotope is directed into the water compartments of the body.[48] Although this assumption is not always true, such measurements can give an excellent indication of approximate amounts of body fat and water.[47,90] Bioelectrical impedance analysis measures the body's impedance to a flow of electrical current as a means of determining total body water. These measurements can then be extrapolated to other body compartments, including total body adipose tissue. More recently, dual photon absorptiometry and dual energy x-ray absorptiometry have been used to measure bone mineral content and amounts of fat and body water.[28,173] The accuracy of the instruments is excellent,

and because of the low amounts of radiation exposure, dual energy x-ray absorptiometry may eventually become the method of choice for measuring pediatric body composition.

NUTRITIONAL REQUIREMENTS

Energy Requirements

The energy needs of infants and children are unique. It is estimated that a premature infant weighing 1 kg has only a 4-day nutritional reserve, and a full-term infant can live for no more than 1 month without nutrition.[83,154] In children, energy is required for the maintenance of body metabolism and for growth. A gross estimate of calorie expenditure can be obtained using the recommended dietary allowance (RDA) for energy requirements, based on the child's age and ideal body weight. Energy requirements vary depending on age and physiologic status of the child (Table 12-1). Periods of active growth and extreme physical activity increase energy requirements. The average distribution of kilocalories in a well-balanced diet is as follows: protein, 15%; fat, 35%; and carbohydrate, 50%.

Although careful clinical examination is important in determining a child's nutritional status, Baker et al.[14] showed that the depleted state cannot be reliably detected on the basis of weight-to-height ratio, triceps skinfold, mid-upper arm circumference, hand strength, albumin concentration, total protein level, or creatinine-height ratio. Actual measurement or estimation of metabolic rate is the best method of following the nutritional status. Commonly used nomograms may significantly underestimate or overestimate energy expenditure.[97,130,138] One of the most accurate methods of measuring energy expenditure is indirect calorimetry,[42] in which carbon dioxide production and oxygen consumption are measured. The sample is best measured in intubated infants yielding a resting energy expenditure (REE). The energy expenditure or metabolic rate, as measured in cubic centimeters of oxygen per minute, can be converted to calories per hour or per day if the substrates are known. All measurements are only approximations of caloric needs; the clinician must make adjustments according to the patient's clinical course. This is an excellent way to monitor patients, particularly those who are in an intensive care setting.[225] In contrast to adults, the rise in REE after

	TABLE 12-1 Kilocalorie and Protein Requirements		
Age (yr)	**Kilocalories (per kg body weight)**	**Protein (g/kg body weight)**	
0-1	90-120	2.0-3.5	
1-7	75-90	2.0-2.5	
7-12	60-75	2.0	
12-18	30-60	1.5	
>18	25-30	1.0	

surgery is much less in children. Mitchell et al.[138] found that the REE of postoperative cardiac patients fell to values below those of normal, healthy children who had not undergone surgery. This finding was confirmed in the study by Letton et al.,[115] who examined energy expenditure in young infants in the postoperative period. These studies suggest that reliance on RDA values may result in the overfeeding of postoperative children (discussed later). Indirect calorimetry, however, may be difficult in young infants with uncuffed endotracheal tubes, where an air leak may lead to significant inaccuracies in results.

Water

The water content of infants is higher than that of adults (75% of body weight versus 65%). Fluids provide the principal source of water; however, some is provided by the oxidation of food and by body tissues. Requirements for water are related to calorie consumption, so infants must consume much larger amounts of water per unit of body weight than adults. In general, calorie requirements (kcal/kg per day) are matched to fluid requirements (mL/kg per day). The daily consumption of fluid by healthy infants is equivalent to 10% to 15% of their body weight, in contrast to only 2% to 4% by adults. In addition, the natural food of infants and children is much higher in water content than that of adults; the fruit and vegetables consumed by infants and children contain about 90% water. Only 0.5% to 3% of fluid intake is retained by infants and children. About 50% is excreted through the kidneys, 3% to 10% is lost through the GI tract, and 40% to 50% is insensible loss.

Protein

The requirement for protein in infants is based on the combined needs of growth and maintenance (see Table 12-1). The average intake of protein should constitute approximately 15% of total calories administered. Two percent of an infant's body weight (compared with 3% of an adult's) consists of nitrogen. Most of the increase in body nitrogen occurs during the first year of life. The nutritional value of protein is based not only on the amount of nitrogen available but also on the amino acid composition of the protein.[103] Protein provides 4 kcal/g of energy and should generally be included in estimates of caloric delivery.

Twenty amino acids have been identified, of which nine are essential in infants (Table 12-2). New tissue cannot be formed unless all the essential amino acids are present in the diet simultaneously; the absence of only one essential amino acid results in a negative nitrogen and protein balance. Protein requirements are thus markedly higher in term neonates and infants (compared with older children), ranging from 2.0 to 3.0 g/kg per day. This estimate is based on several sources. Extrapolation of data on fetal absorption across the placenta during the last trimester indicates that protein needs are 2.2 g/kg per day.[113,238] Delivery of greater amounts of protein to neonates has generally been associated with

TABLE 12-2 Essential Amino Acids	
Threonine	Tryptophan
Leucine	Histidine*
Isoleucine	Tyrosine†
Valine	Cysteine†
Lysine	Proline†
Methionine	Glutamine†
Phenylalanine	Arginine†

*Essential only in infancy.
†May be essential in premature babies.
‡May be essential in times of excess stress and energy demands.

elevated blood urea nitrogen levels. Protein requirements in premature infants are higher than in term infants, ranging from 3.0 to 3.5 g/kg per day.[238] In very-low-birth-weight infants, this requirement may approach 3.85 g/kg per day.[237] Such added protein loads must be balanced against the immaturity of the renal system, and the development of uremia should be monitored. Three amino acids are considered conditionally essential in neonates: histidine, cysteine, and tyrosine.[82,137] It has also been suggested that proline is essential in preterm infants, although this has yet to be confirmed.[179] In addition, taurine is essential for normal neural and retinal development,[236] and taurine supplementation has been shown to decrease the severity of PN-associated cholestasis.[194] Premature infants are at particular risk; thus, specialized crystalline amino acid solutions should be used in premature infants on a prolonged course (>2 weeks) of PN.

Two amino acids that may be beneficial to the integrity of the GI mucosa and the immune status of patients are glutamine and arginine. Although these amino acids are not truly essential, the body may require additional amounts during periods of stress. Glutamine has been shown to prevent TPN-associated atrophy of the intestine in animals and possibly in humans.[191,235] More recently, the efficacy of glutamine in bowel adaptation has been called into question.[34,73,233] Arginine has also been shown to improve nitrogen retention, wound healing, and the immune status.[12,180] However, at least in animal models, early administration of arginine has been shown to worsen prognosis owing to the activation of nitric oxide within the GI tract.[109]

Carbohydrate

Carbohydrates provide a major source of nutrition through parenteral and enteral routes. Carbohydrates can be provided in three forms: monosaccharides (glucose and fructose), disaccharides (lactose, sucrose, and maltose), and complex carbohydrates (starches). Because the body is capable of forming sugars from amino acids, no essential amount of carbohydrate has been defined. However, the addition of small amounts of carbohydrate prevents the breakdown of somatic protein sources and thus acts as a protein-sparing substrate.[104] This effect leads to the suppression of endogenous glucose production and endogenous glucose oxidation, thereby preventing the oxidation of amino acids derived from skeletal muscle. The body has a limited ability to store glucose, although the substrate is essential and is needed almost continuously by the central nervous system. Dextrose is the most common source of carbohydrate, and it yields 3.4 kcal/g. Glucose metabolism may occur aerobically through the tricarboxylic acid cycle, yielding 38 moles of adenosine triphosphate (ATP) per mole of glucose, or anaerobically through the glycolytic cycle, yielding 2 moles of ATP per mole of glucose and producing lactic acid as an end product. Glucose is formed in the liver by means of gluconeogenesis, which uses amino acids from skeletal muscle and lactic acid from the breakdown of glycogen in skeletal muscle through the Cori cycle (once converted to pyruvate). Immediately after a meal, glucose absorption contributes to the bulk of circulating glucose. As soon as 4 hours after a meal, these sources are rapidly depleted, and glycogen from the liver becomes a major source of energy for the next 8 to 12 hours. Newborn infants have relatively limited glycogen reserves (34 g), most of which reside in the liver. Thus, relatively short periods of fasting can lead to a hypoglycemic state.

The primary enteral carbohydrate delivered to neonates and young infants is lactose.[2] Lactose is broken down into glucose and galactose by disaccharidases (e.g., lactase), located along the intestinal epithelial border. Because lactose is the predominant carbohydrate of small children, lactase levels remain sufficiently high in most children until they are at least 2 or 3 years old. Nonlactose formulas that are soy based and contain sucrose or corn syrup may provide adequate amounts of carbohydrates (see the section on enteral feedings). Preterm infants may be unable to digest certain carbohydrates, particularly lactose, because lactase activity in the intestines (via the citric acid cycle) is inadequate. Thus, for premature infants, formulas that have a 50-50 mixture of lactose and glucose polymers are ideal.

Supplementation with inadequate amounts of glucose may lead to a ketotic state, whereby fat and muscles are broken down for gluconeogenesis. Stable infants should receive approximately 40% to 45% of their total caloric intake as carbohydrates. Glucose intolerance does occur and is manifested not only by hyperglycemia but also quite commonly by hypertriglyceridemia (see later). Delivery of carbohydrates greater than the body can use results in hyperglycemia and lipogenesis (discuseed in the section on complications).

Fat

Intravenous fats have the highest caloric density of the three major nutrients (9 kcal/g). In general, intravenous fats should constitute between 30% and 50% of all non-nitrogen calories. Lipids have the advantage of being an excellent source of energy and essential fatty acids. Linoleic acid is essential for neonates, older children, and adults. Deficiencies of linoleic acid may occur rapidly in neonates. Withholding lipids from the PN of a neonate for as few as 3 days may lead to a deficiency of fatty acids.[72,116] In infants, a fatty acid deficiency may result

when less than 1% of the caloric intake is linoleic acid; in general, 2% to 4% of dietary energy should come from essential fatty acids. Manifestations of fatty acid deficiency include scaly skin, hair loss, diarrhea, and impaired wound healing.[66] Absence of trace amounts of linolenic acid may also be the cause of visual and behavioral disorders. Fatty acids are an excellent source of energy to all tissues of the body, except the erythrocytes and the brain. However, the brain can also use fatty acids as an energy source once they are converted to ketones. Fatty acids are carried into the mitochondria for beta oxidation by the carnitine transferase system (see later).

Essentially, two types of fatty acids exist: saturated and unsaturated. Saturated fatty acids lack double carbon bonds and are generally derived from animals. Unsaturated fatty acids have at least one double bond, the position of which is designated by the prefix omega. The two major polyunsaturated fatty acids are linoleic acid, which is an omega-6 fatty acid, and α-linolenic acid, which is an omega-3 fatty acid. Omega-6 fatty acids are usually derived from plants, and omega-3 fatty acids are usually derived from fish oils. Both of these polyunsaturated fats are essential for the development of cell membranes and the central nervous system, as well as for the synthesis of arachidonic acid and related prostaglandins. Thromboxanes derived from omega-6 fatty acids are potential mediators of platelet aggregation, whereas thromboxanes derived from omega-3 fatty acids are potent anticoagulants. Omega-6 fatty acids, which form arachidonic acid, also contribute to the formation of prostaglandin (PG) E_2, a known immunosuppressant, whereas omega-3 fatty acids contribute to the formation of PGE_1 and PGE_3, which do not have an immunosuppressive effect (Fig. 12-1). A 50-50 ratio of omega-6 to omega-3 fatty acids seems to be ideal, based on experimental data from animals that have survived burns.[3] No data are available on the ideal ratio in neonates or children.

Deficiencies can be monitored by calculating a triene-to-tetraene ratio of greater than 0.4 (with normal level ≤ 0.2); where trienes consist of 5,8,11-eicosatrienoic acid and tetraenes consist of linoleic and arachidonic acids and an eicosatrienoic-arachidonic acid.

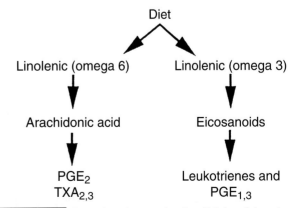

Figure 12-1 Formation of prostaglandins (PGs) and thromboxanes (TXs) derived from omega-3 and omega-6 fatty acids.

Minerals, Trace Elements, and Vitamins

The normal daily requirements of vitamins were recently revised by the Food and Drug Administration.[101] Vitamins are essential components or cofactors of various metabolic reactions. Most commercial infant formulas contain adequate amounts of vitamins to meet known daily requirements. Such requirements were established by the American Medical Association in the 1970s.[7] Infants who receive other types of formula or human milk may require additional vitamin supplementation.

Fat-Soluble Vitamins

Vitamin A

Vitamin A is stored principally in the liver and is involved in the formation of retinoic acid for vision and the coordination of cell cycles. Deficiencies of vitamin A may lead to night blindness, xerophthalmia, poor growth, and impaired resistance to infection. Whether vitamin A can improve bronchopulmonary dysplasia remains uncertain.[102] It is clear, however, that low levels of vitamin A predispose infants to long-term pulmonary disease.[193] Excessive amounts of vitamin A can also be deleterious to infants. As little as 6000 mg of retinol daily can produce anorexia, desquamation of the skin, and increased intracranial pressure.[122]

Vitamin D

Vitamin D is essential for bone formation and mineral homeostasis. A deficiency may occur with fat malabsorption; however, overuse of vitamin D may lead to hypercalcemia.[143] Most formulas contain adequate amounts of vitamin D (approximately 60 IU/100 kcal). There is no evidence that vitamin D supplementation beyond that provided by standard formulas promotes better bone growth.

Vitamin E

Vitamin E seems to have significant antioxidant effects. Vitamin E may prevent the neuropathy seen in infants with biliary atresia, as well as muscle weakness in children with cystic fibrosis.[190] The dose of vitamin E required for full-term infants is approximately 0.7 IU/100 kcal of energy intake. Because of its antioxidant action, vitamin E has been used to decrease lung injury in neonates with bronchopulmonary dysplasia, and it appears that vitamin E is beneficial in this regard.[64] It is less clear whether vitamin E is beneficial in the prevention of retinopathy in premature infants; however, it may reduce the incidence of intraventricular hemorrhage.[156]

Vitamin K

Vitamin K is required at birth to prevent coagulopathy and should be administered soon after delivery.[202] Vitamin K is included in most formulas, but larger amounts may be needed in infants with prolonged episodes of diarrhea. Assessment of deficiency is most readily done by attaining a prothrombin time.

Water-Soluble Vitamins

Deficiencies of water-soluble vitamins are rare in formula-fed and breast-fed babies. B vitamins are needed for carbohydrate, protein, and fat metabolism, as well as oxidation and reduction reactions. Deficiencies may be seen with the short-bowel syndrome and manifest as chelosis and lethargy. An abnormal level of vitamin B_1 (thiamine) is generally the first sign of vitamin B deficiency and can be detected with an erythrocyte transketolase enzyme assay. Vitamin C is required for optimizing several enzyme reactions and has direct antioxidant effects. Excessive amounts of vitamin C may lead to nephrolithiasis and interfere with vitamin B_{12} absorption. Excessive amounts of ascorbic acid during pregnancy may lead to scurvy in normally fed infants.

Trace Elements

Trace elements constitute less than 0.01% of the total body weight in humans.[133] They often function as metalloenzymes, which maximize enzymatic reactions, but they also may act as soluble ionic cofactors or nonprotein organic molecules. Without supplementation, specific deficiencies of many of these factors may manifest clinically in patients maintained on long-term TPN, as well as those with short-bowel syndrome or malabsorptive conditions. Table 12-3 lists the recommended doses of trace elements.

Zinc

Zinc has several biochemical functions, including the formation of metalloenzymes, RNA conformation, and membrane stabilization.[22] In addition, zinc seems to play a critical role in the maintenance of a normal immune system.

TABLE 12–3 Recommended Daily Trace Element Supplements for Pediatric and Adolescent Patients Receiving Total Parenteral Nutrition

Element	Infant* (µg/kg/day)	Adolescent (µg/kg/day)	Consequence of Deficiency
Zinc (sulfate)	250†	50	Dermatitis
Copper (sulfate)	20	20	Anemia, neutropenia
Manganese (sulfate)	1.0	1.0	None identified
Chromium (chloride)	0.20	0.05 to 0.20	Hyperglycenia
Selenium (as selenious acid)	2.0	2.0	Myositis, cardiomyopathy

*Amounts exceed those normally recommended, assuming that a significant proportion of the enteral trace elements will not be absorbed.
†400 µg/kg/day should be added for premature infants.

Deficiencies in zinc can arise from various sources that are common in pediatric surgical patients, including the short-bowel syndrome, thermal burns, peritoneal dialysis, inflammatory bowel disease, and other causes of diarrhea. Clinical manifestations of zinc deficiency include growth retardation, alopecia, skin lesions (acrodermatitis enteropathica), impaired lymphocyte function, and impaired wound healing.[206] Supplementation in premature infants should be a minimum of 400 µg/kg per day. Because GI losses can be higher during episodes of diarrhea and sepsis, higher doses are indicated in these instances. In addition, zinc deficiency may impair recovery of the intestine after massive resection.[204]

Copper

Copper is a critical trace element for metalloenzyme function. The main site of copper storage, distribution, and excretion is the liver. Copper deficiency is common in patients receiving PN formulas that are not supplemented with copper.[99] Manifestations of copper deficiency include a microcytic, hypochromic anemia; neutropenia; and, in children, growth retardation and skeletal demineralization. Removal of copper from infants and children may lead to an aplastic anemic condition, which can be fatal.[195]

Selenium

Over the past two decades, selenium has been acknowledged as an essential trace element. It is a component of a selenoenzyme that helps catalyze glutathione peroxidase, an enzyme necessary to reduce free radicals. The most practical way of measuring selenium levels is by assaying glutathione peroxidase activity in erythrocytes. Selenium levels dramatically decline after as few as 6 weeks of TPN.[79] Without the addition of selenium, deficiencies generally manifest as cardiomyopathy and peripheral myositis with associated muscle tenderness.

Manganese, Chromium, and Molybdenum

Although no clear-cut cases of manganese deficiency have been documented in the literature, manganese is an essential element for many organisms and is believed to be essential for humans as well. Animals that are deficient in manganese show growth retardation and ataxia in the newborn period.[9] Chromium's predominant action seems to be as a potentiator of insulin action, and deficiencies of chromium can lead to poor glucose tolerance.[147] Molybdenum is important in the oxidative metabolism of purines and sulfur-containing compounds.[167] Deficiencies of molybdenum are associated with increases in serum uric acid levels.

ENTERAL NUTRITION

Enteral nutrition (EN) includes oral nutritional supplementation and tube feeding. EN should be the primary source of nutrients if the GI tract is functional. Even when full feedings are not tolerated enterally, the provision of small volumes of "trophic" feedings may prevent further deterioration of intestinal function.

Indications

Infants in a state of good health before surgery or trauma can tolerate 5 to 7 days without significant energy intake without suffering serious systemic consequences, provided that adequate nutritional support is initiated thereafter. Premature infants less than 32 weeks' gestation generally do not have a maturely coordinated suck and swallow reflex. Feedings must therefore be provided enterally either by bolus every 2 to 3 hours or by continuous feedings. Enteral feedings are begun after the resolution of postoperative ileus. There are many formulas available to address various needs (Tables 12-4 and 12-5). Children who have specific underlying diseases associated with malabsorption may benefit from specialized formulas.

Delivery Modalities

Aside from oral intake, a number of modalities are available for enteral delivery. These include nasogastric and nasojejunal feedings. Children receiving gastric feedings tolerate a higher osmolarity and volume than do those being fed into the small bowel. Further, gastric acid may benefit digestion, has a bactericidal effect, and is associated with less-frequent GI complications.[124] Auscultation of air insufflated into the tube is inadequate to verify proper tube placement; confirmation must be obtained by aspiration of GI contents or radiographs.[136] For patients requiring feedings for more than 4 to 8 weeks, a more permanent feeding access (e.g., gastrostomy tube) should be considered. The preoperative assessment usually consists of an upper GI series followed by a 24-hour pH probe study if the results of the upper GI study are abnormal. If either of these studies reveals reflux, a fundoplication should be considered at the time the gastrostomy tube is placed. Assessment of gastric emptying should also be done before surgery.[70,150] The most common procedure for gastrostomy placement is a percutaneous endoscopic gastrostomy (PEG) tube.[76] An improvement in gastrostomy tubes is the gastrostomy "button," made of nonreactive Silastic components. It has a valve placed in a low-profile device that lies almost flush with the abdominal wall, and it can be capped between uses.[75] These buttons can be placed at the same time as the percutaneous endoscopic procedure.[200] It has been reported that the incidence of complications is less with a PEG technique compared with other approaches; however, several complications have been described, including improper placement (i.e., close to the pylorus), inadvertent placement through an adjacent loop of bowel, necrosis of the tract of the gastrostomy tube, and technical failures that require laparotomy.[17]

Use of jejunal tubes is plagued with problems, including involuntary dislodgment of transpylorically placed tubes and catheter obstruction due to inspissation of feedings.

TABLE 12-4 Infant Formulas

Formula	kcal/mL	Protein (g/L)	Protein (% kcal)	Protein Source	Carbohydrate Source	Carbohydrate (% kcal)	Fat Source	Fat (% kcal)	Indications
Similac Special Care (Ross)	0.81	22	11	Nonfat milk, whey	Lactose, corn syrup solids	42	MCT oil, soy oil, coconut oil	47	Prematurity
Neosure (Ross)	0.73	19	10	Nonfat milk, whey	Lactose, corn syrup solids	42	MCT oil, soy oil	48	Prematurity, discharge formula
Enfamil (Mead Johnson)	0.67	14	9	Whey, nonfat milk	Lactose	43	Palm olein, soy oil, coconut oil, sunflower oil	48	Standard
Similac (Ross)	0.67	14	8	Nonfat milk, whey	Lactose	43	Soy oil	49	Standard
	0.81	22	11	Nonfat milk, whey	Lactose	42	Coconut oil	47	
Prosobee (Mead Johnson)	0.67	20	12	Soy isolate, methionine	Corn syrup solids	42	Palm olein, soy oil, coconut oil, sunflower oil	48	Lactose intolerance, galactosemia
Isomil (Ross)	0.67	17	10	Soy isolate, methionine	Corn syrup, sucrose	41	Soy oil, coconut oil	49	Lactose malabsorption, galactosemia
Nutramigen (Mead Johnson)	0.67	19	11	Casein hydrolysate, cystine, tyrosine, tryptophan	Corn syrup solids, modified cornstarch	44	Palm olein, soy oil, coconut oil, sunflower oil	45	Protein intolerance
Pregestimil (Mead Johnson)	0.67	19	11	Casein hydrolysate, cystine, tyrosine, tryptophan	Corn syrup solids, modified cornstarch, dextrose	41	MCT oil, corn oil, soy oil, safflower oil	48	Protein intolerance, cystic fibrosis, neonatal cholestasis, short-bowel syndrome
Alimentum (Ross)	0.67	19	11	Casein hydrolysate, cystine, tyrosine, tryptophan	Sucrose, modified tapioca starch	41	MCT oil, safflower oil, soy oil	48	Protein intolerance, neonatal cholestasis
Neocate (Scientific Hospital Supplies)	0.69	20	12	Free amino acids	Corn syrup solids	47	Safflower oil, corn oil, soy oil	41	Food allergy, protein intolerance, short-bowel syndrome

MCT, medium-chain triglyceride.

Enfamil and Similac both have milk-based proteins and contain lactose as the carbohydrate source. There are only limited reasons to use soy formulas such as Prosobee and Isomil. Both contain corn syrup solids as a carbohydrate source; Isomil also contains sucrose. Soy formulas are indicated to manage galactosemia and primary or secondary lactase deficiency, but they should not be used in patients with a documented allergy or intolerance to milk protein, because one third of such patients are also intolerant of soy. A protein hydrolysate or elemental formula is recommended in infants with a milk protein intolerance. Protein hydrolysates include Nutramigen, Alimentum, and Pregestimil. Alimentum and Pregestimil also provide 50% to 55% of fat as MCTs. If infants have continued symptoms of protein intolerance when ingesting a protein hydrolysate, an amino acid–based formula may be provided. For the infant population, Neocate is the only amino acid–based formula available. Children older than 12 months who continue to be intolerant of milk protein may respond well to Peptamen Jr. (Clintec), which is a whey protein hydrolysate; if an amino acid–based formula is needed in children older than 12 months, options include Neocate 1+ (Scientific Hospital Supplies), L-emental (GalaGen/Nutrition Medical), and Elecare (Ross) (see Table 12-5). Neocate 1+ and Elecare both have long-chain triglycerides. Sixty-eight percent of the fat in L-emental is derived from MCTs.

TABLE 12-5 Pediatric Formulas

Formula	kcal/mL	Protein (g/L)	Protein (% kcal)	Protein Source	Carbohydrate Source	Carbohydrate (% kcal)	Fat Source	Fat (% kcal)	Indications
PediaSure (Ross)	1.0	30	12	Sodium caseinate, whey protein	Hydrolyzed cornstarch, sucrose	44	Safflower oil, soy oil, MCT oil	44	Standard, oral feeds, tube feeds,
Kindercal (Mead Johnson)	1.06	34	13	Sodium caseinate	Maltodextrin, sucrose	50	Canola oil, MCT oil, corn oil, sunflower oil	37	Standard, oral feeds, tube feeds
Boost (Mead Johnson)	1.06	43	17	Milk	Corn syrup, sucrose	53	Canola oil, corn oil, sunflower oil	30	Standard, oral feeds, tube feeds
Peptamen Jr. (Clintec)	1.0	30	12	Hydrolyzed whey	Maltodextrin	55	MCT oil	33	Short-bowel syndrome, cholestasis, pancreatitis
L-emental (GalaGen/ Nutrition Medical)	0.8	24	12	L-Amino acids	Maltodextrin, modified starch	63	MCT oil, soybean oil	25	Short-bowel syndrome, IBD, pancreatitis
Elecare (Ross)	1.0	30	15	L-Amino acids	Corn syrup solids	44	Safflower oil, coconut oil, soy oil	42	Malabsorption, food allergies
Suplena (Ross)	2.5	30	6	Sodium caseinate, calcium caseinate	Hydrolyzed cornstarch, sucrose	51	Safflower oil, soy oil	43	Renal failure

IBD, inflammatory bowel disease; MCT, medium-chain triglyceride.

Short-term complications of surgically placed J-tubes include intra-abdominal abscess and volvulus with bowel infarction. Long-term complications include intestinal obstruction and peritonitis. When using tubes passed distal to the pylorus, continuous drip feedings are initially recommended to prevent the development of diarrhea and other symptoms of dumping. Verification of the location of the tube is mandatory before beginning enteral tube feedings. This requires either aspiration of enteric contents or radiographic confirmation.

Enteral Formulas

The choice of formula depends on the age of the patient and the condition of the GI tract. In general, term infants should be maintained on human milk (see later) or a standard 20 kcal/ounce formula (see Tables 12-4 and 12-5). A lactose-based formula is generally the first choice because it is the most physiologically similar to human milk and is the least expensive. Soy formulas are indicated to manage galactosemia and primary or secondary lactase deficiency. Soy formulas should not be used in patients with a documented allergy or intolerance to milk protein because one third of infants who have an allergen-induced reaction to cow's milk are also intolerant of soy. Therefore, a protein hydrolysate or elemental formula is recommended in infants with a milk protein intolerance. Calories can be added by increasing the volume delivered, increasing the concentration of the formula, or supplementing the feedings. Formula concentrations may be increased to 30 kcal/ounce, but such highly concentrated formulas may be difficult for some infants to digest and have a higher renal solute load; it may take time for an infant to build up a tolerance to the concentrated formula. Higher concentrations have also occasionally been associated with a necrotizing enterocolitis–type process.[31] Formula supplementation can also be achieved by adding a glucose polymer or fats, such as medium-chain triglycerides (MCTs) or vegetable oil. Each 0.5 g of glucose polymer added to an ounce of standard formula increases calories by 0.06 kcal/mL, therefore creating a total caloric delivery of 0.73 kcal/mL. The addition of 0.5 g of oil to the formula increases calories by 0.13 kcal/mL, or a total of 0.8 kcal/mL. Caution must be used when supplementing calories in this fashion, because it may compromise the infant's ability to consume sufficient amounts of protein or minerals if the amount of formula is limited. However, up to 2.0 g of glucose polymer or 1.0 g of oil per ounce of formula can be added safely.

Standard premature infant formulas are milk-based formulas that provide 22 to 24 calories/ounce and are optimized for required vitamins, minerals, and trace elements. A portion of fat is provided as MCTs to compensate for the limited bile salt pool in young infants. MCTs can be absorbed directly through the basolateral surface of the epithelial cell without the need for bile salts. MCTs, however, cannot be used to prevent essential fatty acid deficiency (which requires long-chain triglycerides). The carbohydrate is composed of glucose polymers as well as lactose to optimize carbohydrate absorption in the presence of limited lactase activity. Premature infants

are at increased risk for necrotizing enterocolitis. This risk is not increased with GI priming feeds; however, advancing the rate of feeding too much has been shown to put neonates at increased risk. In general, feeding advancements should not exceed 20 mL/kg per day.[116] Whether feedings are given via bolus or continuous methods does not appear to influence hospital outcome or days required to reach full feeding.[2,189] Finally, premature infants do not fully develop a normal suck and swallow mechanism until after 32 weeks postconceptual age.

If a child is gaining weight poorly, the calorie concentration can be increased by adding relatively less fluid to either the concentrate or the powder. Caution should be used when concentrating these formulas, because rapid advancement in concentration may lead to feeding intolerance as well as rare cases of enterocolitis.[31]

Human Milk

Human milk has a variety of advantages over commercial formulas. The American Academy of Pediatrics advocates nursing until 1 year of age, yet the majority of mothers in the United States stop nursing by the infant's second month of life.[6] Breast-feeding provides both nutrition and passive immunologic protection to the neonate. Breast milk contains 87% water and provides 0.64 to 0.67 kcal/mL. The fat content of breast milk is fairly high at 3.4 g/dL. The protein content of human milk (0.9%) is lower than that of bovine milk or commercial formulas but appears to be much better absorbed because of the higher whey content. Casein, which predominates in bovine milk, is a complex of protein and calcium. The whey fraction contains primarily lactalbumin and lactoferrin, an iron binding protein that is bacteriostatic to *Staphylococcus aureus* and *Escherichia coli* by restricting iron availability.[120] Breast milk also contains elevated levels of cysteine, which may be essential for a neonate, and taurine, which is needed for bile salt excretion and neurologic and retinal development. Despite similar amounts of trace elements, human milk allows a more efficient absorption of these elements compared with commercial formulas. Additionally, ingestion of human milk allows the acquisition of passive immunity via the transfer of both immunoglobulins and lymphocytes from the mother.[162] Although human milk has many advantages, high demands for calcium, phosphorus, electrolytes, vitamins, and trace elements cannot be met with human milk alone. Because of this, human milk fortifiers (one pack per ounce) should be added to breast milk fed to preterm infants. Supplementation should continue until the child achieves the weight of a term infant.

Complications

The GI tract generally tolerates feedings quite well once postoperative ileus has resolved. Not uncommonly, a critically ill child loses a significant portion of the absorptive function, often due to a lactase deficiency. Symptoms generally manifest as cramping, diarrhea, or emesis and often improve with the initiation of a lactose-free diet. Other alterations in the administration of the diet can improve feeding tolerance. First, as previously indicated, the GI tract generally tolerates increased volume more readily than increased osmolarity. Therefore, such adverse symptoms can be avoided by starting with a one-eighth- or one-fourth-strength formula and slowly advancing the concentration. Second, administration of formula by continuous drip may be better tolerated than bolus feedings. The risk of gastroesophageal reflux and dumping symptoms is thereby greatly reduced. Aspiration is a major risk of enteral feedings. Rapid-bolus nasogastric feedings may lead to a high incidence of reflux. Complications can be decreased with the use of a slow, continuous infusion or, preferably, jejunal feedings.[140] However, this latter method has become controversial. Although patients with delayed gastric emptying (e.g., infants with sepsis, recent trauma, electrolyte imbalance, or receipt of opiates) or those who are comatose may be at risk for aspiration, in stable patients, a continuous infusion through a nasogastric tube is associated with no higher incidence of aspiration than is infusion through a nasoduodenal tube.[198] Third, care must be taken to ensure that the enteral formula does not become contaminated, either during preparation or at the bedside. Expiration dates should be observed. Finally, pectin, Metamucil, Lomotil, paregoric, or Imodium may be required for those who have lost a significant amount of bowel length (see the later discussion of short-bowel syndrome). Assessment of adequate carbohydrate absorption can be carried out most readily by measuring stool pH and reducing substances. The presence of a stool pH less than 5.5 or a reducing substance greater than 0.5% indicates the passage of unabsorbed carbohydrates into the stool. Once this is detected, the formula's carbohydrate concentration should be decreased.

PARENTERAL NUTRITION

PN is the intravenous administration of balanced and complete nutrition to support anabolism, prevent weight loss, or promote weight gain. Because acute illness causes mobilization of energy and protein stores, appropriate and timely nutrition should be provided to prevent malnutrition and promote speedy recovery.[146] PN is indicated when oral or enteral feeding is not possible or as supplemental nutrition when enteral feeding fails to meet nutritional needs. PN should be used for the shortest time possible, and oral or enteral feeding should be initiated as soon as clinically feasible. Although enteral feeding can prevent gut atrophy and reduce the risk of PN-associated hepatobiliary complications,[226,227,229] a recent meta-analysis showed that complication rates due to EN and PN are essentially identical.[30]

Indications

TPN is ideal for maintaining nutrition in infants and children who are unable to tolerate enteral feedings. Clinical conditions that are likely to require PN include GI disorders (short-bowel syndrome, malabsorption, intractable diarrhea, bowel obstruction, protracted vomiting, inflammatory bowel disease, enterocutaneous fistula), congenital anomalies (gastroschisis, Hirschsprung's disease, bowel atresia, volvulus, meconium ileus), radiation therapy to the GI tract, chemotherapy resulting in GI dysfunction, and severe respiratory distress syndrome in premature infants. Very-low-birth-weight infants are generally intolerant of enteral feeding and require PN during the first 24 to 48 hours after birth. Signs of starvation may be seen in underfed premature infants in as little as 1 to 2 days. Older children and adults generally do not require TPN unless periods of starvation extend beyond 7 to 10 days. However, young infants require TPN if starvation extends beyond 4 to 5 days.

Venous Access

The type of venous access varies, depending on the nutritional needs of the patient. For infants who will be maintained on TPN for a short period (<10 to 14 days), peripheral TPN is ideal. However, the greatest risk of using peripheral veins is extravasation of the solution, causing an inflammatory response and potential skin necrosis. Since the mid-1990s, a percutaneous intravenous catheter has been used. These catheters are relatively small in diameter (2 French or 22 gauge) and are placed through the child's peripheral veins, in the upper or lower limbs, and passed into the central venous system. Such catheters are extremely well tolerated in adults and children; they can often be maintained for several weeks with reasonably low infection rates.[119,182] Unlike the placement of a Broviac-type catheter, which requires local or general anesthesia, percutaneous intravenous catheters can generally be placed in the neonatal intensive care unit with minimal sedation. Another advantage of these catheters is the avoidance of pneumothorax, because access is through the extremities rather than the chest. The cost of peripheral access devices is considerably less than that of Broviac-type catheters, with comparable rates of infection and complications.[69]

For infants and children who require longer durations of infusion, central venous PN can be administered through a tunneled Silastic catheter (e.g., Broviac 2.7 or 4.0 French), which often has a woven Dacron cuff. Although tunneling of the catheter and cuff has not been shown to reduce catheter sepsis, use of a cuff can prevent accidental dislodgment.[222] The catheter may be placed in the superior or inferior vena cava. The ideal position for the tip of the catheter is the junction of the right atrium and the superior vena cava. The child's facial, external jugular, subclavian, or saphenous vein is an ideal location for access. In children who weigh less than 750 g, the internal jugular or femoral vein may need to be used because of the small caliber of other vessels. A percutaneous polyvinyl chloride central venous line may be used for shorter periods of central intravenous nutrition (e.g., 14 days).

Administration

Neonates are generally maintained on a dextrose and electrolyte solution (e.g., D-10-W, 0.2% normal saline, with 20 mEq KCl/L) at maintenance rates (80 mL/kg per day for the first day and 100 mL/kg per day for the second day) and then begun on PN between 24 and 48 hours after birth. Neonates tend to be somewhat intolerant of large amounts of dextrose or amino acids for the first 2 to 3 days of life. Dextrose solution concentrations are generally initiated at 10% to 12.5%, and the concentration is slowly increased on a daily basis to between 20% and 25%. Monitoring the patient's glucose level and electrolyte balance and checking for glucosuria confirm whether the child can tolerate this level of dextrose administration. PN may be administered via a peripheral or central venous catheter. The risk of developing phlebitis in peripheral veins is greater when the PN solution osmolarity exceeds 600 to 900 mOsm/L.[89] Intravenous solutions with higher osmolarities must be infused through a central vein. The maximum dextrose concentration in peripherally infused solutions in infants and children is 12.5%. Because lipid emulsions are isotonic solutions, co-infusion of lipids with peripheral PN protects the veins and prolongs the viability of peripheral intravenous catheters.[127] Because calcium phosphate precipitates in PN solutions may be life threatening, the Food and Drug Administration has recommended that PN solutions be infused through an in-line filter. A 0.22-μm filter is used for non-lipid-containing PN solutions, whereas a 1.2-μm filter is used for total nutrient admixtures to allow lipid particles (0.5 μm in diameter) to pass through the filter. PN should be initiated as a continuous infusion over 24 hours. For patients receiving long-term PN, the delivery period may be shorter (e.g., 16 hours). Importantly, to avoid hypo- or hyperglycemia, the rate of infusion should be cut in half for 1 to 2 hours before terminating and starting the infusion each day. Additionally, neonates, particularly premature infants, have limited glycogen reserves and generally do not tolerate cycling of PN. Guidelines for writing orders for neonatal PN are given in Figure 12-2.

Maintenance of catheters and prevention of infection require meticulous care, because catheters are a common source of sepsis in neonates.[111] The skin site must be cleansed with an antiseptic solution and dressed in a dry fashion every other day.[169] Tubing and infusion bags are changed every 72 hours, along with a new in-line filter. Tubing used to deliver lipids must be changed every 24 hours.

Composition of Parenteral Formulas

PN is a source of macronutrients (amino acids, dextrose, lipid emulsions), micronutrients (multivitamins, trace minerals), fluids, and electrolytes.

Amino Acids

Pediatric parenteral crystalline amino acid formulas provide essential and nonessential amino acids specifically balanced to meet the needs of the developing child. Neonatal-specific amino acid formulas (Aminosyn-PF, TrophAmine) are designed to closely reproduce the plasma amino acid profile of breast-fed infants. These formulas have led to greater weight gain and improved

nitrogen balance in infants compared with standard amino acid formulas.[19] Some amino acids such as cysteine, tyrosine, glycine, and taurine are considered conditionally essential (see Table 12-2). Taurine supplementation for premature infants is essential to promote bile acid conjugation and to improve bile flow[149] and has been shown to decrease the degree of PN-associated cholestasis.[194] Premature infants are at risk for taurine deficiency as a result of elevated renal taurine losses and their low capacity for taurine synthesis due to low cystathionase enzyme activity.[40,236] Amino acids are a source of energy (4 kcal/g) and nitrogen for protein synthesis. Parenteral amino acids should provide approximately 10% to 15% of total calories. Amino acids are started at 1.0 g/kg per day and advanced to the goal amount over 2 to 3 days. To simulate the intrauterine protein accretion rate, low-birth-weight infants may need up to 3.85 g/kg per day of amino acids.[212,237] Daily amino acid requirements are 2.5 to 3.0 g/kg in term infants, 1.5 to 2.0 g/kg in older children, and 1.0 to 1.5 g/kg in adolescents. Amino acid doses should be adjusted based on the patient's clinical condition and nutritional status. For example, higher amino acid doses are required for wound healing and in patients treated with dialysis or continuous renal replacement therapies to make up for losses through the dialysis membrane and filter.[53,128] Patients with liver failure and hyperammonemia require lower amino acid doses.

Dextrose

Hydrous dextrose is the major source of energy and provides carbon skeletons for tissue accretion. Dextrose also acts as a protein-sparing substrate by preventing the breakdown of somatic protein stores via suppression of gluconeogenesis.[185] In most children and adolescents receiving PN, parenteral dextrose provides 50% to 60% of total calories. The caloric value of hydrous dextrose is 3.4 kcal/g. In infants, PN should be initiated at a dextrose infusion rate of 4.0 to 8.0 mg/kg per minute to maintain adequate serum glucose concentrations. Lower amounts of glucose in young neonates lead to hypoglycemia due to inadequate hepatic production of glucose. Dextrose infusion is thereafter advanced at a daily rate of 2.0 mg/kg per minute until the nutritional goal is achieved. The maximum dextrose infusion rate should not exceed 10 to 14 mg/kg per minute, which can usually be achieved when PN is administered through a central venous catheter.[65,197]

Lipid Emulsions

Intravenous lipid emulsions are a condensed source of energy and essential fatty acids, providing 9 kcal/g of energy. The caloric value of lipid emulsions varies with the concentration; lipid emulsions at 10%, 20%, and 30% concentrations yield 1.1 kcal/mL, 2.0 kcal/mL, and 3.0 kcal/mL, respectively. The intravenous lipid emulsions currently marketed in the United States are made of long-chain triglycerides. Lipids usually provide 30% to 50% of the non-nitrogen caloric needs, or about 20% to 30% of total calories. Typically, lipid emulsions

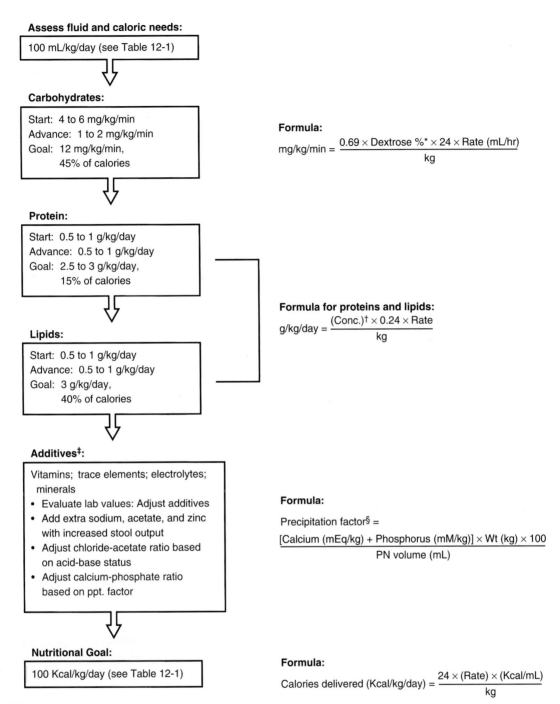

Assess fluid and caloric needs:

100 mL/kg/day (see Table 12-1)

Carbohydrates:

Start: 4 to 6 mg/kg/min
Advance: 1 to 2 mg/kg/min
Goal: 12 mg/kg/min,
      45% of calories

Formula:

$$mg/kg/min = \frac{0.69 \times \text{Dextrose \%}* \times 24 \times \text{Rate (mL/hr)}}{kg}$$

Protein:

Start: 0.5 to 1 g/kg/day
Advance: 0.5 to 1 g/kg/day
Goal: 2.5 to 3 g/kg/day,
      15% of calories

Formula for proteins and lipids:

$$g/kg/day = \frac{(\text{Conc.})^\dagger \times 0.24 \times \text{Rate}}{kg}$$

Lipids:

Start: 0.5 to 1 g/kg/day
Advance: 0.5 to 1 g/kg/day
Goal: 3 g/kg/day,
      40% of calories

Additives‡:

Vitamins; trace elements; electrolytes;
minerals
- Evaluate lab values: Adjust additives
- Add extra sodium, acetate, and zinc
  with increased stool output
- Adjust chloride-acetate ratio based
  on acid-base status
- Adjust calcium-phosphate ratio
  based on ppt. factor

Formula:

Precipitation factor§ =

$$\frac{[\text{Calcium (mEq/kg)} + \text{Phosphorus (mM/kg)}] \times \text{Wt (kg)} \times 100}{\text{PN volume (mL)}}$$

Nutritional Goal:

100 Kcal/kg/day (see Table 12-1)

Formula:

$$\text{Calories delivered (Kcal/kg/day)} = \frac{24 \times (\text{Rate}) \times (\text{Kcal/mL})}{kg}$$

Figure 12–2 How to write orders for parenteral nutrition for a neonate or young infant. Fluids should be adjusted based on the infant's gestational age and body weight. *Dextrose concentration should be used as the percent number (e.g., 20 for 20%). †The concentration in this formula should be written as the percent number (e.g., 4.25 for 4.25%). ‡See the relevant tables for each of these additives. §If the amino acid concentration is greater than 1.5%, the precipitation factor should be less than 3; if the final amino acid concentration is greater than 1% and less than 1.5%, the precipitation factor should be less than 2; if the amino acid concentration is less than 1%, calcium and phosphate should not be added. Adjustments to this formulation are necessary if additives (e.g., cysteine) are placed in the parenteral nutrition.

in infants and children are initiated at a dose of 1.0 g/kg per day and advanced by 1.0 g/kg per day to a maximum of 3.0 g/kg per day. Gradually increasing the daily lipid intake (0.5 or 1.0 g/kg per day) does not seem to improve lipid clearance. However, the lipid emulsion is better cleared[29,96] and lipid utilization is improved[77] when lipids are infused continuously over 24 hours rather than intermittently or for part of the day. There are also differences in the clearance of lipid emulsions. The 20% lipid emulsion is favored over the 10% emulsion because of its better clearance as a result of its lower phospholipid content.[80,205] Because lipid emulsions are derived from vegetable oils, they are also a natural source of variable amounts of vitamin K[114] and vitamin E isomers.[78,196] Hypothetically, because lipid particles are metabolized to fatty acids and monoglycerides, free fatty acids may compete with bilirubin for albumin binding sites, potentially displacing free bilirubin into the serum. Although this led to lipid restrictions in hyperbilirubinemic patients in the past, more recent kinetic studies failed to show that this represents a significant risk of kernicterus, unless the child is at risk for exchange transfusion.[192]

Multivitamins

Pediatric parenteral multivitamins contain a combination of water- and fat-soluble vitamins that are added to the daily PN. Several pediatric multivitamin formulas are available in the United States, but none is specifically designed to meet the needs of premature infants. Pediatric parenteral multivitamins provide low doses of vitamin A and high doses of water-soluble vitamins to premature infants. Higher vitamin A intake may be essential in low-birth-weight infants, who are at increased risk for lung disease.[102] Depletion of water-soluble vitamins occurs rapidly under stressful conditions. Thiamine is a cofactor for normal dextrose metabolism. Dextrose is normally metabolized to pyruvate, which is then converted to acetyl coenzyme A, which undergoes oxidation via the citric acid cycle. If thiamine deficiency occurs, pyruvate is instead converted to lactate, which can result in lactic acidosis.[175] Lactic acidosis has been reported in patients who received dextrose infusions without thiamine supplementation,[16,106] and fatalities from lactic acidosis due to thiamine deficiency were also reported during periodic multivitamin shortages in the United States.

Trace Elements

Standard pediatric trace mineral formulas contain zinc, copper, manganese, and chromium; some formulas have added selenium. Trace element formulas are designed to meet the recommendations of the Nutrition Advisory Group of the American Medical Association and the Society of Clinical Nutrition for daily intravenous supplements of trace minerals in the absence of deficiencies.[7]

Trace element status varies with the patient's underlying clinical condition. For example, zinc losses increase in patients with chronic diarrhea, malabsorption, short-bowel syndrome, and burns.[20,21,129] Zinc deficiency typically manifests as hair loss, a seborrheic type of dermatitis around the nose and mouth, and occasionally a functional ileus. Zinc deficiency is also associated with suboptimal growth, in part due to its effects on the growth hormone–insulin-like growth factor axis.[38,144] Under such conditions, additional zinc is required, which is not normally met by the standard daily trace element additives.

In patients with severe cholestasis, copper and manganese excretion is decreased, because both trace elements are excreted mainly via the bile. As a result, neurotoxicity has been reported with high serum manganese concentrations in patients with cholestasis who were receiving long-term PN.[67,207] Whenever trace elements are restricted or supplemental doses are given, blood trace element concentrations should be measured periodically to avoid deficiencies or toxicities. Trace element deficiencies are not uncommon. Copper deficiency may manifest as hypochromic, normocytic anemia; neutropenia; depigmentation of the skin and hair; hypotonia; psychomotor retardation; and osteoporosis. Fatal pancytopenia due to copper deficiency was reported in a PN-dependent patient with cholestasis who had copper restricted in the PN solution.[195]

Chromium deficiency, although rare, can produce a diabetes-like syndrome. Selenium deficiency, a potential complication of long-term PN support, is manifested by muscular pain and cardiomyopathy. These deficiencies are less commonly observed in patients routinely receiving trace metal additives in the infusate, although levels should be monitored at least on a yearly basis.

Fluids and Electrolytes

PN solution should not be used to manage acute fluid and electrolyte losses. Instead, patients should receive a separate intravenous solution for fluid and electrolyte supplementation (Table 12-6). In the home setting, fluid and electrolyte requirements are incorporated into the PN admixture for convenience of administration. Electrolyte adjustments in PN are based on serum electrolyte concentrations. Adjustments should account for all electrolyte sources and losses, acid-base status, clinical conditions, and medications that affect electrolyte balance.

Sodium

Sodium can be provided in PN solutions in the form of chloride, acetate, or phosphate salts. Neonates and especially premature infants develop a natriuresis during the first 1 to 2 weeks after birth as a result of immature kidney function. Because adequate sodium intake is essential for protein synthesis and tissue development, supplementation is necessary and is guided by serum and urine sodium levels.[41] Premature infants may require as much as 8.0 mEq/kg per day of sodium. The maximum

TABLE 12-6 Daily Electrolyte Requirements for Pediatric Patients

Electrolyte	Daily Maintenance Requirement
For Patients Weighing <10 kg	
Sodium	2.0-5.0 mEq/kg
Potassium	2.0-4.0 mEq/kg
Calcium	0.5-3.0 mEq/kg
Phosphorus	0.5-1.5 mM/kg
Magnesium	0.25-1.0 mEq/kg
For Patients Weighing 10-30 kg	
Sodium	20-150 mEq
Potassium	20-240 mEq
Chloride	20-150 mEq
Acetate	20-120 mEq
Calcium	5-20 mEq
Phosphorus	4-24 mM
Magnesium	4-24 mEq

sodium concentration in PN solutions should not exceed the normal saline solution equivalent (154 mEq/L).

Potassium

Potassium can be provided in PN solutions in the form of chloride, acetate, or phosphate salts. Higher potassium requirements are needed during anabolism[32] and to correct for any GI or renal potassium losses. Potassium concentrations in the PN solution should not exceed 80 mEq/L, and potassium infusion rates in infants and children should not exceed 0.5 mEq/kg per hour.[203] Patients receiving high potassium infusion rates should be in the intensive care unit on a cardiac monitor.

Chloride and Acetate

The chloride-to-acetate ratio in the PN solution can be adjusted based on the patient's acid-base status. Acetate is converted in vivo to bicarbonate at a 1:1 molar ratio. A high acetate–low chloride ratio is indicated to help correct the metabolic acidosis resulting from lower GI fluid and electrolyte losses. High acetate may also be used to help a child compensate for respiratory acidosis. Premature infants are especially at risk for acid-base changes because of inefficient hydrogen ion excretion and bicarbonate reabsorption by the kidneys.[41,95] A low acetate–high chloride ratio minimizes the bicarbonate load in patients with metabolic alkalosis resulting from excessive gastric fluid and electrolyte losses. Caution should be used when adjusting the chloride-to-acetate ratio because dramatic acid-base changes may occur in 2 to 3 days.

Calcium and Phosphate

Calcium and phosphate requirements are greater in infants and children than in adults owing to increased demands for growth. Corticosteroids and loop diuretics, which are commonly used in neonatal and pediatric intensive care patients, can further increase calcium requirements by increasing calcium losses. After birth, hypophosphatemia is commonly observed in premature infants owing to high urinary phosphate excretion.[98] Because phosphates dissociate in monobasic and dibasic forms, depending on the solution's pH, they should be dosed in millimoles (mmol) instead of millequivalents (mEq) to avoid dosing errors. Calcium and phosphate should be provided in adequate ratios and amounts to optimize bone mineralization and prevent metabolic bone disease.[165] Bone mineralization is optimized at an intake ratio of 2.6 mEq of calcium to 1 mmol of phosphorus (1.7 mg calcium to 1 mg phosphorus).[153] Inadequate calcium and phosphorus supplementation is problematic because of solubility limitations; thus, enteral calcium and phosphorus supplementation may be required. Also, cysteine hydrochloride, an acidic compound that can be added to the PN solution, can be used to lower the solution's pH and allow higher delivery of calcium and phosphate amounts. An acidic medium favors the formation of monovalent phosphates instead of the divalent phosphates that would otherwise bind to calcium. Cysteine hydrochloride is added to the neonatal PN solution at a dose of 40 mg/g

of amino acids.[68] Calcium and phosphorus can safely be added to TPN when the concentrations provided satisfy the following equation:

$$\text{Calcium (mEq) + Phosphorus (mM)} \geq 30 \text{ (per 1000 mL of TPN)}$$

The needs for optimal tissue and bone growth may not be met unless calcium and phosphorus are also provided enterally.

Additives

Heparin

Adding heparin to the PN solution at a concentration of 0.5 to 1.0 U/mL[139] maintains the patency of the venous catheter[214] and reduces vein irritation.[231] Further, heparin is a cofactor of lipoprotein lipase, an enzyme released from the vascular endothelium that enhances lipid clearance.[234] Heparin should not be used in patients with bleeding, at risk for bleeding, or with thrombocytopenia.

Histamine$_2$ Receptor Antagonists

Histamine$_2$ receptor antagonists such as ranitidine, famotidine, and cimetidine are compatible with PN and may be added to the PN solution for stress ulcer prophylaxis.

Regular Insulin

Although regular insulin is compatible with the PN solution, insulin therapy is difficult to regulate in infants. Intravenous insulin should therefore be administered as a separate infusion to allow safe titration of the insulin dose.

Iron Dextran

Iron is not routinely added to PN, and iron-deficiency anemia may occur in PN-dependent patients. Iron dextran is the most common parenteral iron available for use when oral iron absorption is unreliable or results in GI intolerance. Because iron can be used as a substrate for bacterial proliferation, iron dextran should be avoided in infected patients. Also, because severe anaphylactic side effects may occur, an intravenous test dose should be administered before the total dose is given. Although not recommended by manufacturers, many qualified groups have used iron dextran safely in patients during the first 4 months of life. Daily iron dextran doses up to 1.0 mg/kg have been added to neonatal PN to prevent iron-deficiency anemia. Iron replacement calculations are given in Table 12-7. The estimated total iron dextran dose can be equally divided into incremental doses and added to the daily supply of non-lipid-containing PN solution until the total replacement dosage is given; iron dextran at therapeutic doses is incompatible with lipid emulsions.[220] A potentially safer intravenous iron preparation is sodium ferric gluconate (Ferrlecit, R&D Laboratories, Marina Del Rey, Calif). It has been used predominantly in renal failure patients but also appears to be effective in children.[145]

TABLE 12-7 Intravenous Iron Replacement Therapy
Calculation for Total Iron Replacement Dose
mL of iron dextran = 0.0476 × weight (kg) × (Hb$_n$ − Hb$_o$) + 1 mL per 5 kg of body weight (up to a maximum of 14 mL)
1 mL of iron dextran = 50 mg of elemental iron
Hb$_n$ = desired hemoglobin (g/dL). The desired hemoglobin is 12 if the patient weighs <15 kg or 14.8 if the patient weighs >15 kg.
Hb$_o$ = measured hemoglobin (g/dL)
Maximal Daily Iron Replacement Dose
Infants weighing <5 kg: 25 mg
Children weighing 5-10 kg: 50 mg
Children weighing >10 kg: 100 mg

Carnitine

Carnitine is a quaternary amine required for the transport of long-chain fatty acids into the mitochondria, where they undergo oxidation.[26] Premature infants are at risk for carnitine deficiency because of their limited carnitine reserves and reduced carnitine synthesis.[181] Decreased fatty acid oxidation and elevated serum triglyceride concentrations have been correlated with low plasma carnitine concentrations.[52] Although many enteral formulations contain carnitine, PN solutions are carnitine free. Supplementation of PN with L-carnitine can normalize plasma carnitine concentrations[27] and improve fatty acid oxidation. Premature infants who develop unexplained hypertriglyceridemia during lipid infusion may benefit from L-carnitine supplementation at a dose of 10 mg/kg per day.[213]

Complications

After almost 40 years' experience with PN, complications continue to be an obstacle in the care of pediatric patients. Major complications of PN can be classified as metabolic, hepatobiliary, and infectious.

Metabolic Complications

Hyperglycemia

Hyperglycemia in patients receiving PN is primarily the result of excessive dextrose infusion. Factors that exacerbate glucose intolerance include sepsis, surgery, diabetes, pancreatitis, prematurity, and corticosteroid therapy. Elevated blood glucose may coincide with PN initiation, but endogenous insulin secretion usually adjusts within 48 to 72 hours. Untreated hyperglycemia causes osmotic diuresis that can lead to hyperosmolar, hyperglycemic, nonketotic dehydration with electrolyte disturbances,[197] impaired phagocytosis,[4] and liver steatosis.[71] Tight control of glucose levels in an intensive care unit setting has been shown to significantly improve the outcome in adults, and this strategy may be applicable to the pediatric population as well.[216]

The first step in managing hyperglycemia is to decrease the dextrose load or reduce the infusion rate. However, this may compromise nutritional intake, because dextrose is the major source of calories in PN. If reducing dextrose does not improve hyperglycemia, insulin therapy is indicated. Because infants have a variable response to insulin therapy,[163] adding insulin to the PN solution should be avoided. Instead, a regular insulin drip should be initiated and titrated based on serial glucose checks.

Hypoglycemia

Hypoglycemia with PN is usually the result of a sudden reduction in the PN infusion rate. In patients who receive PN over a portion of the day (cycled), hypoglycemia can be avoided by gradually reducing the rate over 1 to 2 hours before discontinuation. Premature infants are at increased risk for hypoglycemia owing to their underdeveloped metabolic response[49]; cycling of PN in this group of patients is typically not safe until they are more mature or take a good amount of enteral intake. If discontinuation of PN is unavoidable, intravenous administration of dextrose 10% in water prevents symptomatic hypoglycemia.[13]

Hypertriglyceridemia

High-dextrose infusion is the primary cause of hypertriglyceridemia in PN patients. Excessive carbohydrate intake enhances hepatic and adipose tissue lipogenesis.[1] Other factors that predispose to hypertriglyceridemia in pediatric patients receiving PN include prematurity,[186] lipid overfeeding,[10,11] critical illness, and sepsis.[152] Although the logical response would be to reduce the lipid infusion, a reduction in dextrose is far more effective. If hypertriglyceridemia persists despite reducing the glucose intake, the lipid emulsion dose and rate should be decreased to keep triglyceride levels below 275 mg/dL. A lipid dose of 0.5 to 1.0 g/kg per day in children prevents essential fatty acid deficiency. If a 10% lipid emulsion is used, switching to a 20% emulsion is recommended, owing to its better clearance.[81] Carnitine deficiency may often be a cause of hypertriglyceridemia particularly in preterm infants (see earlier).

Metabolic Acidosis

Metabolic acidosis may result from an excessive chloride or amino acid load in PN. The addition of cysteine hydrochloride to the PN solution to improve calcium and phosphate solubility is another cause of acidemia,[82] which may lead to a leaching of calcium from the infant's bones. Premature infants and patients with liver or renal disease are at increased risk for metabolic acidosis and should be closely monitored for acid-base changes.

Electrolyte Disturbances

Hypokalemia, hypomagnesemia, and hypophosphatemia may result from increased requirements during anabolism and protein synthesis (refeeding syndrome). This is particularly common in severely malnourished patients and should be monitored for as feeding is advanced slowly.[32] Phosphate is also required intracellularly for the generation of high-energy phosphate bonds and bone formation, and an intracellular shift of phosphate occurs with carbohydrate infusion[168]; deficiencies may lead to hypoventilation and coma. Hyperkalemia, hypermagnesemia, and hyperphosphatemia may result from increased intake in combination with decreased renal function and hypercatabolism. Apparent hypocalcemia in malnourished patients is often secondary to a reduced serum albumin concentration, with proportionally low total serum calcium.

Metabolic Bone Disease

Metabolic bone disease, including osteopenia, osteomalacia, and rickets, is a complication in PN-dependent patients. Diagnosis is often difficult and may not be evident until a pathologic fracture is observed. Biochemical markers may reveal elevated serum alkaline phosphatase concentrations, hypercalciuria, low to normal plasma parathyroid hormone, and low 1,25-dihydroxyvitamin D.[55,187] Several factors predispose to PN-associated metabolic bone disease, including calcium and phosphorus deficiency, excessive losses of calcium due to diuretics, excessive vitamin D intake,[188] and aluminum toxicity.[151] Maximizing calcium and phosphorus intake is most important to improve bone mineralization. Calcium deficit is the result of limitations on calcium supplementation and the resultant hypercalciuria from amino acids,[118] with secondary metabolic acidosis.[51] Aluminum, a contaminant of the PN solution, is another possible cause of metabolic bone disease. Aluminum causes bone remodeling by impairing calcium fixation in bones,[219] impairing parathyroid hormone secretion, and reducing the formation of active vitamin D.[107] Premature infants and patients with renal failure are at highest risk for aluminum toxicity owing to their reduced aluminum elimination. Additional vitamin D administration may actually be dangerous, because vitamin D may also play a role in the pathogenesis of metabolic bone disease; however, the exact mechanism is unknown. Withdrawing vitamin D from these patients leads to improvement in bone demineralization, resolution of bone pain, positive calcium balance,[188] and normalization of plasma concentrations of active vitamin D and parathyroid hormone.[221]

Hepatobiliary Complications

Hepatobiliary complications associated with PN include cholestasis, steatosis, and cholelithiasis. Multiple factors may predispose to PN-associated hepatobiliary complications, including prematurity, overfeeding, PN dependence, absence of enteral stimulation for gallbladder contraction, short-bowel syndrome, and recurrent sepsis.[18,210] Cholestasis is the most common hepatobiliary complication in children receiving PN. Jaundice may occur 2 to 3 weeks after PN initiation. A serum conjugated bilirubin concentration of 2.0 mg/dL or greater is commonly used as a biochemical marker of cholestasis.[210] Strategies to prevent or reduce PN-associated cholestasis include initiating enteral feeding, weaning from PN, avoiding overfeeding,[135] balancing calories,[35] cycling PN,[123] and avoiding and promptly treating sepsis.[35] Pharmacologic interventions may include improving bile flow with the administration of bile acids or cholecystokinin; both, however, have been studied in controlled, prospective trials without any proven benefit.[85,211] Oral antibiotics, such as oral gentamicin and metronidazole, have been used to decrease intestinal bacterial overgrowth and reduce bacterial translocation.[218] A rapid rise in direct bilirubin is a strong predictor of impending hepatic failure. Use of a taurine-supplemented PN solution has been shown to decrease the degree of cholestasis in premature infants and those with necrotizing enterocolitis.[194] In infants with short-bowel syndrome, a direct serum bilirubin level greater than 2.5 mg/dL for more than 4 months was associated with 80% mortality,[209] suggesting a potential criterion for referral for transplant evaluation.[33]

Infectious Complications

Sepsis is one of the most frequent and serious complications of centrally infused PN in infants and children.[56] Fever and sudden glucose intolerance are suggestive of sepsis. Persistent hyperglycemia has been shown to increase infection rates, and intensive control is recommended.[217] Microbial culturing of PN should be performed if it is a suspected source of microbial contamination, although this is rare with the use of strict sterile compounding techniques. Catheter-related infections remain the main cause of sepsis in patients receiving PN. Microorganisms can enter the bloodstream (1) along the catheter tract, starting at the skin exit site; (2) via a contaminated intravenous solution; (3) by breaks in sterility at the catheter hub during blood drawing or while cleaning intravenous tubing; or (4) from a distant septic site or the GI tract. The catheter in this case acts as a foreign body focus for bacterial growth. The most important factors in reducing the incidence of septic complications are placement of catheters under strict aseptic conditions and meticulous care of catheter sites. Factors that correlate with catheter-related infections include prolonged catheterization, use of the catheter for multiple purposes, manipulation of the catheter hub, and chronic PN therapy. Most series report an incidence of 0.5 to 2.0 infections per 1000 catheter-days for a nonimmunosuppressed patient with a central venous catheter.[105,232] For immunosuppressed patients (e.g., hematology or oncology patients), a rate of 2 to 3 infections per 1000 catheter-days is generally reported.[54,91] A considerably higher rate of infection is found in children with the short-bowel syndrome—7 to 9 infections per 1000 catheter-days.[37,111,140,157]

Several measures have proved effective in preventing catheter-related infections, including the use of sterile barriers and topical disinfectants during catheter insertion, antimicrobial-coated catheters, and regular catheter flushing. Guidelines for the prevention and management of catheter-related infections have been published elsewhere.[131,148] In general, nonpermanent polyvinyl chloride lines should be removed in cases of catheter sepsis; however, in more than 80% of patients with Silastic catheters (e.g., Broviac or Hickman), the infection can be cleared with intravenous antibiotics. Another method of treating these infections is the antibiotic lock technique; this permits the delivery of markedly higher doses of antibiotics into the catheter, with the antibiotic remaining in the lumen while it is not in use.[50,134] This technique allows the administration of antibiotics that normally have such high minimal inhibitory concentrations that systemic use would result in renal failure (e.g., nafcillin for a staphylococcal infection). Antibiotic lock methods are used routinely in some centers but are probably most useful in patients who may not tolerate an aminoglycoside or vancomycin. Owing to the high failure rate of antibiotics, most patients with catheter subcutaneous tract infections should have the line removed. Most children with fungal infections should also have the catheter removed; there have been reports of fatalities and high failure rates when attempting to salvage the line with antifungal therapy.[43] Trying to maintain a catheter with a candidal infection is associated with a mortality of up to 25%, and there is little chance (13%) of clearing the infection with the line in place.[63] Only a relatively short course (7 to 14 days) of antifungal agents needs to be given after the catheter is removed; however, the results of blood cultures must be negative.[57] For unusual cases in which central venous access has been lost because of previous placement of several catheters, a trial of antifungal agents with the line in place may be attempted. An uncommon fungal organism associated with TPN is *Malassezia furfur*. This organism thrives in a lipid-rich environment, but as long as lipids are withheld, it generally responds to antifungal treatment without catheter removal.

Complications from Overfeeding

Overfeeding can lead to a number of adverse consequences. The administration of excessive dextrose may lead to osmotic diuresis and subsequent dehydration due to serum glucose levels exceeding the renal tubular reabsorption threshold. Immunologic suppression has also been associated with overfeeding and is believed to be due to an inactivation of the complement system, as well as depression of natural killer activation. Overfeeding may also adversely affect the liver, because excessive glucose that is not oxidized is converted into fat (lipogenesis). These changes may lead to elevated serum triglyceride levels and hepatic steatosis. Additionally, overfeeding from carbohydrates associated with lipogenesis leads to high carbon dioxide production, as reflected by an elevated respiratory quotient.[230] Any respiratory quotient value exceeding 1.0 represents overfeeding; this high level may exacerbate ventilatory impairment in a critically ill child because it represents excessive carbon dioxide production. Avoidance of overfeeding may be difficult, emphasizing the importance of estimating nutritional needs in the intensive care unit setting. Caloric needs are best assessed using indirect calorimetry. Overfeeding critically ill patients may also lead to fluid retention, which may further compromise respiratory function.

Technical Complications

In recent years, the incidence of technical complications caused by the placement of central venous lines in infants and children has been greatly reduced by careful attention to technique and radiographic confirmation of catheter position. The incidence of cardiac arrhythmias caused by catheter irritation has been greatly reduced by placing the tip of the catheter at the junction of the superior vena cava and right atrium. Another important point is to ensure that the catheter is not positioned too medially, as this could lead to a pinching of the catheter between the first rib and the clavicle, potentially shearing off the distal catheter into the heart.[87] Even with proper positioning of a silicone catheter, thrombosis of the vein in which the catheter resides can occur, especially in a critically ill patient with sepsis and reduced circulation. Thrombosis of the great vessels requires anticoagulation and catheter removal. Pulmonary embolism and infection of these thrombi have been reported in infants and small children.[208] Thrombolytic therapy has proved effective in clearing the catheter of clots and avoiding the need for catheter replacement.[92] This procedure should be repeated at least twice to ensure the removal of thrombus. Patients with long-term indwelling lines may have occlusion from either lipids or calcium deposits. These patients should receive a trial of ethanol and dilute hydrochloric acid.[223] PN delivery via a peripherally inserted central catheter has greatly increased in the past decade; since 1996, this has become the dominant mode of PN delivery in the United States.[93] This method has the advantage of avoiding many of the complications associated with central venous catheters, and the catheter can often be inserted on the floor with little or no sedation[5,39]; however, thrombotic events are more frequent than with centrally placed catheters.

Monitoring of Laboratory Values

Monitoring of laboratory values is essential, as aberrations in these values are common in pediatric patients, particularly at the initiation of TPN. Table 12-8 gives guidelines for such monitoring. A complete blood count and glucose, blood urea nitrogen, creatinine, and electrolyte (sodium, potassium, chloride, carbon dioxide) levels should be measured at initiation and then at increasing time periods. Liver function tests (alanine aminotransferase, aspartate aminotransferase, lactate dehydrogenase, alkaline phosphatase, and total direct bilirubin) should be performed, and magnesium, albumin, calcium, and phosphorus levels should be checked at initiation and then at progressively increasing intervals. Triglyceride levels should be maintained until the desired level of fat intake is reached.

SPECIAL PROBLEMS IN PEDIATRIC SURGICAL PATIENTS

Pediatric surgical patients respond to the stress of surgery quite differently from older children or adults.[158] The metabolism of children is markedly affected by operative stress. The period of increased energy expenditure,

TABLE 12–8 Guidelines for Blood Laboratory Monitoring in Pediatric Patients Dependent on Total Parenteral Nutrition

	Initial	Daily	Two to Three Times a Week	Weekly	As Indicated
Glucose	X	X	X		
Blood urea nitrogen, creatinine	X	X	X		
Sodium, potassium, chloride, carbon dioxide	X	X	X		
AST, ALT, LDH, alkaline phosphatase, total direct bilirubin, GGTP	X			X	
Magnesium, calcium, phosphorus	X		X		
Albumin, total protein	X			X	
Triglycerides	X*			X	
Hemoglobin, hematocrit, complete blood count, platelets, prothrombin time	X				X
Copper, zinc, selenium, chromium, manganese, iron					X
Total iron binding capacity, ferritin					X
Vitamin concentrations					X
Chemsticks					X
Ammonia					X
Blood cultures					X

*Measured once goal lipid infusion is reached.

ALT, alanine transaminase; AST, aspartate transaminase; GGTP, gamma-glutamyl-transpeptidase; LDH, lactate dehydrogenase.

however, is much shorter than in adults.[94] Induction of anesthesia has profound effects on body metabolism, with agents such as fentanyl having a beneficial effect in reducing the catabolic effect.[8] Moreover, in neonates, protein turnover and catabolism do not seem to be affected by major operative procedures. PN, however, is associated with increased production of oxygen free radicals, which may contribute to suppression of the immune status. Thus, the decision to use PN must take into consideration this potential detriment as well as the potential benefit.

Preoperative Nutritional Support

In malnourished adults, provision of enteral feedings for 2 to 3 weeks preoperatively may reduce postoperative wound infections, anastomotic leakage, hepatic and renal failure, and length of hospital stay. Data on PN support are less clear. A meta-analysis demonstrated only a marginal benefit of preoperative PN. Little benefit, and a possible increase in complications, was noted in mildly or moderately malnourished patients.[108] The most significant benefit has been documented in severely malnourished patients, who developed fewer noninfectious complications if receiving perioperative PN (7 to 15 days before surgery, and 3 days after).[36] However, PN patients were noted to have an increased infection rate that could not be totally explained by the use of central venous catheters. This suggests that the use of PN may actually predispose patients to increased infectious complications. Thus, unless there are clear indications of severe malnutrition (see the earlier discussion of subjective global assessment), a delay in operative management to provide preoperative PN is *not* indicated.[13] An extrapolation of these findings to neonatal patients is difficult because of their limited nutritional stores.

However, because of similarities in the metabolic response to surgery, it seems reasonable to apply these same conclusions to the pediatric population.

Postoperative Nutritional Support

Use of aggressive postoperative support is even more controversial. In adults, the provision of enteral nutrients has been postulated to reduce the rate of sepsis and lower costs. However, nutrient intolerance can be a considerable limitation. Data suggest that when postoperative nutritional support is provided, it should be started early using a combination of PN and EN until the GI tract fully recovers. A controlled study examining the effect of postoperative PN in children demonstrated a positive effect on nitrogen balance and levels of insulin-like growth factor-1; however, no clinical benefit was noted.[126] The effect of PN on postoperative healing has been negligible. In the postoperative period, there are higher infection rates in patients on PN. Meta-analysis studies show that there is an actual adverse effect of postoperative PN.[108] Certainly, prolonged starvation postoperatively places patients at risk.[178] However, in general, postoperative PN should be restricted to those infants who will not tolerate even a short period of starvation or older children who will probably not start EN for at least 5 to 7 days (10 days in adolescents).[13]

Critically Ill Surgical Patients

Nutritional care of critically ill or septic postoperative patients presents a much greater challenge. Clinically, a critically ill child manifests poor enteral feeding, anorexia, and often a paralytic ileus. Insulin resistance results in hyperglycemia and hypertriglyceridemia. Control of this hyperglycemia has been shown to have a significantly beneficial effect in preventing sepsis.[217] Visceral protein stores become progressively reduced over time. Although measurements of albumin may change slowly owing to its long half-life (>8 days), other measures of visceral protein status such as prealbumin levels (half-life of 2 days) better reflect these metabolic derangements. Estimates of energy requirements during this time are important, and these needs are often overestimated in postoperative or septic, critically ill infants. Almost one third of an infant's energy requirement is intended to support growth (30 to 35 kcal/kg per day). Because there is a cessation of growth during sepsis and critical illness, a marked decrease in energy needs may ensue. In one study of critically ill, postoperative infants, the mean measured basal energy expenditure was only 43 kcal/kg per day.[115] However, results are extraordinarily variable, further emphasizing the utility of indirect calorimetry, which can also yield information on the respiratory quotient (see earlier) and aid in the prevention of overfeeding. Although not as well studied in neonates, data from meta-analyses in adult patients suggest that PN is of little proven benefit in most critically ill surgical patients and should be used sparingly in the first few days, until it is determined that the length of starvation will exceed 5 to 7 days.[86]

Biliary Atresia

An infant with biliary atresia, even after a clinically successful hepatic portoenterostomy, typically has a lower than normal amount of bile flow into the intestine, which leads to a profound defect in fat digestion and absorption. Such a deficit may leave the infant with an essential fatty acid deficiency and inadequate absorption of fat-soluble vitamins.[100] This can lead to a lack of bone mineralization and failure to thrive. The essential goal for such an infant is to provide adequate calories using a formula that maximizes fat intake. A commonly used formula in these patients is Pregestimil (Mead Johnson). This formula has a large amount of MCTs and sufficient linoleic acid to prevent fatty acid deficiency in the face of decreased absorption. Use of this formula has been shown to increase growth in such patients.[44] Portagen (Mead Johnson) should not be used in cholestatic infants because it does not provide sufficient essential fatty acids to prevent deficiency. When PN is needed, a standard crystalline amino acid solution should be used; there is no proven benefit to hepatic formulas. Breast-feeding, although generally ideal in infancy, may actually be detrimental in patients with biliary atresia because breast milk has a much higher fat content than commercially available formulas and may not be well tolerated in these children.

Vitamin supplementation is critical in patients with biliary atresia (Table 12-9). Unfortunately, supplemental vitamins are rarely covered by insurance policies, despite the fact that they are medically necessary. Frequent monitoring of vitamin levels is essential to ensure that sufficient supplementation is being achieved. Supplementary water-soluble vitamins in addition to those provided in

TABLE 12–9 Vitamin Therapy in Cholestasis

Vitamin (Trade Name; Manufacturer)	Dose	Supplied as
Vitamin A (Aquasol A; Centeon, LLC)	10,000-15,000 IU/day	3.0-mg tablets 3.0-, 7.5-, or 15-mg capsules 50,000 IU/mL drops*
Vitamin D: 25(OH)D₃ (Calderol; Organon Teknika Corp)	2.0-4.0 µg/kg/day	20- and 50-µg capsules
Vitamin D: 1,25(OH)₂D₃ (Rocaltrol; Roche Labs)	0.01-0.05 µg/kg/day	0.25- and 0.5-µg capsules 0.1 µg/mL liquid
Vitamin E: TPGS (Liqui-E; Twin Labs)	25 IU/kg/day	26.7 IU/mL liquid
Vitamin K	2.5-5.0 mg/day	5-mg tablets

*50,000 IU = 15 mg
TPGS, tocophersolan.

standard infant formulas should be given in a multivitamin preparation. Iron, zinc, and calcium deficiencies should also be carefully screened for. From a practical perspective, it may be difficult and expensive to administer this many vitamins to a small infant. Many use a combination form of fat-soluble vitamins (ADEKs 0.5 mL/kg); however, vitamin K may be inadequate in this formulation, and additional supplementation (2.5 mg/day) should be given. Vitamin levels should be followed, and deficiencies corrected with individual vitamins.

Protein metabolism is impaired in children with biliary atresia; it accounts for 4% to 9% of energy expenditure in healthy infants, but 17% in patients with biliary atresia.[160] Pierro et al.[159] showed that REE was about 29% higher than expected in infants with biliary atresia and that only 35% of the metabolizable energy intake was retained for growth in these children.

Short-Bowel Syndrome

The nutritional support of a child with short-bowel syndrome is complex and requires a multidisciplinary approach, with the pediatric surgeon, pediatric gastroenterologist, pharmacist, and dietitian working together. Although initially the child's sole or main caloric source will be PN, enteral feedings should be started as soon as possible after the onset of short-bowel syndrome. Enteral feedings both stimulate small bowel adaptation and prevent the development of PN-associated cholestasis. The ideal enteral solution is isotonic, and the protein source should be predominantly elemental. Di- and tripeptides have often been advocated because this source of protein is most easily and efficiently absorbed.[215] Although data are limited, others have found better feeding tolerance with the use of an even more elemental (pure amino acid) enteral formulation.[23] The solution should have a fair amount of MCTs, as this source of fat is well absorbed through the basolateral wall of intestinal enterocytes and into the portal venous circulation. However, MCTs contain no essential fatty acids; thus, these fats cannot be the sole source of lipids in these patients. Tables 12-4 and 12-5 list recommended formulas for infants and children, respectively. Despite the use of these elemental formulas for early feedings, more complex diets have the greatest benefit in achieving intestinal adaptation, and a modified regular diet should eventually be instituted.[24]

High stool output is associated with excessive losses of zinc, magnesium, sodium, bicarbonate, and potassium.[201] These losses must be monitored. Total body sodium depletion is associated with failure to thrive, despite the administration of adequate amounts of calories.[183] A simple way to detect such a deficit is to measure a spot urine sodium. A urine sodium level less than 10 mEq/L may indicate total body sodium depletion, and oral supplementation (sodium chloride or sodium bicarbonate, as indicated) should be given on a daily basis.[177] High stool output may be a major obstacle to advancing enteral feedings. The cause of this high output may include infection, malabsorption, rapid transit, and bile acid irritation of the colonic epithelium.[164] The child's stool should be assessed intermittently for infection. Additionally, stool pH, reducing substances, and qualitative fecal fats should be checked. Stool pH less than 5.5 and an elevated reducing substance level (>0.5%) indicates carbohydrate malabsorption. Stool volume should be less than 45 mL/kg/day. Formulas with sucrose as the carbohydrate do not yield a positive reducing substance test, despite carbohydrate malabsorption. Elevation in fecal fats suggests fat malabsorption, which may require modification of the child's enteral diet (i.e., an increase in the percentage of MCTs). An increase in stool alpha$_1$-antitrypsin indicates protein malabsorption, although this is much less commonly encountered. Use of a resin binder (e.g., cholestyramine) markedly reduces bile acid irritation and has proved extremely effective in many infants. However, excessive use of bile acid binders may result in depletion of the circulating bile acid pool, further limiting fatty acid absorption. Because many infants with short-bowel syndrome have dysmotility, only after all other causes have been eliminated (i.e., infections, bacterial overgrowth, bile acid irritation, potentially correctable malabsorption) should an agent to reduce motility be considered.

Obesity

Obesity has become a worldwide problem, with a striking increase in obesity rates reported in North America, Europe, and Asia.[15,45] Rates in the United States demonstrate a threefold increase in obesity over the past 30 years. The implications of this rise in obesity are dramatic. First, more than 50% of children who are diagnosed with obesity will carry that excess weight into adulthood. Second, a number of secondary complications have been identified in these children, including prediabetic condition of syndrome X, type 2 diabetes mellitus, coronary artery disease, and obstructive sleep apnea.[142,161] Additional problems include bone and joint disease and cholelithiasis.

The difficulty in defining obesity has hampered the identification and treatment of many of these children. Although a National Institutes of Health consensus established a body mass index (BMI) of greater than 40 as morbid obesity,[74] BMIs change dramatically during adolescence and do not follow a linear curve. A more consistent definition is based on the number of standard deviations from the mean using Centers for Disease Control and Prevention standardized growth curves.[166] In this regard, "at risk for overweight" is defined as being at the 85th percentile, and "overweight" is defined as being at the 95th percentile.[15] Factors influencing the development of obesity are environmental as well as genetic.[121] The risk of obesity increases to 80% if one parent is obese.[224]

Treatment of this condition is complex, and no ideal method has been advanced. However, it is essential that a team approach be applied[88]; this includes pediatricians, nurses, dietitians, and psychiatric support. The key issues when contemplating surgical intervention for obese adolescents are careful patient evaluation and selection based on sufficient maturity to understand the implications of this lifelong decision, as well as willingness to participate in lifelong follow-up. Vitamin and nutrient deficiencies are common in such patients and require monitoring every 6 months.[112] Levels that are commonly deficient include protein, vitamin B$_{12}$, folate, iron, calcium, vitamin D, and thiamine.

Failure to Thrive

Malnutrition in childhood is associated with poor growth and development. The diagnosis of failure to thrive is based on a weight more than 2 standard deviations below the mean weight percentile (Z score of 2.0), resulting in a child falling on the 2.3 percentile.[170] Failure to thrive may be symmetrical, with height, length, and development of other body organs falling below the fifth percentile, or asymmetrical, with weight below the fifth percentile but length and head circumference within normal limits. In general, patients with symmetrical failure to thrive have more profound malnutrition and suffer from greater neurologic underdevelopment than do those with asymmetrical failure to thrive; the latter patients have relatively normal cognitive development. Recent investigations have shown that abnormal cognitive development in patients with failure to thrive probably results from a poor social environment and is often reversible.[117,199]

The approach to feeding a patient with failure to thrive should include a multidisciplinary assessment of medical, social, and psychological factors. A systematic evaluation to rule out neurologic pathology, swallowing disorders, feeding aversion, malabsorption, and metabolic disorders should be done. A trial of feeding the child in a hospital setting often identifies a problem with the child's home and social environment. Nutritional support for an infant should begin at approximately 50 kcal/kg per day and be increased by 20 to 25 kcal/kg per day as long as GI tolerance to the feeding is adequate. Stool weight should be less than 150 g/day in young infants. Feedings may increase to 150 to 240 kcal/kg per day to achieve adequate catch-up growth.[155] Supplementing the formula with additional potassium (up to 5.0 mEq/kg per day) may also be required during the first week of nutritional rehabilitation. Levels of potassium, magnesium, and phosphate need to be closely monitored because they often drop rapidly after the initiation of feedings. One simple method to calculate caloric needs is that for each gram of weight gain desired per day, five additional calories should be provided.

Handicapped Children

Between 10% and 20% of children in the United States have special health care needs because of chronic illness and developmental disorders.[174] For several of these disorders, pediatric surgeons take an active part in patients' nutritional care; these disorders include neurologic impairment, developmental delay, cerebral palsy, and such genetic syndromes as trisomies 13, 18, and 21 and Cornelia de Lange's and Rett syndromes. Pediatric surgeons are often responsible for providing nutritional access in many of these patients, as well as for maintaining nutritional care before and after surgery. Potential factors that may contribute to poor nutrition in these patients include feeding disorders, uncoordinated tongue movements, poorly coordinated swallowing reflexes, gastroesophageal reflux with associated nutrient loss, and increased energy expenditure caused by muscle spasticity or athetosis (a mixed pattern of too much and too little muscle tone). Because measuring energy expenditure in these children may be impractical, estimates of energy needs can be based on previous studies of REE. Children with spastic-type (hypertonic) cerebral palsy may have lower energy needs than normal; adolescents require a total of approximately 1200 to 1300 kcal/day.[61,110] Children with athetosis may require a higher-than-normal calorie intake—sometimes more than twice the RDA. Children with myelomeningocele are far less active than their peers; for that reason, their energy needs are only 50% to 60% that of normal children (Table 12-10).

If the child's body habitus is markedly abnormal, a more appropriate estimate of energy needs is based on surface area rather than weight. Repeated assessment of the child's growth during nutritional supplementation is essential, because obesity in these children is common. Obesity can impose a considerable burden on the family and caregivers because of the increased difficulty in moving an overweight child.

TABLE 12-10 Guidelines for Estimating Caloric Requirements Based on Height in Children with Developmental Disabilities

Condition	Caloric Recommendation
Ambulatory, ages 5 to 12 yr	13.9 kcal/cm height
Nonambulatory, ages 5 to 12 yr	11.1 kcal/cm height
Cerebral palsy with severely restricted activity	10 kcal/cm height
Cerebral palsy with mild to moderate activity	15 kcal/cm height
Athetoid cerebral palsy, adolescence	Up to 6000 kcal/day
Down syndrome, boys, ages 1 to 14 yr	16.1 kcal/cm height
Down syndrome, girls, ages 1 to 14 yr	14.3 kcal/cm height
Myelomeningocele	Approximately 50% of RDA for age after infancy
	May need as little as 7 kcal/cm height to maintain normal weight
Prader-Willi syndrome	10-11 kcal/cm height (maintenance)
	9 kcal/cm height (to promote weight loss)

RDA, recommended dietary allowance.
From Nelson JK, et al: Mayo Clinic Diet Manual, 7th ed. St Louis, Mosby-Year Book, 1994.

REFERENCES

1. Aarsland A, Chinkes D, Wolfe RR: Hepatic and whole-body fat synthesis in humans during carbohydrate overfeeding. Am J Clin Nutr 1997;65:1774-1782.
2. Akintorin SM, Kamat M, Pildes RS, et al: A prospective randomized trial of feeding methods in very low birth weight infants. Pediatrics 1997;100:E4.
3. Alexander J, Saito H, Trocki O: The importantce of lipid type in the diet after burn injury. Ann Surg 1986;204:1-8.
4. Alexiewicz JM, Kumar D, Smogorzewski M, et al: Polymorphonuclear leukocytes in non-insulin-dependent diabetes mellitus: Abnormalities in metabolism and function. Ann Intern Med 1995;123:919-924.
5. Alhimyary A, Fernandez C, Picard M, et al: Safety and efficacy of total parenteral nutrition delivered via a peripherally inserted central venous catheter. Nutr Clin Pract 1996;11:199.
6. American Academy of Pediatrics: Pediatric Nutrition Handbook, 4th ed. Elk Grove Village, Ill, AAP, 1998.
7. American Medical Association Nutrition Advisory Group: Department of Food and Nutrition: Multivitamin preparations for parenteral use. JPEN J Parenter Enteral Nutr 1979;3:258.
8. Anand K, Sippell M, Aynsley-Green A: Randomised trial of fentanyl anaesthsia in preterm babies undergoing surgery: Effects on the stress response. Lancet 1987;1:243-248.
9. Anderson RA: Selenium, chromium and manganese. In Shils M, Young V (eds): Modern Nutrition in Health and Disease, 7th ed. Philadelphia, Lea & Febiger, 1988, pp 274-277.
10. Andrew F, Chan G, Schiff D: Lipid metabolism in the neonate. I. The effects of Intralipid infusion on plasma triglyceride and free fatty acid concentrations in the neonate. J Pediatr 1976;88:273-278.
11. Andrew F, Chan G, Schiff D: Lipid metabolism in the neonate. II. The effects of Intralipid on bilirubin binding in vitro and in vivo. J Pediatr 1976;88:279-284.
12. Angele M, Smail N, Ayala A, et al: L-Arginine: A unique amino acid for restoring the depressed immune functions following trauma-hemorrhage. J Trauma Injury Infect Crit Care 1999;46:34-41.
13. August D, Teitelbaum DH: Guidelines for the use of parenteral and enteral nutrition in adult and pediatric patients. JPEN J Parenter Enteral Nutr 2002;26:1SA-137SA.

14. Baker J, Detsky A, Wesson D: Nutritional assessment: A comparison of clinical judgement and objective measurements. N Engl J Med 1982;306:969-972.

15. Ball G, Willows N: Definitions of pediatric obesity. CMAJ 2005;172:309-310.

16. Barrett TG, Forsyth JM, Nathavitharana KA, et al: Potentially lethal thiamine deficiency complicating parenteral nutrition in children. Lancet 1993;341:901-902.

17. Beasley SW, Catto-Smith AG, Davidson PM: How to avoid complications during percutaneous endoscopic gastrostomy. J Pediatr Surg 1995;30:671-673.

18. Beath SV, Davies P, Papadopoulou A, et al: Parenteral nutrition-related cholestasis in postsurgical neonates: Multivariate analysis of risk factors. J Pediatr Surg 1996; 31:604-606.

19. Beck R: Use of a pediatric parenteral amino acid mixture in a population of extremely low birth weight neonates: Frequency and spectrum of direct bilirubinemia. Am J Perinatol 1990;7:84-86.

20. Berger MM, Cavadini C, Bart A, et al: Cutaneous copper and zinc losses in burns. Burns 1992;18:373-380.

21. Berger MM, Cavadini C, Chiolero R, Dirren H: Copper, selenium, and zinc status and balances after major trauma. J Trauma Injury Infect Crit Care 1996;40:103-109.

22. Bettger WJ, O'Dell BL: A critical physiological role of zinc in the structure and function of biomembranes. Life Sci 1981;28:1425-1438.

23. Bines J, Francis D, Hill D: Reducing parenteral requirements in children with short bowel syndrome: Impact of an amino acid-based complete infant formula. J Pediatr Gastroenterol Nutr 1998;26:123-128.

24. Bines J, Taylor R, Justice F, et al: Influence of diet complexity on intestinal adaptation following massive small bowel resection in a preclinical model. J Gastroenterol Hepatol 2002;11:1170-1179.

25. Bistrian BR: Nutritional assessment and therapy of protein-calorie malnutrition in the hospital. J Am Diet Assoc 1977;71:393-397.

26. Boehm KA, Helms RA, Christensen ML, et al: Carnitine: A review for the pharmacy clinician. Hosp Pharm 1993; 28:843-850.

27. Bonner CM, DeBrie KL, Hug G, et al: Effects of parenteral L-carnitine supplementation on fat metabolism and nutrition in premature infants. J Pediatr 1995;126:287-292.

28. Braillon PM, Salle BL, Brunet J, et al: Dual energy x-ray absorptiometry measurement of bone mineral content in newborns: Validation of the technique. Pediatr Res 1992; 12:77-80.

29. Brans YW, Andrew DS, Carrillo DW, et al: Tolerance of fat emulsions in very-low-birth-weight neonates. Am J Dis Child 1988;142:145-152.

30. Braunschweig C, Levy P, Sheean P, Wang X: Enteral compared with parenteral nutrition: A meta-analysis. Am J Clin Nutr 2001;74:534-542.

31. Braunschweig CL, Wesley JR, Clark SF, Mercer N: Rationale and guidelines for parenteral and enteral transition feeding of the 3- to 30-kg child. J Am Diet Assoc 1988;88:479-482.

32. Brooks MJ, Melnik G: The refeeding syndrome: An approach to understanding its complications and preventing its occurrence. Pharmacotherapy 1995;15:713-726.

33. Btaiche IF, Khalidi N: Parenteral nutrition-associated liver complications in children. Pharmacotherapy 2002;22: 188-211.

34. Buchman AL: The role of glutamine: Counterpoint. Nutr Clin Pract 2003;18:391-396.

35. Buchmiller CE, Kleiman-Wexler RL, Ephgrave KS, et al: Liver dysfunction and energy source: Results of a randomized clinical trial. JPEN J Parenter Enteral Nutr 1993;17:301-306.

36. Buzby GP, Williford WO, Peterson OL, et al: A randomized clinical trial of total parenteral nutrition in malnourished surgical patients: The rationale and impact of previous clinical trials and pilot study on protocol design. Am J Clin Nutr 1988;47:357-365.

37. Caniano DA, Starr J, Ginn-Pease ME: Extensive short-bowel syndrome in neonates: Outcome in the 1980s. Surgery 1989; 105:119-124.

38. Castillo-Duran C, Rodriguez A, Vengas G, et al: Zinc supplementation and growth of infants born small for gestational age. J Pediatr 1995;127:206-211.

39. Chait PG, Ingram J, Phillips-Gordon C, et al: Peripherally inserted central catheters in children. Radiology 1995; 197:775-778.

40. Chesney RW: Taurine: Is it required for infant nutrition? Am J Nutr 1988;118:6-10.

41. Chevalier RL: Developmental renal physiology of the low birth weight pre-term newborn. J Urol 1996;156:714-719.

42. Chwals WJ, Lally KP, Woolley MM: Indirect calorimetry in mechanically ventilated infants and children: Measurement accuracy with absence of audible airleak. Crit Care Med 1992;20:768-770.

43. Clarke DE, Raffin TA: Infectious complications of indwelling long-term central venous catheters. Chest 1990;97:966-972.

44. Cohen M, Gartner L: The use of medium chain triglycerides in the management of biliary atresia. J Pediatr 1971; 79:379-381.

45. Cole T, Bellizzi M, Flegal K, Dietz W: Establishing a standard definition for child overweight and obesity worldwide: International survey. BMJ 2000;320:1240-1243.

46. Cooper A, Jakobowski D, Spiker J, et al: Nutrition assessment: An integral part of the preoperative pediatric surgical evaluation. J Pediatr Surg 1982;16:554.

47. Coran AG, Drongowski RA: Body fluid compartment changes following neonatal surgery. J Pediatr Surg 1989; 24:829-832.

48. Coran AG, Drongowski RA, Wesley JR: Changes in total body water and extracellular fluid volume in infants receiving total parenteral nutrition. J Pediatr Surg 1984;19:771-776.

49. Cornblath M, Hawdon JM, Williams AF, et al: Controversies regarding the definition of neonatal hypoglycemia: Suggested operational thresholds. Pediatrics 2000;105: 1141-1145.

50. Cowan CE: Antibiotic lock technique. J Intraven Nurs 1992;15:283-287.

51. Cunningham J, Fraher LJ, Clemens TL, et al: Chronic acidosis with metabolic bone disease. Am J Med 1982;73:199-204.

52. Dahlstrom KA, Ament ME, Moukarzel AA, et al: Low blood and plasma carnitine levels in children receiving long-term parenteral nutrition. J Pediatr Gastroenterol Nutr 1990; 11:375-379.

53. Davies SP, Reaveley DA, Brown EA, et al: Amino acid clearances and daily losses in patients with acute renal failure treated by continuous arteriovenous hemodialysis. Crit Care Med 1991;19:1510-1515.

54. Dawson S, Pai MKR, Smith S, et al: Right atrial catheters in children with cancer: A decade of experience in the use of tunnelled, exteriorized devices at a single institution. Am J Pediatr Hematol Oncol 1991;13:126-129.

55. de Vernejoul MC, Messing B, Modrowski D, et al: Multifactorial low remodeling bone disease during cyclic total parenteral nutrition. J Clin Endocrinol Metab 1985;60:109.

56. Donnell S, Taylor N, van Saene H, et al: Infection rates in surgical neonates and infants receiving parenteral nutrition: A five-year prospective study. J Hosp Infect 2002;52:273-280.

57. Donowitz LG, Hendley JO: Short-course amphotericin B therapy for candidemia in pediatric patients. Pediatrics 1995;95:888-891.

58. Dreizen S, Spirakis CN, Stone RE: A comparison of skeletal growth in maturation in under nourished and well nourished girls before and after menarche. J Pediatr 1967;70:256.

59. Dudrick S, Groff D, Wilmore D: Long term venous catheterization in infants. Surg Gynecol Obstet 1969;129:805-808.

60. Dudrick S, Wilmore D, Vars H, Rhoads J: Can intravenous feeding as the sole means of nutrition support growth in the child and restore weight loss in an adult? An affirmative answer. Ann Surg 1969;169:974-984.

61. Eddy T, Nicholson A, Wheeler E: Energy expenditures and dietary intakes in cerebral palsy. Dev Med Child Neurol 1965;7:377-380.

62. Elman R: Amino acid content of blood following intravenous injection of hydrolyzed casein. Proc Soc Exp Biol Med 1937;37:437.

63. Eppes SC, Troutman JL, Gutman LT: Outcome of treatment of candidemia in children whose central catheters were removed or retained. Pediatr Infect Dis J 1989;8:99-104.

64. Falciglia H, Johnson J, Sullivan J, et al: Role of antioxidant nutrients and lipid peroxidation in premature infants with respiratory distress syndrome and bronchopulmonary dysplasia. Am J Perinatol 2003;20:97-107.

65. Farrag HM, Nawrath LM, Healey JE, et al: Persistent glucose production and greater peripheral sensitivity to insulin in the neonate vs the adult. Am J Physiol 1997;272:E86-E93.

66. Feuerstein G, Hallenbeck JM: Leukotrienes in health and disease. FASEB J 1987;1:186-192.

67. Fitzgerald K, Mikalunas V, Rubin H, et al: Hypermanganesemia in patients receiving total parenteral nutrition. JPEN J Parenter Enteral Nutr 1999;23:333-336.

68. Fitzgerald KA, MacKay MW: Calcium and phosphate solubility in neonatal parenteral nutrient solutions containing TrophAmine. Am J Hosp Pharm 1986;43:88-93.

69. Foley MJ: Radiologic placement of long-term central venous peripheral access system ports (PAS Port): Results in 150 patients. J Vasc Interv Radiol 1995;6:255-262.

70. Fonkalsrud EW, Ellis DG, Shaw A, et al: A combined hospital experience with fundoplication and gastric emptying procedure for gastroesophageal reflux in children. J Am Coll Surg 1995;180:449-455.

71. Forsyth JS, Crighton A: Low birthweight infants and total parenteral nutrition immediately after birth. I. Energy expenditure and respiratory quotient of ventilated and non-ventilated infants. Arch Dis Child Fetal Neonatal Ed 1995;73:F4-F7.

72. Friedman Z, Danon A, Stahlman MT, Oates JA: Rapid onset of essential fatty acid deficiency in the newborn. Pediatrics 1976;58:640-649.

73. Fukatsu K, Ueno C, Hashiguchi Y, et al: Glutamine infusion during ischemia is detrimental in a murine gut ischemia/reperfusion model. JPEN J Parenter Enteral Nutr 2003;27:187-192.

74. Gastrointestinal surgery for severe obesity: Proceedings of a National Institutes of Health Consensus Development Conference. Am J Clin Nutr 1992;55:487S-619S.

75. Gauderer ML, Picha GJ, Izant RJ Jr: The gastrostomy "button"—a simple skin-level, non-refluxing device for long-term enteral feedings. J. Pediatr Surg 1984;19:803-805.

76. Gauderer ML, Ponsky JL, Izant RJ Jr: Gastrostomy without laparotomy: A percutaneous endoscopic technique. J Pediatr Surg 1980;15:872-875.

77. Ghisolfi J, Garcia J, Thouvenot JP, et al: Plasma phospholipid fatty acids and urinary excretion of prostaglandins PGE_1 and PGE_2 in infants during total parenteral nutrition, with continuous or sequential administration of fat emulsion. JPEN J Parenter Enteral Nutr 1986;10:631-634.

78. Gutcher GR, Lax AA, Farrell PM: Tocopherol isomers in intravenous lipid emulsions and resultant plasma concentrations. JPEN J Parenter Enteral Nutr 1984;8:269-273.

79. Hankins DA, Riella MC, Scribner BH, Babb AL: Whole blood trace element concentrations during total parenteral nutrition. Surgery 1976;79:674-677.

80. Haumont D, Deckelbaum RJ, Richelle M, et al: Plasma lipid and plasma lipoprotein concentration in low birht weight infants given parenteral nutrition with 20 or 10 percent lipid emulsions. J Pediatr 1989;115:787-793.

81. Haumont D, Richelle M, Deckelbaum RJ, et al: Effect of liposomal content of lipid emulsions on plasma lipid concentrations in low birth weight infants receiving parenteral nutrition. J Pediatr 1992;121:759-763.

82. Heird WC, Gomez MR: Parenteral nutrition in low-birth-weight infants. Annu Rev Nutr 1996;16:471-499.

83. Heird WC, Kashyap S, Gomez MR: Protein intake and energy requirements of the infant. Semin Perinatol 1991; 15:438-448.

84. Hendricks K, Duggan C, Gallagher I: Malnutrition in hospitalized pediatric patients: Current prevalence. Arch Pediatr Asolesc Med 1995;149:1118-1120.

85. Heubi JE, Wiechmann DA, Creutzinger V, et al: Tauroursodeoxycholic acid (TUDCA) in the prevention of total parenteral nutrition-associated liver disease. J Pediatr 2002;141:237-242.

86. Heyland DK, MacDonald S, Keefe L, Drover JW: Total parenteral nutrition in the critically ill patient: A meta-analysis. JAMA 1998;280:2013-2019.

87. Hinke DH, Zandt-Stastny DA, Goodman LR, et al: Pinch-off syndrome: A complication of implantable subclavian venous access devices. Radiology 1990;177: 353-356.

88. Inge T, Zeller M, Garcia V, Daniels S: Surgical approach to adolescent obesity. Adolesc Med Clin 2004;15: 429-453.

89. Isaacs JW, Millikan WJ, Stackhouse J, et al: Parenteral nutrition of adults with 900-milliosmolar solution via peripheral veins. Am J Clin Nutr 1977;30:552-559.

90. Jensen MD: Research techniques for body composition assessment. J Am Diet Assoc 1992;92:454-460.

91. Johnson PR, Decker MD, Edwards KM, et al: Frequency of Broviac catheter infections in pediatric oncology patients. J Infect Dis 1986;154:570-578.

92. Jones GR, Konsler GK, Dunaway RP, et al: Prospective analysis of urokinase in the treatment of catheter sepsis in pediatric hematology-oncology patients. J Pediatr Surg 1993; 28:350-355.

93. Jones K, Kovacevich D, Teitelbaum D: Establishing a comprehensive database for home parenteral nutrition: Six years of data. Nutr Clin Pract 2000;15:279-286.

94. Jones M, Pierro A, Hammond P, Lloyd D: The metabolic response to operative stress in infants. J Pediatr Surg 1993; 28:1258-1263.

95. Kalhoff H, Wiese B, Kunz C, et al: Increased renal net acid excretion in prematures below 1600 g body weight compared with prematures and small-for-date newborns above 2100 g on alimentation with commercial preterm formula. Biol Neonate 1994;66:10-15.

96. Kao LC, Cheng MH, Warburton D: Triglycerides, free fatty acids, free fatty acids/albumin molar ratio, and cholesterol levels in serum of neonates receiving long-term lipid infusions: Controlled trial of continuous vs intermittent regimens. J Pediatr 1984;104:429-435.

97. Kaplan AS, Zemel BS, Neiswender KM, Stallings VA: Resting energy expenditure in clinical pediatrics: Measured versus prediction equations. J Pediatr 1995;127:200-205.

98. Karlen J, Aperia A, Zetterstorm R: Renal excretion of calcium and phosphate in preterm and term infants. J Pediatr 1985;106:814-819.

99. Karpel JT, Peden VH: Copper deficiency in long-term parenteral nutrition. J Pediatr 1972;80:32-34.

100. Kaufman S, Murray N, Wood R: Nutritional support for the infant with extrahepatic biliary atresia. J Pediatr 1987; 110:679-685.

101. Kelly D: Guidelines and available products for parenteral vitamins and trace elements. JPEN J Parenter Enteral Nutr 2002;26:S34-S36.

102. Kennedy KA, Stoll BJ, Ehrenkranz RA, et al: Vitamin A to prevent bronchopulmonary dysplasia in very-low-birth-weight infants: Has the dose been too low? Early Hum Dev 1997;49:19-31.

103. Keshan TH, Miller RG, Jahoor F, Jaksic T: Stable isotopic quantitation of protein metabolism and energy expenditure in neonates on- and post-extracorporeal life support. J Pediatr Surg 1997;32:958-963.

104. Kien L: Carbohydrates. In Tsang RC, Lucas A, Vauy R (eds): Nutritional Needs of the Preterm Infant: Scientific Basis and Practical Guidelines. Baltimore, Williams & Wilkins, 1993, pp 47-63.

105. King DR, Komer M, Hoffman J, et al: Broviac catheter sepsis: The natural history of an iatrogenic infection. J Pediatr Surg 1985;20:728-733.

106. Kitamura K, Takahashi T, Tanaka H, et al: Two cases of thiamine deficiency-induced lactic acidosis during total parenteral nutrition. Tohoku J Exp Med 1993;171:129-133.

107. Klein GL, Berquist WE, Ament ME, et al: Hepatic aluminum accumulation in children on total parenteral nutrition. J Pediatr Gastroenterol Nutr 1984;3:740-743.

108. Klein S, Kinney J, Jeejeebhoy K, et al: Nutrition support in clinical practice: Review of published data and recommendations for future research directions. JPEN J Parenter Enteral Nutr 1997;21:133-156.

109. Kozar R, Verner-Cole E, Schultz S, et al: The immune-enhancing enteral agents arginine and glutamine differentially modulate gut barrier function following mesenteric ischemia/reperfusion. J Trauma 2004;57: 1150-1156.

110. Krick J, Murphy P, Markham J, Shapiro B: A proposed formula for calculating energy needs of children with cerebral palsy. Dev Med Child Neurol 1992;34:481-487.

111. Kurkchubasche AG, Smith SD, Rowe MI: Catheter sepsis in short-bowel syndrome. Arch Surg 1992;127:21-25.

112. Kushner R: Managing the obese patient after bariatric surgery: A case report of severe malnutrition and review of the literature. JPEN J Parenter Enteral Nutr 2000;24:126-132.

113. Lemons J: Fetal-placental nitrogen metabolism. Semin Perinatol 1979;3:177-190.

114. Lennon C, Davidson KW, Sadowski JA, et al: The vitamin K content of intravenous lipid emulsions. JPEN J Parenter Enteral Nutr 1993;17:142-144.

115. Letton RW, Chwals WJ, Jamie A, Charles B: Early postoperative alterations in infant energy use increase the risk of overfeeding. J Pediatr Surg 1995;30:988-993.

116. Leung FY: Nutrient needs and feeding of premature infants: Nutrition Committee, Canadian Paediatric Society. Trace elements in parenteral micronutrition. Can Med Assoc J 1995;152:1765-1785.

117. Levitsky DA, Strupp BJ: Malnutrition and the brain: Changing concepts, changing concerns. J Nutr 1995;125: 2212S-2220S.

118. Lipkin EW, Ott SM, Chesnut CHI: Mineral loss in the parenteral nutrition patient. Am J Clin Nutr 1988;47: 515-523.

119. Lundberg G, Wahlberg E, Rickberg A, Olofsson P: PAS-Port: A new implantable vascular access device for arm placement: Experiences from the first two years. Eur J Surg 1995;161:323-326.

120. Mackie R, Sghir A, Gaskins HR: Developmental microbial ecology of the neonatal gastrointestinal tract. Am J Clin Nutr 1999;69:1035S-1045S.

121. Maffeis C: Childhood obesity: The genetic-environmental interface. Best Pract Res Clin Endocrinol Metab 1999;13: 31-46.

122. Mahoney C, Margolis M, Knauss TA, Labbe R: Chronic vitamin A intoxication in infants fed chicken liver. Pediatrics 1980;65:893-896.

123. Maini B, Blackburn GL, Bistrian BR, et al: Cyclic hyperalimentation: An optimal technique for preservation of visceral proteins. J Surg Res 1976;20:515-525.

124. Marian M: Pediatric nutrition support. Nutr Clin Pract 1993;8:199-209.

125. Marian M, Rappaport W, Cunningham D, et al: The failure of conventional methods to promote spontaneous transpyloric feeding tube passage and the safety of intragastric feeding in the critically ill ventilated patient. Surg Gynecol Obstet 1993;176:475-479.

126. Marvin V, Rebollo M, Castillo-Duran C, et al: Controlled study of early postoperative parenteral nutrition in children. J Pediatr Surg 1999;34:1330-1335.

127. Matsusue S, Nishimura S, Koizumi S, et al: Preventive effect of simultaneously infused lipid emulsion against thrombophlebitis during postoperative peripheral parenteral nutrition. Surg Today 1995;25:667-671.

128. Maxvold N, Smoyer W, Custer J, et al: Amino acid loss and nitrogen balance in critically ill children with acute renal failure: A prospective comparison between classic hemofiltration vs hemofiltration with dialysis. Crit Care Med 2000; 28:1161-1165.

129. McClain CJ: Zinc metabolism in malabsorption syndromes. J Am Coll Nutr 1985;4:49-64.

130. Mendeloff E, Wesley J, Deckert R: Comparison of measured resting energy expenditure (REE) versus estimated energy expenditure (EEE) in infants. JPEN J Parenter Enteral Nutr 1986;10(Suppl):65.

131. Mermel LA: Prevention of catheter-related infections. Ann Intern Med 2000;132:391-402.

132. Merritt RJ, Kalsch M, Roux LD: Significance of hypoalbuminemia in pediatric oncology patients—malnutrition or infection? JPEN J Parenter Enteral Nutr 1985;9:303-306.

133. Mertz W: The essential trace elements. Science 1981;18: 1332-1338.

134. Messing B, Peitra-Cohen S, Debure A, et al: Antibiotic-lock technique: A new approach to optimal therapy for catheter-related sepsis in home-parenteral nutrition patients. JPEN J Parenter Enteral Nutr 1988;12:185-189.

135. Messing B, Zarka Y, Lemann M, et al: Chronic cholestasis associated with long-term parenteral nutrition. Transplant Proc 1994;26:1438-1439.

136. Metheny N, Dettenmeier P, Hampton K, et al: Detection of inadvertent respiratory placement of small-bore feeding tubes: A report of 10 cases. Heart Lung 1990;19:631-638.

137. Miller RG, Jahoor F, Jaksic T: Decreased cysteine and proline synthesis in parenterally fed, premature infants. J Pediatr Surg 1995;30:953-957.

138. Mitchell IM, Davies PSW, Day JME, et al: Energy expenditure in children with congenital heart disease, before and after cardiac surgery. J Thorac Cardiovasc Surg 1994;107: 374-380.

139. Moclair A, Bates I: The efficacy of heparin in maintaining peripheral infusions in neonates. Eur J Pediatr 1995;154: 567-570.

140. Montecalvo M, Steger K, Farber H, et al: Nutritional outcome and pneumonia in critical care patients randomized to gastric versus jejunal tube feedings. Crit Care Med 1992;20:1377-1387.

141. Moukarzel AA, Haddad I, Ament ME, et al: 230 Patient years of experience with home long-term parenteral nutrition in childhood: Natural history and life of central venous catheters. J Pediatr Surg 1994;29:1323-1327.

142. Must A, Jacques P, Dallal G, et al: Long-term morbidity and mortality of overweight adolescents: A follow-up of the Harvard Growth Study of 1922 to 1935. N Engl J Med 1992;327:1350-1355.

143. National Academy of Sciences: Hazards of overuse of vitamin D. Am J Clin Nutr 1975;28:512-516.

144. Ninh N, Maiter D, Veniers J, et al: Failure of exogenous insulin-like growth factor-I to restore normal growth in rats submitted to dietary zinc deprivation. J Endocrinol 1998;159:211-217.

145. Nissenson A, Lindsay R, Swan S, et al: Sodium ferric gluconate complex in sucrose is safe and effective in hemodialysis patients: North American clinical trial. Am J Kidney Dis 1999;35:360-361.

146. Nordenstrom J, Pesson E: Energy supply during total parenteral nutrition—how much and what source? Acta Anaesthesiol Scand 1985;29:95-99.

147. Offenbacher EG, Pi-Sunyer FX: Chromium in human nutrition. Annu Rev Nutr 1988;8:543-563.

148. O'Grady NP, Alexander M, Dellinger EP, et al: Guidelines for the prevention of intravascular catheter-related infections: Centers for Disease Control and Prevention. MMWR Morb Mortal Wkly Rep 2002;51:1-29.

149. Okamoto E, Rassin DK, Zucker CL, et al: Role of taurine in feeding the low-birth-weight infant. J Pediatr 1984;104: 936-940.

150. Okuyama H, Urao M, Starr G, et al: A comparison of the efficacy of pyloromyotomy and pyloroplasty in patients with gastroesophageal reflux and delayed gastric emptying. J Pediatr Surg 1997;32:316-320.

151. Ott SM, Maloney NA, Klein GL, et al: Aluminum is associated with low bone formation in patients receiving chronic parenteral nutrition. Ann Intern Med 1983;98:910-914.

152. Park W, Paust H, Schroder H: Lipid infusion in premature infants suffering from sepsis. JPEN J Parenter Enteral Nutr 1984;8:290-292.

153. Pelegano JF, Rowe JC, Carey DE, et al: Effect of calcium/phosphorus ratio on mineral retention in parenterally fed premature infants. J Pediatr Gastroenterol Nutr 1991;12:351-355.

154. Pereira GR, Zeigler MM: Nutritional care of the surgical neonate. Clin Perinatol 1989;16:233.

155. Peterson KE, Washington J, Rathbun JM: Team management of failure to thrive. J Am Diet Assoc 1984;84:810-815.

156. Phelps DL: The role of vitamin E therapy in high-risk neonates. Clin Perinatol 1988;15:955-963.

157. Piedra P, Dryja D, LaScolea L Jr: Incidence of catheter-associated gram-negative bacteremia in children with short bowel syndrome. J Clin Microbiol 1989;6:1317-1319.

158. Pierro A: Metabolism and nutritional support in the surgical neonate. J Pediatr Surg 2002;37:811-822.

159. Pierro A, Jones MO, Hammond P, et al: A new equation to predict the resting energy expenditure of surgical infants. J Pediatr Surg 1994;29:1103-1108.

160. Pierro A, Koletzko B, Carnielli V: Resting energy expenditure is increased in infants and children with extrahepatic biliary atresia. J Pediatr Surg 1989;24:534-539.

161. Pinhas-Hamiel O, Dolan LM, Daniels SR, et al: Increased incidence of non-insulin-dependent diabetes mellitus among adolescents. J Pediatr 1996;128:608-615.

162. Pittard WBI: Breast milk immunology: A frontier in infant nutrition. Am J Dis Child 1987;133:83-87.

163. Pollack A, Cowett RM, Schwartz R, Oh W: Glucose disposal in low-birth-weight infants during steady-state hyperglycemia: Effects of exogenous insulin administration. Pediatrics 1978;61:546-549.

164. Potter G: Bile acid diarrhea. Dig Dis 1998;16:118-124.

165. Prestridge LL, Schanler RJ, Shulman R, et al: Effect of parenteral calcium and phosphorus on mineral retention and bone mineral content in very low birth weight infants. J Pediatr 1993;122:761-768.

166. Prevention CfDCa: CDC growth charts. In Report no. 314. Atlanta, Department of Health and Human Services, National Center for Health Statistics, 2000.

167. Rajagopalan KV: Molybdenum—an essential trace element. Nutr Rev 1987;45:321-328.

168. Rasmussen A: Carbohydrate induced hypophosphatemia. Acta Anaesthesiol Scand 1985;29:68-70.

169. Reed CR, Sessler CN, Glauser FL, Phelan BA: Central venous catheter infections: Concepts and controversies. Intensive Care Med 1995;21:177-183.

170. Report of the Dietary Guidelines Advisory Committee for the 2000 Dietary Guidelines for Americans, Washington, U.S. Dept. of Health, 2005.

171. Rhoads CM, Parkins W, Tourtelotte D, Vars HM: Method for continuous intravenous administration of nutritive solutions suitable for prolonged metabolic studies in dogs. Am J Physiol 1949;159:409.

172. Rhoads JE, Dudrick SJ: History of intravenous nutrition. In Rombeau JL, Caldwell MD (eds): Clinical Nutrition: Parenteral Nutrition. Philadelphia, WB Saunders, 1986, pp 1-10.

173. Rico H, Revilla M, Villa LF, et al: Body composition in children and Tanner's stages: A study with dual-energy x-ray absorptiometry. Metabolism 1993;42:967-970.

174. Roche A: Growth and assessment of handicapped children. Diet Curr 1970;6:25.

175. Romanski SA, McMahon M, Molly M: Metabolic acidosis and thiamine deficiency. Mayo Clin Proc 1999;74: 259-263.

176. Rose J, Gibbons K, Carlson SE, Koo WWK: Nutrient needs of the preterm infant. Nutr Clin Pract 1993;8:226-232.

177. Sacher P, Hirsig J, Gresser J, Spitz L: The importance of oral sodium replacement in ileostomy patients. Prog Pediatr Surg 1989;24:226-231.

178. Sandstrom R, Drott C, Hyltander A, et al: The effect of postoperative intravenous feeding (TPN) on outcome following major surgery evaluated in a randomized study. Ann Surg 1993;217:185-195.

179. Sangild P, Petersen Y, Schmidt M, et al: Preterm birth affects the intestinal response to parenteral and enteral nutrition in newborn pigs. J Nutr 2002;132:3786-3794.

180. Schilling J, Vranjes N, Fierz W, et al: Clinical outcome and immunology of postoperative arginine, omega-3 fatty acids, and nucleotide-enriched enteral feeding: A randomized prospective comparison with standard enteral and low calorie/low fat IV solutions. Nutrition 1996;12:423-429.

181. Schmidt-Sommerfeld E, Penn D: Carnitine and parenteral nutrition of the neonate. Biol Neonate 1990;58:81-88.

182. Schuman E, Ragsdale J: Peripheral ports are a new option for central venous access. J Am Coll Surg 1995;180: 456-460.

183. Schwarz K, Ternberg J, Bell M, Keating J: Sodium needs of infants and children with ileostomy. J Pediatr 1983;102: 509-513.

184. Sermet-Gaudelus I, Poisson-Salomon A, Colomb V: Simple pediatric nutritional risk score to identify children at risk of malnutrition. Am J Clin Nutr 2000;72:64-70.

185. Shaw JH, Holdaway CM: Protein-sparing effect of substrate infusion in surgical patients is governed by the clinical state, and not by the individual substrate infused. JPEN J Parenter Enteral Nutr 1988;12:433-440.

186. Shennan AT, Bryan MH, Angel A: The effect of gestational age on Intralipid tolerance in newborn infants. J Pediatr 1977;91:134-137.

187. Shike M, Shils ME, Heller A, et al: Bone disease in prolonged parenteral nutrition: Osteopenia without mineralization defect. Am J Clin Nutr 1986;44:89-98.

188. Shike M, Sturtridge WC, Tam CS, et al: A possible role of vitamin D in the genesis of parenteral nutrition-induced metabolic bone disease. Ann Intern Med 1981;95:560-568.

189. Silvestre MAA, Morbach CA, Brans YW, et al: A prospective randomized trial comparing continuous versus intermittent feeding methods in very low birth weight neonates. J Pediatr 1996;128:748-752.

190. Sokol RJ: Vitamin E and neurological deficits. Adv Pediatr 1990;37:119-148.

191. Souba WW, Herskowitz K, Austgen TR, et al: Glutamine nutrition: Theoretical considerations and therapeutic impact. JPEN J Parenter Enteral Nutr 1990;14:237S-243S.

192. Spear ML, Stahl GE, Hamosh M, et al: Effect of heparin dose and infusion rate on lipid clearance and bilirubin binding in premature infants receiving intravenous fat emulsions. J Pediatr 1988;112:94-98.

193. Spears K, Cheney C, Zerzan J: Low plasma retinol concentrations increase the risk of developing bronchopulmonary dysplasia and long-term respiratory disability in very-low-birth-weight infants. Am J Clin Nutr 2004;80:1589-1594.

194. Spencer A, Yu S, Tracy T, et al: Parenteral nutrition-associated cholestasis in neonates: multivariate analysis of the potential protective effect of taurine. JPEN J Parenter Enteral Nutr 2005;29:337-344.

195. Spiegel JE, Willenbucher RF: Rapid development of severe copper deficiency in a patient with Crohn's disease receiving parenteral nutrition. JPEN J Parenter Enteral Nutr 1999;23:169-172.

196. Steephen AC, Traber MG, Ito Y, et al: Vitamin E status of patients receiving long-term parenteral nutrition: Is vitamin E supplementation adequate? JPEN J Parenter Enteral Nutr 1991;15:647-652.

197. Stonestreet BS, Rubin L, Pollak A, et al: Renal functions of low birth weight infants with hyperglycemia and glucosuria produced by glucose infusions. Pediatrics 1980;66:561-567.

198. Strong R, Condon S, Soling M, et al: Equal aspiration rates from postpylorus and intragastric-placed small bore nasoenteric feeding tubes: A randomized prospective study. JPEN J Parenter Enteral Nutr 1992;16:59-63.

199. Strupp BJ, Levitsky DA: Enduring cognitive effects of early malnutrition: A theoretical reappraisal. J Nutr 1995;125:2221S-2232S.

200. Stylianos S, Flanigan LM: Primary button gastrostomy: A simplified percutaneous, open, laparoscopy-guided technique. J Pediatr Surg 1995;30:219-220.

201. Sundaram A, Koutkia P, Apovian C: Nutritional management of short bowel syndrome in adults. J Clin Gastroenterol 2002;34:207-220.

202. Suttie J: Vitamin K responsive hemorrhagic disease of infancy. J Pediatr Gastroenterol Nutr 1990;11:4-6.

203. Taketomo CK, Hodding JH, Kraus DM: In Inc L-C, Hudson OH (eds): Pediatric Dosage Handbook, 8th ed. Hudson, OH, Lexi-Comp, 2001, pp 816-818.

204. Tamada H, Matsuo Y, Nezu R, et al: Zinc deficient diet impairs adaptive changes in the remaining intestine after massive small bowel resection in rats. Br J Surg 1992;79:959-963.

205. Tashiro T, Mashima Y, Yamamori H, et al: Intravenous Intralipid 10% vs 20%, hyperlipidemia, and increase in lipoprotein X in humans. Nutrition 1992;8:155-160.

206. Tasman-Jones C, Kay RG, Lee SP: Zinc and copper deficiency, with particular reference to parenteral nutrition. Surg Annu 1978;10:23-52.

207. Taylor S, Manara AR: Manganese toxicity in a patient with cholestasis receiving total parenteral nutrition [letter]. Anaesthesia 1994;49:1013.

208. Teitelbaum D, Caniano D, Wheller J: Resolution of an infected intracardiac thrombus. J Pediatr Surg 1989;24:1118-1120.

209. Teitelbaum D, Drongowski R, Spivak D: Rapid development of hyperbilirubinemia in infants with the short bowel syndrome as a correlate to mortality: Possible indication for early small bowel transplantation. Transplant Proc 1996;28:2677-2678.

210. Teitelbaum DH: Parenteral nutrition-associated cholestasis. Curr Opin Pediatr 1997;9:270-275.

211. Teitelbaum DH, Tracy TJ, Aouthmany M, et al: Use of cholecystokinin-octapeptide for the prevention of parenteral nutrition-associated cholestasis. Pediatrics 2005;115:1332-1340.

212. Thuren P, Hay WJ: Intravenous nutrition and postnatal growth of the micropremie. Clin Perinatol 2000;27:197-234.

213. Tibboel D, Delemarre FMC, Przyrembel H, et al: Carnitine deficiency in surgical neonates receiving total parenteral nutrition. J Pediatr Surg 1990;25:418-421.

214. Treas LS, Iatinis-Bridges B: Efficacy of heparin in peripheral venous infusion in neonates. J Obstet Gynecol Neonatal Nurs 1992;21:214-219.

215. Tremel H, Kienle B, Weilemann LS, et al: Glutamine dipeptide-supplemented parenteral nutrition maintains intestinal function in the critically ill. Gastroenterology 1994;107:1595-1601.

216. van den Berghe G, Wouters PJ, Bouillon R, et al: Outcome benefit of intensive insulin therapy in the critically ill: Insulin dose versus glycemic control. Crit Care Med 2003;31:359-366.

217. van den Berghe G, Wouters PJ, Weekers F, et al: Intensive insulin therapy in the critically ill patient. N Engl J Med 2001;345:1359-1367.

218. Vanderhoof JA, Langnas AN, Pinch LW, et al: Short bowel syndrome. J Pediatr Gastroenterol Nutr 1992;14:359-370.

219. Vargas JH, Klein GL, Ament ME, et al: Metabolic bone disease of total parenteral nutrition: Course after changing from casein to amino acids in parenteral solutions with reduced aluminum content. Am J Clin Nutr 1988;48:1070-1078.

220. Vaughan LM, Small C, Plunkett V: Incompatibility of iron dextran and a total nutrient admixture. Am J Hosp Pharm 1990;47:1745-1746.

221. Verhage AH, Cheong WK, Allard JP, et al: Increase in lumbar spine bone mineral content in patients on long-term parenteral nutrition without vitamin D supplementation. JPEN J Parenter Enteral Nutr 1995;19:431-436.

222. von Meyenfeldt MM, Stapert J, de Jong PC, et al: TPN catheter sepsis: Lack of effect of subcutaneous tunnelling of PVC catheters on sepsis rate. JPEN J Parenter Enteral Nutr 1980;4:514-517.

223. Werlin SL, Lausten T, Jessen S, et al: Treatment of central venous catheter occlusions with ethanol and hydrochloric acid. JPEN J Parenter Enteral Nutr 1995;19:416-418.

224. Whitaker R, Wright J, Pepe M, et al: Predicting obesity in young adulthood from childhood and parental obesity. N Engl J Med 1997;337:869-873.

225. White MS, Shepherd RW, McEniery JA: Energy expenditure measurements in ventilated critically ill children: Within- and between-day variability. JPEN J Parenter Enteral Nutr 1999;23:300-304.

226. Williamson RC: Intestinal adaptation (first of two parts): Structural, functional and cytokinetic changes. N Engl J Med 1978;298:1393-1402.

227. Williamson RC: Intestinal adaptation (second of two parts): Mechanisms of control. N Engl J Med 1978;298:1444-1450.

228. Wilmore DW, Dudrick SJ: Growth and development of an infant receiving all nutrients exclusively by vein. JAMA 1968;203:860.

229. Wilmore DW, Smith RJ, O'Dwyer ST, et al: The gut: A central organ after surgical stress. Surgery 1988;104:917-923.

230. Wolfe RR, O'Donnell TF, Stone MD, et al: Investigation of factors determining the optimal glucose infusion rate in total parenteral nutrition. Metabolism 1980;29: 892-900.

231. Wright A, Hecker J, McDonald G: Effects of low dose heparin on failure of intravenous infusions in children. Heart Lung 1995;24:79-82.

232. Wurzel CL, Halom K, Feldman JG, Rubin LG: Infection rates of Broviac-Hickman catheters and implantable venous devices. Am J Dis Child 1988;142:536-540.

233. Yang H, Larsson J, Permert J, et al: No effect of bolus glutamine supplementation on the postresectional adaptation of small bowel mucosa in rats receiving chow ad libitum. Dig Surg 2000;17:256-260.

234. Zaidan H, Dhanireddy R, Hamosh M, et al: Lipid clearing in premature infants during continuous heparin infusion: Role of circulating lipase. Pediatr Res 1985;19:23-25.

235. Zeigler T, Young L, Benfell K: Clinical and metabolic efficacy of glutamine-supplemented PN after bone marrow transplantation. Ann Intern Med 1992;116: 821-828.

236. Zelikovic I, Chesney RW, Friedman AL, et al: Taurine depletion in very low birth weight infants receiving total parenteral nutrition: Role of renal immaturity. J Pediatr 1990;116:301-306.

237. Ziegler EE: Protein in premature feeding. Nutrition 1994; 10:69-71.

238. Zlotkin SH, Bryan MH, Anderson GH: Intravenous nitrogen and energy intakes required to duplicate in utero nitrogen accretion in prematurely born human infants. J Pediatr 1981;99:115-120.

Chapter 13

Pediatric Anesthesia

Ira S. Landsman, Mirjana Vustar, and Stephen R. Hays

Dr. Marc Rowe, a leader in pediatric surgery, noted, "no matter how skilled and experienced the pediatric surgeon, safe conduct of the newborn patients through the perioperative period requires an equally competent pediatric anesthesiologist."[242] Anesthetic management of both neonates and older children must take into account the process of rapid growth and development. The child's variable anatomic, physiologic, pharmacologic, and psychological characteristics, as well as the magnitude of the surgical problem, influence anesthetic care. This chapter provides an overview of important issues in pediatric anesthesia and pain management that are directly related to clinical management.

PHYSIOLOGIC CONSIDERATIONS

During the first 3 months of life, circulatory and ventilatory adaptation is completed, thermoregulation processes change, the sizes of body fluid compartments shift toward adult values, skeletal muscle mass increases, and hepatic enzyme systems and renal function mature. Over the next 2 years, the child approaches adult physiologic but not psychological maturity. Between the ages of 6 months and 1 year, infants demonstrate sufficient awareness of their surroundings so that psychological aspects of care become an issue. At that age, sedative drugs may be useful in the child's preoperative preparation. Healthy preschool-aged children (2 to 6 years) present relatively few technical problems to the anesthesiologist, but the child's fear, apprehension, and lack of cooperation are of concern. Treatment of fear and apprehension before surgery in school-aged children (6 to 18 years) may also be necessary.

Newborn infants can feel acute pain and process established pain (postoperative pain). At birth, peripheral nociceptors function similarly to mature receptors.[99] However, the nerves responsible for transmitting the immediate chemical, thermal, and mechanical painful stimuli to the central nervous system (CNS) are not fully mature, nor are the inhibitory pathways from the CNS.[100] In the past, because of their inconsistent response to pain, neonates did not receive adequate analgesia for procedures known to cause pain in adults.[230,279,319]

However, neonates of various gestational ages clearly respond to painful stimuli by measurable physiologic, metabolic, and clinical changes, and analgesia and anesthesia attenuate these changes.[8,9]

Newborns are very sensitive to anesthetic agents and have inefficient mechanisms of drug metabolism and elimination.[39] Until infants are 1 month old, there is a marked interpatient difference in the volume of distribution, sensitivity of the CNS, and quality and quantity of such transport proteins as albumin and α1-acid glycoprotein. These interpatient differences contribute to neonates' varied and often unpredictable responses to anesthetic agents.

After the first several weeks of life, drug metabolism gradually becomes so efficient that many of the opioid agents, such as fentanyl and morphine, have a shorter half-life in infants and young children than in older children and adults. The doses per body weight of intravenous anesthetic agents, such as thiopental and propofol, are higher in the first 6 months of life than during any other period (Fig. 13-1).[145,316] During the first year of life, the concentration of inhalation agent needed to maintain anesthesia is greater than during any other period (Table 13-1, Fig. 13-2). However, the infant's heart is more sensitive to these higher concentrations.

ANESTHETIC RISK

It is part of anesthesiologists' daily practice to estimate the severity of their patients' medical conditions before anesthetizing them. For that purpose, the American Society of Anesthesiologists (ASA) developed its physical status classification in 1941. The ASA classification system does not predict risk, because the type of operative procedure is not taken into consideration.[215] The ASA classification allows the anesthesiologist to tailor the anesthetic based on the patient's underlying condition. The five ASA classes are as follows:

ASA 1: normal healthy patient
ASA 2: patient with mild systemic disease
ASA 3: patient with severe systemic disease
ASA 4: patient with severe systemic disease that is a constant threat to life

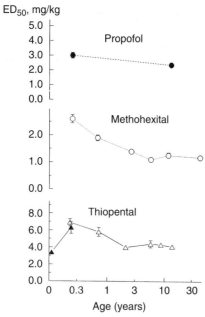

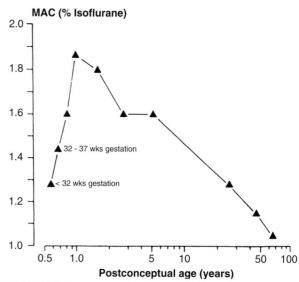

Figure 13-2 Minimum alveolar concentration (MAC) of isoflurane according to gestational age. (From LeDez KM, Lerman J: The minimum alveolar concentration [MAC] of isoflurane in premature neonates. Anesthesiology 1987;67:301.)

Figure 13-1 Estimated ED_{50} (dose of a drug that will induce anesthesia in 50% of patients) plus or minus the standard error in various age groups. Methohexital is indicated by open circles, thiopental by open or filled triangles, and propofol by filled circles. The vertical scales were adapted to yield the same height at ED_{50} for children 7 to 16 years of age. (From University and University Hospital of Lund: Intravenous Induction of Anesthesia in Infants and Children. Lund, Sweden, Studentlitteratur, 1991.)

ASA 5: moribund patient who is not expected to survive without the operation.

Because of the complexity of the child's illness, ASA 3 and 4 patients should have a consultation with an anesthesiologist before the day of surgery.

Death caused by anesthesia alone is uncommon. In the United Kingdom, the overall anesthetic mortality has been

TABLE 13-1 Age versus Mean Minimum Alveolar Concentration of Inhaled Anesthetics in Children

Age (mo)	Halothane*	Isoflurane†	Desflurane‡	Sevoflurane§
1	0.87	1.6	9.16	3.2-3.3
2	1.08	1.9	9.4	3.2-3.3
14	0.97	1.8	8.72	2.5
44	0.91	1.6	8.54	2.5
480	0.76	1.2	7.5	2.5

*From Cook DR, Marcy JH: Pediatric anesthetic pharmacology. In Cook DR, Marcy JH (eds): Neonatal Anesthesia. Pasadena, Calif, Appleton Davies, 1988.
†From Cameron CB, Robinson S, Gregory GA: The minimum anesthetic concentration of isoflurane in children. Anesth Analg 1984;63:418.
‡From Taylor RH, Lerman J: Minimum alveolar concentration of desflurane and hemodynamic responses in neonates, infants, and children. Anesthesiology 1991;75:975.
§From Lerman J, et al: The pharmacology of sevoflurane in infants and children. Anesthesiology 1994;80:814.

estimated as 1:185,000.[48] Children may be at greater risk for anesthesia-related death than adults. The Baltimore Anesthesia Study Commission found the mortality rate for anesthesia in adults to be 3.3:10,000, with a fivefold increased incidence in pediatric patients. Twenty percent of these deaths were in infants younger than 7 days of age. Keenan and Boyan[151] reported a threefold increased risk of cardiac arrest (4.7:10,000) in children younger than 12 years. In a closed claim review by Morray et al.,[202] anesthetic complications and mortality due to respiratory events were higher in children than in adults.

The Pediatric Perioperative Cardiac Arrest Registry was formed in 1994 in an attempt to determine the clinical factors and outcomes associated with cardiac arrest in anesthetized children.[203] Through this registry, it was determined that anesthesia-related cardiac arrest occurred most often in patients younger than 1 year old and in patients with severe underlying disease. Emergency surgery, especially in children with severe underlying disease, was associated with increased mortality if the patient experienced a cardiac arrest during anesthesia. In this study, medication-related problems accounted for 37% of all cardiac arrests and 64% of arrests in ASA 1 and 2 patients. The decreased use of halothane (a potent cardiac depressant) in the United States will improve these statistics when calculated in the future.

Anesthesia mortality tends to be lower in major pediatric centers; for example, between 1966 and 1978, the anesthetic mortality rate at Boston Children's Hospital was 0.8:10,000 in the 0 to 10-year-old group and 0.6:10,000 in the 10- to 20-year-old group. Most deaths occurred in sick patients having emergency surgery. In addition, Keenan et al.[152] suggested that the use of pediatric anesthesiologists for all infants younger than 1 year might decrease anesthetic morbidity in this group.

Auroy et al.[18] observed that a minimum of 200 pediatric cases per year per pediatric anesthesiologist is necessary to reduce the incidence of complications and improve the safety in pediatric practice.

Laryngospasm

Laryngospasm is a common complication of inhalation anesthesia in children. Although the majority of laryngospasm episodes are self-limited or responsive to conservative maneuvers, the anesthesiologist must be prepared to treat laryngospasm with muscle relaxant drugs to restore normal ventilation, because laryngospasm can lead to respiratory failure and cardiac arrest. The incidence of laryngospasm is higher in children than in adults. Olsson and Hallen[212] studied the incidence of laryngospasm in 136,929 patients of all ages over an 11-year period (1967 to 1978) and found an incidence of 8.7 per 1000 patients. The reported laryngospasm incidence during general anesthesia correlated inversely with age, with higher rates in children between the ages of birth and 9 years (17.4 per 1000 patients) and the highest incidence in infants between birth and 3 months (28.2 per 1000 patients). In adolescent patients, a significantly higher laryngospasm incidence was found in males than in females (12.1 versus 7.2 per 1000 patients).[212] The study also showed that children with upper respiratory infections or bronchial asthma had a very high laryngospasm rate (95.8 per 1000 patients).

Treatment of incomplete airway obstruction due to laryngospasm includes removing the irritating surgical stimulus, removing debris from the larynx, and deepening anesthesia. Lung ventilation is facilitated by applying gentle continuous positive airway pressure as 100% oxygen is administered through a tight-fitting facemask. If airway maneuvers do not improve ventilation, a muscle relaxant is required. Intramuscular or intravenous succinylcholine will relax the vocal cords, allowing for adequate lung ventilation.

Postoperative Apnea

Controversy exists over the risk for postoperative apnea in former preterm infants. The conclusions of published studies are limited by their small study sample.[67] Premature infants and full-term babies under 44 weeks' postconceptual age, regardless of whether they have a history of apnea, may develop apnea in the postoperative period.[168,274,312] Postoperative apnea is defined as cessation of breathing or no detectable airflow for 15 seconds or longer, or less than 15 seconds with bradycardia. The cause of this phenomenon is unknown. Recovery from general anesthesia may unmask immature central respiratory regulation or decrease upper airway tone; both factors are believed to be responsible for postoperative apnea.[67]

Although postoperative apnea usually develops in the first 2 hours, it may present as long as 12 hours after anesthesia. Several investigators have tried to establish a postconceptual age after which healthy premature infants with no history of neonatal apnea can be discharged on the day of surgery. Unfortunately, the recommendations vary from 44 weeks[186] to 60 weeks.[107,169,312] The significant variance is based in part on the sophistication of monitoring. The more sophisticated the monitoring, the higher the rate of identified apneic spells. Because considerable controversy exists, each hospital must develop its own policy. It is reasonable to monitor former premature infants for 24 hours if their postconceptual age is 50 weeks or less. Obviously, children with serious medical or neurologic problems or a history of significant and recurrent neonatal apnea are exceptions to this recommendation.

So far, anemia is the only independent risk factor identified that increases the likelihood of postoperative apnea in this at-risk population.[67,309] It has been recommended that anemic preterm infants with hematocrits less than 30% have elective surgery delayed and receive iron supplementation until the hematocrit is greater than 30%. If surgery cannot be deferred, anemic infants must be observed and monitored very carefully for postoperative apnea.

PREANESTHETIC EVALUATION AND PREPARATION

The primary purpose of a preoperative visit is to obtain information about the surgical problem and the medical history and to make an estimate of the patient's response to anesthesia. The preoperative evaluation permits the identification of abnormalities that should be corrected before administration of an anesthetic; these disorders include severe anemia, sickle cell abnormalities, acute systemic infections, and active lower respiratory processes such as asthma, bronchopulmonary dysplasia, and cystic fibrosis.

In addition, the preoperative visit should be used to address the child's and parent's anxiety about the scheduled surgery and anesthesia. Preoperative behavioral evaluation programs are common in major pediatric hospitals. These preparation programs may provide narrative information, hospital tours, role rehearsal, and child life counseling.[147] Outpatient surgery programs may minimize a young child's separation anxiety. Ordinarily, a simple explanation of what the patient can expect before induction of anesthesia reduces the element of surprise and can be used to reinforce preoperative teaching materials. In older children, the preoperative visit allows the anesthesiologist to establish rapport, which fosters trust and may enhance cooperation. In some clinics, parents actively participate in the anesthetic induction process.[29,125] For some parents and preschool-aged children, this joint experience minimizes fear and anxiety; however, for other parents, participation is emotionally traumatic.

Preoperative Oral Fluid Restriction

The patient's stomach must be empty to ensure the safety of anesthesia, but the patient should also be optimally hydrated. These two goals are compatible and

TABLE 13–2 Summary of Fasting Recommendations to Reduce the Risk of Pulmonary Aspiration*

Ingested Material	Minimum Fasting Period (hr)†
Clear liquids‡	2
Breast milk	4
Infant formula	6
Nonhuman milk§	6
Light meal¶	6

*These recommendations apply to healthy patients who are undergoing elective procedures. They are not intended for women in labor. Following these guidelines does not guarantee that complete gastric emptying has occurred.

†Fasting periods apply to all ages.

‡Examples of clear liquids are water, fruit juices without pulp, carbonated beverages, clear tea, and black coffee.

§Because nonhuman milk is similar to solids in terms of gastric emptying time, the amount ingested must be considered when determining an appropriate fasting period.

¶A light meal typically consists of toast and clear liquids. Meals that include fried or fatty foods or meat may prolong gastric emptying time. Both the amount and the type of food ingested must be considered when determining an appropriate fasting period.

Data from ASA Practice Guidelines for Preoperative Fasting and the Use of Pharmacologic Agents to Reduce the Risk of Pulmonary Aspiration: Application to Healthy Patients Undergoing Elective Procedures, A Report by the American Society of Anesthesiologists.

are not difficult to achieve. Patients who are fed at the usual mealtimes and sleep through the night present no particular problems if the operation is scheduled for the early-morning hours.

Numerous studies have failed to document an increased pulmonary aspiration risk when fasting guidelines are relaxed.[137,272] The perioperative fasting guidelines developed by the ASA are listed in Table 13-2.[303] These guidelines allow children to ingest clear liquids up to 2 hours before scheduled surgery. Infants and toddlers can be fed breast milk up until 4 hours before surgery, and infants and young children can be fed formula up until 6 hours before surgery.

If these details are not clearly stated in an itemized fashion with specific times, fluids may inadvertently be withheld from some children, particularly infants, for excessively long periods. Operations should be scheduled according to age, with the youngest patient being the first on the operating schedule. Both the surgeon and the anesthesiologist must be alert to delays and ensure that the infant's fluid restriction is revised accordingly.

Preanesthetic Medications

Various drugs and routes of administration have been described as parts of premedication regimens. In the past, many anesthesiology departments created their own unique mixtures of sedative-hypnotic, narcotic, and antisialagogue medications, which were usually administered by the intramuscular route. The goal of this premedication was to allay anxiety, provide analgesia, decrease autonomic (vagal) reflexes, decrease airway secretions, and reduce the volume and acidity of gastric fluid. The oral or nasal route is now preferred.

Premedication should provide a rapid level of short-term sedation that allows easy separation of the child from the parents and a smooth induction of anesthesia. Because children are usually not in pain before elective surgery, the use of opioids as part of standard premedication is not required. Antisialagogues were useful when diethyl ether and cyclopropane were the commonly used inhalation anesthetics. The newer inhalation agents do not significantly increase the quantity of oral secretions, thereby eliminating the need for anticholinergic premedication.

Midazolam is a popular, short-acting benzodiazepine that is now used frequently for preoperative sedation. It is an anxiolytic, hypnotic, and anticonvulsant agent, with antegrade but not retrograde amnestic properties.[233,292] At physiologic pH, midazolam becomes lipophilic, allowing quick absorption by the gastrointestinal tract and rapid entry into the CNS.[233] Sedative doses of intravenous midazolam can depress the hypoxic ventilatory drive and attenuate reflex cardiorespiratory responses to hypoxemia.[4] When combined with opioids, intravenous midazolam is likely to place unmonitored patients at significant risk for apnea and hypoxemia.[20]

In children, sedation with midazolam can be delivered by the intranasal, oral, rectal, intravenous, or intramuscular route. Walbergh[300] showed that the bioavailability of intranasal midazolam was 51% of the intravenous dose, and the speed of onset was 45% faster than with the rectal route. Wilton et al.[320] reported that intranasal midazolam given to children between 18 months and 5 years of age at a dose of 0.2 mg/kg calmed the patient within 5 to 10 minutes of administration. Tome[288] found that intranasal midazolam at a dose of 0.2 to 0.3 mg/kg produced excellent sedation without prolonging recovery from anesthesia or time to hospital discharge in infants and small children undergoing very short ambulatory surgical procedures. Cardiorespiratory depression has not been encountered when recommended doses of intranasal midazolam (0.2 to 0.3 mg/kg) or oral midazolam (0.5 to 0.75 mg/kg) are administered to otherwise healthy children for preoperative sedation.[83,194,320] Commercially prepared oral midazolam produces satisfactory sedation and anxiolysis within 10 to 20 minutes of consumption.[65] Oral midazolam prepared from the intravenous product has an onset time between 20 and 30 minutes.

Intranasal midazolam can cause mild, transient burning of the nasal mucosa, and amounts greater than 1 mL of a 0.5% solution (5 mg/mL) may produce choking and coughing. If more than 1 mL of 0.5% midazolam is necessary, the oral route is usually better tolerated. Oral midazolam prepared from the intravenous product should be flavored with sweetened clear liquids or syrup to mask the bitter taste. It has been demonstrated that commercially prepared oral midazolam has a more consistent bioavailability and pH characteristics. This stability allows doses as low as 0.25 mg/kg while still producing adequate sedation.[65]

Preoperative medication given to increase the pH of gastric fluid or to promote gastric emptying is not needed in healthy children, because pediatric pulmonary aspiration is rare.[63,284] Clear liquids administered to infants, children, and adults up to 2 hours before surgery do not alter residual gastric volume.[70] In fact, some children who have consumed liquids have a lower residual gastric volume and a higher gastric pH than controls who have had nothing by mouth.

FLUID REQUIREMENTS

Maintenance Fluid Requirements

Various calculations involving body weight, surface area, and calorie expenditure have been used to determine fluid therapy for full-term infants and children.[22,136,243] Body weight and calorie expenditure, as well as estimates of insensible water loss, renal water requirement, stool water loss, and water needed for growth, determine the amount of fluid needed for maintenance. Calorie expenditure is related to size: infants weighing 1 to 10 kg require 100 calories/kg; small children weighing 10 to 20 kg require 1000 calories/day plus 50 calories/day for each kilogram over 10 kg; older children weighing more than 20 kg require 1500 calories/day plus 25 calories/day for each kilogram over 20 kg. For every 100 calories that the patient consumes, 67 mL of water is required for solute excretion; an additional 50 mL per 100 calories is associated with insensible loss, but 17 mL per 100 calories is produced by oxidation. Thus, infants and children need 100 mL of water for each 100 calories expended. Assuming that there are 25 hours in a day, a simple formula can be used to calculate the hourly maintenance fluid needed by healthy full-term infants and children. For children weighing 1 to 10 kg, the hourly maintenance fluid requirement (MFR) is 4 mL/kg per hour. For patients weighing 10 to 20 kg, the hourly MFR is 4 mL/kg per hour for the first 10 kg, plus 2 mL/kg per hour for each kilogram between 10 and 20 kg. For patients weighing more than 20 kg, the MFR is calculated as 4 mL/kg per hour for the first 10 kg, plus 2 mL/kg per hour for the next 10 kg, plus 1 mL/kg per hour for each additional kilogram over 20 kg. For example, a 28-kg child requires 68 mL of maintenance fluid per hour.

For every 100 mL of water given to an infant or child, 3 mEq Na^+, 2 mEq K^+, 2 mEq Cl^-, and 5 g glucose (to prevent ketosis) are required. It is more convenient to equalize the sodium and chloride requirements at 3 mEq. For routine intravenous fluid therapy, 5% dextrose in 0.25% normal saline meets these requirements. However, this is not an ideal fluid for intraoperative use, as noted later.

Premature or Critically Ill Infants

In premature or critically ill infants, many factors influence water and electrolyte balance. The infant's gestational age, postnatal age, weight, renal solute load, and maximum renal concentrating ability are variables. Tissue destruction and catabolism that result from disease, stress, infection, reduced bowel activity, phototherapy, and gastric or intestinal drainage may have marked effects on fluid therapy. These issues have been well reviewed by Rowe,[240] Hammarlund et al.,[123] and Bell and Oh.[22]

Intraoperative Fluid Replacement

Intraoperative fluid replacement involves the initiation of fluid management or, alternatively, a continuation of ongoing therapy. Fluid replacement can be as simple as replacing the deficit from the preoperative fast and providing maintenance fluids, or it can be as complex as correcting preoperative deficits, translocated fluids, and variable blood loss while providing maintenance fluids.

Estimated Fluid Deficit

The fluid deficit incurred during fasting should be replaced during anesthesia. Assuming a child is healthy at the time of fasting, the fluid deficit is estimated by multiplying the hourly MFR by the number of hours the patient has had nothing by mouth (NPO). This deficit can be replaced by infusing half the estimated fluid deficit (EFD) during the first hour of anesthesia and the remaining amount over the next 2 hours.[105] Maintenance fluids should continue in conjunction with replacement fluids. Thus, for an infant undergoing a superficial surgical procedure for 3 hours with minimal or no third-space losses, the amount of fluid needed during surgery is calculated as follows:

$$EFD = Hours\ NPO \times MFR\ (mL/kg/hr)$$
$$First\text{-}hour\ fluids = MFR + \tfrac{1}{2}\ EFD$$
$$Second\text{-}hour\ fluids = MFR + \tfrac{1}{4}\ EFD$$
$$Third\text{-}hour\ fluids = MFR + \tfrac{1}{4}\ EFD$$

Role of Glucose

Surgery may cause the release of stress hormones that decrease insulin sensitivity, so serum glucose levels are usually elevated during surgery. If serum glucose concentrations become too high, glycosuria and osmotic diuresis ensue. Hyperglycemia may contribute to neurologic damage subsequent to episodes of severe ischemia and hypoxia.[113,143,172,208,226,311] Several studies have shown that healthy infants and children remain euglycemic for up to 17 hours after the start of a fast. These studies suggest that healthy infants and children do not require glucose-containing solutions during surgery.[19,311] Frequent monitoring of blood sugar should accompany fluid and glucose therapy in patients who are at high risk for hypoglycemia (e.g., premature infants and those who are small for gestational age, children on total parenteral nutrition, and patients with diabetes).

Choice of Intraoperative Fluid

For most patients, lactated Ringer's solution can be used to provide maintenance and replacement fluids for intraoperative losses. The electrolyte composition of lactated Ringer's is similar to that of serum. Hyponatremia with associated neurologic complications can occur if hypotonic solutions are used for fluid maintenance and replacement of third-space fluid losses.

Most surgical conditions are associated with isotonic transfer of fluids from the extracellular fluid compartment and, to a lesser extent, from the intracellular compartment to a nonfunctional interstitial compartment.[241] This acute sequestration of edematous fluid to a nonfunctional compartment is called third-space loss. Plasma volume may also be compromised. The magnitude of third-space loss varies with the surgical procedure and is usually highest in infants having intra-abdominal surgery. In addition, failure to cover the exposed intestines and the use of heat lamps may increase evaporative losses. In infants, estimated third-space loss is 6 to 10 mL/kg per hour during intra-abdominal surgery, 4 to 7 mL/kg per hour during intrathoracic surgery, and 1 to 2 mL/kg per hour during superficial surgery or neurosurgery. Translocated fluids may represent a large additional functional loss. Thus, clinical signs of the extent of dehydration may be used to estimate the needed fluid replacement. Generally, lactated Ringer's solution is used to restore third-space losses. In cases of massive volume replacement, some advocate using 5% albumin to restore one third to one fourth of the loss. The end point of third-space replacement therapy is maintenance of adequate blood pressure, tissue perfusion, and urine output.

Blood Replacement

Blood replacement depends on the patient's needs, and clear communication between the surgeon and the anesthesiologist is crucial. Accurately measuring blood loss and assessing the limit of safe blood loss in infants are vital parts of any replacement regimen. Weighing sponges and using calibrated miniaturized suction bottles and visual estimates define the magnitude of blood loss. Allowable blood loss is determined by calculating the starting blood volume and hemoglobin or hematocrit of the patient.[38,105] Other factors that should be taken into account to determine allowable blood loss include the patient's age, cardiopulmonary status, and general medical condition. These factors are also used to determine the risk versus benefit of blood transfusion. Normovolemic hemodilution to a predetermined hematocrit can be achieved with crystalloid solutions.

Estimating Allowable Blood Loss

Several methods have been proposed for estimating allowable blood loss (ABL) by calculating the patient's blood volume, weight, and hematocrit. The formulas range from simple to complex, but all involve an estimate of blood volume. Allowable blood loss can be calculated using the following equation:

$$ABL = \text{Weight (kg)} \times EBV \times [Ho - Hl]/H,$$

where EBV is estimated blood volume, Ho is the original hematocrit, Hl is the lowest acceptable hematocrit, and H is the average hematocrit ($[Ho + Hl] \div 2$).

This equation assumes that blood loss and replacement are gradual and exponential. Estimated blood volume is approximately 90 mL/kg for neonates, 80 mL/kg for infants and children, and 65 to 78 mL/kg for adolescents. This equation has general applicability for all age groups.

The ideal fluid to replace blood loss until the lowest acceptable hematocrit is reached is a matter of controversy. Generally, lactated Ringer's solution is given in an amount equal to two to three times the estimated amount of lost blood.

Blood Products

Blood component therapy depends on the clinical setting and the availability of various blood products. Fresh whole blood (i.e., blood that was obtained less than 4 hours previously) has limited availability. Septic infants benefit from the clotting and immune factors, platelets, and white blood cells. If blood loss is predicted to be 40% or more of blood volume, fresh whole blood is helpful in supplying platelets and clotting factors. However, component therapy rather than fresh whole blood is usually used.[47] Packed red blood cells (RBCs) have a hematocrit between 55% and 75% and are relatively hyperkalemic (K ± 15 to 20 mEq/L), acidotic (pH <7.0), and low in ionized calcium. With rapid administration of packed RBCs, each of these factors is significant. The estimated rise in hematocrit for every 10 mL/kg of packed RBCs (assuming a hematocrit of 70%) depends on the patient's age, size, and estimated blood volume (Table 13-3).

When blood loss approaches one blood volume, labile clotting factors are greatly reduced; normal clotting requires 5% to 20% of factor V and 30% of factor VIII. All coagulation factors (except platelets) are present in normal quantities in fresh frozen plasma (FFP). We prefer to provide nearly equal amounts of FFP and packed RBCs to patients with massive blood loss (hematocrit 35% to 40%).

The need for platelets during surgery can be predicted from the preoperative platelet count. Platelets are mobilized from the spleen and bone marrow as bleeding occurs. An infant with a high preoperative platelet count (>250,000/mm^3) may not need a platelet transfusion until two to three blood volumes are lost, whereas an

TABLE 13-3 Estimated Rise in Hematocrit with Increasing Blood Volume

Age	Blood Volume (mL/kg)	Estimated Rise in Hematocrit*
Premature Infants	100	6.30
Term infants	90	7.00
Preschool-aged children	80	7.7
School-aged children	75	8.2
Adults	65	9.3

*The estimated rise in hematocrit for every 10 mL/kg of packed red blood cells (assuming a hematocrit of 70%) depends on the patient's age, size, and estimated blood volume.

infant who has a low count ($<150,000/mm^3$) may need platelets after only one blood volume is lost. Two platelet packs/10 kg increases the platelet count by 10,000 to $15,000/mm^3$.

Rapid administration of cold, citrated blood products can be hazardous; such products must be warmed before infusion. FFP contains the highest amount of citrate per unit volume of any blood product; thus, rapid infusion of FFP causes the greatest change in ionized calcium. Under most circumstances, mobilization of calcium and hepatic metabolism of citrate are sufficiently rapid to prevent precipitous decreases in ionized calcium. However, because infants' calcium stores are small, rapid infusion of FFP can acutely decrease ionized calcium and cause significant decreases in arterial blood pressure.[63,64] Treatment of acute hypocalcemia includes intravenous calcium chloride (10 to 20 mg/kg) or calcium gluconate (30 to 60 mg/kg), which effectively increases ionized calcium and ameliorates hemodynamic changes. Empirical buffering of blood may lead to profound metabolic alkalosis as citrate loads are metabolized.

INHALATION ANESTHETIC AGENTS

Several inhalation agents are available for induction and maintenance of anesthesia. The choice of agent depends on the age of the child and the disease process.

Each agent has general and specific advantages and disadvantages (Table 13-4). None ensure hemodynamic stability. In patients with significant cardiac depression or hemodynamic instability, inhalation agents are generally avoided or used in markedly reduced concentrations. In healthy children, most inhalation agents can be used safely and successfully regardless of age.

To spare children an intravenous injection, anesthesia is often induced by inhalation. However, inhalation anesthesia in children has some risk and is associated with an increased incidence of bradycardia, hypotension, and even cardiac arrest.[151,228] This greater incidence of untoward effects from potent inhalation agents is attributed to age-related differences in uptake, anesthetic requirements, and sensitivity of the cardiovascular system. The uptake of inhalation anesthetics is more rapid in infants and small children than in adults because of major differences in blood-gas solubility coefficients, blood-tissue solubility coefficients, body composition, ratio of alveolar ventilation to functional residual capacity, and distribution of cardiac output.[40,174,177,271,275] Thus, early in the course of anesthetic induction, infants have higher tissue concentrations of the drug than do adults in the brain, heart, and muscle.[59]

Uptake of anesthetic agents can be modified by the presence of cardiac shunts. Right-to-left shunts slow the inhalation induction time of insoluble (nitrous oxide) and moderately soluble (halothane) volatile anesthetics.

TABLE 13-4 Inhalation Anesthetics

Agent	Advantages	Disadvantages and Precautions
Nitrous oxide	Inexpensive Odorless Rapid onset and recovery of clinical effects When combined with potent inhalation anesthetics, side effects of potent agents are reduced Activates the sympathetic nervous system, which attenuates cardiac depression or vasodilatation caused by potent inhalation agents	Should be used as a supplement to other inhalation or intravenous anesthetics to provide complete general anesthesia In critically ill patients, can be a potent vasodilator Expands gas-containing spaces, such as the intestines or middle ear; increases the expansion of pneumothorax and pneumocephalus Exposure to operating room atmosphere contamination may cause neuropathies
Halothane	Nonpungent odor Effective inhalation induction agent Bronchodilator (like all potent inhalation agents)	Causes cardiac depression manifested as bradycardia and decreased myocardial contractility Causes halothane-associated hepatitis (rare in children) Sensitizes the myocardium to the arrhythmogenic properties of epinephrine; however, infants and children require higher doses of epinephrine to stimulate ventricular arrhythmias than do adolescents and adults
Isoflurane	Maintains myocardial contractility and heart rate Minimal sensitization of the myocardium to the arrhythmogenic properties of epinephrine	Pungent odor Not an effective inhalation induction agent Can cause bradycardia in neonates and young infants May cause hypotension by decreasing systemic vascular resistance
Sevoflurane	Nonpungent odor Effective inhalation induction agent Low blood-gas coefficient Maintains myocardial contractility and heart rate Minimal sensitization of the myocardium to the arrhythmogenic properties of epinephrine	More expensive than halothane Metabolized by liver, releasing free fluoride ions; theoretical risk for renal diabetes insipidus Degradation in Baralyme and soda lime, forming potentially toxic metabolites Increased incidence of postanesthesia delirium
Desflurane	Low blood-gas coefficient Maintains myocardial contractility and heart rate Minimal sensitization of the myocardium to the arrhythmogenic properties of epinephrine	Pungent odor Poor inhalation induction agent High incidence of laryngospasm Expensive Increased incidence of postanesthesia delirium

Shunting has a minimal effect when highly soluble agents are used.[276,281] Less soluble agents have a higher concentration in the alveoli than in the blood. Because a right-to-left shunt diverts blood away from the lungs, the amount of agent entering the systemic circulation that is able to reach vessel-rich organs is low. Highly soluble agents, in contrast, have a higher concentration in the blood than in the alveoli. Because most of the agent remains in the blood, the perfusion of the lungs, although limited, still carries large amounts of the agent. The rate of induction remains slow. Under most circumstances, left-to-right shunts do not affect the speed of induction.[281]

Minimum Alveolar Concentration

The minimum alveolar concentration (MAC) is the minimum concentration of an inhaled anesthetic at 1 atmosphere of pressure that prevents skeletal muscle movement in response to a surgical incision in 50% of patients; it is a standard measure of anesthetic potency. The MAC of a volatile anesthetic changes with the patient's age (see Table 13-1). Lerman et al.[178] found that the MAC of halothane in neonates younger than 1 month was 25% lower than in infants 1 month to 1 year of age. LeDez and Lerman[174] showed that premature infants younger than 32 weeks' gestation have a lower MAC for isoflurane than do neonates of longer gestation. For all anesthetic agents, the MAC is highest at 6 to 12 months of age. The increased MAC requirement in conjunction with the rapid uptake of anesthesia makes infants and children very susceptible to anesthetic overdose.[151,228]

Nitrous Oxide

Because nitrous oxide is a nonpotent inhalation agent with a MAC of 105%, it is usually used as an adjunct to the more potent inhalation agents. Nitrous oxide reduces the side effects of these agents by reducing the amount required for effective analgesia. During the induction phase of anesthesia, nitrous oxide hastens the uptake of potent inhalation agents. Eger and Saidman[88] noted that nitrous oxide is more soluble than nitrogen in blood and thus distends any air-containing space, such as the intestines, to which it is carried. As a result, nitrous oxide is usually avoided in patients with closed pneumothorax, intestinal obstruction, or air in the cerebral ventricles. Nitrous oxide has been implicated in lymphocyte depression, testicular damage, birth defects, and miscarriages with chronic exposure, so it is important to adequately scavenge this gas in the operating suite.

Halothane

Halothane was once the most commonly administered anesthetic agent in children because it was less likely than isoflurane and desflurane to cause airway irritation.

However, halothane was not an ideal induction agent because of its potential to cause bradycardia, hypotension, and ventricular ectopy. In many centers, sevoflurane (because of its cardiovascular safety profile) has replaced halothane as the induction agent of choice.[253] Although halothane-associated hepatitis is a concern in adults, it is rare in prepubescent children, even after repeated exposure.[49,301] Warner et al.[302] reported that 60 children had at least 10 episodes of halothane anesthesia without evidence of liver dysfunction.

Halothane causes cardiac depression in animals and humans.[28,44,60,61,89] In addition to the direct actions of this agent on cardiac function, it has interactive effects with catecholamines. Halothane sensitizes the myocardium to the arrhythmogenic properties of epinephrine, although arrhythmias are more common in adults than in children.[144,148,150] Johnston et al.[144] calculated the intravenous dose of epinephrine that would produce three or more premature ventricular beats in 50% of patients anesthetized with enflurane, isoflurane, or halothane (Fig. 13-3). Karl et al.[148] found that no children developed ventricular irritability despite receiving intravenous doses of epinephrine exceeding 1.7 µg/kg. It has also been shown that children undergoing cleft palate repair who were anesthetized with halothane could tolerate 7.8 µg/kg of epinephrine combined with 1% lidocaine without significant cardiac arrhythmias. Tachycardia and hypertension were the most common side effects. Cote[63] has used up to 10 µg/kg of epinephrine added to local anesthetic given over a 20-minute period without significant cardiac arrhythmias.

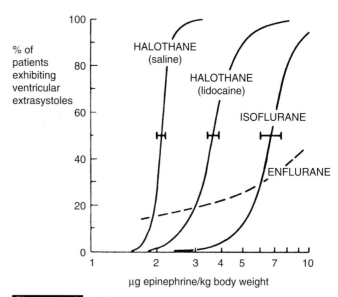

Figure 13–3 In this statistical analysis, the bars indicate the standard deviation from the ED_{50} (the dose of a drug that will induce anesthesia in 50% of patients). The ED_{50} of epinephrine (in µg/kg) is significantly different from that of halothane and isoflurane ($P < 0.01$). Epinephrine injected with lidocaine 0.5% in the halothane group provided significant protection from ventricular extrasystole. (From Johnson RR, Eger EI, Wilson C: A comparative interaction of epinephrine with enflurane, isoflurane, and halothane in man. Anesth Analg 1976;55:709.)

Isoflurane

Isoflurane has a lower solubility coefficient than halothane, so induction and recovery with isoflurane should theoretically be faster than with halothane. However, isoflurane causes moderate to severe airway irritability if used as an induction agent.

The cardiovascular effects of isoflurane in children are well documented. Unlike adults, unpremedicated infants 5 to 26 weeks of age who were anesthetized with isoflurane showed a decrease in heart rate similar to that seen with halothane and a decrease in blood pressure half that seen with halothane.[105] In children older than 2 years who did not receive atropine, isoflurane preserved heart rate and cardiac function better than did halothane.[323] Halothane and isoflurane both reduced blood pressure. Isoflurane reduced peripheral vascular resistance but preserved cardiac output. Gallagher et al.[109] compared the anesthetic effects of halothane and isoflurane on cardiac function in 15 older children using pulsed Doppler echocardiography.[109] Cardiac output, heart rate, and myocardial contractility were preserved with isoflurane, but contractility was decreased with halothane. Kotrly et al.[163] found that isoflurane preserved the baroreceptor response in adults more than did halothane.

Desflurane

Desflurane is a potent inhalation agent. The blood-gas solubility is low and similar to nitrous oxide.[87] Because it is a pungent airway irritant, desflurane results in an unacceptably high incidence of laryngospasm, coughing, and hypoxia when used as an induction agent in children.[282,283,334] Patients anesthetized with desflurane have a faster emergence from general anesthesia. However, desflurane causes a higher incidence of postanesthesia delirium or agitation in children.[310] Cohen et al.[57] concluded that fentanyl supplementation reduces the incidence of severe agitation associated with desflurane anesthesia in children, without delaying emergence.

The cardiovascular profile of desflurane is age dependent.[282] When desflurane was given at a MAC of 1, before incision, the arterial blood pressure decreased approximately 30% compared with awake values, and the heart rate decreased significantly or remained the same. Thus, at a MAC of 1, desflurane, like isoflurane and halothane, seems to attenuate the baroreceptor response in children. Weiskopf et al.[308] also demonstrated that in adults, rapid increases in desflurane from a MAC of 0.55 to 1.66 can transiently increase arterial blood pressure and heart rate; this excitation is associated with an increase in sympathetic and renin-angiotensin system activity.

Sevoflurane

Sevoflurane is a potent inhalation agent with a low blood-gas solubility coefficient; it does not have a pungent odor and is replacing halothane as the inhalation anesthetic of choice for infants and children.[176,270] Clinical studies with sevoflurane in pediatric patients have found shorter times to emergence than with halothane.[81,253] This may be related to the low blood-gas solubility. Sevoflurane has fewer cardiovascular side effects compared with halothane.[139,179,244,253,321,322] Wodey et al.[321] compared cardiovascular changes at equipotent concentrations of sevoflurane and halothane in infants. They concluded that in infants, sevoflurane decreases cardiac output less than halothane, and a minor decrease in contractility is compensated by a greater decrease in systemic vascular resistence (SVR) without a change in heart rate.[321] Unlike halothane, sevoflurane does not increase the sensitivity of the myocardium to the arrhythmogenic effects of epinephrine.[209] Sevoflurane causes a significant decrease in respiratory resistance, and it is an effective bronchodilating agent.[115] Studies show that sevoflurane has an increased incidence of emergence agitation compared with halothane.[293,299] Weldon et al.[314] found that the combination of midazolam premedication and effective postoperative analgesia with caudal block minimizes agitation and excitement in children after sevoflurane anesthesia. Other studies confirmed that adequate analgesia, with ketorolac,[82] fentanyl,[69,106] or clonidine,[165] markedly diminished the incidence of emergence agitation.

The major concern surrounding the use of sevoflurane is that it is metabolized in the liver by the cytochrome system, with the subsequent release of fluoride and the potential for renal diabetes insipidus. However, renal concentrating ability and normal creatinine clearance have been demonstrated in adult volunteers subjected to prolonged sevoflurane exposure. In addition to in vivo metabolism, sevoflurane undergoes degradation by soda lime and Baralyme to produce two potentially toxic olefins, compound A and compound B. Although human exposure to sevoflurane administered by circle absorption systems has not demonstrated toxicity, animal studies have yielded conflicting histologic evidence of chemical-induced toxicity.[34,109,116] Frink et al.[104] concluded that the concentrations of compound A measured in pediatric patients during sevoflurane anesthesia using a 2-L flow circle system were low, and there was no evidence of abnormal renal or hepatic function up to 24 hours after anesthesia.

NEUROMUSCULAR BLOCKING AGENTS

Neuromuscular blocking agents (i.e., muscle relaxants) are used to facilitate endotracheal intubation, to provide surgical relaxation, and to facilitate controlled mechanical ventilation. This is done through blockade of the acetylcholine receptor site on the neuromuscular junction. The use of neuromuscular blocking agents reduces the need for potent inhaled anesthetics or intravenous sedative-hypnotics and thus reduces the incidence of hypotension, bradycardia, and cardiac arrest. Throughout infancy, the neuromuscular junction matures physically and biochemically, the contractile properties of skeletal muscle change, and the amount of muscle in proportion to body weight increases; as a result, the neuromuscular junction is variably sensitive to relaxants.[187] In addition, age-related changes in the volume of distribution of relaxants, their redistribution and clearance, and possibly their rate of metabolism occur. These factors influence the dose-response relationships of relaxants and the duration of neuromuscular blockade.[59,71,117]

When allowances are made for differences in the volume of distribution and for the type and concentration of anesthetic, infants seem to be relatively resistant to succinylcholine and relatively sensitive to nondepolarizing relaxants (Table 13-5). Because of its many untoward effects, succinylcholine, which is a depolarizing relaxant, has fallen into disuse for elective cases.

TABLE 13-5 Muscle Relaxants

Agent	Type	Dose	Metabolism and Excretion	Advantages	Disadvantages and Precautions
Succinylcholine	Short acting; depolarizing	IV: 1.0-2.0 mg/kg IM: younger than 6 mo, 4.0-5.0 mg/kg; older than 6 mo, 3.0-4.0 mg/kg	Pseudocholinesterase	Rapid onset; rapid recovery; may be delivered through intravascular or intramuscular routes	Masseter muscle spasm; trigger for malignant hyperthermia; bradycardia; hyperkalemia leading to life-threatening arrhythmias; myoglobinemia (muscle injury); muscle fasciculations; increased intraocular pressure; prolonged neuromuscular blockade with pseudocholinesterase deficiency. Avoid in patients with muscular dystrophy; multiple trauma >24 hr; burns >24 hr; spinal cord injury >24 hr; malignant hyperthermia susceptible
Mivacurium	Short acting; nondepolarizing	Intubation: 0.2 mg/kg Maintenance: 0.1 mg/kg	Plasma cholinesterase	Recovery time 10 min; infusion possible	Histamine release; unpredictable intubating conditions
Atracurium	Intermediate acting; nondepolarizing	Intubation: 0.5 mg/kg Maintenance: 0.15 mg/kg	Ester hydrolysis; Hoffman degradation	Recovery time 30 min regardless of age; can be used in renal and kidney disease; infusion possible	Histamine release; (metabolite of Hoffman degradation); epileptogenic in high doses
Cisatracurium	Intermediate acting; nondepolarizing	Intubation: 0.1 mg/kg Maintenance: 0.3 mg/kg	Ester hydrolysis; Hoffman degradation	Recovery time 30 min; no cardiovascular effects; infusion possible	
Rocuronium	Intermediate acting; nondepolarizing	Intubation: 0.6 mg/kg (onset 50-80 sec) or 1.2 mg/kg (onset 30 sec) Maintenance: 0.1 mg/kg	Liver and renal	Recovery time 15-40 min (dose dependent); can be used for rapid-sequence intubation; infusion possible	Slight vagolytic
Vecuronium	Intermediate acting; nondepolarizing	Intubation: 0.1 mg/kg Maintenance: 0.02 mg/kg	Renal and liver	Recovery time approx 30 min in children; no histamine release at up to 0.4 mg/kg; no effect on cardiovascular system	Long-acting muscle relaxant in infants; recovery time approx 70 min.
Pancuronium	Long acting; nondepolarizing	Intubation: 0.1 mg/kg Relaxation: 0.02 mg/kg	Renal and liver	Recovery time approx 50 min; inexpensive	Vagolytic; tachycardia; hypertension; histamine release

The degree of neuromuscular blockade should be monitored with a nerve stimulator during the course of the operation, and the patient should be treated with a sufficient dose of the selected agent to achieve the desired degree of block. The paralysis caused by nondepolarizing relaxants should be reversed at the end of each operation unless postoperative mechanical ventilation is planned; anticholinesterase drugs such as neostigmine or edrophonium combined with anticholinergics are given to prevent muscarinic side effects. The effectiveness of reversal is judged by muscle strength, adequacy of ventilation, and response to nerve stimulation. Minimum criteria for withdrawing assisted ventilation should include good muscle tone, flexing of the arms and legs, and adequate respiratory effort. Many anesthesiologists believe that absence of tetanic fade at 50 to 100 Hz may be the best criterion for the adequacy of reversal. Relaxants are also used frequently in the intensive care unit to facilitate controlled mechanical ventilation. Neuromuscular blocking agents have no sedative, hypnotic, or analgesic side effects, but they may indirectly decrease metabolic demand, prevent shivering, decrease nonsynchronous ventilation, decrease intracranial pressure, and improve chest wall compliance. Major organ failure, up-regulation of acetylcholine receptors, malnutrition, electrolyte and acid-base abnormalities, drug interactions, and muscle atrophy can also have a profound influence on the kinetics and dynamics of relaxants. In addition, repeated doses of relaxants over relatively long periods without monitoring of neuromuscular transmission may lead to prolonged muscle weakness despite discontinuation of therapy. Knowledge of neuromuscular pharmacology and its modification by age, concurrent medications, and concurrent disease processes permits a more rational use of neuromuscular blocking agents in intensive care patients.

Complicating Conditions

Myoneuropathies

An unexpectedly prolonged duration of paralysis after the administration of muscle relaxants to intensive care patients is common.[258,286] Individual patients with "intensive care unit neuromuscular syndrome" have had various relaxants administered for different lengths of time, a multitude of underlying critical diseases and coexisting conditions, and a spectrum of muscle weakness. Considerable overlap between this syndrome and disuse atrophy, polyneuropathy of critical illness, and steroid myopathy exists. Some cases seem to represent a pharmacologic overdose, whereas other cases represent specific pathology of the general neuromuscular structures.[175,305] The pathology includes marked atrophy of type I and type II muscle fibers, destruction of muscle, relatively little inflammation, and relatively intact motor and sensory nerves. This syndrome may be related to synergistic dysfunctional up-regulation of acetylcholine receptors caused by critical illness and the administration of muscle relaxants.[175] It has been suggested that reducing the dose of relaxants per unit time

by monitoring neuromuscular transmission may decrease the risk for prolonged paralysis. Lee[175] suggests that periodic interruption of relaxant administration, as well as pharmacodynamic, neurologic, and electrophysiologic studies, may be useful for the early detection of this complication. Prolonged neuromuscular blockade in infants and small children may interfere with normal growth and development of muscle and result in moderate to severe residual weakness that lasts for months. Immobilization-induced atrophy may not be reversible in developing muscle. Thus, recovery of muscle function may be more likely in older infants and children, in whom neuromuscular development has already progressed to a fair degree, than in newborns (especially premature newborns) immobilized shortly after birth.[264]

Malignant Hyperthermia

Malignant hyperthermia (MH) is a life-threatening condition characterized by hyperthermia, hypermetabolism, and muscle injury that occurs in response to a triggering agent. Potent inhalation agents (not nitrous oxide) and the depolarizing muscle relaxant succinylcholine are two potent triggers in children. Triggers that stimulate MH cause excessive release of Ca^{2+} from the sarcoplasmic reticulum of skeletal muscle into the myoplasm, causing a chain of metabolic events that culminates in heat production, cell injury, hyperkalemia, and myoglobinemia.[183] The elevation of intracellular calcium levels observed in human muscle affected by MH is decreased by dantrolene.[183] The mortality rate for untreated MH is greater than 60%; rapid treatment with dantrolene reduces mortality to almost zero.

The incidence of fulminant MH is approximately 1 in 60,000 general anesthesia patients when succinylcholine is used and 1 in 220,000 when it is not used.[213] Most cases of MH occur in patients believed to be healthy. Predisposition to MH is a familial disease of multigenetic inheritance. First-degree relatives are at high risk; second-degree relatives have a lower but significant risk of developing MH in response to the appropriate triggering agents. Patients with Duchenne's muscular dystrophy are believed to be at high risk for developing MH. Other diseases associated with the development of MH are central core disease and King-Denborough syndrome.

The classic signs of MH include tachycardia, ventricular dysrhythmias, tachypnea, a rapid increase in temperature above 39.5°C, rigidity of the jaw or generalized rigidity, metabolic and respiratory acidosis, and decreased mixed venous oxygen saturation. Associated laboratory values include hyperkalemia, hypercarbia, respiratory and metabolic acidosis, increased creatine phosphokinase and lactate, blood clotting abnormalities, and myoglobinuria.

The clinical diagnosis of MH should be considered before signs of hypermetabolism and elevated temperature reach extremes. The early signs of the disorder include tachypnea, tachycardia, increased end tidal carbon dioxide ($ETCO_2$) and ventricular dysrhythmias. These signs must be quickly evaluated because they can have many causes, such as iatrogenic hyperthermia, sepsis, pheochromocytoma, hyperthyroidism, ventilator valve malfunction with rebreathing of carbon dioxide,

TABLE 13–6 Management of Acute Episodes of Malignant Hyperthermia

Stop inhalation anesthetics immediately.

Cancel or conclude surgery as soon as possible.

Hyperventilate with high-flow 100% oxygen.

Administer IV dantrolene (2 mg/kg) and repeat as needed.

Give more dantrolene if signs of the condition reappear.

Initiate cooling with hypothermia blanket, IV cold saline solution (15 mL/kg for 10 min), ice packs in the axillary region and groin, and lavage of body cavities with cold saline solution if core temperature is >37° C. Stop cooling when core temperature falls to 38° C.

Correct metabolic acidosis with 1.0 to 2.0 mEq/kg sodium bicarbonate as an initial dose.

Administer calcium (10 mg/kg calcium chloride) or insulin (0.2 U/kg) in 50% dextrose in water (1 mg/kg) to treat the effects of hyperkalemia.

Administer lidocaine (1 mg/kg) to treat ventricular arrhythmias.

Maintain urine output at 2 mL/kg/hr with furosemide (1 mg/kg) and additional mannitol if needed.

Insert arterial and central venous catheters.

Repeat venous blood gas and electrolyte analysis every 15 min until signs of the disorder resolve and vital signs normalize.

inadequate levels of anesthesia, and faulty temperature and $ETCO_2$ monitors.

Management of an acute episode of MH is outlined in Table 13-6. The cornerstone of treatment is intravenous dantrolene, which must be diluted with sterile, preservative-free, distilled water. The initial intravenous dose is 2.5 mg/kg, although much higher doses may be required. The usual dose limit of 10 mg/kg may be exceeded if necessary.[238] Dosing of dantrolene should be guided by clinical and laboratory signs and done every 5 minutes until metabolic acidosis has resolved. Dantrolene decreases the release of calcium from the sarcoplasmic reticulum by decreasing the mobility of calcium ions or the protein that transports calcium across membranes and is specific for skeletal muscle.[199,227] Dantrolene attenuates muscle hypermetabolism, reducing muscle rigidity and restoring normal muscle function. As skeletal muscle function normalizes, serum potassium decreases and abnormal lactic acid production slows.[247] Patients respond to dantrolene within 20 minutes. The $ETCO_2$ begins to decrease in 6 minutes, and arterial blood gas analysis demonstrates significant resolution of metabolic and respiratory acidosis within 20 minutes.[247] By 45 minutes, metabolic and respiratory acidosis and hyperthermia should be resolved. Dantrolene treatment at higher doses is necessary if metabolic dysfunction persists.[238]

Parents of an affected child may wish to have a muscle biopsy and contracture testing, because negative findings mean that other relatives have no increased risk of MH. Ideally, siblings and first cousins on the affected side should be informed and offered biopsy testing.

In patients with a personal history or a strong family history of MH, surgery can be safely performed under regional or local anesthesia. General anesthesia with nontriggering agents can also be used. All nondepolarizing muscle relaxants and intravenous anesthetic agents are safe to use in patients who are susceptible to MH. Pretreatment with dantrolene is controversial.[102,214] Monitoring for the early signs of MH and initiating quick treatment are the most important aspects of caring for these patients.

LATEX SENSITIVITY

The rate of latex sensitization has been increasing since its first recognition in 1979. Latex anaphylaxis may lead to significant morbidity and occasional mortality. It is essential to identify children at risk for latex sensitization and to take appropriate precautions to prevent intraoperative anaphylaxis. Children with atopic backgrounds and children with spina bifida or genitourinary abnormalities who have undergone multiple surgeries are at increased risk for latex sensitivity. Spina bifida, even in the absence of multiple surgical procedures, seems to be an independent risk factor for latex sensitization.

Severe latex reactions usually occur shortly after parenteral or mucous membrane exposure and include flushing, vasodilatation, severe bronchospasm, and increased vascular permeability with edema and cardiovascular collapse. Mild reactions such as urticaria and angioedema may be masked by the presence of surgical drapes. Therapeutic options include airway maintenance with 100% oxygen, intravenous fluids, and epinephrine to sustain the blood pressure. Epinephrine is the first line of treatment because its mechanism of action sustains blood pressure and stimulates bronchodilatation. Other useful medications include antihistamines (diphenhydramine 0.5 to 1.0 mg/kg intravenously), inhaled bronchodilators, $histamine_2$ blockers, and corticosteroids (methylprednisolone 0.5 mg/kg). Corticosteroids are not the first line of treatment but are beneficial for delayed and late reactions. A latex-free environment is the best way to prevent latex reactions in the operating room.

INTRAVENOUS ANESTHETIC AGENTS

Thiopental

Thiopental is a barbiturate induction agent that can be administered by the intravenous or rectal route. The dose required for intravenous induction varies with age. Westrin et al.[317] concluded that the ED_{50} (the dose of a drug that will induce anesthesia in 50% of patients) for thiopental is 3.4 ± 0.2 mg/kg in neonates and 6.3 ± 0.7 mg/kg in infants 1 to 6 months of age. Jonmarker et al.[145] found that the ED_{50} of an induction dose of thiopental is 7 to 8 mg/kg in infants and 4 to 5 mg/kg in children older than 1 year (Fig. 13-4). These studies confirmed previous findings by Cote et al.[66] and Brett and Fisher,[41] who showed that thiopental requirements are higher in children. Barbiturates decrease cerebral blood flow and intracranial pressure. The direct myocardial depression and venodilatation caused by thiopental are well tolerated by healthy children.[317] In patients who are hemodynamically compromised, however, these cardiovascular effects

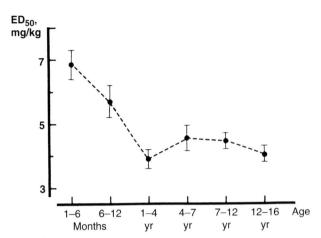

Figure 13–4 Estimated ED_{50} (the dose of a drug that will induce anesthesia in 50% of patients) plus or minus the standard error for thiopental in various age groups. (From Jonmarker C, et al: Thiopental requirements for induction of anesthesia in children. Anesthesiology 1987;67:104.)

can result in significant hypotension. Thiopental should be avoided in children who are dehydrated, have heart failure, or have lost a significant amount of blood. Side effects seen with an induction dose of thiopental include hiccups, cough, and laryngospasm. Valtonen et al.[296] reported these side effects in 20% of children 1 to 6 years of age. Extravasation can cause tissue injury, which is probably secondary to thiopental's alkalinity. Barbiturates also cause histamine release. Anaphylaxis can occur after intravenous injection of thiopental and requires aggressive management with epinephrine, antihistamines, and steroids.

Propofol

Propofol is a sedative-hypnotic, lipophilic intravenous agent used for induction and maintenance of anesthesia. The pharmacokinetics of propofol are characterized by rapid distribution, metabolism, and clearance. After termination of an infusion, redistribution to the peripheral tissues results in a prompt decrease in plasma concentration. Propofol is eliminated by hepatic conjugation to inactive metabolites, and excretion is renal.[333]

Westrin[316] found that unpremedicated infants 1 to 6 months of age require larger induction doses (3.0 ± 0.2 mg/kg) than do children 10 to 16 years of age (2.4 ± 0.1 mg/kg). Similar findings were reported by Aun et al.[16] Hannallah et al.[126] found effective induction doses in unpremedicated children 3 to 12 years of age to be 2.5 to 3.0 mg/kg.[124] Although the mechanisms that contribute to different dose requirements in younger children compared with older children have not been delineated, Westrin[316] hypothesized that because infants have a greater cardiac output in relation to body weight and a larger vessel-rich component, arterial peak concentration reaching the brain may be lower than that achieved in adults.

Administration of opioids in conjunction with propofol reduces the infusion rate necessary for adequate anesthesia.[46] McClune et al.[191] and Short and Chui[266] found that when propofol and midazolam are combined for sedation in adults, the dose of each agent is reduced by 44%. The addition of 0.13 mg/kg of midazolam reduces the necessary propofol infusion rate for general anesthesia by 52%. Propofol possesses antiemetic characteristics, even in subhypnotic doses.[37]

Propofol can induce hypotension, but the mechanism through which this occurs has not been clearly established.[17,124,257] Aun et al.[17] compared the hemodynamic responses to an induction dose of thiopental (5 mg/kg) or propofol (2.5 mg/kg) in 41 healthy children aged 8 months to 12 years. Heart rate, blood pressure, and velocity of flow were measured. The 28% to 31% reduction in mean arterial pressure after propofol was significantly greater than that after thiopental (14% and 21%, respectively). The 10% to 15% reduction in cardiac index was similar for both drugs. The children studied tolerated the hypotensive episodes without requiring pharmacologic intervention. Hannallah et al.[124] noted that, like adults, children anesthetized with propofol have a slower heart rate than those given a volatile agent. Atropine may be useful to attenuate the bradycardia that can develop in young children when propofol and an intravenous opioid are used to maintain anesthesia. Keyl et al.[154] concluded that the vagally mediated heart rate response to cyclic peripheral baroreflex stimulation was markedly depressed during propofol anesthesia, along with an impaired blood pressure response to cyclic baroreceptor stimulation.

Pain at the site of injection occurs in up to 50% of patients receiving propofol through a vein in the dorsum of the hand.[295] Pain on injection of propofol can be attenuated or eliminated by injection through a large antecubital vein or by adding 0.1 mg/kg of lidocaine to every 2 to 3 mg/kg of propofol drawn into the syringe.[112]

MONITORING

Noninvasive Monitoring

The anesthesiologist is concerned with three components of noninvasive monitoring of anesthetized patients. The first is direct observation of the patient and involves no mechanical or electronic instrumentation. The second aspect encompasses the periodic or continuous measurement and recording of vital signs, urine output, blood loss, and fluid and blood replacement, as well as an ever-increasing number of cardiovascular and respiratory parameters. This group of tasks may be subdivided into essential monitoring (i.e., those measurements necessary for the safe conduct of any anesthetic) and specialized monitoring that is required only for certain types of cases. The third aspect includes monitoring the output and performance of the machines and equipment connected to the patient (e.g., thermometers on heating devices, ventilator alarms, and spectrometric analysis of inspired and expired gases).

The ASA has established standards for basic anesthesia monitoring, which include continuous evaluation of the patient's oxygenation, ventilation, circulation, and temperature during the use of all anesthetics. Delivery of an adequate oxygen concentration is ensured by measuring the inspired concentration of oxygen in the patient's breathing system using an oxygen analyzer on the anesthesia machine; blood oxygenation is measured by pulse oximetry. Ventilation is ensured by qualitative clinical signs such as chest excursion, observation of the reservoir breathing bag, and auscultation of breath sounds. Continual monitoring for the presence of carbon dioxide is performed using a quantitative method such as capnography, capnometry, or mass spectroscopy. When ventilation is controlled by a mechanical ventilator, a continuous device that is capable of detecting the disconnection of system components is used. Circulation is monitored by a continuously displayed electrocardiogram, arterial blood pressure, and heart rate determined and evaluated at least every 5 minutes. In addition, adequate circulation is ensured by auscultation of heart sounds, palpation of a pulse, monitoring of a tracing of intra-arterial pressure, ultrasound pulse monitoring, or pulse plethysmography or oximetry. Temperature monitoring is required to aid in the maintenance of appropriate body temperature during all anesthetics.[12]

Temperature Monitoring

The rectum is the most common site for temperature measurement in infants, despite the following disadvantages: (1) potential for perforation of the bowel wall with a stiff thermistor probe wire, (2) potential dislodging of the probe, and (3) excessive warming of the thin tissues of the perianal and coccygeal area by the circulating warm water mattress. A more fundamental objection is that rectal temperatures, in general, do not promptly track rapid temperature changes, such as those that occur during deliberate hypothermia or rewarming. Midesophageal or nasopharyngeal temperature more nearly reflects core temperature, and tympanic temperature theoretically provides ideal information because it most closely reflects the temperature of the brain. The disposable tympanic probes available may be too large for an infant's external auditory canal, however, and the possibility of trauma to the tympanum exists.

During anesthesia and surgery, other temperatures should be monitored, such as the temperature of inspired gases, the warming mattress, and the room. In view of these requirements and the frequent desirability of monitoring more than one site on the patient, a multichannel thermistor thermometer is most useful.

Pulse Oximetry

Continuous, noninvasive monitoring of arterial oxygen saturation (SaO_2) can be accomplished by pulse oximetry. The oximeter is usually placed on a finger or toe, but any site is acceptable as long as a pulsating vascular bed can be interposed between the two elements. Two wavelengths of light chosen for their relative reflectance with oxygenated versus deoxygenated hemoglobin illuminate the tissue under the probe. Through expansion and relaxation, the pulsating vascular bed changes the length of the light path, thereby modifying the amount of light detected. The result is a characteristic plethysmographic waveform, and artifacts from blood, skin, connective tissue, or bone are eliminated. This technique is accurate with oxygen saturations from 70% to 100%. Reduction in vascular pulsation diminishes the instrument's ability to calculate saturations, for example, with hypothermia, hypotension, or the use of vasoconstrictive drugs. In addition to a continuous indication of SaO_2, the pulse oximeter usually provides a continuous readout of pulse rate and amplitude.

Capnography

Capnography is a convenient method to monitor ventilation. In addition, the capnograph is capable of identifying the gases and the concentrations present in a given sample. Usually the profile includes oxygen, carbon dioxide, nitrogen, nitrous oxide, and the major inhaled anesthetic agents.

The accuracy of the displayed inspired and end-tidal values depends on the reliability of the capnographic tracing. In a time capnograph, the curve in Figure 13-5A represents an ideal tracing during quiet respiration with no rebreathing. The presence of a smooth, horizontal alveolar plateau indicates that the maximum value at 4

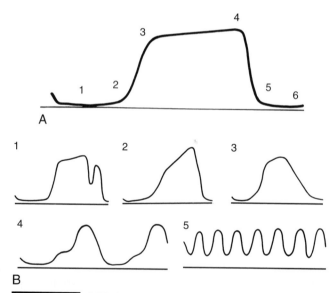

Figure 13–5 *A*, Ideal capnographic tracing: (1) Exhalation begins. (1-2) Anatomic dead space is cleared. (2-3) Dead-space air mixes with alveolar gas. (3-4) Alveolar plateau. (4) End-tidal maximum value; inspiration begins. (4-5) Dead-space air is cleared. (5-6) Inspiratory gas is devoid of carbon dioxide. *B*, Types of capnographic tracings: (1) Efforts at spontaneous breathing with incomplete neuromuscular blockade. (2) Respiratory obstruction. (3) Lack of sustained pressure resulting from a large leak in the breathing system. (4) In the Mapleson D system, when large amounts of fresh gas flow at small tidal volumes, the expired carbon dioxide is diluted, and achievement of a stable alveolar plateau is prevented. (5) The effect of partial rebreathing of carbon dioxide from the expiratory limb of the Mapleson D system, when fresh gas flows at small amounts, is excessively rapid ventilation and small tidal breaths.

represents alveolar gas, which is in equilibrium and close to the arterial carbon dioxide tension. Under such circumstances, and in the absence of maldistribution of ventilation and pulmonary blood flow, the two values should be within 2 to 4 torr of each other. With ventilation-perfusion mismatching, a greater divergence occurs (alveolar-arterial carbon dioxide gradient), especially with the large dead-space ventilation that accompanies pulmonary embolus.

An ideal capnographic tracing cannot always be obtained, but the abnormal curve may be diagnostic or highly suggestive of certain types of problems involving the patient, the anesthetic circuit, or the ventilation technique. The incisura in Figure 13-5B(1) indicates attempts at spontaneous ventilation with inadequate neuro-muscular blockade. The slow, steep expiratory tracing in Figure 13-5B(2) indicates airway obstruction, and the rounded tracing of Figure 13-5B(3) reflects a lack of sustained pressure, similar to that resulting from a large leak in the system. Rapid, shallow, controlled respiration is commonly used in infant anesthesia. As a result, incomplete expiration and partial rebreathing occur, as demonstrated in Figure 13-5B(4). The limitation of a time capnogram is that it is unknown precisely when inspiration and expiration begin, which results in prolongation of the alveolar plateau during inspiratory rebreathing of carbon dioxide. Bhavani-Shankar and Philip[33] suggested that the simultaneous display of flow waveforms allows easy delineation of the inspiratory and expiratory portions of the time capnogram, which facilitates the detection of rebreathing. Further studies are required to predict the clinical benefits of this technology.

Monitoring Neuromuscular Function

The only satisfactory method of monitoring neuromuscular function is stimulation of an accessible peripheral motor nerve and observation or measurement of the response of the skeletal muscle supplied by this nerve. Various nerve stimulators that provide ideal rectangular- or square-wave pulses no longer than 0.2 msec in duration are commercially available. Usually, the ulnar nerve is stimulated at the elbow or wrist with surface electrodes, and the response of the adductor pollicis brevis is noted. Small surface electrodes or needles should be used to minimize the likelihood of direct muscle stimulation. Supramaximal electrical stimuli are necessary to ensure full activation of the nerve. The evoked response to single repeated nerve stimuli at 0.1 Hz or train-of-four stimulation at a low frequency (2 Hz for 2 seconds) allows continuous monitoring of neuromuscular transmission after the administration of muscle relaxants. Tetanic rates of stimulation (50 Hz), train-of-four ratios, or double-burst stimulation allow the assessment of neurotransmission after reversal.

In adults, clinical signs of adequate neuromuscular transmission include the ability to sustain a head lift for 5 seconds in conjunction with a vital capacity of at least 15 to 20 mL/kg or a negative inspiratory force of 30 cm H_2O. Because an infant cannot lift its head for 5 seconds, the ability to flex its arms or legs is a reliable sign of adequate neuromuscular transmission. Because vital capacity cannot easily be determined in infants, inspiratory force is measured instead. The ability to sustain tetany of 30 to 50 Hz for 5 seconds or a near-normal train-of-four ratio (>0.7) is also a reliable sign of adequate neuromuscular transmission.

Invasive Monitoring

The availability of sophisticated noninvasive monitoring devices has reduced the need for invasive monitoring. The need for invasive monitoring is driven more by patient condition than by surgical procedure.[13] Intra-arterial and, to a lesser degree, central venous and pulmonary arterial catheters are required for the continuous measurement of pulse, intravascular pressures, and serial arterial blood gas concentrations, blood chemistry, and coagulation abnormalities intraoperatively and postoperatively for extended periods in critically ill patients.

The most desirable site for arterial sampling is the right radial artery, where the concentration of oxygen tension most closely resembles that of the carotid artery. Postductal arteries have lower oxygen tensions in the presence of right-to-left shunting and may become occluded during such procedures as repair of coarctation of the aorta. When the radial artery is not available, the femoral, dorsalis pedis, or posterior tibial artery may be used. In infants, the brachial and axillary arteries are generally avoided because of the risk of loss of the limb. Femoral artery catheterization may be complicated by joint injury, and cannulation of the superficial temporal artery is associated with a risk of temporal lobe infarction resulting from retrograde perfusion of the vessel during flushing. Despite their accessibility during the first 10 days of life, umbilical arteries are a limited option because the incidence of infection is high. In addition, because of the risk for thrombosis and embolism, the catheter tip must be carefully positioned above the diaphragm or below the third or fourth lumbar vertebra away from the origins of the celiac, mesenteric, and renal arteries. Also, when blood is sampled from below a patent ductus arteriosus in a patient with right-to-left shunting, oxygen saturations in the umbilical arteries may be less than that of the carotid or right radial artery and thus lead to the administration of dangerously high oxygen concentrations.

The indications for central venous catheterization, and especially for flow-directed pulmonary arterial (Swan-Ganz) catheters, are limited in infants and children. The procedure is probably indicated more often for patients in the intensive care unit than for those in the operating room. Central venous catheterization is indicated for patients having operations involving major blood loss, shock, and low-flow states. The preferred route of access for either catheter is the internal jugular vein, although the subclavian or femoral veins are alternatives. Placing the catheter and monitoring the pressure in a major vein returning blood to the heart allow proper maintenance or adjustment of the patient's circulating blood volume.[13] Possible complications include atrial or ventricular arrhythmias, thromboembolic phenomena, hemothorax, pneumothorax, and infection.

PAIN MANAGEMENT

Children of all ages feel pain. Although progress remains to be made, recent interest in and awareness of pediatric pain, along with philosophical shifts and technical advances, have markedly improved pain management for children.[7,140]

Appropriate care of pediatric surgical patients entails pain management tailored to each child's age, emotional and developmental maturity, and surgical procedure. Children's ability to experience pain has often been denied, and their capacity to tolerate potent analgesia has been questioned,[92,255] causing many pediatric patients to undergo surgery without adequate pain management. Historically, up to 40% of children undergoing surgical procedures have reported moderate to severe pain on the first postoperative day.[188] Although many children continue to experience such pain, the evolution of integrated, multidisciplinary approaches has dramatically improved perioperative pain management for children,[223] with preoperative, intraoperative, and postoperative strategies for minimizing pain based on the planned surgical procedure, anticipated severity of postoperative pain, anesthetic technique, and expected course of recovery.[216] Children are reassessed at frequent intervals, and regimens modified as needed.

Children frequently undergo painful interventions other than surgical procedures. Venipuncture, intravenous catheter insertion, and the like characteristically cause brief but significant pain and are often described by children and their families as the most distressing aspect of their illness or hospitalization.[92] Appropriate pain management for children provides adequate analgesia in such settings, enhancing patient cooperation and facilitating the successful completion of procedures.[259] With appropriate intervention, most children should be able to undergo diagnostic and therapeutic procedures with little or no pain and minimal anxiety and stress.

Acute pain is a physiologic response to actual or impending tissue damage and may provide helpful information regarding the location and nature of injury or illness. Accordingly, there is often reluctance to provide potent analgesia to patients with potentially surgical conditions before obtaining a definitive diagnosis. It is now increasingly recognized that this dramatically undertreats pain in such patients, particularly children.[210] Appropriately titrated analgesia not only relieves pain and reduces distress but often allows a more thorough and accurate evaluation, particularly in frightened or uncooperative pediatric patients. Intravenous morphine, for example, provides significant analgesia to children with acute abdominal pain without masking focal tenderness or impairing the clinical diagnosis of appendicitis.[155] The traditional teaching that potent analgesia must be withheld from patients, including children, with potentially surgical diagnoses is invalid and should be abandoned.

Perioperative Planning and General Approach

Perioperative pain management optimizes patient comfort while avoiding excessive sedation or respiratory depression.

Multiple techniques are available, chosen and titrated to effect based on each child's particular needs. Planning begins with the preoperative anesthetic evaluation and continues throughout the surgical procedure and postoperative period.

Numerous nonpharmacologic techniques may augment analgesia, enhance patient cooperation, and minimize pharmacologic therapy.* Nonopioid analgesics most commonly include acetaminophen and various nonsteroidal anti-inflammatory agents; ketamine is increasingly used in certain settings. Oral opioids are often adequate for the treatment of mild to moderate pain, while intravenous opioids are the mainstay of therapy for moderate to severe pain. Persistent requirements for intravenous opioids can be managed with continuous infusion or patient-controlled analgesia modalities. Numerous regional anesthetic techniques may be employed as well.

A useful paradigm for pain management is the World Health Organization's Analgesic Ladder (Fig. 13-6).[327] First proposed in 1986 as a protocol for the management of cancer pain, the Analgesic Ladder has become a popular and effective model for pain management in a variety of settings and can be applied to pediatric surgical patients. There is openness at all levels to adjuvant agents and nonpharmacologic techniques, underscoring that pain is a subjective experience that responds quite differently to various approaches in individual patients. There is a stratified approach to analgesic pharmacology, using nonopioid analgesics for mild pain, lower-potency opioids for moderate pain, and higher-potency opioids for severe pain. Perhaps most importantly, the ultimate goal is complete pain relief.

Development and Physiology

Children of all ages feel pain, but the type and intensity may vary dramatically. Although peripheral nociceptors are fully functional at birth,[99] central modulation and pain perception in children are not well understood. Further, many reflex pathways allowing the expression of nociception are structurally and functionally immature in neonates and young infants.[10] Thus, although peripheral nociceptors register painful stimuli, central processing of pain in these young patients is more variable, and their ability to indicate pain perception is more limited. The response of infants and young children to pain is therefore unpredictable, particularly in premature neonates,[101] which often prevents them from receiving adequate analgesia.

Hypersensitization and Preemptive Analgesia

Acute pain is a physiologic response to actual or impending tissue damage. Untreated, persistent, or severe pain, however, may contribute to potentially detrimental

---

*See references 1, 3, 45, 53, 58, 91, 130, 133, 153, 170, 171, 181, 192, 196, 205, 206, 224, 246, 250, 265.

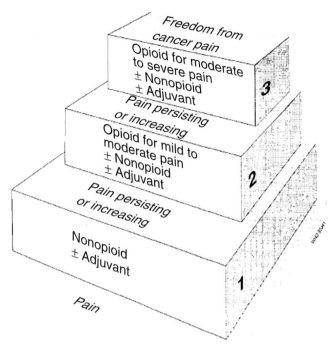

Figure 13–6 First proposed in 1986 as a protocol for managing cancer pain, the Analgesic Ladder has become a popular and effective model for pain management in a variety of settings and can be applied to pediatric surgical patients. (From World Health Organization: Cancer Pain Relief: With a Guide to Opioid Availability, 2nd ed. Geneva, WHO, 1996, p 15.)

pathophysiologic processes.[101,325] Tissue injury and inflammation enhance peripheral nociceptor activity, resulting in hypersensitivity to mechanical and chemical stimuli. In animal models, dorsal horn neurons respond to sustained afferent stimulation with neurophysiologic and morphologic changes consistent with increased excitability. The development of peripheral and central hypersensitization may alter normal sensory perception (dysesthesia), accentuate pain due to noxious stimuli (hyperalgesia), and produce pain in response to normally innocuous processes (allodynia), suggesting that hypersensitization at the cellular and neurophysiologic level correlates with clinical hypersensitivity to pain.

Preemptive analgesia before tissue injury may inhibit stimulation of nociceptive pathways, blunting the neuroendocrine stress response and preventing the development of peripheral and central hypersensitivity.[325] General anesthesia alone is ineffective for such purposes; nonsteroidal anti-inflammatory drugs (NSAIDs), opioids, and a variety of local anesthetic techniques have been studied in animal models, with variable results.[55,56,326] Animal models generally suggest that preemptive analgesia, before noxious stimuli decreases dorsal horn neuron hyperexcitability, blunts observed pain behaviors and lowers clinical analgesic requirements. Human studies, however, have yielded conflicting and frequently negative results, particularly in children.[6,15,96,135,138,166,278] Subjective pain scores, objective assessments, and analgesic requirements are not dramatically affected in most patients by varying the timing of the analgesic technique before or after surgery. Preemptive analgesia as a strategy

for blunting hypersensitization and reducing perioperative pain remains a subject of ongoing investigation and controversy.[73,157,197]

Pain Assessment

Pain assessment in pediatric patients can be challenging. Preverbal or developmentally delayed children may be unable to convey the severity or even the presence of pain to caregivers. In patients of any age, it may be difficult to distinguish pain from agitation. Nonetheless, pain in children should be recognized, assessed, and treated promptly.

Numerous tools have been developed and prospectively validated to allow ongoing quantitative assessment of pain in children of all ages and developmental skills.[23,86] Such instruments generally rely on either subjective self-reporting of pain intensity along a variety of analog scales in patients old enough to understand and cooperate, or objective assessment of various pain-associated behaviors in preverbal, young, or developmentally delayed children. Analog scales use drawings or photographs of faces in varying degrees of distress, with colors, arrows, lines, or numbers (usually 0 to 10) for patients to indicate their level of pain. Children of school age and older are generally capable of using analog scales. In preverbal, young, or developmentally delayed patients, numerous tools allow the quantitative assessment of pain intensity by generating a pain score (again, usually 0 to 10) derived from the objective assessment of various pain-associated behaviors, analogous to the Apgar score used to assess neonatal vigor. Subjective, self-reported analog pain scores and objective, behavioral assessment pain scores in children are often discordant,[30] likely reflecting difficulties in distinguishing pain, agitation, and other causes of distress. The particular pain assessment tool chosen is less important than application of the tool to the appropriate population and consistent use of the tool in each patient over time.

Nonopioid Analgesics

Often overlooked, nonopioid analgesics are important adjunctive agents in pediatric pain management. They are often adequate for mild to moderate pain and may reduce the opioid requirement in cases of moderate to severe pain.[159] Unlike opioids, nonopioid analgesics generally demonstrate a ceiling effect: exceeding recommended doses does not significantly improve analgesia but does increase the risk of side effects and toxicity.[190] Common nonopioid analgesics for children include acetaminophen, various NSAIDs, and, in appropriate settings, ketamine (Table 13-7). Other sedative-hypnotic and induction agents, including chloral hydrate, benzodiazepines, barbiturates, etomidate, and propofol, lack analgesic efficacy.

Acetaminophen

Acetaminophen remains popular for the management of mild to moderate pain in children and as an antipyretic.

TABLE 13-7 Common Nonopioid Analgesics for Children

Drug	Dose	Comments
Acetaminophen	20 mg/kg PO load (max 1000 mg), then 15 mg/kg PO (max 1000 mg) q4h 40 mg/kg PR load (max 1300 mg), then 20 mg/kg PR (max 1300 mg) q4h Max 4 g/24 hr PO or PR	Good antipyretic Hepatic toxicity with overdose
Selected Nonsteroidal Anti-inflammatory Drugs (NSAIDs)		
Choline magnesium trisalicylate	10 mg/kg PO or PR (max 1000 mg) q6h Max 4 g/24 hr	Good antipyretic Only NSAID without platelet dysfunction No association with Reye's syndrome
Ibuprofen	10 mg/kg PO or PR (max 800 mg) q6h Max 4 g/24 hr	Good antipyretic
Ketorolac	0.5 mg/kg IM or IV (max 30 mg) q6h Total duration must be <5 days	Poor antipyretic Potentially significant platelet dysfunction
Ketamine (requires appropriate personnel and monitoring)	4.0-10.0 mg/kg PO (adult dose, 300-500 mg) 3.0-5.0 mg/kg IM (adult dose, 150-300 mg) 0.5-1.0 mg/kg IV (adult dose, 50-100 mg)	Anticholinergic agent; reduces sialorrhea Benzodiazepine; may prevent agitation Increases intracranial pressure; may precipitate seizures

Acetaminophen is a potent inhibitor of cyclooxygenase but has virtually no anti-inflammatory activity and therefore few gastrointestinal, renal, or hematologic complications. The primary toxicity of acetaminophen is hepatic injury, seen with acute and chronic overdose. Acetaminophen may provide complete analgesia for mild to moderate pain and reduces opioid requirements in the treatment of moderate to severe pain, particularly when given on a scheduled basis. Procedural and perioperative analgesia with acetaminophen is enhanced by NSAIDs.[236]

Acetaminophen is available in a variety of oral and rectal preparations in the United States; intravenous preparations are available in other countries. The usual oral dose of acetaminophen is 15 mg/kg (maximum 1000 mg) every 4 hours, although an oral loading dose of 20 mg/kg (maximum 1000 mg) may be given, particularly for procedural or perioperative analgesia. The total dose should not exceed 4 g/day.

Rectal absorption of acetaminophen is slower, and bioavailability is more variable, than with oral administration, requiring higher doses for equivalent analgesia.[245] Although rectal acetaminophen has been shown to reduce pain scores and lower opioid requirements following surgical procedures, including myringotomy tube placement and inguinal hernia repair,[162] at least 40 mg/kg must be given.[236] Maintenance doses of rectal acetaminophen—20 mg/kg (maximum 1300 mg) every 4 hours—may be used in patients unwilling or unable to tolerate oral administration. The total dose should not exceed 4 g/day.

Nonsteroidal Anti-inflammatory Drugs

Like acetaminophen, NSAIDs may provide adequate analgesia for mild to moderate pain and are useful in conjunction with opioids in the management of moderate to severe pain.[160,304] NSAIDs are particularly effective for musculoskeletal pain. Unlike acetaminophen, NSAIDs have significant anti-inflammatory activity, which accounts for possible gastrointestinal, renal, and hematologic side effects. NSAIDs reduce mesenteric and renal perfusion and impair platelet function, potentially causing gastrointestinal ischemia, renal insufficiency, and bleeding. Risk is higher with elevated doses or prolonged administration.

Choline magnesium trisalicylate is the only NSAID that does not cause platelet dysfunction, so it may be useful in patients with coagulopathy or at risk for surgical bleeding. Pediatric aspirin use has declined dramatically since the described association with Reye's syndrome in children with primary varicella.[190] Although choline magnesium trisalicylate is an aspirin derivative, it has no known association with Reye's syndrome; nonetheless, it may be prudent to limit its use in children to patients who have previously had primary varicella or received varicella immunization. Choline magnesium trisalicylate is available in liquid and tablet preparations, and the usual dose is 10 mg/kg (maximum 1000 mg) every 6 hours. The liquid preparation can be given rectally at the same dose to patients unwilling or unable to tolerate oral administration. The total dose should not exceed 4 g/day.

The most widely used oral NSAID in children in the United States is ibuprofen, available in a variety of liquid, tablet, and capsule preparations. Ibuprofen is a moderate-potency analgesic and an excellent antipyretic with an impressive pediatric safety record, but it is still underused for procedural and perioperative pain management in children.[160] The usual oral dose of ibuprofen is 10 mg/kg (maximum 800 mg) every 6 hours. The liquid preparation can be given rectally at the same dose. The total dose should not exceed 4 g/day.

Ketorolac is the only NSAID available for intravenous use as an analgesic. Indomethacin may be given intravenously, but such use is approved only for medical closure of patent ductus arteriosus in infants. Ketorolac is a high-potency NSAID with an analgesic efficacy similar to that of many opioids, and it provides superior perioperative analgesia compared with other NSAIDs or acetaminophen.[204] Ketorolac may be particularly useful in patients who are intolerant of opioids or in procedures that involve a high risk of postoperative nausea and emesis. Initially approved only for intramuscular administration, ketorolac is safe and effective when given intravenously.[232] Oral ketorolac administration is approved for adults but not for children.

The usual dose of ketorolac is 0.5 mg/kg (maximum 30 mg) intramuscularly or intravenously every 6 hours. The volume of distribution and plasma clearance rate of ketorolac in children are roughly twice those in adults, but the overall elimination half-life is similar.[211] As the most potent NSAID, ketorolac also has the highest incidence of side effects; total duration of therapy must not exceed 5 days to avoid potentially serious gastrointestinal and renal complications. Given its ability to compromise mesenteric perfusion, ketorolac should be avoided in infants at risk for necrotizing enterocolitis.

Significant platelet dysfunction may develop after a single dose of ketorolac, and its use in patients at high risk for bleeding is controversial. Initial experience indicated greater intraoperative blood loss during tonsillectomy in children receiving perioperative ketorolac,[245] and retrospective studies reported higher rates of postoperative hemorrhage.[108,146] Other retrospective studies suggested otherwise,[2] and prospective, randomized trials have shown only statistically insignificant trends toward increased bleeding.[21] The product literature warns against using ketorolac in patients at high risk of bleeding; it is probably prudent to avoid administering ketorolac to such patients until more definitive information is available.

Ketamine

Ketamine is a sedative-hypnotic agent similar to phencyclidine. Unlike other sedative-hypnotic agents, ketamine is a potent dissociative analgesic. Although its mechanisms of action are incompletely understood, ketamine is an NMDA receptor antagonist with weak agonist activity at opioid and numerous other receptors. Ketamine produces dose-dependent analgesia and sedation, with induction of general anesthesia at higher doses; amnesia is variable. As with other phencyclidine derivatives, hallucinations and delirium are not uncommon but may be less frequent and less severe in younger patients.[119] Ketamine induces bronchodilatation but also causes sialorrhea, which may be significant. It promotes the release of endogenous catecholamines, with resultant relative preservation of hemodynamic parameters. Ketamine increases intracranial pressure and is a proconvulsant, so it should be used cautiously in patients with intracranial pathology or seizures.

Ketamine is most commonly employed as an intravenous induction agent in small or potentially hemodynamically unstable infants and children, and it may be useful for intramuscular induction in uncooperative patients or those without intravenous access. Ketamine is also used as an adjuvant analgesic in perioperative and intensive care units. More recently, ketamine has been recommended for procedural analgesia and sedation in children in a variety of settings[119,287] and has become particularly popular in pediatric emergency departments, given its favorable safety profile.[219,221] Doses are commonly 0.5 to 1.0 mg/kg intravenously (adult dose, 50 to 100 mg), 3.0 to 5.0 mg/kg intramuscularly (adult dose, 150 to 300 mg), or 4.0 to 10.0 mg/kg orally (adult dose, 300 to 500 mg); rates of adequate analgesia and sedation are high, and rates of serious complications are low. Emergence may be prolonged after oral administration, particularly with higher doses, and agitation during emergence is not uncommon. Concomitant administration of anticholinergic agents such as atropine or glycopyrrolate to prevent sialorrhea is recommended. Concomitant administration of benzodiazepines may decrease the likelihood of hallucinations and delirium. Adequate monitoring and immediate availability of appropriate resuscitation equipment and personnel are mandatory for children receiving ketamine.[85]

Opioid Analgesics

Reluctance to use opioids in children is a common excuse for inadequate pediatric pain management. Opioids are the mainstay of pharmacologic therapy for moderate to severe pain, however, and have established roles in procedural and perioperative pain management for children.[329] Acting on various subtypes of opioid receptors throughout the CNS, opioids cause dose-dependent pain relief and respiratory depression; other side effects include somnolence, miosis, decreased gastrointestinal motility, nausea, and urinary retention. Many opioids induce histamine release, causing urticaria, pruritus, nausea, bronchospasm, and occasionally hypotension. Pruritus is more common, and typically more intense, with neuraxial administration, likely owing to the CNS opioid effect rather than histamine release. Opioid side effects can be managed with a variety of agents (Table 13-8).

The opioid receptor antagonist naloxone rapidly reverses opioid effects. Mild respiratory depression or somnolence can be treated with intravenous naloxone 1.0 µg/kg titrated every 1 to 2 minutes as needed; doses of 10 to 100 µg/kg should be reserved for apnea or coma secondary to opioid overdose. Higher or repeated doses may be necessary. Naloxone may precipitate withdrawal in opioid-dependent patients, and pulmonary edema has been reported with higher doses.

Opioid analgesics do not generally have maximum effective doses. Recommended doses are for initial administration in opioid-naive patients; titration to clinical effect is required, and higher doses may be necessary. Increased dosage requirements (tolerance, tachyphylaxis) are often observed with prolonged administration or persistent pain. Opioid therapy longer than 7 to 10 days may result in physical dependence, requiring weaning before discontinuation to avoid withdrawal.[262] Tolerance and dependence may occur independently. Addiction, a psychopathologic condition of volitional drug-seeking behavior, rarely develops in children receiving appropriately dosed opioids for analgesia and is not a valid reason to withhold therapy.[329]

TABLE 13–8 Agents for Management of Opioid Side Effects

Side Effect	Agent	Dose	Comments
Apnea, coma	Naloxone	10-100 µg/kg IV or IM q1-2min PRN Usual initial max: 400 µg Higher or repeated doses may be required	Resedation may occur Withdrawal in opioid-dependent patients Higher doses may cause pulmonary edema
Mild respiratory depression, mild sedation	Naloxone	1.0 µg/kg IV or IM q1-2min PRN Usual initial max: 400 µg Higher or repeated doses may be required	Resedation may occur
Constipation	Docusate	5.0 mg/kg PO (max 100 mg) bid	Stool softener
Nausea	Metoclopramide	0.1 mg/kg IV (max 10 mg) q6h PRN	Extrapyramidal side effects
	Ondansetron	0.1 mg/kg IV (max 4.0 mg) q6h PRN	Expensive
	Promethazine	0.25-0.5 mg/kg PO, PR, or IV (max 25 mg) q6h PRN	May cause somnolence
Pruritus	Diphenhydramine	0.5-1.0 mg/kg PO or IV (max 50 mg) q6h PRN	May cause somnolence
	Hydroxyzine	0.5-1.0 mg/kg PO or IV (max 50 mg) q6h PRN	May cause somnolence
	Nalbuphine	0.05 µg/kg IV (max 5.0 mg) q4h PRN	For pruritus from neuraxial opioid
	Naloxone	1.0 µg/kg/hr IV infusion	For pruritus from neuraxial opioid

Opioids are commonly administered in conjunction with sedative-hypnotic agents, particularly benzodiazepines, increasing the risk of respiratory depression and desaturation.[20,267,331] Careful titration of doses, appropriate monitoring, and full capability to manage complications, including respiratory depression and apnea, are essential. Appropriate reversal agents should be available.

Opioid use in neonates and young infants has been the subject of much investigation and controversy. Historical studies in rats and humans suggested increased permeability of the neonatal blood-brain barrier to opioids, particularly morphine, and greater clinical respiratory depression.[167,306] It has more recently and more accurately been realized that the pharmacologic properties and clinical effects of morphine,[31,32,52,131,185] fentanyl,[134] and indeed all opioids in human neonates are subject to great individual variability. In general, opioid clearance is decreased and elimination is more prolonged in neonates than in older children, with values approaching adult levels by several months of life. There is no intrinsic reason to withhold opioid therapy from children of any age, provided that doses are individualized to each particular patient and titrated to clinical effect.

Oral Opioids

When pain needs allow and gastrointestinal function permits, oral opioids offer freedom from parenteral therapy. Onset of action is relatively slow, rendering oral opioid therapy unsuitable for the acute management of severe pain. Several lower-potency oral opioids are used commonly in children (Table 13-9), providing adequate analgesia for mild to moderate pain.

Codeine, available in liquid and tablet preparations, commonly in combination with acetaminophen, is usually given at a dose of 1.0 mg/kg (adult dose, 30 to 60 mg) every 4 hours. Codeine has a high rate of gastrointestinal upset. Hydrocodone, available in liquid and tablet preparations, commonly in combination with acetaminophen or an NSAID, is usually given at a dose of 0.2 mg/kg (adult dose, 10 to 15 mg) every 4 hours. Hydrocodone tends to cause less gastrointestinal upset than codeine. Oxycodone is available in tablet

TABLE 13–9 Lower-Potency Oral Opioids for Children

Drug	Dose	Comments
Codeine	1.0 mg/kg PO q4h (adult dose, 30-60 mg)	Tablet and liquid preparations Usually in combination products with acetaminophen High rate of GI side effects
Hydrocodone	0.2 mg/kg PO q4h (adult dose, 10-15 mg)	Tablet and liquid preparations Usually in combination products with acetaminophen or NSAID Moderate rate of GI side effects
Oxycodone	0.1 mg/kg PO q4h (adult dose, 5-10 mg)	Tablet preparations as oxycodone or in combination products with acetaminophen or NSAID Liquid preparation as oxycodone Low rate of GI side effects Sustained-release product available for chronic therapy

GI, gastrointestinal; NSAID, nonsteroidal anti-inflammatory drug.

preparations containing only oxycodone or in combination with acetaminophen or an NSAID; liquid preparations contain only oxycodone. The usual dose of oxycodone is 0.1 mg/kg (adult dose, 5 to 10 mg) every 4 hours. Oxycodone causes little gastrointestinal upset and is generally well tolerated. Sustained-release oxycodone is available for chronic therapy.

Although often given intravenously, higher-potency opioids may also be given orally (Table 13-10). Morphine can be given orally at an initial dose of 0.3 mg/kg (adult dose, 15 to 30 mg) every 3 hours. The histamine release induced by morphine may cause urticaria, pruritus, bronchospasm, and even hypotension at higher doses, although these are less common with oral administration. Sustained-release oral morphine is available for chronic therapy. Hydromorphone can be given orally at an initial dose of 20 to 40 µg/kg (adult dose, 2 to 4 mg) every 3 hours and causes less histamine release than morphine. Meperidine can be given orally at an initial dose of 1.0 mg/kg (adult dose, 50 to 100 mg) every 3 hours but should not be used for prolonged therapy, given the risk of seizures with accumulation of the neurotoxic metabolite normeperidine.[114,201] Normeperidine is excreted renally, so the risk of seizures is increased in patients with renal disease. Methadone can be given orally at a dose of 0.1 mg/kg (adult dose, 5.0 to 10.0 mg) every 6 to 12 hours and is particularly useful for chronic therapy in opioid-dependent patients.[285] Treatment of psychopathologic opioid addiction with methadone may be undertaken only in federally licensed facilities.

Oral transmucosal fentanyl citrate (OTFC) is a formulation of fentanyl in a lozenge attached to a stick. OTFC may provide effective preanesthetic sedation in children,[103,277] as well as analgesia and sedation for painful procedures,[254] although nausea and emesis are common. The usual dose is 5 to 15 µg/kg (adult dose, 400 µg); children may require higher doses than adults. OTFC administration requires appropriate monitoring.[328]

Intravenous Opioids

Intravenous opioids are the mainstay of therapy for moderate to severe pain (see Table 13-10). Subcutaneous or intramuscular administration, although pharmacologically reliable, causes additional pain and distress, particularly in children, and should be avoided.[25,26,248] Side effects are more common and potentially more serious with intravenous opioids, mandating appropriate monitoring and prompt management of complications. Neonates and young infants receiving intravenous opioids should be monitored particularly closely, and doses should be reduced by 25% to 50%. Equipotent doses of opioids entail a similar risk of side effects.[329]

Morphine is the traditional intravenous opioid analgesic, given at an initial dose of 0.1 mg/kg (adult dose, 5 to 10 mg) every 3 hours. Hydromorphone is given at an initial dose of 10 to 20 µg/kg (adult dose, 1 to 2 mg) every 3 hours and causes less histamine release than morphine. Meperidine is given at an initial dose of 1.0 mg/kg (adult dose, 50 to 100 mg) every 3 hours but should not be used for prolonged therapy, given the risk of seizures noted earlier with oral administration.[114,201] Although historically popular, meperidine offers no significant advantages over other opioids and causes no less hepatobiliary spasm at equipotent doses.[262,329] Meperidine is not currently recommended as a first-line analgesic, although it is useful at lower doses for the treatment of shivering. Methadone can be given at an initial dose of 0.05 mg/kg (adult dose, 2.5 to 5 mg) every 6 to 12 hours. Pediatric surgical patients receiving intraoperative methadone require less subsequent analgesia than those receiving intraoperative morphine.[26] The risk

TABLE 13-10 Higher-Potency Opioids for Children

Drug	Dose*	Comments
Fentanyl	5-15 µg/kg PO (adult dose, 400 µg)	Oral preparation for single-dose use
	0.5-1.0 µg/kg IV (adult dose, 50-100 µg) q1h	Rapid infusion may cause chest wall rigidity in infants
	Infusion: 0.5-1.0 µg/kg/hr (adult dose, 50-100 µg/hr)	Transdermal patch not for acute management
	Patch: 25 µg = 1 mg/hr IV morphine	
Hydromorphone	20-40 µg/kg PO (adult dose, 2.0-4.0 mg) q3h	Less histamine release than morphine
	10-20 µg/kg IM, IV, or SC (adult dose 1.0-2.0 mg) q3h	
	Infusion: 4 µg/kg/hr (adult dose, 0.2-0.3 mg/hr)	
Meperidine	1.0 mg/kg PO, IM, IV, or SC (adult dose, 50-100 mg) q3h	Neurotoxic metabolite may cause seizures; higher risk with renal disease
	Infusion: not recommended	No hepatobiliary advantages
Methadone	0.1 mg/kg PO (adult dose, 5-10 mg) q6-12h	Useful for long-term therapy, including palliative care
	0.05 mg/kg IV (adult dose, 2.5-5.0 mg) q6-12h	Treatment of opioid addiction must be in a federally licensed facility
	Infusion: not generally used	
Morphine	0.3 mg/kg PO (adult dose, 15-30 mg) q3h	Histamine release may cause urticaria, pruritus, bronchospasm, hypotension
	0.1 mg/kg IM, IV, or SC (adult dose, 5-10 mg) q3h	
	Infusion: 0.02 mg/kg/hr (adult dose, 1.0-1.5 mg/hr)	High dose and rapid administration increase histamine release
		Sustained-release oral preparation available for chronic therapy

*Recommended doses are for initial administration in opioid-naive patients; titration to clinical effect is required, and higher doses may be necessary. Doses should be reduced 25% to 50% in neonates and young infants.

of respiratory depression and other opioid side effects is also prolonged with methadone.

Fentanyl is commonly used for procedural and perioperative pain management in children because of its rapid onset and short duration of action. The usual initial dose is 0.5 to 1.0 µg/kg intravenously (adult dose, 50 to 100 µg) every hour, with more frequent titration during and immediately after procedures. Fentanyl is highly lipophilic; high-dose, repeated, or sustained administration results in significant tissue accumulation and a markedly prolonged duration of effect.[207] Fentanyl is also available as a transdermal patch that provides continuous transcutaneous absorption, mimicking intravenous infusion; one 25-µg fentanyl patch is roughly equivalent to 1.0 mg/hour intravenous morphine. Onset is slow, and absorption is somewhat variable. Although useful in some settings for the management of chronic pain, transdermal fentanyl is not indicated for acute pain management.[110,329]

Continuous infusion is an effective means of providing analgesia to infants and children requiring more than occasional doses of intravenous opioids. Respiratory depression is uncommon in healthy patients at suggested doses, which neither prevent spontaneous ventilation nor hamper weaning from mechanical ventilatory support.[184] Intravenous infusion doses are as follows: morphine 10 to 20 µg/kg per hour (adult dose, 1.0 to 1.5 mg/hour), hydromorphone 2.0 to 4.0 µg/kg per hour (adult dose, 0.2 to 0.3 mg/hour), and fentanyl 0.5 to 1.0 µg/kg hour (adult dose, 50 to 100 µg/hour). Meperidine infusion is not recommended because of potential neurotoxicity. Methadone infusion is neither necessary nor helpful in most children because of the drug's long half-life. Adequacy of analgesia, level of sedation, and degree of respiratory depression should be followed closely, and the infusion titrated as required. All patients receiving continuous opioid infusions should probably be placed on continuous pulse oximetry, with cardiorespiratory monitoring for neonates and young infants. Doses in opioid-naive neonates and young infants should generally be reduced by 25% to 50%.[95,161]

Patient-Controlled Analgesia

Historically, it has been all too common to provide opioids only after patients feel pain. This can lead to a vicious circle of symptomatic pain followed by frequently delayed administration of medication, with the resultant risk of persistent pain or excessive sedation (Fig. 13-7).[118] This pattern exposes patients to potentially significant opioid side effects while providing only intermittent analgesia. Optimally, opioid levels should be maintained above the threshold for analgesia but below that for obtundation or apnea, preserving a balance between desired efficacy and undesired toxicity (Fig. 13-8).[25] Intermittent bolus dosing of opioids at appropriate intervals before patients develop pain may maintain opioid levels within this analgesic window, but this is time-consuming for staff and entails the risk of drug accumulation. Continuous opioid infusion eventually establishes a pharmacologic steady state but lacks easy short-term adjustment.

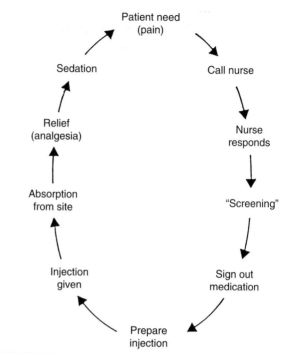

Figure 13-7 Vicious circle of conventional opioid therapy. (From Graves DA, Foster TS, Batenhorst RL, et al: Patient-controlled analgesia. Ann Intern Med 1983;99:360-366.)

A safe, effective, and readily titratable modality for intravenous opioid administration in children is patient-controlled analgesia (PCA).[118,235,318]

With PCA, opioid delivery is controlled by a microprocessor that allows the relatively frequent administration of small doses of drug in response to the patient's request—usually the pressing of a button; an appropriate

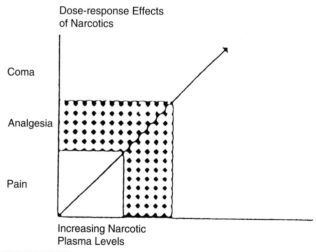

Figure 13-8 Analgesic window of opioid therapy. Idealized dose-response curve shows the continuum from pain to analgesia to coma associated with increasing plasma opioid levels. The shaded area depicts the analgesic window between inadequate pain relief and excessive sedation. (From Berde CB: Pediatric postoperative pain management. Pediatr Clin North Am 1989;36:921-940.)

TABLE 13-11 Patient-Controlled Analgesia Regimens for Children		
Drug	Demand Dose*	Basal Infusion (if used)
Fentanyl	0.5-1.0 µg/kg IV (adult dose, 50-100 µg)	0.5-1.0 µg/kg/hr IV (adult dose, 50-100 µg/hr)
Hydromorphone	4 µg/kg IV (adult dose, 0.2-0.3 mg)	4 µg/kg/hr IV (adult dose, 0.2-0.3 mg/hr)
Meperidine	Not recommended	
Methadone	Not generally used	
Morphine	0.02 mg/kg IV (adult dose, 1.0-1.5 mg)	0.02 mg/kg/hr IV (adult dose, 1.0-1.5 mg/hr)

*Generally every 8-10 min for patient-controlled analgesia; every 15-60 min for nurse- or parent-controlled analgesia. Recommended opioid doses are for initial administration in opioid-naive patients; titration to clinical effect is required, and higher doses may be necessary. Doses should be reduced 25% to 50% in neonates and young infants.

lockout interval is programmed to prevent excessive administration. Analgesia is excellent, and with appropriate doses, serious complications are rare.[26] With proper instruction, most school-age children can safely and effectively use PCA for opioid delivery.[26,111] Nurse- or parent-controlled analgesia can be used for children unable or unwilling to control their own pumps,[5,182,313] although the risk of respiratory depression increases if dosing intervals are not adequately adjusted, particularly in combination with basal infusions.[198]

Morphine is the most common choice for PCA, but hydromorphone or fentanyl can be used (Table 13-11). Meperidine PCA is not recommended because of the increased risk of toxicity with sustained administration. Methadone PCA has been described in pediatric cancer patients with significant opioid requirements and tolerance to other agents,[249] but it is neither necessary nor helpful in most children because of the drug's long half-life. Routine PCA regimens provide morphine 0.02 mg/kg (adult dose, 1.0 to 1.5 mg), hydromorphone 4 µg/kg (adult dose, 0.2 to 0.3 mg), or fentanyl 1.0 µg/kg (adult dose, 50 to 100 µg) every 8 to 10 minutes for patient-controlled administration or every 15 to 60 minutes for nurse- or parent-controlled administration. Longer dosing intervals may be safer in younger or more medically fragile patients. Concomitant basal infusion to ensure ongoing analgesia and sustain drug levels during sleep has been advocated[128] but has not been shown to improve analgesia significantly.[195,315] PCA basal infusions in adults have been shown to increase the risk of respiratory complications,[94,217] but this has not been observed in children. PCA basal infusions in pediatric patients, although safe, appear to offer little analgesic benefit.

Patients receiving PCA should be assessed frequently, and doses and intervals should be adjusted appropriately. Continuous pulse oximetry is recommended for children on any opioid infusion. Cardiorespiratory monitoring may be appropriate in very young or medically fragile patients. Instruction of patients, families, and caregivers regarding appropriate PCA use is essential.

REGIONAL ANESTHESIA

Lidocaine provides dense analgesia but has a relatively short duration of action and often induces motor block. In topical preparations, lidocaine is commonly combined with prilocaine, which may cause methemoglobinemia, particularly in large doses or in small patients. Bupivacaine is widely used in children because of its longer duration of action and relative selectivity for sensory over motor block. It is highly cardiotoxic, however, and thresholds for cardiac and neurologic toxicity are similar; dysrhythmias may occur before obtundation or seizures are noted. Two newer agents, levobupivacaine[121] and ropivacaine,[290] are potentially less toxic alternatives. Levobupivacaine, the L-isomer of bupivacaine, induces conduction block similar to bupivacaine, but with a somewhat higher threshold for cardiac toxicity. Ropivacaine has moderately greater selectivity for sensory over motor block than bupivacaine, with a relatively higher threshold for cardiac toxicity. Use of these newer agents is limited primarily by cost. Adherence to maximum recommended doses (Table 13-12) reduces the risk of toxicity.

Regional anesthesia with local anesthetic can be provided by topical application or direct infiltration at desired sites or by myriad peripheral nerve, plexus, or neuraxial blocks. An advantage of regional anesthesia is that pain relief is often provided without reliance on opioids or other systemic agents, although these may be needed in some children despite apparently successful block.[261] Greater apprehension and variability in developmental and emotional maturity in pediatric patients may explain this unpredictable requirement for supplemental analgesia. Regional anesthesia in children entails a lower risk of adverse effects, including nausea, sedation, and respiratory depression, than does systemic

TABLE 13-12 Maximum Recommended Doses of Local Anesthetics	
Local Anesthetic	Maximum Recommended Dose (mg/kg)*
Bupivacaine	3.0
Levobupivacaine	3.0
Lidocaine	5.0
Prilocaine	7.0
Ropivacaine	4.0

*Addition of a vasoconstrictor such as epinephrine or phenylephrine to local anesthetic solutions may prolong absorption and modestly increase the maximum recommended dose, but this is not reliable.

opioid therapy.[25,78,261,289,291] Regional anesthesia may be particularly advantageous in patients with potentially increased sensitivity to opioids, including neonates and children with chronic respiratory disease. In some settings, regional anesthesia in children has been shown to improve surgical outcomes.[195]

Topical anesthesia can be applied to children without sedation or anesthesia. Infiltration anesthesia can be accomplished in cooperative or older children, or it can be performed during surgical procedures. In contrast to adult practice, peripheral nerve, plexus, and neuraxial blocks in children are most commonly performed after induction of general anesthesia.[75,239] Theoretically, this prevents the detection of complications, including paresthesias, failed block, or injection into undesired sites or structures; fortunately, serious complications of regional techniques in anesthetized children are rare.[25,220,324] Performance of regional anesthesia after induction but before surgical incision offers the advantages of lighter intraoperative anesthesia and more rapid emergence and recovery.[330]

Topical Anesthesia

Numerous formulations of local anesthetics provide cutaneous analgesia without the need for injection (Table 13-13), potentially reducing or eliminating the need for systemic analgesia and sedation.

Eutectic mixture of local anesthetics (EMLA) cream is a combination of 2.5% lidocaine and 2.5% prilocaine. Applied in a thick layer and covered with an occlusive dressing for at least 60 minutes, EMLA provides effective cutaneous analgesia for minor procedures, including circumcision and even chest tube removal.[23,51,122,237,280] Analgesia increases with application up to 4 hours.[62] EMLA cream is easy to apply; patients and families can do so at home. Side effects include erythema, blanching, and rash. The prilocaine component has caused concern about the risk of methemoglobinemia, particularly with generous application or in infants, but this is rare when the product is used appropriately.

Several other preparations of topical anesthetics are available. ELA-Max is an over-the-counter preparation of 4% or 5% liposomal lidocaine.[90] Numby Stuff is a unique system of topical anesthesia employing mild electrical current to promote rapid iontophoretic intradermal transport of a solution of 2% lidocaine and 1:100,000 epinephrine.[14,273] TAC (tetracaine, adrenaline, cocaine) is available in a variety of preparations and provides effective cutaneous analgesia for the repair of superficial lacerations in children.[36,93,132,268]

Infiltration Anesthesia

Infiltration with local anesthetic provides effective analgesia for minor procedures and can be performed in cooperative or older patients without sedation or anesthesia. Any appropriate solution may be used. The acid pH of many local anesthetic solutions enhances solubility and prolongs shelf life but is responsible for much of the pain associated with injection. Buffering pH helps reduce pain in awake patients and may increase efficacy. Addition of 1.0 mEq sodium bicarbonate to 10 mL local anesthetic significantly reduces pain during injection without precipitation of the solution.[54] The bicarbonate is added immediately before use.

Infiltration anesthesia provides adequate analgesia after minor but not major surgical procedures.[74] The technique is straightforward, and the risk of local anesthetic toxicity is low if maximum recommended doses are not exceeded. Wound infiltration during inguinal hernia repair in children provides analgesia similar to that afforded by ilioinguinal-iliohypogastric nerve block[50,231] or caudal block[256] for 2 to 4 hours following the procedure. Longer-term analgesia is inferior, however.[260]

Peripheral Nerve and Plexus Blocks

Successful block of virtually any peripheral nerve or plexus is possible with appropriate equipment and sufficient practitioner interest,[76,260] potentially optimizing analgesia, minimizing opioid requirements, and improving pulmonary function.[189] Peripheral nerve blocks are readily performed in children; several are particularly applicable to pediatric surgical patients. Plexus blocks are performed less frequently in children than in adults, often secondary to practitioner inexperience but also because of logistic challenges in the application of adult techniques to pediatric practice. Intravenous regional anesthesia of the extremity, or Bier block, has been described in children,[80] but its application may be limited by the risk of local anesthetic toxicity. Performance of peripheral nerve and plexus blocks before surgical incision offers the theoretical advantages of preemptive analgesia and lessened overall pain experience, but this has not been reliably demonstrated in clinical practice, particularly in children.[6,15,278] Timing of blocks appears to be less important than their performance.

TABLE 13-13 Topical Anesthetic Formulations

Product	Ingredients	Comments
ELA-Max	Liposomal lidocaine 4% or 5%	Apply for 30 min No dressing required Nonprescription
EMLA	Lidocaine 2.5% + prilocaine 2.5%	Apply for 1-4 hr Requires occlusive dressing Prilocaine may cause methemoglobinemia
Numby Stuff	Iontocaine (lidocaine 2% + epinephrine 1:100,000)	Apply for 10 min Requires specialized electrodes, generator Tingling sensation may frighten some children
TAC	Cocaine 4%-11.8% + tetracaine 0.5%-1% + epinephrine 1:2000-4000	Apply for 20 min Avoid mucous membranes Avoid terminally perfused areas Potential cocaine toxicity

Rectus Block

Recent interest in umbilical surgery in children, particularly the application of laparoscopic techniques, has prompted research on the use of regional anesthesia for such procedures. Terminal cutaneous branches of the lower thoracic intercostal nerves supply the skin of the anterior abdominal midline. Although infiltration anesthesia is readily accomplished in this area, specific nerve block offers the advantage of prolonged analgesia. Rectus sheath block for repair of umbilical and paraumbilical hernias in children has been described[97] and, with minor modifications, has been described as paraumbilical block.[68]

Injection is made halfway between the umbilicus and the lateral linea alba (Fig. 13-9).[68] A blunt bevel needle is introduced through the skin with slight medial angulation until a pronounced give or "pop" is felt as the needle pierces the external rectus sheath. After negative aspiration and a negative test dose to reduce the likelihood of intravascular injection, 0.25 to 0.5 mL/kg of local anesthetic is deposited; little or no resistance should be felt. The needle may be withdrawn and a subcutaneous weal made toward the umbilicus for improved coverage of distal cutaneous braches. Injection is then repeated on the contralateral side. Rectus block can be used at other dermatomal levels for the repair of midline ventral hernias above or below the umbilicus.[76]

Ilioinguinal-Iliohypogastric Block

The ilioinguinal and iliohypogastric nerves are terminal cutaneous branches of the lumbar plexus. The ilioinguinal nerve arises from first lumbar spinal nerve roots and supplies much of the external genitalia and part of the proximal thigh; the iliohypogastric nerve arises from 12th thoracic and 1st lumbar spinal nerve roots to innervate the skin of the anterior abdominal wall above the inguinal ligament. The two nerves are usually blocked in conjunction, providing analgesia for procedures on the ipsilateral groin, including inguinal hernia repair and orchiopexy.[127]

Injection is made 1 to 2 cm medial and 1 to 2 cm superior to the anterior superior iliac spine (Fig. 13-10).[330] A blunt bevel needle is introduced perpendicular to the skin until a distinct give or "pop" is felt as the needle pierces Scarpa's fascia, adherent to the aponeurosis of the external oblique muscle. After negative aspiration and a negative test dose to reduce the likelihood of intravascular injection, 0.5 to 1.0 mL/kg of local anesthetic is deposited; little or no resistance should be felt. The needle may be withdrawn and a subcutaneous weal made toward the umbilicus for improved coverage of distal cutaneous branches of the iliohypogastric nerve. Ilioinguinal-iliohypogastric block provides only cutaneous analgesia; supplemental anesthesia is required for visceral manipulation. Because of this lack of visceral coverage,

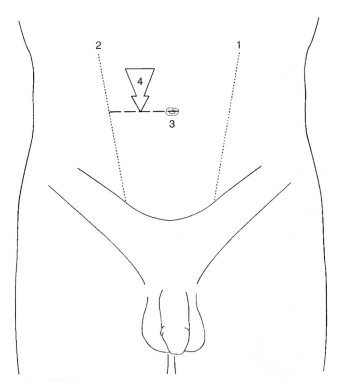

Figure 13–9 Landmarks for rectus block at the umbilicus. Injection is made halfway between the umbilicus and the lateral linea alba. (1 and 2) Left and right lateral lineae albae. (3) Umbilicus. (4) Right-sided injection site. The left-sided injection site is symmetrically located. (From Courreges P, Poddevin F, Lecoutre D: Para-umbilical block: A new concept for regional anaesthesia in children. Paediatr Anaesth 1997;7:211-214.)

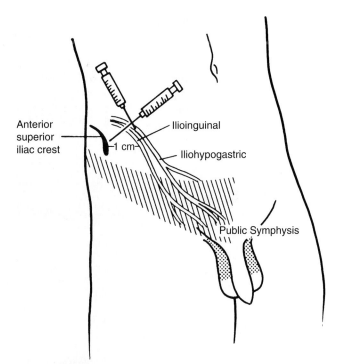

Figure 13–10 Landmarks for ilioinguinal-iliohypogastric block. Injection is made 1 to 2 cm medial and 1 to 2 cm superior to the anterior superior iliac spine. Cutaneous innervation of the ilioinguinal nerve includes much of the external genitalia and part of the proximal thigh; cutaneous innervation of the iliohypogastric nerve includes the skin of the anterior abdominal wall above the inguinal ligament. (From Yaster M, Maxwell LG: Pediatric regional anesthesia. Anesthesiology 1989;70:324-338.)

ilioinguinal-iliohypogastric block is inferior to caudal block at blunting the neuroendocrine stress response to orchiopexy.[269] Bilateral block can be performed, but application may be limited in small children by the dose of local anesthetic required.

Fascia Iliaca Block

The femur and anterior thigh receive innervation from the femoral nerve; the medial and lateral proximal thigh are supplied by the obturator and lateral femoral cutaneous nerves, respectively. Simultaneous block of all three nerves can be accomplished by various techniques, including fascia iliaca block, with resultant analgesia of the proximal leg although sparing the posterior thigh. This block is appropriate for procedures involving the bony femur or soft tissues of the proximal thigh and may be particularly useful in children undergoing quadriceps muscle biopsy for evaluation of myopathy, in whom volatile anesthetic agents are best avoided. Fascia iliaca block is increasingly common in pediatric practice[76,142]; the technical ease is greater and the success rate is higher than for the traditional three-in-one approach.[79]

Injection is made 1 to 2 cm medial and 1 to 2 cm inferior to the anterior superior iliac spine, just inferior to the junction of the middle and lateral thirds of the inguinal ligament (Fig. 13-11).[260] A blunt bevel needle is introduced with slight inferior and lateral angulation, perpendicular to the iliac wing, until two distinct gives or "pops" are felt as the needle pierces first the fascia lata and then the fascia iliaca; the former is usually more pronounced than the latter. Alternatively, the needle may be advanced until encountering the iliac wing and then withdrawn slightly. After negative aspiration and a negative test dose to reduce the likelihood of intravascular injection, 0.5 to 1.0 mL/kg of local anesthetic is deposited; little or no resistance should be felt. Continuous fascia iliac block in children has been described.[218] Bilateral block can be performed, but application may be limited in small children by the dose of local anesthetic required.

Penile Block

Penile block provides analgesia for circumcision and other distal penile procedures, including simple hypospadias repair; caudal block is preferred for more proximal procedures, such as repair of complex hypospadias.[35,141,297,332] In general, penile block has fewer complications than caudal block—in particular, a lower incidence of motor block—but caudal block has a higher success rate and provides more prolonged analgesia. Penile block is not free of risk; puncture of dorsal penile vessels may lead to hematoma,[43] and gangrene of the

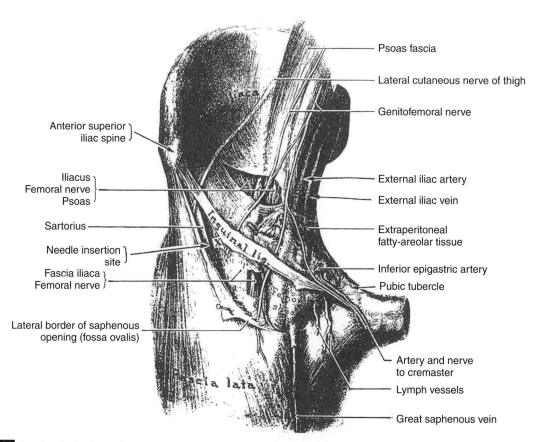

Figure 13-11 Landmarks for fascia iliaca block. Injection is made 1 to 2 cm medial and 1 to 2 cm inferior to the anterior superior iliac spine, just inferior to the junction of the middle and lateral thirds of the inguinal ligament. (From Sethna NF, Berde CB: Pediatric regional anesthesia. In Gregory GA [ed]: Pediatric Anesthesia, 3rd ed. New York, Churchill Livingstone, 1994, pp 281-318.)

glans penis has been reported.[252] Local anesthetic solutions for penile block must not contain epinephrine or other vasoconstrictors.

Injection is made at the base of the penis lateral to the midline at approximately the 10 and 2 o'clock positions (Fig. 13-12).[234,330] Alternatively, a single injection can be made in the midline. A blunt bevel needle is introduced perpendicular to the skin until a distinct give or "pop" is felt as the needle pierces Buck's fascia. After negative aspiration and a negative test dose to reduce the likelihood of intravascular injection, 0.5 to 1.0 mL/kg of local anesthetic, up to 10 mL, is deposited; little or no resistance should be felt. The process is then repeated on the contralateral side. Ring block at the base of the penis superficial to Buck's fascia provides equivalent analgesia and may reduce risk of hematoma.[43]

Neuraxial Block

Neuraxial block involves either spinal or epidural techniques. Spinal block, with injection of anesthetic directly into the cerebrospinal fluid of the spinal subarachnoid space, is performed almost exclusively for procedures in

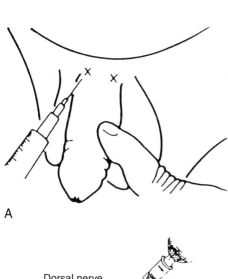

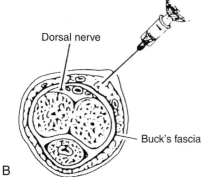

Figure 13-12 Landmarks for penile block. *A,* Injection is made at the base of the penis lateral to the midline at approximately the 10 and 2 o'clock positions. *B,* The dorsal vein, two dorsal arteries, two dorsal nerves, and three corpora of the penis lie beneath Buck's fascia. (*A,* From Yaster M, Maxwell LG: Pediatric regional anesthesia. Anesthesiology 1989;70:324-338. *B,* From Rice LJ, Hannallah RS: Local and regional anesthesia. In Motoyama EK, Davis PJ [eds]: Smith's Anesthesia for Infants and Children, 5th ed. St Louis, CV Mosby, 1990, pp 393-426.)

infants at high risk of apnea following general anesthesia, although continuous spinal techniques are occasionally employed for palliative analgesia. Epidural block, with injection of anesthetic into the potential space between the ligamentum flavum and dura mater, is a far more common technique for procedural and perioperative pain management in children. Anesthetic can be administered as a single injection or by repeated injections or continuous infusion through an indwelling catheter.

Contraindications to neuraxial block include patient or parent refusal, coagulopathy predisposing to neuraxial hematoma, local or systemic infection carrying the risk of neuraxial abscess or meningitis, increased intracranial pressure, and anatomic deformity. Most contraindications are relative; risks and benefits must be weighed in each patient.

Caudal Block

The most common neuraxial block in children is caudal block,[330] in which the epidural space is accessed via the sacral hiatus created by the failure of fusion of the spinous process of the fifth sacral vertebra. The technique is relatively straightforward, the success rate is high, and the complication rate is low.[42,77]

Injection is made between and slightly inferior to the sacral cornua (Fig. 13-13).[330] A blunt bevel needle is introduced with approximately 45 degrees of cephalad angulation until a distinct give or "pop" is felt as the needle pierces the sacrococcygeal ligament, the most inferior aspect of the ligamentum flavum. If bone is encountered, usually representing the posterior aspect of anterior sacral elements, the needle is withdrawn slightly and redirected more parallel to the skin. Correct positioning of the needle tip within the epidural space is confirmed by loss of resistance to injection. After negative aspiration for blood or cerebrospinal fluid and a negative test dose to reduce the likelihood of intravascular injection, the full dose of anesthetic is injected. Serious complications associated with caudal block include intravascular or intraosseous injection, inadvertent dural puncture with resultant spinal anesthesia, injury to pelvic contents, and hematoma; these complications are rare.[225]

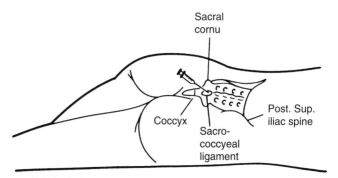

Figure 13-13 Landmarks for caudal block. Injection is made between and slightly inferior to the sacral cornua. (From Yaster M, Maxwell LG: Pediatric regional anesthesia. Anesthesiology 1989;70:324-338.)

Caudal block is most commonly performed as a single injection, with 1.0 mL/kg of anesthetic providing reliable analgesia below the umbilicus in patients less than approximately 30 kg. Perhaps because of their lower overall sympathetic tone, infants and children do not generally demonstrate hemodynamic instability following neuraxial block. Caudal block in pediatric patients induces significant changes in regional blood flow but does not alter heart rate or blood pressure.[173]

The agents administered determine the duration of analgesia following caudal block. Local anesthetic may provide analgesia for several hours and does not cause urinary retention at usual doses.[98] Bupivacaine 0.0625% to 0.25% is used most commonly. The addition of an opioid prolongs analgesia but increases the risk of side effects, particularly respiratory depression. Duration of analgesia and risk of side effects are greater with increasing opioid hydrophilicity, which promotes uptake into the cerebrospinal fluid and enhances distal spread. Caudal fentanyl, a highly lipophilic opioid, can be used for outpatient and ambulatory surgery in children at a dose of 0.5 to 1.0 μg/kg. Caudal morphine, a highly hydrophilic opioid, provides analgesia for more than 12 hours at a dose of 30 to 70 μg/kg but entails a significant risk of side effects, including pruritus and respiratory depression, for up to 24 hours.[164,294] Neuraxial morphine should not be used for outpatient analgesia. Caudal hydromorphone at a dose of 5.0 to 10.0 μg/kg provides more prolonged analgesia than caudal fentanyl, with less risk of respiratory depression than caudal morphine. Caudal administration of clonidine[129,263] and ketamine[307] has been described and may be particularly advantageous in patients with potentially increased sensitivity to opioids, including neonates and children with chronic respiratory disease.

Continuous Techniques

Single-injection caudal block works well for pain anticipated to last less than 24 hours; even caudal morphine does not provide reliable analgesia beyond this time frame. For pain of longer duration, continuous techniques are preferred. Excellent analgesia can be provided by repeated injection or continuous infusion of anesthetic through indwelling epidural catheters, which can be placed via caudal, lumbar, or thoracic approaches to the epidural space in children.[24,84,120] Cervical epidural catheters for palliative care in children have been reported,[222,298] and tunneled catheters for prolonged analgesia have been described.[11]

Epidural catheters can be inserted caudally and threaded to the desired vertebral level, particularly in neonates and young infants, in whom the epidural fat is more gelatinous and the epidural space is largely free of fibrous septa.[77] Distal threading of caudally placed epidural catheters is facilitated by the use of styletted catheters. Epidural catheters can also be placed directly at the desired vertebral level; this is commonly done in patients weighing more than 5 to 10 kg. Epidural catheters placed via a lumbar or thoracic approach do not reliably thread to a distant vertebral level. Catheter direction is unpredictable, and threading more than 3 cm beyond

the needle tip often causes catheter coiling at the level of insertion.[180] Historical concerns over the safety of epidural catheter placement in children under general anesthesia have been largely theoretical, although neurologic complications have been reported.[149] Skin preparation with chlorhexidine rather than iodine-containing solutions confers a lower risk of subsequent catheter colonization.[156] The agent selected for epidural infusion depends on the dermatomal position of the catheter tip relative to the site of pain, as well as on the distribution and intensity of analgesia desired. Numerous combinations of local anesthetic and opioid are commonly used in the United States (Table 13-14); other agents are utilized in other countries.[200,251] Concomitant administration of local anesthetic and opioid is synergistic and enables dose reductions of both agents, minimizing motor block and decreasing the risk of opioid side effects.[27,193] If the epidural catheter tip has been appropriately positioned in close dermatomal proximity to the site of pain, dilute local anesthetic with a lipophilic opioid such as fentanyl may be sufficient. If the epidural catheter tip is at a dermatomal level distant from the painful area, or if this area covers multiple dermatomes, addition of an increasingly hydrophilic opioid such as hydromorphone or morphine may be necessary. Epidural opioids provide excellent analgesia but are associated with side effects, including pruritus, nausea, urinary retention, and respiratory depression; risk of side effects increases with increasing opioid hydrophilicity.[282] Opioid side effects can be managed with a variety of agents (see Table 13-8). Clonidine can be used instead of an opioid for epidural infusion, providing similar analgesia but avoiding opioid side effects.[72,158] This may be particularly advantageous in patients with potentially increased sensitivity to opioids, including neonates and children with chronic respiratory disease.

TABLE 13-14 Agents for Epidural Infusion in Children*

Local Anesthetic†	Opioid†,‡
Bupivacaine 0.0625%-0.1% (max dose 0.4 mg/kg/hr)	Fentanyl 0.5-1.0 μg/kg/hr (adult dose, 50-100 μg/hr)
OR	OR
Levobupivacaine 0.0625%-0.1% (max dose 0.4 mg/kg/hr)	Hydromorphone 2.0-4.0 μg/kg/hr (adult dose, 150-300 μg/hr)
OR	OR
Lidocaine 0.1%-0.5% (max dose 3 mg/kg/hr)	Morphine 3.0-6.0 μg/kg/hr (adult dose, 250-500 μg/hr)
OR	AND/OR
Ropivacaine 0.1%-0.2% (max dose 0.5 mg/kg/hr)	Clonidine 0.25-0.5 μg/kg/hr (adult dose, 25-50 μg/hr)

*Thoracic catheters commonly deliver 0.2-0.3 mL/kg/hr (max 5-10 mL/hr); lumbar catheters, 0.3-0.4 mL/kg/hr (max 10-15 mL/hr); and caudal catheters, 0.4-0.5 mL/kg/hr (max 15-20 mL/hr).

†Recommended local anesthetic and opioid doses should be reduced 25% to 50% in neonates and young infants.

‡Recommended opioid doses are for initial administration in opioid-naive patients; titration to clinical effect is required, and higher doses may be necessary.

Close observation of patients receiving epidural infusions is essential. Continuous pulse oximetry and cardiorespiratory monitoring have been recommended for any child receiving an epidural opioid.[193] Alternatively, all patients receiving epidural infusions may be placed on continuous pulse oximetry, with cardiorespiratory monitoring reserved for patients at increased risk of respiratory depression. Neonates and young infants, children with neurologic or pulmonary disease, and patients receiving a hydrophilic opioid such as morphine may merit more intensive monitoring.[25] Level of consciousness, adequacy of analgesia, degree of motor and sensory block, and presence of side effects should be assessed regularly and frequently for all patients receiving epidural infusions. Continuous neuraxial techniques require significant caregiver diligence and expertise but provide superb analgesia for children with severe pain.

COMMENTS

Appropriate pain management in children requires an understanding of developmental and physiologic issues unique to pediatric patients. A coherent plan encompassing the entire perioperative course should be developed, providing analgesia in proportion to pain and preempting pain whenever possible. Numerous tools are available to perform ongoing quantitative assessment of pain in all children.

Nonpharmacologic techniques may reduce the need for pharmacologic agents, and nonopioid analgesics may reduce the need for opioids. However, opioids are the mainstay of therapy for moderate to severe pain and, in appropriate doses, can be used in patients of any age. Regional anesthesia with local anesthetic optimizes analgesia and reduces the need for systemic agents. Topical and infiltration anesthesia may be provided, or specific peripheral nerve, plexus, or neuraxial blocks may be performed. Pain management is individualized, pain relief is assessed regularly, and regimens are modified as needed to optimize analgesia, minimize side effects, and facilitate recovery.

REFERENCES

1. Adams ML, Brase DA, Welch SP, et al: The role of endogenous peptides in the action of opioid analgesics. Ann Emerg Med 1986;15:1030-1035.
2. Agrawal A, Gerson CR, Seligman I, et al: Postoperative hemorrhage after tonsillectomy: Use of ketorolac tromethamine. Otolaryngol Head Neck Surg 1999;120:335-339.
3. Akman I, Ozek E, Bilgen H, et al: Sweet solutions and pacifiers for pain relief in newborn infants. J Pain 2002;3:199-202.
4. Alexander CM, Gross JB: Sedative doses of midazolam depress hypoxic ventilatory responses in humans. Anesth Analg 1988;67:377-382.
5. Algren J, Deegear C, Skjonsby B, et al: Efficacy and safety of patient-parent, or nurse-controlled analgesia in children. Anesthesiology 1998;89:3.
6. Altintas F, Bozkurt P, Ipek N, et al: The efficacy of pre- versus postsurgical axillary block on postoperative pain in paediatric patients. Paediatr Anaesth 2000;10:23-28.
7. American Academy of Pediatrics Task Force on Pain in Infants, Children, and Adolescents: The assessment and management of acute pain in infants, children, and adolescents. Pediatrics 2001;108:793-797.
8. Anand KJ, Hickey PR: Pain and its effects in the human neonate and fetus. N Engl J Med 1987;317:1321-1329.
9. Anand KJ, Sippell WG, Aynsley-Green A: Randomised trial of fentanyl anaesthesia in preterm babies undergoing surgery: Effects on the stress response. Lancet 1987;1:62-66.
10. Andrews K: The human developmental neurophysiology of pain. In Schechter N, Berde C, Yaster M (eds): Pain in Infants, Children, and Adolescents. Philadelphia, Lippincott Williams & Wilkins, 2003, pp 19-42.
11. Aram L, Krane EJ, Kozloski LJ, et al: Tunneled epidural catheters for prolonged analgesia in pediatric patients. Anesth Analg 2001;92:1432-1438.
12. ASA: ASA House of Delegates standards for basic anesthetic monitoring. 1986.
13. ASA: ASA House of Delegates statement on intravascular catheterizaion procedure. 2000.
14. Ashburn MA, Gauthier M, Love G, et al: Iontophoretic administration of 2% lidocaine HCl and 1:100,000 epinephrine in humans. Clin J Pain 1997;13:22-26.
15. Ates Y, Unal N, Cuhruk H, et al: Postoperative analgesia in children using preemptive retrobulbar block and local anesthetic infiltration in strabismus surgery. Reg Anesth Pain Med 1998;23:569-574.
16. Aun CS, Short SM, Leung DH, et al: Induction dose-response of propofol in unpremedicated children. Br J Anaesth 1992;68:64-67.
17. Aun CS, Sung RY, O'Meara ME, et al: Cardiovascular effects of IV induction in children: Comparison between propofol and thiopentone. Br J Anaesth 1993;70:647-653.
18. Auroy Y, Ecoffey C, Messiah A, et al: Relationship between complications of pediatric anesthesia and volume of pediatric anesthetics. Anesth Analg 1997;84:234-235.
19. Ayers J, Graves SA: Perioperative management of total parenteral nutrition, glucose containing solutions, and intraoperative glucose monitoring in paediatric patients: A survey of clinical practice. Paediatr Anaesth 2001;11:41-44.
20. Bailey PL, Pace NL, Ashburn MA, et al: Frequent hypoxemia and apnea after sedation with midazolam and fentanyl. Anesthesiology 1990;73:826-830.
21. Bailey R, Sinha C, Burgess LP: Ketorolac tromethamine and hemorrhage in tonsillectomy: A prospective, randomized, double-blind study. Laryngoscope 1997;107:166-169.
22. Bell EF, Oh W: Fluid and electrolyte balance in very low birth weight infants. Clin Perinatol 1979;6:139-150.
23. Benini F, Johnston CC, Faucher D, et al: Topical anesthesia during circumcision in newborn infants. JAMA 1993;270:850-853.
24. Berde C, Sethna N, Yemen T, et al: Continuous epidural bupivacaine-fentanyl infusions in children following ureteral reimplantation. Anesthesiology 1990;73(3A):A1128.
25. Berde CB: Pediatric postoperative pain management. Pediatr Clin North Am 1989;36:921-940.
26. Berde CB, Beyer JE, Bournaki MC, et al: Comparison of morphine and methadone for prevention of postoperative pain in 3- to 7-year-old children. J Pediatr 1991;119:136-141.
27. Berde CB, Sethna NF, Levin L, et al: Regional analgesia on pediatric medical and surgical wards. Intensive Care Med 1989;15(Suppl 1):S40-S43.
28. Berry FA: Preoperative assessment and general management of outpatients. Int Anesthesiol Clin 1982;20:3-15.
29. Bevan JC, Johnston C, Haig MJ, et al: Preoperative parental anxiety predicts behavioural and emotional responses to induction of anaesthesia in children. Can J Anaesth 1990;37:177-182.

30. Beyer JE, McGrath PJ, Berde CB: Discordance between self-report and behavioral pain measures in children aged 3-7 years after surgery. J Pain Symptom Manage 1990;5:350-356.

31. Bhat R, Abu-Harb M, Chari G, et al: Morphine metabolism in acutely ill preterm newborn infants. J Pediatr 1992;120:795-799.

32. Bhat R, Chari G, Gulati A, et al: Pharmacokinetics of a single dose of morphine in preterm infants during the first week of life. J Pediatr 1990;117:477-481.

33. Bhavani-Shankar K, Philip JH: Defining segments and phases of a time capnogram. Anesth Analg 2000;91:973-977.

34. Bito H, Ikeda K: Closed-circuit anesthesia with sevoflurane in humans: Effects on renal and hepatic function and concentrations of breakdown products with soda lime in the circuit. Anesthesiology 1994;80:71-76.

35. Blaise G, Roy WL: Postoperative pain relief after hypospadias repair in pediatric patients: Regional analgesia versus systemic analgesics. Anesthesiology 1986;65:84-86.

36. Bonadio WA, Wagner V: Efficacy of TAC topical anesthetic for repair of pediatric lacerations. Am J Dis Child 1988;142:203-205.

37. Borgeat A, Wilder-Smith OH, Saiah M, et al: Subhypnotic doses of propofol possess direct antiemetic properties. Anesth Analg 1992;74:539-541.

38. Bourke DL, Smith TC: Estimating allowable hemodilution. Anesthesiology 1974;41:609-612.

39. Bouwmeester NJ, Hop WC, van Dijk M, et al: Postoperative pain in the neonate: Age-related differences in morphine requirements and metabolism. Intensive Care Med 2003;29:2009-2015.

40. Brandom BW, Brandom RB, Cook DR: Uptake and distribution of halothane in infants: In vivo measurements and computer simulations. Anesth Analg 1983;62:404-410.

41. Brett CM, Fisher DM: Thiopental dose-response relations in unpremedicated infants, children, and adults. Anesth Analg 1987;66:1024-1027.

42. Broadman L, Hanallah R, Norden J, et al: "Kiddie caudals": Experience with 1154 consecutive cases without complications. Anesth Analg 1987;66:S18.

43. Broadman LM, Hannallah RS, Belman AB, et al: Post-circumcision analgesia—a prospective evaluation of subcutaneous ring block of the penis. Anesthesiology 1987;67:399-402.

44. Brower RW, Merin RG: Left ventricular function and compliance in swine during halothane anesthesia. Anesthesiology 1979;50:409-415.

45. Brown JL: Imagination training: A tool with many uses. Contemp Pediatr 1995;12:22-26, 29-30, 32.

46. Browne BL, Prys-Roberts C, Wolf AR: Propofol and alfentanil in children: Infusion technique and dose requirement for total IV anaesthesia. Br J Anaesth 1992;69:570-576.

47. Buchholz DH: Blood transfusion: Merits of component therapy. I. The clinical use of red cells, platelets, and granulocytes. J Pediatr 1974;84:1-15.

48. Buck N, Devlin H, Lunn J: Report on the confidential inquiry into perioperative deaths. Nuffield Provincial Hospitals Trust, London, the King's Fund Publishing House, 1987.

49. Carney FM, Van Dyke RA: Halothane hepatitis: A critical review. Anesth Analg 1972;51:135-160.

50. Casey W, Rice L, Hannallah R, et al: A comparison between bupivacaine instillation versus ilioinguinal/iliohypogastric nerve block for postoperative analgesia following inguinal herniorrhaphy in children. Anesthesiology 1990;72:637-639.

51. Cassidy KL, Reid GJ, McGrath PJ, et al: A randomized double-blind, placebo-controlled trial of the EMLA patch for the reduction of pain associated with intramuscular injection in four- to six-year-old children. Acta Paediatr 2001;90:1329-1336.

52. Chay P, Duffy B, Walker J: Pharmacokinetic-pharmacodynamic relationship of morphine in neonates. Clin Pharmacol Ther 1992;51:334-342.

53. Christensen J, Fatchett D: Promoting parental use of distraction and relaxation in pediatric oncology patients during invasive procedures. J Pediatr Oncol Nurs 2002;19:127-132.

54. Christoph RA, Buchanan L, Begalla K, et al: Pain reduction in local anesthetic administration through pH buffering. Ann Emerg Med 1988;17:117-120.

55. Coderre TJ, Melzack R: Cutaneous hyperalgesia: Contributions of the peripheral and central nervous systems to the increase in pain sensitivity after injury. Brain Res 1987;404:95-106.

56. Coderre TJ, Vaccarino AL, Melzack R: Central nervous system plasticity in the tonic pain response to subcutaneous formalin injection. Brain Res 1990;535:155-158.

57. Cohen IT, Hannallah RS, Hummer KA: The incidence of emergence agitation associated with desflurane anesthesia in children is reduced by fentanyl. Anesth Analg 2001;93:88-91.

58. Collins SK, Kuck K: Music therapy in the neonatal intensive care unit. Neonatal Netw 1991;9:23-26.

59. Cook D: Clinical use of muscle relaxants in infants and children. Anesth Analg 1981;60:335.

60. Cook D, Davis P: Pediatric anesthesia pharmacology. In Lake C (ed): Pediatric Cardiac Anesthesiology. Norwalk, Conn, Appleton & Lange, 1993.

61. Cook DR, Brandom BW, Shiu G, et al: The inspired median effective dose, brain concentration at anesthesia, and cardiovascular index for halothane in young rats. Anesth Analg 1981;60:182-185.

62. Cooper CM, Gerrish SP, Hardwick M, et al: EMLA cream reduces the pain of venipuncture in children. Eur J Anaesthesiol 1987;4:441-448.

63. Cote C (ed): A Practice of Anesthesia for Infants and Children, 2nd ed. Philadelphia, WB Saunders, 1982.

64. Cote C: Calcium chloride versus calcium gluconate: Comparison of ionization and cardiovascular effects in children and dogs. Anesthesiology 1987;66:465.

65. Cote CJ, Cohen IT, Suresh S, et al: A comparison of three doses of a commercially prepared oral midazolam syrup in children. Anesth Analg 2002;94:37-43.

66. Cote CJ, Goudsouzian NG, Liu LM, et al: The dose response of intravenous thiopental for the induction of general anesthesia in unpremedicated children. Anesthesiology 1981;55:703-705.

67. Cote CJ, Zaslavsky A, Downes JJ, et al: Postoperative apnea in former preterm infants after inguinal herniorrhaphy: A combined analysis. Anesthesiology 1995;82:809-822.

68. Courreges P, Poddevin F, Lecoutre D: Para-umbilical block: A new concept for regional anaesthesia in children. Paediatr Anaesth 1997;7:211-214.

69. Cravero JP, Beach M, Thyr B, et al: The effect of small dose fentanyl on the emergence characteristics of pediatric patients after sevoflurane anesthesia without surgery. Anesth Analg 2003;97:364-367.

70. Crawford M, Lerman J, Christensen S, et al: Effects of duration of fasting on gastric fluid pH and volume in healthy children. Anesth Analg 1990;71:400-403.

71. Crumrine RS, Yodlowski EH: Assessment of neuromuscular function in infants. Anesthesiology 1981;54:29-32.

72. Cucchiaro G, Dagher C, Baujard C, et al: Side-effects of postoperative epidural analgesia in children: A randomized study comparing morphine and clonidine. Paediatr Anaesth 2003;13:318-323.

73. Dahl JB, Kehlet H: The value of pre-emptive analgesia in the treatment of postoperative pain. Br J Anaesth 1993;70:434-439.

74. Dahl JB, Moiniche S, Kehlet H: Wound infiltration with local anaesthetics for postoperative pain relief. Acta Anaesthesiol Scand 1994;38:7-14.

75. Dalens B: Regional anesthesia in children. Anesth Analg 1989;68:654-672.

76. Dalens B: "Small blocks" in paediatric patients. Baillieres Clin Anaesthesiol 2000;14:745-758.

77. Dalens B, Hasnaoui A: Caudal anesthesia in pediatric surgery: Success rate and adverse effects in 750 consecutive patients. Anesth Analg 1989;68:83-89.

78. Dalens B, Tanguy A, Haberer JP: Lumbar epidural anesthesia for operative and postoperative pain relief in infants and young children. Anesth Analg 1986;65:1069-1073.

79. Dalens B, Vanneuville G, Tanguy A: Comparison of the fascia iliaca compartment block with the 3-in-1 block in children. Anesth Analg 1989;69:705-713.

80. Davidson AJ, Eyres RL, Cole WG: A comparison of prilocaine and lidocaine for intravenous regional anaesthesia for forearm fracture reduction in children. Paediatr Anaesth 2002;12:146-150.

81. Davis P, et al: Emergency and recovery from sevoflurane in pediatric ambulatory patients: A multicenter study. Anesthesiology 1993;79:A1166.

82. Davis PJ, Greenberg JA, Gendelman M, et al: Recovery characteristics of sevoflurane and halothane in preschool-aged children undergoing bilateral myringotomy and pressure equalization tube insertion. Anesth Analg 1999;88:34-38.

83. DeJong P: Comparison of rectal to intramuscular administration of midazolam and atropine for premedication of children. Acta Anaesthesiol Scand 1988;32:485.

84. Desparmet J, Meistelman C, Barre J, et al: Continuous epidural infusion of bupivacaine for postoperative pain relief in children. Anesthesiology 1987;67:108-110.

85. Drugs AAoPCo: Guidelines for monitoring and management of pediatric patients during and after sedation for diagnostic and therapeutic procedures: Addendum. Pediatrics 2002;110:836-838.

86. Duhn L, Medves J: A systemic integrative review of infant pain assessment tools. Adv Neonatal Care 2004;4:126-140.

87. Eger E, et al: Partition coefficients of I-653 in human blood, saline, and olive oil. Anesth Analg 1987;66:971.

88. Eger EI 2nd, Saidman LJ: Hazards of nitrous oxide anesthesia in bowel obstruction and pneumothorax. Anesthesiology 1965;26:61-66.

89. Eger EI 2nd, Smith NT, Stoelting RK, et al: Cardiovascular effects of halothane in man. Anesthesiology 1970;32:396-409.

90. Eichenfield LF, Funk A, Fallon-Friedlander S, et al: A clinical study to evaluate the efficacy of ELA-Max (4% liposomal lidocaine) as compared with eutectic mixture of local anesthetics cream for pain reduction of venipuncture in children. Pediatrics 2002;109:1093-1099.

91. Eland J: The use of TENS with children. In Schechter N, Berde C, Yaster M (eds): Pain in Infants, Children and Adolescents. Baltimore, Williams & Wilkins, 1993, pp 331-340.

92. Eland J, Anderson J: The experience of pain in children. In Jacox S (ed): Pain: A Sourcebook for Nurses and Other Health Professionals. Boston, Little, Brown, 1977, pp 453-473.

93. Ernst AA, Marvez E, Nick TG, et al: Lidocaine adrenaline tetracaine gel versus tetracaine adrenaline cocaine gel for topical anesthesia in linear scalp and facial lacerations in children aged 5 to 17 years. Pediatrics 1995;95:255-258.

94. Etches RC: Respiratory depression associated with patient-controlled analgesia: A review of eight cases. Can J Anaesth 1994;41:125-132.

95. Farrington EA, McGuinness GA, Johnson GF, et al: Continuous intravenous morphine infusion in postoperative newborn infants. Am J Perinatol 1993;10:84-87.

96. Fassoulaki A, Sarantopoulos C, Zotou M, et al: Preemptive opioid analgesia does not influence pain after abdominal hysterectomy. Can J Anaesth 1995;42:109-113.

97. Ferguson S, Thomas V, Lewis I: The rectus sheath block in paediatric anaesthesia: New indications for an old technique? Paediatr Anaesth 1996;6:463-466.

98. Fisher QA, McComiskey CM, Hill JL, et al: Postoperative voiding interval and duration of analgesia following peripheral or caudal nerve blocks in children. Anesth Analg 1993;76:173-177.

99. Fitzgerald M: Pain and analgesia in neonates. Trends Neurosci 1987;9:254.

100. Fitzgerald M, Anand K: Developmental neuroanatomy and neurophysiology of pain. In Schechter N, Berde C, Yaster M (eds): Pain in Infants, Children, and Adolescents. Baltimore, Williams & Wilkins, 1993.

101. Fitzgerald M, Howard R: The neurobiologic basis of pediatirc pain. In Schechter N, Berde C, Yaster M (eds): Pain in Infants, Children, and Adolescents. Philadelphia, Lippincott Williams & Wilkins, 2003, pp 19-42.

102. Flewellen EH, Nelson TE, Jones WP, et al: Dantrolene dose response in awake man: Implications for management of malignant hyperthermia. Anesthesiology 1983;59:275-280.

103. Friesen RH, Carpenter E, Madigan CK, et al: Oral transmucosal fentanyl citrate for preanaesthetic medication of paediatric cardiac surgery patients. Paediatr Anaesth 1995;5:29-33.

104. Frink EJ Jr, Green WB Jr, Brown EA, et al: Compound A concentrations during sevoflurane anesthesia in children. Anesthesiology 1996;84:566-571.

105. Furman EB, Roman DG, Lemmer LA, et al: Specific therapy in water, electrolyte and blood-volume replacement during pediatric surgery. Anesthesiology 1975;42:187-193.

106. Galinkin J, Fazi L, Cuy R, et al: Use of fentanyl in children undergoing myringotomy and tube placement during halothane and sevoflurane anesthesia. Anesthesiology 2000;93:1378-1383.

107. Galinkin J, Kurth D: Neonatal and pediatric apnea syndromes. Problems in Anesthesia 1988;10:444-454.

108. Gallagher JE, Blauth J, Fornadley JA: Perioperative ketorolac tromethamine and postoperative hemorrhage in cases of tonsillectomy and adenoidectomy. Laryngoscope 1995;105:606-609.

109. Gallagher T, Black S, Black G: Isoflurane does not reduce aortic peak flow velocity in children. Br J Anaesth 1986;58:1116.

110. Gaukroger P: Novel techniques of analgesic delivery. In Schechter N, Berde C, Yaster M (eds): Pain in Infants, Children, and Adolescents. Baltimore, Williams & Wilkins, 1993, pp 195-202.

111. Gaukroger PB, Tomkins DP, van der Walt JH: Patient-controlled analgesia in children. Anaesth Intensive Care 1989;17:264-268.

112. Gehan G, Karoubi P, Quinet F, et al: Optimal dose of lignocaine for preventing pain on injection of propofol. Br J Anaesth 1991;66:324-326.

113. Glauser TA, Rorke LB, Weinberg PM, et al: Acquired neuropathologic lesions associated with the hypoplastic left heart syndrome. Pediatrics 1990;85:991-1000.

114. Goetting MG, Thirman MJ: Neurotoxicity of meperidine. Ann Emerg Med 1985;14:1007-1009.

115. Goff MJ, Arain SR, Ficke DJ, et al: Absence of bronchodilation during desflurane anesthesia: A comparison to sevoflurane and thiopental. Anesthesiology 2000;93:404-408.

116. Gonsowski CT, Laster MJ, Eger EI 2nd, et al: Toxicity of compound A in rats: Effect of increasing duration of administration. Anesthesiology 1994;80:566-573.

117. Goudsouzian NG: Maturation of neuromuscular transmission in the infant. Br J Anaesth 1980;52:205-214.

118. Graves DA, Foster TS, Batenhorst RL, et al: Patient-controlled analgesia. Ann Intern Med 1983;99:360-366.

119. Green SM, Nakamura R, Johnson NE: Ketamine sedation for pediatric procedures. Part 1. A prospective series. Ann Emerg Med 1990;19:1024-1032.

120. Gunter JB, Eng C: Thoracic epidural anesthesia via the caudal approach in children. Anesthesiology 1992;76:935-938.

121. Gunter JB, Gregg T, Varughese AM, et al: Levobupivacaine for ilioinguinal/iliohypogastric nerve block in children. Anesth Analg 1999;89:647-649.

122. Hallen B, Olsson G, Uppfeldt A: Pain-free venipuncture: Effect of timing of application of local anaesthetic cream. Anaesthesia 1984;39:969-972.

123. Hammarlund K, Sedin G, Stromberg B: Transepidermal water loss in newborn infants. VIII. Relation to gestational age and post-natal age in appropriate and small for gestational age infants. Acta Paediatr Scand 1983;72:721-728.

124. Hannallah R, et al: Propofol anesthesia in paediatric ambulatory patients: A comparison with thiopentone and halothane. Can J Anaesth 1983;41:12.

125. Hannallah R, Rosales J: Experience with parent's presence during anesthesia induction in children. Can Anaesthesiol Soc J 1983;30:286.

126. Hannallah RS, Baker SB, Casey W, et al: Propofol: Effective dose and induction characteristics in unpremedicated children. Anesthesiology 1991;74:217-219.

127. Hannallah RS, Broadman LM, Belman AB, et al: Comparison of caudal and ilioinguinal/iliohypogastric nerve blocks for control of post-orchiopexy pain in pediatric ambulatory surgery. Anesthesiology 1987;66:832-834.

128. Hansen LA, Noyes MA, Lehman ME: Evaluation of patient-controlled analgesia (PCA) versus PCA plus continuous infusion in postoperative cancer patients. J Pain Symptom Manage 1991;6:4-14.

129. Hansen T, Henneberg S, Walther-Larsen S, et al: Caudal bupivacaine supplemented with caudal or intravenous clonidine in children undergoing hypospadias repair: A double-blind study. Br J Anaesth 2004;92:223-227.

130. Harrison D, Johnston L, Loughnan P: Oral sucrose for procedural pain in sick hospitalized infants: A randomized-controlled trial. J Paediatr Child Health 2003;39:591-597.

131. Hartley R, Green M, Quinn MW, et al: Development of morphine glucuronidation in premature neonates. Biol Neonate 1994;66:1-9.

132. Hegenbarth MA, Altieri MF, Hawk WH, et al: Comparison of topical tetracaine, adrenaline, and cocaine anesthesia with lidocaine infiltration for repair of lacerations in children. Ann Emerg Med 1990;19:63-67.

133. Hernandez-Reif M, Field T, Largie S, et al: Children's distress during burn treatment is reduced by massage therapy. J Burn Care Rehabil 2001;22:191-195.

134. Hertzka RE, Gauntlett IS, Fisher DM, et al: Fentanyl-induced ventilatory depression: Effects of age. Anesthesiology 1989;70:213-218.

135. Ho JW, Khambatta HJ, Pang LM, et al: Preemptive analgesia in children. Does it exist? Reg Anesth 1997;22:125-130.

136. Holliday M, Segar W: The maintenance need for water in parenteral fluid therapy. Pediatrics 1957;19:823.

137. Hollinger I: Current trends in pediatric anesthesia. Mt Sinai J Med 2002;69:51-54.

138. Holthusen H, Eichwede F, Stevens M, et al: Pre-emptive analgesia: Comparison of preoperative with postoperative caudal block on postoperative pain in children. Br J Anaesth 1994;73:440-442.

139. Holzman RS, van der Velde ME, Kaus SJ, et al: Sevoflurane depresses myocardial contractility less than halothane during induction of anesthesia in children. Anesthesiology 1996;85:1260-1267.

140. Howard RF: Current status of pain management in children. JAMA 2003;290:2464-2469.

141. Irwin MG, Cheng W: Comparison of subcutaneous ring block of the penis with caudal epidural block for post-circumcision analgesia in children. Anaesth Intensive Care 1996;24:365-367.

142. Ivani G, Tonetti F: Postoperative analgesia in infants and children: New developments. Minerva Anestesiol 2004;70:399-403.

143. Jensen BH, Wernberg M, Andersen M: Preoperative starvation and blood glucose concentrations in children undergoing inpatient and outpatient anaesthesia. Br J Anaesth 1982;54:1071-1074.

144. Johnston RR, Eger EI II, Wilson C: A comparative interaction of epinephrine with enflurane, isoflurane, and halothane in man. Anesth Analg 1976;55:709-712.

145. Jonmarker C, Westrin P, Larsson S, et al: Thiopental requirements for induction of anesthesia in children. Anesthesiology 1987;67:104-107.

146. Judkins JH, Dray TG, Hubbell RN: Intraoperative ketorolac and posttonsillectomy bleeding. Arch Otolaryngol Head Neck Surg 1996;122:937-940.

147. Kain ZN, Caldwell-Andrews A, Wang SM: Psychological preparation of the parent and pediatric surgical patient. Anesthesiol Clin North Am 2002;20:29-44.

148. Karl H, et al: Epinephrine-halothane interactions in children. Anesthesiology 1983;58:142.

149. Kasai T, Yaegashi K, Hirose M, et al: Spinal cord injury in a child caused by an accidental dural puncture with a single-shot thoracic epidural needle. Anesth Analg 2003;96:65-67.

150. Katz R, Epstein R: The interaction of anesthetic agents and adrenergic drugs to produce cardiac arrhythmias. Anesthesiology 1968;29:763-784.

151. Keenan R, Boyan C: Cardiac arrest due to anesthesia: A study of incidence and causes. JAMA 1985;253:2373.

152. Keenan R, Shapiro J, Dawson K: Frequency of anesthetic cardiac arrests in infants: Effect of pediatric anesthesiologists. J Clin Anesthesiol 1991;3:433.

153. Kemper KJ, Sarah R, Silver-Highfield E, et al: On pins and needles? Pediatric pain patients' experience with acupuncture. Pediatrics 2000;105:941-947.

154. Keyl C, Schneider A, Dambacher M, et al: Dynamic cardiocirculatory control during propofol anesthesia in mechanically ventilated patients. Anesth Analg 2000;91:1188-1195.

155. Kim M, Strait R, Sato T, et al: A randomized clinical trial of analgesia in children with acute abdominal pain. Acad Emerg Med 2002;9:281-287.

156. Kinirons B, Mimoz O, Lafendi L, et al: Chlorhexidine versus povidone iodine in preventing colonization of continuous epidural catheters in children: A randomized, controlled trial. Anesthesiology 2001;94:239-244.

157. Kissin I: Preemptive analgesia. Anesthesiology 2000;93:1138-1143.

158. Klamt JG, Garcia LV, Stocche RM, et al: Epidural infusion of clonidine or clonidine plus ropivacaine for postoperative analgesia in children undergoing major abdominal surgery. J Clin Anesth 2003;15:510-514.

159. Kokinsky E, Thornberg E: Postoperative pain control in children: A guide to drug choice. Paediatr Drugs 2003;5:751-762.

160. Kokki H: Nonsteroidal anti-inflammatory drugs for postoperative pain: A focus on children. Paediatr Drugs 2003;5:103-123.

161. Koren G, Butt W, Chinyanga H, et al: Postoperative morphine infusion in newborn infants: Assessment of disposition characteristics and safety. J Pediatr 1985;107:963-967.

162. Korpela R, Korvenoja P, Meretoja OA: Morphine-sparing effect of acetaminophen in pediatric day-case surgery. Anesthesiology 1999;91:442-447.

163. Kotrly KJ, Ebert TJ, Vucins E, et al: Baroreceptor reflex control of heart rate during isoflurane anesthesia in humans. Anesthesiology 1984;60:173-179.

164. Krane EJ, Tyler DC, Jacobson LE: The dose response of caudal morphine in children. Anesthesiology 1989;71: 48-52.

165. Kulka PJ, Bressem M, Tryba M: Clonidine prevents sevoflurane-induced agitation in children. Anesth Analg 2001;93:335-338.

166. Kundra P, Deepalakshmi K, Ravishankar M: Preemptive caudal bupivacaine and morphine for postoperative analgesia in children. Anesth Analg 1998;87:52-56.

167. Kupferberg HJ, Way EL: Pharmacologic basis for the increased sensitivity of the newborn rat to morphine. J Pharmacol Exp Ther 1963;141:105-112.

168. Kurth C: Posoperative apnea in premature infants. Anesthesiology 1987;66:488.

169. Kurth CD, LeBard SE: Association of postoperative apnea, airway obstruction, and hypoxemia in former premature infants. Anesthesiology 1991;75:22-26.

170. Kuttner L, Solomon R: Hypnotherapy and imagery for managing children's pain. In Schechter N, Berde C, Yaster M (eds): Pain in Infants, Children, and Adolescents. Philadelphia, Lippincott Williams & Wilkins, 2003, pp 317-328.

171. Lambert SA: The effects of hypnosis/guided imagery on the postoperative course of children. J Dev Behav Pediatr 1996;17:307-310.

172. Lanier WL, Stangland KJ, Scheithauer BW, et al: The effects of dextrose infusion and head position on neurologic outcome after complete cerebral ischemia in primates: Examination of a model. Anesthesiology 1987;66:39-48.

173. Larousse E, Asehnoune K, Dartayet B, et al: The hemodynamic effects of pediatric caudal anesthesia assessed by esophageal Doppler. Anesth Analg 2002;94:1165-1168.

174. LeDez KM, Lerman J: The minimum alveolar concentration (MAC) of isoflurane in preterm neonates, Anesthesiology. 1987;67:301-307.

175. Lee C: Intensive care unit neuromuscular syndrome? Anesthesiology 1995;83:237-240.

176. Lerman J, Davis PJ, Welborn LG, et al: Induction, recovery, and safety characteristics of sevoflurane in children undergoing ambulatory surgery: A comparison with halothane. Anesthesiology 1996;84:1332-1340.

177. Lerman J, Gregory GA, Willis MM, et al: Age and solubility of volatile anesthetics in blood. Anesthesiology 1984;61: 139-143.

178. Lerman J, Robinson S, Willis MM, et al: Anesthetic requirements for halothane in young children 0-1 month and 1-6 months of age. Anesthesiology 1983;59:421-424.

179. Lerman J, Sikich N, Kleinman S, et al: The pharmacology of sevoflurane in infants and children. Anesthesiology 1994;80:814-824.

180. Lim YJ, Bahk JH, Ahn WS, et al: Coiling of lumbar epidural catheters. Acta Anaesthesiol Scand 2002;46: 603-606.

181. Lin Y: Acupuncture. In Schechter N, Berde C, Yaster M (eds): Pain in Infants, Children, and Adolescents. Philadelphia, Lippincott Williams & Wilkins, 2003, pp 426-470.

182. Lloyd-Thomas A, Howard R: A pain service for children. Paediatr Anaesth 1994;4:3-15.

183. Lopez J: Myoplastic free Ca++ during malignant hyperthermia episode in swine. Muscle Nerve 1985;11:82.

184. Lynn AM, Opheim KE, Tyler DC: Morphine infusion after pediatric cardiac surgery. Crit Care Med 1984;12: 863-866.

185. Lynn AM, Slattery JT: Morphine pharmacokinetics in early infancy. Anesthesiology 1987;66:136-139.

186. Malviya S, Swartz J, Lerman J: Are all preterm infants younger that 60 weeks postconceptual age at risk for postanesthetic apnea? Anesthesiology 1993;78:1076.

187. Martin LD, Bratton SL, O'Rourke PP: Clinical uses and controversies of neuromuscular blocking agents in infants and children. Crit Care Med 1999;27:1358-1368.

188. Mather L, Mackie J: The incidence of postoperative pain in children. Pain 1983;15:271-282.

189. Matsota P, Livanios S, Marinopoulou E: Intercostal nerve block with bupivacaine for post-thoracotomy pain relief in children. Eur J Pediatr Surg 2001;11:219-222.

190. Maunuksela E, Olkkola K: Nonsteroidal anti-inflammatory drugs in pediatric pain management. In Schechter N, Berde C, Yaster M (eds): Pain in Infants, Children, and Adolescents. Philadelphia, Lippincott Williams & Wilkins, 2003, pp 171-180.

191. McClune S, McKay A, Wright P: Synergistic interaction between midazolam and propofol. Br J Anaesth 1992; 69:240.

192. McDonnell L, Bowden ML: Breathing management: A simple stress and pain reduction strategy for use on a pediatric service. Issues Compr Pediatr Nurs 1989;12:339-344.

193. McIlvaine WB: Spinal opioids for the pediatric patient. J Pain Symptom Manage 1990;5:183-190.

194. McMillan CO, Spahr-Schopfer IA, Sikich N, et al: Premedication of children with oral midazolam. Can J Anaesth 1992;39:545-550.

195. McNeely JK, Farber NE, Rusy LM, et al: Epidural analgesia improves outcome following pediatric fundoplication: A retrospective analysis. Reg Anesth 1997;22:16-23.

196. Merkel S, Gutstein H, Malviya S: Use of transcutaneous electrical nerve stimulation in a young child with pain from open perineal lesions. J Pain Symptom Manage 1999;18:376-381.

197. Moiniche S, Kehlet H, Dahl JB: A qualitative and quantitative systematic review of preemptive analgesia for postoperative pain relief: The role of timing of analgesia. Anesthesiology 2002;96:725-741.

198. Monitto CL, Greenberg RS, Kost-Byerly S, et al: The safety and efficacy of parent-/nurse-controlled analgesia in patients less than six years of age. Anesth Analg 2000;91:573-579.

199. Morgan KG, Bryant SH: The mechanism of action of dantrolene sodium. J Pharmacol Exp Ther 1977;201:138-147.

200. Moriarty A: Postoperative extradural infusions in children: Preliminary data from a comparison of bupivacaine/diamorphine with plain ropivacaine. Paediatr Anaesth 1999;9:423-427.

201. Morisy L, Platt D: Hazards of high-dose meperidine. JAMA 1986;255:467-468.

202. Morray JP, Geiduschek JM, Caplan RA, et al: A comparison of pediatric and adult anesthesia closed malpractice claims. Anesthesiology 1993;78:461-467.

203. Morray JP, Geiduschek JM, Ramamoorthy C, et al: Anesthesia-related cardiac arrest in children: Initial findings of the Pediatric Perioperative Cardiac Arrest (POCA) Registry. Anesthesiology 2000;93:6-14.

204. Morrison NA, Repka MX: Ketorolac versus acetaminophen or ibuprofen in controlling postoperative pain in patients with strabismus. Ophthalmology 1994;101:915-918.

205. Moss VA: Music and the surgical patient: The effect of music on anxiety. AORN J 1988;48:64-69.

206. Mullooly VM, Levin RF, Feldman HR: Music for postoperative pain and anxiety. J N Y State Nurses Assoc 1988;19:4-7.

207. Murphy MR, Olson WA, Hug CC Jr: Pharmacokinetics of 3H-fentanyl in the dog anesthetized with enflurane. Anesthesiology 1979;50:13-19.

208. Nakakimura K: Glucose administration before cardiac arrest worsens neurologic outcome in cats. Anesthesiology 1990;72:1005.

209. Navarro R, et al: Humans anesthetized with sevoflurane or isoflurane have similar arrhythmic response to epinephrine. Anesthesiology 1994;80:545.

210. O'Donnell J, Ferguson L, Beattie T: Use of analgesia in a paediatric accident and emergency department following limb trauma. Eur J Emerg Med 2002;9:5-8.

211. Olkkola KT, Maunuksela EL: The pharmacokinetics of postoperative intravenous ketorolac tromethamine in children. Br J Clin Pharmacol 1991;31:182-184.

212. Olsson GL, Hallen B: Laryngospasm during anaesthesia: A computer-aided incidence study in 136,929 patients. Acta Anaesthesiol Scand 1984;28:567-575.

213. Ording H: Incidence of malignant hyperthermia in Denmark. Anesth Analg 1985;64:700-704.

214. Ording H, Hedengran AM, Skovgaard LT: Evaluation of 119 anaesthetics received after investigation for susceptibility to malignant hyperthermia. Acta Anaesthesiol Scand 1991;35:711-716.

215. Owens WD: American Society of Anesthesiologists physical status classification system is not a risk classification system. Anesthesiology 2001;94:378.

216. Panel of the Agency for Health Care Policy & Research: Acute Pain Management: Operative or Medical Procedures and Trauma. Clincial Practice Guideline. Rockville, Md, Agency for Health Care Policy & Research, Public Health Service, US Department of Health & Human Services, 1992.

217. Parker RK, Holtmann B, White PF: Effects of a nighttime opioid infusion with PCA therapy on patient comfort and analgesic requirements after abdominal hysterectomy. Anesthesiology. 1992;76:362-367.

218. Paut O, Sallabery M, Schreiber-Deturmeny E, et al: Continuous fascia iliaca compartment block in children: A prospective evaluation of plasma bupivacaine concentrations, pain scores, and side effects. Anesth Analg 2001;92:1159-1163.

219. Petrack E, Marx C, Wright M: Intamuscular ketamine is superior to meperidine, promethazine, and chlorpromazine for pediatric emergency department sedation. Arch Pediatr Adolesc Med 1996;150:676-681.

220. Pietropaoli JA Jr, Keller MS, Smail DF, et al: Regional anesthesia in pediatric surgery: Complications and postoperative comfort level in 174 children. J Pediatr Surg 1993;28:560-564.

221. Pitetti R, Singh S, Pierce M: Safe and efficacious use of procedural sedation and analgesia by nonanesthesiologist in a pediatric emergency department. Arch Pediatr Adolesc Med 2003;157:1090-1096.

222. Plancarte R, Patt R: Intractable upper body pain in a pediatric patient relieved with cervical epidural opioid administration. J Pain Symptom Manage 1991;6:98-99.

223. Polkki T, Pietila A, Vehvilainen-Julkunen K: Hospitalized children's descriptions of their experiences with postsurgical pain relieving methods. Int J Nurs Stud 2003;40:33-44.

224. Pomeranz B: Scientific research into acupuncture for the relief of pain. J Altern Complement Med 1996;2:53-60.

225. Pullerits J, Holzman RS: Pediatric neuraxial blockade. J Clin Anesth 1993;5:342-354.

226. Pulsinelli WA, Waldman S, Rawlinson D, et al: Moderate hyperglycemia augments ischemic brain damage: A neuropathologic study in the rat. Neurology 1982;32:1239-1246.

227. Putney JW, Biancri CP: Site of action of dantrolene in frog sartorius muscle. J Pharmacol Exp Ther 1974;189:202-212.

228. Rackow H, Salanitre E, Green LT: Frequency of cardiac arrest associated with anesthesia in infants and children. Pediatrics 1961;28:697-704.

229. Rauck R, et al: Comparison of the efficacy of epidural morphine given by intermittent injection or continuous infusion for the management of postoperative pain. Reg Anesth 1994;19:316.

230. Rawlings DJ, Miller PA, Engel RR: The effect of circumcision on transcutaneous Po_2 in term infants. Am J Dis Child 1980;134:676-678.

231. Reid MF, Harris R, Phillips PD, et al: Day-case herniotomy in children: A comparison of ilio-inguinal nerve block and wound infiltration for postoperative analgesia. Anaesthesia 1987;42:658-661.

232. Reinhart D, Palladinetti T, Patel M, et al: IV ketorolac vs sufentanil for outpatient ENT surgery, a double-blind, randomized, placebo-controlled study. Anesthesiology 1992;77:3.

233. Reves JG, Fragen RJ, Vinik HR, et al: Midazolam: Pharmacology and uses. Anesthesiology 1985;62:310-324.

234. Rice L, Hannallah R: Local and regional anesthesia. In Motoyama E, Davis P (eds): Smiths' Anesthesia for Infants and Children. St Louis, CV Mosby, 1990, pp 393-426.

235. Rodgers BM, Webb CJ, Stergios D, et al: Patient-controlled analgesia in pediatric surgery. J Pediatr Surg 1988;23:259-262.

236. Romsing J, Moiniche S, Dahl JB: Rectal and parenteral paracetamol, and paracetamol in combination with NSAIDs, for postoperative analgesia. Br J Anaesth 2002;88:215-226.

237. Rosen DA, Morris JL, Rosen KR, et al: Analgesia for pediatric thoracostomy tube removal. Anesth Analg 2000;90:1025-1028.

238. Rosenberg H: International workshop on malignant hyerpyrexia. Anesthesiology 1981;54:530.

239. Ross AK, Eck JB, Tobias JD: Pediatric regional anesthesia: Beyond the caudal. Anesth Analg 2000;91:16-26.

240. Rowe M: Fluid and electrolyte management in pediatric surgery. In Welch K (ed): Pediatric Surgery, vol 2. Chicago, Year Book Medical Publishers, 1986.

241. Rowe MI, Arango A: Colloid versus crystalloid resuscitation in experimental bowel obstruction. J Pediatr Surg 1976;11:635-643.

242. Rowe MI, Rowe SA: The last fifty years of neonatal surgical management. Am J Surg 2000;180:345-352.

243. Roy RN, Sinclair JC: Hydration of the low birth-weight infant. Clin Perinatol 1975;2:393-417.

244. Russell IA, Miller Hance WC, Gregory G, et al: The safety and efficacy of sevoflurane anesthesia in infants and children with congenital heart disease. Anesth Analg 2001;92:1152-1158.

245. Rusy L, Houck C, Sullivan L, et al: A double-blind evaluation of ketorolac tromethamine versus acetaminophine in pediatric tonsillectomy: Analgesia and bleeding, Anesth Analg 1995;80:226-229.

246. Rusy LM, Weisman SJ: Complementary therapies for acute pediatric pain management. Pediatr Clin North Am 2000;47:589-599.

247. Ryan J: Malignant hyperthermia. In Cole E (ed): A Practice of Anesthesia for Infants and Children. Philadelphia, WB Saunders, 1993.

248. Rylance G: Clinical pharmacology: Drugs in children. BMJ (Clin Res Ed) 1981;282:50-51.

249. Sabatowski R, Kasper SM, Radbruch L: Patient-controlled analgesia with intravenous L-methadone in a child with cancer pain refractory to high-dose morphine. J Pain Symptom Manage 2002;23:3-5.

250. Sahler OJ, Hunter BC, Liesveld JL: The effect of using music therapy with relaxation imagery in the management of

patients undergoing bone marrow transplantation: A pilot feasibility study. Altern Ther Health Med 2003;9:70-74.

251. Sanders JC: Paediatric regional anaesthesia: A survey of practice in the United Kingdom. Br J Anaesth 2002;89: 707-710.

252. Sara CA, Lowry CJ: A complication of circumcision and dorsal nerve block of the penis. Anaesth Intensive Care 1985;13:79-82.

253. Sarner JB, Levine M, Davis PJ, et al: Clinical characteristics of sevoflurane in children: A comparison with halothane. Anesthesiology 1995;82:38-46.

254. Schechter N, Weisman S, Rosenblum M, et al: The use of oral transmucosal fentanyl citrate for painful procedures in children. Pediatrics 1995;95:335-339.

255. Schechter NL: The undertreatment of pain in children: An overview. Pediatr Clin North Am 1989;36:781-794.

256. Schindler M, Swann M, Crawford M: A comparison of postoperative analgesia provided by wound infiltration or caudal analgesia. Anaesth Intensive Care 1991;19:46-49.

257. Sebel PS, Lowdon JD: Propofol: A new intravenous anesthetic. Anesthesiology 1989;71:260-277.

258. Segredo V, Caldwell JE, Matthay MA, et al: Persistent paralysis in critically ill patients after long-term administration of vecuronium. N Engl J Med 1992;327:524-528.

259. Selbst S, Zempsky W: Sedation and analgesia in the emergency department. In Schechter N, Berde C, Yaster M (eds): Pain in Infants, Children, and Adolescents. Philadelphia, Lippincott Williams & Wilkins, 2003, pp 651-668.

260. Sethna N, Berde C: Pediatric regional anesthesia. In Gregory G (ed): Pediatric Anesthesia. New York, Churchill Livingstone, 1994, pp 281-318.

261. Shandling B, Steward DJ: Regional analgesia for postoperative pain in pediatric outpatient surgery. J Pediatr Surg 1980;15:477-480.

262. Shannon M, Berde CB: Pharmacologic management of pain in children and adolescents. Pediatr Clin North Am 1989;36:855-871.

263. Sharpe P, Klein JR, Thompson JP, et al: Analgesia for circumcision in a paediatric population: Comparison of caudal bupivacaine alone with bupivacaine plus two doses of clonidine. Paediatr Anaesth 2001;11:695-700.

264. Shear CR: Effects of disuse on growing and adult chick skeletal muscle. J Cell Sci 1981;48:35-54.

265. Shenkman Z, Holzman RS, Kim C, et al: Acupressure-acupuncture antiemetic prophylaxis in children undergoing tonsillectomy. Anesthesiology 1999;90:1311-1316.

266. Short TG, Chui PT: Propofol and midazolam act synergistically in combination. Br J Anaesth 1991;67:539-545.

267. Sievers TD, Yee JD, Foley ME, et al: Midazolam for conscious sedation during pediatric oncology procedures: Safety and recovery parameters. Pediatrics 1991;88:1172-1179.

268. Smith SM, Barry RC: A comparison of three formulations of TAC (tetracaine, adrenalin, cocaine) for anesthesia of minor lacerations in children. Pediatr Emerg Care 1990;6:266-270.

269. Somri M, Gaitini LA, Vaida SJ, et al: Effect of ilioinguinal nerve block on the catecholamine plasma levels in orchidopexy: Comparison with caudal epidural block. Paediatr Anaesth 2002;12:791-797.

270. Splinter W: Halothane: The end of an era? Anesth Analg 2002;95:1471.

271. Splinter WM, Schaefer JD, Zunder IH: Clear fluids three hours before surgery do not affect the gastric fluid contents of children. Can J Anaesth 1990;37:498-501.

272. Splinter WM, Schreiner MS: Preoperative fasting in children. Anesth Analg 1999;89:80-89.

273. Squire S, Kirchhoff K, Hissong K: Comparing two methods of topical anesthesia used before intravenous cannulation in pediatric patients. J Pediatr Health Care 2000;14:68-72.

274. Steward D: Premature infants are more prone to complications following minor surgery than are term infants. Anesthesiology 1982;56:304.

275. Steward DJ, Creighton RE: The uptake and excretion of nitrous oxide in the newborn. Can Anaesth Soc J 1978;25:215-217.

276. Stoelting RK, Longnecker DE: The effect of right-to-left shunt on the rate of increase of arterial anesthetic concentration. Anesthesiology 1972;36:352-356.

277. Streisand JB, Stanley TH, Hague B, et al: Oral transmucosal fentanyl citrate premedication in children. Anesth Analg 1989;69:28-34.

278. Suresh S, Barcelona S, Young N, et al: Does a preemptive block of the great auricular nerve improve postoperative analgesia in children undergoing tympanomastoid surgery? Anesth Analg 2004;98:330-333.

279. Taddio A, Katz J, Ilersich AL, et al: Effect of neonatal circumcision on pain response during subsequent routine vaccination. Lancet 1997;349:599-603.

280. Taddio A, Nulman I, Goldbach M, et al: Use of lidocaine-prilocaine cream for vaccination pain in infants. J Pediatr 1994;124:643-648.

281. Tanner G: Effects of left-to-right mixed left-to-right, and right-to-left shunts on inhalation anesethetic induction in children: A computer model. Anesth Analg 1985;64:101.

282. Taylor RH, Lerman J: Minimum alveolar concentration of desflurane and hemodynamic responses in neonates, infants, and children. Anesthesiology 1991;75:975-979.

283. Taylor RH, Lerman J: Induction, maintenance and recovery characteristics of desflurane in infants and children. Can J Anaesth 1992;39:6-13.

284. Tiret L, Nivoche Y, Hatton F, et al: Complications related to anaesthesia in infants and children: A prospective survey of 40240 anaesthetics. Br J Anaesth 1988;61:263-269.

285. Tobias J, Schleien C, Haun S: Methadone as treatment for iatrogenic narcotic dependency in pediatric intensive care unit patients. Crit Care Med 1990;18:1292-1293.

286. Tobias JD, Lynch A, McDuffee A, et al: Pancuronium infusion for neuromuscular block in children in the pediatric intensive care unit. Anesth Analg 1995;81:13-16.

287. Tobias JD, Phipps S, Smith B, et al: Oral ketamine premedication to alleviate the distress of invasive procedures in pediatric oncology patients. Pediatrics 1992;90:537-541.

288. Tome J: Intranasal midazolam does not delay discharge in patients having ultrashort surgical procedures. Anesth Analg 1993;40:A66.

289. Tree-Trakarn T, Pirayavaraporn S: Postoperative pain relief for circumcision in children: Comparison among morphine, nerve block, and topical analgesia. Anesthesiology 1985;62:519-522.

290. Tsuchiya N, Ichizawa M, Yoshikawa Y, et al: Comparison of ropivacaine with bupivacaine and lidocaine for ilioinguinal block after ambulatory inguinal hernia repair in children. Paediatr Anaesth 2004;14:468-470.

291. Tverskoy M, Cozacov C, Ayache M, et al: Postoperative pain after inguinal herniorrhaphy with different types of anesthesia. Anesth Analg 1990;70:29-35.

292. Twersky R: Midazolam enhances anterograde but not retrograde amnesia in pediatric patients. Anesthesiology 1993;78:51.

293. Uezono S, Goto T, Terui K, et al: Emergence agitation after sevoflurane versus propofol in pediatric patients. Anesth Analg 2000;91:563-566.

294. Valley RD, Bailey AG: Caudal morphine for postoperative analgesia in infants and children: A report of 138 cases. Anesth Analg 1991;72:120-124.

295. Valtonen M, Iisalo E, Kanto J, Rosenberg P: Propofol as an induction agent in children: Pain on injection and pharmacokinetics. Acta Anaesthesiol Scand 1989;33:152-155.

296. Valtonen M, Iisalo E, Kanto J, Tikkanen J: Comparison between propofol and thiopentone for induction of anaesthesia in children. Anaesthesia 1988;43:696-699.

297. Vator M, Wandless J: Caudal or dorsal nerve block? A comparison of two local anaesthestic techniques for postoperative analgesia following day case circumcision. Acta Anaesthesiol Scand 1985;29:175-179.

298. Veyckemans F, Scholtes JL, Ninane J: Cervical epidural analgesia for a cancer child at home. Med Pediatr Oncol 1994;22:58-60.

299. Voepel-Lewis T, Malviya S, Tait AR: A prospective cohort study of emergence agitation in the pediatric postanesthesia care unit. Anesth Analg 2003;96:1625-1630.

300. Walbergh E: Pharmacokinetics of intravenous and intranasal midazolam in children. Anesthesiology 1989;71:A1066.

301. Wark H, O'Halloran M, Overton J: Prospective study of liver function in children following multiple halothane anaesthetics at short intervals. Br J Anaesth 1986;58:1224-1228.

302. Warner LO, Beach TP, Garvin JP, et al: Halothane and children: The first quarter century. Anesth Analg 1984;63:838-840.

303. Warner M, et al: Practice guidelines for preoperative fasting and the use of pharmacologic agents to reduce the risk of pulmonary aspiration: Application to healthy patients undergoing elective procedures. A report by the American Society of Anesthesiologists Task Force on Preoperative Fasting. Anesthesiology 1999;90:896-905.

304. Watcha MF, Jones MB, Lagueruela RG, et al: Comparison of ketorolac and morphine as adjuvants during pediatric surgery. Anesthesiology 1992;76:368-372.

305. Watling S, Dasta J: Prolonged paralysis in intensive care unit patients after the use of neuromuscular blocking agents: A review of the literature. Crit Care Med 1994;22:884.

306. Way WL, Costley EC, Leongway E: Respiratory sensitivity of the newborn infant to meperidine and morphine. Clin Pharmacol Ther 1965;11:454-461.

307. Weber F, Wulf H: Caudal bupivacaine and s(+)-ketamine for postoperative analgesia in children. Paediatr Anaesth 2003;13:244-248.

308. Weiskopf RB, Moore MA, Eger EI 2nd, et al: Rapid increase in desflurane concentration is associated with greater transient cardiovascular stimulation than with rapid increase in isoflurane concentration in humans. Anesthesiology 1994;80:1035-1045.

309. Welborn L, Hannallah R: Anemia and postoperative apnea in former preterm infants. Anesthesiology 1991;74:1003-1006.

310. Welborn LG, Hannallah RS, Norden JM, et al: Comparison of emergence and recovery characteristics of sevoflurane, desflurane, and halothane in pediatric ambulatory patients. Anesth Analg 1996;83:917-920.

311. Welborn LG, McGill WA, Hannallah RS, et al: Perioperative blood glucose concentrations in pediatric outpatients. Anesthesiology 1986;65:543-547.

312. Welborne L: Postoperative apnea in former premature infants: Prospective comparison of spinal and general anesthesia. Anesthesiology 1990;72:838.

313. Weldon B, Connor M, White P: Nurse-controlled versus patient-controlled analgesia following pediatric scoliosis surgery. Anesthesiology 1991;75:3.

314. Weldon BC, Bell M, Craddock T: The effect of caudal analgesia on emergence agitation in children after sevoflurane versus halothane anesthesia. Anesth Analg 2004;98:321-326.

315. Weldon BC, Connor M, White PF: Pediatric PCA: The role of concurrent opioid infusions and nurse-controlled analgesia. Clin J Pain 1993;9:26-33.

316. Westrin P: The induction dose of propofol in infants 1-6 months of age and in children 10-16 years of age. Anesthesiology 1991;74:455-458.

317. Westrin P, Jonmarker C, Werner O: Thiopental requirements for induction of anesthesia in neonates and in infants one to six months of age. Anesthesiology 1989;71:344-346.

318. Wilder R, Berde C, Troshynski T, et al: Patient-controlled analgesia in children and adolescents: Safety and outcome among 1589 patients. Anesthesiology 1992;77:1187.

319. Williamson PS, Williamson ML: Physiologic stress reduction by a local anesthetic during newborn circumcision. Pediatrics 1983;71:36-40.

320. Wilton NC, Leigh J, Rosen DR, et al: Preanesthetic sedation of preschool children using intranasal midazolam. Anesthesiology 1988;69:972-975.

321. Wodey E, Pladys P, Copin C, et al: Comparative hemodynamic depression of sevoflurane versus halothane in infants: An echocardiographic study. Anesthesiology 1997;87:795-800.

322. Wodey E, Senhadji L, Pladys P, et al: The relationship between expired concentration of sevoflurane and sympathovagal tone in children. Anesth Analg 2003;97:377-382.

323. Wolf W, Neal M, Pertson M: The hemodynamic and cardiovascular effects of isoflurane and halothane anesthesia in children. Anesthesiology 1986;64:328.

324. Wood CE, Goresky GV, Klassen KA, et al: Complications of continuous epidural infusions for postoperative analgesia in children. Can J Anaesth 1994;41:613-620.

325. Woolf CJ, Chong MS: Preemptive analgesia—treating postoperative pain by preventing the establishment of central sensitization. Anesth Analg 1993;77:362-379.

326. Woolf CJ, Wall PD: Relative effectiveness of C primary afferent fibers of different origins in evoking a prolonged facilitation of the flexor reflex in the rat. J Neurosci 1986;6:1433-1442.

327. World Health Organization: Cancer Pain Relief: With a Guide to Opioid Availability, 2nd ed. Geneva, WHO, 1996.

328. Yaster M: Pain relief. Pediatrics 1995;95:427-428.

329. Yaster M, Kost-Byerly S, Maxwell L: Opioid agonists and antagonists. In Schechter N, Berde C, Yaster M (eds): Pain in Infants, Children, and Adolescents. Philadelphia, Lippincott Williams & Wilkins, 2003, pp 181-224.

330. Yaster M, Maxwell LG: Pediatric regional anesthesia. Anesthesiology 1989;70:324-338.

331. Yaster M, Nichols DG, Deshpande JK, et al: Midazolam-fentanyl intravenous sedation in children: Case report of respiratory arrest. Pediatrics 1990;86:463-467.

332. Yeoman PM, Cooke R, Hain WR: Penile block for circumcision? A comparison with caudal blockade. Anaesthesia 1983;38:862-866.

333. Zuppa AF, Helfaer MA, Adamson PC: Propofol pharmacokinetics. Pediatr Crit Care Med 2003;4:124-125.

334. Zwass MS, Fisher DM, Welborn LG, et al: Induction and maintenance characteristics of anesthesia with desflurane and nitrous oxide in infants and children. Anesthesiology 1992;76:373-378.

Chapter 14

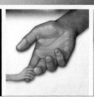

Ethical Considerations

Donna A. Caniano and Carolyn Ells

In his classic text *The Surgeon and the Child*, Potts noted that "the satisfaction of correcting a deformity in a newborn infant lies in the fact that all his life lies before him. Parents hope for miracles, but are grateful for the best that can be given by a mere human being."[19] This profound statement underscores the essence of pediatric surgery, whether repairing a major congenital anomaly, treating a devastating traumatic injury, or resecting a malignancy. Each endeavor offers the pediatric surgeon the joy of providing a child with relief of suffering and the potential for a full and productive life. The ethical challenges faced by pediatric surgeons encompass the basic moral principles of medical practice, issues that are distinctive to the profession of surgery, and other factors that are unique to the care of infants and children. In this chapter we review some of the basic ethical concepts and responsibilities pertinent to pediatric surgical ethics. We also address some new areas of ethical and surgical controversy, including the operative management of children with morbid obesity and sex assignment surgery in infants with intersex conditions.

PEDIATRIC SURGICAL ETHICS

What is distinctive about surgical ethics flows first from what is distinctive about the relationship between surgeons and their patients. Little[11] has identified five pillars that mark the moral domain of the surgeon-patient relationship: rescue, proximity, ordeal, aftermath, and presence. These factors may be present in other therapeutic relationships as well, but they have a special intensity in surgery.

The term *rescue* acknowledges the elements of surrender and dependency that patients and their families experience when surgery is pursued. To be rescued from a serious threat, patients open themselves up to invasive and traumatic surgical remedies over which they have little control. Surgeons and patients and their families (parents in most pediatric surgical encounters) need to work together to confront and negotiate the patient's surrender and dependency within the context of the surgeon's power.

Proximity refers to surgeons' acknowledgment of the close, intimate interactions they have with their patients. Remarkably, surgeons explore the inner bodies of their patients, an aspect of the encounter that differs from other medical interactions. Surgeons see and touch, and incise and suture, parts of patients that the patients themselves can barely imagine. Proximity privileges surgeons with knowledge and an understanding of suffering that patients cannot reciprocate. Patients cannot know their surgeons in this intimate way, nor can they know themselves in the way that their surgeons come to know them.

Surgeons must realize that surgery is an *ordeal* for patients; it is an extreme experience that must be endured. Little[11] has emphasized that surgical patients forgo their autonomy, acknowledge dependency, place trust, face risk, confront embodiment and mortality, lose control over time and space, and experience alienation, pain, fear, discomfort, suffering, and boredom. Depending on the surgical procedure, the patient's sense of personal identity may be irrevocably challenged or changed.

In the *aftermath* of surgery, surgeons must recognize that some patients may have difficulties long after their immediate recovery. Physical and emotional scars, discomfort, risks, and other types of suffering can be reminders of a past illness or injury and signs of vulnerability to future illness or injury. Understanding the aftermath of surgery can help surgeons understand threats to their patients' existential experiences, as well as to their own. In pediatric surgery, aftermath takes on a unique aspect in its dual nature, affecting the child-patient and the parents, both of whom experience the consequences of the surgical encounter.

Presence is both a virtue and a duty for surgeons. They must be a visible and engaged presence throughout the entire surgical experience. In pediatric surgery, this professional obligation extends to the long-term follow-up of their patients, often into young adulthood. For example, pediatric surgeons may be the only specialists who understand the potential long-term complications and functional difficulties that may arise from major neonatal reconstructive operations in the gastrointestinal and hepatobiliary systems. Meeting this duty requires a patient-centered approach to care in which each patient, and his or her particular situation and experience, guides the surgeon in nurturing the surgical relationship and promoting the patient's interests.

Surgeons bring to the surgical relationship the values and ethical principles of their profession, which give priority to the interests and well-being of their patients. In *Surgical Ethics*, McCullough et al.[12] present patients' rights related to the surgical encounter, each of which implies a key professional value. They remind us that patients have the right "not to be killed intentionally or negligently by the surgeon, not to be harmed by intent or negligence of the surgeon ... not to be deceived by the surgeon ... to be adequately informed about the risks and benefits of surgery, to be treated by a knowledgeable, competent practitioner, to have his or her health and well-being more highly valued than the surgeon's own economic interest, and to decide whether to accept treatment under the conditions described."[12]

In pediatric surgery, the professional commitment to fully inform patients, to enable them to choose treatment or nontreatment, and to not deceive them typically requires third parties (in most cases, their parents) to speak, understand, and consent on behalf of infants, children, and adolescents. Although parents are usually the surrogate decision makers for their children, court-appointed guardians or other spokespersons may fulfill this role, depending on relevant laws. In some jurisdictions, and in certain specific circumstances, adolescent patients may be granted authority to make their own decisions about the health care they receive. This situation is particularly applicable to adolescents with chronic illnesses, such as sickle cell disease, cystic fibrosis, and advanced malignancies. However, when an adolescent's consent to or refusal of surgery is in direct opposition to parental wishes, the assistance of social services and legal counsel may be required.

Including the family or surrogate decision makers in the surgical relationship is necessary not just to authorize (or refuse) surgery on behalf of patients. Providing patient-centered care requires an understanding that the patient lives in a family context, which defines, in part, who he or she is as an individual. It also requires acknowledging the greater vulnerability of minor patients who have less of a voice—or often no voice—in treatment decisions and little or no understanding of the surgical process. These patients must be provided with the support they need to optimize their care and the protection they need in light of their vulnerability. Extending the surgical relationship to others helps the surgeon understand the patient and make recommendations that are in the patient's best interests, and it allows others to share in providing the support that these young patients require.

One ethical challenge routinely faced by pediatric surgeons (and surrogate decision makers) is determining the interests of patients whose moral characters and values are not yet substantially (much less fully) formed. The character traits, goals, values, and preferences of minor patients should be factored into plans for their care, but judgment is needed to determine what weight to give them.

Pediatric surgeons should have in their armamentarium various approaches to ethical decision making and problem solving. Baylis and Caniano[1] advocate a team approach to difficult ethical problems encountered in the surgical treatment of infants and children. This approach acknowledges that contemporary health care in tertiary pediatric hospitals relies on several teams: the patient-parent unit, the nursing and allied health care members, and the surgical-medical professionals. The health care team for any given patient must unite around a common moral language and an understanding of the ethical issues relative to the particular situation. For example, the caregivers and decision makers for an extremely premature neonate with multiple congenital anomalies must have practical and cognitive knowledge about the pertinent ethical issues. The team or team leaders must have the capacity to elucidate the values and goals that are important to the parents and other involved family members. The values of the parents and family assume particular relevance when their cultural or religious background differs from that of the health care team in substantive ways. For instance, certain cultural practices may dictate that the authority for medical decision making resides with individuals other than the parents, such as grandparents or community elders. Finally, the team must decide on a specific decision-making method.

Several maxims apply to difficult ethical problems in pediatric surgery: (1) good ethics begin with good facts; (2) rational people may hold opposing and irreconcilable views; (3) generally, the best decisions are those developed by consensus; (4) most decisions do not need to be made in haste; and (5) in cases of severe neonatal and pediatric illness, most decisions are painful, and many do not have happy solutions.

Most ethical dilemmas arise when there is a dispute or disagreement between the surgical-medical professionals and the patient-parents. These disagreements usually center on what constitutes the best interests of the patient (e.g., continued life with the burdens of severe disability) and what describes an acceptable quality of life for the patient. Glover and Caniano[7] have outlined a process for ethical decision making that involves several components, including identifying the decision makers, gathering all the medical-surgical facts with the best available prognostic indications, clarifying the relevant values from the "stakeholders" (usually the parents or close family members, in the case of infants), defining all available treatment and nontreatment options, evaluating all options and making recommendations (usually the responsibility of the pediatric surgeon), and achieving a consensus resolution (an ethics consultant or mediator may be useful in cases of significant dispute). Some of these approaches are addressed later in this chapter, when we discuss some of the newer ethical challenges faced by pediatric surgeons.

INNOVATION AND RESEARCH

Most citizens of progressive societies place great value on innovation in all areas, including medicine. To achieve advances and technical improvements in pediatric surgery, the profession has relied on the individual and collective innovation of its members. Society expects surgeons to pursue innovation and to develop new therapies and treatment techniques. Patients gravitate toward new operations that offer a presumed benefit, as witnessed by the rapid conversion from open to laparoscopic cholecystectomy 2 decades ago. Patients also give great latitude to their surgeons in allowing, or even expecting, them to modify or refine traditional surgical techniques as necessary to complete an operation. McKneally[13] observed that individual surgeons are usually acknowledged for their original thinking and technical accomplishments by having operations named in their honor. Numerous operations in pediatric surgery carry the names of those surgeons who first described them, including Ladd's procedure for midgut volvulus and the Duhamel pull-through for Hirschsprung's disease.

In contrast to other areas of medicine, in which randomized clinical trials precede the introduction of new drugs and treatments, the field of surgery has been free to develop new operations without stringent legal and professional regulations.[6] Although some notable procedures, such as pneumatic reduction of intussusception and the Swenson pull-through for Hirschsprung's disease, were tested in animal models, most operations in pediatric surgery are piloted and perfected on patients. New operations are typically introduced by means of a presentation at a professional meeting of pediatric surgeons and subsequent publication in a peer-reviewed journal. The pediatric surgeon who developed the operation usually reports on his or her experience, in terms of complications and outcomes, in patients treated at a single institution with a variable period of follow-up.

Reasons given for adopting operations in humans without rigorous scrutiny include the following: (1) suitable animal models may be lacking for the particular anatomic condition; (2) the new operation represents an extension of standard, accepted techniques applied in a novel manner; (3) the new operation is meant to benefit an individual patient rather than to learn something; (4) professional standards are lacking for the introduction of new operations; (5) it is often unclear when an operation should undergo clinical trials; and (6) the current system has worked reasonably well for patients in terms of safety and presumed benefit. In fact, numerous operations have been abandoned either because they did not achieve the desired outcome (e.g., sympathectomy for Hirschsprung's disease) or because they had unacceptably high morbidity and mortality rates (e.g., jejunoileal bypass for morbid obesity).

Research is considered to be a systematic investigation designed to develop or contribute generalizable knowledge. In pediatric surgery, an operation may be performed in a novel way to treat a single patient; thus, in a strict sense, such an operation is not research. But, as is often the case, subsequent operations are performed on additional patients, data are collected, and the novel procedure is presented and published. What began as a treatment for a single patient has crossed over into clinical research, making it subject to the ethical standards for human investigation.

In 1966 Beecher published a seminal article in the *New England Journal of Medicine* detailing several examples of medical and surgical treatments that had been published in respected journals yet violated the ethical norms of informed consent and safety.[2] Although the Nuremberg trials following World War II had unveiled the horrors of unethical human experimentation,

mainstream medical research in the United States was largely unregulated, and examples of unethical research practices were problematic. Beecher's report galvanized the public to demand, and the federal government to require, institutional review to ensure the ethical acceptability of all research (medical, behavioral, and surgical) on human subjects.

Through the National Research Act of 1974, the National Commission for the Protection of Human Subjects of Biomedical and Behavioral Research convened a group of respected clinical scientists, physicians, and experts in ethics, religion, and law to review the basic principles that should characterize the conduct of research involving human subjects and to develop guidelines to ensure the conduct of ethical research. The commission issued its summary statement, the Belmont Report,[17] in 1979. The report identified the principles of respect for persons (which it divided into respect for autonomy and protection of the vulnerable), beneficence, and justice as particularly relevant to research ethics. These principles have subsequently become important in clinical practice as well, although their application differs. Within the Belmont Report were two features of critical importance to pediatric surgeons: the role of informed consent for research subjects, and the protection that must be accorded when research is performed on vulnerable subjects, such as children.

Parents and society expect that pediatric surgeons will be conservative guardians in surgical innovation, relying on a long tradition of generally safe operations and of progress in ameliorating the effects of congenital anomalies. Levine[10] has described some newly introduced procedures as *nonvalidated,* a term that acknowledges the ethical and medical hazards of novel operations, which may be obscured by the terminology of innovation. For both pediatric surgeons and parents, the concept of a nonvalidated operation is more transparent and honest; it embodies the fact that the proposed operation has not been subjected to rigorous clinical investigation. The presumption that a given novel operation is superior to its traditional counterpart is, in reality, a presumption only if it lacks an empirical basis. Clinical trials of a nonvalidated operation may reveal that it is superior to, equal to, or worse than conventional procedures. For example, the recent National Institutes of Health–funded clinical trial of fetal endoscopic tracheal occlusion for congenital diaphragmatic hernia was stopped after the enrollment of 24 patients because survival was unexpectedly higher for the infants who received standard care (planned delivery and postnatal care at a tertiary center) compared with those undergoing the fetal intervention.[8]

Lacking rigorous scrutiny, the current system of surgical innovation may hinder the determination of an optimal surgical therapy for a given condition. A compelling argument can be made that pediatric surgeons have an ethical obligation to participate in well-designed prospective, multi-institutional clinical trials that seek to establish the best operations or treatments for their patients.[3] Patients and their families have a right to expect pediatric surgeons to practice competent surgical care that includes the best proven surgical treatments and operations. When pediatric surgeons perform nonvalidated operations on their patients, no matter how well intentioned, they may be providing treatments that are not optimal, because they have not been rigorously tested.

BARIATRIC SURGERY

Obesity among children and adolescents is recognized as a major public health concern in many developed countries. In the United States, obesity affects about 16% of children, one third of whom are considered morbidly obese. Although the causes of this trend are not fully apparent, the decline in physical activity and the high-calorie diets of American children are likely contributing factors.

Obesity in children and adolescents has significant ramifications for the individual and for public health. Because obesity is associated with serious conditions such as hyperlipidemia, hypertension, and type 2 diabetes, the financial and social costs are high. The adverse psychological factors associated with obesity in children and adolescents have not been well studied, but these may have considerable social and financial costs as well. Health care professionals and the broader social community share concerns about the effects of obesity on children and adolescents, in part because of the serious ramifications for their physical and mental health and long-term well-being.

Treatment for morbid obesity includes medical and surgical approaches. The range of success with these approaches varies, and research is needed to better assess them, particularly in a pediatric population. Medical therapy that includes a comprehensive program of exercise and diet has not been successful in adults over the long term. Few children's hospitals have developed comprehensive medical obesity programs; thus, there is scant evidence in the pediatric literature about the outcomes of such programs.

For adults with morbid obesity, surgical therapy is quite popular because it has been successful in achieving weight reduction with acceptable morbidity and mortality rates. Based on the good results in the adult population, it is not surprising that pediatric surgeons are being asked by the public—in particular, eager patients and their parents—to provide bariatric surgery for children and adolescents with morbid obesity (see Chapter 78).

Roux-en-Y gastric bypass and gastric banding, both performed laparoscopically, are the two bariatric operations performed most frequently in adults in North America and Europe. Although both achieve weight loss, gastric banding does not alter the anatomy and is reversible; gastric bypass alters the anatomy in an essentially irreversible manner. Gastric bypass is very effective in achieving weight loss not only because it reduces the size of the stomach but also because it causes malabsorption. Long-term studies in adults indicate that gastric banding is somewhat less effective in achieving major weight loss but is successful in reducing the comorbid conditions of hypertension and diabetes.

There are some ethical concerns about bariatric surgery that pediatric surgeons should consider.[9] Both operations are currently nonvalidated therapies for pediatric patients, and neither safety nor efficacy has been proved by multi-institutional clinical trials in this population. Patients and their surrogate decision makers should understand the nonvalidated nature of these operations before they make an informed choice to have a bariatric operation. Moreover, pediatric surgeons performing these operations should participate, whenever possible, in well-designed clinical studies that seek to define the safety, efficacy, and long-term outcomes of these surgeries in pediatric patients with morbid obesity. As with other nonvalidated treatments, research evaluating the safety and efficacy of bariatric procedures should be designed in a way that does not interfere with the therapeutic objectives of patients.

Because of insufficient research and the relatively recent history of bariatric surgery (isolated case reports in adolescents), the risks and potential benefits of these operations are difficult to assess. Although early results have shown these operations to be safe for adolescents, the long-term outcomes are unknown. The gastric bypass operation raises concerns about chronic nutritional issues, such as vitamin deficiencies, and possible adverse effects over a lifetime. An additional concern is that patients must comply with prescribed dietary restrictions and undergo medical surveillance indefinitely. It is generally well recognized that patients tend to forgo regular checkups over the long term, particularly if they have no physical complaints. Because the long-term risks of these operations for adolescents are unknown, subtle aberrations in physiology that would be detected by close medical supervision might go unnoticed and undiagnosed until they cause serious consequences.

Risks alone do not render a therapy unethical. The ethical assessment of risks involves taking into account the gravity of the risks, the probability that they will occur, and the potential benefits that patients may experience. The potential benefits should be assessed in light of the available evidence and the particular patient's situation. Where there are gaps in research, pediatric surgeons should draw on evidence from the adult population and extrapolate to adolescent patients, as their experience and expertise deem appropriate. In the informed choice process, pediatric surgeons should be honest with patients and their surrogate decision makers about what is known, what is unknown, and the reasoning behind their recommendations regarding a bariatric operation for a particular patient.

For children or adolescents with morbid obesity, bariatric surgery may be viewed as a quick and easy "fix" compared with nonsurgical means of achieving weight loss. Quick and easy solutions are certainly desirable, but if nonsurgical means or less invasive procedures are (or prove to be) safer or more effective, or if they protect important options for children and adolescents (e.g., the ability to make important decisions about their health, bodies, and lives in the future), pediatric surgeons should be wary about agreeing to perform bariatric surgery. Pediatric surgeons, in their role as child advocates, have a professional responsibility to encourage a more balanced reflection and assessment of the therapeutic options for morbid obesity. In general, surgeons should be hesitant to operate on patients who are not capable of making their own informed decisions when the surgery can be safely delayed until they are capable of making such decisions. This is especially true when the surgery has irreversible effects and the safety and efficacy of the surgery are unknown. Pediatric surgeons must consider not only whether bariatric surgery is a potential therapeutic option for a particular patient but also whether it is the *best* option for a particular patient. Although the choice to have or forgo surgery is ultimately up to the patient and his or her surrogate decision makers, the surgeon's recommendations are usually an important factor. For some patients, this may mean recommending a less effective but reversible surgical technique or delaying a decision about surgery until the patient is older and pursuing medical therapy in the meantime.

SEX ASSIGNMENT SURGERY

A variety of conditions in infancy, including ambiguous genitalia, cloacal exstrophy, and penile agenesis, may lead pediatric surgeons to consider sex assignment surgery. During the past decade, the traditional medical and surgical management of newborns with genital ambiguity has become controversial, with individuals who were "reconstructed" in infancy challenging the appropriateness of their treatment and questioning the success of their outcomes. Through advocacy organizations such as the Intersex Society of North America and the Androgen Insensitivity Support Group, adults with intersexuality (most of whom had sex assignment surgery in infancy and childhood) have publicly voiced their extreme dissatisfaction with several aspects of their medical and surgical care.

Intersex is the term now used by medical professionals and the public to refer to congenital conditions that result in nonstandard male or female genital anatomy. A primary assumption underlying sex assignment surgery is that having nonstandard genitalia will cause psychological harm and that this harm can be avoided or reduced by performing surgery to normalize the appearance of the genitals, so that the child can be raised in the gender that corresponds to his or her genital appearance. An infant born with ambiguous genitalia was traditionally considered to have an emergency condition that required prompt diagnosis, exclusion of the life-threatening form of congenital adrenal hyperplasia, and a determination of the appropriate sex of rearing, based largely on anatomic considerations. Neonatologists, pediatric endocrinologists, and pediatric surgeons based their management on the theories of psychosexual development espoused by Money,[16] a renowned psychologist at the Johns Hopkins University. His work defined an individual's *sex* on the basis of the sex organs and an individual's *gender* on the sex role the individual adopted. His theory of psychosexual differentiation held that prenatal influences affect personality traits, including aggressive behavior and maternal feelings, but that the postnatal environment is the primary determinant of gender identity. In essence, Money's theory implied that for humans, behaviors that are denoted male or female are sociocultural constructs rather than biologic imperatives.

For infants with intersexuality, Money's theories had significant implications for decisions about the sex of rearing. First, because the postnatal environment would be critical in determining the infant's gender identity, successful treatment would involve giving unequivocal and clear messages about that gender identity. Second, because gender identity does not depend on the cause of the genital ambiguity, sex and gender assignment should be based on anatomic considerations (and the potential for surgical reconstruction), reproductive potential, and capacity for intercourse. Thus, the individual was assigned a sex and a gender that were medically determined and, in most cases, reinforced by surgical reconstruction in infancy.

Advocates from the intersex organizations, social scientists, and others cite several concerns about early sex assignment surgery. They have identified a paucity of objective, long-term, multi-institutional data on outcome in terms of sexual function, sexual pleasure, and psychosexual identity.[14] Single-institution series involving small numbers of patients who had feminizing surgery in infancy have reported acceptable anatomic, functional, and psychosexual outcomes.[18] Other more recent reports (in which the evaluators were not part of the original pediatric surgical team) indicate that the long-term results of feminizing surgery are not optimal, with functional problems and poor cosmesis.[4,15] A recent study of 14 genetic males with cloacal exstrophy who had female sex assignment surgery in the newborn period found discordant sexual identity in 8 individuals, who reassigned themselves as male.[20] Because there are so few reports on comprehensive outcomes for the various intersex conditions, it is not clear whether the dissatisfaction voiced by those opposed to early sex assignment surgery represents a vocal minority of patients or is reflective of less than optimal results in the majority of patients.

A major ethical concern about the traditional approach involves the paternalistic decision making of medical and surgical professionals. Parents were frequently not given the entire truth about the diagnosis, and if they were, they were told to withhold certain aspects of the condition from the child to lessen gender identity conflicts. Thus, for most individuals with intersexuality, their diagnosis was not revealed to them by their parents or physicians. As adults or adolescents, if they experienced gender identity problems or sexual difficulties and eventually discovered the truth, they expressed tremendous anger and resentment about their treatment as infants and children. In addition to causing disrespect and distrust toward parents and physicians, lying to patients about their intersexuality and withholding their medical histories denies them the opportunity to come to terms with who they are and what has happened to them, to receive psychological counseling, and to seek support from others who have had the same or similar experiences. The ethical duty of informed consent requires that parents of infants with intersexuality be given all relevant information about the diagnosis, treatment options (including no early sex assignment surgery), expected outcomes (including the paucity of comprehensive data on long-term results), and the availability of advocacy organizations and counseling.

In most cases, early sex assignment surgery is not necessary for the infant's physical health. In fact, advocates from the intersex organizations argue that it is not necessary for the child's psychological health either and that it sometimes causes harm. Daaboul and Frader[5] argue that a "middle way" approach should be adopted when making decisions about infants with severely intersexed genitalia and complete discordance with the assigned gender.[5] They note that delaying surgical reconstruction in these infants may cause considerable psychosocial difficulty in the school-age and adolescent years. Further, there are no reliable data on the outcomes of intersex children in developed countries whose genitalia are significantly discordant with their assigned gender. Parents of these severely affected infants should be allowed to make decisions regarding early sex assignment surgery, as long as they have been given full disclosure of the current state of knowledge (or lack thereof) about functional and sexual outcomes.

Adherence to the ethical obligation of full and honest disclosure to the parents of infants with intersexuality should include a willingness by pediatric endocrinologists and pediatric surgeons to honor parental choices, including the rejection of early sex assignment surgery. As long as deferral of surgery carries no risk of physical harm (infection, malignancy in dysgenetic gonads), parents of these infants should be accorded the same authority for decision making that they are given in all other areas of medical treatment.

REFERENCES

1. Baylis F, Caniano DA: Medical ethics and the pediatric surgeon. In Oldham KT, Colombani PM, Foglia RP (eds): Surgery of Infants and Children: Scientific Principles and Practice. Philadelphia, Lippincott-Raven, 1997, p 382.
2. Beecher H: Ethics and clinical research. N Engl J Med 1966;274:1354.
3. Caniano DA: Ethical issues in the management of neonatal surgical anomalies. Semin Perinatol 2004;28:240.
4. Creighton SM, Minto CL, Steele SJ: Objective cosmetic and anatomical outcomes at adolescence of feminizing surgery for ambiguous genitalia done in childhood. Lancet 2001; 358:124.
5. Daaboul J, Frader J: Ethics and the management of the patient with intersex: A middle way. J Pediatr Endocrinol Metab 2001;14:1575.
6. Frader J, Caniano DA: Research and innovation in surgery. In McCullough LB, Jones JW, Brody BA (eds): Surgical Ethics. New York, Oxford University Press, 1998.
7. Glover JJ, Caniano DA: Ethical considerations in newborn surgery. In Puri P (ed): Newborn Surgery. Oxford, Butterworth-Heinemann, 2003.
8. Harrison MR, Keller Rl, Hawgood SB, et al: A randomized trial of fetal endoscopic occlusion for severe fetal congenital diaphragmatic hernia. N Engl J Med 2003;349:1916.
9. Inge TH, Krebs NF, Garcia VF, et al: Bariatric surgery for severely overweight adolescents: Concerns and recommendations. Pediatrics 2003;114:217.
10. Levine RJ: Ethics and Regulation of Clinical Research, 2nd ed. New Haven, Conn, Yale University Press, 1988.
11. Little M: Invited commentary: Is there a distinctively surgical ethics? Surgery 2001;129:668.
12. McCullough LB, Jones JW, Brody BA: Principles and practice of surgical ethics. In McCullough LB, Jones JW, Brody BA (eds): Surgical Ethics. New York, Oxford University Press, 1998.
13. McKneally MF: Ethical problems in surgery: Innovation leading to unforeseen complications. World J Surg 1999;23:786.
14. Meyer-Bahlburg HF: Gender assignment and reassignment in 46,XY pseudohermaphroditism and related conditions. J Clin Endocrinol Metab 1999;84:3455.
15. Minto CL, Liao LM, Woodhouse CRJ, et al: The effect of clitoral surgery on sexual outcome in individuals who have intersex conditions with ambiguous genitalia: A cross-sectional study. Lancet 2003;361:1252.
16. Money J: Gender: History, theory and usage of the term in sexology and its relationship to nature/nurture. J Sex Marital Ther 1985;11:71.
17. National Commission for the Protection of Human Subjects of Biomedical and Behavioral Research: The Belmont Report. OPPR Reports. Washington, DC, US Government Printing Office, 1979.
18. Newman K, Randolph J, Parson S: Functional results in young women having clitoral reconstruction as infants. J Pediatr Surg 1992;27:180.
19. Potts WJ: The Surgeon and the Child. Philadelphia, WB Saunders, 1959, p 3.
20. Reiner WG, Gearhart JP: Discordant sexual identity in some genetic males with cloacal exstrophy assigned to female sex at birth. N Engl J Med 2004;350:333.

Part II

TRAUMA

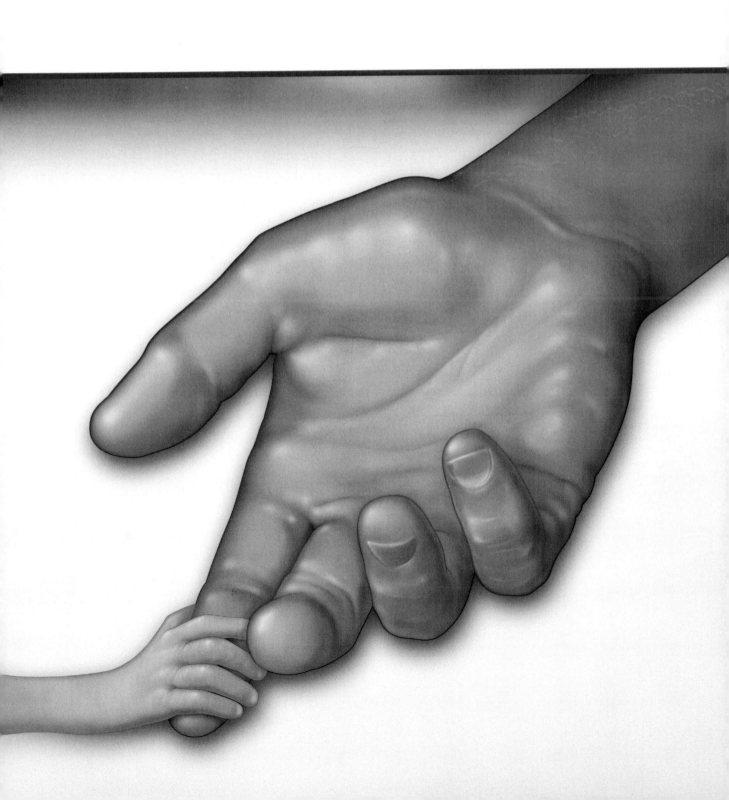

Chapter 15

Accident Victims and Their Emergency Management

Jeffrey R. Lukish and Martin R. Eichelberger

EPIDEMIOLOGY OF CHILDHOOD INJURY

Preventable injuries take an enormous financial and emotional toll on injured children and their families, but also on society as a whole. Unintentional injury is the leading cause of death among children aged 14 and younger in the United States, claiming more than 5600 lives annually or, an average, 15 children each day.[2] In addition, there were nearly 11.8 million medical visits for unintentional injury among American children aged 14 and younger in 2000, or one injury visit for every five children. More than 16% of all hospitalizations for unintentional injuries among children result in permanent disability.[4]

The death rate from unintentional injuries among children aged 14 and younger declined 39% from 1987 to 2000; it declined 42% for children between 1 and 14 years. Nevertheless, unintentional injury continues to be the leading cause of death among children in this age group in the United States. In 2000 the leading cause of fatal unintentional injury among children was motor vehicle occupant injury (28%), followed by drowning (16%) and airway obstruction injury (14%). Falls were the leading cause (36%) of nonfatal injuries seen in hospital emergency rooms in 2001.[20]

Leading causes of unintentional injury–related death vary according to child's age and are dependent on the child's developmental abilities and exposure to potential hazards, in addition to parental perceptions of their child's abilities and injury risk. The smallest decline in the injury death rate occurred among infants younger than 1 year; the decline in that age group was only 10%, compared with 42% in those aged 1 to 4 years, 42% in those 5 to 9 years, and 40% in those 10 to 14 years. Children younger than 1 year have the highest rate of unintentional injury–related death—more than twice that of all children. Airway obstruction is the leading killer in this age group. In children aged 1 to 4 years, drowning accounts for 27% of unintentional injury deaths and is the leading cause of injury-related death. The lowest rate of unintentional death is in the 5- to 9-year age group; the most common cause of death in this age group and in those aged 10 to 14 years is motor vehicle occupant injury (Fig. 15-1).[20]

In all age groups, male children are at higher risk for unintentional injury than are females. This may be due to greater exposure to activities that result in injury, risk taking, and rough play in male children. Race and ethnicity are also important risk factors for unintentional injury in children. American Indian and Alaskan native children have the highest unintentional injury death rate, and African American children have the second highest. These racial and ethnic disparities likely have more to do with living in impoverished communities, a primary predictor of injury, than with biologic differences.[17,20]

Intentional injury and death may result from homicide, child abuse, or suicide. Recognition of this intent requires referral to child protective services for assessment. The resuscitation of these children is frequently a challenge because abuse may be chronic, which results in a child with a limited physiologic reserve (refer to Chapter 24 on child abuse).

RESUSCITATION AND IMPACT ON OUTCOME

Resuscitation of an injured child includes the actions necessary to reverse and control the sudden alterations in physiologic homeostasis that occur as a result of injury. Children are remarkably resilient; however, the initial period of stability has been shown to be significantly shorter as age decreases.[19] Therefore, resuscitation is not complete until injuries have been definitively treated and the child displays physiologic stability without continued intervention.

Differences between children and adults with respect to patterns of injury, physiologic presentation, and management are important, particularly in children younger than 2 years. Physicians who treat injured children must recognize and understand these important distinctions so that the resuscitation process addresses the special needs of the child.

The principle of a trimodal pattern of trauma-related mortality and morbidity in adults must be modified

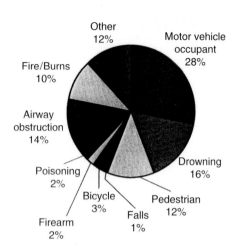

Leading Causes of Fatal
Unintentional Injury
Children 14 and under, 2000

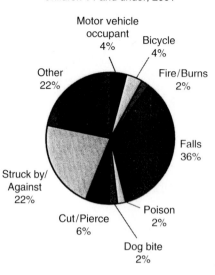

Leading Causes of Nonfatal
Unintentional Injury
Children 14 and under, 2001

Figure 15–1 Percentage of fatal and nonfatal unintentional injuries in children aged 14 years and younger in the United States, 2000-2001. (From National Center for Health Statistics, Centers for Disease Control and Prevention: National Electronic Injury Surveillance System All Injury Program, 2003.)

for children. In the trimodal model, the first mortality peak among injured children occurs within seconds or minutes after injury, due to damage to the central or peripheral nervous system and the central vasculature. Survival can be improved in this group only through prevention efforts. The second mortality peak occurs minutes to hours after injury and is due to mass lesions in the central nervous system (CNS), usually subdural and epidural hematomas; solid organ injury; or collections of fluid in the pleural and pericardial spaces. These injuries require rapid identification and treatment because the time limit for effective resuscitation is shorter in children than in adults by as much as 50%; the Advanced Trauma Life Support protocol focuses on such injuries. Although initial physiologic compensation may have been sufficient to achieve some temporary accommodation, progressive dysfunction and exhausted reserves bring about a critical impairment of oxygen delivery and the child's eventual demise. Advances in the aggressive and systematic delivery of emergency medical services for children have had a salutary effect on preventable death in children. The third mortality peak occurs days to weeks after the initial injury and is the result of complications of injury such as sepsis and systemic inflammatory response syndrome, leading to multiple organ failure syndrome.[18] This late peak in trauma-related mortality is less frequent in younger children.

PRINCIPLES OF RESUSCITATION

Prehospital Care

Systematic management is essential to an injured child's survival. The resuscitation process begins when emergency transport personnel first encounter the child in the field. The fate of any child can turn on the decisions and interventions that transpire during these first crucial moments. The injury-adjusted death rate for children is twice that of adults in the out-of-hospital phase of resuscitation. Similarly, the survival rate for out-of-hospital cardiac arrest in children is only half that of adults.[15] Although part of this discrepancy results from the different causes of cardiac arrest in children and adults, unfamiliarity and inadequate training with children also contributes to poor outcome. The failure rate for resuscitation interventions in the field is twice as high in children as in adults; the failure rate for prehospital endotracheal intubation in children is close to 50%.[11] Unfamiliarity with pediatric resuscitation skills is understandable; although trauma is the most common indication for pediatric ambulance transport, it accounts for less than 10% of total paramedic patient volume in most metropolitan areas.

The most important objectives for emergency personnel in the field are:

1. Recognition and treatment of immediate life-threatening dysfunction.
2. Assessment of the mechanism of trauma and extent of injuries.
3. Documentation of pertinent medical data.
4. Triage to an appropriate-level pediatric trauma facility.

Added to these are the challenges of comforting a terrified and hurt child as well as the distraught parents. Thus, the paramedic's task can be formidable. Consequently, prehospital personnel function best by adopting strict protocols to treat injured children. The priorities and techniques associated with pediatric field resuscitation are similar to those for emergency department care described later.

Primary Survey and Treatment of Life-Threatening Injuries

When an injured child encounters medical personnel, whether in the field or in the emergency room, events should transpire in a rapid sequence designed to recognize and treat acute injuries. This systematic approach allows the standardization of diagnostic and treatment decisions so that individual variations in patterns of injury do not prevent caregivers from recognizing and treating subtle injuries that can have a profound impact on outcome. This systematic framework comprises a primary survey, a resuscitation phase, and a definitive secondary survey. The primary survey is the initial process of identifying and temporizing injuries that are potentially life threatening and follows the ABCDE sequence: airway, breathing, circulation, disability, and exposure. The system relies on simple observations to assess physiologic derangement and immediate intervention to prevent death.

Airway and Cervical Spine Control

Provision of airway control is perhaps the least controversial of all priorities in pediatric trauma management. The inability to establish and maintain a child's airway, leading to hypoxia and inadequate ventilation, continues to be a common cause of cardiorespiratory arrest and death. Significant clinical hypoxia is suspected when oxygen saturation is less than 95%.

Assessment of the airway includes inspection of the oral cavity; manual removal of debris, loose teeth, and soft tissue fragments; and aspiration of blood and secretions with mechanical suction. If a child is neurologically intact, phonates normally, and is ventilating without stridor or distress, invasive airway management is unnecessary. Airway patency can be improved in a spontaneously breathing child by the use of jaw-thrust or chin-lift maneuvers.

An airway that is unsecured because of coma, combativeness, shock, or direct airway trauma requires endotracheal intubation. A nasopharyngeal or oropharyngeal airway can improve management during bag-mask ventilation, but this is a temporizing measure until definitive control is established. In most cases, orotracheal intubation with in-line cervical spine stabilization is the preferred approach to airway control. Although nasotracheal intubation is recommended in nonapneic adults with potential cervical spine injuries, this approach is not indicated and is poorly tolerated in children.

Pediatric airway anatomy is unique and affects management technique. The child's larynx is anatomically higher and more anterior than in the adult, necessitating an upward angulation of the laryngoscope to place the endotracheal tube properly. Removing the anterior half of the rigid cervical collar allows access to the neck for gentle cricoid pressure. The pediatric epiglottis is shorter, less flexible, and tilted posteriorly over the glottic inlet. Because of this, direct control of the epiglottis with a straight blade is usually necessary for proper visualization of the vocal cords. The vocal cords themselves are fragile and easily damaged. The narrowest point in the pediatric airway is the subglottic trachea at the cricoid ring, as opposed to the glottis in adult patients. Therefore, passage of the endotracheal tube through the vocal cords does not guarantee safe advancement into the trachea or avoidance of subglottic injury. Appropriate endotracheal tube selection is an important part of pediatric resuscitation. The internal diameter can range from 3.0 to 3.5 mm in newborns to 4.5 mm at 1 to 2 years of age. After 2 years of age, the internal diameter can be estimated by the following formula: Internal diameter = Age/4 + 4. Approximating the diameter of the patient's little finger is also useful. Because of the narrow subglottic trachea, an uncuffed endotracheal tube is indicated in children 8 years of age or younger (Fig. 15-2).[11,13]

The technique of intubation depends on the urgency of establishing an airway. In a hypotensive, hypoxemic, comatose child, orotracheal intubation is accomplished without delay as an integral part of the resuscitation. In a more elective situation, more attention is given to adequate preoxygenation by bag-mask ventilation with 100% oxygen and premedication. Thoracic trauma can preclude intubation or make attainment of adequate oxygen saturation impossible. Inducing hypocarbia (carbon dioxide partial pressure [$PaCO_2$] 30 to 35 mm Hg) by hyperventilation is advantageous.

Following preoxygenation using mask ventilation, children should receive atropine sulfate (0.01 to 0.02 mg/kg) to ensure that the heart rate remains high during intubation. It is important to maintain an adequate heart rate because this is directly proportional to cardiac output; stroke volume does not change much in children. Also, children should be premedicated with intravenous sedatives and muscle relaxants. Appropriate sedatives include short-acting barbiturates such as thiopental sodium (5.0 mg/kg) if volume status is normal or a benzodiazepine such as midazolam (0.1 mg/kg) if hypovolemia is suspected. Muscle relaxation is achieved with short-acting nondepolarizing agents (vecuronium bromide 0.1 mg/kg) or shorter-acting depolarizing agents (succinylcholine chloride 1.0 mg/kg). The presence of burns and devitalized tissue precludes the use of succinylcholine because of the risk of hyperkalemia. Continuous monitoring of an intubated child with end-tidal CO_2 and pulse oximetry is essential.

In the rare case when tracheal intubation is not possible as a consequence of oral or maxillofacial trauma or congenital anomaly, a surgical airway is indicated. A surgical cricothyrotomy is the preferred approach in children older than 10 years. The cricothyroid membrane is easily exposed through a transverse skin incision to accommodate placement of a small, uncuffed endotracheal tube. Morbidity is lower than with an emergency tracheostomy because of the superficial location of the cricothyroid membrane. The cricothyrotomy should be converted to a formal tracheostomy when the child is stabilized, to avoid subglottic stenosis.

In small children, the cricoid cartilage is a delicate structure and provides the majority of support to the trachea. Injury of this membrane during emergency cricothyrotomy can lead to significant morbidity and lifelong laryngotracheomalacia. To avoid this complication, children younger than 10 years should undergo needle cricothyrotomy and jet insufflation of the trachea. A 16- to 18-gauge intravenous catheter is used to access the tracheal lumen through the cricothyroid membrane and is connected to a 100% oxygen source at a high flow rate of 10 to 12 L/minute. Needle-jet ventilation is limited in children by the hypercarbia that occurs in approximately 30 minutes; therefore, this method is effective for only a short time. Following stabilization of the child, endotracheal intubation or formal tracheostomy is necessary.[13]

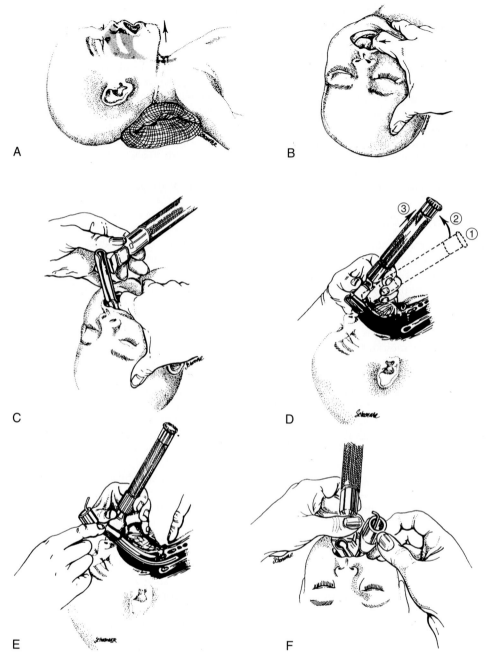

Figure 15–2   Endotracheal intubation. *A,* The pediatric larynx and supraglottic space are anterior and angled cephalad compared with the position in adults. A posterior neck roll optimizes visualization of the vocal cords in children. *B,* The tongue is large relative to the space in a child's oral cavity. The tongue should be moved to one side of the oral cavity to facilitate exposure of the posterior pharynx and supraglottic area. *C,* The laryngoscope blade is inserted from the right side of the mouth and slides back along the vallecula. *D,* With the blade in the proper position and the child's neck slightly extended in the sniffing position, lifting the handle (positions 1, 2, 3) raises the epiglottis and brings the vocal cords into direct vision. *E,* In all except newborns, the straight blade should be placed over the epiglottis to lift it, along with the base of the tongue, to expose the larynx. A stylet with the tip curved within the endotracheal tube facilitates successful intubation. *F,* The endotracheal tube is held in place while the laryngoscope is removed and secured after verification of bilateral breath sounds. (From Eichelberger MR: Pediatric Trauma, Prevention, Acute Care, Rehabilitation. St. Louis, Mosby, 1993.)

Breathing

Compromised breathing and ventilation in an injured child are usually the result of either head injury (impaired spontaneous ventilatory drive) or thoracic injury (impaired lung expansion). Recognition of a head injury is usually obvious, but recognition of a thoracic injury that impairs lung expansion requires a detailed survey. The potential seriousness of these injuries is underscored by the fact that mortality rates for thoracic trauma in children approach 25%.[14]

Following thoracic trauma, air, fluid, or viscera can compromise the pleural space. Compression of the pulmonary parenchyma can result in impaired gas exchange sufficient to produce respiratory distress. In the case of traumatic rupture of the diaphragm, loss of muscular integrity also has a direct effect on lung expansion. The child's mediastinum is extremely mobile; as pressure increases in the pleural space, the mediastinum is displaced to the opposite side, causing compression of the contralateral lung. The distortion of mediastinal vascular structures, along with elevated intrathoracic pressure, can result in a critical reduction in venous return.

Loss of chest wall integrity from flail chest impairs ventilation and oxygenation. Consequently, paradoxical chest wall movement occurs during inspiration, preventing complete lung expansion; assisted positive-pressure breathing is the best treatment. Because of the flexible nature of a child's chest, the force required to fracture multiple ribs is enormous and is transmitted to the underlying lung parenchyma, resulting in a pulmonary contusion. Regions of parenchymal hemorrhage and edema impair ventilation-perfusion matching, and the decrease in pulmonary compliance can dramatically increase the work of breathing; both can precipitate ventilatory failure.

Recognition of ventilatory compromise is usually not difficult, especially with a high index of suspicion. The sound of air movement at the mouth and nares is assessed, as are the rate, depth, and effort of respirations. On inspection, asymmetrical excursion of the chest wall suggests a ventilatory abnormality. Percussion elicits dullness or hyperresonance, depending on the presence of fluid or air in the pleural space, and breath sounds are decreased. With tension hemopneumothorax, mediastinal shift can be detected by tracheal deviation, displacement of the point of maximal cardiac impulse, and distended neck veins caused by impaired venous return.

Mechanical ventilatory failure is life threatening and requires immediate treatment during the primary survey. All children require supplemental oxygen by nasal cannula, mask, or endotracheal tube. Endotracheal intubation and assisted ventilation are sufficient to treat hypoventilation due to head injury, pain from rib fractures, flail chest, and pulmonary contusions. Simple hemopneumothorax may be well tolerated with supplemental oxygen until tube thoracostomy can be performed after the primary survey (Fig. 15-3). In cases of hemopneumothorax that results in compromised ventilation or hypotension, tube thoracostomy is required, often combined with endotracheal intubation and intravenous access for rapid fluid infusion. If tension is present, the hemodynamic derangements can be minimized by needle thoracostomy in the second intercostal space at the midclavicular line, followed by thoracostomy tube placement.

A chest tube of adequate caliber to evacuate blood and air should be inserted into the pleural cavity. The narrow intercostal space of a small child usually limits the size of the tube, but the largest-caliber tube that can be placed should be used. The tube is placed in the midaxillary line at the nipple level (fourth or fifth intercostal space) to avoid intra-abdominal placement through an elevated diaphragm. The tube is directed posterior and cephalad, to evacuate both blood and air, and is connected to a Pleurovac closed-suction drainage system set at –15 cm H_2O (see Fig. 15-3). Persistent hemorrhage

from a thoracostomy tube is uncommon in children; however, drainage of 1 to 2 mL/kg per hour is a sign of significant ongoing bleeding from a vascular or mediastinal injury that may require thoracotomy to identify and control the source.

When endotracheal intubation has been performed, the child's fraction of oxygen in inspired air should be 100%, with a tidal volume of 10 to 12 cc/kg at a rate of 15 to 20 cycles/minute. Oxygenation and ventilation should be manipulated to maintain an arterial oxygen tension (Po_2) greater than 80 mm Hg and a Pco_2 of 30 to 35 mm Hg, with a positive end-expiratory pressure not to exceed 5 cm H_2O. The goal is to prevent secondary brain injury by optimizing oxygenation and cerebral perfusion by minimizing intracranial pressure (ICP). Children with head trauma are best managed by moderate hyperventilation and hypocarbia (Pco_2 30 to 35 mm Hg) to reduce ICP.[6,13,18]

Circulation and Vascular Access

The third priority in the primary survey is the rapid assessment of circulation and the establishment of venous access. Seriously injured children often have normal vital signs, even with significantly decreased circulating volume; their cardiovascular reserve delays the early hemodynamic signs of hypovolemia until relatively late in the resuscitation phase. A high index of suspicion based on the mechanism of injury and continuous careful scrutiny of physiologic parameters and clinical signs are necessary to minimize morbidity.

A reliable sign of adequate perfusion is normal mental status. As the child is resuscitated, clinical signs of the efficacy of resuscitation should be monitored. Improvement in the following parameters is consistent with hemodynamic stability and success of resuscitation:

1. Slowing of the heart rate (<100 beats/minute).
2. Increased pulse pressure (>20 mm Hg).
3. Return of normal skin color and peripheral perfusion.
4. Increased warmth of extremities.
5. Clearing of the sensorium (improving Glasgow Coma Scale score).
6. Increased systolic blood pressure (>80 mm Hg).
7. Urinary output of 1 to 2 mL/kg per hour in infants and 1 mL/kg per hour in adolescents.

After establishment of an adequate airway, provision of venous access in a hypovolemic child is often a challenge. Two functioning catheters are best in all cases of significant injury. Optimally, venous access should be achieved above and below the diaphragm, given the potential for extravasation of resuscitation fluids from occult intra-abdominal venous injuries. Nevertheless, in children, any peripheral venous access is useful.

Two attempts should be made to place large-bore peripheral lines in the upper extremities. If percutaneous placement is unsuccessful, insertion of an intraosseous line is useful in a child younger than 6 years (see later). In children older than 6 years, a venous cutdown performed at the ankle is best. The greater saphenous vein is easily exposed through short transverse incisions 0.5 to 1 cm proximal and anterior to the medial malleolus.

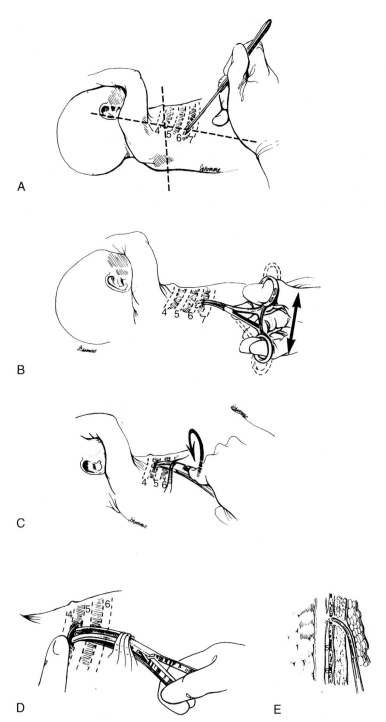

A

B

C

D

E

Figure 15–3   Thoracostomy tube insertion. *A,* An incision is made in the midaxillary line just below the nipple in a male or inframammary fold in a female (fourth intercostal space). *B,* The dissection is carried out in a cephalad direction subcutaneously over two ribs. A long subcutaneous track is preferable in a child to minimize air leak around the tube. *C,* The fourth intercostal space is the ideal place for thoracostomy tube placement. *D,* The entrance into the pleural space should be made just over and superior to the rib to avoid injury to intercostal vessels. *E,* Lateral view of the technique. (From Eichelberger MR: Pediatric Trauma, Prevention, Acute Care, Rehabilitation. St. Louis, Mosby, 1993.)

The exposed vein is suspended over a silk ligature, and the largest appropriate intravenous catheter is introduced into the vessel lumen under direct vision. Transection or ligation of the vein is not necessary (Fig. 15-4).

Central venous catheterization can result in significant complications, such as laceration of the subclavian or femoral artery, making it a less useful technique. The femoral route is preferred because of ease of access. If subclavian venous access is necessary, the child should be placed in the Trendelenburg position with the head maintained in a neutral position without the placement of a posterior shoulder roll. This position provides

optimal cross-sectional area of the subclavian vein in both children and adults.[12]

An intraosseous line is a simple, reliable, and safe route for the administration of fluids, blood products, and medications. The technique is applicable in children 6 years of age and younger because the marrow is well perfused in early childhood. The preferred site for intraosseous insertion is through the flat anteromedial surface of the tibia, about 2 to 3 cm below the tibial plateau. The needle is angled 60 degrees from horizontal and pointed toward the foot. The cortex is penetrated, and the marrow cavity is detected by aspirating blood and particulate material. Alternative sites include the midline distal femur, 3 cm above the condyles directed cephalad in small children, and the distal tibia above the medial malleolus or the proximal humerus in adolescents, although the need for an intraosseous line is rare in this age group. Specially designed intraosseous needles should be available in the pediatric resuscitation room to facilitate this maneuver; however, a 14- to 16-gauge needle can be used. The complication rate is low, but potential complications include osteomyelitis, cellulitis, fracture, growth plate injury, fat embolism, and compartment syndrome.

As soon as vascular access is established, fluid resuscitation with a bolus of fluid is begun. Generally, isotonic crystalloid solution, such as lactated Ringer's solution, is administered in 20 mL/kg increments. If evidence of hypovolemia persists after 40 mL/kg has been given, transfusion of ABO-matched packed red blood cells is initiated in a bolus of 10 mL/kg. Packed red blood cells have the advantages of raising colloid oncotic pressure and effecting a more rapid and sustained intravascular expansion than crystalloid. In addition, the red blood cell provides hemoglobin to increase oxygen carrying capacity. All fluids (crystalloid, colloid, and blood) should be warmed during infusion. This is accomplished by microwaving crystalloid solutions or using a warming device.

It is important to reassess the child's response to resuscitation continually, to characterize the nature and extent of the injuries, and to avoid the complications of excessive fluid resuscitation. As perfusion is restored, the rate of fluid infusion is gradually reduced to avoid unnecessary fluid administration. Pulmonary edema rarely occurs in

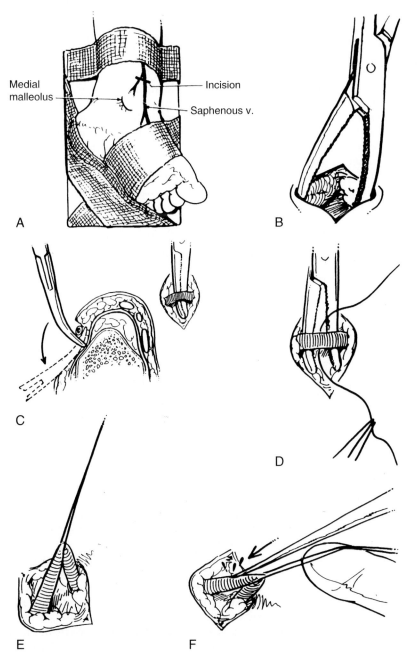

Figure 15-4 Greater saphenous vein cannulation. *A,* Consistent emergency venous access is achieved at the ankle, anterior to the medial malleolus via the saphenous vein. *B,* A transverse incision is made anterior to the medial malleolus (1 cm anterior and 1 cm cephalad). Perpendicular dissection in the incision exposes the saphenous vein. *C,* The vein is dissected circumferentially. *D,* A suture ligature is passed around the vessel. *E* and *F,* Gentle traction on the suture facilitates catheterization of the vein. (From Eichelberger MR: Pediatric Trauma, Prevention, Acute Care, Rehabilitation. St. Louis, Mosby, 1993.)

Medial malleolus — Incision — Saphenous v.

A

B

C

D

E

F

normal lungs, but considerable morbidity results from fluid sequestration in a region of pulmonary or cerebral contusion. If hemodynamic stabilization does not occur with crystalloid and blood resuscitation, hemorrhage is likely from an intra-abdominal or pelvic source, cardiac dysfunction due to tamponade or contusion, tension hemopneumothorax, cerebrospinal injury such as atlanto-occipital dissociation, or profound hypothermia.[7,13]

Disability

A rapid neurologic evaluation is included in the primary survey to identify serious injuries that may have immediate consequences for airway management. A rapid method for describing gross cerebral function is the AVPU mnemonic: alert, voice responsive, pain responsive, or unresponsive. An assessment of pupillary responsiveness and symmetry is also useful. Transtentorial herniation secondary to an expanding intracranial hematoma causes ipsilateral pupillary dilation and loss of light reflex. Direct trauma to the eye is an equally common cause of unilateral anisocoria, but this is usually obvious. Characterization of extremity posturing as decorticate or decerebrate indicates the loss of cortical or global brain function, respectively. In a comatose child with a unilateral fixed and dilated pupil, measures to reduce ICP are imperative. These include early controlled endotracheal intubation to keep the P_{CO_2} regulated (30 to 35 mm Hg) with moderate hyperventilation, which causes cerebral vasoconstriction and decreases cerebral blood flow. This lowers brain volume and ICP, with a resulting increase in cerebral perfusion pressure (CPP). The reverse Trendelenburg position, in which the head is elevated 30 degrees, can also reduce intracranial hypertension but should be used only in children with normal cardiac function.

Exposure

Complete exposure of the child is essential to facilitate a thorough examination and identification of injury. A conscious child does not understand the need for such action, so exposure must be done carefully. A thorough primary survey on a stable child with a normal Glasgow Coma Scale score can be performed without removing all items of clothing simultaneously. Children are particularly apprehensive about pain when exposing an injury that was previously covered, so attention to these special sensitivities frequently results in a more efficient evaluation.

In a child, hypothermia affects physiologic parameters, such as cognitive function, cardiac activity, and coagulation. It is important to maintain core temperature above 35°C to 36°C. A warm resuscitation room preserves core body temperature and minimizes heat loss. Similarly, resuscitation fluid and inhaled gases should be warmed and humidified. Overhead and bed warmers are essential, but a radiant warmer is best for an injured infant.

Resuscitation Phase

The cornerstone of resuscitation is continuous reappraisal of the child's response to therapeutic intervention. Deterioration at any point requires repetition of the primary survey. After the ABCDEs are complete and life-threatening injuries are stable, a gastric tube and urinary catheter should be placed, followed by the drawing of blood for analysis and placement of a cardiac monitor.

In children, acute gastric dilatation can cause both respiratory compromise and vagus-mediated bradycardia. Gastric decompression to evacuate the stomach and reduce the risk of vomiting and aspiration is important in all injured children, especially those with a decreased level of consciousness. Assessment for a stable midface and for the presence of cerebrospinal fluid rhinorrhea is important before the placement of a nasogastric tube for decompression. If the assessment is abnormal, oral gastric tube placement is in order.

A urinary catheter is also placed following a thorough perineal assessment, including a rectal examination. In instances of a high-riding prostate, meatal bleeding, perineal or scrotal ecchymosis, or unstable anterior pelvic fracture, a retrograde urethrogram is indicated before insertion of the catheter.

An electrocardiogram is essential to monitor cardiac rhythm, which is rarely abnormal. Secondary abnormalities are occasionally seen and include sinus bradycardia due to advanced shock; electromechanical dissociation from hypovolemia, tension pneumothorax, or pericardial tamponade; and ventricular fibrillation due to hypothermia or acidosis. Ventricular ectopy, low voltages, and signs of ischemia can accompany myocardial contusion. Beyond evaluating the actual rhythm, diffuse low voltage may be the first indication of hemopericardium.

After vascular access is obtained, blood and urine are obtained for laboratory analyses, including complete blood count and metabolic studies, urinalysis, and arterial blood gas analysis. Blood alcohol level and a toxicology screen are not routine in children but reasonable in adolescents. Blood should also be drawn for type and crossmatch.[5,7]

Neuroresuscitation

Brain injury is the most common cause of acquired disability and mortality during childhood. It is estimated that each year, 1 in 500 children in the United States sustains a brain injury, 7000 children die from head injuries, and 28,000 children become permanently disabled.[1,10] Largely as a result of prevention strategies and regional trauma systems, the overall mortality from severe traumatic brain injury has decreased from approximately 50% in the 1970s to 36% today. In children, the current overall mortality from injury is 3%; the primary cause of death in 70% of cases is central nervous system injury. Overall, the outcome for children older than 3 years is better than for adults with comparable injuries; however, outcome in children younger than 3 years is often poor.[8,13,18]

Traumatic brain injury can be defined as either primary or secondary. Primary brain injury is the structural derangement of cerebral architecture that occurs from direct mechanical impact, resulting in cellular and vascular disruption, infarction, or tissue loss. The child's brain is susceptible to injury of the deep white matter, shear, punctate hemorrhage, brain swelling, and linear nondepressed skull fracture, rather than mass lesions such as subdural and intracerebral hematomas and depressed skull fractures, which are more frequently encountered in adults. Children, however, have a higher incidence of epidural hematoma, perhaps because the thinner, less rigid skull is more apt to fracture and lacerate the meningeal artery. The proportionately larger size of the cranium in children, along with a less muscular and more flexible ligamentous cervical spine, may account for the increased incidence of diffuse axonal injury in injured children.

Primary brain injury responds only to preventive efforts, whereas secondary brain injury is the target of clinical neuroresuscitation. Secondary brain injury occurs as a result of decreased cerebral perfusion following the traumatic event. Both diffuse and regional brain swelling impairs oxygen and substrate delivery largely as a result of increasing ICP and its effect on CPP. CPP, ICP, and mean arterial pressure (MAP) are related by the following equation: CPP = MAP − ICP. Resuscitation should optimize CPP by controlling ICP and maintaining MAP. When ICP exceeds venous outflow pressure (as a result of brain swelling), it acts as a Starling resistor and determines the pressure gradient for cerebral blood flow. Normal CPP values and the ideal range of ICP in children with severe brain injury are not clear.[8] Favorable outcomes in children are possible by maintaining the ICP less than 20 mm Hg in all ages and a CPP greater than 45 mm Hg in children younger than 8 years and 70 to 80 mm Hg in older childen.[3]

Efforts to reduce secondary brain injury focus on maintaining a therapeutic ICP and CPP and normalizing the MAP. The most expeditious method is intubation and controlled hyperventilation, initially reducing Pco_2 to 30 to 35 mm Hg, Po_2 to greater than 100 mm Hg, and pH to 7.40 ± 0.05. Hypocarbia and alkalosis promote cerebral vasoconstriction, limiting cerebral blood volume and lowering ICP. The effect is rapid but can be limited in duration by re-equilibration of cerebrospinal fluid pH balance. The maximal duration of the effect is unknown but may range from several hours to several days. Current therapy maintains Pco_2 in the 30 to 35 mm Hg range. This regimen avoids excessive hyperventilation, which may be deleterious in patients with severe brain injury by converting borderline regions of cerebral ischemia into infarction.[8] A ventriculostomy is usually placed, allowing cerebrospinal fluid to drain to further optimize CPP. A repeat head computed tomography scan is indicated 24 to 48 hours after injury to assess the extent of brain edema, identify new infarcts, or demonstrate the development of a new hematoma or large contusion that may require evacuation. The status of ventilation and fluid hydration should be reassessed and optimized frequently in the first 48 hours.

If these measures fail to control ICP, osmotherapy is undertaken with a rapid bolus intravenous infusion of 20% mannitol at a dose of 0.25 to 0.5 g/kg every 4 to 6 hours. Mannitol is withheld if the serum sodium concentration is greater than 145 mEq/L, serum osmolarity is greater than 310 mOsm, urine output is less than 0.5 mL/kg per hour, or blood pressure is low. Mannitol exerts a therapeutic effect by creating a hyperosmolar environment in the cerebral microcirculation; this improves brain oxygen delivery by exerting a diuresis of free water from the cerebral interstitium, which improves blood flow.[8]

The induction of mild to moderate hypertension may reverse abnormal ICP and raise CPP by improving brainstem microvascular perfusion.[16] Therapy is begun with an intravenous infusion of dopamine at a dose of 5 to 20 μg/kg per minute.

Hyperthermia and seizures are common after traumatic brain injury and can adversely affect efforts to normalize ICP and CPP. Both fever and seizures promote further secondary brain injury by increasing the metabolic demands of the already compromised brain. Therefore, core temperature should be maintained in the normal range (35° C to 36° C) with acetaminophen 10 mg/kg every 4 to 6 hours. Cooling blankets may be necessary for recalcitrant fever. A single seizure in a child following head injury and a subsequent normal neurologic assessment does not require treatment. Seizures that occur within 1 week after injury are treated with phenobarbital in children younger than 1 year and with phenytoin in those older than 1 year. Either drug is administered in a one-time intravenous dose of 10 to 20 mg/kg, followed by daily dosage of 5 mg/kg. Treatment is discontinued after 7 days. Children who develop late seizures require long-term anticonvulsant medication. Whether a comatose child who has not demonstrated seizure activity requires anticonvulsant prophylaxis during the resuscitation process is controversial.

Coagulopathy

Dysfunctional coagulation related to injury occurs in several circumstances: extreme hypothermia, massive transfusion, and severe brain injury. Hypothermia causes excessive bleeding by reducing the efficiency of enzymatic processes that promote coagulation. Massive transfusion, defined as the acute administration of blood products equal to or greater than one blood volume (65 to 80 mL/kg), also causes coagulopathy. Another mechanism results from the storage of blood in anticoagulants containing ethylenediaminetetraacetic acid or citrate (citrate-phosphate-dextrose), both of which chelate calcium and inhibit the calcium-dependent steps of the coagulation cascade. Acute hypocalcemia is another consequence of massive transfusion.

The most common mechanism by which massive transfusion causes coagulopathy is dilutional thrombocytopenia. Coagulopathy due to dilution of other clotting factors is much less common because of a much greater functional reserve of these components. As continued hemorrhage depletes circulating platelets and blood is replaced with red blood cells, a progressive reduction in the platelet count ensues. With acute injury, a reduction in the platelet count to 50,000 can produce surgical bleeding. Platelet levels below 100,000 signify impending coagulopathy, and levels of 50,000 or less require platelet transfusion. Administration of ABO-matched platelets at an initial dose of 0.1 U of concentrate/kg or 4 U/m² of body surface area raises the platelet level by about 40,000.

Severe head injury is also associated with coagulopathy unrelated to platelet dilution. Presumably, large amounts of procoagulant tissue thromboplastin are released from injured areas of the brain, initiating disseminated intravascular coagulation and a consumptive coagulopathy in which all clotting factors and fibrinogen are depleted, as well as platelets. Coagulopathy after head injury is a grim prognostic sign. Treatment requires administration of matched fresh frozen plasma at a dose of 15 to 30 mL/kg. Cryoprecipitate contains large amounts of fibrinogen, factor VIII, factor XIII, and von Willebrand's factor and can be given at a dose of 0.1 U/kg in addition to fresh frozen plasma. Administration of fresh frozen plasma, cryoprecipitate, or both may also be required in the setting of preexisting coagulopathies such as hemophilia, von Willebrand's disease, and advanced liver disease.[13]

PAIN MANAGEMENT

The primary goals of acute pain management are to reduce the stress on the injured child and to improve outcome. Acute pain serves as a noxious stimulus that leads to activation of the physiologic stress response. The result is activation of the neuroendocrine response, which has a profound and deleterious effect on metabolism, thermoregulation, wound healing, and immunity.

The following are critical elements in the management of pain in injured children:

1. An experienced interdisciplinary team, led by a clinician devoted to pain management.
2. A commitment to ensure the least possible pain.
3. Recognition that effective pain management requires constant adjustment.
4. Recognition that anxiety needs to be considered and treated because it may alter the effectiveness of pain treatment.
5. The ability and knowledge to effectively use all pain therapy in real-time coordination with the rest of the child's supportive care and treatment plan.

A team-oriented, protocol-based algorithm that attempts to control pain in this environment will enhance the overall success of the emergency management of these children.[9]

CONCLUSION

A systematic approach to injured children can save lives. Nevertheless, prevention of injury is essential.

The unintentional injury death rate among children has declined nearly 40% during the past 16 years.[20] The most notable progress in prevention has been a 72% decline in childhood deaths from unintentional firearm injuries and a 60% decline in deaths from bicycle-related injuries. The death rate from fire and burn injuries declined 56%, while that from pedestrian injuries dropped 51%. Unfortunately, the motor vehicle occupant death rate, particularly among children aged 5 to 9, has been slow to decline, and the death rate from airway obstruction injury among infants remains unchanged.

Many factors have contributed to the overall dramatic decline in the unintentional childhood injury death rate. It is clear that the highest priority should be on injury prevention, with a particular emphasis on minimizing the injury risk to minorities, younger children, and motor vehicle occupants. Once injury occurs, however, proper resuscitation can save lives.

REFERENCES

1. Centers for Disease Control: Childhood injuries in the United States. Am J Dis Child 1990;144:627-646.
2. Centers for Disease Control and Prevention: Web-based Injury Statistics Query and Reporting System (WISQARS). Fatal Injury Reports 1999-2000. National Center for Injury Prevention and Control, Centers for Disease Control and Prevention. Available at www.cdc.gov/ncipc/wisqars.
3. Chambers IR, Treadwell L, Mendelow AD: Determination of threshold levels of cerebral perfusion pressure and intracranial pressure in severe head injury by using receiver-operating characteristic curves: An observational study in 291 patients. J Neurosurg 2001;94:412-416.
4. Children's Safety Network, Economics and Insurance Resource Center: Special run: Hospitalized unintentional injury among children 15 and under. Feb 2003.
5. Chu UB, Clevenger FW, Imani ER, et al: The impact of selective laboratory evaluation on utilization of laboratory resources and patient call in a level I trauma center. Am J Surg 1996;172:558-562.
6. Committee on Quality Improvement, American Academy of Pediatrics, and Commission on Clinical Policies and Research, American Academy of Family Physicians: The management of minor closed head injury in children. Pediatrics 1999;104:1407-1415.
7. Committee on Trauma of the American College of Surgeons: Advanced Trauma Life Support Instructor Manual. Chicago, American College of Surgeons, 1997.
8. Faillace WJ: Management of childhood neurotrauma. Surg Clin North Am 2002;82:349-363.
9. Golianu B, Krane EJ, Galloway KS, Yaster M: Acute pain in children: Pediatric acute pain management. Pediatr Clin North Am 2000;47:1-24.
10. Kraus JF, Rouk A, Hemyaris P: Brain injury among infants, children, adolescents, and young adults. Am J Dis Child 1990;144:684-691.
11. Losek JD, Bonadio WA, Walsh-Kelly C, et al: Prehospital pediatric endotracheal intubation performance review. Pediatr Emerg Care 1989;5:1.
12. Lukish J, Valladares E, Bulas D, et al: Classical positioning decreases subclavian vein cross sectional area in children. J Trauma 2002;53:272-275.
13. Magnuson DK, Eichelberger MR: Approach to the pediatric trauma patient. In Surgery of Infants and Children. Philadelphia, Lippincott-Raven, 1997, pp 391-414.
14. Peclet MH, Newman KD, Eichelberger MR, et al: Thoracic trauma in children: An indicator of increased mortality. J Pediatr Surg 1990;25:961.
15. Ramenofsky ML, Luterman A, Quindlen E, et al: Maximum survival in pediatric trauma: The ideal system. J Trauma 1984;24:818.
16. Rosner MJ: Pathophysiology and management of increased intracranial pressure. In Andrews BT (ed): Neurosurgical Intensive Care. New York, McGraw-Hill, 1993, pp 57-112.
17. Scheidt PC, et al: The epidemiology of nonfatal injuries among US children and youth. Am J Public Health 1995;85:932-938.
18. Stafford PW, Blineman TA, Nance ML: Practical points in evaluation and resuscitation of the injured child. Surg Clin North Am 2002;82:273-302.
19. Taylor GA, Eichelberger MR: Abdominal CT in children with neurological impairment following blunt trauma. Ann Surg 1989;210:229-233.
20. Wallace AL, Cody BE, Mickalide AD: Report to the Nation: Trends in Unintentional Childhood Injury Mortality, 1987-2000. Washington, DC, National Safe Kids Campaign, May 2003.

Chapter 16

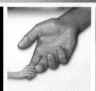

Thoracic Injuries

David E. Wesson

EPIDEMIOLOGY AND PREVENTION

Injuries to the chest wall, diaphragm, lungs, and mediastinal structures occur in about 25% of children treated in level I pediatric trauma centers, usually after high-energy blunt or penetrating trauma. Low-energy mechanisms, such as simple falls from playground equipment, seldom cause chest injury. Thoracic injuries range in severity from minor to rapidly fatal, but virtually all chest injuries can be treated successfully if they are promptly diagnosed. Although chest injuries are less common than injuries to the abdomen, soft tissues, and extra-axial skeleton, they are more lethal. Because of the impact required to cause such injuries, patients have a significant risk of mortality. In fact, thoracic injuries account for a high proportion of all trauma deaths not caused by central nervous system (CNS) injury.

As with most types of pediatric trauma, the male-to-female ratio is between 2:1 and 3:1. Thoracic injuries can be classified by anatomic site (e.g., rib fracture, pulmonary contusion, bronchial laceration), mechanism (blunt or penetrating), or threat to life (immediate or potential). Although most serious blunt injuries to the chest are motor vehicle related in all age groups, the proportion of children injured as pedestrians is much higher than in adults. The causes of penetrating thoracic injuries in teenagers mimic those in adults—mostly knife and gunshot wounds. BBs or pellets fired from air guns, although often considered relatively innocuous, may also cause life-threatening injury.[22] The causes of penetrating injuries in preadolescent children include a number of other unusual mechanisms, such as impalement by shards of broken glass or metal rods.[64]

The most common thoracic injuries seen clinically are listed in Table 16-1.[12] Autopsy series, which include prehospital and emergency department deaths, reveal a higher proportion of rapidly fatal major vascular and cardiac injuries.[3] In adults, rib fractures are by far the most common type of blunt trauma to the chest. In children, pulmonary contusions are the most frequent.[12,58] Tracheobronchial lacerations are more common in children than in adults, whereas the opposite is true for traumatic rupture of the aorta.[82]

The most common thoracic injuries are lung contusion, pneumothorax, hemothorax, and fracture of the ribs, sternum, or scapula. Injuries to the heart, aorta, trachea, bronchi, and diaphragm are much less common but potentially more dangerous. The most common *immediately* life-threatening injuries to the chest are airway obstruction, tension pneumothorax, massive hemothorax, and cardiac tamponade. Open pneumothorax and massive flail chest are rare. The most common *potentially* life-threatening injuries of the chest are myocardial contusion, aortic disruption, ruptured diaphragm, tracheobronchial disruption, and esophageal rupture.

The relative incidence of blunt and penetrating thoracic trauma varies widely, depending on the amount of violence in the community. Peterson et al.[64] reported a large series

TABLE 16–1 Epidemiology of Pediatric Chest Injuries from the National Pediatric Trauma Registry

	Blunt	Penetrating	Total (%)*
Pneumothorax/hemothorax	38	64	41
Pneumothorax	24	23	23
Hemopneumothorax	9	24	11
Hemothorax	5	18	7
Lung	53	29	48
Contusion	49	14	43
Laceration	1	10	3
Heart	5	13	6
Contusion	4	<1	3
Laceration	<1	8	2
Diaphragm	2	15	4
Rib fractures	35	7	30
Aorta	1	1	<1
Bronchus	<1	0	<1
Esophagus	<1	1	<1

*Percentage of the total cases with each type of injury. Overall, 83% of injuries were blunt, 15% were penetrating, and 2% were caused by other mechanisms.
From Cooper A, Barlow B, DiScala C, String D: Mortality and truncal injury: The pediatric perspective. J Pediatr Surg 1994;29:33.

of adults and children with thoracic trauma. Blunt injuries constituted 81% of thoracic injuries in children 12 years of age or younger; penetrating injuries accounted for 58% of chest injuries in adolescents. In Nakayama and Ramenofsky's series,[58] 97% of thoracic injuries in children up to 17 years of age were blunt. Meller et al.[53] reported a series in which nearly all wounded teenagers had penetrating injuries. The National Pediatric Trauma Registry (NPTR) reflects the combined experience of many pediatric trauma centers across North America. From 1985 to 1991, more than 25,000 cases were reported to the NPTR, including 1553 cases of thoracic injury.[12] Eighty-six percent of injuries were blunt (mostly motor vehicle related). The remaining 14% were penetrating (mostly stab or gunshot wounds).

The overall mortality rates for blunt and penetrating cases were almost identical, at 15% and 14%, respectively.[12] Mortality increases with the number of associated injuries. Most of the deaths in the group that had blunt trauma were caused by associated head injuries, whereas most of the deaths in the group with penetrating injuries resulted from the chest injuries themselves. Overall, thoracic injuries were second only to CNS injuries as the cause of death in the NPTR. Most deaths from chest injuries occur at the scene of the accident or in transit to the hospital and result from fatal injuries to vital organs. Patients with thoracic injuries who reach the hospital alive are potentially salvageable.

Although the ratio of blunt to penetrating injuries varies in adults and children, the spectrum of chest injuries and the basic principles of diagnosis and treatment are the same for all ages. The most common injuries—pulmonary contusion, rib fracture, pneumothorax, and hemothorax—can be treated with simple measures such as tube thoracostomy, oxygen, and analgesia. Approximately 20% of patients with these injuries also require endotracheal intubation and mechanical ventilation, often for the management of associated head injuries.

Several thoracic injuries virtually always require operation: major airway lacerations, aortic injuries, structural cardiac and pericardial injuries, and esophageal perforations. One of the greatest challenges in thoracic trauma is to recognize as soon as possible the rare cases that need surgery. In Nakayama's series,[58] 2 of 3 patients with penetrating injuries and only 3 of 83 patients with blunt injuries had chest operations. In Peterson's report,[64] 15% of the children with blunt injuries required thoracotomy (about the same as in adult series), and 40% of those with penetrating injuries required surgery (much higher than in adult series).

Although clinicians are naturally concerned about the treatment of patients, no discussion of chest injuries in children would be complete without mentioning prevention. Motor vehicle accidents and gunshot wounds cause the vast majority of severe pediatric thoracic injuries. These injuries are all preventable. Increasing the use of seat belts and child restraints would substantially reduce the risk of injury to motor vehicle occupants. Reducing the illegal use of firearms would also have major benefits, especially for teenagers. Chest protectors may be effective in reducing the incidence of chest injuries, including commotio cordis, in young athletes.[51,86] In combination, these measures would substantially reduce the incidence and severity of pediatric thoracic trauma and the death and disability that result from it.

CLINICAL PRESENTATION

The pathophysiology of thoracic trauma and the anatomy and physiology on which management strategies are based differ significantly between children and adults. The most important anatomic factors in children are the relatively narrow airway, which is prone to obstruction; the anterior and superior position of the glottis, which makes nasotracheal intubation difficult and therefore inappropriate in an emergency; and the short trachea, which increases the risk of endobronchial intubation. The increased oxygen consumption and low functional residual capacity of children predispose them to hypoxia. Because young children rely largely on the diaphragm to breathe, any increase in intra-abdominal pressure compounds the problem by restricting diaphragmatic excursion.

Children with significant thoracic injuries may present with minimal signs and symptoms. A large adult series from the Maryland Institute of Emergency Medical Services Systems (MIEMSS) found that two thirds of patients with thoracic injuries arrived with stable vital signs.[79] This same finding was reported in children.[53] About 25% of the patients with significant intrathoracic injuries in the MIEMSS series did not have a rib fracture. These "occult" injuries included pneumothorax, hemothorax, myocardial contusion, cardiac rupture, tracheobronchial injury, pulmonary laceration, ruptured diaphragm, and ruptured aorta.

The ribs of a child are more pliable than those of an adult. Consequently, rib fractures are much less common in children. However, it is important to note that because of the elasticity of the chest wall in childhood, severe thoracic injuries may occur without external signs of injury. In Nakayama's series,[58] less than half the children with significant thoracic injuries had rib fractures. The flexibility and compressibility of the chest wall may also explain why traumatic asphyxia is almost unique to children and why major airway trauma is so much more common in children than in adults.

The mediastinal structures are more mobile in children than in adults. Therefore, tension pneumothorax is more likely to shift the mediastinum, compromising ventilation of the contralateral lung and impairing return of venous blood to the heart.

DIAGNOSIS AND INITIAL RESUSCITATION

Diagnosis and initial treatment of patients with traumatic chest injury must occur simultaneously. Although the manifestations of thoracic injury may be immediate or delayed by hours or days, the initial goal is to rule out injuries that are immediately life threatening, such as airway obstruction, tension pneumothorax, massive hemothorax, and cardiac tamponade.

All injury victims should be managed according to the principles of the Advanced Trauma Life Support (ATLS) program of the American College of Surgeons.[1] The overall plan is as follows:

1. Primary survey.
2. Resuscitation of vital functions.
3. Detailed secondary survey.
4. Definitive care.

All children with thoracic trauma must have supplemental oxygen, two large-bore intravenous lines, and a nasogastric tube to prevent gastric distention. A nasogastric tube may also reveal an abnormal position of the esophagus or stomach, indicating aortic injury or a ruptured diaphragm. Children with thoracic trauma should be observed closely. Vital signs and oxygen saturation in arterial blood (SaO$_2$) should be continuously monitored. If the child is intubated, end-tidal carbon dioxide should be monitored continuously or checked frequently. Blood should be available for transfusion. The equipment and skilled personnel needed to address breathing problems and to manage the airway with suction, oral airways, endotracheal tubes, laryngoscopes, and a bag-valve-mask apparatus must always be on hand, especially during transport and diagnostic procedures.

Life-threatening injuries should be identified and treated during the initial resuscitation phase of the ATLS protocol. The first priority is to clear and secure the airway. Endotracheal intubation may be required. After intubation, the position of the endotracheal tube must be checked by observing chest excursion, listening for bilateral air entry, monitoring end-tidal carbon dioxide, and obtaining a chest radiograph. A colorimetric carbon dioxide detector may be used to verify endotracheal tube position, especially in the prehospital setting.[5]

The second priority is to ensure adequate ventilation. Tension pneumothorax, if present, should be treated before a radiograph is obtained. Occasionally, open pneumothorax or massive flail chest requires intubation and assisted ventilation during the initial resuscitation. Persistent shock despite adequate fluid administration usually indicates ongoing blood loss (most likely abdominal). However, if no obvious cause of hypovolemia can be found, the possibility of acute pericardial tamponade should be considered; this condition can be relieved, at least temporarily, by pericardiocentesis.

The indications for urgent thoracotomy may become obvious at any stage (Table 16-2). The most common indications are massive bleeding, massive air leak, and cardiac tamponade. Emergency room (ER) or resuscitative thoracotomy is a controversial technique that does not seem to have clear indications or contraindications. In the report from MIEMSS,[79] none of 39 adult patients who presented without vital signs in the ER survived after emergency thoracotomy. However, emergency thoracotomy may be lifesaving in children, especially those with penetrating cardiac injuries. Powell et al.[66] reported a 26% survival rate in a series of children and adolescents who had ER thoracotomy. These authors recommend thoracotomy in the ER for post-traumatic arrest, or near arrest, in three situations:

1. All cases of penetrating thoracic trauma.
2. Blunt trauma with acute deterioration but signs of life in the ER.
3. Blunt trauma with signs of life at the scene when the scene is in proximity to the hospital.

The incision for emergency thoracotomy should be on the left anterolateral chest wall in the fifth interspace. A rib spreader should be used. If evidence of pericardial tamponade exists, the pericardium should be opened longitudinally, anterior to the phrenic nerve. Cardiac wounds should be controlled by direct pressure and simple suture unless coronary artery damage has occurred, in which case repair may be required. If cardiac tamponade is not present, the aorta should be cross-clamped. If the patient has massive lung injury, the hilum should be clamped or twisted off (see Treatment). Patients who respond to these measures should then have definitive repair performed in the operating room.

In most cases of thoracic trauma, the child is physiologically stable. After initial resuscitation, the next step is the detailed secondary survey. To avoid missing a significant injury, a complete and careful assessment is essential. In nearly all cases, a history that suggests significant impact to the chest can be elicited. Therefore, it is crucial to obtain as much information as possible regarding the details of the accident. Children involved in motor vehicle accidents, occupants and pedestrians alike, require an especially careful assessment. A history of difficulty breathing also indicates significant thoracic injury.

A systematic physical examination of the chest by inspection, percussion, palpation, and auscultation is the next step of the secondary survey. Tachypnea and tenderness and abrasions of the chest wall are predictive of intrathoracic injury.[7,26] One should look for cyanosis, dyspnea, noisy breathing, tracheal deviation, hoarseness or stridor, subcutaneous emphysema, open or sucking chest wounds, reduced or absent breath sounds, venous engorgement, pulsus paradoxus, and hypotension. Dyspnea and cyanosis suggest inadequate oxygenation. Noisy breathing may result from an injury to the airway or the presence of foreign material, such as blood, mucus, or vomitus. Tracheal deviation implies tension pneumothorax or massive hemothorax. Hoarseness, stridor, or other difficulty with phonation suggests direct laryngeal or tracheal injury. Surgical emphysema suggests a tracheal or bronchial laceration or, on rare occasions, an esophageal perforation. Jugular venous engorgement, hypotension, and pulsus paradoxus greater than 10 mm Hg imply cardiac tamponade. The patient should also be checked for signs of acute aortic

---

TABLE 16–2 Indications for Emergency Thoracotomy

Penetrating wound of the heart or great vessels
Massive or continuous intrathoracic bleeding
Open pneumothorax with major chest wall defect
Aortogram indicating injury to the aorta or major branch
Massive or continuing air leak, indicating injury to a major airway
Cardiac tamponade
Esophageal perforation
Diaphragmatic rupture
Impalpable pulse with cardiac massage

coarctation, which can be caused by injury to the thoracic aorta. The most sensitive sign of a significant cardiac injury is hypotension or a large fluid requirement that is not explained by bleeding. A cardiac injury may also cause a loud systolic murmur. Acute congestive heart failure may result from valvular injury or a traumatic ventricular septal defect.

Holmes et al.[32] developed a set of clinical predictors for the presence of chest injuries in a group of children younger than 16 years with blunt torso trauma. The strongest predictors were hypotension, increased respiratory rate, abnormal physical examination of the thorax, associated femur fracture, and a Glasgow Coma Scale score less than 15. Ninety-eight percent of proven cases had at least one of these predictors. Inspection and palpation were the most sensitive, but abnormalities detected on auscultation had the highest positive predictive value. This confirms the importance of clinical assessment in children with blunt trauma. The most common injuries were lung contusion, pneumothorax, and rib fracture, in that order.

In recent years, bedside surgeon-performed ultrasonography (US) has proved helpful in assessing abdominal trauma, and US is now a routine part of the clinical assessment of all major trauma cases.[49] US also has a role in chest trauma. It is sufficiently accurate to be clinically useful in diagnosing pneumothorax, hemothorax, and pericardial effusion.[41,49,62] One recent report documents that surgeon-performed US in the ER is an accurate screening test for the presence of a pneumothorax.[41]

Because it lacks sensitivity and specificity, clinical assessment is routinely supplemented by diagnostic imaging, which is usually the key step in identifying those children who need an operation.[27] Plain chest radiographs are routine, although some authors suggest that they are not necessary in blunt trauma cases when the chest physical examination is completely normal.[7,47] A standard posteroanterior and lateral examination is best, but a supine anteroposterior film will suffice. The chest radiograph should be repeated on arrival at the trauma center, even if the patient has been transferred from another hospital. The important signs of chest injury on plain chest radiographs include subcutaneous emphysema, fractures of the rib or other bony structures, hemothorax, pneumothorax, contusion or other parenchymal lesion (e.g., aspiration pneumonia), mediastinal shift or widening, and diaphragmatic rupture.

Computed tomography (CT) provides greater detail than plain radiographs and is more sensitive in the diagnosis of pneumothorax, rib fracture, and pulmonary contusion. It may also help in the diagnosis of ruptured diaphragm. Because chest films are not 100% sensitive, some groups recommend that CT be used to screen all patients suspected of having a chest injury. The most common injuries identified by CT are pulmonary contusions and lacerations.[50] Many pneumothoraces revealed by CT are either not evident or underestimated on plain films. Manson et al.[50] concluded that plain radiographs, especially those obtained in the trauma resuscitation room, are only "a gross screening examination" for thoracic injury and recommended dynamically enhanced CT in all cases of significant thoracic trauma diagnosed

clinically or by plain radiograph. In such cases, CT provides better definition of the injuries already recognized and may reveal occult injuries not visible on plain radiographs. Exadaktylos et al.[20] support this view. In their experience, CT revealed potentially life-threatening aortic injuries even when the plain chest radiographs were normal. They recommend routine chest CT in all patients with major chest trauma. Renton et al.[70] studied the question of whether CT should replace routine chest radiographs as the initial diagnostic imaging test and concluded that it should not, mainly because the increased cost was not justified by the relatively few changes in management that resulted from the use of CT scans. They estimated that 200 CT scans would have to be done for each clinically significant change in management. In summary, CT should be used liberally in cases of suspected chest injury.

Occasionally, other diagnostic tests, including US, transthoracic or transesophageal echocardiography, bronchoscopy, radionuclide bone scan, angiography, and even video-assisted thoracic surgery are helpful. US is more sensitive than supine anteroposterior chest radiographs and equally sensitive as CT in the diagnosis of traumatic pneumothorax.[72] Recent case reports document the use of video-assisted thoracic surgery to diagnose pericardial rupture and herniation of the heart.[65] In cases of suspected child abuse, a radionuclide bone scan helps detect recent and long-standing rib fractures. Although impractical in most emergencies, magnetic resonance imaging is helpful in defining injuries to the thoracic spine, especially when spinal cord involvement is suspected. It may also help identify diaphragmatic injuries in equivocal cases.[55]

For many years, angiography has been the gold standard for the diagnosis of injuries to the aorta and its main branches. However, there is a clear trend to use helical CT as the initial test for suspected aortic injury, reserving aortography for proven cases to guide the repair or, in some cases, eliminating aortography entirely.

Transthoracic echocardiography is a useful way to diagnose all types of structural heart injury and ventricular dysfunction caused by contusion. It may reveal intracardiac injuries or pericardial tamponade. Transesophageal echocardiography (TEE) is a useful screening test for traumatic rupture of the aorta. It can identify the cause of mediastinal hematomas seen on plain radiographs or CT scans.[46]

Pericardiocentesis may be used for diagnosis when cardiac tamponade is suspected and echocardiography is unavailable. All patients with thoracic trauma should have continuous electrocardiographic monitoring during assessment in the ER. A full 12-lead electrocardiogram should be obtained in cases of suspected cardiac contusion to rule out an arrhythmia. Bronchoscopy should be done in the operating room under general anesthesia in cases of suspected major airway trauma.

TREATMENT

The treatment of thoracic injuries varies from supportive (oxygen, analgesia) to simple interventions (endotracheal intubation, ventilation, tube thoracostomy) to operation (minimally invasive, open thoracotomy with or without cardiopulmonary bypass), depending on the specific structures injured and the severity of the injuries. However, most patients do not require an operation and can be managed with supportive measures, with or without tube thoracostomy.[42]

When an operation is indicated, the ideal location for the incision varies, depending on the preoperative diagnosis. An anterolateral incision in the fifth interspace, which can be extended across the midline, is best in an emergency. A trapdoor incision may be best for vascular injuries in the upper mediastinum. For esophageal injuries, a right posterolateral thoracotomy gives adequate exposure, except for the most distal thoracic esophagus, which is best viewed from the left. Median sternotomy is best for cardiac injuries. Cardiopulmonary bypass is only rarely needed emergently for injuries such as coronary artery laceration and laceration of the thoracic aorta. Intracardiac injuries to the atrioventricular valves or the atrial or ventricular septae do require bypass, but they can be repaired semielectively.

The concept of damage control, which is now well established for intra-abdominal trauma, can also be applied in selected cases of intrathoracic injury. Nonanatomic resection of the lung to control bleeding and massive air leak, pulmonary tractotomy with a GIA stapler for through-and-through wounds of the lung, en masse pneumonectomy, and hilar twist[88] may be lifesaving. The last has been reported in cases of uncontrollable bleeding or air leak from the lung. The inferior pulmonary ligament is divided, and the lower lobe is twisted anteriorly over the upper lobe. This controls the situation so that the patient can be taken back to the intensive care unit (ICU) for stabilization and returned to the operating room later for definitive control, usually by pneumonectomy.

Blunt Injuries

Chest Wall

Soft Tissue

Although seldom clinically important, injuries to the soft tissue of the chest wall suggest the possibility of more serious intrathoracic injuries. Soft tissue injuries to the chest wall should be managed according to accepted principles of wound care.

Rib Fracture

In childhood, the ribs are strong and pliable. Therefore, rib fractures are less common in children than in adults, and flail chest is quite rare. Because rib fractures require a great deal of force, they are an indication of severe injury. Fracture of the first rib suggests the possibility of a major vascular injury, especially to the subclavian artery.[29] First rib fractures may also be complicated by Horner's syndrome and thoracic outlet syndrome.

The goal of treatment is to prevent atelectasis and pneumonia while optimizing patient comfort. The treatment of rib fractures includes rest and analgesia. Oral or intravenous narcotics are usually sufficient for pain control. Intercostal nerve blocks may also be helpful. Children rarely experience pulmonary atelectasis from splinting of the chest wall. Rib fractures usually heal spontaneously within 6 weeks. The overall mortality rate for children with rib fractures in the NPTR was 10%.[12]

Rib fractures in infants and toddlers younger than 3 years old are often caused by child abuse.[24,87] The likelihood of nonaccidental injury in children with one or more rib fractures decreases with increasing age.[87] In cases of child abuse, the typical site of fracture is the neck of the rib near the costotransverse process articulation. Kleinman et al.[40] described fractures of the head of the rib in abused infants; these injuries are usually undetectable on radiographs because the head is cartilaginous. Cystic lesions of the ribs that are located posteriorly are another indication of child abuse,[48] as are multiple rib fractures at varying stages of healing.

Flail Chest

Flail chest is relatively uncommon in children. It occurs when a segment of the chest wall is destabilized by the fracture of several adjacent ribs. The injured chest wall moves paradoxically—in during inspiration and out during expiration. Ventilation is inefficient because of the paradoxical movement. Flail chest is usually associated with a lung contusion. Chest wall splinting and ineffective coughing often compound the primary injury. This leads to consolidation and collapse of the affected lung, which in turn results in ventilation-perfusion mismatch and hypoxia.

Initial treatment of flail chest includes supplemental oxygen, pain relief (intercostal nerve blocks, oral or intravenous narcotics, or an epidural blockade given as a continuous infusion), and physiotherapy. Fluid therapy must be carefully monitored to avoid pulmonary edema, and ICU monitoring is advisable. Children with isolated flail chest and no other significant injuries seldom require ventilation. If respiratory failure develops, endotracheal intubation and positive-pressure ventilation with positive end-expiratory pressure may be required for several days. Tracheotomy is rarely necessary. In the NPTR, the overall mortality rate for patients with flail chest was 40%.[12]

Sternal Fracture

Sternal fractures are less common in young children than in adults because the sternum is cartilaginous.

Pleural Space

Pneumothorax

Pneumothorax can result from an injury to the chest wall, lung parenchyma, tracheobronchial tree, or esophagus. High energy is required to produce a pneumothorax, so it must be considered a marker for other occult injuries.

Simple Pneumothorax: Simple pneumothorax may cause chest pain, respiratory distress, tachypnea, decreased air entry on the affected side, and oxygen desaturation. Careful examination may reveal an abrasion of the chest wall, crepitus, or tracheal shift. However, many patients show no clinical signs or symptoms. This underscores the importance of routine chest radiographs for all trauma cases. The radiographic signs include unilateral or asymmetrical lucency, a sharp outline of the mediastinum, mediastinal shift, and a visible visceral pleural border away from the chest wall. The diagnosis of simple pneumothorax should be confirmed by chest radiograph before treatment.

Simple pneumothoraces should be treated by intercostal chest tube drainage (Fig. 16-1). The best location for chest tube insertion is the fourth or fifth intercostal space (nipple level) in the anterior axillary line. The recommended chest tube sizes are as follows: newborns, 12 to 16 French; infants, 16 to 18 French; school-age children, 18 to 24 French; and adolescents, 28 to 32 French. The chest tube should be connected to an underwater seal on gentle suction and removed when the air leak stops. For most cases, this is the only treatment necessary. A continued or massive air leak suggests injury to the tracheobronchial tree.

A small, asymptomatic pneumothorax may be observed in carefully selected cases. If the patient is to be transferred to another hospital or intubated and ventilated for any reason, or if the pneumothorax exceeds 15%, it should be drained. When in doubt, a chest tube should be inserted.

Open Pneumothorax: Open pneumothorax is rare in children. In cases of open pneumothorax, the intrapleural pressure is equal to that of the atmosphere. As a result, the lung collapses and alveolar ventilation decreases. Sucking wounds should be recognized clinically. They can be treated by inserting a Heimlich valve or applying an occlusive dressing to the wound—taping the dressing on only three sides so that it can act as a flutter valve—and inserting a chest tube in the usual location.

Tension Pneumothorax: Tension pneumothorax may develop when a one-way valve effect occurs, allowing air to enter the pleural space but not to escape (Fig. 16-2). The underlying cause is usually a pulmonary laceration or injury to the trachea or a large bronchus. The intrapleural air pressure exceeds that of the atmosphere, collapses the ipsilateral lung, pushes the mediastinum to the opposite side, flattens the diaphragm, impairs ventilation of the opposite lung, and reduces the return of venous blood to the heart. The pulse and respiratory rate increase, and the patient develops severe distress. The trachea is usually deviated away from the involved side, and the neck veins may become engorged. The ipsilateral side of the chest is hyperresonant to percussion, with diminished breath sounds. Frank cyanosis is a late sign. The most important differential diagnosis is pericardial tamponade. However, this disorder can be distinguished from tension pneumothorax because the trachea is not displaced and the chest is normal to percussion. Tension pneumothorax should be considered when an injured patient, especially one on a

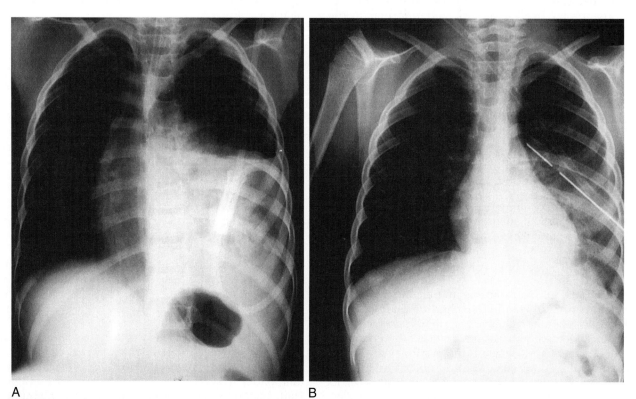

A   B

Figure 16–1 *A,* Left hemopneumothorax; note the nasogastric tube in situ. *B,* The same patient after insertion of an intercostal drain; no other treatment was required. (From Wesson DE: Trauma of the chest in children. Chest Clin North Am 1994;3:423.)

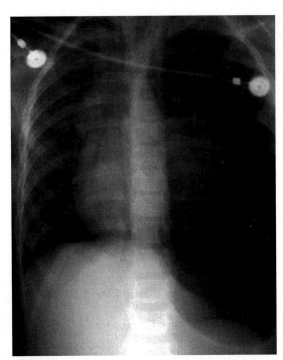

Figure 16–2 Left tension pneumothorax. This photograph demonstrates the classic findings with tension pneumothorax, including mediastinal shift, depression and inversion of the diaphragm, and widening of the interspaces on the involved side. This child had hypotension in addition to respiratory distress because of caval torsion, which was relieved following tube thoracostomy drainage.

mechanical ventilator, suddenly deteriorates for no apparent reason. Both acute gastric dilatation and right mainstem intubation may result in diminished breath sounds on the left and should not be confused with a tension pneumothorax.

The treatment for tension pneumothorax is immediate needle catheter drainage (without waiting for chest radiographs) through either the second intercostal space in the midclavicular line or the fourth or fifth interspace in the axilla, followed by insertion of a chest tube.

Hemothorax

When enough blood is lost into the thorax to cause shock, the term *massive hemothorax* is used. Massive hemothorax is more common after penetrating than blunt trauma.

Hemothorax may result from laceration of an intercostal or internal mammary artery, a lung, or a mediastinal blood vessel. Free bleeding into the pleural space from a major vessel, such as the aorta or one of the pulmonary hilar vessels, is usually rapidly fatal. Most bleeding from the lung stops spontaneously because of the low pressure in the pulmonary circulation. Bleeding from a systemic vessel, such as an intercostal artery, is more likely to cause massive hemothorax, producing signs of hypovolemia, mediastinal shift, diminished breath sounds, and dullness to percussion on the affected side. Hemothorax is often associated with pneumothorax (see Fig. 16-1). The treatment is intercostal drainage to prevent a clotted hemothorax and to monitor the rate and total volume

of blood loss. It is wise to establish two large-bore intravenous catheters; begin treatment for shock, if present; and obtain blood for transfusion before draining a massive hemothorax, because it may precipitate further bleeding. However, drainage and re-expansion of the lung usually stop the bleeding.

In most cases, intercostal drainage is the only treatment needed. However, thoracotomy may be indicated for the following reasons:

1. Initial drainage exceeds 20% to 25% of estimated blood volume.
2. Continued bleeding exceeds 2 to 4 mL/kg per hour.
3. Bleeding is increasing.
4. The pleural space cannot be drained of blood and clots.

Hoth et al.[35] reported an increased likelihood of nontherapeutic exploration when thoracotomy is performed for increased chest tube output in cases of blunt trauma. Autotransfusion may be helpful during surgery for massive intrathoracic bleeding.

Lung

Hematoma and Contusion

Pulmonary contusion is the most common type of blunt injury to the chest in children. Direct force to the lung causes disruption of the parenchyma, bleeding, and edema in a nonanatomic distribution, often without obvious injury to the chest wall. Specific clinical signs or symptoms are seldom evident at presentation, although rib fractures and abrasions over the chest may be present.

Because of the lack of specific physical features, routine chest radiographs are the key to the diagnosis of hematoma and contusion. Pulmonary contusions are usually obvious on plain radiographs taken at admission (Fig. 16-3) and are even more striking on CT, which has shown that they usually lie posteriorly or posteromedially.[50] However, there is no need for CT when a contusion is obvious on plain films. Pulmonary contusions may be progressive, especially when compounded by edema and atelectasis. Children with pulmonary contusions seldom require mechanical ventilation and almost never develop adult respiratory distress syndrome. The differential diagnosis includes aspiration pneumonia, which can result from aspiration at the scene, during transportation, during intubation, or with vomiting after admission. It affects the right lower lobe most frequently.

Patients with extensive lung hematomas or contusions should be monitored carefully with continuous SaO_2 measurements, preferably in an ICU. The treatment for these disorders is supportive, with analgesia, physiotherapy, supplemental oxygen, and fluid restriction. Endotracheal intubation and mechanical ventilation are less likely to be needed for children than for adults. Deterioration after admission is unusual.[8] It is important to guard against overhydration and aspiration of gastric contents. The most common complication is infection of the lung. Most pulmonary hematomas and contusions clear within 10 days unless the lung becomes infected.

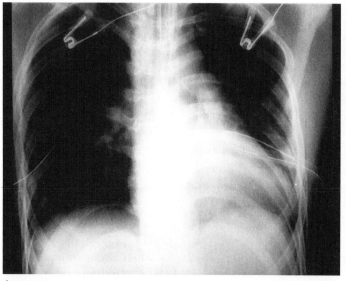

A

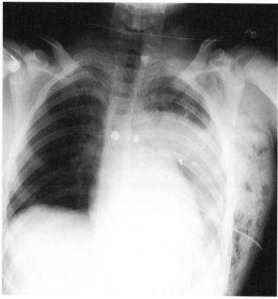

C

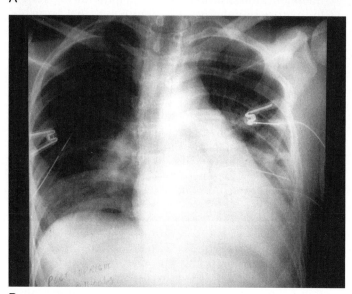

B

Figure 16-3 Pulmonary contusion. *A,* Crush injury with pulmonary contusion; note the multiple rib fractures. *B,* The same patient 2 days later; note the progression of the lesion. *C,* Gunshot wound with pulmonary contusion and subcutaneous emphysema. (From Wesson DE: Trauma of the chest in children. Chest Clin North Am 1993;3:423.)

Pulmonary contusions may be complicated by pneumothorax, hemothorax, or pleural effusion, all of which may require intercostal drainage. These secondary phenomena are much more common in the presence of concomitant fractures of the bones of the chest wall and may be delayed as long as 48 hours. Therefore, serial chest radiographs should be obtained in cases of pulmonary contusion (see Fig. 16-3).

Occasionally, a post-traumatic pneumatocele forms when the injured lung cavitates during healing. Because pneumatoceles usually resolve spontaneously in a few months, treatment is seldom necessary.

Laceration

Pulmonary lacerations are most often seen after penetrating injuries and usually result in a pneumothorax or hemothorax. They may also be caused by rib fractures.

Air embolus is the most serious complication of pulmonary laceration. This diagnosis should be suspected in all children with thoracic trauma who suddenly deteriorate, especially while receiving positive-pressure ventilation in the absence of a pneumothorax. Air embolus may cause focal neurologic deficits. Frothy blood aspirated from an arterial cannula is a telltale sign. Emergency thoracotomy, clamping of the pulmonary hilum, and aspiration of air from the heart or right ventricular outflow tract may be lifesaving.[36]

Trachea and Bronchi

Injuries to the major airways are uncommon in children. Nearly all are caused by blunt trauma.[12] The most common specific lesions are partial or complete transections of one of the main bronchi and tears of the membranous trachea. Airway injuries usually occur within 2 to 3 cm of the carina and may be rapidly fatal if not recognized and treated promptly. Injuries to distal lobar bronchi are also common.

Some patients with major airway injuries die from respiratory failure before reaching the hospital or shortly thereafter. Most present with dyspnea, which is often caused by tension pneumothorax. Other characteristics of patients with major airway injuries are voice disturbance, cyanosis, hemoptysis, massive subcutaneous and mediastinal emphysema, and failure of the lung to expand or continuing large-volume air leak despite properly functioning chest tubes. A lung that fails to expand or a continuous massive air leak after intercostal drainage strongly suggests a major airway injury (Fig. 16-4). Although not common, "dropped lung," in which the lung actually falls to the lower half of the pleural cavity below the level of the injured bronchus, is virtually diagnostic of a major airway injury. Finally, some patients present late with chronic collapse and infection of the involved lung from bronchial obstruction.

Initial management in the trauma room depends on the clinical situation. The initial treatment of airway injuries is to control the airway and breathing according to the ATLS protocol. This may require endotracheal intubation and intercostal drainage. If the patient has a good airway and is well oxygenated, it is prudent not to manipulate the airway by attempting intubation before taking the patient to the operating room. Flexible bronchoscopy may facilitate endotracheal intubation beyond the site of the injury or selective intubation of the uninjured bronchus. High-frequency ventilation with low mean airway pressure may be more effective than conventional methods in the presence of a massive air leak and may help stabilize the patient for surgical repair.[69]

Helical CT may be a good initial test in stable patients with suspected major airway injuries, but bronchoscopy is more reliable. Bronchoscopy is indicated whenever the lung fails to expand or a massive air leak continues after intercostal drainage. It should be performed in the operating room under general anesthesia using a rigid, ventilating bronchoscope. If possible, the patient should be allowed to breathe spontaneously during induction of anesthesia and passage of the bronchoscope. Staff and equipment for thoracotomy must be at hand. In unstable patients or those with possible or confirmed cervical spine injuries, flexible bronchoscopy with the patient awake or through an endotracheal tube may also demonstrate the lesion. At bronchoscopy, a defect in the wall of the airway may be visible. Other bronchoscopic signs of injury include mucosal disruption or exposed cartilage. Bronchography may be needed for distal bronchial injury.

Spontaneous healing is the rule for small lacerations in the membranous trachea and some partial bronchial tears involving up to one third of the circumference. These may be treated nonoperatively. For larger lacerations of the trachea or bronchi, primary surgical repair through a posterolateral thoracotomy is the best way to ensure good long-term results. Distal injuries to a lobar or segmental bronchus may be sealed with fibrin glue or treated by lung resection rather than direct repair. The right side of the chest allows the best exposure of the trachea, carina, and right main bronchus; the left side gives better exposure for injuries to the distal left main bronchus. In the presence of a massive air leak, it may be necessary to clamp the hilum before attempting to repair the airway. Advancing the endotracheal tube or passing a sterile tube across the surgical field into the distal airway may also be helpful during the repair. Simple, interrupted sutures after debridement of the margins work best. Although lobectomy or pulmonary segmentectomy may be necessary, pulmonary resection is done only as a last resort in unstable patients or when the lung is extensively damaged. The late functional results of pulmonary resection or bronchial repair are usually excellent.[59]

Bronchial injuries that are missed initially may seal spontaneously, but there is a risk of stenosis. After months or years, children with spontaneously sealed bronchial injuries may have persistent atelectasis, often with pneumonia or frank bronchiectasis in the involved lung, caused by a bronchial stricture. The diagnosis can be confirmed by bronchography or bronchoscopy. This type of stricture can be dilated in some cases, but open repair or even resection of the involved lung is usually necessary. One report illustrates that late repair of a completely transected mainstem bronchus with preservation of the lung is possible.[78]

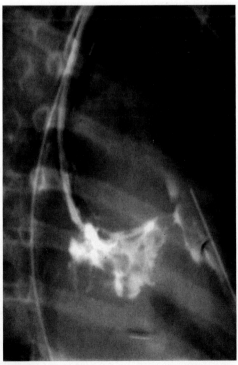

Figure 16–4 This patient had a sustained air leak associated with blunt thoracic injury despite adequate chest tube drainage. Blood was noted in the right upper lobe bronchus, and contrast injection demonstrated the location and extent of the leak, which was controlled by the injection of fibrin glue and chest tube drainage. Operative closure or resection is sometimes required.

Esophagus

The most common causes of esophageal injury are ingestion of caustic liquids and penetrating trauma, which includes iatrogenic instrumentation. Forceful vomiting and retching rarely cause esophageal tears in childhood.

External blunt trauma rarely causes esophageal injury. The mechanism of esophageal injury from blunt trauma is believed to be a sudden increase in intraesophageal pressure caused by expulsion of gas from the stomach through the gastroesophageal junction.

Esophageal perforations cause fever, chest pain, and tachycardia. Occasionally, subcutaneous emphysema develops in the neck. Mediastinal or intrapleural air may be visible on routine chest radiographs or CT. If esophageal injury is suspected, a water-soluble contrast swallow, endoscopy, or both should be done.

When diagnosed within the first 12 hours, esophageal injuries are best treated by primary closure and drainage. When diagnosed later, they may require salivary diversion by means of a cervical esophagostomy and gastrostomy, in addition to thoracic drainage.

Diaphragm

Although rare in children, diaphragmatic injuries can be caused by a forceful impact to the abdomen or by a penetrating missile. It is important to recognize these injuries, because the stomach and bowel may herniate through the defect and strangulate. Ninety percent of diaphragmatic injuries occur on the left side. In blunt trauma, tears are usually in or near the central tendon and oriented radially.

Diaphragmatic injuries are easily missed at initial presentation, especially because they are often associated with other severe injuries. They may be asymptomatic or cause abdominal, thoracic, or ipsilateral shoulder tip pain. Physical examination is rarely helpful in the diagnosis of diaphragmatic injuries. The diagnosis is usually based on the plain chest radiograph, which is the most important diagnostic test (Fig. 16-5). Table 16-3 summarizes the radiographic signs of diaphragmatic injury. Basically, any abnormality of the diaphragm or near the diaphragm on plain chest radiographs should arouse suspicion. Chest radiographs are initially normal in 30% to 50% of cases.[9] Therefore, repeat radiographs should be obtained if a diaphragmatic injury is suspected.

Because other injuries often dominate the clinical picture, delayed diagnosis of a diaphragmatic injury is common. At first, herniation of abdominal viscera into the chest may not have occurred, especially in patients receiving mechanical ventilation. However, the negative intrathoracic pressure of normal breathing may gradually draw the stomach and bowel up into the chest. This can be recognized on plain radiographs, especially if the stomach herniates with a nasogastric tube in place. In the absence of a nasogastric tube, acute dilatation of the herniated stomach may develop, leading to severe respiratory distress.

The diagnosis can be confirmed, if necessary, by upper or lower intestinal radiographic contrast studies. However, these studies may not be possible in patients with multiple acute injuries. Here, CT with multiplanar reconstruction may be helpful. The signs of diaphragmatic injury on CT include discontinuity of the diaphragm, herniation

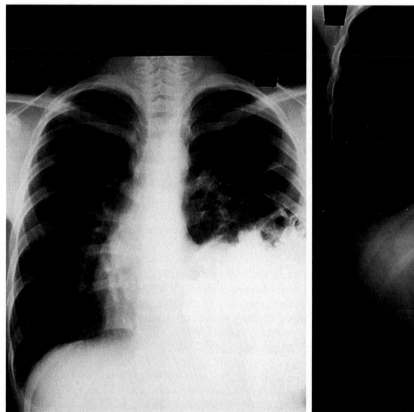
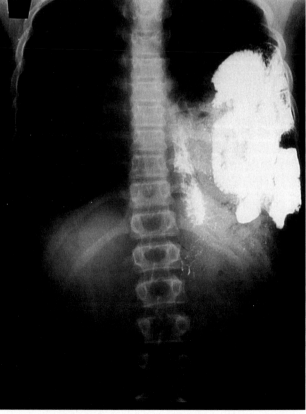

A B

Figure 16-5 Ruptured diaphragm. *A*, Plain chest radiograph. *B*, Herniated bowel on gastrointestinal contrast study.

TABLE 16-3 Radiographic Signs of Diaphragmatic Injury

Obscured hemidiaphragm
Elevated hemidiaphragm
Herniated viscera causing abnormal gas pattern above the
  diaphragm
Tip of nasogastric tube curled up into the chest
Atypical pneumothorax
Platelike atelectasis adjacent to the diaphragm

of intra-abdominal viscera into the chest, and constriction of the stomach as it passes through the defect.[89] In stable patients, magnetic resonance imaging may also help establish the diagnosis.

Some patients present with obstruction or strangulation of the herniated gut late in the course of the disorder. This causes severe abdominal or chest pain (or both), nausea, and vomiting. Primary repair through an abdominal incision is indicated. The usual repair is via open laparotomy, but several recent reports of laparoscopic repair demonstrate the feasibility of this approach.[52,67] Thoracotomy may be required for patients presenting late, because of adhesions in the chest.

Heart and Pericardium

Blunt trauma to the heart can produce several types of injury: concussion, contusion, or frank rupture of myocardium, valve, or septum.[57] Although rare, disruption or thrombosis of a coronary artery may also occur. A tear of the pericardium may allow herniation of the heart into the pleural space, thereby impairing cardiac function and causing a low output state. Occasionally, blunt trauma to the chest produces occult structural cardiac injuries without gross impairment of cardiac function, bleeding, or cardiac tamponade.[18] These injuries include atrial or ventricular septal defects, mitral or tricuspid insufficiency, and ventricular aneurysm formation. Often, the only sign is a new murmur or a change in the electrocardiogram. The diagnosis can be confirmed by echocardiography or cardiac catheterization. These injuries may be repaired electively once the patient is stable.[18] Follow-up echocardiography should be arranged in all cases of known or suspected injury to the heart.

Several case reports have appeared documenting sudden cardiac arrest in children after a direct blow to the chest. The term *commotio cordis* has been applied to this entity.[51,86] Commotio cordis occurs most often during organized sporting events such as baseball. No contusion or other sign of injury can be found at autopsy, and death is usually attributed to ventricular fibrillation.

When performing emergency surgery for cardiac trauma, the surgeon should bear in mind a few simple rules:

1. Prepare and drape the entire chest.
2. Place the incision in the left fourth or fifth interspace in an anterolateral direction (except for stable patients undergoing elective repair of known cardiac injuries, which should be repaired through a median sternotomy).
3. Avoid the phrenic nerve when opening the pericardium.
4. Apply direct pressure to control the bleeding.
5. Suture the heart using pledgets as required.
6. Leave the pericardium open.

Some authors have reported the use of skin staples to control cardiac wounds, but direct suture is preferable. A Foley catheter may be introduced through the defect to control the bleeding during repair.

Although most cardiac injuries can be repaired without cardiopulmonary bypass, this option should be available. During the operation, the surgeon should always check for a thrill, which might indicate a ruptured valve or traumatic ventricular septal defect. It is also important to check for intracardiac lesions by listening for new murmurs and performing echocardiography in the postoperative period. Follow-up echocardiography should also be done after discharge.

Myocardial Contusion

Myocardial contusion is the most common type of blunt cardiac injury. It produces focal damage to the heart that can be identified histologically. It can cause life-threatening arrhythmias and cardiac failure. Treatment is aimed primarily at these complications.

Contusion can be distinguished from concussion and commotio cordis because the latter does not produce any structural change, even at the microscopic level. Contusions are usually, but not always, associated with an injury to the chest wall. Myocardial contusions may be completely silent or cause an arrhythmia (supraventricular tachycardia or ventricular fibrillation) or hypotension secondary to reduced cardiac output.

Unfortunately, although many tests have been proposed, including electrocardiography, echocardiography, myocardial enzyme determinations (CKMB, cardiac troponin I and troponin T), and radionuclide scans, there is no definitive diagnostic test for cardiac contusion.[30,80,81] This makes it difficult to define the indications for any of the currently available diagnostic tests and even more difficult to decide on treatment. Tellez et al.[84] concluded that a "comprehensive diagnostic evaluation of the heart in all children sustaining multiple injuries from blunt trauma cannot be justified." The simplest test is a 12-lead electrocardiogram, which may reveal reversible changes to ST segments and T waves. Echocardiography may show reduced ejection fraction, localized systolic wall motion abnormality, or an area of increased end-diastolic wall thickness and echogenicity. Swaanenburg et al.[80] found that cardiac troponin I and T levels were more accurate and reliable than any of the other diagnostic tests in selecting patients for ICU monitoring. They also recommended a repeat analysis after admission for patients suspected of having myocardial contusion but with normal values at admission.

A prospective study of 41 children with blunt thoracic trauma using a battery of tests, including serum enzyme levels, electrocardiography, echocardiography, and pyrophosphate myocardial scanning, revealed a high incidence of abnormal tests. However, there was little correlation between any of the test results and the clinical course.[45] The authors concluded that myocardial contusion is rarely clinically significant in pediatric thoracic trauma. For practical purposes, significant myocardial contusion can be ruled out when findings on the 12-lead electrocardiogram and echocardiography are normal.

Treatment of myocardial contusion includes inotropic support as indicated, with electrocardiographic monitoring for 12 to 24 hours and frequent blood pressure determinations. Complications tend to occur early in the disorder or not at all.[23] Tellez et al.[84] recommended cardiac monitoring in the ER and ICU to identify arrhythmias and, in patients with arrhythmias and obvious thoracic injuries, serial electrocardiograms and cardiac enzyme tests.

Myocardial Rupture

Rupture of the heart is usually rapidly fatal. In fact, myocardial rupture is the most common cause of death from thoracic injury. In a population-based autopsy series, Bergman et al.[3] found that two thirds of these patients died at the scene of the accident and one third died in the emergency room. Most cases of cardiac rupture result from high-energy impacts, such as those sustained in motor vehicle accidents or falls from great heights. The atria tend to rupture when impact occurs during late systole; ventricles rupture from impact during late diastole. The right ventricle is the most commonly ruptured site.

Children with myocardial rupture usually present with pericardial tamponade (see later). Myocardial necrosis, aneurysm formation, and delayed rupture may also occur.[74] Those with a traumatic atrial septal defect or ventricular septal defect may present with a new murmur without obvious cardiac failure. All patients with chest trauma should be checked carefully for a new murmur before discharge. Any new murmur is an indication for echocardiography. Occasionally, with early diagnosis and repair, patients can survive myocardial rupture.

Valve Injury

Valve injuries are rare but well recognized after blunt trauma.[4,75] Atrioventricular valves are most commonly injured, causing incompetence by damage to the annulus or rupture of the chordae tendinae or papillary muscle (Fig. 16-6). This is one type of blunt cardiac injury that can be repaired semielectively.

Pericardial Tamponade

Pericardial tamponade can result from an accumulation of blood in the pericardial sac after blunt trauma. The full spectrum of pericardial tamponade—pulsus paradoxus and Beck's triad (elevated jugular venous pressure, systemic hypotension, and muffled heart sounds)—rarely develops in patients with acute trauma. Pericardial tamponade is usually associated with tachycardia, peripheral vasoconstriction, jugular venous distention, and persistent hypotension despite aggressive fluid resuscitation.

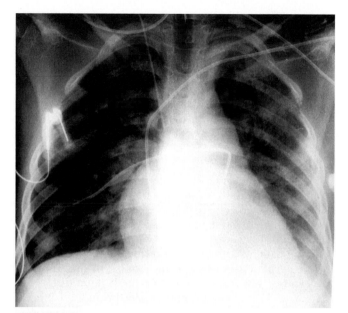

Figure 16-6   Cardiomegaly and pulmonary edema 2 days after blunt chest trauma; note the Swan-Ganz catheter. A torn mitral valve annulus and chordae tendinae were successfully repaired. (From Wesson DE: Trauma of the chest in children. Chest Clin North Am 1993;3:423.)

In fact, pericardial tamponade should be suspected in all cases of unexplained hypotension, especially when it is associated with elevated jugular venous pressure. The best way to confirm the diagnosis is by transthoracic echocardiography, which can be performed by the surgeon at the bedside in conjunction with the focused abdominal sonography for trauma (FAST) examination.[10,62]

Treatment of suspected pericardial tamponade begins with control of the airway and breathing plus restoration and expansion of the circulating blood volume. The diagnosis should be confirmed by echocardiography, which is the single best diagnostic tool. However, if the patient is in severe shock, needle catheter drainage of the pericardial space may be lifesaving (Fig. 16-7). Therefore, in emergency situations or when echocardiography is not available, immediate pericardiocentesis is indicated. The needle should be inserted by the subxiphoid approach at a 45-degree angle upward and toward the left shoulder. A successful tap is confirmed by aspiration of nonclotting blood. A catheter should be inserted and left for repeated aspirations, if necessary, pending definitive treatment. Pericardiocentesis may be complicated by bleeding or damage to the left anterior descending coronary artery. If pericardiocentesis does not stabilize the patient, immediate thoracotomy should be performed to relieve the tamponade and control the bleeding.

Pericardial Laceration

The pericardium may be torn by blunt trauma. The most common site is on the left, anterior to the phrenic nerve. The heart may herniate through the defect and undergo

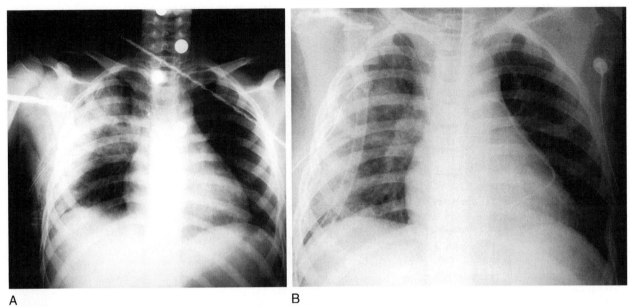

A   B

Figure 16–7   Pericardial tamponade from blunt chest trauma. The patient was a backseat passenger in a high-speed frontal collision. There was a seat-belt mark over the lower sternum. Shock was unresponsive to fluid, and pericardial effusion was demonstrated on transthoracic echocardiography. *A,* Normal heart on plain chest radiograph, with evidence of pulmonary contusion. *B,* Chest radiograph after catheter drainage of bloody pericardial effusion. No further treatment was required. (From Wesson DE: Trauma of the chest in children. Chest Clin North Am 1993;3:423.)

torsion, impairing its function and reducing cardiac output. This type of injury may be recognized on CT or by video-assisted thoracic surgery.[37,85,89]

Aorta

Traumatic rupture of the aorta and its major branches is uncommon in children.[2] Eddy et al.[17] reported that aortic injuries caused 2.1% of all traumatic deaths in children in King County, Washington. Traumatic rupture of the aorta causes a higher proportion of traumatic deaths in adults (approximately 10%) than in children, probably because adult aortas are more brittle and easily torn. Predictors of aortic injury include hypotension, head injury, unrestrained motor vehicle occupant, pelvic fracture, extremity fracture, and other chest injury. However, it is not clear whether mechanism is a reliable predictor. Dyer et al.[16] found it to be "imperfect" and "subjective." Horton et al.[34] found that velocity of 20 miles per hour or greater and near-side passenger compartment intrusion of 15 inches or greater correlated strongly with aortic injury.

Traumatic rupture of the aorta occurs with rapid deceleration, which applies shear stress to the wall of the aorta. The most common sites of injury are near the ligamentum arteriosum, the root of the aorta, or one of the other main branch points, such as the takeoff of the innominate, vertebral, or carotid artery. Tears of the distal arch are usually located on the anteromedial aspect of the aorta and oriented horizontally. Children with Marfan's syndrome are at risk for aortic dissection following blunt trauma to the torso.

Although it is usually rapidly fatal, in some cases, the adventitia and pleura contain the blood and prevent exsanguination. The natural history of patients who do not exsanguinate immediately is unknown, but imminent rupture in these patients is unlikely. Therefore, it is unnecessary to rush them to the operating room before stabilization, a full diagnostic workup, and treatment of other injuries. This may require laparotomy, craniotomy, or both before repair of the aorta.

The management of aortic injuries in children is essentially the same as in adults.[33,38] Diagnosis is difficult because there may be no clinical evidence of thoracic injury. Acute coarctation syndrome—upper limb hypertension, a difference in blood pressure between the upper and lower limbs, and a loud murmur over the precordium or back—is rare. DelRossi et al.[13] reported a series of 27 cases of aortic injury without a single case of coarctation syndrome.

The diagnosis is most often suggested by plain chest radiographs, which are sensitive (false-negative 2% to 7%) but not specific (false-positive 80%). The radiographic signs of traumatic rupture of the aorta are the same as described for adults (Table 16-4, Fig. 16-8).

TABLE 16–4   Radiographic Signs of Aortic Injury

Widened mediastinum (mediastinum-chest ratio >0.25)
Loss or abnormal contour of aortic knob
Depression of left main bronchus (>40 degrees below horizontal)
Deviation of trachea (left margin to right of T4 spinous process)
Deviation of esophagus (nasogastric tube to right of T4 spinous process)
Left pleural cap
Left hemothorax

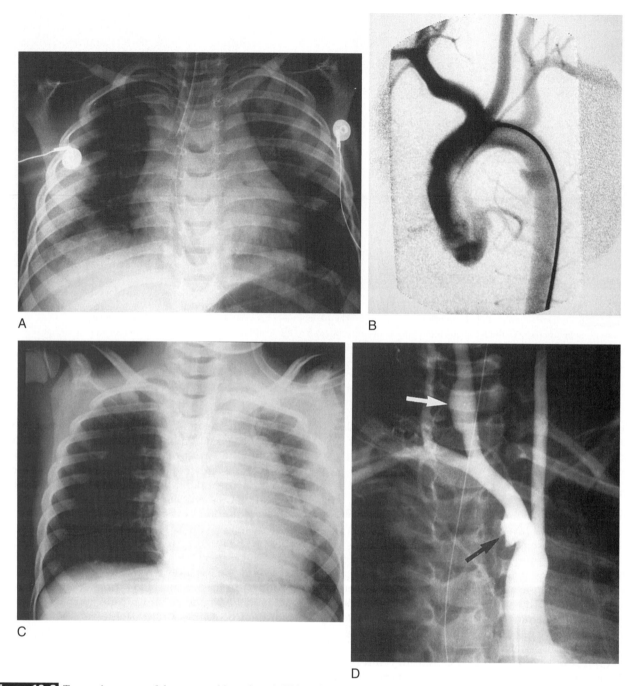

Figure 16–8 Traumatic rupture of the aorta and branches. *A*, Widened mediastinum with deviation of the endotracheal and nasogastric tubes to the right. *B*, In the same patient as in *A*, aortic injury is confirmed by aortogram. *C*, Widened mediastinum in a different patient who sustained blunt trauma to the chest. *D*, In the same patient as in *C*, there is an innominate artery laceration at its origin *(arrow)*. (From Wesson DE: Trauma of the chest in children. Chest Clin North Am 1993;3:423.)

Nearly all reported cases demonstrate widening of the mediastinum (mediastinum-chest ratio >0.25) and an abnormal aortic contour.

Until recently, most authors considered aortography the gold standard diagnostic test. Many now believe that contrast-enhanced multislice helical CT, which is equally sensitive to aortography, is the definitive test for diagnosing aortic injury (Fig. 16-9).[16,25,54,61]

If the helical CT scan is normal, an aortogram is unnecessary. This has substantially reduced the number of negative aortograms done for patients with blunt chest trauma and suspicious plain radiographs. The techniques of helical CT and CT-angiography have been reviewed by Melton et al.[54] and Rubin.[73] Timing of the contrast injection, as well as the volume and rate of infusion, must be carefully controlled to

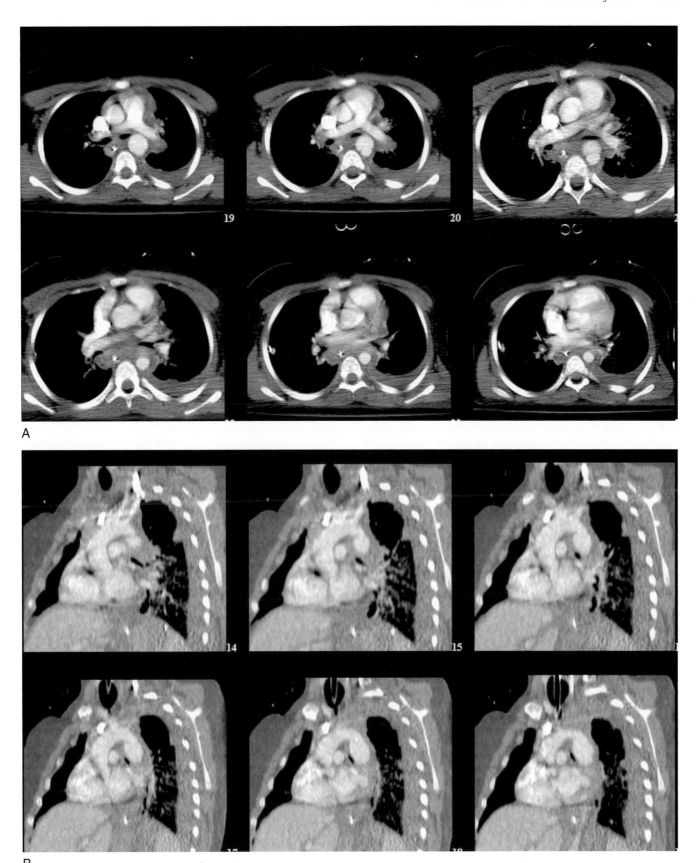

Figure 16–9 Helical computed tomography scan reconstruction showing traumatic rupture of the aorta in a 14-year-old boy. *A*, Transaxial view. Note the periaortic hematoma at the isthmus. *B*, Threé-dimensional reconstruction. Note the interruption of flow at the isthmus.

yield optimal results. Helical CT costs about half as much as aortography.[61]

There is still a role for aortography in equivocal cases or to provide more anatomic detail before repair in proven cases.[11] However, many authorities now argue that helical CT alone is sufficient for the management of aortic injuries.[54]

Transesophageal echocardiography also has a role in the diagnosis of injuries to the descending thoracic aorta, especially for unstable patients in the ICU who are unable to go to the radiology department. It is not useful for injuries of the ascending aorta or its branches. Unfortunately, TEE is operator dependent and not universally available. Le Bret et al.[46] noted three signs on TEE that are sensitive enough to screen patients for aortic injury: increased distance (>3 mm) between the probe and the aorta, double contour of the aortic wall, and US signal between the aorta and the visceral pleura. The sensitivity for diagnosing traumatic rupture of the aorta by TEE was 100% in this report; the specificity was 75%. The authors proposed that TEE be done in all cases of severe chest trauma. TEE is also useful in cases with equivocal findings on CT or aortography to avoid an unnecessary thoracotomy.[63]

Once the diagnosis is proved, treatment options include open repair, endovascular stent-graft, or even nonoperative observation in some cases. Aortic surgery carries a significant risk of complications, including intracranial hypertension, which may exacerbate bleeding; left ventricular strain; renal failure; and spinal cord ischemia. Heparin may increase the likelihood of bleeding at remote sites of injury.

A small intimal flap may heal spontaneously, but surgical repair through a left posterolateral thoracotomy is the treatment of choice, after the patient has been stabilized (the bleeding at other locations should be repaired first). Surgery can be safely delayed pending repair or control of associated severe injuries to the CNS, extensive burns, septic or contaminated wounds, solid organ injuries likely to bleed with heparinization, and respiratory failure.[83] In such cases, beta blockade to control mean arterial blood pressure and ICU monitoring are essential until repair can be safely accomplished. Esmolol is the preferred beta blocker.

Cardiopulmonary bypass (usually left heart bypass) should always be available during repair in case the injury extends to the aortic root. The left lung should be collapsed and retracted. Care is required when dissecting the aorta for cross-clamping to avoid injury to the branches that supply the spinal cord and injury to the vagus nerve and its recurrent branch. Some partial tears can be repaired primarily; however, repair usually requires placement of a woven Dacron graft, especially when the tear is circumferential. There are three basic ways to perform the operation:

1. Clamp and sew.
2. Intraoperative shunt.
3. Mechanical circulatory support.

The simplest is to clamp and sew without a shunt or cardiopulmonary bypass. This is the fastest method and requires the shortest cross-clamp time; it is adequate if the injury is not too extensive. Razzouk et al.[68] reported that the clamp-and-sew technique is feasible in the majority of patients without increased mortality or spinal cord injury. Kwon et al.[43] concur that the clamp technique does not increase mortality or morbidity. However, others strongly disagree. Hochheiser et al.[31] reported a lower incidence of postoperative paraplegia after repair with mechanical circulatory support.

Another option is intraoperative shunting with a heparin-bonded shunt. This may reduce the risk of ischemic damage to the spinal cord without the risks of systemic heparinization; however, there are no controlled studies to prove this.

The third method is to use mechanical circulatory support during the repair. The most common choice is cardiopulmonary bypass from the left superior pulmonary vein or left atrium to the femoral artery.[56] Femoral-femoral bypass with direct perfusion of the distal descending thoracic aorta has also been used. Some authorities believe that cardiopulmonary bypass reduces the risk of paraplegia, but it requires systemic heparinization, which can increase the incidence of intracranial hemorrhage.[44] The rate of paraplegia after repair of traumatic rupture of the aorta is about 5% to 10%. Individual variations in spinal cord blood supply, cross-clamp time, and intraoperative hypotension are important determinants of spinal cord injury.

There have been several recent reports of transfemoral stent insertion (endovascular stent-grafts) for injuries to the thoracic aorta in adults. Early results indicate that the outcome may be better than with standard open repair. Three case series have had remarkably low incidences of paraplegia.[15,39,60] Endovascular stent-grafts have been reported in a small series of children, but there are no reports of long-term results.[38]

Only 1 of 13 patients in Eddy's report,[17] a population-based study that included prehospital deaths, survived traumatic rupture of the aorta. In contrast, DelRossi et al.[13] reported a 75% survival rate in a clinical series. Three of the 21 survivors in DelRossi's series were paraplegic after repair, but two later recovered. DelRossi found no evidence to support one technique of repair over the others. However, Fabian et al.[21] reported that the clamp-and-sew technique is more likely than repair with bypass to result in paraplegia, especially if the cross-clamp time is longer than 30 minutes.

As is true for many types of injury, outcome also depends on associated injuries.[44] Hormuth et al.[33] reported excellent overall results in a series of 11 children with thoracic aortic injuries. They repaired isthmus injuries with left heart bypass and direct perfusion of the distal thoracic aorta, and arch injuries were repaired with hypothermic arrest.

Chylothorax

Injury to the thoracic duct, though rare, causes chylothorax. Most cases resolve spontaneously with nutritional support (total parenteral nutrition or elemental diet with medium-chain triglycerides). Occasionally, ligation of the thoracic duct is necessary.

Traumatic Asphyxia

Traumatic asphyxia, a clinical syndrome that is unique to children, occurs with sudden compression of the abdomen or chest (or both) against a closed glottis.[76] This event causes a rapid rise in intrathoracic pressure, which is transmitted to all the veins that drain into the valveless superior vena cava. Extravasation of blood occurs into the skin of the upper half of the body, the sclerae, and possibly the brain. The brain may also be damaged by hypoxia during and after the injury. The clinical features of this disorder include seizures, disorientation, petechiae in the upper half of the body and conjunctivae, and respiratory failure (Fig. 16-10). Treatment is supportive, and most patients recover uneventfully.

Penetrating Injuries

The initial management of penetrating injuries is the same as for blunt trauma: clear the airway, give oxygen and intravenous fluids, carefully assess the patient, and obtain a plain chest radiograph in every case. An attempt should be made to determine the path of the injury by marking the entry and exit wounds on the plain films. Endotracheal intubation and chest tube insertion should be done as needed during the initial resuscitation. It is important to consider the possibility of a concomitant abdominal injury with any wound below the nipple line. Bronchoscopy is indicated for suspected injury to the major airways; esophagoscopy and water-soluble contrast studies are indicated for suspected esophageal wounds. Echocardiography can be used in stable patients to diagnose suspected heart injuries.

Treatment is also the same as described for blunt trauma. Most patients do not require thoracotomy. The most common indications for surgery are massive bleeding, massive air leak, and pericardial tamponade.

Penetrating injuries are more likely to involve the heart, especially with anterior wounds medial to the midclavicular line. These injuries may cause pericardial tamponade or, if the pericardium has a defect, exsanguinating hemorrhage into the chest. Shock is a clear indication for urgent thoracotomy in cases of penetrating wounds to the chest. However, the management of patients with wounds near the heart who present with normal physiologic parameters is problematic. The most conservative and safest approach is to take all such patients to the operating room for a subxiphoid pericardial window, followed by thoracotomy through a median sternotomy, if necessary. Recent reports suggest that early echocardiography may be a sensitive test for occult cardiac injuries and that this technique can be used to select patients who require a pericardial window, thereby minimizing unnecessary invasive procedures.[10,57,62] In one report, only patients with pericardial effusions on echocardiography underwent subxiphoid pericardial window; if blood was found, a median sternotomy followed. Patients with normal echocardiographs were observed clinically. Harris et al.[28] reported a large experience with penetrating cardiac injuries and recommended cardiac US to diagnose these injuries in stable patients.

When an operation is required for a penetrating cardiac injury, a Foley catheter through the defect may control the bleeding temporarily to facilitate suture of the defect. Median sternotomy is best for known cardiac injuries.

COMPLICATIONS

There is little information in the literature on the morbidity of chest injuries or the complications after surgical management of thoracic injuries in children. The two most common postoperative complications are pulmonary atelectasis and pneumonia. The most serious is paraplegia, which occurs in 5% to 10% of cases of injury to the thoracic aorta.

OUTCOME

The risk for death from thoracic injury varies with the type of injury and the number and severity of associated injuries, particularly to the CNS. Roux and Fisher[71] reported a series of 100 consecutive children with motor vehicle–related chest trauma in South Africa. Ninety-one pedestrians constituted the largest subgroup. The eight patients who died had a mean injury severity score of 34, compared with a score of 25 among the survivors. Seven of the eight children who died had fatal head injuries. Thus, in children with blunt injuries to the chest, the severity of injury and the presence of concomitant head injuries are the main determinants

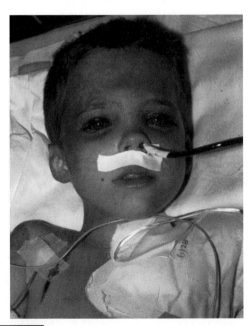

Figure 16–10 Traumatic asphyxia. This child, injured in an auto accident, was restrained but still suffered a severe compression injury of the chest. In addition to petechial hemorrhages over his upper torso, he had 48 hours of mental confusion, indicating that his brain suffered hemorrhage as well.

of survival. In children, death from thoracic injury tends to occur in the first few days after the injury, usually from other injuries and not from respiratory failure or sepsis, as is the case in adults.

The overall mortality for chest injuries was 15% in the NPTR—virtually identical to most adult series.[12] Mortality increases with each individual chest injury: 30% for a ruptured diaphragm, 40% for cardiac injury; and 50% for injury to a major vessel.

The morbidity among survivors is remarkably low. DiScala[14] reported that 90% of survivors in the NPTR had no impairment at the time of discharge.

SUMMARY

The following points summarize the management of thoracic injuries in children:

1. Most thoracic injuries can be diagnosed by a combination of clinical assessment and plain chest radiographs.
2. Most heal with supportive treatment and tube thoracostomy drainage.
3. Life-threatening thoracic injuries are relatively uncommon.
4. A few thoracic injuries require surgery, but even the most severe can be managed successfully if they are recognized and treated expeditiously.

REFERENCES

1. American College of Surgeons: Advanced Trauma Life Support Program for Physicians. Chicago, American College of Surgeons, 1993.
2. Banks E, Chun J, Weaver F: Chronic innominate artery dissection after blunt thoracic trauma: Case report. J Trauma 1995;38:975.
3. Bergman K, Spence L, Wesson D, et al: Thoracic vascular injuries: A post mortem study. J Trauma 1990;30:604.
4. Bertrand S, Laquay N, El Rassi I, et al: Tricuspid insufficiency after blunt chest trauma in a nine-year-old child. Eur J Cardiothorac Surg 1999;16:587.
5. Bhende MS, Thompson AE: Evaluation of an end-tidal CO_2 detector during pediatric cardiopulmonary resuscitation. Pediatrics 1995;95:395.
6. Blackmore CC, Zweibel A, Mann FA: Determining risk of traumatic aortic injury: How to optimize imaging strategy. AJR Am J Roentgenol 2000;174:343.
7. Bokhari F, Brakenridge S, Nagy K, et al: Prospective evaluation of the sensitivity of physical examination in chest trauma. J Trauma 2003;54:1255.
8. Bonadio WA, Hellmich T, Wisconsin M: Post-traumatic pulmonary contusion in children. Ann Emerg Med 1989;8:1050.
9. Brandt M, Luks FI, Spigland NA, et al: Diaphragmatic injury in children. J Trauma 1992;32:298.
10. Carillo EH, Guin BJ, Ali AT, et al: Transthoracic ultrasonography is an alternative to subxiphoid ultrasonography for the diagnosis of hemopericardium in penetrating precordial trauma. Am J Surg 2000;179:34.
11. Chen MY, Miller PR, McLaughlin CA, et al: The trend of using computed tomography in the detection of acute thoracic aortic and branch vessel injury after blunt thoracic trauma: A single-center experience over 13 years. J Trauma 2004;56:783.
12. Cooper A, Barlow B, DiScala C, String D: Mortality and truncal injury: The pediatric perspective. J Pediatr Surg 1994;29:33.
13. DelRossi AJ, Cernaianu AC, Madden LD, et al: Traumatic disruptions of the thoracic aorta: Treatment and outcome. Surgery 1990;108:864.
14. DiScala C: Biannual Report. National Pediatric Trauma Registry, 1995.
15. Dunham MB, Zygun D, Petrasek P, et al: Endovascular stent grafts for acute blunt aortic injury. J Trauma 2004;56:1173.
16. Dyer DS, Moore EE, Ilke DN, et al: Thoracic aortic injury: How predictive is mechanism and is chest computed tomography a reliable screening tool? A prospective study of 1561 patients. J Trauma 2000;48:682.
17. Eddy AC, Rusch VW, Fligner CL, et al: The epidemiology of traumatic rupture of the thoracic aorta in children: A 13-year review. J Trauma 1990;30:989.
18. End A, Rodler S, Oturanlar D, et al: Elective surgery for blunt cardiac trauma. J Trauma 1994;37:798.
19. Eren S, Balci AE, Ulku R, et al: Thoracic firearm injuries in children: Management and analysis of prognostic factors. Eur J Cardiothorac Surg 2003;23:888.
20. Exadaktylos AK, Sclabas G, Schmid SW, et al: Do we really need routine computed tomography scanning in the primary evaluation of blunt chest trauma in patients with "normal" chest radiograph? J Trauma 2001;51:1173.
21. Fabian TC, Richardson JD, Croce MA, et al: Prospective study of blunt aortic injury: Multi-center trial of the American Association for the Surgery of Trauma. J Trauma 1997;42:374.
22. Fernandez L, Radhakrishna J, Gordon RT, et al: Thoracic BB injuries in pediatric patients. J Trauma 1995;38:384.
23. Frame SB, Thompson TC: Blunt cardiac injuries. Adv Trauma Crit Care 1995;10:15.
24. Garcia V, Gottschall CS, Eichelberger MR, et al: Rib fractures in children: A marker of severe trauma. J Trauma 1990;30:695.
25. Gavant ML, Menke PG, Fabian T, et al: Blunt traumatic aortic rupture: Detection with helical CT of the chest. Radiology 1995;197:125.
26. Gittleman MA, Gonzalea-del-Rey J, Brody AS, et al: Clinical predictors for the selective use of chest radiographs in pediatric blunt trauma evaluations. J Trauma 2003;55:670.
27. Hall A, Johnson K: The imaging of paediatric thoracic trauma. Paediatr Respir Rev 2002;3:241.
28. Harris DG, Bleeker CP, Pretorius J, et al: Penetrating cardiac injuries—current evaluation and management of the stable patient. S Afr J Surg 2001;39:90.
29. Harris GJ, Soper RT: Pediatric first rib fractures. J Trauma 1990;30:343.
30. Hirsch R, Landt Y, Porter S, et al: Cardiac troponin I in pediatrics: Normal values and potential use in the assessment of cardiac injury. J Pediatr 1997;130:853.
31. Hochheiser GM, Clark DE, Morton JR: Operative technique, paraplegia, and mortality after blunt traumatic aortic injury. Arch Surg 2002;137:434.
32. Holmes JF, Sokolove PE, Brant WE, et al: A clinical decision rule for identifying children with thoracic injuries after blunt torso trauma. Ann Emerg Med 2002;39:492.
33. Hormuth D, Cefali D, Rouse T, et al: Traumatic disruption of the thoracic aorta in children. Arch Surg 1999;134:759.
34. Horton TG, Cohn SM, Heid MP, et al: Identification of trauma patients at risk of thoracic aortic tear by mechanism of injury. J Trauma 2000;48:1008.

35. Hoth JJ, Scott MJ, Bullock TK, et al: Thoracotomy for blunt trauma: Traditional indications may not apply. Am Surg 2003;69:1108.

36. Hu J, Wall MJ Jr, Estrera AL, et al: Surgical management of traumatic pulmonary injury. Am J Surg 2003; 186:620.

37. Janson JT, Harris DG, Pretorius J, et al: Pericardial rupture and cardiac herniation after blunt chest trauma. Ann Thorac Surg 2003;75:754.

38. Karmay-Jones R, Hoffer E, Meissner M, et al: Management of traumatic rupture of the thoracic aorta in pediatric patients. Ann Thorac Surg 2003;75:1513.

39. Kasirajan K, Heffernan D, Langsfield M: Acute thoracic aortic trauma: A comparison of endoluminal stent grafts with open repair and nonoperative management. Ann Vasc Surg 2003;17:589.

40. Kleinman P, Mark SE, Spevak MR, et al: Fractures of the rib head in abused infants. Radiology 1992;185:119.

41. Knudtson JL, Dort JM, Helmer SD, et al: Surgeon-performed ultrasound for pneumothorax in the trauma suite. J Trauma 2004;56:527.

42. Kulshrestha P, Munshi I, Wait R: Profile of chest trauma in a level I trauma center. J Trauma 2004;57:576.

43. Kwon CC, Gill IS, Fallon WF, et al: Delayed operative intervention in the management of traumatic descending thoracic aortic rupture. Ann Thorac Surg 2002;74:1888.

44. Langanay T, Verhoye JP, Corbineau H, et al: Surgical treatment of acute traumatic rupture of the thoracic aorta—timing reappraisal? Eur J Cardiothorac Surg 2002;21:282.

45. Langer JC, Winthrop AL, Wesson DE, et al: Diagnosis and incidence of cardiac injury in children with blunt thoracic trauma. J Pediatr Surg 1989;24:1091.

46. Le Bret F, Ruel P, Rosier H, et al: Diagnosis of traumatic mediastinal hematoma with transesophageal echocardiography. Chest 1994;105:373.

47. Lomoschitz FM, Eisenhuber E, Linnau KF, et al: Imaging of chest trauma: Radiological patterns of injury and diagnostic algorithms. Eur J Radiol 2003;48:61.

48. Magid N, Glass T: A "hole in a rib" as a sign of child abuse. Pediatr Radiol 1990;20:334.

49. Mandavia DP, Joseph A: Bedside echocardiography in chest trauma. Emerg Med Clin North Am 2004;22:601.

50. Manson D, Babyn PS, Palder S, et al: CT of blunt chest trauma in children. Pediatr Radiol 1995;23:1.

51. Maron BJ, Gohman TE, Kyle SB, et al: Clinical profile and spectrum of commotio cordis. JAMA 2002;287:1142.

52. Matthews BD, Bui H, Harold KL, et al: Laparoscopic repair of traumatic diaphragmatic injuries. Surg Endosc 2003; 17:254.

53. Meller JL, Little AG, Shermeta DW: Thoracic trauma in children. Pediatrics 1984;74:813.

54. Melton SM, Kerby JD, McGiffin D, et al: The evolution of chest computed tomography for the definitive diagnosis of blunt aortic injury: A single-center experience. J Trauma 2004;56:243.

55. Mirvis SE, Shanmuganathan K: MR imaging of thoracic trauma. Magn Reson Imaging Clin N Am 2000;8:91.

56. Moore EE, Burch JM, Moore JB: Repair of the torn descending thoracic aorta using the centrifugal pump for partial left heart by-pass. Ann Surg 2004;240:38.

57. Nagy K, Lohmann C, Kim DO, et al: Role of echocardiography in the diagnosis of occult penetrating cardiac injury. J Trauma 1995;38:859.

58. Nakayama DK, Ramenofsky ML: Chest injuries in childhood. Ann Surg 1989;210:770.

59. Nakayama DK, Rowe MI: Intrathoracic tracheobronchial injuries in childhood. Int Anesthesiol Clin 1988;26:42.

60. Ott MC, Stewart TC, Lawlor DK, et al: Management of blunt thoracic aortic injuries: Endovascular stent versus open repair. J Trauma 2004;56:565.

61. Parker MS, Matheson TL, Rao AV, et al: Making the transition: The role of helical CT in the evaluation of potentially acute thoracic injuries. AJR Am J Roentgenol 2001;176:1267.

62. Patel AN, Brennig C, Cotner J, et al: Successful diagnosis of penetrating cardiac injury using surgeon performed ultrasonography. Ann Thorac Surg 2003;76:2046.

63. Patel HN, Hahn D, Comess KA: Blunt chest trauma: Role of intravascular and transesophageal echocardiography in cases of abnormal thoracic aortogram. J Trauma 2003;55:330.

64. Peterson RJ, Tepas JJ 3rd, Edwards FH, et al: Pediatric and adult thoracic trauma: Age-related impact on presentation and outcome. Ann Thorac Surg 1994;58:14.

65. Place RJ, Cavanaugh DG: Computed tomography to diagnose pericardial rupture. J Trauma 1995;38:882.

66. Powell RW, Gill EA, Jurkovich GJ, et al: Resuscitative thoracotomy in children and adolescents. Am Surg 1988;54:188.

67. Pross M, Manger T, Mirow L, et al: Laparoscopic management of late-diagnosed major diaphragmatic rupture. J Laparoendosc Adv Surg Tech A 2003;10:111.

68. Razzouk AJ, Gundry SR, Wang N, et al: Repair of traumatic aortic rupture: A 25-year experience. Arch Surg 2000; 135:913.

69. Reinoso-Barbero F, Sanabria P, Bueno J, et al: High-frequency ventilation for a child with traumatic bronchial rupture. Anesth Analg 1995;81:183.

70. Renton J, Kincaid S, Ehrlich PF: Should helical CT scanning of the thoracic cavity replace the conventional chest x-ray as a primary assessment tool in pediatric trauma? An efficacy and cost analysis. J Pediatr Surg 2003;38:793.

71. Roux P, Fisher RM: Chest injuries in children: An analysis of 100 cases of blunt chest trauma from motor vehicle accidents. J Pediatr Surg 1992;27:551.

72. Rowan KR, Kirkpatrick AW, Liu D, et al: Traumatic pneumothorax detection with thoracic US: Correlation with chest radiography and CT—initial experience. Radiology 2002;227:305.

73. Rubin GD: CT angiography of the thoracic aorta. Semin Roentgenol 2003;38:115.

74. RuDusky BM: Myocardial contusion culminating in a ruptured pseudoaneurysm of the left ventricle—a case report. Angiology 2003;54:359.

75. Salehian O, Mulji A: Tricuspid valve disruption and ventricular septal defect secondary to blunt chest trauma. Can J Cardiol 2004;20:231.

76. Sarihan H, Abes M, Akyazici R, et al: Traumatic asphyxia in children. J Cardiovasc Surg (Torino) 1997;38:93.

77. Scorpio RS, Wesson DE, Smith CR, et al: Blunt cardiac injuries in children: A postmortem study. J Trauma 1996; 41:306.

78. Shabb BR, Taha M, Nabbout G, et al: Successful delayed repair of a complete transection of the right mainstem bronchus in a five-year-old girl: Case report. J Trauma Injury Infect Crit Care 1995;38:964.

79. Shorr R, Crittenden M, Indeck M, et al: Blunt thoracic trauma: analysis of 515 patients. Ann Surg 1987;206:200.

80. Swaanenburg JC, Klaase JM, DeJongste MJ, et al: Troponin I, troponin T, CKMB-activity and CKMB-mass as markers for the detection of myocardial contusion in patients who experienced blunt trauma. Clin Chim Acta 1998; 272:171.

81. Sybrandy KC, Cramer MJ, Burgersdijk C: Diagnosing cardiac contusion: Old wisdom and new insights. Heart 2002;89:485.

82. Taskinen SO, Salo, JA, Halttunen PE, et al: Tracheobronchial rupture due to blunt chest trauma: A follow-up study. Ann Thorac Surg 1989;48:846.

83. Tatou E, Steinmetz E, Jazayeri S, et al: Surgical outcome of traumatic rupture of the thoracic aorta. Ann Thorac Surg 2000;69:70.

84. Tellez DW, Hardin WD Jr, Takahashi M, et al: Blunt cardiac injury in children. J Pediatr Surg 1987;22:1123.

85. Thomas P, Saux P, Lonjon T, et al: Diagnosis by video-assisted thoracoscopy of traumatic pericardial rupture with delayed luxation of the heart: Case report. J Trauma 1995;38:967.

86. Wang JN, Tsai YC, Chen SL, et al: Dangerous impact—commotio cordis. Cardiology 2000;93:124.

87. Williams RL, Connolloy PT: In children undergoing chest radiography what is the specificity of rib fractures for non-accidental injury? Arch Dis Child 2004;89:490.

88. Wilson A, Wall MJ Jr, Maxson R, et al: The pulmonary hilum twist as a thoracic damage control procedure. Am J Surg 2003;186:49.

89. Worthy S, Kang EY, Hartman TE, et al: Diaphragmatic rupture: CT findings in 11 patients. Radiology 1995; 194:885.

Chapter 17

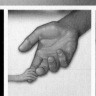

Abdominal Trauma

Steven Stylianos and Richard H. Pearl

Who could have imagined the influence of Simpson's 1968 publication on the successful nonoperative treatment of select children presumed to have splenic injury?[142] Initially suggested in the early 1950s by Warnsborough, then chief of general surgery at the Hospital for Sick Children in Toronto, the era of nonoperative management of splenic injury began with the report of 12 children treated between 1956 and 1965. The diagnosis of splenic injury in this select group was made by clinical findings, along with routine laboratory and plain radiographic findings. Keep in mind that this report predated ultrasonography (US), computed tomography (CT), or isotope imaging. Subsequent confirmation of splenic injury was made in one child who required laparotomy years later for an unrelated condition, when it was found that the spleen had healed in two separate pieces. Nearly 4 decades later, the standard treatment of hemodynamically stable children with splenic injury is nonoperative, and this concept has been successfully applied to most blunt injuries of the liver, kidney, and pancreas as well. Surgical restraint is now the norm, based on an increased awareness of the anatomic patterns and physiologic responses of injured children. Our colleagues in adult trauma care have slowly acknowledged this success and are applying many of the principles learned in pediatric trauma to their patients.[79]

A recent review of the National Pediatric Trauma Registry (NPTR) indicates that 8% to 12% of children suffering blunt trauma have an abdominal injury.[28] Fortunately, more than 90% of them survive. Although abdominal injuries are 30% more common than thoracic injuries, they are 40% less likely to be fatal. The infrequent need for laparotomy in children with blunt abdominal injury has created a debate regarding the role of pediatric trauma surgeons in their treatment. Recent analyses of the NPTR and the National Trauma Data Bank emphasize the overall "surgical" nature of pediatric trauma patients, with more than 25% of injured children requiring operative intervention.[1,141] Clearly, a qualified pediatric trauma surgeon would be the ideal coordinator of such care.

Few surgeons have extensive experience with massive abdominal solid organ injuries requiring immediate surgery. It is imperative that surgeons familiarize themselves with current treatment algorithms for life-threatening abdominal trauma. Important contributions have been made in the diagnosis and treatment of children with abdominal injury by radiologists and endoscopists. The resolution and speed of CT, the screening capabilities of focused abdominal sonography for trauma (FAST), and the percutaneous, angiographic, and endoscopic interventions of nonsurgeon members of the pediatric trauma team have all enhanced patient care and improved outcomes. This chapter focuses on the more common blunt injuries and unique aspects of care in children. Renal and genitourinary injuries are covered separately in Chapter 18.

DIAGNOSTIC MODALITIES

The initial evaluation of an acutely injured child is similar to that of an adult. Plain radiographs of the cervical spine, chest, and pelvis are obtained after the initial survey and evaluation of the ABCs (airway, breathing, and circulation). Other plain abdominal films add little to the acute evaluation of pediatric trauma patients. As imaging modalities have improved, treatment algorithms have changed significantly in children with suspected intra-abdominal injuries. Prompt identification of potentially life-threatening injuries is now possible in the vast majority of children.

Computed Tomography

CT has become the imaging study of choice for the evaluation of injured children owing to several advantages. CT is now readily accessible in most health care facilities; it is a noninvasive, accurate method of identifying and qualifying the extent of abdominal injury; and it has reduced the incidence of nontherapeutic exploratory laparotomy.

Use of intravenous contrast is essential, and "dynamic" methods of scanning have optimized vascular and parenchymal enhancement. The importance of a contrast "blush" in children with blunt spleen and liver injury continues to be debated and is discussed later (Fig. 17-1).[35] Head CT, if indicated, should be performed first without contrast, to avoid concealing a hemorrhagic

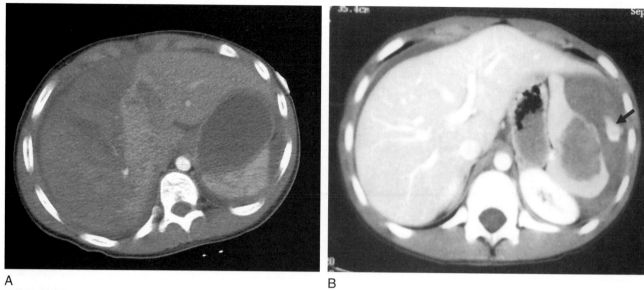

A   B

Figure 17–1 *A,* Abdominal computed tomography scan demonstrating a significant injury to the right hepatic lobe with intravenous contrast "blush." This patient had successful angiographic embolization and avoided operation. *B,* Abdominal computed tomography scan demonstrating a significant injury to the spleen with intravenous contrast "blush" *(arrow).* The patient remained hemodynamically stable and avoided operation.

brain injury. Enteral contrast for enhancement of the gastrointestinal (GI) tract is generally not required in the acute trauma setting and can lead to aspiration.

Not all children with potential abdominal injuries are candidates for CT evaluation. Obvious penetrating injury often necessitates immediate operative intervention. A hemodynamically unstable child should not be taken out of an appropriate resuscitation room for the performance of CT. These children may benefit from an alternative diagnostic study, such as peritoneal lavage or FAST, or urgent operative intervention. The greatest limitation of abdominal CT in trauma is the inability to reliably identify intestinal rupture.[11,15] Findings suggestive but not diagnostic of intestinal perforation are pneumoperitoneum, bowel wall thickening, free intraperitoneal fluid, bowel wall enhancement, and dilated bowel.[59] A high index of suspicion should exist for the presence of bowel injury in a child with intraperitoneal fluid and no identifiable solid organ injury on CT.[127] The diagnosis and treatment of bowel injury are reviewed in detail later.

Focused Abdominal Sonography for Trauma

Clinician-performed sonography for the early evaluation of an injured child is currently being evaluated to determine its optimal use. Examination of Morrison's pouch; the pouch of Douglas; the left flank, including the perisplenic anatomy; and a subxiphoid view to visualize the pericardium is the standard four-view FAST examination (Fig. 17-2). This bedside examination may be a good rapid screening study, particularly in patients too unstable to undergo an abdominal CT scan. Early reports have found FAST to be a helpful screening tool in children, with a high specificity (95%) but low sensitivity (33%) in

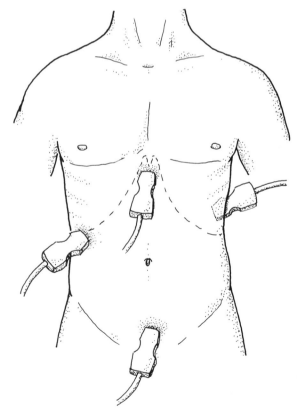

Figure 17–2 Schematic of a focused abdominal sonography for trauma (FAST) examination, with emphasis on views of the subxiphoid, right upper quadrant and Morrison's pouch, left upper quadrant and left paracolic region, and pelvic region and pouch of Douglas. (Original illustration by Mark Mazziotti, MD.)

identifying intestinal injury,[103] and a lack of identifiable free fluid does not exclude a significant injury. FAST may be useful in decreasing the number of CT scans performed for "low-likelihood" injuries. Repetition of the study may be necessary, depending on clinical correlation, and the finding of free fluid in itself is not an indication for surgical intervention. Recently, a simple scoring system for quantifying the amount of hemoperitoneum has been shown to be predictive of the need for laparotomy in a small series of children after blunt abdominal trauma.[101] Prospective validation of such a FAST score is necessary.

Diagnostic Peritoneal Lavage and Laparoscopy

Diagnostic peritoneal lavage (DPL) has been a mainstay in trauma evaluation for more than 3 decades. However, its utility in pediatric trauma is limited. Because up to 90% of solid organ injuries do not require surgical intervention, the finding of free blood in the abdomen by DPL has limited clinical significance. Hemodynamic instability and the need for ongoing blood replacement are the determinants for operation in patients with solid organ injury in the absence of blood in the abdominal cavity. Additionally, the speed and accuracy of CT have further decreased the indications for DPL in pediatric trauma. The sensitivity of CT in diagnosing solid organ injuries and more subtle injuries to the duodenum, pancreas, and intestines continues to improve. This has relegated DPL to the evaluation of patients with clinical findings suggestive of bowel injury and no definitive diagnosis on CT. In this setting, the presence of bile, food particles, or other evidence of GI tract perforation is diagnostic. Recent literature has suggested that laparoscopy can both diagnose and, in some cases, allow definitive surgical management without laparotomy, further limiting the usefulness of DPL. In a study from Dundee, Scotland, comparing DPL and laparoscopy, both tests were highly sensitive (100%), but laparoscopy had a higher specificity (94% versus 83%).[29]

Large prospective trials using laparoscopy in adults have demonstrated increased diagnostic accuracy, decreased nontherapeutic laparotomy rates, and a significant decrease in hospital length of stay, with an attendant reduction in costs. For example, in a report from the University of Tennessee, 55% of patients with abdominal trauma avoided laparotomy after laparoscopic evaluation.[37] Similar work from Jacobi Medical Center in New York City revealed a direct relationship between a reduction in negative laparotomies and increased use of laparoscopy for diagnosis and management.[126] Multiple adult studies have shown the utility of laparoscopy not only in trauma evaluation but also in the definitive management of related injuries. Repairs of gastric and intestinal perforation, bladder rupture, liver laceration, diaphragmatic injury, and splenic injury have all been reported.[21,128,140] The extent of feasible operations is directly related to the surgeon's skill with advanced laparoscopic techniques and the patient's overall stability. At the Children's Hospital of Illinois, our two most recent handlebar injuries causing bowel perforation were successfully treated laparoscopically. As with elective abdominal surgery, the role of laparoscopy in trauma will increase substantially as trauma centers redirect their training of residents to this modality and as more pediatric centers report outcome studies for laparoscopic trauma management in children.[20,44,52]

SOLID ORGAN INJURIES

Spleen and Liver

The spleen and liver are the organs most commonly injured in blunt abdominal trauma, with each accounting for one third of the injuries. Nonoperative treatment of isolated splenic and hepatic injuries in stable children has been universally successful and is now standard practice. However, there is great variation in the management algorithms used by individual pediatric surgeons. Review of the NPTR and recent surveys of the American Pediatric Surgical Association (APSA) membership confirm the wide disparity in practice.[38,133] Controversy also exists regarding the utility of CT grading and the finding of contrast blush as a predictor of outcome in liver and spleen injury.[49,82,89,106] Several recent studies reported contrast blush in 7% to 12% of children with blunt spleen injury (see Fig. 17-1).[25,76,99] The rate of operation in the "blush" group approached or exceeded 20%. The authors emphasized that CT blush was worrisome but that most patients could still be managed successfully without operation. The role of angiographic embolization in pediatric spleen injury has yet to be determined.

Recently the APSA Trauma Committee analyzed a contemporary multi-institution database of 832 children treated nonoperatively at 32 centers in North America from 1995 to 1997 (Table 17-1).[135] Consensus guidelines

TABLE 17-1 Resource Utilization and Activity Restriction in 832 Children with Isolated Spleen or Liver Injury by CT Grade

	Grade I (n = 116)	Grade II (n = 341)	Grade III (n = 275)	Grade IV (n = 100)
Admitted to ICU (%)	55.0	54.3	72.3	85.4
No. hospital days (mean)	4.3	5.3	7.1	7.6
No. hospital days (range)	1-7	2-9	3-9	4-10
Transfused (%)	1.8	5.2	10.1*	26.6*
Laparotomy (%)	0	1.0	2.7†	12.6†
Follow-up imaging (%)	34.4	46.3	54.1	51.8
Activity restriction (mean wk)	5.1	6.2	7.5	9.2
Activity restriction (range wk)	2-6	2-8	4-12	6-12

*Grade III vs grade IV, $p < 0.014$.
†Grade III vs grade IV, $p < 0.0001$.
CT, computed tomography; ICU, intensive care unit.
From Stylianos S, APSA Trauma Committee: Evidence-based guidelines for resource utilization in children with isolated spleen or liver injury. J Pediatr Surg 2000;35:164-169.

TABLE 17-2 Proposed Guidelines for Resource Utilization in Children with Isolated Spleen or Liver Injury by CT Grade

	Grade I	Grade II	Grade III	Grade IV
ICU days	0	0	0	1
Hospital stay (days)	2	3	4	5
Predischarge imaging	None	None	None	None
Postdischarge imaging	None	None	None	None
Activity restriction (wk)*	3	4	5	6

CT, computed tomography; ICU, intensive care unit.

*Return to full-contact, competitive sports (e.g., football, wrestling, hockey, lacrosse, mountain climbing) should be at the discretion of the individual pediatric trauma surgeon. The proposed guidelines for return to unrestricted activity include "normal" age-appropriate activities.

From Stylianos S, APSA Trauma Committee: Evidence-based guidelines for resource utilization in children with isolated spleen or liver injury. J Pediatr Surg 2000; 35:164-169.

on intensive care unit (ICU) stay, length of hospital stay, use of follow-up imaging, and physical activity restriction for clinically stable children with isolated spleen or liver injuries (CT grades I to IV) were defined based on this analysis (Table 17-2). The guidelines were then applied prospectively in 312 children with liver or spleen injuries treated nonoperatively at 16 centers from 1998 to 2000.[136] Patients with other minor injuries such as nondisplaced, noncomminuted fractures or soft tissue injuries were included as long as the associated injuries did not influence the variables in the study. The patients were grouped by severity of injury defined by CT grade. Compliance with the proposed guidelines was analyzed for age, organ injured, and injury grade. All patients were followed for 4 months after injury. It is imperative to emphasize that these proposed guidelines assume hemodynamic stability. The extremely low rates of transfusion and operation document the stability of the study patients.

Specific guideline compliance was 81% for ICU stay, 82% for length of hospital stay, 87% for follow-up imaging, and 78% for activity restriction. There was a significant improvement in compliance from year 1 to year 2 for ICU stay (77% versus 88%, $P < 0.02$) and activity restriction (73% versus 87%, $P < 0.01$). There were no differences in compliance by age, gender, or organ injured. Deviation from the guidelines was the surgeon's choice in 90% of cases and patient-related in 10%. Six patients (1.9%) were readmitted, although none required operation. Compared with the previously studied 832 patients, the 312 patients managed prospectively by the proposed guidelines had a significant reduction in ICU stay ($P < 0.0001$), hospital stay ($P < 0.0006$), follow-up imaging ($P < 0.0001$), and interval of physical activity restriction ($P < 0.04$) within each grade of injury.

From these data it was concluded that prospective application of specific treatment guidelines based on injury severity resulted in conformity in patient management, improved utilization of resources, and validation of guideline safety. Significant reductions in ICU stay,

hospital stay, follow-up imaging, and activity restriction were achieved without adverse sequelae when compared with the retrospective database.

The attending surgeon's decision to operate for spleen or liver injury is best based on evidence of continued blood loss, such as low blood pressure, tachycardia, decreased urine output, and falling hematocrit unresponsive to crystalloid and blood transfusion. The rates of successful nonoperative treatment of isolated blunt splenic and hepatic injury now exceed 90% in most pediatric trauma centers and in adult trauma centers with a strong pediatric commitment (H. N. Lovvorn, personal communication).[87,135,136] A study of more than 100 patients from the NPTR indicated that nonoperative treatment of spleen or liver injury is indicated even in the presence of associated head injury if the patient is hemodynamically stable.[63] Rates of operative intervention for blunt spleen or liver injury were similar with and without an associated closed head injury.

Not surprisingly, adult trauma services have reported excellent survival rates for pediatric trauma patients; however, an analysis of treatment for spleen and liver injuries reveals alarmingly high rates of operative treatment.[42,64,87,113] This discrepancy in operative rates emphasizes the importance of disseminating effective guidelines, because the majority of seriously injured children are treated outside of dedicated pediatric trauma centers. Mooney and Forbes[88] reviewed the New England Pediatric Trauma Database in the 1990s and identified 2500 children with spleen injuries. Two thirds were treated by nonpediatric trauma surgeons, and two thirds were treated in nontrauma centers. After allowing for multiple patient- and hospital-related variables, the authors found that the risk of operation was reduced by half when a surgeon with pediatric training provided care to children with spleen injuries. In a similar review using the KIDS 2000 administrative data set, Rothstein et al.[114] found that despite adjustment for hospital- and patient-specific variables, children treated at an adult general hospital had a 2.8 greater chance ($P < 0.003$), and those treated at a general hospital with a pediatric unit had a 2.6 greater chance ($P < 0.013$), of undergoing splenectomy than those cared for at a freestanding pediatric hospital.

Adult trauma surgeons caring for injured children must consider the anatomic, immunologic, and physiologic differences between pediatric and adult trauma patients and incorporate these differences into their treatment protocols. The major concerns are related to the potential risks of increased transfusion requirements, missed associated injuries, and increased length of hospital stay. Each of these concerns has been shown to be without merit.[78,86,90,95,104,118,133]

Associated Abdominal Injuries

Advocates of surgical intervention for splenic trauma cite their concern about missing associated abdominal injuries if no operation is performed. Morse and Garcia[90] reported successful nonoperative treatment in 110 of 120 children (91%) with blunt splenic trauma, of whom 22 (18%) had associated abdominal injuries. Only 3 of

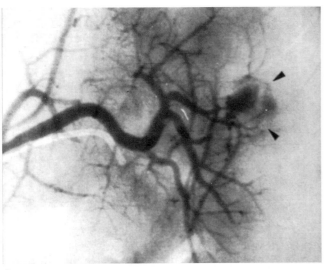
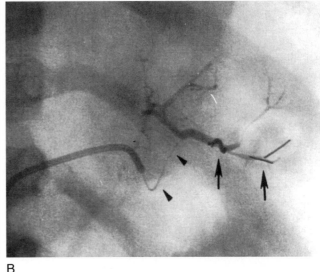

A   B

Figure 17–3 *A*, Splenic pseudoaneurysm after *(arrows)* nonoperative treatment of blunt splenic injury. *B*, Successful angiographic embolization *(arrows* show occlusion of ruptured vessels).

these 120 patients (2.5%) had GI injuries, and each was discovered at early celiotomy done for a specific indication. There was no morbidity from missed injuries or delayed surgery. Similarly, a review of the NPTR from 1988 to 1998 revealed 2977 patients with solid abdominal visceral injuries; only 96 (3.2%) had an associated hollow visceral injury.[95] Higher rates of hollow visceral injury were observed in assaulted patients and in those with multiple solid visceral injuries or pancreatic injuries. Differences in mechanism of injury may account for the much lower incidence of associated abdominal injuries in children with splenic trauma. There is no justification for an exploratory celiotomy solely to avoid missing potential associated injuries in children.

Complications of Nonoperative Treatment

Nonoperative treatment protocols have been the standard for most children with blunt liver and spleen injuries for the past 2 decades. This cumulative experience has allowed us to evaluate both the benefits and the risks of the non-operative approach. Fundamental to the success of a nonoperative strategy is the early, spontaneous cessation of hemorrhage. Transfusion rates for children with isolated spleen or liver injuries have fallen below 10%, confirming the lack of continued blood loss in the majority of patients.[73,82,87,135,136] Despite many favorable observations, isolated reports of significant delayed hemorrhage with adverse outcomes continue to appear.[13,40,46,123] Shilyansky et al.[123] reported two children with delayed hemorrhage 10 days after blunt liver injury. Both children had persistent right upper quadrant and right shoulder pain despite normal vital signs and stable hematocrits. The authors recommended continued in-house observation until symptoms resolve. Other reports have described patients with significant bleeding 38 days after grade II spleen injury and 24 days after grade IV

liver injury.[13,40] These rare occurrences lead to caution when determining a minimum safe interval before the resumption of unrestricted activities.

Routine follow-up imaging studies have identified pseudocysts and pseudoaneurysms following splenic injury (H. N. Lovvorn, personal communication).[41,98] Splenic pseudoaneurysms often cause no symptoms and appear to resolve with time. The true incidence of self-limited, post-traumatic splenic pseudoaneurysms is unknown because routine follow-up imaging after successful nonoperative treatment has been largely abandoned. Once identified, the actual risk of splenic pseudoaneurysm rupture is also unclear. Angiographic embolization techniques can successfully treat these lesions, obviating the need for open surgery and loss of splenic parenchyma (Fig. 17-3). Splenic pseudocysts can achieve enormous size, leading to pain and GI disturbance (Fig. 17-4). Simple percutaneous aspiration leads to a high recurrence rate. Laparoscopic excision and marsupialization are highly effective (Fig. 17-5).

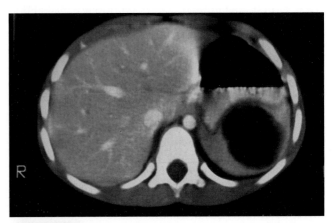

Figure 17–4 Computed tomography scan of post-traumatic splenic pseudocyst.

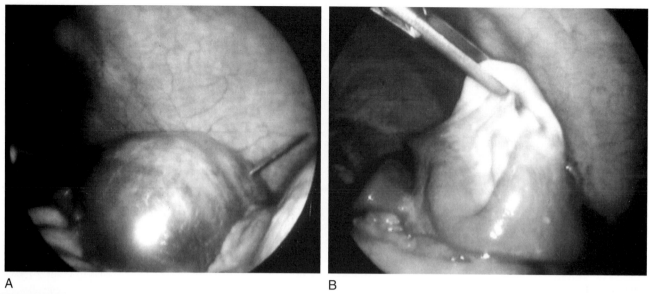

A   B

Figure 17–5   *A,* Laparoscopic view of splenic pseudocyst capsule. *B,* Appearance of cyst wall after laparoscopic aspiration and before marsupialization.

Sequelae of Damage-Control Strategies

Even the most severe solid organ injuries can be treated without surgery if there is a prompt response to resuscitation.[108] In contrast, emergency laparotomy, embolization, or both are indicated in patients who are hemodynamically unstable despite fluid and red blood cell transfusion. Most spleen and liver injuries requiring operation are amenable to simple methods of hemostasis using a combination of manual compression, direct suture, topical hemostatic agents, and mesh wrapping.[14,72] In young children with significant hepatic injury, the sternum can be divided rapidly to expose the suprahepatic or intrapericardial inferior vena cava, allowing for total hepatic vascular isolation (Fig. 17-6).[150] Children can tolerate periods of vascular isolation for 30 minutes or longer as long as their blood volume is replenished. With this exposure, the liver and major perihepatic veins can be isolated and the bleeding controlled, permitting direct suture repair or ligation of the offending vessel. Although the cumbersome and dangerous technique of atriocaval shunting has been largely abandoned, newer endovascular balloon catheters can be useful for temporary vascular occlusion to allow access to the juxtahepatic vena cava.[4]

The early morbidity and mortality of severe hepatic injuries are related to the effects of massive blood loss and replacement with large volumes of cold blood products. The consequences of prolonged operations with massive blood product replacement include hypothermia, coagulopathy, and acidosis. Although the surgical team may keep pace with blood loss, life-threatening physiologic and metabolic consequences are inevitable, and many of these critically ill patients are unlikely to survive once their physiologic reserves have been exhausted. A multi-institutional review identified exsanguination as the cause of intraoperative death in 82% of 537 patients at eight academic trauma centers.[57] The mean pH was 7.18 and the mean core temperature was 32°C before death.

Moulton et al.[93] reported survival in only 5 of 12 (42%) consecutive operative cases of retrohepatic vascular or severe parenchymal liver injury in children.

Maintenance of physiologic stability during the struggle for surgical control of severe bleeding is a formidable challenge even for the most experienced surgical team, particularly when hypothermia, coagulopathy, and acidosis occur. This triad creates a vicious circle in which each derangement exacerbates the others, and the

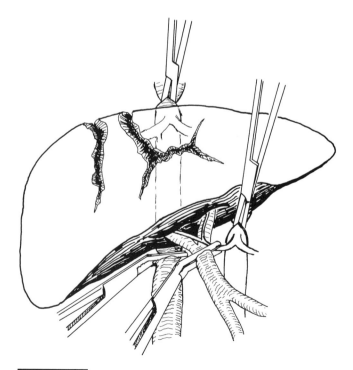

Figure 17–6   Total hepatic vascular isolation with occlusion of the porta-, supra-, and infrahepatic inferior vena cava and supraceliac aorta (optional). (Original illustration by Mark Mazziotti, MD.)

physiologic and metabolic consequences often preclude completion of the procedure. Lethal coagulopathy from dilution, hypothermia, and acidosis can rapidly occur.[145] Experimental studies have defined the alterations in pro- and anticoagulant enzyme processes, platelet activation, and platelet adhesion defects with varying degrees of hypothermia.[147] The infusion of activated recombinant factor VII in patients with massive hemorrhage has been promising in several case reports.[68]

Increased emphasis on physiologic and metabolic stability in emergency abdominal operations has led to the development of staged, multidisciplinary treatment plans, including abbreviated laparotomy, perihepatic packing, temporary abdominal closure, angiographic embolization, and endoscopic biliary stenting.[5,32,45,69,149] Asensio et al.[6] reported on 103 patients with mostly penetrating grade IV or V hepatic injuries treated between 1991 and 1999. Mean blood loss was estimated at 9.4 L, and mean volume infusion in the operating room was 15 L. Packing of the hepatic injuries was used in 50% of patients at the first operation. Forty percent of patients who survived the initial operative control of hemorrhage had postoperative angiographic embolization (Fig. 17-7). Survival was 63% in grade IV patients and 24% in grade V patients, emphasizing the lethality of such injuries despite a well-choreographed, staged, multidisciplinary approach. Trauma surgeons treating critically injured children must familiarize themselves with these lifesaving techniques.

Abbreviated laparotomy with packing for hemostasis, allowing resuscitation before planned reoperation, is an alternative in unstable patients in whom further blood loss would be untenable. This "damage-control" philosophy is a systematic, phased approach to the management of exsanguinating trauma patients.[8,119,143] The three phases of damage control are detailed in Table 17-3. Although controversial, several resuscitative end points

TABLE 17-3 "Damage-Control" Strategy in Exsanguinating Trauma Patients	
Phase 1	Abbreviated laparotomy for exploration
	Control of hemorrhage and contamination
	Packing and temporary abdominal wall closure
Phase 2	Aggressive ICU resuscitation
	Core rewarming
	Optimization of volume and oxygen delivery
	Correction of coagulopathy
Phase 3	Planned reoperation(s) for packing change
	Definitive repair of injuries
	Abdominal wall closure

ICU, intensive care unit.

have been proposed beyond the conventional vital signs and urine output, including serum lactate, base deficit, mixed venous oxygen saturation, and gastric mucosal pH. Once a patient is rewarmed, coagulation factors are replaced, and oxygen delivery is optimized, he or she can be returned to the operating room for pack removal and definitive repair of injuries. A review of nearly 700 adult patients treated by abdominal packing from several institutions demonstrated hemostasis in 80%, survival of 32% to 73%, and abdominal abscess rates of 10% to 40%.[26,53] Although abdominal packing with planned reoperation has been used with increasing frequency in adults during the past 2 decades, there is little published experience in children.[30,36,56,80,115,132,134,138] Nevertheless, we believe that this technique has a place in the management of children with massive intra-abdominal bleeding, especially after blunt trauma.

We reported a 3-year-old child who required abdominal packing for a severe liver injury, making closure of the abdomen impossible.[138] A Silastic "silo" was constructed

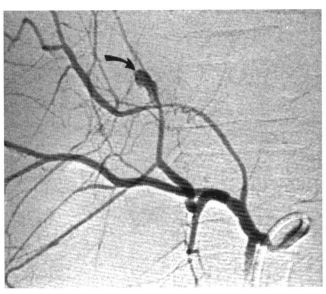

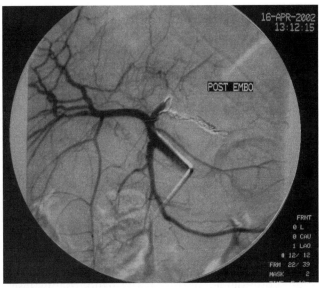

A   B

Figure 17-7 *A,* Hepatic artery angiogram in a patient with persistent hemorrhage after initial damage-control laparotomy. The bleeding vessel is identified *(curved arrow). B,* Successful embolization was performed.

to accommodate the bowel until the packing could be removed. The patient made a complete recovery. The combined technique of packing and a silo allowed time for correction of the hypothermia, acidosis, and coagulopathy, without compromise of respiratory mechanics. One review reported 22 infants and children (age 6 days to 20 years) with refractory hemorrhage who were treated with abdominal packing.[134] The anatomic site of hemorrhage was the liver or hepatic veins in 14, retroperitoneum or pelvis in 7, and pancreatic bed in 1. Primary fascial closure was accomplished in 12 patients (55%), and temporary skin closure or prosthetic material was used in the other 10. Packing controlled hemorrhage in 21 of 22 patients (95%). Removal of the packing was possible within 72 hours in 18 patients (82%). No patient rebled after the packing was removed; however, 2 patients died with the packing in place. Seven patients (32%) developed an abdominal or pelvic abscess, and all were successfully drained by laparotomy (6 patients) or percutaneously (1 patient); 6 of the 7 patients with abdominal sepsis survived. Overall, 18 patients (82%) survived. Two deaths were due to multisystem organ failure, one to cardiac failure from complex cardiac anomalies, and one to exsanguination after blunt traumatic liver injury. There were no differences in the volume of intraoperative blood product transfusion, time to initiate packing, physiologic status, or type of abdominal closure between survivors and nonsurvivors.

Although the success of abdominal packing is encouraging, it may contribute to significant morbidity, such as intra-abdominal sepsis, organ failure, and increased intra-abdominal pressure. Intra-abdominal packs are contaminated by skin and gut flora, but these organisms are not those implicated in subsequent patient sepsis.[48] Adams et al.[2] evaluated fluid samples from 28 patients with abdominal packing and found peritoneal endotoxin and mediator accumulation even when cultures were sterile. The authors concluded that laparotomy pad fluid accumulating after damage-control laparotomy can contribute to neutrophil dysfunction by enhancing neutrophil respiratory burst and inhibiting neutrophil responses to specific chemotactic mediators needed to fight infection. Thus, the known propensity of such patients to both intra-abdominal and systemic infection may be related to changes in neutrophil receptor status and effector function related to the accumulation of inflammatory mediators in the abdomen. Early washout, repetitive packing, and other efforts to minimize mediator accumulation deserve consideration.

It is essential to emphasize that the success of the abbreviated laparotomy and planned reoperation depends on an early decision to employ this strategy before irreversible shock occurs. When employed as a desperate, last-ditch resort after prolonged attempts at hemostasis have failed, abdominal packing has been uniformly unsuccessful. Physiologic and anatomic criteria have been identified as indications for abdominal packing. Most of these focus on intraoperative parameters, including pH (~7.2), core temperature (<35°C), and coagulation values (prothrombin time >16 seconds), in a patient with profuse hemorrhage requiring large volumes of blood product transfusion.

The optimal time for re-exploration is controversial, because neither the physiologic end points of resuscitation nor the increased risk of infection with prolonged packing are well defined. The obvious benefits of hemostasis provided by packing are also balanced against the potential deleterious effects of increased intra-abdominal pressure on ventilation, cardiac output, renal function, mesenteric circulation, and intracranial pressure. Timely alleviation of the secondary abdominal compartment syndrome may be a critical salvage maneuver for patients. Temporary abdominal wall closure at the time of packing can prevent the abdominal compartment syndrome. We recommend temporary abdominal wall expansion in all patients requiring packing until hemostasis is obtained and visceral edema subsides.

A staged operative strategy for unstable trauma patients represents advanced surgical care and requires sound judgment and technical expertise. Intra-abdominal packing for control of exsanguinating hemorrhage is a lifesaving maneuver in highly selected patients in whom coagulopathy, hypothermia, and acidosis render further surgical procedures unduly hazardous. Early identification of patients likely to benefit from abbreviated laparotomy techniques is crucial for success.

Abdominal Compartment Syndrome

The abdominal compartment syndrome is a term used to describe the deleterious effects of increased intra-abdominal pressure.[116] The syndrome includes respiratory insufficiency from worsening ventilation-perfusion mismatch, hemodynamic compromise from preload reduction due to inferior vena cava compression, impaired renal function from renal vein compression, decreased cardiac output, intracranial hypertension from increased ventilator pressures, splanchnic hypoperfusion, and abdominal wall overdistention. The causes of intra-abdominal hypertension in trauma patients include hemoperitoneum, retroperitoneal or bowel edema, and use of abdominal or pelvic packing. The combination of tissue injury and hemodynamic shock creates a cascade of events, including capillary leak, ischemia-reperfusion, and release of vasoactive mediators and free radicals, which combine to increase extracellular volume and tissue edema. Experimental evidence indicates that there are significant alterations in cytokine levels in the presence of sustained intra-abdominal pressure elevation.[100,112] Once the combined effects of tissue edema and intra-abdominal fluid exceed a certain level, abdominal decompression must be considered.

The adverse effects of abdominal compartment syndrome have been acknowledged for decades; however, abdominal compartment syndrome has only recently been recognized as a life-threatening but potentially treatable entity.[122,149] The incidence of this complication has increased markedly in recent years due to high-volume resuscitation protocols. Measurement of intra-abdominal pressure can be useful in determining the contribution of abdominal compartment syndrome to altered physiologic and metabolic parameters.[19,31,54] Intra-abdominal pressure can be determined by measuring bladder pressure. This involves instilling 1 mL/kg of saline into the Foley catheter and connecting it to a pressure transducer or manometer via a three-way stopcock. The symphysis pubis is used as the zero reference point, and the pressure is measured in centimeters of water or millimeters of mercury. Intra-abdominal pressures in the range of 20 to 35 cm H_2O or 15 to 25 mm Hg have been identified as an indication to decompress the abdomen. Many prefer to intervene according to alterations in other physiologic and metabolic parameters rather than a specific pressure measurement. Chang et al.[19] reported 11 adult trauma patients with abdominal compartment syndrome in whom abdominal decompression using pulmonary artery catheters and gastric tonometry improved preload, pulmonary function, and visceral perfusion. Anecdotally, decompressive laparotomy has been used successfully to reduce refractory intracranial hypertension in patients with isolated brain injury without overt signs of abdominal compartment syndrome.[85]

Experience with abdominal decompression for abdominal compartment syndrome in children is limited.[31,34,97,122,134,138] Nonspecific abdominal CT findings in children with abdominal compartment syndrome include narrowing of the inferior vena cava, direct renal compression or displacement, bowel wall thickening with enhancement, and a rounded appearance of the abdomen.[34] Neville et al.[97] reported the use of patch abdominoplasty in 23 infants and children, only 3 of whom were trauma patients. These authors found that patch abdominoplasty for abdominal compartment syndrome effectively decreased airway pressures and oxygen requirements. Failure to respond with a decrease in airway pressures or fraction of inspired oxygen was an ominous sign in their series. Several authors have found that abdominal decompression resulted in decreased airway pressures, increased oxygen tension, and increased urine output in children with abdominal compartment syndrome.[31,97,122]

Many materials have been suggested for use in temporary patch abdominoplasty, including Silastic sheeting, Gore-Tex sheeting, intravenous bags, cystoscopy bags, ostomy appliances, and various mesh materials (Fig. 17-8). The vacuum-pack technique, used successfully in adults, seems promising.[8,80,139]

Bile Duct Injury

Nonoperative management of pediatric blunt liver injury is highly successful but is complicated by a 4% risk of persistent bile leakage.[10,117] Radionuclide scanning is recommended when biliary tree injury is suspected.[120] Delayed views may show a bile leak even if early views are normal. Several reports have highlighted the benefits of endoscopic retrograde cholangiopancreatography (ERCP) with placement of transampullary biliary stents for biliary duct injury following blunt hepatic trauma. Although ERCP is invasive and requires conscious sedation, it can pinpoint the site of injury and allow treatment of the injured ducts without open surgery (Fig. 17-9). Endoscopic transampullary biliary decompression is a recent addition to the treatment options for patients with persistent bile leakage. The addition of sphincterotomy during ERCP for persistent bile leakage following blunt liver injury has been advocated to decrease intrabiliary pressure and encourage internal decompression.[22,92,121] It is important to note that endoscopic biliary stents may migrate or become obstructed and require specific treatment.

INJURIES TO THE DUODENUM AND PANCREAS

In contrast to the liver and spleen, injuries to the duodenum and pancreas are much less frequent, accounting for less than 10% of intra-abdominal injuries in children sustaining blunt trauma. Isolated duodenal and pancreatic injuries occur in approximately two thirds of cases, with combined injuries to both organs occurring in the remainder. The severity of the duodenal or pancreatic injury and associated injuries determines the necessity for operative versus nonoperative management. The "protected" retroperitoneum both limits the chance of injury and increases the difficulty of early diagnosis. Added to this diagnostic dilemma is the frequency of associated intra-abdominal or multisystem injuries, which can mask subtle physical and radiographic diagnostic signs of injury to the duodenum and pancreas.

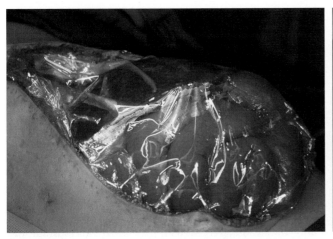
A

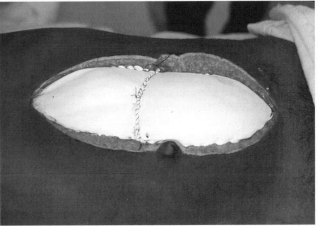
B

Figure 17–8 *A,* Abdominal wall expansion with Silastic sheeting. *B,* Abdominal wall expansion with a Gore-Tex patch.

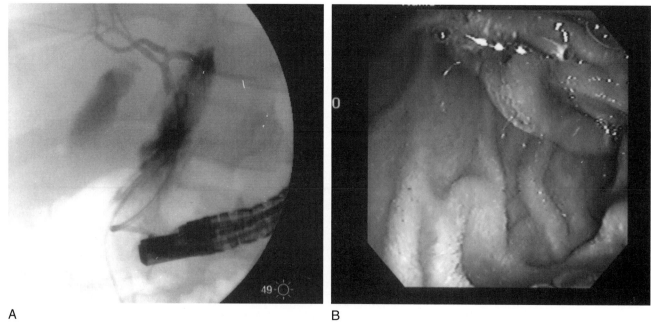

A   B

Figure 17–9 *A*, Endoscopic retrograde cholangiopancreatography demonstrating several bile leaks after blunt liver injury. *B*, Endoscopic view of transampullary biliary stent.

Duodenum

In a report on blunt duodenal rupture, Ballard et al.[7] reviewed a 6-year statewide (Pennsylvania) experience. Of 103,864 patients registered from 28 trauma centers, blunt injury to the duodenum occurred in 206 (0.2%), of whom only 30 (14%) had full-thickness rupture. The mechanism of injury was car crash in 70%, which included both adults and children. Of those without significant head injury (26 of 30), 92% either reported abdominal pain or had tenderness or rebound on physical examination. CT was performed in 18 patients; retroperitoneal air or extravasation of contrast was seen in only 26% of scans; an equal number were interpreted as normal. Mortality was 13% and was not affected by a delay in diagnosis or treatment. This study emphasizes the difficulty of analyzing this injury owing to the low numbers reported by individual centers (and surgeons). Additionally, the investigators reviewed the range of repairs performed—from duodenal closure to the Whipple procedure—but commented that no definitive recommendations could be made because of the small number of patients and the many centers reporting.

In contrast, a group from Toronto reported a single-center experience in a series of 27 children (mean age, 7 years) sustaining blunt duodenal injuries and treated over a 10-year period (1986 to 1996).[124] Thirteen children had duodenal perforations (mean age, 9 years), and 14 sustained duodenal hematomas (mean age, 5 years). Associated injuries were seen in 19 patients (10 pancreas, 5 spleen, 4 liver, 2 long bone fracture, 1 central nervous system, 1 renal contusion, 1 jejunal perforation, and 1 gastric rupture). Seventeen patients were transferred from other facilities, with a 4-hour median time to transfer. The median interval from injury to surgery in those sustaining perforation was 6 hours. A comparison of the clinical

presentation, laboratory evaluation, and radiographic findings in those with duodenal hematoma versus perforation is presented in Table 17-4. Most patients had abdominal CT scans performed with oral and intravenous contrast (Figs. 17-10 and 17-11). A comparison of CT findings in these patient groups is presented in Table 17-5. These data

TABLE 17–4 Presenting Symptoms and Signs in Children with Duodenal Hematoma and Duodenal Perforation

Patient Characteristic	Duodenal Hematoma	Duodenal Perforation
Number	14	13
Age (yr)	5	9*
ISS score	10	25*
Seat belt worn: no. (%)	6 (100)	5 (71)
Presentation		
Pain or tenderness: no. (%)	10 (71)	12 (92)
		11 (85)
Bruising: no. (%)	6 (43)	
GCS score	15	15
Associated injuries		
Pancreatic: no. (%)	7 (50)	3 (23)
Lumbar spine: no. (%)	1 (7)	4 (31)
Total: no. (%)	11 (79)	8 (62)
Laboratory evaluation		
Hgb: mg %/Hct	12.3/0.36	12.1/0.37
Amylase: units (%)	678 (64)	332 (46)

*Statistically significant difference.
GCS, Glasgow Coma Scale; Hct, hematocrit; Hgb, hemoglobin; ISS, Injury Severity Scale.
From Shilyansky J, Pearl RH, Kroutouro M, et al: Diagnosis and management of duodenal injuries in children. J Pediatr Surg 1997;32:880-886.

Figure 17–10 Abdominal compated tomography findings in an 8-year-old girl who sustained a duodenal hematoma after a fall at a playground. *A,* The *arrow* points to the markedly narrowed duodenal lumen. *B to D,* The *arrows* point to the large intramural hematoma. The child was treated with nasogastric suction and total parenteral nutrition. She was eating a regular diet 24 days after her injury.

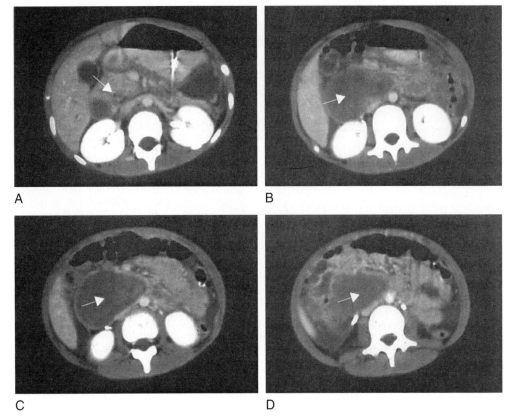

Figure 17–11 Abdominal computed tomography findings in a 4-year-old boy with duodenal perforation caused by a motor vehicle accident. *A,* The *arrow* points to the disrupted duodenal wall. *B to D, Small arrows* point to extravasated retroperitoneal enteral contrast. In *C,* the *large arrow* points to extraluminal retroperitoneal air. A large defect involving the second and third portions of the duodenum was found. Primary repair, pyloric exclusion, tube duodenostomy, and gastrojejunostomy were performed. The child resumed eating 5 days after injury and went home 4 days later.

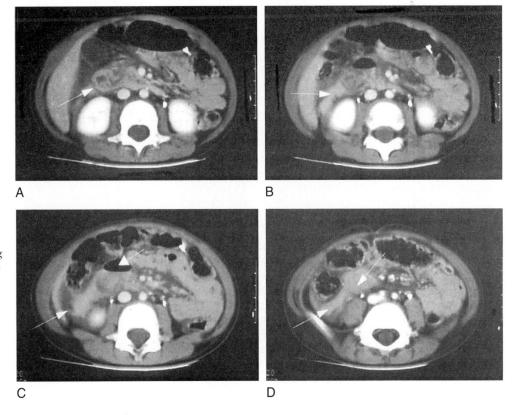

TABLE 17-5 Comparison of Computed Tomography Findings in Children with Duodenal Hematoma and Duodenal Perforation

Finding	Duodenal Hematoma (n = 10) No. (%)	Duodenal Perforation (n = 9) No. (%)
Free air	1 (10)*	2 (22)
Free fluid	8 (80)	9 (100)
Retroperitoneal fluid	9 (90)	9 (100)
Bowel wall and peritoneal enhancement	2 (20)	4 (44)
Duodenal caliber change	4 (40)	3 (33)
Thickened duodenum	10 (100)	8 (89)
Mural hematoma	10 (100)	0
Retroperitoneal air	0	8 (89)
Retroperitoneal contrast†	0	4 (57)
Retroperitoneal air or contrast	0	9 (100)

*The child had an associated jejunal perforation.

†Enteral contrast was not administered in two children.

From Shilyansky J, Pearl RH, Kroutouro M, et al: Diagnosis and management of duodenal injuries in children. J Pediatr Surg 1997:32:880-886.

demonstrate that the clinical presentation is strikingly similar in both groups, with only age and injury severity score achieving statistical significance (but of little clinical relevance in individual patients). However, extravasation of air or enteral contrast into the retroperitoneal, periduodenal, or prerenal space was found in every child with a duodenal perforation (9 of 9) but in none of the 10 who had duodenal hematoma. The authors noted that few previous reports in the literature described these specific CT findings with duodenal injuries in general, and in particular, no previous series of pediatric patients had been reported. This experience and a 1986 report from the same center[146] summarize a total of 24 patients with duodenal hematoma, all treated nonoperatively. The CT scans (or upper GI contrast studies in equivocal cases) showing duodenal narrowing, corkscrewing, or obstruction without extravasation were diagnostic in all cases. In the current series of 14 patients treated nonoperatively, the duration of nasogastric decompression was 12 days (mean), and the length of total parenteral nutrition administration was 18 days (mean). Symptoms resolved in 13 of 14 patients an average of 16 days after injury. The remaining child developed a chronic fibrous stricture requiring operative duodenoplasty 49 days after injury. This child also had a pancreatic contusion.

Desai et al.[33] from St. Louis Children's Hospital reviewed their experience with 24 duodenal injuries from blunt abdominal trauma.[33] There were 19 duodenal hematomas (15 diagnosed by CT, and 4 by upper GI studies), 17 of which were treated nonoperatively. In those with perforation, 4 of 5 were amenable to simple suture repair. The experiences from Salt Lake City and Pittsburgh emphasize an alarming finding that a common cause of duodenal trauma is child abuse, especially in younger patients.[24,43] Therefore, isolated duodenal injures should

raise suspicion if the history or mechanism of injury described is inconsistent with the actual injury.

In all these series, patients sustaining duodenal perforation were treated operatively in a variety of ways, depending on the injury severity and the surgeon's preference. We recommend primary closure of a duodenal perforation (whenever possible). Primary closure can be combined with duodenal drainage and either pyloric exclusion with gastrojejunostomy (Fig. 17-12) or gastric drainage with feeding jejunostomy. These surgical options decrease the incidence of duodenal fistula, reduce the time to GI tract alimentation, and shorten hospital stay. When faced with complicated duodenal trauma, an effective combination is the three-tube technique: duodenal closure (primary repair, serosal patch, or anastomosis) with duodenal drainage tube for decompression (tube 1), pyloric exclusion with an absorbable suture via gastrotomy and gastric tube placement (tube 2), and feeding jejunostomy (tube 3). Several closed suction drains are placed adjacent to the repair. When the duodenum is excluded (via an absorbable suture for temporary closure of the pylorus), complete healing of the injury routinely occurs before the spontaneous reopening of the pyloric channel (Fig. 17-13). However, no matter what repair the surgeon selects, a summary of the literature demonstrates that protecting the duodenal closure

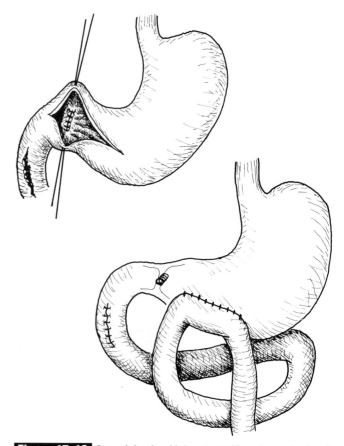

Figure 17-12 Lateral duodenal injury treated by primary duodenal repair and pyloric exclusion consisting of closing the pylorus with an absorbable suture and gastrojejunostomy. Closed suction drainage of the repair is not depicted. (Original illustration by Mark Mazziotti, MD.)

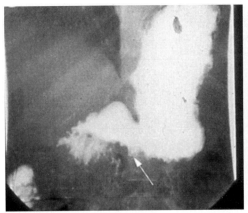
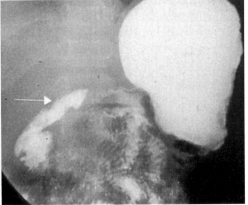

Figure 17–13 Upper gastrointestinal study of a 7-year-old girl with duodenal perforation resulting from a motor vehicle accident. Primary repair, pyloric exclusion, retrograde tube duodenostomy, gastrojejunostomy, and feeding gastrostomy were performed. The child tolerated jejunal feeds 6 days after the injury and oral feeds 12 days after the injury. *A,* Six weeks postinjury, an upper gastrointestinal study demonstrated spontaneous closure of the gastrojejunostomy *(arrow)*. *B,* A patent pylorus is evident *(arrow)*.

A   B

(drain and exclusion) and a route for enteral feeding (gastrojejunostomy or feeding jejunostomy) reduces morbidity and hospital length of stay.[39,70]

The surgical options are listed in Table 17-6 and illustrated in Figures 17-12 and 17-14. Of note, pancreaticoduodenectomy (the Whipple procedure) is rarely required. Although occasionally reported in the literature, pancreaticoduodenectomy should be reserved for the most severe injuries to the duodenum and pancreas in which the common blood supply is destroyed and reconstruction is impossible.

Pancreas

Injuries to the pancreas are slightly more frequent than duodenal injuries, with estimated ranges from 3% to 12% in children sustaining blunt abdominal trauma.[71] As with duodenal injuries, individual centers frequently have small patient numbers and thus are unable to evaluate their results critically. Recently, two centers (Toronto and San Diego) reported their experience with divergent methods of managing blunt traumatic pancreatic injuries in a series of reports.[16,17,61,75,125,144] Here, we compare these papers and excerpt other authors' experience to make management recommendations.

Canty and Weinman (San Diego)[17] reported 18 patients with major pancreatic injuries over a 14-year period.

The mechanism of injury was car or bike crashes. Sixteen of the 18 patients had CT scans on admission. Of these, 11 suggested injury; in 5, the injury was missed. Distal pancreatectomy was performed in 8 patients (44%). In 5 of 6 patients with either proximal duct injuries or injuries missed on the initial CT scan, pseudocysts developed;

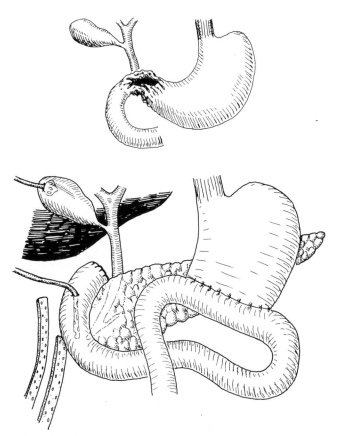

Figure 17–14 Duodenal diverticularization for combined proximal duodenal and pancreatic injury. Resection and closure of the duodenal stump, tube duodenostomy, tube cholecystostomy, gastrojejunostomy, and multiple closed suction drains are depicted. A feeding jejunostomy should be strongly considered (not depicted). (Original illustration by Mark Mazziotti, MD.)

TABLE 17–6 Surgical Options in Duodenal Trauma
Repair of the duodenum
Diversion of the gastrointestinal tract (pyloric exclusion or duodenal diverticularization)
Gastric decompression (gastric tube insertion or gastrojejunostomy)
Gastrointestinal tract access for feeding (jejunostomy tube or gastrojejunal anastomosis)
Decompression of the duodenum (duodenostomy tube)
Biliary tube drainage
Wide drainage of the repaired area (lateral duodenal drains)

pseudocysts also occurred in 2 other children who had minimal initial symptoms and no admission CT scans. Of these 7 pseudocysts, 2 resolved and 5 were treated by cystogastrostomy. Two patients, treated more recently, received ERCP with duct stenting and experienced resolution of symptoms and complete healing. The authors concluded that distal injuries should be treated with distal pancreatectomy, proximal injuries with observation, and pseudocysts with observation or cystogastrostomy. They also concluded that acute ERCP management with stent placement is safe and effective, and that CT is suggestive but not always diagnostic for the type and location of pancreatic injuries.[16,17,61]

The experience summarized in three reports from Toronto is markedly different.[75,125,144] The extensive CT findings suggestive of pancreatic injury are detailed in Table 17-7. In the first brief report, 2 patients with documented duct disruption (by ERCP or catheter-gram) had complete duct healing without operative intervention.[75] This was followed by a summary report of 35 consecutive children treated over 10 years (1987 to 1996).[125] Twenty-three had early diagnosis (<24 hours), whereas diagnosis was delayed (2 to 14 days) in 12 patients. Twenty-eight children were treated nonoperatively, and the other 7 had operations for other injuries. In the 28 cases treated nonoperatively, CT was diagnostic, revealing five patterns of injury: contusion, stellate fragmentation, partial fracture, complete transection, and pseudocyst (Fig. 17-15). The patients were placed in three clinical groups based on

TABLE 17-7 Summary of Associated CT Findings in Children with Pancreatic Injuries

Associated Finding	No. of Children
Intraperitoneal fluid	21
Lesser sac fluid	20
Focal peripancreatic fluid	20
Retroperitoneal fluid	20
Right anterior pararenal fluid	16
Left anterior pararenal fluid	15
Thickened Gerota's fascia (right and left)	16
Mesenteric fluid or hematoma	13
Left posterior pararenal fluid	9
Fluid separating SV and pancreas	7
Fluid surrounding SMV and PV	7
Fluid separating pancreas and duodenum	6

CT, computed tomography; PV, portal vein; SMV, superior mesenteric vein; SV, splenic vein.
Data from references 75, 125, 144.

CT grade (Table 17-8). In these 28 patients, pseudocysts occurred in 10 (2 of 14 in group 1, 5 of 11 in group 2, and 3 of 3 in group 3). No patients in group 1 required drainage, whereas 4 in group 2 and all 3 in group 3 required intervention. These drainage procedures occurred 10 to 14 days after injury. Average time for the

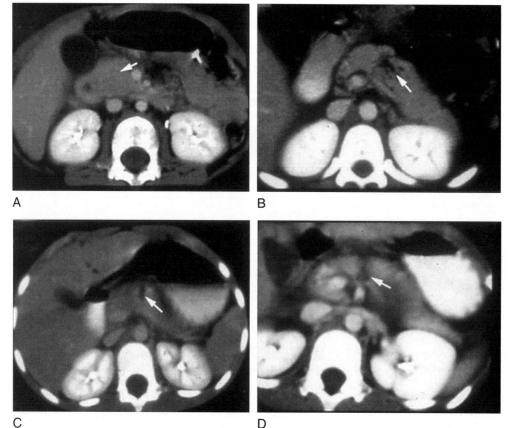

Figure 17–15 Computed tomography findings in children with pancreatic trauma. *A,* Contusion. *B,* Stellate fragmentation. *C,* Partial fracture. *D,* Transection.

TABLE 17-8 Proposed Classification of CT Findings in Children with Pancreatic Injuries

Group (Clinical)	Grade (CT)	Pancreatic Injury	Description	No. of Children
1	I	Contusion	Diffuse or focal swelling of the pancreas	14
2	II	Stellate fragmentation	Fluid or blood dissecting within pancreatic parenchyma	2
	III	Partial fracture	Incomplete separation of two portions of the pancreas	1
3	IV	Complete transection	Complete separation of two portions of the pancreas	8
	V	Pseudocyst	Persistent peripancreatic fluid collection	3

Data from references 75, 125, 144.

initiation of oral feeding was 15 days (11 days for group 1, 15 days for group 2, and 23 days for group 3). Mean hospital stay for all patients treated nonoperatively was 21 days.

A comparison of the San Diego and Toronto protocols is depicted in Figure 17-16. The striking differences in these series are the 100% diagnostic sensitivity of CT in Toronto versus 69% in San Diego and the 44% operative rate in San Diego versus 0% in Toronto. A subsequent study from Toronto reviewed the follow-up on 10 patients with duct transections.[144] Four of these children (40%) developed pseudocysts, three of which were drained percutaneously (Fig. 17-17). The mean hospital stay was 24 days, and all recovered. Follow-up CT in eight of nine patients revealed atrophy of the distal pancreas in six and completely normal glands in two. There was no exocrine or endocrine dysfunction in a mean of 47 months of follow-up. The authors concluded that following nonoperative management of pancreatic blunt trauma, atrophy (distal) or recanalization occurs in all cases with no long-term morbidity.

Reports from Dallas and Seattle favor early distal pancreatectomy for transection to the left of the spine to shorten hospital stay.[81,83] However, long-term sequelae of adhesive intestinal obstruction and endocrine and exocrine dysfunction were not assessed. Other reports document the efficacy of magnetic resonance pancreatography as a diagnostic tool, early ERCP intervention for diagnosis and treatment with ductal stenting, and the use of somatostatin to decrease pancreatic secretions and promote healing.[12,51,65,111,130] Of note, a large single-center series from Japan reported nonoperative management in 19 of 20 children with documented pancreatic injury (9 contusions, 6 lacerations, and 5 main duct disruptions).[67] In all cases, recovery was complete without surgery. That center's experience with pseudocyst formation and treatment and overall outcome virtually mirrors that of the Toronto report.

These reports from major pediatric trauma centers are clearly in conflict. Some favor and document the efficacy and safety of observational care for virtually all pancreatic injuries, including duct disruption; others advocate aggressive surgical management with debridement or resection. Because proponents supply compelling data for each of these treatments, algorithms reflecting individual hospital or surgeon preference will probably determine which treatment plan is selected. However, it is clear that with simple transection of the pancreas at or to the left of the spine, spleen-sparing distal pancreatectomy

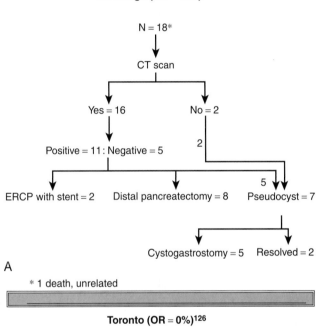

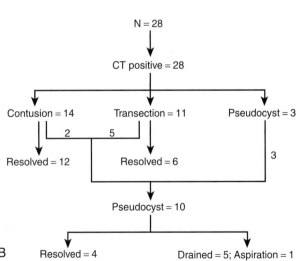

Figure 17-16 Comparison of protocols in the management of blunt pancreas injury in children. *A*, San Diego. *B*, Toronto. CT, computed tomography; ERCP, endoscopic retrograde cholangiopancreatography; OR, operating room. (*A*, from Canty TG Sr, Weinman D: Management of major pancreatic duct injuries in children. J Trauma 2001;50:1001-1007. *B*, from Shilyansky J, Sen LM, Kreller M, et al: Nonoperative management of pancreatic injuries in children. J Pediatr Surg 1998;33:343-345.)

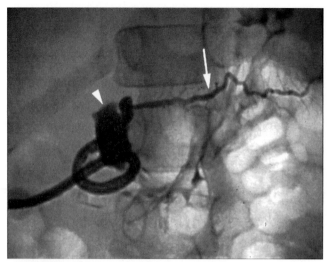

Figure 17–17 Contrast study through a percutaneous drain placed into a pancreatic pseudocyst *(arrowhead)* after blunt trauma in a child. Communication with the main pancreatic duct *(arrow)* is demonstrated. The pseudocyst resolved without fistula formation or operative intervention.

can provide definitive care for this isolated injury, with short hospitalization and acceptable morbidity (Fig. 17-18).

With this controversy in mind, we favor conservative therapy whenever possible, including the following:

1. Early spiral CT with oral and intravenous contrast in all patients who, by history, physical examination, or mechanism of injury, may have blunt trauma to the pancreas.
2. Documentation of injuries and early ERCP to provide duct stenting in selected cases.
3. Nonoperative management with total parenteral nutrition.
4. Expectant management of pseudocyst formation.
5. Percutaneous drainage for symptomatic, infected, or enlarging pseudocyst.

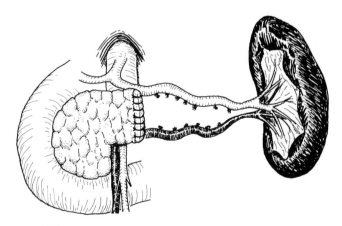

Figure 17–18 Spleen-sparing distal pancreatectomy. (Original illustration by Mark Mazziotti, MD.)

INJURIES OF THE STOMACH, SMALL INTESTINE, AND COLON

Injuries to the stomach, small intestine, and colon are easier to diagnose and manage than those previously discussed. In blunt trauma there are three different mechanisms that cause distinct patterns of injury to these organs. First is a crush injury that occurs as the stomach, jejunum, ileum, or transverse colon is compressed violently against the spine. Hematomas, lacerations, or partial or complete transections can occur, with instantaneous or delayed perforation or obstruction. Second, burst injury occurs when rapid compressive forces are applied to a filled and distended hollow viscus, without direct mechanical compression. Shoulder- and seat-belt injuries to the GI tract can occur in this fashion. Third is shear injury caused by rapid acceleration-deceleration of an organ that is tethered at one end, such as the ligament of Treitz, ileocecal region, or rectosigmoid junction. With deceleration, the injury is caused by the tearing of tissue at the point of fixation.

Regardless of the mechanism of injury, a perforated viscus causes rapid contamination of the abdominal cavity. On the initial trauma assessment, virtually all neurologically intact patients have some symptoms (pain) and physical findings (tenderness, guarding, rebound). In fact, many reports have documented that the initial and serial physical examinations have a higher degree of diagnostic specificity than US or CT for these injuries.[23,60,91] In a series from New Mexico reporting 48 patients with small bowel injury, all conscious patients had abnormal physical findings either on presentation or after serial physical examinations.[91] Other diagnostic tests (US, CT, DPL, lab tests) were of comparatively less value. These findings were confirmed by a similar series from North Carolina involving 32 children with intestinal injury confirmed at laparotomy; 94% had physical findings suggestive of intestinal injury on admission, with 84% having diffuse abdominal tenderness (peritoneal signs).[60] Prompt diagnosis of these injuries is possible when free air and GI contrast extravasates into the abdominal cavity at the time of the initial injury. However, when partial-thickness lacerations, hematomas, or avulsed mesenteric blood vessels occur, progression to full-thickness defects with leakage can be delayed over hours to days (Fig. 17-19). A high index of suspicion is indicated, along with the liberal use of serial physical examinations.

Injuries to the stomach and small intestine are straightforward to repair. A full stomach usually ruptures at the greater curvature with a blowout or stellate configuration. Debridement with direct repair is virtually always sufficient. Small intestinal injuries run the gamut from simple laceration to transection to complete avulsion with larger segments of compromised bowel. However, unless the contamination is massive (or other injuries require extensive repair), debridement or resection with anastomosis is usually sufficient. In colon injures, particularly if there is a delay in diagnosis and significant fecal contamination, colostomy with a defunctionalized distal mucous fistula or Hartmann's pouch is in order. If isolated colon injuries occur and are repaired

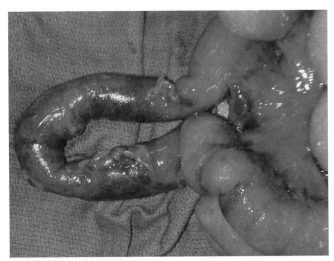

Figure 17–19 Small bowel mesentery avulsion with ischemic bowel.

early, on-table bowel irrigation, bowel anastomosis, and perioperative antibiotic coverage are safe and effective and avoid the complications caused by stomas and reoperation. The critical factors with injuries to the intraperitoneal GI tract are early recognition of the injury; prompt resuscitation; expeditious surgery, with complete removal of contaminated and devitalized tissue; reconstruction or diversion of the GI tract, as clinically indicated; and broad-spectrum antibiotics, with the duration of therapy dependent on the degree of contamination and postoperative clinical course (e.g., normalization of white blood cell count, absence of fever, return of GI tract function).

Seat-Belt Sign

Frequent physical examinations and vigilance are required for the subset of injuries caused by lap-belt restraints when children are passengers in high-speed automobile crashes.[23] These children present with visible seat-belt signs on physical examination of the abdomen (Fig. 17-20).

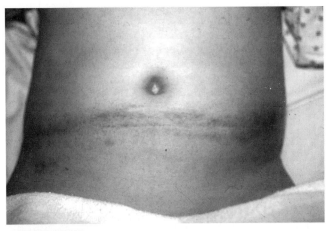

Figure 17–20 Seat-belt sign across the lower abdomen.

Multiple studies have documented increased abdominal injuries to both solid and hollow organs with this finding.[18,131,148] An interesting triad of injuries has been noted: abdominal wall contusions or herniation, Chance fractures of the lumbar spine, and isolated jejunal or ileal perforations. One report reviewed 95 patients admitted with abdominal trauma, all of whom were wearing seat belts at the time of injury; in 60 of 95 there was a seat-belt sign.[148] Nine of the 60 patients with the seat-belt sign had intestinal injuries, compared with none of the 35 without the seat-belt sign. The more common injuries described earlier can distract both the patient and the trauma team, causing delay in the diagnosis of serious vascular injuries involving the aorta and iliac vessels.[94,107]

In recent reports from Philadelphia, a database created by the State Farm Insurance Company was used to review 147,985 children who were passengers in motor vehicle crashes.[77,96] In that series, 1967 children (1.33%) had abdominal bruising from seat-belt restraints. Although abdominal wall bruising was infrequent, those with this finding were 232 times more likely to have a significant intra-abdominal injury than were those without a bruise. These data further revealed that 1 of 9 children with an abdominal seat-belt sign had a significant intra-abdominal injury. Therefore, although the seat-belt sign is rare, CT scanning (admission and serial) is mandated when it is present. Optimal ($n = 881$) and suboptimal ($n = 1086$) use of seat-belt restraints was noted. After adjusting for age and seating position, optimally restrained children were more than three times less likely (odds ratio 3.51) than suboptimally restrained children to suffer an abdominal injury.

Imaging for Gastrointestinal Injury

Imaging of the GI tract has evolved over the past decade, with spiral CT or FAST examinations done by surgeons in the emergency department directly impacting diagnostic accuracy and decision making. Some of the strengths and weaknesses of CT diagnosis have already been discussed. However, the ability to diagnose and treat blunt abdominal trauma in children has clearly been enhanced by this modality. Two studies from Toronto examined these issues. The first, in 1992, reviewed 12 patients with blunt abdominal trauma evaluated by CT.[50] It found that bowel wall enhancement was a sign of either global GI tract ischemia associated with fatal central nervous system injury or, when seen with bowel wall thickening and free peritoneal fluid, bowel perforation. A follow-up study in 1996 reviewed 43 patients evaluated over 10 years with surgically confirmed GI tract perforation.[59] Extraluminal air was seen in 47%, with one false-positive. Five CT findings were found to be suggestive but not diagnostic of GI tract perforation: extraluminal air, free intraperitoneal fluid, bowel wall thickening, bowel wall enhancement, and bowel dilatation. In every patient who had all five of these findings, bowel perforation was confirmed. However, this occurred in only 18% of the study population. All patients had at least one of these five specific CT findings. There were no false-negative studies.

As mentioned previously, although CT scanning is a reliable modality for assessing GI tract perforations, it should not replace and does not improve on diligent serial clinical evaluations. A similar study from Calgary reviewed 145 children with blunt abdominal trauma.[47] CT scans were interpreted as positive for GI tract injury in 20 and negative in 152 (several children had more than one study). The sensitivity of abdominal CT scan was determined to be 0.93 for mesenteric or intestinal injuries requiring surgery, with a negative predictive value of 0.99 in this study population. Therefore, CT rarely misses significant mesenteric or intestinal injuries.

The significance of isolated free intraperitoneal fluid in the absence of solid organ injury has frequently been heralded as a sign of intestinal trauma. Hulka et al.[58] reported a series of 259 CT scans (all with oral and intravenous contrast) and found only 24 patients (9%) with isolated free intraperitoneal fluid. Among the 16 patients with only a "small amount" of isolated fluid, only 2 required laparotomy. However, 4 of 8 patients (50%) with fluid in more than one location had a bowel injury requiring exploration. These authors also noted that enteral contrast is rarely present to aid in the diagnosis of bowel injury. Similar findings were reported by Holmes et al.,[55] with small quantities of intraperitoneal fluid having little clinical significance. In their report, only 8% of abdominal CT scans were positive for isolated intraperitoneal fluid, and in only 17% of these cases was there an identifiable injury. This represented only 7 of the 542 children (1.3%) studied.

Finally, FAST was found to be useful as a screening tool, with high specificity (95%) but low sensitivity (33%) in evaluating intestinal injury.[103] In that study of 89 FAST-negative children, only 20 went on to have CT scans performed, all at the surgeon's request. Without this finding, they all might have had abdominal CT scans. Clearly, FAST can decrease the number of unnecessary CT scans performed, but it cannot detect the specific abdominal organs injured. FAST is therefore of limited value in assessing these injuries. Finally, to come full circle, in a large study from Pittsburgh, 350 children with abdominal trauma were reviewed, with 30 requiring laparotomy (8.5%).[3] There were five false-negative CT scans (26%) in 19 patients who underwent delayed laparotomy (3.5 hours or longer after injury). Those authors concluded that serial physical examination, not CT scanning, is the gold standard for diagnosing GI tract perforations in children. We concur.

INJURIES TO THE PERINEUM, ANUS, AND GENITALIA

Children present with injuries to the perineum, anus, and external genitalia primarily from two mechanisms: accidental falls and sexual abuse. Accidental injuries are sustained by falling onto blunt or sharp objects in a straddled fashion. These injuries are characterized by bruising, contusion, laceration, or penetration, depending on the object struck and the height of the fall. Accidental injuries frequently involve the external genitalia, urethra, perineal body, and anus but rarely involve the rectum.

Conversely, injuries sustained by sexual abuse are commonly rectal or vaginal penetrations from violent, nonconsensual acts or the purposeful insertion of objects into these orifices. Therefore, when examining a child with injuries to the perineum, isolated rectal or vaginal trauma should always be considered child abuse until proved otherwise; conversely, polytrauma to the perineum with genital, perineal, and anal involvement is typically accidental.[62,110]

Diagnosis of the extent of perineal injury frequently requires examination under anesthesia by means of proctoscopy, sigmoidoscopy, and retrograde urethrogram. After assessing the degree of injury, surgical strategies include repair of urethral injuries (directly or via stenting), urinary diversion with a suprapubic cystostomy, repair of rectal tears, rectal irrigation, placement of drains when required, and, in more complex injuries, fecal diversion by colostomy. After recovery, detailed radiologic confirmation of complete healing (e.g., by intravenous pyelogram, cystogram, urethrogram, contrast enemas) must be performed before reconstruction of fecal continuity or removal of urinary stents or urinary undiversion.

Although rare, pediatric fatalities have been reported with rectal impalement from abuse.[102] Neonatal rectovaginal injuries have also been reported as an infrequent but life-threatening complication of traumatic delivery.[74] However, more commonly, rectal insertion of thermometers, Hegar dilators, or enema tubes can cause significant rectal injuries in newborns, requiring surgical repair. We recently treated a 3-day-old infant with perforation of the rectosigmoid junction from frequent enemas required for the treatment of obstipation from cystic fibrosis; laparotomy and colostomy were required. Therefore, in newborns, apparently innocuous rectal manipulation can cause severe injuries requiring surgical evaluation and intervention.

DIAPHRAGMATIC INJURIES

Traumatic injury to the diaphragm is infrequently observed, even at the largest pediatric trauma centers. At Children's Hospital of Illinois, only two traumatic diaphragmatic injuries were treated from 1998 to 2002 out of more than 800 admissions requiring level I pediatric trauma evaluation. At the Hospital for Sick Children in Toronto, only 15 children with this injury were seen from 1977 to 1998.[66,109] In a similar report covering 1992 to 2002 at Denver Children's Hospital, 1397 children were admitted and observed for blunt abdominal trauma, 387 had intra-abdominal injuries, but there were only 6 diaphragmatic ruptures (0.5%).[9] The injury is caused by massive compressive forces to the abdominal cavity, creating acceleration of abdominal contents cephalad, rupturing the diaphragmatic muscle. Occasionally, penetrating trauma causes this injury; however, in these cases, the injury is often found incidentally at exploration for other injuries. In the series reported from Toronto, 13 of 15 patients had diaphragmatic rupture from blunt trauma; the mean age was 7.5 years, with the right and left diaphragm equally involved.[109] The diagnosis was made with only a chest radiograph in more than half the patients. Three injuries were missed at the initial evaluation. Owing to the force required to cause this injury, multiple associated injuries should be expected. In this report, 81% of patients had multiple injuries, including liver laceration (47%), pelvic fracture (47%), major vascular injury (40%), bowel perfusion (33%), long bone fracture (20%), renal laceration (20%), splenic laceration (13%), and closed head injury (13%). As expected, there were many complications, five deaths, and a mean hospital stay of 20 days. Emergent surgery in children with this constellation of associated injuries should include palpation of both diaphragms as a routine part of the abdominal exploration. Direct suture repair is usually possible after debridement of any devitalized tissue. Pledgeted sutures can be used to buttress the repair and prevent tearing of the muscle, making the closure more secure. If sufficient diaphragm tissue is destroyed, a tension-free closure with a 2-mm Gore-Tex patch can be used, similar to the repair of congenital diaphragmatic hernias in newborns. Reports of laparoscopic or thoracoscopic repair of this injury include delayed repairs on stable patients without associated injuries.[84,105] Delayed diagnosis of this injury in infants has been reported, as has renal avulsion into the chest through a traumatically ruptured diaphragm.[27,129,137] Owing to the infrequent presentation of this injury, one must have a high index of suspicion when the mechanism of injury and the degree and location of other injuries support the possibility of diaphragmatic injury.

SUMMARY

Recent advances in the treatment of trauma and the provision of critical care in children have resulted in improved outcomes following major injuries. It is imperative that pediatric surgeons familiarize themselves with current treatment algorithms for life-threatening abdominal trauma. Important contributions have been made in the diagnosis and treatment of children with abdominal injury by radiologists and endoscopists. Clinical experience and published reports addressing specific concerns about the nonoperative treatment of children with solid organ injuries and recent radiologic and endoscopic contributions have made pediatric trauma care increasingly nonoperative. Although the trend is in this direction, the pediatric surgeon should remain the physician of record in the multidisciplinary care of critically injured children. The decision not to operate is always a surgical decision.

REFERENCES

1. Acierno SP, Jurkovich GJ, Nathens AB: Is pediatric trauma still a surgical disease? Patterns of emergent operative intervention in the injured child. J Trauma 2004;56: 960-966.
2. Adams JM, Hauser CJ, Livingston DH, et al: The immunomodulatory effects of damage control abdominal packing on local and systemic neutrophil activity. J Trauma 2001;50:792-800.
3. Albanese CT, Meza MP, Gardner MJ, et al: Is computed tomography a useful adjunct to the clinical examination for the diagnosis of pediatric gastrointestinal perforation from blunt abdominal trauma in children? J Trauma 1996;40:417-421.
4. Angeles AP, Agarwal N, Lynd C: Repair of a juxtahepatic inferior vena cava injury using a simple endovascular technique. J Trauma 2004;56:918-921.
5. Asensio JA, Demetriades D, Chahwan S: Approach to the management of complex hepatic injuries. J Trauma 2000;48:66-69.
6. Asensio JA, Roldan G, Petrone P, et al: Operative management and outcomes in 103 AAST-OIS grades IV and V complex hepatic injuries: Trauma surgeons still need to operate, but angioembolization helps. J Trauma 2003; 54:647-654.
7. Ballard RB, Badellino MM, Enyon CA, et al: Blunt duodenal rupture: A 6 year statewide review. J Trauma 1997;43:729-733.
8. Barker DE, Kaufman HJ, Smith LA, et al: Vacuum pack technique of temporary abdominal closure: A 7-year experience with 112 patients. J Trauma 2000;48:201-207.
9. Barsness KA, Bensard DD, Ciesla D, et al: Blunt diaphragmatic rupture in children. J Trauma 2004;56:80-82.
10. Bass BL, Eichelberger MR, Schisgall R: Hazards of nonoperative therapy of hepatic trauma in children. J Trauma 1984;24:978-982.
11. Bensard DD, Beaver BL, Besner GE, et al: Small bowel injury in children after blunt abdominal trauma: Is diagnostic delay important? J Trauma 1996;41:476-483.
12. Boman-Vermeeren JM, Vermeeren-Walters G, Broos P, et al: Somatostatin in the treatment of a pancreatic pseudocyst in a child. J Pediatr Gastroenterol Nutr 1996;23:422-425.
13. Brown RL, Irish MS, McCabe AJ, et al: Observation of splenic trauma: When is a little too much? J Pediatr Surg 1999;34:1124-1126.
14. Brunet C, Sielezneff I, Thomas P, et al: Treatment of hepatic trauma with perihepatic mesh. J Trauma 1994;37:200-204.
15. Bulas DI, Taylor GA, Eichelberger MR: The value of CT in detecting bowel perforation in children after blunt abdominal trauma. AJR Am J Roentgenol 1989;153:561-564.
16. Canty TG Sr, Weinman D: Treatment of pancreatic duct disruption in children by an endoscopically placed stent. J Pediatr Surg 2001;36:345-348.
17. Canty TG Sr, Weinman D: Management of major pancreatic duct injuries in children. J Trauma 2001;50:1001-1007.
18. Chandler CF, Lane JS, Waxman KS: Seatbelt sign following blunt trauma is associated with increased incidence of abdominal injury. Am Surg 1997;63:885-888.
19. Chang MC, Miller PR, D'Agostino R, et al: Effects of abdominal decompression on cardiopulmonary function and visceral perfusion in patients with intra-abdominal hypertension. J Trauma 1998;44:440-445.
20. Chen MK, Schropp KP, Lobe TE: The use of minimal access surgery in pediatric trauma: A preliminary report. J Laparoendosc Surg 1995;5:295-301.
21. Chen RJ, Fang JF, Lin BC, et al: Selective application of laparoscopy and fibrin glue in the failure of nonoperative management of blunt hepatic trauma. J Trauma 1998;44:691-695.
22. Church NG, May G, Sigalet DL: A minimally invasive approach to bile duct injury after blunt liver trauma in pediatric patients. J Pediatr Surg 2002;37:773-775.
23. Ciftci AO, Tanyel FC, Salman AB, et al: Gastrointestinal tract perforation due to blunt abdominal trauma. Pediatr Surg Int 1998;13:259-264.
24. Clendenon JN, Meyers RL, Nance ML, et al: Management of duodenal injuries in children. J Pediatr Surg 2004; 39:964-968.

25. Cloutier DR, Baird TB, Gormley P, et al: Pediatric splenic injuries with a contrast blush: Successful nonoperative management without angiography and embolization. J Pediatr Surg 2004;39:969-971.

26. Cogbill TH, Moore EE, Jurkovich GJ: Severe hepatic trauma: A multicenter experience with 1335 liver injuries. J Trauma 1988;28:1433-1438.

27. Cohen Z, Gabriel A, Izrachi S, et al: Traumatic avulsion of kidney into the chest through a ruptured diaphragm in a boy. Pediatr Emerg Care 2000;3:180-181.

28. Cooper A, Barlow B, DiScala C, et al: Mortality and truncal injury: The pediatric perspective. J Pediatr Surg 1994;29:33-38.

29. Cuschieri A, Hennessy TP, Stephens RB, et al: Diagnosis of significant abdominal trauma after road traffic accidents: Preliminary results of a multicentre clinical trial comparing mini-laparoscopy with peritoneal lavage. Ann R Coll Surg Engl 1988;70:153-155.

30. Davies MRQ: Iatrogenic hepatic rupture in the newborn and its management by pack tamponade. J Pediatr Surg 1997;32:1414-1419.

31. DeCou JM, Abrams RS, Miller RS, et al: Abdominal compartment syndrome in children: Experience with three cases. J Pediatr Surg 2000;35:840-842.

32. Denton JR, Moore EE, Codwell DM: Multimodality treatment for grade V hepatic injuries: Perihepatic packing, arterial embolization, and venous stenting. J Trauma 1997;42:964-968.

33. Desai KM, Dorward IG, Minkes RK, et al: Blunt duodenal injuries in children. J Trauma 2003;54:640-646.

34. Epelman M, Soudack M, Engel A, et al: Abdominal compartment syndrome in children: CT findings. Pediatr Radiol 2002;32:319-322.

35. Eubanks JW, Meier DE, Hicks BA, et al: Significance of "blush" on computed tomography scan in children with liver injury. J Pediatr Surg 2003;38:363-366.

36. Evans S, Jackson RJ, Smith SD: Successful repair of major retrohepatic vascular injuries without the use of shunt or sternotomy. J Pediatr Surg 1993;28:317-320.

37. Fabian TC, Croce MA, Stewart RM, et al: A prospective analysis of diagnostic laparoscopy in trauma. Ann Surg 1993;217:557-565.

38. Fallat ME, Casale AJ: Practice patterns of pediatric surgeons caring for stable patients with traumatic solid organ injury. J Trauma 1997;43:820-824.

39. Fang JF, Chen RJ, Ling BC: Controlled reopen suture technique for pyloric exclusion. J Trauma 1998;45:593-596.

40. Fisher JC, Moulton SL: Nonoperative management and delayed hemorrhage following pediatric liver injury. J Pediatr Surg 2004;39:619-622.

41. Frumiento C, Sartorelli K, Vane DW: Complications of splenic injuries: Expansion of the nonoperative theorem. J Pediatr Surg 2000;35:788-791.

42. Frumiento C, Vane DW: Changing patterns of treatment for blunt splenic injuries: An 11-year experience in a rural state. J Pediatr Surg 2000;35:985-989.

43. Gaines BA, Shultz BS, Morrison K, et al: Duodenal injuries in children: Beware of child abuse. J Pediatr Surg 2004;39:600-602.

44. Gandhi RR, Stringel G: Laparoscopy in pediatric abdominal trauma. JSLS 1997;1:349-351.

45. Ginzburg E, Klein Y, Sutherland M, et al: Prolonged clamping of the liver parenchyma: A salvage maneuver in exsanguinating liver injury. J Trauma 2004;56:922-923.

46. Goettler CE, Stallion A, Grisoni ER, et al: Delayed hemorrhage after blunt hepatic trauma. J Trauma 2002;52:556-559.

47. Graham JS, Wong AL: A review of computed tomography in the diagnosis of intestinal and mesenteric injury in pediatric blunt abdominal trauma. J. Pediatr Surg 1996;31:754-756.

48. Granchi TS, Abikhaled JA, Hirshberg A, et al: Patterns of microbiology in intra-abdominal packing for trauma. J Trauma 2004;56:45-51.

49. Hackam DJ, Potoka D, Meza M, et al: Utility of radiographic hepatic injury grade in predicting outcome for children after blunt abdominal trauma. J Pediatr Surg 2002;237:386-389.

50. Hara H, Babyn PS, Bourgeois D: Significance of bowel wall enhancement on CT following blunt abdominal trauma in childhood. J Comput Assist Tomogr 1992;16:94-98.

51. Harrell DJ, Vitale GC, Larson GM: Selective role for endoscopic retrograde cholangiopancreatography in abdominal trauma. Surg Endosc 1998;12:400-404.

52. Hawegawa T, Miki Y, Yoshioka Y, et al: Laparoscopic diagnosis of blunt abdominal trauma in children. Pediatr Surg Int 1997;12:132-136.

53. Hirshberg A, Mattox KL: Planned re-operation for severe trauma. Ann Surg 1995;222:3-8.

54. Hobson KG, Young KM, Ciraulo A, et al: Release of abdominal compartment syndrome improves survival in patients with burn injury. J Trauma 2002;53:1129-1134.

55. Holmes JF, London KL, Brant WE, et al: Isolated intraperitoneal fluid on abdominal computed tomography in children with blunt trauma. Acad Emerg Med 2000;7:335-341.

56. Horwitz JR, Black T, Lally KP: Venovenous bypass as an adjunct for the management of a retrohepatic venous injury in a child. J Trauma 1995;39:584-585.

57. Hoyt DB, Bulger EM, Knudson MM: Death in the operating room: An analysis of a multi-center experience. J Trauma 1994;37:426-432.

58. Hulka F, Mullins RJ, Leonardo V, et al: Significance of peritoneal fluid as an isolated finding on abdominal computed tomographic scans in pediatric trauma patients. J Trauma 1998;44:1069-1072.

59. Jamieson DH, Babyn PS, Pearl R: Imaging gastrointestinal perforation in pediatric blunt abdominal trauma. Pediatr Radiol 1996;26:188-194.

60. Jerby BL, Attorri RJ, Morton D Jr: Blunt intestinal injury in children: The role of the physical examination. J Pediatr Surg 1997;32:580-584.

61. Jobst MA, Canty TG Sr, Lynch FP: Management of pancreatic injury in pediatric blunt abdominal trauma. J Pediatr Surg 1999;34:818-824.

62. Kadish HA, Schunk JE, Britton H: Pediatric male rectal and genital trauma: Accidental and nonaccidental injuries. Pediatr Emerg Care 1998;14:95-98.

63. Keller MS, Sartorelli KH, Vane DW: Associated head injury should not prevent nonoperative management of spleen or liver injury in children. J Trauma 1996;41:471-475.

64. Keller MS, Vane DW: Management of pediatric blunt splenic injury: Comparison of pediatric and adult trauma surgeons. J Pediatr Surg 1995;30:221-225.

65. Kim HS, Lee DK, Kim IW, et al: The role of retrograde pancreatography in the treatment of traumatic pancreatic duct injury. Gastrointest Endosc 2001;54:45-55.

66. Koplewitz BZ, Ramos C, Manson DE, et al: Traumatic diaphragmatic injuries in infants and children: Imaging findings. Pediatr Radiol 2000;30:471-479.

67. Kouchi K, Tanabe M, Yoshida H, et al: Nonoperative management of blunt pancreatic injury in children. J Pediatr Surg 1999;34:1736-1738.

68. Kularni R, Daneshmand A, Guertin S, et al: Successful use of activated recombinant factor VII in traumatic liver injuries in children. J Trauma 2004;56:1348-1352.

69. Kushimoto S, Arai M, Aiboshi J, et al: The role of interventional radiology in patients requiring damage control laparotomy. J Trauma 2003;54:171-176.

70. Ladd AP, West KW, Rouse TM, et al: Surgical management of duodenal injuries in children. Surgery 2002;132:748-753.

71. Lane MJ, Mindelzun RE, Jeffery RB: Diagnosis of pancreatic injury after blunt abdominal trauma. Semin Ultrasound CT MR 1996;17:177-182.

72. Lange DA, Zaret P, Merlotti GJ, et al: The use of absorbable mesh in splenic trauma. J Trauma 1988;28:269-275.

73. Lenwand MJ, Atkinson CC, Mooney DP: Application of the APSA evidence-based guidelines for isolated liver or spleen injuries: A single institution experience. J Pediatr Surg 2004;39:487-490.

74. Lickstein DA, Moriary KP, Feins NR: Neonatal rectovaginal tear during cesarean section. J Pediatr Surg 1998;33:1315-1316.

75. Lucaya J, Vasques E, Caballerro F, et al: Nonoperative management of traumatic pancreatic pseudocysts associated with pancreatic duct laceration in children. Pediatr Radiol 1998;28:5-8.

76. Lutz N, Mahboubi S, Nance ML, et al: The significance of contrast blush on computed tomography in children with splenic injuries. J Pediatr Surg 2004;39:491-494.

77. Lutz N, Nance ML, Kallan MJ, et al: Incidence and clinical significance of abdominal wall bruising in restrained children involved in motor vehicle crashes. J Pediatr Surg 2004;39:972-975.

78. Lynch JM, Ford H, Gardner MJ: Is early discharge following isolated splenic injury in the hemodynamically stable child possible? J Pediatr Surg 1993;28:1403-1407.

79. Malhotra AK, Fabian TC, Croce MA, et al: Blunt hepatic injury: A paradigm shift from operative to nonoperative management in the 1990s. Ann Surg 2000;231:804-813.

80. Markley MA, Mantor PC, Letton RW, et al: Pediatric vacuum packing wound closure for damage-control laparotomy. J Pediatr Surg 2002;37:512-514.

81. McGahren ED, Magnuson D, Schauer RT, et al: Management of transection of the pancreas in children. Aust N Z J Surg 1995;65:242-246.

82. Mehall JR, Ennis JS, Saltzman DA, et al: Prospective results of a standardized algorithm based on hemodynamic status for managing pediatric solid organ injury. J Am Coll Surg 2001;193:347-353.

83. Meier DR, Coln CD, Hicks BA, et al: Early operation in patients with pancreas transection. J Pediatr Surg 2001;36:341-344.

84. Meyer G, Huttl TP, Hatz RA, et al: Laparoscopic repair of traumatic diaphragmatic hernias. Surg Endosc 2000;14:1010-1014.

85. Miglietta MA, Salzano LJ, Chiu WC, et al: Decompressive laparotomy: A novel approach in the management of severe intracranial hypertension. J Trauma 2003;55:551-555.

86. Miller K, Kou D, Stallion A, et al: Pediatric hepatic trauma: Does clinical course support intensive care unit stay? J Pediatr Surg 1998;33:1459-1462.

87. Mooney DP, Birkmeyer NJO, Udell JV: Variation in the management of pediatric splenic injuries in New Hampshire. J Pediatr Surg 1998;33:1076-1080.

88. Mooney DP, Forbes PW: Variation in the management of pediatric splenic injuries in New England. J Trauma 2004;56:328-333.

89. Moore EE, Cogbill TH, Jurkovich GJ: Organ injury scaling: Spleen and liver (1994 revision). J Trauma 1995;38:323-324.

90. Morse MA, Garcia VF: Selective nonoperative management of pediatric blunt splenic trauma: Risk for missed associated injuries. J Pediatr Surg 1994;29:23-27.

91. Moss RL, Musemeche CA: Clinical judgment is superior to diagnostic tests in the management of pediatric small bowel injury. J Pediatr Surg 1996;8:1178-1181.

92. Moulton SL, Downey EC, Anderson DS: Blunt bile duct injuries in children. J Pediatr Surg 1993;28:795-797.

93. Moulton SL, Lynch FP, Canty TG: Hepatic vein and retrohepatic vena caval injuries in children: Sternotomy first? Arch Surg 1991;126:1262-1266.

94. Muniz AE, Haynes JH: Delayed abdominal aortic rupture in a child with a seat-belt sign. J Trauma 2004;56:194-197.

95. Nance ML, Keller MS, Stafford PW: Predicting hollow visceral injury in the pediatric blunt trauma patient with solid visceral injury. J Pediatr Surg 2000;35:1300-1303.

96. Nance ML, Lutz N, Arbogast KB, et al: Optimal restraint reduces the risk of abdominal injury in children involved in motor vehicle crashes. Ann Surg 2004;239:127-131.

97. Neville HL, Lally KP, Cox CS: Emergent abdominal decompression with patch abdominoplasty in the pediatric patient. J Pediatr Surg 2000;35:705-708.

98. Norotsky MC, Rogers FB, Shackford SR: Delayed presentation of splenic artery pseudoaneurysms following blunt abdominal trauma: Case reports. J Trauma 1995;38:444-447.

99. Nwomeh BC, Nadler EP, Meza MP, et al: Contrast extravasation predicts the need for operative intervention in children with blunt splenic trauma. J Trauma 2004;56:537-541.

100. Oda J, Ivatury RR, Blocher CR, et al: Amplified cytokine response and lung injury by sequential hemorrhagic shock and abdominal compartment syndrome in a laboratory model of ischemia-reperfusion. J Trauma 2002;52:625-632.

101. Ong AW, McKenney MG, McKenney KA, et al: Predicting the need for laparotomy in pediatric trauma patients on the basis of the ultrasound score. J Trauma 2003;54:503-508.

102. Orr CJ, Clark MA, Hawley DA, et al: Fatal anorectal injuries: A series of four cases. J Forensic Sci 1995;40:219-221.

103. Patel JC, Tepas JJ: The efficacy of focused abdominal sonography for trauma (FAST) as a screening tool in the assessment of injured children. J Pediatr Surg 1999;34:44-47, 52-54.

104. Pearl RH, Wesson DE, Spence LJ: Splenic injury: A five year update with improved results and changing criteria for conservative management. J Pediatr Surg 1989;24:428-431.

105. Pitcher G: Fiber-endoscopic thoracoscopy for diaphragmatic injury in children. Semin Pediatr Surg 2001;10:17-19.

106. Potoka DA, Schall LC, Ford HR: Risk factors for splenectomy in children with blunt splenic trauma. J Pediatr Surg 2002;37:294-299.

107. Prince JS, LoSasso BE, Senac MO: Unusual seat-belt injuries in children. J Trauma 2004;56:420-427.

108. Pryor JP, Stafford PW, Nance ML: Severe blunt hepatic trauma in children. J Pediatr Surg 2001;36:974-979.

109. Ramos CT, Koplewitz BZ, Babyn PS, et al: What have we learned about traumatic diaphragmatic hernias in children? J Pediatr Surg 2000;35:601-604.

110. Reinberg O, Yazbeck S: Major perineal trauma in children. J Pediatr Surg 1989;24:982-984.

111. Rescorla FJ, Plumley DA, Sherman S, et al: The efficacy of early ERCP in pediatric pancreatic trauma. J Pediatr Surg 1995;30:336-340.

112. Rezende-Neto JB, Moore EE, de Andrade MVM, et al: Systemic inflammatory response syndrome secondary to abdominal compartment syndrome: Stage for multiple organ failure. J Trauma 2002;53:1121-1128.

113. Rhodes M, Smith S, Boorse D: Pediatric trauma patients in an "adult" trauma center. J Trauma 1993;35:384-393.

114. Mooney DP, Rothstein DH, Forbes PW: Variation in the management of pediatric splenic injuries in the United States. J Trauma Surg (in press).

115. Rotondo MF, Schwab CW, McGonigal MD: Damage control: An approach for improved survival in exsanguinating penetrating abdominal injury. J Trauma 1993;35:375-383.

116. Saggi BH, Sugerman HJ, Ivatury RR, et al: Abdominal compartment syndrome. J Trauma 1998;45:597-609.

117. Scioscia PJ, Dillon PW, Cilley RE: Endoscopic sphincterotomy in the management of posttraumatic biliary fistula. J Pediatr Surg 1994;29:3-6.

118. Shafi S, Gilbert JC, Carden S: Risk of hemorrhage and appropriate use of blood transfusions in pediatric blunt splenic injuries. J Trauma 1997;42:1029-1032.

119. Shapiro MB, Jenkins DH, Schwab CW, et al: Damage control: Collective review. J Trauma 2000;49:969-978.

120. Sharif K, Pimpalwar AP, John P, et al: Benefits of early diagnosis and preemptive treatment of biliary tract complications after major blunt liver trauma in children. J Pediatr Surg 2002;37:1287-1292.

121. Sharpe RP, Nance ML, Stafford PW: Nonoperative management of blunt extrahepatic biliary duct transection in the pediatric patient. J Pediatr Surg 2002;37:1612-1616.

122. Sharpe RP, Pryor JP, Gandhi RR, et al: Abdominal compartment syndrome in the pediatric blunt trauma patient treated with paracentesis: Report of two cases. J Trauma 2002;53:380-382.

123. Shilyansky J, Navarro O, Superina RA, et al: Delayed hemorrhage after nonoperative management of blunt hepatic trauma in children: A rare but significant event. J Pediatr Surg 1999;34:60-64.

124. Shilyansky J, Pearl RH, Kroutouro M, et al: Diagnosis and management of duodenal injuries in children. J Pediatr Surg 1997;32:880-886.

125. Shilyansky J, Sen LM, Kreller M, et al: Nonoperative management of pancreatic injuries in children. J Pediatr Surg 1998;33:343-345.

126. Simon RJ, Rabin J, Kuhls D: Impact of increased use of laparoscopy on negative laparotomy rates after penetrating trauma. J Trauma 2002;53:297-302.

127. Sivit CJ, Taylor GA, Bulas DI, et al: Blunt trauma in children: Significance of peritoneal fluid. Radiology 1991;178:185-188.

128. Smith RS, Fry WR, Morabito DJ, et al: Therapeutic laparoscopy in trauma. Am J Surg 1995;170:632-637.

129. Sola JE, Mattei P, Pegoli W Jr, et al: Rupture of the right diaphragm following blunt trauma in an infant: Case report. J Trauma 1994;36:417-420.

130. Soto JA, Alvarez O, Munera F, et al: Traumatic disruption of the pancreatic duct: Diagnosis with MR pancreatography. AJR Am J Roentgenol 2001;176:175-178.

131. Stassen NA, Lukan JK, Carrillo EH, et al: Abdominal seat belt marks in the era of focused abdominal sonography for trauma. Arch Surg 2002;137:718-723.

132. Strear CM, Graf JL, Albanese CT, et al: Successful treatment of liver hemorrhage in the premature infant. J Pediatr Surg 1998;33:849-851.

133. Stylianos S: Controversies in abdominal trauma. Semin Pediatr Surg 1995;4:116-119.

134. Stylianos S: Abdominal packing for severe hemorrhage. J Pediatr Surg 1998;33:339-342.

135. Stylianos S, APSA Trauma Committee: Evidence-based guidelines for resource utilization in children with isolated spleen or liver injury. J Pediatr Surg 2000;35:164-169.

136. Stylianos S, APSA Trauma Study Group: Prospective validation of evidence-based guidelines for resource utilization in children with isolated spleen or liver injury. J Pediatr Surg 2002;37:453-456.

137. Stylianos S, Bergman KS, Harris BH: Traumatic renal avulsion into the chest: Case report. J Trauma 1991;31:301-302.

138. Stylianos S, Jacir NN, Hoffman MA, et al: Pediatric blunt liver injury and coagulopathy managed with packs and silo. J Trauma 1990;30:1409-1410.

139. Suliburk JW, Ware DN, Balogh Z, et al: Vacuum-assisted wound closure achieves early fascial closure of open abdomens after severe trauma. J Trauma 2003;55:1155-1160.

140. Taner AS, Topgul K, Kucukel F, et al: Diagnostic laparoscopy decreases the rate of unnecessary laparotomies and reduces hospital costs in trauma patients. J Laparoendosc Adv Surg Tech A 2001;11:207-211.

141. Tepas JJ, Frykberg ER, Schinco MA, et al: Pediatric trauma is very much a surgical disease. Ann Surg 2003;237:775-781.

142. Upadhyaya P, Simpson JS: Splenic trauma in children. Surg Gynecol Obstet 1968;126:781-790.

143. Vargo D, Sorenson J, Barton R: Repair of grade VI hepatic injury: Case report and literature review. J Trauma 2002;53:823-824.

144. Wales PW, Shuckett B, Kim PC: Long term outcome of non-operative management of complete traumatic pancreatic transection in children. J Pediatr Surg 2001;36:823-827.

145. Watts DD, Trask A, Soeken K, et al: Hypothermic coagulopathy in trauma: Effect of varying levels of hypothermia on enzyme speed, platelet function, and fibrinolytic activity. J Trauma 1998;44:846-854.

146. Winthrop AL, Wesson DE, Filler RM: Traumatic duodenal hematoma in the pediatric patient. J Pediatr Surg 1986;21:757-760.

147. Wolberg AS, Meng ZH, Monroe DM, et al: A systematic evaluation of the effect of temperature on coagulation enzyme activity and platelet function. J Trauma 2004;56:1221-1228.

148. Wotherspoon S, Chu K, Brown AF: Abdominal surgery and the seat-belt sign. Emerg Med 2001;13:61-65.

149. Yang EY, Marder SR, Hastings G, et al: The abdominal compartment syndrome complicating nonoperative management of major blunt liver injuries: Recognition and treatment using multimodality therapy. J Trauma 2002;52:982-986.

150. Yellin AE, Chaffee CB, Donovan AJ: Vascular isolation in treatment of juxtahepatic venous injuries. Arch Surg 1971;102:566-573.

Chapter 18

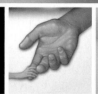

Genitourinary Tract Trauma

Rebeccah L. Brown and Victor F. Garcia

EPIDEMIOLOGY

Injury is the leading cause of death in children and young adults in the United States, with injury to the kidney from either blunt or penetrating trauma being the most common genitourinary tract injury.[21,122] Almost 50% of genitourinary tract injuries involve the kidney.[121] Blunt abdominal trauma is responsible for 90% of pediatric genitourinary tract injuries,[21] with the kidney being injured in 10% to 20% of all blunt trauma cases.[121,122] The kidney is the most commonly injured solid organ, injured more frequently than the liver, spleen, or pancreas.[21,43,130] Serious renal injuries are most often associated with injuries to other organs, with multiple organ involvement occurring in 80% of those with penetrating trauma and 75% of those sustaining blunt trauma.[172] The majority of associated injuries are closed-head injuries and extremity fractures.[7,43,145] Associated abdominal injuries occur in 42% to 74% of patients, primarily involving the spleen and liver in blunt trauma and the bowel in penetrating trauma.[102,104,122,179,182] The majority of isolated renal injuries can be classified as relatively minor injuries.[40] Mortality is rare due to isolated renal trauma and is more often attributed to the combined effects of major multisystem trauma.

MECHANISMS OF INJURY

Most blunt renal injuries are due to sudden deceleration forces. Confined within Gerota's fascia, the kidney may be crushed against the ribs or the vertebral column, resulting in laceration or contusion. Direct injury to the renal parenchyma and collecting system may also occur from penetration of sharp, bony fragments of adjacent fractured ribs. Rapid deceleration may cause arterial or venous injury from stretching of the fixed renal vascular pedicle.[21] Because the intima of the renal artery is less elastic than that of the media and adventitia, it is predisposed to laceration, which may lead to subintimal dissection and arterial thrombosis.[69] Mechanisms of blunt renal injury include pedestrian/motor vehicle crashes (60%), falls (22.5%), sports injuries (10%), assault (3.5%), and other causes (4%).[175] Most children who sustain renal injury in motor vehicle accidents are unrestrained[122]; however, violent deceleration with severe flexion-extension as seen with seatbelts is a well-recognized mechanism of renal injury associated with a higher risk of renal pedicle avulsion and ureteropelvic junction (UPJ) injury. Interestingly, bicycle crashes are the most common sports-related cause of renal injury in children and are associated with a significant risk of high-grade renal injury.[75] Although there is a perception among pediatric surgeons and urologists that contact sports such as football, hockey, and martial arts incur the greatest risk for renal injury in children,[175] a review by McAleer and colleagues[123] demonstrated that bicycle crashes accounted for 24% of injuries compared with only 5% for contact sports. This may have some impact on the type of counseling that should be provided regarding activity for children after severe renal injury and for those with solitary kidneys. Penetrating genitourinary tract injuries are becoming more common and should be suspected with any penetrating injuries to the chest, abdomen, flank, and lumbar regions.[28,65] Iatrogenic injuries are uncommon and generally readily diagnosed. A significant risk of trauma occurs with needle puncture of the kidney for biopsy or endourologic access; endoscopic access of the urethra, bladder, or ureter; and procedures done on viscera adjacent to the genitourinary system. The most common iatrogenic injury is to the ureter during gynecologic and oncologic procedures.

ANATOMIC CONSIDERATIONS

Children are considered to be at increased risk for genitourinary tract trauma owing to unique anatomic differences between children and adults.[21,109,139] In children, the kidneys are larger relative to the size of the child's body and positioned lower in the abdomen, making them more exposed and vulnerable to injury. They are also less protected because of decreased perirenal fat, weaker abdominal wall musculature, and a poorly ossified thoracic rib cage. Because many pediatric kidneys retain their fetal lobulations, the risk for renal parenchymal disruption and lower pole amputation is increased. Furthermore, the renal capsule and Gerota's fascia are less developed than in adults, creating a greater potential for laceration, nonconfined bleeding, and urinary extravasation. Because of the relative mobility of a child's kidney, rapid deceleration is more likely to result in renal pedicle injury and UPJ disruption. In a comparative series of children and adults who sustained blunt renal trauma, Brown and colleagues[21] concluded that although the likelihood of major renal injury was significantly higher in the pediatric population, the severity of trauma was significantly lower.

For similar reasons, preexisting renal disease or congenital renal anomalies may predispose children to an increased risk of genitourinary tract injury from blunt trauma. The reported incidence of preexisting renal disease or congenital genitourinary anomalies in children sustaining renal trauma varies from 1% to 23%.[19,38,45,67,121,122,135,146] Underlying congenital anomalies associated with hydronephrosis (UPJ obstruction), abnormal kidney position (horseshoe kidneys, crossed fused renal ectopia), or abnormal kidney consistency (polycystic kidney disease, urinary reflux) may predispose the kidney to significant injury despite relatively minor forces.[45] Gross hematuria associated with an ostensibly minor trauma should alert the physician to the possibility of an underlying pathologic lesion of the urinary tract and should prompt further radiologic imaging. Although underlying congenital genitourinary anomalies may have an increased risk of injury in children, they do not appear to be associated with any increased morbidity or long-term disability.[123]

CLINICAL FEATURES

The evaluation of possible injury to the genitourinary tract is a part of the systematic and expeditious assessment required in all seriously injured patients. The mechanism of injury is important to know in order to assess the risk of injury. Direct blows to the abdomen or flank and significant deceleration forces as may occur in motor vehicle accidents and falls should alert the physician to the possibility of renal injury. Penetrating injuries to the abdomen, flank, back, chest, and pelvis should also raise suspicion for injury to the genitourinary tract. Although the presence of abdominal or flank tenderness and flank ecchymosis or mass suggests renal injury, up to 25% of patients with severe renal injury have unremarkable abdominal examinations. Indeed, only 55% of children with significant renal injuries present with tenderness over the injured kidney. Conversely, only about half of children with renal tenderness on examination have a condition more serious than minor renal trauma.[167]

Perineal ecchymosis, swelling, laceration, and bleeding are highly suggestive of genitourinary trauma. The presence of blood at the urinary meatus or a boggy mass or upward displacement of the prostate on digital rectal examination in boys requires formal urethrography to evaluate for possible injury to the urethra before any attempts at urethral catheterization.

Gross hematuria is indicative of genitourinary trauma and mandates further radiologic imaging. Conversely, the absence of hematuria, either gross or microscopic, does not exclude the possibility of significant genitourinary trauma. In fact, complete avulsion of the renal vascular pedicle

and disruption of the UPJ have both been described in the absence of hematuria.[14,35-38,43,131,158,166,179]

Whereas fractures of the lower ribs and lumbar spine may be associated with renal trauma, fractures of the pelvis may be associated with bladder and urethral injuries. Eight percent of patients with a pelvic fracture have associated lower urinary tract injuries. The comparative incidence of lower urinary tract injury with various types of pelvic fractures is 27% in patients with symphysiolysis, 17% in patients with pelvic fracture, and 2% in patients with a fracture of the pubis.[196] In a study by Aihara and associates,[3] certain types of pelvic fractures were found to be associated with increased risk for rectal, bladder, or urethral injuries. Rectal injury was associated with widening of the symphysis pubis. Bladder injuries were most commonly associated with widening of the sacroiliac joint, symphysis pubis, and fractures of the sacrum, with widening of the symphysis pubis being the strongest predictor of bladder injury. Urethral injuries were most commonly associated with widening of the symphysis pubis and fractures of the inferior pubic ramus. Fractures involving these locations should heighten suspicion of associated rectal and lower urinary tract injuries and prompt directed diagnostic studies.

Gross hematuria in the presence of a pelvic fracture strongly suggests a bladder perforation. Any degree of hematuria in the presence of a pelvic fracture is an indication for cystography. Ninety-five percent of patients with bladder injuries have gross hematuria, and the remaining patients have microscopic hematuria.

DIAGNOSTIC EVALUATION

A urine sample should be obtained in all trauma patients to assess for potential injury to the genitourinary tract. Gross hematuria is highly indicative of trauma to the genitourinary tract, although it does not necessarily correlate with severity of injury. In the absence of gross hematuria, the urine dipstick is a safe and reliable method to screen for the presence of hematuria. The false-positive rate is 4.3%.[58] Dipstick results that are negative for hematuria do not need the added expense of microscopic analysis. However, if hematuria is revealed by dipstick evaluation, the specimen should be examined microscopically for more accurate quantification.[44,58] It should be noted that microscopic hematuria can be associated with such procedures as atraumatic passage of a urethral catheter. However, in this instance, the degree of hematuria is minimal, and more than 5 red blood cells (RBCs) per high-powered field (HPF) should be considered abnormal.[44,178]

A critical issue in the management of suspected genitourinary tract injury is the need for and extent of radiographic evaluation. Although most would agree that gross hematuria is an indication for formal diagnostic evaluation, much controversy exists as to whether microscopic hematuria as an isolated finding on urinalysis in pediatric trauma patients warrants further radiologic imaging.*

It remains unclear what degree of microscopic hematuria, if any, warrants radiographic evaluation in children.

---

*See references 7, 8, 22, 30, 71, 90, 91, 102, 112, 114, 121, 133, 140, 145, 167, 170, 174, 182, and 183.

Several studies have attempted to answer the question as to whether the adult criteria for imaging of renal trauma, including findings of gross hematuria, shock, major associated injuries, and significant deceleration injury, can be applied to children. Although degrees of microhematuria ranging from *any* degree of microhematuria[112,183] to 20 RBCs per HPF[91] to 50 RBCs per HPF[145] have been reported as significant in the literature, a careful analysis of published reports on 382 children with renal injuries reveals that the application of adult criteria for imaging would have identified 98% to 100% of all renal injuries.[174]

It is generally accepted that abdominal trauma associated with shock warrants radiographic evaluation of the genitourinary system. Several authors have found that young adults with a history of blunt trauma and microscopic hematuria *without* shock, associated major intra-abdominal injuries, or a history of rapid deceleration can be managed safely without renal imaging.[29,128,138,152] However, up to 25% of patients with any degree of hematuria *and* shock have significant renal injury.[89,131,152] One of the pitfalls in applying adult criteria for the imaging of renal trauma to children, especially with regard to the presence or absence of shock, is that children are unique in their ability to maintain normal blood pressure in the face of significant hypovolemia and blood loss. In fact, only 5% of children with major renal injury have clinical signs of shock.[101,167] Therefore, hypotension itself is not a reliable indicator of the severity of renal injury in the pediatric population.[167,183] Tachycardia typically precedes hypotension as an early indicator of shock in children and may be a worrisome sign. Accordingly, the decision on imaging in children, as in adults, should be based not on isolated findings but rather on the whole clinical picture, including mechanism of injury (direct blow, major deceleration, or flexion-extension injury), vital signs (tachycardia or hypotension), physical examination findings (abdominal/flank tenderness or contusion), urinalysis (microhematuria or gross hematuria), and associated injuries. In most cases, microhematuria is not an isolated finding. Most children with microhematuria will have some other parameter, such as mechanism of injury, physical findings, or other associated injuries, that would warrant further imaging, therefore decreasing the likelihood of missed injury.

Abdominal computed tomography (CT) is the standard for radiographic evaluation of abdominal trauma in children and is the most accurate imaging and staging modality for evaluation of renal injury.[18,102,121,201] CT is highly sensitive and specific for detection of parenchymal contusions/lacerations, perinephric/retroperitoneal hematoma, urinary extravasation, and segmental or major arterial injuries; delineation of nonviable, nonperfused tissue or segmental infarction; and demonstration of other associated intra-abdominal injuries. With the advent of the newer, faster helical CT scanners, it is essential to obtain delayed images during the nephrogram phase (>80 seconds) to detect renal parenchymal and venous injury as well as during the excretory phase (2 to 10 minutes) to avoid missing urine or blood extravasation. Extravasated urine accumulates, whereas extravasated arterial contrast dilutes out after the bolus of contrast agent is stopped.[133,176]

CT has replaced the intravenous pyelogram (IVP) in the hemodynamically stable patient. However, a one-shot IVP still remains useful in the hemodynamically unstable patient before emergent surgical exploration to determine the presence of two functional kidneys, the presence and extent of urinary extravasation, and the presence of renal pedicle injury. In children, 2 to 3 mL/kg of nonionic contrast is injected intravenously, followed by an abdominal radiograph immediately and 10 minutes later.[133] It should be recognized that the IVP provides only very basic information and is not useful in staging of renal injuries. In fact, some studies have shown that as many as 20% of patients with significant renal injuries will have a normal IVP. Likewise, nonvisualization of the kidney on IVP does not necessarily correlate with arterial occlusion or injury. Other factors, including renal contusion with vascular spasm, overhydration, and hypotension or hypoperfusion, may produce similar findings in up to half of patients.[48]

Arteriography has been largely supplanted by CT and CT angiography for the diagnosis and staging of renal injury. More invasive than CT, arteriography requires the expertise of an experienced interventional radiologist and may be associated with a formidable risk for arterial injury in small children whose vessels may be prohibitively small, fragile, and difficult to access or cannulate. The current role of arteriography is in the diagnosis of delayed or ongoing renal hemorrhage, renovascular injury, or delayed arteriovenous fistula or pseudoaneurysm formation where interventional techniques such as selective embolization[61,64,93,116,137,184] or endovascular stenting[23,111,134] may be therapeutic.

Ultrasound, although utilized extensively in Europe for the assessment of acute renal trauma, has not found widespread acceptance in the United States. In the United States, ultrasonography in the trauma patient is mostly limited to the Focused Assessment with Sonography for Trauma (FAST) examination, which is performed primarily to detect the presence of free intraperitoneal fluid. The FAST examination has not been particularly useful in children except perhaps in the hemodynamically unstable patient with an associated closed-head injury to rapidly exclude the presence of intra-abdominal hemorrhage. In the hemodynamically stable child, CT provides more useful information. Ultrasound is not particularly sensitive for detecting parenchymal injuries, except in the most experienced hands, and only with close color and pulsed Doppler interrogation can a vascular injury be diagnosed. Therefore, its utility in the acute setting at present remains quite limited.

It is critical to remember that CT and IVP are not sensitive for bladder laceration unless the bladder is fully distended. Haas and coworkers[86] compared the accuracy of routine helical CT versus conventional cystography in 15 patients with suspected bladder injury. Cystography accurately diagnosed and classified the injury in all 15 patients, whereas CT was only about 60% accurate. Consequently, cystography is the imaging modality of choice when bladder injury is suspected. For conventional cystography, after a scout film is obtained, a small amount of contrast medium is infused, followed by a second radiograph to check for gross extravasation. If gross extravasation is seen, a Foley catheter is inserted and placed to drainage. If extravasation is not seen, then the remainder of the contrast medium is instilled and radiographs are obtained in the anteroposterior, oblique, and lateral projections. It is essential for the bladder to be fully distended to avoid missing small-to-moderate tears of the bladder wall. The bladder of adolescents should be filled with 300 to 400 mL of contrast medium. The bladder of smaller children should be filled by gravity infusion until the patient becomes uncomfortable or the bladder capacity is reached. In children younger than 2 years of age, the bladder capacity is 7 mL × weight (kg). In children 2 to 11 years of age, the bladder capacity is age in years plus 2 × 30 mL.[68,106]

As part of the cystogram, all the contrast medium is drained from the bladder and a postevacuation radiograph is taken. Up to 15% of extraperitoneal bladder ruptures are identified only on the radiograph taken after evacuation. The extent of extravasation seen with extraperitoneal bladder rupture may be limited to the pelvic area or be quite dramatic, extending into a pelvic hematoma or coursing along the lateral pelvic wall. Extravasation from an intraperitoneal bladder rupture flows into the peritoneum, outlining the bowel with contrast agent.

More recently, CT cystography has been found to be faster and equally accurate for defining and staging bladder injuries provided that the basic principles for conventional cystography, including complete distention of the bladder and imaging both before and after evacuation, are followed. Simply clamping a Foley catheter after intravenous contrast agent administration for CT is not adequate and will result in an unacceptably high rate of missed injuries.[113,156]

Retrograde pyelography plays a role in the assessment of ureteral and renal pelvic integrity when UPJ injury is suspected. Failure of opacification of the distal ureter on CT should raise suspicion for a ureteral injury[187]; and if insufficient detail is provided by CT, then retrograde pyelography is indicated.

Retrograde urethography is indicated when urethral injury is suspected. A Foley catheter with a minimally inflated balloon is inserted into the fossa navicularis of the distal urethra, and approximately 30 mL of contrast medium is instilled under fluoroscopic vision. A normal retrograde urethrogram should demonstrate complete filling of the intact urethra with passage of contrast medium into the bladder. The presence of filling defects or extravasation of the contrast agent indicates urethral disruption. In the presence of hematuria, a cystogram should follow the retrograde urethrogram, even if the retrograde urethrogram is normal, because 10% to 15% of patients with urethral disruption from a pelvic fracture will have a concomitant bladder injury.[48]

INJURY GRADING AND SCORING SYSTEMS FOR GENITOURINARY INJURIES

In 1989, the American Association for the Surgery of Trauma (AAST) Injury Scaling Committee devised and published a classification or grading system for genitourinary tract injuries (Table 18-1) to standardize injury descriptions for research and data collection purposes. Figure 18-1 is an illustrative depiction of this grading system. Injuries are graded on scale from I to V ranging from the most minor injury (grade I) to the most complex (grade V). For the kidney, this grading system has proved highly applicable, and a study by Santucci and associates[173] of 2467 renal trauma patients validated its usefulness as a measure of the seriousness of renal injury and as a predictor of the need for surgery. For example, patients with a grade I injury require observation only, whereas those with a grade V injury are more likely to require nephrectomy. Those with intermediate injuries (grades II to IV) require individualized therapy, with a trend toward more invasive therapy as injury grade increases. It should be noted, however, that this study was composed primarily of adult patients. Thus, extrapolation of results from this series may not be entirely applicable to children. Furthermore, the AAST system has been criticized for grouping complex parenchymal injury with major renovascular injury in the grade IV and V categories, because management may be quite different for the same grades of injury. Modifications addressing this issue have been proposed for future iterations of the scaling system. The AAST scaling systems for ureteral, bladder, and urethral injury (see Table 18-1) have not gained as widespread acceptance and have been used less consistently.

MANAGEMENT OF SPECIFIC INJURIES

Kidney

Blunt Injuries

As with traumatic injuries to the spleen and liver, the majority of blunt renal trauma in children can be safely managed nonoperatively.* Almost 85% of pediatric renal injuries are considered relatively minor, with grade I and II contusions and minor parenchymal lacerations predominating. These lower grade renal injuries will invariably heal without further sequelae. Major parenchymal injuries occur in 10% to 15%, whereas major disruption of the renal pedicle occurs in the remaining 5% of children.[48,179]

Children with microscopic hematuria and a minor renal injury diagnosed and graded by CT may require brief hospitalization for observation or may be discharged home with clear follow-up instructions. Children with higher-grade renal injury by CT and/or gross hematuria are hospitalized and placed at bed rest with close monitoring of vital signs and serial physical examinations and blood cell counts. Traditionally, ambulation is begun once the patient is fully resuscitated and hemodynamically stable, blood cell counts have stabilized, and gross hematuria has resolved. It is not unusual for patients with gross hematuria to occlude their bladder outlet or Foley catheter with clot. Decreased urine output, bladder distention, or bladder spasms should alert the clinician

---

*See references 2, 7, 8, 43, 88, 109, 112, 118, 120, 168, 171, 179, and 197.

TABLE 18–1	Urologic Injury Scale of the American Association for the Surgery of Trauma

Grade*	Injury Description†
Renal Injury Scale	
I Contusion	Microscopic or gross hematuria; urologic studies normal
Hematoma	Subcapsular, nonexpanding without parenchymal laceration
II Hematoma	Nonexpanding perirenal hematoma confined to the renal retroperitoneum
Laceration	<1 cm parenchymal depth of renal cortex without urinary extravasation
III Laceration	>1 cm parenchymal depth of renal cortex without collection system rupture or urinary extravasation
IV Laceration	Parenchymal laceration extending through the renal cortex, medulla, and collecting system
Vascular	Main renal artery or vein injury with contained hemorrhage
V Laceration	Completely shattered kidney
Vascular	Avulsion of renal hilum that devascularizes kidney
Ureter Injury Scale	
I Hematoma	Contusion of hematoma without devascularization
II Laceration	≤50% transection
III Laceration	>50% transection
IV Laceration	Complete transection with 2 cm devascularization
V Laceration	Avulsion of renal hilum that devascularizes kidney
Bladder Injury Scale	
I Hematoma	Contusion, intramural hematoma
Laceration	Partial thickness
II Laceration	Extraperitoneal bladder wall laceration ≤2 cm
III Laceration	Extraperitoneal (>2 cm) or intraperitoneal (≤2 cm) bladder wall lacerations
IV Laceration	Intraperitoneal bladder wall laceration >2 cm
V Laceration	Intra- or extraperitoneal bladder wall laceration extending into the bladder neck or ureteral orifice (trigone)
Urethral Injury Scale	
I Contusion	Blood at urethral meatus; urethrography normal
II Stretch injury	Elongation of urethra without extravasation on urethrography
III Partial disruption	Extravasation of urethrographic contrast medium at injury site, with contrast visualized in the bladder
IV Complete disruption	Extravasation of urethrographic contrast medium at injury site without visualization in the bladder; <2 cm of urethral separation
V Complete disruption	Complete transection with >2 cm urethral separation, or extension into the prostate or vagina

*Advance one grade for multiple injuries to the same organ.
†Based on most accurate assessment at autopsy, laparotomy, or radiologic study.
From Moore EE, Shackford SR, Pachter HL, et al: Organ injury scaling: Spleen, liver, and kidney. J Trauma 1989;29:1664.

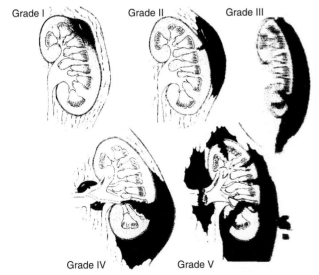

Grade I Grade II Grade III

Grade IV Grade V

Figure 18–1 Artist's rendition of the American Association for the Surgery of Trauma grading system for genitourinary tract trauma. (Reproduced with permission from Coburn M: Genitourinary trauma. In Moore E, Feliciano DV, Mattox KL [eds]: Trauma, 5th ed. New York, McGraw-Hill, 2004.)

to this possibility. Placement of a Foley catheter or irrigation or replacement of an existing Foley catheter should remediate the problem. Although it is generally suggested that patients maintain a decreased level of activity until the microscopic or gross hematuria resolves, there are no evidence-based guidelines in the literature addressing appropriate length or type of activity restrictions for renal trauma. The period of time at which healing is adequate to allow return to full activity without risk has not yet been defined. Prospective studies are warranted.

Although there is little controversy regarding management of the lower grade, less complex renal injuries in hemodynamically *stable* patients or the management of high grade, complex renal injuries in hemodynamically *unstable* patients, the management of those with intermediate injuries remains less well defined. Although the AAST grading scale appears to have some predictive value on the need for surgery, indications for surgery are based more on hemodynamic stability of the patient and associated injuries, rather than on grade of renal injury based on imaging criteria. The only absolute indication for surgery is hemodynamic instability with ongoing bleeding and transfusion requirements. Radiographic signs of ongoing renal bleeding include an expanding or uncontained retroperitoneal hematoma or complete avulsion of the main renal artery or vein with extravasation as demonstrated by CT or arteriography.[94]

Although significant renal injury with urinary extravasation has in the past been considered a relative, if not absolute, indication for renal exploration, more recent studies would suggest that most of these types of injuries can be successfully managed nonoperatively in the hemodynamically stable patient.[120,148,161,171] Matthews and associates[120] reported spontaneous resolution of urinary extravasation in 27 of 31 patients (87%), while the remaining 4 patients required ureteral stents due to persistent extravasation. Similarly, Russell and coworkers[171] reported management of 15 pediatric patients with grade IV renal injuries with urinary extravasation—9 patients (60%) required observation only; 1 required emergent partial nephrectomy due to hypotension and ongoing bleeding; and 5 developed urinomas, 2 of whom were treated with percutaneous drainage and 3 of whom required ureteral stents. Although complications can occur with nonoperative management, most complications associated with urinary extravasation are easily treated by percutaneous drainage[171] or endoscopic stent placement,[120,161,171] thereby achieving higher rates of renal salvage.

Patients with major renal trauma associated with enteric or pancreatic injury may be at increased risk for serious infectious complications, such as perinephric abscess and infected urinoma. In a study comparing nonoperative versus surgical management of patients with major renal lacerations with a devitalized fragment after blunt abdominal trauma, Husmann and associates[98] found that renal exploration and surgical repair significantly improves the prognosis only in those patients with concomitant intraperitoneal injuries. Therefore, operative exploration of the kidney should be considered in children with major blunt renal injuries with a devascularized segment in association with intestinal perforation or complex pancreatic injury to reduce the incidence of serious infectious complications.

Nonoperative management of hemodynamically stable children with complex higher grade blunt renal injury has become the standard of care in most centers. Most pediatric and adult series report successful nonoperative management of even the most complex injuries, including shattered but perfused kidneys and complex lacerations with extensive perinephric hematoma and urinary extravasation.[6,171] Proponents of nonoperative management of these patients note that in the absence of prospective studies comparing immediate exploration versus expectant management, no reliable data are available to suggest that surgery done early in the course of injury reduces the long- or short-term complications. The risk for nephrectomy associated with immediate exploration is avoided, and delayed surgery is only necessary in 0% to 13% of patients.[7,8,112,171,179,197] With recent advances in interventional radiology techniques and equipment, the need for delayed open surgery has diminished significantly.[78] An algorithm for the management of renal injuries in children is presented in Figure 18-2.

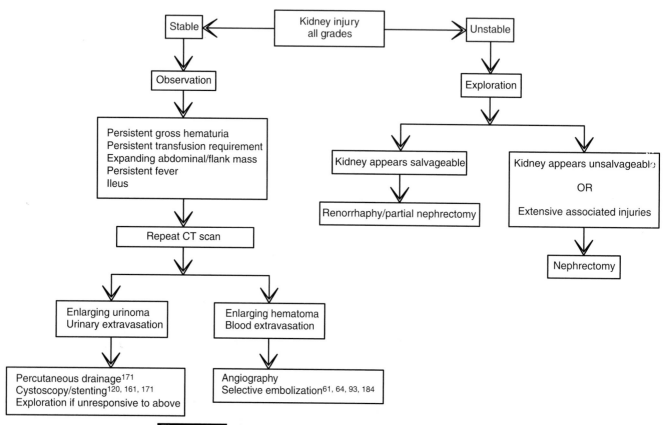

Figure 18–2   Algorithm for the management of renal injuries in children.

Collective review of 10 retrospective pediatric series of blunt renal trauma published over the past 13 years (1991-2004)* consists of 668 patients with the following grades of injury: grade I (342); grade II (46); grade III (64); grade IV (85); grade V (24); grades IV and V (16); grades I and II (50); grades I to III (18); and grades II and III (23). Operative intervention for renal injury was required in 45 patients (6.7%), including 31 nephrectomies (4.6%), 11 partial nephrectomies (1.6%), 1 renorrhaphy, and 2 nephrostomies. All patients with grades I and II renal injuries were successfully managed nonoperatively. Only 2 patients with grade III renal injuries required operative intervention: 1 with nephrectomy and 1 with a partial nephrectomy. Forty-one of 125 (33%) children with grade IV and V renal injuries required operative intervention, including 30 nephrectomies (13 grade IV; 15 grade V; 2 grades IV and V); 10 partial nephrectomies (8 grade IV, 1 grade V, and 1 grades IV and V), 1 renorrhaphy (grades IV and V), and 2 nephrostomies (grades IV and V). The indication for operative intervention in almost all cases was hemodynamic instability with ongoing bleeding, with most requiring emergent operations within 24 hours of admission. The percentage of patients requiring operative intervention for renal injury ranged from 1.7%[112] to 12.7%,[118] with the vast majority being those with high-grade (IV to V) complex injuries. Nonoperative management was successful in 93% of *all* patients with blunt renal trauma, 97% of those with grade III renal injuries, 75% of those with grade IV renal injuries, and 33% of those with grade V renal injuries.

Penetrating Injuries

Penetrating renal injuries are rare in children. Although most gunshot wounds to the abdomen will require abdominal exploration, retroperitoneal dissection and exploration is indicated only if preoperative or intraoperative assessment suggests a major renal injury with extravasation outside of Gerota's fascia, there is suspicion for significant nonurologic retroperitoneal injury (great vessels, duodenum, pancreas, colon), and/or inspection reveals an expanding or pulsatile retroperitoneal hematoma.[191] McAninch and coworkers[128] classified gunshot wounds involving the kidney into five categories: (1) contusions (18.4%), (2) minor lacerations (13.8%), (3) major lacerations (50.5%), (4) vascular injuries (6.9%), and (5) lacerations combined with vascular injury (10.3%). The majority of patients had multiple injuries, with 95% requiring associated procedures. The nephrectomy rate was 13.8%. Although many of the kidneys removed were potentially salvageable, most were removed because of the patient's precarious hemodynamic status.

For renal-proximity stab wounds, nonoperative treatment is appropriate in hemodynamically stable patients without associated injuries who have been staged appropriately by triple-contrast CT.[68,198] However, a high index of suspicion for missed ureteral and other associated injuries must be maintained if a nonoperative pathway is chosen.

In a retrospective review by McAninch and coworkers,[127] 55% of renal stab wounds and 24% of renal gunshot wounds were successfully managed nonoperatively with an acceptable complication rate. In the hemodynamically unstable patient with penetrating trauma or those with a retroperitoneal hematoma at laparotomy, a one-shot IVP may be useful to identify renal injury and confirm the presence and function of two renal units to further guide management.

Renovascular Injuries

Major renovascular injuries are rare in children. Carroll and colleagues[31] and Turner and associates[190] reported penetrating trauma as a cause of renovascular injuries in 64% and 68% of their patients, respectively. Conversely, Cass and coworkers[39] identified blunt external trauma as the cause of renovascular injury in 76% of patients. Regardless of the mechanism, these patients tend to have high injury severity scores, large transfusion requirements, and associated life-threatening multisystem injury,[31,39,179] the management of which supersedes that of renal injury. Knudson and colleagues[105] reported that factors associated with a poor outcome after renovascular injuries include blunt trauma, grade V injury, and attempted arterial repair. Grade V injuries are frequently associated with severe major parenchymal injuries, which contribute to poor function of the revascularized kidney. Patients with grade V injuries with severe parenchymal disruption may be better served by immediate nephrectomy, provided that a functional contralateral kidney is present. Bruce and associates[23] compared 12 patients with blunt renal artery injuries who underwent operative intervention (9 nephrectomies; 3 revascularizations) with 16 patients who were managed nonoperatively, 1 of whom underwent endovascular stent placement. They concluded that nonoperative management of unilateral blunt renal artery injuries is safe and often successful, with a 6% risk of developing post-traumatic renovascular hypertension.

The pathogenesis of renovascular injuries due to blunt trauma is thought to be caused by rapid deceleration, which results in stretching of the renal vasculature, disruption of the arterial intima, and arterial thrombosis.[31] Blunt arterial injury occurs more commonly on the left side than on the right side[31,33,34,190] because the right renal artery is longer than the left and may be better able to withstand the stretching caused by deceleration.[31]

Although hematuria may be absent or microscopic in 13% to 56% of patients with renovascular injuries,[31,39,65,128,179] most patients have other symptoms or signs that raise suspicion for a major renal injury and prompt further diagnostic imaging.[31,179]

Renovascular injury is suggested on CT by (1) lack of renal enhancement or excretion, often in the presence of normal renal contour; (2) vein enhancement; (3) central hematoma; (4) abrupt cutoff of an enhanced renal artery; and (5) nonopacification of the pelvicaliceal system.[31,179]

The approach to this type of injury depends on the time to diagnosis, the type and extent of the vascular injury, and the extent of the associated injuries.[31,105,179]

---

*See references 7, 8, 21, 43, 112, 118, 158, 171, 174, and 179.

Repair of the right renal vein may be difficult owing to its short length and proximity to the inferior vena cava. Nonetheless, injuries to the main renal vein can be repaired in most cases.[31] Laceration of the left renal vein at its origin can be managed by ligation because collateral circulation supplied by gonadal and adrenal veins usually allows for adequate venous drainage.[31,83]

Segmental arteries are difficult to repair and may best be managed by ligation with accompanying partial nephrectomy if the area of infarction encompasses more than 15% of the kidney.[90] However, others suggest that nonoperative management should be considered in any patient with segmental artery occlusion that is not associated with uncontrolled retroperitoneal hemorrhage, extensive urinary extravasation, or other intra-abdominal indications for surgery. This management strategy has been associated with an acceptably low incidence of complications.[11,31]

Arterial repair is most appropriate and most successful for renovascular injuries caused by penetrating trauma. Notwithstanding occasional reports of successful revascularization in patients 19 hours after injury,[82] the success of the procedure greatly diminishes after 8 hours of renal ischemia.[31,69,82,147,177] Ivatury and coworkers[99] reviewed 40 penetrating renovascular injuries and concluded that salvage of a kidney with a renovascular injury is determined primarily by the nature and extent of associated injuries. Furthermore, they reported that while attempts at renal artery repair are often futile, renal vein injuries are more amenable to repair and have a better prognosis. Nephrectomy, however, remains the procedure of choice in the hemodynamically unstable patient with multiple trauma.

Blunt injuries to the main renal artery are associated with lowest success rate for complete renal preservation.[31,179,190] Haas and associates[85] reviewed the management of 12 patients with complete renal artery occlusion secondary to blunt trauma. Renal artery revascularization was attempted in 5 patients with a median warm ischemia time of 5 hours (range: 4.5 to 36 hours). Although four of five revascularizations were deemed technically successful at the time of operation, 3 patients demonstrated no function and 1 showed minimal function on postoperative renal function scans. Two patients required delayed nephrectomy due to complications, and of the 7 patients who underwent nonoperative management, 3 patients developed significant hypertension requiring nephrectomy for blood pressure control. Based on these results, the authors are unable to advocate emergency revascularization for unilateral renal artery occlusion in the presence of a normal functional contralateral kidney unless the patient is hemodynamically stable and warm ischemia time is less than 5 hours. Patients with unilateral injury, complete arterial thrombosis, extensive associated injuries, and a prohibitively long period of renal ischemia may be managed either by primary nephrectomy or expectant nonoperative management depending on the hemodynamic stability of the patient. There are reports of successful endovascular stenting for traumatic renal artery dissection and thrombosis in both children[134] and adults.[23,111] An attempt should be made to revascularize all patients with bilateral renal artery injury or solitary kidneys.[31,46,160] An algorithm for the management of renovascular injuries is presented in Figure 18-3.

Complications

Although most renal injuries in children can be managed nonoperatively, nonoperative management is not without complications. If a nonoperative course is chosen, the patient must be carefully monitored. Falling blood counts, ongoing transfusion requirements, and persistent gross hematuria may be indicative of ongoing bleeding. A repeat CT scan or arteriogram is warranted. An arteriogram may be especially useful since some injuries with ongoing bleeding may be amenable to selective embolization to control the bleeding. Indeed, the success of nonoperative management may be enhanced by angiographic embolization in select patients.[64] However, profuse bleeding not amenable to embolization requires emergent operative exploration.

Prolonged ileus, fevers, and expanding abdominal/flank mass or discomfort may be indicative of persistent urinary extravasation or urinoma, which is the most common complication after renal trauma. Russell and associates[171] reported that about two thirds of all urinomas in children will spontaneously resolve. Accordingly, small, noninfected, stable collections require no treatment other than observation, whereas larger, expanding collections may be managed by percutaneous drainage[171] or endoscopic placement of ureteral stents.[120,161,171] Broad-spectrum antibiotics are also administered intravenously.

Delayed renal bleeding is unusual and most commonly occurs within 2 weeks of injury. However, Teigen and coworkers[184] reported two children who developed massive life-threatening hemorrhage several weeks after the initial injury diagnosed by arteriography and successfully treated by percutaneous transcatheter embolization.

Perinephric abscesses may be associated with ileus, high fevers, and sepsis. CT is diagnostic. Most of these abscesses are successfully treated with intravenous broad-spectrum antibiotics and percutaneous drainage. Multiloculated abscesses not amenable to percutaneous drainage may require operative drainage.

Late complications may include hydronephrosis, arteriovenous fistula, pseudoaneurysm, pyelonephritis, calculus formation, and delayed renal hypertension. Posttraumatic arteriovenous fistula and pseudoaneurysm may be successfully managed by percutaneous endovascular embolization.[116,137] The incidence of renal hypertension after trauma is quite low, occurring in fewer than 5% of patients.[85,141,142,194] The incidence is thought to be even lower in children. Although hypertension usually occurs anywhere from 2 weeks to several months after injury,[85,142,194] long-term follow-up is essential because onset may be delayed up to 10 to 15 years after injury.[160]

Follow-Up/Outcomes

Evidence-based guidelines for follow-up of children after renal injury are conspicuously lacking in the literature. In a retrospective study, Abdalati and associates[1]

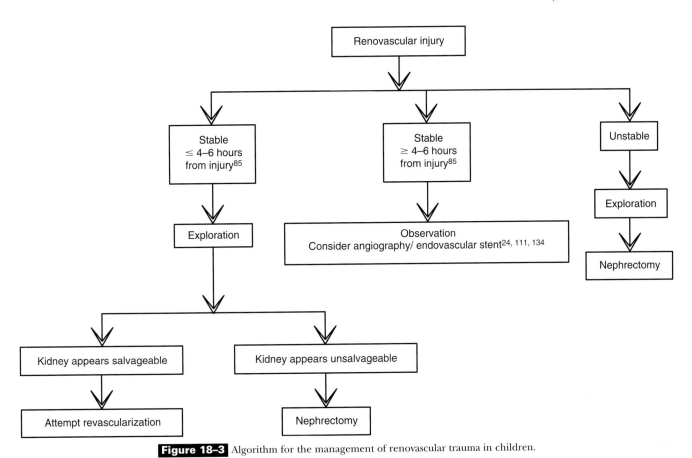

Figure 18–3 Algorithm for the management of renovascular trauma in children.

correlated initial CT grading of renal injury with frequency of complications and time course of healing in 35 patients. From this study, they concluded that grades I and II injuries healed completely and required clinical but not radiologic follow-up. Grade III injuries were associated with the highest risk of complications (30%), with healing taking up to 4 months to complete. Thus, it was recommended that grade III injuries be followed by sequential imaging with CT, scintigraphy, and/or ultrasound for 3 to 4 months until complete healing was documented. Grade IV injuries were often associated with some degree of renal loss and required radiologic follow-up to assess complications and residual renal function. Although CT provides important information regarding healing and the presence of complications, quantitative dimercaptosuccinic acid (DMSA) scintigraphy is a more useful tool to assess residual renal function after injury.[143] A study by Keller and coworkers[103] evaluated the functional outcome of non-operatively managed renal injuries in 17 children as measured by blood urea nitrogen (BUN), creatinine, blood pressure, and DMSA renal scan after radiographic evidence of complete healing. Similar to the findings of Abdalati and associates,[1] complete healing was documented radiographically within 3 months in all cases. They concluded that functional outcome correlates with injury grade, with grades II to IV injuries retaining near normal function and grade V injuries demonstrating significant loss of renal function due to scarring

and parenchymal volume loss. Despite diminished function on DMSA renal scans, all children were asymptomatic, normotensive, and had normal BUN and creatinine levels. Larger prospective clinical and radiologic outcome studies are warranted to further assess time to healing, incidence of complications, residual function, and long-term outcomes after renal trauma to provide the physician with a more evidence-based approach to appropriate follow-up and counseling for the injured child. At present, it is generally recommended that children with more severe renal injuries be followed with serial blood pressure monitoring and CT and DMSA at 3 to 6 months postinjury. Further imaging is also indicated for onset of any urologic symptoms or development of hypertension.

Operative Management of Renal Trauma

Although most cases of renal trauma in children may be successfully managed nonoperatively, the surgeon should be familiar with techniques of operative management as well. As discussed previously, operative management of renal trauma is generally reserved for hemodynamically unstable patients or those patients with severe associated injuries. The patient is usually explored through a generous midline abdominal incision. Although traditionally it has been taught that the surgeon should first gain proximal control of the renal artery and vein before entering Gerota's fascia or the hematoma in order to reduce blood loss and decrease the nephrectomy rate,[125] this approach has recently been challenged. In both retrospective studies[4,56] and a prospective, randomized clinical trial[81] it was concluded that vascular control of the renal hilum before opening Gerota's fascia has no effect on the nephrectomy rate, transfusion requirements, or blood loss but does significantly prolong operative times by up to an hour or more. The nephrectomy rate appears to depend more on the degree of injury rather than on the type of renal vascular control.[4]

No matter what the approach, the kidney is exposed and vascular control is obtained at the hilum. With exsanguinating hemorrhage, rapid mobilization of the kidney with digital control of the hilum may be necessary. The left renal vein can be ligated because collateral drainage is provided by the left adrenal and gonadal veins. However, trauma to the right renal vein requires repair. Segmental arteries may be ligated and partial nephrectomy performed if the area of infarction encompasses more than 15% of the kidney.[90] If the patient is hemodynamically stable, the kidney itself is salvageable, and the period of warm ischemia after injury is acceptable, renal artery repair and revascularization may be attempted. Otherwise, a nephrectomy should be performed.

If it appears salvageable, the damaged kidney is debrided to viable tissue and intrarenal hematomas are evacuated. Hemostasis should be obtained with absorbable sutures placed in a figure-of-eight pattern. The open collecting system should be closed with fine, absorbable, monofilament sutures, because woven sutures may cut through renal tissue.[126] Internal stents may be required if the ureter or renal pelvis has been injured.

The renal capsule should be closed to approximate the renal margins. If the capsule is destroyed, the lacerated margins should be covered with omental pedicle grafts, retroperitoneal fat, or polyglycolic acid mesh.[90,126] Approximation and covering of renal tissue aids in hemostasis and wound healing and prevents delayed bleeding and extravasation of urine.[126]

Ureter

Ureteral injury is uncommon and assumes secondary importance in children with potentially life-threatening injuries. Nonetheless, delays in diagnosis and treatment are associated with major morbidity and a significant risk for life-threatening urosepsis later during the course of injury.[14,26,76,96] Boone and colleagues[14] reported the risk for urologic complications to be 13% when blunt UPJ disruption was diagnosed within 24 hours compared with 54% with delayed diagnosis. The risk for renal loss was 4.5% to 9% with early diagnosis compared with 32% to 33% with delayed diagnosis.[14,96]

Ureteral trauma is classified by the anatomic location of the injury and by the extent of mural damage (see Table 18-1).[144] Blunt ureteral injuries are rare, occurring in less than 1% of patients with blunt abdominal trauma. Direct injuries may result from crush injuries or severe hyperextension or flexion injuries. Direct compression against a transverse process or vertebral body has been described,[199] and an association with traumatic paraplegia has been noted.[100] Patients with congenital ureteral

obstruction are also predisposed to injury of the collecting system.[89] Surgical repair is unlikely to be successful if the underlying obstruction is not recognized and treated.

Indirect mechanisms of ureteral injury in children include falls or rapid deceleration. As noted by Boone and colleagues,[14] the UPJ is particularly prone to disruption secondary to these mechanisms. Howerton and associates[96] reviewed 54 cases of ureteral avulsion within 4 cm of the UPJ and found that this type of injury was three times more common in children than in adults. Similarly, the right kidney was injured three times more often than the left.

Penetrating trauma involving the ureter occurs in approximately 4% of patients and is most often caused by a stab or gunshot wound. Although this type of injury is most commonly seen in adults, it occurs in a significant percentage of children as well.[181] In the largest series to date, Perez-Brayfield and coworkers[157] reviewed 118 patients with gunshot wounds to the ureter managed by a variety of surgical procedures, depending on the location and severity of the defect. They reported a 20% incidence of complications and concluded that a high index of suspicion is necessary to avoid missing these injuries.

Iatrogenic injuries to the ureter in children occur most commonly during ureteroscopic and percutaneous endourologic procedures. Open surgical procedures, such as those involving resection of an abdominal or pelvic tumor or colectomy, may also be associated with ureteral trauma. Radiation injury is also occasionally encountered.

The paucity of early signs and symptoms makes the nonoperative diagnosis of ureteral injuries difficult. Boone and colleagues[14] encountered gross hematuria in 27% of patients with UPJ disruption, whereas an additional 26% of patients had microscopic hematuria with shock. Absence of hematuria was noted in about one third of patients. As reviewed by Brandes and coworkers,[16] 23% to 37% of ureteral injuries reported in the literature have conspicuous absence of significant hematuria. Flank tenderness, ecchymosis, and mass effect are encountered in only approximately 7% of patients with proximal ureteral injury.[14] Patients occasionally present with anuria if the injury is bilateral or involves a solitary kidney.

Imaging modalities for diagnosis of ureteral trauma include CT and IVP. Up to 75% of ureteral injuries are missed by IVP.[16,165] Ureteral injuries may be difficult to diagnose by CT as well. With the faster helical CT scanners currently in use, it is critical to obtain delayed images during the excretory phase (2 to 10 minutes) so that ureteral extravasation is not missed. Failure of opacification of the ureter should also raise suspicion for ureteral injury.[187] Retrograde pyelography is quite sensitive and should be performed in hemodynamically stable patients suspected to have a ureteral injury.

Delayed diagnosis of ureteral injury occurs in approximately half of patients owing to the subtle nature of the clinical findings, frequent absence of hematuria, lack of sensitivity of radiologic imaging techniques, and high incidence of multisystem injury with concomitant patient instability.[14,165] Ureteral injuries may be heralded by sepsis, vascular collapse, or drainage of urine from surgical wounds. Periureteral fibrosis, phlegmon, and abscess are common. Other complications include obstruction from stenosis and renal failure.

In contrast to management of renal injuries, nonoperative management has limited application for ureteral injuries. Minor ureteral injuries with limited extravasation may be managed nonoperatively with a retrograde stent. However, most patients with ureteral injuries fare better with early operative repair. If the diagnosis is delayed significantly, temporary stenting or percutaneous nephrostomy diversion followed by interval operative reconstruction may be indicated, owing to the increased inflammation, friability, and complications associated with attempts at repair more than 3 to 5 days after injury.

The treatment of ureteral injuries is dictated primarily by the location and mechanism of injury, amount of tissue loss, and the condition of the local tissues. Ureteral injury associated with a severely damaged or shattered kidney is best managed by nephrectomy. In the absence of or with limited renal injury, attempts at primary ureteral repair should be attempted. Disruption of the UPJ is generally manageable by dismembered pyeloplasty. If damage to the renal pelvis is extensive, it should be surgically debrided and closed and ureteral continuity should be restored by ureterocalicostomy. Midureteral injuries are repaired by limited debridement to viable tissue and a spatulated end-to-end anastomosis using fine absorbable suture. Injuries to the pelvic ureter are often amenable to a simple ureteral reimplantation. Occasionally, a psoas hitch or Boari flap is required for a tension-free anastomosis.[84] Ureteral stents are used routinely.

Patients with ureteral trauma from a bullet wound require that the ureter be debrided until the edges bleed freely. Intravenous fluorescein and a Wood's lamp are occasionally useful to predict viability. Peristalsis is not a reliable sign of viability. A spatulated end-to-end anastomosis is performed, and stenting is mandatory. Unstable patients with multiple injuries are best managed by exteriorization of the transected ureter as an intubated ureterostomy or by simple ureteral ligation with intraoperative or postoperative percutaneous nephrostomy. Simple ureteral ligation is also an excellent form of management for unstable patients in whom the length of the ureteral defect precludes primary repair. Definitive reconstruction of a long ureteral defect is done on an elective basis once the patient is stable.[12,165,181] Options include renal mobilization (which can yield 3 to 5 cm),[181] the Boari flap or psoas hitch,[15] and autotransplantation.[12,193] Additionally, transureteroureterostomy and ileal interposition can be done.[181]

Delayed diagnosis associated with significant adjacent visceral injury (i.e., duodenal or pancreatic injury) may be particularly problematic. Such injuries are marginally amenable to reconstruction. Percutaneous antegrade ureteral stenting with later, elective surgical correction of stenosis or fistula, if encountered, is the preferred method of management.[186] This may also be the best approach to management of ureteral injury associated with infected urinoma, abscess, delayed diagnosis, or ureteral contusions complicated by urinary extravasation.

Bladder

Anatomy

Although the bladder in children is located in the extraperitoneal space of Retzius, it is considered an intra-abdominal organ.[53] As the bony pelvis grows, the bladder assumes a pelvic position and is increasingly protected from injury. The anatomic attachments of the bladder influence the pattern of injury seen after some forms of trauma. The bladder is bound laterally by the internal obturator muscles and the umbilical ligaments.[53] At its base the bladder is attached to the urogenital diaphragm. Denonvillier's or the rectovesical fascia binds it posteriorly. Unlike the rest of the bladder, the dome is mobile and distensible.[154]

Causes

The bladder may be injured by blunt or penetrating trauma. Although penetrating injury to the bladder can be caused by any injury to the lower abdomen, the most common cause of unintentional injury is iatrogenic.[52,62,80] Migration or erosion of drains, ventriculoperitoneal shunts, intrauterine devices, and Foley catheters are rare causes of unintentional injury to the bladder.[25,50,53,202] Intentional penetrating injuries are most commonly caused by gunshot wounds, which are usually associated with other intra-abdominal injuries.

Blunt trauma accounts for 80% of injuries to the bladder. The susceptibility of the bladder to injury is somewhat dependent on the amount of urine contained at the time of injury.[154] Motor vehicle crashes are the most common cause of blunt trauma to the bladder.[53] Pelvic fractures with sharp bony fragments may lacerate the bladder (usually near the bladder neck), and shearing forces can tear the bladder at its moorings.[53,151] A forceful, direct blow to the abdomen may rupture the dome of the bladder, even without an associated pelvic fracture.[53,180]

Because of its relatively protected position within the pelvis, considerable blunt force is required to cause bladder injury. Not surprisingly, serious injuries to other intra-abdominal organs are seen in almost half of patients with bladder injuries.[70] While 75% to 95% of bladder injuries are associated with pelvic fractures,[27,70,151,180] only 4% to 20% of patients with pelvic fractures have concomitant bladder injuries.[13,24,72,163]

Classification and Definitions

Bladder injuries due to blunt trauma may be further classified as contusions, and extraperitoneal and intraperitoneal ruptures. Extraperitoneal bladder ruptures occur in 60% to 65% of cases; intraperitoneal ruptures occur in 25% of cases; and a combination of the two occurs in 10% to 15% of cases.[95] The AAST grading scale for bladder injuries is shown in Table 18-1.

Contusions are disruptions in the bladder muscularis without loss of continuity of the bladder wall, whereas ruptures are complete disruptions of the bladder wall.[53] Contusions typically resolve without intervention.

Extraperitoneal bladder ruptures are usually associated with pelvic fractures.[42,52,54] Nineteen percent of patients (mostly male) with extraperitoneal bladder ruptures have a concomitant urethral injury, and 8% have an associated intraperitoneal injury.[53,54]

In contrast to extraperitoneal ruptures, intraperitoneal ruptures are infrequently associated with pelvic fractures (Fig. 18-4). These injuries are often caused by compression (burst-type injury) from a suprapubic blow to a distended bladder or sudden, forceful deceleration.[42,52,188] Intraperitoneal ruptures most commonly occur at the dome of the bladder, whereas extraperitoneal ruptures are usually caused by bony perforation or shearing forces.[41,55] In infants and young children, the bladder is an intraperitoneal organ, and if it is ruptured it will often cause intraperitoneal extravasation of urine.[122] Occasionally, bladder ruptures may result from an extensive hematoma of the bladder wall or, in neonates, from manipulation of an umbilical artery catheter.[20,60]

Management

Bladder Contusions

Most bladder contusions heal spontaneously without intervention. If the sacral innervation of the bladder is intact, patients with bladder contusions have excellent outcomes. Patients with a large pelvic hematoma that causes considerable bladder distortion may have difficulty voiding and may benefit from Foley catheter drainage.

Intraperitoneal Rupture

Intraperitoneal ruptures are frequently associated with other significant injuries, necessitating a thorough and deliberate evaluation of the patient. The weakest and most mobile part of the bladder, the dome, is the most common site of intraperitoneal rupture. This type of injury occurs more commonly in children.[53,122]

Intraperitoneal bladder ruptures are best managed by early operative repair. Protracted extravasation of urine into the peritoneal cavity can lead to life-threatening metabolic, septic, and mechanical derangements.[27,60,92] Patients presenting more than 24 hours after intraperitoneal rupture of the bladder may have elevated BUN, creatinine, and potassium levels; a decreased serum sodium concentration; and a laboratory profile similar to that of patients with acute renal failure.[92]

The bladder should be approached through a lower midline abdominal incision to avoid lateral contained hematoma. If necessary, the rent in the dome of the bladder can be widened to facilitate a thorough examination of the inner aspect of the bladder. Associated extraperitoneal tears can be closed from within by a single running layer of absorbable suture; however, the surgeon must ensure that the patency of the ureteral orifices is preserved. An intravenous injection of indigo carmine may help verify the location and integrity of the ureteral orifices. The dye should be seen effluxing from the ureteral orifices within 10 minutes. Lacerations extending into the bladder neck should be carefully repaired to reconstruct the sphincteric components and reduce the likelihood of later urinary incontinence. Intraperitoneal bladder injuries are repaired with absorbable suture in two layers.

After the bladder is repaired, a closed-suction drain is placed and brought out through a separate stab incision. Although in the past most surgeons would insert a large-bore suprapubic cystostomy tube instead of or in addition to a transurethral catheter for urinary drainage after repair of an intraperitoneal bladder rupture, more recent literature would suggest that transurethral catheter drainage is not only adequate, but preferable. For any degree of bladder injury, transurethral catheters are equally effective, are associated with fewer complications, and may be removed sooner than suprapubic catheters.[95,185,192]

Urinary drainage is generally maintained for 5 to 10 days. Most surgeons will obtain a cystogram before removal of the urinary drainage catheter to evaluate the integrity of the repair. If no extravasation is documented, then the urinary catheter and closed-suction drain can be removed.

Extraperitoneal Rupture

The preferred management of extraperitoneal rupture is transurethral catheter drainage alone. This approach is safe and effective and obviates the need for bladder exploration, manipulation of the extraperitoneal hematoma, and converting a closed pelvic fracture into an open one. At times, the degree of extravasation of contrast medium may be alarming. However, because it is dependent not only on the size of the tear but also on the amount of contrast medium instilled,[53,55] the degree of extravasation alone may not indicate the severity or extent of the tear in the bladder.[27,35-37,54] In most

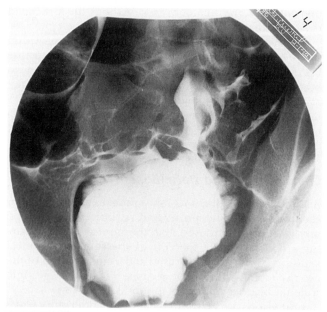

Figure 18–4 Voiding cystourethrography demonstrating intraperitoneal rupture of the bladder. The patient also had bilateral fractures of the superior ischial and inferior pubic rami.

instances, the tear heals completely and transurethral catheter drainage is successful even with extensive urinary extravasation.[41,42,55] Almost 90% of extraperitoneal bladder ruptures heal within 10 days and the remainder within 3 weeks.[55] Operative intervention is rarely required.

Penetrating Injuries

Because of the high likelihood of associated injuries, which often take priority in management, patients with penetrating injuries to the bladder generally require exploratory laparotomy. The peritoneal cavity is opened in the midline, and injuries to the intra-abdominal viscera and major vasculature are addressed first.

Attention is then directed to the bladder, and the extent of injury is determined. All devitalized bladder tissue and debris from clothing or bony spicules are removed.[27] The integrity of the ureters can be confirmed with intravenous injection of indigo carmine. A diligent search should be made for extravasation, and, if necessary, the ureters should be intubated.

Bladder mobilization is unnecessary and invites precipitous bleeding. Large, nonexpanding hematomas should be left undisturbed. The bladder should be entered through the dome. Extraperitoneal defects should be closed intravesically with a single layer of running absorbable suture. A watertight closure is ideal but not essential. With adequate bladder drainage, even a tenuous closure can heal satisfactorily. Intraperitoneal defects should be closed in two layers with absorbable suture. Closed-suction drains are placed as previously described, and transurethral catheter drainage is maintained for 5 to 10 days.

Urethra

Although urethral trauma is a secondary consideration in children with potential life-threatening trauma, such injuries account for a disproportionate degree of long-term morbidity. It remains unclear whether delayed or immediate repair is superior, and there are no prospective, randomized studies addressing the issue. The majority of the available data are based on retrospective series in adults. The only available pediatric series are limited by small numbers of patients. Data from adult studies may not be applicable to children owing to anatomic differences. For example, in contrast to adults, the posterior urethra is not protected by the prostate in children and may be injured at any level.

Blunt trauma with disruption of the bony pelvis accounts for most posterior urethral injuries in children. About 5% of males with a fractured pelvis will also have an injury to the posterior urethra.[153] Of these cases, 10% to 20% will have an associated bladder rupture.[55] Motor vehicle accidents account for 90% of urethral injuries, and the remaining 10% result from falls, crush injuries, or sporting injuries. A lateral pelvic force without pelvic fracture rarely results in urethral disruption. Penetrating injuries involving the posterior urethra including stab wounds, gunshot wounds, and iatrogenic causes are rare.

Anterior urethral injuries are often encountered after straddle injuries, such as a fall astride a fence, kicks, or bicycle injuries. Penetrating trauma to the anterior urethra is rare but may be seen with gunshot or stab wounds. Urethral instrumentation, penile surgery, and injuries from sexual intercourse and masturbation may also result in anterior urethral trauma.

The diagnosis of urethral trauma is relatively straightforward. Symptoms of urethral injury may include the inability to void or the sensation of voiding without passing urine. Blood at the urinary meatus or gross hematuria after trauma strongly suggests urethral injury. Physical examination of the penis, scrotum, and perineum may reveal swelling and ecchymosis. The integrity of and boundaries of Buck's, Colles', and Scarpa's fascias indicate the region injured. Digital rectal examination may reveal upward displacement of the prostate or a boggy mass. This, however, may be difficult to assess in young children, so urethral imaging is required to confirm the diagnosis.

If there is suspicion of a urethral injury, blind passage of a transurethral urinary catheter should not be attempted because there is a risk of creating a false passage with the catheter and converting a partial disruption into a complete one. Retrograde urethrography is the imaging modality of choice for diagnosis of urethral trauma. Findings of elongation, filling defect, or extravasation indicate urethral injury. If urethral integrity is demonstrated by retrograde urethrography, the catheter is then advanced and a cystogram is performed to exclude concomitant bladder injury.

Table 18-1 outlines the classification of urethral injuries that includes contusions, stretch injuries, partial disruptions, and complete disruptions. A filling defect caused by contusion and hematoma or an elongated urethra without extravasation on retrograde urethrography indicates grade I or II injury. Urethral extravasation with bladder continuity indicates partial disruption (grade III). Urethral extravasation with no admission of contrast agent into the proximal urethra or bladder suggests complete disruption (grade IV). Spasm of the periurethral musculature can mimic complete disruption. Figure 18-5 provides an example of injury to the bulbous urethra.

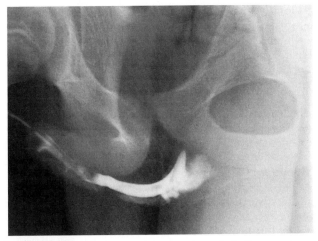

Figure 18–5 Extravasation of contrast from the bulbous urethra due to penoscrotal urethral disruption. The posterior membranous and prostatic urethra is intact.

The long-term sequelae of urethral trauma can be devastating and may include impotence, retrograde ejaculation, incontinence, and urethral strictures. Some of these complications may be a direct consequence of the trauma itself or may be related to surgical attempts at repair.

A diagnosis of anterior urethral injury is suggested if the retrograde urethrogram reveals only minimal extravasation with good urethral continuity and if the patient is able to void. Grade I or II injuries to the anterior urethra usually heal spontaneously without insertion of any indwelling urinary catheters, as long as the patient is able to void. Intermediary grade anterior urethral injuries may be managed by an indwelling transurethral Foley catheter, whereas more complex injuries are best managed in the initial stages by placement of a suprapubic catheter. Delayed urethral strictures occur commonly, and most are amenable to urethroplasty.

Penetrating injuries to the anterior urethra may be managed by exploration and primary repair or suprapubic urinary diversion. Husmann and colleagues[97] reviewed management of 17 patients with partial transection of the anterior urethra due to low-velocity gunshot wounds and concluded that patients were best managed by aggressive wound debridement, corporeal repair, primary suture repair of the urethra, and placement of a suprapubic catheter. Strictures developed much less frequently with this approach (1 of 8) compared with suprapubic diversion and transurethral catheter stenting (7 of 9).

In children, the majority of posterior urethral injuries may be managed nonoperatively. Grade I or II injuries, which may allow spontaneous voiding, are managed without surgery and without an indwelling urinary catheter. Patients who are unable to void are managed by insertion of a small, transurethral Foley catheter. Grade III injuries with minimal extravasation may also be managed by passing a small, transurethral Foley catheter under fluoroscopic guidance immediately after the retrograde urethrogram. If the catheter does not pass easily, however, a suprapubic tube should be placed.

Options for repair of more complex posterior urethral injuries include primary surgical repair with anastomosis of the disrupted urethral ends, delayed primary surgical repair, primary surgical catheter realignment, primary endoscopic and radiologic realignment, or suprapubic cystostomy with delayed urethroplasty.

Primary surgical repair involves evacuation of the pelvic hematoma, mobilization of the prostate and urethra, and direct end-to-end anastomosis between the prostatic and membranous urethra. Problems with this approach include increased risk of uncontrolled bleeding due to exploration of the injury site with release of the tamponade effect of the hematoma; increased risk of impotence due to dissection of the periprostatic and periurethral tissues; and increased risk of incontinence due to damage to the intrinsic urethral sphincter mechanism by dissection, mobilization, and debridement of torn urethral ends.[51,53,56,57,108,195] To minimize these complications, Mundy[150] advocated delaying primary surgical repair

until 7 to 10 days after injury once the patient was more stable, the operative view was less obscured by bleeding, and before the onset of fibrosis.

Primary surgical catheter realignment was first introduced by Ormond and Cothran in 1934 with multiple variations in technique over the ensuing years.[59,66,73,107] Despite not requiring direct suturing of the disrupted urethral ends, this technique still requires an open procedure with entry into and evacuation of pelvic hematoma with all of the attendant risks of primary surgical repair. More recently, innovative combined transurethral and transvesical endoscopic and interventional radiologic techniques have been introduced to achieve primary alignment without the risk of exploring the disrupted urethra.[47,49,74,77,115,132,164,169] Furthermore, because there is no manipulation of periprostatic tissues and no additional trauma to the cavernous nerves, there should be no additional risk of erectile dysfunction other than that caused by the injury itself. These minimally invasive techniques have produced encouraging results so far, but clinical experience is limited to small series. Postoperative outcomes of these small series indicate that 88% to 100% of patients are continent, 14% to 39% of patients have some degree of erectile dysfunction, and about half require subsequent internal urethrotomies.

Concerns about the impact of primary open surgical repair or catheter realignment on potency and urinary continence led to the introduction of an alternative treatment approach, namely suprapubic cystostomy with delayed urethroplasty. First advocated by Johanson of Sweden in 1953, no attempt is made to explore the urethra but rather the urinary stream is simply diverted via a suprapubic cystostomy tube. A stricture is considered inevitable and is repaired several months later. This approach has gained widespread acceptance and is considered a standard approach to the management of complex posterior urethral disruptions. Advantages of this approach include avoiding entry into a fresh pelvic hematoma with risk of blood loss and infection, speed and simplicity of suprapubic tube insertion, and decreased incidence of impotence and incontinence due to avoidance of dissection of the prostate and urethra.[73] Disadvantages include prolonged need for a suprapubic tube with risk of infection and stone formation as well as the nearly 100% risk for urethral strictures, which may be quite complex and difficult to repair even in the delayed setting.[107] Tunc and colleagues[189] reviewed 77 cases of delayed repair of traumatic posterior urethral injuries and demonstrated adequate urethral continuity in 95%, postoperative incontinence in 9%, and postoperative erectile dysfunction in 16%. They concluded that delayed posterior urethroplasty is a successful treatment option with acceptable morbidity.

After extensive literature review regarding different approaches to management of complex posterior urethral injuries, Holevar and associates[95] concluded that these injuries may be treated with either primary endoscopic realignment or suprapubic cystostomy with delayed urethroplasty with similar results.

Urethral trauma in females is rare.[32,162] The usual mechanism of injury involves pelvic fracture incurred during a motor vehicle accident. Straddle injury occasionally results in damage to the urethra. Female urethral injuries may be distal avulsion from the perineal attachment or proximal disruptions and lacerations. The latter type of injury is characteristically associated with other pelvic injuries, including vaginal and bladder neck lacerations.

Perry and colleagues[159] reviewed the evaluation of urethral injuries in females with pelvic fractures. Blood at the vaginal introitus mandates a meticulous vaginal examination. The urinary meatus must also be carefully examined and its patency confirmed by passage of a catheter. However, it is important to note that catheters can often be passed into the bladder even in the presence of a significant urethral injury. Development of vulval edema after removal of the catheter warrants prompt investigation. Because urethrography in young girls is difficult and unreliable, urethroscopy is the preferred diagnostic modality. Delays in diagnosis of urethral injury in girls occur frequently and have devastating consequences.[159] Such injury is misdiagnosed in about 50% of cases and can result in life-threatening sepsis and necrotizing fasciitis. Therefore, one should have a low threshold for performing urethroscopy when urethral injury is suspected in a young girl.

Treatment is dictated by the extent and location of injury. Urethral injuries that extend into the bladder neck require meticulous repair with reapproximation of the bladder outlet and urethra. Such injuries are encountered about two thirds of the time.[121,122,126,129] Associated vaginal injuries are repaired primarily. Urethral crush injuries that do not involve the bladder neck are managed by extended transurethral Foley catheterization (6 to 8 weeks) or, if necessary, suprapubic catheter drainage. Significant long-term complications associated with pediatric female urethral trauma are common and include urethral stenosis, urethrovaginal fistula, incontinence, and vaginal stenosis.[63]

Clearly every effort must be made to promptly detect and aggressively manage this uncommon injury.

External Genitalia

Girls

Blunt genital trauma in girls is fairly common. The presenting symptoms are usually the presence of blood in the underpants or on the perineum shortly after injury.[117] Blunt genital trauma most commonly results from straddle injury. The most common types of injury, in decreasing order of frequency, are lacerations or contusions of the perineal body, vagina, labia, urethra, and rectum. Due to the extreme difficulty of performing a thorough genitourinary examination in an awake, uncomfortable, anxious, and embarrassed child, the majority of patients are best evaluated in the operating room under general anesthesia. Indeed, as many as 76% of patients will have more extensive injuries than can be appreciated in the emergency department.[117]

Management of female genital trauma is dictated by the type and extent of injury. Necrotic, contused tissue should be debrided. Lacerations are primarily repaired after hemostasis is achieved. Absorbable sutures are used to preclude the need for removal. Urethroscopy and proctoscopy may be necessary to more thoroughly evaluate the injury.

Boys

The most common injury to the penis is iatrogenic injury during circumcision.[80] Complications of circumcision include penile amputation, urethral fistulization, laceration of the glans penis, and inaccurate removal of the foreskin resulting in phimosis degloving injury. Most of these injuries are avoidable with use of proper technique.

Penile injury resulting from blunt or penetrating trauma is rare in children. Urethral lacerations should be managed as described in the previous section. The findings of an expanding hematoma, palpable corporal defect, and excessive bleeding suggest cavernosal injuries. When possible, these injuries should be repaired primarily.[17] Urinary diversion with a suprapubic tube is occasionally necessary.[79] The preferred method of management of gunshot wounds with a limited extent of injury is debridement of superficial wounds, repair of the cavernosal defects, and primary repair of the urethral injury.[87]

Penile erectile dysfunction (impotence) can occur after blunt pelvic and perineal trauma.[149] The dysfunction results from shearing of the penile blood vessels in the pelvis. Penile revascularization may restore potency.[119] Priapism may also occur after blunt trauma. For this disorder, selective angiography is helpful to diagnose the injury and to embolize the arteriovenous fistula causing the priapism. Doppler ultrasonography is also useful to characterize and localize the lesion.[138]

Injury resulting from zipper entrapment of the penis can be addressed, in many cases, in the emergency department but may require a general anesthetic for release of the penis.[200] Penile strangulation injuries due to constricting bands are managed by removal of the constricting band in as atraumatic a manner as possible. In children, hair tourniquets are common sources of constriction and may be quite difficult to remove. Severe strangulation injuries may result in necrosis of the distal penile skin, glans, cavernosum, or urethra. Conservative debridement and urinary diversion may be required.[48]

Scrotal injuries may result from penetrating trauma, blunt trauma, or both. High-resolution ultrasonography is very useful in the evaluation of these injuries.[10] Ultrasonography of penetrating injuries can identify testicular rupture and extratesticular soft tissue abnormalities as well as the presence and location of foreign bodies.[110] This technique is also useful in distinguishing less serious injuries, such as scrotal hematomas, hydroceles, and hematoceles, from surgical emergencies, such as testicular rupture and infarction. It should be noted that epididymal rupture is not as easily identified on ultrasonography.[155] Patients with hematoceles should be considered for exploration to evacuate the blood from the tunica vaginalis testis because this approach reduces morbidity and hastens recovery. Testicular disruption is managed by debridement and primary closure.[5]

REFERENCES

1. Abdalati H, Bulas K, Sivit C, et al: Blunt renal trauma in children: Healing of renal injuries and recommendations for imaging follow-up. Pediatr Radiol 1994;24:573.

2. Ahmed S, Morris LL: Renal parenchymal injuries secondary to blunt abdominal trauma in childhood: A 10-year review. Br J Urol 1982;54:470.

3. Aihara R, Blansfield JS, Milham FH, et al: Fracture locations influence the likelihood of rectal and lower urinary tract injuries in patients sustaining pelvic fractures. J Trauma 2002;52:205.

4. Altala A, Miller FB, Richardson JD, et al: Preliminary vascular control for renal trauma. Surg Gynecol Obstet 1991; 173:386.

5. Altarac S: Management of 53 cases of testicular trauma. Eur Urol 1994;25:119.

6. Altman AL, Haas C, Dinchman KH, et al: Selective non-operative management of blunt grade 5 renal injury. J Urol 2000;164:27-30.

7. Bass DH, Semple PL, Cywes S: Investigation and management of blunt renal injuries in children: A review of 11 years' experience. J Pediatr Surg 1991;26:196.

8. Baumann L, Greenfield, Aker J, et al: Nonoperative management of major blunt renal trauma in children: In-hospital morbidity and long-term followup. J Urol 1992;148:691.

9. Beaver BL, Colombani PM, Fal A, et al: The efficacy of computed tomography in evaluating abdominal injuries in children with major head trauma. J Pediatr Surg 1987; 22:1117.

10. Berman JM, Beidle TR, Kunberger LE, Letourneau JG: Sonographic evaluation of acute intrascrotal pathology. AJR Am J Roentgenol 1996;166:857.

11. Bertini JE Jr, Flechner SM, Miller P, et al: The natural history of trauma branch renal artery injury. J Urol 1986; 135:228.

12. Bodie B, Novick AC, Rose M, Strafton RA: Long-term results with renal autotransplantation for ureteral replacement. J Urol 1986;136:1187.

13. Bond SJ, Gotschall CS, Eichelberger MR: Predictors of abdominal injury in children with pelvic fracture. J Trauma 1991;31:1169.

14. Boone TB, Gilling PJ, Husmann DA: Ureteropelvic junction disruption following blunt abdominal trauma. J Urol 1993; 150:33.

15. Bracken RB, Sheldon CA: Psoas hitch, Boari flap and transureteroureterostomy. In Fowler JE Jr (ed): Mastery of Surgery: Urologic. Boston, Little, Brown, 1992.

16. Brandes SB, Chelsky MJ, Buckman RF, Hanno PM: Ureteral injuries from penetrating trauma. J Trauma 1994;36:766.

17. Brandes SB, Buckman RF, Chelsky MJ, Hanno PM: External genitalia gunshot wounds: A ten-year experience with 56 cases. J Trauma 1995;39:266.

18. Bretan APN Jr, McAninch JW, Federle MP, et al: Computerized tomographic staging of renal trauma: 85 consecutive cases. J Urol 1986;136:561.

19. Brower P, Paul J, Brosman SA: Urinary tract abnormalities presenting as a result of blunt abdominal trauma. J Trauma 1978;18:719.

20. Brown D, Maghill HL, Block DL: Delayed presentation of traumatic intraperitoneal bladder rupture. Pediatr Radiol 1986;16:253.

21. Brown SL, Elder JS, Spirnak JP: Are pediatric patients more susceptible to major renal injury from blunt trauma? A comparative study. J Urol 1998;160:138.

22. Brown SL, Haas C, Dinchman KH, et al: Radiologic evaluation of pediatric blunt renal trauma in patients with microscopic hematuria. World J Surg 2001;25:1557.

23. Bruce LM, Croce MA, Santaniello JM, et al: Blunt renal artery injury: Incidence, diagnosis, and management. Am Surg 2001;67:550.

24. Burgess AR, Eastridge BJ, Young JW, et al: Pelvic ring disruption: Effective classification systems and treatment protocols. J Trauma 1990;30:848.

25. Burnett DG: Near bladder perforation in urethra-catheter extrusion: An unusual complication of cerebrospinal fluid-peritoneal shunting. J Urol 1982;127:543.

26. Campbell EW, Filderman PS, Jacobs SC: Ureteral injury due to blunt and penetrating trauma. Urology 1992;40:216.

27. Carroll PR, McAninch JW: Major bladder trauma: Mechanism of injury and a unified method of diagnosis and repair. J Urol 1984;132:254, 1984.

28. Carroll PR, McAninch JW: Operative indications in penetrating renal trauma. J Trauma 1985;25:587, 1985.

29. Carroll PR, McAninch JW: Current management of blunt renal trauma. Urol Ann 1987;1:171.

30. Carroll PR, McAninch JW: Staging renal trauma. Urol Clin North Am 1989;16:193.

31. Carroll PR, et al: Renovascular trauma: Risk assessment, surgical management, and outcome. J Trauma 1990;20:547.

32. Carter CT, Schafer N: Incidence of urethral disruption in females with traumatic pelvic fractures. Am J Emerg Med 1993;11:218.

33. Cass AS, Susset J, Khan A, et al: Renal pedicle injury in the multiple injured patient. J Urol 1979;122:728.

34. Cass AS: Immediate radiological evaluation and early surgical management of genitourinary injuries from external trauma. J Urol 1979;122:772.

35. Cass AS: Immediate surgical management of severe renal injuries in multiple injured patients. Urology 1983;21:140.

36. Cass AS: Renal trauma in the multiple-injured child. Urology 1983;21:487.

37. Cass AS: Blunt renal pelvic and ureteral injury in multiple-injured patients. Urology 1983;22:268.

38. Cass AS: Blunt renal trauma in children. J Trauma 1983; 23:123.

39. Cass AS, Bubrick M, Luxenberg M, et al: Renal pedicle injury in patients with multiple injuries. J Trauma 1985; 23:892.

40. Cass AS, Luxenberg M, Gleich P, et al: Clinical indications for radiographic evaluation of blunt renal trauma. J Urol 1986;136:370.

41. Cass AS, Luxenberg M: Features of 164 bladder ruptures. J Urol 1987;138:743.

42. Cass AS: Diagnostic studies and bladder rupture: Indications and techniques. Urol Clin North Am 1989;16:267.

43. Ceylan H, Gunsar C, Etensel B, et al: Blunt renal injuries in Turkish children: A review of 205 cases. Pediatr Surg Int 2003;19:710.

44. Chandhoke PJ, McAninch JW: Detection and significance of microscopic hematuria in patients with blunt renal trauma. J Urol 1988;140:16.

45. Chopra P, St-Vil D, Yazbeck S: Blunt renal trauma—blessing in disguise? J Pediatr Surg 2002;37:779.

46. Clark DE, Georgitis JW, Ray RS: Renal arterial injuries caused by blunt trauma. Surgery 1981;90:87.

47. Clark WR, Patterson DE, Williams HJ Jr: Primary radiologic realignment following posterior urethral disruption. Urology 1992;39:182.

48. Coburn M: Genitourinary trauma. In Moore E, Feliciano DV, Mattox KL (eds): Trauma, 5th ed. New York, McGraw-Hill, 2004.

49. Cohen JK, Berg G, Carl GH, et al: Primary endoscopic realignment following posterior urethral disruption. J Urol 1991;146:1548.

50. Cohen MS, et al: Bladder perforation after orthopedic hip surgery. Urology 1977;9:291.

51. Coffield KS, Weems WL: Experience with management of posterior urethral injury associated with pelvic fracture. J Urol 1977;117:722.

52. Corriere JN Jr, Sandler CM: Management of the ruptured bladder: Seven years experience with 111 cases. J Trauma 1986;26:830.

53. Corriere JN Jr: Trauma to the lower urinary tract. In Gillenwater JY, et al (eds): Adult and Pediatric Urology. Chicago, Year Book Medical, 1987.

54. Corriere JN Jr, Sandler CM: Mechanisms of injury patterns of extravasation and management of extraperitoneal bladder rupture due to blunt trauma. J Urol 1988;139:43.

55. Corriere JN Jr, Sandler CM: Management of extraperitoneal bladder rupture. Urol Clin North Am 1989;16:275.

56. Corriere JN Jr, McAndrew JD, Benson GS: Intraoperative decision making in renal trauma surgery. J Trauma 1991;31:1390.

57. Crassweller PO, Farrow GA, Robson CJ, et al: Traumatic rupture of the supramembranous urethra. J Urol 1977;118:770.

58. Daum GS, Krolikowski FJ, Reuter KL, et al: Dipstick evaluation of hematuria in abdominal trauma. Am J Clin Pathol 1988;89:538.

59. DeWeerd JH: Immediate realignment of posterior urethral injury. Urol Clin North Am 1977;4:75.

60. Diamond DA, Ford C: Neonatal bladder rupture: A complication of umbilical artery catheterization. J Urol 1989;142:1543.

61. Dinkel HP, Danuser H, Triller J: Blunt renal trauma: Minimally invasive management with microcatheter embolization experience in nine patients. Radiology 2002;223:723.

62. Dmochowski R, Crondell SS, Corriere JN Jr: Bladder injury in uroascites from umbilical artery catheterization. Pediatrics 1986;77:421.

63. Dorai CDRT, Boucaut HAP, Dewan PA: Urethral injuries in girls with pelvic trauma. Eur Urol 1993;24:371.

64. Eastham JA, Wilson TG, Larsen DW, et al: Angiographic embolization of renal stab wounds. J Urol 1992;148:268.

65. Eastham JA, Wilson TG, Ahlering TE: Urological evaluation and management of renal-proximity stab wounds. J Urol 1993;150:1771.

66. Elliott DS, Barrett DM: Long-term follow-up and evaluation of primary realignment of posterior urethral disruptions. J Urol 1997;157:814.

67. Esho JO, Ireland GW, Cass AS: Renal trauma and preexisting lesions of kidney. Urology 1973;1:134.

68. Fairhurst JJ, Rubin CM, Hyde I, et al: Bladder capacity in infants. J Pediatr Surg 1991;26:55.

69. Fay R, Brosman S, Lindstrom R, Cohen A: Renal artery thrombosis: A successful revascularization by autotransplantation. J Urol 1974;111:572.

70. Flancbaum L, Morgan AS, Fleisher M, et al: Blunt bladder trauma: Manifestation of severe injury. Urology 1988;31:220.

71. Fleisher G: Prospective evaluation of selective criteria for imaging among children with suspected blunt renal trauma. Pediatr Emerg Care 1989;5:8.

72. Flint L, Babikan G, Anders M, et al: Definitive control of mortality from severe pelvic fracture. Ann Surg 1990;211:703.

73. Follis HW, Koch MO, McDougal WS: Immediate management of prostatomembranous urethral disruptions. J Urol 1992;147:1259.

74. Gelbard MK, Heyman AM, Weintraub P: A technique for immediate realignment and catheterization of the disrupted prostatomembranous urethra. J Urol 1989;142:52.

75. Gerstenbluth RE, Spirnak JP, Elder JS: Sports participation and high grade renal injuries in children. J Urol 2002;168:2575.

76. Ghali AM, El Malik EM, Ibrahim AI, et al: Ureteric injuries: Diagnosis, management, and outcome. J Trauma 1999;46:150.

77. Gheiler EL, Frontera JR: Immediate primary realignment of prostatomembranous urethral disruptions using endourologic techniques. Urology 1997;49:596.

78. Gill B, Palmer L, Reda E, et al: Optimal renal preservation with timely percutaneous intervention: A changing concept in the management of blunt renal trauma in children in the 1990s. Br J Urol 1994;74:370.

79. Gomez RG, Castanheira AC, McAninch JW: Gunshot wounds to the male external genitalia. J Urol 1993;150:1147.

80. Gonzales ET Jr, Guerriero WG: Genitourinary trauma in children. In Kelalis PP, King LR, Bellman AB (eds): Clinical Pediatric Urology. Philadelphia, WB Saunders, 1985.

81. Gonzales RP, Falimirski M, Holevar MR, et al: Surgical management of renal trauma: Is vascular control necessary? J Trauma 1999;47:1039.

82. Guerriero WG, Carlton SE Jr, Scott R Jr, et al: Renal pedicle injuries. J Trauma 1971;1:53.

83. Guerriero WG: Penetrating renal injuries in the management of renal pedicle injury. Urol Clin North Am 1977;4:3.

84. Guerriero WG: Ureteral injury. Urol Clin North Am 1989;16:237.

85. Haas CA, Dinchman KH, Nasrallah PF, et al: Traumatic renal artery occlusion: A 15 year review. J Trauma 1998;45:557.

86. Haas CA, Brown SL, Spirnak JP: Limitations of routine spiral computerized tomography in the evaluation of bladder trauma. J Urol 1999;162:51.

87. Hall SJ, Wagner JR, Edelstein RA, et al: Management of gunshot wounds to the penis and anterior urethra. J Trauma 1995;38:439.

88. Haller JA Jr, Papa P, Drugas G, Colombani P: Nonoperative management of solid organ injuries in children. Is it safe? Ann Surg 1994;219:625.

89. Hardeman S, Husmann DA, Chinn HK, et al: Blunt urinary tract trauma: Identifying those patients who require radiological studies. J Urol 1989;141:1095.

90. Herschorn S, Kodona RT, Abara EO: Genitourinary trauma. In McMurtry R, McMillan GA (eds): Management of Blunt Trauma. Baltimore, Williams & Wilkins, 1990.

91. Herschorn S, Raadomski SB, Shoskes DA, et al: Evaluation and treatment of blunt renal trauma. J Urol 1991;146:274.

92. Heyns CF, Rimington PD: Intraperitoneal rupture of the bladder causing the biochemical features of renal failure. Br J Urol 1987;60:217.

93. Heyns CF, Van Vollenhoven P: Increasing role of angiography and segmental artery embolization in the management of renal stab wounds. J Urol 1992;147:1231.

94. Holcroft HW, Trunkey DD, Minagi H, et al: Renal trauma and retroperitoneal hematomas: Indications for exploration. J Trauma 1975;15:1045.

95. Holevar M, Ebert J, Luchette F, et al: Practice management guidelines for the management of genitourinary trauma. On Internet site for Eastern Association for the Surgery of Trauma, Copyright 2004.

96. Howerton RA: Proximal ureteral avulsion from blunt abdominal trauma. Milit Med 1991;156:311.

97. Husmann DA, Boone TB, Wilson WT: Management of low velocity gunshot wounds to the anterior urethra: The role of primary repair versus urinary diversion alone. J Urol 1993;150:70.

98. Husmann DA, Gilling PJ, Perry MO, et al: Major renal lacerations with a devitalized fragment following blunt abdominal trauma: A comparison between nonoperative (expectant) versus surgical management. J Urol 1993; 150:1774.

99. Ivatury RR, Zubowski R, Stahl WM: Penetrating renovascular trauma. J Trauma 1989;29:1620.

100. Javadpour N, Guinan P, Bush IM: Renal trauma in children. Surg Gynecol Obstet 1973;136:237.

101. Jetvich MJ, Montero GG: Injuries to renal vessels by blunt trauma in children. J Urol 1969;102:493.

102. Karp MP, Jewett TC Jr, Kuhn JP, et al: The impact of computed tomography scanning on the child with renal trauma. J Pediatr Surg 1986;21:617.

103. Keller MS, Eric Coln C, Garza JJ, et al: Functional outcome of nonoperatively managed renal injuries in children. J Trauma 2004;57:108-110.

104. Knudson MM, McAninch JW, Gomez R, et al: Hematuria as a predictor of abdominal injury after blunt trauma. Am J Surg 1992;164:482.

105. Knudson MM, Harrison PB, Hoyt DB, et al: Outcome after major renovascular injuries: A Western Trauma Association multicenter report. J Trauma 2000;49:1116.

106. Koff SA: Estimating bladder capacity in children. Urology 1983;21:248.

107. Koraitim MM: Pelvic fracture urethral injuries: Evaluation of various methods of management. J Urol 1996;156:1288.

108. Koraitim MM: Pelvic fracture urethral injuries: The unresolved controversy. J Urol 1999;161:1433.

109. Kuszmarov IW, Morehouse DD, Gibson S: Blunt renal trauma in the pediatric population: A retrospective study. J Urol 1981;126:648.

110. Learch TJ, Hansch LP, Ralls PW: Sonography in patients with gunshot wounds of the scrotum: Imaging findings and their value. AJR Am J Roentgenol 1995;165:879.

111. Lee JT, White RA: Endovascular management of blunt traumatic renal artery dissection. J Endovasc Ther 2002; 9:354.

112. Levy JB, Baskin LS, Ewalt DH, et al: Nonoperative management of blunt pediatric major renal trauma. Urology 1993;42:418.

113. Lis LE, Cohen AJ: CT cystography in the evaluation of bladder trauma. J Comput Assist Tomogr 1990;14:386.

114. Livene PM, Gonzales ET: Genitourinary trauma in children. Urol Clin North Am 1985;12:53.

115. Londergan TA, Gundersen LH, Van Every MJ: Early fluoroscopic realignment for traumatic urethral injuries. Urology 1997;49:101.

116. Lupattelli T, Garaci FG, Manenti G, et al: Giant high-flow renal arteriovenous fistula treated by percutaneous embolization. Urology 2003;61:837.

117. Lynch JM, Gardner MJ, Albanese CT: Blunt urogenital trauma in prepubescent female patients: More than meets the eye. Pediatr Emerg Care 1995;11:372.

118. Margenthaler JA, Weber TR, Keller MS: Blunt renal trauma in children: Experience with conservative management at a pediatric trauma center. J Trauma 2002; 52:928.

119. Matthews LA, Herbener TE, Seftel AD: Impotence associated with blunt pelvic and perineal trauma: Penile revascularization as a treatment option. Semin Urol 1995; 13:66.

120. Matthews LA, Smith EM, Spirnak JP: Nonoperative treatment of major blunt renal lacerations with urinary extravasation. J Urol 1997;157:2056.

121. McAleer IM, Kaplan G, Sherz HC, et al: Genitourinary trauma in the pediatric patient. Urology 1993;42:563.

122. McAleer IM, Kaplan GW: Pediatric genitourinary trauma. Urol Clin North Am 1995;22:177.

123. McAleer IM, Kaplan GW, LoSasso BE: Congenital urinary tract anomalies in pediatric renal trauma patients. J Urol 2002;168:1808.

124. McAleer IM, Kaplan GW, LoSasso BE: Renal and testis injuries in team sports. J Urol 2002;168:1805.

125. McAninch JW, Carroll PR: Renal trauma: Kidney preservation through improved vascular control—A refined approach. J Trauma 1984;22:285.

126. McAninch JW: Genitourinary trauma. In Moore EE, Mattox KL, Feliciano DV (eds): Trauma. East Norwalk, CT, Appleton & Lange, 1991.

127. McAninch JW, Carroll P, Klosterman P, et al: Renal reconstruction after injury. J Urol 1991;145:932.

128. McAninch JW, Carroll PR, Armenkas NA, et al: Renal gunshot wounds: Methods of salvage and reconstruction. J Trauma 1993;35:279.

129. McAninch JW, Morey AF, Bruce JE: Efficacy of radiographic imaging in pediatric blunt renal trauma. Proc Am Urol Assoc Suppl 1996;155:526A.

130. Medica J, Caldamone A: Pediatric renal trauma: Special considerations. Semin Urol 1995;13:73.

131. Mee SL, McAninch JW, Rovinson AL, et al: Radiographic assessment of renal trauma: A 10-year prospective study of patient selection. J Urol 1989;141:1095.

132. Melekos MD, Pantazakos A, Daouaher H, et al: Primary endourologic re-establishment of urethral continuity after disruption of the prostatomembranous urethra. Urology 1992;39:135.

133. Mercader VP, Gatenby RA, Curtis BR: Radiographic assessment of genitourinary trauma. Trauma 1996;13:129.

134. Merrott T, Portier F, Galinier P, et al: Trauma of the renal pedicle in children: Report of 2 cases of late revascularization with endovascular prosthesis. Prog Urol 2000; 10:277.

135. Mertz JHO, Wishard WN JR, Nourse MH, et al: Injury to the kidney in children. JAMA 1963;183:830.

136. Miller SF, Chait PG, Burrows PE, et al: Post-traumatic arterial priapism in children: Management with embolization. Radiology 1995;196:59.

137. Miller DC, Forauer A, Faerber GJ: Successful angioembolization of renal artery pseudoaneurysms after blunt abdominal trauma. Urology 2002;59:444.

138. Miller KS, McAninch JW: Radiographic assessment of renal trauma: Our 15-year experience. J Urol 1995;154:352.

139. Monstrey SJ, vander Staak FH, vander Werken C, et al: Urinary tract injuries in children: Are they different from adults? Z Kinderchir 1988;43:31.

140. Monstrey SJ, vanderWerken C, Debruyne FM, et al: Rational guidelines in renal trauma assessment. Urology 1988;31:469.

141. Monstrey SJ, Beerthuizen GI, vander Werken C, et al: Renal trauma and hypertension. J Trauma 1989;29:65.

142. Montgomery RC, Richardson JD, Harty JI: Post-traumatic renovascular hypertension after occult renal injury. J Trauma 1998;45:106.

143. Moog R, Becmeur F, Dutson E: Functional evaluation by quantitative dimercaptosuccinic acid scintigraphy after kidney trauma in children. J Urol 2003;169:641.

144. Moore EE, Shackford SR, Pachter HL, et al: Organ injury scaling: Spleen, liver, and kidney. J Trauma 1989; 29:1664.

145. Morey AF, Bruce JE, McAninch JW: Efficacy of radiographic imaging in pediatric blunt renal trauma. J Urol 1996;156:2014.

146. Morse TS, Smith JP, Howard WHR, et al: Kidney injuries in children. J Urol 1967;98:539.

147. Morton JR, Crawford ES: Bilateral traumatic renal artery thrombosis. Ann Surg 1972;176:62.

148. Moudounie SM, Patard JJ, Manunta P, et al: A conservative approach to blunt renal lacerations with urinary extravasation and devitalized renal segments. Br J Urol 2001;87:290.

149. Munarriz RM, Yan OR, Znehra A, et al: Blunt trauma: The pathophysiology of the hemodynamic injury. J Urol 1995;153:1831.

150. Mundy AR: The role of delayed primary repair in the acute management of pelvic fracture injuries of the urethra. Br J Urol 1991;68:273.

151. Murphy JP: Genitourinary trauma. In Ashcraft KW (ed): Pediatric Urology. Philadelphia, WB Saunders, 1990.

152. Nicolaisen GS, McAninch JW, Marshall GA, et al: Renal trauma: Re-evaluation of the indications for radiographic assessment. J Urol 1985;133:183.

153. Noe HN, Jerkins GR: Genitourinary trauma. In Kelalis PP, Kemp LR, Belman AB (eds): Clinical Pediatric Urology. Philadelphia, WB Saunders, 1992.

154. Oliver JA, Taguchi Y: Rupture of the full bladder. Br J Urol 1964;36:524.

155. Patil MG, Onuora VC: The value of ultrasound in the evaluation of patients with blunt scrotal trauma. Injury 1994;25:177.

156. Peng MY, Parisky YR, Cornwell EE, et al: CT cystography versus conventional cystography in evaluation of bladder injury. AJR Am J Roentgenol 1999;173:1269.

157. Perez-Brayfield MR: Gunshot wounds to the ureter: A 40 year experience at Grady Memorial Hospital. J Urol 2001;166:119.

158. Perez-Brayfield MR, Gatti JM, Smith EA, et al: Blunt traumatic hematuria in children: Is a simplified algorithm justified? J Urol 2002;167:2543.

159. Perry MO, Husmann DA: Urethral injuries in female subjects following pelvic fractures. J Urol 1992;147:139.

160. Peterson NE: Review article: Traumatic bilateral renal infarction. J Trauma 1989;29:158.

161. Philpott JM, Nance ML, Carr MC, et al: Ureteral stenting in the management of urinoma after severe blunt renal trauma in children. J Pediatr Surg 2003;38:1096.

162. Pode D, Shapiro A: Traumatic avulsion of the female urethra: Case report. J Trauma 1990;30:235.

163. Poole GV, Ward EF, Griswold JA, et al: Complications of pelvic fractures from blunt trauma. Ann Surg 1992;58:225.

164. Porter JR, Takayama TK, Defalco AJ: Traumatic posterior urethral injury and early realignment using magnetic urethral catheters. J Urol 1997;158:425.

165. Presti JC, Carroll PR, McAninch JW: Ureteral and pelvic injuries from external trauma: Diagnosis and management. J Trauma 1989;29:370.

166. Pumberger W, Stoll E, Metz S: Ureteropelvic junction disruption following blunt abdominal trauma. Pediatr Emerg Care 2002;18:364.

167. Quinlan DM, Gearhart JP: Blunt renal trauma in childhood. Features indicating severe injury. Br J Urol 1990; 66:526.

168. Radmayr C, Oswald J, Muller E, et al: Blunt renal trauma in children: 26 years clinical experience in an alpine region. Eur Urol 2002;42:297.

169. Rehman J, Samadi D, Ricciardi R Jr, et al: Early endoscopic realignment as primary therapy for complete posterior urethral disruptions. J Endourol 1998;12:283.

170. Rober PE, Smith JB, Pierce JM: Gunshot injuries of the ureter. J Trauma 1990;30:83.

171. Russell TS, Gomelsky A, McMahon DR, et al: Management of grade IV renal injury in children. J Urol 2001;66:1049.

172. Sagalowsky AI, McConnell JD, Peters PC: Renal trauma requiring surgery: An analysis of 185 cases. J Trauma 23:128, 1983.

173. Santucci RA, McAninch JW, Safir M, et al: Validation of the American Association for the Surgery of Trauma organ injury severity scale for the kidney. J Trauma 2001; 50:195.

174. Santucci RA, Langenburg SE, Zachareas MJ: Traumatic hematuria in children can be evaluated as in adults. J Urol 2004;171:822.

175. Sharp DS, Ross JH, Kay R: Attitudes of pediatric urologists regarding sports participation in children with a solitary kidney. J Urol 2002;168:1811.

176. Shuman WP: CT of blunt abdominal trauma in adults. Radiology 1997;205:297.

177. Skinner D: Traumatic renal artery thrombosis: A successful thrombectomy and revascularization. Ann Surg 1973; 172:264.

178. Sklar DP, Diven B, Jones J: Incidence and magnitude of catheter-induced hematuria. Am J Emerg Med 1986; 4:14.

179. Smith EM, Elder JS, Spirnak JP: Major blunt renal trauma in the pediatric population: Is a nonoperative approach indicated? J Urol 1993;149:546.

180. Snyder H, Caldamone AA: Genitourinary injuries. In Welch KJ, Randolph JG, Ravitch MM (eds): Pediatric Surgery, 4th ed. Chicago, Mosby Year Book, 1986.

181. Spirnak JP, Persky L, Resnick MI: The management of civilian ureteral gunshot wounds: A review of 18 patients. J Urol 1985;134:733.

182. Stalker HP, Kaufman RA, Stedje K: The significance of hematuria in children after blunt abdominal trauma. AJR Am J Roentgenol 1990;154:569.

183. Stein JP, Kaji DM, Eastham J, et al: Blunt renal trauma in the pediatric population: Indications for radiographic evaluation. Urology 1994;44:406.

184. Teigen CL, Venbrux AC, Quinlan DM, Jeffs RD: Late massive hematuria as a complication of conservative management of blunt renal trauma in children. J Urol 1992;147:1333.

185. Thomae KR, Kilambi NK, Poole GV: Method of urinary diversion in nonurethral traumatic bladder injuries. Retrospective analysis of 70 cases. Am Surg 1998;64:77-80.

186. Toporoff B, Sclafani S, Scalea T, et al: Percutaneous antegrade ureteral stenting as an adjunct for treatment of complicated ureteral injuries. J Trauma 1992;32:534.

187. Townsend M, DeFalco AJ: Absence of ureteral opacification below ureteral disruption: A sentinel CT finding. AJR Am J Roentgenol 1995;164:253.

188. Tso EL, Beaver BL, Haller JJ Jr: Abdominal injuries in the restrained pediatric passenger. J Pediatr Surg 1993; 28:915.

189. Tunc HM, Tefekli AH, Kaplancan T, et al: Delayed repair of post-traumatic posterior urethral distraction injuries: Long-term results. Urology 2000;55:837.

190. Turner WW Jr, Snyder WH III, Fry WJ: Mortality and renal salvage after renovascular trauma: A review of 94 patients treated in a 20 year period. Am J Surg 1983;146:848.

191. Velmahos GC, Degiannis E: The management of urinary tract injuries after gunshot wounds of the anterior and posterior abdomen. Injury 1997;28:535.

192. Volpe MA, Pachter EM, Scalea TM, et al: Is there a difference in outcome when treating traumatic intraperitoneal bladder rupture with or without a suprapubic tube? J Urol 1999;161:1103.

193. Wazzan W, Azoury B, Heinady K, et al: Missile injuries of the upper ureter treated by delayed renal autotransplantation and ureteropyelostomy. Urology 1993;42:725.

194. Weaver FA, Kuehne JP, Papanicolau G: A recent institutional experience with renovascular hypertension. Am Surg 1996;62:241.

195. Weems WL: Management of genitourinary injuries in patients with pelvic fractures. Ann Surg 1979;189:717.

196. Werkman HA, Jansen C, Klein JP, et al: Urinary tract injuries in multiply-injured patients: A rational guideline for the initial assessment. Injury 22:471, 1991.

197. Wessel LM, Scholz S, Jester I, et al: Management of kidney injuries in children with blunt abdominal trauma. J Pediatr Surg 2000;35:1326.

198. Wessells H, McAninch JW, Meyer A, et al: Criteria for non-operative treatment of significant penetrating renal lacerations. J Urol 157:24, 1997.

199. Whitesides E, Kozlowdki DL: Ureteral injury from blunt abdominal trauma: Case report. J Trauma 1994;36:745.

200. Wyatt JB, Scobie WG: The management of penile zipper entrapment in children. Injury 1994;25:59.

201. Yale-Loehr AJ, Kramer SS, Quinlan DM, et al: CT of severe renal trauma in children: Evaluation and course of healing with conservative therapy. AJR Am J Roentgenol 1989; 152:109.

202. Zakin D: Perforation of the bladder by the intrauterine device. Obstet Gynecol Surv 1984;39:59.

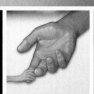

Chapter 19

Musculoskeletal Trauma

Richard S. Davidson and Michelle S. Caird

Musculoskeletal trauma is the most common medical emergency in children. The number of cases continues to increase in association with the popularity of motor vehicles, all-terrain vehicles, and power lawn mowers. In a child with multiple injuries, optimal treatment requires a cooperating team of medical professionals with diverse specialties who understand the priorities of each team member. As in all other pediatric specialties, it is important to remember that children are not "little adults." Priority management need not compromise complete patient management.

This chapter reviews the important differences between the musculoskeletal systems of children and adults, and it highlights the principles of evaluation and management in children with musculoskeletal injuries. The treatment of high-priority musculoskeletal injuries is specifically discussed, including open fractures, compartment syndrome, femoral neck fractures, mangled extremities, spine trauma, and suspected child abuse. For details on the management of specific musculoskeletal fractures and injuries of childhood, readers should refer to textbooks on children's fractures.[16,25,27]

MUSCULOSKELETAL SYSTEMS OF CHILDREN AND ADULTS

Differences in the musculoskeletal anatomy and biomechanics of children and adults determine the unique patterns of musculoskeletal injury seen in childhood. Injuries to growing bones are a double-edged sword: they can have a remarkable capacity for healing and remodeling, but they are also subject to the problems of overgrowth and growth disturbance, which can have lifelong consequences.

Anatomy

The major anatomic distinctions of skeletally immature bones are the physis and the periosteum. Each long bone in a child contains the epiphysis, physis, metaphysis, and diaphysis (Fig. 19-1). The epiphysis is the area beyond the physis, or primary growth plate, which contains the articular cartilage. The secondary center of ossification arises within the epiphysis and progressively enlarges as the cartilage ossifies during skeletal maturation. The physis provides longitudinal growth and converts the newly formed cartilage into bone in the metaphysis. The diaphysis, or shaft, is surrounded by periosteum, which generates new bone and provides circumferential bone growth. By adulthood, the growth plate closes, and there is limited potential for remodeling.

Biomechanics

Skeletally immature bones are porous, less brittle, and better able to tolerate deformation than are mature bones. Pores stop the progression of a fracture line but weaken the bone under a compressive force. As a result, a greater variety of fractures is seen in children than in adults. A child's bone can bend without fracture (Fig. 19-2); it can buckle under compression; it can fracture like a "green stick," with an incomplete crack on the tension side and a bend on the compression side; and it can fracture completely.

The thick periosteum that surrounds the diaphysis of the bone can minimize or prevent displacement of diaphyseal fractures. The periosteum tears on the tension side of a fracture but often remains intact on the compression side. The intact periosteum can then function as a hinge or a spring, increasing deformity. Depending on the injury, the periosteum may simplify or complicate reduction of a fracture (Fig. 19-3).

In the complex of bone, ligaments, and cartilage in a child, the physis is the weakest part and therefore is the most likely site of failure. An angular force to a joint in a young child is most likely to cause a fracture along the growth plate, whereas in an adolescent or an adult, a ligamentous injury or dislocation would occur. Frankel and Nordin[15] provide extensive information on the biomechanics of bone. In a fall on an outstretched hand, a young child is unlikely to sprain a wrist; more commonly, a child sustains a fracture with a displaced distal radius growth plate. Similarly, instead of spraining an ankle, a child is more likely to sustain a physeal fracture of the distal fibula. Under low-energy forces, these injuries are unlikely to lead to growth disturbance.

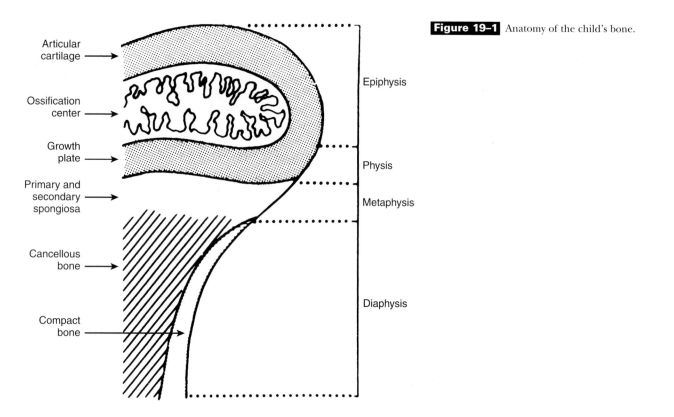

Figure 19-1 Anatomy of the child's bone.

The Salter-Harris classification system of fractures involving the physis can guide proper management (Fig. 19-4).[28] Type 1 fractures extend along the entire physis. Type 2 fractures involve part of the growth plate and part of the metaphysis; these fractures are seldom associated with growth arrest except when they occur in the distal femur

Bend

Buckle

Greenstick

Complete

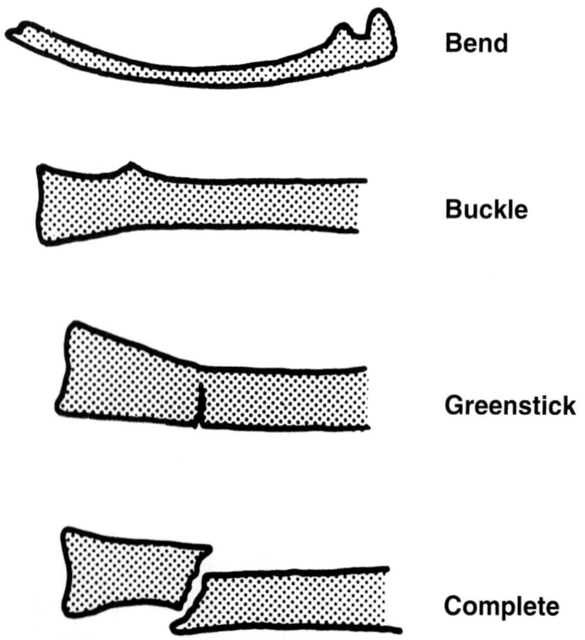

Figure 19-2 Fracture types in children. (From Rang M: Children's Fractures. Philadelphia, JB Lippincott, 1974.)

and proximal tibia. Type 3 fractures involve part of the physis and pass across the epiphysis into the joint. Because of the possibility of incongruity of the joint, type 3 fractures often require open reduction and fixation. Type 4 fractures occur longitudinally, crossing the physis from the metaphysis into the epiphysis. This type of fracture is commonly associated with subsequent formation of a bony bar across the physis, which causes partial growth arrest with subsequent angulation. Open reduction and internal fixation are usually required for type 4 fractures, because joint incongruity and fusion across the physis are common. Type 5 fractures are diagnosed retrospectively, when all or part of the physis fails to grow. It is hypothesized that injury to the physis results from direct compression or local vascular insult. Growth disturbance may result in loss of longitudinal growth or angular deformities. Damage to the physis in high-energy injuries can lead to asymmetrical growth in any of the fracture types.

Physiology

The physiologic differences between the musculoskeletal systems of children and adults are found in healing and remodeling. Growing bones are also at risk for the unique problems of overgrowth and growth disturbance.

Healing in children is rapid and age dependent. A newborn may achieve clinically stable union of a fracture in 1 week, whereas a similar fracture in an adolescent may take 6 weeks to heal. In children, the rapid healing process partially results from the thick periosteum, which may form its own bone bridge. Except for displaced

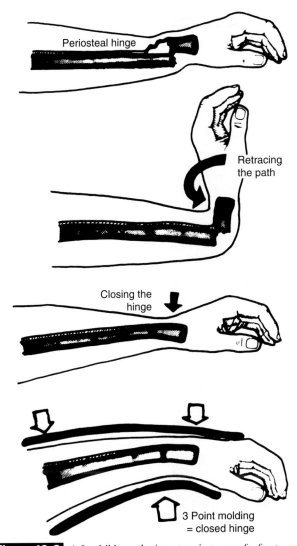

Periosteal hinge

Retracing
the path

Closing the
hinge

3 Point molding
= closed hinge

Figure 19–3 *A,* In children, the intact periosteum of a fracture prevents reduction by traction. *B,* By retracing the path of injury, the fracture can be reduced. *C,* Closing the hinge. *D,* A cast with three-point molding holds the hinge closed and keeps the fracture reduced. (From Rang M: *Children's Fractures.* Philadelphia, JB Lippincott, 1974.)

intra-articular fractures or fractures with gross soft tissue interposition, nonunion of fractures is rare in children.

The bones of children have great potential for remodeling, but the limitations must be understood. Remodeling potential is better in younger patients, in deformities closer to the physes, and where angulation is in the plane of motion of the nearest joint. Remodeling does not effectively correct angulation perpendicular to joint motion or rotation. These deformities should be reduced before healing begins (Fig. 19-5).

Growth stimulation may follow fractures of long bones. This can be especially apparent in the lower extremity. The inequality in leg length that results from such stimulation is less important in children younger than 2 years and in adolescents. For children of other ages, an average 1-cm increase can be expected in femur fractures.[11,29,32] Although discrepancies in leg length are unpredictable, it is often possible to reduce the ultimate inequality by allowing the fracture to heal with a 1-cm overlap in an otherwise anatomic alignment. Most of the growth stimulation occurs within the first year after injury, so follow-up visits for 1 year are recommended, even after uneventful healing.

Damage to the physis can produce severe shortening, angular deformity, or both. Although this may be caused by the initial trauma, it can also result from failure to obtain anatomic reduction of a physeal fracture or from repeated or overzealous attempts at reduction (Fig. 19-6). When major (>2 cm) limb length discrepancies in the lower extremities are evident, treatment depends on the amount of remaining skeletal growth and the projected difference in limb lengths. Treatment may involve timed ablation of the growth plate on the normal limb, shortening osteotomy of the normal limb, or lengthening of the short limb. Angular deformities can also be addressed, taking into consideration the patient's skeletal age and the severity of the deformity.

EVALUATION OF MUSCULOSKELETAL INJURIES

Clinical Assessment

The initial assessment of children with multiple injuries may be difficult. Details of the incident may be missing, and the patient's history may be incomplete. The Advanced Trauma Life Support (ATLS) system of assessment involves a primary evaluation to identify and immediately address life-threatening injuries, followed by a secondary

Figure 19–4 Salter-Harris classification of epiphyseal fractures. Type 1 involves the entire physis. Type 2 involves part of the growth plate and part of the metaphysis. Type 3 involves part of the physis and passes across the epiphysis into the joint. Type 4 is longitudinal, crossing the physis from the metaphysis into the epiphysis. Type 5 is diagnosed retrospectively when the physis fails to grow. See text for clinical implications of each fracture type.

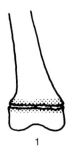
1

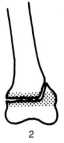
2

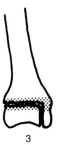
3

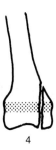
4

5

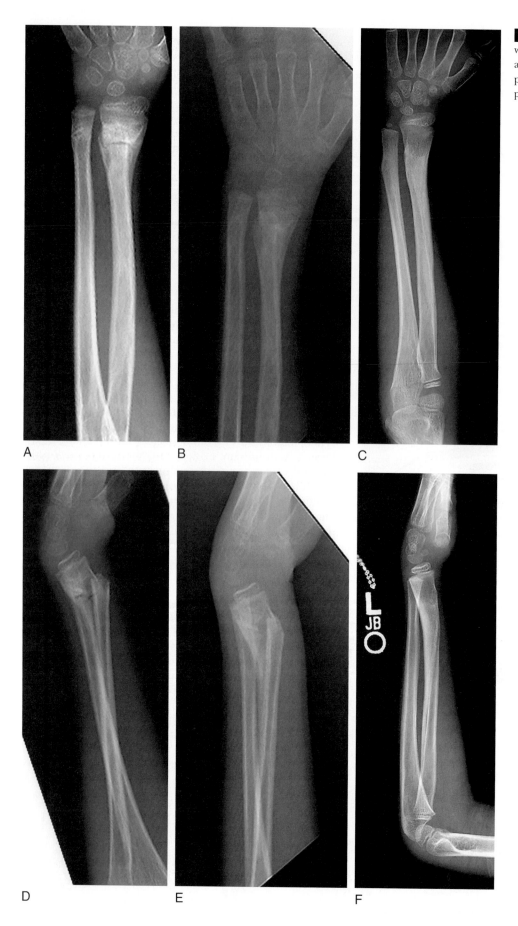

A

B

C

D

E

F

Figure 19–5 Seven-year-old boy with eight degrees of remodeling of a forearm fracture over a 9-month period. *A* to *C*, Anteroposterior plane. *D* to *F*, Lateral plane.

Figure 19-6 Anteroposterior radiograph of the knees in a 13-year-old boy shows growth disturbance of the left distal femoral growth plate after a fracture (on right in photo).

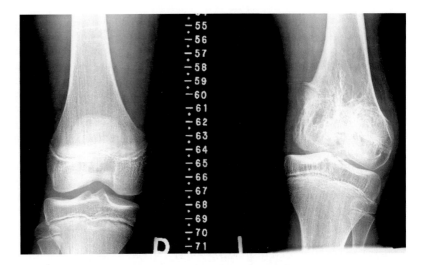

evaluation to find and treat other significant injuries. The injuries identified in the secondary evaluation must also be treated in a timely manner to prevent devastating lifelong consequences. Postponing the management of serious musculoskeletal injury for an extended period can be associated with a poor prognosis for return to normal function.

The musculoskeletal examination begins with observation of the patient for sites of deformity, swelling, contusions, abnormal color, and open fractures. If a fracture is suspected, confirmatory diagnostic studies may be integrated into the complete physical examination. If such studies cannot be done, it must be assumed that a fracture exists, and the suspected site must be splinted until the fracture is confirmed or ruled out. Splinting may also reduce discomfort and limit further damage to soft tissue. A complete neurovascular examination is essential in any case of suspected limb or spine injury. When an uncooperative patient will not allow an adequate physical examination or, in the case of comatose patients or preverbal

children, cannot provide a history, judicial use of special diagnostic studies can be critical.

Radiographic Assessment

Plain radiography is the first and most widely used test to identify skeletal injury in children, but it can also be a major source of misdiagnosis in this age group. Cartilage, which makes up a large percentage of the child's skeleton, is radiolucent but can fracture. Ossification centers appear at different ages in different locations. The timing of their appearance and their location vary greatly and can suggest fractures. Confusion most frequently occurs in the elbow, knee, and cervical spine. Comparison of the injured and uninjured limbs can be useful. Plain radiographic soft tissue signs, such as the posterior fat pad sign in elbow injuries, are associated with a high likelihood of underlying fracture (Fig. 19-7).[30]

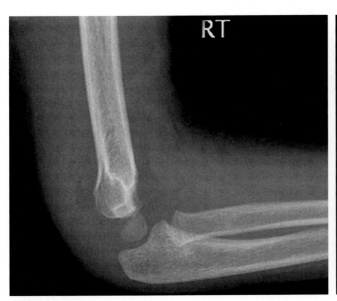

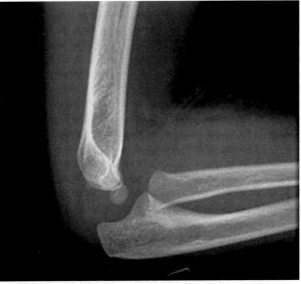

A   B

Figure 19-7 Lateral elbow radiographs of a 2-year-old boy with a mildly displaced supracondylar humerus fracture and posterior fat pad sign (A) and a normal age-matched elbow (B).

A number of imaging studies are available for the assessment of pediatric musculoskeletal injuries and are injury and age specific. Radiographs may confirm fractures. Ultrasonography is a readily available, noninvasive imaging test that can be used to evaluate the unossified epiphysis, especially in injuries about the elbow.[8] Magnetic resonance imaging (MRI) may also be helpful, especially in evaluating the injured spine, but it may require general anesthesia in a young or uncooperative patient. Computed tomography (CT) scanning is useful in periarticular fractures in children approaching skeletal maturity. For example, ankle physeal fractures in children with partially closed physes are best delineated with CT scan.[22] Arteriography may be required to assess vascular injury associated with a fracture. Rarely, proximal tibial physeal fractures and distal humerus fractures through the supracondylar region can be associated with disruption of the blood supply to the distal limb. These injuries require emergent treatment, and an intraoperative arteriogram may also be needed. Joint aspiration can identify blood and fat, which indicate an intra-articular fracture that would not be identified on radiographs. Finally, arthrography and arthroscopy may define intra-articular injury to the cartilage and ligaments.

MANAGEMENT OF MUSCULOSKELETAL INJURIES

Immediate Treatment

Priority treatment cannot interfere with complete treatment of an injured child. Proper timing and coordination of management with other disciplines are imperative. Traction or splinting often adequately stabilizes the musculoskeletal injury until other tests and treatments have been completed. Immobilization may also reduce the need for pain medications, which can mask the symptoms of other disorders, such as intra-abdominal injuries, and inhibit diagnosis.

Although there are many types of splints, ranging from plaster to traction bows, the basic principles of fracture management remain the same. The injured part should be splinted as it is found, and the joints above and below the injury should be immobilized without compromising the circulation of the soft tissues. Portable traction splints or custom-molded, well-padded plaster or fiberglass splints can be used in the initial management of fractures. Failure to immobilize the fracture can cause further soft tissue damage from sharp bone ends, crushing of entrapped neurovascular elements, or reopening of clotted vessels.

Definitive Fracture Management

Adequate stabilization of fracture fragments prevents further soft tissue injury, frequently decreases pain, and facilitates wound care and patient mobilization. Techniques of definitive stabilization in children include splinting, casting, skeletal traction, external fixation, pinning, flexible intramedullary nailing, and plating.

The choice of fixation method depends on the child's age, the location of the fracture, the presence and extent of soft tissue injury, and the presence of multitrauma.

Metaphyseal undisplaced or impacted fractures are likely to heal faster than diaphyseal or displaced fractures. Fractures with devitalized bone or soft tissues take longer to heal. Radiographic evaluation in conjunction with clinical judgment and experience is needed when determining the healing time of fractures in children.

Fragments of bone must be held together until they are sufficiently strong to withstand the forces specific to the bone. A satisfactory position must be obtained, without harming adjacent tissue, before the fracture becomes fixed. Fractures in newborns and infants begin to heal within a few days, but fractures in adolescents can be moved freely for 10 to 14 days. Excessive cast padding, resolution of swelling, or a poorly applied cast may permit progressive malposition within the cast. Fractures should be followed with frequent radiographs until union is secure, to avoid displacement. Unstable fractures should be imaged before consolidation to evaluate for loss of alignment. This allows for easy repeat reduction.

In children, the thick periosteum tears on the tension side of a fracture but often remains intact on the compression side. The intact periosteum can then function as a hinge, increasing the success of closed reduction of displaced fractures by three-point molding (see Fig. 19-3). Reduction must be performed gently. Forceful and repeated manipulation of physeal fractures can produce iatrogenic damage and growth disturbances. Entrapment of soft tissue occasionally prevents reduction of an otherwise stable fracture (Fig. 19-8) and requires open reduction and immobilization in a cast.

In some cases, internal fixation with crossed pins, plates and screws, intramedullary nails, or external fixation with pins in metal outriggers or rods may be useful (Fig. 19-9). The benefits of each of these devices must be weighed against the future need for operative removal and the possible disturbance to the growth plate. Specific indications for internal and external fixation may include fractures with significant soft tissue injury, fractures in

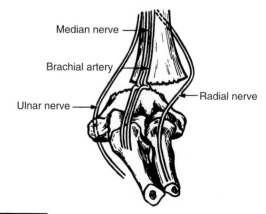

Figure 19–8 Supracondylar elbow fracture. Soft tissue may become entrapped between bone fragments in these types of fractures.

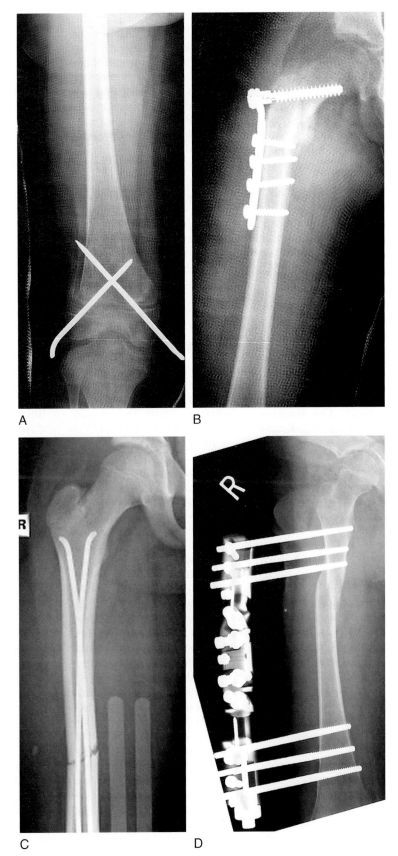

Figure 19–9 Anteroposterior radiographs of right femur fractures fixed with a variety of fixation methods. *A*, Salter-Harris type 2 fracture with crossed pins in a 9-year-old girl. *B*, Intertrochanteric fracture with screws and side plate in a 7-year-old boy. *C*, Transverse shaft fracture with elastic intramedullary nails in a 13-year-old boy. *D*, Subtrochanteric fracture with external fixator in an 8-year-old boy.

children with closed head injury, those associated with neurovascular injury, and fractures that fail nonoperative treatment. Comminuted and oblique fractures and those with complete tears of the periosteum may be too unstable for cast immobilization. In cases of intra-articular fractures, such as Salter-Harris types 3 and 4, open reduction and internal fixation are frequently necessary to avoid incongruity of the joint or growth disturbances. Fractures associated with neurovascular injury requiring repair should be stabilized first.

HIGH-PRIORITY MUSCULOSKELETAL INJURIES

Although many musculoskeletal injuries in children can be treated on an urgent rather than an emergent basis, the discussion of some high-priority musculoskeletal injuries in children is warranted. Even in nonurgent cases, it is important to remember that injuries to growing bones can have lifelong consequences.

Open Fractures and Traumatic Arthrotomies

Open fractures are true orthopedic emergencies because a delay in treatment can lessen the chance of saving the limb. These injuries frequently result from high-energy trauma. The fractures communicate with the outside environment and are at increased risk for infection. The cornerstones of management include recognition, administration of appropriate antibiotics, stabilization of the fracture, and prompt irrigation and adequate debridement of wounds. Open fractures may require multiple surgical procedures to achieve adequate soft tissue coverage and fracture healing.

When a laceration or abrasion is noted in proximity to a fracture, an open fracture must be suspected. Radiographic evidence of air shadows around the fracture may confirm the diagnosis. A sharp fragment of bone can tear through the skin, and the elastic properties of a child's bone can readily straighten the fracture fragments after the force is discontinued. The protruding point of bone can then draw back under the skin, taking debris and bacteria with it into the deep tissues. Minimal signs of injury do not necessarily mean a minimal chance of infection. Wounds should not be probed in the emergency department, where the risk of iatrogenic contamination is high and the likelihood of adequate debridement is low; if necessary, such procedures should be done in the operating room.

The Gustilo system classifies open fractures according to the size and extent of soft tissue damage.[17] Type I is an open fracture with a clean wound smaller than 1 cm. Type II is an open fracture with a laceration longer than 1 cm without extensive soft tissue damage, flaps, or avulsions. Type III is an open fracture with extensive soft tissue injury and is further divided into three subtypes; type IIIA has adequate soft tissue coverage of a fractured bone despite extensive laceration of soft tissue, type IIIB involves extensive soft tissue injury with periosteal stripping that requires grafting or a flap for coverage, and type IIIC is an open fracture associated with arterial injury that requires repair. The risk of infection is related to the severity of the injury: 2% in type I open fractures, 2% to 10% in type II open fractures, and up to 50% in type III open fractures.[17]

Wounds should initially be dressed with sterile gauze soaked with antiseptic. Hemorrhage should be controlled by direct pressure. Patients should receive tetanus prophylaxis and antibiotics at recognition of the injury. First-generation cephalosporins cover the gram-positive organisms found in type I and type II injuries. An aminoglycoside is added for type III injuries, and ampicillin or penicillin is added for farm injuries to fight potential anaerobic infection.

Each wound must be adequately debrided and copiously irrigated with the patient under general anesthesia. Wounds may need to be re-evaluated after 2 or more days for additional debridement. Primary closure or delayed primary closure may be appropriate for some open fractures, whereas grafting or flap coverage is needed for larger soft tissue defects. The goal of debridement is removal of devitalized tissue to avoid the catastrophic consequences of an infection, which may include limb loss or chronic osteomyelitis. Adequate immobilization is necessary for soft tissue healing. For small lacerations, immobilization in a cast that has been windowed for wound inspection may suffice. For larger lacerations, external fixation is often necessary to provide stable fixation with access to the wound.

Joint penetration by a foreign body can cause a diagnostic dilemma. Radiographs can be helpful if they reveal an "air arthrogram." Injection of sterile normal saline into the joint can also be diagnostic. If the liquid exits the wound or laceration, joint penetration has occurred and requires irrigation and debridement in the operating room.

Compartment Syndrome

Compartment syndrome occurs when pressure is elevated within a confined fascial space. This causes circulatory compromise and can progress to tissue necrosis. Closed fractures and crush injuries with associated edema may cause compartment syndrome. Forearm and leg compartments are most often involved. Ischemic injury starts when tissue pressure is 30 mm Hg below mean arterial pressure.[20] The pressure within the compartments surrounding a fracture should be measured if compartment syndrome is suspected. Commercially available tissue pressure monitors or other measuring devices, including electronic arterial pressure monitoring devices, can be used.

The diagnosis of compartment syndrome in children can be difficult. Adults with compartment syndrome verbalize extreme pain and demonstrate pain with passive stretch of the muscles within the affected compartments, whereas children often have difficulty communicating their discomfort. The classic signs of compartment syndrome are the five Ps—pain, pallor, paresthesia, paralysis, and pulselessness. These signs are rather unreliable in children and may manifest late in the process. An increasing analgesia requirement is an important sign of compartment syndrome in children.[2]

With early recognition and timely management, full recovery can be achieved. All external compression is removed from the limb, compartment pressures are measured, and, if elevated, the compartments are surgically decompressed. In the forearm, volar and dorsal fasciotomies are required. In the leg, all four compartments (anterior, lateral, deep posterior, and superficial posterior) must be released. This can be accomplished with two incisions. Without prompt intervention, the result is irreversible damage to soft tissues with loss of function, subsequent contractures, and deformity.[34]

Femoral Neck Fracture

Although rare in children, fractures of the femoral neck and intertrochanteric region require attention (Fig. 19-10). These fractures frequently result from high-energy impact, including traffic accidents and falls from a height,[6] and are associated with a high complication rate from avascular necrosis, coxa vara, nonunion, delayed union, and premature physeal closure.[4,9] The upper end of the femur lies within the joint capsule. After roughly 4 years of age, blood is supplied primarily by retinacular vessels that course from distal in the neck to proximal in the head. Delay in treatment of a fracture at the neck is associated with increased risk of avascular necrosis of the head and destruction of the joint and can cause lifelong disability. Early decompression of the hip joint, reduction of the fracture, and internal fixation can minimize the complications.[6]

Mangled Extremities

Severely traumatized or mangled extremities in children must be assessed and treated through a multidisciplinary approach on a case-by-case basis. They may involve extensive injury to or segmental loss of skin, muscle, bone, and neurovascular structures. Some limbs may be unsalvageable owing to extensive damage, some can be reconstructed with a resulting dysfunctional limb, and others can be salvaged with a good outcome. The Mangled Extremity Severity Score rates injuries based on objective criteria at initial presentation, including skeletal and soft tissue injury, limb ischemia, shock, and patient age. Although originally developed in a primarily adult population,[18] it can be a useful adjunct to managing lower extremity trauma in children.[12]

Segmental bone loss is rare in children and does not necessitate amputation. If periosteum can be preserved, the potential to reform bone is extensive. Proper techniques of debridement and stabilization, along with adequate time, may produce good results in children. External fixation techniques can allow for bone transport and osteogenesis to replace lost bone and axial deformity.

Power lawn mower injuries are uncommon, preventable injuries that cause significant morbidity in children.[10,13,23] Direct contact with the blade leads to laceration of tissue, amputation, or devitalizing shredding of the extremity. Such injury can result in damage to the vasculature and growth plate, joint stiffness, infection, or amputation. If salvage is undertaken, treatment follows that of open fractures.

In the case of amputation, preservation of bony length and retention of all viable soft tissue are important for the ultimate functional outcome. Amputation through the diaphysis of a child's bone frequently results in overgrowth of the bony stump through the skin. This is especially true of the fibula, tibia, and humerus and can necessitate cutting back the bone every few years.

Spine Trauma

Injuries of the spine in children can be divided into those affecting the cervical spine and those in the thoracic and lumbar spine (see also Chapter 21). Just as in other parts

Figure 19–10 Anteroposterior pelvis radiograph of a 14-year-old boy shows a left femoral neck fracture that required internal fixation.

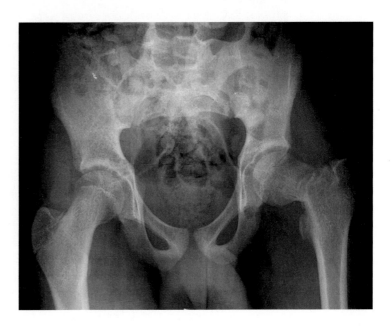

or

Figure 19–11 A pediatric backboard should have a torso mattress or an occiput recess to accommodate the child's relatively large head and avoid potentially dangerous cervical spine flexion.

of the body, patterns of injury to the spine in children differ from those in adults. Radiographic imaging can be challenging. Principles of immobilization are different for children as well.

Cervical spine injuries in children differ from those in adults.[7] Children have greater ligamentous laxity and weaker neck musculature. In addition, they have large heads relative to body size; this effect is more pronounced in younger children. Cervical spine injuries in children tend to occur higher in the neck and can be primarily ligamentous or apophyseal without bony fracture.[19] When immobilizing a child on a backboard, the relatively large head should be considered; a child's backboard splint should have a recess for the occiput or a mattress for the torso to maintain the alignment of the cervical spine, avoiding flexion of the neck (Fig. 19-11).[21]

Radiographic evaluation of the pediatric cervical spine can be challenging. Pseudosubluxation, or the apparent forward displacement of C2 on C3 and, less commonly, C3 on C4, is a well-described plain radiographic finding in normal children younger than 8 years.[5] Other sources

of difficulty in interpreting radiographs include incomplete ossification, epiphyseal variation, and elasticity of the disks and vertebral bodies relative to the neural structures, which allows extensive injury to the soft tissues without evidence of abnormality on plain radiographs or SCIWORA (spinal cord injury without radiographic abnormality). MRI is helpful in evaluating soft tissues in cases of possible cervical spine ligamentous injury in children.[14]

Injuries to the thoracic and lumbar spine are rare in children. The growth of vertebral bodies occurs through the apophyses or growth centers on the cranial and caudal ends of the bodies. With compression injury, adolescents are at risk for traumatic displacement of the vertebral apophysis and the attached disk into the spinal canal, especially in the lumbar region.[33] Symptoms are similar to those seen in central disk herniation, including muscle weakness and absent reflexes. This injury requires recognition and emergent surgical decompression.

Lap-belt injuries occur in children when they violently flex over the seat belt and the posterior spine is distracted.[31] A fracture propagates from the posterior portions of the vertebra to the disks or vertebral body in the front (Fig. 19-12). In addition to the vertebral injury, children can sustain abdominal and aortic injuries. Such injuries should be suspected when an abdominal contusion, or the telltale seat-belt sign, is evident in a trauma patient. These injuries require immobilization and possible internal fixation if the injury is ligamentous.

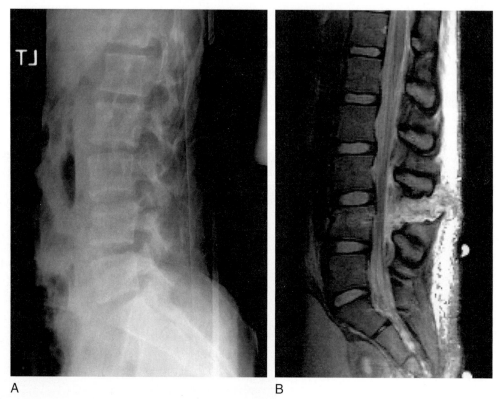

A   B

Figure 19–12 Lap-belt injury of L4 in a 15-year-old girl without neurologic injury. *A,* Lateral lumbar spine radiograph shows fracture of both the L4 body and the posterior spine. *B,* Sagittal magnetic resonance image of the lumbar spine shows the extensive bony and soft tissue injury.

Child Abuse

The maltreatment of children is a complex medical and social problem, and its recognition is key to management (see also Chapter 24). Fractures before walking age in the absence of metabolic disease or child abuse are rare. Fractures are the second most common manifestation of child abuse after skin lesions.[24] Suspicion of abuse must be raised when there is a discrepancy between history and injury, when multiple fractures are present in different stages of healing, or when bruising, metaphyseal fractures, or long bone fractures appear in children younger than 1 year.[3,26] No social stratum is free of this problem.

REFERENCES

1. Akbarnia B, Torg JS, Kirkpatrick J: Manifestations of the battered child syndrome. J Bone Joint Surg Am 1974; 56:1159.
2. Bae DS, Kadiyala RK, Waters PM: Acute compartment syndrome in children: Contemporary diagnosis, treatment, and outcome. J Pediatr Orthop 2001;21:680.
3. Blakemore LC, Loder RT, Hensinger RN: Role of intentional abuse in children 1 to 5 years old with isolated femoral shaft fractures. J Pediatr Orthop 1996;16:585.
4. Canale ST, Bourland WL: Fracture of the neck and intertrochanteric region of the femur in children. J Bone Joint Surg Am 1977;59:431.
5. Cattell HS, Filtzer DL: Pseudosubluxation and other normal variations in the cervical spine in children. J Bone Joint Surg Am 1965;47:1295.
6. Cheng JCY, Tang N: Decompression and stable internal fixation of femoral neck fractures in children can affect the outcome. J Pediatr Orthop 1999;19:338.
7. Copley LA, Dormans JP: Cervical spine disorders in infants and children. J Am Acad Orthop Surg 1998;6:204.
8. Davidson RS, Markowitz RI, Dormans JP, et al: Ultrasonographic evaluation of the elbow in infants and young children after suspected trauma. J Bone Joint Surg Am 1994;76:1804.
9. Davison BL, Weinstein SL: Hip fractures in children: A long-term follow-up study. J Pediatr Orthop 1992;12:355.
10. Dormans JP, Azzoni M, Davidson RS, et al: Major lower extremity lawn mower injuries in children. J Pediatr Orthop 1995;15:78.
11. Edvardsen P, Syversen SM: Overgrowth of the femur after fracture of the shaft in childhood. J Bone Joint Surg Br 1976;58:339.
12. Fagelman MF, Epps HR, Rang M: Mangled extremity severity score in children. J Pediatr Orthop 2002;22:182.
13. Farley FA, Senunas L, Freenfield ML, et al: Lower extremity lawn-mower injuries in children. J Pediatr Orthop 1996;19:669.
14. Flynn JM, Closkey RF, Mahboubi S, et al: Role of magnetic resonance imaging in the assessment of pediatric cervical spine injuries. J Pediatr Orthop 2002;22:573.
15. Frankel VH, Nordin M: Basic Biomechanics of the Skeletal System. Philadelphia, Lea & Febiger, 1980.
16. Green NE, Swiontkowski MF: Skeletal Trauma in Children, 3rd ed. Philadelphia, WB Saunders, 2003.
17. Gustilo RB, Anderson JT: Prevention of infection in the treatment of one thousand and twenty-five open fractures of long bones. J Bone Joint Surg Am 1976;58:453.
18. Helfet DL, Howey T, Sanders R, et al: Limb salvage versus amputation: Preliminary results of the mangled extremity severity score. Clin Orthop 1990;256:80.
19. Henrys P, Lyne ED, Lifton C, et al: Clinical review of cervical spine injuries in children. Clin Orthop 1977; 129:172.
20. Heppenstall RB, Sapega AA, Scott R, et al: The compartment syndrome: An experimental and clinical study of muscular energy metabolism using phosphorus nuclear magnetic resonance spectroscopy. Clin Orthop 1988; 226:138.
21. Herzenberg JE, Hensinger RN, Dedrick DK, et al: Emergency transport and positioning of young children who have an injury of the cervical spine: The standard backboard may be hazardous. J Bone Joint Surg Am 1989;71:15.
22. Karrholm J, Jansson LI, Laurin S: Computed tomography of intraarticular supination—eversion fractures of the ankle in adolescents. J Pediatr Orthop 1981;1:181.
23. Loder RT, Brown KL, Zaleske DJ, et al: Extremity lawn-mower injuries in children: Report by the Research Committee of the Pediatric Orthopaedic Society of North America. J Pediatr Orthop 1997;17:360.
24. McMahon P, Grossman W, Gaffney M, et al: Soft tissue injury as an indication of child abuse. J Bone Joint Surg Am 1995;77:1179.
25. Ogden JA: Skeletal Injury in the Child, 3rd ed. New York, Springer, 2000.
26. Rex C, Kay PR: Features of femoral fractures in nonaccidental injury. J Pediatr Orthop 2000;20:411.
27. Rockwood CA Jr, Wilkins KD, Beaty JH, et al: Fractures in Children, 5th ed. Philadelphia, Lippincott Williams & Wilkins, 2001.
28. Salter RB, Harris WR: Injuries involving the epiphyseal plate. J Bone Joint Surg Am 1963;45:587.
29. Shapiro F: Fractures of the femoral shaft in children: The overgrowth phenomenon. Acta Orthop Scand 1981; 52:649.
30. Skaggs DL, Mirzayan R: The posterior fat pad sign in association with occult fracture of the elbow in children. J Bone Joint Surg Am 1999;81:1429.
31. Smith WS, Kauffer H: Patterns and mechanisms of lumbar injuries associated with lap seat belts. J Bone Joint Surg Am 1969;51:239.
32. Stephens MM, Hsu LC, Leong JC: Leg length discrepancy after femoral shaft fractures in children: Review after skeletal maturity. J Bone Joint Surg Br 1989;71:615.
33. Techakapuch S: Rupture of the lumbar cartilage plate into the spinal canal in an adolescent: A case report. J Bone Joint Surg Am 1981;45:481.
34. Whitesides TE, Heckman MM: Acute compartment syndrome: Update on diagnosis and treatment. J Am Acad Orthop Surg 1996;4:209.

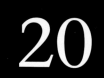
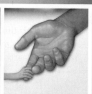

Chapter 20

Hand, Soft Tissue, and Envenomation Injuries

Michael L. Bentz and Delora Mount

Evaluation of pediatric hand and soft tissue injuries requires a systematic approach that includes all relevant organ systems at the site of trauma.[1] A high index of suspicion is necessary to make an accurate diagnosis and exclude subtle problems, particularly in toddlers and infants who are unable to cooperate with a detailed examination. Injuries are triaged according to their threat to life. After such triage has taken place, the more peripheral and often more dramatic and distracting injuries can be better defined.[6] The history is important to define baseline function, previous injuries, right- or left-hand dominance, and the mechanism and timing of injury. The initial physical examination must define vascularity and perfusion because an ischemic or poorly perfused extremity necessitates emergent surgical intervention. Other findings can be handled in a less urgent fashion, after an orderly assessment is complete. The patient should be examined in a well-lighted area with the parents present to exert a calming influence over a frightened child and thus increase the reliability of findings. This chapter focuses on the acute evaluation and management of hand, soft tissue, and envenomation injuries to provide a foundation for the accurate triage of injured children.[5,14]

HAND AND SOFT TISSUE INJURIES

Evaluation

Vascularity

The goal of the initial examination is to determine the presence or extent of vascular injury, hypoperfusion, or ischemia. Symptoms of ischemia include pallor, paresthesia, paralysis, pain, and lack of pulse. The digits should be pink and warm if the patient has not had hypothermic exposure or proximal tourniquet application. Normal capillary refill time is 3 seconds and is most accurately tested by compressing the lateral aspect of the distal phalanx adjacent to the nail plate. A delayed refill time indicates impaired arterial inflow, whereas a rapid refill

time suggests venous hypertension or insufficiency. The pulse should be palpated bilaterally at the radial, ulnar, and brachial arteries. Percutaneous Doppler ultrasonography can be used to qualitatively and quantitatively define inflow if the pulse cannot be detected or if it is asymmetrical. Allen's test is important to define the relative contributions of the radial and ulnar arteries to the palmar arches of the hand. The ulnar artery is the dominant source of inflow to the hand and continues into a patent palmar arch in 85% of uninjured hands.[7] Significant bleeding noted during the initial evaluation is managed by firm manual compression or, if the time until definitive intervention is expected to be prolonged, by proximal tourniquet application. A hemostat or clamp should not be placed blindly into the wound, because lack of blood flow may injure adjacent neural structures. Impaled or retained foreign objects should be left in situ until definitive management is possible because they may staunch the flow of blood from a vascular injury.

Peripheral Nerves

Peripheral nerves should be evaluated after vascular inflow has been assessed. Isolated nerve injuries cause predictable neurologic deficits that manifest as abnormalities in sensation or motor function, depending on the location of injury.[18] Vascular injuries can also cause neurologic deficits, particularly in subacute wounds; therefore, the evaluation of nerve and vascular injuries should generally occur in tandem. A clear concept of cross-sectional anatomy is helpful in visualizing potential at-risk structures. Evaluating the nerve function at the distal aspect of the hand can be used to screen for a more proximal nerve injury.

The median nerve is responsible for sensation to the three and a half volar radial digits. The function of this nerve can be tested by a pinprick or, more objectively, by two-point tactile discrimination. Median nerve motor function can be tested by palpating the contraction of the abductor pollicis brevis and opponens pollicis muscles as the patient forms an "O" with the index finger

Figure 20–1 The ability to form an "O" with the index finger and thumb, with palpable contraction of the thenar muscles, indicates an intact median nerve.

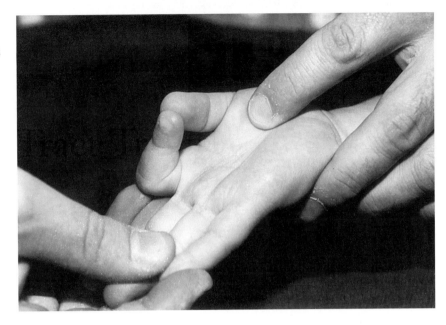

and thumb (Fig. 20-1). The ulnar nerve supplies sensation to the one and a half ulnar digits. Motor function of this nerve is most accurately tested by palpating the contraction against the force of the first dorsal interosseous muscle while the fingers are spread (Fig. 20-2). There is no radial nerve motor innervation of the intrinsic hand muscles, so the motor function of the radial nerve is best screened by wrist and digit extension (Fig. 20-3). The radial nerves provide sensation to the three and a half dorsal radial digits of the hand to the level of the distal phalanges, although overlap is common. Serial examination can be quite helpful, and cooperation and a focused effort are essential for a reliable evaluation. Further, neurologic findings associated with compartment syndrome evolve over time and may not be obvious during the initial examination.[13]

Skeleton, Tendons, and Ligaments

Although some skeletal injuries are obvious on routine examination, most require radiographic evaluation. Physical examination findings of fracture include deformity, crepitus, ecchymosis, pain, instability, and swelling. Anteroposterior, lateral, and oblique radiographs should be obtained for all but the most minor injuries to evaluate for fractures, dislocations, and foreign objects. Familiarity with the Salter-Harris classification of pediatric fractures is important because the specific fracture patterns offer prognostic information relevant to subsequent growth (see Chapter 19).[16,23] The presentation of fractures has been well documented.[12,19] The examination and radiographic appearance are combined to accurately describe the fracture. Open fractures have an associated

Figure 20–2 Digit spread with palpable contraction of the first dorsal interosseous muscle is consistent with an intact ulnar nerve.

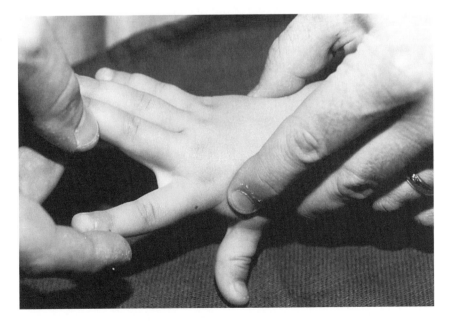

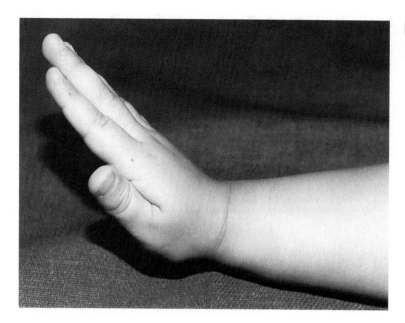

Figure 20–3 Digit and wrist extension demonstrates radial nerve integrity because no muscles in the hand are innervated by radial nerves.

full-thickness soft tissue injury, whereas closed fractures do not. Simple fractures result in two bone fragments, whereas comminuted fractures involve several fragments. Greenstick fractures involve one cortex and are particularly relevant in children because of their malleable bones. The description of a fracture should also include information regarding length (shortened, elongated, normal), angulation (volar, dorsal, radial, ulnar), rotation (present or absent), and displacement as a percentage of normal alignment.

Tendon injuries can be very difficult to diagnose, particularly in young or uncooperative children. In such cases, surgical exploration is necessary to definitely confirm certain injuries. The posture of the hand at rest gives information regarding tendon integrity. In a relaxed position, the hand should form a gentle cascade; this position results from passive tension of the tendons. With compression of the distal forearm, all digits should adopt flexion posturing as a result of the tenodesis effect. A digit that remains extended out of the cascade suggests disruption of the flexor mechanism (Fig. 20-4). The flexor digitorum superficialis tendon to each of the four fingers is tested by holding the adjacent digits in a fixed position and allowing metacarpophalangeal joint flexion (Fig. 20-5). The flexor digitorum profundus and flexor pollicis longus tendons are evaluated by holding the middle phalanx and observing distal interphalangeal joint flexion.

Ligament injuries can be difficult to diagnose, particularly in the presence of associated soft tissue or skeletal injuries.[24] Abnormal joint stability is an indicator of disruption of the ligaments.[12] If the opposite side is uninjured, joint stability should be compared with that side as an indicator of preinjury status. Plain and stress radiographs of an avulsion fracture at the site of ligament insertion can confirm clinical findings.

Soft Tissue

A thorough determination of soft tissue injuries is important for a knowledgeable evaluation of wound healing,[25]

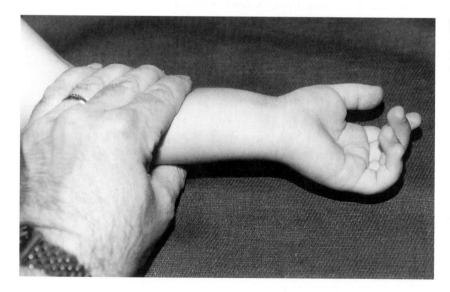

Figure 20–4 Forearm compression has failed to cause flexion of the index finger in this patient; this suggests flexor mechanism discontinuity to the index finger.

Figure 20–5 Function of the flexor digitorum superficialis tendon is tested by demonstrating isolated metacarpophalangeal and proximal interphalangeal joint flexion. Flexor digitorum profundus tendon function is tested by holding the middle phalanx fixed and observing distal interphalangeal joint flexion.

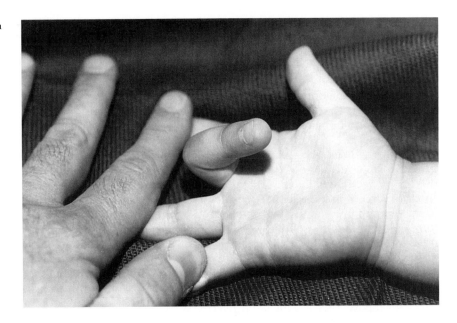

but even more so for the evaluation of long-term function and outcome of primary or secondary reconstructive surgery. The amount of soft tissue present in the area of a wound determines the feasibility of primary repair of vascular, neural, and osteoligamentous injuries, and an adequate amount is required for proper healing. The size (measured objectively), shape, location, and general configuration of each wound is recorded, and the mechanism of injury and preinjury status of the patient are established. Obvious foreign objects are removed, although projectiles impaled through an extremity are left in situ until they can be managed definitively. Exposed vital structures as well as associated fractures and tendon injuries are noted.

Early Treatment

Vascular

Ischemia is one of the few surgical emergencies associated with upper limb trauma. Revascularization is a top priority after the correction of life-threatening injuries. Because irreversible changes start to occur after 4 hours of ischemia, expeditious surgical intervention is mandatory, especially if the ischemic tissue involves muscle. Primary vascular repair is the most effective procedure and is ideally accomplished by debridement, mobilization, and primary anastomosis of injured segments. Reversed vein grafts, which are frequently done with foot, forearm, saphenous, or cephalic veins, should be used liberally if tension or lack of tissue prevents easy approximation of adjacent segments. In general, all arteries and veins proximal to the elbow should be repaired. Repair of arterial injuries below the elbow should also be considered to prevent cold intolerance; however, only about half of these repairs remain patent.[10] If necessary, the radial artery can be ligated primarily. Once repairs are complete, fasciotomy should be considered if ischemia has been prolonged,

soft tissue damage is significant, or adequate postoperative monitoring is not available.[13] Serial examination should then be pursued in an effort to make an early diagnosis of recurrent ischemia or postsurgical thrombosis or bleeding. The role of anticoagulation therapy in this setting is controversial and is based on the surgeon's preference and experience.

Peripheral Nerves

Injury to the peripheral nerves is not an emergency and can frequently be addressed when an adjacent vascular injury is being repaired. When a wound is clean, uninfected, and well vascularized, primary nerves should be repaired in an end-to-end fashion. Such repair can be facilitated through the mobilization of proximal and distal injured segments, which can reduce tension and augment blood flow. If mobilization of the injured segments cannot adequately repair the defect, interpositional nerve grafts can be used for definitive reconstruction. In such cases, early secondary repair in the first 10 days after injury is optimal. To ensure that the injured area remains intact, the involved limb should be splinted to minimize further proximal migration of the transected nerve before surgery and to relieve anastomotic tension.

Skeleton, Tendons, and Ligaments

When injuries to the skeleton, tendons, or ligaments are diagnosed, restoration of normal or acceptable anatomy followed by appropriate immobilization is indicated. In children, an injury that is suspected but not objectively defined is particularly common. Hand fractures may not be evident on radiographs for several weeks. In this situation, presumptive treatment should be carried out, which usually involves immobilization of the potentially injured area, despite equivocal physical examination or radiographic findings. Immobilization is rarely contraindicated in children because it allows protection from further injury, improves pain control, and maintains local anatomy. Use of a splint (instead of a cast) is ideal because it allows swelling into a nonfixed space and limits the possibility of vascular compromise during the acute injury and postreduction periods.

Anatomic reduction of fractures and dislocations can be done at the time of injury or in the following week, with good functional results.[29] In the acute setting, excellent anesthesia can be obtained by performing a hematoma block. This is accomplished by injecting 2 to 3 mL of lidocaine 1% without epinephrine into the fracture site. Reduction in the subacute setting most commonly requires a traditional digital block. Particularly in smaller children, it must be kept in mind that the limiting dose of plain lidocaine is 4 mg/kg of body weight. A description of the reduction maneuvers for specific types of fractures is beyond the scope of this chapter, but in general, gentle manual traction or finger-trap distraction with simultaneous rotation or derotation allows improvement in many types of fractures and dislocations.[8] Postreduction radiographs should be obtained in most if not all patients before or after immobilization. The specific position of immobilization is less critical for children than adults because children are less prone to stiffening and tightening of the ligaments. The "position of safety" can always be used at least initially for splinting: the wrist is placed in 30 to 45 degrees of extension, the metacarpophalangeal joints are placed in 70 degrees of flexion, and the interphalangeal joints are left straight. Serial physical and radiographic examinations are tailored to the specific injury and clinical course.

Soft Tissue

After soft tissue and associated vital structure injuries are documented, irrigation of all significant wounds should be performed with normal saline solution, after which foreign objects are removed and tissue that is clearly devitalized is debrided. These procedures may require a local anesthetic, which should be given only after a thorough neurologic examination has been completed. Simple lacerations and small surface-area avulsions can be closed primarily using the same layered closure method used for deep or gaping wounds under tension. Suture choice depends on the location, size, and cause of the wound, as well as the patient's age. A smaller child who requires sedation for the primary wound repair will be hypersensitive to suture removal, when sedation is usually not available. In such cases, absorbable sutures reinforced with Steri-strips and an adhesive are ideal. Permanent sutures should be used in older or cooperative patients to minimize the inflammatory response and avoid early scarring. The potential for scarring depends on the location of the wound and the mechanism of injury. Scarring can be minimized through judicious wound closure.

Open wounds that cannot be closed primarily require more elaborate intervention. To bridge the gap between injury and wound closure, the wound must be managed and protected. Normal saline wet-to-wet dressings are a simple and effective way to provide limited debridement, allow the initiation of granulation, and prevent desiccation.

Povidone-iodine dressings should be reserved for short-term use in infected wounds. Acetic acid solution (0.25%) is appropriate for wounds that have culture documentation of infection with *Pseudomonas* species. Quantitative wound biopsies should be reserved for nonthermal burns.

If the skin defect is only partial thickness and no vital structures are exposed, split-thickness skin grafting or skin distraction is appropriate. Split-thickness skin grafts are used for larger wounds, less cosmetically significant wounds, or those in which the wound bed may not be optimal because of infection, inflammation, or ischemia. Full-thickness skin grafts contract less after revascularization and thus are ideal for cosmetically significant areas or those where wound contraction is undesirable. Local skin flaps can also be used in such settings, offering a cosmetically favorable replacement of like tissue. These skin flaps can be random if they have no specific blood supply or axial if the blood is supplied by a specific vessel.[17] Regional muscle flaps can be used almost anywhere in the body, especially when highly vascularized tissue of significant bulk is required to cover exposed critical structures and fill dead space. Similar to axial pattern skin flaps, these muscle flaps are used on the basis of a known blood supply, which makes their dissection reliable and safe. Finally, when local tissue is not available or is inadequate to provide wound closure, microvascular free tissue transfer is indicated using specific donor "free flaps" to accomplish specific tasks.

Amputations

Traumatic amputations in children should be considered for replantation by a qualified microsurgical team, given the excellent results obtained when compared with adult series.[15] To optimize the chance of success, the amputated part should be wrapped in saline-moistened gauze, sealed in a plastic bag, and placed in a bag of ice and saline solution; the part must not contact the ice directly.

ENVENOMATION INJURIES

Snakebites

More than 2700 species of snakes exist; 115 of these species are indigenous to the United States, and only 19 of the 115 species are poisonous.[9] Pit vipers, which are named for the pit located between their eyes and nostrils, account for most bites. Pit vipers include rattlesnakes, copperheads, and cottonmouths.[28] Coral snakes represent the other poisonous family. Most bites occur during the summer months in the morning, late afternoon, or evening. Not all bites are associated with envenomation. Signs of envenomation include pain, edema, ecchymosis, nausea, vomiting, hypotension, disseminated intravascular coagulopathy, hemolysis, mental status changes, seizures, and death.[21] The severity of signs is proportional to the degree of envenomation. Early intervention includes reassurance and support, immobilization, limb elevation, venous tourniquet application, and rapid transfer to the nearest medical facility. Cryotherapy and wound incision and suction are no longer recommended. Mild pit viper envenomations (characterized by mild pain, local edema, lack of systemic signs, and normal laboratory values) require up to 5 vials of antivenin; moderate envenomations (severe pain, extending edema, nausea, vomiting, neurologic signs, and abnormal laboratory values) require 10 to 15 initial vials of antivenin, with retreatment as necessary; and severe envenomations (rapid progression of local, systemic, and laboratory abnormalities) require an initial dose of 15 to 20 vials of antivenin.[21] Antivenin is administered intravenously only after a skin test has been done to rule out the possibility of an anaphylactic reaction. The initial dose for children is one and a half to two times that of adults because of the smaller circulating blood volume and relative venom concentration.[2,19] Initial dosing should be followed by aggressive intravenous hydration. Fasciotomy should be considered but is seldom required.[26] Initial management of bites from snakes from other countries is similar, although antivenin use requires adjustment, depending on the type of snake.[27] In addition to its use for pit vipers from North America, antivenin is effective for bites from fer-de-lance, bushmaster, and cantil snakes, which are found in Central and South America. Australian species frequently known to cause envenomations include the common brown snake, mainland tiger snake, lowland copperhead, and red-bellied black snake.

Other Bite Injuries

Gila monsters, which are found in the southwestern United States, and their relative the Mexican beaded lizard are active in late spring. These lizards inject venom as long as they cling to the victim. Wounds show edema, but tissue loss is less pronounced than that associated with envenomation by pit vipers; however, systemic signs can ultimately be similar. These injuries are managed by removing the animal from its victim, followed by local and systemic supportive care. Antivenin is not available. Radiographs should be obtained to exclude retained teeth.[11]

Black widow spiders are venomous New World spiders; the females are black with an hourglass-shaped red mark on the abdomen.[3] Local signs of a bite can be limited, followed by systemic neuromuscular symptoms of diffuse rigidity and spasm that potentially lead to respiratory arrest approximately 1 hour later. Envenomations by black widow spiders are managed by local care, fluid and cardiovascular support, parenteral calcium gluconate, muscle relaxation, and antivenin.[2,5,11,22]

Scorpion stings in children have serious sequelae. Bark scorpions are the only toxic species in the United States; however, others are common in Mexico and equatorial countries. Local signs of envenomation are minimal, whereas systemic neuromuscular findings are present in the sympathetic and parasympathetic systems. Children are particularly susceptible to the severe cardiorespiratory and neuromuscular dysfunction associated with envenomation. Therapy of scorpion stings includes local wound care, topical ice, specific antivenin, and systemic support, including ventilation, control of

tachyarrhythmias, and sedation. Treatment is similar to that for spider bites, although scorpion stings are generally less serious.[20]

Finally, human bite wounds can pose some of the most challenging definitive management problems among all bite-induced injuries.[4] Based on the quantitative and qualitative characteristics of oral flora, including the principal pathogen *Eikenella corrodens,* aggressive primary intervention is mandatory to achieve a satisfactory outcome in all these injuries. Thorough irrigation of penetrating bite wounds is mandatory, as well as broad-spectrum antibiotic coverage, followed by frequent wound checks.

REFERENCES

1. Ablove RH, Moy OJ, Peimer CA: Pediatric hand disease: Diagnosis and treatment. Pediatr Clin North Am 1998;45:1507-1524.
2. Allen C: Arachnid envenomations. Emerg Clin North Am 1992;10:269-298.
3. Banner W: Bites and stings in the pediatric patient. Curr Probl Pediatr 1988;18:1-69.
4. Bhende MS, Dandrea LA, Davis, HW: Hand injuries in children presenting to a pediatric emergency department. Ann Emerg Med 1993;22:1519-1523.
5. Binder LS: Acute arthropod envenomation: Incidence, clinical features and management. Med Toxicol Adverse Drug Exp 1989;4:163-173.
6. Buncke GM, Buntic RF, Romeo O: Pediatric mutilating hand injuries. Hand Clin 2003;19:121-131.
7. Coleman SS, Anson BJ: Arterial patterns in the hand based on a study of 650 specimens, Surg Gynecol Obstet 1961;113:409-424.
8. Eaton RG, Littler JW: Joint injuries and their sequelae. Clin Plast Surg 1976;3:85-98.
9. Forks TP: Evaluation and treatment of poisonous snakebites. Am Fam Physician 1994;50:123-130.
10. Gelberman RH, et al: The results of radial and ulnar arterial repair in the forearm: Experience in three medical centers. J Bone Joint Surg Am 1982;64:383-387.
11. Hassen LB: Reptile and arthropod envenomations. Occup Med 1991;6:447-461.
12. Hastings H, Simmons BP: Hand fractures in children: A statistical analysis. Clin Orthop 1984;188:120-130.
13. Holden CEA: Compartmental syndromes following trauma. Clin Orthop 1975;113:95-102.
14. Innis PC: Office evaluation and treatment of finger and wrist injuries in children. Curr Opin Pediatr 1995;7:83-87.
15. Jaeger SH, Tsai TM, Kleinert HE: Upper extremity replantation in children. Orthop Clin North Am 1981;12:897-907.
16. Leclercq C, Korn W: Articular fractures of the finger in children. Hand Clin 2000;16:523-534.
17. McGregor IA, Morgan G: Axial and random pattern flaps. Br J Plast Surg 1973;16:202-213.
18. Moberg E: Evaluation of sensibility in the hand. Surg Clin North Am 1960;40:357-362.
19. Nofsinger CC, Wolfe SW: Common pediatric hand fractures. Curr Opin Pediatr 2002;14:42-45.
20. Rimsza ME, Zimmerman DR, Bergeson PS: Scorpion envenomation. Pediatrics 1980;66:298-302.
21. Rudolph R, et al: Snakebite treatment at a southeastern regional referral center. Am Surg 1995;61:767-772.

22. Russell FE: Venomous arthropods. In Schacter LA, Hansen R (eds): Pediatric Dermatology. New York, Churchill Livingstone, 1988.

23. Salter RB, Harris WR: Injuries involving the epiphyseal plate. J Bone Joint Surg Am 1963;45:587-622.

24. Simmons BP, Lovallo JL: Hand and wrist injuries in children. Clin Sports Med 1988;7:495-512.

25. Stewart GM, Quan L, Horton MA: Laceration management. Pediatr Emerg Care 1993;9:247-250.

26. Stewart RM, et al: Antivenin and fasciotomy/debridement in the treatment of the severe rattlesnake bite. Am J Surg 1989;158:543-547.

27. Tibballs J: Diagnosis and treatment of confirmed and suspected snake bite: Implications from an analysis of 46 paediatric cases. Med J Aust 1992;156:270-274.

28. Weber RA, White RR: Crotalidae envenomation in children. Ann Plast Surg 1993;31:141-145.

29. Wood VE: Fractures of the hand in children. Orthop Clin North Am 1976;7:527-542.

Chapter 21

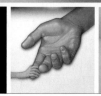
Central Nervous System Injuries

Thomas G. Luerssen

Injuries to the brain and spinal cord continue to be the major cause of mortality and morbidity from childhood trauma. Despite 25 years of intensive clinical research, no specific medical therapy for any traumatic neurologic injury has yet been defined. Nevertheless, there has been a steady and substantial advance in our understanding of the natural history of brain and spinal cord injuries; moreover, there have been changes in management that have clearly resulted in improved outcomes.

We have now entered the era of "evidence-based medicine" whereby recommendations for disease and injury management are supposed to be derived from critical analysis of available scientific research. In the past decade, management strategies for central nervous system (CNS) injuries have been subjected to this type of analysis. These efforts have resulted in the publication of practice management guidelines.[2,21,63,87] Analysis of the clinical evidence and development of these recommendations represent a substantial amount of work by many of the leading experts in the field. Unfortunately, these reviews also uncovered a remarkable lack of strong scientific evidence on which to develop recommendations, especially in the pediatric age group, so most of the available recommendations regarding the diagnosis and treatment of neurologic injuries can be supported only by the lowest degree of medical certainty. Nevertheless, these published practice parameters are useful summaries of the current understanding of the various treatments of brain and spinal cord injury. These publications are referenced frequently in this chapter, and interested readers are encouraged to review these practice parameters and the citations of the analyzed literature that serve as the basis for the recommendations.

BASIC STRATEGY FOR TREATMENT OF CENTRAL NERVOUS SYSTEM INJURY

One of the most enduring concepts underlying the management of brain and spinal cord injury is that of primary and secondary injury.[124] The primary neurologic injury involves the immediate disruption of neuronal, axonal, and supportive structures and vascular tissues.

The magnitude and location of the primary injury, along with the variety of irreversible cellular processes that immediately ensue, something that has been referred to as "delayed primary injury," are directly related to the mechanism of injury. These immediate tissue disruptions are also considered to be self-limited and are, by definition, essentially untreatable. Given all of this, one can easily see that the primary brain injury is the major determinant of injury outcome.

Obviously, the primary injury can be devastating and, in many high-energy mechanisms, immediately lethal. In persons not immediately killed by an injury, the primary injury triggers a cascade of intracellular and extracellular biochemical changes, both in the region of the injury and systemically, many of which are deleterious and cause acceleration and augmentation of the initial injury. These reactive processes represent the onset of what has been termed the "secondary injury." These secondary reactive processes can begin at almost any time after the injury and can persist for some time. The secondary injury not only results in new damage, both in the region of the primary injury and in areas of previously uninjured brain or spinal cord, but also causes deleterious effects in other organs and body systems.

Systemic reactions commonly seen after brain or spinal cord injury include hypotension and hypoxia. It has clearly been shown that even brief and mild episodes of either hypoxia or hypotension can have profoundly deleterious effects on the outcome of both brain and spinal cord injury.[28,123,141] Although it is well known that spinally injured patients can be rendered hypotensive by an isolated injury, it is now also clear that isolated brain injury can cause systemic hypotension. Multiple injuries, occult organ injuries, or other causes of exsanguination that result in hypovolemia are not required for this hypotensive response to occur. Of the early systemic complications, it appears that hypotension is much more deleterious to an acutely injured brain than hypoxia is. This is probably also true for an acutely injured spinal cord. Finally, it is clear that these complications can occur very early, frequently, and in many cases so briefly that they are either undetected or unreported, even in modern intensive care units.[12,88]

There are also other common systemic responses, many of which occur shortly after an injury but can also cause further injury even days after the institution of therapy. Hyperthermia, either from fever or as a result of overly aggressive warming, is harmful to an injured brain.[168] Hyperglycemia, which is commonly seen in the stress response and can be aggravated by fluid administration or attempted nutrition, is also believed to be deleterious to acutely injured neurons.[18,27,149]

Tissue disruptions, commonly referred to as cerebral or spinal cord contusions, cause reactive changes in the tissues immediately surrounding the area of injury. A variety of tissue factors are released, such as those in the kallikrein-kinin system, and these factors can cause disturbances in microcirculation and the blood-brain or blood–spinal cord barrier that ultimately result in the complex entity that has generally been referred to as post-traumatic edema.[113] There are hypermetabolic responses related to neural tissue injury that may outstrip the local or regional substrate supply.[13] Excitotoxic amino acids such as glutamate and aspartate are released from injured neurons.[56] Post-traumatic seizures, especially prolonged subclinical seizures, may contribute to this response in the injured brain.[172] Along with the reactive biochemical changes, expanding local hemorrhages caused by direct vascular injury can lead to further compression of adjacent vessels and result in an ischemic penumbra around the acute injury.

Although the systemic and biochemical processes of secondary injury are complex, it appears that the pathophysiologic end point of all of them is ischemic damage. Ischemic neuronal damage is almost universally seen in the neuropathologic examination of patients who have suffered traumatic brain and spinal cord injury.[70,164]

Even though numerous biochemical cascades have been identified and physiologically characterized, and many have been the target of pharmaceutical intervention, no drug has yet been shown to be specifically effective for the treatment of CNS injury. Trials of high-dose steroids, calcium channel blockers, free radical scavengers, and glutamate antagonists have been generally negative, although small and specific subgroups of patients were identified in post hoc analyses that may have benefited from one or another of these therapies. More concerning is that some groups of patients were apparently harmed by the administration of some of these agents.[32] Despite this lack of development of a specific therapy, 20 years of clinical trials involved in the assessment of these agents have shown steady improvement in neurologic outcomes, more so in the arena of brain injury than in spinal cord injury. This trend toward improved outcome is almost certainly due to the realization that many of the ischemic processes can be prevented by aggressive application of systemic manipulation, beginning with the resuscitation phase of the injury and continuing through the period of acute therapy.

The essential therapeutic strategies for brain and spinal cord injury are based on preventing ischemic injury by the aggressive support of intravascular volume and blood pressure at all times. The historical idea of restricting fluids in head-injured patients is no longer accepted. The early use of vasopressors is encouraged. Reduction of focal vascular compression by removal of mass lesions and aggressive prevention and management of reactive brain or cord swelling to protect perfusion are procedures that are aimed at minimizing local and general ischemic injury. These three relatively simplistic concepts—support of systemic blood pressure, reduction of intracranial pressure to ensure cerebral perfusion, and removal of compressive lesions plus prevention of deleterious complications—are now the mainstay of management of brain and spinal cord injuries.

IMMEDIATE ISSUES: RESUSCITATION AND TRANSPORT OF INJURED CHILDREN

Effective supportive and preventive therapy should begin as quickly after the injury as possible. Goals of the initial resuscitation are twofold: prevention of as much secondary injury as possible and prevention of any new primary injury before undertaking neurodiagnostic studies. One can accomplish the first goal by ensuring oxygenated perfusion of the brain and spinal cord by restoring and maintaining age-appropriate normal blood pressure and volume as early as possible. This action, coupled with restoring and maintaining normal ventilation, is, at least at this time, more important than the administration of any drug. The exact means of accomplishing this goal, that is, the type of resuscitation fluid or the means of ensuring ventilation, is probably less important than accomplishing the goal itself. Most current studies indicate that isotonic or slightly hypertonic saline solution is an appropriate fluid for resuscitating and maintaining blood pressure in neurologically injured patients,[21,29,181] although the use of colloids and more highly concentrated hypertonic solutions is also being investigated.

Tissue oxygenation is important, and therefore adequate airway and ventilation support is required. Early intubation by experienced personnel with appropriate analgesia and sedation will certainly accomplish this goal. However, the role of intubation of injured children (and adults) in the field is still controversial.[77] It appears that this maneuver is associated with a relatively high complication rate and may not be warranted in many situations.[2,65,127,174]

For patients with possible spinal injuries, prevention of further injury begins with stabilization of the spine. This maneuver involves much more than the application of a collar or securing a child to a rigid board. It is important that normal anatomic alignment be maintained. Very young children have proportionately larger heads and therefore have a tendency toward cervical flexion when lying supine.[33] A cervical collar alone does not completely immobilize an injured spine in a child.[83] Specific attention should be directed to immobilizing the spine in an anatomic position, including ensuring a normal relative position of the head to the body. Young children require some additional elevation of the body so that the head falls back to a truly neutral position. Once these parameters have been achieved, that is, stabilization of the spine in an anatomic position and establishment of systemic blood pressure and respiration support, an injured child may be transported for definitive diagnosis and treatment of the injury.

TRAUMATIC BRAIN INJURY

Epidemiology

Despite the frequency of head injury in children, epidemiologic data in this area are relatively limited. A study in the United Kingdom indicated that 40% of all patients seen in emergency departments for the treatment of head injuries were children.[17] It is important, however, to distinguish between "head injury" and "brain injury" in discussing outcomes and therapy, although it is probably equally important to group these entities in discussing mechanisms and prevention. Accordingly, population-based studies indicate an average incidence of clinically important head injury in children of about 185 per 100,000, with the incidence generally dropping with increasing age.[19,96] Boys are injured at a rate approximately twice that of girls.

Overall, 85% of the brain injuries sustained in childhood are mild and not life threatening.[97,111] Although severe brain injuries are rare, they still constitute a major concern in pediatric trauma management. Reports from pediatric trauma centers have indicated that well over half of all deaths resulting from blunt trauma in children are caused by a brain injury.[121,171]

The severity and mechanism of brain injury seem to be linked to outcomes. The mechanism of injury is also age dependent. The most common mechanism resulting in head injury in children is a fall, but the usual falls in childhood are not associated with severe injuries. The major cause of severe brain injury in young children seems to be abuse. In older children, severe brain injury is most commonly seen in relation to motor vehicle accidents.

Many accidental brain injuries that occur in children are preventable. Proper use of occupant restraints in motor vehicles can prevent up to 90% of the serious injuries to young children.[147] The implementation of a mandatory child restraint law in Michigan reduced the number of motor vehicle–related injuries in children by 25%.[116] Wearing helmets for bicycle riding, as well as for other recreational activities such as skateboarding, skating, skiing, and horseback riding, should decrease the risk for brain injury,[129,148,167] although educational programs regarding helmet use have had only limited success thus far.[64] Many falls are preventable. Vigilance regarding open windows and stairways, including the use of gates or bars, substantially reduces the occurrence of these injuries.

The Spectrum of Traumatic Brain Injury

There are many ways to undertake an overview of the major types of traumatic brain injury. The author has come to prefer one that includes a relationship of injury types, mechanism, and natural history. The simplest way to do this is by categorizing major injury types as either focal or diffuse. Accepting the caveat that many traumatic injuries are "mixtures" of focal and diffuse injury, one can still base individual management strategies on the initial appearance of the type of brain injury.

Focal or Diffuse Brain Injury?

Focal injuries include contusions, lacerations, traumatic hematomas, and localized damage caused by expanding masses and shifts and distortions of the brain. Diffuse injuries include the spectrum of diffuse axonal injury (DAI), which encompasses what is commonly called cerebral concussion, as well as other diffuse insults such as global ischemia, systemic hypoxia, diffuse brain swelling, and diffuse vascular injury. Focal injuries are usually immediately apparent on admitting computed tomography (CT) scans. Nonetheless, they may be clinically asymptomatic. In contrast, diffuse injuries may show much less striking changes on early neuroimaging studies, even though the patient may exhibit profound alterations in consciousness and neurologic function. Focal injuries are more likely to require therapeutic surgical procedures, whereas diffuse injuries may require extensive diagnostic studies to determine the type and magnitude of the injury. Diffuse injuries are also more likely to require prolonged monitoring of intracranial pressure (ICP) to guide therapy. It is useful to discuss the characteristics of these types of injuries individually, but it is important to remember that in many cases, especially with more severe injuries, both injury types may be present.

Focal Brain Injury

Most focal brain injuries are associated with impact-related mechanisms. Because short falls are the most common cause of accidental head injury in childhood, cranial impacts and their resulting focal injuries are also common. Furthermore, impact mechanisms are associated with skull fractures, which are also commonly seen in the pediatric age group. In fact, about 20% of head-injured children who are admitted to the hospital have skull fractures.[105] Despite the frequency of skull fracture in childhood, the majority of children with this injury will not require any intervention or suffer any complication directly related to the fracture. Therefore, the clinical importance of most skull fractures is that the fracture serves as an indicator of both the mechanism and severity of the head injury. Most studies of the importance of skull fractures have determined that the finding of a skull fracture in a head-injured patient is statistically associated with a higher likelihood that an expanding intracranial hematoma or a significant brain injury is also present.[25,82,101,105,166] Furthermore, complex skull fractures, or the occurrence of multiple fractures, is generally associated with higher-energy mechanisms and therefore more severe injuries to the brain.

As indicated earlier, most focal brain injuries are immediately apparent on initial neuroimaging studies and, depending on the size and location, result in focal neurologic dysfunction. The most common focal injury resulting from nonpenetrating mechanisms is a cerebral contusion (Fig. 21-1). It is generally a surface lesion

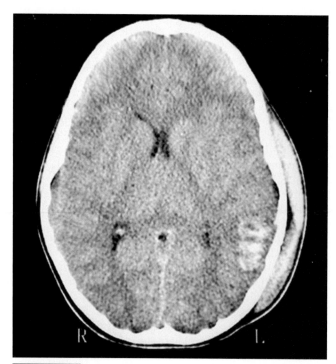

Figure 21–1 This cerebral contusion underlying a linear skull fracture (not demonstrated) was the result of a cranial impact, as demonstrated by the overlying soft tissue swelling and hemorrhage. The patient had no neurologic deficit.

related to cranial impact or brain movement over irregular intracranial surfaces or along the edges of dura. The clinical manifestation of cerebral contusions depends mostly on the extent of the initial injury, the amount of associated hemorrhage resulting in a mass effect, and the location of the contusion in the brain. Even though cerebral contusions may result in localized swelling, isolated lesions are not generally life-threatening. Many cerebral contusions are neurologically silent, only to be discovered on the initial CT scan underlying a skull fracture or along the anterior cranial base. When these injuries are symptomatic, they usually cause a focal neurologic deficit or seizures. The latter are thought to occur commonly in adults with acute cerebral contusions.[38] However, the incidence of seizures in children with cerebral contusions appears to be no greater than that in children with either normal CT scans or epidural hematomas.[73]

Traumatic intracerebral hematomas are unusual lesions in the pediatric age group. The pathogenesis of these hemorrhages is unclear, but it seems likely to be related to disruption of central arterial blood vessels. Accordingly, these lesions are associated with more severe mechanisms of injury and with more profound neurologic dysfunction. In many cases these lesions are part of a larger picture of DAI, which is discussed later. Traumatic intracerebral hematomas are distinguished from hemorrhagic contusions by their lack of contact with the surface of the brain.[67] They can be quite large and, because of the location, can leave a child with a profound neurologic deficit. Surgical evacuation can be considered if ICP is high, but in the author's experience,

neurologic outcomes are not improved by evacuation of these hematomas.

Children seem to be uniquely prone to non-missile-associated penetrating injuries of the skull and brain. These injuries are usually the result of a fall onto or being struck by sharp objects such as nails, pencils, sharp sticks, or lawn toys (Fig. 21-2). One of the major dangers of these injuries is that unless the offending object remains embedded, the entry wound may be hidden or seem trivial.[22,44,126] Anterior penetration of the skull base can be transorbital, via the orbital roof, or through the nose or mouth. Thus, direct evidence of cranial penetration may not be visible or may be masked by local swelling.

Penetrating injuries can result in focal contusions, intracerebral hemorrhages, and cerebral lacerations, but these lesions are usually silent because of their locations and small size. Deeper penetrations are more likely to be symptomatic, not only because the tissue injury is more extensive but also because of the potential for injuring major vessels. Many penetrating injuries become symptomatic in delayed fashion because of expansion of intracerebral hemorrhage, recognition of a cerebrospinal fluid (CSF) fistula, or the development of symptoms indicating infection. Therefore, a very high index of suspicion is required, and careful radiologic studies are called for whenever there is a possibility of subtle cranial penetration. Wood, glass, and residual bits of debris may be difficult to detect on routine imaging studies, including CT.[76]

Cranial penetrating injury is also strongly associated with direct cerebrovascular injury.[51] Magnetic resonance imaging (MRI) with the addition of magnetic resonance angiography (MRA) or the increasingly useful modality of CT angiography (CTA) should be considered whenever there is evidence of deep cranial penetration or if substantial subarachnoid or focal intracerebral hemorrhage is present.

Diffuse Brain Injuries

The majority of brain injuries occurring in childhood are diffuse injuries. Diffuse brain injuries are characterized by general disturbances in neuronal function that begin immediately at the time of injury. Despite this, brain structure is generally preserved on admitting CT scans. Diffuse injuries occur as a direct result of energy dissipation within the substance of the brain or as a result of systemic insults. All these injuries exist on a continuum from extremely mild, and apparently completely reversible, to lethal. Frequently, the different types of diffuse brain injury occur together or in sequence and can act synergistically to affect neurologic status and the outcome.

Diffuse primary brain injuries are generally the result of angular or translational acceleration (or deceleration), with the amount of tissue disruption being roughly proportional to the amount of energy dissipated in the brain substance.[68] As the amount of neuronal disruption increases, the depth and duration of neurologic dysfunction increase and the neurologic outcome worsens. There is a strong association with the appearance of certain hemorrhages on CT scan, specifically, subarachnoid hemorrhage, small but widespread

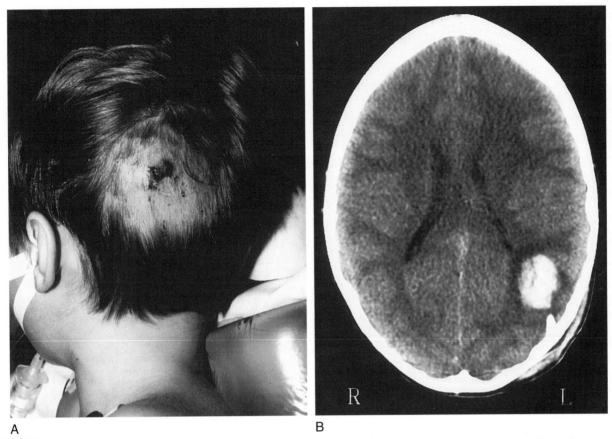

A   B

Figure 21-2 The occult injury frequently seen with low-velocity cranial penetration in young children is demonstrated. The patient was struck in the left parietal region by a lawn dart, and loss of consciousness did not occur. The lawn dart fell out immediately. The injury was misinterpreted as a minor scalp laceration and was closed with butterfly bandages. Three days later, fever and headache developed. A, Appearance of the entry wound before surgical exploration. B, Computed tomography shows a compound fracture and intracerebral hematoma. During surgery, hair, dirt, and bone fragments were removed from the cerebral cortex.

intracerebral hemorrhages, and intraventricular hemorrhage (Fig. 21-3).[1] Finally, although the occurrence of traumatic, surgically accessible masses is not characteristic of diffuse brain injury, subdural hematomas are seen commonly along with DAI, and some of these subdural hematomas are large enough that surgical evacuation may be a necessary component of initial therapy. However, these subdural hemorrhages are better viewed as another marker of the diffuse brain injury rather than as a mass that should be treated in isolation, such as an epidural hematoma or hemorrhagic contusion.

Like all brain injuries, diffuse primary brain injuries occur within a spectrum of severity. At one end of the spectrum is a very mild, transient physiologic disturbance in neurologic function that includes the syndromes commonly associated with "cerebral concussion," whereas at the other end is the progressively more damaging and ultimately lethal entity that is now called "diffuse axonal injury."

The modern view of cerebral concussion is based on the pioneering work of Ommaya and Gennarelli,[130,131] which defines concussive brain injuries as a graded set of clinical syndromes showing increasing disturbances in the level and content of consciousness. This definition allows the inclusion of specific post-traumatic disturbances that are commonly seen in children after so-called mild head injuries, including confusion without amnesia, confusion associated with amnesia of varying depth and duration, and the classic loss of consciousness with and without transient sensorimotor paralysis or disturbances in respiration or circulation.

As the amount of energy in the injury mechanism increases, tissue disruption occurs and results in DAI. It is now clear that the most common cause of prolonged coma from mechanical brain injury is DAI. Patients who have suffered DAI are unconscious from the time of injury and remain so for a prolonged period.[66] It is not uncommon to note pupillary changes, skewed gaze, and decerebration. This constellation of symptoms had been called "brainstem contusion" in the era before MRI, and although isolated brainstem contusion can certainly occur, it is extremely rare. Instead, most patients in coma who appear to have brainstem dysfunction after closed head injury have suffered DAI.

The findings on initial CT scanning depend on the severity of the injury and the degree of associated hemorrhage. In some cases the initial CT scan may be normal. Subsequently, the characteristic lesions may be discovered

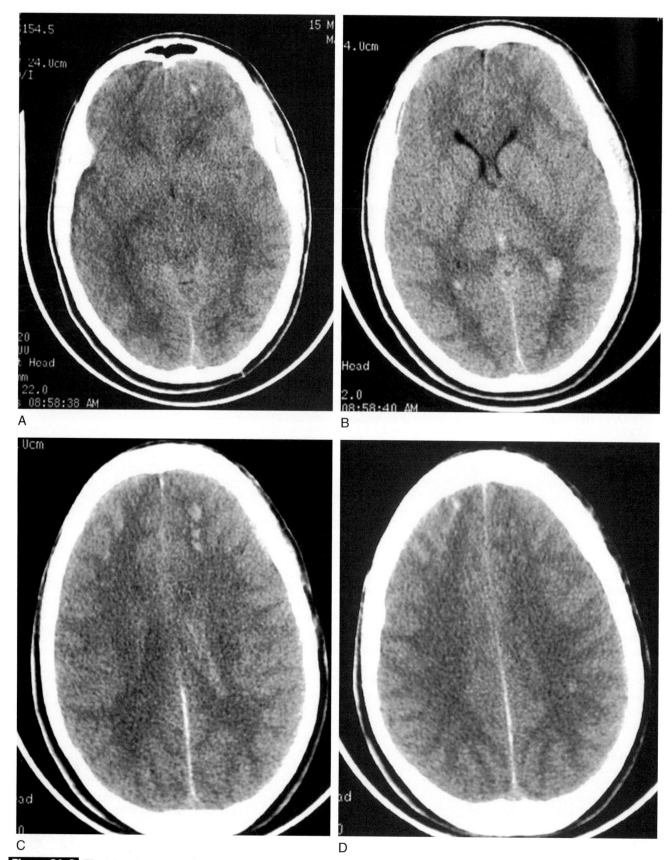

A

B

C

D

Figure 21–3 The "classic" appearance of diffuse axonal injury on an admitting computed tomographic scan includes subarachnoid and intraventricular hemorrhage, brain swelling, and small petechial hemorrhages throughout the brain.

on MRI and can vary from some transient signal changes in the deep white structures to widespread hemorrhagic and nonhemorrhagic shearing injury. The characteristic CT scan appearance of DAI is multiple petechial hemorrhages in the deep white matter and central structures. However, the finding of intraventricular hemorrhage or focal subarachnoid hemorrhage specifically located in the prepontine cistern is also strongly suggestive of DAI.

Gunshot Wounds

Injuries from firearms are a major public health problem in children. Because of the way these injuries are reported, it is difficult to determine the overall incidence of this injury in children. However, recent reports indicate that 10% of all childhood injury deaths are related to firearms, a number exceeded only by deaths from motor vehicle accidents, drowning, and house fires.[62,176] From the standpoint of management and outcome, there is little to differentiate gunshot injuries in children from those in adults. Poor outcome is related to the depth of coma, bilateral or transventricular injury, elevated ICP, and large intracerebral hemorrhages.[138] Nonetheless, most authorities recommend aggressive treatment of all patients except those with clearly nonsurvivable injuries,[90] although substantial neurologic and cognitive deficits can be expected.[55,125]

Injuries caused by nonpowder firearms, such as BB and pellet guns, are three times more frequent than true gunshot wounds in children,[176] with adolescent males having the highest risk for injury.[122] These injuries are generally less severe and therefore associated with lower mortality rates. Surgical treatment is not usually required for BB gun injuries. Pellet rifle injuries, because they are higher-velocity and larger-caliber missile injuries, are more severe and are probably best treated as true gunshot wounds.

Crush Injuries

Young children are susceptible to the unusual static loading-type crushing injury to the skull. These injuries occur as a result of a heavy object's falling on a child or being run over by a vehicle. Crush injuries are dramatic in both clinical and radiographic findings (Fig. 21-4), but neurologic outcomes can be quite good.[48] Multiple skull fractures are typical and include complex basilar skull fractures and facial fractures. CSF leaks and cranial nerve palsies are commonly seen. The mechanism of injury and the clinical findings would suggest overwhelming injury and a poor outcome. However, despite the initial appearance of the injury, many times major cortical structures are preserved. Therefore, if the child has survived the initial injury, aggressive multidisciplinary management can result in satisfactory long-term functional outcomes.

Inflicted Injuries

By far, the most common cause of severe and life-threatening brain injury in infants is inflicted injury (also see Chapter 24). All physicians involved in the care of injured children should be familiar with the clinical manifestations and characteristic radiographic findings of inflicted injuries. This entity has recently been reviewed in detail.[37,47] Infants with an alteration in consciousness, with or without a new onset of seizures, retinal hemorrhages, and acute intracranial hemorrhages on CT scan, are likely to have suffered nonaccidental injuries, especially if the history of the injury is unknown or reported

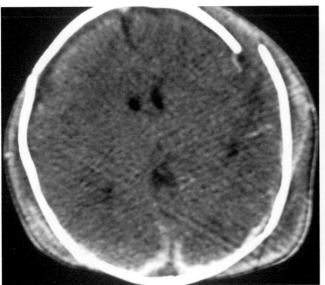

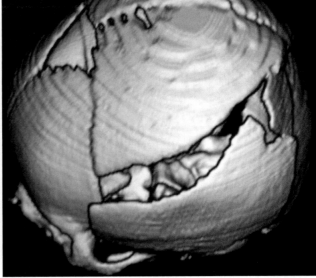

A   B

Figure 21–4 Crushing-type injury in an infant. This computed tomographic (CT) scan (*A*) and 3-D reconstruction (*B*) show a cranial "burst" injury. Despite intracranial hemorrhage and dural laceration, the structure of the brain is preserved and decompressed. The child required dural and cranial reconstruction but recovered with minimal deficits.

to be minor. The additional finding of new or healing skeletal fractures or other solid organ injuries is pathognomonic for this injury. Comprehensive multidisciplinary evaluation by physicians with expertise in child abuse is indicated for all infants who are suspected to have been abused.

Initial Assessment of Brain-Injured Children

The purpose of the initial assessment of a brain-injured patient is twofold. First and most important, one establishes a working diagnosis of the type and severity of the injury in order to direct the selection of initial therapies, as well as the planning and coordination of other diagnostic studies and the management of any associated systemic injuries. Second, one establishes a baseline to measure the effects, both positive and deleterious, of the therapies or interventions.

Historically, the main focus of the initial assessment of brain-injured patients was determining the severity of the injury by assessing the level of consciousness. The most widely used evaluation instrument for this purpose is the Glasgow Coma Scale.[165] This score, as it was designed, correlates well with outcome.[21] However, with the improvements in transport and field resuscitation of severely injured patients, which usually requires the prehospital administration of analgesics and sedation, neurologic assessment to determine the type and severity of brain injury becomes less useful.[161] Furthermore, there is a small, but important group of brain-injured patients who have little or no impairment in consciousness but subsequently deteriorate because of mass lesions or brain swelling.[86,95,114]

Recently, it has become clear that certain findings on CT also correlate well with outcome after brain injury. This radiographic assessment can be obtained rapidly and is not affected by any ongoing therapies. Regardless of the apparent level of consciousness, the early radiographic identification of injury types and the institution of appropriate management or monitoring have substantially improved the overall outcome after traumatic brain injury. Furthermore, it is now clear that a head-injured patient with a completely normal CT scan has an exceedingly low risk for either deterioration or poor outcome. In the author's experience, the CT scan has become the most important element of the early diagnosis of brain injury, especially in young children.

The important CT scan findings involve not only the detection of potentially surgically accessible mass lesions but also the search for and detection of the constellation of findings typically seen with diffuse brain injury: subarachnoid, intraventricular, or intraparenchymal hemorrhage and what may be very subtle early signs of brain swelling, including compression of the perimesencephalic cisterns or shift or compression of the ventricular system. Early identification of the presence of diffuse brain injury on the CT scan is more important than the clinical impression of injury severity. These findings should influence the expectations for outcome and the decisions for monitoring and therapy. The severity of diffuse brain injury can be graded by the appearance of the admitting CT scan. As shown in Figure 21-5, these specific findings correlate well with outcome,[21] and therefore one can make immediate management decisions.

Most current practice parameters regarding the evaluation of head-injured patients include recommendations

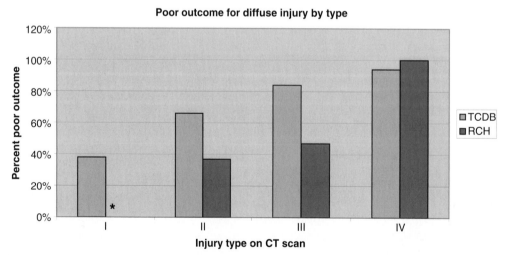

Poor outcome for diffuse injury by type

Figure 21–5 Effect of the appearance of the admission computed tomographic scan on outcome after injury. The data for this graph were generated from information reported from the Traumatic Coma Data Bank (TCDB)[117] and from unpublished data on 1000 consecutive pediatric patients admitted for brain injury to the James Whitcomb Riley Hospital for Children, Indianapolis, IN (RCH). Poor outcome is defined as severely disabled, vegetative survival, or death according to the Glasgow Outcome Scale.[139]
Definitions:
   Diffuse injury I: No visible intracranial pathology seen on computed tomography.
   Diffuse injury II: Cisterns are present with a midline shift of 0 to 5 mm or the presence of lesion densities (or both); no high- or mixed-density lesions larger than 25 cc.
   Diffuse injury III: Cisterns compressed or absent with a midline shift of 0 to 5 mm; no high- or mixed-density lesion larger than 25 cc.
   Diffuse injury IV: Midline shift greater than 5 mm; no high- or mixed-density lesion larger than 25 cc.

for an early diagnostic CT scan.[2,5,21,29,77] Essentially, all potentially severely injured patients, that is, those with an alteration in consciousness, should undergo CT scanning as soon as they are physiologically stable and can be safely transported and maintained in the scanner. For head-injured children with apparently minor trauma, current recommendations allow for clinical assessment and a period of observation without undertaking any neuroimaging, so long there is a clear history of a low-energy mechanism and, at most, only a brief loss of consciousness. One should add that these children should also be completely asymptomatic and neurologically normal and have no complicating medical disorders. On the other hand, any child with a history of more than a few seconds of unconsciousness, a seizure, or clinical signs of cranial impact, skull fracture, cranial penetration, or CSF leak or any child with headache, persistent vomiting, lethargy, or irritability should undergo CT scanning as soon as possible.[78,134] Finally, children who have been injured via high-energy mechanisms that result in apparently isolated chest, abdominal, or skeletal injuries should undergo a CT scan of the brain before the administration of an anesthetic or the institution of narcotic analgesia or sedation that would preclude accurate ongoing neurologic examination.

It should be clear from the previous discussion that plain skull radiography has only a limited and secondary role in the initial evaluation of head injury. CT scanning will detect most clinically important skull fractures. Conversely, skull radiographs provide only limited information about the type and location of any brain injury. MRI is more sensitive than CT scanning for detecting most brain pathology and has supplanted CT as the study of choice for many neurologic disorders. However, for acute traumatic brain injury, all necessary information for making management decisions is still provided by CT scanning. In most circumstances, CT scanning is still more quickly and easily obtained and is less costly than MRI.

Finally, while acknowledging the expanding primary role of neuroimaging in the diagnosis and management of traumatic brain injury, a careful physical and neurologic examination is still extremely important. The entire head should be inspected for indications of impact, scalp injury, cranial deformities, and cranial or orbital penetration. Documentation of cranial nerve function, especially pupillary size, shape, and reactivity, is necessary and will serve as comparison for serial examinations. Evidence of anterior basilar skull fractures, manifested by periorbital ecchymoses, nasal hemorrhage, or CSF rhinorrhea, is a contraindication to the placement of nasogastric tubes until the integrity of the anterior cranial skull base can be determined. Retroauricular bruising, hemotympanum, otorrhagia, and CSF otorrhea are indicative of temporal bone fractures that may not be immediately evident on standard screening CT and may result in the delayed appearance of cranial neuropathy. In the event of possible inflicted injury, dilated funduscopic examination by an ophthalmologist is recommended.[6] Documentation of the level of consciousness and any apparent motor or sensory deficits, along with notation of the presence of confounders to the examination such as intubation, medications, swelling, splints, and other factors, is still a necessary element of the initial evaluation of a head-injured patient.

Early Management of Severe Brain Injury

As stated previously, the primary objective of resuscitation of a brain-injured patient is to preserve cerebral perfusion during transport and evaluation. The ongoing objective of therapy for severe brain injury is to optimize the perfusion of injured and uninjured brain and create a milieu that minimizes the chance for additional secondary injury and maximizes the amount of neuronal recovery. One must do this while avoiding or reversing deleterious processes that would result in further neuronal injury or the expansion of hemorrhagic masses, including systemic complications that directly affect an injured brain such as sepsis, acute lung injury, hyperglycemia, and coagulopathy.

A variety of treatment strategies have been propounded for the treatment of traumatic brain injury. Most of these therapies involve systemic manipulations to achieve what is believed to be either a therapeutic or a protective response. All the "newer" therapies have theoretical attractions, and their proponents report outcomes that appear to be better than those of historical controls. However, at least so far, when these therapies have been tested directly against what could be termed "standard therapies," no benefits have been demonstrated. Consequently, the treatment recommendations currently in place are essentially descriptions of how to apply the historically "standard" therapies of controlled ventilation, fluid management, sedation, and control of blood pressure and ICP.

To do this one must understand as much as possible about the patient's intracranial dynamics and optimize cerebral perfusion by removing surgically accessible masses and managing ICP by safely manipulating, as much as possible, cerebral blood volume (arterial and venous), CSF volume, and brain volume.[112] For severely injured and some less severely injured patients, institution and manipulation of therapies are guided by the placement of an ICP monitor. ICP monitoring provides the basis for making many of the important management decisions for brain-injured patients.[107,120]

The application of individual medical therapies is beyond the scope of this chapter. However, it is important to realize that each of the current therapies for elevated ICP has both general and specific effects and that each has complications associated with its use. The historically common administration of high-dose steroids to brain-injured patients is no longer considered to be beneficial and may, in fact, be harmful. Accordingly, the current guidelines do not recommend that *any* specific therapy, for instance, hyperventilation, osmotic diuretics, or other medications, be administered "prophylactically" or universally for brain-injured patients. It is also suggested that specific therapies be applied in a logical sequence and guided by ICP monitoring and frequent reassessment of response to therapy.

The basic level of therapy for severe traumatic brain injury includes controlled ventilation with maintenance of normal oxygenation and $PaCO_2$ concentrations.

Intubated patients should have adequate sedation and analgesia at all times. Intravascular volume should be supported at all times with blood and fluids to maintain normal hematocrit and electrolyte concentrations. Fluid restriction is not recommended. Hypotonic fluids should be avoided to prevent any trend toward hyponatremia. The head of the bed may be elevated to reduce intracranial venous pressure, as long as normal central venous pressure is maintained by adequate volume replacement. For many severe diffuse brain injuries, this level of therapy may be all that is necessary.

Escalated therapies include the use of CSF drainage, usually by way of a ventricular catheter, osmotic diuresis with mannitol, and mild hyperventilation. Whenever escalation of therapy is considered, one must also escalate the physiologic monitoring for treatment effect and complications. Table 21-1 summarizes the author's approach to escalating medical therapy for brain injury, based on current treatment guidelines. A small percentage of patients require even more intensive therapy for

elevated ICP, including high-dose barbiturates, intensive osmotic therapy, or intensive hyperventilation. These therapies have a higher complication rate and should therefore be used only when absolutely necessary and by physicians with experience in neurologic critical care.

Surgical decision making for severely injured patients is usually straightforward. Clearly, cranial penetrating injuries, including compound skull fractures, require urgent surgical attention. The removal of large, surgically accessible mass lesions may be the first step in the overall therapeutic management of a severe brain injury. Other than that, the initial surgical procedures may be limited to the placement of an ICP monitor, a ventricular catheter, or both. These procedures can be performed at the bedside if necessary. In many cases, such as closed depressed fractures, burst fractures, or comminuted cranial and craniofacial fractures, surgical correction can be performed when the patient is stable or improving from the neurologic injury.

Typically, the major surgical therapy for brain injury involves the removal of traumatic intracranial hematomas. The overall incidence of surgically accessible hematomas in children is substantially lower than that in adults, and the distribution of hematoma types is different. Subdural hematomas are most common in infants, but are rarely of a size that requires surgical removal. As discussed at the outset of this chapter, acute subdural hematomas in older children are generally more indicative of a severe diffuse injury (Fig. 21-6). Extradural hematomas are the

TABLE 21–1 Medical Therapies for Traumatic Brain Injury	
Treatment	**Monitoring**
Evaluation and Resuscitation	
Restoration of normal blood pressure	Systemic blood pressure and oxygenation
Intubation and ventilation	Neurologic examination
	End-tidal CO_2
Basic-Level Therapy	
Elevation of head of bed	Systemic blood pressure and oxygenation
Keep head in neutral position	Intracranial pressure
Sedation and muscular paralysis	Arterial Po_2, Pco_2, and pH
Mechanical ventilation to maintain $Paco_2$ at 35-40 mm Hg	Weight, urine output, pulse, and pulse pressure
Maintain normal to slightly increased intravascular volume	Hemogram, serum electrolytes, glucose, and blood urea nitrogen
Normal fluid and electrolyte status (no fluid restriction); avoid anemia, hyperglycemia	Monitor and aggressively treat for fever and sepsis
Body temperature normal to slightly hypothermic	Computed tomography
Escalated Therapy	
Ventricular cerebrospinal fluid drainage	Ventricular catheter
Mannitol	Central venous pressure
Moderate hyperventilation to maintain $Paco_2$ at 30-35 mm Hg	Serum osmolality and electrolytes
Intensive Therapy for Refractory Intracranial Pressure	
High-dose barbiturate therapy	Continuous or compressed spectral electroencephalography
Lumbar cerebrospinal fluid drainage if indicated	Barbiturate levels
Profound hyperventilation	Jugular venous oxygen saturation, monitors of cerebral blood flow

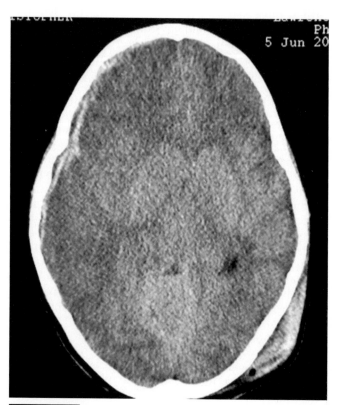

Figure 21–6 Acute subdural hematoma. The hemorrhage overlying the hemisphere (*left* side of the image) seems small. Note, however, the extensive shift of the brain and the hemispheric swelling, which are indicative of severe diffuse injury.

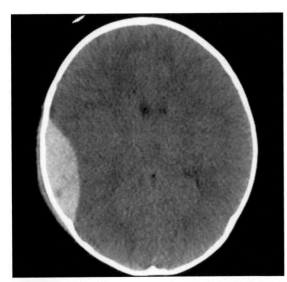

Figure 21-7 Acute extradural hematoma. Note the thickness of the hemorrhagic mass, but also note the lack of shift in comparison to what is demonstrated with a subdural hematoma in Figure 21-6. This lack of swelling and shift is an indication of an uninjured brain responding normally to the expanding mass. As long as this mass is removed before the onset of coma, mortality and morbidity are essentially nil.

more common surgically accessible masses in children, especially older children who have suffered a cranial impact (Fig. 21-7). Small epidural hematomas over the cerebral convexity are likely to resolve without surgical removal. Those that occur in more limited "spaces," such as the temporal fossa or the posterior fossa, are more concerning, and even small epidural hematomas in these locations may need to be removed. Large hemorrhagic contusions or traumatic intracerebral hematomas are very rare in the pediatric age group.[111]

Given this, the decision for removal of a traumatic intracranial hematoma should be part of an overall treatment strategy for the brain injury. Clearly, removal of a large extradural hematoma may be the only therapy needed. On the other hand, in the setting of diffuse brain injury, removal of what would otherwise be considered a nonsurgical intracranial mass can result in substantial improvement in the intracranial volume/pressure relationships that are essential to maintaining adequate cerebral perfusion. Expanding on this concept is the recent rediscovery of "therapeutic decompressive craniectomy." There is a growing, yet completely anecdotal literature about the role of cranial decompressive surgery in the overall management of severe traumatic brain injury.[2,59] The procedure clearly increases available "volume" and lowers ICP. However, it is not clear whether decompressive craniectomy provides an additional or unique benefit over standard medical therapy. It is also not clear when in the course of injury management that this surgical option should be undertaken.

Management of "Minor" Brain Injuries

The vast majority of children with head injury have trivial, minor, or minimal primary brain injuries. These children are destined to recover completely, usually without any intervention whatsoever. However, within this large group there exists a small fraction of patients who are harboring an enlarging hematoma or who are in the early stages of brain swelling. These patients are at increased risk for delayed but rapid deterioration that will result in death or disability. The focus of the evaluation of an apparently minor brain injury is to identify patients who are at risk for neurologic deterioration or delayed complications and to prevent either from occurring.[134] In many ways, diagnosis and management of these patients are more challenging and important than managing severe injuries because successful intervention results almost universally in good outcomes.[95,114]

Recommendations about this issue have been published.[5,156] As with other types of brain injury, early CT scanning is the lynchpin to accurate diagnosis and recognition of brain-injured patients at risk for deterioration.[42,82,106,128] Identification of cisternal compression, hemorrhagic shear and contusion, or small traumatic hematomas indicates that the patient is at risk for deterioration regardless of the level of consciousness. These patients are candidates for frequent reassessment, including repeat neuroimaging, ICP monitoring, and even the early application of therapies to control intracranial dynamics.[110,118] Attention to intravenous fluid management appears to be of major importance because many of the children with apparently trivial brain injuries seem to deteriorate in the face of even mild hyponatremia.[84,159] Therefore, maintenance fluids for these patients, as for most patients with brain injury, should be normal saline or its equivalent.[181] There should also be close attention to maintaining normal intravascular volume and serum electrolyte status.

Although the identification of patients at risk for deterioration includes the appearance of certain abnormalities on CT scanning, an even more important finding from the burgeoning literature about CT scanning and head injury is emerging. Specifically, the finding of a completely normal CT scan in a mildly injured patient is associated with essentially no risk for life-threatening deterioration.[36,160] Given that additional information from a normal CT scan, a child with a history of an accidental minor head injury who does not have a skull fracture, does not have a history of seizures, and is asymptomatic may be released to competent caretakers and not be admitted for observation.

For adolescents who suffer cerebral concussion as a result of sporting activities, there are now published guidelines describing the evaluation and management of such individuals, along with recommendations about when athletes may return to sporting activities after a concussion.[4,23,92,175]

Early Complications of Head Injury

Acute complications of head injury include those related to skull fractures, infectious processes associated with cranial penetration and CSF fistulas, and acute neurologic complications such as post-traumatic epilepsy. As with most aspects of head injury management, recognition of patients with injuries that put them at risk for these complications, followed by appropriate diagnostic studies, monitoring, and when possible, intervention, is key to optimizing outcome.

Complications of Skull Fractures

Simple nondepressed or minimally depressed skull fractures will heal spontaneously. Widely diastatic or cranial burst fractures[45] in young children are indications of dural injury and are not likely to heal without surgical reconstruction. With modern neuroimaging, early identification of these injuries allows early elective repair, thereby avoiding the complication usually referred to in the literature as a "growing skull fracture."[140,177] The typical syndrome of an enlarging skull defect and progressive neurologic deterioration, both of which are related to craniocerebral erosion and an enlarging leptomeningeal cyst that appears over the course of months to years after the injury,[177] is completely avoidable with early repair of the dura and skull. However, focal brain injury is commonly seen with severely depressed, diastatic, and cranial burst fractures, and these patients will have an increased incidence of seizures and focal neurologic deficits.

Basilar Skull Fractures

The major issue of acute clinical importance for patients with presumed basilar fractures is that these fractures are potentially compound and therefore place the patient at increased risk for infection. The obvious indication of CSF leaking from the nose or ear is present in only 10% to 20% of cases.[31,89] Therefore, other signs of basilar fracture must be searched for because these fractures are easily missed on routine neuroimaging studies. Such signs include bilateral orbital ecchymoses or swelling, signs of midface or orbital fracture, hemotympanum, otorrhagia, and Battle's sign. These patients are at increased risk for the development of meningitis for several weeks after the injury. Given this and in view of the fact that compounding of basilar fractures probably occurs more often than not without any evidence of CSF fistulas, it is necessary that parents and caretakers of children who are thought to have sustained a basilar fracture be counseled not only about the importance of recognizing CSF rhinorrhea or otorrhea if it should occur at home but also about the urgent importance of seeking immediate medical attention for children who have signs or symptoms even remotely suggestive of bacterial meningitis up to several weeks after the injury. Despite the increased risk for bacterial meningitis, the administration of prophylactic antibiotics has not been shown to be beneficial.[53,94,146] Some centers are administering pneumococcal vaccine to patients with presumed basilar skull fractures, although it is not yet clear that such vaccination reduces the occurrence of pneumococcal meningitis.

Basilar skull fractures are also associated with cranial neuropathies. The olfactory nerve is the most commonly injured of all cranial nerves and is especially at risk in patients with anterior basilar fractures. Fractures that occur more posteriorly along the skull base or that include the orbit and midface place the optic nerves at risk. Visual loss may be acute or delayed, and ophthalmologic evaluation and follow-up are warranted. Basilar fractures involving the petrous bone can result in auditory, vestibular, or facial nerve injury, or any combination of these injuries. These patients may need otologic evaluation and audiometric studies.[108]

Direct Cerebrovascular Injuries

Although traumatic intracranial aneurysms are exceedingly rare after closed head injury, more than 20% of all post-traumatic aneurysms occur in the pediatric age group.[20] Penetrating injuries, especially stab wounds and deep penetrations, have a high incidence of vascular injury associated with them. Suspicion is raised when a large amount of subarachnoid hemorrhage or a focal intracerebral hemorrhage is seen on the CT scan. CTA or MRA (or both) can screen for injury, but in some cases diagnostic angiography should be performed. If the studies are not conclusive, early repeat imaging is warranted.

Post-traumatic Seizures

One of the most common complications of brain injury, even mild brain injury, is epilepsy. Most studies indicate that the incidence of post-traumatic seizures is substantially higher in children than in adults.[9,115] Risk factors associated with post-traumatic epilepsy include younger age and increasing injury severity.[30,73] However, it is not clear that infants with inflicted injuries, who would have a very high incidence of early epilepsy, were excluded from these studies.[109] If one removes this particular group from the analysis, the incidence of post-traumatic epilepsy in children appears to be relatively low.

A distinction must be made between early and late post-traumatic seizures. Early seizures are generally defined as those that occur within the first week after injury. For pediatric patients, this definition would include the so-called impact-related seizure that occurs in up to 10% of mildly head-injured children.[50,73,104] These seizures are usually self-limited and the CT scan is normal. Treatment is not recommended, and the long-term outcome is good.[41,81] This particular syndrome is almost never seen in head-injured adults, in whom early epilepsy is strongly associated with structural brain injury or subdural hematoma.

For severely head-injured children, that is, children in coma or with structural injury on the admitting CT scan, there is limited and conflicting information regarding the clinical significance and management of early and late post-traumatic epilepsy.[30,170,179] Current recommendations indicate that all patients with severe injury who experience recurrent seizures should be treated with anticonvulsant medication. Phenytoin is the most widely recommended drug for this purpose.[2,26] There is some evidence that prophylactic administration of phenytoin to severely head-injured patients reduces the incidence of *early* post-traumatic seizures, although it is not clear that outcomes after the injury are improved by this therapy.[21] On the other hand, there is strong evidence that routine administration of anticonvulsants to severely head-injured patients neither reduces the incidence of *late* epilepsy nor improves the outcome of the injury. Therefore, administration of anticonvulsants as seizure prophylaxis beyond the first week after the injury is not recommended.[2,21,26]

Postconcussion Syndromes

A syndrome of neurologic dysfunction that seems to be unique to young children has been called the "pediatric concussion syndrome." Shortly after what would seem like a mild cranial impact injury the child exhibits the acute onset of pallor, diaphoresis, and impaired responsiveness. CT scans are normal and the syndrome appears to resolve as rapidly as it occurs. The underlying mechanism is unknown, although it has been suggested that it may be a variation of post-traumatic epilepsy.[152]

Other much more rarely occurring transient neurologic disturbances have been reported after mild head injury in children, including transient cortical blindness, speech arrest, ataxia, receptive dysphasia, and prolonged disorientation.[91,178] CT scans are, again, normal, and the symptoms resolve spontaneously. The etiology is not clear.

Outcomes after Traumatic Brain Injury

There is substantial variability in the reporting of outcomes after childhood head injury. With the exception of infants suffering inflicted head injuries, the overall mortality from head injury in children is roughly half that reported for head injury of similar severity in adults.[21] In larger series of patients, mortality for head injury in children is generally less than 5% for all levels of injury severity and lower than 20% in children defined as having "severe" injuries based on either the Glasgow Coma Scale or other injury severity scoring systems.[102,111,170] Factors related to poor outcomes include high-energy mechanisms, structural injury, swelling and shift on admitting CT scans, persistent or resistant elevations in ICP, the presence of chest or abdominal injuries, and systemic complications.

Traumatic brain injury is the leading cause of acquired disability in childhood.[99] For children who survive traumatic brain injury, neurologic and cognitive outcomes are related to the child's age, the severity of injury, and the amount of permanent structural injury to the brain.[8,14,60,102,119] Children who have suffered severe brain injury are likely to have persistent adverse effects on intellectual function, memory, attention, language, and behavior.[103] It is likely that these deficits have ongoing and perhaps compounding effects on learning and socialization. Consequently, it is possible that the overall neurobehavioral outcomes for significant childhood head injury are worse for children than for similarly injured adults.

Outcomes after inflicted brain injuries deserve separate discussion. This particular injury is associated with the highest mortality and morbidity of childhood head injuries. The reported mortality approaches 40%.[46,49] Morbidity is also high, especially if the infant shows evidence of cerebral infarction or hypoxic-ischemic injury.

Outcomes after Mild Brain Injuries

Mild brain injury, that is, a brain injury with a limited effect on consciousness and with preservation of brain structure, is by far the most common CNS injury in the pediatric age group. Over three quarters of all childhood head injuries are classified as mild.[100,111] Only recently has attention turned to the long-term outcomes after cerebral concussion in children.[154] Although there is still variability in defining mild head injury and the spectrum of severity within that taxonomy,[150,157,169] two general concepts appear to be emerging in the available literature. First, somatic complaints such as headache, visual disturbances, light and noise intolerance, and dizziness and emotional disturbances such as depression, anxiety or irritability, and cognitive impairment, including poor school performance, are common in mildly brain-injured children in the days and weeks immediately after the injury.[57] Second, so long as the child did not suffer any cognitive or behavioral disturbances before the brain injury, all of the early postconcussion symptoms just described appear to resolve completely in no more than a few months.[169]

SPINAL CORD INJURY

Spinal cord injuries in children are rare, but the consequences of such injuries can be devastating. As with traumatic brain injury, modern neuroimaging has contributed considerably to the diagnosis and management of traumatic myelopathy. As discussed at the beginning of this chapter, the major therapeutic efforts for spinal cord injury are the same as for brain injury and are aimed at preventing new primary injury and ameliorating the secondary injury. The first objective is accomplished by maintaining anatomic alignment of the vertebral column during the period of resuscitation and evaluation. The second objective is much more difficult,[3] but begins with supporting blood pressure and oxygenation.

In general, the diagnostic and therapeutic algorithms for children with spinal and spinal cord injury are similar to those used to manage adult patients. Guidelines for the management of spinal cord injury have been published recently and summarize current knowledge.[87] However, there are important differences in clinical manifestations, anatomy, radiographic findings, and management of spinal injuries in children, especially very young children. This section concentrates on these issues.

Epidemiology

Less than 10% of spinal cord injuries or approximately 1000 new spinal cord injuries occur each year in children.[93] Vertebral column injuries that do not involve the spinal cord are much more common. In a series of 122 children, only half the children with vertebral injuries had neurologic deficits.[72]

The mechanisms and pattern of injury are related to both age and gender. In very young children, the male-to-female ratio is roughly equal. In older children, the more "adult" distribution appears, with a male-to-female ratio of about 4:1. Approximately half of pediatric spinal injuries are the result of motor vehicle accidents. A quarter of injuries are the result of diving accidents. Clearly, prevention efforts directed at these two mechanisms alone would dramatically reduce the rate of spinal injury in children. The remaining major mechanisms of injury are falls and sporting activities, each of which accounts for about 10% of reported injuries. Younger children are more likely to be injured as the result of a fall, whereas older children are more likely to be injured in diving accidents or sports.[7,133]

Younger children tend to have spinal column injuries in the cervical region, whereas older children tend to have a distribution of spinal injuries similar to adults.[151] Children are more likely to experience spinal cord injury without apparent vertebral fractures or dislocations. These characteristics are generally thought to be related to the anatomic properties of the juvenile spine and are independent of the mechanism of injury. The pediatric spine has several properties that essentially allow significant, self-reducing displacement of the vertebral column. These properties include increased elasticity of the joint capsules and ligaments, shallow and horizontally oriented facet joints, anterior wedging of the vertebral bodies, and poorly developed uncinate processes.[11,58] Furthermore, young children have disproportionately larger heads and weaker cervical musculature. All of these elements permit a wider range of flexion and extension and rostrocaudal distraction. The fulcrum of motion is higher in the juvenile spine, which explains the greater incidence of rostral injuries in children. This tendency decreases and the incidence of more characteristic vertebral fracture and dislocation increases with increasing age.[10] Finally, it is important to remember that 10% to 15% of spinal injuries in children involve "skip" injuries with vertebral or cord injuries at multiple levels.[72,74] Therefore, depending on the mechanism of injury, when a child is determined to have spinal cord injury or vertebral disruption, the entire spinal axis should be surveyed for other injuries.

Injuries to the thoracic and lumbar spine are uncommon in children. Less than 20% of all spinal injuries in children occur below the cervical spine.[143] Major mechanisms involve falls from heights and high-energy motor vehicle accidents, including the characteristic spinal distraction injury resulting from automobile lap belts.[71]

The Clinical Spectrum of Spine and Spinal Cord Injury

Because spinal cord injury is rare in children, it may be overlooked, especially in the very young and those with multiple injuries. As discussed in the next section, the presence of apparently normal plain radiographic studies will not completely rule out either vertebral

instability or spinal cord injury. Therefore, one must have an increased index of suspicion based on injury mechanism and the neurologic findings. High-energy mechanisms such as motor vehicle accidents and falls from heights are more likely to cause spinal or spinal cord injury. An unconscious patient of any age should be assumed to have a spinal cord injury until a complete assessment is possible.

The clinical indicator of spinal injury in awake patients is pain and muscular spasm or guarding against movement. Any child complaining of neck or back pain or stiffness after an injury needs a complete assessment of the integrity and stability of the spine. Children can suffer torticollis as the result of atlantoaxial rotatory subluxation. Rotatory subluxation can occur as the result of apparently minor injury or even a coughing spell. Such children are usually neurologically normal. Plain radiographs can be deceiving, but CT scan of the spine in the axial plane is diagnostic.[162]

The cardinal sign of a spinal cord injury is neurologic dysfunction below an anatomic spinal motor or sensory level. Complete or severe incomplete cord injuries with motor dysfunction are readily detectable in conscious patients. A spinal cord injury is generally manifested as symmetrical flaccid paralysis with sensory loss at the same anatomic level. There are strong indirect indicators of spinal cord injury in a comatose patient or those with multiple injuries. Cervical spinal cord injuries can cause profound systemic hypotension, a syndrome known as "neurogenic shock" and caused by disruption of sympathetic pathways below the level of injury. Unlike the more common hypovolemic shock, neurogenic shock is suggested by the finding of bradycardia in the face of hypotension. These patients are also vasodilated despite being hypothermic. Hypovolemic shock results in hypotension, tachycardia, and vasoconstriction. Other systemic findings suggesting spinal cord injury include paradoxical respiration, priapism, Horner's syndrome, and an inability to sweat.

Less severe injuries may result in transient neurologic dysfunction, dysesthesias, focal weakness, sensory loss, or dissociation of motor and sensory function such as in Brown-Séquard or other central cord syndromes. Any history of transient neurologic dysfunction involving the limbs or bladder, regardless of duration and apparent complete recovery, must be taken as strong evidence of spinal cord injury.

Spinal Cord Injury without Radiographic Abnormality

Spinal cord injury without radiographic abnormality (SCIWORA) was defined by Pang and Wilberger in 1982 to describe patients who exhibit objective findings of traumatic myelopathy with no evidence of fracture or ligamentous instability on routine screening plain radiography or CT scanning.[137] SCIWORA is essentially an injury of children, especially younger children, and is probably directly related to the biomechanical properties of the juvenile spine outlined earlier. As with vertebral injury, there is a tendency toward more rostral injury with younger age. Younger children suffering SCIWORA are more likely to have severe or complete cord injuries than older children are. Severe spinal cord injury in older children is more typically associated with a vertebral injury than with SCIWORA.[72,132,136]

Diagnosis of this syndrome is complicated by the frequent occurrence of delayed neurologic deficits. Many children with this injury will demonstrate neurologic deficits hours to days after the reported injury and in the absence of any further injury.[136] The mechanism of this delayed deterioration is unknown, but Pang has speculated that there is repeated injury to an already mildly injured spinal cord, either because of the innate normal flexibility of the spine or because of subtle ligamentous injury with increased segmental movement at the injury site.[135] This argument is supported by the observation that recurrent SCIWORA may occur in about 20% of children who are not immobilized and that immobilization of the cervical spine markedly reduces the incidence of this phenomenon.[142]

Finally, this syndrome was initially described before the widespread use of MRI for the diagnosis of spinal disease. Although it is still true that these children do not have evidence of bony injury or overt instability on plain spine radiographs or CT scans, most (but not all) patients will have evidence of spinal cord or ligamentous or other soft tissue injury on MRI.[34,43,69] Therefore, it is essential that all physicians who provide early evaluations of injured children be aware of this disorder and continue to consider the possibility of spinal or spinal cord injury, even when the initial radiographic studies may be reported as normal.

Initial Assessment of Spine or Spinal Cord Injury

Detection of spinal injury in a child can be challenging. As with brain injury, the initial clinical findings will guide the decision for selecting diagnostic imaging. Unlike brain injury, plain spine radiography is still an important initial tool for assessment of a spinally injured patient. Any child who has neck pain, muscular guarding of spinal movement, or a neurologic deficit or who has multiple injuries from a high-energy mechanism, especially one that includes "distraction" of the spine, such as would occur with a seat-belted passenger in a motor vehicle collision, has a spinal injury until proved otherwise.

Older children who are normally conscious can express appropriate clinical symptoms and signs that indicate spinal or neural injury. Current recommendations indicate that an older child who is awake and conversant and who has no neurologic deficit, or a history of one, or any pain or tenderness along the posterior spinal midline needs no further radiographic assessment or other diagnostic studies.[87] Such is not the case for younger children, who are at higher risk for occult spinal and spinal cord injury simply because they are unable to express complaints of pain.[98] Therefore, a lower threshold for radiographic screening must apply to younger children.

There are now fairly well proven "decision rules" for performing screening radiographic studies, specifically, anteroposterior, lateral, and open-mouth odontoid views in adult patients.[79,80] These studies indicate that there is extremely low probability of injury and low yield on radiographic studies if patients exhibit the following five criteria: no midline cervical tenderness, no focal neurologic deficit, normal alertness, no intoxication, and no painful distracting injury. The application of these decision rules to pediatric patients suggested similar findings, although the number of very young children in the study cohort was limited.[173] Accordingly, the caveats about young children also apply to this recommendation.

Radiographic surveys of the spine in pediatric patients are complicated by the normal anatomic variations in the juvenile spine that are described in the preceding section. Growth centers and synchondroses can be mistaken for traumatic injuries. The increased normal flexibility of the spine commonly appears as "pseudosubluxation."[24,158] Most pseudosubluxation occurs between the second and third vertebral bodies, with allowable displacement of up to 4 mm in children younger than 8 years. This movement, along with the normal anterior movement between the atlas and the dens,[163] can be mistaken for ligamentous injury. Therefore, spinal radiographic studies obtained in children must be interpreted with caution and with complete familiarity with developmental anatomy of the spine.

Flexion-extension radiographs can be used to rule out ligamentous injury of the cervical spine in awake and cooperative patients. However, most studies investigating the utility of dynamic radiographs have indicated that instability is not likely to be detected on these studies if routine static studies show normal alignment in the neutral position.[52,145]

CT scanning of the spine is extremely helpful for detecting subtle fracture, soft tissue swelling, and rotatory subluxation, as well as for defining congenital abnormalities and developmentally normal variations that may mimic fractures on plain radiographs. Furthermore, CT is a rapid and accurate way to detect compromise of the spinal canal or nerve root foramina after traumatic injury. However, many spinal injuries are ligamentous and may be missed if CT scanning is the only study performed. Therefore, CT should be viewed as an adjunctive study to plain radiography, not a substitute.

MRI is now the best study to image the injured spinal cord and to detect subtle ligamentous and other soft tissue injuries. As discussed earlier, many, but not all patients with SCIWORA will show abnormalities on MRI that confirm the clinical diagnosis. Findings on MRI correlate with outcome after spinal cord injury.[35,69,155] However, it is not clear that the management decisions required for spinal cord injury in children have been altered by any findings on MRI.[87]

Early Management of Spinal Cord Injury

As with traumatic brain injury, aggressive support of systemic perfusion and oxygenation is of paramount importance. Because children will tend to have more rostral cervical cord injuries, impaired respiratory function is likely to be a concern. Furthermore, gastric dilatation commonly accompanies acute spinal injuries, and this can add a substantial mechanical barrier to effective respiration. Therefore, early nasogastric decompression of the stomach should be considered. For midlevel and higher cervical injuries, elective intubation may be needed to support respiration until a comprehensive assessment of the injury is completed. Endotracheal intubation of a spinally injured child is technically challenging and should be performed by an expert without manipulating the relative position of the head and neck.

Restoration and support of systemic blood pressure will result in maintenance of perfusion of the injured spinal cord. Patients with severe cord injuries, especially in the cervical portion, are at most risk for systemic hypotension. Although the initial resuscitation can be undertaken with intravascular volume loading, neurogenic hypotension should be treated with vasopressors. Resuscitation and maintenance of normal blood pressure in a patient with a spinal cord injury are complicated and may be aided by invasive monitoring of central venous pressure.

The pharmacotherapy of spinal cord injury has been the subject of active research and scientific controversy. After completion and reporting of the second National Spinal Cord Injury Study (NASCIS-II),[15] it was recommended that all patients with acute spinal cord injuries be administered high-dose methylprednisolone. The recommendations did not officially extend to pediatric patients, but most centers applied these treatment recommendations to all age groups. Despite a subsequent study[16] that appeared to confirm the initial findings, the methodology and conclusions of these studies have been seriously questioned.[85,87] At this time, the administration of high-dose steroids to spinally injured patients, including children, is listed as a treatment option that should be undertaken only with the knowledge that evidence suggesting harmful side effects is more consistent than any suggestion of clinical benefit.[87]

Early surgical therapy is rarely needed. Most pediatric fractures and dislocations can be reduced and maintained in anatomic alignment with a variety of orthotic devices, including a halo brace. Early surgical reduction and fusion are considered only for cases in which clear neurologic deterioration is occurring in the face of irreducible subluxation or compression from bone fragments, extruded disk material, or an enlarging hematoma. These issues are unusual in young children. Adolescents suffer injury types similar to adults and can be treated according to the surgical recommendations available for adult patients.[87] There is limited scientific information about the advisability and outcomes of operative management of spinal injury in young children, although recent reports indicate that surgical instrumentation is becoming more common.[54,61] Anatomic reduction of deformity, stabilization of clearly unstable injuries, and decompression of neural elements are indications cited for surgical treatment of spinal injury in children. Most of these goals can be accomplished nonoperatively. Current recommendations indicate that most vertebral injuries in young children should initially be treated nonoperatively, with surgical management reserved for persistent or progressive deformity or ligamentous instability.[87]

Complications

Children are subject to all the complications associated with spinal injury, including skin breakdown, infections, deep venous thrombosis, autonomic dysreflexia, contractures, spasticity, neurogenic bladder and bowel, and progressive spinal deformity.[180] However, the single major acute complication of spinal cord injury in children is respiratory compromise. The most common cause of death in the acute phase of injury is respiratory failure.[40] Aggressive pulmonary care is essential, and ventilatory support may be necessary until the accessory muscles of respiration can strengthen. Many of the other complications can be avoided or minimized by the early intervention of physiatrists and other rehabilitation specialists.

The incidence of venous thromboembolism in spinally injured children has been reported, probably incorrectly, to be roughly similar to that in adults.[180] However, series involving only pediatric patients indicate that this complication is extremely rare.[144] Therefore, specific recommendations for prophylaxis of this possible complication vary widely. For adults and, presumably, older children and adolescents, thromboprophylaxis consisting of low-molecular-weight or low-dose heparin in combination with rotating beds, pneumatic compression stockings, or electrical stimulation is recommended for up to 12 weeks after the injury.[87,180]

Outcomes

The mortality associated with spinal cord injury in children has been reported to be 28%, which is significantly higher than the mortality rate for this injury reported in adults.[75,135] The majority of these deaths appeared to occur at the scene and would not be affected by current management strategies. For survivors of spinal injury, outcomes are related to the level and severity of injury. Complete injuries remain complete, and although limited functional improvement may be seen over time, full recovery is not expected.[72,74,132,136] Children with incomplete spinal cord injuries have a good chance of showing significant functional improvement, even to complete recovery.[72,74]

The cost of long-term care for these injuries is staggering. The lifetime cost of care for a child with a spinal cord injury ranges in the millions of dollars.[39,133,153] This cost must be added to the loss of productivity that accompanies these devastating injuries. The adult employment rate for individuals suffering childhood spinal cord injury is about 50%.[180] Factors associated with successful employment were younger age at injury, less severe neurologic impairment, better education, longer duration of living with the sequelae of the injury, and ability to drive independently.

REFERENCES

1. Adams JH: Brain damage in fatal non-missile head injury in man. In Braakman R (ed): The Handbook of Clinical Neurology, vol 13, Head Injury. New York, Elsevier, 1990, p 43.
2. Adelson PD, Bratton SL, Carney NA, et al: Guidelines for the acute medical management of severe traumatic brain injury in infants, children and adolescents. Crit Care Med 2003;31:S417.

3. Amar AP, Levy ML: Pathogenesis and pharmacological strategies for mitigating secondary damage in acute spinal cord injury. Neurosurgery 1999;44:1027.

4. American Academy of Neurology: Practice parameter: The management of concussion in sports (summary statement). Neurology 1997;48:581.

5. American Academy of Pediatrics: The management of minor closed head injury in children. Pediatrics 1999;104:1407.

6. American Academy of Pediatrics: Shaken baby syndrome: Rotational cranial injuries—technical report. Pediatrics 2001;108:206.

7. Anderson JM, Schutt AH: Spinal injury in children: A review of 156 cases seen from 1950 through 1978. Mayo Clin Proc 1980;55:499.

8. Anderson V, Catroppa C, Morse S, et al: Recovery of intellectual ability following traumatic brain injury in childhood: Impact of injury severity and age at injury. Pediatr Neurosurg 2000;32:282.

9. Annegers JF, Hauser WA, Coan SP, Rocca WA: A population-based study of seizures after traumatic brain injuries. N Engl J Med 1998;338:20.

10. Apple JS, Kirks DR, Merten DF, Martinez S: Cervical spine fractures and dislocations in children. Pediatr Radiol 1987;17:45.

11. Bailey DK: The normal cervical spine in infants and children. Radiology 1952;59:712.

12. Bekar, A, Ipekoglu Z, Tureyen K, et al: Secondary insults during intrahospital transport of neurosurgical intensive care patients. Neurosurg Rev 1998;21:98.

13. Bergsneider M, Hovda DA, Shalmon E, et al: Cerebral hyperglycolysis following severe traumatic brain injury in humans: A positron emission tomography study. J Neurosurg 1997;86:241.

14. Berryhill P, Lilly MA, Levin HS, et al: Frontal lobe changes after severe diffuse closed head injury in children: A volumetric study of magnetic resonance imaging. Neurosurgery 1995;37:392.

15. Bracken MB, Shepard MJ, Collins WF, et al: A randomized, controlled trial of methylprednisolone or naloxone in the treatment of acute spinal cord injury: Results of the second National Acute Spinal Cord Injury Study. N Engl J Med 1990;322:1405.

16. Bracken MB, Shepard MJ, Holford TR, et al: Administration of methylprednisolone for 24 or 48 hours or tirilizad mesylate for 48 hours in the treatment of acute spinal cord injury. Results of the third National Acute Spinal Cord Injury randomized controlled trial. National Acute Spinal Cord Injury Study. JAMA 1997;277:1597.

17. Brookes M, MacMillan R, Cully S, et al: Head injuries in accident and emergency departments. How different are children from adults? J Epidemiol Commun Health 1990;44:747.

18. Bruno A, Biller J, Adams HP, et al: Acute blood glucose levels and outcome from ischemic stroke: Trial of ORG 10172 in Acute Stroke Treatment (TOAST) investigators. Neurology 1999;59:280.

19. Bruns J, Hauser WA: The epidemiology of traumatic brain injury: A review. Epilepsia 2003;44:2.

20. Buckingham MJ, Crone KR, Ball WS, et al: Traumatic intracranial aneurysms in childhood: Two cases and a review of the literature. Neurosurgery 1988;22:398.

21. Bullock RM, Chesnut RM, Clifton GL, et al: Guidelines for the management of severe traumatic brain injury. J Neurotrauma 2000;17:451.

22. Caldicott DG, Pearce A, Price R, et al: Not just another 'head lac' ... low-velocity, penetrating intra-cranial injuries: A case report and review of the literature. Injury 2004;35:1044.

23. Cantu RC: Return to play guidelines after a head injury. Clin Sports Med 1998;17:45.

24. Cattell HS, Filtzer DL: Pseudosubluxation and other normal variations in the cervical spine in children. A study of one hundred and sixty children. J Bone Joint Surg Am 1965;47:1295.

25. Chan KH, Mann KS, Yue CP, et al: The significance of skull fracture in acute traumatic intracranial hematomas in adolescents: A prospective study. J Neurosurg 1990;72:189.

26. Chang BS, Lowenstein DH: Practice parameter: Antiepileptic drug prophylaxis in severe traumatic brain injury. Neurology 2003;60:10.

27. Cherian L, Goodman JC, Robertson CS: Hyperglycemia increases brain injury caused by secondary injury after cortical impact in rats. Crit Care Med 1997;25:1378.

28. Chesnut RM: Avoidance of hypotension: Conditio sine qua non of successful severe head injury management. J Trauma (Suppl) 1997;42:S4.

29. Chesnut RM: Management of brain and spine injuries. Crit Care Clin 2004;20:25.

30. Chiaretti A, De Benedictus R, Polidori G, et al: Early post-traumatic seizures in children with head injury. Childs Nerv Syst 2000;16:862.

31. Cooper PR: Cerebrospinal fluid fistulas and pneumocephalus. In Barrow DL (ed): Complications and Sequelae of Head Injury. Park Ridge, IL, American Association of Neurological Surgeons, 1992, p 1.

32. CRASH Trial Collaborators: Effect of intravenous corticosteroids on death within 14 days in 10008 adults with clinically significant head injury (MRC CRASH trial): Randomized placebo-controlled trial. Lancet 2004;364:1321.

33. Curran C, Dietrich AM, Bowman MJ, et al: Pediatric cervical spine immobilization: Achieving neutral position? J Trauma 1995;39:729.

34. Dare AO, Dias MS, Li V: Magnetic resonance imaging correlation in pediatric spinal cord injury without radiographic abnormality. J Neurosurg 2002;97(Suppl):33.

35. Davis PC, Reisner A, Hudgins PA, et al: Spinal injuries in children: Role of MR. AJNR Am J Neuroradiol 1993;14:607.

36. Davis RL, Mullen N, Makela M, et al: Cranial computed tomography scans in children after minimal head injury with loss of consciousness. Ann Emerg Med 1994;24:640.

37. Deputy S: Shaking-impact syndrome of infancy. Semin Pediatr Neurol 2003;10:112.

38. De Santis A, Cappricci E, Granata G: Early post traumatic seizures in adults: Study of 84 cases. J Neurosurg Sci 1979;23:207.

39. De Vivo MJ: Causes and cost of spinal cord injury in the United States. Spinal Cord 1997;35:809.

40. De Vivo MJ, Black KJ, Stover SL: Causes of death during the first 12 years after spinal cord injury. Arch Phys Med Rehabil 1993;74:248.

41. Dias MS, Carnevale F, Li V: Immediate posttraumatic seizures: Is routine hospitalization necessary? Pediatr Neurosurg 1999;30:232.

42. Dias MS, Lillis KA, Calvo C, et al: Management of accidental minor head injuries in children: A prospective outcomes study. J Neurosurg (Pediatrics) 2004;101:38.

43. Dickman CA, Zabramski JM, Hadley MN, et al: Pediatric spinal cord injury without radiographic abnormalities: Report of 26 cases and review of the literature. J Spinal Disord 1991;4:296.

44. DiRoio C, Jourdan C, Mottolese C, et al: Craniocerebral injury resulting from transorbital stick penetration in children. Childs Nerv Syst 2000;16:503.

45. Donahue DJ, Sanford RA, Muhlbauer MS, et al: Cranial burst fracture in infants: Acute recognition and management. Childs Nerv Syst 1995;11:692.

46. Duhaime AC, Christian C, Moss E, et al: Long-term outcome in infants with shaking-impact syndrome. Pediatr Neurosurg 1996;24:292.

47. Duhaime AC, Christian CW, Roarke LB, Zimmerman RA: Nonaccidental head injury in infants—the "shaken-baby syndrome." N Engl J Med 1998;338:1822.

48. Duhaime AC, Eppley M, Margulies S, et al: Crush injuries to the head in children. Neurosurgery 1995;37:401.

49. Duhaime AC, Gennarelli TA, Thibault LT, et al: The shaken baby syndrome: A clinical, pathological, and biomechanical study. J Neurosurg 1987;66:409.

50. Duhaime AC, Sutton LN: Delayed sequelae of pediatric head injury. In Barrow DL (ed): Complications and Sequelae of Head Injury. Park Ridge, IL, American Association of Neurological Surgeons, 1992, p 169.

51. du Trevou MD, van Dellen JR: Penetrating stab wounds to the brain: The timing of angiography in patients presenting with the weapon already removed. Neurosurgery 1992;31:905.

52. Dwek JR, Chung CB: Radiography of cervical spine injury in children: Are flexion-extension radiographs useful for acute trauma? AJR Am J Roentgenol 2000;174:1617.

53. Einhorn A, Mizrahi EM: Basilar skull fractures in children. The incidence of CNS infection and the use of antibiotics. Am J Dis Child 1978;132:1121.

54. Eleraky MA, Theodore N, Adams M, et al: Pediatric cervical spine injuries: Report of 102 cases and review of the literature. J Neurosurg 2000;92(Suppl):12.

55. Ewing-Cobbs L, Thompson NM, Miner ME, et al: Gunshot wounds to the brain in children and adolescents: Age and neurobehavioral development. Neurosurgery 1994;35:225.

56. Faden AI, Demediuk P, Panter SS, et al: The role of excitatory amino acids and NMDA receptors in traumatic brain injury. Science 1989;244:798.

57. Farmer MY, Singer HS, Mellitus ED, et al: Neurobehavioral sequelae of minor head injuries in children. Pediatr Neurosci 1987;13:304.

58. Fesmire FM, Luten RC: The pediatric cervical spine: Developmental anatomy and clinical aspects. J Emerg Med 1989;7:133.

59. Figaji AA, Fieggen AG, Peter JC: Early decompressive craniotomy in children with severe traumatic brain injury. Childs Nerv Syst 2003;19:666.

60. Filley CM, Cranberg LD, Alexander MP, Hart EJ: Neurobehavioral outcome after closed head injury in childhood and adolescence. Arch Neurol 1987;44:194.

61. Finch GD, Barnes MJ: Major cervical spine injuries in children and adolescents. J Pediatr Orthop 1998;18:811.

62. Fingerhut LA, Kleinman JC, Godfrey E, et al: Firearm mortality among children, youth, and young adults 1-34 years of age, trends and current status: United States, 1979-88. Monthly Vital Stat Rep 1991;39(Suppl):1.

63. Gabriel EJ, Ghajar J, Jagoda A, et al: Guidelines for prehospital management of traumatic brain injury. J Neurotrauma 2002;19:113.

64. Garton HJL, Luerssen TG: Head injuries. In Biller J, Bogousslavsky J (eds): Clinical Trials in Neurologic Practice. Boston, Butterworth Heinemann, 2001, p 77.

65. Gausche M, Lewis RJ, Stratton SJ, et al: Effect of out-of-hospital pediatric endotracheal intubation on survival and neurological outcome: A controlled clinical trial. JAMA 2000;283:783.

66. Gennarelli TA, Adams JH, Graham DI: Diffuse axonal injury—a new conceptual approach to an old problem. In Baethmann A, Go KG, Unterberg A (eds): Mechanisms of Secondary Brain Damage. New York, Plenum Press, 1986, p 15.

67. Gennarelli TA, Segawa H, Wald V, et al: Physiological response to angular acceleration of the head. In Grossman RG, Gildenberg, PL (eds): Head Injury: Basic and Clinical Aspects. New York, Raven Press, 1982, p 129.

68. Gennarelli TA, Thibault LE: Biological models of head injury. In Becker DP, Povlishok JT (eds): Central Nervous System Trauma Status Report 1985. Bethesda, MD, NINCDS/NIH, 1985, p 391.

69. Grabb PA, Pang D: Magnetic resonance imaging in the evaluation of spinal cord injury without radiographic abnormality in children. Neurosurgery 1994;35:406.

70. Graham DI: The pathology of brain ischemia and possibilities for therapeutical intervention. Br J Anaesth 1985;57:3.

71. Greenwald TA, Mann DC: Pediatric seatbelt injuries: Diagnosis and treatment of lumbar flexion-distraction injuries. Paraplegia 1994;32:743.

72. Hadley MN, Zabramski JN, Browner CM, et al: Pediatric spinal trauma: Review of 122 cases of spinal cord and vertebral column injuries. J Neurosurg 1988;68:18.

73. Hahn YS, Fuchs S, Flannery AM, et al: Factors influencing posttraumatic seizures in children. Neurosurgery 1988;22:864.

74. Hamilton MG, Myles ST: Pediatric spinal injury: Review of 174 hospital admissions. J Neurosurg 1992;77:700.

75. Hamilton MG, Myles ST: Pediatric spinal injury: Review of 61 deaths. J Neurosurg 1992;77:705.

76. Hansen JE, Gudeman SK, Holgate RC, Saunders RA: Penetrating intracranial wood wounds: Clinical limitations of computed tomography. J Neurosurg 1988;68:752.

77. Haydel MJ, Preston CA, Mills TJ, et al: Indications for computed tomography in patients with minor head injury. N Engl J Med 2000;343:100.

78. Haydel MJ, Shembekar AD: Prediction of intracranial injury in children aged five years and older with loss of consciousness after minor head injury due to nontrivial mechanisms. Ann Emerg Med 2003;42:507.

79. Hoffman JR, Mower WR, Wolfson AB, et al: Validity of a set of clinical criteria to rule out injury to the cervical spine in patients with blunt trauma. N Engl J Med 2000;343:94.

80. Hoffman JR, Wolfson AB, Todd K, et al: Selective cervical spine radiography in blunt trauma: Methodology of the National Emergency X-Radiography Utilization Study (NEXUS). Ann Emerg Med 1998;32:461.

81. Holmes JF, Palchak MJ, Conklin MJ, Kuppermann N: Do children require hospitalization after immediate posttraumatic seizures? Ann Emerg Med 2004;43:706.

82. Hsiang JNK, Yeung T, Yu ALM, et al: High risk mild head injury. J Neurosurg 1997;87:234.

83. Huerta C, Griffith R, Joyce SM: Cervical spine stabilization in pediatric patients: Evaluation of current techniques. Ann Emerg Med 1987;16:1121.

84. Humphreys R, Hendrick EB, Hoffman H: The head-injured child "who talks and dies." A preventable problem? In Marlin A (ed): Concepts in Pediatric Neurosurgery X. Basel, Karger, 1990, p 196.

85. Hurlbert RJ: Methylprednisolone for acute spinal cord injury: An inappropriate standard of care. J Neurosurg 2000;93(Suppl):1.

86. Iverson GL, Lovell MR, Smith S, Franzen MD: Prevalence of abnormal CT-scans following mild head injury. Brain Inj 2000;14:1057.

87. Joint Section on Disorders of the Spine and Peripheral Nerves of the American Association of Neurological Surgeons and the Congress of Neurological Surgeons: Guidelines for the management of acute cervical spine and spinal cord injuries. Neurosurgery 2002;50(Suppl):S166.

88. Jones PA, Andrews PJD, Midgley S, et al: Measuring the burden of secondary insults in head-injured patients during intensive care. J Neurosurg Anesthesiol 1994;6:4.

89. Kadish HA, Schunk JE: Pediatric basilar skull fracture: Do children with normal neurologic findings and no intracranial injury require hospitalization? Ann Emerg Med 1995;26:37.

90. Kaufman HH: Treatment of civilian gunshot wound to the head. Neurosurg Clin N Am 1991;2:387.

91. Kaye EM, Herskowitz J: Transient post-traumatic cortical blindness: Brief v prolonged syndromes in childhood. J Child Neurol 1986;1:206.

92. Kelly JP, Nichols JS, Filley KO, et al: Concussion in sports: Guidelines for the prevention of catastrophic outcome. JAMA 1991;266:2867.

93. Kewalramani LS, Kraus JF, Sterling HM: Acute spinal cord lesions in a pediatric population: Epidemiological and clinical features. Paraplegia 1980;18:206.

94. Klastersky J, Sadeghi M, Brihaye J: Antimicrobial prophylaxis in patients with rhinorrhea or otorrhea. A double-blind study. Surg Neurol 1976;6:111.

95. Klauber MR, Marshall LF, Luerssen TG, et al: Determinants of head injury mortality: Importance of the low risk patient. Neurosurgery 1989;24:31.

96. Kraus JF: Epidemiological features of brain injury in children: Occurrence, children at risk, causes and manner of injury, severity and outcomes. In Broman SH, Michel ME (eds): Traumatic Head Injury in Children. New York, Oxford University Press, 1995, p 22.

97. Kraus JF, Rock A, Hemyari P: Brain injuries among infants, children, adolescents and young adults. Am J Dis Child 1990;144:684.

98. Laham JL, Cotcamp DH, Gibbons PA, et al: Isolated head injury versus multiple trauma in pediatric patients: Do the same indications apply? Pediatr Neurosurg 1994;122:431.

99. Lazar MF, Menaldino S: Cognitive outcome and behavioral adjustment in children following traumatic brain injury: A developmental perspective. J Head Trauma Rehabil 1995;10:55.

100. Lescohier I, DiScala C: Blunt trauma in children: Causes and outcomes of head versus intracranial injury. Pediatrics 1993;91:721.

101. Levi L, Guilburd JN, Linn S, Feinsod M: The association between skull fracture, intracranial pathology and outcome in pediatric head injury. Br J Neurosurg 1991;5:617.

102. Levin HS, Aldrich EF, Saydjari C, et al: Severe head injury in children: Experience of the Traumatic Coma Data Bank. Neurosurgery 1992;31:435.

103. Levin HS, Ewing-Cobbs L, Eisenberg HM: Neurobehavioral outcome of pediatric closed head injury. In Michel ME, Broman SH (eds): Traumatic Head Injury in Children. New York, Oxford University Press, 1995, p 70.

104. Lewis RJ, Lee L, Inkelis SH, Gilmore D: Clinical predictors of post traumatic seizures in children with head trauma. Ann Emerg Med 1993;22:1114.

105. Lloyd DA, Carty H, Patterson M, et al: Predictive value of skull radiography for intracranial injury in children with blunt head injury. Lancet 1997;349:821.

106. Lobato R, Rivas J, Gomez P, et al: Head-injured patients who talk and deteriorate into coma: Analysis of 211 cases studied with computerized tomography. J Neurosurg 1991;75:256.

107. Luerssen TG: Intracranial pressure: Current status in monitoring and management. Semin Pediatr Neurol 1997;4:146.

108. Luerssen TG: Skull fractures after closed head injury. In Albright LA, Pollack IF, Adelson PD (eds): Principles and Practice of Pediatric Neurosurgery. New York, Thieme, 1999, p 813.

109. Luerssen TG, Huang JC, McLone DG, et al: Retinal hemorrhages, seizures and intracranial hemorrhages: Relationships and outcomes in children suffering traumatic brain injury. In Marlin AE (ed): Concepts in Pediatric Neurosurgery XI. Basel, Karger, 1991, p 87.

110. Luerssen T, Hults K, Klauber M, et al: Improved outcome as a result of recognition of absent and compressed cisterns on initial CT scans. In Hoff J, Betz A (eds): Intracranial Pressure VII. Berlin, Springer-Verlag, 1989, p 598.

111. Luerssen TG, Klauber MR, Marshall LF: Outcome from head injury related to patient's age: A longitudinal prospective study of adult and pediatric head injury. J Neurosurg 1988;68:409.

112. Luerssen TG, Wolfla CE: Pathophysiology and management of increased intracranial pressure in children. In Andrews BT, Hammer GB (eds): Pediatric Neurosurgical Intensive Care. Park Ridge, IL, American Association of Neurological Surgeons, 1997, p 37.

113. Maier-Hauff K, Baethmann AJ, Lange M, et al: The kallikrein-kinin system as mediator in vasogenic brain edema. Part 2—studies on kinin formation in focal and perifocal brain tissue. J Neurosurg 1984;61:97.

114. Mandera M, Wencel T, Bazowski P, Krauze J: How should we manage children after mild head injury? Childs Nerv Syst 2000;16:156.

115. Mansfield RT: Head injury in children and in adults. Crit Care Clin 1997;13:611.

116. Margolis LH, Wagenaar AC, Liu W: The effects of a mandatory child restraint law on injuries requiring hospitalization. Am J Dis Child 1988;142:1099.

117. Marshall LF, Marshall SB, Klauber LF, et al: A new classification of head injury based on computerized tomography. J Neurosurg 1991;75(Suppl):S14.

118. Marshall LF, Toole BA, Bowers SB: The National Traumatic Coma Data Bank Part 2: Patients who talk and deteriorate: Implications for treatment. J Neurosurg 1983;59:285.

119. Mataro M, Poco MA, Sahuquillo J, et al: Neuropsychological outcome in relation to the Traumatic Coma Data Bank classification of computed tomography imaging. J Neurotrauma 2001;18:869.

120. Mayer SA, Chong JY: Critical care management of increased intracranial pressure. J Intensive Care Med 2002;17:55.

121. Mayer T, Walker ML, Johnson D, et al: Causes of morbidity and mortality in severe pediatric trauma. JAMA 1981;245:719.

122. McNeill AM, Annest JL: The ongoing hazard of BB and pellet gun–related injuries in the United States. Ann Emerg Med 1995;26:187.

123. Megur K, Tator CH: Effect of multiple trauma on mortality and neurological recovery after spinal cord or cauda equina injury. Neurol Med Chir 1988;28:34.

124. Miller JD, Sweet RC, Narayan R, Becker DP: Early insults to the injured brain. JAMA 1978;240:439.

125. Miner ME, Ewing-Cobbs L, Kopaniky DR, et al: The results of treatment of gunshot wounds to the brain in children. Neurosurgery 1990;26:20.

126. Mono J, Hollenberg RD, Harvey JT: Occult transorbital intracranial penetrating injuries. Ann Emerg Med 1986;15:589.

127. Murray JA, Demetirades D, Berne TV, et al: Prehospital intubation in patients with severe head injury. J Trauma 2000;49:1065.

128. Nagy K, Joseph K, Krosner S, et al: The utility of head computed tomography after minimal head injury. J Trauma 1999;46:268.

129. Nelson DE, Bixby-Hammett D: Equestrian injuries in children and young adults. Am J Dis Child 1992;146:611.

130. Ommaya AK: Biomechanics of head injury: Experimental aspects. In Nahum AM, Melvin J (eds): The Biomechanics

of Trauma. Norwalk, CN, Appleton-Century-Crofts, 1985, p 245.

131. Ommaya AK, Gennarelli TA: Cerebral concussion and traumatic unconsciousness: Correlation of experimental and clinical observations of blunt head injuries. Brain 1974;97:633.

132. Osenbach RK, Menezes AH: Spinal cord injury without radiographic abnormality in children. Pediatr Neurosci 1989;15:168.

133. Osenbach RK, Menezes AH: Pediatric spinal cord and vertebral column injury. Neurosurgery 1992;30:385.

134. Palchak MJ, Holmes JF, Vance CW, et al: A decision rule for identifying children at low risk for brain injuries after blunt head trauma. Ann Emerg Med 2003;42:492.

135. Pang D: Spinal cord injuries. In McLone DG (ed): Pediatric Neurosurgery, 4th ed. Philadelphia, WB Saunders, 2001, p 660.

136. Pang D, Pollack IF: Spinal cord injury without radiographic abnormality in children—the SCIWORA syndrome. J Trauma 1989;29:654.

137. Pang D, Wilberger JE: Spinal cord injury without radiographic abnormalities in children. J Neurosurg 1982;57:114.

138. Paret G, Barzilai A, Lahat E, et al: Gunshot wounds in brains of children: Prognostic variables in mortality, course, and outcome. J Neurotrauma 1998;15:967.

139. Pettigrew LEL, Wilson JTL, Teasdale G: Assessing disability after head injury: Improved use of the Glasgow Outcome Scale. J Neurosurg 1998;89:939.

140. Pezzotta S, Silvani V, Gaetani P, et al: Growing skull fractures in childhood. J Neurosurg Sci 1985;29:129.

141. Pigula FA, Wald SL, Shackford SR, Vane DW: The effect of hypotension and hypoxia on children with severe head injuries. J Pediatr Surg 1993;28:310.

142. Pollack IF, Pang D, Sclabassi R: Recurrent spinal cord injury without radiographic abnormalities in children. J Neurosurg 1988;69:177.

143. Proctor MR: Spinal cord injury. Crit Care Med 2002;30(Suppl):S489.

144. Radecki RT, Gaebler-Spira D: Deep vein thrombosis in the disabled pediatric population. Arch Phys Med Rehabil 1994;75:248.

145. Ralston ME, Chung K, Barnes PD, et al: Role of flexion-extension radiographs in blunt pediatric cervical spine injury. Acad Emerg Med 2001;8:237.

146. Rathore MH: Do prophylactic antibiotics prevent meningitis after basilar skull fracture? Pediatr Infect Dis J 1991;10:87.

147. Rivara FP: Epidemiology and prevention of pediatric traumatic brain injury. Pediatr Ann 1994;23:12.

148. Rivara FP, Thompson DC, Thompson RS, et al: The Seattle Children's bicycle helmet campaign: Changes in helmet use and head injury admissions. Pediatrics 1994;93:567.

149. Rovlias A, Kotsou S: The influence of hyperglycemia on neurological outcome in patients with severe head injury. Neurosurgery 2000;46:335.

150. Ruff RM, Jurica P: In search of a unified definition for mild traumatic brain injury. Brain Inj 1999;13:943.

151. Ruge JR, Sinson GP, McLone DG: Pediatric spinal injury: The very young. J Neurosurg 1988;68:25.

152. Ryan CA, Edmonds J: Seizure activity mimicking brain stem herniation in children following head injuries. Crit Care Med 1988;16:812.

153. Sadowsky CL, Margherita A: The cost of spinal cord injury care. Spine 1999;13:593.

154. Satz P, Zaucha K, McCleary C, et al: Mild head injury in children and adolescents: A review of studies (1970-1995). Psychol Bull 1997;122:107.

155. Schaefer DM, Flanders AE, Olsterholm JL, et al: Prognostic significance of MRI in acute phase of spinal injury. J Neurosurg 1992;76:218.

156. Schutzman SA, Barnes P, Duhaime AC, et al: Evaluation and management of children younger than two years old with apparently minor head trauma: Proposed guidelines. Pediatrics 2001;107:983-993.

157. Servadei F, Teasdale G, Merry G, et al: Defining acute mild head injury in adults: A proposal based on prognostic factors, diagnosis, and management. J Neurotrauma 2001;18:657.

158. Shaw M, Burnett H, Wilson A, Chan O: Pseudosubluxation of C2 on C3 in polytraumatized children: Prevalence and significance. Clin Radiol 1999;54:377.

159. Snoek J, Minderhoud J, Wilmink J: Delayed deterioration following mild head injury in children. Brain 1984;107:15.

160. Stein SC, Ross SE: The value of computed tomographic scans in patients with low-risk head injuries. Neurosurgery 1990;26:638.

161. Stocchetti N, Pagan F, Calappi E, et al: Inaccurate early assessment of neurological severity in head injury. J Neurotrauma 2004;21:1131.

162. Suback BR, McLaughlin MR, Albright AL, Pollack IF: Current management of pediatric atlantoaxial rotatory subluxation. Spine 1998;23:2174.

163. Sullivan CR, Bruwer AJ, Harris LE: Hypermobility of the cervical spine in children. A pitfall in the diagnosis of cervical dislocation. Am J Surg 1958;95:636.

164. Tator CH, Koyanagi I: Vascular mechanisms in the pathophysiology of human spinal cord injury. J Neurosurg 1997;86:483.

165. Teasdale G, Jennett B: Assessment of coma and impaired consciousness: A practical scale. Lancet 1974;2:81.

166. Teasdale GM, Murray G, Anderson E, et al: Risks of acute traumatic intracranial hematoma in children and adults: Implications for managing head injuries. BMJ 1990;300:363.

167. Thompson DC, Rivara FP, Thompson R: Helmets for preventing head and facial injuries in bicyclists (Cochrane Review). In The Cochrane Library, Issue 2, 2002. Oxford, Update Software.

168. Thompson HJ, Tkacs NS, Saatman KE, et al: Hyperthermia following traumatic brain injury: A critical evaluation. Neurobiol Dis 2003;12:163.

169. Thompson MD, Irby JW: Recovery from mild head injury in pediatric populations. Semin Pediatr Neurol 2003;10:130.

170. Tilford JM, Simpson PM, Yeh TS, et al: Variations in therapy and outcome for pediatric head trauma patients. Crit Care Med 2001;29:1056.

171. Vane DW, Keller MS, Sartorelli KH, Miceli AP: Pediatric trauma: Current concepts and treatments. J Intensive Care Med 2002;17:230.

172. Vespa PM, Nuwer MR, Nenov V, et al: Increased incidence and impact of nonconvulsive and convulsive seizures after traumatic brain injury as detected by continuous electroencephalographic monitoring. J Neurosurg 1999;91:750.

173. Viccellio P, Simon H, Pressman BD, et al: A prospective multicenter study of cervical spine injury in children. Pediatrics 2001;108:E20.

174. Wang HE, Peitzman AB, Cassidy LD, et al: Out-of-hospital endotracheal intubation and outcome after traumatic brain injury. Ann Emerg Med 2004;44:439.

175. Warren WL, Bailes JE: On the field evaluation of athletic head injuries. Clin Sports Med 1998;17:13.

176. Wilson MH, Baker SP, Teret SP, et al: Saving Children: A Guide to Injury Prevention. New York, Oxford University Press, 1991, p 149.

177. Winston K, Beatty RM, Fischer EG: Consequences of dural defects acquired in infancy. J Neurosurg 1983;59:839.
178. Yamamoto LG, Bart RD: Transient blindness following mild head trauma. Clin Pediatr (Phila) 1988;27:479.
179. Young KD, Okada PJ, Sokolove PE, et al: A randomized, double-blinded, placebo controlled trial of phenytoin for the prevention of early posttraumatic seizures in children with moderate to severe blunt head injury. Ann Emerg Med 2004;43:435.
180. Zidek K, Srinivasan R: Rehabilitation of a child with a spinal cord injury. Semin Pediatr Neurol 2003;10:140.
181. Zornow MH, Prough DS: Fluid management in patients with traumatic brain injury. New Horizons 1995;3:488.

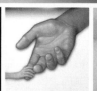

Chapter 22

Vascular Injury

Joseph J. Tepas III

Principles of polysystem injury management have undergone significant change during the past decade. The evolution of damage-control surgery; the progress in understanding traumatic stress, especially as related to the management of systemic inflammatory response syndrome; and the emergence of increasingly sophisticated imaging technology have all contributed to a more precise and effective system of care for the severely injured. Included in this evolution has been continued refinement of the principles of evaluating and managing vascular injuries.[15] Validation of the predictive accuracy of clinical examination and better definition of indications for arteriography have led to more timely operative intervention based on effective resuscitation, accurate assessment of associated injuries, and anticipation of reperfusion injury.[13,17] With the emergence of endovascular technology, acute management of some vascular injuries may well move from the operating room to the angiography suite. At the heart of managing vascular injuries, however, is the technical repair of damaged blood vessels and restoration of peripheral perfusion. Although the basic surgical skills required are similar for patients of all ages, infants and children have unique characteristics that can present significant challenges.[9,21,31,32,39]

EPIDEMIOLOGY

In the adult population, most vascular injury is the result of penetrating trauma.[4] This is not so for infants and children.[20,30] Blunt injury predominates in the pediatric population, with almost half of all vascular injuries in children resulting from this type of mechanism. Table 22-1 lists

the mechanism and mortality for 1368 children with at least one vascular injury recorded in the National Pediatric Trauma Registry (NPTR) between 1989 and 2001. Although this represents only 1.3% of registry cases, the 13% crude mortality rate (compared with a 2.9% rate for the entire registry) demonstrates the lethality of these injuries and the variability of outcome based on body region affected (Table 22-2).

As in the adult population, vascular trauma can be divided into injuries that involve major truncal vessels and extremity injuries that disrupt peripheral perfusion. In children, the latter are commonly associated with skeletal fractures rather than penetrating injury. In fact, the incidence of vascular injury occurring in children with penetrating extremity trauma is remarkably low. Victoroff et al.[46] reviewed their experience with 75 children sustaining 76 penetrating extremity injuries (gunshot wounds) treated at National Children's Medical Center from 1985 to 1989. There were no documented vascular injuries and only two nerve injuries caused by bullets or bullet fragments. The greater majority of injuries were minor musculoskeletal disruption from which recovery was quick and complete. Data from the NPTR listed in Table 22-2 indicate a similarly low mortality for extremity injuries, but with a significantly higher rate

TABLE 22–1 Injury Mechanism in 1368 Children in National Pediatric Trauma Registry II and III

Mechanism	Proportion (%)	Mortality (%)
Penetrating	52	10
Blunt	47	17
Crush	1	8

TABLE 22–2 Distribution of 1628 Vascular Injuries in 1368 Children in National Pediatric Trauma Registry II and III

Region	ICD-9-CM	Total No.	No. Lived	No. Died (%)	% Operated
Neck	900-901	249	196	53 (21)	41
Chest	901-902	161	98	63 (39)	70
Abdomen, pelvis	902-903	374	248	126 (34)	50
Upper extremity	903-904	497	494	3 (1)	21
Lower extremity	904-905	326	318	8 (3)	36

ICD-9-CM, International Classification of Diseases, 9th ed, Clinical Modification.

of vascular operative intervention, as indicated by International Classification of Diseases, 9th edition, Clinical Modification (ICD-9-CM) operative codes 35.00 through 39.

Vascular injury in childhood has two distinct components. In addition to the inury resulting from external mechanical force, the increasing use of complex endovascular diagnostic and therapeutic procedures continues is associated with a low but consistent incidence of iatrogenic damage to vascular structures.[24,34,39] With increasing refinement of technique and improved technology, however, this appears to be decreasing.[39]

EVALUATION

General principles of assessment of acute vascular disruption are based on clinical evaluation. Regardless of cause, suspicion of vascular injury should stimulate a logical system of clinical assessment based first on the patient's history. During the initial clinical assessment, two immediate questions must be answered: (1) Is there evidence of disruption of the integrity of the circulatory system? (2) Is perfusion adequate? Despite the implied causal relationship of these two points, each can be deranged without immediate effect on the other. Prolonged postinjury spasm, a common characteristic of childhood vascular trauma, may cause peripheral ischemia in an otherwise anatomically intact vascular tree. Conversely, effective collateral circulation, enhanced by the absence of obliterative vascular disease, may sustain distal circulation despite deranged proximal flow. Thus, not every disruption of vascular flow produces immediate peripheral ischemia, and evidence of acute ischemia may not necessarily portend operative vascular injury. Regardless of circumstances, confirmation or restoration of cellular perfusion is the immediate priority in assessing any child with a vascular injury.[32]

Numerous investigators have validated the predictive accuracy of thorough clinical examination and, in the process, have refined the indications for arteriography.[13,16] The latter issue is especially important in pediatric patients because of the increased potential for additional iatrogenic injury. Frykberg et al.[16] demonstrated the predictive accuracy of "hard" signs of injury and recommended immediate operative intervention for any patient with active bleeding, expanding hematoma, pulse deficit, or bruit or thrill. Nonexpanding hematoma, hypotension, peripheral nerve deficit, or a history of bleeding from the wound were considered "soft" signs that required only clinical observation. Long-term follow-up of this population has confirmed the predictive accuracy of this approach and has validated the authors' initial recommendation that routine arteriography is not necessary for the management of proximity injury.[5,17] For children, the issue of angiography is even more relevant because of the risk of iatrogenic injury to tiny vessels, contrast toxicity, and the increased frequency of persistent spasm as the major cause of ischemia. Reichard et al.[38] analyzed the predictive accuracy of clinical signs in their review of 75 children with vascular injury treated on the pediatric trauma service

at Cook County Hospital. Part of their report included a comparison to 12 children managed by an "adult" protocol that required arteriography. None of the studies performed for proximity alone was abnormal. All 10 children with vascular injury had hard signs. Four of 77 children with no vascular injury also manifested at least one hard sign, yielding a 100% sensitivity and 95% specificity of physical examination. Of note is that these data validate similar recommendations published by Meagher et al.[30] in 1979 and emphasize that arteriography for acute injury should be considered only if the risk of performance is outweighed by a risk of ischemia that cannot be defined by history and clinical signs.[6,29,40] This is especially so when considering "one-shot" emergency department arteriography, despite recent reports of the safety and efficacy of this approach.[23] For chronic injury, however, arteriography is considered essential for accurate planning of revascularization.

Duplex Doppler, B-mode ultrasonography, multidetector computed tomography-angiography, and magnetic resonance angiography are newly established technologies in clinical imaging. The first two are reasonably portable and can define flow and flow velocity. Their role in the diagnosis of acute injury, however, has not been well established. The last two are the result of continued evolution of computer-enhanced imaging. They offer the capability of visualizing vascular anatomy and flow without direct invasion of the arterial tree.[44] Recent reports have demonstrated the value of these modalities in diagnosing suspected vascular injuries in children. Three-dimensional reconstructions can precisely define both the level of injury and the efficiency of collateral circulation (Fig. 22-1). Although noninvasive techniques avoid cannulation of the arterial tree, a higher volume of contrast material may be required. Patient selection must therefore consider the risk of arterial injury versus the potential toxicity of the contrast agent.

Children usually do not suffer from atherosclerotic vascular disease. Because their vessels are elastic, they usually stretch and transiently deform, rather than rupture, in response to the application of force. The immediate effect of this is an increased potential for flow disruption secondary to intimal tears. The effect of such decreased flow may be acute ischemia or marginal insufficiency that stimulates increased collateralization. Whereas the former should be easily discernible on clinical examination, the latter can be very subtle and clinically silent. Therefore, functional and anatomic integrity of the circulation must be clinically confirmed and documented in every injured child. Of equal importance is the understanding that the unexplainable absence of palpable pulses, especially in the lower extremities, may be the result of preexisting rather than acute injury. If perfusion pressure is suddenly lowered because of other acute injuries, collateral circulation may become inadequate, and symptoms of progressive ischemia may emerge. In their analysis of the predictive accuracy of clinical findings of pediatric vascular injury, Reichard et al.[38] extol the accuracy of the ankle-brachial index (ABI) as indicative of inadequate peripheral perfusion. Their data suggest that an ABI less than 0.99 indicates clinically critical vascular injury, reinforcing

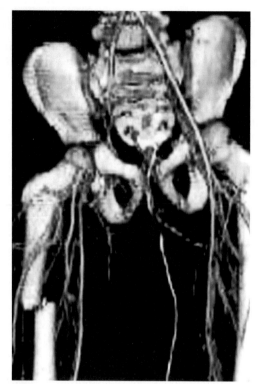

Figure 22–1 Computed tomographic angiogram from a 5-year-old hit by a car. He underwent repair of transposition of the great vessels as an infant and was noted to have a pulseless right foot. Evaluation demonstrated a clinically silent femoral artery disruption.

intensive care nursery discharge data that suggest that the true incidence of vascular injury is higher than previously believed. In fact, findings reported by Seibert et al.[43] suggest that assessment of the peripheral pulses and measurement of the ABI should be part of the routine postdischarge assessment of any baby treated with an umbilical artery catheter.

TRAUMATIC INJURIES

Traumatic injuries can be divided into those involving the trunk (neck and torso) and those involving the extremities (upper or lower). Each area presents unique challenges to accurate diagnosis and timely management.

Truncal Injuries

Cervical vascular injuries appear to be rare in childhood. To test their proposed algorithm for the diagnosis of blunt cervical vascular injury, Rozycki et al.[41] reviewed injuries associated with a cervicothoracic seat-belt sign in 797 motor vehicle crash victims treated over 17 months by the Grady Memorial Hospital Trauma Service. The 3% of patients with carotid injury were all adults. No injuries were missed, and none were noted in children. With the gradual increase in compliance with child-restraint laws, the potential association between seat-belt marks and significant vascular injury will require continued

close follow-up. Cox's[2] review of the operative management of 36 children with vascular injuries included 9 children with 11 carotid or jugular injuries. Eight of these were penetrating neck injuries. Mortality occurred in only two of the three hemodynamically unstable children.

Torso vascular injuries are relatively rare in childhood. This is probably the result of the greater elasticity of young, healthy vessels. Although children are not immune to thoracic vascular disruption, most series that include pediatric patients demonstrate a low incidence compared with adults. Clinical reports of aortic injuries in children suggest that the natural history is no different from that of adults. Mortality is extremely high, especially for those children with a presenting systolic blood pressure below 90 mm Hg. Eddy et al.[8] reviewed the King County coroner's records over a 12-year period (1975 to 1987), and found 13 cases of aortic disruption in children. Only three of these children reached a hospital alive, and just one survived. Experience in the NPTR is somewhat more heartening, in that 26 of 54 children (48%) with aortic ruptures survived to hospital discharge. This representative sample from multiple contributing hospitals in North America is similar to that reported from a single institution by Cox et al.,[2] suggesting that the outcome from this catastrophic injury may be better than that consistently reported for adults. Major thoracic venous injuries are even less common and are usually associated with major pulmonary disruption.

Because of the preponderance of blunt injury in the pediatric population, especially as a result of vehicle-related mishaps, abdominal vascular injuries can and do occur.[7] Arterial disruption is far less common than venous disruption. Hypotension progressing to frank shock is the most common associated finding, making the decision to explore the abdomen relatively straightforward, expect when a solid viscus injury is the most likely cause. Fayiga et al.[11] reviewed 18 years of experience in the operative management of pediatric blunt vascular injuries. Twenty-one major abdominal venous injuries were present in 17 patients and were lethal in 11 (65%). None of the abdominal venous injuries was recognized before laparotomy. As in numerous other series, survival was directly related to hemodynamic stability at presentation. Most complications were related to nonvascular injuries. The majority of vascular injuries were repaired directly, which parallels the experience from a similar series of 16 abdominal vascular injuries reported by Cox et al.,[2] wherein interposition grafts were required to repair only one aortic disruption and one superior mesenteric artery transection.

Extremity Injuries

The vast majority of lower extremity vascular injuries are the result of blunt mechanisms, are arterial, and are commonly associated with skeletal fracture.[9,14,22] Popliteal injuries, in particular, are often the result of sports and cycling mishaps. Initial assessment must confirm the presence of palpable distal pulses and adequate capillary perfusion. Immediate reduction of displaced fracture fragments or subluxated joints often results in restoration of palpable distal pulses. If the duration of ischemia has been longer than 6 hours, the possibility of evolving compartment syndrome should prompt the consideration of fasciotomy.[45] Interposition of reversed contralateral saphenous vein remains the treatment of choice for all disrupted segments. Synthetic material should be considered only as a last resort when autologous vessel cannot be harvested and fabricated into a patch or conduit.[31] Anastomoses are constructed using monofilament simple sutures.[32] As the repair is being completed, the distal clamp is first released to confirm adequate backflow. The proximal clamp is then released to flush any residual air or clot before the final sutures are tied. Vasospasm, if significant, can usually be reduced by gentle mechanical dilation using coronary artery dilators. Veins should be repaired before arteries. Children who have undergone repair of venous injuries should be anticoagulated for 48 hours postoperatively. Some authors use heparin; others simply use dextran solutions for 2 to 3 days postoperatively. Reed et al.[37] reported their experience with seven children with popliteal artery injuries who underwent immediate operative repair. Four had blunt and three had penetrating injuries. Associated morbidity included three fractures, four severe soft tissue wounds, and one nerve injury. All patients underwent angiography. Three angiograms were intraoperative, so presumably the four preoperative studies were required to confirm the diagnosis. Treatment included two primary repairs and four vein graft bypasses. Anastomoses were spatulated and sutured in an interrupted fashion. One child required fasciotomy. There were no deaths, amputations, or reoperations. At the time of their report (1990), follow-up ranged between 10 and 42 months. All patients had normal Doppler pressures or distal pulses. These data illustrate the relationship between prompt, aggressive treatment and successful outcome. Other investigators report similar recommendations and emphasize that the high proclivity for prolonged vasospasm makes arterial anastomosis in childhood especially challenging.[11]

The vast majority of extremity vascular injuries in children are associated with axial skeletal disruption. In its most severe form, this combination of bone and soft tissue destruction can result in what has been called the "mangled extremity." It is usually characterized by major soft tissue avulsion that can be associated with significant tissue loss. Initial assessment must consider tissue viability, anticipated limb function, and the need for amputation of a potential source of massive tissue necrosis and sepsis. The Mangled Extremity Severity Score (MESS) has been proposed as an accurate system of evaluation and prediction of limb salvage (Table 22-3). Although originally devised for adults, Fagelman et al.[10] demonstrated that the MESS had a predictive accuracy of 93% when retrospectively applied to 36 injured children. Vascular disruption associated with fractures must be addressed immediately so that subsequent axial skeletal repair will produce a viable extremity. Restoration of flow may be accomplished by temporary bypass until fracture fixation is achieved. When possible, venous repair should precede arterial repair.

TABLE 22-3 Mangled Extremity Severity Score (MESS)

Factor	Score
Skeletal/soft tissue injury	
Low-energy (stab, simple fracture, pistol gunshot wound)	1
Medium energy (open or multiple fractures, dislocation)	2
High energy (high-speed crash, rifle gunshot wound)	3
Very high energy (high-speed injury, gross contamination)	4
Limb ischemia	
Reduced/absent pulse, normal perfusion	1*
Pulseless, paresthesias, poor capillary refill	2*
Cool, insensate, paralyzed, numb	3*
Shock	
Systolic blood pressure always >90 mm Hg	1
Transient hypotension	2
Persistent hypotension	3
Age (yr)	
<30	1
30-50	2
>50	3

*Score doubled for ischemia >6 hr.
MESS >7 = 100% prediction for amputation.

Devitalized tissue must be debrided, and fasciotomy should be considered. Nerve function must be evaluated and documented before debating amputation. Although it is true that children recover amazingly well from what may initially appear to be devastating injuries, being permanently crippled by an insensate, immobile extremity is a poor alternative to an active life with a functional and properly fitted prosthesis. The decision to amputate is therefore based on an assessment of limb viability and a prediction of limb functionality. The MESS serves as a reasonable guideline, but the ultimate decision rests with the surgeon, the child's parents, and, when possible, the child.

Upper extremity vascular injury is usually associated with supracondylar fractures. Axillary stretch injuries, especially when associated with high-energy forces, such as vehicular ejection, may disrupt arterial or venous structures, producing a hematoma that is not as precisely definable as those seen with more distal injuries. In addition to signs of obvious blood loss, diffuse edema of the axilla or shoulder region and diminution of peripheral pulses should prompt angiographic confirmation of both the existence and the anatomic configuration of the injury.

Supracondylar fractures may disrupt brachial arterial flow by direct injury or by compression, with or without prolonged spasm. As with the lower extremity, definitive management begins with an assessment of the adequacy of perfusion and confirmation of the vessel's integrity. Of interest is a recent report that describes use of the ipsilateral basilic vein as an ideal interposition graft for the reconstruction of vessels in which segmental loss has occurred.[27] Salvage from damage of upper extremity injuries is generally good, with return of functionality related to the nature of the associated musculoskeletal and neurologic disruption. The incidence of compartment syndrome as a result of prolonged ischemia in the upper extremity is reported to be significantly lower than that for lower extremity injuries; however, careful follow-up for adequate perfusion and avoidance of postischemia muscle contracture must be part of long-term management.

IATROGENIC INJURY

Despite the evolution of increasingly sophisticated methods of imaging for infants and children, the potential for damage to the vascular integrity of a small child or tiny infant remains ever present. There have been numerous reports over the past decade describing this particular problem.[1,12,34,36] Many have been case reports of complications from some usually innocuous maneuver of routine care. Demircin et al.,[3] for example, reported an infant with brachial artery pseudoaneurysm resulting from inadvertent puncture during antecubital venipuncture. The lesion was repaired by direct suture under proximal compression. Gamba et al.[19] reviewed their experience with iatrogenic vascular lesions in low-birth-weight neonates. Of 335 infants encountered between 1987 and 1994, 9 (2.6%) were diagnosed with vascular injury. Mean birth weight was 880 g (range, 590 to 1450 g), although the mean weight at diagnosis was 1825 g (range, 1230 to 2730 g). Injuries were associated with venipuncture in seven of the nine cases and included six femoral arteriovenous fistulas, two of which were bilateral. One carotid lesion and five femoral arteriovenous fistulas were repaired using microvascular technique. Outcome as determined by follow-up clinical examination and Doppler flow studies was excellent, leading the authors to emphasize the role of aggressive medical and microsurgical management of these injuries. In 1981 O'Neill et al.[35] reviewed their experience with the surgical management of 41 infants with major thromboembolic problems associated with umbilical artery catheters. Although most complications were related to emboli distal to the femoral artery, eight infants required emergency operative intervention for acute aortic obstruction. Four infants underwent transverse aortic thrombectomies, three of whom recovered completely. As principles of umbilical artery catheter management have become better established, these problems appear to have become less frequent.

The increasing use of extracorporeal membrane oxygenation has raised the question of the potential need to reconstruct cervical vessels, especially when the process of oxygenation support involves the use of both the carotid artery and the jugular vein. LaQuaglia et al.[26] described their experience in nine children with iatrogenic arterial injuries repaired with microsurgery. An operating microscope was routinely used, and repair was performed using 9-0 to 11-0 nylon suture. Spasm was controlled with topical 2% lidocaine or papaverine. As microsurgical technique continues to evolve and better suture materials become available, this approach will become an increasingly valuable adjunct to the management of major injuries to tiny vessels.

The femoral artery remains the most common site of iatrogenic injury. As noted earlier in the discussion of traumatic injury, efficient collateralization of the pelvis and gluteal region may result in these lesions remaining clinically silent throughout most of childhood. Lin et al.[28] analyzed 1674 diagnostic or therapeutic catheterizations performed in 1431 infants between 1986 and 2001. Thirty-six procedures were required in 34 children. The authors stratified complications into nonischemic, acute femoral ischemia, and chronic femoral ischemia. Nonischemic lesions included pseudoaneurysms ($n = 4$), arteriovenous fistulas ($n = 5$), and groin hematomas ($n = 5$). All were repaired directly, using interrupted polydioxanone (PDS) or polypropylene (Prolene) sutures. Acute femoral ischemic lesions were the most common and required a variety of procedures from thrombectomy to patch repair. Chronic femoral ischemia was defined as evidence of flow disruption noted after 30 days post procedure. Seven children presented with clinical signs an average of 193 days (range, 31 to 842) after the index procedure. All seven were symptomatic with claudication, leg length discrepancy, or gait disturbance. Operative repair consisted of revascularization using reversed saphenous vein for ileofemoral bypass in five children and femorofemoral bypass in one child. Only one child required patch angioplasty. The authors' analysis of potential contributory factors identified a statistically significant predictive relationship for patient age younger than 3 years, more than three previous catheterizations, performance of a therapeutic versus simple diagnostic maneuver, and use of guiding catheters larger than 6 French. The value of this study lies both in the identification of potentially predictive factors and in the documentation of the relatively short time required for chronic ischemia to become symptomatic. Children at risk of vascular injury with any abnormal clinical finding must be followed for at least 5 years, and preferably through the start of adolescence. Limb length discrepancy as a result of disruption of a major vascular structure may not become manifest until years after the precipitating event.[48] Recent reports have suggested that operative revascularization of iatrogenic injury before adolescence corrects some limb length discrepancy; however, these have been relatively small series and do not represent a consensus.

As is the case with the management of traumatic injury, the high proclivity for spasm and the need to differentiate prolonged spasm from arterial disruption are challenging components of the initial assessment. Prolonged spasm is thought to be the result of intimal injury, which causes derangement of nitric oxide production and disrupts the control of arterial wall tension.[18,33] When endothelial-medial contact is lost, as can be caused by shearing friction from an oversized or overzealously placed catheter, underlying vascular smooth muscle is incapable of relaxation.[25] Angiographic confirmation of spasm requires the additional risk of the very mechanism suspected of causing the problem. Computed tomography-angiography or magnetic resonance arteriography may be the solution to this clinical conundrum, although the dose and concentration of contrast must be carefully considered when comparing risk and benefit. The role of spasm in causing gangrene is controversial, despite case reports suggesting cause and effect.[42]

From a clinical perspective, once spasm has been confirmed to be the sole cause of diminished peripheral perfusion, management must focus on the confirmation of evidence of tissue viability and absence of signs of evolving compartment syndrome or peripheral ischemia. Assuming that the basic cause of acute spasm is at least partly related to intimal injury, the risk of thrombosis must be a primary consideration. Over the past few years, routine anticoagulation therapy has been supplemented by thrombolytic agents, especially urokinase.[20] Recommended doses of urokinase vary and tend to be empirical. Up to 6000 U/kg per hour have been used in infants, with good success and no complications. Most recently, a report by Zenz et al.[49] on the use of tissue plasminogen activator suggested that more rapid restoration of flow could be achieved with this drug.

Digital Ischemia Syndrome

Intravenous catheter–related, ipsilateral digital ischemia may suddenly develop in infants or small children with an acute infectious disease, usually associated with dehydration and hypovolemia. In a review of 104 cases, Villavicencio et al.[47] reported primary involvement of the hand in 68.2% of patients and of the foot in the remainder. The age of the patients ranged from 29 days to 36 months (mean age, 14 months). The infectious process was of respiratory origin in 27.8% of cases, localized to the gastrointestinal tract in 60.5%, and localized to other areas in 11.5%. The most frequently cultured microorganisms were *Escherichia coli*, *Salmonella*, *Shigella*, *Streptococcus*, *Staphylococcus*, *Klebsiella*, and *Pseudomonas*. Digital cyanosis usually occurs shortly after venous cannulation and is probably the result of venospasm provoked by the presence of an indwelling catheter. As described earlier, damaged endothelium may stimulate vasoconstriction. Immobilization causes constriction of the limbs and impairs the muscle action that is necessary to assist venous return. Persistence of these conditions increases extravascular pressure and gradually produces microcirculatory failure, leading to necrosis, which begins at the most distal areas of the digits.

Treatment begins with the prompt recognition of persistent cyanosis, correction of the underlying systemic disorder, and immediate removal of the catheter. Anticoagulation should be initiated immediately. Lesions should be gently washed daily in warm water, and the involved limb should be actively and passively exercised through the full range of motion. Direct heating should be avoided because ischemic tissue burns at lower temperatures than normal. Small pieces of cotton should be placed between fingers or toes, and all lesions should be covered with sterile, dry dressings. Areas of dry gangrene do not require surgical removal. If some question of infection trapped under an eschar exists, the area can be gently elevated at its corners to allow adequate drainage. As is the case with arterial lesions, amputation should not be considered until clear demarcation has occurred.

SUMMARY

Vascular injury in the pediatric population is considerably different from that encountered in adults. Traumatic injury presents a unique set of characteristics that reflect the epidemiology of pediatric trauma and, if carefully managed, can exploit the intrinsically healthy status of the child's vascular system. Iatrogenic injury is the price of miniaturization. It is a recognized trade-off for the dramatic advances that have made many lifesaving procedures possible. Attention to detail in those most at risk may not eliminate the problem but will at least reduce the incidence and raise awareness. Accurate diagnosis, timely revascularization, and aggressive management of reperfusion are essential for complete recovery and normal long-term growth. The key to success is a high index of suspicion, recognition of the unique characteristics discussed ealier, and aggressive operative intervention using the high level of precision that is the cornerstone of success in the surgical care of children.

REFERENCES

1. Chaikof EL, Dodson TF, Salam AA, et al: Acute arterial thrombosis in the very young. J Vasc Surg 1992;16: 428-435.
2. Cox CS Jr, Black CT, Duke JH, et al: Operative treatment of truncal vascular injuries in children and adolescents. J Pediatr Surg 1998;33:462-467.
3. Demircin M, Peker O, Tok M, et al: False aneurysm of the brachial artery in an infant following attempted venipuncture. Turk J Pediatr 1996;38:389-391.
4. Dennis JW, Frykberg ER, Crump JM, et al: New perspectives on the management of penetrating trauma in proximity to major limb arteries. J Vasc Surg 1990;11:84-92.
5. Dennis JW, Frykberg ER, Veldenz HC, et al: Validation of nonoperative management of occult vascular injuries and accuracy of physical examination alone in penetrating extremity trauma: 5- to 10-year follow-up. J Trauma 1998; 44:242 (discussion).
6. Dennis JW, Jagger C, Butcher JL, et al: Reassessing the role of arteriogram in the management of posterior knee dislocations. J Trauma 1993;35:692-695.
7. de Virgilio C, Mercado PD, Arnell T, et al: Noniatrogenic pediatric vascular trauma: A ten-year experience at a level I trauma center. Am Surg 1997;63:781-784.
8. Eddy AC, Rusch VW, Marchioro T, et al: Treatment of traumatic rupture of the thoracic aorta: A 15-year experience. Arch Surg 1990;125:1351 (discussion 1355).
9. Eren N, Ozgen G, Ener BK, et al: Peripheral vascular injuries in children. J Pediatr Surg 1991;26:1164-1168.
10. Fagelman MF, Epps HR, Rang M: Mangled extremity severity score in children. J Pediatr Orthop 2002;22:182-184.
11. Fayiga YJ, Valentine RJ, Myers SI, et al: Blunt pediatric vascular trauma: Analysis of forty-one consecutive patients undergoing operative intervention. J Vasc Surg 1994; 20:419 (discussion 424).
12. Flanigan DP, Keifer TJ, Schuler JJ, et al: Experience with iatrogenic pediatric vascular injuries: Incidence, etiology, management, results. Ann Surg 1983;198:430-442.
13. Francis H, Thal ER, Weigelt JA, et al: Vascular proximity: Is it a valid indication for arteriography in asymptomatic patients? J Trauma 1991;31:512-514.

14. Friedman RJ, Jupiter JB: Vascular injuries and closed extremity fractures in children. Clin Orthop 1984;188:112-119.

15. Frykberg ER: Advances in diagnosis and treatment of extremity vascular trauma. Surg Clin North Am 1995;75:207-223.

16. Frykberg ER, Crump JM, Dennis JW, et al: Nonoperative observation of clinically occult arterial injuries: A prospective evaluation. Surgery 1991;109:85-96.

17. Frykberg ER, Dennis JW, Bishop K, et al: The reliability of physical examination in the evaluation of penetrating extremity trauma for vascular injury: Results at one year. J Trauma 1991;31:502-511.

18. Furchgott RF, Zawadzki JV: The obligatory role of endothelial cells in the relaxation of arterial smooth muscle by acetylcholine. Nature 1980;288:373-376.

19. Gamba P, Tchaprassian Z, Verlato F, et al: Iatrogenic vascular lesions in extremely low birth weight and low birth weight neonates. Vasc Surg 1997;26:643-646.

20. Giacoia GP: High-dose urokinase therapy in newborn infants with major vessel thrombosis. Clin Pediatr 1993;32:231-237.

21. Harris LM, Hordines J: Major vascular injuries in the pediatric population. Ann Vasc Surg 2003;17:266-269.

22. Hoover JD, Almond PS: Isolated pediatric peripheral vascular injury caused by blunt trauma: A new occurrence. J Trauma 2004;56:198-200.

23. Itani KM, Rothenberg SS, Brandt ML, et al: Emergency center arteriography in the evaluation of suspected peripheral vascular injuries in children. J Pediatr Surg 1993;28:677-680.

24. Klein MD, Coran AG, Whitehouse WM Jr, et al: Management of iatrogenic arterial injuries in infants and children. J Pediatr Surg 1982;17:933-939.

25. Kuo PC, Schroeder RA: The emerging multifaceted roles of nitric oxide. Ann Surg 1995;221:220-235.

26. LaQuaglia MP, Upton J, May JW Jr: Microvascular reconstruction of major arteries in neonates and small children. J Pediatr Surg 1991;26:1136-1140.

27. Lewis HG, Morrison CM, Kennedy PT, et al: Arterial reconstruction using the basilic vein from the zone of injury in pediatric supracondylar humeral fractures: A clinical and radiological series. Plast Reconstr Surg 2003;111:1159 (discussion 1164).

28. Lin Ph, Dodson TF, Bush RL, et al: Surgical intervention for complications caused by femoral artery catheterization in pediatric patients. J Vasc Surg 2001;34:1071-1078.

29. McCorkell SJ, Harley JD, Morishima MS, et al: Indications for angiography in extremity trauma. AJR Am J Roentgenol 1985;145:1245-1247.

30. Meagher DP Jr, Defore WW, Mattox KL, et al: Vascular trauma in infants and children. J Trauma 1979;19:532-536.

31. Milas ZL, Dodson TF, Ricketts RR: Pediatric blunt trauma resulting in major arterial injuries. Am Surg 2004;70:443-447.

32. Mills RP, Robbs JV: Paediatric arterial injury: Management options at the time of injury. J R Coll Surg Edinb 1991;36:13-17.

33. Moncada S, Higgs A: The L-arginine:nitric oxide pathway. N Engl J Med 1993;329:2002-2012.

34. Nehler MR, Taylor LM Jr, Porter JM: Iatrogenic vascular trauma. Semin Vasc Surg 1998;11:283-293.

35. O'Neill JA, Neblett WW, Born ML: Management of major thromboembolic complications of umbilical artery catheters. J Pediatr Surg 1981;16:972-978.

36. Pigula FA, Buenaventura P, Ettedgui JA, et al: Management of retroperitoneal arterial injury after heart catheterization in children. Ann Thorac Surg 2000;69:1582-1584.

37. Reed MK, Lowry PA, Myers SI: Successful repair of pediatric politeal artery trauma. Am J Surg 1990;160:287-290.

38. Reichard KW, Hall JR, Meller JL, et al: Arteriography in the evaluation of penetrating pediatric extremity injuries. J Pediatr Surg 1994;29:19-22.

39. Reichard KW, Reyes HM: Vascular trauma and reconstructive approaches. Semin Pediatr Surg 1994;3:124-132.

40. Reid JD, Weigelt JA, Thal ER, et al: Assessment of proximity of a wound to major vascular structures as an indication for arteriography. Arch Surg 1998;123:942-946.

41. Rozycki GS, Tremblay L, Feliciano DV, et al: A prospective study for the detection of vascular injury in adult and pediatric patients with cervicothoracic seat belt signs. J Trauma 2002;52:618 (discussion 623).

42. Russo VJ: Traumatic arterial spasm resulting in gangrene. J Pediatr Orthop 1985;5:486-488.

43. Seibert JJ, Northington FJ, Miers JF, et al: Aortic thrombosis after umbilical artery catheterization in neonates: Prevalence of complications of long-term follow-up. AJR Am J Roentgenol 1991;156:567-569.

44. Soares G, Ibarra R, Ferral H: Abnominal aortic injury in a child: intravenous digital substraction angiogram (IVDSA) for the diagnosis of pediatric vascular trauma. Pediatr Radiol 2003;33:563-566.

45. Uslu MM, Altun NS, Cila E, at al: Relevance of mangled extremity severity score to compartment syndromes. Arch Orthop Trauma Surg 1995;114:229-232.

46. Victoroff BN, Robertson WW Jr, Eichelberger MR, et al: Extremity gunshot injuries treated in an urban children's hospital. Pediatr Emerg Care 1994;10:1-5.

47. Villavicencio JL, Gonzalez-Carna JL: Acute vascular problems of children. Curr Probl Surg 1985;22:1-85.

48. Whitehouse WM, Coran AG, Stanley JC, et al: Pediatric vascular trauma: Manifestations, management, and sequelae of extremity arterial injury in patients undergoing surgical treatment. Arch Surg 1976;111:1269-1275.

49. Zenz W, Muntean W, Beitzke A, et al: Tissue plasminogen activator (Alteplase) treatment for femoral artery thrombosis after cardiac catheterisation in infants and children. Br Heart J 1993;70:382-385.

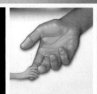

Chapter 23

Burns

Dai H. Chung, Arthur P. Sanford, and David N. Herndon

In 1944 Lund and Browder[69] developed a diagram that allowed a quantifiable assessment of the percentage of total body surface area (TBSA) burned. While treating victims of the Coconut Grove fire in Boston in 1946, Cope and Moore[18] were able to quantify the amount of fluid required to maintain the central electrolyte composition after "burn shock." In the 1960s the discovery of efficacious topical antimicrobial agents, such as 0.5% silver nitrate,[75] mafenide acetate (Sulfamylon),[68] and silver sulfadiazine (Silvadene),[30] had a significant impact on reducing the incidence of burn wound sepsis. These and other advances in burn care during the past several decades have resulted in an overall improved survival rate for major burn patients. In recent years, continued progress has been made in several areas of burn care. Early surgical excision of eschar and grafting have significantly minimized the incidence of burn wound sepsis and shortened the total length of hospital stay. Treatment with anabolic agents restores net positive nitrogen balance during the prolonged postburn hypermetabolic period. Acute recognition of inhalation injury and effective treatment have also improved the overall outcome for burn patients. These are but a few of the significant advances that have led to a further decline in burn-related deaths.[8] Today, the overall increased survival rate among major burn victims is most evident in the pediatric population, where the mortality rate is 50% in children 14 years and younger with 98% TBSA burns; in other age groups it is 50% for those with 75% TBSA burns.[42]

Although the overall incidence of burn injuries has declined as a result of preventive measures and legislation, more than 1 million burn injuries still occur each year in the United States. Fortunately, most of these burn injuries are minor, but approximately 45,000 patients suffer moderate to severe burns that require hospitalization. Of these cases, 67% are young males, and 40% are children younger than 15 years.[3] As the second leading cause of accidental death in children younger than 5 years, burns resulted in 532 pediatric deaths in 2001. In 2002 an estimated 92,500 children younger than 14 years were treated in hospital emergency rooms for burn-related injuries (58,100 with thermal burns and 22,600 with scald burns).[12] Of the children aged 4

and younger who are hospitalized for burn-related injuries, 65% have scald burns, 20% have contact burns, and the remainder have flame burns. The majority of scald burns in infants and toddlers are from hot foods and liquids. Hot grease spills are notorious for causing deep burns to the involved areas. Hot tap-water burns, which can easily be prevented by installing special faucet valves so that water does not leave the tap at a temperature above 120°F (48.8°C), frequently result in large burned areas in children.[2] Children also suffer product-related contact burns from curling irons, ovens, steam irons, and fireworks. Contact with the electrical current in wall outlets also causes a significant percentage of injuries, as does contact with electrical cords. Child abuse also represents a significant cause of burns in children (Fig. 23-1). Burns with bilateral symmetry or a stocking-glove distribution, particularly to the dorsum of hands, along with a delay in seeking medical attention, should raise the suspicion of child abuse. In the adolescent age group, flame burns are more common, frequently occurring as a result of experimenting with fire and volatile agents.

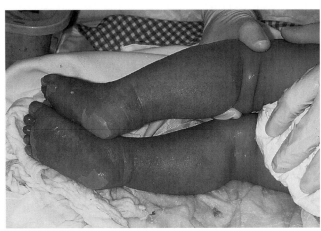

Figure 23–1 Scald burn of lower extremities in an infant. Bilateral stocking distribution with well-demarcated margins is consistent with a burn injury resulting from child abuse.

PATHOPHYSIOLOGY

As the largest organ in the body, the skin maintains fluid and electrolyte homeostasis, guards against harmful environmental insults, and acts as a barrier to infection. Other important functions include thermoregulation, metabolism of vitamin D production, and processing of neurosensory inputs. The total surface area of skin ranges from 0.2 to 0.3 m² in a typical newborn and 1.5 to 2.0 m² in an adult, making up nearly 15% of total body weight. Anatomically, the epidermis is composed primarily of epithelial cells, specifically keratinocytes. The process of epidermal maturation from the basal layer of keratinocytes to desquamation generally takes about 2 to 4 weeks. The dermis is made up of fibroblasts, which produce collagen and elastin, and is subdivided into a superficial papillary dermis and a deep reticular dermis. The papillary dermis and reticular dermis are separated by a plexus of nerves and blood vessels. The reticular dermis and fatty layer contain skin appendages, such as hair follicles, sweat glands, and sebaceous glands. Therefore, burns involving the deep dermis are generally insensate to touch and painful stimuli.

Thermal injury results in coagulation necrosis of the epidermis and varying degrees of injury to the underlying tissue. The extent of burn injury depends on the temperature, duration of exposure, skin thickness, ability of the skin to dissipate heat, and specific heat of the causative agent. For example, the specific heat of fat is higher than that of water; therefore, grease burns often result in much deeper burns than do scald burns from water with the same temperature and duration of exposure. Thermal energy is easily transferred from high-energy molecules to those of lower energy during contact, through the process of heat conduction. The skin generally provides a barrier to the transfer of energy to deeper tissues; therefore, much of the burn injury is confined to this layer. However, local tissue response to the zone of initial burn injury can lead to progressive destruction of surrounding tissue.

The area of cutaneous burn injury is divided into three zones: coagulation, stasis, and hyperemia (Fig. 23-2). The zone of coagulation comprises the initial burn eschar, where cells become irreversibly damaged and necrotic at the time of injury. The area immediately surrounding the necrotic area is a zone of stasis, where most cells are initially viable but tissue perfusion becomes progressively impaired from the local release of inflammatory mediators such as thromboxane A_2, arachidonic acid, oxidants, and cytokines.[95] Their influence on the microcirculation results in the formation of platelet thrombus, neutrophil adherence, fibrin deposition, and vasoconstriction, which lead to cell necrosis. However, adequate wound care and resuscitation may reverse this process and prevent extensive cell necrosis. Thromboxane A_2 inhibitors can significantly improve dermal blood flow to decrease the zone of stasis.[19] Antioxidants as well as bradykinin antagonists also improve local blood flow.[20,79] Inhibition of neutrophil adherence to endothelium with anti-CD18 or anti-intercellular adhesion molecule monoclonal antibodies improves tissue perfusion in animal models.[11,72] Peripheral to the zone of stasis lies the zone of hyperemia, which is characterized by vasodilatation and increased blood flow as part of the inflammatory response.

The burn-induced inflammatory response is not limited to the local wound in burns involving greater than 40% TBSA. A massive systemic release of thromboxane A_2, along with other inflammatory mediators (bradykinin, leukotrienes, catecholamines, activated complement, vasoactive amines), imposes a major physiologic burden on the cardiopulmonary, renal, and gastrointestinal (GI) systems.[97] Decreased plasma volume due to increased capillary permeability and subsequent plasma leak into the interstitial space can lead to depressed cardiac function. As a result of low cardiac output, renal blood flow can decrease, leading to a diminished glomerular filtration rate. Activation of other stress-induced hormones and mediators, such as angiotensin, aldosterone, and vasopressin, can further compromise renal blood flow, resulting in oliguria.[78] If not properly treated, this condition can progress to acute tubular necrosis and renal failure, which is associated with a poor outcome for burn patients.[61] Atrophy of small bowel mucosa occurs as a result of increased epithelial apoptosis and decreased epithelial proliferation.[16,17,100] Intestinal permeability to macromolecules, which are normally repelled by an intact mucosal barrier, increases after a burn injury.[13,67,87] Transient mesenteric ischemia is thought to be an important contributing factor to increased intestinal permeability, which can result in a more frequent incidence of bacterial translocation and subsequent endotoxemia. Burn injury also causes a global depression of immune function. Macrophage production is decreased; neutrophils are impaired in terms of their functions such

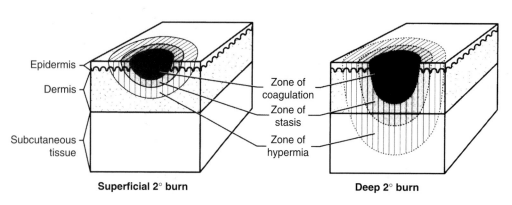

Epidermis
Dermis
Subcutaneous tissue

Zone of coagulation
Zone of stasis
Zone of hypermia

Superficial 2° burn

Deep 2° burn

Figure 23-2 Three zones of burn injury: coagulation, stasis, and hyperemia.

as diapedesis, chemotaxis, and phagocytosis; cytotoxic T-lymphocyte activity is decreased. These impaired functions of neutrophils, macrophages, and T lymphocytes contribute to an increased risk for infectious complications after burns.[5,6,32,57,64,101]

MANAGEMENT

First Aid

A burn patient must immediately be removed from the source of burn injury, and potential life-threatening injuries must be quickly assessed and addressed independent of the cutaneous burns, as in the case of a multiple trauma victim. Burned clothing and metal jewelry are removed. Immediate cooling by pouring cold water onto the surface of burn wounds must be used with caution to avoid hypothermia. After the removal of clothing, the patient should be kept warm in blankets. With chemical burns, wounds should be irrigated with copious amounts of water, taking care not to spread the chemical to adjacent uninvolved areas. Attempts to neutralize chemicals are contraindicated, as this process may produce additional heat and increase the burn injury.

As with any trauma patient, burn patients are quickly assessed through primary and secondary surveys. In the primary survey, airway, breathing, and circulation are assessed, and any potential life-threatening conditions are identified and treated quickly. Symptoms such as wheezing, tachypnea, and hoarseness indicate impending major airway problems; the airway must be rapidly secured with intubation and 100% oxygen support. Oxygen saturation is monitored using a pulse oximeter, and chest expansion is observed to ensure equal air movement. However, adequate oxygen saturation does not mean that the airway is protected, because children have the ability to compensate until just before catastrophic airway collapse occurs. Circumferential full-thickness burns to the chest can significantly impair respiratory function by constricting the trunk and preventing adequate chest expansion. If necessary, escharotomy should be performed to allow better chest expansion and subsequent ventilation. Blood pressure may be difficult to obtain in burned patients with charred extremities. Pulse rate can be used as an indirect measure of intravascular volume; the presence of tachycardia is an indication of the continued need for aggressive fluid resuscitation.

Burn depth is categorized according to the involved layers of skin: epidermis, papillary dermis, reticular dermis, subcutaneous fat, and underlying structures (Fig. 23-3). First-degree burns are confined to the epidermis, which is intact, erythematous, and painful to touch. The application of topical ointment containing aloe vera and the administration of oral nonsteroidal anti-inflammatory agents constitute standard treatment. First-degree burns (e.g., sunburn) heal spontaneously without scarring in 7 to 10 days. Second-degree burns are divided into superficial and deep, based on the depth of dermal involvement. Superficial second-degree burns are limited to the papillary dermis and are typically erythematous and painful with blisters. These burns spontaneously

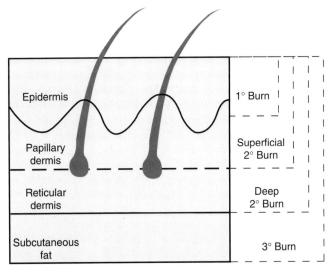

Figure 23-3   Burn depth. First-degree burns are confined to the epidermis. Superficial second-degree burns involve the papillary dermis, and deep second-degree burns involve reticular dermis. Third-degree burns are full-thickness injuries through the epidermis and dermis. (Adapted from Wolf S, Herndon DN: Burns. In Townsend CM Jr [ed]: Textbook of Surgery, 17th ed. Philadelphia, WB Saunders, 2004, p 571.)

re-epithelialize in 10 to 14 days from retained epidermal structures and may leave only slight skin discoloration. Deep second-degree burns extend into the reticular layer of the dermis. The deep epidermal appendages allow some of these wounds to heal slowly over several weeks, usually with significant scarring. Third-degree burns are full-thickness injuries resulting in complete destruction of the epidermis, dermis, and dermal appendages and are characterized by a dry, leathery eschar that is insensate to any stimuli. Without any residual epidermal or dermal appendages, such burn wounds heal by re-epithelialization from the edges. Fourth-degree burns, typically resulting from profound thermal or electrical injury, involve organs beneath the layers of the skin, such as muscle and bone.

An accurate and rapid determination of burn depth is vital to the proper management of burn injuries. In particular, the distinction between superficial and deep dermal burns is critical, as this dictates whether the burn can be managed without surgical procedures. Unfortunately, the determination of whether an apparent deep dermal burn will heal in 3 weeks is only about 50% accurate, even when made by an experienced surgeon. Early excision and grafting provide better results than nonoperative therapy for such indeterminate burns. More precise, objective methods to determine burn depth include techniques such as laser Doppler flowmetry and fluorescein to determine blood flow; ultrasonography to detect denatured collagen; and light reflectance of the wound.[9,60,80,81] Ultimately, burn wound biopsy is the most precise diagnostic tool[53]; however, it is not clinically useful because it is invasive and indicates only the static condition of the wound. It also requires an experienced pathologist to interpret histologic findings. Despite these modern technologies, clinical observation is still the most reliable method of determining burn depth.

Full-thickness circumferential burns to the extremities produce a constricting eschar, which may result in vascular compromise to the distal tissues, including nerves. Accumulation of tissue edema beneath the nonelastic eschar impedes venous outflow, resulting in a compartment syndrome and eventually affecting arterial flow. When distal pulses are absent on palpation or Doppler examination, escharotomies of the extremities are performed to avoid vascular compromise of the limb tissues, after confirmation of the absence of a central circulation problem. Using either a scalpel or electrocautery, escharotomies are performed at the bedside along the lateral and medial aspects of the involved extremities (Fig. 23-4). When the hands are involved, incisions are carried down onto the thenar and hypothenar eminences and along the dorsolateral aspects of the digits, taking care to avoid injury to the neurovascular bundle. Because injuries requiring escharotomy are typically full thickness, minimal bleeding is encountered. If vascular compromise has been prolonged, reperfusion after an escharotomy may cause reactive hyperemia and further edema formation in the muscle compartments. Ischemia-reperfusion injury also releases free oxygen radicals, resulting in transient hypotension. If increased compartment pressures are noted, fasciotomy should be performed immediately to avoid permanent ischemic injuries to the nerves and soft tissues.

Intravenous (IV) access should be established immediately to infuse lactated Ringer's solution according to resuscitation guidelines. Peripheral IV access is preferred, but femoral venous access is an ideal alternative in patients with massive burns. If the only IV access available is through burned tissue, this route should be chosen for immediate resuscitation and later changed to a more appropriate site under sterile conditions. When vascular access is problematic in small children with burned extremities, the intraosseous route is an alternative in those younger than 6 years. A nasogastric tube is placed in all patients with major burns to combat the onset of gastric ileus. Almost immediate enteral nutrition can be initiated via a transpyloric feeding tube. A Foley catheter is placed to accurately monitor urine output as a measure of end-organ perfusion. Admission laboratory studies should include complete blood count, type and crossmatch for packed red blood cells, chemistry, urinalysis, coagulation profile, and chest radiograph. If inhalation injury is suspected, arterial blood gas with carboxyhemoglobin level should also be determined to guide respiratory therapy.

Burn size is generally assessed by the "rule of nines" in adolescents and adults. Each upper extremity and the head are 9% of the TBSA, and the lower extremities and the anterior and posterior trunks are 18% each. The perineum, genitalia, and neck make up the remaining 1% of the TBSA. A quick estimate of burn size can also be obtained by using the patient's palm to represent 1% of TBSA and transposing that measurement onto the wound. However, use of the rule of nines can be misleading in children because of their different body proportions. In children, the head and neck constitute a relatively larger portion of the TBSA, and the lower extremities account for a smaller portion. For example, an infant's head constitutes 19% of TBSA, compared with 9% in an adult. Thus, a modified rule of nines, based on the anthropomorphic differences of infancy and childhood, is generally used to assess pediatric burn size (Fig. 23-5). Table 23-1 can be used to estimate the percentage of TBSA burned, based on the patient's age and the body part burned.

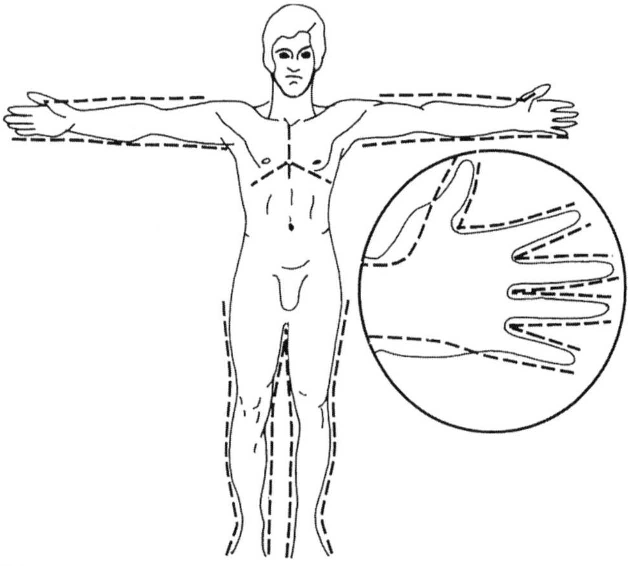

Fluid Resuscitation

Appropriate fluid resuscitation should begin promptly upon securing IV access. Peripheral IV access is sufficient in the majority of small to moderate burns. Saphenous vein cutdowns are useful in cases of difficult access; in children, however, percutaneous femoral central venous access may be easier and more reliable. There are many fluid resuscitation guidelines for delivering various concentrations of colloid and crystalloid solutions. The Parkland formula (4 mL of lactated Ringer's solution per kilogram of body weight per percentage of TBSA burned) is most widely used, but children's fluid resuscitation requirements should be based on body surface area rather than weight. Because children have a greater body surface area in relation to weight, weight-based formulas can underresuscitate children with minor burns and may grossly overresuscitate those with extensive burns.[36] TBSA can be rapidly estimated from height and weight using standard nomograms (Fig. 23-6). The Galveston formula (Shriners Hospital for Children) uses 5000 mL/m² burned plus 2000 mL/m² TBSA of lactated Ringer's solution given over the first 24 hours after the injury, with half the volume administered during the first 8 hours and the remaining half over the next 16 hours (Table 23-2).

Figure 23–4 Escharotomies. The incisions are made on the medial and lateral aspects of the extremity. Hand escharotomies are performed on the medial and lateral digits and on the dorsum of the hand. (From Eichelberger MR [ed]: Pediatric Trauma: Prevention, Acute Care, Rehabilitation. St Louis, Mosby, 1993, p 569.)

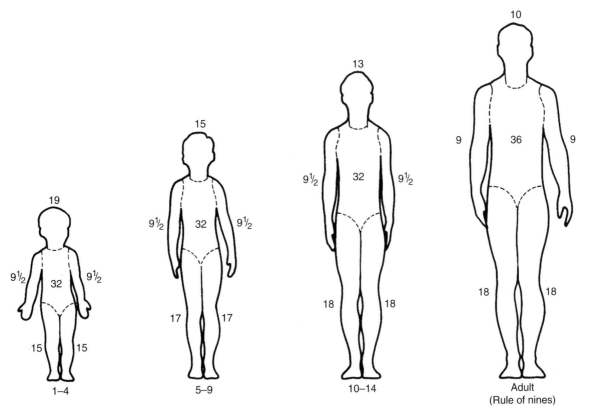

Figure 23–5 Modified "rule of nines" for pediatric patients. (From Herndon DN [ed]: Total Burn Care, 2nd ed. Philadelphia, WB Saunders, 2002, p 429.)

Regardless of which guidelines are used, the primary goal of fluid resuscitation is to achieve adequate organ tissue perfusion. Fluid administration should be titrated to maintain a urine output of greater than 1 mL/kg per hour. Approximately 50% of administered fluid is sequestered in nonburned tissues in 50% TBSA burns, owing to the increased capillary permeability that occurs, particularly in the first 6 to 8 hours after injury.[21] During this period, large molecules leak into the interstitial space to increase extravascular colloid osmotic pressure. Therefore, to maintain intravascular osmotic pressure, albumin is added 12 hours after the injury. After the first 24 hours, 3750 mL/m² burned of lactated Ringer's solution is given to replace evaporative fluid loss, plus 1500 mL/m² TBSA per 24 hours for maintenance. A dextrose-containing solution, such as 5% dextrose with one quarter to one half normal saline, is used as the primary solution. Children younger than 2 years are susceptible to hypoglycemia due to limited glycogen stores; therefore, lactated Ringer's solution with 5% dextrose is given during the first 24 hours after burns.

TABLE 23–1 Estimated Percentage of Total Body Surface Area Burned Based on Age and Area Burned

Area	<1 Year	1-4 Years	5-9 Years	10-14 Years	15 Years	Adult
Head	19	17	13	11	9	7
Neck	2	2	2	2	2	2
Anterior trunk	13	13	13	13	13	13
Posterior trunk	13	13	13	13	13	13
Buttock	2.5	2.5	2.5	2.5	2.5	2.5
Genitalia	1	1	1	1	1	1
Upper arm	4	4	4	4	4	4
Lower arm	3	3	3	3	3	3
Hand	2.5	2.5	2.5	2.5	2.5	2.5
Thigh	5.5	6.5	8	8.5	9	9.5
Leg	5	5	5.5	6	6.5	7
Foot	3.5	3.5	3.5	3.5	3.5	3.5

Burn size estimates based on the area burned are more precise than the rule of nines for pediatric patients.

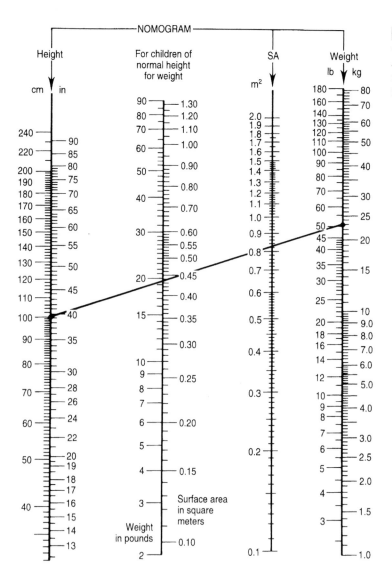

NOMOGRAM

Figure 23–6 Standard nomogram for the determination of body surface area based on height and weight. A straight line drawn between the height and weight measurements determines the total body surface area in square meters.

Children often do not exhibit clinical signs of hypovolemia until more than 25% of the circulating volume is depleted and complete cardiovascular collapse is imminent. Tachycardia reflects a compensatory response to hypovolemia, but caution is needed to avoid overinterpreting this finding, because reflex tachycardia due to postinjury catecholamine response is common. A lethargic child with decreased capillary refill and cool, clammy extremities needs prompt attention. Measurement of arterial blood pH and base deficit values can also reflect the adequacy of fluid resuscitation. Hyponatremia is a frequent complication in pediatric burn patients

TABLE 23–2 Acute Burn Fluid Resuscitation Guidelines		
Formula	**First 24 Hours**	**Thereafter**
Parkland	Lactated Ringer's solution 4 mL/kg/% TBSA burned; 50% total volume during first 8 hr after injury and remaining 50% over subsequent 16 hr	5% dextrose with Na$^+$, K$^+$, and albumin to maintain normal serum electrolytes and colloid oncotic pressure
Brooke	Lactated Ringer's solution (with colloid 0.5 mL/kg/% TBSA burned) 2 mL/kg/% TBSA burned; 50% total volume during first 8 hr after injury and remaining 50% over subsequent 16 hr	Titrate to maintain urine output 0.5-1.0 mL/kg/hr
Galveston	Lactated Ringer's solution (12.5 g albumin/L added 12 hr after injury) 5000 mL/m^2 burned + 2000 mL/m^2 total; 50% total volume during first 8 hr after injury and remaining 50% over subsequent 16 hr	3750 mL/m^2 burned + 1500 mL/m^2 total; substitute IV fluid volume with enteral formula

TBSA, total body surface area.

after aggressive fluid resuscitation. Frequent monitoring of serum chemistry with appropriate correction is required to avoid severe electrolyte imbalance. A serious complication such as central pontine myelinolysis can occur as a result of careless, rapid correction of hypernatremia.[1]

Hypertonic saline resuscitation can be beneficial in treating burn-induced shock.[74,96] This process maintains intravascular volume more effectively by removing fluid from the interstitial space through osmosis, thus decreasing generalized tissue edema. However, it is not widely used because of the potential risk of hypernatremia, hyperosmolarity, renal failure, and alkalosis.[55,97] Some favor the use of a modified hypertonic solution—adding an ampule of sodium bicarbonate to each liter of lactated Ringer's solution during the first 24 hours of resuscitation.[26]

After initial first aid and the start of appropriate fluid resuscitation, transferring the patient to a tertiary burn center should be considered. Burn units with experienced multidisciplinary teams are best prepared to treat patients with major burns. In addition to physicians and nurses, respiratory and rehabilitation therapists play a critical role in the management of acute burns. Any patient who sustains a "major burn injury," as defined by the American Burn Association (Table 23-3), should be transferred to a nearby burn center for further care.

Topical Antimicrobials

Proper wound care is guided by an accurate assessment of burn depth and size. First-degree burns require no dressing, but the involved areas should be kept out of direct sunlight. They are generally treated with topical ointments for symptomatic pain relief. Superficial second-degree burns are treated with daily dressing changes and topical antimicrobials. They can also be treated with simple application of petroleum gauze or synthetic dressings to allow rapid, spontaneous re-epithelialization. Deep second- and third-degree burns require excision of eschar and skin grafting.

TABLE 23-3 American Burn Association Criteria for Major Burn Injury

Second- and third-degree burns >10% TBSA in patients aged <10 or >50 yr
Second- and third-degree burns >20% TBSA in other age groups
Third-degree burns >5% TBSA in any age group
Burns involving the face, hands, feet, genitalia, perineum, and skin overlying major joints
Significant chemical burns
Significant electrical burns, including lightning injury
Inhalation injury
Burns with significant concomitant trauma
Burns with significant preexisting medical disorders
Burns in patients requiring special social, emotional, and rehabilitative support (including suspected child abuse and neglect)

TBSA, total body surface area.

TABLE 23-4 Topical Antimicrobial Agents

Antimicrobial Agent	Characteristics
Silver sulfadiazine (Silvadene)	Broad-spectrum activity and painless; does not penetrate eschar; impairs epithelialization; leukopenia
Mafenide acetate (Sulfamylon; 10% cream or 5% soaks)	Broad-spectrum activity, including *Pseudomonas*; penetrates eschar; painful in second-degree burns; may cause metabolic acidosis (inhibits carbonic anhydrase inhibitor) and inhibition of epithelialization
Silver nitrate (0.5%)	Broad-spectrum activity; does not penetrate eschar; discolors contacted areas; may cause hyponatremia, methemoglobinemia
Bacitracin/Polysporin	Painless, but limited antimicrobial activity
Nystatin	Inhibits fungal growth; frequently used in combination with Silvadene
Mupirocin (Bactroban)	Effective against *Staphylococcus*
Povidone-iodine	Broad-spectrum activity, but possible systemic absorption
Dakin solution (0.025%)	Effective against almost all microbes

Table 23-4 lists topical antimicrobial agents used for the management of burn wounds. None of these agents effectively prevents the colonization of organisms that are commonly harbored in the eschar, but they maintain the bacterial quantity at less than 10^2 to 10^5 colonies per gram of tissue. Routine punch quantitative wound biopsy can indicate impending burn wound sepsis and possible failure of skin graft from infection.

Silver sulfadiazine (Silvadene) is the most commonly used topical agent for burn wound dressings. Although it does not penetrate eschar, it has a broad spectrum of efficacy and soothes the pain associated with second-degree burns. Silver sulfadiazine on fine mesh gauze can be used separately or in combination with other antimicrobial agents, such as nystatin. This combination, providing additional antifungal coverage, has significantly reduced the incidence of *Candida* infection in burned patients.[22,24] The most common side effect is leukopenia; however, this is caused by margination of white blood cells and is only transient.[59] When the leukocyte count falls below 3000 cells/mm^3, changing to another topical antimicrobial quickly resolves this complication.

Mafenide acetate (Sulfamylon) is more effective in penetrating eschar and is therefore frequently used in third-degree burns. Fine mesh gauze impregnated with Sulfamylon (10% water-soluble cream) is applied directly to the burn wound. Compared with silver sulfadiazine, Sulfamylon has a much broader spectrum of efficacy, including coverage against *Pseudomonas* and *Enterococcus*. It is also available in a 5% solution to soak burn wounds, eliminating the need to perform frequent dressing changes. Sulfamylon is a potent carbonic anhydrase inhibitor, so it can cause metabolic acidosis. This side effect can usually be avoided by limiting its use to only 20% TBSA at any one time and rotating application sites every several hours with another topical agent, such as Silvadene. Additionally, it is painful when applied, limiting its use in an outpatient setting, especially with children.

In addition to 5% Sulfamylon solution, 0.5% silver nitrate and 0.025% sodium hypochlorite (Dakin solution) are available. These solutions are generally poured onto gauze dressings on the wound, avoiding the need for frequent dressing changes and the potential loss of grafts or healing cells. Silver nitrate is painless on application and has broad coverage, but its side effects include electrolyte imbalance (hyponatremia, hypochloremia) and dark gray or black stains. A new commercially available dressing containing biologically active silver ions (Acticoat) retains the effectiveness of silver nitrate without the side effects. Dakin solution is effective against most microbes, including *Pseudomonas*. However, it requires frequent dosing because of the inactivation of hypochlorite when it comes in contact with protein; it can also retard healing cells.[38]

Petroleum-based antimicrobial ointments such polymyxin B, bacitracin, and Polysporin are painless and transparent, allowing easier monitoring of burn wounds. These agents are generally effective only against gram-positive organisms, and their use is limited to facial burns, small areas of partial-thickness burns, and healing donor sites. Like Silvadene, these petroleum-based agents can be used in combination with nystatin to suppress skin *Candida* colonization.

Wound Dressings

Superficial second-degree burns can be managed using various methods. Topical antimicrobial dressings using Silvadene are most commonly used, but synthetic dressings such as Biobrane and Opsite offer the unique advantage of eliminating frequent, painful dressing changes and tissue fluid loss. The general principle of these synthetic products is to provide sterile coverage of superficial second-degree burn wounds to allow rapid, spontaneous re-epithelialization of the involved areas.

Biobrane is a thin, synthetic material composed of an inner layer of nylon coated with porcine collagen and an outer layer of rubberized silicone. It is pervious to air but not to fluids and is available in simple sheets or preshaped gloves (Fig. 23-7).[66] After placement on clean, fresh, superficial second-degree burn wounds using Steri-strips and bandages, the Biobrane dressing dries up, becoming adherent to burn wounds within 24 to 48 hours. Once the dressing is adherent, the covered areas are kept open to air and examined closely for the first few days to detect any signs and symptoms of infection. As epithelialization occurs beneath the Biobrane, the sheet is easily peeled off the wound. If serous fluid accumulates beneath the Biobrane, sterile needle aspiration can preserve its use. However, if foul-smelling exudate is detected, the Biobrane should be removed and topical antimicrobial dressings applied. Alternatively, Opsite or Tegaderm can be used to cover superficial second-degree burn wounds. Commonly used as postoperative dressings in surgical patients, both are relatively inexpensive, are easy to apply, and provide

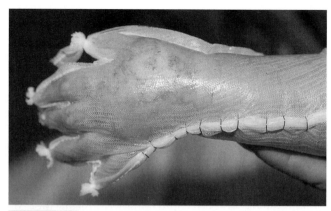

Figure 23–7   Biobrane glove. Biobrane is an ideal synthetic wound coverage material for superficial second-degree burns. It promotes rapid re-epithelialization without painful dressing changes.

an impervious barrier to the environment. Their transparent nature allows easy monitoring of covered second-degree burn wounds. Despite lacking any special biologic factors (e.g., collagen and growth factors) to enhance wound healing, they promote a spontaneous re-epithelialization process. Biobrane and Opsite are preferred to topical antimicrobial dressings when dealing with small, superficial second-degree burn wounds, especially in outpatient settings, to avoid the pain associated with dressing changes. TransCyte, composed of human fibroblasts that are then cultured on the nylon mesh of Biobrane, is another option.

Synthetic and biologic dressings are also available to provide coverage for full-thickness burn wounds. Integra, which is made of a collagen matrix with an outer silicone sheet, is a synthetic dermal substitute for the treatment of full-thickness burn wounds. After the collagen matrix engrafts into the wound in approximately 2 weeks, the outer silicone layer is replaced with epidermal autografts. Epidermal donor sites heal rapidly without significant morbidity, and Integra-covered wounds scar less; however, they are susceptible to wound infection and must be monitored carefully. Alloderm is another dermal substitute with decellularized preserved cadaver dermis. These synthetic dermal substitutes have tremendous potential for minimizing scar contractures and improving cosmetic and functional outcome. Temporary wound coverage can be achieved using biologic dressings, such as xenografts from swine and allografts from cadaver donors. Particularly useful when dealing with large TBSA burns, biologic dressings can provide immunologic and barrier functions of normal skin. The areas of xenograft and allograft are eventually rejected by the immune system and sloughed off, leaving healthy recipient beds for subsequent autografts. Although extremely rare, the transmission of viral diseases from allograft is a potential concern.

Excision and Grafting

Early excision with skin grafting has been shown to decrease operative blood loss and length of hospital stay and ultimately improve the overall survival of burn patients.[42,46] Typically, tangential excision of a full-thickness burn wound is performed within 3 days of injury, after relative hemodynamic stability has been achieved. The accurate determination of burn depth is vital to proper management. In particular, distinguishing between superficial and deep thermal burns is critical, as this dictates whether the burn wound can be treated with dressing changes alone or requires surgical excision. Eschar is sequentially shaved using a powered dermatome (Zimmer) or knife blades (Watson, Weck) until a viable tissue plane is achieved. Early excision of eschar (usually <24 hours after burns) generally decreases operative blood loss, owing to the actions of vasoconstrictive substances such as thromboxane and catecholamines. Once the burn wound becomes hyperemic 48 hours after injury, bleeding during excision of the eschar can be excessive. Tourniquet and subcutaneous injections of epinephrine-containing solution can lessen the blood loss, but these techniques may hinder the surgeon's ability to differentiate viable from nonviable tissue.[70] A topical hemostatic agent such as thrombin can also be used, but it is expensive and not very effective against excessive bleeding from open wounds. In patients with deep full-thickness burns, electrocautery is used to rapidly excise eschar with minimal blood loss. More importantly, the earlier the excision, the less blood loss is anticipated in burns greater than 30% of TBSA.[23] However, with scald burns it is more difficult to assess the burn depth initially; therefore, such burns require a more conservative approach, with delayed excision.

Ideally, the excised burn wound is covered with autografts. Burns wounds less than 20% to 30% of TBSA can be closed at one operation with split-thickness autografts. Split-thickness autografts are harvested using dermatomes, and donor sites are dressed with petroleum-based gauze, such as Xeroform or Scarlet Red. Opsite can also be used to cover donor sites. Sheet autografts are preferred for a better long-term aesthetic outcome, but narrowly meshed autografts (1:1 or 2:1) have the advantages of limiting the total surface area of donor harvest and allowing better drainage of fluid at the grafted sites. With massive burns, the closure of burn wounds is achieved by a combination of widely meshed autografts (4:1 to 6:1) with allograft (2:1) overlay (Fig. 23-8). Repeat grafting is required for large burns, with sequential harvesting of split-thickness autograft from limited donor sites until the entire burn wound is closed. As the meshed autografts heal, allografts slough off, but the formation of significant scar is a major disadvantage of this technique. Therefore, the use of widely meshed graft is avoided in the face and functionally important hands. A full-thickness graft that includes both dermal and epidermal components provides the best outcome in wound coverage, with diminished contracture and better pigment match. However, its use is generally limited to small areas, owing to the lack of abundant full-thickness donor skin.

The limitation of donor sites in massively burned patients is partially addressed with the use of systemic recombinant human growth hormone. Administration of growth hormone results in accelerated donor site healing, allowing more frequent donor site harvest.[39,44] In one study, growth hormone hastened donor site healing time by an average of 2 days, which ultimately shortened the length of hospital stay from 0.8 to 0.54 day per percent of TBSA burned.[39] These effects of growth hormone are thought to be due to stimulation of insulin-like growth factor-1 (IGF-1) release, along with the induction of IGF-1 receptors in the burn wound.[44] Insulin given alone can also decrease donor site healing time from 6.5 to 4.7 days.[82] Decreasing the time between each harvest by 1 day can significantly impact the total length of hospital stay in massively burned patients who require multiple grafting procedures. Administration of growth hormone in burned children was also associated with a 23% reduction in total cost of hospital care for a typical 80% TBSA burn.[39]

Recently, the use of cultured keratinocytes from the patient's own skin has generated considerable interest as a potential solution for massively burned patients with limited donor sites.[31,86,91] The concept of using cultured skin to provide complete coverage is appealing, but there are several problems to overcome before it can be widely used. Cultures of keratinocytes grow slowly and, once grafted, are very susceptible to mechanical trauma, resulting in only 50% to 70% graft take. Although a recent report showed that patients with greater than 80% TBSA burns receiving conventional treatment had shorter hospital stays than patients receiving cultured epithelial grafts,[4] the latter technology is a potentially attractive concept to treat massively burned patients.

HYPERMETABOLIC RESPONSE

Burn patients demonstrate a dramatic increase in metabolic rate. Better understanding of the mechanisms involved in the hypermetabolic response in burn injuries is one of the factors responsible for decreased mortality from massive burns over the last 3 decades. The hypermetabolic response—which is generally greater with increasing burn size but reaches a plateau at 40% TBSA burns[43]—is characterized by increased energy expenditure, oxygen consumption, proteolysis, lipolysis, and nitrogen losses. These physiologic changes are induced by the up-regulation of catabolic agents such cortisol, catecholamine, and glucagon, which act synergistically to increase the production of glucose, a principal fuel

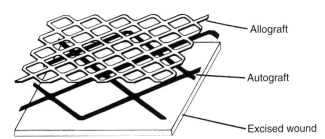

Figure 23-8 Wound coverage with 4:1 meshed autograft and 2:1 meshed allograft overlay. (From Eichelberger MR [ed]: Pediatric Trauma: Prevention, Acute Care, Rehabilitation. St Louis, Mosby, 1993, p 581.)

Allograft

Autograft

Excised wound

during acute inflammation.[89] Cortisol stimulates gluconeogenesis and proteolysis and sensitizes adipocytes to lipolytic hormones. Catecholamines stimulate the rate of glucose production through hepatic gluconeogenesis and glycogenolysis, as well as the promotion of lipolysis and peripheral insulin resistance, in which serum insulin levels are elevated but cells become resistant.[58] The increase in glucagon, which is stimulated by catecholamines, further promotes gluconeogenesis.

A significant protein catabolism occurs in severe burns. Cortisol is catabolic and is partially responsible for the loss of tissue protein and the negative nitrogen balance. In addition, burn injury is associated with decreased levels of anabolic hormones, such as growth hormone and IGF-1, which contributes significantly to net protein loss. The synthesis of protein (which is essential for the production of collagen for wound healing), antibodies, and leukocytes to participate in the immune response requires a net positive nitrogen balance. Excess catecholamines in postburn patients also contribute to persistent tachycardia and lipolysis. The consequences of these physiologic insults are cardiac failure and fatty infiltration of the liver.

Growth hormone and IGF-1 levels are decreased after burn injury. Pharmacologic agents have been used to attenuate catabolism and stimulate growth despite a burn injury.[77] Growth hormone, insulin, IGF-1, IGF-binding protein-3, testosterone, and oxandrolone improve nitrogen balance and promote wound healing.[28,37,47,82,99] Exogenous administration of recombinant human growth hormone, which increases protein synthesis, has been shown to improve nitrogen balance, preserve lean muscle mass, and increase the rate of wound healing.[44,98] The anabolic action of growth hormone appears to be mediated by an increase in protein synthesis, whereas IGF-1 decreases protein degradation. Growth hormone also enhances wound healing by stimulating hepatic and local production of IGF-1 to increase circulating and wound site levels.[39] Plasma growth hormone levels, which are decreased following severe burns, can be restored by the administration of recombinant growth hormone (0.2 mg/kg per day) in massively burned children to accelerate skin graft donor site wound healing and shorten hospital stay by more than 25% (Fig. 23-9).[34] The treatment of severely burned children with recombinant human growth hormone has been shown to be safe and efficacious. Growth hormone given during acute hospitalization maintains growth in severely burned children.[83] Height velocity improved during the first 2 years after burn injury in growth hormone–treated patients when compared with control patients. Recombinant human growth hormone also stimulates bone formation and muscle protein synthesis by up-regulation of IGF-1, successfully abating muscle catabolism and osteopenia.[63]

In severely burned patients, muscle anabolism can result from the administration of submaximal dosages of insulin by stimulating muscle protein synthesis. Insulin administration has also been demonstrated to improve skin graft donor site healing and wound matrix formation.[27] Testosterone production is greatly decreased after severe burn injury, which may last for months in postpubertal males. Increased protein synthesis with

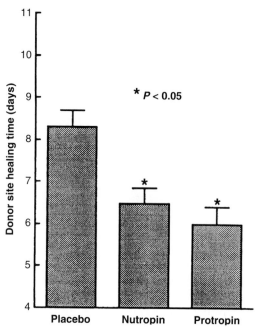

Figure 23-9   Donor site healing time for groups receiving either placebo (normal saline, $n = 26$) or recombinant growth hormone (Nutropin 0.2 mg/kg/day, $n = 20$; or Protropin 0.2 mg/kg/day, $n = 20$). A significant reduction in average healing time is noted with both forms of recombinant growth hormone when compared with control patients (mean ± SEM; * $P < 0.05$ versus placebo). (From Gilpin DA, Barrow RE, Rutan RL, et al: Recombinant human growth hormone accelerates wound healing in children with large cutaneous burns. Ann Surg 1994;220:19.)

testosterone administration is accompanied by a more efficient utilization of intracellular amino acids derived from protein breakdown and an increase in the inward transport of amino acids. An increase in net protein synthesis is attainable in adults with large burns by restoring testosterone concentrations to the physiologic range.[28] An analogue of testosterone with less androgenic effect, oxandrolone, has been used in acute and rehabilitating adult burn patients, with promising results with regard to weight gain. Oxandrolone alone has been shown to enhance protein synthesis efficiency, which improves muscle protein metabolism in severely burned children.[90]

The use of a beta blocker, propranolol, has been shown to lower resting heart rate and left ventricular work and to decrease peripheral lipolysis while maintaining lean body mass,[7] without adversely affecting cardiac output or the ability to respond to cold stress.[14,25,54] Recently, beta blockade using propranolol during hospitalization has been shown to attenuate hypermetabolic response and reverse muscle protein catabolism in burned children (Fig. 23-10).[43] Propranolol was given at a standard starting dose (1.98 mg/kg per day) and then titrated to decrease heart rate approximately 20% from baseline values. After 2 weeks of treatment, resting energy expenditure and oxygen consumption had increased in the control group. In contrast, patients in the propranolol group had significant decreases in these variables. Concurrently with the decline in energy expenditure, beta blockade also improved the kinetics of skeletal

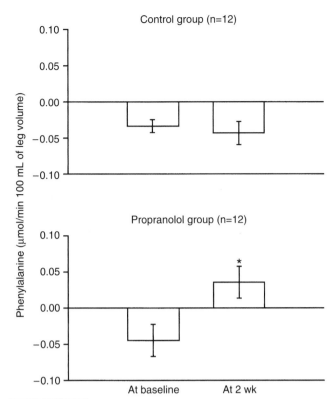

Figure 23–10 Mean change from baseline in the net balance of muscle protein synthesis and breakdown during 2 weeks of treatment with propranolol. Values were obtained from a 5-hour kinetic study using isotopically labeled phenylalanine. Asterisk (*) indicates a significant difference between the two groups ($P = 0.001$ by t-test) and a significant difference between the baseline value and the value at 2 weeks ($P = 0.002$ by paired t-test). (From Herndon DN, Hart DW, Wolf SE, et al: Reversal of catabolism by beta-blockade after severe burns. N Engl J Med 2001;345:1223.)

muscle protein. The muscle protein net balance improved by 82% compared with pretreatment baseline values, whereas it decreased only 27% in untreated controls.[43] Further, administering propranolol to burned children also receiving human growth hormone has salutary cardiovascular effects, decreases the release of free fatty acids from adipose tissue, and increases the liver's efficiency in handling secreted free fatty acids and very-low-density lipoproteins. Administration of propranolol has also been shown to decrease peripheral lipolysis and fat deposition in the liver of burn patients.[43]

Ketoconazole is an inhibitor of steroid ring synthesis and blocks the production of cortisol, indicating a potential use in the modulation of hypermetabolism. Difficulties with ketoconazole include its poor absorption in the pH-neutral stomach of ulcer prophylaxis patients. Even when accounting for this difficulty, we have found no effect on metabolic rate or protein synthesis with the oral administration of ketoconazole (unpublished data). Insulin, propranolol, and oxandrolone are the most cost-effective agents for the treatment of the hypermetabolic responses to trauma. Further, the role of nutrition in supporting the hypermetabolic response to trauma is often overlooked, but it clearly plays a part.

NUTRITION

The metabolic rate of patients with burns increases from 1.5 times the normal rate in a patient with 25% TBSA burns to 2 times the normal rate in those with 40% TBSA burns.[35] Children are particularly vulnerable to protein-calorie malnutrition because of their proportionally less body fat and smaller muscle mass, in addition to increased metabolic demands. This malnutrition is associated with dysfunction of various organ systems, including the immune system, and delayed wound healing. Therefore, optimal nutritional support must be provided to maintain and improve vital organ functions. Feeding tubes are generally placed under fluoroscopic guidance immediately after the initial evaluation of burns, and enteral nutrition is started within hours after injury. Early enteral feedings have been shown to decrease the level of catabolic hormones, improve nitrogen balance, maintain gut mucosal integrity, and decrease overall hospital stay.[15,73,88] Although hyperalimentation can deliver sufficient calories, its use in burn patients has been associated with deleterious effects on immune function; small bowel mucosal atrophy, with an increased incidence of bacterial translocation; and a decrease in survival.[41,48] Enteral nutrition is always preferred to parenteral nutrition and is associated with a decreased metabolic rate and lower incidence of sepsis in burn patients.

Several formulas are used to calculate caloric requirement in burn patients. Both the Curreri formula (25 kcal/kg plus 40 kcal/% TBSA burned) and the modified Harris-Benedict formula (calculated or measured resting metabolic rate times injury factor) use the principle of providing maintenance calories plus the additional calories required related to the burn size. Similar to fluid resuscitation guidelines, caloric requirements based on total and burned body surface area rather than weight are more appropriate for pediatric burn patients (Table 23-5).[50-52] The exact nutrient requirements of burn patients are not clear, but it is generally accepted that maintenance of energy requirement and replacement of protein losses are vital. The recommended enteral tube feedings should have 20% to 40% of the calories as protein, 10% to 20% as fat, and 40% to 70% as carbohydrates. Milk is one of the least expensive and best tolerated forms of nutrition, but sodium supplementation may be needed to avoid dilutional hyponatremia. There are also various commercially available enteral formulas, such as Vivonex and PediaSure, to choose from.

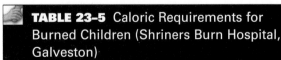

TABLE 23–5 Caloric Requirements for Burned Children (Shriners Burn Hospital, Galveston)

Age Group	Daily Caloric Requirements
Infant and toddler	2100 kcal/m² total + 1000 kcal/m² burned
Child	1800 kcal/m² total + 1300 kcal/m² burned
Adolescent	1500 kcal/m² total + 1500 kcal/m² burned

PHARMACOTHERAPY

Analgesia

Burn wound treatment and rehabilitation therapy produce pain in patients of all ages. Infants and children do not express their pain in the same way adults do and may display fear, anxiety, agitation, tantrums, depression, and withdrawal. With older children, allowing them to participate in their own wound care can give them some sense of control and alleviate fear and pain. Various combinations of analgesics and anxiolytic medications are used effectively during procedures and dressing changes (Table 23-6). Successful pain management of burned children requires an understanding that pain is associated with the burn depth and phase of wound healing. Pain management protocols should be tailored to control background pain as well as particular procedure-related painful stimuli. Physical therapy, which is vital to optimize good functional outcome, can be provided more effectively with appropriate pain control; however, absolute caution must be exercised to prevent any potential complications due to overmedication at the time of exercise therapy. In children as young as 5 years old, patient-controlled analgesia may be an ideal option to provide a steady-state background infusion of narcotic with an additional bolus regimen.[71] Burn injuries are traumatic for burned children as well as for their families. Burn care professionals must do everything they can to make the experience as tolerable as possible while assisting burn patients to a successful recovery.

Sedatives and Anxiolytics

Ketamine is a commonly used procedural sedative-anesthetic in burn patients. Derived from phencyclidine, it is characterized by dissociative anesthesia and has excellent analgesic properties. Given at a dose of 1.0 to 2.0 mg/kg intravenously or 5.0 to 7.0 mg/kg intramuscularly, the effect is rapid, but with a relatively short duration of action. In addition, ketamine is frequently used as an anesthetic agent for operative procedures, without compromising airway reflexes. The use of ketamine is contraindicated in patients with increased intracranial pressure.

Benzodiazepines are commonly used to control burn-related anxiety as well as to enhance the effects of narcotics for pain control. Lorazepam (Ativan) at a dosage of 0.03 mg/kg orally or intravenously is an effective anxiolytic agent. It is also useful as a hypnotic agent to improve patient restfulness in the acute care setting. Diazepam (Valium) has a longer duration of action than lorazepam, making it useful in more chronic settings. Diazepam also improves muscle relaxation, which can facilitate rehabilitative therapy. Midazolam (Versed) has a rapid onset of action; peak plasma levels are achieved within 30 minutes, with a half-life of 2 to 5 hours. It is commonly used to achieve the desired level of sedation for procedures and dressing changes. Because it induces anterograde amnesia, it is commonly used as a premedication on the day of surgery.

Antibiotics

The use of perioperative IV antibiotics has had a tremendous impact in improving the survival of major burn patients in the past 2 decades. Bacteria colonized in a burn eschar can potentially shed systemically at the time of eschar excision, contributing to sepsis and other organ system infection. Empirically, a broad-spectrum IV antibiotic regimen (e.g., vancomycin, third-generation cephalosporins, and penicillins) is given perioperatively to patients with greater than 40% TBSA burns to protect against *Streptococcus, Staphylococcus aureus,* and *Pseudomonas*. The antibiotic regimen is subsequently modified, depending on sensitivities identified by quantitative cultures of the excised eschar. In acute burns, a gram-positive coccus is generally the predominant organism involved, but colonization with gram-negative organisms and even fungi is frequently encountered in chronic burn wounds, and these organisms must be covered with appropriate IV antibiotics during excision and grafting. In addition to burn wound sepsis, graft loss may be attributed to the presence of an infected wound at the time of skin grafting or colonization of the grafted bed shortly after surgery. The most common organisms responsible for graft loss are beta-hemolytic streptococci (*S. pyogenes, S. agalactiae,* or *S. viridans*). They are generally sensitive to third-generation cephalosporins and fluoroquinolones. The emergence of multiresistant bacteria, such as methicillin-resistant *S. aureus,* has become a serious problem for burn centers. Therefore, IV antibiotics should be used with diligence, but only for perioperative coverage and treatment of an identified source of infection.

TABLE 23-6 Pharmacotherapy Agents

Agent	Dose	Indication
Morphine sulfate	0.05-0.1 mg/kg IV or 0.3 mg/kg PO	Acute pain; procedures and dressing changes
Meperidine	1.0-2.0 mg/kg PO or IV	Acute pain; procedures and dressing changes
Ketamine	1.0-2.0 mg/kg IV or 5.0-7.0 mg/kg IM	Surgery; procedures and dressing changes
Diazepam	1.0-2.0 mg PO or IV	Preoperative; anxiety
Chloral hydrate	250-500 mg PO	Preoperative; insomnia
Midazolam	0.25-0.5 mg/kg PO or IV	Anxiety; used in combination with narcotics
Lorazepam	0.03 mg/kg PO or IV	Background anxiety

INHALATION INJURY

Inhalation injury is a major cause of death in burn patients. The mortality rate for children with isolated cutaneous burns is 1% to 2% but increases to approximately

40% in the presence of inhalation injury.[49,92] Inhalation injury is caused primarily by inhaled toxins such as fumes, gases, and mists. Although the supraglottic region can be injured by both thermal and chemical insults, tracheobronchial and lung parenchymal injuries rarely occur as a result of direct thermal damage because the heat disperses rapidly in the larynx. Hypoxia, increased airway resistance, decreased pulmonary compliance, increased alveolar epithelial permeability, and increased pulmonary vascular resistance may be triggered by the release of vasoactive substances (thromboxane A_2, C_{3a}, and C_{5a}) from damaged epithelium.[93] Neutrophil activation plays a critical role in this process, and pulmonary function has been shown to improve with the use of a ligand binding to E-selectins (inhibiting neutrophil adhesion) and anti-interleukin-8 (inhibiting neutrophil chemotaxis). Another significant form of respiratory tract pathology is the sloughing of ciliated epithelial cells from the basement membrane, resulting in exudate formation. The exudate, which consists of lymph proteins, coalesces to form fibrin casts. These fibrin casts are frequently resistant to routine pulmonary toilet and can create a "ball-valve" effect in localized areas of lung, eventually causing barotrauma.

The diagnosis is usually made based on clinical history and physical examination findings during the initial evaluation. Victims trapped in a house fire with excessive smoke and fumes are likely to have sustained severe inhalation injury. Facial burns with singed hair and carbonaceous sputum suggest the presence of inhalation injury. Hoarseness and stridor suggest significant airway obstruction, so the airway should be secured immediately with endotracheal intubation. Patients who present with disorientation and obtundation are likely to have elevated carbon monoxide levels (carboxyhemoglobin >10%). Cyanide toxicity as a result of the combustion of common household items may also contribute to unexplained metabolic collapse. Diagnostic tools, such as bronchoscopy and xenon-133 scanning, are more than 90% accurate in determining the presence of inhalation injury. Fiber-optic bronchoscopic examination of the airway at the bedside (avoiding the need to transport critically injured burn patients to the nuclear medicine department) is usually sufficient to identify airway edema and inflammatory changes of the tracheal mucosa such as hyperemia, mucosal ulceration, and sloughing. It remains the gold standard to confirm the presence of inhalation injury.[56] Ventilation scan with xenon 133 can also identify regions of inhalation injury by assessing respiratory exchange and excretion of xenon by the lungs.[76]

The treatment of inhalation injury begins at the scene of the burn accident. The administration of 100% oxygen rapidly decreases the half-life of carbon monoxide. The airway must be secured with intubation in patients exhibiting signs and symptoms of imminent respiratory failure. Aggressive pulmonary toilet with physiotherapy and frequent suctioning is vital to prevent any serious respiratory complications. Humidified air is delivered at high flow, and bronchodilators and racemic epinephrine are used to treat bronchospasm. IV heparin has been shown to reduce tracheobronchial cast formation, improve minute ventilation, and lower peak inspiratory pressures after smoke inhalation. Inhalation treatments such as 20% acetylcysteine nebulized solution (3 mL every 4 hours) plus nebulized heparin (5000 to 10,000 units with 3 mL normal saline every 4 hours) are effective in improving the clearance of tracheobronchial secretions and minimizing bronchospasm, thereby significantly decreasing reintubation rates and mortality.[10,62]

The presence of inhalation injury generally requires increased fluid resuscitation, up to 2 mL/kg per percent TBSA burned more than would be required for the same size burn without an inhalation injury. In fact, pulmonary edema that is associated with inhalation injury is not prevented by fluid restriction; rather, inadequate resuscitation may increase the severity of pulmonary injury by the sequestration of polymorphonuclear cells.[40] Steroids have not been shown to be of any benefit in inhalation injury. Prophylactic IV antibiotics are not indicated but are started if there is a clinical suspicion of pneumonia. Early pneumonia is usually the result of gram-positive organisms such as methicillin-resistant *S. aureus*, whereas later infection is caused by gram-negative organisms such as *Pseudomonas*. Serially monitored sputum cultures and bronchial washings should guide antibiotic therapy.

NONTHERMAL INJURIES

Chemical Burns

Children often accidentally come in contact with various household cleaning products. Treatment of chemical burns involves the immediate removal of the causative agent and lavage with copious amounts of water, taking care to avoid hypothermia and to ensure that the effluent does not contact uninjured areas. Fluid resuscitation is also started. Decontamination is not performed in a tub; rather, the wounds are irrigated toward a drain, such as in a shower. After copious irrigation, wounds should be covered with topical antimicrobial dressing, and appropriate surgical plans should be made. Rapid recognition of the offending chemical agent is crucial to proper management.[29] When in doubt, the local poison control center should be contacted to identify the chemical composition of the product involved.

The common offending chemical agents can be classified as alkali or acid. Alkalis, such as lime, potassium hydroxide, sodium hydroxide, and bleach, are among the most common agents involved in chemical injuries. Mechanisms of alkali-induced burns are saponification of fat, resulting in increased cell damage from heat, extraction of intracellular water, and formation of alkaline proteinates with hydroxyl ions. These ions induce further chemical reaction in the deeper tissues. Attempts to neutralize alkalis are not recommended, because the chemical reaction can generate more heat and add to the injury. Acid burns are not as common. Acids induce protein breakdown by hydrolysis, resulting in the formation of an eschar, and therefore do not penetrate as deeply as alkaline burns. Formic acid injuries are rare but can result in multiple systemic effects, such as metabolic acidosis, renal failure, intravascular hemolysis, and acute respiratory distress syndrome. Hydrofluoric acid burns are managed differently from other acid burns.[94] After copious local irrigation with water, fluoride ions must be neutralized with topical application of 2.5% calcium gluconate gel. If not appropriately treated, free fluoride ions can cause liquefaction necrosis of the affected tissues, including bones. Because of potential hypocalcemia, patients should be closely monitored for prolonged QT intervals.

Electrical Burns

Electrical burns are rare in children, accounting for only 3% to 5% of all admitted burn patients. Electrical burns are categorized as either high- or low-voltage injuries.[50] High-voltage injuries are characterized by varying degrees of local burns and destruction of deep tissues.[65,84] Electrical current enters a part of the body and travels through tissues with the lowest resistance, such as nerves, blood vessels, and muscles. Heat generated as electrical current passes through deep tissues with relatively high resistance, such as bones, and damages adjacent tissues that may not be readily visible. Skin is mostly spared owing to its high resistance to electrical current. Primary and secondary surveys, including electrocardiograms, should be completed. If the initial electrocardiogram is normal, no further monitoring is necessary; however, any abnormal findings require continued monitoring for 48 hours and appropriate treatment of dysrhythmias when detected.[85]

The key to the management of electrical burns lies in the early detection and proper treatment of injuries to deep structures. Edema formation and subsequent vascular compromise are common in extremities. Fasciotomies are frequently necessary to avoid potential limb loss. If myoglobin is present in urine, vigorous hydration, with the administration of sodium bicarbonate to alkalinize the urine and mannitol to achieve diuresis and to act as a free radical scavenger, is indicated. Repeated wound exploration and debridement of affected areas are required before ultimate wound closure because there is a component of delayed cell death and thrombosis. The mechanism of electrical burn injury is to overwhelm the cellular systems that operate at millivolt or milliamp levels, so cells that survive the initial injury may slowly die over a week's time as ion gradients deteriorate and thrombosis of the microvasculature proceeds. Electrical injuries may also have a thermal, nonconductive component as the electricity flashes. This is treated as if it were a conventional thermal burn. Low-voltage injury is similar to thermal injury without the transmission of electrical current to deep tissues and usually requires only local wound care.

OUTPATIENT BURNS

The majority of pediatric burns are minor, often resulting from scalds involving less than 10% TBSA or contact with hot objects causing small, isolated areas of thermal injury. Such burns are usually partial-thickness skin injuries and can be treated on an outpatient basis. After an initial assessment, the burn wound is gently washed with water and a mild soap with appropriate pain control. Blisters can be left intact when they are small and unlikely to rupture spontaneously, especially on the palms of the hand, because they provide a natural barrier against the environment and are beneficial to avoid daily dressing changes. Spontaneous resorption of the fluid occurs in approximately 1 week with the re-epithelialization process. Larger areas of blisters should be debrided, and topical antimicrobial dressings applied. Silvadene is most commonly used owing to its broad-spectrum antimicrobial properties, as well as its soothing effect on superficial second-degree burns. However, because silver sulfadiazine can impede epithelization, its use should be discontinued when healing partial-thickness wounds are devoid of necrotic tissue and evidence of re-epithelialization is noted. Alternatively, antimicrobial dressings with triple antibiotic ointment (neomycin, bacitracin, and polymyxin B sulfate) or Polysporin, which has no negative effect on epithelialization, are commonly used. For small, superficial partial-thickness burns, nonmedical white petrolatum-impregnated fine mesh or porous mesh gauze (Adaptic), or fine mesh absorbent gauze impregnated with 3% bismuth tribromophenate in a nonmedicinal petrolatum blend (Xeroform), is usually sufficient, without the need for topical antimicrobials. Superficial burns of the face can be treated with the application of triple antibiotic ointment without any dressings.

The frequency of dressing change varies from twice daily to once a week, depending on the size and depth of the burn and the amount of drainage. Those who advocate twice-daily dressing changes base their care on the use of topical antimicrobials whose half-life is about 8 to 12 hours. Others who use petrolatum-based or bismuth-impregnated gauze recommend less frequent dressing changes—once every 3 to 5 days. The use of synthetic wound dressings is ideal for the outpatient treatment of superficial partial-thickness burns.[33] When applied appropriately to fresh, partial-thickness wounds, Biobrane adheres to the wound rapidly and is very effective in promoting re-epithelialization in 1 to 2 weeks (see Fig. 23-7). Although daily dressing changes are eliminated, Biobrane-covered wounds should still be monitored closely for signs of infection.

REHABILITATION

Acute Therapy

Rehabilitation therapy is an essential component of burn care. During the acute phase of burn care, splints are used to prevent joint deformities and contractures. Made of thermoplastic materials, which are amenable to heat manipulation, splints are fitted individually to each patient. Application of splints at all times except during exercise periods can prevent the severe contractures that occur in patients with large burns. Patients are mobilized out of bed immediately after the graft takes, and aggressive physical therapy is provided.

After the acute phase, hypertrophic scar formation is a major concern. Burn depth, patient age, and genetic factors all play an important role in hypertrophic scar formation. In general, deep second-degree burn wounds, requiring 3 weeks or more to heal, produce hypertrophic scarring. Children are more prone to hypertrophic scar formation than adults are, probably because of the high rate of cell mitosis associated with growth. Constant pressure applied 24 hours a day is the most effective method to minimize hypertrophic scar formation; pressure garments should be worn until scars mature. Scar maturation usually occurs 6 to 18 months after injury; in younger patients, scars mature at a much slower rate. In addition to splints and pressure garments, exercise therapy is a crucial component of rehabilitation therapy. Families should receive thorough instruction on a program of range-of-motion exercises and muscle strengthening.

Extended Therapy

Burn survivors and their families need rehabilitation therapy for extended periods on both a physical and a psychological level. All must deal with feelings ranging from guilt to post-traumatic stress. In one study, a group of surgeons reviewed the images of 12 burn survivors with 80% or greater TBSA burned and 70% third-degree burns, and predicted their status with respect to scarring and future employability. They predicted that all the patients would experience difficult psychological adjustments, and that many would require multiple operations in the reconstructive phase.[45] In reality, the patients received twice as many operations as predicted, yet three quarters of these children demonstrated normal adjustment and emotional growth. When this longitudinal study was followed for additional 10 years, the children's emotional assessment scores were equal to those of their uninjured peers. That so few of these survivors developed serious psychological and social difficulties is a striking testament to human resilience.

REFERENCES

1. Ayus JC, Arieff AI: Hyponatremia and myelinolysis. Ann Intern Med 1997;127:163.
2. Baptiste MS, Feck G: Preventing tap water burns. Am J Public Health 1980;70:727.
3. Barillo DJ, Goode R: Fire fatality study: Demographics of fire victims. Burns 1996;22:85.
4. Barret JP, Wolf SE, Desai MH, et al: Cost-efficacy of cultured epidermal autografts in massive pediatric burns. Ann Surg 2000;231:869.
5. Bjerknes R, Vindenes H, Laerum OD: Altered neutrophil functions in patients with large burns. Blood Cells 1990; 16:127.
6. Bjerknes R, Vindenes H, Pitkanen J, et al: Altered polymorphonuclear neutrophilic granulocyte functions in patients with large burns. J Trauma 1989;29:847.
7. Breitenstein E, Chiolero RL, Jequier E, et al: Effects of beta-blockade on energy metabolism following burns. Burns 1990;16:259.
8. Brigham PA, McLoughlin E: Burn incidence and medical care use in the United States: Estimates, trends, and data sources. J Burn Care Rehabil 1996;17:95.
9. Brink JA, Sheets PW, Dines KA, et al: Quantitative assessment of burn injury in porcine skin with high-frequency ultrasonic imaging. Invest Radiol 1986;21:645.
10. Brown M, Desai M, Traber LD, et al: Dimethylsulfoxide with heparin in the treatment of smoke inhalation injury. J Burn Care Rehabil 1988;9:22.
11. Bucky LP, Vedder NB, Hong HZ, et al: Reduction of burn injury by inhibiting CD18-mediated leukocyte adherence in rabbits. Plast Reconstr Surg 1994;93:1473.
12. Burn Injury Fact Sheet. Washington, DC, National Safe Kids Campaign; 2004.
13. Carter EA, Gonnella A, Tompkins RG: Increased transcellular permeability of rat small intestine after thermal injury. Burns 1992;18:117.
14. Chance WT, Nelson JL, Foley-Nelson T, et al: The relationship of burn-induced hypermetabolism to central and peripheral catecholamines. J Trauma 1989;29:306.
15. Chiarelli A, Enzi G, Casadei A, et al: Very early nutrition supplementation in burned patients. Am J Clin Nutr 1990; 51:1035.
16. Chung DH, Evers BM, Townsend CM Jr, et al: Burn-induced transcriptional regulation of small intestinal ornithine decarboxylase. Am J Surg 1992;163:157.
17. Chung DH, Evers BM, Townsend CM Jr, et al: Role of polyamine biosynthesis during gut mucosal adaptation after burn injury. Am J Surg 1993;165:144.
18. Cope O, Moore FD: The redistribution of body water. Ann Surg 1947;126:1016.
19. DelBeccaro EJ, Robson MC, Heggers JP, et al: The use of specific thromboxane inhibitors to preserve the dermal microcirculation after burning. Surgery 1980;87:137.
20. Demling RH, LaLonde C: Early postburn lipid peroxidation: Effect of ibuprofen and allopurinol. Surgery 1990; 107:85.
21. Demling RH, Mazess RB, Witt RM, et al: The study of burn wound edema using dichromatic absorptiometry. J Trauma 1978;18:124.
22. Desai MH, Herndon DN: Eradication of *Candida* burn wound septicemia in massively burned patients. J Trauma 1988;28:140.
23. Desai MH, Herndon DN, Broemeling L, et al: Early burn wound excision significantly reduces blood loss. Ann Surg 1990;211:753.
24. Desai MH, Rutan RL, Heggers JP, et al: *Candida* infection with and without nystatin prophylaxis: An 11-year experience with patients with burn injury. Arch Surg 1992; 127:159.
25. Drost AC, Burleson DG, Cioffi WG Jr, et al: Plasma cytokines following thermal injury and their relationship with patient mortality, burn size, and time postburn. J Trauma 1993;35:335.
26. Du GB, Slater H, Goldfarb IW: Influences of different resuscitation regimens on acute early weight gain in extensively burned patients. Burns 1991;17:147.
27. Ferrando AA, Chinkes DL, Wolf SE, et al: A submaximal dose of insulin promotes net skeletal muscle protein synthesis in patients with severe burns. Ann Surg 1999;229:11.
28. Ferrando AA, Sheffield-Moore M, Wolf SE, et al: Testosterone administration in severe burns ameliorates muscle catabolism. Crit Care Med 2001;29:1936.
29. Fitzpatrick KT, Moylan JA: Emergency care of chemical burns. Postgrad Med 1985;78:189.
30. Fox CL Jr, Rappole BW, Stanford W: Control of *Pseudomonas* infection in burns by silver sulfadiazine. Surg Gynecol Obstet 1969;128:1021.

31. Gallico GG 3rd, O'Connor NE, Compton CC, et al: Permanent coverage of large burn wounds with autologous cultured human epithelium. N Engl J Med 1984;311:448.

32. Gamelli RL, He LK, Liu H: Macrophage suppression of granulocyte and macrophage growth following burn wound infection. J Trauma 1994;37:888.

33. Gerding RL, Emerman CL, Effron D, et al: Outpatient management of partial-thickness burns: Biobrane versus 1% silver sulfadiazine. Ann Emerg Med 1990;19:121.

34. Gilpin DA, Barrow RE, Rutan RL, et al: Recombinant human growth hormone accelerates wound healing in children with large cutaneous burns. Ann Surg 1994; 220:19.

35. Goran MI, Peters EJ, Herndon DN, et al: Total energy expenditure in burned children using the doubly labeled water technique. Am J Physiol 1990;259(4 Pt 1):E576.

36. Graves TA, Cioffi WG, McManus WF, et al: Fluid resuscitation of infants and children with massive thermal injury. J Trauma 1988;28:1656.

37. Hart DW, Wolf SE, Ramzy PI, et al: Anabolic effects of oxandrolone after severe burn. Ann Surg 2001;233:556.

38. Heggers JP, Sazy JA, Stenberg BD, et al: Bactericidal and wound-healing properties of sodium hypochlorite solutions: The 1991 Lindberg Award. J Burn Care Rehabil 1991; 12:420.

39. Herndon DN, Barrow RE, Kunkel KR, et al: Effects of recombinant human growth hormone on donor-site healing in severely burned children. Ann Surg 1990;212:424.

40. Herndon DN, Barrow RE, Linares HA, et al: Inhalation injury in burned patients: Effects and treatment. Burns Incl Therm Inj 1988;14:349.

41. Herndon DN, Barrow RE, Stein M, et al: Increased mortality with intravenous supplemental feeding in severely burned patients. J Burn Care Rehabil 1989;10:309.

42. Herndon DN, Gore D, Cole M, et al: Determinants of mortality in pediatric patients with greater than 70% full-thickness total body surface area thermal injury treated by early total excision and grafting. J Trauma 1987;27:208.

43. Herndon DN, Hart DW, Wolf SE, et al: Reversal of catabolism by beta-blockade after severe burns. N Engl J Med 2001;345:1223.

44. Herndon DN, Hawkins HK, Nguyen TT, et al: Characterization of growth hormone enhanced donor site healing in patients with large cutaneous burns. Ann Surg 1995;221:649.

45. Herndon DN, LeMaster J, Beard S, et al: The quality of life after major thermal injury in children: An analysis of 12 survivors with greater than or equal to 80% total body, 70% third-degree burns. J Trauma 1986;26:609.

46. Herndon DN, Parks DH: Comparison of serial debridement and autografting and early massive excision with cadaver skin overlay in the treatment of large burns in children. J Trauma 1986;26:149.

47. Herndon DN, Ramzy PI, DebRoy MA, et al: Muscle protein catabolism after severe burn: Effects of IGF-1/IGFBP-3 treatment. Ann Surg 1999;229:713.

48. Herndon DN, Stein MD, Rutan TC, et al: Failure of TPN supplementation to improve liver function, immunity, and mortality in thermally injured patients. J Trauma 1987;27:195.

49. Herndon DN, Thompson PB, Traber DL: Pulmonary injury in burned patients. Crit Care Clin 1985;1:79.

50. Hildreth MA, Herndon DN, Desai MH, et al: Caloric needs of adolescent patients with burns. J Burn Care Rehabil 1989;10:523.

51. Hildreth MA, Herndon DN, Desai MH, et al: Current treatment reduces calories required to maintain weight in pediatric patients with burns. J Burn Care Rehabil 1990;11:405.

52. Hildreth MA, Herndon DN, Desai MH, et al: Caloric requirements of patients with burns under one year of age. J Burn Care Rehabil 1993;14:108.

53. Ho-Asjoe M, Chronnell CM, Frame JD, et al: Immunohistochemical analysis of burn depth. J Burn Care Rehabil 1999;20:207.

54. Honeycutt D, Barrow R, Herndon D: Cold stress response in patients with severe burns after beta-blockade. J Burn Care Rehabil 1992;13(2 Pt 1):181.

55. Huang PP, Stucky FS, Dimick AR, et al: Hypertonic sodium resuscitation is associated with renal failure and death. Ann Surg 1995;221:543.

56. Hunt JL, Agee RN, Pruitt BA Jr: Fiberoptic bronchoscopy in acute inhalation injury. J Trauma 1975;15:641.

57. Hunt JP, Hunter CT, Brownstein MR, et al: The effector component of the cytotoxic T-lymphocyte response has a biphasic pattern after burn injury. J Surg Res 1998;80:243.

58. Jahoor F, Herndon DN, Wolfe RR: Role of insulin and glucagon in the response of glucose and alanine kinetics in burn-injured patients. J Clin Invest 1986;78:807.

59. Jarrett F, Ellerbe S, Demling R: Acute leukopenia during topical burn therapy with silver sulfadiazine. Am J Surg 1978;135:818.

60. Jerath MR, Schomacker KT, Sheridan RL, et al: Burn wound assessment in porcine skin using indocyanine green fluorescence. J Trauma 1999;46:1085.

61. Jeschke MG, Barrow RE, Wolf SE, et al: Mortality in burned children with acute renal failure. Arch Surg 1998;133:752.

62. Kimura R, Traber LD, Herndon DN, et al: Treatment of smoke-induced pulmonary injury with nebulized dimethylsulfoxide. Circ Shock 1988;25:333.

63. Klein GL, Wolf SE, Goodman WG, et al: The management of acute bone loss in severe catabolism due to burn injury. Horm Res 1997;48(Suppl 5):83.

64. Klimpel GR, Herndon DH, Stein MD: Peripheral blood lymphocytes from thermal injury patients are defective in their ability to generate lymphokine-activated killer (LAK) cell activity. J Clin Immunol 1988;8:14.

65. Laberge LC, Ballard PA, Daniel RK: Experimental electrical burns: Low voltage. Ann Plast Surg 1984;13:185.

66. Lal S, Barrow RE, Wolf SE, et al: Biobrane improves wound healing in burned children without increased risk of infection. Shock 2000;14:314.

67. LeVoyer T, Cioffi WG Jr, Pratt L, et al: Alterations in intestinal permeability after thermal injury. Arch Surg 1992;127:26.

68. Lindberg RB, Moncrief JA, Switzer WE, et al: The successful control of burn wound sepsis. J Trauma 1965;5:601.

69. Lund CC, Browder NC: The estimation of areas of burns. Surg Gynecol Obstet 1944;79:352.

70. Marano MA, O'Sullivan G, Madden M, et al: Tourniquet technique for reduced blood loss and wound assessment during excisions of burn wounds of the extremity. Surg Gynecol Obstet 1990;171:249.

71. McDonald AJ, Cooper MG: Patient-controlled analgesia: An appropriate method of pain control in children. Paediatr Drugs 2001;3:273.

72. Mileski W, Borgstrom D, Lightfoot E, et al: Inhibition of leukocyte-endothelial adherence following thermal injury. J Surg Res 1992;52:334.

73. Mochizuki H, Trocki O, Dominioni L, et al: Mechanism of prevention of postburn hypermetabolism and catabolism by early enteral feeding. Ann Surg 1984;200:297.

74. Monafo WW: The treatment of burn shock by the intravenous and oral administration of hypertonic lactated saline solution. J Trauma 1970;10:575.

75. Moyer CA, Brentano L, Gravens DL, et al: Treatment of large human burns with 0.5 per cent silver nitrate solution. Arch Surg 1965;90:812.

76. Moylan JA Jr, Wilmore DW, Mouton DE, et al: Early diagnosis of inhalation injury using 133 xenon lung scan. Ann Surg 1972;176:477.

77. Murphy KD, Lee JO, Herndon DN: Current pharmacotherapy for the treatment of severe burns. Expert Opin Pharmacother 2003;4:369.

78. Myers SI, Minei JP, Casteneda A, et al: Differential effects of acute thermal injury on rat splanchnic and renal blood flow and prostanoid release. Prostaglandins Leukot Essent Fatty Acids 1995;53:439.

79. Nwariaku FE, Sikes PJ, Lightfoot E, et al: Effect of a bradykinin antagonist on the local inflammatory response following thermal injury. Burns 1996;22:324.

80. O'Reilly TJ, Spence RJ, Taylor RM, et al: Laser Doppler flowmetry evaluation of burn wound depth. J Burn Care Rehabil 1989;10:1.

81. Park DH, Hwang JW, Jang KS, et al: Use of laser Doppler flowmetry for estimation of the depth of burns. Plast Reconstr Surg 1998;101:1516.

82. Pierre EJ, Barrow RE, Hawkins HK, et al: Effects of insulin on wound healing. J Trauma 1998;44:342.

83. Ramirez RJ, Wolf SE, Barrow RE, et al: Growth hormone treatment in pediatric burns: A safe therapeutic approach. Ann Surg 1998;228:439.

84. Robson MC, Murphy RC, Heggers JP: A new explanation for the progressive tissue loss in electrical injuries. Plast Reconstr Surg 1984;73:431.

85. Robson MC, Smith DJ: Care of the thermal injured victim. In Jurkiewicz MJ, Krizek TJ, Mathes SJ, et al (eds): Plastic Surgery: Principles and Practice. St Louis, CV Mosby, 1990.

86. Rue LW 3rd, Cioffi WG, McManus WF, et al: Wound closure and outcome in extensively burned patients treated with cultured autologous keratinocytes. J Trauma 1993;34:662.

87. Ryan CM, Yarmush ML, Burke JF, et al: Increased gut permeability early after burns correlates with the extent of burn injury. Crit Care Med 1992;20:1508.

88. Saito H, Trocki O, Alexander JW, et al: The effect of route of nutrient administration on the nutritional state, catabolic hormone secretion, and gut mucosal integrity after burn injury. JPEN J Parenter Enteral Nutr 1987;11:1.

89. Shamoon H, Hendler R, Sherwin RS: Synergistic interactions among antiinsulin hormones in the pathogenesis of stress hyperglycemia in humans. J Clin Endocrinol Metab 1981;52:1235.

90. Sheffield-Moore M, Urban RJ, Wolf SE, et al: Short-term oxandrolone administration stimulates net muscle protein synthesis in young men. J Clin Endocrinol Metab 1999;84:2705.

91. Sheridan RL, Tompkins RG: Cultured autologous epithelium in patients with burns of ninety percent or more of the body surface. J Trauma 1995;38:48.

92. Thompson PB, Herndon DN, Traber DL, et al: Effect on mortality of inhalation injury. J Trauma 1986;26:163.

93. Traber DL, Herndon DN, Stein MD, et al: The pulmonary lesion of smoke inhalation in an ovine model. Circ Shock 1986;18:311.

94. Trevino MA, Herrmann GH, Sprout WL: Treatment of severe hydrofluoric acid exposures. J Occup Med 1983;25:861.

95. Vo LT, Papworth GD, Delaney PM, et al: A study of vascular response to thermal injury on hairless mice by fibre optic confocal imaging, laser Doppler flowmetry and conventional histology. Burns 1998;24:319.

96. Warden GD: Burn shock resuscitation. World J Surg 1992;16:16.

97. Warden GD: Fluid resuscitation and early management. In Herndon DN (ed): Total Burn Care. Philadelphia, WB Saunders, 1996, p 53.

98. Wilmore DW, Moylan JA Jr, Bristow BF, et al: Anabolic effects of human growth hormone and high caloric feedings following thermal injury. Surg Gynecol Obstet 1974;138:875.

99. Wolf SE, Barrow RE, Herndon DN: Growth hormone and IGF-I therapy in the hypercatabolic patient. Baillieres Clin Endocrinol Metab 1996;10:447.

100. Wolf SE, Ikeda H, Matin S, et al: Cutaneous burn increases apoptosis in the gut epithelium of mice. J Am Coll Surg 1999;188:10.

101. Zedler S, Faist E, Ostermeier B, et al: Postburn constitutional changes in T-cell reactivity occur in CD8+ rather than in CD4+ cells. J Trauma 1997;42:872.

Chapter 24

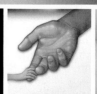

Child Abuse and Birth Injuries

Dennis W. Vane

CHILD ABUSE

Child abuse encompasses physical abuse, sexual abuse, emotional abuse, and neglect. This maltreatment of children has become a significant focus of attention in our society. The media routinely publish accounts of the alleged traumatic and sometimes fatal abuse of children among all socioeconomic classes and levels of celebrity. The myth that child abuse and other violence in the home occur only among the poor and the uneducated has been debunked. Child abuse is a worldwide problem that affects all levels of society. Prevention and effective treatment depend on the timely detection of epidemiologic situations that lend themselves to the maltreatment of children.

Unfortunately, the "minor" status of children leads to the justifiable issue of the relative rights of parents and guardians. Religious and societal "norms" have created barriers to the identification of victims in many nations. Around the globe, relatively few nations have addressed this problem at all.[3] In the United States and Canada, legislation aimed at identifying child abuse and neglect was enacted beginning in the 1960s.[71] Since that time, the reporting of child abuse to civil authorities has been mandated for almost all professionals dealing with children. The legislation protects the reporting individual from liability (usually by using the phrase "suspicion of" or "injuries consistent with"), supersedes all professional-client privilege, and sometimes even imposes penalties for failure to report abuse.[47]

Epidemiology

Estimates in the United States indicate that approximately 1.4 million children under the age of 18 suffer some sort of maltreatment every year.[54] This represents between 2% and 3% of the population. In about 160,000 children, this maltreatment is considered physically serious or life threatening. Between 1000 and 2000 deaths are attributed to child abuse each year in the United States, and 80% of those children are younger than 5 years. Forty percent of the deaths occur in the first year of life.[48] Although deaths occur predominantly in the younger

age groups, maltreatment of children generally increases with age. In teenagers, the incidence of abuse is thought to be twice that in preschool children.[54]

Patterns of child abuse occur with differing frequencies over the social strata. Sexual and emotional abuse have no socioeconomic associations, whereas physical abuse and neglect are more frequently associated with poverty.[54] Often several types of abuse are perpetrated on the same child or within the same family. Additionally, abuse commonly occurs in families with other forms of intrafamilial violence, such as spousal abuse and violence among siblings.[49]

Child abuse is a self-perpetuating social and economic problem. Problems with substance abuse and depression are reportedly two to three times more likely in abused children than in the general population, and abused children are likely to be far more physically aggressive with their peers.[22,32] It is estimated that approximately 30% of abuse victims eventually abuse their own children.[20] Some authors have suggested that this perpetual cycle of abuse is attributable in part to changes in the neuroendocrine system influencing arousal, learning, growth, and the individual's pain threshold.[20]

What is clear is that the incidence of child abuse is significantly underreported, because professional contact or recognition is often required to identify abuse in the first place. Physicians must recognize not only abuse that has already occurred but also the factors indicating a high potential for abuse if this dramatic worldwide problem is to be prevented.

Presentation

Physicians must be aware that abused children are often withdrawn and avoid eye contact with their interviewers. Interviewers must be cognizant of the fact that children often respond with answers that they think will please the interviewer, so care must be taken not to influence the child's responses. Young children are prone to associative fabrication, which may influence or even alter reality. The clinical history in suspected child abuse cases should include a detailed history of the family situation, unrelated caregivers, substance abuse in the household, and any history of past abuse. Even with these indicators, child abuse is extremely hard to accurately diagnose.

Given the wide spectrum of abuse, presenting symptoms vary accordingly. In the youngest victims, the diagnosis often depends on physical signs such as bruising, patterned burn injuries, retinal hemorrhages, and long bone fractures. Among all children, presentations that should raise a high level of suspicion in the clinician include multiple injuries in different stages of healing; injuries not consistent with the history provided by the caregiver; a history that changes when retold, particularly when the incident was "unwitnessed"; and injuries to the perineum. Wisslow[71] provided an excellent summary of the presenting physical injuries in cases of child abuse and neglect (Table 24-1). In children, essentially any injury can be the result of abuse; however, particular injuries and injury patterns have a high degree of association with abuse.

Traumatic Brain Injury

Head injury is perhaps the most common injury associated with child abuse, and it is certainly the most devastating.

Penetrating head injury is relatively rare in abuse victims, and most head injuries occur in younger children.[36] Blunt injury most commonly manifests as "shaken baby syndrome" or, more accurately, "shaken impact syndrome," in which the insult is caused by an acceleration and deceleration of the brain within the cranial compartment due to violent shaking (Fig. 24-1). Recent studies indicate that some sort of contact with an object is necessary for the classic brain injury to occur, but that object may be relatively soft and produce no external indication of trauma.[21] Angular forces created during shaking and eventual percussion against an object result in rotation of the brain within the skull. This causes diffuse axonal injury and tearing of the subdural bridging veins, often resulting in subdural hematoma. Spontaneous subdural hematoma or its occurrence from unintentional trauma is uncommon in children, so its presence should raise the suspicion of child abuse. Acute contact with stationary objects results in the characteristic multiple skull fractures associated with repetitive injury. Secondary brain injury is also frequently associated with abuse, resulting in intracranial hemorrhage, anoxia secondary to apnea, hypoperfusion, cardiac arrest, and potentially herniation of the brainstem.[35] Brain injury secondary to

---

 TABLE 24-1   Signs and Symptoms Suggesting Child Abuse or Neglect

Subnormal growth
   Weight, height, or both less than 5th percentile for age
   Weight less than 5th percentile for height
   Decreased velocity of growth
Head injuries
   Torn frenulum of upper or lower lip
   Unexplained dental injury
   Bilateral black eyes with history of single blow or fall
   Traumatic hair loss
   Retinal hemorrhage
   Diffuse or severe central nervous system injury with history of minor to moderate fall (<3 m)
Skin injuries
   Bruise or burn shaped like an object
   Bite marks
   Burn resembling a glove or stocking or with some other distribution suggestion an immersion injury
   Bruises of various colors (in different stages of healing)
   Injury to soft tissue areas that are normally protected (thighs, stomach, upper arms)
Gastrointestinal or genitourinary injuries
   Bilious vomiting
   Recurrent vomiting or diarrhea witnessed only by parent
   Chronic abdominal or perineal pain with no identifiable cause
   History of genital or rectal pain
   Injury to genitals or rectum
   Sexually transmitted disease
Bone injuries
   Rib fracture in the absence of major trauma, such as a motor vehicle accident
   Complex skull fracture after a short fall (<1.2 m)
   Metaphyseal long bone fracture in an infant
   Femur fracture (any configuration) in a child younger than 1 yr
   Multiple fractures in various stages of healing
Laboratory studies
   Implausible or physiologically inconsistent laboratory results (polymicrobial contamination of body fluids, sepsis with unusual organisms,
     electrolyte disturbances inconsistent with the child's clinical state or underlying illness, wide and erratic variations in test results)
   Positive toxicologic tests in the absence of a known ingestion or medication
   Bloody cerebrospinal fluid (with xanthochromic supernatant) in an infant with altered mental status and no history of trauma

From Wisslow LS: Child abuse and neglect. N Engl J Med 1995;332:1425-1431.

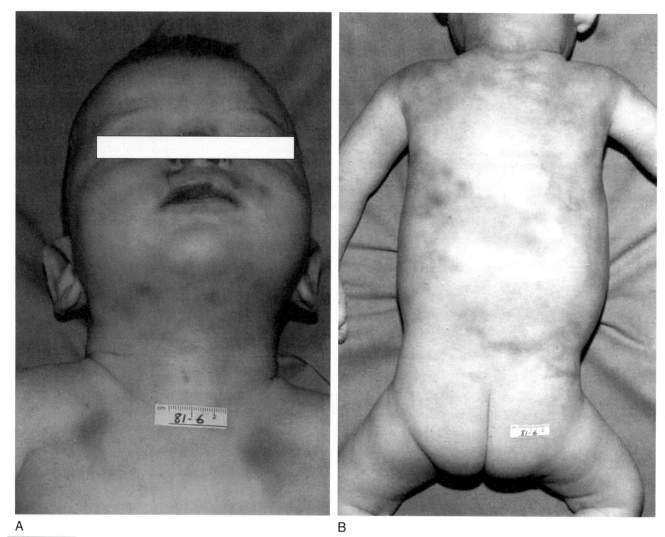

A   B

Figure 24–1 *A* and *B*, Shaken baby syndrome is often recognizable by external bruising about the chest, shoulders, and neck caused by the fingers and hands.

abuse carries a reported mortality rate of 15% to 38%, which is significantly higher than that of similar injuries caused by unintentional trauma.[21] Nonfatal outcomes in abused children with traumatic brain injuries are also significantly worse than in those whose injuries were sustained unintentionally.[24] Nonenhanced computed tomography is considered the most appropriate diagnostic tool for the identification of intentional head injury. Intracranial lesions are easily identified, as are the often associated skull fractures.[58]

Although most commonly seen in younger children, head injury associated with child abuse occurs in older children as well. Whereas external signs of trauma are infrequent in younger children, older children usually present with visible injuries secondary to violent external trauma. These injuries are often severe, with poor outcomes.[43]

The identification of retinal hemorrhage has been deemed almost pathognomonic of child abuse[13]; however, recent studies indicate that retinal hemorrhage occurs in cases of nonintentional injury as well, including normal vaginal delivery, which can cause compression of the baby's soft skull.[18,25] The presence of retinal hemorrhage from nonintentional injury is so rare, however, that it should stimulate a high level of suspicion for child abuse. When it is identified, the physician should begin an appropriate workup to investigate that possibility.

Fractures

It is postulated that approximately 80% of child abuse cases in the United States are identified radiographically.[12] Fractures secondary to child abuse can be found in any age group, although fractures in older children are more commonly from high-impact unintentional injury.[10] The presence of a long bone fracture in any child younger than 2 years has a high association with intentional injury.[14,16] Investigators have historically associated several fracture types with abuse, but it is probably more accurate to state that all fracture types can be associated with multiple causes. Spiral fractures, once reported as the most common type of fracture in abuse victims, have been replaced in more recent studies with single transverse fractures.[46] Spiral fractures are the result of torsional force applied to the extremity secondary to rotation of some sort. Transverse fractures are the result of a direct injury to the bone. This information should be used by the evaluating physician in conjunction with the history of injury to determine whether the history coincides with the presenting injury.

Diaphyseal fractures of the long bones are the most common fractures associated with child abuse, particularly those of the tibia, femur, and humerus. If the child is not ambulatory, the association between these fractures and abuse is extremely high.[46] Epiphyseal-metaphyseal fractures, although much less common than diaphyseal injuries, are reportedly far more specific for intentional injury.[17] The forces required to sustain these injuries greatly exceed the forces normally associated with falls and other minor trauma. Epiphyseal-metaphyseal fractures are also commonly known as corner fractures or bucket-handle fractures.

Type 1 fractures of the femur and humerus have a high association with abuse when encountered outside of the neonatal period.[26] This is particularly true if the history of injury does not contain significant high-force violent trauma. These injuries require considerable force to occur and, when nonintentional, are commonly associated with significant soft tissue damage and other injuries. Other types of Salter-Harris injuries do not appear to have a strong association with intentional abuse.

Clavicular fractures can also be associated with abuse, but there is a low specificity. Clavicular fractures of either end rather than the midshaft are usually the result of significant traction or the trauma of shaking.[50] Rib fractures, in contrast, have an extremely high association with abuse. It is postulated that the relatively elastic rib cage in children prevents most fractures secondary to accidental trauma. When fractures of the ribs do occur, the association with abuse is high—up to 82%.[8]

Spinal fractures are rare in children, as is cord injury. The difficulty in diagnosing vertebral body injuries and the relatively protected spine make any association with abuse difficult to determine. Suffice it to say that any injury of the spine or spinal cord requires an extremely violent force, and the cause must be carefully investigated.

It is critical for any physician treating children to investigate all fractures, particularly in the younger age groups. Minimal trauma does not commonly cause fractures, except when associated with other pathology. Getting an accurate history is critical. The presence of multiple fractures associated with a history of minimal trauma always requires an investigation for potential child abuse. The identification of multiple fractures, particularly when the age of the fractures is different, is almost pathognomonic of abuse. When abuse is suspected, skeletal surveys are indicated. The American College of Radiology has published standards for these surveys.[6]

Burns

Burns are a fairly common indication of child abuse, representing approximately 20% of pediatric burn injuries. Abuse victims often have characteristic patterns of burn infliction that physicians should be aware of.[45] Common patterns include circumferential burns,

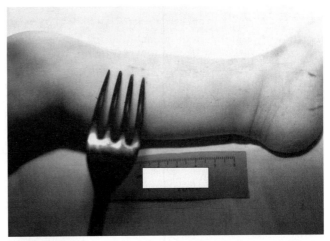

Figure 24–2   Punctate injuries or burns of the extremities caused by a recognizable object such as a fork indicate child abuse.

particularly when the burns are on more than one extremity; "pattern" burns or branding; burns to the buttocks, genitalia, or perineum; and punctate or cigarette burns (Fig. 24-2). Burn victims who are abused are usually younger than unintentional burn victims and have a history of being burned in the bathroom.[33] The demographics of intentionally burned children are striking. These children are often being raised by single mothers or are in foster care, they are in homes where other children have previously been removed because of abuse, and there is an almost 40% chance that past abuse has already been investigated.[33]

With burns, the history of injury is critical and is often inconsistent with the burn pattern. The burn itself often exhibits uncharacteristic features, such as lack of splash marks from falling liquids, consistent depth throughout the burn rather than the normal "feathering" of depth, and larger surface areas than expected based on the history. These burns, which are often the result of immersion, present with clear lines of demarcation, indicating that the child was unable to move during the incident and was probably restrained. Inflicted burns to the buttocks and perineum often occur in children being toilet trained when a caregiver becomes frustrated over an "accident." The depth of burn is also important. It takes approximately 1.5 seconds to cause a second-degree burn in adult skin immersed in water at 150° F. That is certainly more time than anyone would keep his or her hands immersed volitionally.

A complete history and physical examination are necessary in any child seen for burns or the suspicion of abuse. Other signs of abuse are often discernible, such as healed or healing fractures or possibly perineal injuries. Additionally, recent data indicate that some burn injuries mimic chronic skin conditions.[31] Thus, a high level of suspicion must be maintained when clinicians see lesions that do not present in characteristic locations or do not respond to normal therapy. Given the high incidence of recurrence in burn injury, physicians must ensure that the child is discharged to a safe environment.

Thoracoabdominal Injury

Fortunately, significant thoracoabdominal injury secondary to child abuse is uncommon, estimated to occur in about 5% of abused children.[61] Unfortunately, thoracoabdominal injury is the second leading cause of death in these children, following head injury.[55] Any type of blunt or penetrating abdominal injury can be caused intentionally.[15,19,38,56,61] Injuries commonly result from severe blows to the abdomen or chest cavity, and as previously stated, rib fractures in children should raise the suspicion of abuse.[8] Most important, the clinician must ascertain the history of injury to determine whether the injury is consistent with the mechanism described. For example, recent reports indicate that a simple fall down a flight of stairs does not generate the force or dynamics necessary for a hollow viscus perforation.[34] Similarly, significant head injury requires a mechanism generating more force than simply rolling out of bed.

Injuries to the perineum should always lead to a consideration of child abuse. Aside from burns to the perineum, discussed previously, injuries resulting from abuse tend to be penetrating in nature. Rectal or vaginal trauma resulting in laceration should routinely be investigated, as should lacerations in the penile and scrotal region. Abuse may involve retained foreign bodies as well. The physician should always investigate anal and vaginal orifices that appear to be dilated, particularly those that may result in incontinence. Signs of abuse to the perineum are often chronic, and areas of scar and old lacerations should be noted.

The radiographic and diagnostic workup for children suffering thoracoabdominal abuse is identical to that for unintentional injury. Recommendations for appropriate scans and diagnostics have been updated by the American Academy of Pediatrics.[5] Management of these injuries is also the same as for unintentional thoracoabdominal injuries.[37,64]

BIRTH INJURIES

Birth injury is estimated to occur in 6 to 8 of every 1000 live births in the United States, but it is responsible for around 2% of the perinatal mortality.[65] Injury most commonly occurs in babies with macrosomia but can also be associated with fetal organomegaly, mass lesions, prematurity, protracted labor, precipitous delivery, breech presentation, and cephalopelvic dissociation. The development and widespread use of prenatal ultrasonography, along with other advances in perinatal care, have allowed the early identification of many of these factors, along with recommendations for the delivery of such high-risk infants.[28]

Soft Tissue Injury

The most common birth injury encountered is injury to the soft tissue. This can present as a hematoma (often cephalohematoma), simple cutaneous bruising, or fat necrosis manifesting as subcutaneous masses. These lesions resolve spontaneously within months and require no treatment other than reassurance of the parents.

Less commonly, lacerations secondary to instrumentation may occur. These lacerations can usually be closed with adhesive strips or cutaneous glue rather than sutures. Suturing may be necessary, however, when adhesive closure cannot achieve the appropriate cosmetic result. Fine material should always be used, and healing is usually excellent. Lacerations are rarely deep, but if they are, standard precautions for wound exploration should be followed.

Torticollis has been ascribed to birth trauma or intrauterine malpositioning.[63] The cause is debatable, because torticollis has been found in infants who were delivered by cesarean section as well as in those delivered vaginally. The classic presentation is a small, firm mass in the body of the sternocleidomastoid muscle. The head is tilted toward the mass, with the face classically turned to the contralateral side. Physical therapy performed by the parents is successful in the vast majority of cases, and surgical intervention is rarely indicated. Facial asymmetry may result in untreated lesions.

Fractures

The most common fracture associated with birth trauma is clavicular, occurring in about 2.7 of every 1000 births.[57] The fracture is noticed when the infant does not move the arm or swelling occurs over the clavicle. The fracture is commonly in the midshaft and generally requires no treatment, although some authors recommend figure-of-eight splints or pinning the baby's shirtsleeve to the chest on the affected side.[41] Occasionally, because of shoulder dystocia, the clavicle may be intentionally fractured.[9]

Fractures of the humerus usually occur in either the shaft or the proximal epiphysis. Epiphyseal fractures are difficult to diagnose because of a lack of ossification points in the neonatal epiphysis. Associated neurologic findings may be noted with fractures of the humerus, including Erb's palsy and radial nerve palsy.[9,44] Shoulder dislocation is most likely not related to birth trauma but rather to intrauterine causes or therapy for Erb's palsy.[7] Distal fractures and dislocations of the radial head may also occur and are often associated with breech delivery.[1,66] Proximal fractures of the humerus can be successfully treated by bandaging the arm to the chest in a neutral position for epiphyseal injuries and by strapping the arm to the chest with an abduction device or possibly a posterior splint for shaft fractures.[52]

Birth trauma can cause fractures of the femur at almost any location. Breech delivery and high birth weight are predisposing factors.[67] Presentation consists of abnormal rotation of the lower extremity, pain, or swelling. Treatment involves application of a traction device, spica cast, or both.[68] Reduction should be close to anatomic, because overgrowth and remodeling of the femur are not usually dramatic.[51]

Neurologic Injury

Brachial plexus injury is the most common neurologic birth injury.[30] Approximately 21% of these injuries are associated with a shoulder dystocia at birth. Erb's palsy

(C3 to C5) is the most common of the brachial plexus injuries and usually resolves spontaneously, with little residual effect. Presentation involves a lack of motion of the affected shoulder, with the limb adducted and internally rotated to the prone position. Distal sensation and hand function are usually normal. Even after aggressive physical therapy, about 2% of cases are permanent.[29] Lower injuries of the C6 to T1 cervical roots (Klumpke's palsy) present with a lack of hand and wrist function. These lesions may be accompanied by Horner's syndrome, with the associated physical findings. Microsurgical repair has been described for recalcitrant brachial plexus injuries, with relatively good success, but this should be reserved only for infants failing aggressive physical therapy.[60] Phrenic nerve paralysis is a commonly associated finding and should be investigated whenever brachial plexus injury is identified. Isolated brachial plexus injury can cause significant shoulder abnormalities, and therapy should not be delayed.[4]

Phrenic nerve injury can also occur in isolation.[65] Treatment of phrenic nerve injury depends on the severity of the respiratory embarrassment experienced by the child. Asymptomatic injuries should not be treated; injuries resulting in respiratory impairment should be treated with diaphragmatic plication or other procedures designed to reduce the paradoxical movement of the diaphragm with respiration.[42]

Certainly the most devastating neurologic birth injuries involve the central nervous system. Lesions of the cervical spine are rare but are devastating when they occur. The cause of injury is usually a vaginal delivery with a breech or transverse lie.[2] As with all cervical spine injuries, high lesions require mechanical ventilation, and lower lesions have devastating physical sequelae. Survival is poor in neonates with complete transection. Partial injury may mimic cerebral palsy.[40]

Subdural, subarachnoid, intraventricular, and intraparenchymal bleeds have also been associated with birth trauma. Outcome is dependent on the extent of the lesion and the presentation. Usually these lesions are secondary to vacuum extraction,[23,70] which is also implicated as the cause of subgaleal cephalohematoma. Although most hematomas resolve without incident or sequelae, approximately 25% have been reported to cause death in affected neonates.[69] Traction injury to the internal carotid artery has also been reported in difficult births. Outcome from these injuries is varied and depends on the extent of vascular damage and collateral perfusion.[62] Similarly, direct injury to the optic nerve has been described.[39]

The most common central nervous system injury during childbirth is anoxic brain damage and the resultant "cerebral palsy." The cause is controversial, but difficult delivery is a common association.

Treatment of neurologic birth trauma is usually expectant, with aggressive physical therapy. Recalcitrant peripheral injuries have responded to surgical repair.

Thoracoabdominal Injury

Injuries to the chest are believed to be the result of pressure on the thoracic cavity. Pneumothorax, pneumomediastinum, and chylothorax have been described.[53,69]

Perforation of the esophagus or cricopharyngeus can also occur. In most cases of birth trauma to the chest, expectant observation is indicated. The clinical course dictates the need for operative intervention. High perforations of the esophagus and cricopharyngeus can usually be treated by observation or occasionally drainage.[65] Lower lesions require drainage or operative repair. With early identification, results are excellent. Perforation of the esophagus can also result from placement of a gastric tube in the neonatal period.

Liver hematoma is the most common intra-abdominal injury secondary to birth trauma (Fig. 24-3). The usual presentation is anemia, but it can also be shock.[27] Diagnosis is usually made by ultrasonography, but a thorough investigation may be necessary to rule out other hepatic masses in a newborn. Treatment is usually expectant and includes volume resuscitation and correction of any hypothermia or coagulopathy. Occasionally, operative intervention is necessary when the baby is unstable or continued hemorrhage occurs. Hemostatic agents appear to be more helpful than attempts at suture repair in stopping hepatic bleeding in newborns.[11] In any case, control of hepatic hemorrhage is very difficult in this age group.

Splenic injury is rare and presents much like hepatic injury. Intra-abdominal blood may be the only presenting sign, and as in hepatic injury, other pathology must be ruled out.[59] Treatment includes expectant observation and correction of coagulopathy or hypothermia. Operative intervention is difficult and usually results in splenectomy. Hemostatic agents may also be useful.

As with splenic injury, injury to the adrenal glands is uncommon because of the relative protection provided by the thoracic ribs. The presentation may be hemorrhage or adrenal insufficiency in severe cases. Injury can also be identified from calcifications found on a radiograph taken later in life. As with all intra-abdominal solid organs, investigation of hematomas requires a workup to rule out other pathology, such as underlying tumor.

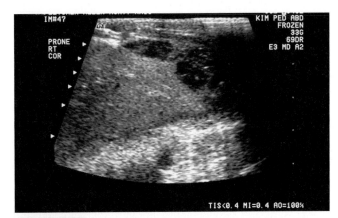

Figure 24-3 Ultrasonography of the abdomen clearly demonstrates this hepatic hematoma caused by birth trauma, which resolved spontaneously. Lesions like this can be followed by ultrasonography; if they persist, other causes such as neoplasm must be investigated.

REFERENCES

1. Akbarnia BA, Silberstein MJ, Rend RJ, et al: Arthrography in the diagnosis of fractures in the distal end of the humerus in infants. J Bone Joint Surg Am 1986;68:599-601.

2. Allen JP: Birth injury to the spinal cord. Northwest Med 1986;69:323-326.

3. Al-Moosa A, Al-Shaiji J, Al-Fadhli A, et al: Pediatricians' knowledge, attitudes and experience regarding child maltreatment in Kuwait. Child Abuse Negl 2003;27:1161-1178.

4. Al-Qattan MM: Classification of secondary shoulder deformities in obstetric brachial plexus palsy. J Hand Surg [Br] 2003;28:483-486.

5. American Academy of Pediatrics: Diagnostic imaging of child abuse. Pediatrics 2000;105:1345-1348.

6. American College of Radiology: Standards for Skeletal Surveys in Children. American College of Radiology, 1997.

7. Babbitt DP, Cassidy RH: Obstetrical paralysis and dislocation of the shoulder in infants. J Bone Joint Surg Am 1968;50:1447-1452.

8. Barsness KA, Cha E, Bensard DD, et al: The positive predictive value of rib fractures as an indicator of nonaccidental trauma in children. J Trauma 2003;54:1107-1110.

9. Bianco AJ, Schlein AP, Kruse RI, et al: Birth fractures. Minn Med 1972;55:471-474.

10. Blakemore LC, Loder RT, Hensinger RN: Role of intentional abuse in children 1 to 5 years old with isolated femoral shaft fractures. J Pediatr Orthop 1996;16:585-588.

11. Blocker SH, Ternberg JL: Traumatic liver laceration in the newborn: Repair with fibrin glue. J Pediatr Surg 1986;21:369-371.

12. Brown T: Radiography's role in detecting child abuse. Radiol Technol 1995;66:389-390.

13. Budenz DL, Farber MG, Mirchandani HG, et al: Ocular and optic nerve hemorrhages in abused infants with intracranial injuries. Ophthalmology 1994;101:559-565.

14. Caffey J: Multiple fractures in the long bones of infants suffering from chronic subdural hematoma. AJR Am J Roentgenol 1946;56:163-173.

15. Cameron CM, Lazoritz S, Calhoun AD: Blunt abdominal injury: Simultaneously occurring liver and pancreatic injury in child abuse. Pediatr Emerg Care 1997;13:334-336.

16. Cameron JM, Rae LJ: Atlas of the Battered Child Syndrome. Edinburgh, Churchill Livingstone, 1975.

17. Chapman S: Radiological aspects of non-accidental injury. J R Soc Med 1990;83:67-71.

18. Choi HJ, Lee SY, Yang H, et al: Retinal haemorrhage in vivax malaria. Trans R Soc Trop Med Hyg 2004;98:387-389.

19. Coant PN, Kornberg AE, Brody AS, et al: Markers for occult liver injury in cases of physical abuse in children. Pediatrics 1992;89:274-278.

20. De Bellis MD, Putnam FW: The psychobiology of child maltreatment. Child Adolesc Psychiatr Clin N Am 1994;3:663-678.

21. Deputy S: Shaking-impact syndrome of infancy. Semin Pediatr Neurol 2003;10:112-119.

22. Dodge KA, Bates JE, Petit GS: Mechanisms in the cycle of violence. Science 1990;250:1678-1683.

23. Dwyer D: Problems after vacuum-assisted childbirth. Nursing 2002;32:74.

24. Ewing-Cobbs L, Kramer L, Prasad M, et al: Neuroimaging: Physical and developmental findings after inflicted and noninflicted traumatic brain injury in young children. Pediatrics 1998;102:300-307.

25. Forbes BJ, Christian CW, Judkins AR, et al: Inflicted childhood neurotrauma (shaken baby syndrome): Ophthalmic findings. J Pediatr Ophthalmol Strabismus 2004;41:80-88.

26. Forlin E, Guille J, Kumar S, et al: Transepiphyseal fractures on the neck of the femur in very young children. J Pediatr Orthop 1992;12:164-168.

27. French CE, Waldstein G: Subcapsular hemorrhage of the liver in the newborn. Pediatrics 1982;69:204-208.

28. Friesen CD, Miller AM, Rayburn WF: Influence of spontaneous or induced labor on delivering the macrosomic fetus. Am J Perinatol 1995;12:63-66.

29. Gherman RB, Ouzounian JG, Goodwin TM: Brachial plexus palsy: An in utero injury? Am J Obstet Gynecol 1999;180:1303-1307.

30. Gherman RB, Ouzounian JG, Satin AJ, et al: A comparison of shoulder dystocia-associated transient and permanent brachial plexus palsies. Obstet Gynecol 2003;102:544-548.

31. Heider TR, Priolo D, Hultman CS, et al: Eczema mimicking child abuse: A case of mistaken identity. J Burn Care Rehabil 2002;23:357-359.

32. Holmes SJ, Robins LN: The role of parental disciplinary practices in the development of depression and alcoholism. Psychiatry 1988;51:24-36.

33. Hultman CS, Priolo D, Cairns BA, et al: Return to jeopardy: The fate of pediatric burn patients who are victims of abuse and neglect. J Burn Care Rehabil 1998;19:367-376.

34. Huntimer CM, Muret-Wagstaff S, Leland NL: Can falls on stairs result in small intestine perforations? Pediatrics 2000;106:301-305.

35. Johnson DL, Boal D, Baule R: The role of apnea in nonaccidental head injury. Pediatr Neurosurg 1995;23:305-310.

36. Keenan HT, Runyan DK, Marshall SW: A population-based study of inflicted traumatic brain injury in young children. JAMA 2003;290:621-626.

37. Keller MS: Blunt injury to solid abdominal organs. Semin Pediatr Surg 2004;13:106-111.

38. Keller MS, Stafford PW, Vane DW: Conservative management of pancreatic trauma in children. J Trauma 1997;42:1097-1100.

39. Khalil SK, Urso RG, Mintz-Hittner HA: Traumatic optic nerve injury occurring after forceps delivery of a term newborn. J Pediatr Ophthalmol Strabismus 2003;7:146-147.

40. Koch BM: Neonatal spinal cord injury. Arch Phys Med Rehabil 1979;60:378-381.

41. Kogutt MS, Swischuk LE, Fagan CJ: Patterns of injury and significance of uncommon fractures in the battered child syndrome. Radiology 1974;121:143-149.

42. Langer JC, et al: Plication of the diaphragm for infants and young children with phrenic nerve palsy. J Pediatr Surg 1988;23:749-751.

43. Lee ACW, Ou Y, Fong D: Depressed skull fractures: A pattern of abusive head injury in three older children. Child Abuse Negl 2003;27:1323-1329.

44. Lemperg R, Liliequist B: Dislocation of the proximal epiphysis of the humerus in newborns. Acta Paediatr Scand 1970;59:377-380.

45. Lenoski EF, Hunter KA: Specific patterns of inflicted burn injuries. J Trauma 1977;17:842-846.

46. Loder RT, Bookout C: Fracture patterns in battered children. J Orthop Trauma 1991;5:428-433.

47. Ludwig S, Kornberg AE (eds): Child Abuse: A Medical Reference, 2nd ed. New York, Churchill Livingstone, 1992.

48. McClain PW, Sacks JJ, Froehlke RG, et al: Estimates of fatal child abuse and neglect, United States, 1979 through 1988. Pediatrics 1993;91:338-343.

49. McKibben L, De Vos E, Newberger EH: Victimization of mothers of abused children: A controlled study. Pediatrics 1989;84:531-535.

50. Merten DF, Radkowski MA, Leonidas JC: The abused child: A radiological appraisal. Radiology 1983;146:377-381.

51. Mitchell WC, Coventry MB: Osseous injuries in the newborn. Minn Med 1959;42:1-4.

52. Moucha CS, Mason DE: Distal humeral epiphyseal separation. Am J Orthop 2003;32:497-500.

53. Nakagawa H, Yamauchi M, Kusuyama T, et al: Cervical emphysema secondary to pneumomediastinum as a complication of childbirth. Ear Nose Throat J 2003;82: 948-951.

54. National Center on Child Abuse and Neglect: Study Findings: Study of National Incidence and Prevalence of Child Abuse and Neglect: 1988. Washington, DC, Department of Health and Human Services, 1988.

55. National Pediatric Trauma Registry. Boston, Tufts University.

56. Ng CS, Hall CM, Shaw DG: The range of visceral manifestations of non-accidental injury. Arch Dis Child 1997;77: 167-174.

57. Oppenheim WL, Davis A, Growdon WA, et al: Clavicle fractures in the newborn. Clin Orthop 1990;250:176-180.

58. Pärtan G, Pamberger P, Blab E, et al: Common tasks and problems in paediatric trauma radiology. Eur J Radiol 2003;48:103-124.

59. Perdomo Y, Fiore N, Reyna T: Splenic injury presenting with isolated scrotal findings in a stable newborn. J Pediatr Surg 2003;38:1673-1675.

60. Piatt JH: Birth injuries of the brachial plexus. Pediatr Clin North Am 2004;51:421-440.

61. Purdue GF, Hunt JL: Burn injuries. In Ludwig S, Kornberg AE (eds): Child Abuse: A Medical Reference, 2nd ed. New York, Churchill Livingstone, 1992, pp 105-116.

62. Robertson WC, Pettigrew LC: "Congenital" Horner's syndrome and carotid dissection. J Neuroimaging 2003;13: 367-370.

63. Sanerkin BG, Edwards P: Birth injury to the sternocleidomastoid muscle. J Bone Joint Surg Br 1066;48:441.

64. Sartorelli KH, Vane DW: The diagnosis and management of children with blunt injury of the chest. Semin Pediatr Surg 2004;13:98-105.

65. Schullinger JN: Birth trauma. Pediatr Clin North Am 1993;40:1351-1358.

66. Siffert RS: Displacement of the distal humeral epiphysis in the newborn infant. J Bone Joint Surg Am 1963;45:165-169.

67. Theodorou SD, Ierodiaconou MN, Mitsou A: Obstetrical fracture-separation of the upper femoral epiphysis. Acta Orthop Scand 1982;53:239-243.

68. Towbin R, Crawford AH: Neonatal traumatic proximal femoral epiphysiolysis. Pediatrics 1979;63:456-459.

69. Uchil D, Arulkumaran S: Neonatal subgaleal hemorrhage and its relationship to delivery by vacuum extraction. Obstet Gynecol Surv 2003;58:687-693.

70. Whitby EH, Griffiths PD, Rutter S, et al: Frequency and natural history of subdural haemorrhages in babies and relation to obstetric factors. Lancet 2003;362:846-851.

71. Wissow LS: Child abuse and neglect. N Engl J Med 1995;332:1425-1431.

Part III

MAJOR TUMORS OF CHILDHOOD

Chapter 25

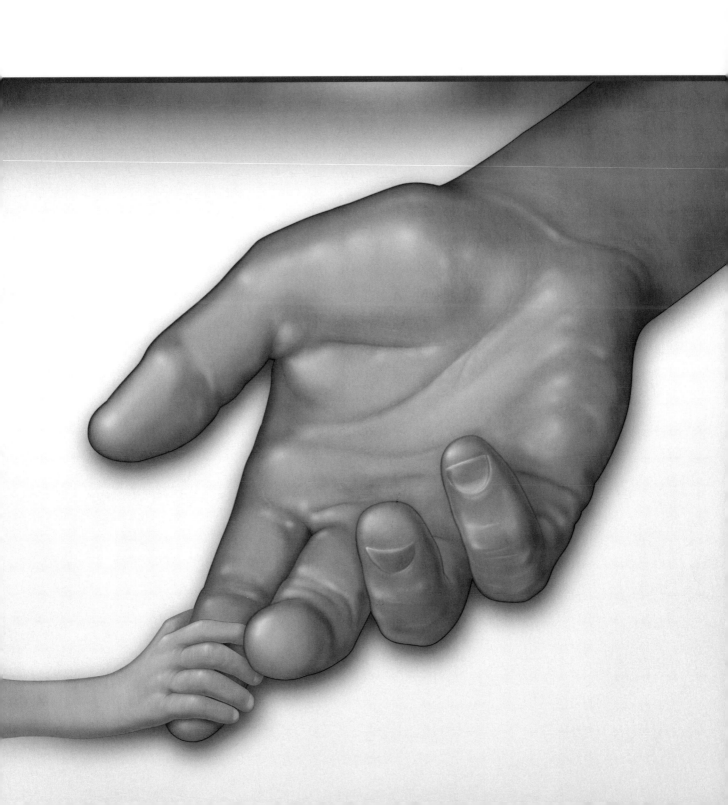

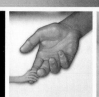

Principles of Pediatric Oncology, Genetics of Cancer, and Radiation Therapy

Matthew J. Krasin and Andrew M. Davidoff

A number of milestones in the evolution of cancer therapy have come from the field of pediatric oncology. The first clear evidence that chemotherapy could provide effective treatment for childhood malignancy occurred in 1950, when Farber[41] reported temporary cancer remission in children with acute lymphoblastic leukemia (ALL) treated with the folic acid antagonist aminopterin.[41] The first successful use of a multidisciplinary approach to cancer treatment occurred in the 1950s and 1960s through the collaborative efforts of pediatric surgeons, radiation therapists, and pediatric oncologists aiming to improve the treatment of Wilms' tumor in children.[60] Such a multidisciplinary approach is now used throughout the field of oncology. The successful use of a combination of chemotherapeutic agents to cure Hodgkin's disease and ALL during the 1960s led to the widespread use of combination chemotherapy to treat virtually all types of pediatric cancers. Since the late 1980s, neuroblastoma has been the paradigm for the use of therapies of variable intensity, depending on risk stratification determined by clinical and biologic variables, including molecular markers. Other advances in pediatric oncology have included the development of interdisciplinary, national cooperative clinical research groups to critically evaluate new therapies, the efficacy of dose-intensive chemotherapy programs in improving the outcome of advanced-stage solid tumors, and the supportive care necessary to make the latter approach possible. The development and application of these principles and advances have led to substantially increased survival rates for children with cancer and profound improvements in their quality of life.

Additionally, advances in molecular genetic research in the past 2 decades have led to an increased understanding of the genetic events in the pathogenesis and progression of human malignancies, including those of childhood. A number of pediatric malignancies have served as models for molecular genetic research. Chromosomal structural changes, activating or inactivating mutations of relevant genes or their regulatory elements, gene amplification, and gene imprinting may each play a role in different tumor types. In some instances, these genetic events occur early in tumorigenesis and are specific for a particular tumor type, such as chromosomal translocation t(11;22)(q24;q12) in Ewing's sarcoma; other aberrations occur in a variety of different tumor types and are almost always associated with additional genetic changes, such as chromosome 1p deletion in neuroblastoma and Wilms' tumor. Some alterations involve oncogenes—genes that, when activated, lead directly to cancer—whereas others involve tumor suppressor genes, whose inactivation allows tumor progression. The result of alterations in these genetic elements, regardless of the mechanism, is disruption of the normal balance between proliferation and death of individual cells. These discoveries have highlighted the utility of molecular analysis for a variety of purposes, including diagnosis, risk stratification, and treatment planning; the understanding of syndromes associated with cancer; genetic screening and genetic counseling; and prophylactic treatment, including surgical intervention. Soon, treatment regimens are likely to be individualized on the basis of the molecular biologic profile of a patient's tumor. In addition, molecular profiling will lead to the development of new drugs designed to induce differentiation of tumor cells, block dysregulated growth pathways, or reactivate silenced apoptotic pathways.

EPIDEMIOLOGY AND SURVIVAL STATISTICS

Cancer in children is uncommon; it represents only about 2% of all cancer cases. Nevertheless, after trauma, it is the second most common cause of death in children older than 1 year. Each year, approximately 130 new cases of cancer are identified per million children younger than 15 years (or about 1 in 7000). This means that in the United States, about 9000 children younger than 15 years are diagnosed with cancer each year, in addition

TABLE 25–1 Frequency of Cancer Diagnoses in Childhood

Type of Cancer	Percentage of Total
Leukemia	30
Brain tumors	22
Lymphoma	15
Neuroblastoma	8
Sarcoma	7
Wilms' tumor	6
Germ cell tumors	5
Osteosarcoma	4
Retinoblastoma	2
Liver tumors	1

to 4000 patients aged 15 to 19 years.[152] Leukemia is the most common form of cancer in children, and brain tumors are the most common solid tumor of childhood (Table 25-1). Lymphomas are the next most common malignancy in children, followed by neuroblastoma, soft tissue sarcomas, Wilms' tumor, germ cell tumors, osteosarcoma, and retinoblastoma. A slightly different distribution is seen among 15- to 19-year-olds, in whom Hodgkin's disease and germ cell tumors are the most frequently diagnosed malignancies; non-Hodgkin lymphoma, nonrhabdomyosarcoma soft tissue sarcoma, osteosarcoma, Ewing's sarcoma, thyroid cancer, and melanoma also occur with an increased incidence.

In general, the incidence of childhood cancer is greatest during the first year of life, peaks again in children aged 2 to 3 years, and then slowly declines until age 9. The incidence then steadily increases again through adolescence. Each tumor type shows a different age distribution pattern, however. Variations by gender are also seen. For example, Hodgkin's disease, ALL, brain tumors, neuroblastoma, hepatoblastoma, Ewing's sarcoma, and rhabdomyosarcoma are more common in boys than in girls younger than 15 years, whereas only osteosarcoma and Ewing's sarcoma are more common in boys than in girls older than 15 years. However, girls in the older age group have Hodgkin's disease and thyroid cancer more frequently than boys do. Distribution also varies by race: white children generally have a 30% greater incidence of cancer than do black children. This difference is particularly notable for ALL, Ewing's sarcoma, and testicular germ cell tumors.

The probability of surviving childhood cancer has improved greatly since Farber induced the first remissions in patients with ALL. In the early 1960s, approximately 30% of children with cancer survived their disease. By the mid-1980s, about 65% of children with cancer were cured, and by the mid-1990s, the cure rate had increased to nearly 75%.[122] These great strides resulted from three important factors: (1) the sensitivity of childhood cancer, at least initially, to available chemotherapeutic agents; (2) the treatment of childhood cancer in a multidisciplinary fashion; and (3) the treatment of most children in major pediatric treatment centers in the context of a clinical research protocol using the most current and promising therapy. Although progress in the treatment of some tumor types such as ALL and Wilms' tumor has been outstanding, progress in the treatment of others, such as metastatic neuroblastoma and rhabdomyosarcoma, has been modest. Therefore, there is still a need for significant improvement in the treatment of childhood cancer.

MOLECULAR BIOLOGY OF CANCER

During normal cellular development and renewal, cells evolve to perform highly specialized functions to meet the physiologic needs of the organism. Development and renewal involve tightly regulated processes that include continued cell proliferation, differentiation to specialized cell types, and programmed cell death (apoptosis). An intricate system of checks and balances ensures proper control over these physiologic processes. The genetic composition (genotype) of a cell determines which pathway or pathways will be followed in exerting that control. In addition, the environment plays a crucial role in influencing cell fate: cells use complex signal transduction pathways to sense and respond to neighboring cells and their extracellular milieu.

Cancer is a genetic disease whose progression is driven by a series of accumulating genetic changes influenced by hereditary factors and the somatic environment. These genetic changes result in individual cells acquiring a phenotype that provides them with a survival advantage over surrounding normal cells. Our understanding of the processes that occur in malignant cell transformation is increasing; many discoveries in cancer cell biology have been made by using childhood tumors as models. This greater understanding of the molecular biology of cancer has also contributed significantly to our understanding of normal cell physiology.

Normal Cell Physiology

Cell Cycle

Genetic information is stored in cells and transmitted to subsequent generations of cells through nucleic acids organized on chromosomes as genes. A gene is a functional unit of heredity that exists on a specific site or locus on a chromosome, is capable of reproducing itself exactly at each cell division, and is capable of directing the synthesis of an enzyme or other protein. The genetic material is maintained as DNA formed into a double helix of complementary strands. The backbone of each strand is made up of linked sugar and phosphate groups to which complementary bases—a purine (adenine or guanine) and a pyrimidine (cytosine or thymine)—are connected by hydrogen bonds. DNA normally exists in a tightly wound complex maintained by histone proteins in the nucleus. Unwinding of the DNA is required for its activation. The complementary nature of the two DNA strands allows DNA to be exactly replicated during cell division: each strand serves as a template for the synthesis of the second strand. The cell must ensure that synthesized DNA (3 billion base pairs) has been accurately copied. DNA replication errors that go uncorrected potentially alter the function of normal cell regulatory proteins.

Protein synthesis begins with the transcription of a single strand of messenger RNA (mRNA) from a DNA template. RNA contains the pyrimidine uracil, instead of the DNA base thymine, and a pentose sugar, ribose, instead of the deoxyribose sugar found in DNA. After transcription, the mRNA undergoes modifications that affect its sequence, length, physical form, and stability. Following this, translation of the mRNA template into the sequence of amino acids that constitutes a polypeptide occurs. Additional post-translational modifications can then be made to these newly synthesized proteins. These proteins, whose sequence is dictated by the DNA of a given cell, are responsible for an enormous range of activities within the cell and direct, in particular, the cell's division cycle, by which cells proliferate.

The molecular machinery used to control the cell cycle is highly organized and tightly regulated (Fig. 25-1).[134] Normal growth results from the progression of cells

through cycles of DNA replication (S phase) and cell division or mitosis (M phase). These two phases of the cell cycle are separated by two intervening growth phases (G_1 and G_2). Cells can also temporarily leave the cell cycle and enter a resting state called G_0. Signals that stimulate or inhibit cellular growth converge on a set of evolutionarily conserved enzymes that drive cell cycle progression. Two classes of proteins, cyclins and cyclin-dependent kinases, form complexes that mediate progression through the cell cycle by sequentially phosphorylating target proteins. Cyclin-dependent kinase inhibitors regulate the activity of the cyclin-dependent kinases and serve as a "braking" system for the cell cycle machinery. In addition, various "checkpoints" exist to halt progression through the cell cycle during certain environmental situations or times of genetic error resulting from inaccurate synthesis or damage. Two of the most well-studied participants in the cell cycle checkpoint system are p53 and retinoblastoma (RB) proteins.[135] In normal circumstances, cells divide and terminally differentiate, thereby leaving the cell cycle, or they enter a resting state. Inactivation of the effectors of cell cycle regulation or the bypassing of cell cycle checkpoints can result in dysregulation of the cell cycle—a hallmark of malignancy.

Signal Transduction

Signal transduction pathways regulate all aspects of cell function, including metabolism, cell division, death, differentiation, and movement. Multiple extracellular and intracellular signals for proliferation or quiescence must be integrated by the cell, and it is this integration of signals from multiple pathways that determines the response of a cell to competing and complementary signals. Extracellular signals include growth factors, cytokines, and hormones; the presence or absence of adequate nutrients and oxygen; and contact with other cells or an extracellular matrix. Signaling mediators often bind to membrane-bound receptors on the outside of the cell, but they may also diffuse into the cell and bind receptors in the cytoplasm or on the nuclear membrane. Binding of a ligand to a receptor stimulates the activities of small-molecule second messengers—proteins necessary to continue the transmission of the signal. Signaling pathways ultimately effect the activation of nuclear transcription factors that are responsible for the expression or silencing of genes encoding proteins involved in all aspects of cellular physiology.

Receptors with tyrosine kinase activity are among the most important transmembrane receptors. They are composed of an extracellular ligand-binding domain, a transmembrane domain, and an intracellular, cytoplasmic, tyrosine kinase domain. The binding of ligand to a receptor may cause a conformational change in the receptor or lead to the linking of the receptor to one or more other receptors. Either event results in activation of the receptor. The tyrosine kinase domain, in particular, is responsible for conveying signals intracellularly by phosphorylating internal substrates directly or by activating associated tyrosine kinases.

Several important transmembrane receptors with protein kinase activity have been identified and grouped

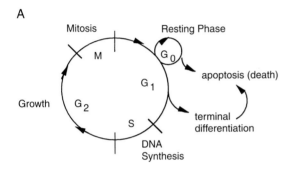

A

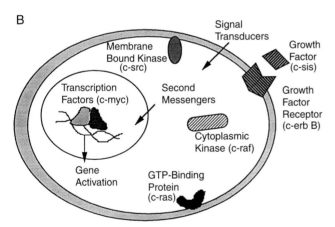

B

Figure 25-1 *A,* The cell cycle. Normal cell growth proceeds in an orderly fashion, with cells proceeding through the cycle of DNA replication (S) and mitosis (M). These cycles are separated by two intervening phases of growth (G_1 and G_2). Cells are signaled to leave the cycle to enter a resting state, to differentiate, or to die. *B,* Cell signal transduction. Proto-oncogene products (examples in parentheses) are involved in all aspects of signal transduction that move the cell through the cell cycle. The process begins when extracellular growth factors bind to a transmembrane growth factor receptor, thereby inducing the protein kinase activity of the receptor. Other proteins bind to the phosphorylated receptor and transmit a signal to the nucleus through membrane-bound and cytoplasmic messengers. This activates nuclear transcription factors, which bind to DNA and affect the transcription of growth-related genes. GTP, guanosine triphosphate.

in families on the basis of structural similarities.[148] These families include the epidermal growth factor receptors (EGFRs), fibroblast growth factor receptors, insulin-like growth factor (IGF) receptors, platelet-derived growth factor (PDGF) receptors, transforming growth factor receptors, and neurotrophin receptors (Trks). Abnormalities of members of each of these families are often found in pediatric malignancies and therefore are thought to play a role in their pathogenesis. Characteristic abnormalities of these receptors often form the basis of both diagnostic identification of certain tumor types and, more recently, targeted therapy for tumors with these specific abnormalities.

Programmed Cell Death

Multicellular organisms have developed a highly organized and carefully regulated mechanism of cell suicide in order to maintain cellular homeostasis. Normal development and morphogenesis are often associated with the production of excess cells, which are removed by the genetically programmed process called apoptosis. Cells undergoing apoptosis have distinct morphologic features (plasma membrane blebbing, reduced volume, nuclear condensation), and their DNA is subjected to endonucleolytic cleavage.

Apoptosis is initiated by the interaction of "death ligands," such as tumor necrosis factor-α (TNF-α), Fas, and TNF-related apoptosis-inducing ligand (TRAIL), with their respective receptors. This interaction is followed by aggregation of the receptors and recruitment of adapter proteins to the plasma membrane, which activate caspases.[105] Caspases are a large family of proteases that function in both the initiation of apoptosis in response to proapoptotic signals and the subsequent effector pathway that disassembles the cell. Thus, apoptosis limits cellular expansion and counters cell proliferation. Because cell survival signals may also be activated through pathways mediated by nuclear factor κB, the fate of a cell is determined by the balance between death signals and survival signals.[85] Other signals arising from cellular stress (e.g., DNA damage, hypoxia, oncogene activation) may also effect cell cycle arrest or apoptosis.

An alternative to cell death mediated by receptor-ligand binding is cellular senescence, which is initiated when chromosomes reach a critical length. Eukaryotic chromosomes have DNA strands of unequal length, and their ends, called telomeres, are characterized by species-specific nucleotide repeat sequences. Telomeres stabilize the ends of chromosomes, which are otherwise sites of significant instability.[133] Over time and with each successive cycle of replication, chromosomes are shortened by failure to complete replication of their telomeres. Thus, telomere shortening acts as a biologic clock, limiting the life span of a cell. Germ cells, however, avoid telomere shortening by using telomerase, an enzyme capable of adding telomeric sequences to the ends of chromosomes. This enzyme is normally inactivated early in the growth and development of an organism. Persistent activation or the reactivation of telomerase in somatic cells appears to contribute to the immortality of transformed cells.

Malignant Transformation

Alteration or inactivation of any of the components of normal cell regulatory pathways may lead to the dysregulated growth that characterizes neoplastic cells. Malignant transformation may be characterized by cellular dedifferentiation or failure to differentiate, cellular invasiveness and metastatic capacity, or decreased drug sensitivity. Tumorigenesis reflects the accumulation of excess cells that results from increased cell proliferation and decreased apoptosis or senescence. Cancer cells do not replicate more rapidly than normal cells, but they show diminished responsiveness to regulatory signals. Positive growth signals are generated by proto-oncogenes, so named because their dysregulated expression or activity can promote malignant transformation. These proto-oncogenes may encode growth factors or their receptors, intracellular signaling molecules, and nuclear transcription factors (Table 25-2). Conversely, tumor suppressor genes, as their name implies, control or restrict cell growth and proliferation. Their inactivation, through various mechanisms, permits the dysregulated growth of cancer cells. Also important are the genes that regulate cell death. Their inactivation leads to resistance to apoptosis and allows the accumulation of additional genetic aberrations.

Cancer cells carry DNA that has point mutations, viral insertions, or chromosomal or gene amplifications, deletions, or rearrangements. Each of these aberrations can alter the context and process of normal cellular growth and differentiation. Although genomic instability is an inherent property of the evolutionary process and normal development, it is through genomic instability that the malignant transformation of a cell may arise. This inherent instability may be altered by inheritance or exposure to destabilizing factors in the environment. Point mutations may terminate protein translation, alter protein function, or change the regulatory target sequences that control gene expression. Chromosomal alterations create new genetic contexts within the genome and lead to the formation of novel proteins or to the dysregulation of genes displaced by aberrant events.

Genetic abnormalities associated with cancer may be detected in every cell in the body or only in the tumor cells. Constitutional or germline abnormalities either are inherited or occur de novo in the germ cells (sperm or oocyte). Interestingly, despite the presence of a genetic abnormality that might affect growth regulatory pathways in all cells, people are generally predisposed to the development of only certain tumor types. This selectivity highlights the observation that gene function contributes to growth or development only within a particular milieu or physiologic context. Specific tumors occur earlier and are more often bilateral when they result from germline mutations than when they result from sporadic or somatic alterations. Such is often the case in two pediatric malignancies, Wilms' tumor and retinoblastoma. These observations led Knudson[81] to propose a "two-hit" mechanism of carcinogenesis in which the first genetic defect, already present in the germline, must be complemented by an additional spontaneous

TABLE 25-2 Proto-oncogenes and Tumor Suppressor Genes in Pediatric Malignancies

Oncogene Family	Proto-oncogene	Chromosome Location	Tumor
Growth factors and receptors	Erb B2	17q21	Glioblastoma
	Trk	9q22	Neuroblastoma
Protein kinase	Src	7p11	Rhabdomyosarcoma, osteosarcoma, Ewing's sarcoma
Signal transducers	H-ras	11p15.1	Neuroblastoma
Transcription factors	c-myc	18q24	Burkitt's lymphoma
	N-myc	2p24	Neuroblastoma

Syndrome	Tumor Suppressor Gene	Chromosome Location	Tumor
Familial polyposis coli	APC	5q21	Intestinal polyposis, colorectal cancer
Familial retinoblastoma	RB	13q24	Retinoblastoma, osteosarcoma
WAGR*	WT1	11p13	Wilms' tumor
Denys-Drash†	WT1	11p13	Wilms' tumor
Beckwith-Wiedemann‡	WT2 (?)	11p15	Wilms' tumor, hepatoblastoma, adrenal
Li-Fraumeni	p53	17q13	Multiple (see text)
Neurofibromatosis type 1	NF1	17q11.2	Sarcomas, breast cancer
Neurofibromatosis type 2	NF2	22q12	Neurofibroma, neurofibrosarcoma, brain tumor
Von Hippel-Lindau	VHL	3p25-26	Renal cell cancer, pheochromocytoma, retinal angioma, hemangioblastoma

*Wilms' tumor, aniridia, genitourinary abnormalities, mental retardation.
†Wilms' tumor, pseudohermaphroditism, mesangial sclerosis, renal failure.
‡Multiple tumors, hemihypertrophy, macroglossia, hyperinsulinism.

mutation before a tumor can arise. In sporadic cancer, cellular transformation occurs only when two (or more) spontaneous mutations take place in the same cell.

Much more common, however, are somatically acquired chromosomal aberrations, which are confined to the malignant cells. These aberrations affect growth factors and their receptors, signal transducers, and transcription factors. The general types of chromosomal alterations associated with malignant transformation are shown in Figure 25-2. Although a low level of chromosomal instability exists in a normal population of cells, neoplastic transformation occurs only if these alterations affect a growth-regulating pathway and confer a growth advantage.

DNA Content

Normal human cells contain two copies of each of 23 chromosomes; a normal "diploid" cell therefore has 46 chromosomes. Although cellular DNA content, or ploidy, is accurately determined by karyotypic analysis, it can be estimated by the much simpler method of flow cytometric analysis. Diploid cells have a DNA index of 1.0, whereas near-triploid cells have a DNA index ranging from 1.26 to 1.76. The majority (55%) of primary neuroblastoma cells are triploid or near triploid (e.g., having between 58 and 80 chromosomes), whereas the remainder are near diploid (35 to 57 chromosomes) or near tetraploid (81 to 103 chromosomes).[76] Neuroblastomas consisting of near-diploid or near-tetraploid cells usually have structural genetic abnormalities (e.g., chromosome 1p deletion and amplification of the MYCN oncogene), whereas those consisting of near-triploid cells are characterized by three almost complete haploid sets of

chromosomes with few structural abnormalities.[16] Importantly, patients with near-triploid tumors typically have favorable clinical and biologic prognostic factors and excellent survival rates compared with those who have near-diploid or near-tetraploid tumors.[92]

Chromosomal Translocations

Many pediatric cancers, specifically hematologic malignancies and soft tissue neoplasms, have recurrent, nonrandom abnormalities in chromosomal structure, typically chromosomal translocations (Table 25-3). The most common result of a nonrandom translocation is the fusion of two distinct genes from different chromosomes. The genes are typically fused within the reading frame and express a functional, chimeric protein product that has transcription factor or protein kinase activity. These fusion proteins contribute to tumorigenesis by activating genes or proteins involved in cell proliferation. For example, in Ewing's sarcoma the consequence of the t(11;22)(q24;q12) translocation is a fusion of EWS, a transcription factor gene on chromosome 22, and FLI-1, a gene encoding a member of the ETS family of transcription factors on chromosome 11.[97] The resultant chimeric protein, which contains the DNA binding region of FLI-1 and the transcription activation region of EWS, has greater transcriptional activity than does EWS alone.[98] The EWS–FLI-1 fusion transcript is detectable in approximately 90% of Ewing's sarcomas. At least four other EWS fusions have been identified in Ewing's sarcoma; fusion of EWS with ERG (another ETS family member) accounts for an additional 5% of cases.[137] Alveolar rhabdomyosarcomas have characteristic translocations between the long arm of chromosome 2 (75% of cases) or the short

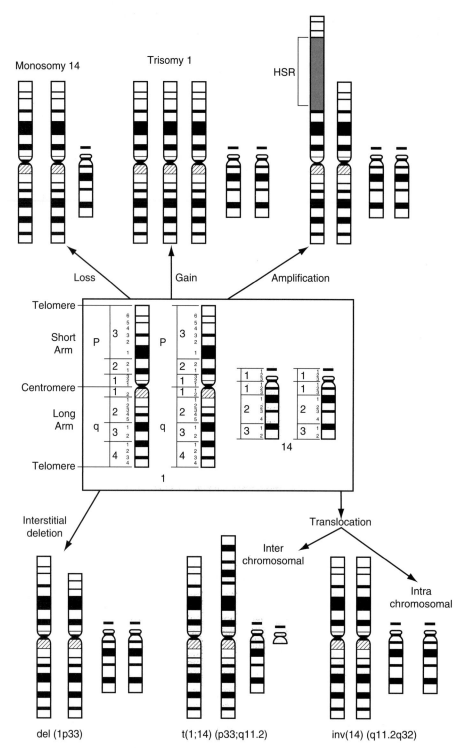

Figure 25–2 Spectrum of gross chromosomal aberrations using chromosomes 1 and 14 as examples. HSR, homogeneously staining regions. (From Look AT, Kirsch IR: Molecular basis of childhood cancer. In Pizzo PA, Poplack DG [eds]: Principles and Practices of Pediatric Oncology. Philadelphia: Lippincott-Raven, 1997, p 38.)

arm of chromosome 1 (10% of cases) and the long arm of chromosome 13. These translocations result in the fusion of *PAX3* (at 2q35) or *PAX7* (at 1p36) with *FKHR*, a gene encoding a member of the forkhead family of transcription factors.[53] The *EWS–FLI-1* and *PAX7–FKHR* fusions appear to confer a better prognosis for patients with Ewing's sarcoma and alveolar rhabdomyosarcoma, respectively.[8,33]

Translocations that generate chimeric proteins with increased transcriptional activity also characterize desmoplastic small round cell tumor,[88] myxoid liposarcoma,[120] extraskeletal myxoid chrondrosarcoma,[27] malignant melanoma of soft parts,[154] synovial sarcoma,[28] congenital fibrosarcoma,[149] cellular mesoblastic nephroma,[127] and dermatofibrosarcoma protuberans.[109]

TABLE 25–3 Common, Recurrent Translocations in Soft Tissue Tumors

Tumor	Genetic Abnormality	Fusion Transcript
Ewing's sarcoma, primitive neuroectodermal tumor	t(11;22)(q24;q12)	FLI1-EWS
	t(21;22)(q22;q12)	ERG-EWS
	t(7;22)(p22;q12)	ETV1-EWS
	t(17;22)(q12;q12)	E1AF-EWS
	t(2;22)(q33;q12)	FEV-EWS
Desmoplastic small round cell tumor	t(11;22)(p13;q12)	WT1-EWS
	t(11;22)(q24;q12)	FLI1-EWS
Synovial sarcoma	t(X;18)(p11.23;q11)	SSX1-SYT
	t(X;18)(p11.21;q11)	SSX2-SYT
Alveolar rhabdomyosarcoma	t(2;13)(q35;q14)	PAX3-FKHR
	t(1;13)(p36;q14)	PAX7-FKHR
Malignant melanoma of soft part (clear cell sarcoma)	t(12;22)(q13;q12)	ATF1-EWS
Myxoid liposarcoma	t(12;16)(q13;p11)	CHOP-TLS(FUS)
	t(12;22)(q13;q12)	CHOP-EWS
Extraskeletal myxoid chondrosarcoma	t(9;22)(q22;q12)	CHN-EWS
Dermatofibrosarcoma protuberans and giant cell fibroblastoma	t(17;22)(q22;q13)	COL1A1-PDGFB
Congenital fibrosarcoma and mesoblastic nephroma	t(12;15)(p13;q25)	ETV6-NTRK3
Lipoblastoma	t(3;8)(q12;q11.2)	?
	t(7;8)(q31;q13)	?

From Davidoff AM, Hill DA: Molecular genetic aspects of solid tumors in childhood. Semin Pediatr Surg 2001;10:106-118.

Proto-oncogene Activation

Proto-oncogenes are commonly activated in transformed cells by point mutations or gene amplification. The classic example of proto-oncogene activation by a point mutation involves the cellular proto-oncogene *RAS*. RAS-family proteins are associated with the inner, cytoplasmic surface of the plasma membrane and function as intermediates in signal transduction pathways that regulate cell proliferation. Point mutations in *RAS* result in constitutive activation of the RAS protein and, therefore, the continuous activation of the RAS signal transduction pathway. Activation of RAS appears to be involved in the pathogenesis of a small percentage of pediatric malignancies, including leukemia and a variety of solid tumors.

Gene amplification (i.e., selective replication of DNA sequences) enables a tumor cell to increase the expression of crucial genes whose products are ordinarily tightly controlled. The amplified DNA sequences, or amplicons, may be maintained episomally (i.e., extrachromosomally) as double minutes—paired chromatin bodies lacking a centromere—or as intrachromosomal, homogeneously staining regions. In about one third of neuroblastomas, for example, the transcription factor and proto-oncogene *MYCN* is amplified. *MYCN* encodes a 64-kDa nuclear phosphoprotein (MycN) that forms a transcriptional complex by associating with other nuclear proteins expressed in the developing nervous system and other tissues.[82] Increased expression of MycN increases the rates of DNA synthesis and cell proliferation and shortens the G_1 phase of the cell cycle.[94] The *MYCN* copy number in neuroblastoma cells can be amplified 5- to 500-fold and is usually consistent among primary and metastatic sites and at different times during tumor evolution and treatment.[15] This consistency suggests that *MYCN* amplification is an early event

in the pathogenesis of neuroblastoma. Because gene amplification is usually associated with advanced stages of disease, rapid tumor progression, and poor outcome, it is a powerful prognostic indicator.[17,132] The cell surface receptor gene *ERBB2* is another proto-oncogene that is commonly overexpressed due to gene amplification, an event that occurs in breast cancer, osteosarcoma, and Wilms' tumor.[114]

Comparative genomic hybridization studies have shown that a gain of genetic material on the long arm of chromosome 17 (17q) is perhaps the most common genetic abnormality in neuroblastomas: such gain occurs in approximately 75% of primary tumors.[146] Chromosome 17q gain is strongly associated with other known prognostic factors but may be a powerful independent predictor of adverse outcome.[13] Gain of 17q most often results from an unbalanced translocation of this region to other chromosomal sites, most frequently 1p or 11q. The term *unbalanced* indicates that extra copies of 17q are present, in addition to the normal chromosome 17. Although it is unclear what the crucial gene or genes are on 17q and how extra copies of 17q contribute to the malignant phenotype of neuroblastoma, the existence of 17q amplification in neuroblastoma suggests the presence of a proto-oncogene on 17q.

Inactivation of Tumor Suppressor Genes

Tumor suppressor genes, or antioncogenes, provide negative control of cell proliferation. Loss of function of the proteins encoded by these genes, through deletion or mutational inactivation of the gene, liberates the cell from growth constraints and contributes to malignant transformation. The cumulative effect of genetic lesions that activate proto-oncogenes or inactivate tumor suppressor genes is a breakdown in the balance between cell proliferation and cell loss due to differentiation or apoptosis. Such imbalance results in clonal overgrowth of a specific cell lineage. The first tumor suppressor gene to be recognized was the retinoblastoma susceptibility gene, *RB*. This gene encodes a nuclear phosphoprotein that acts as a "gatekeeper" of the cell cycle. *RB* normally permits cell cycle progression through the G_1 phase when it is phosphorylated, but it prevents cell division when it is unphosphorylated. Inactivating deletions or point mutations of *RB* cause the protein to lose its regulatory capacity. The nuclear phosphoprotein p53 has also been recognized as an important tumor suppressor gene, perhaps the most commonly altered gene in all human cancers. Inactivating mutations of the *p53* gene also cause the p53 protein to lose its ability to regulate the cell cycle. The *p53* gene is frequently inactivated in solid tumors of childhood, including osteosarcoma, rhabdomyosarcoma, brain tumors, anaplastic Wilms' tumor, and a subset of chemotherapy-resistant neuroblastoma.[7,78,86] In addition, heritable cancer-associated changes in the *p53* tumor suppressor gene occur in families with Li-Fraumeni syndrome, an autosomal dominant predisposition for rhabdomyosarcoma, other soft tissue and bone sarcomas, premenopausal breast cancer, brain tumors, and adrenocortical carcinomas.[95] Other tumor suppressor genes include Wilms' tumor 1 (*WT1*), neurofibromatosis 1 (*NF1*), and von Hippel-Lindau (*VHL*).

Other tumor suppressor genes are presumed to exist but have not been definitively identified. For example, early karyotype analyses of neuroblastoma-derived cell lines found frequent deletion of the short arm of chromosome 1.[18] Deletion of genetic material in tumors suggests the presence (and subsequent loss) of a tumor suppressor gene, but no individual tumor suppressor gene has been identified on chromosome 1p. Functional confirmation of the presence of a 1p tumor suppressor gene came from the demonstration that transfection of chromosome 1p into a neuroblastoma cell line results in morphologic changes of differentiation and ultimately cell senescence.[5] Approximately 20% to 35% of primary neuroblastomas exhibit 1p deletion, as determined by fluorescent in situ hybridization (FISH), and the smallest common region of loss is located within region 1p36.[51] Deletion of 1p is also common in Wilms' tumor.[62]

Metastasis

Metastasis is the spread of cancer cells from a primary tumor to distant sites and is the hallmark of malignancy. The development of tumor metastases is the main cause of treatment failure and a significant contributing factor to morbidity and mortality resulting from cancer. Although the dissemination of tumor cells through the circulation is probably a frequent occurrence, the establishment of metastatic disease is a very inefficient process. It requires several events, including the entry of the neoplastic cells into the blood or lymphatic system, the survival of those cells in the circulation, their avoidance of immune surveillance, their invasion of foreign (heterotopic) tissues, and the establishment of a blood supply to permit expansion of the tumor at the distant site.

Simple, dysregulated cell growth is not sufficient for tumor invasion and metastasis. Many tumors progress through distinct stages that can be identified by histopathologic examination, including hyperplasia, dysplasia, carcinoma in situ, invasive cancer, and disseminated cancer. Genetic analysis of these different stages of tumor progression suggests that uncontrolled growth results from progressive alteration in cellular oncogenes and inactivation of tumor suppressor genes, but these genetic changes driving tumorigenicity are clearly distinct from those that determine the metastatic phenotype.

Histologically, invasive carcinoma is characterized by a lack of basement membrane around an expanding mass of tumor cells. Matrix proteolysis appears to be a key part of the mechanism of invasion by tumor cells, which must be able to move through connective tissue barriers, such as the basement membrane, to spread from their site of origin. The proteases involved in this process include the matrix metalloproteinases and their tissue inhibitors. The local environment of the target organ may profoundly influence the growth potential of extravasated tumor cells.[44] The various cell surface receptors that mediate interactions between tumor cells and between tumor cells and the extracellular matrix include cadherins, integrins (transmembrane proteins formed by the noncovalent association of α and β subunits), and CD44, a transmembrane glycoprotein involved in cell adhesion to hyaluronan.[144] Tumor cells must decrease their adhesiveness to escape from the primary tumor, but at later stages of metastasis, the same tumor cells need to increase their adhesiveness during arrest and intravasation to distant sites.

Angiogenesis

Angiogenesis is the biologic process of new blood vessel formation. This complex, invasive process involves multiple steps, including proteolytic degradation of the extracellular matrix surrounding existing blood vessels, chemotactic migration and proliferation of endothelial cells, the organization of these endothelial cells into tubules, the establishment of a lumen that serves as a conduit between the circulation and an expanding mass of tumor cells, and functional maturation of the newly formed blood vessel.[50,123] Angiogenesis involves the coordinated activity of a wide variety of molecules, including growth factors, extracellular matrix proteins, adhesion receptors, and proteolytic enzymes. Under physiologic conditions, the vascular endothelium is quiescent and has a very low rate of cell division, such that only 0.01% of endothelial cells are dividing.[50,70,123] However, in response to hormonal cues or hypoxic or ischemic conditions, the endothelial cells can be activated to migrate, proliferate rapidly, and create lumens.

Angiogenesis occurs as part of such normal physiologic activities as wound healing, inflammation, the female reproductive cycle, and embryonic development. In these processes, angiogenesis is tightly and predictably regulated. However, angiogenesis can also be involved in the progression of several pathologic processes in which there is a loss of regulatory control, resulting in persistent growth of new blood vessels. Such unabated neovascularization occurs in rheumatoid arthritis, inflammatory bowel disease, hemangiomas of childhood, ocular neovascularization, and the growth and spread of tumors.[49]

Compelling data indicate that tumor-associated neovascularization is required for tumor growth, invasion, and metastasis.[9,47,48,116] A tumor in the prevascular phase (i.e., before new blood vessels have developed) can grow to only a limited size, approximately 2 to 3 mm³. At this point, rapid cell proliferation is balanced by equally rapid cell death by apoptosis, and a nonexpanding tumor mass results. The switch to an angiogenic phenotype with tumor neovascularization results in a decrease in the rate of apoptosis, thereby shifting the balance to cell proliferation and tumor growth.[71,91] This decrease in apoptosis occurs, in part, because the increased perfusion resulting from neovascularization permits improved nutrient and metabolite exchange. In addition, the proliferating endothelium may supply, in a paracrine manner, a variety of factors that promote tumor growth, such as IGF-I and IGF-II.[64]

In experimental models, increased tumor vascularization correlates with increased tumor growth, whereas restriction of neovascularization limits tumor growth. Clinically, the onset of neovascularization in many human tumors is temporally associated with increased tumor growth,[138] and high levels of angiogenic factors are commonly detected in blood and urine from patients with advanced malignancies.[107] In addition, the number and density of new microvessels within primary tumors have been shown to correlate with the likelihood of metastasis, as well as the overall prognosis for patients with a wide variety of neoplasms, including pediatric tumors such as neuroblastoma and Wilms' tumor.[1,101]

It has become increasingly evident that the regulation of tumor angiogenesis is complex: new blood vessel formation occurs as the result of competing pro- and antiangiogenic signals originating in multiple tissues.[23] Specific genetic events in certain cancers, such as altered expression of the *p53* tumor suppressor gene[32,153] or the human *EGFR* gene,[89,113,151] not only affect the cell cycle but also play a role in angiogenesis by modulating key signals (e.g., up-regulating the expression of vascular endothelial growth factor [VEGF] or down-regulating the expression of the endogenous angiogenesis inhibitor thrombospondin 1).

Metastasis also appears to be dependent on angiogenesis.[45,91] This dependence is probably due to several factors. First, new blood vessels in the primary tumor provide increased opportunities for the shedding of tumor cells into the circulation. Also, disruption of the basement membrane by proteases released by the proliferating endothelial cells may contribute to the metastatic potential of a tumor.[19,128] Finally, successful growth of metastatic cells in foreign target organs depends on the stimulation and formation of new blood vessels, perhaps even when cells metastasize to the bone marrow.

MOLECULAR DIAGNOSTICS

The explosion of information about the human genome has led not only to an improved understanding of the molecular genetic basis of tumorigenesis but also to the development of a new discipline: the translation of these molecular events into diagnostic assays. The field of molecular diagnostics has developed from the need to identify abnormalities of gene or chromosome structure in patient tissues and as a means of supporting standard histopathologic and immunohistochemical diagnostic methods. In most instances, the result of genetic testing confirms light microscopic and immunohistochemistry-based diagnosis. In some instances, however (e.g., primitive, malignant, small round cell tumor; poorly differentiated synovial sarcoma; lipoblastic tumor), molecular analysis is required to make a definitive diagnosis.

The molecular genetic methods most commonly used to analyze patient tumor material include direct metaphase cytogenetics or karyotyping, FISH, and reverse transcriptase polymerase chain reaction (RT-PCR). Additional methods, such as comparative genomic hybridization, loss of heterozygosity analysis, and complementary DNA (cDNA) microarray analysis, may eventually become part of the routine diagnostic repertoire but are currently used as research tools at referral centers and academic institutions. Each standard method is summarized in Table 25-4. As with any method, molecular genetic assays have advantages and disadvantages, and it is important to understand and recognize their limitations. It is also necessary to know the specific type of material required for each molecular assay. Surgeons can best appreciate the fine balance between minimizing the trauma and tissue disruption associated with a biopsy procedure and obtaining enough tissue for diagnosis, molecular genetic studies, and tissue banking for future analysis.

The value of molecular genetic analysis of patient tissue is not limited to aiding histopathologic diagnosis. Many of the most important markers provide prognostic information as well. *MYCN* amplification in neuroblastomas,[16] for example, is strongly associated with biologically aggressive behavior. Amplification of this gene can be detected by routine metaphase cytogenetics or by FISH, and current neuroblastoma protocols include the presence or absence of *MYCN* amplification in their stratification schema. Some fusion gene variants are also thought to influence prognosis. In initial studies, two examples noted to confer relatively favorable prognoses are the type 1 variant fusion of *EWS–FLI1* in Ewing's sarcoma or primitive neuroectodermal tumor[33] and the *PAX7–FKHR* fusion in alveolar rhabdomyosarcoma.[8] Complementary DNA microarray technology is likely to lead to the discovery of many more prognostically relevant genes.

New technologies are emerging that permit accurate, high-throughput analysis or "profiling" of tumor tissue: gene expression can be analyzed by using RNA microarrays, and proteins by using proteomics. These approaches identify a unique "fingerprint" of a given tumor that can provide diagnostic or prognostic information. Proteomic analysis can also identify unique proteins in patients' serum or urine; such a profile can be used for early tumor detection, to distinguish risk categories, and to monitor for recurrence.

Microarray analysis has also been used to characterize the response of tumor cells to stimuli such as stress, hypoxia, and therapy by analyzing a tumor cell's entire complement of RNA. The commercial availability of

TABLE 25–4 Comparison of Cytogenetic and Molecular Methods Used in the Pathologic Diagnosis of Soft Tissue Tumors

Method	Purpose	Advantages	Disadvantages
Cytogenetics	Low-resolution analysis of metaphase chromosomes of cells grown in culture	Does not require a priori knowledge of genetic abnormalities Available in most diagnostic centers	Requires fresh, sterile tumor tissue for growth in culture Low sensitivity; detects only large structural abnormalities No histologic correlation Slow and technically demanding (may take several weeks to perform)
In situ hybridization	Detection of translocations, amplifications, and gene deletions by hybridization of nucleic acid probes to specific DNA or mRNA sequences	Can be applied to chromosomal preparations as well as cytologic specimens, touch preparations, and paraffin sections Morphologic correlation is possible Multiple probes can be assayed at the same time Rapid (usually only 2 days)	Cannot detect small deletions or point mutations Interpretation can be difficult, especially with formalin-fixed, paraffin-embedded material Only a limited number of specific nucleic acid probes are available commercially
PCR and RT-PCR	Extremely sensitive detection of DNA sequences and mRNA transcripts for the demonstration of fusion genes, point mutations, and polymorphisms	Highest sensitivity and specificity of all molecular diagnostic techniques DNA sequencing of PCR products can confirm results and provide additional information Requires minimal tissue Versatile; can be applied to fresh tissue as well as formalin-fixed, paraffin-embedded tissue Morphologic correlation is possible Presence of normal tissue usually does not affect test results Rapid (usually 3-5 days)	Formalin-fixation diminishes sensitivity Combinatorial variability within fusion gene partners requires appropriate redundant primer design to avoid false-negative test results Extreme sensitivity requires exacting laboratory technique to avoid false-positive test results

mRNA, messenger RNA; PCR, polymerase chain reaction; RT-PCR, reverse transcriptase polymerase chain reaction.
From Davidoff AM, Hill DA: Molecular genetic aspects of solid tumors in childhood. Semin Pediatr Surg 2001;10:106-118.

various precoated kits and their ease of use have led to widespread application of this approach. The procedure involves the hybridization of complementary strands of labeled DNA or RNA from tumors with known genes or oligonucleotides derived from the genome. The known genes or oligonucleotides are attached to a solid support, the microarray. Hybridization is detected by fluorescence. Once the quality and consistency of sample material can be refined and data management and statistical analyses validated and standardized, gene profiling microarrays will probably be used routinely to analyze pediatric malignancies.

CHILDHOOD CANCER AND HEREDITY

Advances in molecular genetic techniques have also improved our understanding of cancer predisposition syndromes. Constitutional gene mutations that are hereditary (i.e., passed from parent to child) or non-hereditary (i.e., de novo mutations in the sperm or oocyte before fertilization) contribute to an estimated 10% to 15% of pediatric cancers.[119] Constitutional chromosomal abnormalities are the result of an abnormal number or structural rearrangement of the normal

46 chromosomes and may be associated with a predisposition to cancer. Examples are the predisposition to leukemia seen with trisomy 21 (Down syndrome) and to germ cell tumors with Klinefelter's syndrome (47XXY). Structural chromosomal abnormalities include interstitial deletions resulting in the constitutional loss of one or more genes.

Wilms' tumors may be sporadic, familial, or associated with specific genetic disorders or recognizable syndromes. A better understanding of the molecular basis of Wilms' tumor has been achieved largely through the study of the latter two types of tumors. The WAGR syndrome (Wilms' tumor, aniridia, genitourinary abnormalities, and mental retardation) provides an easily recognizable phenotype for grouping children likely to have a common genetic abnormality. Constitutional deletions from chromosome 11p13 are consistent in children with WAGR syndrome[121] and also occur in approximately 35% of those with sporadic Wilms' tumor.[31] A study of a large series of patients identified the gene deleted from chromosome 11p13 as *WT1*.[22] This gene encodes a nuclear transcription factor that is essential for normal kidney and gonadal development[118] and appears to act as a tumor suppressor, but its precise role is unclear at this time. Aniridia in patients with WAGR syndrome is thought to occur after the loss of one copy of the *PAX6* gene located close to *WT1* on chromosome 11.[143] Denys-Drash syndrome, which is characterized by a very high risk of Wilms' tumor, pseudohermaphroditism, and mesangial sclerosis leading to early renal failure, is associated with germline mutations in the DNA binding domain of *WT1*.[112] The mutated WT1 protein appears to function by a dominant negative effect. Only 6% to 18% of sporadic Wilms' tumors have *WT1* mutations.[112,147]

In another subset of patients with Wilms' tumor, there is loss of genetic material in a region distal to the *WT1* locus toward the telomeric end of chromosome 11 (11p15).[30] It has therefore been suggested that there is a second Wilms' tumor susceptibility gene, tentatively named *WT2*, in 11p15. Loss of heterozygosity at this locus has also been described in patients with Beckwith-Wiedemann syndrome, a congenital overgrowth syndrome characterized by numerous growth abnormalities as well as a predisposition to a variety of malignancies, including Wilms' tumor.[83] (See Chapter 27.)

Neurofibromatosis type 1 (NF1) is one of the most common genetic disorders. The NF1 protein normally inhibits the proto-oncogene *RAS*, but in patients with NF1, mutation of one copy of the gene combined with deletion of the other permits uncontrolled *RAS* pathway activation. These patients are then susceptible to myelogenous disorders, benign tumors, gliomas, and malignant peripheral nerve sheath tumors. An inherited predisposition to pediatric cancers is also associated with Li-Fraumeni syndrome (which results from inactivating mutations of the *p53* gene and puts patients at risk for osteosarcoma, rhabdomyosarcoma, adrenocortical carcinoma, and brain tumors, among other tumors), familial retinoblastoma (which results from inactivating mutations of the *RB* gene and puts patients at risk for osteosarcoma as well as retinoblastoma), familial adenomatous polyposis, and multiple endocrine neoplasia syndromes. Another set of inherited risk factors is represented by mutations of DNA repair genes (so-called caretaker genes), as seen in xeroderma pigmentosa and ataxia-telangiectasia.[80] Understanding these complex syndromes and their pathogenesis is important in efforts to screen for early detection and, possibly, for prophylactic therapy.

GENETIC SCREENING

Along with an increased understanding of the molecular basis of hereditary childhood cancer has come the opportunity to identify children who are at high risk of malignancy and, in some cases, to intervene before the cancer develops or when it is still curable. Two examples include familial adenomatous polyposis and familial thyroid cancer.

Familial adenomatous polyposis is an autosomal dominant inherited disease in which hundreds to thousands of adenomatous intestinal polyps develop during the second and third decades of life. Mutations of the adenomatous polyposis coli *(APC)* gene on chromosome 5q21 occur in approximately 80% of kindreds of persons who have the disease.[108,117] These mutations initiate the adenomatous process by allowing clonal expansion of individual cells that, over time, acquire additional genetic abnormalities that lead to the development of invasive colorectal carcinoma.[55] Prophylactic colectomy is recommended for patients with this germline mutation, although the most appropriate timing for this intervention in children with familial adenomatous polyposis is controversial. These patients are also at increased risk of hepatoblastoma.[79]

Medullary thyroid carcinoma (MTC) is a rare malignancy that may occur sporadically or as part of two syndromes: multiple endocrine neoplasia (type 2A or 2B) syndrome or familial MTC syndrome. In children, MTC is much more likely to occur in association with a familial syndrome. An apparently 100% association between germline *RET* mutations[104] and MTC guides the recommendation for prophylactic thyroidectomy in affected patients. There is no effective adjuvant treatment other than surgery for MTC, highlighting the need for early intervention. Patients with germline *RET* mutations should also be screened for pheochromocytoma, which occurs in 50% of patients with multiple endocrine neoplasia type 2A, and hyperparathyroidism, which occurs in 35% of such patients.[72] In addition, patients who are at risk for MTC or have newly diagnosed MTC, as well as their relatives, should be screened for the germline *RET* mutation so that appropriate surgical and genetic counseling can be given.

GENERAL PRINCIPLES OF CHEMOTHERAPY

Cytotoxic agents were first noted to be effective in the treatment of cancer in the 1960s, after alkylating agents such as nitrogen mustard gas, used during World War II, were observed to cause bone marrow hypoplasia. Chemotherapy is now an integral part of nearly all cancer treatment regimens. The overriding goal of cancer chemotherapy is to maximize tumoricidal effect (efficacy) while minimizing adverse side effects (toxicity). This goal can be difficult to achieve, however, because the dose at which tumor cells are affected is often similar to the dose that affects normal proliferating cells, such as those in the bone marrow and gastrointestinal tract. Despite the early promise of chemotherapy and the observation that most tumor types are initially sensitive to chemotherapy, often exquisitely so, the successful use of chemotherapy is often thwarted by two factors: the development of resistance to the agent and the agent's toxicity to normal tissues. Nevertheless, chemotherapy remains an integral part of therapy when used as an adjunct to treat localized disease or as the main component to treat disseminated or advanced disease.

A number of principles and terms are essential to the understanding of chemotherapy as a therapeutic anticancer modality. *Adjuvant chemotherapy* refers to the use of chemotherapy for systemic treatment following local control of a clinically localized primary tumor, generally by surgical resection or radiation therapy. The goal in this setting is to eliminate disease that is not detectable by standard investigative means at or beyond the primary tumor's site. *Neoadjuvant chemotherapy* refers to chemotherapy delivered before local therapeutic modalities, generally in an effort to improve their efficacy; to treat micrometastatic disease as early as possible, when distant tumors are smallest; or to achieve both of these aims. *Induction chemotherapy* refers to the use of chemotherapeutic agents as the primary treatment for advanced disease. In general, chemotherapy given to children with solid tumors and metastatic disease at the time of first examination has a less than 40% chance of effecting long-term, disease-free survival. Exceptions include Wilms' tumor with favorable histologic features, germ cell tumors, and paratesticular rhabdomyosarcoma, but most children with metastatic disease are at high risk of disease recurrence or progression. *Combination chemotherapy* refers to the use of multiple agents, which generally have different mechanisms of action and nonoverlapping toxicities, that provide effective, synergistic antitumor activity and minimal side effects. The efficacy of combination chemotherapy is explained by the Goldie-Coldman hypothesis,[56] which states that a tumor's response to an individual drug reflects the individual tumor cells' sensitivity to that drug. The chance of a tumor developing a resistance phenotype depends on the rate of mutation and the number of tumor cells or tumor size. Once a single tumor cell becomes resistant to a given agent, the tumor can no longer be cured by that agent. Combining agents with different mechanisms of action decreases the likelihood that a tumor cell will develop resistance to any or all agents and is therefore more likely to effect a cure.

Pharmacokinetics describes the relationship between time and the plasma concentration of a drug, and drug exposure is quantified by calculating the area under the curve of the graph of drug concentration against time. The pharmacokinetics of a drug is influenced by its absorption, distribution, metabolism, clearance, half-life, and excretion and by the presence of active metabolites. The interpretation of pharmacokinetic data requires an understanding of the relation between plasma concentration of the drug and its anticancer effect. The dose-response curve for a given agent is usually sigmoidal, with a threshold level, lag phase, linear response, and plateau. The slope of the linear phase is often quite steep, and this steepness implies a significant loss of efficacy with a slight dose reduction. Therefore, the delivery of a maximum tolerated dose, to ensure that the dose range of the linear phase has been exceeded, has become a basic principle of chemotherapy. Dose intensity can be maximized by increasing the total dose of an agent or by shortening the interval between doses. Inappropriate dose reduction may lead to residual tumor cells not being eliminated. The *therapeutic index* is the ratio of beneficial to harmful effects.

An emerging theory regarding optimal chemotherapeutic dosages that is somewhat counter to the long-standing and widely used approach of maximum tolerated dose is metronomic dosing. This new approach, which entails the continuous delivery of a low dose of chemotherapeutic agents, may be effective for two reasons. First, because most agents are cell-cycle specific (i.e., they kill only cells that are at specific points in the cell cycle), only a fraction of tumor cells is susceptible at any given time. Therefore, a longer duration of exposure to an agent may result in more tumor cells being susceptible. Second, metronomic dosing may allow the agent to target the endothelial cells that constitute the expanding tumor vasculature, as well as the tumor cells themselves. The traditional scheduling of cytotoxic therapy—the administration of a maximum tolerated dose, followed by a rest period to allow the recovery of affected normal tissue (notably the bone marrow and gastrointestinal tract)—may also permit the recovery and proliferation of the more slowly dividing endothelial cells in a tumor bed and thereby permit tumor regrowth.[20] A metronomic schedule in which cytotoxic drugs are administered continuously or at least more frequently, without a treatment-free interval, and at a lower total dose may therefore be more effective at controlling tumor progression, even if the tumor cells themselves are resistant to the drug.[20] This approach appears to be true for cytotoxic drugs and antiangiogenic agents.

The rational design of chemotherapy treatment programs and clinical trials involves an understanding of the mechanisms of action of these agents, their metabolism, and their toxicity profiles. Most agents used to treat tumors in children affect the synthesis or function of nucleic acids (DNA or RNA) in malignant and normal cells. Therefore, these agents can kill tumor cells but can also affect normal tissue. The mechanisms of action and side effects of commonly used agents are listed in Table 25-5. Alkylating agents interfere with cell growth by covalently cross-linking DNA and are not cell-cycle specific. Antitumor antibiotics intercalate into the double helix of DNA and break the DNA strands. Antimetabolites are truly cell-cycle specific because they interfere with the use of normal substrates for DNA and RNA synthesis, such as purines and thymidine. The plant alkaloids can inhibit microtubule function (vinca alkaloids, taxanes) or DNA topoisomerases (camptothecins inhibit topoisomerase I; epipodophyllotoxins inhibit topoisomerase II), and these actions also lead to breaks in DNA strands. Topoisomerases are a class of enzymes that alter the supercoiling of double-stranded DNA. They act by transiently cutting one (topoisomerase I) or both (topoisomerase II) strands of the DNA to relax the DNA coil and extend the molecule. The regulation of DNA supercoiling is essential to DNA transcription and replication, when the DNA helix must unwind to permit the proper function of the enzymatic machinery involved in these processes. Thus, topoisomerases maintain the transcription and replication of DNA.

The common toxic effects of these agents are also listed in Table 25-5. Most toxicity associated with chemotherapy is reversible and resolves with cessation of treatment. Other side effects may be reversed by giving specific antidotes such as leucovorin for toxicity associated with methotrexate. Leucovorin acts in the same way in the body as folic acid does, but it does not negate the therapeutic efficacy of methotrexate. However, some chemotherapeutic agents may have lifelong effects. Of particular concern is that certain drugs can lead to a second malignancy. Most notable is the development of leukemia after the administration of the epipodophyllotoxins and cyclophosphamide.[145]

TABLE 25–5 Common Chemotherapeutic Agents

Class of Drug	Agent	Synonyms	Brand Name	Mechanism of Action	Common Toxic Effects	Site of Activation	Method of Elimination	Susceptible Solid Tumors
Alkylating agents	Carboplatin	CBCDCA	Paraplatin	Platination, intra- and interstrand DNA cross-linking	A, H, M (esp. thrombocytopenia), N/V		Renal	BT, GCT, NBL, STS
	Cisplatin	CDDC	Platinol	Platination, intra- and interstrand DNA cross-linking	A, N/V, R (significant), ototoxicity, neuropathy		Renal	BT, GCT, NBL, OS
	Cyclophosphamide	CTX	Cytoxan	Alkylation, intra- and interstrand DNA cross-linking	A, N/V, SIADH, M, R, cardiac, cystitis	Liver	Hepatic, renal (minor)	Broad, BMT
	Ifosfamide	IFOS	Ifex	Alkylation, intra- and interstrand DNA cross-linking	A, CNS, N/V, M, R, cardiac, cystitis	Liver	Hepatic, renal (minor)	Broad
	Dacarbazine		DTIC	Methylation	H, N/V, M, hepatic vein thrombosis	Liver	Renal	NBL, STS
	Temozolomide	TMZ	Temodar	Methylation	CNS, N/V, M	Spontaneous	Renal	BT
	Nitrogen mustard	Mechlorethamine	Mustargen	Alkylation, intra- and interstrand DNA cross-linking	A, M (significant), N/V, mucositis, vesication, phlebitis, diarrhea		Spontaneous hydrolysis	BT
	Melphalan	L-PAM	Alkeran	Alkylation, intra- and interstrand DNA cross-linking	M, N/V, mucositis, diarrhea		Spontaneous hydrolysis	NBL, RMS, BMT
	Busulfan		Busulfex	Alkylation, intra- and interstrand DNA cross-linking	A, H, M, N/V, P, mucositis		Renal	BMT
Antimetabolites	Cytarabine	Ara-C	Cytosar	Inhibits DNA polymerase, incorporated into DNA	M, N/V, diarrhea, CNS	Target cell	Biotransformation	Limited
	Fluorouracil	5-FU	Several	Inhibits thymidine synthesis, incorporated into DNA/RNA	CNS, N/V, M, cardiac, diarrhea, mucositis, skin, ocular	Target cell	Biotransformation, renal (minor)	Gastrointestinal carcinomas, liver tumors
	Mercaptopurine	6-MP	Purinethol	Inhibits thymidine synthesis, incorporated into DNA/RNA	H, M, mucositis	Target cell	Biotransformation, renal (minor)	Limited
	Methotrexate	MTX	Trexall	Blocks folate metabolism, inhibits purine synthesis	CNS, H, M, R, mucositis, skin		Renal, hepatic (minor)	OS
Antibiotics	Dactinomycin	Actinomycin D	Cosmegen	DNA intercalation, strand breaks	A, H, M, N/V, mucositis, vesication		Hepatic	RMS, W
	Bleomycin	BLEO	Blenoxane	DNA intercalation, strand breaks	P, skin, mucositis		Hepatic, renal	GCT
	Anthracyclines Daunomycin	Daunorubicin	Cerubidine	DNA intercalation, strand breaks, free radical formation	A, M, N/V, cardiac, diarrhea, vesication, potentiates XRT reaction		Hepatic	Limited

Continued

TABLE 25–5 Common Chemotherapeutic Agents—Cont'd

Class of Drug	Agent	Synonyms	Brand Name	Mechanism of Action	Common Toxic Effects	Site of Activation	Method of Elimination	Susceptible Solid Tumors
	Adriamycin	Doxorubicin	Adriamycin	DNA intercalation, strand breaks, free radical formation	A, M, N/V, cardiac, diarrhea, mucositis, vesication, potentiates XRT reaction		Hepatic	Broad
Plant alkaloids								
Epipodophyllotoxins								
	Etoposide	VP-16	VePesid	Topoisomerase II inhibitor, DNA strand breaks	A, M, N/V, mucositis, neuropathy, diarrhea		Renal	Broad
	Teniposid	VM-26	Vumon	Topoisomerase II inhibitor, DNA strand breaks	A, M, N/V, mucositis, neuropathy, diarrhea		Degraded	Broad
Vinca alkaloids								
	Vincristine	VCR	Oncovin	Inhibits tubulin polymerization, blocks mitosis	A, SIADH, neuropathy, vesicant		Hepatic	Broad
	Vinblastine	VLB	Velban	Inhibits tubulin polymerization, blocks mitosis	A, M, mucositis, vesication		Hepatic	GCT
Taxanes								
	Paclitaxel		Taxol	Interferes with microtubule formation	A, M, cardiac, mucositis, CNS, neuropathy			
	Docetaxel		Taxotere	Interferes with microtubule formation	A, neutropenia, cardiac, mucositis, CNS, neuropathy			
Camptothecins								
	Topotecan	TPT	Hycamtin	Topoisomerase I inhibitor, DNA strand breaks	A, H, M, N/V, mucositis, diarrhea, skin		Renal	NBL, RMS
	Irinotecan	CPT-11	Camptosar	Topoisomerase I inhibitor, DNA strand breaks	A, H, M, N/V, diarrhea	Liver, gastrointestinal tract	Hepatic, renal (minor)	NBL, RMS
Miscellaneous	L-Asparaginase	Erwinia	Elspar	L-Asparagine depletion, inhibits protein synthesis	CNS, H, coagulopathy, pancreatitis, anaphylaxis		Degraded	Limited
	Corticosteroids			Nuclear receptor–mediated apoptosis	Avascular necrosis, hyperglycemia, hypertension, myopathy, pancreatitis, peptic ulcers, psychosis, salt imbalance, weight gain	Liver	Hepatic, renal (minor)	BT

Toxic effects: A, alopecia; CNS, central nervous system toxicity; H, hepatotoxicity; M, myelosuppression; N/V, nausea and vomiting; P, pulmonary toxicity; R, renal toxicity; SIADH, syndrome of inappropriate antidiuretic hormone; XRT, radiotherapy. Solid tumors: BMT, conditioning for bone marrow transplantation; BT, brain tumor; EWS, Ewing's sarcoma; GCT, germ cell tumors; NBL, neuroblastoma; OS, osteosarcoma; RMS, rhabdomyosarcoma; STS, soft tissue sarcoma; W, Wilms' tumor.

Finally, understanding the metabolism of chemotherapeutic agents is important. Certain agents require metabolism at a specific site or organ for their activation or are eliminated from the body by a specific organ (see Table 25-5). The processes of activation and elimination require normal organ function (e.g., the liver for cyclophosphamide); therefore, children with liver or kidney failure may not be able to receive certain agents.

Risk Stratification

Major advances in the variety of chemotherapeutic agents and dosing strategies used to treat pediatric cancers in the past 30 years are reflected in improved patient survival rates. Regimen toxicity (including late effects, which are particularly important in the pediatric population) and therapeutic resistance are the two main hurdles preventing further advancement. As more information about diagnostically and prognostically useful genetic markers becomes available, therapeutic strategies will change accordingly. With molecular profiling, patients can be categorized to receive a particular treatment on the basis of not only the tumor's histopathologic and staging characteristics but also its genetic composition. Some patients whose tumors show a more aggressive biologic profile may require dose intensification to increase their chances of survival. Patients whose tumors do not have an aggressive biologic profile may benefit from the lower toxicity of less intensive therapy. Such an approach may allow the maintenance of high survival rates while minimizing long-term complications of therapy in these patient populations.

The paradigm for the use of different therapeutic intensities on the basis of risk stratification drives the management of pediatric neuroblastoma. There is increasing evidence that the molecular features of neuroblastoma are highly predictive of its clinical behavior. Most current studies of the treatment of neuroblastoma are based on risk groups that take into account both clinical and biologic variables. The most important clinical variables appear to be age and stage at diagnosis, and the most powerful biologic factors appear to be *MYCN* status, ploidy (for patients younger than 1 year), and histopathologic classification. These variables currently define the Children's Oncology Group risk strata and therapeutic approach. At one extreme, patients with low-risk disease are treated with surgery alone; at the other extreme, patients at high risk for relapse are treated with intensive multimodality therapy that includes multiagent, dose-intensive chemotherapy; radiation therapy; and stem cell transplantation. Other factors such as 17q gain, 1p deletion, caspase 8 inactivation, and TrkA/B expression are currently being evaluated and may help further refine risk assessment in the future. The management of other solid pediatric tumors is also shifting to risk-defined treatment. For example, the next protocol for the management of patients with Wilms' tumor is likely to include risk stratification and therapy adjustment based on molecular analysis of the primary tumor for 16q and 1p deletions.

Targeted Therapy

Another major change in the approach to the treatment of cancer has been the concept of targeted therapy. Until recently, the development of anticancer agents was based on the empirical screening of a large variety of cytotoxic compounds without particular regard to disease specificity or mechanism of action. Now, one of the most exciting prospects for improving the therapeutic index of anticancer agents, as well as overcoming the problem of therapy resistance, involves targeted therapy. As the molecular bases for the phenotypes of specific malignancies are being elucidated, potential new targets for therapy are becoming more clearly defined. The characterization of pathways that define malignant transformation and progression has focused new agent development on key pathways involved in the crucial processes of cell-cycle regulation, receptor signaling, differentiation, apoptosis, invasion, migration, and angiogenesis, which may be perturbed in malignant tissues. Information about the molecular profile of a given tumor type can be assembled from a variety of emerging methods, including immunohistochemistry, FISH, RT-PCR, cDNA microarray analysis, and proteomics. This information can then be used to develop new drugs designed to counter the molecular abnormalities of the neoplastic cells. For example, blocking oncogene function or restoring suppressor gene activity may provide tumor-specific therapy. In addition, molecular profiling may lead to the development of drugs designed to induce differentiation of tumor cells, block dysregulated growth pathways, or reactivate silenced apoptotic pathways.

Some agents target alterations in the regulation of cell proliferation. Herceptin (trastuzumab) is a monoclonal antibody that binds to the cell surface growth factor receptor ERBB2 with high affinity and acts as an antiproliferative agent when used to treat ERBB2-overexpressing cancer cells.[99] It is currently being tested against ERBB2-positive tumors such as osteosarcoma and Wilms' tumor. Pediatric high-grade gliomas that overexpress EGFR may be amenable to a similar therapeutic agent, gefitinib (Iressa), a small-molecule inhibitor of EGFR (ERBB1).[14] In addition, small-molecule tyrosine kinase inhibitors, such as imatinib (Gleevec), designed to block aberrantly expressed growth-promoting tyrosine kinases—ABL in chronic myelogenous leukemia[142] and c-KIT in gastrointestinal stromal tumors[21]—are being evaluated in clinical trials. Imatinib may also be useful in treating pediatric tumors in which PDGF signaling plays a role in tumor cell survival and growth. Other kinase inhibitors, such as flavopiridol, target cyclin-dependent kinases that modulate the cell cycle,[77] whereas rapamycin (sirolimus) inhibits the mammalian target of rapamycin (mTOR), a protein whose activation[129] normally leads to increased translation of proteins necessary for cell proliferation. Inhibitors of farnesyl transferase (the enzyme responsible for the activation of RAS), such as R115777, are also being tested in clinical trials. Although activating mutations are very common in adult malignancies, they are rare in pediatric tumors. However, the RAS pathway is occasionally activated by upstream growth factors or oncogenic proteins in such pediatric diseases as juvenile myelomonocytic leukemia, certain brain tumors, and NF1, so agents such as R115777 are being tested against these conditions as well. Also of potential therapeutic utility are small-molecule inhibitors that recognize antigenic determinants on unique fusion peptides or one of the fusion peptide partners in tumors that have chromosomal translocations (e.g., sarcomas). Tumors that depend on autocrine pathways for growth (e.g., overproduction of IGF-II in rhabdomyosarcoma or PDGF in dermatofibrosarcoma protuberans) may be sensitive to receptor blocking mediators (e.g., antibodies to the IGF-II or PDGF receptor).

Other agents target alteration of the cell death and differentiation pathways. Caspase 8 is a cysteine protease that regulates programmed cell death, but in tumors such as neuroblastoma, DNA methylation and gene deletion combine to mediate the complete inactivation of caspase 8, almost always in association with *MYCN* amplification.[140] Methylation of cytosine residues in genomic DNA is quite common and usually occurs at cytosine residues adjacent to guanosine. DNA methylation is important in the transcriptional repression or silencing of certain genes, particularly developmentally regulated genes. Caspase 8-deficient tumor cells are resistant to apoptosis mediated by death receptors and doxorubicin; this resistance suggests that caspase 8 may be acting as a tumor suppressor. However, brief exposure of caspase 8-deficient cells to demethylating agents, such as decitabine, or to low levels of interferon-γ can lead to the re-expression of caspase 8 and the resensitization of the cells to chemotherapeutic drug-induced apoptosis. Histone deacetylase also seems to have a role in gene silencing associated with resistance to apoptosis[69]; therefore, histone deacetylase inhibitors such as depsipeptide are also being tested for the treatment of certain pediatric malignancies. Finally, cells with alterations in programmed cell death as a result of the persistence or reactivation of telomerase activity, which somatic cells normally lose after birth, can be targeted by various telomerase inhibitors.

An example of targeting cell differentiation comes from neuroblastoma, in which different neurotrophin receptor pathways appear to mediate the signal for both cellular differentiation and malignant transformation of sympathetic neuroblasts to neuroblastoma cells. Neurotrophins are expressed in a wide variety of neuronal tissues and other tissues that require innervation. They stimulate the survival, maturation, and differentiation of neurons and exhibit a developmentally regulated pattern of expression.[6,90] Neurotrophins and their Trk tyrosine kinase receptors are particularly important in the development of the sympathetic nervous system and have been implicated in the pathogenesis of neuroblastoma. Three receptor-ligand pairs have been identified: TrkA, TrkB, and TrkC, which are the primary receptors for nerve growth factor, brain-derived neurotrophic factor (BDNF), and neurotrophin 3 (NT-3), respectively.[6] TrkA appears to mediate the differentiation of developing neurons or neuroblastoma in the presence of nerve growth factor ligand and to mediate apoptosis in the absence of nerve growth factor.[90] Conversely, the TrkB-BDNF pathway appears to promote neuroblastoma cell survival through autocrine or paracrine signaling, especially in *MYCN*-amplified tumors.[106] TrkC is expressed in approximately 25% of neuroblastomas and is strongly associated with TrkA expression.[139] Studies are ongoing to test agonists of TrkA in an attempt to induce cellular differentiation. Conversely, blocking the TrkB-BDNF signaling pathway with Trk-specific tyrosine kinase inhibitors such as CEP-751 may induce apoptosis by blocking crucial survival pathways.[40,106] This targeted approach has the attractive potential for increased specificity and lower toxicity than conventional cytotoxic chemotherapy.

INHIBITION OF ANGIOGENESIS

Because tumor growth and spread appear to be dependent on angiogenesis, inhibition of angiogenesis is a logical anticancer strategy. This approach is particularly appealing for several reasons. First, despite the extreme molecular and phenotypic heterogeneity of human cancer, it is likely that most, if not all, tumor types, including hematologic malignancies, require neovascularization to achieve their full malignant phenotype. Therefore, antiangiogenic therapy may have broad applicability for the treatment of cancer. Second, the endothelial cells in a tumor's new blood vessels, although rapidly proliferating, are inherently normal and mutate slowly. They are therefore unlikely to evolve a phenotype that is insensitive to an angiogenesis inhibitor, unlike the rapidly proliferating tumor cells, which undergo spontaneous mutation at a high rate and can readily generate drug-resistant clones. Finally, because the new blood vessels induced by a tumor are sufficiently distinct from established vessels to permit highly specific targeting,[3,131] angiogenesis inhibitors should have a high therapeutic index and minimal toxicity. The combination of conventional chemotherapeutic agents with angiogenesis inhibitors appears to be particularly effective.

The first clinical demonstration that an angiogenesis inhibitor could cause regression of a tumor came with the use of interferon-α in a patient treated for life-threatening pulmonary hemangioma.[150] An increasing number of natural and synthetic inhibitors of angiogenesis, which inhibit different effectors of angiogenesis, have since been identified, and many of these agents have been tested in clinical trials. Minimal toxicity has been observed for these agents. Examples include drugs that directly inhibit endothelial cells, such as thalidomide and combretastatin; drugs that block activators of angiogenesis, such as bevacizumab (Avastin), a recombinant humanized anti-VEGF antibody, or "VEGF trap"; drugs that inhibit endothelium-specific survival signaling, such as Vitaxin, an anti-integrin antibody; and drugs with nonspecific mechanisms of action, such as celecoxib and interleukin-12 (IL-12). The National Cancer Institute has set up a Web site that lists all the ongoing clinical trials of angiogenesis inhibitors (http://www.cancer.gov/clinical-trials/developments/anti-angio-table).

Because antiangiogenic therapy may be only tumoristatic, tumor progression may resume when the growth restrictions of angiogenesis inhibition are discontinued.

Therefore, chronic delivery of antiangiogenic agents may be required. Gene therapy, with its potential for sustained expression, may provide a more practical method than chronic protein administration for the long-term delivery of angiogenesis inhibitors.[43]

IMMUNOTHERAPY

The immune system has evolved as a powerful means to detect and eliminate molecules or pathogens that are recognized as "foreign." However, because tumors arise from host cells, they are generally relatively weakly immunogenic. In addition, malignant cells have evolved several mechanisms that allow them to elude the immune system. These mechanisms include the ability to down-regulate the cell surface major histocompatibility complex molecules required for activation of many of the immune effector cells, to produce immunosuppressive factors, and to variably express different proteins that might otherwise serve as targets for the immune system in a process known as antigenic drift. Nevertheless, because of the large number of mutations and chromosomal aberrations occurring in cancer cells, which results in the expression of abnormal, new, or otherwise silenced proteins, it is likely that most if not all cancers contain unique, tumor-associated antigens that can be recognized by the immune system. Examples include the fusion proteins commonly found in pediatric sarcomas and the embryonic neuroectodermal antigens that continue to be produced by neuroblastomas.

Recruiting the immune system to help eradicate tumor cells is an attractive approach for several reasons. First, circulating cells of the immune system have ready access to even occult sites of tumor cells. Second, the immune system has powerful effector cells capable of effectively and efficiently destroying and eradicating targets, including neoplastic cells. Initial efforts to recruit the immune system to recognize and destroy tumor cells by using cytotoxic effector mechanisms that are T-cell dependent or independent focused on recombinant cytokines. Cytokines act by directly stimulating the immune system[66] or by rendering the target tumor cells more immunogenic. More recently, however, since the discovery that gene transfer can be used to markedly increase the immunogenicity of a tumor, tumor cell-based vaccine approaches have been used. For example, tumor cells transfected with genes that encode cytokines show a substantial increase in their immunogenicity, which allows them to act as an antitumor vaccine when injected into a host.[4,10,42,57,141] Transduced tumor cells appear to be much more immunogenic than low doses of cytokines injected directly into lesions. Because the cytokines are produced locally by the transduced tumor cells, there are none of the adverse effects associated with the administration of cytokines at the high systemic doses needed to induce antitumor responses. This gene transfer approach also permits tumor cell targeting without the identification of specific tumor-associated antigens.

Because of the concern that tumor cells may not present antigens appropriately to host immune effector cells, alternative vaccine strategies have been used in which tumor lysates or antigenic peptides are delivered to autologous dendritic cells—the immune system's antigen-presenting cells. This approach can expand specific T-cell populations and mediate tumor regression.[54] An extension of this approach using gene-modified, cytokine-expressing dendritic cells is being evaluated in preclinical studies.[136] Other preclinical studies have shown that the tumor antigen-specific immune response can be further enhanced by the administration of immunostimulatory CpG oligodeoxynucleotides after vaccination with cytokine-expressing tumor cells.[130]

Neuroblastoma has been the most popular target for immunotherapy in the pediatric population. Clinical trials of the treatment of neuroblastoma by transferring cytokine genes into autologous or allogeneic tumor cells have shown that gene-modified, cytokine-expressing tumor cell vaccines have little toxicity and can induce an antitumor immune response.[11,12,126] Neuroblastoma cells are sensitive to antibody-dependent cell-mediated cytotoxicity, as well as to complement-dependent cytotoxicity.[25] Although a particular neuroblastoma antigen has not been defined, murine monoclonal antibodies have been raised against the ganglioside GD2, a predominant antigen on the surface of neuroblastoma cells. These antibodies elicited therapeutic responses,[26,65] but with substantial toxicity, particularly neuropathic pain.[111] Because the induction of antibody-dependent cell-mediated cytotoxicity with anti-GD2 antibodies is enhanced by cytokines such as granulocyte-macrophage colony-stimulating factor[111] and interleukin-2 (IL-2),[67] current antineuroblastoma antibody trials are evaluating the use of a humanized, chimeric anti-GD2 antibody (ch14.18) with these cytokines and a fusion protein (hu14.18:IL2) that consists of the humanized 14.18 antibody linked genetically to human recombinant IL-2.

GENERAL PRINCIPLES OF RADIATION THERAPY

Radiation therapy is one of the three primary modalities used to manage pediatric cancers in the modern era. Its use, alone or combined with surgery and systemic chemotherapy, forms the basis of management of many forms of childhood malignancy. Radiation therapy is delivered to an estimated 2000 or more children per year for the primary treatment of tumor types as diverse as leukemia, brain tumors, sarcomas, Hodgkin's disease, neuroblastoma, and Wilms' tumor.[36] Delivery of radiation therapy in the pediatric setting differs from that in the adult setting because of the balance between curative therapy and an anticipated long life span during which long-term morbidity may result from the therapy.

Clinical Considerations

Radiation therapy for the management of pediatric cancer is most frequently combined with surgery and chemotherapy as part of a multidisciplinary treatment plan. Although radiation therapy is used as a single modality in adult oncology, the sensitive nature of pediatric tumors requires the use of a combined therapy approach to maximize tumor control while minimizing the long-term side effects of treatment. Radiation may be delivered preoperatively, postoperatively (relative to a definitive surgical resection), or definitively without surgical management. Systemic therapy may also be integrated into this management approach.

Definitive Irradiation

Definitive radiation therapy is an alternative to surgical resection of primary solid tumors. It is often the only local therapeutic approach for children and adolescents with leukemia or lymphoma.[37,52] Although it is considered the only treatment option for unresectable tumors, definitive radiation therapy may be used as an alternative to surgical resection to allow the preservation of an organ or function while maintaining excellent local tumor control. Definitive radiation therapy for rhabdomyosarcoma has been used as an alternative to surgical resection, which has potentially greater morbidity; it has achieved high rates of local tumor control while allowing preservation of function.[38] The Ewing's sarcoma family of tumors may also be considered candidates for definitive radiation therapy as an alternative to surgery. With careful patient selection, excellent local tumor control rates can be maintained while reducing or avoiding the morbidity associated with difficult surgical resections.[84,125]

Preoperative Irradiation

Preoperative radiation therapy may be used in several situations. Targeting of a localized tumor is straightforward in the preoperative setting, when the tumor has clearly defined margins undisturbed by a surgical procedure. The volume of normal, healthy tissues receiving high doses of radiation may be reduced, because the areas at risk for disease involvement can be better defined. Preoperative radiation therapy has been used in the management of Wilms' tumor to decrease the chance of tumor rupture[75] and in the management of nonrhabdomyosarcoma soft tissue sarcoma and Ewing's sarcoma to facilitate surgical resection.[34,110] One of the limitations of preoperative radiation, however, particularly in patients with sarcoma, may be the slightly higher incidence of postoperative wound complications.[110]

Postoperative Irradiation

Postoperative radiation therapy combined with surgical resection is the most common application of adjuvant radiation treatment in the United States. Despite some degree of difficulty in targeting, a postoperative approach allows a review of the histologic studies of the complete tumor specimen, including identification of the tumor margins and the response to any previous therapy. Wound healing complications appear to be reduced with this approach, and the radiation dose can be more accurately tailored to the pathologic findings after primary resection.

Interactions of Chemotherapy and Radiation

Most children's cancers are managed with systemic chemotherapy. In children receiving radiation therapy as well as systemic chemotherapy, issues of enhanced local efficacy and enhanced local or regional toxicity need to be considered. Solid tumors that are frequently treated with combined chemotherapy and radiation therapy include Wilms' tumor, neuroblastoma, and sarcomas. These tumors are subdivided into those in which chemotherapy is given concomitantly with radiation therapy[38,61] and those in which it is given sequentially, before or after radiation therapy.[59,75,96] When delivering radiation therapy concurrently with or temporally close to a course of chemotherapy, several issues must be considered.

Chemotherapeutic Enhancement of Local Irradiation

Several systemic chemotherapeutic agents used against pediatric tumors may enhance the efficacy of radiation therapy when delivered concomitantly. Cisplatin, 5-fluorouracil, mitomycin C, and gemcitabine, for example, are well-known radiation sensitizers.[2,46,124] Concomitant delivery of any of these drugs with radiation therapy may require that they be administered at a dose and schedule different from those typically used when the drugs are delivered alone. Despite the potential of increased toxicity, significant improvements in local tumor control have been shown in randomized studies of concomitant drug and radiation therapy.[2,46]

Irradiation Combined with Agents Having Limited or No Sensitizing Effect

In the management of pediatric malignancies, radiation is often combined with systemic therapy not to increase its local efficacy but to allow continued delivery of systemic therapy to control micrometastatic or metastatic disease. Agents combined with radiation therapy in this setting are common in the management of pediatric sarcomas and include ifosfamide and etoposide, which are delivered concurrently with radiation therapy for Ewing's sarcoma, and vincristine and cyclophosphamide, which are delivered concurrently with radiation therapy for rhabdomyosarcoma.[38,61] Although local toxicity may be increased by such an approach, this risk is often outweighed by the benefit of continuously delivered systemic therapy, particularly in tumors associated with a high incidence of micrometastatic disease.

Agents That Increase Radiation Toxicity

Several agents significantly increase the local toxicity of radiation. For this reason, these agents are not given concomitantly with irradiation and are often withheld for a period after the completion of radiation therapy. The two most notable agents are doxorubicin and actinomycin, both of which can induce significant skin and mucosal toxicity when delivered concurrently with radiation therapy.[24,29] The camptothecins (including irinotecan and topotecan) also potentiate mucosal toxicity when delivered concurrently with radiation therapy.[58,100] Although this increase in toxicity suggests a possible increase in local efficacy, this benefit has not been noted with current treatment approaches and chemotherapeutic dosing guidelines. For this reason, these agents are avoided during the delivery of radiation therapy and are withheld for 2 to 6 weeks after the completion of treatment.

The current era of systemic therapy continues to broaden with the availability of many new agents that target molecular pathways. It is important to consider the possibility of new toxicities when combining novel agents with a known therapy such as radiation.

Delivery of Fractionated Radiation Therapy

Conventional, external beam irradiation is delivered in a fractionated form. Fractionation implies daily doses of radiation delivered 5 days per week and amounting to the prescribed dose for a particular tumor type. Radiation delivered once daily at a fraction size between 1.5 and 2.0 Gy on 5 days per week is considered "conventionally" fractionated. This daily dose is well tolerated by normal tissues adjacent to the tumor and appears to effect local tumor control in many tumor systems.

There has been interest in the hyperfractionation of radiation therapy to treat pediatric malignancies, most notably brain tumors and solid tumors, to try to overcome the biologic resistance of malignancies.[38,87] Although the efficacy of altered fractionation is unproved in the management of children's cancers, there are several reasons to consider alternative treatment schedules with a documented efficacy equivalent to that of conventional fractionation. Hyperfractionation, with a dose of less than 1.5 Gy per fraction, may allow the delivery of standard total doses of radiation but with fewer late effects. Accelerated hyperfractionated radiation therapy, in which the overall treatment time is compressed, may have the benefit of allowing a short course of radiation therapy between other therapies, including systemic therapy or bone marrow transplantation. This approach has been used in children with neuroblastoma[87] and is currently being investigated in the management of Hodgkin's disease in patients undergoing bone marrow transplantation. Alterations of treatment fractionation continue to be studied in the pediatric setting, but their potential benefit must be weighed against the difficulties of delivering multiple treatments per day, particularly to young children who require general anesthesia for treatment.

Radiation Therapy Treatment Techniques

Traditional Radiation Therapy

The planning and delivery of traditional, or conventional, radiation therapy are based on nonvolumetric imaging studies (i.e., conventional radiographs). Patients are positioned in a manner that allows the orientation of radiation beams from the conventional directions: anterior, posterior, and lateral. Limitations of this approach are related to the ability of conventional radiographs to accurately convey the location of tumor-bearing tissue. Although treatment beams are oriented around the tumor, adjacent normal tissues also receive high doses of radiation. Depending on the accuracy of the delineation of adjacent normal tissues on radiographs, the dose to those tissues may not be known. Radiation is delivered via a photon beam generated by a linear accelerator.

Image-Guided Radiation Therapy

Image-guided radiation therapy comprises a group of techniques that deliver radiation to a defined volume usually delineated by computed tomography (CT) or magnetic resonance imaging (MRI). Relatively low doses may be incidentally delivered to surrounding normal tissues. Radiation therapy may be described as image guided when four criteria are met: (1) three-dimensional imaging data (CT or MRI) are acquired with the patient in the treatment position; (2) imaging data are used to delineate and reconstruct the tumor volume and normal tissues in three dimensions; (3) radiation beams can be freely oriented in three dimensions in the planning and delivery processes, and structures traversed by the beam can be visualized with the eye of the beam; and (4) the distribution of doses received by the tumor volume and any normal tissue is computable on a point-by-point basis in three-dimensional space. Several different methods of delivering image-guided photon radiation are currently in use and are discussed here.

Conformal Radiation Therapy

The delivery of three-dimensional conformal radiation therapy allows specific targeting of tumor volumes on the basis of imaging studies performed with the patient in the treatment position. This method of delivery uses multiple fields or portals, with each beam aperture shaped to the tumor volume, and is performed daily. Beam modifiers such as wedges are used to conform the radiation beam to the tumor and to ensure that the tumor volume receives a homogeneous dose. Conformal radiation therapy has been intensively studied in adults with head and neck cancer, lung cancer, and prostate cancer and has been shown to excel when the target volume is convex and crucial structures do not invaginate the target volume. Available data demonstrate that it has low toxicity despite high doses of radiation to the target volume.[103]

Intensity-Modulated Radiation Therapy

Intensity-modulated radiation therapy is another method of delivering external beam radiation that requires imaging of the patient in the treatment position and delineation of target volumes and normal tissues. Radiation is delivered to the target as multiple small fields that do not encompass the entire target volume but collectively deliver the prescribed daily dose. Intensity-modulated radiation therapy differs from conformal radiation therapy in that it (1) increases the complexity and time required for the planning and delivery of treatment; (2) increases the amount of quality-assurance work required before treatment is delivered; (3) increases dose heterogeneity within the target volume, such that some intralesional areas receive a relatively high dose; and (4) can be used to treat concave targets while sparing crucial structures that invaginate the target volume. The last point holds promise for better protecting normal tissue and reducing late toxic effects. Preliminary data from adult patients given intensity-modulated radiation therapy demonstrate its potential for reducing treatment toxicity when applied to pediatric brain tumors and other adult tumors.[73]

Brachytherapy

Brachytherapy is a method of delivering radiation to a tumor or tumor bed by placing radioactive sources within or adjacent to the target volume, usually at the time of surgical resection and under direct vision. Planning of the dose to be delivered to the target volume is accomplished after resection and may use CT or MRI studies; the appropriate strength of the radioactive source is determined prospectively. Sources commonly used in children include iridium 192 and iodine 125. Brachytherapy may consist of either low dose-rate treatments (approximately 40 to 80 cGy per hour) or high dose-rate treatments (approximately 60 to 100 cGy per minute). Low dose-rate treatments are delivered over a period of days, often while the patient remains hospitalized, whereas high dose-rate treatments are divided into fractions and delivered on several days over 1 to 2 weeks. The primary advantage of brachytherapy is that a radiation source can be placed into or adjacent to the tumor, often at the time of resection. Preoperative planning and cooperation between the surgical and radiation oncology teams are necessary to ensure the appropriate and accurate implementation of brachytherapy. Nonrhabdomyosarcoma soft tissue sarcomas and some rhabdomyosarcomas are the pediatric tumors most commonly treated with brachytherapy.[102,115] Most other pediatric solid tumors are not amenable to brachytherapy, however, because of the tumor's behavior (e.g., radioresistance) or its anatomic location (e.g., retroperitoneal).

Other Delivery Methods

Several other means of delivering radiation to primary tumor sites are used in adult and pediatric oncology. Intraoperative radiation therapy has been used intermittently after resection in the management of localized tumors.[63] Although of limited availability in the United States, intraoperative radiation therapy has the distinct advantage of allowing the operative tumor bed to be visible in the operating theater while radiation is delivered, thereby enhancing the accuracy of delivery and providing the opportunity to displace or temporarily move mobile crucial structures (e.g., bowel, bladder) from the field of delivery. The primary limitation of intraoperative radiation therapy is that it can deliver only a single fraction of radiation, usually in the 10 to 20 Gy range.

Radiation tolerances of normal tissues that cannot be removed from the treatment field must be respected and may limit the ability to deliver an effective treatment dose.

Proton radiation therapy and other approaches using heavy charged particles have been investigated at a limited number of centers. The primary benefit of therapy with proton or other heavy charged particle beams is the capacity to end the radiation beam at a specific and controllable depth. This may allow the protection of healthy, normal tissues directly adjacent to tumor-bearing tissues.[74] However, the use of proton therapy is limited because of the expense of constructing a suitable treatment facility; only a small number of institutions are so equipped. Although interest in proton therapy decreased in the late 1990s, it has now resumed, and several new facilities are currently under construction in the United States. With appropriately designed studies and comparisons with current state-of-the-art image-guided therapy delivered with photon beams, a determination of the potential benefits of this treatment modality may be made.

Palliative Radiation Therapy

For many patients, the management of cancer, particularly pediatric cancer, focuses on curative therapy incorporating surgery, radiation therapy, and chemotherapy in a multidisciplinary plan. Despite substantial success in the management of pediatric cancer, many children experience disease recurrence and ultimately die from their malignancy. Although it is far less frequently discussed, palliative radiation therapy is often a valid intervention.[68] Implicit in the concept of palliative radiation therapy is that its purpose is to treat a symptom. The ultimate goal of a palliative approach is to maintain quality of life for patients who will not survive their disease while minimizing the number of disruptive interventions they must undergo. Radiation oncologists are often asked to palliate symptoms from painful sites of disease, particularly those with bony involvement, and symptoms resulting from compression of vital structures, including spinal cord, peripheral nerves, and respiratory tract. Delivery of radiation in this setting is identical to that of curative radiation, with radiation delivered on a daily basis. Close attention is paid to the symptoms being palliated, while treatment-related effects are minimized. A palliative course of therapy is highly individualized, and its success or failure depends on the histologic diagnosis, previous therapy, duration of symptoms, and symptom being treated.

Acute and Late Toxicities of Radiation Therapy

The treatment-related effects of radiation therapy, both acute and chronic, are well described for pediatric and adult patients, but unfortunately, their incidence and relation to the dose and volume of treatment are poorly characterized.[39] Historically, treatment-related effects have been classified as acute or late; an arbitrary time point of 90 days after the completion of treatment defines the division between the two classifications. Current guidelines for assessing adverse events related to treatment no longer recognize this arbitrary distinction, but the use of early and late time points is instructive in the discussion of radiation-related effects. Essentially all such effects originate from within the confines of the treatment beams, usually the high-dose regions of treatment. The most common early and late treatment-related effects arising from radiation are listed in Table 25-6. Despite the arbitrary nature of the division into early and late effects, this classification distinguishes effects from which the patient is likely to recover completely from those that are likely to be permanent. Early treatment-related effects, if managed appropriately, will resolve as normal, healthy tissues adjacent to the tumor-bearing tissues gradually recover from the effects of radiation. The period of recovery can range from days to months, but the patient is often left with minimal sequelae. Treatment-related effects that are observed later, after the completion of radiation therapy, are more likely to be chronic or permanent. They appear to be related to the normal healing response of healthy irradiated tissue, resulting in the formation of an unwanted effect such as fibrosis. Many late treatment effects can be managed but are not reversible. For children receiving curative therapy, long-term effects are a primary concern and are best managed with a preventive approach. Some of the long-term effects of treatment in children should be ameliorated by limiting the volume of normal tissue irradiated at high doses and by implementing approaches that minimize the radiation dose to adjacent healthy tissues.

TABLE 25-6 Treatment-Related Adverse Events in Children Treated with Radiation

Organ/Site	Acute	Chronic
Skin	Erythema	Atrophy
	Desquamation	Hyperpigmentation
Subcutaneous tissue	Edema	Fibrosis
Mucosa	Mucositis	Ulceration
Central nervous system	Edema	Necrosis
	Headache	Myelitis
		Decline in cognition
Eye	Conjunctivitis	Cataract
		Retinopathy
		Dry eye
Thyroid	—	Hypothyroidism
Heart	—	Pericarditis
		Myocarditis
Lung	Pneumonitis	Pulmonary fibrosis
Bowel	Nausea	Necrosis
	Diarrhea	
Kidney	—	Nephritis
		Renal insufficiency
Bladder	Dysuria	Hemorrhagic cystitis
	Urgency	
	Frequency	
Muscle	Edema	Fibrosis
		Hypoplasia
Bone	—	Premature physis closure
		Hypoplasia

GENERAL PRINCIPLES OF STEM CELL TRANSPLANTATION

Infusion or transplantation of hematopoietic cells capable of reconstituting the hematopoietic system is used in two broad instances. First, hematopoietic stem cell transplantation (HSCT) can be used to replace missing or abnormal components of a defective hematopoietic system. Second, HSCT can be used to reconstitute elements of the hematopoietic system destroyed by intensive chemotherapy or radiation therapy for solid tumors or disorders of the hematopoietic system itself. The transplanted cells can be the patient's own (i.e., autologous), in which case the cells are obtained before the administration of myelosuppressive therapy, or they may come from a donor (i.e., allogeneic) who is generally an HLA-identical sibling, a mismatched family member, or a partially matched unrelated donor. The latter two circumstances require immunosuppressive and graft engineering strategies to permit successful engraftment and avoid graft-versus-host disease. Hematopoietic progenitor cells are usually obtained from the bone marrow or peripheral blood. They are the crucial component of the transplant because they are capable of self-renewal and, therefore, long-term production of cells of the various hematopoietic lineages. Occasionally, when available, banked umbilical cord blood may be used as the source of hematopoietic stem cells (HSCs). In general, although autologous cells are the safest to use for HSCT, they may be contaminated with tumor cells. Graft-versus-host disease, which may occur with allogeneic HSCT, can be life threatening, but a modest graft-versus-host reaction may be beneficial if directed against the host's tumor cells.

Bone marrow is normally harvested from the posterior iliac crest to a total volume of 10 to 20 mL/kg body weight of the recipient. Peripheral blood stem cells are harvested after their mobilization with recombinant granulocyte colony-stimulating factor, given daily for up to a week before harvest. The exact nature of the crucial cellular component responsible for the reconstitution of the hematopoietic system is unknown, but the number of cells having the surface marker CD34 has been shown to be related to the rate of engraftment.[35] Before HSCT, the recipient receives a preparative (or "conditioning") chemotherapeutic regimen. This treatment serves several purposes, including killing residual tumor cells, providing immunosuppression for allogeneic HSCT, and providing "space" in the marrow into which transplanted HSCs can engraft. Before reinfusion, the HSC product may be manipulated ex vivo to enrich it for putative progenitor cells (e.g., CD34+ or CD133+ cells), using positive or negative selection methods, to facilitate hematopoietic reconstitution; to remove donor T lymphocytes, thereby decreasing the risk of graft-versus-host disease in allogeneic HSCT; or to purge contaminating tumor cells from the product used in autologous HSCT.

Complications of HSCT can be significant. The most common early complication is infection, which results from the transient but profound immunosuppression of the patient, combined with the breakdown of mucosal barriers. Another common complication is veno-occlusive disease, which is characterized clinically by painful enlargement of the liver, jaundice, and fluid retention. Ultrasound examination shows reversal of flow in the portal vein. Liver biopsy samples show a classic histologic appearance of obliterated hepatic venules and necrosis of centrilobular hepatocytes. There is no specific treatment for this condition; only supportive care can be given, and mild or moderate veno-occlusive disease is self-limited. Other acute complications of HSCT include graft-versus-host disease, a process mediated by donor T cells targeting host cells with antigenic disparities, and graft failure. Late complications include chronic graft-versus-host disease, endocrine insufficiency, secondary malignancies, growth failure, and other sequelae related to the use of total-body irradiation as part of some preparatory regimens. Nevertheless, despite the toxicity, HSCT is now an integral part of successful therapy for many high-risk malignancies in children.

CLINICAL TRIALS

As previously stated, the past 40 years have seen a significant increase in overall survival rates for children with cancer. This increase has been achieved through the development of new drugs and treatment approaches, improved supportive care, and better diagnostic modalities to permit earlier cancer detection. The benefits of these advances have been confirmed by carefully designed and analyzed clinical trials. Because childhood cancer is relatively rare, excellent organization and planning of these trials are essential. In the United States and other participating countries, clinical trials are largely conducted by the Children's Oncology Group, with smaller pilot studies being run by large individual institutions or small consortia.

Clinical trials are generally divided into three phases. Phase I studies are designed to evaluate the potential toxicity of a new diagnostic or therapeutic agent. Small numbers of patients are usually required for a phase I study, which typically uses a dose-escalating design in which cohorts of patients are observed for signs of toxicity before they advance to higher doses. The end point of this type of study is generally a determination of the safety of the agent or the maximum tolerated dose (or both). However, the increasing number of biologic reagents being introduced and tested may require a shift to the assessment of the optimal biologic dose. Enrollment in a phase I toxicity study is often restricted to patients whose disease has not responded to conventional or "standard-of-care" therapy. Phase II trials are conducted to determine whether a new agent or treatment approach is sufficiently efficacious to warrant further study. Phase II agents are often given to newly diagnosed patients before they begin or just after they complete standard therapy. The testing of new agents in an "upfront window" (i.e., before standard therapy) has been shown not to have an adverse effect on the efficacy of delayed standard therapy. Finally, phase III studies are designed to compare the efficacy of an experimental therapy with that of standard therapy. They are best done as prospective, randomized trials, but often, because of small patient numbers, a phase III study is done by comparing the efficacy of an experimental therapy with that of standard therapy given to historic control subjects. It is through such systematic assessment of the risks and benefits of new therapies that approaches are rejected or accepted as the new standard of care and the field of pediatric oncology is advanced.

CONCLUSION

Advances in molecular genetic research in the past 2 decades have led to increased understanding of the genetic events in the pathogenesis and progression of human malignancies, including those of childhood. A number of pediatric malignancies serve as models for the molecular genetic approach to cancer. The pediatric experience highlights the utility of molecular analysis for a variety of purposes. Demonstration of tumor-specific translocations by cytogenetics, FISH, and RT-PCR confirms histopathologic diagnoses. Detection of chromosomal abnormalities, gene overexpression, and gene amplification is used in risk stratification and treatment planning. Elucidation of pathways involving tumor suppressor genes has increased our understanding of syndromes associated with cancer and has led the way for genetic screening and counseling and prophylactic surgical intervention. And in the near future, translation of the molecular profile of a given tumor will form the basis of a new therapeutic approach. Treatment will be tailored such that patients with biologically high-risk tumors receive intensified regimens to achieve a cure, whereas patients with biologically low-risk tumors may experience a cure and benefit from the lower toxicity of nonintensive therapy. Elucidation of the complex molecular pathways involved in tumorigenesis will also encourage the production of targeted anticancer agents with high specificity, efficacy, and therapeutic index.

REFERENCES

1. Abramson LP, Grundy PE, Rademaker AW, et al: Increased microvascular density predicts relapse in Wilms' tumor. J Pediatr Surg 2003;38:325-330.
2. Al Sarraf M, LeBlanc M, Giri PG, et al: Chemoradiotherapy versus radiotherapy in patients with advanced nasopharyngeal cancer: Phase III randomized intergroup study 0099. J Clin Oncol 1998;16:1310-1317.
3. Arap W, Pasqualini R, Ruoslahti E: Cancer treatment by targeted drug delivery to tumor vasculature in a mouse model. Science 1998;279:377-380.
4. Asher AL, Mule JJ, Kasid A, et al: Murine tumor cells transduced with the gene for tumor necrosis factor-alpha: Evidence for paracrine immune effects of tumor necrosis factor against tumors. J Immunol 1991;146:3227-3234.
5. Bader SA, Fasching C, Brodeur GM, et al: Dissociation of suppression of tumorigenicity and differentiation in vitro effected by transfer of single human chromosomes into human neuroblastoma cells. Cell Growth Differ 1991;2:245-255.
6. Barbacid M: Neurotrophic factors and their receptors. Curr Opin Cell Biol 1995;7:148-155.
7. Bardeesy N, Falkoff D, Petruzzi MJ, et al: Anaplastic Wilms' tumour, a subtype displaying poor prognosis, harbours p53 gene mutations. Nat Genet 1994;7:91-97.

8. Barr FG: The role of chimeric paired box transcription factors in the pathogenesis of pediatric rhabdomyosarcoma. Cancer Res 1999;59:1711s-1715s.

9. Bicknell R, Harris AL: Mechanisms and therapeutic implications of angiogenesis. Curr Opin Oncol 1996;8:60-65.

10. Blankenstein T, Qin ZH, Uberla K, et al: Tumor suppression after tumor cell-targeted tumor necrosis factor alpha gene transfer. J Exp Med 1991;173:1047-1052.

11. Bowman L, Grossmann M, Rill D, et al: IL-2 adenovector-transduced autologous tumor cells induce antitumor immune responses in patients with neuroblastoma. Blood 1998;92:1941-1949.

12. Bowman LC, Grossmann M, Rill D, et al: Interleukin-2 gene-modified allogeneic tumor cells for treatment of relapsed neuroblastoma. Hum Gene Ther 1998;9:1303-1311.

13. Bown N, Cotterill S, Lastowska M, et al: Gain of chromosome arm 17q and adverse outcome in patients with neuroblastoma. N Engl J Med 1999;340:1954-1961.

14. Bredel M, Pollack IF, Hamilton RL, et al: Epidermal growth factor receptor expression and gene amplification in high-grade non-brainstem gliomas of childhood. Clin Cancer Res 1999;5:1786-1792.

15. Brodeur GM, Hayes FA, Green AA, et al: Consistent N-myc copy number in simultaneous or consecutive neuroblastoma samples from sixty individual patients. Cancer Res 1987;47:4248-4253.

16. Brodeur GM, Maris JM, Yamashiro DJ, et al: Biology and genetics of human neuroblastomas. J Pediatr Hematol Oncol 1997;19:93-101.

17. Brodeur GM, Seeger RC, Schwab M, et al: Amplification of N-myc in untreated human neuroblastomas correlates with advanced disease stage. Science 1984;224:1121-1124.

18. Brodeur GM, Sekhon G, Goldstein MN: Chromosomal aberrations in human neuroblastomas. Cancer 1977;40:2256-2263.

19. Brooks PC, Silletti S, von Schalscha TL, et al: Disruption of angiogenesis by PEX, a noncatalytic metalloproteinase fragment with integrin binding activity. Cell 1998;92:391-400.

20. Browder T, Butterfield CE, Kraling BM, et al: Antiangiogenic scheduling of chemotherapy improves efficacy against experimental drug-resistant cancer. Cancer Res 2000;60:1878-1886.

21. Buchdunger E, Cioffi CL, Law N, et al: Abl protein-tyrosine kinase inhibitor STI571 inhibits in vitro signal transduction mediated by c-kit and platelet-derived growth factor receptors. J Pharmacol Exp Ther 2000;295:139-145.

22. Call KM, Glaser T, Ito CY, et al: Isolation and characterization of a zinc finger polypeptide gene at the human chromosome 11 Wilms' tumor locus. Cell 1990;60:509-520.

23. Carmeliet P, Jain RK: Angiogenesis in cancer and other diseases. Nature 2000;407:249-257.

24. Cassady JR, Richter MP, Piro AJ, et al: Radiation-Adriamycin interactions: preliminary clinical observations. Cancer 1975;36:946-949.

25. Cheung NK: Immunotherapy: Neuroblastoma as a model. Pediatr Clin North Am 1991;38:425-441.

26. Cheung NK, Burch L, Kushner BH: Monoclonal antibody 3F8 can effect durable remissions in neuroblastoma patients refractory to chemotherapy: A phase II trail. In Evans AE, D'Angio GJ, Kundson AG (eds): Advances in Neuroblastoma Research, 3rd ed. Hoboken, NJ: Wiley-Liss, 1991, p 395.

27. Clark J, Benjamin H, Gill S, et al: Fusion of the EWS gene to CHN, a member of the steroid/thyroid receptor gene superfamily, in a human myxoid chondrosarcoma. Oncogene 1996;12:229-235.

28. Clark J, Rocques PJ, Crew AJ, et al: Identification of novel genes, SYT and SSX, involved in the t(X;18)(p11.2;q11.2) translocation found in human synovial sarcoma. Nat Genet 1994;7:502-508.

29. Cohen IJ, Loven D, Schoenfeld T, et al: Dactinomycin potentiation of radiation pneumonitis: A forgotten interaction. Pediatr Hematol Oncol 1991;8:187-192.

30. Coppes MJ, Bonetta L, Huang A, et al: Loss of heterozygosity mapping in Wilms' tumor indicates the involvement of three distinct regions and a limited role for nondisjunction or mitotic recombination. Genes Chromosomes Cancer 1992;5:326-334.

31. Coppes MJ, Haber DA, Grundy PE: Genetic events in the development of Wilms' tumor. N Engl J Med 1994;331:586-590.

32. Dameron KM, Volpert OV, Tainsky MA, et al: Control of angiogenesis in fibroblasts by p53 regulation of thrombospondin-1. Science 1994;265:1582-1584.

33. de Alava E, Kawai A, Healey JH, et al: *EWS-FLI1* fusion transcript structure is an independent determinant of prognosis in Ewing's sarcoma. J Clin Oncol 1998;16:1248-1255.

34. Delaney TF, Spiro IJ, Suit HD, et al: Neoadjuvant chemotherapy and radiotherapy for large extremity soft-tissue sarcomas. Int J Radiat Oncol Biol Phys 2003;56:1117-1127.

35. Diaz MA, Vicent MG, Garcia-Sanchez F, et al: Long-term hematopoietic engraftment after autologous peripheral blood progenitor cell transplantation in pediatric patients: Effect of the CD34+ cell dose. Vox Sang 2000;79:145-150.

36. Donaldson SS, Halperin EC: Subspecialty training and certification for radiation oncology. J Am Coll Radiol 2004;1:488-492.

37. Donaldson SS, Hudson MM, Lamborn KR, et al: VAMP and low-dose, involved-field radiation for children and adolescents with favorable, early-stage Hodgkin's disease: Results of a prospective clinical trial. J Clin Oncol 2002;20:3081-3087.

38. Donaldson SS, Meza J, Breneman JC, et al: Results from the IRS-IV randomized trial of hyperfractionated radiotherapy in children with rhabdomyosarcoma—a report from the IRSG. Int J Radiat Oncol Biol Phys 2001;51:718-728.

39. Emami B, Lyman J, Brown A, et al: Tolerance of normal tissue to therapeutic irradiation. Int J Radiat Oncol Biol Phys 1991;21:109-122.

40. Evans AE, Kisselbach KD, Yamashiro DJ, et al: Antitumor activity of CEP-751 (KT-6587) on human neuroblastoma and medulloblastoma xenografts. Clin Cancer Res 1999;5:3594-3602.

41. Farber S: Chemotherapeutic studies of tumors, including leukemia, in children. Am J Dis Child 1950;79:961-962.

42. Fearon ER, Pardoll DM, Itaya T, et al: Interleukin-2 production by tumor cells bypasses T helper function in the generation of an antitumor response. Cell 1990;60:397-403.

43. Feldman AL, Libutti SK: Progress in antiangiogenic gene therapy of cancer. Cancer 2000;89:1181-1194.

44. Fidler IJ: The organ microenvironment and cancer metastasis. Differentiation 2002;70:498-505.

45. Fidler IJ, Ellis LM: The implications of angiogenesis for the biology and therapy of cancer metastasis. Cell 1994;79:185-188.

46. Flam M, John M, Pajak TF, et al: Role of mitomycin in combination with fluorouracil and radiotherapy, and of salvage chemoradiation in the definitive nonsurgical treatment of epidermoid carcinoma of the anal canal: Results of a phase III randomized intergroup study. J Clin Oncol 1996;14:2527-2539.

47. Folkman J: What is the evidence that tumors are angiogenesis dependent? J Natl Cancer Inst 1990;82:4-6.

48. Folkman J: The role of angiogenesis in tumor growth. Semin Cancer Biol 1992;3:65-71.

49. Folkman J: Clinical applications of research on angiogenesis. N Engl J Med 1995;333:1757-1763.

50. Folkman J, D'Amore PA: Blood vessel formation: What is its molecular basis? Cell 1996;87:1153-1155.

51. Fong CT, Dracopoli NC, White PS, et al: Loss of heterozygosity for the short arm of chromosome 1 in human neuroblastomas: Correlation with N-myc amplification. Proc Natl Acad Sci U S A 1989;86:3753-3757.

52. Friedmann AM, Hudson MM, Weinstein HJ, et al: Treatment of unfavorable childhood Hodgkin's disease with VEPA and low-dose, involved-field radiation. J Clin Oncol 2002; 20:3088-3094.

53. Galili N, Davis RJ, Fredericks WJ, et al: Fusion of a fork head domain gene to PAX3 in the solid tumour alveolar rhabdomyosarcoma. Nat Genet 1993;5:230-235.

54. Geiger JD, Hutchinson RJ, Hohenkirk LF, et al: Vaccination of pediatric solid tumor patients with tumor lysate-pulsed dendritic cells can expand specific T cells and mediate tumor regression. Cancer Res 2001;61:8513-8519.

55. Giardiello FM: Gastrointestinal polyposis syndromes and hereditary nonpolyposis colorectal cancer. In Rustgi AD (ed): Gastrointestinal Cancers: Biology, Diagnosis, and Therapy. Philadelphia: Lippincott-Raven, 1995, pp 367-377.

56. Goldie JH, Coldman AJ: A mathematic model for relating the drug sensitivity of tumors to their spontaneous mutation rate. Cancer Treat Rep 1979;63:1727-1733.

57. Golumbek PT, Lazenby AJ, Levitsky HI, et al: Treatment of established renal cancer by tumor cells engineered to secrete interleukin-4. Science 1991;254:713-716.

58. Graham MV, Jahanzeb M, Dresler CM, et al: Results of a trial with topotecan dose escalation and concurrent thoracic radiation therapy for locally advanced, inoperable nonsmall cell lung cancer. Int J Radiat Oncol Biol Phys 1996;36:1215-1220.

59. Green DM: The treatment of stages I-IV favorable histology Wilms' tumor. J Clin Oncol 2004;22:1366-1372.

60. Green DM, Jaffe N: Wilms' tumor—model of a curable pediatric malignant solid tumor. Cancer Treat Rev 1978; 5:143-172.

61. Grier HE, Krailo MD, Tarbell NJ, et al: Addition of ifosfamide and etoposide to standard chemotherapy for Ewing's sarcoma and primitive neuroectodermal tumor of bone. N Engl J Med 2003;348:694-701.

62. Grundy P, Coppes MJ, Haber D: Molecular genetics of Wilms' tumor. Hematol Oncol Clin North Am 1995;9: 1201-1215.

63. Haas-Kogan DA, Fisch BM, Wara WM, et al: Intraoperative radiation therapy for high-risk pediatric neuroblastoma. Int J Radiat Oncol Biol Phys 2000;47:985-992.

64. Hamada J, Cavanaugh PG, Lotan O, et al: Separable growth and migration factors for large-cell lymphoma cells secreted by microvascular endothelial cells derived from target organs for metastasis. Br J Cancer 1992;66:349-354.

65. Handgretinger R, Baader P, Dopfer R, et al: A phase I study of neuroblastoma with the anti-ganglioside GD2 antibody 14.G2a. Cancer Immunol Immunother 1992;35: 199-204.

66. Hank JA, Robinson RR, Surfus J, et al: Augmentation of antibody dependent cell mediated cytotoxicity following in vivo therapy with recombinant interleukin 2. Cancer Res 1990;50:5234-5239.

67. Hank JA, Surfus J, Gan J, et al: Treatment of neuroblastoma patients with antiganglioside GD2 antibody plus interleukin-2 induces antibody-dependent cellular cytotoxicity against neuroblastoma detected in vitro. J Immunother 1994;15:29-37.

68. Harris MB: Palliative care in children with cancer: Which child and when? J Natl Cancer Inst Monogr 2004;144-149.

69. Henderson C, Brancolini C: Apoptotic pathways activated by histone deacetylase inhibitors: Implications for the drug-resistant phenotype. Drug Resist Update 2003;6:247-256.

70. Hobson B, Denekamp J: Endothelial proliferation in tumours and normal tissues: Continuous labelling studies. Br J Cancer 1984;49:405-413.

71. Holmgren L, O'Reilly MS, Folkman J: Dormancy of micrometastases: Balanced proliferation and apoptosis in the presence of angiogenesis suppression. Nat Med 1995; 1:149-153.

72. Howe JR, Norton JA, Wells SA Jr: Prevalence of pheochromocytoma and hyperparathyroidism in multiple endocrine neoplasia type 2A: Results of long-term follow-up. Surgery 1993;114:1070-1077.

73. Huang E, Teh BS, Strother DR, et al: Intensity-modulated radiation therapy for pediatric medulloblastoma: Early report on the reduction of ototoxicity. Int J Radiat Oncol Biol Phys 2002;52:599-605.

74. Hug EB, Sweeney RA, Nurre PM, et al: Proton radiotherapy in management of pediatric base of skull tumors. Int J Radiat Oncol Biol Phys 2002;52:1017-1024.

75. Jereb B, Burgers JM, Tournade MF, et al: Radiotherapy in the SIOP (International Society of Pediatric Oncology) nephroblastoma studies: A review. Med Pediatr Oncol 1994;22:221-227.

76. Kaneko Y, Kanda N, Maseki N, et al: Different karyotypic patterns in early and advanced stage neuroblastomas. Cancer Res 1987;47:311-318.

77. Kaur G, Stetler-Stevenson M, Sebers S, et al: Growth inhibition with reversible cell cycle arrest of carcinoma cells by flavone L86-8275. J Natl Cancer Inst 1992;84:1736-1740.

78. Keshelava N, Zuo JJ, Waidyaratne NS, et al: p53 mutations and loss of p53 function confer multidrug resistance in neuroblastoma. Med Pediatr Oncol 2000;35:563-568.

79. Kingston JE, Herbert A, Draper GJ, et al: Association between hepatoblastoma and polyposis coli. Arch Dis Child 1983;58:959-962.

80. Kinzler KW, Vogelstein B: Familial cancer syndromes: The role of caretakers and gatekeepers. In Vogelstein B, Kinzler KW (eds): The Genetic Basis of Human Cancer. New York: McGraw-Hill, 1998, pp 241-599.

81. Knudson AG Jr: Mutation and cancer: Statistical study of retinoblastoma. Proc Natl Acad Sci U S A 1971;68: 820-823.

82. Kohl NE, Kanda N, Schreck RR, et al: Transposition and amplification of oncogene-related sequences in human neuroblastomas. Cell 1983;35:359-367.

83. Koufos A, Grundy P, Morgan K, et al: Familial Wiedemann-Beckwith syndrome and a second Wilms' tumor locus both map to 11p15.5. Am J Hum Genet 1989;44:711-719.

84. Krasin MJ, Rodriguez-Galindo C, Davidoff AM, et al: Efficacy of definitive irradiation and multi-agent systemic therapy for localized Ewing's sarcoma family of tumors (ESFT). Int J Radiat Oncol Biol Phys 2003;57:S197.

85. Kucharczak J, Simmons MJ, Fan Y, et al: To be, or not to be: NF-kappaB is the answer—role of Rel/NF-kappaB in the regulation of apoptosis. Oncogene 2003;22:8961-8982.

86. Kusafuka T, Fukuzawa M, Oue T, et al: Mutation analysis of p53 gene in childhood malignant solid tumors. J Pediatr Surg 1997;32:1175-1180.

87. Kushner BH, Wolden S, LaQuaglia MP, et al: Hyperfractionated low-dose radiotherapy for high-risk neuroblastoma after intensive chemotherapy and surgery. J Clin Oncol 2001;19:2821-2828.

88. Ladanyi M, Gerald W: Fusion of the *EWS* and *WT1* genes in the desmoplastic small round cell tumor. Cancer Res 1994;54:2837-2840.

89. Laughner E, Taghavi P, Chiles K, et al: HER2 (neu) signaling increases the rate of hypoxia-inducible factor 1alpha (HIF-1alpha) synthesis: Novel mechanism for HIF-1-mediated vascular endothelial growth factor expression. Mol Cell Biol 2001;21:3995-4004.

90. Levi-Montalcini R: The nerve growth factor 35 years later. Science 1987;237:1154-1162.
91. Liotta LA, Steeg PS, Stetler-Stevenson WG: Cancer metastasis and angiogenesis: An imbalance of positive and negative regulation. Cell 1991;64:327-336.
92. Look AT, Hayes FA, Nitschke R, et al: Cellular DNA content as a predictor of response to chemotherapy in infants with unresectable neuroblastoma. N Engl J Med 1984;311:231-235.
93. Look AT, Kirsch IR: Molecular basis of childhood cancer. In Pizzo PA, Poplack DG (eds): Principles and Practices of Pediatric Oncology. Philadelphia: Lippincott-Raven, 1997, p 38.
94. Lutz W, Stohr M, Schurmann J, et al: Conditional expression of N-myc in human neuroblastoma cells increases expression of alpha-prothymosin and ornithine decarboxylase and accelerates progression into S-phase early after mitogenic stimulation of quiescent cells. Oncogene 1996;13:803-812.
95. Malkin D, Li FP, Strong LC, et al: Germ line p53 mutations in a familial syndrome of breast cancer, sarcomas, and other neoplasms. Science 1990;250:1233-1238.
96. Matthay KK, Villablanca JG, Seeger RC, et al: Treatment of high-risk neuroblastoma with intensive chemotherapy, radiotherapy, autologous bone marrow transplantation, and 13-cis-retinoic acid: Children's Cancer Group. N Engl J Med 1999;341:1165-1173.
97. May WA, Gishizky ML, Lessnick SL, et al: Ewing sarcoma 11;22 translocation produces a chimeric transcription factor that requires the DNA-binding domain encoded by FLI1 for transformation. Proc Natl Acad Sci U S A 1993;90:5752-5756.
98. May WA, Lessnick SL, Braun BS, et al: The Ewing's sarcoma EWS/FLI-1 fusion gene encodes a more potent transcriptional activator and is a more powerful transforming gene than FLI-1. Mol Cell Biol 1993;13:7393-7398.
99. McNeil C: Herceptin raises its sights beyond advanced breast cancer. J Natl Cancer Inst 1998;90:882-883.
100. Mehta VK, Cho C, Ford JM, et al: Phase II trial of preoperative 3D conformal radiotherapy, protracted venous infusion 5-fluorouracil, and weekly CPT-11, followed by surgery for ultrasound-staged T3 rectal cancer. Int J Radiat Oncol Biol Phys 2003;55:132-137.
101. Meitar D, Crawford SE, Rademaker AW, et al: Tumor angiogenesis correlates with metastatic disease, N-myc amplification, and poor outcome in human neuroblastoma. J Clin Oncol 1996;14:405-414.
102. Merchant TE, Parsh N, del Valle PL, et al: Brachytherapy for pediatric soft-tissue sarcoma. Int J Radiat Oncol Biol Phys 2000;46:427-432.
103. Merchant TE, Zhu Y, Thompson SJ, et al: Preliminary results from a phase II trial of conformal radiation therapy for pediatric patients with localised low-grade astrocytoma and ependymoma. Int J Radiat Oncol Biol Phys 2002;52:325-332.
104. Mulligan LM, Kwok JB, Healey CS, et al: Germ-line mutations of the RET proto-oncogene in multiple endocrine neoplasia type 2A. Nature 1993;363:458-460.
105. Nagata S: Apoptosis by death factor. Cell 1997;88:355-365.
106. Nakagawara A, Azar CG, Scavarda NJ, et al: Expression and function of Trk-B and BDNF in human neuroblastomas. Mol Cell Biol 1994;14:759-767.
107. Nguyen M, Watanabe H, Budson AE, et al: Elevated levels of the angiogenic peptide basic fibroblast growth factor in urine of bladder cancer patients. J Natl Cancer Inst 1993;85:241-242.
108. Nishisho I, Nakamura Y, Miyoshi Y, et al: Mutations of chromosome 5q21 genes in FAP and colorectal cancer patients. Science 1991;253:665-669.
109. O'Brien KP, Seroussi E, Dal Cin P, et al: Various regions within the alpha-helical domain of the COL1A1 gene are fused to the second exon of the PDGFB gene in dermatofibrosarcomas and giant-cell fibroblastomas. Genes Chromosomes Cancer 1998;23:187-193.
110. O'Sullivan B, Davis AM, Turcotte R, et al: Preoperative versus postoperative radiotherapy in soft-tissue sarcoma of the limbs: A randomised trial. Lancet 2002;359:2235-2241.
111. Ozkaynak MF, Sondel PM, Krailo MD, et al: Phase I study of chimeric human/murine anti-ganglioside G(D2) monoclonal antibody (ch14.18) with granulocyte-macrophage colony-stimulating factor in children with neuroblastoma immediately after hematopoietic stem-cell transplantation: A Children's Cancer Group Study. J Clin Oncol 2000;18:4077-4085.
112. Pelletier J, Bruening W, Kashtan CE, et al: Germline mutations in the Wilms' tumor suppressor gene are associated with abnormal urogenital development in Denys-Drash syndrome. Cell 1991;67:437-447.
113. Petit AM, Rak J, Hung MC, et al: Neutralizing antibodies against epidermal growth factor and ErbB-2/neu receptor tyrosine kinases down-regulate vascular endothelial growth factor production by tumor cells in vitro and in vivo: Angiogenic implications for signal transduction therapy of solid tumors. Am J Pathol 1997;151:1523-1530.
114. Pinthus JH, Fridman E, Dekel B, et al: ErbB2 is a tumor associated antigen and a suitable therapeutic target in Wilms' tumor. J Urol 2004;172:1644-1648.
115. Pisters PW, Harrison LB, Leung DH, et al: Long-term results of a prospective randomized trial of adjuvant brachytherapy in soft tissue sarcoma. J Clin Oncol 1996; 14:859-868.
116. Pluda JM: Tumor-associated angiogenesis: Mechanisms, clinical implications, and therapeutic strategies. Semin Oncol 1997;24:203-218.
117. Powell SM, Petersen GM, Krush AJ, et al: Molecular diagnosis of familial adenomatous polyposis. N Engl J Med 1993;329:1982-1987.
118. Pritchard-Jones K, Fleming S, Davidson D, et al: The candidate Wilms' tumour gene is involved in genitourinary development. Nature 1990;346:194-197.
119. Quesnel S, Malkin D: Genetic predisposition to cancer and familial cancer syndromes. Pediatr Clin North Am 1997;44:791-808.
120. Rabbitts TH, Forster A, Larson R, et al: Fusion of the dominant negative transcription regulator CHOP with a novel gene FUS by translocation t(12;16) in malignant liposarcoma. Nat Genet 1993;4:175-180.
121. Riccardi VM, Sujansky E, Smith AC, et al: Chromosomal imbalance in the aniridia-Wilms' tumor association: 11p interstitial deletion. Pediatrics 1978;61:604-610.
122. Ries LG: Childhood cancer mortality. In Ries LG, Smith MA, Gurney JG, et al (eds): Cancer Incidence and Survival among Children and Adolescents: United States SEER Program 1975-1995. National Cancer Institute, 1999, pp 165-169.
123. Risau W: Mechanisms of angiogenesis. Nature 1997;386:671-674.
124. Robinson BW, Ostruszka L, Im MM, et al: Promising combination therapies with gemcitabine. Semin Oncol 2004;31:2-12.
125. Rodriguez-Galindo C, Spunt SL, Pappo AS: Treatment of Ewing sarcoma family of tumors: Current status and outlook for the future. Med Pediatr Oncol 2003;40:276-287.
126. Rousseau RF, Haight AE, Hirschmann-Jax C, et al: Local and systemic effects of an allogeneic tumor cell vaccine combining transgenic human lymphotactin with interleukin-2 in patients with advanced or refractory neuroblastoma. Blood 2003;101:1718-1726.

127. Rubin BP, Chen CJ, Morgan TW, et al: Congenital mesoblastic nephroma t(12;15) is associated with *ETV6-NTRK3* gene fusion: Cytogenetic and molecular relationship to congenital (infantile) fibrosarcoma. Am J Pathol 1998; 153:1451-1458.

128. Ruegg C, Yilmaz A, Bieler G, et al: Evidence for the involvement of endothelial cell integrin alphaVbeta3 in the disruption of the tumor vasculature induced by TNF and IFN-gamma. Nat Med 1998;4:408-414.

129. Sabers CJ, Martin MM, Brunn GJ, et al: Isolation of a protein target of the FKBP12-rapamycin complex in mammalian cells. J Biol Chem 1995;270:815-822.

130. Sandler AD, Chihara H, Kobayashi G, et al: CpG oligonucleotides enhance the tumor antigen-specific immune response of a granulocyte macrophage colony-stimulating factor-based vaccine strategy in neuroblastoma. Cancer Res 2003;63:394-399.

131. Schnitzer JE: Vascular targeting as a strategy for cancer therapy. N Engl J Med 1998;339:472-474.

132. Seeger RC, Brodeur GM, Sather H, et al: Association of multiple copies of the N-myc oncogene with rapid progression of neuroblastomas. N Engl J Med 1985;313: 1111-1116.

133. Sharpless NE, DePinho RA: Telomeres, stem cells, senescence, and cancer. J Clin Invest 2004;113:160-168.

134. Sherr CJ: The Pezcoller lecture: Cancer cell cycles revisited. Cancer Res 2000;60:3689-3695.

135. Sherr CJ, McCormick F: The RB and p53 pathways in cancer. Cancer Cell 2002;2:103-112.

136. Shimizu T, Berhanu A, Redlinger RE Jr, et al: Interleukin-12 transduced dendritic cells induce regression of established murine neuroblastoma. J Pediatr Surg 2001;36: 1285-1292.

137. Sorensen PH, Lessnick SL, Lopez-Terrada D, et al: A second Ewing's sarcoma translocation, t(21;22), fuses the EWS gene to another ETS-family transcription factor, ERG. Nat Genet 1994;6:146-151.

138. Srivastava A, Laidler P, Davies RP, et al: The prognostic significance of tumor vascularity in intermediate-thickness (0.76-4.0 mm thick) skin melanoma: A quantitative histologic study. Am J Pathol 1988;133:419-423.

139. Svensson T, Ryden M, Schilling FH, et al: Coexpression of mRNA for the full-length neurotrophin receptor Trk-C and Trk-A in favourable neuroblastoma. Eur J Cancer 1997;33: 2058-2063.

140. Teitz T, Wei T, Valentine MB, et al: Caspase 8 is deleted or silenced preferentially in childhood neuroblastomas with amplification of MYCN. Nat Med 2000;6:529-535.

141. Tepper RI, Mule JJ: Experimental and clinical studies of cytokine gene-modified tumor cells. Hum Gene Ther 1994;5:153-164.

142. Thiesing JT, Ohno-Jones S, Kolibaba KS, et al: Efficacy of STI571, an abl tyrosine kinase inhibitor, in conjunction with other antileukemic agents against bcr-abl-positive cells. Blood 2000;96:3195-3199.

143. Ton CC, Hirvonen H, Miwa H, et al: Positional cloning and characterization of a paired box- and homeobox-containing gene from the aniridia region. Cell 1991;67: 1059-1074.

144. Toole BP: Hyaluronan and its binding proteins, the hyaladherins. Curr Opin Cell Biol 1990;2:839-844.

145. van Leeuwen FE: Risk of acute myelogenous leukaemia and myelodysplasia following cancer treatment. Baillieres Clin Haematol 1996;9:57-85.

146. Vandesompele J, Van Roy N, Van Gele M, et al: Genetic heterogeneity of neuroblastoma studied by comparative genomic hybridization. Genes Chromosomes Cancer 1998;23:141-152.

147. Varanasi R, Bardeesy N, Ghahremani M, et al: Fine structure analysis of the WT1 gene in sporadic Wilms' tumors. Proc Natl Acad Sci U S A 1994;91:3554-3558.

148. Vogelstein B, Kinzler KW: Cancer genes and the pathways they control. Nat Med 2004;10:789-799.

149. Wai DH, Knezevich SR, Lucas T, et al: The *ETV6-NTRK3* gene fusion encodes a chimeric protein tyrosine kinase that transforms NIH3T3 cells. Oncogene 2000;19: 906-915.

150. White CW, Sondheimer HM, Crouch EC, et al: Treatment of pulmonary hemangiomatosis with recombinant interferon alfa-2a. N Engl J Med 1989;320:1197-1200.

151. Xiong S, Grijalva R, Zhang L, et al: Up-regulation of vascular endothelial growth factor in breast cancer cells by the heregulin-beta1-activated p38 signaling pathway enhances endothelial cell migration. Cancer Res 2001;61:1727-1732.

152. Young JL Jr, Ries LG, Silverberg E, et al: Cancer incidence, survival, and mortality for children younger than age 15 years. Cancer 1986;58:598-602.

153. Zhang L, Yu D, Hu M, et al: Wild-type p53 suppresses angiogenesis in human leiomyosarcoma and synovial sarcoma by transcriptional suppression of vascular endothelial growth factor expression. Cancer Res 2000;60: 3655-3661.

154. Zucman J, Delattre O, Desmaze C, et al: EWS and ATF-1 gene fusion induced by t(12;22) translocation in malignant melanoma of soft parts. Nat Genet 1993;4:341-345.

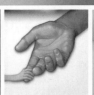

Chapter 26

Biopsy Techniques for Children with Cancer

James D. Geiger and Douglas C. Barnhart

The importance of biopsy techniques has increased as the use of preoperative chemotherapy has become common for many childhood cancers. In the past, definitive diagnosis was made at the time of surgical resection of the primary tumor. Currently, many children undergo percutaneous or open incisional biopsy rather than initial resection. Moreover, with a better understanding of the molecular changes associated with these malignancies, definitive diagnosis and accurate staging can be accomplished with smaller specimens. This should lead to less morbidity associated with the diagnosis of solid malignancies in children.

There has been a progression toward less invasive techniques to obtain a diagnosis—from complete surgical extirpation to incisional biopsy to percutaneous needle biopsy and minimal-access surgery. This change in practice has been driven not only by the evolution of surgical technique but also by an improved understanding of the molecular markers used for both diagnosis and risk stratification in pediatric solid malignancies. Ironically, this progression has complicated rather than simplified the selection of biopsy techniques in individual cases, because multiple factors must be considered. Percutaneous needle biopsy,[19,34] minimal-access surgical biopsy,[24] and open biopsy are all safe and effective ways of obtaining an initial diagnosis as well as verifying recurrent or metastatic disease. However, the success of these techniques is obviously dependent on individual institutional experience, which must be considered when selecting a biopsy technique. In addition, it is critical to realize that many of the advances in risk stratification and improved therapy for pediatric malignancies have been facilitated by the development of large tumor banks and the associated biology studies. Without large biopsy specimens, these tumor banks and the development of research cell lines would not have been possible. For a number of tumors, including neuroblastoma, the collection of such specimens is important to further our understanding of the disease.

There has been significant progress toward risk-stratified treatment regimens.[18] As this stratification becomes more complex, the type of information needed from biopsy specimens also becomes more individualized. In order to select the biopsy method that will be the least morbid yet yield all the information necessary to stratify an individual patient, the surgeon must be knowledgeable about the stratification schema that will be used for multimodality therapy. This concept can be exemplified by considering two patients with abdominal masses suggestive of neuroblastoma, both of whom have apparent metastatic disease in the bone marrow, and their treatment under the current Children's Oncology Group (COG) schema.[57] The first patient is younger than 1 year, and this child's treatment group could be low, intermediate, or high risk. This determination requires *N-myc* amplification status, International Neuroblastoma Pathology Classification status, and DNA ploidy, which necessitates sampling of the primary lesion. In contrast, an older child with a similar presentation would be classified as high risk. Therefore, one could consider confirming the diagnosis and assigning a risk group based on bone marrow biopsies alone. Clearly, knowledge of multimodality therapy is essential in the selection of a biopsy technique.

HANDLING OF SPECIMENS

Historically, most diagnoses were based on the histologic appearance of tumor tissue on permanent sections using hematoxylin and eosin stains. This was supplemented by the use of immunohistochemistry, which could similarly be performed on formalin-fixed specimens. There has been extensive progress in the molecular diagnosis of childhood malignancies, including recognition of genetic aberrations that have both diagnostic and prognostic significance.[9,39,41] Techniques used to detect these changes include reverse transcriptase-polymerase chain reaction,[11] fluorescent in situ hybridization, microarray analysis,[39] and flow cytometry. Inappropriate specimen handling can preclude the completion of these analyses. For example, phenotypic classification of lymphoma cannot be performed using flow cytometry on formalin-fixed lymph nodes. Given the rapidly evolving field of molecular diagnosis, it is essential that the surgeon consult with the pathologist regarding specimen handling before performing the biopsy.

PERCUTANEOUS NEEDLE BIOPSY

Fine-needle aspiration was first introduced as a technique for obtaining specimens for cytopathology by Grieg and Gray in 1904.[17] Jereb et al.[29] reported success with the use of needle biopsy for the diagnosis of pediatric solid tumors in 1978. Subsequently, extensive experience from multiple institutions has confirmed the accuracy and safety of both needle aspiration and core needle biopsy techniques. The appeal of these techniques is that they permit diagnosis without a significant delay in the institution of multimodality therapy and, in some situations, can be performed as outpatient procedures.

Needle biopsies are often performed under either general anesthesia or sedation. In selected older children, some sites may be biopsied under local anesthesia alone using these methods.[54]

Percutaneous needle biopsies may be performed by palpation in the extremities and other superficial locations, such as lymph nodes. Deeper biopsies require either ultrasonography or computed tomography (CT) guidance. Ultrasonography can be supplemented with Doppler mode; it allows the clear identification of large vessels and other structures and provides real-time visualization as the needle is advanced.[51] Some core needle devices also deposit a small air bubble, which allows verification of the site that was biopsied. CT permits clear visualization of the aerated lung[10] and is not obscured by bowel gas. It also allows for measurement and planning of the depth of biopsy.[19] Decision making regarding image guidance occurs in conjunction with the radiologist; ideally, biopsies should be performed with both modalities.

FINE-NEEDLE ASPIRATION BIOPSY

Fine-needle aspiration biopsy (FNAB) has the obvious appeal of being the least invasive biopsy technique. It is typically performed using a 22- to 25-gauge needle with multiple passes into the lesion if necessary. Successful diagnosis using FNAB requires coordination with an experienced cytopathologist; to improve the diagnostic yield, the specimens should be examined immediately after they are taken. Additional aspirations may be taken if initial samples are inadequate.[52] Large series with fine-needle aspirates in both children and adults have confirmed the safety of the technique.[16,31]

Historically, diagnosis using FNAB was based primarily on cytologic appearance with conventional stains and light microscopy. In adult patients with a higher prevalence of carcinomas, FNAB is a popular method of confirming the presence of malignancy in suspicious lesions. In adults, a diagnosis of carcinoma and determination of the primary site are often sufficient to make initial treatment decisions. However, given the fact that multimodality therapy is histiotype specific in pediatric patients, FNAB is used less frequently in children. The recent application

of molecular techniques and electron microscopy to supplement light microscopy has increased the histiotype specificity of FNAB and may lead to its increased application in pediatric solid malignancies.[20,30]

The most straightforward application of FNAB is the verification of metastatic or recurrent disease in the setting of a previously characterized primary tumor.[26] In this context, documenting the presence of malignant cells is often sufficient to guide further clinical decisions. This least invasive biopsy method is particularly appealing in patients who may already be immunologically or otherwise physiologically compromised.

There is an increasing body of literature to support the use of FNAB in the diagnosis of sarcomas. Fine-needle aspirates have provided a definitive diagnosis of osteosarcoma in 65%[12] to 92%[32] of patients; this technique is as accurate in children as it is in adults. The use of FNAB in soft tissue tumors has been facilitated by the recognition of cytogenetic abnormalities and fusion proteins that are specific to these tumor types.[30,31] However, caution should be exercised when using FNAB in this setting, because the reported series come from a limited number of institutions with extensive experience in the interpretation of this cytology.

FNAB has not been widely used for the diagnosis of small round blue cell tumors of childhood. However, with the increasing availability of ancillary studies such as electron microscopy, immunocytochemistry, DNA ploidy, cytogenetics, and fluorescent in situ hybridization, its use may become more common.[3] Use of FNAB for the evaluation of head and neck masses in children has been reported to have good sensitivity and specificity.[35,37] The results of these series should be interpreted with caution, however, because the majority of these aspirates diagnosed reactive lymphadenopathy; the number of new malignant diagnoses was small. Additionally, false-negative results occurred frequently in patients who were ultimately diagnosed with lymphoma in other series (not specifically isolated to the head and neck).[52]

CORE NEEDLE BIOPSY

The obvious advantage of core needle biopsy over FNAB is that it provides a large enough sample to allow histologic examination rather than only cytologic examination. Additionally, it can provide sufficient tissue for molecular evaluation. Despite the widespread use of this technique in adults, its application in children is not as common. Several series have reported the efficacy and safety of this technique in more than 280 children.[19,34,51,54]

Various core needle devices may be used, typically ranging in size from 14 gauge[34] to 18 gauge.[19] Needles are designed so that a cutting sheath advances over the core of the needle to obtain a tissue biopsy that is protected within the sheath as the needle is withdrawn. This cutting sheath may be advanced either manually (e.g., Tru-Cut by Allegiance) or by a spring-loaded firing system (e.g., Monopty by Bard) (Fig. 26-1). There are no data directly comparing the quality of specimens obtained with these two types of systems in pediatric malignancies. The faster deployment of the spring-loaded systems may

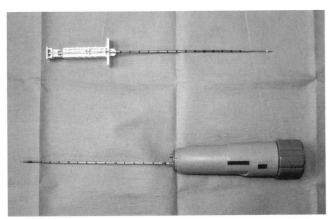

Figure 26-1 Two commonly used core needle biopsy devices. The upper device is a 14-gauge Tru-Cut needle (Allegiance). It is advanced into the region of interest, and then the inner needle is advanced. The outer sheath is manually advanced over the inner needle to obtain a core. The lower device is a 16-gauge Monopty biopsy device (Bard). It is spring-loaded and is activated after the tip is advanced into the region of interest. The spring-loaded mechanism automatically sequentially advances the obturator and the cannula.

result in less crush artifact, which has been demonstrated in pediatric kidney biopsies.[54] Regardless of the system used, visual inspection of the core biopsy is necessary to verify adequate sampling. Many patients in these series required only a single pass to acquire adequate tissue. Repeated passes were made if inadequate initial samples were obtained.

Success with core needle biopsy has been demonstrated in a wide variety of anatomic locations, including the neck, mediastinum, lung, peritoneal cavity, liver, retroperitoneum, kidney, adrenal gland, pelvis, and extremities.[19,34,51,54] The diagnostic accuracy in malignant disease observed in four series is summarized in Table 26-1. The sensitivity of the biopsy technique is acceptable, but there were clearly problematic cases in which the incorrect diagnosis was made. These inaccuracies may have been avoidable with additional clinical history[19] or additional sampling. In some of the discordant cases, the uncertainty of the diagnosis was recognized immediately and addressed with repeat percutaneous or open biopsy. Core needle biopsy tends to be more accurate in detecting metastasis or recurrence than for obtaining the initial diagnosis.

No patients in these series suffered procedure-related death or required operative intervention for procedural complications. One series reported a significant decrease in hematocrit requiring transfusion in 3% of core needle biopsy procedures, and 10% of patients undergoing a transthoracic biopsy required a thoracostomy tube.[51]

Given the risk of pneumothorax and the variability of lesion position with respiration, core needle biopsy of pulmonary lesions merits special consideration. Connolly et al.[10] reported their experience with core needle biopsy of small lung lesions in children in 1999. Biopsies were performed under CT guidance with a coaxial needle system while the child was under general anesthesia. All imaging studies and biopsies were performed on complete exhalation. Adequate core tissue samples were obtained for diagnosis in 83% of patients, with the average size of the lesion being 9 mm. When adequate cores were not obtained, aspiration cytology was performed and raised the overall diagnostic yield to 94%. Twenty-seven percent of patients had small pneumothoraces, but none were symptomatic or required drainage.

Needle track tumor recurrence represents an oncologic complication specific to this biopsy technique. Estimates of this complication in adults vary widely, ranging from 3.4% in hepatocellular carcinoma[33] to 0.01% in thoracic tumors.[5] The incidence of this complication is influenced by several factors. Immunologic, chemotherapeutic, and radiotherapeutic effects decrease the likelihood of needle track recurrence. The larger needles used for core needle biopsies are associated with a greater risk than are the fine needles used for aspiration.[21] There are two reported cases of needle track recurrence in children with Wilms' tumors.[4]

MINIMAL-ACCESS SURGERY

The widespread use of minimal-access surgery, including laparoscopy and thoracoscopy, has had a significant impact on general pediatric surgery over the last 15 years. Both techniques are now being used in cancer diagnosis and therapy. Gans and Berci[14] reported their initial experience with multiple endoscopic techniques in children in 1971. Interestingly, one of the chief applications of peritonoscopy that they advocated was to guide the biopsy of metastatic implants. The application of both laparoscopy and thoracoscopy has now grown to include the initial diagnosis of childhood malignancies and the assessment of refractory or metastatic disease.

	No. of Patients		
Author/Year	(Total/Malignancy)	Sensitivity (%)	Comments
Klose et al[34]/1991	39/16	100	Correct histiogenetic classification in all tumors
Somers et al[54]/1993	25/23	88	4 discordant cases, including neuroblastoma diagnosed as ganglioneuroma
Skoldenberg et al[51]/2002	110/84	82	16 cases failed to yield diagnosis due to inadequate specimen
Guimaraes et al[19]/2003	54/54	82	In 4 cases, initial interpretation was changed, including Wilms' tumor diagnosed as neuroblastoma

TABLE 26-1 Diagnostic Accuracy of Core Needle Biopsy

Laparoscopy

Laparoscopy affords several advantages in the evaluation of the abdominal cavity in children with cancer. First, it provides the opportunity to examine the entire peritoneal cavity and perform a systematic examination of all peritoneal surfaces. The entire length of the bowel can be examined, along with its mesentery and lymph nodes. Multiple biopsies can easily be obtained. The second chief advantage of laparoscopy is the decreased physiologic stress it produces in these children, who may already be critically ill. Finally, as in all minimally invasive procedures, postoperative pain is reduced and recovery is hastened.[28] The chief disadvantages of laparoscopy are the limited ability to assess retroperitoneal structures and the loss of tactile evaluation of deep lesions.

Diagnostic laparoscopy and biopsy have been used in several settings in the management of children with solid malignancies.[24,48] Biopsies obtained using laparoscopic techniques have a high rate of success in yielding diagnostic tissue.[24,47] Laparoscopy allows the surgeon to obtain larger tissue samples than may be obtained with core needle biopsy. This is particularly relevant if larger samples are required for biologic studies. In the initial diagnosis, laparoscopy aids in identifying the site of origin of large abdominal masses. Laparoscopy is superior to CT in assessing intraperitoneal neoplasms and for the evaluation of ascites.[7] For example, laparoscopy allows the direct determination of whether a pelvic mass arises from the ovary or the bladder neck, which may be difficult to distinguish by radiologic studies. Direct visualization via laparoscopy has been used to assess the resectability of hepatoblastoma.[24] During the course of treatment, laparoscopy may be used to assess for new metastatic disease or to assess for initial tumor response as a second-look procedure.

One area of concern about the use of laparoscopy in cancer patients is port site recurrence. This complication has been observed in a variety of adult malignancies, most notably in adenocarcinoma of the colon and gallbladder.[40] This complication is most frequently reported after resection of an unexpected gallbladder carcinoma.[49] Cases of port site recurrence have also occurred in adults after the resection of liposarcoma[25] and cervical carcinoma.[2] More recent reports cite a very low rate of port site recurrence in adult patients with upper gastrointestinal[50] and renal malignancies.[15] Data are relatively limited concerning this issue in children. The COG retrospective study of 85 children noted no port site recurrences.[24] In a survey of Japanese pediatric laparoscopic surgeons, there were no port site recurrences following 85 laparoscopic and 44 thoracoscopic procedures.[27] It should be noted, however, that 104 of these tumors were neuroblastomas, with many being detected by mass screening; the general applicability of these data may therefore be limited. Given the differences in tumor biology between adult adenocarcinomas and pediatric neoplasms, which often have a marked response to neoadjuvant therapy, it is difficult to generalize from the adult literature. Certainly, additional surveillance for port site recurrence of pediatric tumors is merited.

Laparoscopy in children is typically performed under general anesthesia to facilitate tolerance of pneumoperitoneum. The only absolute contraindication to laparoscopic evaluation is cardiopulmonary instability that would prevent safe insufflation of the peritoneal cavity. The supine position is used most commonly and affords a complete view of the peritoneal cavity. To facilitate visualization, a 30-degree laparoscope is used, along with at least two additional ports for manipulation and retraction. Ascites should be collected for cytologic analysis, and all peritoneal surfaces should be inspected. Incisional biopsies can be performed using laparoscopic scissors. Hemostasis is achieved using a combination of electrocautery and hemostatic agents (as discussed later in the section on open incisional biopsy) or by tissue approximation via laparoscopic suturing. Biopsy specimens are typically retrieved using a specimen bag. This reduces the chance of specimen destruction during retrieval and may decrease the risk of port site recurrence. Cup biopsy forceps can be used to obtain specimens as well. Core needle biopsies can be directed by laparoscopy and used to sample retroperitoneal, intraperitoneal, or hepatic masses. For deep-seated tumors, such as intrahepatic lesions, laparoscopic ultrasonography can be used to guide biopsy procedures and to compensate for the inability to palpate tissues.[8,38]

Complications associated with the laparoscopic diagnosis and treatment of solid tumors in children are infrequent. The need to convert to an unplanned open operation has similarly been low.[24,28,48]

Thoracoscopy

Thoracoscopy was first reported by Jacobus in 1910 as a technique for the lysis of pleural adhesions resulting from tuberculosis. The initial experience with its use in children was reported by Rodgers and Talbert in 1976.[45] They described nine children, including two oncology patients (Ewing's sarcoma and recurrent Hodgkin's lymphoma). Since this initial report, thoracoscopy has become widely used for the evaluation of thoracic lesions in children, for several reasons. Primarily, postoperative pain associated with thoracoscopic biopsy or resection is markedly decreased compared with conventional open thoracotomy. Moreover, thoracoscopy allows near-complete visualization of all parietal and visceral pleural surfaces, which cannot be accomplished with a thoracotomy. Additionally, in most children, the mediastinum does not contain a significant amount of adipose tissue and therefore can be inspected thoracoscopically.

Although primary neoplasms of the lung are rare in children, pulmonary lesions are often a confounding issue in the treatment of children with cancer.[56] The most common tumor to have early pulmonary metastases is Wilms' tumor. Pulmonary metastases are also common with bone and soft tissue sarcomas, hepatic tumors, teratocarcinomas, and melanomas. Thoracoscopy is frequently used to evaluate for metastases either at the time of initial diagnosis or after follow-up imaging. A common clinical scenario is difficulty in distinguishing an opportunistic

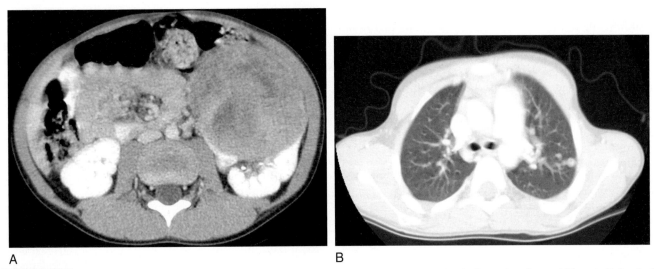

Figure 26–2 Computed tomography (CT) scans obtained at the time of diagnosis of a new abdominal mass in a 5-year-old boy. *A,* Abdominal and pelvic CT scans show a large left-sided renal mass. *B,* Chest CT scan demonstrates a single 8-mm pulmonary nodule in the left upper lobe. No other pulmonary lesions were identified. At the time of nephrectomy, a thoracoscopic excisional biopsy of the lung lesion was performed. Final pathology of the kidney demonstrated a stage II favorable-histology Wilms' tumor, and the lung pathology showed a hyalinized granuloma.

infection from new metastatic lung disease during the course of therapy. In areas with endemic granulomatous disease, thoracoscopy can also be helpful at the time of diagnosis (Fig. 26-2). The diagnostic accuracy of thoraco-scopic biopsies in this setting is very high.[44,47,48,56]

Mediastinal lesions can also be biopsied or resected using thoracoscopy.[42,44] Thoracoscopy provides clear visualization of both the anterior and posterior medi-astinum, even in small children, and we prefer it over mediastinoscopy for the evaluation of mediastinal lesions in children.

The only absolute contraindications to thoracoscopy are complete obliteration of the pleural space and inability to tolerate single-lung ventilation when complete collapse of the lung is required.

Thoracoscopy in children is typically performed under general anesthesia with mechanical ventilation. Visualization is facilitated by single-lung ventilation, if possible, and supplemented with insufflation. In older children, this may be accomplished with a double-lumen endotracheal tube. In smaller children, the left lung can be isolated by right mainstem bronchial intubation. Left mainstem intubation is difficult, and the tube frequently dislodges into the right side with positioning. Right lung deflation is performed by endotracheal intubation and right bronchial occlusion with either a dedicated bronchial blocker or a Fogarty catheter placed using rigid bronchoscopy. Fogarty catheter size is based on age: #3 for patients 4 years and younger and #5 for those aged 5 to 12 years.[55] This may be inflated and deflated during the procedure as needed. If selective ventilation is difficult to achieve or poorly tolerated by the patient, low-pressure insufflation (5 to 10 cm of water pressure) with carbon dioxide will assist with visualization. The anesthesiologist must monitor for any adverse effects from this controlled tension pneumothorax. It can

be rapidly evacuated if necessary but is typically well tolerated.

Typically, the child is placed in lateral thoracotomy posi-tion. Hyperextension of the chest increases the intercostal space and facilitates movement of the thoracoscopy ports. This positioning should be adjusted for mediastinal lesions. For anterior lesions, a more supine position is used; for posterior lesions, the patient is positioned more prone. The initial port is placed at the midaxillary line using blunt dissection. Additional ports are placed under thoracoscopic guidance at sites based on the location of the lesion of interest. A 30-degree thoracoscope is help-ful in achieving complete visualization of all pleural surfaces. Complete inspection is also facilitated by the use of multiple port sites.

Careful correlation to cross-sectional imaging is essen-tial to successful thoracoscopic sampling, particularly of smaller lesions. Pleura-based or subpleural pulmonary lesions are often apparent when the lung is deflated. These can be resected using endoscopic stapling devices and retrieved using specimen bags. Identification of deeper lesions is more challenging. After complete collapse of the lung, palpation of the parenchyma allows the identification of larger lesions. Biopsy of smaller lesions can be based on anatomic location if CT localization is specific, such as apical, lingular, or basilar lesions. CT-guided localization may be performed preoperatively with placement of a fine wire[23] or injection of methylene blue[43] or stained autolo-gous blood.[36] These localization techniques have been very effective in obtaining accurate diagnoses in children.[36,43] Intrathoracic ultrasonography may be helpful in localizing deeper parenchymal lesions.[53] However, this technique is not widely used, and assessment of its efficacy in children is limited. In the future, image-guided biopsies will likely be accomplished with intraoperative magnetic resonance imaging or CT guidance.

After sampling of the tissues is completed, the pneumothorax can be evacuated with a small catheter placed on water seal. Unless extensive pulmonary biopsies are performed or the lung is otherwise diseased, a thoracostomy tube is not required. Most children can be discharged the next day, and chemotherapy can be started promptly.[36]

Thoracoscopic techniques are highly effective in achieving a diagnosis. Most pediatric series report success in obtaining accurate diagnostic tissue in almost all cases.[24,44,48,56] Complications during diagnostic thoracoscopy are rare. Pneumothorax or persistent air leak may occur in children with underlying parenchymal lung disease or those requiring high-pressure ventilatory support. There is the potential for injury to subdiaphragmatic organs during initial trocar placement owing to elevation of the diaphragm during single-lung ventilation.

OPEN INCISIONAL BIOPSY

Incisional biopsy remains the gold standard with regard to the quality of tissue sampling if complete excision will not be performed. Laparotomy or thoracotomy allows large samples to be obtained under direct vision, which can provide improved diagnosis compared with needle biopsies. For example, in the National Wilms' Tumor Study Group-4, open biopsy was more successful than core needle biopsy at identifying anaplasia.[22] Correlation with preoperative imaging allows multiple samples to be obtained if there is inhomogeneity within the tumor that causes concern about sampling error.

The ability to obtain larger specimens is beneficial not only in providing tissue for molecular diagnosis and prognosis but also in providing samples for tissue banking and creation of cell lines. Samples obtained from these biopsies provided the clinical material that allowed the development of the molecular diagnostic and prognostic techniques referred to earlier. Further stratification of risk, to allow more precise risk-based therapy, remains a major focus for pediatric oncology trials. Finally, specimens that are tissue-banked from these larger specimens can be used for investigational therapies, such as vaccines, in individual patients.

There are several important factors when performing an open biopsy. The initial biopsy should take into consideration the ultimate operative treatment of the tumor. For example, the incision for biopsy of an extremity mass should be oriented parallel to the axis of the limb, and care should be taken to avoid undermining subcutaneous or fascial planes. This allows subsequent wide local excision to be performed, with minimal additional resection of tissue owing to the biopsy. Likewise, testicular masses should be biopsied only through an inguinal approach; a scrotal biopsy incision could require the addition of a hemiscrotectomy to the subsequent orchiectomy. Laparotomy for biopsy should be planned to allow subsequent resection through extension of the same incision.

Significant distortion of anatomic relations can occur with large retroperitoneal tumors, and attention must be paid to avoid injury to structures such as the ureters, bile duct, or major vascular structures that may be distracted over the mass. The most common intra-abdominal tumors in children tend to be vascular, and bleeding from the biopsy site is the most common serious complication. Strategies to reduce perioperative hemorrhage include normalization of coagulation parameters preoperatively and adequate operative exposure. Cauterization of the tumor capsule may help control bleeding, but we have found that direct pressure after packing the biopsy site with oxidized cellulose, combined with procoagulants (described later), is more efficient than generous cautery of the biopsy base. If possible, closure of the tumor capsule can aid with hemostasis.

Supplements to achieve hemostasis can include topical agents, fibrin sealants, and recombinant factor VIIa. Commercially available topical products include gelatin foam pads, microfibrillar collagen, and oxidized cellulose, which is available as fabric and cottonoid. Fibrin sealants are composed of fibrinogen, thrombin, and calcium; mixture of these components as they are delivered to the tissue results in the rapid formation of a fibrin clot.[46] Recombinant factor VIIa was originally developed to treat patients with hemophilia who had developed inhibitors; however, it has increasingly been used to treat patients with severe bleeding without a preexisting bleeding disorder. There are numerous reports of its use in trauma and a randomized trial showing its efficacy in radical prostatectomy.[13] Its effective use to control hemorrhage after biopsy of a hepatoblastoma has been reported,[6] and we have had success in controlling bleeding from a hepatic metastasis from Wilms' tumor. This is an expensive therapy, and although its risks are poorly characterized, initial experience suggests a low rate of thromboembolic complications.[1]

One of the important roles of a surgeon is providing adequate tissue for diagnosis and risk stratification. Traditionally, the open biopsy served this purpose extremely well and can be accomplished with low morbidity. In the future, the need for open biopsy will diminish with further advances in molecular diagnosis that require only small tumor specimens or perhaps no biopsy of the primary tumor at all. A thorough understanding of the potential diagnoses and their treatment, as well as coordination between the surgeon and oncologist, is critical to determining the appropriate approach in each individual patient.

REFERENCES

1. Abramowicz, M: Novoseven for nonhemophilia hemostasis. Med Lett 2004;46:1181.
2. Agostini A, et al: Port site metastasis after laparoscopy for uterine cervical carcinoma. Surg Endosc 2003;17:1663-1665.
3. Akhtar M, et al: Fine-needle aspiration biopsy diagnosis of small round cell tumors of childhood: A comprehensive approach. Diagn Cytopathol 1999;21:81-91.
4. Aslam A, Spicer RD: Needle track recurrence after biopsy of non-metastatic Wilms' tumor. Pediatr Surg Int 1996;11:416-417.
5. Ayar D, et al: Needle-track metastasis after transthoracic needle biopsy. J Thorac Imaging 1998;13:2-6.

6. Barro C, et al: Successful use of recombinant factor VIIa for severe surgical liver bleeding in a 5-month-old baby. Haemophilia 2004;10:183-185.

7. Barth RA, et al: A comparison study of computed tomography and laparoscopy in the staging of abdominal neoplasms. Dig Dis Sci 1981;26:253-256.

8. Berber E, Siperstein AE: Laparoscopic ultrasound. Surg Clin North Am 2004;84:1061-1084.

9. Bown N: Neuroblastoma tumour genetics: Clinical and biological aspects. J Clin Pathol 2001;54:897-910.

10. Connolly BL, et al: CT-guided percutaneous needle biopsy of small lung nodules in children. Pediatr Radiol 1999;29:342-346.

11. Dagher R, et al: Molecular confirmation of Ewing sarcoma. J Pediatr Hematol Oncol 2001;23:221-224.

12. Dodd LG, et al: Utility of fine-needle aspiration in the diagnosis of primary osteosarcoma. Diagn Cytopathol 2002;27:350-353.

13. Friederich PW, et al: Effect of recombinant activated factor VII on perioperative blood loss in patients undergoing retropubic prostatectomy: A double-blind placebo-controlled randomised trial. Lancet 2003;361:201-205.

14. Gans SL, Berci G: Advances in endoscopy of infants and children. J Pediatr Surg 1971;6:199-233.

15. Gill IS, et al: Laparoscopic radical nephrectomy in 100 patients: A single center experience from the United States. Cancer 2001;92:1843-1855.

16. Gonzalez-Campora R: Fine needle aspiration cytology of soft tissue tumors. Acta Cytol 2000;44:337-343.

17. Grieg ED, Gray AC: Lymphatic glands in sleeping sickness. BMJ 1904;1:1252.

18. Grosfeld JL: Risk-based management of solid tumors in children. Am J Surg 2000;180:322-327.

19. Guimaraes AC, et al: Computed tomography-guided needle biopsies in pediatric oncology. J Pediatr Surg 2003;38:1066-1068.

20. Gurley AM, et al: The utility of ancillary studies in pediatric FNA cytology. Diagn Cytopathol 1992;8:137-146.

21. Haddad FS, Somsin AA: Seeding and perineal implantation of prostatic cancer in the track of the biopsy needle: Three case reports and a review of the literature. J Surg Oncol 1987;35:184-191.

22. Hamilton TE, et al: Open biopsy is superior to needle for detection of anaplasia in patients with Wilms' tumor. Paper presented at the American Pediatric Surgical Association meeting, 2004.

23. Hanninen EL, et al: Computed tomography-guided pulmonary nodule localization before thoracoscopic resection. Acta Radiol 2004;45:284-288.

24. Holcomb GW 3rd, et al: Minimally invasive surgery in children with cancer. Cancer 1995;76:121-128.

25. Horiguchi A, et al: Port site recurrence after laparoscopic resection of retroperitoneal liposarcoma. J Urol 1998;159:1296-1297.

26. Howell LP: Changing role of fine-needle aspiration in the evaluation of pediatric masses. Diagn Cytopathol 2001;24:65-70.

27. Iwanaka T, et al: No incidence of port-site recurrence after endosurgical procedure for pediatric malignancies. Pediatr Surg Int 2003;19:200-203.

28. Iwanaka T, et al: Endosurgical procedures for pediatric solid tumors. Pediatr Surg Int 2004;20:39-42.

29. Jereb B, Us-Krasovec M, Jereb M: Thin needle biopsy of solid tumors in children. Med Pediatr Oncol 1978;4:213-220.

30. Kilpatrick SE, Garvin AJ: Recent advances in the diagnosis of pediatric soft-tissue tumors. Med Pediatr Oncol 1999;32:373-376.

31. Kilpatrick SE, et al: Is fine-needle aspiration biopsy a practical alternative to open biopsy for the primary diagnosis of sarcoma? Experience with 140 patients. Am J Clin Pathol 2001;115:59-68.

32. Kilpatrick SE, et al: The role of fine needle aspiration biopsy in the diagnosis and management of osteosarcoma. Pediatr Pathol Mol Med 2001;20:175-187.

33. Kim SH, et al: Needle-tract implantation in hepatocellular carcinoma: Frequency and CT findings after biopsy with a 19.5-gauge automated biopsy gun. Abdom Imaging 2000;25:246-250.

34. Klose KC, et al: CT-guided percutaneous large-bore biopsies in benign and malignant pediatric lesions. Cardiovasc Intervent Radiol 1991;14:78-83.

35. Liu ES, et al: Fine needle aspiration biopsy of pediatric head and neck masses. Int J Pediatr Otorhinolaryngol 2001;60:135-140.

36. McConnell PI, Feola GP, Meyers RL: Methylene blue-stained autologous blood for needle localization and thoracoscopic resection of deep pulmonary nodules. J Pediatr Surg 2002;37:1729-1731.

37. Mobley DL, Wakely PE Jr, Frable MA: Fine-needle aspiration biopsy: Application to pediatric head and neck masses. Laryngoscope 1991;101:469-472.

38. Montorsi M, et al: Laparoscopy with laparoscopic ultrasound for pretreatment staging of hepatocellular carcinoma: A prospective study. J Gastrointest Surg 2001;5:312-315.

39. Mora J, Gerald WL, Cheung NK: Evolving significance of prognostic markers associated with new treatment strategies in neuroblastoma. Cancer Lett 2003;197:119-124.

40. Paolucci V, et al: Tumor seeding following laparoscopy: International survey. World J Surg 1999;23:989-995, discussion 996-997.

41. Pappo AS, et al: Biology and therapy of pediatric rhabdomyosarcoma. J Clin Oncol 1995;13:2123-2139.

42. Partrick DA, Rothenberg SS: Thoracoscopic resection of mediastinal masses in infants and children: An evaluation of technique and results. J Pediatr Surg 2001;36:1165-1167.

43. Partrick DA, et al: Successful thoracoscopic lung biopsy in children utilizing preoperative CT-guided localization. J Pediatr Surg 2002;37:970-973, discussion 970-973.

44. Rao BN: Present day concepts of thoracoscopy as a modality in pediatric cancer management. Int Surg 1997;82:123-126.

45. Rodgers BM, Talbert JL: Thoracoscopy for diagnosis of intrathoracic lesions in children. J Pediatr Surg 1976;11:703-708.

46. Rousou J, et al: Randomized clinical trial of fibrin sealant in patients undergoing resternotomy or reoperation after cardiac operations: A multicenter study. J Thorac Cardiovasc Surg 1989;97:194-203.

47. Saenz NC, et al: The application of minimal access procedures in infants, children, and young adults with pediatric malignancies. J Laparoendosc Adv Surg Tech A 1997;7:289-294.

48. Sailhamer E, et al: Minimally invasive surgery for pediatric solid neoplasms. Am Surg 2003;69:566-568.

49. Schaeff B, Paolucci V, Thomopoulos J: Port site recurrences after laparoscopic surgery: A review. Dig Surg 1998;15:124-134.

50. Shoup M, et al: Port site metastasis after diagnostic laparoscopy for upper gastrointestinal tract malignancies: An uncommon entity. Ann Surg Oncol 2002;9:632-636.

51. Skoldenberg EG, et al: Diagnosing childhood tumors: A review of 147 cutting needle biopsies in 110 children. J Pediatr Surg 2002;37:50-56.

52. Smith MB, et al: A rational approach to the use of fine-needle aspiration biopsy in the evaluation of primary and recurrent neoplasms in children. J Pediatr Surg 1993;28:1245-1247.

53. Smith MB, et al: A prospective evaluation of an endoscopic ultrasonic probe to detect intraparenchymal malignancy at pediatric thoracoscopy. J Laparoendosc Surg 1996;6: 233-237.

54. Somers JM, et al: Radiologically-guided cutting needle biopsy for suspected malignancy in childhood. Clin Radiol 1993;48:236-240.

55. Tan GM, Tan-Kendrick AP: Bronchial diameters in children— use of the Fogarty catheter for lung isolation in children. Anaesth Intensive Care 2002;30:615-618.

56. Waldhausen JH, Tapper D, Sawin RS: Minimally invasive surgery and clinical decision-making for pediatric malignancy. Surg Endosc 2000;14:250-253.

57. Weinstein JL, Katzenstein HM, Cohn SL: Advances in the diagnosis and treatment of neuroblastoma. Oncologist 2003;8:278-292.

Chapter 27

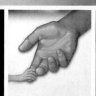

Wilms' Tumor

Edward P. Tagge, Patrick B. Thomas, and H. Biemann Othersen, Jr.

Wilms' tumor continues to be a subject of intense interest, involving both clinical and basic science investigations. With the aid of five cooperative protocols by the National Wilms' Tumor Study Group (NWTSG), there has been marked improvement in survival. In the fourth NWTSG study (NWTS-4), the 2-year relapse-free survival rate for children with low-risk Wilms' tumor exceeded 91%.[60] However, there continue to be a variety of unsolved problems. Anaplastic tumors, clear cell sarcomas of the kidney, and rhabdoid tumors of the kidney are still relatively resistant to therapy. Ten percent of patients have poor prognostic variables, including unfavorable histology, chromosomal loss on 1p and 16q, and diploidy. Patients with lung or liver metastases, major tumor spillage during resection, remote lymph node involvement, and bilateral tumors all have worse outcomes. In addition, there is an increasing appreciation of the long-term morbidity of successful cancer therapy in children. Finally, the underlying molecular basis of Wilms' tumor is quite complex and remains unclear.

This chapter briefly summarizes the new information available, focusing on the conclusions of NWTS-4, a preliminary discussion of the results of NWTS-5, and an overview of future directions in Wilms' tumor management.

HISTORY

Pathologic descriptions of the tumor now known as nephroblastoma were written as early as 1872.[44] In 1879 Osler realized that physicians were reporting renal tumors in children and giving them different names, though they were all describing the same type of solid tumor.[104] The classic article was presented in 1899 when Wilms (a surgeon) reviewed the literature and added seven cases of his own, describing the clinical picture that now bears his name.[139] Initially, surgical excision was the only therapeutic option, but the prognosis was grim. However, in 1916 radiation therapy was added by Friedlander,[50] and Ladd improved the surgical technique, increasing the survival rate to 20%.[83] Chemotherapy with actinomycin D and vincristine was eventually added, and this combination of surgical excision, postoperative irradiation, and chemotherapy ushered in the modern era, with a 2-year survival rate of 81% reported.[47]

Because Wilms' tumor is an infrequent occurrence in the United States, it was realized that collaborative research was mandatory to obtain statistically significant numbers of patients. Thus the NWTSG was established in 1969. The original membership included institutions from the Children's Cancer Study Group, the Pediatric Division of the Southwest Oncology Group, and the Pediatric Division of the Cancer and Leukemia Group B. The initial goals of the NWTSG were to improve the survival of children with Wilms' tumor and other renal tumors, to study the long-term outcome of children treated successfully by identifying adverse effects, to study the epidemiology and biology of Wilms' tumor, and to make information regarding successful treatment strategies for Wilms' tumor available to physicians around the world. The therapeutic studies conducted by the NWTSG eventually involved more than 250 pediatric oncology treatment centers in the United States, Canada, and several other countries. During its final years, approximately 450 to 500 patients with Wilms' tumor were entered annually, including 70% to 80% of all cases in the United States.

In 2001 the NWTSG merged with the Children's Cancer Group, the Pediatric Oncology Group (POG), and the Intergroup Rhabdomyosarcoma Study Group to form a new national organization, the Children's Oncology Group (COG). Patient entry into the NWTSG clinical trial protocols was completed in 2002, and future clinical trials will be conducted by the renal disease committee of the COG. The "NWTS" designation will still be used for the continuing study of late effects.

EPIDEMIOLOGY

Worldwide, Wilms' tumor affects approximately 1 child per 10,000 younger than 15 years.[16,19] Wilms' tumor represents approximately 6% of childhood cancers in the United States, and the total incidence is estimated at 450 to 500 cases a year.[34] Incidence rates appear to be slightly elevated for blacks (both American and African) in comparison to whites but are only half as great among Asians.

Several case-control studies have suggested that paternal occupation, maternal hormone exposure during pregnancy, or genetic predisposition may increase the risk for Wilms' tumor.

The median age at onset is 38 months in the NWTS series, with the onset in girls occurring on average 6 months later than in boys. Patients with bilateral tumors, aniridia, cryptorchism or hypospadias, Beckwith-Wiedemann syndrome, or intralobar nephrogenic rests tend to be diagnosed much younger than average (median age, 17 to 27 months). Those with familial disease or multicentric tumors have intermediate age-at-onset distributions, whereas those with perilobar nephrogenic rests are diagnosed at older ages.

Wilms' tumor shows a strong association with certain congenital anomalies: WAGR syndrome (Wilms' tumor, aniridia, genitourinary malformations, and mental retardation), Beckwith-Wiedemann syndrome (an overgrowth syndrome characterized by exomphalos, visceromegaly, macroglossia, and hyperinsulinemic hypoglycemia), and hemihypertrophy.[98] Urologic anomalies, such as lobular nephromegaly, hypospadias, and cryptorchidism, are often seen with Wilms' tumor.

WAGR syndrome is a rare genetic disorder and is associated with a defect in chromosome 11p13. Most children with WAGR syndrome are diagnosed at birth because the aniridia is usually obvious. However, less than 1% of children with Wilms' tumor have WAGR syndrome.

Aniridia is a severe eye disease characterized by iris hypoplasia; both sporadic cases and familial cases with an autosomal dominant inheritance exist. Some of the sporadic cases are caused by large chromosomal deletions involving the Wilms' tumor gene (WAGR syndrome), resulting in an increased risk of developing Wilms' tumor. A recent review of cancer and aniridia cases found that patients with sporadic aniridia have a relative risk of 67 (confidence interval, 8.1 to 241) of developing Wilms' tumor.[66]

Denys-Drash syndrome is characterized by pseudohermaphroditism, progressive glomerulopathy, and Wilms' tumor. Genetically it is associated with mutations of the Wilms' tumor 1 *(WT1)* gene. More than 90% of patients with Denys-Drash syndrome who carry constitutional intragenic *WT1* mutations are at high risk for the development of Wilms' tumor. In fact, prophylactic bilateral nephrectomy in two patients with missense mutations in the *WT1* gene was recently reported.[75]

A small percentage of Wilms' tumors are familial in nature. The pattern of transmission for hereditary Wilms' tumor is likely autosomal dominant, with incomplete and variable penetrance.[18,112] Although some familial cases involve mutations in *WT1*, more are associated with the familial Wilms' tumor genes *FWT1* at 17q and *FWT2* at 19q, for which fine-scale mapping is currently in progress.

MOLECULAR BIOLOGY AND GENETICS

The development of Wilms' tumor is thought to involve changes in a number of genes that function to control normal kidney development and growth.[32] Roughly 2% of children diagnosed with Wilms' tumor have a relative who was also diagnosed with Wilms' tumor. The occurrence of these rare Wilms' tumor families suggests that an altered gene is important in the development of this nephroblastic tumor. Other factors point to the importance of an underlying genetic predisposition. Wilms' tumors can occur bilaterally in approximately 5% to 10% of affected children.[29] In addition, nephrogenic rests, potentially premalignant lesions, are found within the kidneys of 30% to 40% of children with Wilms' tumors.

Wilms' tumor is an important model for the study of fundamental mechanisms of carcinogenesis. Statistical evidence to support the involvement of a tumor suppressor gene in the pathogenesis of Wilms' tumor was initially provided by Knudson and Strong in 1972.[82] According to Knudson's hypothesis of tumor suppressor genes, patients with a familial cancer syndrome inherit one chromosome with an inactive tumor suppressor gene locus because of germline mutation. The counterpart tumor suppressor gene on the remaining paired chromosome is subsequently inactivated by a somatic mutation, leading to the formation of cancer. Knudson extended his famous two-hit model of carcinogenesis, originally proposed for retinoblastoma, to Wilms' tumor. In this model, children who were susceptible to retinoblastoma or Wilms' tumor were born with a constitutional DNA mutation in one allele of a presumed tumor suppressor gene—so-called loss of heterozygosity (LOH). Thus, only one new genetic event, the deletion or inhibition of the paired allele, would be needed for tumorigenesis to occur. This condition would increase the likelihood of bilateral tumor formation and an earlier age of onset compared with sporadic cases. Subsequent review of chromosomal LOH revealed that the maternal allele was lost in 52 of 53 tumors demonstrating this trait.[30] This surprising fact implies that chromosomal loss from a tumor is not a random event and that the alleles of the Wilms' tumor suppressor locus are not equivalent. This functional difference between the maternal and paternal alleles of a gene is termed genomic imprinting.

However, the genetics of Wilms' tumor are even more complex than originally believed. More recent evidence suggests that some bilateral and multifocal Wilms' tumors may arise from somatic mosaicism rather than a germline mutation, contradicting the central tenet of the two-hit model.[6] The biologic pathways leading to the development of Wilms' tumor involve several genetic loci, including two genes on chromosome 11p—one on chromosome 11p13 (the Wilms' tumor suppressor gene *WT1*), and the other on chromosome 11p15 (the putative Wilms' tumor suppressor gene *WT2*). In addition, loci at 1p, 7p, 16q, and 17p (the *p53* tumor suppressor gene) are believed to harbor genes involved in the biology of Wilms' tumor. More recent studies have localized two familial predisposition genes on chromosomes 19 and 17, but their actual identification is still ongoing. It is also known that predisposition in some families is due to neither *WT1* nor the chromosome 19 or 17 genes, implying that other Wilms' tumor predisposition genes exist.

WT1

The mapping of the genetic loci associated with Wilms' tumor resulted from a combination of clinical observations, karyotype analyses, and molecular genetic studies. In 1964 Miller et al.[98] reported an association between aniridia and Wilms' tumor. Subsequently, the rare complex of developmental anomalies known as the WAGR syndrome was described, in which more than 30% of affected children developed Wilms' tumor.[101] Karyotypic analysis of those children demonstrated a deletion in the short arm of one copy of chromosome 11 at band 13.[116] The observation that the rare WAGR syndrome was invariably associated with interstitial deletions of chromosome 11p13, and that tumor tissue at this same locus often displayed LOH, ultimately led to the cloning of the first Wilms' tumor gene *WT1*.[20,52] *WT1* is a complex gene encoded by 10 exons. Cells that express *WT1* produce four distinct *WT1* messenger RNAs (mRNAs), which reflect alternative splicing patterns of the transcription products of the *WT1* gene. The WT1 protein is between 45 and 49 kD in size, depending on which mRNA splice variant is translated into protein. The carboxyl terminus of the WT1 protein contains four zinc finger domains, which is a protein motif known to facilitate binding to DNA in a sequence-specific pattern. This implies that *WT1* is a transcriptional factor regulating yet unknown targeted genes. *WT1* has important functions during genitourinary development, evidenced by its highly restricted temporal and spatial expression in glomerular precursors and by the failure of kidney development in *WT1*-null mice. In addition to its function in genitourinary development, a role in hematopoiesis is suggested by *WT1*'s aberrant expression in a subset of acute human leukemias. *WT1* is also expressed in mesothelial cells; a specific oncogenic chromosomal translocation fusing the N-terminal domain of the Ewing's sarcoma gene *EWS* to the three C-terminal zinc fingers of *WT1* underlies desmoplastic small round cell tumor.[86]

Ninety percent of patients with the even rarer Denys-Drash syndrome harbor germline mutations in *WT1*. Most are missense mutations resulting in single amino acid substitutions. Microscopic examination of the kidney in patients with the WAGR and Denys-Drash syndromes often reveals intralobar nephrogenic rests.[8] The existence of dominant negative mutations of *WT1* is supported by the observation of specific constitutional mutations of *WT1* in children with Denys-Drash syndrome.[31,109] Unlike children with the WAGR syndrome, in whom large deletions on 11p13 are seen,[109] those with Denys-Drash syndrome have only point mutations of the *WT1* gene.[108] Interestingly, the phenotypic effects of these constitutional *WT1* mutations are far more severe than those resulting from complete deletion of *WT1*, suggesting that the altered WT1 protein in patients with Denys-Drash syndrome is dysfunctional and acts in a dominant-negative fashion.[4,89]

WT1 is mutated in approximately 20% of all patients with Wilms' tumors. The frequency of germline *WT1* mutations in patients with bilateral Wilms' tumor and of detectable *WT1* mutations in Wilms' tumor specimens is low. Linkage at the *WT1* locus has been excluded in most familial cases.[77] Inherited *WT1* alterations have also been observed in a few small families with Wilms' tumor, but studies of large families have demonstrated that their inherited predisposition to Wilms' tumor is not due to an altered *WT1* gene. A recent review of cancer cases and aniridia in Denmark found that patients with sporadic aniridia have a relative risk of 67 (confidence interval, 8.1 to 241) of developing Wilms' tumor.[66] However, patients with the WAGR syndrome or Denys-Drash syndrome each account for less than 1% of all children with Wilms' tumor. The role of *WT1* mutations in patients with unilateral Wilms' tumor not associated with congenital syndromes seems to be limited, because less than 15% have mutations of *WT1*.[51]

WT2

In a subset of Wilms' tumors, LOH has been demonstrated for markers at the 11p15 locus, with maintenance of heterozygosity for the 11p13 locus.[72,114] Karyotypes of Wilms' tumors have demonstrated DNA loss at the 11p15 locus. Here, several genes *(IGF2, p57KIP2, H19, KVLQT1)* that regulate somatic growth are subject to dysregulated imprinting, including the gene for Beckwith-Wiedemann syndrome (BWS). This is the location for the putative second Wilms' tumor gene, *WT2*, which has yet to be cloned.[85]

BWS may result from overexpression of a gene at 11p15 that normally has only the paternal copy of the gene expressed (a process called genomic imprinting). In fact, karyotypic analysis has demonstrated a constitutional duplication of the paternal 11p15 chromosomal fragment in some children with BWS. Other children with the syndrome have two grossly normal copies of chromosome 11, both inherited from the father (thus there is no maternal copy)—a phenomenon called uniparental isodisomy.[68,71] It is believed that inheritance of two copies of the paternal gene for BWS would double the expression of this gene, resulting in the overgrowth features.

Much interest has centered on insulin-like growth factor 2 (IGF2), which resides at 11p15, as the candidate *WT2* gene because it is subjected to genomic imprinting. However, to date, no direct evidence has implicated this factor in the pathogenesis of BWS or Wilms' tumor. Investigators in Japan identified a paternally expressed imprinted gene, *PEG8/IGF2AS*, in this locus.[103] It is transcribed in the opposite direction to the *IGF2* transcripts, and some genomic regions are shared with the *IGF2* gene. Interestingly, *PEG8/IGF2AS* and *IGF2* were found to be overexpressed in Wilms' tumor samples, at levels 10 to 100 times greater than in normal kidney tissue neighboring the tumors. These findings imply that *PEG8/IGF2AS* may be a marker for Wilms' tumor and also suggest the possibility that *PEG8/IGF2AS* is one of the candidate Wilms' tumor genes.

Additional Wilms' Tumor Loci

The existence of an additional Wilms' tumor locus on the long arm of chromosome 16 (16q) has been suggested by tumor LOH for 16q in approximately 20% of Wilms' tumor specimens (compared with a 5% background rate).[28,78,95] Preliminary analysis by Grundy et al.[69] in 232 patients with Wilms' tumor suggested the LOH for l6q was a statistically important adverse prognostic factor. When compared with patients without LOH, the relapse rate was 3.3 times higher ($P = 0.01$), and the mortality rate was 12 times higher ($P < 0.01$), in patients with LOH for 16q. The same study also reported LOH for 1p in 12% of Wilms' tumor patients, along with relapse and mortality rates that were three times higher than for patients without 1p LOH (not statistically significant). Because of these data, NWTS-5 studied the effect of LOH for 16q and 1p on the prognosis for Wilms' tumor patients.

Linkage analyses in four large families with an inherited susceptibility to Wilms' tumor have implicated the existence of yet another Wilms' tumor gene.[67,77] Genes at 11p13, 11p15, and 16q have been determined not to play a role in the Wilms' tumors of those families, and detailed linkage analyses will be required to determine the chromosomal location of the familial Wilms' tumor gene.

Glypican-3 (GPC3) is a heparan sulfate proteoglycan that can bind to growth factors, such as IGF2. One report noted increased expression of GPC3 in Wilms' tumor and hepatoblastoma, suggesting a growth-promoting or neutral activity for this gene.[132] Another study determined the presence of sequence variants of GPC3 in tumor and normal tissue from 41 male patients with Wilms' tumor.[138] Two nonconservative single base changes were present in tumor tissue only, implying a possible role for GPC3 in Wilms' tumor development.

Investigators from Columbia University performed a survey of gene expression in Wilms' tumor using oligonucleotide microarrays,[87] identifying 357 genes differentially expressed between Wilms' tumors and fetal kidneys. Wilms' tumors systematically overexpressed genes corresponding to the earliest stage of metanephric development and underexpressed genes corresponding to later stages. This signature set was enriched in genes encoding transcription factors PAX2[131] and HOXA11, as well as the metastasis-associated transcription factor E1AF.

CLINICAL PRESENTATION

In the past, most children presented with an asymptomatic abdominal mass, usually noted by a family member (Fig. 27-1). The availability of modern imaging techniques, such as ultrasonography (US) and computed tomography (CT), has allowed the early evaluation of abdominal pain and the discovery of nonpalpable renal masses. Early symptoms include microscopic hematuria (in one third of patients) and other urinary disturbances, malaise, weight loss, and anemia. Occlusion of the left renal vein by tumor extension may obstruct the left spermatic vein, with a resultant varicocele. In addition, tumor thrombus may progress up the inferior vena cava into the heart (right atrium) and cause cardiac malfunction. Occasionally, an acute abdominal crisis occurs after rupture of a Wilms' tumor as a result of a relatively minor abdominal injury.

The physical examination should include careful palpation of the abdomen and measurement of blood pressure.

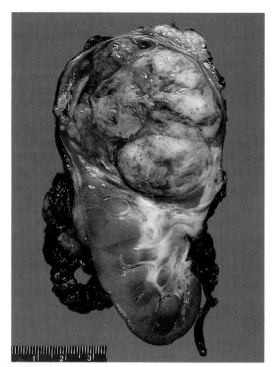

Figure 27–1 Large tumor mass in the superior portion of the kidney. The tumor bulge was felt by a visiting grandmother.

Wilms' tumor usually presents with a round, smooth, palpable flank mass. Patients with Wilms' tumor may have hypertension secondary to tumor production of renin or renal vascular compression by the mass. Finally, it is important to identify genitourinary anomalies and the presence of aniridia or hemihypertrophy.

DIAGNOSIS

No definitive diagnostic blood or urine test for Wilms' tumor exists, although there has been interest in the diagnostic utility of vascular endothelial growth factor (VEGF),[81] hyaluronan,[92] and basic fibroblastic growth factor (bFGF).[2] Advances in imaging technology have improved the ability to detect Wilms' tumor and its precursor, nephroblastomatosis, as well as the spread of tumor to other organs.[55] However, in terms of imaging, there is still wide variation in clinical practice compared with the guidelines recommended by the NWTSG. The preferred radiologic method for evaluating children with suspected Wilms' tumor is CT (Fig. 27-2), with US particularly suited for the detection of venous extension. Magnetic resonance imaging (MRI) identifies blood vessel involvement, although it is not one of the NWTSG-recommended preoperative studies (Fig. 27-3). CT of the abdomen may also identify lesions in the contralateral kidney or liver. A plain chest radiograph is taken to evaluate for pulmonary metastasis. CT of the chest is controversial because lesions not visible on radiographs but seen on CT are difficult to interpret. A recent study looked at whether identifying minimal pulmonary metastatic disease by chest CT in patients with Wilms' tumors and normal

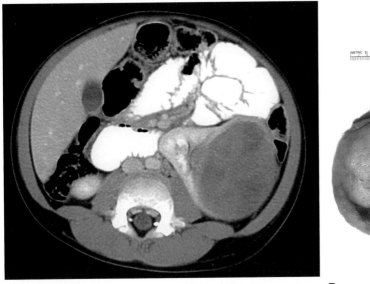

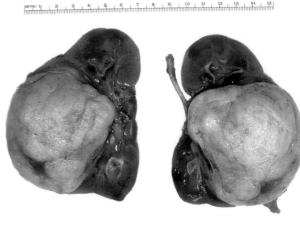

A   B

Figure 27-2 *A,* Abdominal computed tomography scan demonstrating a large tumor mass in the left kidney. *B,* Bivalved left kidney with tumor.

chest radiographs could predict children at increased risk of pulmonary relapse.[105] A retrospective analysis of 449 children entered into the United Kingdom Children's Cancer Study Group (UKCCSG) Second Wilms' Tumor Study between July 1986 and September 1991 was performed.

When only stage I patients were analyzed, there was a significant difference between the pulmonary relapse rate of 43% (3 of 7) in the CT-positive group and 10% (5 of 48) in the CT-negative group ($P = 0.02$). Importantly, 4 of 8 patients with stage I disease with pulmonary relapse died.

SCREENING

Children with BWS and idiopathic hemihypertrophy are at increased risk for developing Wilms' tumor. A recent report evaluating patients from the BWS Registry and previously published studies noted that children with BWS and hemihypertrophy benefited from US screening at intervals of 4 months or less,[24] although false-positive screening examinations did result in unnecessary surgery. The National Institutes of Health performed a cost-benefit analysis of screening for Wilms' tumor and hepatoblastoma in children with BWS.[96] Assuming that US examinations were performed three times a year from birth until age 7 years, screening a child with BWS from birth until age 4 years resulted in a cost per life-year saved of $9,642; continuing until age 7 years resulted in a cost per life-year saved of $14,740.

PATHOLOGY

The classic Wilms' tumor is composed of the three components seen in normal kidney differentiation: blastema, tubules, and stroma (Fig. 27-4). These components are believed to recapitulate the differentiation of the normal nephron unit. Classic Wilms' tumors are known to be heterogeneous with respect to component proportions and to exhibit aberrant adipose tissue, skeletal muscle, cartilage, and bone. Wilms' tumors may also contain only

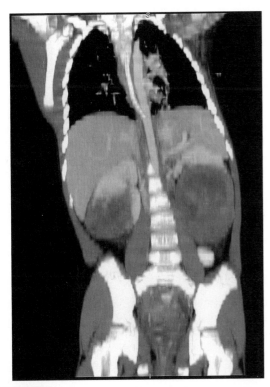

Figure 27-3 Coronal section of a magnetic resonance image demonstrating bilateral Wilms' tumors almost totally replacing normal kidney tissue. No vascular involvement was noted on this study.

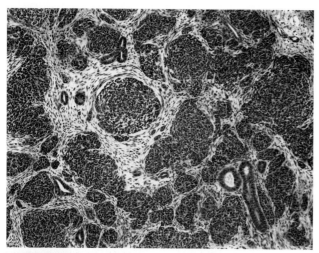

Figure 27–4 Medium-power microscopic view (×100; H&E stain) of Wilms' tumor with tripartite histology. Epithelial elements consist of tubules (lower right-hand portion of image) and abortive tubular structures. The majority of the slide contains cellular blastema with small round primitive cells with scant cytoplasm. The mesenchymal elements have a looser spindle cell configuration.

one of these components (monophasic Wilms' tumors); such tumors can be difficult to distinguish from other childhood tumors.

Other renal tumors that may be clinically confused with Wilms' tumors are congenital mesoblastic nephroma, clear cell sarcoma of the kidney, and rhabdoid tumor of the kidney. Congenital mesoblastic nephromas are low-grade spindle cell tumors that recur locally but rarely metastasize. Clear cell sarcomas and rhabdoid tumors initially were believed to be variants of Wilms' tumors, and they were included as "unfavorable histology" in NWTS-1. However, with better histologic, immunohistochemical, and molecular characterization of these two tumors, it has been found that neither has a relationship to Wilms' tumors. Indeed, both types of tumors have distinct histopathologic characteristics, aggressive behavior, and a poor response to treatment.

Although Wilms' tumors have an excellent prognosis, each of the three cellular components can exhibit focal or diffuse anaplasia, which is a major indicator of a poor outcome. The presence of anaplasia is currently the only criterion for "unfavorable histology" in a Wilms' tumor. Anaplasia denotes the presence of gigantic polypoid nuclei within the tumor sample. Recognition of this change requires both (1) nuclei with major diameters at least three times those of adjacent cells, with increased chromatin content; and (2) the presence of multipolar or otherwise recognizably polypoid mitotic figures. The criteria distinguishing focal from diffuse anaplasia were recently modified. The original definition of focal anaplasia was based on the amount of anaplasia present. Any tumor with anaplastic nuclear changes present in less than 10% of microscopic fields was originally designated as having focal anaplasia. This criterion permitted inclusion when anaplasia was present throughout the tumor, albeit at low density, and cases of anaplasia in extrarenal sites or in metastatic deposits. The new definition emphasizes the

distribution of anaplasia and requires that anaplastic nuclear changes be confined to sharply restricted foci within the primary tumor. The overall incidence of anaplasia varies from 3.2% to 7.3%.[14,141] Anaplasia is rarely seen in tumors of patients younger than 2 years at diagnosis; its incidence increases to about 13% in patients older than 5 years.[57] A higher incidence has recently been reported in female patients and in non-Caucasian patients.[14,141] Anaplastic Wilms' tumors frequently show aneuploidy and mutations in the tumor suppressor gene *p53*.[113]

Clear Cell Sarcoma of the Kidney

Also known as "bone metastasizing renal tumor of childhood,"[94] clear cell carcinoma of the kidney is a distinctive renal neoplasm of childhood that has a propensity for a more widespread pattern of metastases than Wilms' tumor, including bone, brain, and soft tissue. This tumor has a high rate of recurrence and mortality, and it is essential that this entity be recognized to facilitate the early administration of more effective chemotherapy regimens than those employed for Wilms' tumor. There are several variants of clear cell sarcoma of the kidney, including the classic pattern, the hyalinizing pattern, and the epithelioid pattern.

Rhabdoid Tumor of the Kidney

Rhabdoid tumor of the kidney is a distinctive renal neoplasm most often encountered in infants younger than 1 year; it is uncommon in patients older than 5 years.[6,137] It is extremely aggressive and is the most prognostically unfavorable pediatric renal neoplasm. The most distinctive features of rhabdoid tumor of the kidney are large cells with large, vesicular nuclei (Fig. 27-5); a prominent single nucleolus; and the presence of cytoplasmic inclusions composed of whorled masses of intermediate filaments. Another distinctive feature is the aggressive, invasive pattern of this lesion (Fig. 27-6). Rhabdoid tumor of the kidney has a diverse immunohistochemical profile, and the same cell can be positive for many supposedly incompatible epitopes for epithelial, myogenous, neural, and mesenchymal cell types. Features that are helpful in identifying rhabdoid tumor of the kidney include the presence of hypercalcemia and widespread lymphogenous and hematogenous metastases in an infant.

Nephrogenic Rests

In a kidney with Wilms' tumor, associated renal developmental abnormalities called nephrogenic rests (nephroblastomatosis) are often present (Fig. 27-7). These rests are small foci of persistent primitive blastemic cells that are normally found in neonatal kidneys.[9] The kidneys of virtually all children with inherited susceptibility to Wilms' tumor contain nephrogenic rests, thereby providing evidence of a constitutional defect in kidney development. In addition, 25% to 40% of children with sporadic

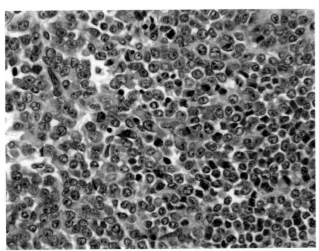

Figure 27-5   High-power microscopic view (×400) of tumor cells with eccentric nuclei and prominent, glassy, inclusion-like eosinophilic cytoplasm. These features merit the descriptor "rhabdoid" (muscle like).

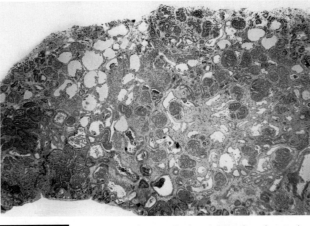

Figure 27-7   Low-power microscopic view (×20) of nephrogenic rest, with aggregates of primitive metanephric tissue with dark-staining blastema and primitive tubule formation. Normal tubules are present in the lower left portion of the image.

Wilms' tumor have nephrogenic rests within the nearby "normal" kidney tissue.[9]

A report from our group noted that the same somatic mutation of *WT1* was present in the Wilms' tumor and in the nearby nephrogenic rests, providing molecular evidence that nephrogenic rests may be premalignant lesions.[107] The association between nephrogenic rests and the genetic loci implicated in Wilms' tumor may also be reflected in the anatomic location of these premalignant lesions.[7,9] Nephrogenic rests developing at the periphery of the renal lobe (perilobar nephrogenic rests) are usually found in children with BWS. Intralobar nephrogenic rests, which may arise anywhere in the renal lobe, are typically found in children with aniridia or other features associated with *WT1*.[9] These observations suggest that the various Wilms' tumor genes may be involved in distinct developmental pathways in the kidney and that their inactivation may interrupt normal kidney development at specific times.

STAGING

The following staging system was used in the NWTS-5 protocol and was modified from previous NWTSG trials.

Stage I: The tumor is limited to the kidney and is completely resected. It did not rupture and was not biopsied before removal. The renal capsule has an intact outer surface. The vessels of the renal sinus are not involved, and there is no evidence of tumor at or beyond the margins of resection.

Stage II: The tumor extends beyond the kidney but is completely resected. There is regional extension of tumor (i.e., penetration of the renal capsule or extensive invasion of the renal sinus). The blood vessels outside the renal parenchyma, including those of the renal sinus, contain tumor. The tumor was biopsied (except for fine-needle aspiration) before removal, or there was spillage of tumor before or during surgery that is confined to the flank and does not involve the peritoneal surface. There is no evidence of tumor at or beyond the margins of resection.

Stage III: Residual nonhematogenous tumor is present, confined to the abdomen. Any one of the following may occur:

1. Lymph nodes within the abdomen or pelvis are found to be involved by tumor (renal hilar, para-aortic, or beyond).
2. The tumor has penetrated through the peritoneal surface.
3. Tumor implants are found on the peritoneal surface.

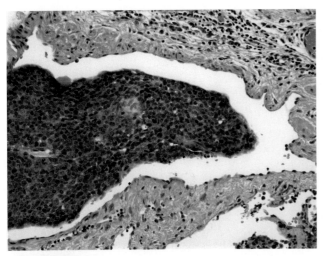

Figure 27-6   Medium-power microscopic view (×100) showing "tongue" of tumor within a vascular channel, an indicator of extensive angiolymphatic invasion.

4. Gross or microscopic tumor remains postoperatively (e.g., tumor cells are found at the margin of surgical resection on microscopic examination).

5. The tumor is not completely resectable because of local infiltration into vital structures.

6. Tumor spill, not confined to the flank, occurred either before or during surgery.

Stage IV: Hematogenous metastases (e.g., lung, liver, bone, brain) or lymph node metastases outside the abdominopelvic region are present. Pulmonary nodules not detected on chest radiographs but visible on chest CT do not mandate treatment with whole-lung irradiation, and such patients are treated according to the stage of the renal tumor.

Stage V: Bilateral renal involvement is present at diagnosis. An attempt should be made to stage each side according to the foregoing criteria, based on the extent of disease before biopsy.

TREATMENT

All children with Wilms' tumor should have the benefit of therapy from a team of pediatric physicians consisting of radiologists, pathologists, oncologists, surgeons, anesthesiologists, and radiotherapists. Cosentino et al.[33] reported their 25-year experience with Wilms' tumor at Children's Memorial Hospital in Chicago. They noted an increased survival in patients who were treated primarily at their specialized children's hospital compared with those who had surgical excision of Wilms' tumor by general surgeons and general urologists followed by subsequent referral.

Operative Therapy

Despite the advances in multimodal treatment of Wilms' tumor, surgical staging and tumor resection remain the central components of therapy[123] (Fig. 27-8). The surgeon must remove the tumor, determine the intra-abdominal stage by lymph node sampling, and carefully examine the liver and the contralateral kidney. Even if the tumor is considered nonresectable, an open biopsy furnishes an adequate sample of the tumor and allows intra-abdominal staging.

The surgical guidelines for management of a possible Wilms' tumor have been clearly outlined. A large transabdominal, transperitoneal incision is recommended for adequate exposure. Thoracic extension may occasionally be necessary. The celiotomy must be large enough to avoid excessive tumor manipulation, which has been associated with increased intraoperative tumor spill. Complete exploration of the abdomen is required. The contralateral kidney should be palpated before nephrectomy to exclude bilateral Wilms' tumors. Gerota's fascia must be incised, the kidney turned to visualize its posterior surface, and any suspicious areas biopsied. Then the lateral peritoneal reflection over the tumor is opened, and the colon is reflected medially. The renal vein and inferior vena cava are palpated carefully to rule out extension of the tumor into the vein. Ideally, this determination should be made by preoperative US. If tumor extension is present, this should be removed en bloc with the kidney. Patients with extension of tumor thrombus above the level of the hepatic veins are probably best managed with preoperative chemotherapy to facilitate shrinkage of the intravascular thrombus.

An attempt should be made to first expose and ligate the renal vessels to lessen the chance of hematogenous

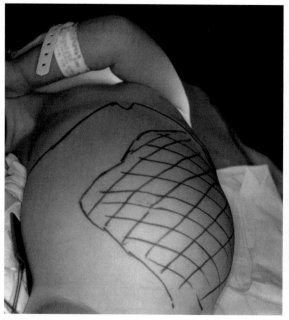
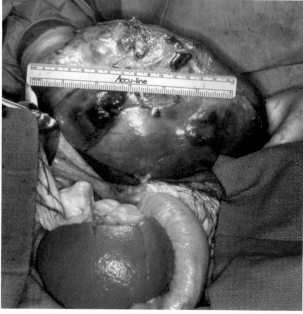

A   B

Figure 27–8   *A,* Schematic of the extent of a large Wilms' tumor. *B,* Large tumor and left kidney after removal.

spread of tumor cells; however, initial ligation should not be performed if it would be technically difficult or dangerous. The analysis of surgical factors in NWTS-1 and NWTS-2 showed that delayed ligation of the renal vein did not produce any deleterious effects.[84] However, intraoperative pulmonary embolism has been reported, and early vein ligation may avert this complication.[127] Care should be taken to avoid rupture of the tumor capsule and tumor spill. The adrenal gland may be left in place if it is not abutting the tumor; if it is (as with superior pole lesions), the adrenal gland should be removed with the neoplasm. The ureter is ligated and divided as low as possible because of the risk of urothelial tumor extension. The tumor and the uninvolved portion of the kidney are mobilized and removed intact. Tumors that involve contiguous structures should be biopsied and staged. These patients can be treated with chemotherapy to shrink the tumor, thereby allowing nephrectomy with preservation of the contiguous organs. Radical en bloc resection of nonessential structures (e.g., tail of the pancreas, segment of diaphragm) should be undertaken only if the surgeon is sure that all disease can be completely removed. If residual neoplasm must be left behind, a biopsy should be done, and the site identified with metallic clips. The use of titanium clips is strongly recommended, as ferromagnetic clips can interfere with CT. Clips are best applied by placing a nonabsorbable suture in the structure to be marked and attaching the clip to the suture.

Partial nephrectomy is generally not indicated in patients with unilateral Wilms' tumor. Exceptions include children with synchronous or metachronous bilateral disease or solitary kidneys. The recommended approach for these patients is initial biopsy followed by combination chemotherapy before definitive surgical resection.

The surgeon should assign a local-regional stage to the tumor based solely on the operative findings. The presence or absence of disease in hilar and regional lymph nodes is an extremely important factor in accurate staging and choice of appropriate therapy. Routine lymph node sampling from the iliac, para-aortic, and celiac areas must be done for accurate staging. Involved or suspicious lymph nodes should be excised, but formal lymph node dissection is not recommended. For accurate staging, it is also important to determine the extent of any peritoneal soilage. The peritoneum is considered "soiled" if there has been a biopsy, there is tumor spill, or the tumor has ruptured. Preoperative incisional or percutaneous needle biopsy using either the anterior or posterior approach is considered local spillage. Incisional biopsy during operation before nephrectomy is considered local spillage unless, in the surgeon's judgment, the entire peritoneal cavity has been soiled in the process (diffuse spill). Tumors are sometimes adherent to adjacent structures (e.g., colon, spleen, diaphragm). Tumors and adherent tissues that are removed en bloc entail no tumor spill. Those that are removed as separate specimens—the neoplastic tissue having been cut across in the process—are considered to involve tumor spill (local or diffuse). When tumor rupture occurs preoperatively and tumor cells are disseminated throughout the peritoneal cavity, the patient's disease is classified as stage III, and radiation therapy must be delivered to the entire peritoneal surface (abdomen and pelvis).

Tumors may be inoperable because of size, extension into the suprahepatic portion of the inferior vena cava, or other reasons. Past experience in the NWTSG and studies conducted by the Societe Internationale d'Oncologie Pediatrique (SIOP) have shown that pretreatment with chemotherapy almost always reduces the bulk of the tumor and renders it resectable.[22,54,56,117,133] It is recommended that all patients undergo initial exploration to assess operability and obtain a biopsy specimen of the tumor, because the staging error rate in nonbiopsied renal masses is 5% to 10%. Patients who are staged by imaging studies alone are also at risk for understaging or overstaging, leading to inappropriate treatment. Once there is adequate reduction in the tumor's size to facilitate nephrectomy, definitive resection should be completed. In general, radiographic re-evaluation should be performed at week 5. Radiographic evidence of persistent disease can occasionally be misleading, because the tumor's failure to shrink could be due to predominance of skeletal muscle or benign elements. If the tumor remains inoperable, biopsy of both the primary tumor and accessible metastatic lesions should be performed. Patients with progressive disease have a very poor prognosis and require treatment with a different, more intensive chemotherapy regimen.[121]

Chemotherapy

Because patients in the United States are treated based on NWTSG protocols, the recently completed NWTS-5 chemotherapy regimens are applied in this section. As a rule, chemotherapy follows radical nephrectomy and lymph node sampling, except in the case of bilateral disease or inoperable tumors. The specific treatment plan varies by stage, patient age, tumor weight, and histology.

TABLE 27-1 National Wilms' Tumor Study-5: Stage I with Favorable or Anaplastic Histology or Stage II with Favorable Histology: Chemotherapy Regimen EE-4A

Week	0	1	2	3	4	5	6	7	8	9	10	11	12	13	14	15	16	17	18
	A			A			A			A			A			A			A
		V	V	V	V	V	V	V	V	V	V		V*			V*			V*

A, dactinomycin (45 µg/kg); V, vincristine (0.05 mg/kg); V*, vincristine (0.067 mg/kg).

TABLE 27–2 National Wilms' Tumor Study-5: Stages III and IV with Favorable Histology or Stages II to IV with Focal Anaplasia: Chemotherapy Regimen DD-4A

Week	0	1	2	3	4	5	6	7	8	9	10	11	12	13	14	15	16	17	18	19	20	21	22	23	24
	A			D+			A			D+			A			D*			A			D*			A
		V	V	V	V	V	V	V	V	V	V	V	V*			V*			V*			V*			V*
	XRT																								

A, dactinomycin (45 µg/kg IV); D*, doxorubicin (1.0 mg/kg IV); D+, doxorubicin (1.5 mg/kg IV); V, vincristine (0.05 mg/kg IV); V*, vincristine (0.067 mg/kg IV); XRT, radiation therapy.

Patients fitting into the following scenarios are treated with nephrectomy and chemotherapy regimen EE-4A (Table 27-1), using dactinomycin and vincristine:

Stage I, favorable histology, age younger than 24 months, tumor weight less than 550 g.
Stage I, favorable histology, age older than 24 months, tumor weight greater than 550 g.
Stage I, focal or diffuse anaplasia.
Stage II, favorable histology.

Patients fitting into the following scenarios are treated with nephrectomy, abdominal irradiation, and triple-drug chemotherapy regimen DD-4A (Table 27-2):

Stage III, favorable histology.
Stage II or III, focal anaplasia.
Stage IV, favorable histology or focal anaplasia. (Pulmonary nodules not detected on chest radiographs but visible on CT do not mandate treatment with whole-lung irradiation. The decision to administer whole-lung irradiation is at the discretion of the investigator.)

Patients fitting into the following scenarios are treated with nephrectomy, abdominal irradiation using 1080 cGy, and four-drug chemotherapy regimen I (Table 27-3):

Stages II to IV, diffuse anaplasia.
Stages I to IV, clear cell sarcoma of the kidney.

There is no universal agreement about the timing of chemotherapy and surgery for resectable unilateral Wilms' tumor.[54] For more than 30 years, SIOP has recommended that the diagnosis of Wilms' tumor be based on imaging and metabolic exclusion of neuroblastoma, or preoperative percutaneous biopsy, and that treatment start with preoperative chemotherapy to improve the stage distribution and decrease the complication rate. Initial SIOP studies disclosed that preoperative chemotherapy and radiotherapy reduced the incidence of tumor spill at surgery.[40] Subsequent authors have continued to emphasize the benefits of this approach, stating that preoperative chemotherapy results in easier operations with significantly fewer tumor ruptures and a favorable stage distribution, without putting the patient at increased risk of postoperative morbidity or reduced survival.[22,56] A recent prospective SIOP study compared 4-week and 8-week preoperative chemotherapy in patients older than 6 months with unilateral Wilms' tumor.[133] No advantage was found with prolonged preoperative treatment for any of the following factors: percent stage I, intraoperative tumor rupture rate (1% versus 3%), 2-year event-free survival (84%), and 5-year overall survival (92% versus 87%).

The NWTSG does not recommend preoperative needle biopsy of unilateral Wilms' tumor because the sample is small, intra-abdominal staging cannot be done, and needle biopsy may cause local spread, intratumor bleeding, or, rarely, rupture. In addition, NWTSG studies have not shown intraoperative rupture to be a major problem, and treatment without pathologic confirmation may cause diagnostic error. This concern was emphasized by Zoeller et al.,[140] who reported both emergency surgery

TABLE 27–3 National Wilms' Tumor Study-5: Stages II to IV with Diffuse Anaplasia or Stages I to IV with Clear Cell Sarcoma of the Kidney: Chemotherapy Regimen I

Week	0	1	2	3	4	5	6	7	8	9	10	11	12	13	14	15	16	17	18	19	20	21	22	23	24
	D						D						D						D						D
		V	V		V	V	V	V	V		V	V	V*	V*					V*						V*
				C			C*			C			C*			C			C*			C			C*
				E						E						E						E			
	XRT																								

C, cyclophosphamide (14.7 mg/kg/day × 5 IV); C*, cyclophosphamide (14.7 mg/kg/day × 3 IV); D, doxorubicin (1.5 mg/kg IV); E, etoposide (3.3 mg/kg/day × 5 IV); V, vincristine (0.05 mg/kg IV); V*, vincristine (0.067 mg/kg IV); XRT, radiation therapy.

performed because of tumor rupture and incorrect diagnosis of renal cell carcinoma in a small cohort of children treated by the SIOP protocol.

In the United States, extensive experience has accumulated using preoperative therapy for children with Wilms' tumor. However, preoperative chemotherapy is considered most appropriate for children with bilateral tumors in whom parenchyma-sparing procedures are desirable,[117] patients with inoperable tumors, and those with extensive intravascular tumor extension. The NWTSG concern is that patients staged by imaging studies alone are at risk for understaging or overstaging. If one chooses to give preoperative therapy based on imaging alone (with or without a needle biopsy), the local tumor should be considered a stage III lesion, and treatment should include regimen DD-4A for patients with favorable or focal anaplasia histology or unknown histology and regimen I for patients with diffuse anaplasia histology.

The UKCCSG Wilms' Tumor Study 3 has adopted preoperative chemotherapy for Wilms' tumors but requires a prechemotherapy biopsy for histologic diagnosis. A recent review of the usefulness and safety of prechemotherapy biopsy noted that biopsy material was not diagnostic in 4% of patients, and in 12% the biopsy revealed tumors other than Wilms' tumor.[135] Of the 182 children who had percutaneous cutting needle biopsy, a fall in hemoglobin (20% of cases) and local pain (19%) were the most common complications. One child required emergency nephrectomy due to massive intratumoral bleeding, another had tumor rupture and subsequently died, and a third developed a needle tract tumor recurrence 8 months after the biopsy.

Radiotherapy

Since the early decades of the 20th century, radiation therapy has played an important role in the management of Wilms' tumor. In the past, high radiation doses and eccentric field arrangements were responsible for significant late toxicity; however, examination of long-term survivors and information obtained from the NWTSG and SIOP studies have allowed us to tailor radiation fields and doses to provide high levels of local tumor control with minimal late effects.[39]

Patients with stage I and II tumors with favorable histology do not require abdominal irradiation. Children with stage I anaplastic Wilms' tumor do not receive abdominal irradiation, but those with stages II to IV do. All patients with clear cell sarcoma of the kidney receive postoperative radiotherapy.

All stage III patients are given postoperative irradiation totaling 1080 cGy in 6 fractions. Tumor bed irradiation is used when only hilar lymphadenopathy is present or when there is residual disease confined to the flank. The field is extended across the midline to include all the vertebral bodies at the levels concerned, but not far enough to overlap any portion of the contralateral kidney. The portals are extended (e.g., for the entire length of the para-aortic chains) when these nodes are involved. Total abdominal irradiation is given when there is diffuse peritoneal seeding, gross tumor spillage within the abdominal cavity during surgery, or preoperative intraperitoneal rupture. For stage IV patients, infradiaphragmatic irradiation is given if the primary tumor would have qualified as stage III; otherwise, no abdominal radiotherapy is administered. When stage IV patients have pulmonary metastases, both lungs are treated, regardless of the number and location of visible metastases. The portals cover both lungs, specifically including the apices and posterior inferior portions, and 1200 cGy is administered in 8 fractions.

TREATMENT CHALLENGES

Intracaval and Atrial Extension

Tumors that extend into the renal vein or vena cava present particular problems.[25] Preoperative US usually demonstrates the extent of any problem accurately. Pulmonary tumor embolus is a risk, and infracardiac caval occlusion and exploration are recommended. When the proximal extent of the thrombus can be clearly established, the vena cava is occluded above that point and opened, and the tumor thrombus is removed. Some prefer to open the cava without proximal occlusion and insert a large-bore, open-ended suction tube into the vein and advance it as the tumor is sucked out. If the tumor is adherent to the wall of the vena cava, removal by balloon catheter is required. A recent report illustrated an unusual case in which the tumor within the cava was tightly adherent to the venous wall and required complete excision of the vena cava and left renal vein and a portion of the iliac system.[115] Free-floating and adherent tumors are classified as stage II, but if the tumor invades the wall of the vein, it should be considered stage III.[49]

Most authors agree that tumor growth into the suprahepatic vena cava and atrium requires cardiopulmonary bypass when managed surgically.[23] However, if the tumor can be localized and controlled below the atrium, resection without the use of cardiopulmonary bypass may limit morbidity. Lodge et al.[90] described a technique in which tumor thrombectomy was performed without the use of cardiopulmonary bypass. They used transesophageal echocardiography to localize the tumor thrombus and an upper midline extension of the transverse abdominal incision to obtain intrapericardial control of the inferior vena cava (Fig. 27-9A) before extracting the tumor thrombus from the infrahepatic vena cava (Fig. 27-9B).

Previous data showed that primary surgical removal of tumors with intracaval extension is associated with an increased incidence of surgical complications.[119] This was particularly true for those patients with extension above the level of the hepatic veins or even farther into the right atrium. These extensive tumors can be managed with preoperative chemotherapy to facilitate shrinkage of the intravascular thrombus.[120] Preoperative therapy allows the caval tumor extension to shrink or even totally disappear, thereby obviating the need for cardiopulmonary bypass for removal of the tumor thrombus.

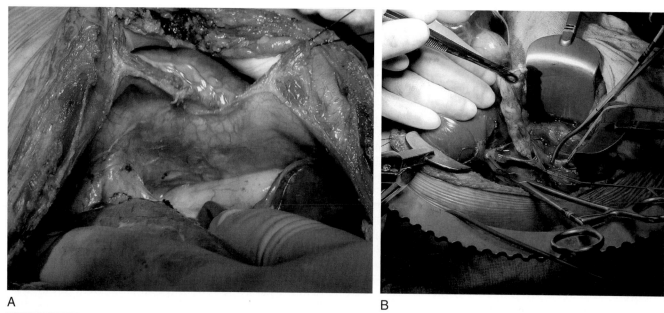

A B

Figure 27–9 *A*, Close-up intraoperative procedure. The surgeon's hand is displacing the liver down, exposing the suprahepatic inferior vena cava below the diaphragm. Just above that, the diaphragm has been incised, along with the pericardium, in anticipation of intrapericardial control of the inferior vena cava. *B*, Intraoperative picture of extraction of tumor embolus from the vena cava below the liver.

A recent review detailed the outcomes of children who had intravascular extension into the inferior vena cava or atrium.[125] Of 2731 patients in NWTS-4, 165 (6%) had intravascular extension of Wilms' tumor. The level of extension was the inferior vena cava in 134 (4.9%) and the atrium in 31 (1.1%). Sixty-nine patients (55 with inferior vena cava extension and 14 with atrial extension) received preoperative therapy. Complications during preoperative chemotherapy were seen in five patients. The intravascular extension of the tumor regressed in 39 of 49 children with comparable pre- and post-therapy radiographic studies, including 7 of 12 in whom the tumor regressed from an atrial location, thus obviating the need for cardiopulmonary bypass. Surgical complications occurred in 36.7% of the children in the atrial group and 17.2% in the inferior vena caval group. The frequency of surgical complications was 26% in the primary resection group versus 13.2% in the group undergoing preoperative therapy. When all the complications of therapy were considered, the incidence of complications among those receiving preoperative therapy was not statistically different from the incidence among those undergoing primary resection. The difference in 3-year relapse-free survival (76.9% for 165 patients with intravascular extension; 80.3% for 1622 patients with no extension) was not statistically significant. Thus, preoperative treatment facilitated resection by decreasing the extent of the tumor thrombus, but the overall frequency of complications was similar in both groups.

Bilateral Tumor

Patients who present with bilateral Wilms' tumor (stage V) account for approximately 5% of all cases (Fig. 27-10).

The surgical management of these patients remains controversial. Some groups have advocated bilateral nephrectomy followed by transplantation. Another approach uses ex vivo tumor dissection followed by autotransplantation in an attempt to preserve functioning renal tissue.[41] However, reviews of children treated with preoperative chemotherapy based on NWTS regimens indicate that they have an excellent prognosis; survival rates for those having a favorable histology exceed 80% at 2 years[11,13] and 70% at 10 years after diagnosis.[100] However, there is an increased risk of renal failure in these patients. Concerns regarding the impact of hyperfiltration injury on patients

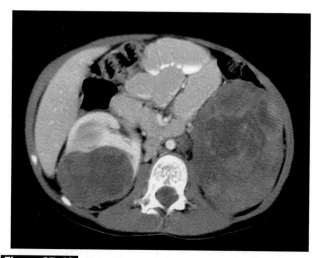

Figure 27–10 Abdominal computed tomography scan showing bilateral Wilms' tumor. The darker-appearing tumor tissue has totally replaced the left kidney and is in the posterior portion of the right kidney.

with less than 50% of the renal parenchyma remaining after resection, and the presence of renal failure in 5.4% of long-term survivors of bilateral Wilms' tumor, have resulted in a more conservative surgical approach in these patients. Identifying these patients at the time of initial diagnosis is important to facilitate renal-sparing surgery. The study by Coppes et al.[27] identified the joint presence of perilobar nephrogenic rests and intralobar nephrogenic rests, or the presence of perilobar nephrogenic rests in children diagnosed during the first year of life, as important risk factors. These features did not predict all future events, however, and further study is warranted.

Patients treated by preoperative chemotherapy have an equivalent survival to those undergoing initial radical surgery, but more renal units can be preserved in those given preoperative chemotherapy. Thus, radical excision of the tumor should not be attempted at the initial operation. Partial nephrectomy or wedge excision can be performed at the initial operation only if all tumor can be removed, with preservation of the majority of renal parenchyma on both sides. Bilateral biopsies should be obtained to confirm the presence of Wilms' tumor in both kidneys and define the histologic type. Discordant pathology may be observed in 4% of cases. Suspicious lymph nodes should be biopsied, and a surgical stage assigned to each side.

For patients fitting the following scenarios, chemotherapy regimen EE-4A (see Table 27-1) should be administered after the initial surgical biopsy and staging:

Bilateral stage I with favorable histology or focal or diffuse anaplasia.
Bilateral tumors, one or both kidneys evaluated as stage II, with favorable histology.

For patients fitting the following scenarios, chemotherapy regimen DD-4A (see Table 27-2) is used:

Bilateral stage II with focal anaplasia.
Bilateral stage III or IV with favorable histology or focal anaplasia.
Patients with bilateral stage II, III, or IV tumor with diffuse anaplasia are treated initially with regimen I (see Table 27-3).

The response to therapy should be evaluated after week 5 by CT scan to assess the reduction in tumor volume and the feasibility of partial resection. At the time of the second-look procedure, partial nephrectomy should be done only if it will not compromise tumor resection and only if negative margins can be obtained. If there is extensive tumor involvement precluding partial resection in one kidney, complete excision of tumor from the least involved kidney is performed. If this procedure leaves a viable and functioning kidney, radical nephrectomy is performed to remove the opposite kidney. If there is a possibility that the remaining kidney can be salvaged, only a biopsy should be obtained, and the extent of disease delineated with titanium clips. Additional chemotherapy is then given, and the patient is reassessed before week 12. If there is persistent disease, the patient should receive radiation therapy.

Approximately 1% of children with unilateral Wilms' tumor develop contralateral disease. Coppes et al.[27] assessed the demographic and histologic features associated with metachronous bilateral Wilms' tumor by reviewing all children registered during the first four NWTSs.[27] Fifty-eight of 4669 registered children developed metachronous bilateral Wilm's tumor. The cumulative incidence of contralateral disease 6 years after initial diagnosis decreased from greater than 3% in NWTS-1 to approximately 1.5% in the three subsequent studies ($P = 0.08$). Patients with nephrogenic rests had a significantly increased risk of metachronous disease; this was particularly true for young children (20 of 206 aged younger than 12 months, compared with 0 of 304 aged older than 12 months).

A report from the Children's Hospital of Philadelphia reviewed the experience with renal salvage procedures in patients with bilateral Wilms' tumor.[26] From 1982 to 1997, 23 children with bilateral Wilms' tumor were treated with partial nephrectomy, including 7 who were also treated with brachytherapy. Anaplasia was the most significant factor associated with an unfavorable outcome ($P = 0.003$). The authors concluded that (1) preoperative chemotherapy followed by nephron-sparing surgery is indicated in patients with bilateral Wilms' tumor, except those with diffuse anaplasia, and (2) brachytherapy should be considered for local disease involving chemoresistant tumors.

Tumor in Horseshoe Kidney

Wilms' tumor arising within a horseshoe kidney presents a difficult diagnostic and therapeutic challenge (Fig. 27-11A). The incidence of horseshoe kidneys in the general population is 1 in 400.[76] Neville et al.[102] described 41 of 8617 patients (0.48%) enrolled in the NWTSG from 1969 to 1998 who developed a Wilms' tumor in a horseshoe kidney, suggesting that Wilms' tumor is 1.96 times more common in patients with horseshoe kidney than in the general population. In their study, horseshoe kidney was not recognized preoperatively in 13 patients, 10 of whom were evaluated with CT. Primary surgical resection was performed in 26 patients, and 15 children were treated with preoperative chemotherapy after biopsy. Surgical complications occurred in 14.6% of patients, including two urine leaks, two ureteral obstructions, and one ureteral injury. Although 37% of Wilms' tumors arising in a horseshoe kidney were judged inoperable at initial exploration, all were amenable to resection after chemotherapy.

Present NWTSG recommendations are as follows: At initial exploration, if the tumor is resectable and involves only one side of the horseshoe kidney, resection is recommended. In bilateral cases, accurate surgical staging should be performed via biopsies of all tumors and any suspicious lymph nodes. The patient should then receive stage-appropriate adjuvant therapy, followed by second-look surgery approximately 6 weeks later to assess tumor response and perform definitive resection if possible (Fig. 27-11B). Despite the frequency of tumor entrance into the collecting system in these difficult cases, the overall incidence of surgical complications in patients with horseshoe kidneys is similar to that reported for other NWTS patients.[119,122]

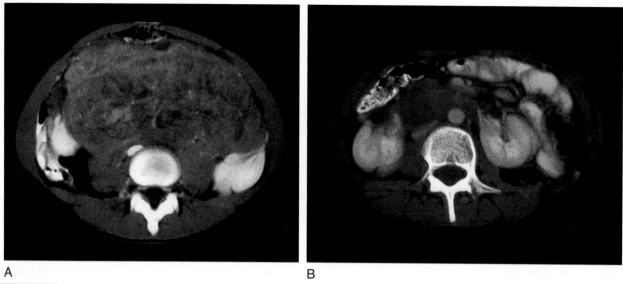

A   B

Figure 27–11 *A*, Massive midline Wilms' tumor in a horseshoe kidney. *B*, Same tumor after preoperative chemotherapy. There has been marked shrinkage, making the tumor amenable to resection, leaving two functioning renal units on both sides of the spine.

Partial Nephrectomy

Partial nephrectomy for unilateral disease remains controversial. A SIOP report examined the experience with partial nephrectomy for children with renal tumors.[21] Surgical criteria for partial resection included tumor confined to one pole of the kidney and occupying less than a third of the kidney, no invasion of the renal vein or collecting system, and clear margins around the tumor. Using these criteria, 13 of 90 cases were suitable for partial nephrectomy. Of these 13 patients, 5 underwent partial nephrectomy. None of the 5 patients had a positive margin or recurrent local disease, and ipsilateral renal function was preserved in all cases.

Recurrent Disease

Shamberger et al.[124] reviewed the data for the 100 NWTS-4 patients (out of 2482) who developed local recurrence. The greatest relative risk for local recurrence was observed in patients with stage III disease, unfavorable histology, and tumor spill during surgery. Multiple regression analysis indicated that tumor spill and the absence of lymph node biopsy were associated with an increased relative risk of recurrence. Survival after local recurrence was poor, with a 2-year survival rate of 43%. Survival was also dependent on initial stage; those who received more therapy before relapse had a worse prognosis. This study demonstrated that tumor spill results in an increased risk of local relapse and reaffirmed the importance of lymph node sampling so that tumors are neither understaged nor undertreated.

A recent retrospective review of 54 patients with recurrent Wilms' tumor observed that the 5-year overall survival estimates were 63.6% for patients treated after 1984, compared with 20.6% for patients treated before 1984.[42]

No patient with recurrent anaplastic histology survived. Only three patients received high-dose chemotherapy with autologous stem cell rescue, indicating significant progress in the treatment of recurrent favorable-histology Wilms' tumor using salvage regimens with conventional chemotherapy.

Early recognition of recurrence may improve outcome. Researchers from the United Kingdom recently studied serum VEGF levels in 13 children with Wilms' tumor.[12] Before surgery, the median VEGF level was 20 ng/mL; by the week after operation, levels had fallen to 1.9 ng/mL ($P < 0.001$, ANOVA). Six months after tumor resection, three of the children had died. A VEGF level greater than 10 ng/mL 3 months after surgery suggested tumor recurrence in the three patients who died.

PROGNOSTIC FACTORS

Histology

Early on, the prognostic importance of Wilms' tumor histology was appreciated, with the 12% of Wilms' tumors with "unfavorable histology" accounting for more than half of the deaths. In the late 1970s, patients with stage II to IV Wilms' tumor with diffuse anaplasia were noted to have a poor prognosis with conventional therapy.[10,14,141] A preliminary analysis of the results of NWTS-3 suggested that the addition of cyclophosphamide to the standard three drugs—vincristine, dactinomycin, and doxorubicin—improved the relapse-free survival.[35] After revising the definition of focal and diffuse anaplasia, Faria et al.[48] noted that the addition of cyclophosphamide had a dramatic effect on the 4-year relapse-free percentage of patients with diffuse anaplasia. No such effect was identified in patients with focal anaplasia[58]; their prognosis was similar to that of similarly staged patients with favorable histology. Patients with stage IV disease and diffuse anaplasia had a 4-year relapse-free survival rate of 16.7%, despite treatment with the four-drug regimen, indicating a need for further intensification of therapy.

Recently, mutational analysis of 140 Wilms' tumors showed an association between Wilms' tumors with anaplastic features and the occurrence of *p53* mutations.[3] However, because a *p53* mutation had also been identified in a Wilms' tumor with favorable histologic features, it remained to be determined whether *p53* alterations can be used as a molecular marker for anaplastic Wilms' tumors or as a marker for an adverse outcome. To address that question, investigators studied 97 Wilms' tumors for *p53* expression and correlated expression with outcome.[130] They detected *p53* in 13 of 97 tumors and found that it was associated with disease relapse (39% versus 17%; $P = 0.06$) but not anaplasia. Among *p53*-negative patients, only 5% had metastatic disease, compared with 31% of *p53*-positive patients ($P = 0.038$). Overall survival at 1 year was 94% for *p53*-negative patients and 85% for *p53*-positive patients ($P = 0.34$).

In 2002, SIOP noted that certain histologic features that remain after preoperative chemotherapy, such as blastema, are of prognostic significance, whereas others are not. Therefore, in the next SIOP trials and study, a revised classification of renal tumors will be followed for treatment purposes: completely necrotic (low-risk tumors), blastemic (high-risk tumors), and others (intermediate-risk tumors).[136]

DNA Content

Increased tumor cell DNA content has been correlated with a more favorable prognosis in children with a variety of tumors, including embryonal rhabdomyosarcoma,[106] neuroblastoma,[91] and acute lymphoblastic leukemia.[134] For Wilms' tumor, however, the data have been mixed; aneuploidy was associated with a worse prognosis among patients with favorable-histology Wilms' tumors in one series[70] but not in another.[5] More recently, possible chromosomal prognostic factors have been identified by Grundy et al.,[69] who evaluated DNA gain and loss for several chromosomal segments. In a study of 232 children registered during NWTS-3 and NWTS-4, LOH of 16q markers was present in 17.2% of tumor tissue and was associated with a statistically significantly worse 2-year relapse-free and overall survival. LOH of chromosome 1p markers, present in tumor tissue from 11% of children with Wilms' tumor, was associated with poorer relapse-free and overall survival rates, which were of borderline statistical significance ($P = 0.08$ and 0.12, respectively). In contrast, LOH for 11p markers or duplication of 1q, present in 33% and 25% of cases, respectively, was not associated with any difference in outcome. Study of the prognostic significance of tumor cell DNA content was continued in NWTS-5, with the hope that newly confirmed DNA variables will facilitate the tailoring of treatment to anticipated outcome.

Conflicting data were presented by 13 member laboratories of the U.K. Cancer Cytogenetics Group.[15] In a review of 127 abnormal karyotypes, univariate survival analysis showed no significant adverse effects for karyotype complexity, 1p loss, or 11p loss. The poor outcome of cases with 16q loss was of borderline significance, and the association between relapse risk and gain of 1q material was not significant. Only monosomy 22 was a significant marker of poor outcome (13 cases showing 50% relapse-free survival at 5 years, compared with 79% survival for the remaining 114 cases; $P = 0.02$).

Hing et al.[73] undertook an analysis of comparative genomic hybridization of 58 samples of favorable-histology Wilms' tumors taken at initial diagnosis or relapse. Gain of 1q was significantly more frequent in the relapse group (27 of 46 [59%] versus 5 of 21 [24%]; $P = 0.019$). This result suggests that identifying 1q gain at diagnosis could be used to select patients with an increased risk of relapse who might benefit from early treatment intensification. Lu et al.[93] confirmed this study, noting that in 18 cases of Wilms' tumor with favorable histology, relative overexpression of genes on the long arm of chromosome 1 was seen in all tumors that relapsed, but in none that remained in remission.

Gene Expression

Examining the expression of tyrosine kinase (Trk) receptors in 39 children with Wilms' tumor, Eggert et al.[46] noted that children with high levels of full-length TrkB mRNA (TrkBfull) had a significantly greater risk of death than children whose tumors had little or no TrkBfull expression ($P = 0.02$). The 5-year relapse-free survival was 100% for patients with low tumor expression of TrkBfull, compared with 65% for those with high tumor expression of TrkBfull ($P < 0.003$). Conversely, children with tumors that expressed high mRNA levels of a functionally inactive truncated TrkB receptor (TrkBtrunc) had a greater 5-year relapse-free survival than did children with low levels of TrkBtrunc (95% versus 68%; $P = 0.005$).

Ghamen et al.[53] evaluated the prognostic value of various apoptosis-associated regulatory proteins, such as Bcl-2, Bax, and Bcl-X, in a group of 61 Wilms' tumors. An increased expression of Bcl-2 was observed in the blastemic component of increasing pathologic stages, while a gradual decline of Bax expression was observed. Univariate analysis showed that blastemic Bcl-2 expression and the Bcl-2/Bax ratio were indicative of clinical progression, and blastemic Bcl-2 expression was a prognostic marker for clinical progression, independent of stage.

Growth Factors

Previous reports noted that the sera and urine of children with Wilms' tumor often contain increased concentrations of hyaluronan. Using a mouse heterotransplant model, Lovvorn et al.[92] noted that the sera of mice supporting tumor growth had a median hyaluronan concentration of 9379 µg/L, compared with a median concentration of 416 µg/L in animals not supporting tumor growth.[92] The highest serum hyaluronan concentrations were detected in animals harboring blastema-predominant tumors with an unfavorable histology. Complete resection of established tumors also resulted in the return of serum hyaluronan to preheterotransplant concentrations.

Lin et al.[88] measured bFGF levels in preoperative and postoperative urine samples from 97 patients with Wilms' tumor. Urinary bFGF was elevated in 42% of preoperative samples, and higher-stage tumors resulted in higher preoperative levels. Patients with relapse or persistent disease had significantly elevated postoperative bFGF levels.

Kayton et al.[81] detected VEGF with increasing frequency and quantity in a mouse model of Wilms' tumor. Lung metastases occurred in 8 of 10 animals with VEGF-positive tumors but in only 3 of 11 animals with VEGF-negative tumors, an association that was statistically significant. VEGF was found in 10 of 12 clinical Wilms' tumor specimens tested.

Davidoff et al.[38] developed adeno-associated virus vectors containing the soluble, truncated form of VEGF receptor-2 (Flk-1), a known inhibitor of endothelial cell activation. Significant antitumor efficacy was observed in two murine models of pediatric kidney tumors. Tumor development was prevented in 10 of 15 mice (67%), with significant growth restriction of tumors in the remaining mice.

OUTCOMES

NWTSG Results

Five therapeutic studies have been completed: NWTS-1 (1969-1974), NWTS-2 (1975-1979), NWTS-3 (1980-1985), NWTS-4 (1986-1995), and NWTS-5 (1995-2002). Five-year survival percentages for patients enrolled in NWTS protocols were 79.7% for 1969-1974 enrollees, 81.6% for 1975-1979, 86.3% for 1980-1984, 88.6% for 1985-1989, and 90.4% for 1990-1995. These are among the highest for all childhood cancers.

The major conclusions of NWTS-1, -2, and -3 were as follows:

1. Postoperative irradiation therapy of the renal bed is not necessary for stage I tumors or for stage II tumors with favorable histology.
2. Survival of patients with stage III, favorable-histology tumors is best when therapy consists of dactinomycin, vincristine, and doxorubicin combined with 1000 cGy radiation therapy to the flank, or dactinomycin and vincristine combined with 2000 cGy radiation therapy.
3. Cyclophosphamide does not improve the prognosis when added to the treatment of stage IV favorable-histology tumors.

As a result of these studies, the 2-year survival rate of children diagnosed with Wilms' tumor rose from 20%[47] to 90%.[35-37]

NWTS-4 found that pulse-intensive actinomycin D and doxorubicin dosing is as efficacious as and less toxic than the traditional divided-dose method; it is also more cost-effective, saving an estimated $790,000 a year.[60,61] NWTS-4 also revealed that 6 months of treatment for stage II to IV favorable-histology tumors is equivalent to 15 months of treatment. Ritchey et al.[122] examined the incidence of surgical complications among patients enrolled in NWTS-4. In a random sample of 534 patients, 68 patients (12.7%) experienced 76 complications. Intestinal obstruction was the most common complication (5.1% of patients), followed by extensive hemorrhage (1.9%), wound infection (1.9%), and vascular injury (1.5%). Intravascular extension into the inferior vena cava, nephrectomy performed through a flank or paramedian incision, and tumor diameter 10 cm or greater were also associated with an increased risk of surgical complications. NWTS-4 also demonstrated that surgical rupture of the tumor must be prevented, because spills produce an increased risk of local relapse.[124]

NWTS-5 (also know as POG 9440 and CCG 4941) opened in July 1995 and closed in June 2002. It had a variety of objectives, including to (1) evaluate the importance of various biologic prognostic factors; (2) decrease the morbidity of treatment by limiting initial therapy; (3) improve the survival of patients with unfavorable-histology tumors, including Wilms' tumor with diffuse anaplasia, clear cell sarcoma of the kidney, and malignant rhabdoid tumor of the kidney; and (4) study the biology and pathology of patients who present with bilateral Wilms' tumor. The results from NWTS-5 with regard to the genetic implications for clinical outcome are still being analyzed and have not been published.

Of particular interest in NWTS-5 was the management of small stage I tumors. Green and Jaffe,[63] in a 1979 review, had suggested that nephrectomy might be adequate therapy for patients younger than 24 months with tumors weighing less than 550 g. A subsequent review of children treated during NWTS-1, -2, and -3 supported the hypothesis that NWTS regimens had not improved the excellent prognosis among this group of children.[59] Thus a "surgery only" arm was developed for investigation in NWTS-5. By March 31, 1998, 69 patients had been entered in the surgery-only treatment arm. Nine patients relapsed: three in the tumor bed or abdomen, one in the pleural space, four in bilateral lungs, and one in the contralateral kidney. The relapse-free survival percentage at 2 years was 82.1%, far below the established relapse-free survival percentage cutoff of 95%. Thus the surgery-only trial was suspended.

European Results

Results from Europe have been similar to NWTS results. For instance, the results of the UKCCSG Second Wilms' Tumor Study were reported in 2000.[99] Four-year event-free survival was as follows: stage I with favorable histology, 94%; stage II with favorable histology, 91%; and stage III with favorable histology, 84%. The outlook for patients with anaplastic or rhabdoid variants was poor. A recent Italian review of 98 nephroblastoma patients treated in three consecutive SIOP trials resulted in a 5-year cure rate of 90%.[79] Clinical course was influenced mainly by diffuse anaplasia and, to a minor extent, by lymph node involvement. A total of 2535 cases registered in 34 population-based cancer registries in 16 European countries were included in a recent EURO-CARE report.[110] The overall, 5-year survival of all children diagnosed from 1985 to 1989 was 83%. There was significantly lower survival among patients registered in the formerly socialist countries of Estonia, Poland, and Slovakia; overall European survival was slightly lower compared with results reported from the United States and Australia.

Specialized Tumors

A review of 4669 patients treated with NWTS-3 and NWTS-4 protocols yielded 53 children with BWS.[111] BWS patients were more likely to present with lower-stage tumors ($P = 0.0001$). The overall survival rate at 4 years for BWS patients was nearly identical to that of patients without BWS (89% versus 90%). Twenty-one percent of patients with BWS had bilateral disease. BWS patients enrolled in NWTS-4 had smaller tumors than those enrolled in NWTS-3 ($P = 0.02$), suggesting that US screening may be efficacious.

Argani et al.[1] reviewed 351 cases of clear cell sarcoma of the kidney, including 182 cases entered in NWTS-1 to -4. Overall survival was 69%, and multivariate analysis revealed four independent prognostic factors for survival: treatment with doxorubicin, stage, age at diagnosis, and tumor necrosis.

The results for children with the WAGR syndrome were analyzed and reported by Breslow et al.[17] Of the 8533 patients enrolled between 1969 and 2002 by the NWTSG, 64 patients (0.75%) had the WAGR syndrome. Comparing WAGR and non-WAGR patients, the average birth weights (2.94 and 3.45 kg), median ages at diagnosis (22 and 39 months), percentage with bilateral disease (17% and 6%), metastatic disease (2% and 13%), favorable-histology tumors (100% and 92%), and intralobar nephrogenic rests (77% and 22%) all differed. Survival estimates for WAGR and non-WAGR patients were similar at 4 year (95% versus 92%) but significantly different at 27 years (48% versus 86%). Five late deaths among WAGR patients were from end-stage renal disease.

Treatment Morbidity and Mortality

An increasing number of children with Wilms' tumor can expect to be cured, reflecting the undisputed progress made in the treatment of children with this renal cancer. However, there is an increasing awareness of the late effects of cancer therapy.[45] The standardized mortality ratio observed in the Childhood Cancer Survivor Study was 9.6 overall and 14.1 for the 5-year survivors of Wilms' tumor. Cumulative mortality was 1.8%, 3.1%, and 5.0% at 10, 15, and 20 years, respectively.[97] Some of the effects occur immediately after treatment (e.g., after the administration of certain chemotherapy) and are usually transient, but they may become permanent. Although children seem to tolerate acute toxicities of therapy better than adults do, the growing child may be more vulnerable to the delayed adverse sequelae of cancer therapy, such as effects on growth, fertility, and neuropsychological function.

Wilms' tumor patients have known risk factors for cardiac, renal, and pulmonary toxicity. NWTS-1 demonstrated that the risk of congestive heart failure persisted for 8 to 12 years or more from the time of anthracycline treatment. Patients treated in NWTS-1 to -4 were reviewed to determine the frequency of congestive heart failure and the risk factors for it following Wilms' tumor treatment with doxorubicin.[62] The cumulative frequency of congestive heart failure was 4.4% at 20 years among patients treated initially and 17.4% at 20 years among those treated for relapsed Wilms' tumor. The relative risk of congestive heart failure was increased in females and by cumulative doxorubicin dose, lung irradiation, and left abdominal irradiation. A more recent report noted that the most important predictor of worsening cardiac performance was total anthracycline dose: patients receiving less than 240 mg/m² showed no cardiac deterioration more than 10 years after the end of treatment.[129]

Children with Wilms' tumor are also at risk for renal dysfunction from a variety of factors, including radiation therapy, use of nephrotoxic chemotherapy agents, a theoretical risk due to hyperfiltration,[43] and the possible involvement of a genetic component (e.g., patients with Denys-Drash syndrome). In 1996 Ritchey et al.[118] reported the spectrum of renal failure in 55 of 5823 patients treated in NWTS-1 to -4, noting that the risk of renal failure at 16 years was 0.6% for all unilateral-disease patients and 13% for bilateral-disease patients.

Survivors of childhood cancer are also at increased risk of developing a second malignant neoplasm, both leukemias and solid tumors. The cumulative risk at 20 years varies between 3% and 10% over several studies and is 5 to 20 times greater than that expected in the general population.[65,128] The incidence of second malignancies following Wilms' tumor in NWTS patients was initially reported in 1988; 15 second malignancies were identified among 2438 patients, and the observed-to-expected ratio, or standardized incidence ratio, was 8.5.[18] These results were updated in 1996, and a similar standardized incidence ratio of 8.4 was observed, with 43 second malignant neoplasms occurring. Three breast cancers were found, and the relative risk in multivariate analysis was 12. To help characterize cases of secondary acute myelogenous leukemia on NWTSG protocols, Shearer et al.[126] reviewed the 7 patients with that disease among the 43 identified as having second malignant neoplasms. All patients received chemotherapy regimens that included doxorubicin[10] or etoposide,[1] and 6 were treated with infradiaphragmatic irradiation. The median latency period from initial diagnosis of the renal neoplasm to development of secondary acute myelogenous leukemia was 3 years (range, 1.2 to 4 years).

Radiation therapy has a variety of adverse effects. One study, designed to estimate the reduction in adult stature induced by radiation therapy of the spine in children treated for Wilms' tumor, noted that height reductions were dependent on dose, portal size, and age at treatment.[74] Younger children were more often affected.

Observed height deficits were 4.1 cm for 57 patients who received 15 to 24 Gy at a mean age of 55 months; there was no height deficit among 16 children who received doses less than 15 Gy at a mean age of 83 months. Another retrospective study was undertaken to determine the possible effect of radiation therapy, chemotherapy, or both on live births, birth weight, and frequency of congenital malformations in pediatric Wilms' tumor survivors.[64] A questionnaire was distributed among survivors of Wilms' tumor treated in NWTS-1 to -4. Respondents reported 427 pregnancies. Women who received flank radiation therapy were at increased risk of fetal malposition and premature labor, and the offspring of these women were at risk for low birth weight, premature birth, and the occurrence of congenital malformations. Importantly, fertility can be preserved in children with Wilms' tumor after upper abdominal radiation therapy (10 to 20 Gy) that does not include the entire pelvis.[80]

FUTURE DIRECTIONS

For the first time since 1969, the NWTS is not conducting a clinical trial of treatment protocols. Current and future efforts are focused on using the large cohort of former Wilms' tumor patients to study the long-term effects of diagnosis and treatment in survivors and to better understand the pathogenesis and cause of Wilms' tumor. The NWTS is currently conducting a Late Effects Study (LATE, also known as POG 9442 and CCG 4941L), which opened in October 1995, designed to identify treatment-related conditions that may develop in participants who were originally treated in one of the five clinical trials. LATE is a federally funded, multi-institutional observational study that follows participants and their children throughout their lives to continue monitoring treatment results and possible late effects. The specific study objectives include the following:

1. Determine the incidence of life-threatening medical conditions in survivors of Wilms' tumor.
2. Determine mortality rates in former Wilms' tumor patients.
3. Determine the risk of serious pregnancy complications and other adverse reproductive events in survivors of Wilms' tumor.
4. Determine the frequency of Wilms' tumor and other cancers in the children and other family members of Wilms' tumor patients.
5. Identify the most informative subgroups of Wilms' tumor patients for use by molecular biologists and epidemiologists.

By identifying the treatment and host factors associated with excess mortality, interventions may be developed to target those at highest risk. Now that 90% of children with Wilms' tumor are being cured, it is most important to focus attention on the duration and quality of life in the survivors. Future Wilms' tumor protocols will be done through the COG. These protocols are still in development at the time of this writing.

REFERENCES

1. Argani P, Perlman EJ, Breslow NE, et al: Clear cell sarcoma of the kidney: A review of 351 cases from the National Wilms' Tumor Study Group Pathology Center. Am J Surg Pathol 2000;24:4-18.
2. Argenta PA, Lin RY, Sullivan KM: Basic fibroblast growth factor is a Wilms' tumor marker. Surg Forum 1994; 45:789.
3. Bardeesy N, Falkoff D, Petruzzi MJ, et al: Anaplastic Wilms' tumour, a subtype displaying poor prognosis, harbours p53 mutations. Nat Genet 1994;7:91-97.
4. Bardeesy N, Zabel B, Schmitt K, et al: WT1 mutations associated with incomplete Denys-Drash syndrome define a domain predicted to behave in a dominant-negative fashion. Genomics 1994;21:663-664.
5. Barrantes JC, Muir KR, Toyn CE, et al: Thirty-year population-based review of childhood renal tumours with an assessment of prognostic features including tumour DNA characteristics. Med Pediatr Oncol 1993;21: 24-30.
6. Beckwith JB: Wilms' tumor and other renal tumors of childhood: A selective review from the National Wilms' Tumor Study Pathology Center. Hum Pathol 1983;14: 481-492.
7. Beckwith JB: Precursor lesions of Wilms' tumor: Clinical and biological implications. Med Pediatr Oncol 1993; 21:158-168.
8. Beckwith JB: Nephrogenic rests and the pathogenesis of Wilms' tumor: Developmental and clinical considerations. Am J Med Genet 1998;79:268-273.
9. Beckwith JB, Kiviat NB, Bonadio JF: Nephrogenic rests, nephroblastomatosis, and the pathogenesis of Wilms' tumor. Pediatr Pathol 1990;10:1-36.
10. Beckwith JB, Palmer NF: Histopathology and prognosis of Wilms' tumors: Results from the First National Wilms' Tumor Study. Cancer 1978;41:1937-1948.
11. Bishop HC, Tefft M, Evans AE, et al: Survival in bilateral Wilms' tumor—review of 30 National Wilms' Tumor Study cases. J Pediatr Surg 1977;12:631-638.
12. Blann AD, Li JL, Li C, et al: Increased serum VEGF in 13 children with Wilms' tumour falls after surgery but rising levels predict poor prognosis. Cancer Lett 2001;173: 183-186.
13. Blute ML, Kelalis PP, Offord KP, et al: Bilateral Wilms' tumor. J Urol 1987;138:968-973.
14. Bonadio JF, Storer B, Norkool P, et al: Anaplastic Wilms' tumor: Clinical and pathologic studies. J Clin Oncol 1985; 3:513-520.
15. Bown N, Cotterill SJ, Roberts P, et al: Cytogenetic abnormalities and clinical outcome in Wilms' tumor: A study by the UK Cancer Cytogenetics Group and the UK Children's Cancer Study Group. Med Pediatr Oncol 2002; 38:11-21.
16. Breslow N, Olshan A, Beckwith JB, et al: Epidemiology of Wilms' tumor. Med Pediatr Oncol 1993;21:172-181.
17. Breslow NE, Norris R, Norkool PA, et al: Characteristics and outcomes of children with the Wilms' tumor-aniridia syndrome: A report from the National Wilms' Tumor Study Group. J Clin Oncol 2003;21:4579-4585.
18. Breslow NE, Olson J, Moksness J, et al: Familial Wilms' tumor: A descriptive study. Med Pediatr Oncol 1996; 27:398-403.
19. Bunin GR, Meadows AT: Epidemiology and Wilms' tumor: Approaches and methods. Med Pediatr Oncol 1993;21: 169-171.

20. Call KM, Glaser T, Ito CY, et al: Isolation and characterization of a zinc finger polypeptide gene at the human chromosome 11 Wilms' tumor locus. Cell 1990;60:509-520.
21. Canning DA: Is partial nephrectomy appropriate treatment for unilateral Wilms' tumor? J Urol 1999;161:367.
22. Capra ML, Walker DA, Mohammed WM, et al: Wilms' tumor: A 25-year review of the role of preoperative chemotherapy. J Pediatr Surg 1999;34:579-582.
23. Chiappini B, Savini C, Marinelli G, et al: Cavoatrial tumor thrombus: Single-stage surgical approach with profound hypothermia and circulatory arrest, including a review of the literature. J Thorac Cardiovasc Surg 2002;124:684-688.
24. Choyke PL, Siegel MJ, Craft AW, et al: Screening for Wilms' tumor in children with Beckwith-Wiedemann syndrome or idiopathic hemihypertrophy. Med Pediatr Oncol 1999;32:196-200.
25. Clayman RV, Sheldon CA, Gonzales R: Wilms' tumor: An approach to vena caval intrusion. Prog Pediatr Surg 1983;15:285-290.
26. Cooper CS, Jaffe WI, Huff DS, et al: The role of renal salvage procedures for bilateral Wilms' tumor: A 15-year review. J Urol 2000;163:265-268.
27. Coppes MJ, Arnold M, Beckwith JB, et al: Factors affecting the risk of contralateral Wilms' tumor development: A report from the National Wilms' Tumor Study Group. Cancer 1999;85:1616-1625.
28. Coppes MJ, Bonetta L, Huang A, et al: Loss of heterozygosity mapping in Wilms' tumor indicates the involvement of three distinct regions and a limited role for nondisjunction or mitotic recombination. Genes Chromosomes Cancer 1992;5:326-334.
29. Coppes MJ, de Kraker J, van Dijken PJ, et al: Bilateral Wilms' tumor: Long-term survival and some epidemiological features. J Clin Oncol 1989;7:310-315.
30. Coppes MJ, Haber DA, Grundy PE: Genetic events in the development of Wilms' tumor. N Engl J Med 1994;331:586-590.
31. Coppes MJ, Huff V, Pelletier J: Denys-Drash syndrome: Relating a clinical disorder to genetic alterations in the tumor suppressor gene WT1.J Pediatr 1993;123:673-678.
32. Coppes MJ, Pritchard-Jones K: Principles of Wilms' tumor biology. Urol Clin North Am 2000;27:423-433.
33. Cosentino CM, Raffensperger JG, Luck SR, et al: A 25-year experience with renal tumors of childhood. J Pediatr Surg 1993;28:1350-1355.
34. Crist WM, Kun LE: Common solid tumors of childhood. N Engl J Med 1991;324:461-471.
35. D'Angio GJ, Breslow N, Beckwith JB, et al: Treatment of Wilms' tumor: Results of the Third National Wilms' Tumor Study. Cancer 1989;64:349-360.
36. D'Angio GJ, Evans AE, Breslow N, et al: The treatment of Wilms' tumor: Results of the National Wilms' Tumor Study. Cancer 1976;38:633-646.
37. D'Angio GJ, Evans A, Breslow N, et al: The treatment of Wilms' tumor: Results of the Second National Wilms' Tumor Study. Cancer 1981;47:2302-2311.
38. Davidoff AM, Nathwani AC, Spurbeck WW, et al: rAAV-mediated long-term liver-generated expression of an angiogenesis inhibitor can restrict renal tumor growth in mice. Cancer Res 2002;62:3077-3083.
39. Davies-Johns T, Chidel M, Macklis RM: The role of radiation therapy in the management of Wilms' tumor. Semin Urol Oncol 1999;17:46-54.
40. de Kraker J, Voute PA, Lemerle J, et al: Preoperative chemotherapy in Wilms' tumour: Results of clinical trials and studies on nephroblastomas conducted by the International Society of Paediatric Oncology (SIOP). Prog Clin Biol Res 1982;100:131-144.
41. Desai D, Nicholls G, Duffy PG: Bench surgery with autotransplantation for bilateral synchronous Wilms' tumor: A report of three cases. J Pediatr Surg 1999;34:632-634.
42. Dome JS, Liu T, Krasin M, et al: Improved survival for patients with recurrent Wilms' tumor: The experience at St. Jude Children's Research Hospital. J Pediatr Hematol Oncol 2002;24:192-198.
43. Donckerwolcke RM, Coppes MJ: Adaptation of renal function after unilateral nephrectomy in children with renal tumors. Pediatr Nephrol 2001;16:568-574.
44. Eberth DJ: Myoma sarcomatodes renum. Virchows Arch Pathol Anat Physiol 1872;10:518-521.
45. Egeler RM, Wolff JE, Anderson RA, et al: Long-term complications and post-treatment follow-up of patients with Wilms' tumor. Semin Urol Oncol 1999;17:55-61.
46. Eggert A, Grotzer MA, Ikegaki N, et al: Expression of the neurotrophin receptor TrkB is associated with unfavorable outcome in Wilms' tumor. J Clin Oncol 2001;19:689-696.
47. Farber S: Chemotherapy in the treatment of leukemia and Wilms' tumor. JAMA 1966;198:826-836.
48. Faria P, Beckwith JB, Mishra K, et al: Focal versus diffuse anaplasia in Wilms' tumor—new definitions with prognostic significance: A report from the National Wilms' Tumor Study Group. Am J Surg Pathol 1996;20:909-920.
49. Federici S, Galli G, Ceccarelli PL, et al: Wilms' tumor involving the inferior vena cava: Preoperative evaluation and management. Med Pediatr Oncol 1994;22:39-44.
50. Friedlander A: Sarcoma of the kidney treated by roentgen ray. Am J Dis Child 1916;12:328-331.
51. Gessler M, Konig A, Arden K, et al: Infrequent mutation of the WT1 gene in 77 Wilms' tumors. Hum Mutat 1994;3:212-222.
52. Gessler M, Poustka A, Cavenee W, et al: Homozygous deletion in Wilms' tumours of a zinc-finger gene identified by chromosome jumping. Nature 1990;343:774-778.
53. Ghanem MA, Van der Kwast TH, Den Hollander JC, et al: The prognostic significance of apoptosis-associated proteins BCL-2, BAX and BCL-X in clinical nephroblastoma. Br J Cancer 2001;85:1557-1563.
54. Godzinski J, Tournade MF, de Kraker J, et al: The role of preoperative chemotherapy in the treatment of nephroblastoma: The SIOP experience. Societe Internationale d'Oncologie Pediatrique. Semin Urol Oncol 1999;17:28-32.
55. Goske MJ, Mitchell C, Reslan WA: Imaging of patients with Wilms' tumor. Semin Urol Oncol 1999;17:11-20.
56. Graf N, Tournade MF, de Kraker J: The role of preoperative chemotherapy in the management of Wilms' tumor: The SIOP studies. International Society of Pediatric Oncology. Urol Clin North Am 2000;27:443-454.
57. Green DM, D'Angio G J, Beckwith B, et al: Wilms' tumor (nephroblastoma, renal embryoma). In Pizzo PA, Poplack DG (eds): Principles and Practices of Pediatric Oncology, 2nd ed. Philadelphia, JB Lippincott, 1993 pp 713-738.
58. Green DM, Beckwith JB, Breslow NE, et al: Treatment of children with stages II to IV anaplastic Wilms' tumor: A report from the National Wilms' Tumor Study Group. J Clin Oncol 1994;12:2126-2131.
59. Green DM, Breslow NE, Beckwith JB, et al: Treatment outcomes in patients less than 2 years of age with small, stage I, favorable-histology Wilms' tumors: A report from the National Wilms' Tumor Study. J Clin Oncol 1993;11:91-95.

60. Green DM, Breslow NE, Beckwith JB, et al: Comparison between single-dose and divided-dose administration of dactinomycin and doxorubicin for patients with Wilms' tumor: A report from the National Wilms' Tumor Study Group. J Clin Oncol 1998;16:237-245.

61. Green DM, Breslow NE, Beckwith JB, et al: Effect of duration of treatment on treatment outcome and cost of treatment for Wilms' tumor: A report from the National Wilms' Tumor Study Group. J Clin Oncol 1998;16:3744-3751.

62. Green DM, Grigoriev YA, Nan B, et al: Congestive heart failure after treatment for Wilms' tumor: A report from the National Wilms' Tumor Study Group. J Clin Oncol 2001;19:1926-1934.

63. Green DM, Jaffe N: The role of chemotherapy in the treatment of Wilms' tumor. Cancer 1979;44:52-57.

64. Green DM, Peabody EM, Nan B, et al: Pregnancy outcome after treatment for Wilms' tumor: A report from the National Wilms' Tumor Study Group. J Clin Oncol 2002;20: 2506-2513.

65. Green DM, Zevon MA, Reese PA, et al: Second malignant tumors following treatment during childhood and adolescence for cancer. Med Pediatr Oncol 1994;22:1-10.

66. Gronskov K, Olsen JH, Sand A, et al: Population-based risk estimates of Wilms' tumor in sporadic aniridia: A comprehensive mutation screening procedure of PAX6 identifies 80% of mutations in aniridia. Hum Genet 2001;109:11-18.

67. Grundy P, Koufos A, Morgan K, et al: Familial predisposition to Wilms' tumour does not map to the short arm of chromosome 11. Nature 1988;336:374-376.

68. Grundy P, Telzerow PE, Paterson MC, et al: Chromosome 11 uniparental isodisomy predisposing to embryonal neoplasms. Lancet 1991;338:1079-1080.

69. Grundy PE, Telzerow PE, Breslow N, et al: Loss of heterozygosity for chromosomes 16q and 1p in Wilms' tumors predicts an adverse outcome. Cancer Res 1994;54:2331-2333.

70. Gururangan S, Dorman A, Ball R, et al: DNA quantitation of Wilms' tumour (nephroblastoma) using flow cytometry and image analysis. J Clin Pathol 1992;45:498-501.

71. Henry I, Bonaiti-Pellie C, Chehensse V, et al: Uniparental paternal disomy in a genetic cancer-predisposing syndrome. Nature 1991;351:665-667.

72. Henry I, Grandjouan S, Couillin P, et al: Tumor-specific loss of 11p15.5 alleles in del 11p13 Wilms' tumor and in familial adrenocortical carcinoma. Proc Natl Acad Sci U S A 1989;86:3247-3251.

73. Hing S, Lu YJ, Summersgill B, et al: Gain of 1q is associated with adverse outcome in favorable histology Wilms' tumors. Am J Pathol 2001;158:393-398.

74. Hogeboom CJ, Grosser SC, Guthrie KA, et al: Stature loss following treatment for Wilms' tumor. Med Pediatr Oncol 2001;36:295-304.

75. Hu M, Zhang GY, Arbuckle S, et al: Prophylactic bilateral nephrectomies in two paediatric patients with missense mutations in the WT1 gene. Nephrol Dial Transplant 2004;19:223-226.

76. Huang EY, Mascarenhas L, Mahour GH: Wilms' tumor and horseshoe kidneys: A case report and review of the literature. J Pediatr Surg 2004;39:207-212.

77. Huff V, Compton DA, Chao LY, et al: Lack of linkage of familial Wilms' tumour to chromosomal band 11p13. Nature 1988;336:377-378.

78. Huff V, Reeve AE, Leppert M, et al: Nonlinkage of 16q markers to familial predisposition to Wilms' tumor. Cancer Res 1992;52:6117-6120.

79. Jenkner A, Camassei FD, Boldrini R, et al: 111 Renal neoplasms of childhood: A clinicopathologic study. J Pediatr Surg 2001;36:1522-1527.

80. Kalapurakal JA, Peterson S, Peabody EM, et al: Pregnancy outcomes after abdominal irradiation that included or excluded the pelvis in childhood Wilms' tumor survivors: A report from the National Wilms' Tumor Study. Int J Radiat Oncol Biol Phys 2004;58:1364-1368.

81. Kayton ML, Rowe DH, O'Toole KM, et al: Metastasis correlates with production of vascular endothelial growth factor in a murine model of human Wilms' tumor. J Pediatr Surg 1999;34:743-747.

82. Knudson AG, Strong LC: Mutation and cancer: A model for Wilms' tumor of the kidney. J Natl Cancer Inst. 1972;48:313-324.

83. Ladd WE, White RR: Embryoma of the kidney (Wilms' tumor). JAMA 1941;117:1859-1863.

84. Leape LL, Breslow NE: The surgical treatment of Wilms' tumor: Results of the National Wilms' Tumor Study. Ann Surg 1978;187:351-356.

85. Lee MP, DeBaun MR, Mitsuya K, et al: Loss of imprinting of a paternally expressed transcript, with antisense orientation to KVLZT1, occurs frequently in Beckwith-Wiedemann syndrome and is independent of insulin-like growth factor II imprinting. Proc Natl Acad Sci U S A 1999;96: 5203-5208.

86. Lee SB, Haber DA: Wilms' tumor and the WT1 gene. Exp Cell Res 2001;264:74-99.

87. Li CM, Guo M, Borczuk A, et al: Gene expression in Wilms' tumor mimics the earliest committed stage in the metanephric mesenchymal-epithelial transition. Am J Pathol 2002;160:2181-2190.

88. Lin RY, Argenta PA, Sullivan KM, et al: Diagnostic and prognostic role of basic fibroblast growth factor in Wilms' tumor patients. Clin Cancer Res 1995;1:327-331.

89. Little MH, Williamson KA, Mannens M, et al: Evidence that WT1 mutations in Denys-Drash syndrome patients may act in a dominant-negative fashion. Hum Mol Genet 1993; 2:259-264.

90. Lodge AJ, Jaggers J, Adams D, et al: Vascular control for resection of suprahepatic intracaval Wilms' tumor: Technical considerations. J Pediatr Surg 2000;35: 1836-1837.

91. Look AT, Hayes FA, Shuster JJ, et al: Clinical relevance of tumor cell ploidy and N-myc gene amplification in childhood neuroblastoma. A Pediatric Oncology Group Study. J Clin Oncol 1991;9:581-591.

92. Lovvorn HN 3rd, Savani RC, Ruchelli E, et al: Serum hyaluronan and its association with unfavorable histology and aggressiveness of heterotransplanted Wilms' tumor. J Pediatr Surg 2000;35:1070-1078.

93. Lu YJ, Hing S, Williams R, et al: Chromosome 1q expression profiling and relapse in Wilms' tumour. Lancet 2002;360:385-386.

94. Marsden HB, Lawler W: Bone-metastasizing renal tumor of childhood. Br J Cancer 1978;38:437-441.

95. Maw MA, Grundy P, Millow LJ, et al: A third Wilms' tumor locus on chromosome 16q. Cancer Res 1992;52: 3094-3098.

96. McNeil DE, Brown M, Ching A, et al: Screening for Wilms' tumor and hepatoblastoma in children with Beckwith-Wiedemann syndrome: A cost-effective model. Med Pediatr Oncol 2001;37:349-356.

97. Mertens A, Neglia J, Yasui Y, et al: Mortality rates and causes of death among 5-year survivors of childhood and adolescent cancer. Proc Am Soc Clin Oncol 1999;19:569a.

98. Miller RW, Fraumeni JG, Manning MD: Association of Wilms' tumor with aniridia, hemihypertrophy and other congenital abnormalities. N Engl J Med 1964;270: 922-930.

99. Mitchell C, Jones PM, Kelsey A, et al: The treatment of Wilms' tumour: Results of the United Kingdom Children's Cancer Study Group (UKCCSG) second Wilms' tumour study. Br J Cancer 2000;83:602-608.

100. Montgomery BT, Kelalis PP, BLute ML, et al: Extended followup of bilateral Wilms' tumor: Results of the National Wilms' Tumor Study. J Urol 1991;146:514-518.

101. Narahara K, Kikkawa K, Kimira S, et al: Regional mapping of catalase and Wilms' tumor-aniridia, genitourinary abnormalities, and mental retardation triad loci to the chromosome segment 11p1305-p1306. Hum Genet 1984;66:181-185.

102. Neville H, Ritchey ML, Shamberger RC, et al: The occurrence of Wilms' tumor in horseshoe kidneys: A report from the National Wilms' Tumor Study Group (NWTSG). J Pediatr Surg 2002;37:1134-1137.

103. Okutsu T, Kuroiwa Y, Kagitani F, et al: Expression and imprinting status of human PEG8/IGF2AS, a paternally expressed antisense transcript from the IGF2 locus, in Wilms' tumors. J Biochem 2000;127:475-483.

104. Osler W: Two cases of striated myo-sarcoma of the kidney. J Anat Physiol 1879;14.

105. Owens CM, Veys PA, Pritchard J, et al: Role of chest computed tomography at diagnosis in the management of Wilms' tumor: A study by the United Kingdom Children's Cancer Study Group. J Clin Oncol 2002;20:2768-2773.

106. Pappo AS, Crist WM, Kuttesch J, et al: Tumor-cell DNA content predicts outcome in children and adolescents with clinical group III embryonal rhabdomyosarcoma. J Clin Oncol 1993;11:1901-1905.

107. Park S, Bernard A, Bove KE, et al: Inactivation of WT1 in nephrogenic rests, genetic precursors to Wilms' tumour. Nat Genet 1993;5:363-367.

108. Pelletier J, Bruening W, Kashtan CE, et al: Germline mutations in the Wilms' tumor suppressor gene are associated with abnormal urogenital development in Denys-Drash syndrome. Cell 1991;67:437-447.

109. Pelletier J, Bruening W, Li FP, et al: WT1 mutations contribute to abnormal genital system development and hereditary Wilms' tumour. Nature 1991;353:431-434.

110. Plesko I, Kramarova E, Stiller CA, et al: Survival of children with Wilms' tumour in Europe. Eur J Cancer 2001;37:736-743.

111. Porteus MH, Narkool P, Neuberg D, et al: Characteristics and outcome of children with Beckwith-Wiedemann syndrome and Wilms' tumor: A report from the National Wilms' Tumor Study Group. J Clin Oncol 2000;18:2026-2031.

112. Rahman N, Arbour L, Houlston R, et al: Penetrance of mutations in familial Wilms' tumor gene FW1. J Natl Cancer Inst 2000;96:650-652.

113. Re GG, Hazen-Martin DJ, Sens DA, et al: Nephroblastoma (Wilms' tumor): A model system of aberrant renal development. Semin Diagn Pathol 1994;11:126-135.

114. Reeve AE, Sih SA, Raizis AM, et al: Loss of allelic heterozygosity at a second locus on chromosome 11 in sporadic Wilms' tumor cells. Mol Cell Biol 1989;9:1799-1803.

115. Renaud EJ, Liu D, Pipe SW, et al: Inferior vena cavectomy for nonexcisable Wilms' tumor thrombus. J Pediatr Surg 2001;36:526-529.

116. Riccardi VM, Sujansky E, Smith AC, et al: Chromosomal imbalance in the aniridia-Wilms' tumor association: 11p interstitial deletion. Pediatrics 1978;61:604-610.

117. Ritchey ML: The role of preoperative chemotherapy for Wilms' tumor: The NWTSG perspective. National Wilms' Tumor Study Group. Semin Urol Oncol 1999;17:21-27.

118. Ritchey ML, Green DM, Thomas PR, et al: Renal failure in Wilms' tumor patients: A report from the National Wilms' Tumor Study Group. Med Pediatr Oncol 1996;26:75-80.

119. Ritchey ML, Kelalis PP, Breslow N, et al: Surgical complications after nephrectomy for Wilms' tumor. Surg Gynecol Obstet 1992;1992:507-514.

120. Ritchey ML, Kelalis PP, Haase GM, et al: Preoperative therapy for intracaval and atrial extension of Wilms' tumor. Cancer 1993;71:4104-4110.

121. Ritchey ML, Pringle K, Breslow N, et al: Management and outcome of inoperable Wilms' tumor: A report of National Wilms' Tumor Study-3. Ann Surg 1994;220:683-690.

122. Ritchey ML, Shamberger RC, Haase G, et al: Surgical complications after primary nephrectomy for Wilms' tumor: Report from the National Wilms' Tumor Study Group. J Am Coll Surg 2001;192:63-68.

123. Ross JH, Kay R: Surgical considerations for patients with Wilms' tumor. Semin Urol Oncol 1999;17:33-39.

124. Shamberger RC, Guthrie KA, Ritchey ML, et al: Surgery-related factors and local recurrence of Wilms' tumor in National Wilms' Tumor Study 4. Ann Surg 1999;229:292-297.

125. Shamberger RC, Ritchey ML, Haase GM, et al: Intravascular extension of Wilms' tumor. Ann Surg 2001;234:116-121.

126. Shearer P, Kapoor G, Beckwith JB, et al: Secondary acute myelogenous leukemia in patients previously treated for childhood renal tumors: A report from the National Wilms' Tumor Study Group. J Pediatr Hematol Oncol 2001;23:109-111.

127. Shurin SB, Gauderer MW, Dahms BB, et al: Fatal intraoperative pulmonary embolization of Wilms' tumor. J Pediatr 1982;101:559-562.

128. Smith MB, Xue H, Strong LC, et al: Forty-year experience with second malignancies after treatment of childhood cancer: Analysis of outcome following the development of the second malignancy. J Pediatr Surg 1993;28:1342-1348.

129. Sorensen K, Levitt GA, Bull C, et al: Late anthracycline cardiotoxicity after childhood cancer: A prospective longitudinal study. Cancer 2003;97:1991-1998.

130. Sredni ST, de Camargo B, Lopes LF, et al: Immunohistochemical detection of p53 protein expression as a prognostic indicator in Wilms' tumor. Med Pediatr Oncol 2001;37:455-458.

131. Tagge EP, Hanson P, Re GG, et al: Paired box gene expression in Wilms' tumor. J Pediatr Surg 1994;29:134-141.

132. Toretsky JA, Zitomersky NL, Eskenazi AE, et al: Glypican-3 expression in Wilms' tumor and hepatoblastoma. J Pediatr Hematol Oncol 2001;23:496-499.

133. Tournade MF, Com-Nougue C, de Kraker J, et al: Optimal duration of preoperative therapy in unilateral and non-metastatic Wilms' tumor in children older than 6 months: Results of the Ninth International Society of Pediatric Oncology Wilms' Tumor Trial and Study. J Clin Oncol 2001;19:488-500.

134. Trueworthy R, Shuster JJ, Look T, et al: Ploidy of lymphoblasts is the strongest predictor of treatment outcome in B-progenitor cell acute lymphoblastic leukemia of childhood: A Pediatric Oncology Group Study. J Clin Oncol 1992;10:606-613.

135. Vujanic GM, Kelsey A, Mitchell C, et al: The role of biopsy in the diagnosis of renal tumors of childhood: Results of the UKCCSG Wilms' tumor study 3. Med Pediatr Oncol 2003;40:18-22.

136. Vujanic GM, Sandstedt B, Harms D, et al: Revised International Society of Paediatric Oncology (SIOP) working classification of renal tumors of childhood. Med Pediatr Oncol 2002;38:79-82.

137. Weeks DA, Beckwith JB, Mierau GW, et al: Rhabdoid tumor of kidney: A report of 111 cases from the National Wilms' Tumor Study Pathology Center. Am J Surg Pathol 1989;13:439-458.

138. White GR, Kelsey AM, Varley JM, et al: Somatic glypican 3 (GPC3) mutations in Wilms' tumour. Br J Cancer 2002; 86:1920-1922.

139. Wilms M: Die Mischgeschwuelste der Niere. In Leipzig, 1899, Arthur Georgi.

140. Zoeller G, Pekrun A, Lakomek M, et al: Wilms' tumor: The problem of diagnostic accuracy in children undergoing preoperative chemotherapy without histological tumor verification. J Urol 1994;151:169-171.

141. Zuppan CW, Beckwith JB, Luckey DW: Anaplasia in unilateral Wilms' tumor: A report from the National Wilms' Tumor Study Pathology Center. Hum Pathol 1988;19:1199-1209.

Chapter 28

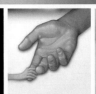

Neuroblastoma

Jay L. Grosfeld

Neuroblastoma is one of the most common solid tumors in infancy and childhood. This neoplasm, of neural crest origin, may arise in the adrenal medulla and along the sympathetic ganglion chain from the neck to the pelvis. The clinical course is quite variable, as this highly malignant tumor demonstrates unusual behavior. Although instances of spontaneous regression and tumor maturation from a malignant to a benign histologic form have been observed,[27,43,63,76,83,144,147] the disease is progressive in many cases. Survival in children with other malignancies, such as Wilms' tumor, rhabdomyosarcoma, acute lymphocytic leukemia, germ cell tumors, Hodgkin's disease, and non-Hodgkin's lymphoma, has been significantly improved by the aggressive use of combined treatment modalities, but the outlook for many children with advanced neuroblastoma remains dismal.[25,27,67,74,77,83,116] This neoplasm exhibits great heterogeneity in its behavior and represents a significant challenge to practitioners caring for affected children.

Primitive neuroblasts can be identified in the fetal adrenal gland in the 10th to 12th intrauterine week. The nodules increase in number by 20 weeks' gestation but gradually diminish in number toward the end of gestation. Neuroblastoma in situ in the adrenal gland is seen in 1 of every 260 neonates who die of congenital heart disease and in as many as 1 in 39 infants in the first 3 months of life who die from other causes. The clinical incidence of the tumor is approximately 1 in 7500 to 10,000 children.[13,27,73,74] Neuroblastoma is responsible for 10% of all childhood tumors and 15% of all cancer deaths. The exact cause remains unknown. There are 700 cases diagnosed annually in the United States. Approximately 40% of cases are diagnosed by age 1 year, 75% by 7 years, and 98% by 10 years.[27] More than half the patients are younger than 2 years at the time of diagnosis.[78] Neuroblastoma is slightly more common in boys than in girls, with a ratio of 1.2:1.0.[27,74] It is the most common intra-abdominal malignancy in newborns. Although a decrease in cancer incidence and mortality has been observed in adults, the incidence of cancer in infants in the United States increased from 189 cases per million to 220 cases per million from 1980 to 1990.[115] Male infants have an increased rate of central nervous system tumors, neuroblastoma, and retinoblastoma, while girls have an increased rate of teratoma and hepatoblastoma.[115] The embryonal nature of neuroblastoma has been well documented by its identification on prenatal ultrasonography, and the tumor has been known to rarely invade the placenta during the antenatal period.[3,12,56,101,109,146,171,226] More than 55 cases of antenatally discovered neuroblastoma have been reported in the literature since the original description by Fenart et al. in 1983.[65] The masses are usually identified during ultrasound examinations performed after 32 weeks' gestation. The earliest reported instance was observed at 18 weeks.[103]

Mothers of infants with congenital neuroblastoma occasionally experience flushing and hypertension during pregnancy as a result of catecholamine released from the fetal tumor in utero. The neoplasm has been described in twins on many occasions, and familial occurrences in both mother and child and father and son have been reported.[37,70,171] Concordance for neuroblastoma in twins during infancy indicates that hereditary factors may be predominant, whereas discordance in older twins suggests that a random mutation may be more important. The median age for the occurrence of familial neuroblastoma is 9 months, in contrast to 18 months in the general population. Maris et al.[145] observed that 20% of patients with familial neuroblastoma have bilateral or multifocal tumors and reported evidence for a hereditary neuroblastoma predisposition locus on chromosome 16p12-13. Neuroblastoma has been observed in infants with Beckwith-Wiedemann syndrome (BWS), neurofibromatosis (von Recklinghausen's disease), Hirschsprung's disease, central hypoventilation syndrome (Ondine's curse), fetal alcohol syndrome, and in offspring of mothers taking phenytoin (fetal hydantoin syndrome) for seizure disorders.[7,59,119,161,206] Although it is unlikely that environmental factors play an important role in causing this tumor, neuroblastoma has been noted among infants of mothers receiving medical therapy for vaginal infection during pregnancy and with paternal occupational exposure to electromagnetic fields.[27]

Neuroblastoma may occur at any site where neural crest tissues are found in the embryo. The neuroblast is derived from primordial neural crest cells that migrate from the mantle layer of the developing spinal cord. Tumors may arise in the neck, posterior mediastinum,

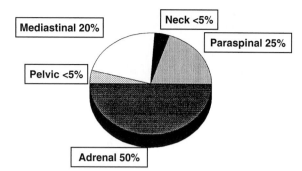

Figure 28–1 Distribution of cases of neuroblastoma at each of the primary tumor sites. Primary tumors most commonly occur in the adrenal gland.

retroperitoneal (paraspinal) ganglia, adrenal medulla, and pelvic organ of Zuckerkandl.[73,74,79,83] In 75% of cases, the tumor is located in the retroperitoneum, in either the adrenal medulla (50%) or the paraspinal ganglia (25%). In 20% of cases, the primary tumor is in the posterior mediastinum. Less than 5% of tumors occur in the neck or pelvis (Fig. 28-1).[27,73,74,83] Primary intracranial cerebral neuroblastoma also occurs.[46,246] In addition, a teratoma in an infant may occasionally contain foci of neuroblastoma. Rare cases of neuroblastoma arising in the bladder have also been reported.[60] The fate of the neuroblasts can follow one of three clinical pathways: (1) spontaneous regression, (2) maturation by differentiation from neuroblastoma to a benign ganglioneuroma, or most frequently, (3) rapid progression to a highly malignant tumor that is often resistant to treatment.

MASS SCREENING

In an effort to identify early cases of neuroblastoma that were amenable to cure, mass screening programs were initiated in Japan in 1985, evaluating urinary vanillylmandelic acid (VMA) and homovanillic acid (HVA) levels in infants at 6 months of age. These studies identified a large number of infants with neuroblastoma. The survival in these cases was exceptionally high compared with the survival in patients who present with clinical disease diagnosed by conventional methods. The Japanese screening effort doubled the actual incidence of neuroblastoma in infants younger than 1 year but neither decreased the number of cases observed in older children nor improved the survival of children older than 1 year.[19,27,199,200] Sawada et al.[199,200] reported a 96% survival rate in 170 cases of neuroblastoma identified by screening. These observations suggest that neuroblastomas identified by screening were most likely biologically favorable tumors that spontaneously regressed.[199] However, a small number of screened patients have had tumors with unfavorable biologic markers and a poor prognosis, and a few screened patients who tested negative at age 6 months later (at 12 to 18 months of age) developed highly aggressive neuroblastomas.[106]

In general, mass screening has provided important information regarding the natural history of this enigmatic tumor and has identified a group of tumors that clearly regress and represent a biologically favorable form of tumor, in contrast to that noted in older children.[147] Prospective, population-based, controlled screening trials in Quebec minimized the rate of false-positive cases but had an overall sensitivity of only 45%. The results were similar to the findings in Japan.[237] A German study offered screening to 2.6 million infants between 9 and 18 months of age. This effort identified 149 cases of neuroblastoma in 1800 screened infants, demonstrating a predictive value of 8%.[202] The German investigators estimated that two thirds of the tumors detected by screening would have regressed spontaneously. The potential risks were highlighted by the fact that all three children who died in the group detected by screening had localized disease and succumbed from complications of treatment. These studies in North America and Europe suggest that screening may result in an overdiagnosis of neuroblastoma and the institution of unnecessary therapies.[201] However, the results observed in screening studies are valuable and should help minimize treatment in a substantial subset of infants diagnosed with early-stage neuroblastoma that has an excellent chance of either maturing or spontaneously regressing.[239] In a limited trial of expectant observation in 11 patients with localized disease detected by mass screening, all tumors decreased in size during the observation period.[239] Oue et al.[169] observed 22 patients with tumors that were identified by screening; 13 (59%) spontaneously regressed, and 9 underwent resection for increasing size. Although none had N-*myc* amplification, other unfavorable biologic factors were noted in 8 babies, including diploidy, unfavorable histology, and chromosomal deletion (1p), yet all the babies survived.[169] Some have suggested that there are compelling medical and psychological reasons (especially among parents in false-positive cases) for the cessation of neuroblastoma screening.[54,238] Following the cessation of screening elsewhere in the world, the Ministry of Health in Japan discontinued its mass screening program in April 2004.[169]

CLINICAL PRESENTATION

Neuroblastoma is a tumor with multiple clinical manifestations related to the site of the primary tumor, the presence of metastases, and the production of certain metabolic tumor by-products. Fifty percent to 75% of reported cases present with an abdominal mass. The tumor may be hard, nodular, fixed, and painful on palpation. Generalized symptoms including weight loss, failure to thrive, abdominal pain and distention, fever, and anemia.[27,73,74,83] Hypertension is found in 25% of cases and is related to the production of catecholamines by the tumor. Instances of hypercalcemia have been observed in association with neuroblastoma, and hemoperitoneum caused by sudden spontaneous rupture of the neoplasm has also been reported.[8,24]

Neoplasms arising in the upper mediastinum or neck may involve the stellate ganglion and cause Horner's syndrome, characterized by ptosis, miosis, enophthalmos, anhidrosis, and heterochromia of the iris on the affected side.[73,74,83] Metastases to the bony orbit may produce

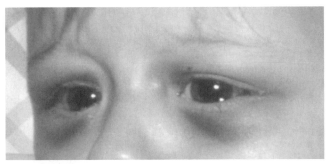

Figure 28-2 Child with bilateral orbital ecchymoses ("panda eyes" or "raccoon eyes") resulting from orbital metastases from neuroblastoma.

proptosis or bilateral orbital ecchymosis—often referred to as "panda eyes" or "raccoon eyes" (Fig. 28-2). The latter finding in a child without a history of trauma should always raise the index of suspicion for the presence of a malignancy. Mediastinal tumors may be associated with respiratory distress, due to the tumor's interference with lung expansion, and dysphagia caused by extrinsic pressure on the esophagus (Fig. 28-3).[5,66,74,243] Mediastinal and paraspinal retroperitoneal lesions may manifest with paraplegia related to tumor extension through an intervertebral foramen, resulting in a dumbbell- or hourglass-shaped lesion that may cause extradural compression of the spinal cord.[73,118,174,198,242] In a few patients, cauda equina syndrome has also been observed. Pelvic tumors may be associated with bladder and bowel dysfunction. Anemia is often related to bone marrow invasion by the tumor. Excessive catecholamine production by the tumor may result in flushing, sweating, and irritability. Acute cerebellar ataxia, characterized by opsomyoclonus and nystagmus ("dancing eye syndrome"), has been observed.[9,121,195,196,207] Two thirds of these cases have occurred in infants with mediastinal neuroblastoma. The involuntary muscular contractions and random eye movements are unrelated to metastases. The cause of this unusual presentation of neuroblastoma is unknown.

An autoimmune phenomenon related to an antigen-antibody complex has been suggested.[9,195,207] Of interest is the fact that these unusual neurologic symptoms may persist even after tumor resection. Poor school performance and learning deficits are not uncommon in these children.[195,196]

Infants with neuroblastoma, ganglioneuroblastoma, and, occasionally, benign ganglioneuroma may present with intractable diarrhea characterized by watery, explosive stools and hypokalemia.[42,58,127] The diarrhea is related to the production of vasoactive intestinal polypeptide (VIP) by the tumor.[42,58,74,127] These tumors often have somatostatin receptors.

Neuroblastoma may spread by direct extension into surrounding structures, lymphatic infiltration, or hematogenous metastases. Regional and distant lymph nodes, liver, bone marrow, and bone cortex are frequently involved.[72,74,77,83,91,165] Patients with bone cortex metastases have an ominous prognosis. Bone metastases occur in sites containing red marrow and involve the metaphyseal areas of long bones in addition to the skull, vertebral column, pelvis, ribs, and sternum.[27,74,77,83] Bone lesions may cause extreme pain. In some cases, the clinical presentation may be characterized by a child's refusal to walk because of leg pain due to bone metastases. Occasionally, patients with advanced disease present with a bleeding diathesis related to thrombocytopenia from extensive involvement of bone marrow and interference with hepatic production of clotting factors by liver metastases. Multiple subcutaneous skin nodules and hepatomegaly may occur in infants with stage IV-S neuroblastoma. Hematogenous metastases to the brain, spinal cord, and heart are unusual. Brain metastases usually manifest in older children with headaches and seizures.[25,110] Lung metastases are found on chest radiographs in only 4% of patients.[222] This may be the result of direct extension to the lung from mediastinal lymph nodes or diffuse hematogenous spread, presenting with a radiographic pattern that may be confused with pulmonary edema or interstitial pneumonia.[222] Occasionally, lung involvement by intralymphatic metastases (not seen on chest radiographs) is noted at autopsy.

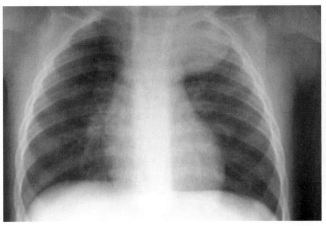
A

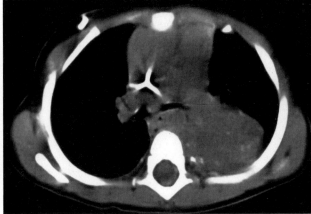
B

Figure 28-3 *A*, Plain chest radiograph shows the presence of a left upper thoracic tumor. *B*, Computed tomography scan documents a mass in the posterior mediastinum that contains calcium, suggestive of a neuroblastoma.

DIAGNOSIS

Diagnosis of neuroblastoma is made through a variety of imaging and isotopic studies, serum and urine determinations, and histologic and genetic evaluation of tumor tissue. On the plain abdominal radiograph, approximately 50% of cases may show finely stippled tumor calcification.[73,74,77] Radiographs also may show displacement of bowel gas by a mass. Paraspinal widening is commonly found with celiac axis tumors. Chest radiographs may show a posterior mediastinal tumor or paraspinal widening above the diaphragm from extension of an abdominal tumor. Computed tomography (CT) can demonstrate tumor calcification in approximately 80% of cases (Fig. 28-4).[1,73] With CT studies using contrast enhancement, one can often distinguish kidney and liver from adrenal and paraspinal lesions and evaluate for intracranial extension of skull metastases.[1,22,74] Magnetic resonance imaging (MRI) is extremely useful in detecting intraspinal tumor extension and, in some instances, the tumor's relationship to major vascular structures. Helical (spiral) CT with three-dimensional reconstruction is also a useful method of evaluating this latter relationship. The workup of patients with retroperitoneal tumors includes an initial upright radiograph of the abdomen, an ultrasound examination to distinguish a cystic from a solid lesion, and an evaluation for potential obstruction or compression of the inferior vena cava. As a rule, obstruction of the inferior vena cava in patients with neuroblastoma suggests the presence of an initially unresectable lesion.[74,75] Abdominal CT is performed with intravenous contrast material so that an intravenous urogram can be acquired during the same study.[75] In most instances, paraspinal or adrenal neuroblastoma causes lateral or downward displacement of the ipsilateral kidney or ureter (or both). A separate intravenous urogram is not necessary. A long bone survey, isotopic bone scintigraphy (using the bone-seeking isotopes technetium and metaiodobenzylguanidine [MIBG]), and multiple bone marrow aspirates are also obtained.[74,75,77,93] MIBG also images the primary tumor in the adrenal medulla. Isotopic bone scans show a close correlation with the radiographic skeletal survey and are occasionally more sensitive.[93] False-positive bone scans can occur in cases of recent bone trauma or inflammation. The bone-seeking isotopes are picked up by metastatic foci in the bone and by the punctate calcifications in the primary tumor (Fig. 28-5).[73,74] Demonstration of the bone-seeking isotope in a retroperitoneal or posterior mediastinal mass suggests that the lesion is a neuroblastoma. Although angiography was once performed to evaluate many childhood tumors, this test is rarely used today because vascular structures can be readily identified by other imaging studies such as helical CT or magnetic resonance angiography (Fig. 28-6).

Pelvic neuroblastoma may manifest with both urinary symptoms and constipation. The tumor, usually palpable on rectal examination, must be differentiated from presacral teratoma, yolk sac tumor, nonosseous Ewing's tumor, and pelvic rhabdomyosarcoma.[74,83]

Because neuroblastoma is a tumor derived from neural crest cells, it may secrete hormonal products and is likely a member of the amine precursor uptake and decarboxylation (APUD) family of tumors. More than 90% of children with neuroblastoma have tumors that produce high levels of catecholamines or their by-products. Quantification of catecholamine by-product secretion is best done by 24-hour urine collection.[136] Adrenaline, noradrenaline, dopamine, metanephrine, HVA, VMA, and vanillylglycolic acid levels are determined. Children with immature, more undifferentiated tumors tend to excrete higher levels of certain by-products (e.g., HVA).[73] Patients with more mature tumors excrete more VMA. In rare instances, however, the tumor does not secrete excessive catecholamines. Prasad et al.[177] suggested that these are parasympathetic neuroblastomas that secrete increased levels of acetylcholine and fail to metabolize tyrosine to dopamine. Patients with advanced malignancy have elevated urine concentrations of cystathionine and homoserine; increased serum levels of neuron-specific enolase, ferritin, and lactic dehydrogenase; and, in 25%

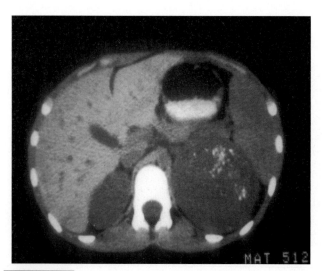

Figure 28–4   Adominal computed tomography shows a retroperitoneal mass with stippled calcification, consistent with neuroblastoma.

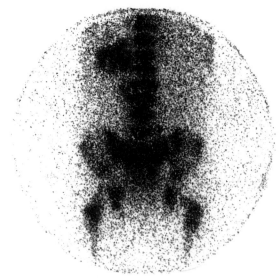

Figure 28–5   I[123]-MIBG scintiscan shows the presence of bone metastases and uptake of the isotope in a primary tumor in the adrenal gland.

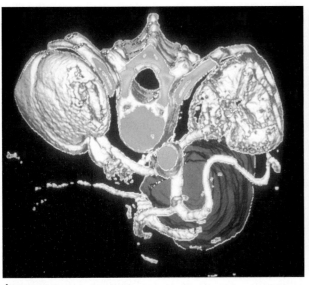
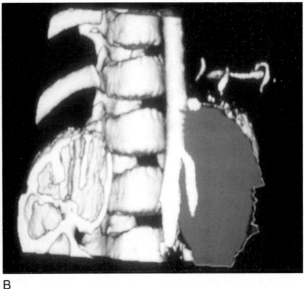

A   B

Figure 28-6 Helical computed tomography scan with three-dimensional reconstruction of a neuroblastoma arising near the celiac axis. *A,* Anterior view indicates that the tumor does not involve the branches of the celiac axis. *B,* Lateral view demonstrates that the superior mesenteric artery passes through the tumor. *(See color plate.)*

of cases, sera positive for carcinoembryonic antigen.[87,167,216,228,244] Although these observations are of historical interest, none of these serum levels are independent prognostic factors, nor are they currently used to determine treatment. Although histologic examination of tissue is the key to the conclusive diagnosis of neuroblastoma, in advanced disease, rosettes of tumor cells in bone marrow aspirate and increased urinary excretion of VMA or other catecholamine by-products are often indicative of the diagnosis. Immunologic analysis of bone marrow aspirate may be more sensitive than conventional analysis in detecting tumor cells.[156] Serial immunocytologic analysis of peripheral blood samples have also identied circulating neuroblasts, documenting tumor dissemination.

STAGING

Various staging schemes for neuroblastoma were used in the past, including Evans's criteria from the Children's Cancer Group (CCG),[62] the St. Jude staging system[91] used by the Pediatric Oncology Group (POG), a TNM (tumor, lymph node, metastasis) status system employed by the International Union Contra Cancer in Europe, and the Japanese Neuroblastoma Study Group staging system. These staging criteria were in basic agreement regarding localized, completely resected lesions; instances of metastasis to the bone cortex; and infants with Evans's stage IV-S tumors. They disagreed on other aspects of staging, including Evans's stage III cases and the importance of lymph node involvement. In 1988 an international staging system was devised that established a common set of criteria that could be used worldwide and would permit the accrual of large numbers of cases and valid comparisons of data (Table 28-1).[29] The International Neuroblastoma Staging System (INSS) uses certain features of the POG and CCG systems and identifies distinct prognostic groups. These criteria were revised by Brodeur et al. in 1993.[28] In 2001 the CCG and POG merged with the National Wilms' Tumor

TABLE 28-1 International Neuroblastoma Staging System

Stage	Description
I	Localized tumor confined to area of origin; complete excision, with or without microscopic residual disease; ipsilateral and contralateral lymph nodes negative (nodes attached to primary tumor and removed en bloc with it may be positive)
IIA	Unilateral tumor with incomplete gross excision; ipsilateral and contralateral lymph nodes negative
IIB	Unilateral tumor with complete or incomplete excision; positive ipsilateral, nonadherent regional lymph nodes; contralateral lymph nodes negative
III	Tumor infiltrating across the midline with or without lymph node involvement; or unilateral tumor with contralateral lymph node involvement; or midline tumor with bilateral lymph node involvement or bilateral infiltration (unresectable)
IV	Dissemination of tumor to distant lymph nodes, bone, bone marrow, liver, or other organs
IV-S	Localized primary tumor as defined for stage I or II with dissemination limited to liver, skin, or bone marrow (limited to infants younger than 1 yr)

From Brodeur GM, Pritchard J, Berthold F, et al: Revision of the international criteria for neuroblastoma diagnosis, staging and response to treatment. J Clin Oncol 1993;11:1466-1477; Brodeur GM, Seeger RC, Barrett A, et al: International criteria for diagnosis, staging, and response to treatment in patients with neuroblastoma. J Clin Oncol 1988;6:1874-1881.

Study and Rhabdomyosarcoma Study Group to form the Children's Oncology Group (COG), which now employs the INSS for all cases of neuroblastoma. At my institution, 266 cases of neuroblastoma were staged as follows: 14 (5.2%) stage I, 52 (19.6%) stage II, 62 (23.4%) stage III, 117 (44%) stage IV, and 21 (7.8%) stage IV-S.

PATHOLOGY AND HISTOLOGY

The pathologic classification of neuroblastoma has been revised, and histologic features of the tumor have been established that have important prognostic value.[111,211,212] The most useful system developed is the Shimada classification, which divides neuroblastic tumors into age-related favorable and unfavorable histologic categories based on whether the tumor exhibits a stroma-rich or stroma-poor appearance (Table 28-2).[211] Stroma-rich tumors are characterized by extensive Schwannian stroma and signs of neuroblastic differentiation (i.e., developed nuclear and cytoplasmic features of ganglion cells). Stroma-poor tumors contain immature, undifferentiated neural crest cells and have a high mitotic karyorrhexis index (MKI). The MKI refers to nuclear fragmentations and is determined by the sum of the number of necrotic tumor cells, the number of cells with mitosis, and the number of cells with malformed, lobulated, or pyknotic nuclei per 5000 cells examined. The MKI varies with age; a high MKI value in infants younger than 18 months is greater than 200/5000 cells, and for those older than 18 months it is greater than 100/5000 cells. All patients older than 5 years have unfavorable histology. Stroma-poor tumors often have N-*myc* amplification,

a high MKI, and a dismal outcome. A report by Shimada et al.[212] documented that both histology and N-*myc* amplification provided prognostic information that was independent of staging. Neuroblastomas with N-*myc* amplification have a characteristic histopathologic phenotype and a rapidly progressive clinical course.

The International Neuroblastoma Pathology Classification (INPC) adopted the Shimada classification with some minor modifications.[208-210,213] This age-linked classification is both prognostically significant and biologically relevant. The current system subdivides the undifferentiated subtype into undifferentiated and poorly differentiated tumors; changes the name of stroma-rich, well-differentiated tumors to ganglioneuroma maturing; and adds a descriptive Schwannian, stroma-dominant character to ganglioneuroma.[208] Age remains a critical prognostic factor, and the grade of differentiation and MKI have different prognostic effects, depending on the patient's age at diagnosis. Although the presence of calcification was thought to favorably influence survival, further studies demonstrated that calcification does not have an independent prognostic impact.[111,208] Favorable Shimada histology was associated with an 85% survival rate, compared with 41% for unfavorable histologic types. All ganglioneuroblastoma nodular (GNBn) cases were initially classified as unfavorable tumors. Umehara et al.[230] were the first to define subsets of these specific neoplasms that exhibit different behavior. Peuchmaur et al.[173] recently revised the INPC by dividing GNBn cases into two prognostic subsets—favorable and unfavorable. The favorable type was associated with an 86% event-free survival, whereas the unfavorable type (two thirds of cases) had only a 32% event-free survival. Children with the favorable subset of GNBn have an overall survival of greater than 90%, compared with 33.2% for the unfavorable GNBn subset (Fig. 28-7).[172] Large cell neuroblastoma has been identified as a distinct phenotype with aggressive clinical behavior.[229] These tumors have unfavorable histologic features, including monomorphous undifferentiated neuroblasts, a low incidence of calcification, and a high MKI. Immunohistochemical studies showed that large cell neuroblastoma cells stained positive for neuron-specific enolase, prodrug gene products, and tyrosine hydroxylase and were negative for CD99.[229]

On gross examination, neuroblastoma usually appears as a highly vascular purple-gray mass that is often solid but occasionally cystic. The tumor has an easily ruptured, friable pseudocapsule that may lead to significant hemorrhage during operative manipulation. The tumor is often necrotic, especially the undifferentiated form. Mature tumors (ganglioneuromas) have a more solid consistency and frequently have a fleshy white color. The histologic pattern may be quite variable. Primitive stroma-poor neuroblastomas may be indistinguishable from other small, blue round cell tumors such as Ewing's tumor, rhabdomyosarcoma, or primitive neuroectodermal tumors. The neuroblast is a small round cell consisting predominantly of the nucleus without much cytoplasm. Immature, undifferentiated tumors are characterized by closely packed small spheroid cells without any special arrangement or differentiation.[142] Nuclei may appear cone shaped and are hyperchromic. Rosette formation

TABLE 28-2 Modified Shimada Pathologic Classification of Neuroblastic Tumors

Appearance	Favorable Histology	Unfavorable Histology
Stroma rich	Well differentiated (ganglioneuroma) Ganglioneuroblastoma, intermixed	Ganglioneuroblastoma, nodular
Stroma poor (i.e., neuroblastoma)		
Age <18 mo	MKI <4%	MKI >4% or undifferentiated
Age 18-60 mo	MKI <2% and differentiating	MKI >2% or undifferentiated or poorly differentiated
Age >5 yr	None	All

MKI, mitotic karyorrhexis index.
From Shimada H, Chatten J, Newton WA Jr, et al: Histopathologic prognostic factors in neuroblastoma: Definition of subtypes of ganglioneuroblastoma and an age-linked classification of neuroblastoma. J Natl Cancer Inst 1984;73:405-416; Shimada H, Stram DO, Chatten J, et al: Identification of subsets of neuroblastomas by combined histopathologic and N-myc analysis. J Natl Cancer Inst 1995;87:1470-1476.

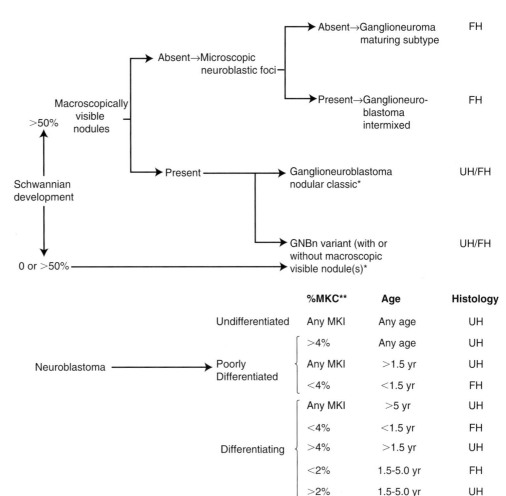

Figure 28-7 International Neuroblastoma Pathology Classification. FH, favorable histology; GNBn, ganaglioneuroblastoma nodular; MKI, mitotic karyorrhexis index; %MKC, mitotic and karyorrhectic cells; UH, unfavorable histology; * classic GNBn (single, macroscopically visible, usually hemorrhagic nodule in stroma-rich, stroma-dominant tissue background; ** MKC 2%, 100 of 5000 cells; MKC 4%, 200 of 5000 cells. (From Peuchmaur M, d'Amore ES, Joshi VV, et al: Revision of the International Neuroblastoma Pathology Classification: Confirmation of favorable and unfavorable prognostic subsets in ganglioneuroblastoma, nodular. Cancer 2003;98:2274-2281.)

may be observed and is considered a sign of early tumor differentiation (Fig. 28-8). The center of each rosette is formed by a tangle of fine nerve fibers. More mature-appearing, stroma-rich tumors may contain cells that resemble normal ganglion cells, with an admixture of histologic components characterized by abundant nerve filaments, neuroblastic rosettes, and ganglion cells all seen in a single microscopic field.[70,137] On electron microscopy, neurofibrils and electron-dense, membrane-bound neurosecretory granules may be observed. The neurosecretory granules may be the site of conversion of dopamine to norepinephrine. These ultrastructural findings and genetic identification of the tumor tissue can usually separate neuroblastoma from other small cell tumors. Instances of spontaneous maturation from a highly malignant, undifferentiated neuroblastoma to a ganglioneuroblastoma and subsequently a benign ganglioneuroma have been observed. Ambros et al.[11] reported that maturing neuroblastomas consist of both Schwann cells and neuronal cells, including ganglion cells. Schwann cells have normal numbers of chromosomes and triploid flow cytometry, in contrast to other neuronal cells, including ganglion cells.[11] These observations suggest that Schwann cells may be a reactive population of normal cells that invade a neuroblastoma recruited or attracted by trophic factors and may be responsible for tumor maturation and serve as an anti-neuroblastoma agent.[10,11,26] Schwann cells also produce angiogenesis inhibitors that induce endothelial cell apoptosis and may limit tumor growth by restricting angiogenesis.[27,40]

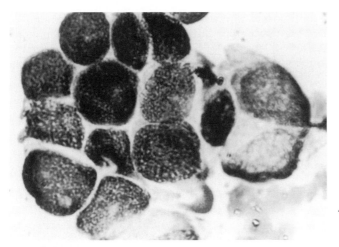

Figure 28-8 Histologic appearance of rosettes of neuroblastoma cells from a bone marrow aspirate, an early sign of tumor differentiation.

BIOLOGIC AND GENETIC ALTERATIONS

Unique oncogenes are observed in tumors, such as N-*myc* and *ras* oncogenes.[25,27] Amplification of N-*myc* (>10 copies) is associated with advanced disease, tumor progression, and a poor outcome, especially in children older than 1 year.[25,27,29,152,158,212] Overexpression of N-*myc* probably impairs differentiation and promotes the proliferation of immature neural crest–derived cells.[25,26] The N-*myc* proto-oncogene is located on the short arm of chromosome 2p24. Double minutes and long, nonbanding staining regions have been observed at this site and may represent amplified cellular genes. Approximately 30% of patients with neuroblastoma have tumors with N-*myc* amplification. More than 90% of patients with N-*myc* amplification have rapidly progressive disease and are reistant to therapy. DNA flow cytometry studies evaluating tumor ploidy indicate that children with diploid tumors have a worse outcome than those with aneuploid (hyperdiploidy or triploidy) tumors.[27,74] N-*myc* amplification is commonly associated with chromosome 1p deletion and diploidy.[30,89] Diploid tumors are commonly associated with an unbalanced gain of chromosome 17q, even in the absence of N-*myc*.[11,27,30,144] Allelic loss of 11q and 14q and gains of 4q, 6q, 11q, and 18q have also been observed (Table 28-3).[27]

High expression of the neurotropin Trk-A (a high-affinity nerve growth factor receptor) is associated with a good prognosis and is inversely related to N-*myc*.[157,158] Trk-A is observed in young infants and in those with stage I and stage IV-S tumors and indicates a very favorable outcome.[157,158] Trk-A is associated with neural cell differentiation and tumor regression and may play a role in angiogenic inhibition. The low-affinity nerve growth factor receptor gene is another proto-oncogene that has a prognostic effect similar to Trk-A and probably influences cellular maturation.[25,27,120] In contrast, high expression of Trk-B with its ligand BDNF may provide an autocrine survival pathway in unfavorable tumors, particularly those with N-*myc* amplification.[27,100,159] These patients have more advanced disease, are usually older than 1 year, and have a dismal outcome.[27,100,159] Trk-C expression has also been identified in neuroblastoma and is usually observed in lower-stage tumors that do not express N-*myc*.[27,240]

Another gene has been cloned, the multidrug resistance (MDR)-associated protein gene, that is associated with chemotherapy resistance, overexpression of N-*myc*, and a poor outcome.[166] Similarly, elevated P-glycoprotein levels are associated with progressive disease and a poor outcome.[35,235] Telomerase is increased in tumor cells and maintains cell viability by preserving the telomeres that protect the end of chromosomes.[27,191] There is an inverse relationship between telomerase levels and outcome in neuroblastoma and a direct correlation between telomerase levels and N-*myc* amplification.[27] CD44 is a glycoprotein found on the cell surface of a number of tumors, including neuroblastoma. High expression of CD44 is associated with a favorable outcome. In contrast, nm23 overexpression is observed in instances of advanced and aggressive neuroblastoma.[140] The ganglioside GD2 is found on human neuroblastoma cell membranes, and increased levels are associated with active disease and tumor progression. Gangliosides inhibit the tumor-specific immune response.[152]

TABLE 28-3 Genetic Alterations in Neuroblastoma

Genetic Feature	Associated Factors	Risk Group
N-*myc* amplification (2p24 locus)	Diploidy or tetraploidy Allelic loss of 1p, high Trk-B, advanced disease (stage III, IV)	High
Allelic gain		
17q gain	More aggressive tumor associated with N-*myc* amplification	High
Gain at 4q, 6p, 7q, 11q, 18q observed	Occurs concurrently with N-*myc* amplification	Risk related to N-*myc*
Allelic loss		
1p36	Often associated with N-*myc* 70%-80% are near diploid tumors associated with disease progression	High
11q	Few associated with N-*myc* amplification	Intermediate; decreased survival in patients without N-*myc* amplification
	Correlates with LOH 14q	
14q	Correlates with LOH 11q, inverse relationship with 1p and N-*myc*	Intermediate
Predisposition		
16p12-13	Familial neuroblastoma	Low
	Multifocal and bilateral neuroblastoma	
Association		
Chromosome 10 (Ret-oncogene)	Hirschsprung's disease	Variable
11p15.5	Beckwith-Wiedemann syndrome	Low

LOH, loss of heterozygosity.

Note: This table does not include changes in the genetic expression of Trk-A, -B, and -C; the multidrug-resistant protein gene; telomerase; or others that are covered elsewhere in this chapter.

Evaluation of the relationship between tumor angiogenesis and outcome in infants with neuroblastoma demonstrates that increased tumor vascularity characterized by microvessel density correlates with advanced disseminated disease and the likelihood of metastases.[47,49,57,153] Angiogenesis is controlled by the balance of humoral stimulators, inhibitors, and signal transduction pathways.[40] Angiogenesis is associated with N-*myc* amplification, unfavorable histology, and poor outcome. Neuroblastoma produces angiogenic factors that induce blood vessel growth, including vascular endothelial growth factor (VEFG), platelet-derived growth factor (PDGF-A), stem cell factor, and their respective receptors Flk-1, PDGFR, and C-*kit*.[15] Komuro et al.[122] demonstrated that high VEGF-A expression correlated with stage IV disease and suggested that it could be a target for antiangiogenic therapy. Kaicker et al.[112] noted that VEGF antagonists inhibit neoangiogenesis and tumor growth in experimental neuroblastoma in athymic mice with xenograft neuroblastoma cell line NGP. They also found that thalidomide suppressed angiogenesis and reduced microvessel density but not tumor growth. Kim et al.[117] and Rowe et al.[193] also demonstrated inhibition of tumor growth in experimental neuroblastoma models using antiangiogenic strategies. Imatinib mesylate, a compound used to treat patients with gastrointestinal stromal tumors, has been shown to decrease the growth of neuroblastoma in vivo and in vitro, decrease cell viability, and increase apoptosis (by ligand-stimulated phosphorylation of C-*kit* and PDGFR) in a severe combined immunodeficiency (SCID) mouse model.[15] Davidoff et al.[49] demonstrated that gene therapy using in situ tumor cell transduction with retroviral vectors can deliver angiogenesis inhibitors for the Flk-1 receptor and restrict tumor-induced angiogenesis and tumor growth.

The Bcl-2 family of proteins is responsible for relaying apoptotic signals that influence tumor cell regression and is expressed in most neuroblastomas. The *Bcl-2* gene produces a protein that prevents neuronal cell death (apoptosis). The level of Bcl-2 expression is high in advanced cases associated with a poor outcome and low in cases demonstrating tumor apoptosis (regression) and differentiation. High Bcl-2 expression may also play a role in acquired resistance to chemotherapy.[55] Subgroups of the Bcl-family include Bcl-xL, which inhibits apoptosis, and Bcl-xS, which induces natural cell death. VEGF upregulates Bcl-2 expression and promotes neuroblastoma cell survival by altering apoptosis and its regulation proteins.[14] Elevated caspase levels (enzymes responsible for apoptotic signaling) are associated with an improved outcome in neuroblastomas that demonstrate favorable biologic features.[27]

RISK-BASED MANAGEMENT

For many years, the choice of therapy in neuroblastoma varied with the extent of disease at the time of diagnosis, the patient's age, and the stage.[23,27,41,62] Total excision or excision of as much tumor as possible in localized cases resulted in the best outcomes.[61,73] Stage I lesions were managed by operation alone.[74,83] Patients with stage II disease had operative resection, but many had microscopic residual disease or tumor that extended into an intervertebral foramen, making complete resection impossible. Some of these patients received localized radiotherapy. Others received only operation, despite the presence of residual tumor; these patients had only a 75% to 80% cure rate.[74,124,164]

Because of the wide variability in tumor behavior in stage II patients with residual disease and the poor survival of those with more advanced tumors (stages III and IV), it became apparent that additional information was required to determine the appropriate treatment. During the past 2 decades, a number of biologic and genetic factors have been identified that are important prognostic indicators and currently influence therapy. Based on the impact of the new INSS, the use of the INPC, and the identification of numerous biologic and genetic characteristics as risk factors and predictors of outcome, a risk-based management system has been developed to determine treatment.[27,74,208-210,213] Newer treatment protocols individualize treatment using risk factors as predictors of outcome in an effort to maximize survival, minimize long-term morbidity, and improve the quality of life. Current protocols are now based on low-, intermediate-, and high-risk tumor categorization (Table 28-4). Good outcomes are associated with stage I, II, and IV-S patients who are younger than 1 year and have hyperdiploid DNA flow cytometry, favorable histology, less than one copy of N-*myc*, high Trk-A expression, and absence of chromosome 1p abnormalities. In contrast, a poor prognosis is likely in children older than 1 year with advanced tumors (stages III and IV), more than 10 copies of N-*myc*, low Trk-A expression, diploid DNA ploidy, allelic loss of 1p36, and unfavorable histology.

For low-risk patients, surgical excision of the tumor is usually curative and avoids the risks associated with chemotherapy. Intermediate-risk patients are usually treated with surgery and standard chemotherapy. The poor prognosis in high-risk patients justifies a much more intense treatment regimen, including combination chemotherapy followed by complete surgical excision (if possible), radiation therapy to achieve local control, myeloablative treatments, and bone marrow rescue.

OPERATIVE MANAGEMENT

Complete surgical removal of the primary tumor remains an essential component of treatment in the vast majority of cases. Operative procedures are performed using endotracheal general anesthesia and careful monitoring. Appropriate large-bore intravenous catheters are placed in the upper limbs. Adequate intravenous access is important because these tumors are quite vascular, and blood loss may be excessive. Body temperature, oxygen saturation, electrocardiogram, and pulse rate are monitored. The blood pressure must also be carefully monitored intraoperatively to detect sudden hypertension caused by excessive catecholamine release from the tumor.

In patients with primary tumors located in the retroperitoneum, the operation is performed through a long, transverse transperitoneal-supraumbilical incision.

TABLE 28-4 Neuroblastoma Risk Groups

INSS Stage	Age	N-*myc* Status*	INPC (Histology)	DNA Ploidy†	Risk Group
I	0-21 yr	Any	Any	Any	Low
IIA/IIB	>365 days	Any	Any	Any	Low
	365 days-21 yr	Nonamplified	Any	—	Low
	365 days-21 yr	Amplified	Favorable	—	Low
	365 days-21 yr	Amplified	Unfavorable	—	High
III	<365 days	Nonamplified	Any	Any	Intermediate
	<365 days	Amplified	Any	Any	High
	>365 days-21 yr	Nonamplified	Favorable	—	Intermediate
	>365 days-21 yr	Nonamplified	Unfavorable	—	High
	>365 days-21 yr	Amplified	Any	—	High
IV	<365 days	Nonamplified	Any	Any	Intermediate
	<365 days	Amplified	Any	Any	High
	>365 days-21 yr	Any	Any	—	High
IV-S	<365 days	Nonamplified	Favorable	>1	Low
	<365 days	Nonamplified	Any	=1	Intermediate
	<365 days	Nonamplified	Unfavorable	Any	Intermediate
	<365 days	Amplified	Any	Any	High

*N-*myc* nonamplified =1 copy, amplified >1 copy.
†DNA index >1 (aneuploid) or =1 (diploid).
INPC, International Neuroblastoma Pathology Classification; INSS, International Neuroblastoma Staging System.
Modified from Children's Oncology Group protocols by LaBerge JM: Neuroblastoma. In O'Neill JA Jr, Grosfeld JL, Fonkalsrud EW, Coran AG (eds): Principles of Pediatric Surgery, 2nd ed. St Louis, Mosby, 2003.

In some cases, a bilateral subcostal chevron incision or a thoracoabdominal incision may be required. The peritoneal space is entered, and on either side, the colon is reflected medially and inferiorly by incising the attachments to the lateral abdominal wall. The spleen and pancreas are mobilized and displaced upward and medially for left-sided tumors. For right-sided tumors, the duodenum and head of the pancreas can be mobilized and retracted medially and the liver attachments divided to improve exposure (Fig. 28-9). In most children with localized disease, all or most of the tumor can be removed successfully. The patient's condition should not be jeopardized by an overzealous surgical attempt at initial resection. En bloc contiguous resection of normal surrounding structures, such as the spleen, stomach, pancreas, and colon, can almost always be avoided. In some cases, it is impossible to separate an adrenal or paraspinal neuroblastoma from the ipsilateral kidney, and nephrectomy may be necessary. It is important to excise any suspicious para-aortic and perirenal lymph nodes for staging purposes. A routine retroperitoneal lymph node dissection is usually not performed. The margins of the tumor resection are marked with titanium clips to guide the port if radiation is required and will reduce the scatter effect noted with other types of metal clips on follow-up CT scan.

Because neuroblastoma may have a friable pseudocapsule, careful handling of the tumor during dissection is important to avoid tumor spill and hemorrhage. Neuroblastoma often adheres to or surrounds the great vessels, and special care should be taken to identify and spare the blood supply to important visceral structures, such as the branches of the celiac axis and superior mesenteric artery. Primary adrenal tumors may be fed by a number of small arteries. The major venous drainage is usually constant, directly to the inferior vena cava on the right side and into the left renal vein and subdiaphragmatic vessels on the left. Although there is no good evidence that partial excision and reduction of tumor bulk favorably affect the prognosis for this highly malignant childhood neoplasm, an improved response to adjunctive therapy has been observed when tumor resection has been accomplished.[74,83,134] Overly aggressive palliative debulking that places the child at risk for life-threatening hemorrhage is not indicated. Following a good response to initial chemotherapy, the tumor often shrinks and can be removed during a delayed primary resection or at a second-look operative procedure.[75,78,83,85,134] Inferiorly located paraspinal and primary pelvic tumors often require careful dissection to separate the lesion from the bifurcation of the aorta and inferior vena cava. The tumor frequently extends into the intervertebral foramina (Fig. 28-10).

Minimally invasive surgical techniques have also been employed for selected cases of neuroblastoma.[102] Adrenal tumors initially detected by mass screening have been excised laparoscopically by a number of investigators.[123,160] Yamamoto et al.[239] described three cases of adrenal neuroblastoma in which the lesions were less than 20 mm in diameter. They used a five-trocar technique and kept the intra-abdominal pressure for the pneumoperitoneum less than 4 mm Hg. The well-encapsulated tumors were completely excised; they were placed in a plastic bag and removed through the 10-mm trocar site. All had favorable histology, and none had N-*myc* amplification. No recurrences were observed. Kouch et al.[125] described laparoscopic resection of six adrenal tumors less than 4 cm in size. There were no conversions

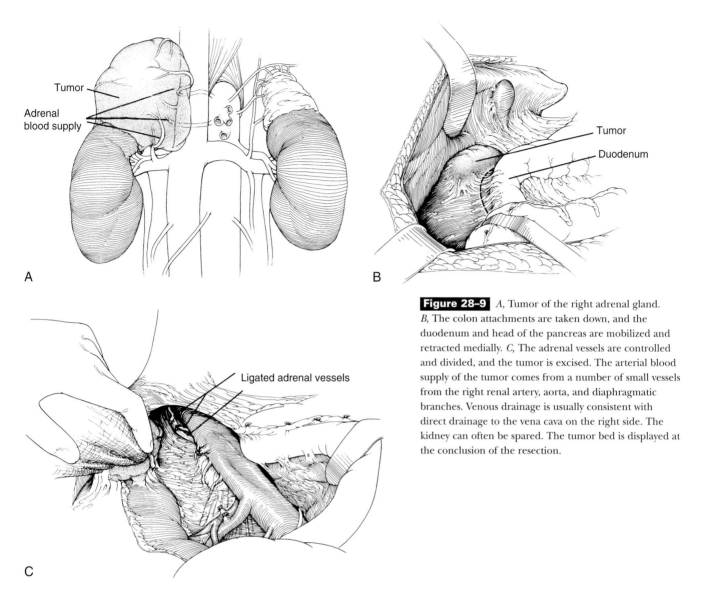

A

Tumor

Adrenal
blood supply

B

Tumor

Duodenum

Ligated adrenal vessels

C

Figure 28–9 *A,* Tumor of the right adrenal gland. *B,* The colon attachments are taken down, and the duodenum and head of the pancreas are mobilized and retracted medially. *C,* The adrenal vessels are controlled and divided, and the tumor is excised. The arterial blood supply of the tumor comes from a number of small vessels from the right renal artery, aorta, and diaphragmatic branches. Venous drainage is usually consistent with direct drainage to the vena cava on the right side. The kidney can often be spared. The tumor bed is displayed at the conclusion of the resection.

or tumor recurrence in the abdomen or at the port sites. Iwanaka et al.[107] used laparoscopy for tumor biopsy in advanced cases of neuroblastoma and compared the minimally invasive resection of tumors to open excision via laparotomy. There was no significant difference in the length of procedure or blood loss; however, time to start chemotherapy, interval to postoperative oral intake, and length of hospital stay were less following laparoscopic tumor resection.[107,108] De Lagausie et al.[52] described nine cases of adrenal neuroblastoma treated by the laparoscopic approach. Two were detected prenatally, and seven were noted postnatally, including three with stage IV disease. The mean age was 38 months (range, 2 months to 9 years). Complete excision was accomplished in eight children, and one had to be converted to an open procedure. In three cases, one or more lymph nodes were also excised. There were no deaths and one port site infection. These and other reports suggest that in selected cases, laparoscopic biopsy and tumor excision are both safe and effective.[52]

Mediastinal tumors are usually approached through a standard posterolateral thoracotomy incision. Excision of the pleura and the endothoracic fascia around the tumor usually allows entry into an appropriate dissection plane. Mobilization of the tumor from the rib edges is accomplished with both sharp and blunt dissection. It is important to identify and either ligate or clip specific intercostal blood vessels feeding and draining the tumor. The tumor may be attached to a number of sympathetic ganglia and intercostal nerves and often extends, in one or more areas, into the intervertebral foramina (Fig. 28-11).[4,66,155,243] It may be impossible to remove every bit of tumor at the foraminal sites. Small primary tumors have been successfully removed by thoracoscopic techniques. Thoracoscopy is also useful in obtaining tissue for biopsy.

In patients with neurologic symptoms (including paraplegia) associated with dumbbell tumors, prompt MRI and an urgent laminotomy to excise extradural tumor and relieve cord compression are recommended before attempting intrathoracic resection of the tumor. The mediastinal resection can be delayed a short time to allow the patient's neurologic symptoms to improve. If extradural tumor is present on imaging studies but the patient is asymptomatic, chemotherapy is initiated and

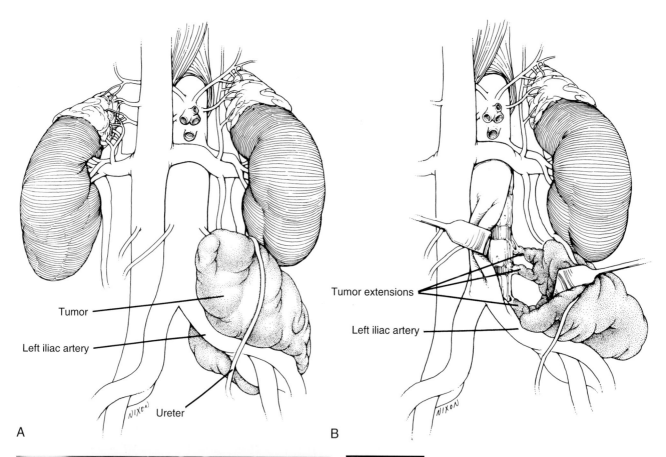

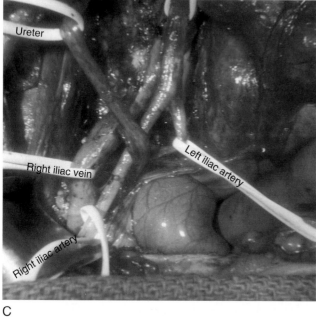

Figure 28–10 *A,* Lower retroperitoneal paraspinal neuroblastoma and its relationship to the bifurcation of the aorta and ureter. *B,* Tumor may extend into the vertebral foramina. *C,* Photograph of the operative field after resection of a right-sided pelvic neuroblastoma. Note the vascular loops placed around the iliac arteries, right iliac vein, and ureter to facilitate a safe dissection. *(C, see color plate.)*

may shrink the tumor and avoid the need for laminotomy or laminectomy. The choice of therapy for intraspinal tumor extension is still somewhat controversial. Plantaz et al.[174] reviewed 42 patients in France and recommended initial chemotherapy followed by surgical removal of residual disease. Yiin et al.[242] described 13 cases of neuroblastoma with symptomatic spinal cord compression and neurologic deficits. All the patients were treated initially with chemotherapy: three recovered, four improved, and six worsened and became paraplegic. Two of the six recovered after laminectomy. Those authors recommended spinal cord decompression for patients who have neurologic deterioration on chemotherapy. Sandberg et al.[198] described the treatment

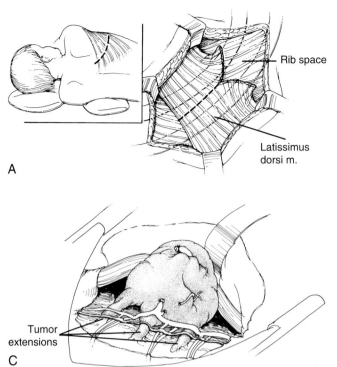

A

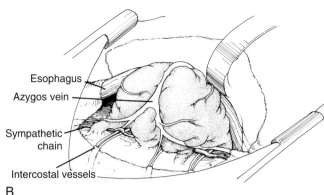

B

C

Figure 28–11 *A*, Right posterolateral thoracotomy incision used for the excision of a posterior mediastinal neuroblastoma. *B*, Relationship of the tumor to surrounding tissues. *C*, The tumor is mobilized and retracted anteriorly, exposing numerous intervertebral extensions. The tumor extensions are divided at the vertebral foramina, leaving small remnants of residual tumor behind. This does not adversely influence the outcome.

of 46 patients with epidural or neural foraminal tumor involvement. Nine were low-risk patients with normal neurologic examinations who remained neurologically intact following operation or chemotherapy. Four low-risk patients with high-grade spinal cord compression improved or remained stable after surgical intervention, but two who were treated with chemotherapy had worsening deficits. Eleven of 12 high-risk patients with normal neurologic examinations and without radiographic high-grade spinal cord compression were treated with chemotherapy and had no neurologic deterioration. Of 16 high-risk patients with high-grade spinal cord compression, 7 of 10 treated initially with chemotherapy and all 6 who underwent initial surgery improved or remained stable. Spinal deformities occurred in 12.5% (2 of 16) treated nonoperatively and in 30% (9 of 30) who underwent operation. The authors concluded that patients with high-risk tumors and spinal involvement but normal neurologic examinations should be offered chemotherapy, with the understanding that a small percentage may require operations for progressive neurologic deficits. Chemotherapy may be avoided in patients with low-risk tumors who can be offered a potentially curative procedure. Patients and their families should be made aware that operative intervention may be associated with subsequent spinal deformity in as many as 30% of cases.[198]

Cervical neuroblastoma is often localized and has a favorable outcome.[82] Haddad et al.,[86] in a study of 43 cervical neuroblastomas, identified four risk factors that were associated with increased operative morbidity: adherence to vascular structures, tumor size, friability, and dumbbell tumors. Imaging studies may show a solid mass with vascular displacement and narrowing.[2] Tumors arising in the neck or upper mediastinum often involve

the stellate ganglion. If not present preoperatively, resection may result in postoperative Horner's syndrome.[2,73] This is a relatively minor consequence outweighed by complete tumor excision and survival, but the patient's family should be made aware of this possible complication. Special attention should be given to protecting the brachial plexus and the phrenic, vagus, and recurrent laryngeal nerves. Whether additional therapy is necessary for stage II tumors depends on the patient's risk assessment based on age, tumor histology, and presence of adverse biologic and genetic factors (e.g., >10 copies of N-*myc*, chromosome 1p deletion, diploid flow cytometry, unfavorable histology).[74] Thirteen percent of stage II cases have high-risk prognostic factors and require aggressive chemotherapy.

Patients with more advanced disease (stage III) often require more aggressive treatment, including operative resection (if possible), multiagent chemotherapy, and initial local irradiation. Stage III tumors in the pelvis or near the celiac axis are often unresectable initially. After chemotherapy, however, the tumor frequently becomes small enough to be excised at a second-look operation.[74,83] Patients with stage III disease have an improved outlook after complete resection.[74,85] The type of adjunctive therapy depends on tumor resectability, histology, and biologic and genetic characteristics affecting risk for that specific neoplasm. Completely resected tumors with favorable prognostic factors may require less intensive chemotherapy. In contrast, patients with incomplete tumor resection are usually treated with local irradiation to the tumor bed and more dose-intensive chemotherapy regimens. Those with high-risk unresponsive tumors may benefit from intensive cytoablative chemotherapy followed by autologous bone marrow transplantation (BMT).[31,84,148,149] High-risk stage III cases can usually be predicted by the presence of adverse biologic features, such as age older than 1 year, unfavorable tumor histology, and more than 10 copies of N-myc.[148,149] The marrow is purged for tumor cells with multiple monoclonal antibodies before BMT.[151] Employment of BMT early in the management of unresponsive tumors with high-risk biologic factors results in a better outcome than if BMT is attempted as a last-ditch effort in patients with progressive disease.[149,151,178] In recent years, the use of autologous stem cell transplantation has replaced traditional BMT in many childhood cancer facilities.

The CCG compared initial resection at diagnosis with delayed primary resection and second-look procedures for initially inoperable stage IV tumors. Complete resection was possible in 62% of the initial group, 77% of delayed primary operations, and 66% of second-look procedures.[84] The risk of concomitant nephrectomy and the incidence of postoperative complications were lower in children in the delayed primary resection group.[84] Because there was no difference in survival among the three groups (40% among complete responders at 3 years), delayed primary resection after chemotherapy was considered the procedure of choice in children with stage IV tumors. The role of primary tumor resection in patients with stage IV disease is unsettled. In patients who respond completely or partially to chemotherapy, it has been my practice to perform a delayed primary or second-look operation to remove all possible residual tumor. There are conflicting reports concerning the efficacy of complete resection in stage IV disease. Haase et al.,[84] reporting for the CCG, described a survival advantage for stage IV patients with complete resection following delayed primary excision after chemotherapy. In contrast, reports by Kiely[116] and Shorter et al.[215] suggest that there is no survival advantage for stage IV patients with complete resection. However, LaQuaglia et al.,[134] in a report of 70 stage IV patients, noted that gross tumor resection and a higher-intensity chemotherapy protocol resulted in improved overall survival. Although some studies have shown an improved survival in stage IV

patients with a complete response to chemotherapy and tumor resection,[78,84,218] data concerning the biologic characteristics of the surviving patients were often lacking, and an independent effect of gross tumor resection could not be demonstrated.[134] More recently, LaQuaglia et al.[135] reviewed 141 INSS stage IV patients and reaffirmed that the rate of gross tumor resection improved with more intense chemotherapy. The probability of local tumor progression was 50% in unresected patients, compared with 10% in those with gross total resection. The overall survival rate was 50% in resected patients, versus 11% in patients with unresected tumors.[135] Aggressive surgical management is occasionally associated with late complications in survivors, including ipsilateral atrophy of the kidney following adrenal resection and ejaculatory problems following pelvic tumor excision.[126] Of interest is the very favorable outlook noted in patients with stage III and IV tumors arising in the pelvis following complete tumor resection.[74,84]

NEUROBLASTOMA IN INFANCY

Infants younger than 1 year at diagnosis have a significantly improved outcome. At the Riley Hospital for Children, the survival rate was 76% for infants younger than 1 year and only 32% for older patients (Fig. 28-12).[76] This favorable outlook for patients younger than 1 year extends across all stages, including infants with stage IV metastatic disease. The incidence of stage IV lesions in infants younger than 1 year is 30%, compared with 60% to 70% in older patients.[76]

Although resection of the primary tumor in stage IV disease is controversial, in my personal experience, the only infant survivors had excision of the primary tumor.[76] Similarly, a CCG report described 7 of 11 infants with stage IV disease who had complete delayed primary tumor resection and remained disease free for more than 5 years.[84,85] Infants with stage IV disease respond better to chemotherapy than older children do; 50% of

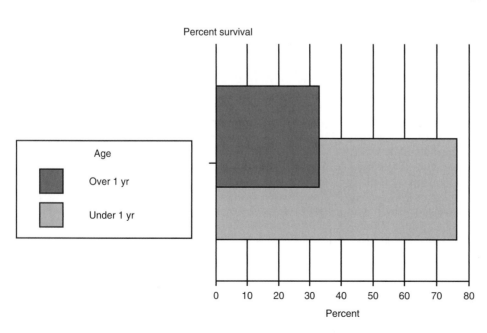

Figure 28-12 Bar graph demonstrates the improved survival in infants with neuroblastoma who are younger than 1 year.

infants have a complete response to treatment, compared with 22% of older children.[85] This observation suggests that resolution of metastases may have a greater impact on length of survival than the surgical excision does. Further, this implies that surgical resection is beneficial in some infants and should be attempted when disseminated disease is controlled by chemotherapy.

Paul et al.[170] documented a 75% 5-year survival rate in 24 stage IV patients younger than 1 year, compared with a 10% survival rate for older patients with stage IV tumors. Patients were treated with nitrogen mustard, vincristine, dacarbazine, doxorubicin, cyclophosphamide, and cisplatin without BMT. Schmidt et al.[204] observed a 93% survival rate in infants younger than 1 year with stage IV disease without N-*myc* amplification; however, those with more than 10 copies of the N-*myc* oncogene had rapidly progressive disease and often succumbed despite chemotherapy.[204] Therefore, more intensive chemotherapy regimens and BMT may be necessary to attain a cure, especially in highly selected infants presenting with adverse biologic markers.

STAGE IV-S

The most unusual group of patients with neuroblastoma are those infants younger than 1 year with stage IV-S disease, characterized by hepatomegaly, subcutaneous nodules, and positive bone marrow, that would otherwise be classified as stage I or II primary tumor. Stage IV-S cases account for approximately 30% of patients with neuroblastoma

recognized in the first year of life.[76] Treatment of these patients is somewhat controversial. Some infants may die as a result of complications of stage IV-S disease rather than tumor progression.

Complications of severe hepatomegaly include respiratory insufficiency, caused by significant elevation of the diaphragm by the large, tumor-filled liver; coagulopathy; and renal compromise due to compression by the mass (Fig. 28-13).[21,45,50,76,236] Vomiting may occur because of a change in the gastroesophageal angle related to the diaphragmatic elevation, resulting in gastroesophageal reflux, protein-calorie malnutrition, and aspiration pneumonia. Total parenteral nutrition may be a useful therapeutic adjunct.[188,189,231] Most fatalities in stage IV-S cases occur in infants younger than 2 months with severe symptoms related to hepatomegaly, who do not tolerate therapy as well as older infants do.[76,162] Symptomatic hepatomegaly caused by tumor infiltration may benefit from low-dose irradiation to the liver in the range of 600 to 1200 Gy, administered in doses of 100 to 150 Gy/day.[21,76,83] Although some early reduction in the size of the liver is seen, and peripheral edema may resolve in a few weeks, complete resolution may take 6 to 15 months.[76] Resolution of the liver mass is probably related more to the natural course of stage IV-S disease than to radiotherapy. Administration of low-dose cyclophosphamide 5 mg/kg per day is a reasonable treatment alternative. Although some investigators advocate the insertion of a Dacron-reinforced Silastic sheet to create a temporary ventral abdominal wall hernia to accommodate the enlarged liver and reduce intra-abdominal pressure, I have not

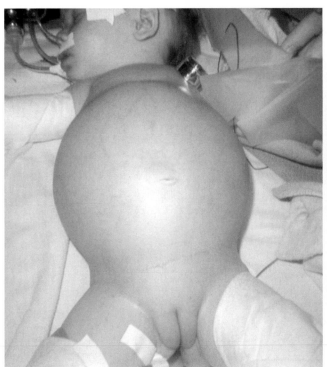

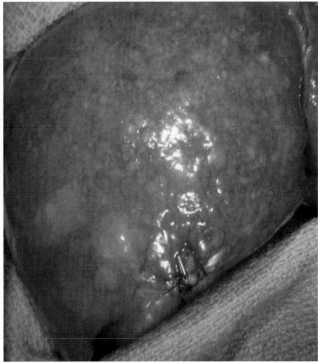

A
B

Figure 28-13 *A*, Six-week-old infant presented with abdominal distention and hepatomegaly. *B*, Appearance of the liver at laparotomy. There were multiple metastatic nodules, and the biopsy confirmed the diagnosis of stage IV-S neuroblastoma.

found this technique to be effective.[205] Mortality due to septic complications after insertion of an external Silastic sheet has been observed.[21,76] To reduce the risk of infection, Lee and Applebaum[139] recommend the use of an internal polytetrafluoroethylene patch to create a temporary ventral hernia. The graft can be removed in stages as the bulk of the hepatic mass regresses over time.

Survival of these unusual infants with remote metastases is greater than 80%, often without specific treatment. Table 82-5 summarizes the results reported in 12 studies of stage IV-S neuroblastoma, with an overall 86% survival rate. Most patients with stage IV-S disease (>90%) have favorable genetic and biologic factors, including high Trk-A expression, no N-*myc* amplification, favorable histology, and no evidence of allelic loss of chromosome 1p. This suggests that the majority of stage IV-S tumors undergo spontaneous regression. Although most patients with stage IV-S disease do well, Wilson et al.[236] reported 18 cases with a heterogeneous tumor presentation and a survival rate of only 50%, including three patients with N-*myc* amplification. The presence of adverse genetic and biologic prognostic factors suggests that this subset of patients (<10%) requires more aggressive therapy. Of interest is that infants with multiple subcutaneous nodules seem to have the most favorable outlook. This may be due to increased immunologic activity as a result of tumor being present in multiple sites.[76] Increased uptake of major histocompatibility complex (MHC) class I antigen by neuroblastoma cells in vitro and in vivo may influence the outcome favorably.[220] Infants with stage IV-S disease have normal levels of MHC class I surface antigen expression, whereas those with stages I to IV have low levels.[220] Sugio et al.[224] reported that down-modulation of MHC class I antigen expression is associated with increased amplification of the N-*myc* oncogene in patients with advanced disease.

In 2002 Nickerson et al.[162] described 80 infants with stage IV-S disease from the CCG. Fifty-eight cases were managed without specific therapy. All 44 asymptomatic patients survived without treatment. Symptomatic patients were treated with cyclophosphamide 5 mg/kg per day for 5 days and hepatic radiation at a dose of 4.5 Gy over 3 days. Five of six deaths occurred in symptomatic infants younger than 2 months. Event-free 5-year survival was 86%, and overall survival was 92%. Early intervention is indicated in stage IV-S patients with life-threatening complications (e.g., hepatosplenomegaly, coagulopathy, renal failure).[76,162] Surgical resection did not alter outcome. More aggressive chemotherapy is also required in those cases in which the tumor demonstrates more than 10 copies of N-*myc*, chromosome 1p deletion, or other adverse biologic markers.[76,162,203] Amplification of N-*myc* may be observed in 1 of 12 patients with stage IV-S tumors who develop progressive disease and succumb, despite having a favorable prognostic stage. In 2003 Schleiermacher et al.,[203] in a report concerning 94 babies with stage IV-S neuroblastoma in France, observed an 88% overall survival and recommended a more intensive regimen using cisplatin and etoposide for those who require therapy. Some infants with stage IV-S have survived without resection of the primary tumor (in some, the primary tumor may not be identified). Knowing that resection of the primary tumor may have some benefit in infants with stage IV tumors, resection of the primary neoplasm should be accomplished when feasible, especially in high-risk stage IV-S cases with any unfavorable characteristics.[76]

CYSTIC NEUROBLASTOMA

Cystic neuroblastomas are relatively rare and are often identified on prenatal ultrasound examinations.[227] They characteristically occur in the adrenal gland, and almost all are diagnosed in early infancy (Fig. 28-14). Few are calcified, and only 10% are associated with elevation of

TABLE 28-5 Survival in Stage IV-S Neuroblastoma		
Author (Year)	No. of Patients	No. of Survivors (%)
D'Angio et al (1971)[45]	16	14 (88)
Breslow et al (1971)[23]	19	18 (95)
Nitschke et al (1980)[165]	11	11 (100)
Nickerson et al (1985)[163]	35	31 (89)
Blatt et al (1987)[21]	11	8 (73)
Wilson et al (1991)[236]	18	9 (50)
Suarez et al (1991)[223]	34	28 (75)
DeBernardi et al (1992)[50]	76	63 (83)
Grosfeld et al (1993)[76]	21	17 (81)
Hatchitanda et al (1996)[88]	45	36 (80)
Nickerson et al (2000)[162]	80	74 (92)
Schleiermacher et al (2003)[203]	94	83 (88)
Total	460	392 (85)

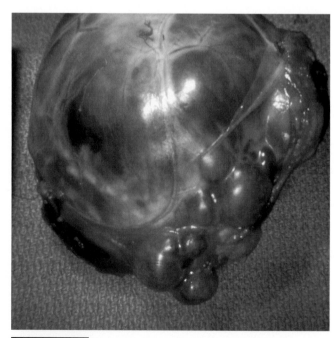

Figure 28–14 Photograph of a cystic neuroblastoma of the adrenal gland in a 5-month-old baby that required complete excision. The patient was managed by surgery alone and is a long-term survivor.

urinary VMA and HVA levels.[187] They are associated with a benign behavior and a favorable outcome. There is some evidence that these lesions have a tendency to regress and undergo spontaneous involution.[103] Some investigators have recommended observation alone, with close serial sonogram monitoring of the mass during the first few months of life to be sure that the tumor mass shrinks, indicating tumor regression. Operative resection should be reserved for those tumors that fail to regress or that increase in size. When resection is indicated, surgery is the only therapy recommended. The COG has initiated a prospective study of observation only for cases of cystic neuroblastoma. It uses strict criteria in terms of tumor volume (<16 mL if solid or <65 mL if cystic), taking into account the fact that neonates with cystic neuroblastoma may have large tumors but an excellent prognosis.

MULTIFOCAL AND BILATERAL NEUROBLASTOMA

Bilateral neuroblastoma is relatively uncommon and occurs more often in familial cases in young infants who may have alterations at the predisposition locus on chromosome 16p12-13.[145] In the past, therapy has included observation alone; unilateral resection, with observation of the second (smaller) lesion or enucleation; and bilateral adrenalectomy and hormonal support. I have treated three children with bilateral tumors (one occurring metachronously) with bilateral adrenal excision. All three are long-term survivors maintained on hormonal support. Some bilateral tumors resolve spontaneously, while others persist and enlarge, requiring surgical intervention. The prognosis is good, and most of the children survive. Occasionally these infants have other sites of multifocal disease. Tumor enucleation has been performed in cases with favorable biologic markers to preserve adrenal function. Hiyama et al.[98] described multifocal neuroblastoma in 8 of 106 cases (7.5%).[98] Seven of eight had favorable histology, and all expressed Trk-A1 mRNA and the Ha-ras p21 protein. None of the patients expressed N-*myc* amplification or had elevated telomerase levels. Four had near triploid DNA flow cytometry, and all eight had a proliferative index (percentage of cells in the S-phase) of less than 25%. Four were treated with multistage resections. Five had bilateral neuroblastoma and were treated with tumor enucleation. All survived and are free of recurrence, and none require steroid replacement. The authors reviewed 53 additional multifocal cases and noted that 18 had a family history of neuroblastoma and 25 were detected incidentally. Because of the excellent prognosis in patients with favorable biologic features, Hiyama's group recommended conservative surgical excision (enucleation) using minimally invasive surgical techniques.[98]

CHEMOTHERAPY

Although multiagent chemotherapy has significantly improved the survival rate in many tumors (e.g., Wilms' tumor), chemotherapy has no such effect in infants and children with resectable localized neuroblastoma with favorable biologic and genetic characteristics. For stage I and most stage II patients, surgery alone is all that is necessary.[61,74,83] Stage II patients with poor prognostic biologic and genetic factors, however, are at higher risk and should be treated more aggressively with multiagent chemotherapy, including cisplatin, doxorubicin (Adriamycin), cyclophosphamide, and etoposide (VP-16). For advanced cases (stages III and IV), the mainstay agents throughout the 1970s and early 1980s included cyclophosphamide, vincristine, and dacarbazine.[61,64,67] Treatment failures received doxorubicin and teniposide (VM-26).

Although these chemotherapy protocols did not effectively increase the cure rate of stage IV patients, such treatment reduced the size of the primary tumor, often cleared the bone marrow of tumor cells, and occasionally was associated with histologic maturation from malignant neuroblastoma to benign ganglioneuroma.[67,77] Unfortunately, only 40% of patients with stage IV disease demonstrated a complete response to chemotherapy; 30% had a partial response, and 30% were unresponsive.[67] When the clinical estimation of response was subjected to confirmation by laparotomy, many patients thought to be responders to chemotherapy actually had persistent tumor not identified by preoperative testing.[75,78,218]

Numerous studies confirmed the limited effectiveness of chemotherapy regimens in patients with metastatic disease.[67,165] Using cell kinetic data, Hayes et al.[92] demonstrated that the proliferating fraction of the tumor cell population in neuroblastoma is exceedingly small. A large pool of nonproliferating resting cells is resistant to chemotherapy. Timed sequential administration of cell cycle–specific and nonspecific drugs (cyclophosphamide and doxorubicin, or cisplatin with teniposide or doxorubicin) was subsequently tested and resulted in improved response rates.[72,90] This improvement led to more aggressive, more intensive treatment programs using multiple agents, including cyclophosphamide, doxorubicin, cisplatin, teniposide, and etoposide.[165] Myeloablative therapy using near-lethal doses of phenylalanine mustard (melphalan) with autologous bone marrow rescue also improved the tumor response rate.[178] A combination of melphalan, doxorubicin, teniposide, and low-dose total-body irradiation followed by autologous BMT resulted in a 40% relapse-free rate and, if deaths due to toxicity were excluded, a 34% 2-year survival rate in stage IV patients.[44]

Based on these findings, treatment for stage IV and for advanced stage III disease became more aggressive. More dose-intensive chemotherapy, using combinations of cyclophosphamide, doxorubicin, cisplatin, teniposide or etoposide, and vincristine, was employed.[62,132,149] Surgery and regional and total-body irradiation of residual disease in the tumor bed were added.[84,151] An alternative treatment relied on myeloablative chemotherapy using escalating doses of drugs given by constant infusion, followed by autologous (purged) bone marrow infusion but without total-body irradiation.[151] Newer chemotherapeutic agents, including ifosfamide, carboplatin, and epirubicin, were brought into use.[233] The addition of 13-*cis*-retinoic acid (isotretinoin), a biologic response modifier that causes tumor differentiation and decreases bone marrow tumor involvement, was shown to be useful.[151,184,233] Reynolds et al.,[183,185] in a phase III randomized trial in high-risk patients, showed that high-dose pulse therapy with 13-*cis*-retinoic acid given after completion of intensive chemoradiation (with or without auotologous BMT) significantly improved event-free survival. In phase I studies, the cytotoxic synthetic retinoid 4-HPR (fenretinide) achieved multilog cell kills in neuroblastoma cell lines resistant to trans- and 13-*cis*-retinoic acid and was better tolerated when ceramide modulators were used to reduce toxicity. Fenretinide has also been shown to exhibit antiangiogenic properties.[186]

Other high-intensity, compressed chemotherapy protocols include the use of high-dose cyclophosphamide, carboplatin, and etoposide with granulocyte colony-stimulating factor to mobilize peripheral blood stem cells and enhance hematopoietic reconstitution of neutrophils and platelets. The stem cells are harvested by leukapheresis for later reinfusion. Mesna is used to avoid high-dose cyclophosphamide-induced hemorrhagic cystitis. After dose-intense induction, surgical intervention is employed to resect the primary tumor and any bulky metastases. Peripheral blood stem cell infusion is used to reconstitute the marrow after myeloablative treatment. Immunoglobulin G levels are monitored and replaced with gamma globulin. Sulfamethoxazole and fluconazole are given prophylactically to avoid opportunistic *Pneumocystis carinii* and fungal infection.

With regard to BMT, patients who receivied purged autologous cells responded better than those getting allogeneic cells, mainly because of a higher toxic death rate and an increased incidence of graft-versus-host disease in the latter group.[148] Patients with high-risk stage IV disease have a better outcome with BMT, especially if they have amplification of the N-*myc* oncogene.[148,150,151] These newer chemotherapy pilot programs resulted in improved survival of stage III patients older than 2 years at diagnosis from 36% to 86%; survival of stage IV patients (older than 1 year) increased from 11% to 37% at 3 years of age and was 23% at 6 years of age.[148,149] There is a high risk of Epstein-Barr virus–associated lymphoproliferative disease with highly immunosuppressive therapies.[176] Allogeneic BMT, especially when supported by T-cell-depleted stem cell products, is a risk factor. Although the risk after autologous BMT is low (3.5%), there is an increased risk when sequentially high-dose chemotherapy is supported by CD34+-selected peripheral blood stem cells. Median time to lymphoproliferative disease was 3 months post transplant. All patients with lymphoproliferatiave disease were in the selected CD34+ group; treatment was with rituximab and ganciclovir. In many centers, peripheral blood stem cell transplantation has replaced autologous BMT as the method of choice. Obtaining blood can be accomplished on an outpatient basis with less pain and anxiety, and stem cell transplantation is associated with fewer complications and less toxicity. Tumor cells can be purged from the sample. Kanold et al.[114] reported that ex vivo expansion of autologous perihperal blood CD34+ cells provided a purge effect in children with neuroblastoma, documented

by screening the number of tyrosine hydroxylase mRNA transcripts.

RADIATION THERAPY

In general, the role of radiation therapy in the management of neuroblastoma has become more limited in recent years. Once a mainstay of treatment, radiation therapy is used primarily (1) to control local disease in instances of incomplete tumor resection or local recurrence, (2) to reduce the tumor burden in preparation for BMT, and (3) for palliation in patients with refractory end-stage disease or painful metastases.[53,81,113,143]

External beam radiation is associated with considerable toxicity in growing children, resulting in growth disturbance, bony deformity, endocrine deficiency, hypoplastic soft tissue changes, skin atrophy, and, of greater concern, secondary malignancies in the radiation portal. Techniques used to decrease radiation-induced toxicity include hyperfractionating the radiation dose, which usually does not reduce the desired antitumor effect, and avoiding the simultaneous administration of chemotherapy agents that may enhance the radiation effect.[133] Brachytherapy and intraoperative radiotherapy can better confine the radiation effect to the target tissue and spare surrounding normal tissues.[80,138] Although early local control can be achieved, only 38% of stage IV patients given intraoperative radiotherapy survived after 3 years. Some patients still require supplemental external beam radiation, and postoperative ureteral stricture, renal artery stenosis, and neuropathies have been described.[83] Haas-Kogan et al.[80] described an experience using intraoperative radiotherapy in 23 cases of high-risk neuroblastoma and noted that this technique was effective only in patients who had gross total resection of the primary tumor.[80] All patients with partial tumor resection had recurrence, despite radiotherapy, and subsequently died. There are few data to support the efficacy of this therapy. Intraoperative radiotherapy is sometimes cumbersome to perform, especially in institutions that do not have an operative suite in the radiotherapy department or radiation therapy equipment (including linear accelerators) in the operating room. Under these circumstances, after attempted tumor resection, the patient has to be transported under general anesthesia for the treatment to take place.

Children with refractory advanced neuroblastoma with widespread involvement often suffer severe pain due to metastases. Kang et al.[113] employed targeted radiotherapy using submyeloablative doses of I^{131}-MIBG to achieve disease palliation. The treatment stabilized disease, relieved pain, or improved performance status, with 31% of patients showing an objective response to treatment. They concluded that this modality is useful for treating end-stage neuroblastoma. Targeted radiation therapy with MIBG has also been used in combination with myeloablative chemotherapy and proton beam radiation for recurrent and refractory neuroblastoma. Proton beam therapy has the advantage of delivering radiation more precisely than conventional methods. As it becomes more widely available, it may play a greater role in the management of children with neuroblastoma requiring radiation treatment.[27]

Deutsch and Tersak[53] decribed the use of radiotherapy (300 to 1000 cGy) for palliative treatment of symptomatic metastases to bone. The most common treatment sites were the skull, spine, hip, and femur. Twenty-nine percent of patients survived 1 year or longer (range, 1 to 52 months). Only 8% survived more than 3 years.

IMMUNOTHERAPY

In the 1970s and 1980s, it was observed that tumor regression in neuroblastoma suggests that an immunologic mechanism may be involved, resulting from an unusual tumor-host relationship.[6,17,20,170] Lymphocytes from children with neuroblastoma were observed to inhibit colonies of neuroblasts in culture but not cells from other tumors.[20] Sera from patients with progressive disease contain a blocking antibody that prevents a lymphocyte-mediated cytotoxic response and inhibits lymphocyte blastogenesis to phytohemagglutinins.[94,95] Lymphocytes from patients with neuroblastoma also have a decreased systemic and in situ natural killer activity.[71] In experimental studies, operative electrocoagulation[245] and hyperthermia resulting from high-intensity focused ultrasonography induced immunity in mice with neuroblastoma. A major problem is that advanced neuroblastoma cells are MHC class I deficient and evade immunorecognition.

Although immunotherapy evolved slowly, this has changed with the production of recombinant interleukin-2 (IL-2), a cytokine that can mediate immunoreactivity and cancer regression.[192] IL-2 is produced by helper T lymphocytes. The interaction of antigens with T lymphocytes activates lymphoid cells to express receptors for IL-2. Stimulation of IL-2 secretion leads to expansion of immune cells and effective immunity. Newer molecular biologic techniques have been developed to identify genes that encode cancer antigens and their immunogenic peptides. Immune cells can be generated against the antigens present on cancer cells that are the potential targets of immune therapy.[192]

Vertuani et al.[232] reported that retinoids and T-cell-based immunotherapy may be an effective combination for the treatment of neuroblastoma. Retinoids serve as multistep modulators of the MHC class I presentation pathway and sensitize neuroblastomas to cytotoxic lymphocytes.[183,185,232] The use of tumor cell vaccines derived from irradiated cells transduced with IL-2 or interferon, targeted I[121]-MIBG therapy, and I[131]-labeled anti-GD2 antibody therapy have been attempted alone or in combination with BMT; however, data are not yet available to document the efficacy of these treatments.[148] Raffaghello et al.[180] employed an anti-GD2 antibody in nude mice with neuroblastoma and noted increased long-term survival and decreased metastatic spread in a dose-dependent manner in treated mice compared with controls. Cheung et al.[39] suggested that immunotherapy using ganglioside GD2 monoclonal antibody should be directed at minimal disease and must be used in conjunction with

dose-intensive chemotherapy to be effective. Kushner et al.[130] described the management of seven patients who relapsed with widespread disease after initial treatment with surgery alone for locoregional neuroblastoma. They received dose-intensive chemotherapy, anti-GD2 3F8 antibody, and targeted radiotherapy using I[131]-labeled 3F8 if they had assessable disease, or 3F8, granulocyte-macrophage colony-stimulating factor, and 13-*cis*-retinoic acid if they were in remission. Five of the seven patients remained in remission from 4 to 8 years later.[130] The same group reported that high-dose cyclophosphamide, irinotecan, and topotecan were effective in achieving remission and inducing an immunologic state conducive to antibody-based passive immunotherapy (using 3F8 antibody) in resistant neuroblastoma.[131]

Dendritic cells are potential targets for immunotherapy. They can enhance growth and differentiation of CD40-activated B lymphocytes, directly affect natural killer cell function, and act as antigen presenters.[181] Redlinger et al.[182] noted that advanced neuroblastoma impairs dendritic cell differentiation and function in adoptive immunotherapy. It has been shown that in neuroblastoma, gangliosides inhibit dendritic cell function. IL-12 is a potent proinflammatory cytokine that enhances the cytotoxic activity of T lymphocytes and resting natural killer cells.[182] In a murine model of neuroblastoma, Shimizu et al.[214] demonstrated that IL-12 transduced dendritic cell vaccine (with an adenoviral vector expressing IL-12) resulted in a complete and sustained antitumor response. Tumor regression was associated with a high infiltration of dendritic cells and viable T cells.

PROGNOSIS

For many years, the age of the patient and the stage of disease at the time of diagnosis were the two key independent variables determining prognosis in children with neuroblastoma. Evans et al.[62,63] and others found that infants younger than 1 year and those with stage I, II, or IV-S disease had a significantly better outcome.[45,77,83,124,206] Patients older than 1 year and those with advanced disease (stages III and IV) did poorly. The worst survival data were observed in patients older than 1 year with stage IV disease and metastases to cortical bone.[23,27,73,77,83]

The site of the primary tumor was also considered predictive of survival by some investigators. Patients with tumors in cervical, pelvic, and mediastinal locations had an improved outlook compared with children with retroperitoneal (paraspinal or adrenal) tumors. Breslow and McCann[23] and Koop and Schnaufer,[124] however, suggested that the improved outlook in these cases can be explained by the patient's age and stage of disease. Despite these conflicting views, Filler et al.,[66] Young,[243] and Adams et al.[4] reported that site is a beneficial prognostic indicator for mediastinal lesions, and Haase et al.[83] noted the same for pelvic tumors regardless of other factors.

Some early reports concerning neuroblastoma suggested that the more mature and differentiated the tumor, the better the prognosis.[142] Others noted that a more mature histology may be associated with the same dismal outcome as in patients with undifferentiated neuroblasts.[124] In patients with metastatic disease, the presence of more mature elements seemed to improve the outlook and was associated with increased survival.[67,77,218] Shimada et al.[211] subsequently classified the histopathology of neuroblastoma into favorable and unfavorable types, characterized by a stroma-rich appearance for the former and a stroma-poor appearance for the latter. The Shimada classification was also age related. The impact of Shimada histology class on prognosis proved to be important, especially when associated with other prognostic biologic variables, particularly amplification of the N-*myc* oncogene and allelic loss on the short arm of chromosome 1 (1p36).[212] The current INPC (which embraced and modified the Shimada classification) further divided cases into subsets of favorable and unfavorable histologic types and is a highly significant independent predictor of prognosis.[104,173,208,212,213] N-*myc* amplification is seen in approximately 30% of neuroblastoma cases and has an important role in modulating the malignant phenotype in neuroblastoma.[27,148,157] The prognostic value of N-*myc* is independent of stage and age. N-*myc* is associated with a poor response to treatment, rapidly progressive disease, and a dismal outcome. Although attempts to stimulate tumor maturation with nerve growth factor, adrenergic agonists, papaverine, prostaglandins, exogenous cyclic adenosine monophosphate, and hyperthermia were successful in the laboratory setting, there was minimal clinical evidence of their usefulness.[36,73,97,137,234] The use of retinoids as a promoter of differentiation, however, has rekindled interest in this concept and has been successful in prolonging survival in advanced cases during clinical trials.[151] The addition of *cis*-retinoic acid to the treatment protocol for high-risk cases of neuroblastoma following BMT or peripheral stem cell transplantation is now standard practice.[27]

Nakagawara et al.[157,158] reported that high levels of the proto-oncogene Trk-A, a receptor for the neurotrophin nerve growth factor, were associated with excellent survival in infants with neuroblastoma. Trk-A receptor is activated by nerve growth factor and may have an important role in spontaneous regression and tumor differentiation.[157,158] Trk-A is associated with younger patients, lower-stage disease, and absence of N-*myc* expression. Trk-A also down-regulates angiogenic factor expression and the number of microvessels in neuroblastoma tumor cell lines. Multivariate analysis, however, suggests that N-*myc* is a more important independent prognostic factor. In contrast, Trk-B, another neurotropin receptor, is often associated with N-*myc* amplification and, due to its ligand BDNF, may provide a tumor cell survival or growth advantage.[159] The Trk-B–BDNF pathway also contributes to enhanced angiogenesis, tumorigenicity, cell survival, and drug resistance.[27,100] Trk-C (similar to Trk-A) is identified in lower-stage tumors without N-*myc* amplification.[27] The Bcl-2 oncoprotein is responsible for relaying apoptotic signaling and is expressed by most neuroblastomas. Increased Bcl-2 expression in neuroblastoma is

associated with inhibition of chemotherapy-induced apoptosis and a poor outcome.[14,27,32,55] Decreased expression of caspases (enzymes resoponsible for executing the apoptotic signal) is also associated with a dismal outcome. In contrast, increased expression of caspases in neuroblastomas with favorable biologic features is associated with an improved outcome. Tumors with high CD44 cell surface expression are usually well differentiated and result in improved survival.

Cellular DNA content is a predictor of response to chemotherapy in infants with unresectable neuroblastoma. Flow cytometry studies show that hyperdiploidy and triploidy are associated with a favorable outcome, whereas diploid tumors have a poor outcome. Similar to N-*myc*, DNA ploidy is of prognostic value independent of stage and age, and the two factors (N-*myc* and ploidy) together provide important complementary prognostic information for infants.[11,27] DNA ploidy flow cytometry correlates well with response to chemotherapy and outcome.

The survival rate for patients who present with opsoclonus and nystagmus ("dancing eye syndrome") is approximately 90%. This syndrome is seen more frequently (>60%) in patients with primary mediastinal tumors, in patients with stage I or II disease, and in infants younger than 1 year.[9,207] In addition, these tumors are often more histologically mature. Presence of the dancing eye syndrome in patients who present with advanced tumors and N-*myc* overexpression, however, is associated with a poor outcome.[99] Despite tumor resection and adrenocorticotropic hormone treatment, the neurologic symptoms in survivors (including learning disabilities and attention deficits) may persist for many years.[121,195,196]

The outlook is also improved for patients who present with the hypokalemic watery diarrhea syndrome associated with a VIP-producing neurogenic tumor.[42,58,127] Serum VIP levels can serve as a tumor marker in these cases, in which the tumor often does not secrete catecholamines. These patients frequently have tumors that are more mature and well differentiated (e.g., ganglioneuroblastoma). VIP production has also been observed in cases of benign ganglioneuroma, again suggesting that these lesions have a more benign behavior. Somatostatin receptors are expressed more frequently in tumor tissue from patients with lower-stage disease and favorable histology without N-*myc* amplification. These observations suggest that somatostatin receptor expression is a favorable prognostic factor.[154,179]

Children with advanced neuroblastoma frequently show evidence of protein-calorie malnutrition associated with immunoincompetence, based on anergy to a variety of skin test antigens.[188,189] Rickard et al.[189] demonstrated that patients with stage IV neuroblastoma who were malnourished at diagnosis had more treatment delays and a significantly worse outcome than adequately nourished counterparts with similar disease severity. These observations suggest that a nutritional assessment at diagnosis should be a component of the patient's staging.[188] In addition, Van Eys et al.[231] and Rickard et al.[188,189] showed that significant nutritional depletion occurs with multimodal cancer therapy and that total parenteral nutrition can replete and maintain the patient's nutritional status during intensive tumor therapy. In a recent study, Sala et al.[197] reported that the incidence of malnutrition in children with advanced neuroblastoma was 50%. They stressed the importance of nutritional status and its possible influence on the course of the disease and survival. Of interest is a study from Toronto, Canada, that implies that mandatory folic acid fortification of flour—initially intended to reduce the incidence of neural tube defects—was associated with a 60% decrease in the incidence of neuroblastoma in the province of Ontario.[69]

Previously, Laug et al.[136] demonstrated that stage IV patients with a high urinary HVA/VMA ratio have a significantly worse outlook. A greater production of HVA may be indicative of a primitive and immature tumor with more malignant potential. Hann et al.[87] reported that 63% of patients with stage IV disease had high serum ferritin levels, which was predictive of a poor prognosis, especially in girls older than 2 years. A number of studies showed that neuroblastic tumors produce increased serum levels of neuron-specific enolase.[167,228] Zeltzer et al.[244] documented that neuron-specific enolase levels are elevated in 96% of patients with metastatic disease and that high serum levels are associated with a poor prognosis, particularly in infants. Elevated serum lactic dehydrogenase levels are also associated with a poor prognosis in localized neuroblastoma.[216] The prognostic role of the multidrug resistance gene *(MDR-1)* in neuroblastoma is controversial.[16,166] High levels of the MDR-associated protein gene (located on chromosome 16), however, is associated with a poor outcome. This effect is independent of stage, N-*myc*, and Trk-A status.[166] Although these earlier observations were of interest and shed light on the behavior of this enigmatic neoplasm, in the present era, age, INSS stage, N-*myc* status, allelic loss at the 1p36 locus, unbalanced 17q gain, and INPC are now considered the key predictors of outcome for neuroblastoma. The current survival rates are greater than 90% for low-risk cases, 70% to 75% for intermediate-risk cases, and 25% to 30% for high-risk cases. The overall survival at 3 years is 50%.[27]

SUMMARY AND FUTURE DIRECTIONS

This common pediatric malignancy remains an enigma because of the high variability in tumor behavior. The primitive neuroblastic tumor may follow one of three possible pathways: spontaneous regression (apoptosis), differentiation and maturation to a benign ganglioneuroma, or, more commonly, tumor proliferation and rapid malignant progression. Fetal ultrasonography and infant screening programs have clearly demonstrated that some tumors spontaneously regress. Age-related histopathologic studies have clarified that some tumors (favorable histology) differentiate and mature, whereas others (unfavorable histology) are undifferentiated neoplasms that respond poorly to treatment and have a rapidly progressive course and fatal outcome.

Recognition of important biologic (and genetic) characteristics can categorize these tumors into risk groups (low, intermediate, and high) that determine future treatment protocols. Risk-based management permits individualized care for each patient based on age, INSS stage, INPC histology, and biologic and genetic characteristics that affect the behavior of each tumor.[27,74,213] This avoids unnecessary and potentially harmful treatment in patients categorized as having low-risk tumors who may do well with surgery alone (and occasionally observation alone in highly selected cases). It allows the physician to reserve the most aggressive treatment protocols for children with the highest-risk tumors and the most guarded prognosis. At present, the outlook is best in low-risk patients: infants younger than 1 year, patients with localized tumors that can be completely excised (stages I and II) with favorable INPC histology and low-risk biologic and genetic factors, and infants with stage IV-S disease. Infants with cystic neuroblastomas detected on prenatal sonograms also have a very favorable outcome. In patients with stage IV-S disease and those with cystic, multifocal, or bilateral tumors and favorable biologic characteristics, observation alone may be reasonable. Close sonographic monitoring of these cases in the first year of life is important to be sure that the tumor shrinks and undergoes regression. Increase in tumor size is an indication for operative intervention. Intermediate-risk cases include stage III patients (according to the INSS) without adverse biologic risk factors and stage IV patients younger than 1 year without biologic risk factors. Problem areas that continue to require special attention include (1) infants older than 1 year; (2) high-risk patients, including stage II patients older than 1 year with high N-*myc* expression and unfavorable histology and those with advanced disease (stages III and IV) and adverse prognostic biologic and genetic variables; and (3) the prevention and treatment of complications of aggressive multimodal therapy. The last include conventional and total-body irradiation damage, immunosuppression, cardiac and renal toxicity, scoliosis, adverse effect on growth and development, delayed sexual maturation, learning disabilities, and the occurrence of second neoplasms, including renal tumors.[27,68,194]

A better understanding of factors influencing tumor regression and differentiation and tumor-host immune interactions is required. In children with high-risk tumors, identifying additional tumor markers and targeting effective monoclonal antibodies against the tumor; developing improved techniques to clear the bone marrow of tumor cells; employing new and more effective chemotherapy programs (with or without total-body irradiation); hematologic rescue with autologous purged peripheral blood stem cell infusions; and using growth factors (e.g., granulocyte colony-stimulating factor) and other biologic tumor modulators (*cis*-retinoic acid) to protect against infection and promote regression and differentiation may control the progression of disease and improve the outlook for this highly malignant tumor. Despite some improvements in outcome using high-intensity treatments, the outlook for patients with advanced disease remains dismal, with less than half surviving. Alternative treatment protocols using novel and less toxic biologically based therapies (targeted proapoptotic, antiangiogenic, and immunotherapies) will no doubt be tested in the next few years in an attempt to improve the outcome of children with advanced neuroblastoma and diminish the toxicity associated with the current high-intensity but relatively ineffective treatment programs. Molecular profiling of the genetic changes that occur in neuroblastoma will likely permit a more concise classification system to predict outcome and further define the choice of specific therapy, which may include targeting the genes, proteins, and signaling pathways responsible for malignant progression of the tumor.[27]

REFERENCES

1. Abrams HL, Siegelman SS, Adams DF, et al: Computed tomography versus ultrasound of the adrenal gland: A prospective study. Radiology 1982;143:121-128.
2. Abramson SJ, Berdon WE, Ruzal-Shapiro C, et al: Cervical neuroblastoma in eleven infants—a tumor with favorable prognosis: Clinical and radiologic (US, CTR, MRI) findings. Pediatr Radiol 1993;23:253-257.
3. Acharya S, Jayabose S, Kogan S, et al: Prenatally diagnosed neuroblastoma. Cancer 1997;80:304-310.
4. Adams GA, Shochat SJ, Smith EI et al: Thoracic neuroblastoma: A pediatric oncology group study. J Pediatr Surg 1993;28:372-377.
5. Adkins ES, Sawin R, Gerbing RB, et al: Efficacy of complete resection for high risk neuroblastoma: A Children's Cancer Group study. J Pediatr Surg 2004;39:931-936.
6. Akeson R, Seeger RC: Interspecies neural membrane antigens on cultured human and murine neuroblastoma cells. J Immunol 1977;118:1995-2003.
7. Allen RW Jr, Ogden B, Bentley FL, Jung AL: Fetal hydantoin syndrome: Neuroblastoma and hemorrhagic disease in a neonate. JAMA 1980;44:1464-1465.
8. Al-Rashid RA, Cress C: Hypercalcemia associated with neuroblastoma. Am J Dis Child 1979;133:838-841.
9. Altman A, Baehner RL: Favorable prognosis for survival in children with coincident opsomyoclonus and neuroblastoma. Cancer 1976;37:846-852.
10. Ambros IM, Attarbashi A, Rumpler S, et al: Neuroblastoma cells provoke Schwann cell proliferation in vitro. Med Pediatr Oncol 2001;36:163-168.
11. Ambros IM, Zellner A, Roald B, et al: Role of ploidy, chromosome 1p, and Schwann cells in the maturation of neuroblastoma. N Engl J Med 1996;334:1505-1511.
12. Anders D, Kindermann G, Pfeifer U: Metastasizing fetal neuroblastoma with involvement of the placenta simulating fetal erythroblastosis. J Pediatr 1973;82:50-53.
13. Beckwith JB, Perrin EV: In-situ neuroblastoma: A contribution to the natural history of neural crest tumors. Am J Pathol 1963;43:1089-1104.
14. Beirle EA, Strande LK, Chen MK: VEGF upregulates bcl-2 expression and is associated with decreased apoptosis in neuroblastoma cells. J Pediatr Surg 2002;7:467-471.
15. Beppu K, Jaboine J, Merchant MS, et al: Effect of imatinib mesylate on neuroblastoma tumorigenesis and VEGF expression. J Natl Cancer Inst 2004;96:46-55.
16. Bernardi J, et al: Prognostic value of MDR1 gene expression in neuroblastoma: Results of a multivariate analysis. Prog Clin Biol Res 1994;385:111.
17. Bernstein I , Hellstrom KE, Wright PW, et al: Immunity to tumor antigens: Potential implications in human neuroblastoma. J Natl Cancer Inst 1976;57:711-715.
18. Berthold F, Kassenböhmer R, Zieschang J: Multivariate evaluation of prognostic factors in localized neuroblastoma. Am J Hematol Oncol 1994;16:107-115.
19. Bessho F, Hashizume K, Nakajo T, et al: Mass screening in Japan increased the detection of infants with neuroblastoma without a decrease in cases in older children. J Pediatr 1991;119:237-241.
20. Bill AH: Immune aspects of neuroblastoma: Current information. Am J Surg 1971;122:142-147.
21. Blatt JB, Deutsch M, Wollman MR: Results of therapy in stage IV-S neuroblastoma with massive hepatomegaly. Int J Radiat Oncol Biol Phys 1987;13:1467-1471.
22. Blatt JB, Fitz G, Mirro J: Recognition of central nervous system metastases in children with metastatic primary extracranial neuroblastoma. Pediatr Hematol Oncol 1997;14:233-241.
23. Breslow N, McCann B: Statistical estimation of prognosis for children with neuroblastoma. Cancer Res 1971;31:1098-1103.
24. Brock CE, Ricketts RR: Hemoperitoneum from spontaneous rupture of neonatal neuroblastoma. Am J Dis Child 1982;136:370-371.
25. Brodeur GM: Molecular basis for heterogeneity in human neuroblastoma. Eur J Cancer 1995;31A:505-510.
26. Brodeur GM: Schwann cells as antineuroblastoma agents. N Engl J Med 1996;334:1537-1539.
27. Brodeur GM: Neuroblastoma: Biological insights into a clinical enigma. Nat Rev Cancer 2003;3:203-216.
28. Brodeur GM, Pritchard J, Berthold F, et al: Revision of the international criteria for neuroblastoma diagnosis staging and response to treatment. J Clin Oncol 1993;11:1466-1477.
29. Brodeur GM, Seeger RC, Barrett A, et al: International criteria for diagnosis of staging and response to treatment in patients with neuroblastoma. J Clin Oncol 1988;6:1874-1881.
30. Caron H, van Sluis B, de Kraker J, et al: Allelic loss of chromosome 1p as a predictor of unfavorable outcome in patients with neuroblastoma. N Engl J Med 1996;334:225-230.
31. Castel V, Bedal MD, Bezanilla JL, et al: Treatment of stage III neuroblastoma with emphasis on intensive induction chemotherapy: A report from the Neuroblastoma Group of the Spanish Society of Pediatric Oncology. Med Pediatr Oncol 1995;34:29-35.
32. Castel VP, Heidelberger KP, Bromberg J, et al: Expression of the apoptosis-suppressing protein bcl-2 in neuroblastoma is associated with unfavorable histology and N-myc amplification. Am J Pathol 1993;143:1543-1550.
33. Castleberry RP, Pritchard J, Ambros P, et al: The International Neuroblastoma Risk Groups (INRG): A preliminary report. Eur J Cancer 1997;33:2113-2116.
34. Castleberry RP, Shuster JJ, Smith EI: Pediatric Oncology Group experience with the International Staging System criteria for neuroblastoma. J Clin Oncol 1994;12:2378-2381.
35. Chan HS, Haddad G, Thorner PS, et al: P-glycoprotein expression as a predictor of the outcome of therapy for neuroblastoma. N Engl J Med 1991;325:1608-1614.
36. Chang THT, Prasad KN: Differentiation of mouse neuroblastoma cells in-vitro and in-vivo, induced by cyclic adenosine monophosphate (cAMP). J Pediatr Surg 1976;11:847-858.
37. Chatten J, Voorhees ML: Familial neuroblastoma: Report of a kindred with multiple disorders including

neuroblastoma in four siblings. N Engl J Med 1967;277: 1230-1236.

38. Cheung NK: Monclonal antibody-based therapy for neuroblastoma. Curr Oncol Rep 2000;2:547-551.

39. Cheung NK, Kushner BH, Yeh SD, et al: 3F8 Monoclonal antibody treatment of patients with stage 4 neuroblastoma: A phase II study. Int J Oncol 1998;12:1299-1306.

40. Chlenski A, Liu S, Cohn SL: The regulation of angiogenesis in a neuroblastoma. Cancer Lett 2003;197:47-52.

41. Coldman AJ, Fryer CJ, Elwood JM, Sonley MJ: Neuroblastoma: Influence of age at diagnosis, stage, site and sex on prognosis. Cancer 1980;46:1896-1901.

42. Cooney DR, Voorhees ML, Fisher JE, et al: Vasoactive intestinal polypeptide producing neuroblastoma. J Pediatr Surg 1982;17:821-825.

43. Cushing H, Wolbach SB: Transformation of malignant paravertebral sympathicoblastoma into benign ganglioneuroma. Am J Pathol 1927;3:203.

44. D'Angio GJ, Evans AE: Experience with cyclic low-dose total body irradiation for metastatic neuroblastoma [abstract]. Proc Am Soc Clin Oncol 1982;23:52.

45. D'Angio GJ, Evans AE, Koop CE: Special pattern of widespread neuroblastoma with a favorable prognosis. Lancet 1971;1:1046-1049.

46. Dastur DK: Cerebral ganglioglioneuroblastoma: An unusual brain tumor of the neuron series. J Neurol Neurosurg Psychiatry 1982;45:139-142.

47. Davidoff AM, Kandel JJ: Antiangiogenic therapy for the treatment of pediatric solid malignancies. Semin Pediatr Surg 2004;13:53-60.

48. Davidoff AM, Leary MA, Ng CT, et al: Retroviral vector producer cell mediated angiogenesis inhibition restricts neuroblastoma growth in-vivo. Med Pediatr Oncol 2000;35:638-640.

49. Davidoff AM, Leary MA, Ng CY, et al: Gene therapy mediated expression by tumor cells of the angiogenesis inhibitor Flk-1 results in inhibition of neuroblastoma growth in-vivo. J Pediatr Surg 2001;36:30-36.

50. DeBernardi B, Pianca C, Boni L, et al: Disseminated neuroblastoma (stage IV and IV-S) in the first year of life: Outcome related to age and stage. Italian Cooperative Group on Neuroblastoma. Cancer 1992;70:1625-1633.

51. DeBernardi B, Conte M, Mancini A, et al: Localized resectable neuroblastoma: Results of the 2nd study of the Italian Cooperative Group for Neuroblastoma. J Clin Oncol 1995;13:884-893.

52. de Lagausie P, Berribi D, Michon J, et al: Laparoscopic adrenal surgery for neuroblastoma in children. J Urol 2003;170:932-935.

53. Deutsch M, Tersak JM: Radiotherapy for symptomatic metastases to bone in children. Am J Clin Oncol 2004;27:128-131.

54. Dobrovoljski G, Kerbl R, Strobl C, et al: False-positive results in neuroblastoma screening: The parents' view. J Pediatr Hematol Oncol 2003;25:14-18.

55. Dole M, Nunez G, Merchant AK, et al: Bcl-2 inhibits chemotherapy induced apoptosis in neuroblastoma. Cancer Res 1994;54:3253-3259.

56. Dreyfus M, Neuhart D, Baldauf JJ, et al: Prenatal diagnosis of cystic neuroblastoma. Fetal Diagn Ther 1994;9:269-272.

57. Eggert A, Ikegaki N, Kwiatkowski J, et al: High-level expression of angiogenic factors is associated with advanced tumor stage in human neuroblastomas. Clin Cancer Res 2000;6:1900-1908.

58. El-Shafie M, Samuel D, Klippel CH, et al: Intractable diarrhea in children with VIP-secreting ganglioneuroblastoma. J Pediatr Surg 1983;18:34-36.

59. Emery LG, Shields M, Shah MR, et al: Neuroblastoma associated with Beckwith-Wiedemann syndrome. Cancer 1983;52:176-179.

60. Entz-Werle N, Marcellin L, Becmeur F, et al: The urinary bladder: An extremely rare location of pediatric neuroblastoma. J Pediatr Surg 2003;38:E10-E12.

61. Evans AE, Albo V, D'Angio GJ, et al: Cyclophosphamide treatment of patients with localized and regional neuroblastoma: A randomized study. Cancer 1976;38:655-660.

62. Evans AE, D'Angio GJ, Randolph JG: A proposed staging for children with neuroblastoma. Cancer 1971;27: 374-378.

63. Evans AE, Gerson J, Schnaufer L: Spontaneous regression of neuroblastoma. Natl Cancer Inst Monogr 1976;44:49-54.

64. Evans AE, Heyn RN, Newton WA Jr, Leikin SL: Viscristine sulfate and cyclophosphamide for children with metastatic neuroblastoma. JAMA 1969;207:1325-1327.

65. Fenart D, Deville A, Donzeau M, Bruneton JN: Neuroblastome retroperitoneal diagnostique in utero. J Radiol 1983;64:359-361.

66. Filler RM, Traggis DG, Jaffe N, Vawter GF: Favorable outlook for children with mediastinal neuroblastoma. J Pediatr Surg 1972;7:136-143.

67. Finklestein JZ, Klemperer, MA, Evans AE, et al: Multiagent chemotherapy for children with metastatic neuroblastoma: A report from the Children's Cancer Study Group. Med Pediatr Oncol 1979;6:179-188.

68. Fleitz JM, Wooten-Gorges SC, Wyatt-Ashmead J, et al: Renal cell carcinoma in long-term survivors of advanced stage neuroblastoma early in childhood. Pediatr Radiol 2003; 33:540-545.

69. French AE, Grant R, Weitzman S, et al: Folic acid food fortification is associated with a decline in neuroblastoma. Clin Pharmacol 2003;74:288-294.

70. Gerson JM, Chatten J, Eisman S: Familial neuroblastoma—a follow-up. N Engl J Med 1974;190:487.

71. Gerson JM, Herberman RB: Systemic and in-situ natural killer activity in patients with neuroblastoma. In Evans AE (ed): Advances in Neuroblastoma Research. New York, Raven Press, 1980.

72. Green AA, Hayes FA, Hustu HO: Sequential cyclophosphamide and doxorubicin for induction and complete remission in children with disseminated neuroblastoma. Cancer 1981;48:2310-2317.

73. Grosfeld JL: Neuroblastoma: A 1990 overview. Pediatr Surg Int 1991;6:9-13.

74. Grosfeld JL: Risk based management of childhood solid tumors. J Am Coll Surg 1999;189:407-425.

75. Grosfeld JL, Ballantine TVN, Baehner RL: Experience with "second-look" operations in pediatric solid tumors. J Pediatr Surg 1978;13:275-280.

76. Grosfeld JL, Rescorla FJ, West KW, Goldman J: Neuroblastoma in the first year of life: Clinical and biologic factors influencing outcome. Semin Pediatr Surg 1993;2:37-46.

77. Grosfeld JL, Schatzlein M, Ballantine TVN, et al: Metastatic neuroblastoma: Factors influencing survival. J Pediatr Surg 1978;13:59-65.

78. Grosfeld JL, West KW, Weber TR: The role of second-look procedures in the management of retroperitoneal tumors in children. J Pediatr Hematol Oncol 1984;6:441-447.

79. Haas D, Ablin AR, Miller C, et al: Complete pathologic maturation and regression of stage IV-S neuroblastoma without treatment. Cancer 1988;62:818-825.

80. Haas-Kogan DA, Fisch BM, Wara WB, et al: Introperative radiation therapy for high risk neuroblastoma. Int J Radiat Oncol Biol Phys 2000;47:985-992.

81. Haas-Kogan DA, Swift PS, Eslch M, et al: Impact of radiotherapy for high risk neuroblastoma: A Children's Cancer Group study. Int J Radiat Oncol Biol Phys 2003; 56:28-39.

82. Haase GM: Head and neck neuroblastomas. Semin Pediatr Surg 1994;3:194-202.

83. Haase GM, LaQuaglia MP: Neuroblastoma. In Ziegler M, Azizkhan RG, Weber TR (eds): Operative Pediatric Surgery. New York, McGraw-Hill, 2003, pp 1181-1191.

84. Haase GM, O'Leary MC, Ramsay NK, et al: Aggressive surgery combined with intensive chemotherapy improves survival in poor risk neuroblastoma. J Pediatr Surg 1991; 26:1119-1123.

85. Haase GM, Wong KY, deLorimier AA, et al: Improvement in survival after excision of the primary tumor in stage III neuroblastoma. J Pediatr Surg 1989;24:194-200.

86. Haddad M, Triglia JM, Helardot P, et al: Localized cervical neuroblastoma: Prevention of surgical complications. Int J Pediatr Otorhinolaryngol 2003;67:1361-1367.

87. Hann JL, et al: Serum ferritin levels as a guide to prognosis in stage IV neuroblastoma [abstract]. Proc Am Soc Clin Oncol 1983;24:72.

88. Hatchitanda Y, Hata J: Stage IV-S neuroblastoma: A clinical, histological and biological analysis. Hum Pathol 1996;27:1135-1138.

89. Hayashi Y, Kanmda N, Inaba T, et al: Cytogenetic findings and prognosis in neuroblastoma with emphasis on marker chromosome 1. Cancer 1989;63:125-132.

90. Hayes FA, Green AA, Casper J, et al: Clinical evaluation of sequentially scheduled cisplatin and VM-26 in neuroblastoma: Response and toxicity. Cancer 1981;48:1715-1718.

91. Hayes FA, Green AA, Hustu HO, Kumar ML: Surgicopathologic staging of neuroblastoma: Prognostic significance of regional lymph node metastases. J Pediatr 1983;102:59-62.

92. Hayes F, Green AA, Mauer AM, et al: Correlation of cell kinetics and clinical response to chemotherapy in disseminated neuroblastoma. Cancer Res 1977;37:3766-3770.

93. Heisel MA, Miller JH, Reid BS, Siegel SE: Radionuclide bone scan in neuroblastoma. Pediatrics 1983;71:206-209.

94. Hellstrom I, Hellstrom KE, Pierce GE, Bill AH: Demonstration of cell bound humoral immunity against neuroblastoma cells. Proc Natl Acad Sci U S A 1968;60: 1231-1238.

95. Hellstrom KE, Hellstrom I: Lymphocyte mediated cytotoxicity and blocking serum activity to tumor antigens. Adv Immunol 1974;18:209-217.

96. Helson L, Ghavimi F, Wu CJ, et al: Carcinoembryonic antigen in children with neuroblastoma. J Natl Cancer Inst 1976;57:725-726.

97. Helson L, Helson C, Peterson RF, Das SK: A rationale for the treatment of metastatic neuroblastoma. J Natl Cancer Inst 1976;57:727-729.

98. Hiyama E, Yokoyama T, Hiyama K et al: Multifocal neuroblastoma: Biologic behavior and surgical aspects. Cancer 2000;88:1955-1963.

99. Hiyama E, Yokoyama T, Ichikawa T, et al: Poor outcome in patients with advanced stage neuroblastoma and coincident opsomyoclonus syndrome. Cancer 1994;74: 1821-1826.

100. Ho R, Eggert A, Hishiki T, et al: Resistance to chemotherapy mediated by TrkB in neuroblastoma. Cancer Res 2002;62:6462-6466.

101. Ho TC, Estroff JA, Kozakewich H, et al: Prenatal detection of neuroblastoma: A ten year experience from the Dana-Farber Cancer Institute and Children's Hospital. Pediatrics 1993;92:358-364.

102. Holcomb GW: Minimally invasive surgery for solid tumors. Semin Surg Oncol 1999;7:184-192.

103. Holgersen LO, Subramanian S, Kirpekar M, et al: Spontaneous resolution of antenatally diagnosed adrenal masses. J Pediatr Surg 1996;31:153-155.

104. Ikeda H, Iehara T, Tsuchida Y, et al: Experience with the International Neuroblastoma Staging System and pathology classification. Br J Cancer 2002;86:1110-1116.

105. Ikeda H, Suzuki N, Takahashi A, et al: Surgical treatment of neuroblastomas in infants under 12 months of age. J Pediatr Surg 1998;33:1246-1250.

106. Ishimoto K, Kiyokawa H, Fujita H, et al: Problems of mass screening for neuroblastoma: Analysis of false negative cases. J Pediatr Surg 1990;25:398-401.

107. Iwanaka T, Arai M, Ito M, et al: Surgical treatment for abdominal neuroblastoma in the laparoscopic era. Surg Endosc 2001;15:751-754.

108. Iwanaka T, Arai M, Kawashima H, et al: Endosurgical procedures for pediatric solid tumors. Pediatr Surg Int 2004;20:39-42.

109. Jennings RW, LaQuaglia MP, Leong K, et al: Fetal neuroblastoma: Prenatal diagnosis and natural history. J Pediatr Surg 1993;28:1168-1174.

110. Jiang TH, Yang CP, Hung IJ, et al: Brain metastases in children with neuroblastoma—a single institution experience. Med Pediatr Oncol 2003;41:570-571.

111. Joshi VV, Cantor AB, Altschuler G, et al: Age-linked prognostic categorization based on a new histologic grading system of neuroblastoma. Cancer 1992;69:2183-2196.

112. Kaicker S, McCRudden KW, Beck L, et al: Thalidomide is anti-angiogenic in a xenograft model of neuroblastoma. Int J Oncol 2003;23:1651-1655.

113. Kang TI, Brophy P, Hickeson M, et al: Targeted radiotherapy with submyeloablative doses of I[131]-MIBG is effective for disease palliation in highly refractory neuroblastoma. J Pediatr Hematol Oncol 2003;25:769-763.

114. Kanold J, Halle P, Tchirkov A, et al: Ex-vivo expansion of autologous PB CD34+ cells provide a purge effect in children with neuroblastoma. Bone Marrow Transplant 2003;32:485-488.

115. Kenney LB, Miller BA, Gloeker-Reis LA, et al: Increased incidence of cancer in infants in the United States 1980-1990. Cancer 1998;82:1396-1400.

116. Kiely EM: The surgical challenge of neuroblastoma. J Pediatr Surg 1994;29:128-133.

117. Kim ES, Soffer SZ, Huang J, et al: Distinct response of experimental neuroblastoma to combination antiangiogenic strategies. J Pediatr Surg 2002;37:518-522.

118. King D, Goodman J, Hawk T, et al: Dumbbell neuroblastoma in children. Arch Surg 1975;110:888-891.

119. Kinney H, Faix R, Brazy J: The fetal alcohol syndrome and neuroblastoma. J Pediatr 1980;66:130-132.

120. Kogner P, Barbani G, Dominici C, et al: Co-expression of messenger RNA for Trk protooncogene and low affinity nerve growth factor receptors in neuroblastoma with favorable prognosis. Cancer Res 1993;53:2044-2050.

121. Koh PS, Raffensperger J, Berry S, et al: Long-term outcome in children with opsoclonus myoclonus and ataxia and coincident neuroblastoma. J Pediatr 1994;125: 712-716.

122. Komuro H, Kaneko S, Kaneko M, et al: Expression of angiogenic factors and tumor progression in human neuroblastoma. J Cancer Res Clin Oncol 2001;127:739-743.

123. Komuro H, Makino S, Tahara K: Laparoscopic resection of an adrenal neuroblastoma detected by mass screening that grew in size during the observation period. Surg Endosc 2000;14:297.

124. Koop CE, Schnaufer L: The management of abdominal neuroblastoma. Cancer 1975;35:905-909.
125. Kouch K, Yoshida H, Matsunaga T, et al: Extirpation of mass screened adrenal neuroblastoma by retroperitoneoscopy. Surg Endosc 2003;17:1769-1772.
126. Kubota M, Yagi M, Kanada S, et al: Long-term follow up and status of patients with neuroblastoma after undergoing either aggressive surgery or chemotherapy: A single institutional study. J Pediatr Surg 2004;39:1328-1332.
127. Kudo K, Kitajima S, Munakata H, Yagihashi S: WDHA syndrome caused by VIP-producing ganglioneuroblastoma. J Pediatr Surg 1982;17:426-428.
128. Kumar AM, Wrenn EL Jr, Fleming ID, et al: Preoperative therapy for unresectable malignant tumors in children. J Pediatr Surg 1975;10:657-670.
129. Kushner BH, Cheung NK, LaQuaglia MP, et al: Survival from locally invasive or widespread neuroblastoma without cytotoxic therapy. J Clin Oncol 1996;14:373-381.
130. Kushner BH, Kramer K, LaQuaglia MP, Cheung NK: Curability of recurrent disseminated disease after surgery alone for loco-regional neuroblastoma using intensive chemotherapy and anti-GD-2 immunotherapy. J Pediatr Hematol Oncol 2003;25:512-514.
131. Kushner BH, Kramer K, Modak S, Cheung NK: Campothecin analogs (irinotecan or topotecan) plus high dose cyclophosphamide as preparative regimens for antibody based immunotherapy in resistant neuroblastoma. Clin Cancer Res 2004;10:84-87.
132. Kushner BH, LaQuaglia MP, Bonilla MA, et al: Highly effective induction therapy for stage IV neuroblastomas in children over 1 year of age. J Clin Oncol 1994;12:2607-2613.
133. Kushner BH, Wolden S, LaQuaglia MP, et al: Hyperfractionated low dose radiotherapy for high-risk neuroblastoma after intensive chemotherapy and surgery. J Clin Oncol 2001;19:2821-2828.
134. LaQuaglia MP, Kushner BH, Heller G, et al: Stage 4 neuroblastoma diagnosed at more than 1 year of age: Gross total resection and clinical outcome. J Pediatr Surg 1994;29:1162-1165.
135. LaQuaglia MP, Kushner BH, Su W, et al: The impact of gross total resection on local control and survival in high-risk neuroblastoma. J Pediatr Surg 2004;39:412-417.
136. Laug WE, Siegel SE, Shaw KN, et al: Initial urinary catecholamine metabolite concentrations and prognosis in neuroblastoma. Pediatrics 1978;62:77-83.
137. Lazo J, Ruddon RW: Neurite extension and malignancy of neuroblastoma cells after treatment with PGE_1 and papaverine. J Natl Cancer Inst 1977;59:137-143.
138. Leavey PJ, Odom LF, Poole M, et al: Intraoperative radiation therapy in pediatric neuroblastoma. Med Pediatr Oncol 1997;28:424-428.
139. Lee EW, Applebaum H: Abdominal expansion as a bridging technique in stage IV-S neuroblastoma with massive hepatomegaly. J Pediatr Surg 1994;29:1470-1471.
140. Leone A, Seeger RC, Hong CM, et al: Evidence for nm23 RNA overexpression, DNA amplification and mutation in aggressive neuroblastoma. Oncogene 1993;8:855-865.
141. Luttikhuis ME, Powell JE, Rees SA, et al: Neuroblastoma with chromosome 11q loss and single copy MYCN comprise a biologically distinct group of tumours with adverse prognosis. Br J Cancer 2001;85:531-537.
142. Mäkinen J: Microscopic patterns as a guide to prognosis of neuroblastoma in childhood. Cancer 1972;29:1637-1646.
143. Marcus KJ, Shamberger R, Litman H, et al: Primary tumor control in patients with stage 3/4 unfavorable neuroblastoma treated in tandem double stem cell transplants. Pediatr Hematol Oncol 2003;25:934-940.
144. Maris JM, Matthay KK: The molecular biology of neuroblastoma. J Clin Oncol 1999;17:2264-2279.
145. Maris JM, Weiss MJ, Mosse Y, et al: Evidence for a hereditary neuroblastoma predisposition locus at 16p12-13. Cancer Res 2002;62:6651-6658.
146. Martinez-Mora J, Castellvi A, Coroleu W, et al: Cystic adrenal neuroblastoma: Prenatal diagnosis by ultrasonography. Med Pediatr Oncol 1995;24:109-115.
147. Matsumura M, Tsunoda A, Nishi T, et al: Spontaneous regression of neuroblastoma detected by mass screening. Lancet 1991;338:447-448.
148. Matthay KK: Progress in the treatment of advanced stage neuroblastoma. Pediatric Neoplasms, Postgraduate Course, 82nd Clinical Congress, American College of Surgeons, San Francisco, Oct 1996.
149. Matthay KK, Perez C, Seegar RC, et al: Treatment and outcome for stage III neuroblastoma based on prospective biology staging: A Children's Cancer Group study. J Clin Oncol 1998;16:1256-1264.
150. Matthay KK, Seeger RC, Reynolds CP, et al: Allogeneic vs autologous purged bone marrow transplantation for neuroblastoma: A report from the Children's Cancer Group study. J Clin Oncol 1994;12:2382-2389.
151. Matthay KK, Villlablanca JG, Seegar RC, et al: Treatment of high risk neuroblastoma with intensive chemotherapy, radiotherapy, autologous bone marrow transplantation, and 13-cis-retinoic acid: A Children's Cancer Group study. N. Engl J Med 1999;341:1165-1173.
152. McKallip R, Li R, Ladisch S: Tumor gangliosides inhibit the tumor specific immune response. J Immunol 1999;163:3718-3726.
153. Meitar D, Crawford SE, Rademaker AW, et al: Tumor angiogenesis correlates with metastatic disease, N-myc amplification and poor outcome in human neuroblastoma. J Clin Oncol 1996;14:405-414.
154. Moertel CL, Reubi JC, Scheithauer BS, et al: Expression of somatostatin receptors in childhood neuroblastoma. Am J Clin Pathol 1994;102:752-756.
155. Molofsky WJ, Chutorian AM: Non-surgical treatment of intraspinal neuroblastoma. Neurology 1981;31:1170-1173.
156. Moss TJ, Reynolds CP, Sather HN, et al: Prognostic value of immunocytologic detection of bone marrow metastases in neuroblastoma. N Engl J Med 1991;324:219-226.
157. Nakagawara A, Arima M, Azar CG, et al: Inverse relationship between Trk expression and N-myc amplification in human neuroblastoma. Cancer Res 1992;52:1364-1368.
158. Nakagawara A, Arima-Nakagawara M, Scavarda MG, et al: Association between high levels of expression of the Trk gene and favorable outcome in human neuroblastoma. N Engl J Med 1993;328:847-854.
159. Nakagawara A, Azar CG, Scavardo NJ, et al: Expression and function of Trk-B and BDNF in human neuroblastomas. Mol Cell Biol 1994;14:759-767.
160. Nakajima K, Fukuzawa M, Fukui Y, et al: Laparoscopic resection of mass screened adrenal neuroblastoma in an 8 month old infant. Surg Laparosc Endosc 1997;7:498-500.
161. Nemecek ER, Sawin RW, Park J: Treatment of neuroblastoma in patients with neurocristopathy syndromes. J Pediatr Hematol Oncol 2003;25:159-162.
162. Nickerson HJ, Matthay KK, Seegar RC, et al: Favorable biology and outcome of stage IV-S neuroblastoma with

supportive care or minimal therapy: A Children's Cancer Group study. J Clin Oncol 2000;18:477-486.

163. Nickerson HJ, Nesbit ME, Grosfeld JL, et al: Comparison of stage IV and IV-S neuroblastoma in the first year of life. Med Pediatr Oncol 1985;13:261-268.

164. Ninane J, Pritchard J, Morris Jones PH, et al: Stage II neuroblastoma: Adverse prognostic significance of lymph node involvement. Arch Dis Child 1982;57:438-442.

165. Nitschke R, Cangir A, Crist W, Berry DH: Intensive chemotherapy for metastatic neuroblastoma: A Southwest Oncology Group study. Med Pediatr Oncol 1980;8:281-288.

166. Norris MD, Bordow SD, Marshall GM, et al: Expression of the gene for multidrug resistance associated protein and outcome in patients with neuroblastoma. N Engl J Med 1996;334:231-238.

167. Odelstad L, Pahlman S, Lackgren G, et al: Neuron specific enolase: A marker for differential diagnosis of neuroblastoma and Wilms' tumor. J Pediatr Surg 1982;17:381-385.

168. Oue T, Fukuzawa M, Kusafuka T, et al: In situ detection of DNA fragmentation and expression of bcl-2 in human neuroblastoma: Relation to apoptosis and spontaneous regression. J Pediatr Surg 1996;31:251-257.

169. Oue T, Inoue M, Yoneda A, et al: Profile of neuroblastoma detected by mass screening, resected after observation without treatment: Results of the Wait and See pilot study. J Pediatr Surg 2005;40:359-363.

170. Paul SR, Tarbell NJ, Korf B, et al: Stage IV neuroblastoma in infants: Long-term survival. Cancer 1991;67:1493-1497.

171. Pegelow CH, Ebbin AJ, Powars D, Towner JW: Familial neuroblastoma. J Pediatr 1975;87:763-765.

172. Perkins DG, Kopp CM, Haust MD: Placental infiltration in congenital neuroblastoma. Histopathology 1980;4:383-389.

173. Peuchmaur M, d'Amore ES, Joshi VV, et al: Revision of the International Neuroblastoma Pathology Classification: Confirmation of favorable and unfavorable prognostic subsets in ganglioneuroblastoma, nodular. Cancer 2003;98:2274-2281.

174. Plantaz D, Rubie H, Michon J, et al: The treatment of neuroblastoma with intraspinal extension with chemotherapy followed by surgical removal of residual disease: A prospective study of 42 patients—results of the NBL 90 study of the French Society of Pediatric Oncology. Cancer 1996;3:521-525.

175. Ponzoni M, Bocca P, Chiesa V, et al: Differential effects of N-4-hydroxyphenylretinamide and retinoic acid on neuroblastoma cells: Apoptosis and differentiation. Cancer Res 1995;55:853-861.

176. Powell JL, Buniz NJ, Callahan C, et al: An unexpectedly high incidence of Epstein-Barr virus lymphoproliferative disease after CD34+ selected autologous peripheral blood stem cell transplant in neuroblastoma. Bone Marrow Transplant 2004;33:651-657.

177. Prasad KN, Mandal B, Kumar S: Demonstration of cholinergic cells in human neuroblastoma and ganglioneuroma. J Pediatr 1973;82:677-679.

178. Pritchard J, McElwain TJ, Graham-Pole J: High dose melphalan with autologous bone marrow for treatment of advanced neuroblastoma. Br J Cancer 1982;45:86-94.

179. Qualman SJ, O'Diorisio MS, Fleshman DJ, et al: Neuroblastoma: Correlation of neuropeptide expression in tumor tissue with other prognostic factors. Cancer 1992;70:2005-2012.

180. Raffaghello L, Marimpietri D, Pagnan G, et al: Anti-GD2 monoclonal antibody immunotherapy: A promising strategy in the prevention of neuroblastoma relapse. Cancer Lett 2003;197:205-209.

181. Redlinger RE, Shimizu T, Remy T, et al: Cellular mechanisms of interleukin-12 mediated neuroblastoma regression. J Pediatr Surg 2003;38:199-204.

182. Redlinger RE Jr, Mailliard RB, Barksdale EM: Neuroblastoma and dendritic cell function. Semin Pediatr Surg 2004;13:61-71.

183. Reynolds CP: Differentiating agents in pediatric malignancies: Retinoids in neuroblastoma. Curr Oncol Rep 2000;2:511-518.

184. Reynolds CP, Kane DJ, Einhorn PA, et al: Response of neuroblastoma to retinoic acid in vitro and in vivo. Prog Clin Biol Res 1996;366:203-211.

185. Reynolds CP, Matthay KK, Villablanca JG, et al: Retinoid therapy of high risk neuroblastoma. Cancer Lett 2003;197:185-192.

186. Ribatti D, Raffaghello L, Marimpietri D, et al: Fenretinide as an anti-angiogenic agent in neuroblastoma. Cancer Lett 2003;197:181-184.

187. Richards ML, Gundersen AE, Williams MS: Cystic neuroblastoma of infancy. J Pediatr Surg 1995;30:1354-1357.

188. Rickard KA, Detamore CM, Coates TD, et al: Effect of nutrition staging on treatment delays and outcome in stage IV neuroblastoma. Cancer 1983;52:587-598.

189. Rickard KA, Grosfeld JL, Kirksey A, et al: Reversal of protein-energy malnutrition in children during treatment of advanced neoplastic disease. Ann Surg 1979;190:771-781.

190. Rill DR, Santana VM, Roberts WM, et al: Direct demonstration that autologous bone marrow transplantation for solid tumors can return a multiplicity of tumorigenic cells. Blood 1994;84:380-383.

191. Riley RD, Heney D, Jones DR, et al: A systematic review of molecular and biological tumor markers in neuroblastoma. Clin Cancer Res 2004;10:4-12.

192. Rosenberg SA: Development of effective immunotherapy for the treatment of patients with cancer. J Am Coll Surg 2004;198:685-696.

193. Rowe DH, Huang J, Li J, et al: Suppression of primary tumor growth in a mouse model of human neuroblastoma. J Pediatr Surg 2000;35:977-981.

194. Rubino C, Adjadj E, Guerin S, et al: Long-term risk of second malignant neoplasms after neuroblastoma in childhood: Role of treatment. Int J Cancer 2003;107:791-796.

195. Rudnick C, Khakoo Y, Antunes NL: Opsoclonus-myoclonus-ataxia syndrome in neuroblastoma: Clinical outcome and antineural antibodies—a report from the Children's Cancer Group study. Med Pediatr Oncol 2001;36:612-622.

196. Russo C, Cohn SL, Petruzzi MJ, et al: Long term neurologic outcome in children with opsoclonus-myoclonus associated with neuroblastoma: A report from the Pediatric Oncology Group. Med Pediatr Oncol 1997;28:284-288.

197. Sala A, Pencharz P, Barr RD: Children, cancer and nutrition—a dynamic triangle in review. Cancer 2004;100:677-687.

198. Sandberg DI, Bilsky MH, Kushner BH, et al: Treatment of spinal involvement in neuroblastoma patients. Pediatr Neurosurg 2003;39:291-298.

199. Sawada T, Sugimoto T, Kawakatsu H, et al: Mass screening for neuroblastoma in Japan. Pediatr Hematol Oncol 1991;8:93-109.

200. Sawada T, Todo S, Fujita K, et al: Mass screening of neuroblastoma in infancy. Am J Dis Child 1982;136:710-712.

201. Schilling FH, Parker C: Mass screening in neuroblastoma: The European experience. In Brodeur GM, Sawada T,

Tsuchida Y, Vote PA (eds): Neuroblastoma. Amsterdam, Elsevier, 2000, pp 281-292.

202. Schilling FH, Spix C, Berthold F, et al: German neuroblastoma mass screening study at 12 months of age: Statistical aspects and preliminary results. Med Pediatr Oncol 1998; 31:435-441.

203. Schleiermacher G, Rubie H, Hartmann O, et al: Treatment of stage 4s neuroblastoma—report of 10 years experience of the French Society of Paediatric Oncology (SFOP). Br J Cancer 2003;89:470-476.

204. Schmidt ML, Lukens JN, Seeger RC, et al: Biologic factors determine prognosis in infants with stage IV neuroblastoma: A prospective Children's Cancer Group study. J Clin Oncol 2000;18:1260-1268.

205. Schnaufer L, Koop CE: Silastic abdominal pouch for temporary hepatomegaly in stage IV-S neuroblastoma. J Pediatr Surg 1975;10:73-75.

206. Seeler RA, Israel JN, Royal JE, et al: Ganglioneuroblastoma and fetal hydantoin-alcohol syndrome. Pediatrics 1979; 63:524-527.

207. Senelick RC, Bray PF, Lahey ME, et al: Neuroblastoma and myoclonic encephalopathy: Two cases and a review of the literature. J Pediatr Surg 1973;8:623-632.

208. Shimada H: The International Neuroblastoma Pathology Classification. Pathologica 2003;95:240-241.

209. Shimada H, Ambros IM, Dehner LP, et al: Terminology and morphologic criteria of neuroblastic tumors: Recommendations by the International Neuroblastoma Pathology Committee. Cancer 1999;86:349-363.

210. Shimada H, Ambros IM, Dehner LP, et al: The International Neuroblastoma Pathology Classification (the Shimada system). Cancer 1999;86:364-372.

211. Shimada H, Chatten J, Newton WA Jr, et al: Histopathologic prognostic factors in neuroblastoma: Definition of subtypes of ganglioneuroblastoma and an age-linked classification of neuroblastoma. J Natl Cancer Inst 1984;73:405-416.

212. Shimada H, Stram DO, Chatten J, et al: Identification of subsets of neuroblastomas by combined histopathologic and N-myc analysis. J Natl Cancer Inst 1995;87:1470-1476.

213. Shimada H, Umehara S, Monobe Y, et al: International Neuroblastoma Pathology Classification for prognostic evaluation of patients with peripheral neuroblastic tumors: A report from the Children's Cancer Group. Cancer 2001;92:2451-2461.

214. Shimizu T, Berhanu A, Redlinger RE Jr, et al: Interleukin-12 transduced dendritic cells induce regression of established murine neuroblastoma. J Pediatr Surg 2001;36:1285-1292.

215. Shorter NA, Davidoff AM, Evans AE, et al: The role of surgery in the management of stage IV neuroblastoma: A single institution study. Med Pediatr Oncol 1995;24:287-291.

216. Shuster JJ, McWilliams, MB, Castleberry R, et al: Serum lactate dehydrogenase in childhood neuroblastoma: A POG recursive partitioning study. Am J Clin Oncol 1992; 15:295-303.

217. Shusterman S, Grupp SA, Maris JM: Inhibition of tumor growth in a human neuroblastoma xenograft model with TNP-470. Med Pediatr Oncol 2000;35:673-676.

218. Sitarz A, Finkelstein J, Grosfeld JL, et al: An evaluation of the role of surgery in disseminated neuroblastoma: A report from the Children's Cancer Study Group. J Pediatr Surg 1983;18:147-151.

219. Spurbeck WW, Davidoff AM, Lobe TE, et al: Minimally invasive surgery in pediatric cancer patients. Ann Surg Oncol 2004;11:340-343.

220. Squire R, Fowler CL, Brooks SP, et al: The relationship of class I MHC antigen expression to stage IV-S disease

and survival in neuroblastoma. J Pediatr Surg 1990;25: 381-386.

221. Stevens MM: Stage IV-S neuroblastoma: Disseminated malignancy with a favorable prognosis—three case reports. Aust Paediatr J 1979;15:39-43.

222. Stigall R, Smith WL, Francken EA, et al: Intrapulmonic metastatic neuroblastoma. Ann Radiol 1979;22:223-227.

223. Suarez A, Hartmann O, Vassal G, et al: Treatment of stage IV-S neuroblastoma: A study of 34 cases treated from 1982-1987. Med Pediatr Oncol 1991;19:473-477.

224. Sugio K, Nakagawara A, Sasazuki T: Association of expression between N-myc gene and major histocompatibility complex class I gene in surgically resected neuroblastoma. Cancer 1991;67:1384-1388.

225. Suzuki T, Bogenmann, Shimada H, et al: Lack of high affinity nerve growth factor receptors in aggressive neuroblastoma. J Natl Cancer Inst 1993;5:377-384.

226. Suzuki T, Yokota J, Mugishima H, et al: Frequent loss of heterozygosity on chromosome 14q in neuroblastoma. Cancer Res 1989;49:1095-1098.

227. Tanaka S, Tajiri T, Noguchi S, et al: Prenatally diagnosed cystic neuroblastoma: A report of 2 cases. Asian J Surg 2003;26:225-227.

228. Tapia F, Polak JM, Barbosa AJ, et al: Neuron specific enolase is produced by neuroendocrine tumors. Lancet 1981;1:808-811.

229. Tornoczky T, Kalman E, Kajtar PG, et al: Large cell neuroblastoma: A distinct phenotype of neuroblastoma with aggressive clinical behavior. Cancer 2004;100:390-397.

230. Umehara S, Nakagawara A, Matthay KK, et al: Histopathology defines prognostic subsets of ganglioneuroblastoma nodular. Cancer 2000;89:1150-1161.

231. Van Eys J, Copeland EM, Cangir A, et al: A clinical trial of hyperalimentation in children with metastatic malignancies. Med Pediatr Oncol 1980;8:63-73.

232. Vertuani S, De Geer A, Levitsky V, et al: Retinoids act as multistep modulators of the major histocompatibility class I presentation pathway and sensitize neuroblastomas to cytotoxic lymphocytes. Cancer Res 2003;63:8006-8013.

233. Villablanca JG, Khan AA, Avramis VI, et al: Phase I trial of 13 cis-retinoic acid in children with neuroblastoma following bone marrow transplantation. J Clin Oncol 1995;13:894-901.

234. West KW, Weber TR, Grosfeld JL: Synergistic effect of hyperthermia, papaverine and chemotherapy in murine neuroblastoma. J Pediatr Surg 1980;15:913-917.

235. White L: P-glycoprotein expression and progression of neuroblastoma. N Engl J Med 1992;326:1162-1163.

236. Wilson PC, Coppes MJ, Solh H, et al: Neuroblastoma stage IV-S a heterogenous disease. Med Pediatr Oncol 1991;19:467-472.

237. Woods W, Gaor N, Shuster JT, et al: Screening of infants and mortality due to neuroblastoma. N Engl J Med 2002; 346:1041-1046.

238. Woods WG: Screening for neuroblastoma: The final chapter. J Pediatr Hematol Oncol 2003;25:3-4.

239. Yamamoto K, Hanada R, Kikuchi A, et al: Spontaneous regression of localized neuroblastoma detected by mass screening. J Clin Oncol 1998;16:1265-1269.

240. Yamashiro DJ, Nakagawara A, Ikegaki N, et al: Expression of TrkC in favorable human neuroblastoma. Oncogene 1996;12:37-41.

241. Yanik GA, Levine JE, Mattay KK, et al: Pilot study of metiodobenzylguanidine in combination with myeloablative chemotherapy and autologous stem cell support for the treatment of neuroblastoma. J Clin Oncol 2002; 20:2142-2149.

242. Yiin J, Chang CS, Jan YJ, Wang YC: Treatment of neuro-blastoma with intraspinal extension. J Clin Neurosci 2003; 10:579-583.

243. Young DG: Thoracic neuroblastoma/ganglioneuroma. J Pediatr Surg 1983;18:37-41.

244. Zeltzer PM, Marangos PJ, Parama AM, et al: Raised neuron specific enolase in the serum of children with metastatic neuroblastoma: A report from the Children's Cancer Study Group. Lancet 1983;2:361-363.

245. Ziegler MM, Vega A, Koop CE: Electrocoagulation induced immunity—an explanation for regression of neuroblastoma. J Pediatr Surg 1980;15:34-37.

246. Zimmerman RA, Bilaniuk CT: CT of primary and second-ary craniocerebral neuroblastoma. AJR Am J Roentgenol 1980;135:1239-1242.

Chapter 29

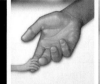

Nonmalignant Tumors of the Liver

Philip C. Guzzetta, Jr.

Primary liver tumors constitute less than 3% of tumors seen in the pediatric population, and only one third of those tumors are benign.[2,17,30,69] Despite the rarity of benign liver tumors, recommendations for diagnostic evaluation and management can be made, based on the experience gained from centers with a relatively large number of patients. Benign tumors may be epithelial (focal nodular hyperplasia, hepatocellular adenoma), mesenchymal (infantile hepatic hemangioendothelioma, cavernous hemangioma, mesenchymal hamartoma), or other (teratoma, inflammatory pseudotumor). Nonparasitic cysts, although not technically neoplasms, are also discussed in this chapter.

One of the more interesting aspects of benign liver tumors in children is their predilection to occur in patients with other conditions. Hepatocellular adenomas have long been associated with the use of oral contraceptives in adults. Children are at risk for hepatocellular adenoma when they have received androgen therapy for aplastic anemia, have chronic iron overload from transfusion in β-thalassemia, or have received corticosteroids after renal transplantation.[8] Patients with type I glycogen storage disease are at increased risk for hepatocellular adenoma[5] and focal nodular hyperplasia[48]; liver hamartomas may occur in children with tuberous sclerosis.[33]

CLINICAL PRESENTATION

Most children with benign liver tumors present with a painless right upper quadrant abdominal mass or hepatomegaly. Symptoms of gastrointestinal compression, such as constipation, anorexia, or vomiting, may also be present. If the mass is painful, the pain is usually dull and aching and is caused by expansion of the liver capsule or compression of the normal surrounding structures. Jaundice and weight loss are uncommon except in infants with infantile hepatic hemangioendothelioma (IHH), and those signs should raise the suspicion that the lesion is malignant. Acute abdominal pain may be caused by bleeding into the mass or into the peritoneum, particularly in hepatocellular adenomas, although this problem is rarely seen in children. Children may present with congestive heart failure (CHF) and thrombocytopenia,

which is known as Kasabach-Merritt syndrome when associated with a vascular anomaly such as IHH.[35] Cutaneous hemangiomas are seen in about half the children with IHH,[25,55,59] and the rapid liver enlargement with IHH can cause abdominal compartment syndrome and respiratory distress.[52] CHF without significant thrombocytopenia can also be seen with liver arteriovenous malformation (AVM)[20] or mesenchymal hamartoma.[60] Fetal hydrops has been identified by prenatal ultrasonography in some fetuses with IHH[21] or mesenchymal hamartoma.[34]

DIAGNOSIS

Laboratory Tests

Serum alpha fetoprotein (AFP) is present in very high concentrations at birth (48,000 ± 35,000 ng/mL) and rapidly declines to adult levels of less than 10 ng/mL by 8 months of age (Table 29-1).[73] Thus, in infants younger than 8 months, AFP levels must be interpreted in the context of this dramatic change. Markedly elevated AFP

TABLE 29–1 Normal Serum Alpha Fetoprotein (AFP) Levels of Infants, by Age

Age	No. of Patients	AFP Level ± SD (ng/mL)
Premature	11	138,734 ± 41,444
Newborn	55	48,406 ± 34,718
Newborn-2 wk	16	33,113 ± 32,503
2 wk-1 mo	43	9452 ± 12,610
1 mo	12	2645 ± 3080
2 mo	40	323 ± 278
3 mo	5	88 ± 87
4 mo	31	74 ± 56
5 mo	6	46.5 ± 19
6 mo	9	12.5 ± 9.8
7 mo	5	9.7 ± 7.1
8 mo	3	8.5 ± 5.5

From Wu JT, Book L, Sudar K: Serum alpha fetoprotein (AFP) levels in normal infants. Pediatr Res 1981; 5:50.

levels in a child with a liver mass almost certainly means that the mass is malignant, although milder elevation may be encountered with some benign lesions such as mesenchymal hamartoma[31] or teratoma.[66] As mentioned previously, significant thrombocytopenia associated with a liver mass is usually part of the Kasabach-Merritt syndrome due to IHH. Hypothyroidism may also occur in IHH[27]; thyroid function tests should be done routinely in these children, because hypothyroidism significantly impacts their management.[42]

Imaging Techniques

The initial imaging study in a child presenting with an abdominal mass should be a supine radiograph of the abdomen, looking for calcifications within the mass. The next imaging study should be an abdominal sonogram with Doppler spectral analysis, followed by computed tomography (CT) with intravenous contrast (Fig. 29-1).[6] Magnetic resonance imaging (MRI) may be indicated, depending on the sonogram and CT scan results, especially when surgical resection is planned and more detailed information about the vascular anatomy relative to the tumor is desired. Arteriography is reserved for children with IHH or, rarely, mesenchymal hamartoma[45] with CHF, in whom embolization of the tumor blood supply is needed for treatment. Liver-spleen radionuclide scans are seldom helpful in differentiating liver masses and thus are unnecessary in centers that have CT and MRI. The use of percutaneous biopsy under sonogram or CT guidance in children with benign tumors is generally discouraged (unless excision of the tumor would pose a major risk to the child), because establishing a diagnosis on the basis of a small sample may be problematic for the pathologist, and because resection is the proper therapy for most of these tumors. The findings on imaging studies are discussed in the sections on each individual tumor.

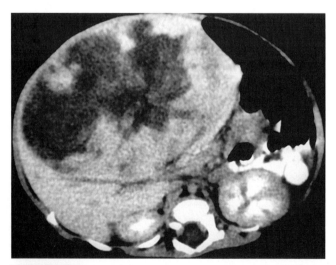

Figure 29-1   Contrast-enhanced abdominal computed tomography scan of a 6-month-old female infant with a large hemangioendothelioma of the left hepatic lobe. Note the central area of necrosis.

VASCULAR TUMORS

Infantile Hepatic Hemangioendothelioma

IHH is by far the most common benign liver tumor in children. Increasingly, IHH is being diagnosed prenatally, and similar to affected neonates, the fetus may be asymptomatic or profoundly ill.[21,55] Symptomatic children present before 6 months of age 80% of the time, with many presenting in the newborn period.[25,55,59] The most common physical finding is hepatomegaly. The disease has a wide range of severity, with some children being asymptomatic and others having life-threatening CHF, abdominal compartment syndrome, and severe thrombocytopenia. In most series, the female-to-male ratio is 2:1, and about half the children have a cutaneous hemangioma as well as IHH.[11,25,59] In infants, IHH, can be reliably diagnosed by abdominal sonogram and dynamic contrast-enhanced CT. Lesions are usually present throughout the liver but may be localized to a few hepatic segments.[68] On ultrasonography, multifocal, echolucent nodules usually have high-flow vessels, while solitary lesions have a more heterogeneous echogenicity.[6] Before the administration of intravenous contrast, these lesions have low attenuation on CT; with contrast, they enhance diffusely or centripetally.[6] MRI of IHH reveals the extent of disease, the flow characteristics, and the flow structure.[6] Despite the high rate of accuracy in diagnosing IHH by imaging techniques, AFP and catecholamine levels should be obtained, because occasionally a hepatoblastoma or stage IV-S neuroblastoma is misdiagnosed as IHH.[29]

Dehner and Ishak[12] identified two microscopic patterns of IHH. Type 1, the more common histologic pattern, is characterized by an orderly arrangement of dilated and compressed endothelium-lined vascular spaces supported by reticulin fibers with benign cytologic features. In their review, 17 of 23 lesions were type 1. Type 2 lesions have a more aggressive histologic appearance, with more complex and irregular branching structures within the vascular lumens. Endothelial cells are more hyperchromatic and pleomorphic than in type 1 lesions, although mitoses are uncommon. In Dehner and Ishak's series, the mortality rate was higher for patients with type 2 than type 1 tumors, but more recent series report a favorable outcome regardless of type. Thus, the histopathology of the tumor does not seem to correlate with prognosis.

Management of these tumors depends on the severity of symptoms and the location of the lesion. When the lesion is asymptomatic and little hepatomegaly is present, observation is the appropriate therapy, as long as the diagnosis can be made with a high degree of certainty on the basis of noninvasive radiographic studies. Unless there is serious concern that the lesion is malignant, percutaneous or open biopsy is discouraged because of the risk of significant hemorrhage.

Treatment of a symptomatic child is directed first toward pharmacologic control of the tumor with corticosteroids,[25,55,59] interferon (IFN),[9,18] vincristine,[47] or cyclophosphamide.[28] Despite initial enthusiasm for IFN therapy for IHH, there are concerns about serious side effects with both IFN-alpha 2a[3] and IFN-alpha 2b.[6] In addition, the therapy takes weeks to months to be effective, which is too long in critically ill neonates to be clinically useful. The success rate of any medical therapy is difficult to assess because of the wide disparity in disease severity and the fact that the usual single-center experience is fewer than 20 patients. In my experience, however, very ill neonates with CHF and thrombocytopenia due to diffuse or multifocal lesions are seldom improved with medical therapy alone. Embolization is most effective in children with disease restricted to only a few of the eight hepatic segments,[68] but some success has been reported in children with diffuse IHH as well.[6] Diffuse IHH lesions frequently have extrahepatic arterial collaterals arising from the superior mesenteric, phrenic, intercostal, and internal mammary arteries, as well as some blood supply from the portal venous system.[6,20] This makes complete elimination of the blood flow by embolization virtually impossible.

Although hepatic artery ligation was recommended as treatment for IHH in the past, it prevents effective embolization and thus should be avoided. If disease progression occurs despite embolization, hepatic resection[11,55] or even liver transplantation[11,36] may be needed if the child is to survive. Radiation therapy has been used to treat these lesions,[52,53] but the long-term effect of hepatic radiation in an infant is unknown, and there is one disturbing report that described three children with angiosarcoma of the liver who had previously been treated for IHH with radiation therapy.[19] Estimates of survival rates with IHH are unreliable because of the variability of the disease and the wide range of treatment approaches, but in children younger than 6 months with CHF, reported survival rates are between 45% and 90% for this "benign" tumor.[11,25,55]

Hemangioma

Hemangioma is the most common vascular liver tumor in adults; in children, however, hemangiomas are usually incidental findings in asymptomatic patients.[12] Hemangiomas have widely dilated, nonanastomotic vascular spaces lined with flat endothelial cells and supported by fibrous tissue on microscopic examination.[12] Review of the literature on hemangioma in children is problematic, because some authors have called the lesions hemangiomas when the patient's age and clinical presentation were more consistent with hemangioendothelioma.[10] In addition, because the preferred treatment for these lesions is not surgical, there is usually no specimen for the accurate assessment of histopathology. In children, the risk of hemorrhage with hemangiomas is low; thus, unless the patient is having pain or disability from hepatomegaly, no treatment is recommended. In contrast, adults with giant hemangiomas (>4 cm in diameter) are generally treated by resection.[1,57]

Arteriovenous Malformation

An AVM may occur within the liver parenchyma or outside the liver between the hepatic artery and the portal venous system. Similar to patients with hemangioendotheliomas, patients with hepatoportal AVMs usually present before 6 months of age, many in the newborn period, with hepatomegaly, CHF, and a bruit over the liver.[14] In older children and adults, hepatic AVM may occur as part of hereditary hemorrhagic telangiectasia, also known as Osler-Weber-Rendu disease.[6,7] Angiography is diagnostic, and embolization is therapeutic in some patients, but it is necessary to eliminate the extensive collaterals for successful closure of the AVM.[6,14] Fatal complications from the embolization of liver AVMs have been reported.[71] Steroids have no place in the management of these lesions, and AVMs not managed successfully with embolization may be controlled with hepatic arterial ligation.[23,24]

Mesenchymal Hamartoma

Mesenchymal hamartoma (MH) usually presents as a painless right upper quadrant abdominal mass in a child younger than 2 years.[13,37,64] Some patients may have evidence of CHF,[45,60] and, similar to IHH, MH has been diagnosed prenatally.[34] Edmondson[17] proposed that MH arises from a mesenchymal rest that becomes isolated from the normal portal triad architecture and differentiates independently. The tumor grows along bile ducts and may incorporate normal liver tissue. Because the blood vessels and bile ducts are components of the mesenchymal rest, the biologic behavior of the tumor varies with the relative predominance of these tissues within the loose connective tissue stroma (mesenchyma) that surrounds them. Thus, the tumor may present as a predominantly cystic structure (Fig. 29-2) that enlarges rapidly because of fluid accumulation,[61] or it may be predominantly vascular and present with CHF.[60]

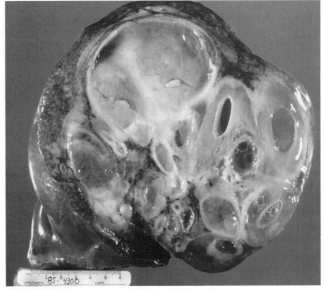

Figure 29–2 Cross section of a pathology specimen of a left hepatic lobectomy for mesenchymal hamartoma in a 10-month-old male infant.

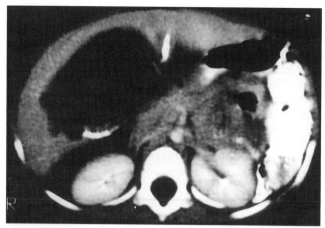

Figure 29–3 Contrast-enhanced abdominal computed tomography scan of a recurrent mesenchymal hamartoma of the right hepatic lobe, previously treated by unroofing. It was subsequently managed successfully by partial right hepatic lobectomy.

Von Schweinitz et al.[67] suggested that fat-storing (Ito) cells of the immature liver may be involved in the development of MH.

Serum AFP levels are usually normal in children with MH, but they may be mildly elevated.[31,40] The radiographic features of these tumors are consistent and distinguishing; abdominal sonography and CT demonstrate a single, usually large, fluid-filled mass with fine internal septations and no calcifications.[62]

Management must be tempered by the understanding that MH usually follows a benign course,[4] although there have been reports of malignant transformation.[46,50] In general, complete operative resection is the procedure of choice, if it can be accomplished safely. Huge lesions or those that involve both lobes may be treated by unroofing and marsupializing the cysts, although the lesion may recur after incomplete resection (Fig. 29-3).

MH is an entity distinct from the liver hamartomas associated with tuberous sclerosis. The latter are smaller, multifocal lesions that may be associated with angiomyolipomas in other locations, such as the kidney; they are rarely symptomatic and usually present in children older than 2 or 3 years. These hamartomas have little clinical significance, but their presence may be helpful in diagnosing tuberous sclerosis.[33]

Hepatocellular Adenoma

Although isolated lesions are encountered in childhood, hepatocellular adenoma (HCA) is most commonly observed in adults in association with the use of anabolic corticosteroids or estrogen. HCA has been described in children treated with anabolic steroids and multiple blood transfusions for chronic anemia,[8] and it is expected in children with type I glycogen storage disease.[26] Bianchi[5] proposed several mechanisms for the development of HCA in patients with type I glycogen storage disease, including (1) regional imbalance in insulin and glucagon metabolism, because these hormones are important in the regulation of hepatocyte proliferation and regeneration; (2) response to glycogen overload; and (3) oncogene activation.

Microscopic examination of these adenomas reveals hepatocytes in sheets and cords oriented along sinusoids without a ductal component. The cells have glycogen-filled cytoplasm and small nuclei without mitoses. Adjacent liver and vessels are compressed but not invaded. Children usually do not have coexisting cirrhosis.[8] The histologic pattern is similar to that of a well-differentiated hepatocellular carcinoma, and development of hepatocellular carcinoma within an unresected HCA has been reported.[32,65]

In children, HCA generally presents as an asymptomatic hepatic mass. The mass is solid on ultrasonography and CT. Liver enzyme and AFP levels are normal. A feature unique to this lesion is its propensity for intraperitoneal hemorrhage from spontaneous rupture. In adults, intraperitoneal bleeding is almost always seen in patients receiving estrogen therapy, and tumor regression may occur with the cessation of hormone administration. In patients with glycogen storage disease and HCA, tumor regression may occur with the correction of metabolic disturbances.[5] Because of the known association between HCA and hepatocellular carcinoma, resection of HCA is recommended when it occurs in a child who is not receiving steroids and does not have glycogen storage disease. If resection cannot be accomplished without substantial risk, observation of the lesion while monitoring the serum AFP level may be appropriate. If the AFP level begins to increase or the lesion is significantly symptomatic, and if the risk of resection is unacceptably high, liver transplantation may be the best alternative.

Focal Nodular Hyperplasia

Focal nodular hyperplasia (FNH) in children presents as an irregularly shaped, nontender liver mass. It is frequently found incidentally at laparotomy for another cause or on radiographic studies performed for another indication. The female-to-male ratio for FNH is approximately 4:1.[63] FNH is occasionally seen with vascular malformations and hemangiomas in the liver,[70] and it has been postulated that the lesions represent an unusual response to injury or ischemia.[17] On abdominal sonography, the lesions may be isoechoic, hypoechoic, or hyperechoic to normal liver parenchyma and may be multiple in 10% to 15% of patients. The classic central scar may not be seen on ultrasonography. CT typically shows a hypervascular lesion with a dense stellate central scar. Conventional arteriography or magnetic resonance angiography shows a hypervascular mass with feeding arteries entering the periphery and converging on the central portion of the tumor. Some cases of fibrolamellar hepatocellular carcinoma are radiographically indistinguishable from FNH, which is a cause for concern if the diagnosis is being made without a biopsy.[43] There are reports of adult patients who have FNH and hepatocellular carcinoma simultaneously.[44]

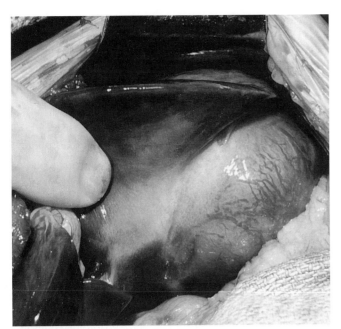

Figure 29–4 Surgical view of focal nodular hyperplasia within the left lobe of the liver in a 2-year-old child treated by left lateral lobectomy.

On gross examination, the lesions are nonencapsulated, occasionally pedunculated, and quite firm (Fig. 29-4). Microscopic examination shows proliferation of hepatocytes and bile ducts and the pathognomonic central fibrosis. These lesions rarely become malignant, and hemorrhage is rare. Therefore, expectant therapy is appropriate when removal might be associated with significant morbidity, the child is asymptomatic, and the diagnosis has been made conclusively by radiographic studies, normal AFP levels, and biopsy.[51]

OTHER TUMORS

Teratoma

There have been fewer than 25 case reports of hepatic teratoma in children.[66,72] These children are invariably younger than 1 year, and calcification is usually present within the lesion, helping to differentiate it from other tumors. Some of these lesions have met the criteria for an intrahepatic fetus in fetu.[41] Serum AFP levels may be elevated with a teratoma, but only mildly elevated in comparison to the levels seen with hepatoblastoma. Resection is the procedure of choice for a teratoma because of the risk of malignancy in any immature elements of the tumor.

Inflammatory Pseudotumor

Inflammatory pseudotumor of the liver is rare. These lesions are generally seen in children older than 3 years but have been reported in younger children as well.

Because this lesion is predominantly solid, it is difficult to differentiate it from other benign or malignant tumors by imaging studies. Invariably, the serum AFP level is normal. Fever, leukocytosis, and high C-reactive protein level in a child with a solid liver mass and normal AFP level are suggestive of an inflammatory pseudotumor of the liver. This lesion is thought to be an inflammatory reaction to some insult, although the instigating cause is usually unknown. Because it is difficult to diagnose this lesion without a large biopsy or resection of the lesion, most children undergo resection, which is curative.[22,54]

Nonparasitic Cysts

Nonparasitic cysts of the liver are rare and occur more commonly in adults than in children. Although they may be present and symptomatic at birth, most of these cysts are asymptomatic and are identified incidentally at autopsy or laparotomy. Symptoms are related to abdominal distention or displacement of adjacent structures. These lesions occur with equal frequency in males and females.[15] Nonparasitic cysts are generally unilocular and lined by cuboidal or columnar epithelium, characteristic of bile ducts. The cyst fluid is typically clear or brown, and bile is rarely present. Pathologic studies suggest that nonparasitic cysts arise from congenital or secondary obstruction of peribiliary glands. These glands normally arise from the ductal plate at the hepatic hilum around the seventh week of gestation and continue to proliferate until adolescence.[15] Symptomatic cysts can be effectively treated by simple unroofing, marsupialization,[38] or sclerotherapy.[49] If biliary communication is suspected, cholangiography may identify the source and allow the communicating ductule to be oversewn.

Cystic dilatation of the intrahepatic ducts may also present as a mass, although jaundice and cholangitis are often associated with this problem. Resection of the affected lobe is the preferred therapy.[39] If MH appears to be completely cystic on imaging, it may be misdiagnosed as a nonparasitic cyst. Post-traumatic bile cysts result from ductal disruption and intrahepatic accumulation of bile. These lesions can be treated by percutaneous drainage or, in some cases, by biliary sphincterotomy to reduce the bile duct pressure and lessen the biliary leak.[58] Resection is rarely necessary for post-traumatic cysts. Multiple parenchymal cysts associated with hereditary polycystic kidney disease are generally asymptomatic and so small that they do not require intervention.

Epidermoid cysts differ from other nonparasitic cysts, in that the lining epithelium is squamous rather than cuboidal. This histologic characteristic has led to the theory that these lesions may be foregut bud anomalies trapped in the hepatic substance. Although these lesions are rare, there has been a report of malignant degeneration. Thus, resection is the appropriate management.[56]

ACKNOWLEDGMENT

The author thanks W. Raleigh Thompson, MD, for his contribution to this chapter in the fifth edition of this book.

REFERENCES

1. Baer HU, Dennison AR, Moulton W, et al: Enucleation of giant hemangiomas of the liver. Ann Surg 1992;216:673.

2. Baggenstoss AH: Pathology of tumors of liver in infancy and childhood. In Pack G, Islami A (eds): Tumors of the Liver. New York: Springer-Verlag, 1970, p 240.

3. Barlow CF, Priebe CJ, Mulliken JB, et al: Spastic diplegia as a complication of interferon alpha-2a treatment of hemangiomas of infancy. J Pediatr 1998;132:527.

4. Barnhart DC, Hirschl RB, Garver KA, et al: Conservative management of mesenchymal hamartoma of the liver. J Pediatr Surg 1997;32:1495.

5. Bianchi L: Glycogen storage disease I and hepatocellular tumors. Eur J Pediatr 1993;152:S63.

6. Burrows PE, Dubois J, Kassarjian: Pediatric hepatic vascular anomalies. Pediatr Radiol 2001;31:533.

7. Buscarini E, Buscarini L, Danesino C, et al: Hepatic vascular malformations in hereditary hemorrhagic telangiectasia: Doppler sonographic screening in a large family. J Hepatol 1997;26:111.

8. Chandra RS, Kapur SP, Kelleher J, et al: Benign hepatocellular tumors in the young: A clinicopathologic spectrum. Arch Pathol Lab Med 1984;108:168.

9. Chang E, Boyd A, Nelson CC, et al: Successful treatment of infantile hemangiomas with interferon-alpha-2b. J Pediatr Hematol Oncol 1997;19:237.

10. Cohen RC, Myers NA: Diagnosis and management of massive hepatic hemangiomas in childhood. J Pediatr Surg 1986;21:6.

11. Daller JA, Bueno J, Gutierrez J, et al: Hepatic hemangioendothelioma: Clinical experience and management strategy. J Pediatr Surg 1999;34:98.

12. Dehner LP, Ishak KG: Vascular tumors of the liver in infants and children. Arch Pathol 1971;92:101.

13. DeMaioribus CA, Lally KP, Sim K, et al: Mesenchymal hamartoma of the liver. Arch Surg 1990;125:598.

14. Dickman PS, Meza MP, Newman B: Hepatic vascular malformations. Pediatr Pathol Lab Med 1995;15:155.

15. Donovan MJ, Kozakewich H, Perez-Atayde A: Solitary nonparasitic cysts of the liver: The Boston Children's Hospital experience. Pediatr Pathol Lab Med 1995;15:419.

16. Dubois J, Hershon L, Carmant L, et al: Toxicity profile of interferon alfa-2b in children: A prospective evaluation. J Pediatr 1999;135:782.

17. Edmondson HA: Differential diagnosis of tumors and tumor like lesions of liver in infancy and childhood. Am J Dis Child 1956;91:168.

18. Ezekowitz RAB, Mulliken JB, Folkman J: Interferon alfa-2a therapy for life-threatening hemangiomas of infancy. N Engl J Med 1992;326:1456.

19. Falk H, Herbert JT, Edmonds L, et al: Review of four cases of childhood hepatic angiosarcoma—elevated environmental arsenic exposure in one case. Cancer 1981;47:382.

20. Fellows KE, Hoffer FA, Markowitz RI, et al: Multiple collaterals to hepatic infantile hemangioendotheliomas and arteriovenous malformations: Effect on embolization. Radiology 1991;181:813.

21. Gembruch U, Baschat AA, Gloeckner-Hoffmann K, et al: Prenatal diagnosis and management of fetuses with liver hemangiomata. Ultrasound Obstet Gynecol 2002; 19:454.

22. Hata Y, Sasaki F, Matuoka S, et al: Inflammatory pseudotumor of the liver in children: Report of cases and review of the literature. J Pediatr Surg 1992;27:1549.

23. Hazebroek FWJ, Tibboel D, Robben SGF, et al: Hepatic artery ligation for hepatic vascular tumors with arteriovenous and arterioportal venous shunts in the newborn: Successful management of two cases and review of the literature. J Pediatr Surg 1995;30:1127.

24. Heaton ND, Davenport M, Karani J, et al: Congenital hepatoportal arteriovenous fistula. Surgery 1995;117:170.

25. Holcomb GW, O'Neill JA, Mahboudi S, et al: Experience with hepatic hemangioendothelioma in infancy and childhood. J Pediatr Surg 1988;23:661.

26. Howell RR, Stevenson RE, Ben-Menachem Y, et al: Hepatic adenomata with type 1 glycogen storage disease. JAMA 1976;236:1481.

27. Huang SA, Tu HM, Harney JW, et al: Severe hypothyroidism caused by type 3 iodothyronine deiodinase in infantile hemangiomas. N Engl J Med 2000;343:185.

28. Hurvitz SA, Hurvitz CH, Sloninsky L, et al: Successful treatment with cyclophosphamide of life threatening diffuse hemangiomatosis involving the liver. J Pediatr Hematol Oncol 2000;22:527.

29. Ingram JD, Yerushalmi B, Connell J, et al: Hepatoblastoma in a neonate: A hypervascular presentation mimicking hemangioendothelioma. Pediatr Radiol 2000;30:794.

30. Ishak KG: Primary hepatic tumors in childhood. In Popper H, Schaffner F (eds): Progress in Liver Diseases, vol 5. New York, Grune & Stratton, 1976, p 636.

31. Ito H, Kishikawa T, Toda T, et al: Hepatic mesenchymal hamartoma of an infant. J Pediatr Surg 1984;19:315.

32. Janes CH, McGill DB, Ludwig J, et al: Liver cell adenoma at the age of 3 years and transplantation 19 years later after development of carcinoma: A case report. Hepatology 1993;17:583.

33. Jozwiak S, Pedich M, Rajszys P, et al: Incidence of hepatic hamartomas in tuberous sclerosis. Arch Dis Child 1992; 67:1363.

34. Kamata S, Nose K, Sawai T, et al: Fetal mesenchymal hamartoma of the liver: Report of a case. J Pediatr Surg 2003;38:639.

35. Kasabach HH, Merritt KK: Capillary hemangioma with extensive purpura: Report of a case. Am J Dis Child 1940;59:1063.

36. Kasahara M, Kiuchi T, Haga H, et al: Monosegmental living-donor liver transplantation for infantile hepatic hemangioendothelioma. J Pediatr Surg 2003;38:1108.

37. Lack EE: Mesenchymal hamartoma of the liver: A clinical and pathologic study of nine cases. Am J Pediatr Hematol Oncol 1986;8:91.

38. Litwin DEM, Taylor BR, Greig P, et al: Nonparasitic cysts of the liver: The case for conservative surgical management. Ann Surg 1987;205:45.

39. Longmire WP, Mandiola SA, Gordon HE: Congenital cystic disease of the liver and biliary system. Ann Surg 1971;174:711.

40. Luks FI, Yazbeck S, Brandt ML, et al: Benign liver tumors in children: A 25 year experience. J Pediatr Surg 1991; 26:1326.

41. Magnus KG, Millar AJW, Sinclair-Smith CC, et al: Intrahepatic fetus-in-fetu: A case report and review of the literature. J Pediatr Surg 1999;34:1861.

42. Mason KP, Koka BV, Eldredge EA, et al: Perioperative considerations in a hypothyroid infant with hepatic haemangioma. Paediatr Anaesth 2001;11:228.

43. Meyers RL, Scaife ER: Benign liver and biliary tract masses in infants and toddlers. Semin Pediatr Surg 2000;9:146.

44. Muguti G, Tait N, Richardson A, et al: Hepatic focal nodular hyperplasia: A benign incidentaloma or a marker of serious hepatic disease? HPB Surg 1992;5:171.

45. Mulrooney DA, Carpenter B, Georgieff M, et al: Hepatic mesenchymal hamartoma in a neonate: A case report and review of the literature. J Pediatr Hematol Oncol 2001; 23:316.

46. O'Sullivan MJ, Swanson PE, Knoll J, et al: Undifferentiated embryonal sarcoma with unusual features arising within mesenchymal hamartoma of the liver: Report of a case and review of the literature. Pediatr Dev Pathol 2001;4:482.

47. Perez J, Pardo J, Gomez C: Vincristine—an effective treatment of corticoid-resistant life- threatening infantile hemangiomas. Acta Oncol 2002;41:197.

48. Pizzo CJ: Type I glycogen storage disease with focal nodular hyperplasia of the liver and vasoconstrictive pulmonary hypertension. Pediatrics 1980;65:341.

49. Raboei E, Luoma R: Definitive treatment of congenital liver cyst with alcohol. J Pediatr Surg 2000;35:1138.

50. Ramanujam TM, Ramesh JC, Goh DW, et al: Malignant transformation of mesenchymal hamartoma of the liver: Case report and review of the literature. J Pediatr Surg 1999;34:1684.

51. Reymond D, Plaschkes J, Ridolfi Luthy A, et al: Focal nodular hyperplasia of the liver in children: Review of follow-up and outcome. J Pediatr Surg 1995;30:1590.

52. Ricketts RR, Stryker S, Raffensperger JG: Ventral fasciotomy in the management of hepatic hemangioendothelioma. J Pediatr Surg 1982;17:187.

53. Rotman M, John M, Stowe S, et al: Radiation treatment of pediatric hepatic hemangiomatosis and coexisting cardiac failure. N Engl J Med 1980;302:852.

54. Sakai M, Ikeda H, Suzuki N, et al: Inflammatory pseudotumor of the liver: Case report and review of the literature. J Pediatr Surg 2001;36:663.

55. Samuel M, Spitz L: Infantile hepatic hemangioendothelioma: The role of surgery. J Pediatr Surg 1995;30:1425.

56. Schullinger JN, Wigger HJ, Price JB, et al: Epidermoid cysts of the liver. J Pediatr Surg 1983;18:240.

57. Schwartz SI, Husser WC: Cavernous hemangioma of the liver: A single institution report of 16 resections. Ann Surg 1987;205:456.

58. Scioscia PJ, Dillion PW, Cilley RE, et al: Endoscopic sphincterotomy in the management of posttraumatic biliary fistula. J Pediatr Surg 1994;29:3.

59. Selby DM, Stocker JT, Waclawiw MA, et al: Infantile hemangioendothelioma of the liver. Hepatology 1994;20:39.

60. Smith WL, Ballantine TVN, Gonzalez-Crussi F: Hepatic mesenchymal hamartoma causing heart failure in the neonate. J Pediatr Surg 1978;13:183.

61. Srouji MN, Chatten J, Schulman WM, et al: Mesenchymal hamartoma of the liver in infants. Cancer 1978;42:2483.

62. Stanley P, Hall TR, Woolley MM, et al: Mesenchymal hamartomas of the liver in childhood: Sonographic and CT findings. AJR Am J Roentgenol 1986;147:1035.

63. Stocker JT, Ishak KG: Focal nodular hyperplasia of the liver: A study of 21 pediatric cases. Cancer 1981;48:336.

64. Stocker JT, Ishak KG: Mesenchymal hamartoma of the liver: Report of 30 cases and review of the literature. Pediatr Pathol 1983;1:245.

65. Tesluk H, Lawrie J: Hepatocellular ademona: Its transformation to carcinoma in a user of oral contraceptives. Arch Pathol Lab Med 1981;105:296.

66. Todani T, Tabuchi K, Watanabe Y, et al: True hepatic teratoma with high alpha fetoprotein in serum. J Pediatr Surg 1977;12:591.

67. von Schweinitz D, Gomez Dammeier B, Gluer S: Mesenchymal hamartoma of the liver—new insight into histogenesis. J Pediatr Surg 1999;34:1269.

68. Warmann S, Bertram H, Kardorff R, et al: Interventional treatment of infantile hepatic hemangioendothelioma. J Pediatr Surg 2003;38:1177.

69. Weinberg AG, Finegold MJ: Primary hepatic tumors of childhood. Hum Pathol 1983;14:512.

70. Whelan TJ, Baugh J, Chandor S: Focal nodular hyperplasia of the liver. Ann Surg 1973;177:150.

71. Whiting JH, Korzenik JR, Miller FJ, et al: Fatal outcome after embolotherapy for hepatic arteriovenous malformations of the liver in two patients with hereditary hemorrhagic telangiectasia. J Vasc Interv Radiol 2000;11:855.

72. Witte DP, Kissane JM, Askin FB: Hepatic teratomas in children. Pediatr Pathol 1983;1:81.

73. Wu JT, Book L, Sudar K: Serum alpha fetoprotein (AFP) levels in normal infants. Pediatr Res 1981;15:50.

Chapter 30

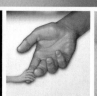

Liver Tumors

James B. Atkinson and Daniel A. DeUgarte

Malignant liver neoplasms account for 1% of all pediatric malignancies and are the third most common intra-abdominal neoplasm after neuroblastoma and nephroblastoma. The two primary malignant neoplasms of the liver are hepatoblastoma and hepatocellular carcinoma. Survival has significantly improved for hepatoblastoma with the advent of new chemotherapy protocols and advances in liver surgery. The prognosis for hepatocellular carcinoma remains poor. Complete resection is required for cure.

EPIDEMIOLOGY

Hepatoblastoma and hepatocellular carcinoma have a different incidence, age distribution, genetic basis, and associated risk factors (Table 30-1). From 1979 to 1996, the incidence of hepatoblastoma rose from 0.6 to 1.2 per million U.S. residents younger than 20 years, and that of hepatocellular carcinoma decreased from 0.45 to 0.29 per million.[14] Hepatoblastoma and hepatocellular carcinoma both occur more frequently in males.[14,50] Hepatoblastoma usually occurs in children aged 6 months to 3 years, whereas hepatocellular carcinoma occurs in older children and adults.

TABLE 30–1 Comparison of Hepatoblastoma and Hepatocellular Carcinoma

	Hepatoblastoma	Hepatocellular Carcinoma
Incidence	1.2 cases per million[12]	0.29 cases per million[12]
Age distribution	6 mo to 3 yr	>5 yr
Risk factors	Beckwith-Weidemann syndrome	Hepatitis B virus
	Familial adenomatous polyposis	Cirrhosis
	Hemihypertrophy	Liver disease
	Low birth weight[26,54]	
5-yr survival	52% to 75%[12,40,47,55]	18% to 28%[11,26]

Hepatoblastoma is associated with Beckwith-Wiedemann syndrome, familial adenomatous polyposis, hemihypertrophy, and low birth weight.[16,23,44,60,66] The most common genetic aberrations involve chromosomes 1p, 1q, 2q, 4q, 7q, 8q, 12p, 17q, 20, 22q, Xp, and Xq.[68,71,75] Hepatoblastoma has also been associated with stabilizing mutations of β-catenin and activation of Wnt/β-catenin signaling.[6] Up-regulation of insulin-like growth factor 2 has also been observed in hepatoblastomas and may be mediated by the overexpression of PLGA1 oncogene, a transcriptional activator on the 8q chromosome.[78] Cytogenetic abnormalities have not led to the identification of a causal factor nor been shown to influence prognosis. The cause of hepatoblastoma remains unclear, but recent theories suggest that hepatoblastoma is derived from a pluripotent hepatic stem cell or oval stem cell that can differentiate into both hepatocytes and biliary epithelial cells. Both hepatoblastoma cells and oval stem cells express markers for these two lineages. Further, the structural features of hepatoblastoma resemble those found in distinct phases of hepatogenesis.[61,79]

The association between very low birth weight (VLBW) and hepatoblastoma may be explained by a higher likelihood of genetic abnormalities or the susceptibility of the immature liver to the effects of intensive perinatal therapy (e.g., oxygen, diuretics, radiation). In one study, hepatoblastoma patients had a longer duration of and more aggressive perinatal therapy than did birth weight–matched controls.[54] VLBW infants may also be at higher risk of developing advanced hepatoblastoma.[26] Some reports have suggested that infants with VLBW or other conditions associated with hepatoblastoma might benefit from screening with serial ultrasound examinations and serum alpha fetaprotein (AFP) monitoring to increase the likelihood of early detection.[11] However, a cost-benefit analysis of screening for hepatoblastoma in high-risk patients must be performed before it is applied routinely.

Hepatocellular carcinoma occurs predominantly in the setting of underying liver disease and cirrhosis. In young children, hepatocellular carcinoma has been associated with tyrosinemia and other inherited metabolic disorders.[76] The incidence of hepatocellular carcinoma in the United States is higher in Asians and foreign-born children.[10,14] In Taiwan, hepatocellular carcinoma occurs

in children as young as 5 months and often is associated with maternal transmission of hepatitis B virus.

502

predominantly in hepatitis B viral carriers.[14] Hepatitis B vaccinations led to a significant decrease in the rate of hepatocellular carcinoma.[8,36,46] A Taiwanese study comparing hepatocellular carcinoma in children and adults demonstrated that hepatitis B viral infection was always present in children (100% versus 80%), the frequency of liver cirrhosis was similar (70%), and the rate of resectability was lower in children (18% versus 56%).[10]

CLINICAL FEATURES AND LABORATORY DATA

Most patients with liver tumors present with an abdominal mass, and more than two thirds of liver tumors are malignant.[17] Although most patients are asymptomatic, some note abdominal distention, anorexia, weight loss, pain, nausea, and fatigue. An abdominal computed tomography (CT) or ultrasound scan is obtained, which usually reveals a solid liver mass. Laboratory studies should include complete blood cell count, chemistry panel, liver function tests, coagulation profile, and serum AFP levels. Thrombocytosis is present in 60% of cases.[73] Anemia and elevated serum transaminase levels are occasionally observed.[57] Diagnosis is ultimately made with biopsy. An algorithm for the diagnosis and treatment of malignant liver neoplasms is presented in Figure 30-1.

The most sensitive laboratory test for hepatoblastoma and hepatocellular carcinoma is serum AFP level. AFP is produced in the fetal liver and yolk sac, and levels decline to adult values during the first 6 months after birth. Although AFP can be used effectively as a tumor marker, it is nonspecific. Serum AFP levels are elevated in over 90% of hepatoblastomas and in approximately 70% of hepatocellular carcinomas.[13,31] Falsely elevated serum AFP levels can be noted in hepatitis, cirrhosis, hemangioendothelioma, germ cell tumor, testicular tumor and gallbladder carcinoma. Normal AFP levels have been observed with both well-differentiated and immature hepatoblastomas and frequently occur with the fibrolamellar variants of hepatocellular carcinoma.[12,13,72] Serum AFP levels can be used to monitor chemotherapeutic efficacy and to detect disease recurrence. Rarely, hepatoblastoma may secrete β-human chorionic gonadotropin, associated with sexual precocity.

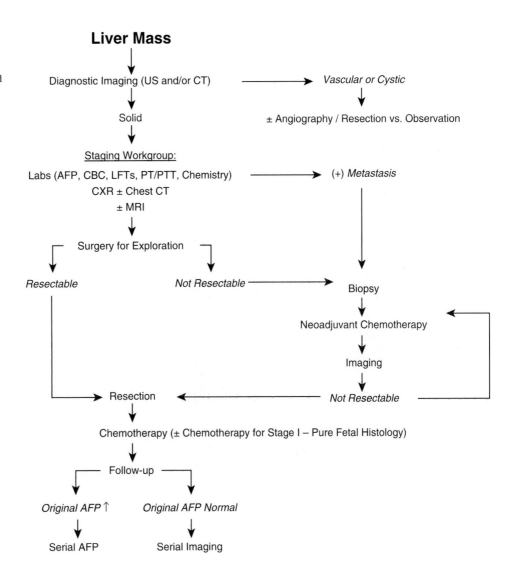

Figure 30-1 Algorithm for the diagnosis and treatment of a liver mass. AFP, alpha fetoprotein; CBC, complete blood count; CT, computed tomography; CXR, chest radiograph; LFT, liver function tests; MRI, magnetic resonance imaging; PT/PTT, prothrombin time/partial thromboplastin time; US, ultrasound.

Liver Mass

Diagnostic Imaging (US and/or CT) → *Vascular or Cystic*

↓ *(Vascular or Cystic)*
± Angiography / Resection vs. Observation

Solid

↓

Staging Workgroup:
Labs (AFP, CBC, LFTs, PT/PTT, Chemistry) → (+) *Metastasis*
CXR ± Chest CT
± MRI

↓

Surgery for Exploration

Resectable — *Not Resectable* → Biopsy

Neoadjuvant Chemotherapy

↓

Imaging

↓

Not Resectable

Resection ←

Chemotherapy (± Chemotherapy for Stage I – Pure Fetal Histology)

↓

Follow-up

Original AFP ↑   *Original AFP Normal*

↓   ↓

Serial AFP   Serial Imaging

IMAGING

Imaging is helpful both for diagnostic purposes and to assess tumor resectability. Ultrasonography or CT of the abdomen is performed initially to assess the tumor.[23] A chest radiograph or CT scan of the chest should also be obtained to rule out metastatic disease. Ultimately, imaging should delineate the size and location of tumors, evaluate for metastatic disease, and determine whether vascular invasion of the portal vein, hepatic veins, or inferior vena cava is present. Although advances in imaging have improved the ability to predict resectability, the ultimate assessment is made in the operating room by the surgeon.

Ultrasonography is helpful for the initial evaluation and to assess vascular involvement. Liver lesions can be categorized sonographically as solid, cystic, or vascular. Malignant liver neoplasms are usually well-defined hyperechoic (solid) lesions on ultrasonography.[15] Color Doppler ultrasonography is helpful in diagnosing venous thrombosis and vascular shunts within the tumor.[63] It has also been used intraoperatively to aid in determining vascular involvement and tumor resectability.

CT with intravenous and gastrointestinal contrast enhancement is useful to delineate tumor type, size, and location and to detect regional lymphadenopathy. Abdominal CT usually reveals a mass with low attenuation. Helical CT with three-dimensional reconstruction can be performed in complex cases that require nonstandard resections.

Magnetic resonance imaging (MRI) and magnetic resonance angiography are especially helpful in determining the tumor's relationship to the hepatic vasculature and biliary anatomy. Liver tumors have homogeneous hypointensity on T1-weighted images and hyperintensity on T2-weighted images.[5] Three-dimensional reconstruction can significantly enhance the surgeon's ability to predict resectability (Fig. 30-2).

Angiography was used in the past to delineate the anatomy of the hepatic vasculature, but with the availability of MRI and contrast-enhanced CT, it is rarely required for the diagnostic evaluation of malignant liver neoplasms. Angiography is used in some cases to perform selective chemoembolization as a therapeutic intervention.

DIFFERENTIAL DIAGNOSIS AND HISTOLOGY

Diagnosis is ultimately made with biopsy using percutaneous, laparoscopic, or open approaches. Fine-needle aspiration can be sufficient for diagnosis. Some groups permit the initiation of neoadjuvant chemotherapy based on clinical criteria when those clinical features are highly suggestive of hepatoblastoma or hepatocellular carcinoma.[13] However, given the significant error rate in clinical diagnosis, we strongly advocate biopsy in all cases.[19]

The distribution of malignant and benign primary hepatic tumors of children is shown in Table 30-2. Hepatoblastoma and hepatocellular carcinoma are of

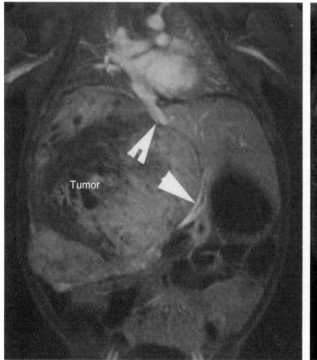
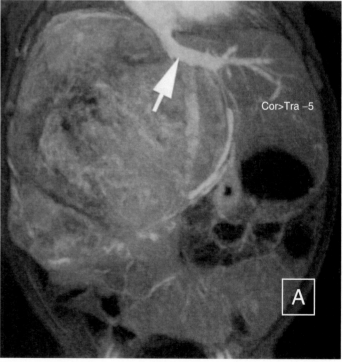

A   B

Figure 30–2 *A,* Magnetic resonance imaging of a 6-month-old child demonstrates a 10-cm right hepatic mass. *B,* Magnetic resonance angiography with three-dimensional reconstruction allows image rotation and delineation of vascular anatomy. Compression of the intrahepatic vena cava demonstrates unresectability.

TABLE 30-2 Incidence of Primary Hepatic Tumors in Childhood	
Tumor	**% of Patients**
Malignant	
Hepatoblastoma	43
Hepatocellular carcinoma	23
Sarcoma	6
Benign	
Benign vascular tumor	13
Mesenchymal hamartoma	6
Adenoma	2
Focal nodular hyperplasia	2
Other	5

Adapted from Weinberg AG, Finegold MJ: Primary hepatic tumors of childhood. Hum Pathol 1983;14:512-537.

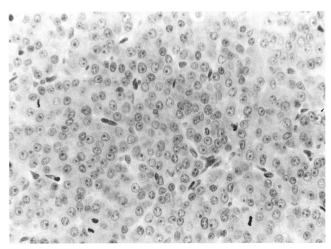

Figure 30-3 Photomicrograph demonstrates pure fetal histology (PFH) with minimal mitotic activity (<2 mitoses/10 400× microscopic fields). In stage I hepatoblastoma, PFH has been associated with significantly improved event-free survival.

epithelial origin and account for more than 90% of malignant liver neoplasms.[76] Primary liver neoplasms can also be of mesenchymal origin; of these, sarcomas are the most common. Undifferentiated embryonal sarcomas and rhabdomyosarcoma usually occur in children aged 5 to 10 years. They are associated with a normal serum AFP level and are vimentin positive on staining.[74] Other reported malignancies include the malignant transformation of mesenchymal hamartoma,[58] angiosarcoma, cholangiocarcinoma, rhabdoid tumor,[59] immature teratoma, and choriocarcinoma.[69] Metastatic disease to the liver is relatively uncommon in children.

Histologic classification of hepatoblastomas has minimal predictive value in determining prognosis. Uniform criteria have not been established, but most pediatric pathologists have simplified the classification into epithelial and mixed (epithelial and mesenchymal) types. The epithelial type is subdivided into fetal, embryonal, macrotrabecular, and small cell undifferentiated types.[60] Small cell undifferentiated histology may confer an unfavorable outcome.[22] Conversely, pure fetal histology (PFH) with minimal mitotic activity (<2 mitoses/10 400× microscopic fields) has been associated with significantly improved event-free survival (Fig. 30-3).[49,76] In fact, adjuvant chemotherapy is no longer routinely recommended by the Children's Oncology Group for children who undergo complete resection of hepatoblastomas with PFH.

With respect to hepatocellular carcinoma, it has been proposed by some investigators that patients with a fibrolamellar variant may have a higher resection rate and improved survival than those with the typical variant.[12,33] However, Katzenstein et al.[30] observed that although the median survival may be longer, no difference is noted when a stage-for-stage comparison is made between the fibrolamellar variant and other cell types.

STAGING

Multiple staging systems have been proposed to classify both hepatoblastoma and hepatocellular carcinoma. The system currently used by the Pediatric Oncology Group (POG) in the United States and the German Cooperative Pediatric Liver Tumor Study Group is shown in Table 30-3.[21,49] This classification scheme is based on the postoperative extent of disease. Approximately 5% of hepatoblastomas that are completely resected (stage I) have PFH with low mitotic activity.[49] Residual disease is defined as microscopic (stage II), macroscopic (stage III), or extrahepatic or metastatic (stage IV). Approximately 20% of hepatoblastomas have distant metastasis at the time of diagnosis.[21,49,56,65] Hepatocellular carcinoma usually presents at a more advanced stage than hepatoblastoma does.[13,29] Although the POG staging system is useful in determining the postoperative prognosis, it does not provide information on the preoperative extent of disease.

To assess tumor response and resectability before and after neoadjuvant chemotherapy, the International Society of Pediatric Oncology (SIOP) developed the PRETEXT (pretreatment extent of disease) staging system.[13,57] The PRETEXT system is based on radiologic findings and describes both the number and the location of involved liver sectors and takes into account invasion of the hepatic and portal veins as well as extrahepatic and metastatic disease (Fig. 30-4). For example, a group III, p, m tumor has three out of four sectors involved by tumor, with ingrowth of the portal vein and metastasis.

TABLE 30-3 Staging for Hepatoblastoma and Hepatocellular Carcinoma	
Stage	**Description**
I*	Complete resection
II	Microscopic residual tumor
III	Macroscopic residual tumor
IV	Distant metastasis

*Stage I hepatoblastoma can be subdivided into (1) pure fetal histology with minimal mitotic activity and (2) all other histologic types.

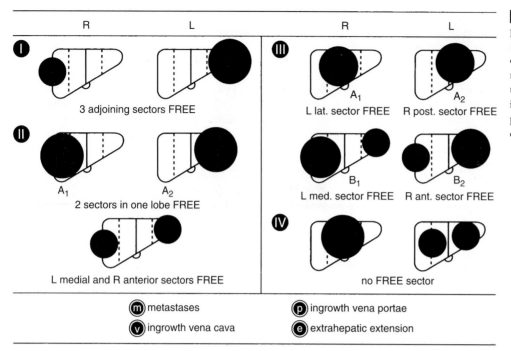

Figure 30-4 The SIOP pretreatment grouping system (PRETEXT) describes the extent of liver involvement based on the number of sectors involved and takes into account metastasis (m), ingrowth of vena cava (v) and portal vein (p), and extrahepatic extension (e).

This staging system has allowed oncologists to compare tumor response to different neoadjuvant regimens. Other classification schemes that have been developed for hepatoblastoma include those by the Japanese Society of Pediatric Surgeons and TNM classifications.[62]

In children, hepatocellular carcinoma also has been investigated using the POG and PRETEXT staging systems.[13,29] In adults, the Okuda and Barcelona Clinic classifications[38,48] have been used to take into account both the extent of tumor involvement and the severity of liver disease.

SURGERY

The primary goal of surgery is complete anatomic resection. Resectability can be compromised by multifocality, bilobar involvement, portal vein or vena cava thrombosis, vascular invasion, para-aortic lymphadenopathy, extension to the hepatic hilum, and distant metastasis. In centrally located tumors, hepatic vein involvement may preclude safe resection. In general, nonanatomic liver resections should be avoided because of a higher rate of incomplete tumor resection and local relapse.[20] When histology demonstrates microscopic residual disease following resection, reoperation should be strongly considered to extend the margins of resection when anatomically feasible.

Successful hepatic resection requires careful planning and supportive care. An experienced pediatric anesthesiologist is essential. The first step in the operative procedure is placement of reliable large-bore venous catheters, arterial monitoring lines, and supplemental peripheral venous catheters. The patient should be positioned such that the surgeon has access to the neck, chest, abdomen, and groins. In the event that additional access or more extensive exposure is needed, these areas will be easily accessible within the sterile field. The Trendelenburg position lowers the caval and hepatic venous pressures and minimizes the risk of air embolism.

An initial subcostal incision can be used to evaluate the tumor's location and extent. The remainder of the abdomen is searched for any evidence of metastatic disease not detected by preoperative studies. Once a decision is made to proceed with resection, the incision is extended across the abdomen. In older children, a midline extension toward the xiphoid provides even wider exposure of the liver and tumor.

The liver and tumor are completely mobilized from all anatomic attachments. The triangular ligament is divided from the left hepatic vein to its termination at the left diaphragm. The right lobe of the liver is then retracted from the right diaphragm, and the bare attachments are divided by cautery. As the liver is delivered through the incision, the remaining attachments of the right adrenal gland and several branches of the infrahepatic vena cava are divided to completely mobilize the liver.

Additional mobilization of the infrahepatic vena cava is then performed such that the vena cava above the origin of the renal veins to the junction with the hepatic parenchyma is encircled and controlled with a vessel loop. With complete mobilization of the liver, a final assessment of the plan for resection is made. The portal structures can be palpated bimanually through the foramen of Winslow for evidence of tumor invasion and the presence of frequently encountered vascular anomalies. The retrohepatic vena cava should be assessed for location within the hepatic parenchyma or evidence of tumor invasion. Finally, a careful assessment of the relationship between the tumor and the hepatic veins should be made. The accuracy of this assessment may be enhanced by preoperative images and intraoperative ultrasonography. Unexpected invasion of the remaining solitary hepatic vein is the most common cause of positive resection margins, severe intraoperative hemorrhage, and postoperative liver failure due to acute portal hypertension from hepatic vein injury (Budd-Chiari syndrome). Once this assessment is completed, the mobilized tumor and liver can be evaluated for the required resection. Options include a standard right or left hepatic lobectomy, extended right or left lobectomy, or, in rare cases, a central or segmentally based anatomic resection.

The sequence of the dissection is similar in all cases. Once the tumor and liver have been mobilized and the surgeon determines that the tumor is resectable, attention is directed to a vascular dissection of the portal structures. The hepatic artery, common bile duct, and portal vein are identified near the duodenum and distal to the branching of the pancreaticoduodenal artery. The gallbladder is dissected from the liver, and the cystic duct is ligated. A vascular dissection of the common duct, hepatic artery, and portal vein is then performed, with identification and ligation of the structures supplying the intended segment or lobe of the liver and tumor. As the hepatic arterial and portal venous branches are ligated, a line of demarcation appears to guide the parenchymal dissection.

Once the portal dissection is complete, attention is directed to the retrohepatic inferior vena cava. The liver and tumor are rotated to the left, exposing the course of the vena cava. A tedious and careful dissection of the vena cava is performed beginning distally and working superiorly toward the hepatic veins. Myriad small paired branches can be identified, dissected, and ligated as the vena cava is freed from the hepatic parenchyma. In difficult cases, the Pringle maneuver, clamping across the remaining portal vasculature and clamping the supra- or infradiaphragmatic vena cava, may facilitate dissection. Clamping of the portal structures should be limited to 15 minutes, with the total clamp time not to exceed 60 minutes. At the conclusion of this portion of the surgery, the vena cava will be entirely free except for the major hepatic veins.

The final portion of the vascular dissection is the identification and division of the appropriate hepatic veins. The right, middle, and left hepatic veins originate very close to the surface of the liver. The course of the veins is extremely short until they combine into the structure of the atrium of the heart. Before beginning the resection, it is critical that involvement at the hepatic veins has been accurately assessed. Intraoperative ultrasonography can be of great assistance in planning the surgical approach to these important structures. Because the veins branch rapidly after entering the substance of the liver, it is technically much safer to divide them in the parenchyma if the tumor margins allow the use of this technique. Marking the surface of the liver with cautery just distal to the hepatic veins to be divided guides

parenchymal dissection and is safer than attempting extrahepatic ligation of the veins.

When the tumor or anatomy does not permit intraparenchymal division of the hepatic veins, wide exposure and careful dissection should be used to isolate and divide the veins. Frequently, this can be delayed until most of the parenchyma has been divided and the specimen is nearly ready for delivery to the pathologist. The surgeon should not hesitate to obtain supradiaphragmatic control of the vena cava when control of the hepatic veins is difficult to achieve.

Upon completion of the vascular dissection, a line of demarcation should be visible to guide the parenchymal dissection. Cautery may be used to circumferentially mark the line of resection 3 to 5 mm in deep. Particular care should be taken to mark the course of the parenchymal dissection in the area of the previously dissected portal structures and through the previously identified path to control the hepatic veins. The anesthesiologist should be alerted at this point to prepare for the potential blood loss associated with parenchymal dissection. The parenchymal dissection in the classic operation may proceed with blunt and finger fracture technique or by passing ligatures around bundles of hepatic parenchyma, tying the suture, and cutting through the parenchyma to reveal the vascular and biliary structures. Depending on surgeon preference, the Harmonic Scalpel (Ethicon Endosurgery, Cincinnati, Ohio), the Integra Selector (Integra, Plainsboro, N.J.), or the TissueLink device (TissueLink, Dover, N.H.) may be used to facilitate dissection. Although these devices aid in a precise dissection, the key to a successful and relatively blood-free parenchymal dissection is a complete vascular dissection before dividing the parenchyma.

Knowledge of the three-dimensional segmental anatomy of the liver described by Couinard (Fig. 30-5) is essential in planning liver resections (Fig. 30-6). Segmentectomy involves resection of a single segment. A right hepatic lobectomy involves resection of segments V, VI, VII, and VIII and ligation of the right hepatic artery, right portal

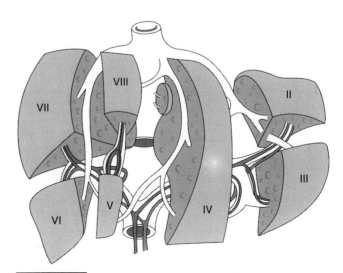

Figure 30–5 The anatomy of the liver is divided into segments as described by Couinard.

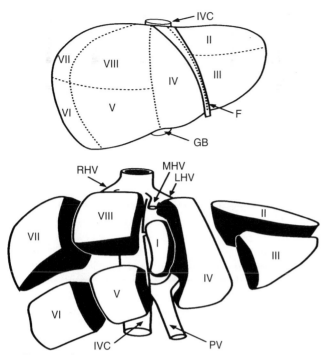

Figure 30–6 Standard anatomic liver resections are based on the segmental anatomy of the liver. Left lobectomy (formerly left lateral segmentectomy) excises segments II and III; left hepatectomy, segments II, III, and IV; extended left hepatectomy, segments II, III, IV, V, and VIII (and occasionally I); right hepatectomy, segments V, VI, VII, and VIII; and extended right hepatic lobectomy (formerly right trisegmentectomy), segments IV, V, VI, VII, and VIII (and occasionally I). GB, gallbladder; IVC, inferior vena cava; LHV, left hepatic vein; MHV, middle hepatic vein; PV, portal vein; RHV, right hepatic vein.

vein, right hepatic biliary duct, and right hepatic vein. The liver parenchyma is divided through the median portal fissure on a line between the gallbladder fossa and the vena cava. The large distal branch and the smaller branches of the middle hepatic vein supplying these segments must also be divided. An extended right hepatic lobectomy (right trisegmentectomy) includes resection of segments I, IV, and V through VIII. The right and middle hepatic veins are divided. The liver parenchyma is divided along the falciform ligament and left portal fissure. In addition, the branches of the left hepatic artery, portal vein, and hepatic biliary duct to segments I and IV are ligated.

Left lobectomy involves resection of segments II, III, and IV and ligation of the left hepatic artery, left portal vein, left hepatic biliary duct, and left hepatic vein. The liver parenchyma is divided through the median portal fissure. The branches of the middle hepatic vein to segment IV are also divided. A left lateral segmentectomy involves resection of segments II and III. The branches of the left hepatic artery, portal vein, and hepatic biliary duct to these segments are ligated. An extended left hepatic lobectomy (left trisegmentectomy) involves resection of segments I through IV, V, and VIII. The liver

parenchyma is divided along the right portal fissure. The left hepatic artery, left portal vein, left hepatic biliary duct, and left and middle hepatic veins are ligated. The branches of the right hepatic artery, right portal vein, and right hepatic biliary duct to segments V and VIII are also ligated.

When only segments IV, V, and VIII are involved with tumor, central hepatic resection (mesohepatectomy) can be performed.[34] Branches to the left portal vein to segment IV are divided in the umbilical fissure. The middle hepatic vein and right anterior sectoral pedicles are ligated. Central hepatic resection offers the advantage of preserving normal hepatic parenchyma (either segments I-II or VI-VII), which would ordinarily be removed in a standard anatomic resection (i.e., extended right or left lobectomy).

When the tumor is not resectable using standard anatomic resections, novel techniques have been used. Hepatic vein reconstruction using portal vein or synthetic graft has been performed when the hepatic vein or vena cava is involved by tumor.[9] When all hepatic veins are involved, one approach is to rely on venous outflow through the inferior hepatic vein, allowing resection of all segments except V and VI (we have no personal experience with this technique).[67]

In the most challenging cases, tumor resection can be performed ex vivo (on the back table) using methods developed for liver transplantation. Blood flow to the heart is preserved with venovenous bypass. Following hepatectomy, the liver is infused with University of Wisconsin solution and placed in an ice bath. Back-table tumor resection and hepatic vein–vena cava reconstruction are performed before reimplantation.[24]

Upon completion of the resection, adequate hemostasis is achieved. Special attention is given to the raw surface of the remaining liver for both bleeding and bile leak. Drains are placed in the suprahepatic and subhepatic spaces. Complications following hepatic resection include bleeding, subphrenic abscess, biliary fistula, wound infection, and biliary obstruction.

Several advances in anesthesia and surgical technique have improved resection rates and decreased perioperative mortality to less than 5%. When the operation is complicated by severe bleeding, total vascular isolation can be achieved by clamping the supra-and infrahepatic inferior vena cava in combination with the Pringle maneuver.[37] Bleeding can then be controlled before proceeding with resection. Vascular staplers can be used to transect hepatic vessels, resulting in reduced operative time and blood loss.[77] Vascular staplers, ultrasonic dissection, laser, Harmonic Scalpel, finger fracture, sharp dissection, and Kelly clamp have all been used to divide liver parenchyma. Argon beam coagulation and fibrin glue can be used to help control bleeding from the residual liver tissue. Laparoscopic liver resections have also been described in adults[45] and have potential applications in children.

Standard anatomic resections can lead to the loss of a significant percentage of liver parenchyma: right extended lobectomy, 85%; right lobectomy, 65%; left lobectomy, 35%; segmental or wedge resection, 3% to 15%.

Most children with otherwise normal liver parenchyma can easily adapt to major resections with compensatory hyperplasia of the remaining liver. However, neonates have immature livers and are particularly susceptible to developing postoperative hepatic insufficiency manifested by hypoglycemia, hypoalbuminemia, and hypoprothrombinemia. Maintenance intravenous fluids contain 10% dextrose. Supplemental albumin and vitamin K can be administered for the first postoperative week. Oral feedings can usually be resumed in 2 to 3 days. Chemotherapy is usually withheld for 3 weeks in patients who have had extensive resections or compromised liver function to permit adequate liver replication to occur.

LIVER TRANSPLANTATION

Ultimately, up to 6% of patients with hepatoblastoma will require orthotopic liver transplantation (Fig. 30-7).[23,54] Liver transplantation should be considered for every child presenting with involvement of all four sectors of the liver or involvement of three sectors when complete tumor excision by partial hepatectomy is unlikely. A contraindication to liver transplantation is the presence of extrahepatic disease following chemotherapy.

Several reports describe favorable outcomes following liver transplantation in children.[1,3,32,51,52,54,61] In patients who undergo primary liver transplantation for hepatoblastoma following neoadjuvant chemotherapy, 10-year survival rates of 85% have been achieved.[51] Tumor recurrence appears to be more frequent in children with a previous attempt at hepatic resection. In patients who undergo "rescue" liver transplantation following partial hepatectomy, the 5-year overall survival is 30% to 50%. Positive margins after an initial attempt at resection is associated with a particularly poor prognosis. These results suggest that heroic attempts at partial hepatectomy should be avoided, and liver transplantation should be considered when the potential for complete resection is in question.[51]

For hepatocellular carcinoma, liver transplantation has the theoretical advantage of removing not only the tumor but also the entire diseased preneoplastic liver. Most centers restrict transplantation for hepatocellular carcinoma to patients with single tumors 5 cm or smaller or three nodules 3 cm or smaller.[39] The overall 5-year survival rate following liver transplantation for hepatocellular carcinoma is 60% to 70% in adult series.[48]

The scarcity of cadaveric donors, especially in the pediatric age group, has led to the use of segmental grafts from living donors or split-liver cadaveric donors. Living, related donor transplantation for tumors has been associated with improved graft survival and outcome.[76] Total hepatectomy in these patients should include removal of the retrohepatic inferior vena cava. This need has discouraged the use of split livers in this population. In cases in which a segmental graft is used, reconstruction of the vena cava can be achieved with either a preserved allogeneic iliac vein or the internal jugular vein procured from the living donor.[8,41] Disadvantages of transplantation include the associated expense and risks

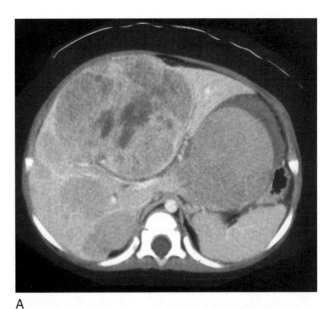

A

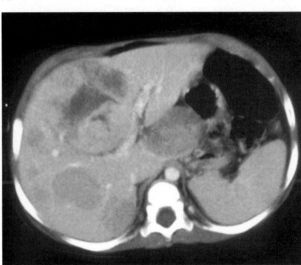

B

Figure 30–7 Computed tomography scan demonstrates a multifocal hepatoblastoma. Despite a good response to chemotherapy, liver transplantation is the only hope for cure.

of lifelong immunosuppression, which may enhance tumor recurrence or secondary malignancies.

ADJUVANT THERAPY

Although cure ultimately requires complete resection, chemotherapy remains the mainstay of adjuvant therapy for hepatoblastoma and hepatocellular carcinoma. Neoadjuvant chemotherapy has been advocated for the purposes of downstaging disease, improving the likelihood of complete resection, and ultimately improving long-term survival.[16] The disadvantage of neoadjuvant therapy is that nonresponders can experience disease progression, and ultimately the tumor can be upstaged or become unresectable. Therefore, imaging and serum

AFP levels should be performed routinely to assess for response when neoadjuvant therapy is used.

There are several chemotherapeutic regimens. Regimens with cisplatin, vincristine, and 5-fluorouracil have had comparable results to those with cisplatin and doxorubicin, with fewer side effects.[29,49] The SIOP advocates cisplatin and doxorubicin and attributes better tolerance of this regimen to lower doses of doxorubicin.[13] A German study group utilizes cisplatin, ifosfamide, and doxorubicin as its chemotherapeutic regimen.[21] Results were similar to SIOP's, but toxicity was potentially greater. Etoposide (VP-16) and carboplatin are used for recurrent or unresponsive disease. Early reports suggest that irinotecan may be a promising chemotherapeutic agent in refractory or relapsed hepatoblastoma.[31,55] Use of antiangiogenic agents, including anti-vascular endothelial growth factor antibody and topotecan, resulted in reduction of tumor volume in experimental liver tumors.[42,43]

Neoadjuvant therapy has had a significant impact in improving resectability in hepatoblastoma, but outcomes are less favorable in children with hepatocellular carcinoma. Up to 50% to 70% of stage III hepatoblastomas can be rendered resectable after neoadjuvant chemotherapy.[49] In stage III hepatocellular carcinoma, however, resection can be achieved in only 10% to 36% of patients following chemotherapy (Fig. 30-8).[13,29]

Radiation therapy has a limited role in the management of hepatoblastoma and hepatocellular carcinoma. Current cooperative trials provide for permissive use of radiation therapy in children with residual disease. However, the ultimate goal remains complete surgical resection as the only effective for cure.

In the hope of avoiding the systemic side effects of standard adjuvant therapies, novel and less toxic treatment modalities have been sought. One proposed strategy that selectively targets tumor cells is suicide gene therapy.[27] This strategy involves the expression of a gene that converts a membrane-permeable nontoxic prodrug into a toxic agent (suicide drug) in tumor cells only. For example, in vivo models for hepatocellular carcinoma have used a replication-deficient adenovirus carrying suicide genes such as *Escherichia coli* cytosine.[7,28,47] A transcriptional control element like that for AFP is used to selectively express the suicide gene in tumor cells.

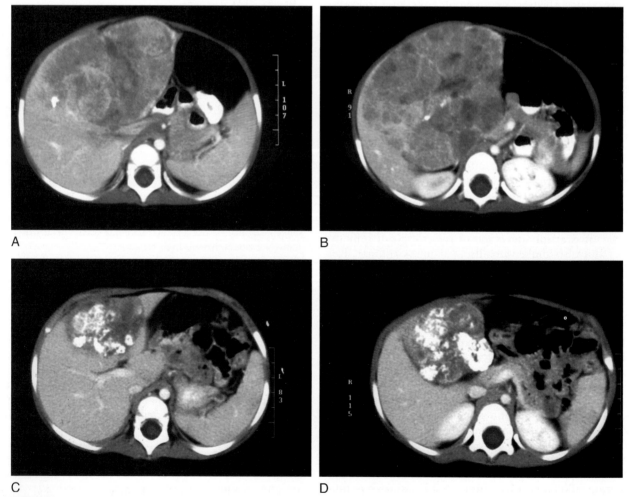

A   B   C   D

Figure 30–8 Neoadjuvant chemotherapy can significantly decrease tumor size and ultimately make lobectomy easier and safer. Prominent calcification is seen after chemotherapy, and the right portal vein is noted to be patent.

ABLATIVE THERAPIES

Patients with lesions that cannot be anatomically resected and those who are not candidates for transplantation can be considered for local ablative therapies, including chemoembolization, radiofrequency ablation, percutaneous injection of ethanol, and cryoablation.[2,35,64] Ablative therapies offer palliation and may prolong survival but rarely achieve a cure. Alternatively, ablative therapies can act as a bridge to transplantation until a suitable donor becomes available.

Radiofrequency ablation uses a needle electrode inserted into the tumor that delivers alternating current in the range of radiofrequency waves to cause focal thermal injury. Larger lesions require multiple overlapping applications, each lasting 10 to 20 minutes.

Cryoablation uses direct freezing and thawing to cause cell death by protein denaturation, cell membrane disruption, and hypoxia. Intraoperatively, the Pringle maneuver can be performed to decrease the warming effects of larger blood vessels passing through or near the site to be ablated. Usually, two freeze cycles lasting 15 to 20 minutes each are followed by spontaneous thaw cycles. The goal of ablative therapies is to incorporate a 1-cm rim of normal tissue. This can be confirmed sonographically by the presence of echogenic microbubbles with radiofrequency ablation or a round, echogenic expanding rim with cryoablation.

Intrahepatic arterial chemoembolization has the potential to improve chemotherapeutic response and allow for contralateral liver hyperplasia. The procedure involves angiographic placement of a catheter into the main feeding artery of the tumor. Doxorubicin (Adriamycin) dispersed in lipiodol and cisplatin is infused, and embolization is then performed with Gelfoam.[53] Drug levels within the tumor can reach 50 to 400 times that used in conventional chemotherapy without an increase in systemic toxicity. Reports concerning chemoembolization in children have been limited, but subsequent surgical resectability has been achieved in some cases.[4,40,53] Complications of chemoembolization include hepatic artery thrombosis and gastric ulceration. Chemoembolization can also be used before transplantation when systemic neoadjuvant chemotherapy has failed.[4]

PROGNOSIS AND FOLLOW-UP

The 5-year survival rate for hepatoblastoma has markedly improved from 35% 3 decades ago to 75% in some series.[14,17,50,57,65] The prognosis for hepatocellular carcinoma remains dismal, with 5-year overall survival rates of less than 18% to 28%.[13,29] Lesions that are successfully resected have a better prognosis, with 91% to 100% 5-year survival in hepatoblastoma and 30% to 54% for hepatocellular carcinoma.[10,13,49,57,73] Results for estimated 5-year event-free survival reported by the Intergroup Hepatoma Study are summarized in Table 30-4. The German Cooperative Pediatric Liver Tumor Study Group had similar results for disease-free survival in hepatoblastoma (mean follow-up 58 months): 89% ($n = 27$) for stage I,

TABLE 30-4 Estimated Five-Year Event-Free Survival for Hepatoblastoma and Hepatocellular Carcinoma

Stage	Hepatoblastoma	Hepatocellular Carcinoma
I (pure fetal histology)	100% (n = 9)	
I (other histologic types)	91% (n = 43)	
I (hepatocellular carcinoma)		88% (n = 8)
II	100% (n = 7)	— (n = 0)
III	64% (n = 83)	8% (n = 25)
IV	25% (n = 40)	0% (n = 13)

Data adapted from Ortega JA, Dougless EC, Feusner JH, et al: Randomized comparison of cisplatin/vincristine/Auorouracil and cisplatin/continuous infusion doxorubicin for treatment of pediatric hepatoblastoma: A report from the Children's Cancer Group and the Pediatric Oncology Group. J Clin Oncol 2000;18:2665-2675; and Katzenstein HM, Krailo MD, Malogolowkin MH, et al: Hepatocellular carcinoma in children and adolescents: Results from the Pediatric Oncology Group and the Children's Cancer Group Intergroup Study. J Clin Oncol 2002;20: 2789-2797.

100% ($n = 3$) for stage II, 68% ($n = 25$) for stage III, and 21% ($n = 14$) for stage IV.[21]

The primary predictor for poor prognosis in hepatoblastoma and hepatocellular carcinoma is metastatic disease.[10,13,21] Multifocality, size, and lack of response to chemotherapy are also predictive of poor prognosis in hepatocellular carcinoma.[13] Although metastatic disease portends a worse prognosis, some metastatic lesions have a complete response to chemotherapy. Pulmonary resection should be considered in selected patients with lung lesions that persist after chemotherapy.

Following hepatic resection, most patients receive postoperative chemotherapy. Patients should be followed closely to ensure that serum AFP levels return to normal and that the neoplasm does not recur. In those patients who present with normal AFP levels, serial ultrasonography or CT can be performed to screen for recurrence.

CONCLUSION

Advances in anesthesia, surgical technique, and chemotherapy have led to a significant improvement in the prognosis of children with hepatoblastoma. Outcomes for hepatocellular carcinoma remain poor. Liver transplantation is useful in patients with unrectable tumors. Continued cooperation of multi-institutional pediatric cancer study groups will be required to achieve additional advances in the treatment of malignant liver neoplasms.

ACKNOWLEDGMENT

We are grateful to Marcio Malogolowkin, MD, chair of the Liver Tumor Subcommittee of the Children's Oncology Group and director of the Bone and Soft Tissue Tumor Program at Children's Hospital, Los Angeles, for his review of the manuscript.

REFERENCES

1. Achilleos OA, Buist LJ, Kelly DA, et al: Unresectable hepatic tumors in childhood and the role of liver transplantation. J Pediatr Surg 1996;31:1563-1567.
2. Ahrar K, Gupta S: Hepatic artery embolization for hepatocellular carcinoma: Technique, patient selection, and outcomes. Surg Oncol Clin N Am 2003;12:105-126.
3. Al-Qabandi W, Jenkinson H, Buckels JA, et al: Orthotopic liver transplantation for unresectable hepatoblastoma: A single center's experience. J Pediatr Surg 1999;34:1261-1264.
4. Arcement CM, Towbin RB, Meza MP, et al: Intrahepatic chemoembolization in unresectable pediatric liver malignancies. Pediatr Radiol 2000;30:779-785.
5. Boechat MI, Kangarloo H, Ortega J, et al: Primary liver tumors in children: Comparison of CT and MR imaging. Radiology l988;169:727-732.
6. Buendia MA: Genetic alterations in hepatoblastoma and hepatocellular carcinoma: Common and distinctive aspects. Med Pediatr Oncol 2002;39:530-535.
7. Cao G, Kuriyama S, Gao J, et al: Gene therapy for hepatocellular carcinoma based on tumour-selective suicide gene expression using the alpha-fetoprotein (AFP) enhancer and a housekeeping gene promoter. Eur J Cancer 2001;37:140-147.
8. Chang MH, Chen CJ, Lai MS, et al: Universal hepatitis B vaccination in Taiwan and the incidence of hepatocellular carcinoma in children. N Engl J Med 1997;336:1855-1859.
9. Chardot C, Saint-Martin C, Gilles A, et al: Living related liver transplantation and vena cava reconstruction after total hepatectomy including vena cava for hepatoblastoma. Transplantation 2002;73:90-92.
10. Chen JC, Chen CC, Chen WJ, et al: Hepatocellular carcinoma in children: Clinical review and comparison with adult cases. J Pediatr Surg 1998;33:1350-1354.
11. Clericuzio CL, Chen E, McNeil DE, et al: Serum alpha-fetoprotein screening for hepatoblastoma in children with Beckwith-Wiedemann syndrome or isolate hemihyperplasia. J Pediatr 2003; 143:270-272.
12. Craig JR, Peters RL, Edmondson HA, et al: Fibrolamellar carcinoma of the liver; a tumor of adolescents and young adults with distinctive clinico-pathologic features. Cancer l980;46:372-379.
13. Czauderna P, Mackinlay G, Perilongo G, et al: Hepatocellular carcinoma in children: Results of the first prospective study of the International Society of Pediatric Oncology group. J Clin Oncol 2002;20:2798-2804.
14. Darbari A, Sabin KM, Shapiro CN, et al: Epidemiology of primary hepatic malignancies in US children. Hepatology 2003;38:560-566.
15. de Campo M, de Campo JF: Ultrasound of primary hepatic tumours in children. Pediatr Radiol 1988;19:19-24.
16. Evans AE, Land VJ, Newton WA, et al: Combination chemotherapy (vincristine, Adriamycin, cyclophosphamide, and 5-fluorouracil) in the treatment of children with malignant hepatoma. Cancer 1982;50:821-826.
17. Exelby PR, Filler RM, Grosfeld JL: Liver tumors in children with particular reference to hepatoblastoma and hepatocellular carcinoma: American Academy of Pediatrics Surgical Section Survey—1974. J Pediatr Surg 1975;10:329-337.
18. Feusner J, Plaschkes J: Hepatoblastoma and low birth weight: A trend or chance observation? Med Pediatr Oncol 2002;39:508-509.
19. Finegold MJ: Chemotherapy for suspected hepatoblastoma without efforts at surgical resection is a bad practice. Med Pediatr Oncol 2002;39:484-486.
20. Fuchs J, Rydzynski J, Hecker H, et al: The influence of preoperative chemotherapy and surgical technique in the treatment of hepatoblastoma—a report from the German Cooperative Liver Tumour Studies HB 89 and 94. Eur J Pediatr Surg 2002;12:255-261.
21. Fuchs J, Rydzynski J, Von Schweinitz D, et al: Pretreatment prognostic factors and treatment results in children with hepatoblastoma: A report from the German Cooperative Pediatric Liver Tumor Study HB 94. Cancer 2002;95:172-182.
22. Haas JE, Feusner JH, Finegold MJ: Small cell undifferentiated histology in hepatoblastoma may be unfavorable. Cancer 2001;92:3130-3134.
23. Helmberger TK, Ros PR, Mergo PJ, et al: Pediatric liver neoplasms: A radiologic-pathologic correlation. Eur Radiol 1999;9:1339-1347.
24. Hemming AW, Reed AI, Langhan MR, et al: Hepatic vein reconstruction for resection of hepatic tumors. Am Surg 2002;235:850-858.
25. Hughes LJ, Michels VV: Risk of hepatoblastoma in familial adenomatous polyposis. Am J Med Genet 1992;43:1023-1025.
26. Ikeda H, Hachitanda Y, Tanimura M, et al: Development of unfavorable hepatoblastoma in children of very low birth weight: Results of a surgical and pathologic review. Cancer l998;82:1789-1796.
27. Kanai F: Transcriptional targeted gene therapy for hepatocellular carcinoma by adenovirus vector. Mol Biotechnol 2001;18:243-250.
28. Kanai F, Lan KH, Shiratori Y, et al: In vivo gene therapy for alpha-fetoprotein-producing hepatocellular carcinoma by adenovirus-mediated transfer of cytosine deaminase gene. Cancer Res l997;47:561-565.
29. Katzenstein HM, Krailo MD, Malogolowkin MH, et al: Hepatocellular carcinoma in children and adolescents: Results from the Pediatric Oncology Group and the Children's Cancer Group Intergroup Study. J Clin Oncol 2002;20:2789-2797.
30. Katzenstein HM, Krailo MD, Malogolowkin MH, et al: Fibrolamellar hepatocellular carcinoma in children and adolescents. Cancer 2003;97:2006-2012.
31. Katzenstein HM, Rigsby C, Shaw PH, et al: Novel therapeutic approaches in the treatment of children with hepatoblastoma. J Pediatr Hematol Oncol 2002;24:751-755.
32. Koneru B, Flye MW, Bussutil RW, et al: Liver transplantation for hepatoblastoma: The American experience. Ann Surg 1991;213:118-121.
33. Lack EE, Neave C, Vawter GF: Hepatocellular carcinoma: Review of 32 cases in childhood and adolescence. Cancer 1983;52:1510-1515.
34. LaQuaglia MP, Shorter NA, Blumgart LH: Central hepatic resection for pediatric tumors. J Pediatr Surg 2002;37:986-989.
35. Lau WY, Leung TW, Yu SC, et al: Percutaneous local ablative therapy for hepatocellular carcinoma: A review and look into the future. Ann Surg 2003;237:171-179.
36. Lee CL, Ko YC: Hepatitis B vaccination and hepatocellular carcinoma in Taiwan. Pediatrics 1997;99:351-353.
37. Liu DC, Vogel AM, Gulec S, et al: Hepatectomy in children under total hepatic occlusion. Am Surg 2003;69:539-541.
38. Llovet JM, Bru C, Bruix J: Prognosis of hepatocellular carcinoma: The BCLC staging classification. Semin Liver Dis 1999;19:329-338.

39. Llovet JM, Burroughs A, Bruix J: Hepatocellular carcinoma. Lancet 2003;362:1907-1917.
40. Malogolowkin MH, Stanley P, Steele DA, et al: Feasibility and toxicity of chemoembolization for children with liver tumors. J Clin Oncol 2000; 18:1279-1284.
41. Martinez JA, Rigamonti W, Rahier J, et al: Preserved vascular homograft for revascularization of pediatric liver transplant: A clinical, histological, and bacteriological study. Transplantation 1999;68:672-677.
42. McCrudden KW, Hopkins B, Frischer J, et al: Anti-VEGF antibody in experimental hepatoblastoma: Suppression of tumor growth and altered angiogenesis. J Pediatr Surg 2003;38:308-314.
43. McCrudden KW, Yokoi A, Thosani A, et al: Topotecan is anti-angiogenic in experimental hepatoblastoma. J Pediatr Surg 2002;37:857-861.
44. Molmenti EP, Wilkinson K, Molmenti H, et al: Treatment of unresectable hepatoblastoma with liver transplantation in the pediatric population. Am J Transplant 2002;2:535-538.
45. Morino M, Morra I, Rosso E, et al: Laparoscopic vs open hepatic resection: A comparative study. Surg Endosc 2003; 17:1914-1918.
46. Ni Y-H, Change M-H, Huang L-M, et al: Hepatitis B virus infection in children and adolescents in a hyperendemic area: 15 years after mass hepatitis B vaccination. Ann Intern Med 2001;135:796.
47. Ohashi M, Kanai F, Tateishi K, et al: Target gene therapy for alpha-fetoprotein-producing hepatocellular carcinoma by E1B55k-attenuated adenovirus. Biochem Biophys Res Commun 2001;282:529-535.
48. Okuda K, Ohtsuki T, Obata H, et al: Natural history of hepatocellular carcinoma and prognosis in relation to treatment: Study of 850 patients. Cancer 1985;56:918-928.
49. Ortega JA, Douglass EC, Feusner JH, et al: Randomized comparison of cisplatin/vincristine/fluorouracil and cisplatin/continuous infusion doxorubicin for treatment of pediatric hepatoblastoma: A report from the Children's Cancer Group and the Pediatric Oncology Group. J Clin Oncol 2000;18:2665-2675.
50. Ortega JA, Krailo MD, Hans JE, et al: Effective treatment of unresectable or metastatic hepatoblastoma with cisplatin and continuous infusion doxorubicin chemotherapy: A report from the Children's Cancer Study Group. J Clin Oncol 1991;9:2167.
51. Otte JB, Aronson DC, Brown J, et al: Liver transplantation for hepatoblastoma: Results from the International Society of Pediatric Oncology (SIOP) study SIOPEL-1 and review of the world experience. Pediatr Blood Cancer 2004; 42:74-83.
52. Otte JB, Aronson D, Vraux H, et al: Preoperative chemotherapy, major liver resection, and transplantation for primary malignancies in children. Transplant Proc 2001; 28:2393.
53. Oue T, Fukuzawa M, Kusafuka T, et al: Transcather arterial chemoembolization in the treatment of hepatoblastoma. J Pediatr Surg 1998;33:1771-1775.
54. Oue T, Kubota A, Okuyama H, et al: Hepatoblastoma in children of extremely low birth weight: A report from a single perinatal center. J Pediatr Surg 2003;38:134-137.
55. Palmer RD, Williams DM: Dramatic response of multiply relapsed hepatoblastoma to irinotecan (CPT-11). Med Pediatr Oncol 2003;41:78-80.
56. Perilongo G, Brown J, Shafford E, et al: Hepatoblastoma presenting with lung metastases: Treatment results of the first cooperative, prospective study of the International Society of Pediatric Oncology on childhood liver tumors. Cancer 2000;89:1845-1853.
57. Pritchard J, Brown J, Shafford E, et al: Cisplatin, doxorubicin, and delayed surgery for childhood hepatoblastoma: A successful approach—results of the first prospective study of the International Society of Pediatric Oncology. J Clin Oncol 2000;18:3819-3828.
58. Ramanujam TM, Ramesh JC, Goh DW, et al: Malignant transformation of mesenchymal hamartoma of the liver: Case report and review of the literature. J Pediatr Surg 1999:34:1684-1686.
59. Ravindra KV, Cullinane C, Lewis IJ, et al: Long-term survival after spontaneous rupture of a malignant rhabdoid tumor of the liver. J Pediatr Surg 2002;10:1488-1490.
60. Rowland JM: Hepatoblastoma: Assessment of criteria for histologic classification. Med Pediatr Oncol 2002;39:478-483.
61. Ruck P, Xiao JC: Stem-like cells in hepatoblastoma. Med Pediatr Oncol 2002;39:504-507.
62. Sasaki F, Matsunaga T, Iwafuchi M, et al: Outcome of hepatoblastoma treated with the JPLT-1 (Japanese Study Group for Pediatric Liver Tumor) Protocol-1: A report from the Japanese Study Group for Pediatric Liver Tumor. J Pediatr Surg 2002;37:851-856.
63. Sato M, Ishida H, Konno K, et al: Liver tumors in children and young patients: Sonographic and color Doppler findings. Abdom Imaging 2000;25:596-601.
64. Scaife CL, Curley SA: Complication, local recurrence, and survival rates after radiofrequency ablation for hepatic malignancies. Surg Oncol Clin N Am 2003;12:243-255.
65. Schnater JM, Aronson DC, Plaschkes J, et al: Surgical view of the treatment of patients with hepatoblastoma: Results from the first prospective trial of the International Society of Pediatric Oncology Liver Tumor Study Group. Cancer 2002;94:1111-1120.
66. Sindhi R, Rosendale J, Mundy D, et al: Impact of segmental grafts on pediatric liver transplantation: A review of the United Network for Organ Sharing Scientific Registry Data (1990-1996). J Pediatr Surg 1999;34:107-111.
67. Superina RA, Bambini D, Filler RM, et al: A new technique for resecting "unresectable" liver tumors. J Pediatr Surg 2000;35:1294-1299.
68. Surace C, Leszl A, Perilongo G, et al: Fluorescent in situ hybridization (FISH) reveals frequent and recurrent numerical and structural abnormalities in hepatoblastoma with no informative karyotype. Med Pediatr Oncol 2002; 39:536-539.
69. Szavay PO, Wermes C, Fuchs J, et al: Effective treatment of infantile choriocarcinoma in the liver with chemotherapy and surgical resection: A case report. J Pediatr Surg 2000; 35:1134-1135.
70. Tanimura M, Matsui I, Abe J, et al: Increased risk of hepatoblastoma among immature children with a lower birth weight. Cancer Res 1998;58:3032-3035.
71. Terracciano LM, Bernasconi B, Ruck P, et al: Comparative genomic hybridization analysis of hepatoblastoma reveals high frequency of X-chromosome gains and similarities between epithelial and stromal components. Hum Pathol 2003;34:864-871.
72. Tsuchida Y, Ikeda H, Suzuki N, et al: A case of well-differentiated, fetal-type hepatoblastoma with very low serum-alpha-fetoprotein. J Pediatr Surg 1999;12:1762-1764.
73. von Schweinitz D, Hadam MR, Welte K, et al: Production of interleukin-1β and interleukin-6 in hepatoblastoma. Int J Cancer 1993;53:728.
74. Webber EM, Morrison KB, Pritchard SL, et al: Undifferentiated embryonal sarcoma of the liver: Results of clinical management in one center. J Pediatr Surg 1999;34:1641-1644.

75. Weber RG, Pietsch T, von Schweinitz D, et al: Characterization of genomic alterations in hepatoblastomas: A role for gains on chromosomes 8q and 20 as predictors of poor outcome. Am J Pathol 2000;157:571-578.

76. Weinberg AG, Finegold MJ: Primary hepatic tumors of childhood. Hum Pathol 1983;14:512-537.

77. Yanaga K, Nishizaki T, Yamamoto K, et al: Simplified inflow control using stapling devices for major hepatic resection. Arch Surg 1996;131:104-106.

78. Zatkova A, Rouillard JM, Hartmann W, et al: Amplification and overexpression of the IGF2 regulator PLAG1 in hepatoblastoma. Genes Chromosomes Cancer 2004;39: 126-137.

79. Zimmerman A: Pediatric liver tumors and hepatic ontogenesis: Common and distinctive pathways. Med Pediatr Oncol 2002;39:492-503.

Chapter 31

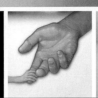

Gastrointestinal Tumors

Patrick A. Dillon and Robert P. Foglia

Primary gastrointestinal (GI) tumors are relatively uncommon in infants and children. GI malignancies account for approximately 1.2% of all pediatric cancer cases.[4] The clinical presentation and histopathology of GI tumors in children can differ significantly from those seen in adults. In addition, the discovery of genetic markers and the use of immunohistochemistry have allowed a more thorough identification of these tumors, although these same advances have made it difficult to assess their true incidence.

The most common presenting symptoms are nonspecific and include abdominal pain, vomiting, and rectal bleeding. The duration of symptoms is often several weeks before diagnosis, and emergent surgery for intestinal obstruction may be required.[4,50] Although not a common diagnosis, the possibility of a GI malignancy should be considered in any child with signs and symptoms of intestinal obstruction, intractable abdominal pain, and alteration in bowel habits or GI bleeding. In addition, children with bowel disorders should receive a detailed and vigorous diagnostic evaluation, including contrast studies, ultrasonography, computed tomography (CT), and endoscopy to both confirm the diagnosis and detect the extent of disease.[31]

GASTROINTESTINAL STROMAL TUMORS

Epidemiology

Gastrointestinal stromal tumors (GISTs) are rare tumors of the GI tract. The incidence is difficult to determine, owing to changes in nomenclature, cellular origin, and diagnostic criteria. Classification has also been hindered by published reports that contain only a few patients, the mixing of benign and malignant tumors, and failure to separate primary and recurrent GISTs.[12] In addition, GISTs have been grouped together, regardless of anatomic location, making prediction of their clinical behavior difficult.[57]

The median age at presentation is between the 5th and 6th decades of life; these tumors are considered rare in patients younger than 40 years. Gender distribution is equal. The most common site of origin is the stomach (50% to 70%), followed by the small intestine (20% to 30%), colon or rectum (10%), and esophagus (5%). The mesentery or omentum may occasionally be the site of origin for GIST.[39,43]

GIST is currently classified as a mesenchymal tumor of the GI tract and is thought to originate from the interstitial cell of Cajal, an intestinal pacemaker cell.[34] Historically, smooth muscle tumors such as leiomyomas and leiomyosarcomas and neural tumors such as schwannomas and malignant peripheral nerve sheath tumors have been categorized as GISTs. However, histologic and immunohistochemical features now distinguish GISTs from tumors of smooth muscle origin.

Association with Other Conditions

In 1977 Carney et al.[7] reported the rare association of gastric leiomyosarcoma, functioning extra-adrenal paraganglioma, and pulmonary chondroma in unrelated young women. The patients' young age, the multifocal locations, and the multiple organ involvement raised the possibility of an inherited disorder, but thus far, no genetic link has been identified.[6] A primary feature of Carney's triad is gastric stromal tumors. These tumors are usually located along the lesser curve or antrum and produce few local symptoms; continued growth can lead to mucosal ulceration and GI bleeding, and serosal involvement is common. The multifocal nature of the tumor can lead to local recurrence as well as widespread but slowly progressive metastatic lesions. Traditional adjuvant therapy has been unsuccessful in treating metastatic disease.[6] Despite the possible development of additional gastric tumors in the remaining stomach, less than total gastrectomy, if feasible, is likely the best initial operation to avoid the complications of total gastrectomy, particularly in teenage patients. Patients treated in this manner should be advised that new gastric tumors may develop and should be re-examined at 3-year intervals. Evaluation for adrenal tumors in patients with gastric stromal sarcomas or pulmonary chondromas (or both) should be considered, and a family history should be obtained from patients with Carney's triad. However, family screening and genetic counseling for the disorder are not currently recommended.[6]

A subset of GIST has been identified and is commonly referred to as GI autonomic nerve tumor (GANT). There have been very few cases of GANT reported in the pediatric population. However, in small series of pediatric patients, there is a female predominance, and symptoms may include abdominal pain, fullness, emesis, and a palpable abdominal mass.[33] GANT can arise in any part of the GI tract, with the small intestine being the most common site in adults. As is the case with GIST, when GANT occurs in children, it tends to favor the stomach as the primary site of origin.[33] The majority of pediatric patients have localized disease at the time of diagnosis, and surgical resection of the tumor is the treatment of choice. Currently there appears to be no defined role for chemotherapy or radiation. In children, localized disease and small tumor size at the time of diagnosis likely aid in the more favorable long-term prognosis compared with adults. Immunocytochemical and ultrastructural evaluation is required to differentiate these tumors from GIST, and established criteria for malignancy are not currently available for the pediatric population.[33]

Clinical Presentation

At the time of presentation, most patients have experienced some symptoms, most often generalized abdominal pain, dyspepsia, and occult GI bleeding. Iron-deficiency anemia, which can be present in children, should prompt an investigation to rule out the GI tract as the source of the anemia.[33] Less commonly, patients present with a palpable abdominal mass or intestinal obstruction.[46] Standard imaging studies to assist in the diagnosis include plain radiographs and CT; there also appears to be a potential role for whole-body fluorodeoxyglucose positron emission tomography.[13] Endoscopy can be helpful in identifying a tumor mass, especially if the tumor is located in the stomach or the proximal small intestine.

Pathology

GISTs are defined as cellular spindle cell, epithelioid, or occasionally pleomorphic mesenchymal tumors of the GI tract that express the KIT (CD117, stem cell factor receptor) protein, as detected using immunohistochemistry. Additional cell type markers such as CD34, smooth muscle actin, desmin, and S-100 protein are used to establish a diagnosis of GIST.[39] Attempts to predict the outcome of GIST rely on traditional pathologic criteria such as size, stage, extent of tumor invasion into mucosa or surrounding organs, mitotic index, and nuclear pleomorphism. Although these criteria have been useful in predicting GIST behavior, no single feature is consistently reliable when it comes to predicting outcome.[27] Morphologic features that are associated with malignant gastric stromal tumors include tumor size greater than 7 cm, high cellularity, mucosal invasion, and mitotic count greater than 5 mitoses per 50 high-powered fields. All these

factors must be considered when distinguishing benign from malignant gastric stromal tumors.[57] Recently, a mutation in the *c-kit* gene on exon 11 was identified in GIST. Patients found to have this mutation showed an increased risk of recurrence and higher mortality compared with GIST patients without the *c-kit* mutation.[43]

Treatment

Complete surgical resection of GISTs, along with any possible pseudocapsules, is the recommended approach. Although wide margins are not thought to be necessary, en bloc resection may require complete or partial organ removal to achieve clear margins.[18] Achieving negative pathologic margins is generally not difficult, because GISTs tend to hang from, and do not diffusely infiltrate, the organ of origin. Consequently, wedge resection of the stomach or segmental resection of the intestine provides adequate therapy; wide resection has no known benefit.[49] In addition, because the status of the microscopic margins does not appear to be important for survival, vital structures should not be sacrificed if gross tumor clearance has already been attained.[12] GIST rarely metastasizes to lymph nodes, so lymphadenectomy is seldom warranted.[46]

The high rate of local and distant recurrence underscores the need for adjuvant therapy. GIST has traditionally been resistant to radiotherapy and all previously available systemic treatments. However, the ability of imatinib to reduce tumor size significantly has changed the management of GIST. Imatinib is a signal transduction inhibitor that exerts its activity in GIST through the blockade of the adenosine triphosphate binding site of KIT, a transmembrane receptor protein-tyrosine kinase. Imatinib has been successful in treating patients with chronic myeloid leukemia and other Philadelphia chromosome–positive leukemias. The use of imatinib for GIST patients is based on the hypothesis that imatinib can block the constitutive activity of KIT receptor tyrosine kinase in the cells of GISTs.[13] With the use of imatinib, surgical resection may be possible for GIST patients with widespread metastatic disease who would otherwise not be candidates for surgery. This therapy may also decrease the incidence of postoperative GIST recurrence and spread and thereby extend lives. Although the trials of adjuvant and neoadjuvant imatinib are ongoing, it appears reasonable to suggest that surgery be considered the first option for patients with resectable GISTs, followed by enrollment in a clinical trial of imatinib as a postoperative adjuvant in cases of incomplete resection, tumor spillage, or other high-risk factors. For cases of recurrent or metastatic GIST, a trial of imatinib, followed by surgical resection, should be considered.

Survival

The long-term survival following surgical resection of GIST varies in published series and is especially difficult to determine in children, because most reports either contain small numbers of patients or include primarily adult patients (Table 31-1). Moreover, given the recent

TABLE 31–1 Five-Year Survival of Patients with Gastrointestinal Stromal Tumors Following Surgical Resection

Institution	Years Covered	No. of Patients Evaluated	No. of Patients Completely Resected (%)	5-Year Survival (%)
Mayo Clinic	1950-1974	108	52 (48)	50
MSKCC	1949-1973	38	20 (53)	65
MCV	1951-1984	51	30 (59)	63
MDACC	1957-1997	191	99 (52)	48
MGH	1962-1986	55	40 (73)	35
MSKCC	1982-1998	200	80 (40)	54

MCV, Medical College of Virginia; MDACC, MD Anderson Cancer Center; MGH, Massachusetts General Hospital; MSKCC, Memorial Sloan-Kettering Cancer Center.

changes in the recognition and pathologic categorization of these tumors, many older series may contain tumors that are not actually GISTs. Despite these obstacles, several factors appear to be useful in predicting long-term outcome following surgical resection: tumor size, mitotic index, and location (Table 31-2). Improved survival is noted when tumors are less than 5 cm, compared with those 5 to 10 cm; in turn, this intermediate group of tumors has a better prognosis than those greater than 10 cm. Low-grade tumors have a mitotic index of less than 10 per 50 high-powered fields, whereas high-grade tumors have an index of greater than 10 per 50 high-powered fields. Tumor location has also been found to predict prognosis, with gastric tumors having an improved survival compared with GISTs in other locations.[46]

ESOPHAGEAL AND GASTRIC CANCER

Esophageal or gastric cancer in a child is extremely rare. According to Surveillance, Epidemiology, and End Results (SEER) data from the National Cancer Statistics Branch, esophageal carcinoma was diagnosed in 10,441 patients between 1988 and 1996. Of those patients, only three (0.03%) were between 10 and 19 years of age, and no patients were younger than 10 years.[20]

TABLE 31–2 Prognostic Factors for Gastrointestinal Stromal Tumors

Factor	Benign*	Malignant
Size	<5 cm	>5 cm
Cellularity	Low	High
Nuclear pleomorphism	Absent to minimal	May be prominent
Necrosis	Absent	Present
Mitosis	<0-1 per 30-50/ HPF	1-5 or more per 10/HPF
Infiltrative growth attern	Absent	May invade adjacent structures
Metastasis	Absent	Present
c-kit Mutation	Absent	Frequently present

*No single feature is absolutely predictive of benign behavior. Tumor size, mitotic rate, and presence or absence of necrosis appear to be the most important factors in predicting behavior.
HPF, high-powered field, 400×.

Despite the rarity of esophageal cancer, there are known risk factors associated with a predisposition for tumor development. With regard to esophageal adenocarcinoma, the development of Barrett's esophagus secondary to chronic gastroesophageal reflux disease (GERD) is the primary risk factor. Pediatric populations that appear to be at increased risk for the development of Barrett's esophagus secondary to chronic GERD include children with severe neurologic deficits, such as cerebral palsy, and those with congenital defects involving the esophagus, such as esophageal atresia and tracheoesophageal fistula.[19] The overall incidence of Barrett's esophagus has been estimated by Hassall[28] to be 0.02% among young patients with severe GERD and associated risk factors; the incidence of Barrett's changes is probably even lower for those without risk factors. Nevertheless, adenocarcinoma of the esophagus has been documented in adolescents with long-standing GERD, and surveillance with upper endoscopy and multiple stepwise biopsies may benefit those children who have the mucosal changes of Barrett's esophagus.[29]

Barrett's changes can also be seen with the retained cervical esophagus following esophageal replacement surgery. A history of this type of surgery requires the control of gastric pH and long-term surveillance endoscopy with biopsy of the retained upper esophageal segment. Depending on the technique and approach, esophageal replacement surgery for patients with esophageal atresia may result in retention of the distal esophageal segment. This remnant can cause severe chronic esophagitis and Barrett's changes requiring surgical resection. Because Barrett's esophagus is a premalignant lesion and can lead to the development of esophageal adenocarcinoma, the distal segment of esophagus should be removed at the time of esophageal replacement surgery.[48] There have also been case reports of esophageal carcinomas arising in children after chemical injuries to the esophagus. Endoscopic follow-up with biopsies should be considered for patients with Barrett's esophagus and for those with chemical injuries to monitor for the development of malignant changes.[47]

Between 1997 and 2001, the SEER database reported a gastric cancer incidence of 0.1% for patients younger than 20 years from a total of 15,274 cases reported.[55] Despite the rarity of gastric adenocarcinoma in children, there are several case reports of adenocarcinoma of the stomach in children as young as 2½ years.[17] The tumors can arise from any anatomic location in the stomach[38]; symptoms may be quite vague but can include epigastric pain, weight loss, vomiting, and anemia. In addition, symptoms associated with esophageal achalasia have been reported in conjunction with gastric adenocarcinoma.[1,17]

CARCINOID TUMORS

Epidemiology

Carcinoid tumors originate from neuroendocrine cells found along the primitive GI tract. These neoplasms originate from the same progeny cells as other GI cells and are part of the amine precursor uptake and decarboxylation (APUD) system.[59] Pediatric carcinoid tumors can occur in the GI tract—stomach, small intestine, appendix (most common), and rectum—as well as in extraintestinal sites such as the lung. Although carcinoid tumors of the appendix are rare in children and adolescents, they are nevertheless the most common GI tumor among this age group.[10,40] The incidence is difficult to assess in the pediatric population because most large series include retrospective data that may exclude certain types of carcinoid tumor, but the reported incidence appears to be in the range of 0.08% to 0.169%,[16,52] or approximately 1.14 per million children per year,[42] with a slight female predominance.[23,40]

Diagnosis

Pediatric carcinoid tumors are often discovered during an operation for presumed appendicitis or incidentally during surgery unrelated to the carcinoid tumor. Although clinical signs consistent with acute appendicitis or suggestive of a gynecologic pathology may result in exploration, true inflammatory changes of the appendix are often not seen.[10] The lack of inflammation may be the result of appendiceal carcinoid tumors typically being located in the distal portion of the appendix; thus, proximal obstruction of the appendiceal lumen is not seen (Fig. 31-1).[16,23]

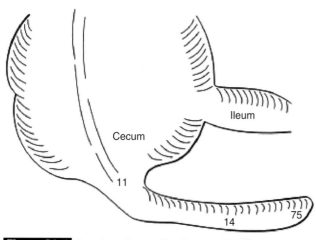

Figure 31-1   Location of appendiceal carcinoids (%).

Although symptoms may be atypical and carcinoid size can be variable, there is no report of carcinoid syndrome associated with carcinoid tumors confined to the appendix.[16,52]

In contrast to patients with appendiceal or incidental carcinoid tumors, pediatric patients with extra-appendiceal carcinoid tumors, such as in the lung or liver, are often symptomatic and have diffuse disease at the time of diagnosis. Broaddus et al.[5] reported that 46% of their patients with extra-appendiceal carcinoids had recurrent tumor or metastasis following the initial diagnosis or disseminated disease at the time of diagnosis.

Treatment

For pediatric carcinoid tumors limited to the appendix, surgical resection of the appendix is the treatment of choice and often results in a cure. Long-range follow-up reveals either minimal or no recurrence of disease and a rare likelihood of metastatic disease.[10,40,60] The most important factor in surgical decision making for carcinoid tumors of the appendix is the size of the tumor. For carcinoids less than 2 cm in diameter, appendectomy alone is usually adequate. Histologic evidence of invasion into the mesoappendix and tumors that involve the base of the appendix are indications for performance of a right hemicolectomy, regardless of tumor diameter. Carcinoid tumors larger than 2 cm in diameter, those with high-grade malignancies, and goblet cell adenocarcinoids are also indications to proceed with a right hemicolectomy.[23]

Pathology

Important pathologic tumor characteristics include size, histologic subtype, mesoappendiceal involvement, and lymph node status. Carcinoids can also be graded as benign, borderline malignant, low-grade malignant, or high-grade malignant, although a more precise and uniform classification system may identify patients who would benefit from more aggressive surgery.[58] Van Eeden et al.[58] attempted to address this issue by requesting that the World Health Organization apply the current classification of lung neuroendocrine tumors to all neuroendocrine tumors of the GI tract as well.

COLORECTAL ADENOCARCINOMA

Adenocarcinoma of the colon and rectum is the most common cancer of the GI tract, with an annual incidence in the United States of approximately 148,300 cases and 56,600 deaths. The lifetime risk of colorectal cancer in the general population is 5% to 6%.[30] Colorectal cancer is the second most common cancer of the alimentary tract in children, following liver tumors. Colorectal cancer is rare in children, however, with an incidence between 1.3 and 2 cases per million lives.[41,56] Although cancer of the colon has been diagnosed in a child as young as 9 months old, most pediatric cases occur in the second decade of life; the median age at

TABLE 31-3 Predisposing Factors for Colorectal Cancer in Children

Familial polyposis syndromes
Inflammatory bowel disease, especially ulcerative colitis
Hereditary nonpolyposis syndromes
Previous ureterosigmoidostomy
Chronic parasitic infection
Previous radiation therapy
Diet high in fat and low in fiber
Possible exposure to environmental chemicals and radiation

diagnosis is 15 to 19 years.[35,45,53] The development of carcinoma of the colon appears to be associated with several predisposing factors (Table 31-3). These include a diet high in fat and cholesterol and low in fiber, exposure to environmental chemicals and radiation, polyposis syndromes, inflammatory bowel disease, hereditary nonpolyposis syndromes, urinary diversion with a previous ureterosigmoidostomy, chronic parasitic infection, and previous radiation therapy.

The cause of the tumor can be categorized as sporadic in approximately 75% of patients, familial in approximately 10% to 20% of patients who have at least two first-degree relatives with colon cancer (but no defined genetic pattern), genetic (polyposis syndromes) in approximately 1% of patients, inflammatory bowel disease in approximately 1%, and hereditary nonpolyposis syndromes in approximately 5% to 6%.

Although diet has a putative role in the development of colon cancer in adults, no similar studies have been done to support this role in children. Various environmental factors are associated with tumor formation. In one study, exposure to herbicides was found in 10 of 13 children who developed colon cancer.[44]

Colorectal cancer differs greatly between adults and children. These differences include the presenting signs and symptoms, primary site of the tumor, pathologic findings, stage, and prognosis.

Association with Other Conditions

Because the sporadic form of pediatric colorectal carcinoma accounts for approximately 75% of cases, this suggests that 25% of childhood cases have some associated predisposing condition. Sporadic colon cancer in young patients appears to be an aggressive disease whose morphology and natural history differ from those of familial adenomatous polyposis, hereditary nonpolyposis colorectal cancer, and adult colon cancer. Tumor development most likely occurs secondary to tumor suppressor gene involvement, loss of heterozygosity, or a mutational event.[11]

Several genetic disorders carry a significant risk for the subsequent development of colon carcinoma and are characterized as polyposis syndromes. They include Gardner's syndrome (adenomatous polyps and soft tissue and bone tumors), Turcot's syndrome (familial adenomatous polyps and central nervous system tumors), and familial polyposis coli. Both Gardner's syndrome and familial polyposis are autosomal dominant disorders and are associated with adenomatous polyps in both the colon and the small intestine.

Bassey[3] has shown that the incidence of colon carcinoma in patients with familial polyposis is 50% by 28 years of age and that the eventual likelihood of colon cancer approaches 100%. Patients who have an APC mutation or who have one or more first-degree relatives with familial adenomatous polyposis are at high risk, and screening with flexible sigmoidoscopy should begin by age 10 to 12 years. Patients with colonic polyps, a verified APC germline mutation, or both require annual endoscopic examination. As patients reach their teens and 20s, the increased number of polyps may prevent adequate and safe colonoscopic polypectomy. When this occurs, prophylactic surgery should be performed to remove the affected colon. Surgical options include subtotal colectomy with end ileostomy or ileorectal anastomosis followed by annual endoscopy of the remaining rectum. Currently, many patients are candidates for total abdominal proctocolectomy with a restorative small bowel pouch anal anastomosis.

Peutz-Jeghers syndrome is associated with the appearance of hamartomatous polyps. The incidence of colon carcinoma in patients with Peutz-Jeghers syndrome is 2% to 3%. Likewise, juvenile polyposis seems to have an increased potential for the development of colon carcinoma.[9,24,54]

Recommendations for colon resection are based on the likelihood of the development of malignancy. The entire surface of the colon can be carpeted with thousands of polyps in these patients. Realistically, the ability to carry out surveillance and identify suspicious lesions is low. There is little question that colectomy is the appropriate treatment for patients with familial polyposis, Gardner's syndrome, and Turcot's syndrome. Because of the relatively low incidence of malignancy with Peutz-Jeghers syndrome and juvenile polyposis, surveillance is a reasonable strategy.

There is a clear-cut and progressively increasing likelihood of the development of colon carcinoma in patients with ulcerative colitis. This risk is approximately 20 times greater than that in the general population and is related to the total length of time a patient has ulcerative colitis.[24] After the first 10 years with ulcerative colitis, the likelihood of cancer development increases from 1% to 2% per year.[15] Several important features noted in patients with ulcerative colitis who develop colon carcinoma include occurrence at a young age, prevalence of multiple sites of malignancy, and a higher likelihood of malignancy in patients with colitis involving the entire colon than in those with only left-sided colitis.[25]

Crohn's disease is another type of inflammatory bowel disease in which the risk for colon cancer is up to 20 times greater than that in the general population.[61] The likelihood of malignancy is related in part to the amount of bowel involved. However, cancer can develop in areas of colon that appear grossly normal,[36] which in some ways makes the diagnosis of a malignancy in a patient with Crohn's disease more difficult than in a patient with ulcerative colitis. Therefore, regular surveillance protocols and random biopsies are especially important. In patients with inflammatory bowel disease, a contrast enema and colonoscopy are the mainstays of surveillance. Biopsies should be performed on any suspicious areas and randomly during the colonoscopy.

Hereditary nonpolyposis colorectal cancer, or Lynch syndrome, has an autosomal dominant inheritance and is the most common form of hereditary colorectal cancer.[8,37] It accounts for approximately 1% to 3% of all cases of colorectal cancer and is five times more prevalent than familial polyposis-related colon cancer.[8,22] This type of colorectal cancer usually presents with proximal colon lesions (approximately 70% are proximal to the splenic flexure), and patients develop cancer at a younger age (mean, approximately 45 years) than patients with colorectal cancer in general.[22,37] Hereditary nonpolyposis colorectal cancer is also notable for the development of synchronous and metachronous extracolonic cancers, such as carcinoma of the endometrium, ovary, stomach, small bowel, pancreas, hepatobiliary tract, brain, and upper uroepithelial tract.[37]

Ureterosigmoidostomy performed for urinary diversion in patients with bladder exstrophy and other genitourinary anomalies is associated with colon cancer. Eraklis and Folkman[21] reported that 5% of patients with a ureterosigmoidostomy developed colon cancer, in each case at the site of the ureteral implant. Experimental data have implicated chronic inflammation caused by the mixture of feces and urine at the implant site as a cause of the cancer, especially when the urine has been infected. Patients with this type of urinary diversion warrant close follow-up and should undergo annual sigmoidoscopy.

Children with a primary cancer treated with radiation are at risk for the subsequent development of colorectal carcinoma in the radiation field. LaQuaglia et al.[35] described one patient who had resection of a Wilms' tumor, received radiation to the retroperitoneal area, and subsequently developed cancer of the left colon. Others have reported two cases of colorectal cancer as a second malignancy following treatment of a retroperitoneal rhabdomyosarcoma and a Wilms' tumor, both treated with resection and radiation therapy.[14] The first child was a 1-year-old boy whose retroperitoneal rhabdomyosarcoma was treated with preoperative radiation, surgery, and chemotherapy. At 2 years of age he developed radiation colitis and, subsequently, adenomatous polyps. At age 11 years a rectal adenocarcinoma developed (Fig. 31-2). The second child had a Wilms' tumor treated at 9 months of age with surgery and radiation therapy. He also developed radiation colitis and, subsequently, multifocal adenocarcinoma of the colon 42 years later. Results of immunohistochemical studies were positive for the p53 antigen in both tumors in the latter patient and in the adenomas of the first patient. It is speculated that the radiation caused a p53 mutation, which led to the neoplasia.

Diagnosis

In children with colorectal tumors, common presenting symptoms include abdominal pain in almost all patients;

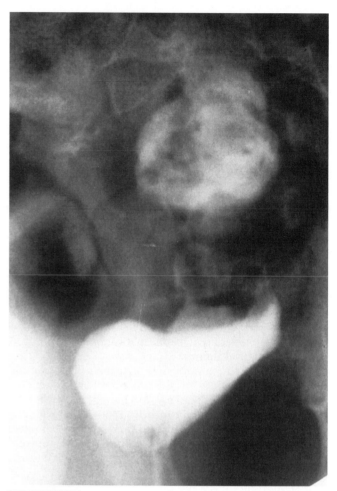

Figure 31–2 Contrast enema in an 11-year-old boy who had previously been treated with radiation for a retroperitoneal rhabdomyosarcoma. The radiograph shows almost complete obstruction in the rectum.

nausea and vomiting in 40% to 70%; and a change in bowel habits and the development of constipation, particularly with left-sided lesions. Physical findings that are often noted in these patients include abdominal distention, tenderness, and a mass. More than half these children have chemical evidence of blood in the stool. A history of rectal bleeding may be elicited in approximately one third of patients and is more prevalent in those with cancer of the left colon and rectum. Significant weight loss affects 20% to 30% of patients.

The median length of time from the onset of symptoms to presentation is often several months; at least one report cited almost a year between the onset of symptoms and the diagnosis.[53] Diagnosis can be delayed if the patient's symptoms are attributed to more common pediatric conditions such as appendicitis, intussusception, or gastroenteritis.[31] Another possible explanation for the delay in diagnosis may be adolescents' tendency to hide symptoms owing to embarrassment.[51] Rectal bleeding, which may also be a sign of benign pathology such as polyps or hemorrhoids, should raise the suspicion for a colorectal malignancy; early diagnosis depends on a high index of suspicion.[32] Steinberg et al.[53] considered a

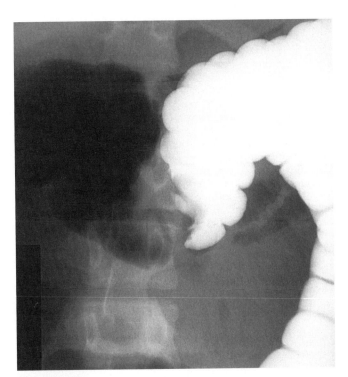

Figure 31–3 Contrast enema in a 14-year-old patient who presented with a 1-month history of abdominal pain and constipation. Complete obstruction in the transverse colon is demonstrated.

delayed diagnosis to have occurred if the patient's symptoms had been present for longer than 3 months; they found that five of nine patients with colon cancer had had symptoms for 3 to 36 months (mean, 11 months) before the diagnosis of cancer. This delay in diagnosis may be an important factor contributing to the advanced stage of disease in many of these children. On the basis of the signs and symptoms at presentation, two scenarios can develop. In the first, the clinical diagnosis is an acute surgical abdomen caused by appendicitis or peritonitis. In this case, the child is often taken directly to the operating room. The second, more common scenario occurs when intestinal obstruction is diagnosed. Radiographic evaluation usually demonstrates a mass lesion in the colon, and a contrast enema identifies the point of obstruction (Fig. 31-3). Depending on the location of the lesion, sigmoidoscopy or colonoscopy allows biopsy and diagnosis. In adults, most lesions are rectosigmoid in location and can be identified by sigmoidoscopy. In contrast, childhood colorectal cancer is relatively evenly distributed throughout the colon; one third of tumors are located in the right colon.[35,45] Colonoscopy is often the technique of choice to obtain a biopsy for diagnosis.

Pathologic Characteristics

Two characteristics of colorectal tumors differ markedly in children and adults: stage and histologic type of adenocarcinoma. Approximately 40% of adults with colon cancer have tumors in which regional lymph nodes are involved or have distant metastases (Dukes' stage C or D lesions).

In children, more than 80% of tumors are Dukes' stage C or D.[35,45,53] In addition, the histologic finding of a mucinous type of adenocarcinoma is found in over half the children with colorectal tumors. The mucinous subtype has an aggressive course and is known to metastasize early.[56] This is at least one order of magnitude greater than the approximate 5% incidence of mucinous adenocarcinoma in adults with colon cancer. There is no obvious reason why this mucinous histologic type is seen so frequently in childhood colon carcinoma. The synergy of the more advanced stage of disease at the time of diagnosis and the increased frequency of a mucinous subtype (which carries a poor prognosis) contributes to the poor prognosis in these patients.

The microsatellite status of the lymph nodes is thought to identify distinct pathways of genetic development in pediatric patients with colorectal cancer. Patients with colorectal cancer and high-frequency microsatellite instability were more likely to have multiple synchronous or metachronous colorectal cancers and were diagnosed at a younger age than those with microsatellite stability.[26] Microsatellite instability is not, however, predictive of a family history of colorectal cancer or of unique phenotypic features.[11]

The utility of carcinoembryonic antigen (CEA) has been well established in adults with colon cancer, but there is little evidence of a similar utility in pediatric patients. Rao et al.[45] identified 4 of 20 patients with Dukes' stage C or D lesions who had normal antigen levels at the time of diagnosis.[45] In a longitudinal evaluation of these children, CEA levels correlated with an increase or decrease in tumor burden in 60% of patients; unfortunately, the other 40% had normal antigen levels despite progressive disease. At this time, CEA levels have not been shown to correlate well with response to treatment in children.

Treatment

The primary treatment for colon cancer in children is surgical resection consisting of a wide excision of the involved colon, the mesentery, and the lymphatic drainage area. Unfortunately, resection for cure is possible in only 40% to 69% of pediatric patients; these percentages are much lower than those in adults with colon cancer.[35,45] The ovaries and the omentum are common sites of metastasis. If resection for cure is performed, omentectomy and, in female patients, oophorectomy are appropriate.

No specific chemotherapy protocols are available for these children. In most studies, some type of chemotherapy was given, and radiation therapy has been used in selected patients. Although anecdotal case reports indicate that one or both of these methods may result in success, no data document the benefit of either chemotherapy or radiation therapy for cure or palliation.

The overall rate and duration of survival among children with colon carcinoma are dismal; studies often show that less than 5% of patients survive 5 years.[2] More recently, LaQuaglia et al.[35] reported survival in 8 of 29 patients (28%) with a median follow-up of 4.7 years.

Survival was directly related to complete resection. In patients who had resection for cure, predictors of survival included node involvement or high histologic grade. The primary aim of treatment in pediatric colon cancer is complete resection during the initial surgery. With the poor survival even in patients who have undergone complete resection, adjuvant chemotherapy is appropriate. The use of chemotherapy, combined with second-look surgery in selected cases, may improve survival.

Summary

The biology of colon carcinoma in children is, in many ways, different from that in adults. The presentation, histologic type, stage, and prognosis differ sharply. Most cases of childhood colorectal cancer derive from previous adenomas. Kindreds with an increased likelihood to form adenomas are thus at increased risk for colorectal carcinoma. This information suggests that genetics may play a greater role than was previously thought and that fewer cases are truly sporadic. Attention focused on the molecular genetics of colon carcinoma in children should lead to a better understanding of this disease. In turn, this will identify patients at high risk and may result in earlier diagnosis and intervention and staging at a lower level, which may enhance survival.

REFERENCES

1. Aichbichler BW, Eherer AJ, Petritsch W, et al: Gastric adenocarcinoma mimicking achalasia in a 15-year-old patient: A case report and review of the literature. J Pediatr Gastroenterol Nutr 2001;32:103-106.
2. Andersson A, Bergdahl L: Carcinoma of the colon in children: A report of six new cases and a review of the literature. J Pediatr Surg 1976;11:967-971.
3. Bassey HJR: Familial Polyposis Coli. Baltimore, Johns Hopkins University Press, 1975.
4. Bethel CA, Bhattacharyya N, Hutchinson C, et al: Alimentary tract malignancies in children. J Pediatr Surg 1997;32:1004-1008.
5. Broaddus RR, Herzog CE, Hicks MJ: Neuroendocrine tumors (carcinoid and neuroendocrine carcinoma) presenting at extra-appendiceal sites in childhood and adolescence. Arch Pathol Lab Med 2003;127:1200-1203.
6. Carney JA: Gastric stromal sarcoma, pulmonary chondroma, and extra-adrenal paraganglioma (Carney triad): Natural history, adrenocortical component, and possible familial occurrence. Mayo Clin Proc 1999;74:543-552.
7. Carney JA, Sheps SG, Go VL, Gordon H: The triad of gastric leiomyosarcoma, functioning extra-adrenal paraganglioma and pulmonary chondroma. N Engl J Med 1977;296:1517-1518.
8. Chung DC, Rustgi AK: The hereditary nonpolyposis colorectal cancer syndrome: Genetics and clinical implications. Ann Intern Med 2003;138:560-570.
9. Coburn MC, Pricolo VE, DeLuca FG, Bland KI: Malignant potential in intestinal juvenile polyposis syndromes. Ann Surg Oncol 1995;2:386-391.
10. Corpron CA, Black CT, Herzog CE, et al: A half century of experience with carcinoid tumors in children. Am J Surg 1995;170:606-608.
11. Datta RV, LaQuaglia MP, Paty PB: Genetic and phenotypic correlates of colorectal cancer in young patients. N Engl J Med 2000;342:137-138.
12. DeMatteo RP, Lewis JJ, Leung D, et al: Two hundred gastrointestinal stromal tumors: Recurrence patterns and prognostic factors for survival. Ann Surg 2000;231:51-58.
13. Demetri GD, von Mehren M, Blanke CD, et al: Efficacy and safety of imatinib mesylate in advanced gastrointestinal stromal tumors. N Engl J Med 2002;347:472-480.
14. Densmore TL, Langer JC, Molleston JP, et al: Colorectal adenocarcinoma as a second malignant neoplasm following Wilms' tumor and rhabdomyosarcoma. Med Pediatr Oncol 1996;27:556-560.
15. Devroede GJ, Taylor WF, Sauer WG, et al: Cancer risk and life expectancy of children with ulcerative colitis. N Engl J Med 1971;285:17-21.
16. Doede T, Foss HD, Waldschmidt J: Carcinoid tumors of the appendix in children: Epidemiology, clinical aspects and procedure. Eur J Pediatr Surg 2000;10:372-377.
17. Dokucu AI, Ozturk H, Kilinc N, et al: Primary gastric adenocarcinoma in a 2.5-year-old girl. Gastric Cancer 2002;5:237-239.
18. Eisenberg BL, Judson I: Surgery and imatinib in the management of GIST: Emerging approaches to adjuvant and neoadjuvant therapy. Ann Surg Oncol 2004;11:465-475.
19. El Serag HB, Bailey NR, Gilger M, Rabeneck L: Endoscopic manifestations of gastroesophageal reflux disease in patients between 18 months and 25 years without neurological deficits. Am J Gastroenterol 2002;97:1635-1639.
20. Eloubeidi MA, Desmond R, Arguedas MR, et al: Prognostic factors for the survival of patients with esophageal carcinoma in the US: The importance of tumor length and lymph node status. Cancer 2002;95:1434-1443.
21. Eraklis AJ, Folkman MJ: Adenocarcinoma at the site of ureterosigmoidostomies for exstrophy of the bladder. J Pediatr Surg 1978;13:730-734.
22. Fitzgibbons RJ Jr, Lynch HT, Stanislav GV, et al: Recognition and treatment of patients with hereditary nonpolyposis colon cancer (Lynch syndromes I and II). Ann Surg 1987;206:289-295.
23. Goede AC, Caplin ME, Winslet MC: Carcinoid tumour of the appendix. Br J Surg 2003;90:1317-1322.
24. Greenstein AJ, Sachar DB, Smith H, et al: Cancer in universal and left-sided ulcerative colitis: Factors determining risk. Gastroenterology 1979;77:290-294.
25. Greenstein AJ, Slater G, Heimann TM, et al: A comparison of multiple synchronous colorectal cancer in ulcerative colitis, familial polyposis coli, and de novo cancer. Ann Surg 1986;203:123-128.
26. Gryfe R, Kim H, Hsieh ETK, et al: Tumor microsatellite instability and clinical outcome in young patients with colorectal cancer. N Engl J Med 2000;342:69-77.
27. Haider N, Kader M, McDermott M, et al: Gastric stromal tumors in children. Pediatr Blood Cancer 2004;42:186-189.
28. Hassall E: Co-morbidities in childhood Barrett's esophagus. J Pediatr Gastroenterol Nutr 1997;25:255-260.
29. Hassall E, Dimmick JE, Magee JF: Adenocarcinoma in childhood Barrett's esophagus: Case documentation and the need for surveillance in children. Am J Gastroenterol 1993;88:282-288.
30. Jemal A, Thomas A, Murray T, Thun M: Cancer statistics, 2002. CA Cancer J Clin 2002;52:23-47.
31. Karnak I, Ciftci AO, Senocak ME, Buyukpamukcu N: Colorectal carcinoma in children. J Pediatr Surg 1999;34:1499-1504.
32. Karnak I, Kale G, Tanyel FC, Buyukpamukcu N: Malignant stromal tumor of the colon in an infant: Diagnostic difficulties and differential diagnosis. J Pediatr Surg 2003;38:245-247.

33. Kerr JZ, Hicks MJ, Nuchtern JG, et al: Gastrointestinal autonomic nerve tumors in the pediatric population: A report of four cases and a review of the literature. Cancer 1999;85:220-230.

34. Kindblom LG, Remotti HE, Aldenborg F, Meis-Kindblom JM: Gastrointestinal pacemaker cell tumor (GIPACT): Gastrointestinal stromal tumors show phenotypic characteristics of the interstitial cells of Cajal. Am J Pathol 1998; 152:1259-1269.

35. LaQuaglia MP, Heller G, Filippa DA, et al: Prognostic factors and outcome in patients 21 years and under with colorectal carcinoma. J Pediatr Surg 1992;27:1085-1089.

36. Leichtner AM: Intestinal neoplasms. In Walker WA, et al (eds): Pediatric Gastrointestinal Disease. Philadelphia, BC Decker, 1991.

37. Lynch HT, de la Chapelle A: Hereditary colorectal cancer. N Engl J Med 2003;348:919-932.

38. McGill TW, Downey EC, Westbrook J, et al: Gastric carcinoma in children. J Pediatr Surg 1993;28:1620-1621.

39. Miettinen M, Lasota J: Gastrointestinal stromal tumors—definition, clinical, histological, immunohistochemical, and molecular genetic features and differential diagnosis. Virchows Arch 2001;438:1-12.

40. Moertel CL, Weiland LH, Telander RL: Carcinoid tumor of the appendix in the first two decades of life. J Pediatr Surg 1990;25:1073-1075.

41. Odone V, Chang L, Caces J, et al: The natural history of colorectal carcinoma in adolescents. Cancer 1982;49:1716-1720.

42. Parkes SE, Muir KR, al Sheyyab M, et al: Carcinoid tumours of the appendix in children 1957-1986: Incidence, treatment and outcome. Br J Surg 1993;80:502-504.

43. Pidhorecky I, Cheney RT, Kraybill WG, Gibbs JF: Gastrointestinal stromal tumors: Current diagnosis, biologic behavior, and management. Ann Surg Oncol 2000; 7:705-712.

44. Pratt CB, Rivera G, Shanks E, et al: Colorectal carcinoma in adolescents: Implications regarding etiology. Cancer 1977;40(5 Suppl):2464-2472.

45. Rao BN, Pratt CB, Fleming ID, et al: Colon carcinoma in children and adolescents: A review of 30 cases. Cancer 1985;55:1322-1326.

46. Roberts PJ, Eisenberg B: Clinical presentation of gastrointestinal stromal tumors and treatment of operable disease. Eur J Cancer 2002;38(Suppl 5):S37-S38.

47. Schettini ST, Ganc A, Saba L: Esophageal carcinoma secondary to a chemical injury in a child. Pediatr Surg Int 1998;13:519-520.

48. Shamberger RC, Eraklis AJ, Kozakewich HP, Hendren WH: Fate of the distal esophageal remnant following esophageal replacement. J Pediatr Surg 1988;23:1210-1214.

49. Shiu MH, Farr GH, Papachristou DN, Hajdu SI: Myosarcomas of the stomach: Natural history, prognostic factors and management. Cancer 1982;49:177-187.

50. Skinner MA, Plumley DA, Grosfeld JL, et al: Gastrointestinal tumors in children: An analysis of 39 cases. Ann Surg Oncol 1994;1:283-289.

51. Soper RT: Gastrointestinal neoplasms. In: Ashcraft KW, Holder TM (eds): Pediatric Surgery. Philadelphia, W.B. Saunders, 1993, pp 464-469.

52. Spunt SL, Pratt CB, Rao BN, et al: Childhood carcinoid tumors: The St Jude Children's Research Hospital experience. J Pediatr Surg 2000;35:1282-1286.

53. Steinberg JB, Tuggle DW, Postier RG: Adenocarcinoma of the colon in adolescents. Am J Surg 1988;156:460-462.

54. Stemper TJ, Kent TH, Summers RW: Juvenile polyposis and gastrointestinal carcinoma: A study of a kindred. Ann Intern Med 1975;83:639-646.

55. Surveillance, Epidemiology, and End Results (SEER) Program. SEER 1975-2001. SEER Stat Database. Bethesda, Md, National Cancer Institute, DCCPS, Surveillance Research Program, Cancer Statistics Branch, 2004.

56. Symonds DA, Vickery AL: Mucinous carcinoma of the colon and rectum. Cancer 1976;37:1891-1900.

57. Trupiano JK, Stewart RE, Misick C, et al: Gastric stromal tumors: A clinicopathologic study of 77 cases with correlation of features with nonaggressive and aggressive clinical behaviors. Am J Surg Pathol 2002;26:705-714.

58. Van Eeden S, Quaedvlieg PF, Taal BG, et al: Classification of low-grade neuroendocrine tumors of midgut and unknown origin. Hum Pathol 2002;33:1126-1132.

59. Van Gompel JJ, Sippel RS, Warner TF, Chen H: Gastrointestinal carcinoid tumors: Factors that predict outcome. World J Surg 2004;28:387-392.

60. Volpe A, Willert J, Ihnken K, et al: Metastatic appendiceal carcinoid tumor in a child. Med Pediatr Oncol 2000; 34:218-220.

61. Weedon DD, Shorter RG, Ilstrup DM, et al: Crohn's disease and cancer. N Engl J Med 1973;289:1099-1103.

Chapter 32

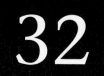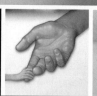

Rhabdomyosarcoma

Richard J. Andrassy

Rhabdomyosarcoma (from the Greek *rhabdos*, meaning "rod"; *mys*, "muscle"; and *sarkos*, "flesh") is a primary malignancy in children and adolescents that arises from embryonic mesenchyma with the potential to differentiate into skeletal muscle. Rhabdomyosarcoma (RMS) accounts for more than 50% of all soft tissue sarcomas in children and is thus the most common soft tissue sarcoma. Sarcomas in adults arise mostly in the extremities, whereas RMS in children can occur anywhere there is skeletal muscle, as well as in sites with no skeletal muscle (e.g., urinary bladder, bile ducts). RMS can arise at any site and in any tissue except bone. The most common sites are the head and neck region and the genitourinary tract, with only 20% occurring in the extremities.

The original distinction of soft tissue sarcomas and bone sarcomas from epithelial and hematopoietic tumors is attributed to Virchow, who in the mid-1850s propounded a theory of "cellular pathology" that ascribed the origin of tumors to specific types of cells.[99] The first case of RMS was described by Webner in 1854 in a 21-year-old patient with a tongue tumor.[97] In 1946 Stout[106] reported a series of adults with a malignant condition of the trunk and limbs. In 1954 Pack et al.[79] described a group of children with RMS of the skeletal muscle. In 1958 Horn et al.[50] proposed a classification of this tumor into four subgroups: embryonal, alveolar, botryoid, and pleomorphic. During those early years, surgery was the only therapy available, and radical excision was the standard. Survival rates were poor except in selected sites where total excision was possible by means of radical surgery, such as amputation or pelvic exenteration. Survival rates of 7% to 70% were seen, depending on site.[78]

In 1950 Stobbe et al.[105] demonstrated improved outcomes in head and neck sites when radiation therapy was added after incomplete resection of RMS. In 1961 Pinkel et al.[83] advocated adjuvant chemotherapy after complete surgical excision and postoperative radiation therapy, which was the beginning of the multimodal approach to solid tumors.

Recognizing the value of this multimodal approach, as well as the relative rarity of these tumors, the leadership of three cooperative pediatric cancer research groups in the United States (the Children's Cancer Study Group and the pediatric sections of the Cancer and Leukemia Group B and the Southwest Oncology Group), in concert with the National Cancer Institute, formed the Intergroup Rhabdomyosarcoma Study (IRS) Group in 1972 to investigate the therapy and biology of RMS and undifferentiated sarcoma in previously untreated patients younger than 21 years old. Since then, five successive clinical protocols involving almost 5000 patients have been completed: IRS-I (1972 to 1978), IRS-II (1978 to 1984), IRS-III (1984 to 1991), IRS-IV Pilot (for patients with advanced disease only; 1987 to 1991), and IRS-IV (1991 to 1997).[1,2,6-8,11,18] Based on lessons learned from these studies, IRS-V was opened in 1997 for patients with low-risk disease (i.e., with a good prognosis for survival) and expanded in 1999 to other patients.

Although the trend has been toward far less mutilating surgery, the surgeon plays an important role in initial biopsy and staging, primary re-excision, appropriate wide local resection, and second-look operations. The surgeon should be an early participant in the multimodal approach to treatment.

EPIDEMIOLOGY

RMS is the third most common solid tumor in infants and children, after neuroblastoma and Wilms' tumor. There are approximately 250 to 300 new cases per year in the United States. There is a slightly greater incidence in males compared with females (3:2) and in Caucasians compared with non-Caucasians (12:5). The peak age at presentation is bimodal, with the primary peak occurring between 2 and 5 years of age and the secondary peak between 15 and 19 years.

Patients with RMS appear to have a higher incidence of other congenital anomalies.[98] Both RMS and Wilms' tumor are associated with an increased incidence of genitourinary anomalies. RMS is also linked to anomalies of the central nervous system.[98] Patients with von Recklinghausen's neurofibromatosis have an increased risk of RMS.[42,101]

The Li-Fraumeni familial cancer syndrome, first reported in 1969, includes soft tissue sarcomas occurring in siblings and cousins; parents and other relatives have a variety of malignancies, including RMS, adrenocortical carcinoma, glioblastoma, breast cancer, and lung cancer.[61,62] This syndrome is an autosomal dominant disorder and is frequently associated with a germline mutation of p53.[66] Breast cancer in mothers is the major associated malignancy in families of children with soft tissue malignancy.[107] A review of the mothers of 13 children with RMS showed that their risk of breast cancer was 3 to 13.5 times greater than that of controls.[13]

Other somewhat weaker associations with fetal alcohol syndrome, maternal exposure to marijuana or cocaine, x-ray exposure, and employment as a health care worker have been suggested.[39,40,95]

RMS has also been observed in association with Beckwith-Wiedemann syndrome, a fetal overgrowth syndrome associated with abnormalities on chromosome 11p15, where the gene for insulin-like growth factor II (IGF-II) is located.[28]

The two histologic subtypes of RMS—embryonal and alveolar—have distinct genetic alterations that may play a role in the pathogenesis of these tumors. In alveolar RMS, there is a characteristic translocation between the long arm of chromosome 2 and the long arm of chromosome 13, referred to as t(2;13) (q35;q14). This translocation fuses the *PAX3* gene (believed to regulate transcription during early neuromuscular development) with the *FKHR* gene (a member of the forkhead family of transcription factors). It is believed that this fusion transcription factor may inappropriately activate the transcription of genes that contribute to a transformed phenotype. The variant t(1;13) (p36;q14) fuses the *PAX7* gene located on chromosome 1 with *FKHR*. Patients with tumors expressing the *PAX-FKHR* fusion tend to be younger and are more likely to present with an extremity lesion, suggesting a distinct clinical phenotype. Polymerase chain reaction assays are now available that allow confirmation of the diagnosis of alveolar RMS based on the presence of these fusion genes.[28,63,72,110]

Embryonal RMS is known to involve loss of heterozygosity at the 11p15 locus, with loss of maternal genetic information and duplication of paternal genetic information. This is the location of the *IGF-II* gene. IGF-II has been demonstrated to stimulate the growth of RMS cells, whereas the blockade of this factor using monoclonal antibodies inhibits tumor growth both in vitro and in vivo.[113] Several other solid neoplasms are associated with genomic deletions on the short arm of chromosome 11, including Wilms' tumor, hepatoblastoma, and neuroblastoma.

The MyoD family of genes codes for DNA binding proteins that regulate the transcription of DNA sequences encoding myogenic proteins such as desmin, creatine kinase, and myosin.[59,112] In RMS, the down-regulation of this gene does not occur, so that MyoD1 expression remains at high levels in tumor cells.[108] The biologic significance of this overexpression is not clear; however, the detection of high levels of the MyoD1 gene product may be used to diagnose RMS.[102]

The change in a cell's DNA content has been described in a variety of tumors and may have some prognostic significance. The DNA content of embryonal RMS tumors ranges between diploid and hyperdiploid (1.1 to 1.8 times the normal amount of DNA). It has been reported that diploid embryonal RMS tumors may have a worse prognosis than hyperdiploid tumors. Near tetraploidy was associated with alveolar histology.[28,53]

RAS oncogene mutations have been described in RMS cell lines and tumor specimens. It is not known whether these alterations are involved in RMS tumor pathogenesis or reflect secondary abnormalities that occur during tumor progression.[28]

Aberrant expression of the *MET* oncogene in embryonal and alveolar RMS tumor samples and established cell lines has been described. MET encodes the receptor for HGF/scatter factor, which is known to control cell motility and invasion in epithelial cells. It is hypothesized that the overexpression of MET may provide RMS cells with the same property as embryonal myoblasts, allowing them to migrate into surrounding connective tissues.[31]

PATHOLOGY

RMS cells arise from undifferentiated mesodermal tissue and fall into the broader category of the small, round, blue cell tumors of childhood. The differentiation of specific tumor type is accomplished by a combination of light microscopy, immunohistochemical techniques, electron microscopy, and molecular genetic techniques. The characteristic feature that permits a tumor to be classified as RMS is the identification of a myogenic lineage. Typically, this consists of the light microscopic identification of cross-striations that are characteristic of skeletal muscle or rhabdomyoblasts.[4,113] Skeletal muscle or muscle-specific proteins can be identified by immunohistochemical staining.

Histologically, RMS is classified as a small, round, blue cell tumor of childhood, a category that also includes neuroblastoma, Ewing's sarcoma, small cell osteogenic sarcoma, non-Hodgkin's lymphoma, and leukemia. Each of the two major subtypes of RMS has a characteristic histologic appearance. Embryonal RMS is the most common histologic subtype, constituting more than 30% of all newly diagnosed tumors. This embryonal subtype, particularly the botryoid and spindle cell variants, was thought to have a much better prognosis, but there is now controversy whether the histologic subtype or the site of the tumor is the strongest indicator of prognosis.

Botryoid RMS, described as a "cluster of grapes," is seen in cavitary structures and has a good prognosis. The spindle cell variants arise disproportionately in the paratesticular region but may also be seen in the head and neck, especially the orbit, and the extremities.[19,60] These subtypes are almost always associated with limited disease, behave less aggressively than the classic embryonal tumors, and have an extremely good prognosis; however, both types account for only 5% to 6% of all RMS.[60]

The pathologic description of RMS as a tumor of myogenic lineage was first advanced in 1958 by Horn et al.[50] These investigators proposed the first classification scheme that divided RMS into four different pathologic types (embryonal, botryoid, alveolar, and pleomorphic). This system has been used for decades and was modified into a "universal" system by an international group of pediatric pathologists in 1994. This system ascribes prognostic significance to each histologic subtype by classifying

TABLE 32-1 Histologic Variants of Childhood Rhabdomyosarcoma: International Rhabdomyosarcoma Pathologic Classification

I. Favorable prognosis
   a. Botryoid
   b. Spindle cell
II. Intermediate prognosis
   a. Embryonal
   b. Pleomorphic (rare)
III. Poor prognosis
   a. Alveolar (including solid variant)
   b. Undifferentiated

From Asmar L, et al: Agreement among and within groups of pathologists in the classification of rhabdomyosarcoma and related childhood sarcomas: Report of an international study of four pathology classifications. Cancer 1994;74:2579.

them into groups with favorable, intermediate, and poor prognoses (Table 32-1).[11]

The alveolar variant accounts for approximately 20% of tumors and frequently arises in the extremities, trunk, or perineum; these tumors have an unfavorable prognosis.[11] The alveolar variant is characterized by a prominent alveolar arrangement of stroma and dense, small, round tumor cells resembling those of lung tissue. A subtype is the "solid" alveolar RMS, characterized by an architecture of dense cellular sheets lacking any intercellular stroma but with cytologic features identical to those found in the classic alveolar tumors. Undifferentiated sarcoma is a poorly defined category of sarcomatous tumor whose cells show no evidence of myogenesis or other differentiation.[75,76] The distribution of histologic subtypes is shown in Table 32-2.

A number of monoclonal antibodies have been shown to react with elements of RMS and have been useful in its diagnosis. These include antibodies to desmin, muscle-specific actin, sarcomeric actin, and myoglobin. All have been used to confirm the myogenic lineage of cells and, when used in combination, have very good specificity and sensitivity.[121] MyoD1 was mentioned earlier; other nonmyogenic protein products that can be identified in these tumors include cytokeratin, neuron-specific enolase, S-100 protein, and Leu-7.

TABLE 32-2 Histologic Distribution of Patients with Rhabdomyosarcoma in Intergroup Rhabdomyosarcoma Study-III

Histologic Type	Percentage
Embryonal	53
Alveolar	19
Undetermined	18
Undifferentiated	7
Botryoid	5
Extraosseous Ewing's	3

From Newton WA, et al: Pathology of rhabdomyosarcoma and related tumors. In Maurer HM, Ruymann FB, Pochedly C (eds): Rhabdomyosarcoma and Related Tumors in Children and Adolescents. Boca Raton, Fla, CRC Press, 1991.

CLINICAL PRESENTATION

The clinical presentation of RMS depends on the site of origin of the primary tumor, the age of the patient, and the presence or absence of metastatic disease. The majority of symptoms are related to compression of local structures; occasionally, there is mild pain. There are no classic paraneoplastic syndromes associated with RMS.

The head and neck region is the most common site of presentation and accounts for about 35% of patients in the IRS studies.[25] The head and neck sites are divided into the orbits (10%), parameningeal tissues (middle ear, nasal cavity and paranasal sinuses, nasopharynx, and infratemporal fossa; 15%), and nonparameningeal tissues (scalp, face, oral cavity, oropharynx, hypopharynx, and neck; 10%). These tumors are most commonly of the embryonal subtype and rarely spread to regional lymph nodes.[56,85,89] Orbital tumors produce proptosis and, occasionally, ophthalmoplegia. Those arising from parameningeal sites often produce nasal, aural, or sinus obstruction, with or without a mucopurulent or sanguineous discharge. Head and neck RMS arising from sites other than the orbit or parameningeal sites often presents as a painless, enlarging mass that tends to remain localized.[114] Parameningeal tumors may extend into the cranium, with resultant cranial nerve palsy and meningeal symptoms.

Genitourinary RMS accounted for 26% of all primary tumors in IRS-III.[25] These tumors are considered as two distinct entities: bladder-prostate tumors (10%) and nonbladder-prostate tumors (16%). The latter occur in paratesticular sites, perineum, vulva, vagina, and uterus. Paratesticular RMS may present as a painless swelling in the scrotum or inguinal canal and may initially be thought to be a hernia, hydrocele, or varicocele. Bladder tumors produce hematuria and urinary obstruction. Prostate tumors can produce large pelvic masses resulting in urinary frequency or constipation if significant compression of the bladder or intestinal tract occurs. RMS can also arise in the male or female genital tracts. Vaginal tumors tend to occur in very young children and present with a mass or vaginal bleeding and discharge. Uterine tumors generally present in older girls and are quite extensive by the time of diagnosis. Paratesticular RMS has a high predilection for lymph node spread to the retroperitoneum, especially in boys older than 10 years.[121] Vaginal tumors rarely spread to regional lymph nodes.

Extremity RMS occurs in approximately 20% of patients.[7,74] These tumors present with a mass and have a high incidence of regional lymph node spread (50%).[7,74] The majority of these tumors are of the alveolar subtype and, because of site and possibly histology, are more aggressive.

Approximately 15% of children with RMS present with metastatic disease, and their prognosis has not improved significantly over the last 15 years, despite changes in therapy.[25,96] Isolated lung metastases appear to be rare and should be biopsied to prove disease.

Neonatal presentation of RMS is extremely rare, with only 14 cases (0.4% of patients in IRS-I through -IV) being reported.[64] They tend to be embryonal-botryoid or undifferentiated in histology.

DIAGNOSIS

The diagnosis of RMS is usually made by direct open biopsy. There are no helpful markers or specific imaging studies. The pathologist is expected to identify the histologic subgroups of RMS to allow adequate staging and to direct therapy. For this purpose, several grams of tissue are needed. Biopsies of genitourinary RMS are frequently performed using the endoscope. Needle biopsies that are performed to establish the diagnosis of prostatic RMS are difficult to interpret and must include several cores. Trunk and extremity RMS should have excisional or incisional biopsy, with the incision placed so that it will not interfere with the incision required for subsequent wide local excision. This usually means an axial incision in extremities. Wide local excision with clear margins is the ultimate goal. Regional lymph nodes are evaluated, depending on the location of the primary tumor. Trunk and extremity lesions have a high incidence of lymph node involvement, and sentinel lymph node mapping is advised.[73,74]

Patients with RMS require a complete workup before definitive surgery. The preoperative evaluation includes imaging, blood work, and bone marrow evaluation. The complete preoperative or pretreatment evaluation is outlined in Table 32-3.

The most important part of the diagnostic process is obtaining adequate tissue for histologic and cytologic diagnosis and classification. This procedure is generally accomplished by open incisional biopsy under general anesthesia.

Staging and Clinical Grouping

Pretreatment staging for RMS is performed to stratify the extent of the disease for the purpose of determining the appropriate treatment regimen as well as to compare outcome. This classification is a modification of the TNM staging system and is based on primary tumor site, primary tumor size, clinical regional node status, and distant metastatic spread (Table 32-4).[58,74]

Pretreatment size is determined by external measurement or by magnetic resonance imaging or computed tomography (CT), depending on the anatomic location. The staging is "clinical" and should be done by the responsible surgeon based on preoperative imaging and physical findings. Intraoperative or pathologic results do not affect the stage but do affect the clinical group.

The IRS clinical grouping system is based on the pretreatment and operative outcome (Table 32-5). Its basic premise is that total tumor extirpation at the original site is the best hope for cure, and it stratifies patients

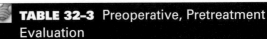

TABLE 32-3 Preoperative, Pretreatment Evaluation

History and physical examination (height, weight)
Measurement of lesion (physical or imaging)
Complete blood count, differential, platelets
Urinalysis
Electrolytes, creatinine, calcium, phosphorus
Alkaline phosphatase, lactate dehydrogenase, bilirubin, serum glutamic-pyruvic transaminase
Bone marrow biopsy or aspirate
Chest radiograph
Magnetic resonance imaging (MRI) or computed tomography (CT) of primary tumor
CT of chest
MRI or CT of head (for head tumors)
Bone scan
Cerebrospinal fluid cytology (for parameningeal tumors)
Electrocardiogram or echocardiogram (selective)

TABLE 32-4 Pretreatment Staging Classification

Stage	Sites	Tumor	Size	Nodes	Metastasis
I	Orbit	T_1 or T_2	a or b	N_0 or N_x	M_0
	Head and neck (excluding parameningeal)				
	Bladder-nonprostate				
II	Bladder-prostate	T_1 or T_2	a	N_0 or N_x	M_0
	Extremity				
	Cranial parameningeal				
	Other (includes truncal, retroperitoneal, perineal, biliary, intrathoracic)				
III	Bladder-prostate	T_1 or T_2	a	N_1	
	Extremity		b	N_0, N_1, N_x	M_0
	Cranial parameningeal				
	Other (as in stage II)				
IV	All	T_1 or T_2	a or b	N_0, N_1, N_x	M_1

Tumor: T_1, confined to anatomic site of origin: (a) 5 cm diameter in size, (b) >5 cm diameter in size; T_2, extension and/or fixation to surrounding tissue: (a) 5 cm diameter in size, (b) > 5 cm diameter in size.
Regional nodes: N_0, regional nodes not clinically involved; N_1, regional nodes clinically involved by neoplasm; N_x, clinical status of regional nodes unknown (especially sites that preclude lymph node evaluation).
Metastasis: M_0, no distant metastasis; M_1, metastasis present.

TABLE 32–5 Intergroup Rhabdomyosarcoma Study Clinical Grouping System

Group I: Localized disease, completely resected.
   (Regional nodes not involved—lymph node biopsy or sampling is highly advised [9602] or required [9803, 9802], except for head and neck lesions.)
   (a) Confined to muscle or organ of origin.
   (b) Contiguous involvement—infiltration outside the muscle or organ of origin, such as through fascial planes.
   Note: This includes both gross inspection and microscopic confirmation of complete resection. Any nodes that may be inadvertently taken with the specimen must be negative. If the latter are involved microscopically, the patient is placed in group IIb or IIc.
Group II: Total gross resection with evidence of regional spread.
   (a) Grossly resected tumor with microscopic residual disease (surgeon believes that all the tumor has been removed, but the pathologist finds tumor at the margin, and additional resection to achieve a clean margin is not feasible [9602] or reasonable [9803, 9802]). No evidence of gross residual tumor. No evidence of regional node involvement. Once radiotherapy and chemotherapy have been started, re-exploration and removal of the area of microscopic residual do not change the patient's group.
   (b) Regional disease with involved nodes, completely resected with microscopic residual.
   Note: Complete resection with microscopic confirmation of no residual disease makes this different from groups IIa and IIc. Additionally, in contrast to group IIa, regional nodes (which are completely resected) are involved, but the most distal node is histologically negative.
   (c) Regional disease with involved nodes, grossly resected, but with evidence of microscopic residual or histologic involvement of the most distal regional node (from the primary site) in the dissection.
   Note [9602 only]: The presence of microscopic residual disease makes this group different from group IIb, and nodal involvement makes this group different from group IIa.
Group III: Incomplete resection with gross residual disease.
   (a) After biopsy only.
   (b) After gross or major resection of the primary tumor (>50%).
Group IV: Distant metastatic disease present at onset (lung, liver, bone, bone marrow, brain, distant muscle and nodes).
   Note [9602 only]: The above excludes regional lymph nodes and adjacent organ infiltration, which places the patient in a more favorable grouping (see group II).
   The presence of positive cytology in cerebrospinal fluid or pleural or abdominal fluids or implants on pleural or peritoneal surfaces or in the omentum are regarded as indications for placement in group IV.

Numbers in brackets are the specific study number under the IRS protocols.

according to tumor resectability. This has led, in the past, to aggressive and often mutilating procedures. This system does not take into account the biologic nature or natural history of the tumor, nor does it account for the experience and the aggressiveness of the operating surgeon.

With the more frequent use of biopsy and neoadjuvant chemotherapy, there has been a "shift" from group I or II to group III, with biopsy followed by neoadjuvant therapy. Group assignment is based on intraoperative findings and postoperative pathologic status and includes final pathologic verification of margins, residual tumor, node involvement, and cytologic examination of pleural and peritoneal fluid, when applicable. Both clinical grouping and pretreatment staging have been shown to correlate with outcome.[4,27,74]

Based on the findings from IRS-I through -IV, risk groups have been established for treatment in IRS-V, which combines group, stage, and histology subtype to allocate patients to three different therapeutic protocols according to risk of recurrence (Table 32-6). Low-risk patients have an estimated 3-year failure-free survival (FFS) rate of 88%; intermediate-risk patients have an estimated 3-year FFS rate of 55% to 76%, and high-risk patients have a 3-year FFS rate of less than 30%. Multidisciplinary treatment is recommended, as defined by histologic subtype, primary site, extent of disease at diagnosis, and response to treatment. The goal is to achieve local control with preservation of form and function.[92]

TREATMENT

The approach to the treatment of RMS has been multimodal for more than 30 years. The advances in understanding the biology and treatment of this disease can

TABLE 32–6 Intergroup Rhabdomyosarcoma Study-V Risk Groups

Risk Group	Stage	Clinical Group, Node Status, Site
Low	I	I, II; N_0; all favorable sites (orbit, head and neck, nonparameningeal, genitourinary, nonbladder-prostate)
	I	III; N_0, N_x; orbit only
	II	I; N_0, N_x; all other (unfavorable) sites; tumor =5 cm in widest diameter
Intermediate	I	II; N_1; all favorable sites (see above)
	I	III; N_0, N_x, N_1; all favorable sites except orbit
	II	II, III; N_0, N_x, N_1; all other sites
	III	II, III; N_0, N_x, N_1; all other sites
High	IV	IV; N_0, N_x, N_1; any site with metastatic disease, including tumor cells in cerebrospinal, pleural, or peritoneal fluid or omental implants

N_0, regional nodes not clinically involved; N_1, regional nodes clinically involved by neoplasm; N_x, clinical status of regional nodes unknown (especially sites that preclude lymph node evaluation).

largely be attributed to the IRS (I-V). The surgical treatment for RMS has become progressively less mutilating or surgically aggressive while maintaining the excellent survival statistics of earlier studies.

The surgical treatment of RMS is site specific and is discussed later by individual site. The general principles include complete wide excision of the primary tumor and surrounding uninvolved margins while preserving cosmesis and function.

The initial biopsy is generally incisional except in small lesions, where excisional biopsy is possible. Some lesions have a pseudocapsule that may allow the lesion to be shelled out, giving the surgeon the false notion that he or she has removed the entire lesion. Many sites have gross or microscopic residual tumor, and pretreatment re-excision is warranted if this can be done without mutilation.[43]

Biopsy of any lesion may involve reoperation and wide excision. Longitudinal incisions are frequently better than horizontal incisions on areas such as an extremity. A biopsy to confirm malignancy requires that the biopsy tract be excised at the time of reoperation; if the biopsy site is inappropriately placed, this excision may require much larger incisions or resections than necessary.

Solid tumor biopsies are traditionally divided into excisional biopsies, in which the entire tumor is included in the specimen, and incisional biopsies, in which only a portion of the tumor is included. In an excisional biopsy, margins should be carefully marked to allow re-resection should the biopsy reveal a positive margin on review. Ideally, excisional biopsies are planned to allow resections that will leave behind only negative margins. If such an excisional biopsy would result in too large a resection, incisional biopsy is more appropriate.

If biopsy margins are not carefully marked on both the specimen and the operative field (usually by sutures or clips), the surgeon's ability to subsequently obtain negative margins is severely compromised. For example, an inappropriate approach to biopsy may lead to further difficulties in the case of testicular masses. Any testicular mass should be approached through an inguinal rather than a scrotal incision so that proximal control of the cord can be obtained and a wide local excision performed without seeding the scrotum with tumor. The proximal spermatic cord should be examined for free margins. Higher excision may be necessary if tumor is still present. Biopsy of the tumor through the scrotum may lead to further scrotal resection and increased risk of local recurrence.

Secondary excision after initial biopsy and neoadjuvant therapy has a better outcome than does partial or incomplete excision. There has been a shift of patients into clinical group III, but chemotherapy followed by delayed or second-look surgery allows a better prognosis with less mutilating surgery. Biopsy of regional nodes, or sentinel lymph node mapping, is warranted in selected sites, such as the extremity.

In some patients with extremity or trunk RMS, initial tumor resection is thought to be complete, but histopathologic review reveals microscopic residual disease corresponding to clinical group IIa in the surgical margins. In many of these patients, primary re-excision (PRE) is possible, achieving wider disease-free margins. Hays et al.[43]

demonstrated the benefits of PRE. In IRS-I and IRS-II, 154 patients with extremity or trunk RMS were initially placed in clinical group IIa; then 41 patients underwent successful PRE and were converted to clinical group I before the onset of adjuvant therapy. These patients were compared with 113 patients who had microscopic residual disease and did not undergo PRE and with 73 patients who were free of disease after the initial resection (clinical group I). Among the 41 PRE patients, the 3-year Kaplan-Meier survival estimate was 91%, compared with 74% for group IIa patients not undergoing PRE and 74% for group I patients. This approach may be applicable to tumors in other locations as well. PRE should be considered, even if the margins are apparently normal, if the initial resection was not a "cancer" operation (i.e., malignancy was not suspected at the initial excision).[21,43]

Second-look operations have been used for several pediatric tumors to evaluate therapeutic response and to remove any residual tumor after completing initial therapy. The use of second-look operations was evaluated in IRS-III and shown to be beneficial in clinical group II RMS patients.[115,117-119] The performance of a second-look operation changed the response status in a significant number of patients; 12% of presumed complete-response patients were found to harbor residual tumor, and 74% of both partial- and no-response patients were recategorized as complete responders after operation. The survival rate of these recategorized patients was similar to that of patients confirmed to be complete responders at re-exploration.[117,118]

The general surgical principles learned from IRS-I through -IV and thus considered in IRS-V include the following: (1) Patients with localized, completely resected disease (group I) generally have the best prognosis for 5-year FFS and overall survival. Patients with metastases at diagnosis (group IV) have the worst outlook, and those with group II and III disease have an intermediate prognosis. Thus, it is preferable to try to remove all visible tumor, if doing so is feasible without excessive morbidity. (2) When a lesion has been resected, primary re-resection is indicated if the primary operation was not a cancer operation for malignancy. Any question about margin status warrants re-resection. Group I (totally resected) patients with embryonal RMS are not subjected to postoperative radiation therapy.[123] (3) It is desirable to preserve organ function and thus spare such structures as the eye, vagina, and bladder. Also, patients with tumor at or near these sites have a good prognosis. Primary chemotherapy followed by radiation therapy is the recommended approach. Delayed excision of initially unresected tumor may improve the prognosis by changing a partial response into a complete response after initial shrinkage of the tumor by chemotherapy, with or without radiation therapy.[117] (4) There is a relationship between age at diagnosis and likelihood of regional lymph node involvement in boys with nonmetastatic paratesticular RMS. Event-free survival in IRS-IV was better for boys younger than 10 years because the nodal relapse rate was lower than in those aged 10 years and older. We now recommend performing a modified ipsilateral retroperitoneal lymph node dissection in older boys who have no clinical evidence of regional node involvement. If the nodes are uninvolved, cyclophosphamide and radiation therapy are withheld; if tumor is present in the nodes, cyclophosphamide and radiation therapy are given, in addition to vincristine and actinomycin D.[120,121]

Other considerations for IRS-V include a more aggressive approach to evaluating lymph nodes. In the earlier studies,[56,57] lymph node involvement was thought to be rare at most sites, because the nodes were rarely evaluated. More recent studies suggest that the incidence of involved lymph nodes in patients with primary tumors of the extremity may be higher than initially suspected.[68] Sentinel lymph node mapping, using a vital dye such as Lymphazurin blue along with radiolabeled technetium sulfur colloid, can localize the regional node most likely to contain tumor cells.[73] The surgeon removes the indicated sentinel node, and the pathologist can thoroughly investigate the presence or absence of tumor in that node. The sentinel node reflects the status of the nodal basin. If the node is positive, the nodal basin is irradiated. The utility of sentinel lymph node mapping is being evaluated in IRS-V.

For patients whose tumors are initially deemed unresectable, a second-look procedure should be considered after initial chemotherapy. Imaging studies have not been consistently reliable in determining the actual response to treatment. In IRS-III, 75% of children with group III tumors and evidence of partial or no response on imaging studies either had a pathologically complete response or were converted to such a response by resection of all remaining tumor. Most (but not all) patients who showed a complete response on imaging studies were confirmed as having such a response by secondary surgery. Survival was better in those patients who converted to a complete response. Secondary surgery is less beneficial in children with stage IV disease. Second-look surgery is least useful for tumors in the head and neck but is appropriate for tumors in the trunk and limbs. The trend toward improved survival in patients converted to a complete response by means of second-look operations has been enduring.[117,118]

CHEMOTHERAPY

Before multimodal therapy, surgery alone for RMS resulted in survival rates of less than 20%. Local micrometastatic disease, nodal disease, or unrecognized or untreated distant disease frequently led to early recurrence and subsequent death mainly due to advanced metastatic disease.

The development of adjuvant and later neoadjuvant chemotherapy has led to a marked increase in survival. The IRS Group studies have shown progressively better survival rates with less mutilating surgery and less chemotoxicity.[24,25,69,70,83]

Agents with known activity in the treatment of RMS include vincristine (V), actinomycin D (A), doxorubicin, cyclophosphamide (C), ifosfamide (I), and etoposide (E). Melphalan and cisplatin were evaluated for their potential role in patients with locally extensive or metastatic disease and did not improve outcome compared with other options in the randomized trials involving patients with clinical group III or IV disease.[25,100]

VAC has been the gold standard for combination chemotherapy in the treatment of most cases of RMS. Consecutive large randomized trials have led to modifications of this combination tailored to specific subgroups based on clinical group and site of disease. In patients with clinical group I embryonal tumors, results of IRS-III showed equivalent survival for patients treated with VA only versus VAC.[25] In IRS-IV, patients with clinical group I paratesticular or orbital disease were treated with VA alone for 2 years. In an IRS-V pilot study, VA chemotherapy alone was given to patients with "low-risk" disease, including those with stage I, clinical group I or II (N_0) orbital, head and neck (nonparameningeal), or genitourinary tract (nonbladder-prostate) disease; those with stage II, clinical group I disease; and those with stage I, clinical group III (orbit only N_0) disease.[28,92]

When evidence of the efficacy of etoposide and ifosfamide for RMS was recognized,[71] this was incorporated into a randomized treatment protocol in IRS-IV. Randomization of VAC versus VAI versus VIE was done for nonmetastatic RMS. Data from IRS-IV indicate that the current standard combination of VAC, with cyclophosphamide at 2.2 g/m² per dose with granulocyte colony-stimulating factor, is equally efficacious with regard to FFS and overall survival, as are VAI and VIE.[26]

Therapy for patients with intermediate-risk disease may be improved by the introduction of new agents. Dose intensification using known active chemotherapeutic agents should also be considered. Preliminary IRS-IV results have shown an improvement in FFS for intermediate-risk embryonal RMS, probably related to an increased cyclophosphamide dose.[2] Escalation of cyclophosphamide from 0.9 g/m² in IRS-III to 2.2 g/m² in IRS-IV improved the FFS of patients with embryonal RMS but not those with alveolar RMS or undifferentiated RMS.[2]

Data from IRS-I, IRS-II, and IRS-III in 1431 patients indicate that there is no benefit to adding doxorubicin to VAC in patients with group III and group IV disease, whether analyzed together or within group III and group IV categories individually.[25,69,70,92] The addition of doxorubicin and cisplatin with or without etoposide to the VAC regimen did not improve the outcome for patients with advanced disease in IRS-III.[25,69,70]

Patients with metastatic disease have a poor prognosis despite aggressive therapy. Intensive, multiagent combinations have been used in an attempt to improve survival. The International Society of Pediatric Oncology (SIOP) reported a 53% response rate to a combination of carboplatin, epirubicin, and vincristine in previously untreated patients with metastatic RMS.[33]

The use of methotrexate in front-line treatment regimens offers the potential advantages of relative lack of additive myelosuppression and a different mechanism of action. In a phase II trial, Pappo et al.[81] reported a 33% response rate to high-dose methotrexate in patients with previously untreated, advanced-stage RMS.

Topotecan, a campotothecin analogue that acts as an inhibitor of topoisomerase I, is being examined for its potential role in RMS (inhibition of topoisomerase I inhibits DNA repletion). The IRS Group reported a 45% response rate to topotecan used in a window setting in newly diagnosed patients with nonparameningeal metastatic RMS.[82,111] An IRS-V pilot for metastatic RMS is currently evaluating topotecan in combination with cyclophosphamide in an up-front window before VAC and radiation therapy. It appears to be active in newly diagnosed patients with metastatic RMS and can be given in combination with VAC.[82]

Autologous bone marrow transplantation has been used in several of the childhood solid tumors. To date, it has not been of value in patients with metastatic RMS.[51,54]

In summary, the recommendations for IRS-V, which is presently ongoing, are as follows:

Low-risk patients are those with localized embryonal RMS in favorable sites (stage I) or in unfavorable sites (stages II and III) that has been grossly removed. Those with the best prognosis are placed in subgroup A and receive VA with or without radiation therapy. The others, placed in subgroup B, receive VAC with or without radiation therapy.

Intermediate-risk patients are those with localized alveolar RMS or undifferentiated sarcoma (stages I to III) or embryonal RMS (stages II and III) with gross residual disease (group III) or embryonal RMS with metastases (group IV) younger than 10 years at diagnosis. They are randomized to receive VAC or VAC alternating with vincristine and cyclophosphamide plus topotecan, along with radiation therapy.

High-risk patients have embryonal RMS diagnosed at 10 years of age or older, or alveolar RMS or undifferentiated sarcoma at any age younger than 21 years, with metastases at diagnosis (group IV). They receive a trial of irinotecan[34] over 6 weeks, followed by VAC. Irinotecan is continued at intervals for those who responded to it initially but is omitted for nonresponders. High-risk patients with cranial parameningeal tumors and meningeal impingement at diagnosis receive VAC without irinotecan.

RADIOTHERAPY

Radiotherapy is tailored for specific sites and is based on extent of disease. In some sites, such as the head and neck or pelvis, tumors often cannot be completely removed surgically. Radiation therapy may be used in conjunction with chemotherapy to eradicate residual tumor cells. The guidelines for radiation doses have changed over successive IRS Group studies. The dosage is now tailored to the amount of residual disease (gross or microscopic) and the tumor response.

In IRS-IV, radiation therapy was defined by clinical group. Patients with completely resected clinical group I, TNM stage I and II tumors received no radiotherapy. Patients with completely resected group I, stage II tumors and those with group II tumors received conventional external beam radiation to a total dose of 4140 cGy. Clinical group III patients were randomized to receive 5040 cGy external beam radiation or hyperfractionated radiotherapy to a dose of 5940 cGy. Based on IRS-IV, there is no indication that giving hyperfractionated radiotherapy with 59.4 Gy in two daily fractions of 1.1 Gy, with a 6-hour interfractional interval, results in a better local-regional control rate among children with group III tumors than that obtained with 50.4 Gy in 1.8 fractions daily.[29,30]

There is no evidence of a benefit in giving radiation to patients with completely resected, local lesions (group I), provided the histologic subtype is embryonal RMS.[123] Graded doses of irradiation are appropriate for all other patients, based on the patient's group at the time of study entry. Volumes to be irradiated include the pretreatment primary tumor and the regional lymph node area, if involved. Patients with group IV disease receive radiation therapy to both the primary site and the sites of metastases, within the limits of bone marrow tolerance.

An analysis of patients with group II disease in IRS-I through -IV showed improved outcome in IRS-III and -IV, perhaps due to intensified therapy.[103]

Local failure rates for patients with group III disease in IRS-III and -IV were reviewed in 2000 by the IRS Statistical Office. The rates have remained stable or improved. In IRS-IV, local failure rates were 2% in orbit primary sites, 16% in cranial parameningeal sites, and 12% in other head or neck sites. Local failure rates were 7% in extremity sites, 19% in genitourinary sites, and 14% in other sites.

Current IRS Group results suggest that most patients with cranial parameningeal sarcoma, including those with localized intracranial extension contiguous with the primary tumor at diagnosis, can be successfully managed with systemic chemotherapy and radiation therapy. Radiation therapy is directed to the primary tumor, including any extension, along with a 2-cm margin, including the adjacent meninges. Whole-brain irradiation and intrathecal anticancer agents are not necessary in the absence of diffuse meningeal involvement, such as multiple intracranial metastases.[89,91]

A summary of the recommendations for radiation therapy in IRS-V include the following: Patients with completely excised embryonal RMS (group I) receive no radiation therapy. However, patients with completely excised (group I) alveolar RMS and undifferentiated sarcoma receive radiation therapy to the primary site.[123] Other patients receive radiation therapy as a function of group, histologic subtype, and status of regional lymph nodes or distant metastases. Patients with metastases receive radiation therapy to the primary tumor and to sites of metastases within the limits of bone marrow tolerance.[92]

MANAGEMENT BY SITE

Head and Neck

Head and neck lesions include superficial head and neck, orbit, parotid, buccal, laryngeal, and oropharyngeal locations. The multidisciplinary approach to therapy has allowed less aggressive surgical procedures while maintaining an excellent prognosis at this site. Wide excision is appropriate when feasible, but the possibility of achieving wide margins is restricted to small superficial lesions.[47]

Tumors of the orbit have an excellent response to therapy because the tumor is usually confined to the bony orbit and there is a paucity of lymphatics. Abramson et al.[1] demonstrated that radiation therapy plus chemotherapy is the most effective treatment for orbital RMS; this type of therapy ended the need for orbital exenteration. Survival of more than 90% of patients is standard with VA chemotherapy and radiation therapy.[25,32,114] Metastatic spread to regional nodes is seen in less than 3% of patients.[56] Cervical lymph node biopsy or sentinel lymph node mapping does not appear to be warranted unless nodes are clinically involved. Patients with nodal involvement should be treated with the IRS intermediate-risk protocol. Thus, except for small lid lesions, the role of surgery for orbital primary tumors is limited to biopsy alone.[32,52,114,116] Orbital exenteration has been used selectively in recurrent disease.

Nonorbital, nonparameningeal sites include superficial and deep tumors that do not impinge on the meninges. For some tumors, such as parotid, laryngeal, oropharyngeal, and other deep tumors, surgery is limited to biopsy followed by chemotherapy and radiation therapy for tumor eradication.[116] This treatment regimen has led to survival rates of 83%.[3,38]

The need for alkylating agents in orbital and nonorbital head and neck sites has been questioned.[7,52,114,116] In IRS-III, patients with orbital and nonparameningeal head and neck tumors who received intensive VA chemotherapy and radiation therapy had the same rate of survival (90%) as did patients in IRS-II who received those therapies in conjunction with alkylating agents.[24,25] The present recommendation for this low-risk group is to receive VA with or without radiation therapy.[27]

Parameningeal tumors are associated with a poor prognosis because of the propensity for extension and the presence of abundant lymphatics.[3,20,56,116] In addition, parameningeal RMS often occurs in hidden sites, which frequently results in delayed diagnosis.[32,114,116] Fifteen percent of patients with parameningeal RMS present with metastatic disease.[25] Bone erosion is a predictor of local relapse.[67] More intensive treatment of parameningeal RMS, including VAC chemotherapy, intrathecal chemotherapy, and radiation therapy to the entire cranial neuraxis, has resulted in increased survival.[86] In patients receiving this intensified therapy, the tumor-free survival rate increased from 33% to 57%, and the failure rate for local tumor control fell from 28% to 6%.[86] The value of prophylactic radiation therapy to the central nervous system has been questioned.[35] In IRS-III, radiation therapy and intrathecal chemotherapy were based on the degree of meningeal involvement, and most patients received less radiation therapy than that used in IRS-II. There was no decrease in progression-free survival among patients in IRS-III compared with those in IRS-II.[24,25]

Craniofacial resection for anterior skull-based tumors of the nasal areas, paranasal sinuses, temporal fossa, and other such sites should be reserved for surgical teams with expertise in its performance and for secondary procedures when tumor persists after initial chemotherapy and radiation therapy. In some reports, no viable tumor could be found in the resected specimens, despite a residual mass effect on imaging studies.[109,117,118] Other studies suggested a good correlation between evidence of stable residual disease on CT and subsequent local relapse and death.[36] This is being investigated further.

Genitourinary Sites

The genitourinary sites include the bladder, prostate, paratesticular areas, vagina, uterus, vulva, and, rarely, kidneys or ureter. RMS is the most common malignancy of the pelvic structures in children. Tumors in these locations are considered in two different categories on account of their different prognoses: bladder-prostate versus vulvovagina, uterus, and paratesticular. These sites accounted for approximately 25% of cases in IRS-III.[25] In 6% of those patients with pelvic tumors in IRS-I and -II, the exact site of origin within the pelvis could not be defined. Tumors in the vagina and testicular areas have a good prognosis and are more commonly of embryonal histology, often with the botryoid (vaginal) or spindle cell (paratesticular) variant.

Bladder RMS and prostate RMS can be difficult to distinguish from each other because of their anatomic proximity and the tumor's tendency to grow to a large size before diagnosis. When this determination is possible, however, it is evident that patients with bladder tumors have a better prognosis than those with tumors arising from the prostate.[115] The majority of tumors in these areas are embryonal (71%) or botryoid (20%); 2% are of alveolar histology.[75]

In IRS-III it was found that children with tumors of the bladder or prostate who received more intensive chemotherapy and earlier radiation therapy had a survival rate only slightly lower than that of patients with head and neck tumors. This finding contrasts with that of IRS-II.[24,25,69,70,87]

Bladder or prostate tumors commonly arise near the area of the trigone and produce symptoms of bladder outlet obstruction or hematuria. Diagnosis is usually made by cystoscopic evaluation and biopsy, as well as CT or magnetic resonance imaging. Previously, the initial management of these tumors in children was usually anterior or total pelvic exenteration, followed by chemotherapy and radiation; this treatment produced very good long-term survival rates, approaching 85% in some series, but it also necessitated a permanent urinary conduit and, in some cases, colostomy.[87,90] Today, bladder salvage is an important goal, and less aggressive surgical procedures are common.[44-46,49] Neoadjuvant chemotherapy and radiation have decreased the rate of exenterative cystectomy from greater than 50% to approximately 30%.[44-46] In IRS-III 50% of patients with bladder RMS received cisplatin in addition to vincristine-doxorubicin (Adriamycin)-cyclophosphamide or VAC and irradiation. Of 171 children with primary bladder lesions enrolled in IRS-I through -III, 40 underwent partial cystectomy after receiving neoadjuvant chemotherapy and radiation. Relapse occurred in nine patients (seven locally). The Kaplan-Meier estimate of survival rate with a functioning bladder among all children with bladder or prostate tumors in IRS-III was 60%. Long-term survival was in excess of 80%.[44-46]

Exenteration is no longer the primary treatment for RMS of the prostate. This site accounted for about 5% of newly diagnosed cases in IRS-III. The mean age at the time of diagnosis was 5.3 years. Most tumors were relatively large, had embryonal histology, and were clinically localized but unresectable without major loss of organ function. The 44 patients with group III tumors (gross residual disease) were treated according to the IRS-III protocol. Forty-three of them underwent biopsy only, and one patient had subtotal resection as the initial procedure. The average number of surgical procedures per patient was two (range, one to five). Six of the 44 patients had no additional surgery. The second-look procedures performed in the other 38 patients included exenteration,[14] prostatectomy,[4] cystoscopic or perineal needle biopsy,[9] laparotomy with biopsy,[6] and subtotal excision with bladder salvage.[3] Additional surgery was required for four patients for evaluation of residual mass, postoperative fistula, ureteral stricture, or small bowel obstruction. Six patients with relapse or residual disease underwent additional chemotherapy and late exenteration,[3] prostatectomy,[1] or biopsy.[2] Four of the six were cured, one received treatment for a second malignancy, and the other had residual disease after exenteration. Thus, 36 of the 44 patients with group III tumors were cured (minimum follow-up, 6 years; range, 6 to 11 years), compared with 23 of 47 patients in IRS-II. The bladder salvage rate for those cured of their disease was also better (64% versus 57%). Conservative, delayed surgery, performed after intensive chemotherapy with or without radiotherapy, yields a better cure rate while maintaining a high rate of bladder salvage in children with group III prostatic RMS.[65]

Paratesticular Sites

Paratesticular RMS represents 7% of all childhood RMS and 12% of childhood scrotal tumors.[120] Most paratesticular RMS is embryonal, nonmetastatic, and highly curable with multimodal therapy including surgery, multiagent chemotherapy, and, for patients with retroperitoneal lymph node involvement or incompletely resected disease, radiation therapy.[80]

Most tumors present as a painless scrotal mass and are often easily resected (group I). Survival rates exceed 90% for group I and II patients.[60,96] Lesions adjacent to the testis or spermatic cord should be removed by orchiectomy and resection of the entire spermatic cord through an inguinal incision with proximal control of the spermatic cord. The contralateral testis may be transposed to the adjacent thigh, temporarily, when scrotal radiotherapy is required. Open scrotal biopsy or tumor spillage should be avoided, because inguinal recurrence may follow; spillage or open biopsy requires scrotectomy with or without radiation. If biopsy is warranted before orchiectomy, the following steps should be followed: (1) achieve atraumatic high control of the spermatic cord; (2) mobilize the testis and cord, carefully isolated from the operative field; (3) keep the biopsy site closed and the testes covered while awaiting the frozen section report; (4) change gowns and gloves and the instruments that were used for biopsy; (5) if the biopsy report is positive, remove the

testes and the entire cord, including the atraumatic clamp, together; (6) thoroughly irrigate the field. Patients with spillage are considered clinical group IIa regardless of the completeness of resection.[41]

The incidence of nodal metastatic disease for paratesticular RMS has been reported to be as high as 26% to 43%.[37,77,86,120] During IRS-III, all patients were required to undergo ipsilateral retroperitoneal lymph node dissection. During IRS-IV, the retroperitoneal lymph nodes were evaluated with CT. In this study, only those patients with lymph node involvement on CT required surgical evaluation of the lymph nodes. This led to the "down-grouping" of about 15% of patients from group II (lymph nodes positive) to group I (total resection, no nodal disease). This effect was higher in adolescents (>30%). This change led to fewer patients receiving radiation to the retroperitoneum, but also a poorer FFS in IRS-IV and a higher relapse rate. For patients younger than 10 years, long-term survival rate did not differ between IRS-III and -IV and was excellent (IRS-III, 100%; IRS-IV, 98%). However, treatment in about 30% of adolescents assigned to group I tumor status in IRS-IV failed; those patients required retreatment, with poor salvage. In IRS-IV, among patients given retroperitoneal lymph node radiation and intensive three-agent chemotherapy, including alkylating agents, survival at 3 years was 100%. Based on these data, the IRS Group resumed recommending retroperitoneal lymph node dissection for all patients older than 10 years.

This remains controversial, because SIOP no longer recommends retroperitoneal lymph node dissection for any patients. Olive et al.[77] found that chemotherapy was effective in eradicating occult micrometastases; thus, they concluded that lymph node dissection was not necessary in completely resected paratesticular RMS treated with multiagent chemotherapy.

Retroperitoneal lymph node dissection is associated with significant long-term complications. Heyn et al.[48] found it to be associated with intestinal obstruction, loss of ejaculatory function, and lower extremity lymphedema.

There are risks associated with using the more intensive chemotherapy protocol as well. Cyclophosphamide is an N-phosphorylated cyclic derivative of nitrogen mustard. Side effects of cyclophosphamide include immunosuppression, pulmonary fibrosis, sterility, and testicular atrophy in men.[122]

Present recommendations are that all patients with paratesticular RMS should have thin-cut abdominal and pelvic CT scans with double contrast to evaluate for evidence of nodal involvement. Patients aged 10 years and older receive ipsilateral retroperitoneal nerve-sparing template node dissection. Patients with group II disease receive intensified treatment (e.g., VAC and retroperitoneal lymph node radiation).[16] Disease in children younger than 10 years can be staged with abdominal thin-cut (5-mm slices) CT, reserving ipsilateral node dissection for those with positive scans. Patients with group I disease should receive VA chemotherapy without radiation. Inguinal nodes are rarely involved and are biopsied only if clinically positive or if the scrotum is invaded by tumor. Inguinal nodes are not considered regional; when they are positive, this places the patient in stage IV (clinical group IV).

Vulva, Vagina, and Uterus

Vulvovaginal and uterine RMS is the most common malignancy of the pediatric female genital system. This tumor generally presents in the first few years of life with vaginal bleeding, discharge, or a vaginal mass. If the tumor arises from the vulva, it consists of a firm nodule embedded in the labial folds, or it may be periclitoric in location. Diagnosis is made with incisional or excisional biopsy. Vaginal lesions generally have embryonal or botryoid embryonal histology and have an excellent prognosis.[4,6,9] Vulvar lesions may have alveolar histology, but because most are localized, they also have a good prognosis. Vaginal lesions usually arise from the anterior vaginal wall in the area of the embryonic vesicovaginal septum (urogenital sinus). The bladder, prostatic utricle, prostate, and lower vagina all arise from the urogenital sinus. These are common sites for RMS in both sexes.

Before 1972, pelvic exenteration was the accepted surgical approach for vaginal RMS. Beginning in 1972, the IRS Group began to enter patients in prospective clinical trials. The first eight patients with nonmetastatic vaginal RMS underwent primary surgical intervention, followed by postoperative chemotherapy with VAC. Three patients also received radiotherapy. Because vaginal RMS appeared to be responsive to chemotherapy, IRS-II consisted of a primary chemotherapy regimen followed by delayed surgical intervention with or without radiation. Fourteen of 20 patients (70%) eventually underwent surgical resection.[9]

During IRS-III, these patients were given primary chemotherapy consisting of VAC plus doxorubicin and cisplatin after initial biopsy (clinical group III). Only 7 of 23 patients (30%) underwent surgical resection after primary chemotherapy. Six of the seven patients had no viable tumor in the resected specimen, and one had maturing rhabdomyoblasts. The presence of rhabdomyoblasts may not signify persistent active disease.[49] At M. D. Anderson Cancer Center, we continued chemotherapy without resection when rhabdomyoblasts were found. No viable tumor or rhabdomyoblasts were found after further chemotherapy or subsequent biopsy in these patients. Only six patients in IRS-III underwent radiotherapy.[6]

During IRS-IV, only 3 of 21 patients (14%) underwent surgical resection after primary chemotherapy. Three patients had only rhabdomyoblasts, and one patient who underwent early second-look surgery had rhabdomyoblasts and a small amount of viable tumor. No patient in IRS-IV had a cystectomy, and all but one patient are still alive with no evidence of disease.

Early IRS Group studies suggested that patients with primary tumors of the uterus were a distinct group, distinguished from those with vaginal tumors by older age, propensity to local recurrence, and poorer prognosis. Early surgical treatment was radical. Beginning in 1984 (IRS-III), these patients were treated with neoadjuvant chemotherapy consisting of doxorubicin, cisplatin, vincristine, dactinomycin, and cyclophosphamide. These therapies allowed for less extensive resection and less irradiation, with excellent local and distant control of disease. Survival continues to improve with less radical surgical intervention.[22]

For tumors of the vagina, vulva, and uterus, the general principles followed in IRS-V include biopsy and staging, followed by chemotherapy as directed by stage and group (i.e., risk category). Second- and third-look operations with biopsy and cystoscopy are common. Distal vaginal lesions may be polypoid or localized and are amenable to primary resection or delayed resection. Rarely is vaginectomy or hysterectomy indicated, except for recurrent or persistent viable tumor. Lymph node involvement is very rare. Oophorectomy is not done except for direct involvement with advanced or recurrent disease.

A primary chemotherapy approach with the gold standard of VAC, followed by local resectional therapy and occasional use of radiotherapy when indicated, has produced excellent results.[10] Patients aged 1 to 9 years fared the best (5-year survival of 98%); patients outside of this age range benefited from the intensified therapy used in IRS-III or -IV (5-year survival of 67% in IRS-I and -II, versus 90% in IRS-III and -IV).[10]

Trunk

Primary RMS of the trunk may occur in paraspinal sites, the thoracic or chest wall, the abdominal wall, intraabdominal sites, or the pelvis or retroperitoneum. These tumors tend to have a higher incidence of alveolar histology and a somewhat worse prognosis in some sites.[8,88] These lesions present differently, depending on site, and are discussed separately.

Paraspinal Sites

Paraspinal RMS presents as an enlarging mass in the paravertebral muscle area. This is usually diagnosed by incisional biopsy and must be distinguished from extraosseous Ewing's sarcoma, which is more common in this site in our experience. For all truncal tumors, the biopsy should be performed in the long axis of the tumor (i.e., parallel to the ribs), to allow for wide local excision and rib resection as necessary.

Most patients with paraspinal lesions require chemotherapy before resection, and many require postoperative radiation therapy. Wide local excision is frequently done in conjunction with a plastic surgeon, who can assist in flap closure of the defect. In small children, it may be wise to eliminate radiation therapy close to the spine whenever feasible.

Abdominal Wall

This location is relatively rare (<1% of all patients) and requires excisional or incisional biopsy, followed by wide local complete resection or neoadjuvant chemotherapy, followed by second-look surgery. In a review of IRS patients, FFS at 5 years was 65%.[12] Older patients with alveolar histology and larger tumors had a worse prognosis.

Chest Wall

Chest wall and intrathoracic locations are rare sites of pediatric sarcomas. Of 2747 patients registered in IRS-I, -II, and -III, only 105 had primary tumors of the chest wall, pleura, lung, or heart. It has been suggested that these sites have a poor prognosis owing to histology, advanced stage at presentation, and difficulty of local resection. Early studies showed high rates of local and distant relapse.[88] A review of IRS-II and -III[8] included 84 patients with thoracic sarcomas: 76 chest wall tumors, 3 lung tumors, 4 pleural tumors, and 1 that arose from the heart. Sixty patients (71%) achieved a complete response. Thirty-nine patients had a local relapse, and 22 patients had a distant relapse. Forty-two percent of patients survived. Progression-free survival was not significantly associated with histology, site, clinical group, or IRS number. Overall survival was significantly associated with clinical group, size, and local or distant recurrence but not histology or IRS number by univariate analysis. In a multivariate analysis, only clinical group and local and distant recurrence showed statistical significance. Thus, if survival is to be improved, local tumor control with negative margins must be achieved. Clinical group II patients were treated with radiation therapy and had a better survival rate than did those in clinical group I (totally resected and thus no radiation therapy), indicating that the resection may have left microscopic or even gross residual disease. Either second-look surgery or consideration of local radiation therapy for possible residual disease in clinical group I may be indicated to improve survival.[8]

Specific surgical management of chest wall RMS includes initial biopsy (longitudinal to ribs) and staging. Following neoadjuvant chemotherapy, the tumor is resected to clear margins, and attached pleura or lung is removed as necessary. If needed, wide local resection can be followed by chest wall reconstruction, usually with a synthetic material covered by a myocutaneous flap. Frequently, tumor size reduction allows resection with primary closure.

Retroperitoneal and Pelvic Sites

RMS of the retroperitoneum and pelvis usually presents as a large, bulky tumor whose exact site of origin is difficult to determine.[23] Frequently, these tumors invade or involve vital organs or vessels; thus, only biopsy can be performed at the initial exploration. Early IRS Group studies indicated a poor prognosis for these sites.[23] Blakely et al.[14] reported on 94 patients with group III disease from IRS-III and IRS-IV Pilot and found a 57% FFS rate at 4 years. They found that age younger than 10 years at diagnosis and embryonal histology were favorable prognostic factors, as was the performance of a debulking procedure before instituting chemotherapy and radiation therapy.[14] Recently Raney et al.[93] reported on the results of 56 patients with localized retroperitoneal and pelvic RMS. Fifty-four of these patients had gross residual disease (clinical group III) at the completion of the initial diagnostic procedure. Two patients underwent grossly complete surgical excision with microscopic involved margins without (group IIa) or with (group IIc) tumor-involved regional lymph nodes that were removed before beginning chemotherapy. Only 15 patients (27%) had 50% or more of the tumor removed before beginning chemotherapy and were classified as debulked; the other 41 patients were classified as having biopsy only. Among the 15 patients who underwent debulking of the tumor before chemotherapy or radiotherapy, there have been no treatment failures thus far. In contrast, 15 of the 41 patients who underwent biopsy only developed recurrent sarcoma. Thus, it appears that debulking may be of value when it can be achieved safely and with minimum morbidity. Otherwise, an alternative would be delayed primary excision after shrinkage with chemotherapy.

Biliary Sites

Patients with biliary RMS do relatively well with chemotherapy and radiotherapy without aggressive surgical resection.[84,104] Most patients have the botryoid variant of embryonal RMS, which responds well to chemotherapy. Although these tumors present with significant obstructive jaundice, biopsy followed by neoadjuvant chemotherapy commonly reduces the jaundice without the need for resection or internal or external biliary drainage. Surgical resection or bypass involves significant complications. Spunt et al.[104] reported on 25 patients treated in IRS-I through -IV and found that total resection was rarely possible, external biliary drains were frequently associated with infection, and tumors responded well to combination chemotherapy without aggressive surgical intervention.

Perineal and Perianal Sites

RMS of the perineum or anus is a rare sarcoma of childhood with a relatively poor prognosis. Blakely et al.[15] reported on 71 patients treated in IRS-I through -IV. The majority (64%) were at an advanced stage (clinical groups III and IV) at initial presentation, and 50% had positive regional lymph node involvement. The 5-year FFS for all patients was 45%, and the overall survival rate was 49%. Characteristics that were associated with significantly improved survival were primary tumor size less than 5 cm, lower (less advanced) clinical group and stage, negative lymph node status, and age younger than 10 years. When the extent of disease was controlled for multivariate analysis, only age younger than 10 years predicted an improved outcome. The 5-year overall survival rate for patients younger than 10 years was 71%, versus 20% for older patients (P < 0.001). Because of the high incidence of regional lymph node involvement, biopsy of clinically suspicious nodes should be done, and sentinel lymph node mapping for nonclinically suspicious nodes should be entertained.

Extremities

Primary tumors of the extremity accounted for 19% of RMS in IRS-III[7] and 20% in IRS-IV.[74] Despite the intensive efforts of the IRS Group, the outcome of extremity RMS remains suboptimal compared with that of RMS in other sites. Improvements in survival have been seen with subsequent studies, but estimated 5-year survival is about 74% for patients without distant metastatic disease.[7] Analysis of these studies suggests that the improvement is attributable to the intensification of therapy for patients with a poorer prognosis, while allowing a decrease in therapy for those with a good prognosis. Various prognostic factors have been suggested for extremity RMS in children. The elements of the Lawrence-Gehan[58] staging system used in IRS-IV are local tissue invasiveness, tumor size, presence of nodal and distant metastases, and site. Because the extremities are relatively unfavorable sites, no extremity tumors are classified as stage I by this system. A total of 139 patients were entered in IRS-IV with extremity RMS and were assigned a preoperative stage and a clinical group, as follows: stage II ($n = 34$), stage III ($n = 73$), stage IV ($n = 32$); group I ($n = 31$), group II ($n = 21$), group III ($n = 54$); group IV ($n = 33$). Three-year FFS was 55%, and the overall survival rate was 70%. FFS was significantly worse for patients with advanced disease. Totally resected patients (group I) had a 3-year FFS of 91%.[74]

Initial treatment consists of biopsy, either incisional or excisional. This should be done in a longitudinal or axial direction to allow for wide local excision. If wide local excision can be accomplished without mutilation, this should be considered. The standard 2-cm margins are arbitrary and are not practical in children. There is little evidence that a clear margin of only a few millimeters involves a higher risk for recurrence than do larger margins. Amputation is rarely indicated except for larger recurrent or persistent disease. Excision of the entire muscle from origin to insertion, as recommended in the past, is not necessary. The importance of complete resection is emphasized, because survival is markedly improved with total excision or microscopic residual only. Careful determination of margin status is extremely important, and re-resection at initial or subsequent operation is warranted. Hays et al.[43] demonstrated that patients with node-negative extremity and trunk sarcomas who underwent re-excision for microscopic residual tumor had a survival rate that was significantly higher than those who did not have re-excision or were reported to have no residual tumor after initial resection. It is our policy to recommend re-excision for all patients referred to our institution after previous resection, no matter what was previously reported. We have found residual and even gross disease in patients reported to have complete resection (probably because the surgeon was unaware that cancer was present).

Lymph node involvement with extremity RMS in IRS-I and -II was only 12%,[5,7,56,57] because few patients actually had lymph node biopsy. LaQuaglia et al.[55] reported a 40% incidence of positive nodes. In a review of IRS-IV, Andrassy et al.[7] demonstrated that 39% of patients who underwent evaluation of their lymph nodes had histologic confirmation of disease. Neville et al.,[74] in a review of IRS-IV data, found that 50% of biopsied lymph nodes contained disease. Of the patients whose lymph nodes were clinically negative but were biopsied anyway, 17% were found to have microscopic disease. The finding of histologically positive lymph nodes is a statistically significant predictor of FFS. Although lymph node dissection has not improved the survival rate, positive regional nodes should be irradiated to prevent local recurrence. We have used and recommended lymphatic mapping with sentinel node biopsy to evaluate the regional nodes.[73,74] If sentinel lymph node mapping is not available, aggressive sampling is warranted.

COMPLICATIONS

Complications of treatment for RMS are varied and extensive. These include chemotherapy toxicity and death, radiation-related acute and long-term complications, and the standard surgical complications of biopsy and resection. Discussion of the specific complications and their treatment is beyond the scope of this chapter. Long-term follow-up of all patients is warranted for delayed complications and second malignancies.[94]

TREATMENT OF METASTATIC DISEASE

Metastatic disease most commonly involves the lung (58%), bone (33%), regional lymph nodes (33%), liver (22%), and brain (20%).[21] Of the patients enrolled in IRS-III,[25] 14% were clinical group IV at the time of diagnosis. Primary sites more likely to have metastases include the extremities (23%), parameningeal sites (13%), and retroperitoneal, trunk, gastrointestinal, and intrathoracic sites. Primary sites with a low incidence of metastases include the orbit (1.8%), nonparameningeal or nonorbital head and neck (4.5%), and genitourinary sites.[97] Metastatic disease is the single most important predictor of clinical outcome in patients with RMS. The 3-year FFS is only 25% in patients with metastatic disease.[25,70] As mentioned previously, regional node metastases vary with the site of the primary tumor (highest in the extremities) and also affect survival.

The lung is the most common site of metastatic disease. Patients with only lung metastases appear to have a somewhat better prognosis than do those with metastases in multiple sites or metastases to bone or liver.[96] Patients with only lung metastases also have a greater incidence of favorable histology and a smaller number of extremity primary tumors.[96] Because RMS is highly chemosensitive, resection of numerous metastases is not indicated. In our experience, an isolated single metastasis to the lung has a better prognosis than do multiple metastases. For this reason, it is worthwhile to biopsy a single metastasis to confirm histology. The better prognosis may well be related to the treatment of nonmetastatic lung lesions other than RMS. Persistent or recurrent disease after chemotherapy may warrant resection both for diagnosis and possibly to decrease the tumor burden. Overall, there has been little improvement in the survival of patients with metastatic disease. They are presently categorized in stage IV, group IV and are considered high risk.

Aggressive chemotherapy and radiation in an attempt to improve survival is being studied. During IRS-IV, 127 eligible patients were treated for metastatic disease with one of two regimens that incorporated a window of either ifosfamide and etoposide with vincristine, dactinomycin, and cyclophosphamide or vincristine, melphalan, and VAC. The estimated overall survival and FFS was 39% and 25%, respectively, at 3 years. Overall survival at 3 years was influenced by histology (47% for embryonal versus 34% for all others) and number of metastatic sites. By multivariate analysis, the presence of two or fewer metastatic sites was the only significant predictor.[17]

OUTCOME

The overall trend has been an increase in survival for each subsequent IRS Group study. The survival rate depends on clinical group, stage, and primary site. The overall 5-year survival rate in IRS-III was 71%; it was 90% for clinical group I, 80% for clinical group II, 70% for clinical group III, and 30% for clinical group IV. The survival rate by pretreatment staging classification was 80% for stage I, 68% for stage II, 49% for stage III, and 21% for stage IV.[124]

Overall, FFS rates for the patients treated in IRS-IV did not differ from those of similar patients treated in IRS-III; the estimated 3-year FFS rate was 76% in IRS-III and 77% in IRS-IV. Three-year FFS rates were improved for patients with embryonal RMS treated in IRS-IV compared with IRS-III (83% versus 74%). The improvement seemed to be restricted to patients with stage II or stage II-III, group I-II embryonal RMS. The sites of treatment failure were local in 93 patients (51%), regional in 30 (17%), and distant in 58 (32%). Salvage therapy after relapse differed by group. Forty-one percent of patients with group I-II tumors were alive 3 years after relapse, compared with 22% of those with group III tumors.[27]

REFERENCES

1. Abramson DH, et al: The treatment of orbital rhabdomyosarcoma with irradiation and chemotherapy. Ophthalmology 1979;86:1330.
2. Anderson GJ, et al: Rhabdomyosarcoma of the head and neck in children. Arch Otolaryngol Head Neck Surg 1990; 116:428.
3. Anderson JR, et al: Improved outcome for patients with embryonal histology but not alveolar histology rhabdomyosarcoma: Results from Intergroup Rhabdomyosarcoma Study IV (IRS-IV). Proc Soc Clin Oncol 1998;17:526a.
4. Andrassy RJ: Rhabdomyosarcoma. Semin Pediatr Surg 1997;6:17.
5. Andrassy RJ: Advances in the surgical management of sarcomas in children. Am J Surg 2002;184:484.
6. Andrassy RJ, et al: Conservative surgical management of vaginal and vulvar pediatric rhabdomyosarcoma: A report from the Intergroup Rhabdomyosarcoma Study-III. J Pediatr Surg 1995;30:1034.
7. Andrassy RJ, et al: Extremity sarcomas: An analysis of prognostic factors from the Intergroup Rhabdomyosarcoma Study (IRS) III. J Pediatr Surg 1996;31:191.
8. Andrassy RJ, et al: Thoracic sarcomas in children. Ann Surg 1998;227:170.
9. Andrassy RJ, et al: Progress in the surgical management of vaginal rhabdomyosarcoma: A 25-year review from the Intergroup Rhabdomyosarcoma Study Group. J Pediatr Surg 1999;34:731.
10. Arndt CA, et al: What constitutes optimal therapy for patients with rhabdomyosarcoma of the female genital tract? Cancer 2001;91:2454.
11. Asmar L, et al: Agreement among and within groups of pathologists in the classification of rhabdomyosarcoma and related childhood sarcomas: Report of an international study of four pathology classifications. Cancer 1994;74:2579.
12. Beech TR, et al: What comprises appropriate therapy for children/adolescents with rhabdomyosarcoma arising in the abdominal wall? A report from the Intergroup Rhabdomyosarcoma Study Group. J Pediatr Surg 1999;34:668.
13. Birch JM, et al: Excess risk of breast cancer in the mothers of children with soft tissue sarcomas. Br J Cancer 1984; 49:325.
14. Blakely ML, et al: Does debulking improve survival rate in advanced-stage retroperitoneal embryonal rhabdomyosarcoma? J Pediatr Surg 1999;5:736.
15. Blakely ML, et al: Prognostic factors and surgical treatment guidelines for children with rhabdomyosarcoma of the perineum or anus: A report of Intergroup Rhabdomyosarcoma Studies I through IV, 1972 through 1997. J Pediatr Surg 2003;38:347.
16. Breneman JC, et al: The management of pediatric genitourinary rhabdomyosarcoma. In Vogelzang NJ, et al (eds): The Comprehensive Textbook of Genitourinary Oncology. Baltimore, Williams & Wilkins, 1996.
17. Breneman JC, et al: Prognostic factors and clinical outcomes in children and adolescents with metastatic rhabdomyosarcoma: A report from the Intergroup Rhabdomyosarcoma Study IV. J Clin Oncol 2003;21:78.
18. Burger RA, et al: Extent of surgery in rhabdomyosarcoma of urogenital structures. Eur Urol 1989;16:114.
19. Cavazzana AO, et al: Spindle cell rhabdomyosarcoma. Am J Surg Pathol 1992;16:229.
20. Coene IMJH, et al: Rhabdomyosarcoma of the head and neck in children. Clin Otolaryngol 1992;17:291.
21. Cofer BR, et al: Rhabdomyosarcoma. In Andrassy RJ (ed): Pediatric Surgical Oncology. Philadelphia, WB Saunders, 1998.
22. Corpron CA, et al: Conservative management of uterine pediatric rhabdomyosarcoma: A report from the Intergroup Rhabdomyosarcoma Study III and IV Pilot. J Pediatr Surg 1995;30:942.
23. Crist WM, et al: Soft tissue sarcomas arising in the retroperitoneal space in children: A report from the Intergroup Rhabdomyosarcoma Study. Cancer 1985;56:2125.
24. Crist WM, et al (for the IRS Committee): Prognosis in children with rhabdomyosarcoma: A report of IRS-I and IRS-II. J Clin Oncol 1990;8:443.
25. Crist WM, et al: Intergroup Rhabdomyosarcoma Study (IRS) III. J Clin Oncol 1995;13:610.
26. Crist WM, et al: Preliminary results for patients with local/regional tumors treated on the Intergroup Rhabdomyosarcoma Study-IV (1991-1997). Proc Am Soc Clin Oncol 1999; 18:18.
27. Crist WM, et al: Intergroup Rhabdomyosarcoma Study-IV: Results for patients with nonmetastatic disease. J Clin Oncol 2001;19:3091.
28. Dagher R, et al: Rhabdomyosarcoma: An overview. Oncologist 1999;4:34.
29. Donaldson S, et al: Hyperfractionated radiation in children with rhabdomyosarcoma: Results of an Intergroup Rhabdomyosarcoma Pilot Study. Int J Radiat Oncol Biol Phys 1995;32:903.
30. Donaldson SS, et al: Results from the Intergroup Rhabdomyosarcoma Study-IV randomized trial of hyperfractionated radiation in children with rhabdomyosarcoma. Int J Radiat Oncol Biol Phys 2000;48:178.

31. Ferracini R, et al: Retrogenic expression of the MET proto-oncogene correlates with the invasive phenotype of human rhabdomyosarcomas. Oncogene 1996;12:1697.

32. Fiorillo A, et al: Multidisciplinary treatment of primary orbital rhabdomyosarcoma: A single institution experience. Cancer 1991;67:560.

33. Frascella E, et al: Response of previously untreated metastatic rhabdomyosarcoma to combination chemotherapy with carboplatin, epirubicin, and vincristine. Eur J Cancer 1996;32A:821.

34. Furman W, et al: A phase I study of irinotecan (CPT-11) in children with relapsed solid tumors. Proc Am Soc Clin Oncol 1998;17:187a.

35. Gasparini M, et al: Questionable role of CNS radioprophylaxis in the therapeutic management of childhood rhabdomyosarcoma with meningeal extension. J Clin Oncol 1990;8:1854.

36. Gilles R, et al: Head and neck rhabdomyosarcomas in children: Value of clinical and CT findings in the detection of local regional relapses. Clin Radiol 1994;49:412.

37. Goldfarb B, et al: The role of retroperitoneal lymphadenectomy in localized paratesticular rhabdomyosarcoma. J Urol 1994;152:785.

38. Gross M, et al: Therapy of rhabdomyosarcoma of the larynx. Int J Pediatr Otorhinolaryngol 1988;15:93.

39. Grufferman A, et al: In utero x-ray exposure and risk of childhood rhabdomyosarcoma. Paper presented at the Fourth Annual Meeting of the Society for Epidemiologic Research, June 11, 1991, Buffalo, NY.

40. Grufferman S, et al: Parents' use of recreational drugs and risk of rhabdomyosarcoma in their children. Cancer Causes Control 1993;4:217.

41. Hamilton CR, et al: The management of paratesticular rhabdomyosarcoma. Clin Radiol 1989;40:314.

42. Hartley AN, et al: Patterns of cancer in the families of children with soft tissue sarcoma. Cancer 1993;72:923.

43. Hays DM, et al: Primary re-excision for patients with "microscopic residual" following initial excision of sarcomas of trunk and extremity sites. J Pediatr Surg 1989;24:5.

44. Hays DM, et al: Partial cystectomy in the management of rhabdomyosarcoma of the bladder: A report from the Intergroup Rhabdomyosarcoma Study. J Pediatr Surg 1990;25:719.

45. Hays DM, et al: Retention of functional bladders among patients with vesicle/prostatic sarcomas in the Intergroup Rhabdomyosarcoma Studies (IRS) (1978-1990) [abstract]. Med Pediatr Oncol 1991;19:423.

46. Hays DM, et al: Children with vesical rhabdomyosarcoma (RMS) treated by partial cystectomy, with neoadjuvant or adjuvant chemotherapy with or without radiotherapy. J Pediatr Hematol Oncol 1995;17:46.

47. Healy GB, et al: The role of surgery in rhabdomyosarcoma of the head and neck in children. Arch Otolaryngol Head Neck Surg 1991;117:1185.

48. Heyn R, et al (for the IRS Committee): Late effects of therapy in patients with paratesticular rhabdomyosarcoma. J Clin Oncol 1992;10:614.

49. Heyn R, et al: Preservation of the bladder in patients with rhabdomyosarcoma. J Clin Oncol 1997;15:69.

50. Horn RC, et al: Rhabdomyosarcoma: A clinicopathological study and classification of 39 cases. Cancer 1958;11:181.

51. Horowitz ME, et al: Total-body irradiation and autologous bone marrow transplant in the treatment of high-risk Ewing's sarcoma and rhabdomyosarcoma. J Clin Oncol 1993;11:1911.

52. Kao GD, et al: The sequelae of chemoradiation therapy for head and neck cancer in children: Managing impaired growth, development and other side effects. Med Pediatr Oncol 1993;21:60.

53. Kilpatrick SE, et al: Relationship of DNA ploidy to histology and prognosis in rhabdomyosarcoma. Cancer 1994;74:3227.

54. Koscielniak E, et al: Do patients with metastatic and recurrent rhabdomyosarcoma benefit from high-dose therapy with hematopoietic rescue? Report of the German/Austrian Pediatric Bone Marrow Transplantation Group. Bone Marrow Transplant 1997;19:227.

55. LaQuaglia MP, et al: Factors predictive of mortality in pediatric extremity rhabdomysarcoma. J Pediatr Surg 1990;25:238.

56. Lawrence W Jr, et al: Lymphatic metastasis with childhood rhabdomyosarcoma. Cancer 1987;60:910.

57. Lawrence W Jr, et al: Surgical lessons from the Intergroup Rhabdomyosarcoma Study (IRS) pertaining to extremity tumors. World J Surg 1988;12:676.

58. Lawrence W Jr, et al: Pretreatment TNM staging of childhood rhabdomyosarcoma: A report of the Intergroup Rhabdomyosarcoma Study Group, Children's Cancer Study Group, Pediatric Oncology Group. Cancer 1997;80:1165.

59. Leader M, et al: Myoglobin: An evaluation of its role as a marker of rhabdomyosarcomas. Br J Cancer 1989;59:106.

60. Leuschner I, et al: Spindle cell variants of embryonal rhabdomyosarcoma in the paratesticular region: A report of the Inergroup Rhabdomyosarcoma Study. Am J Sur Pathol 1993;17:221.

61. Li FP, et al: Soft tissue sarcomas, breast cancer and other neoplasms: A familial syndrome? Ann Intern Med 1969;71:747.

62. Li FP, et al: A cancer family syndrome in twenty-four kindreds. Cancer Res 1988;48:5358.

63. Li M, et al: Molecular genetics of Beckwith-Wiedemann syndrome. Curr Opin Pediatr 1997;9:623.

64. Lobe TE, et al: Neonatal rhabdomyosarcoma: The IRS experience. J Pediatr Surg 1994;29:1167.

65. Lobe TE, et al: The argument for conservative, delayed surgery in the management of prostatic rhabdomyosarcoma. J Pediatr Surg 1996;31:1084.

66. Malkin D, et al: Germ line p53 mutations in a familial syndrome of breast cancer, sarcomas, and other neoplasms. Science 1990;250:1233.

67. Mandell LR, et al: The influence of extensive bone erosion on local control in non-orbital rhabdomyosarcoma of the head and neck. Int J Radiat Oncol Biol Phys 1989;17:649.

68. Mandell LR, et al: Prognostic significance of regional lymph node involvement in childhood extremity rhabdomyosarcoma. Med Pediatr Oncol 1990;18:466.

69. Maurer HM, et al: The Intergroup Rhabdomyosarcoma Study-I: A final report. Cancer 1988;61:209.

70. Maurer HM, et al: The Intergroup Rhabdomyosarcoma Study-II. Cancer 1993;71:1904.

71. Miser JS, et al: Ifosfamide with mesna uroprotection and etoposide: An effective regimen in the treatment of recurrent sarcomas and other tumors of children and young adults. J Clin Oncol 1987;5:1191.

72. Morison IM, et al: Insulin-like growth factor 2 and overgrowth: Molecular biology and clinical implications. Mol Med Today 1998;4:110.

73. Neville HL, et al: Lymphatic mapping with sentinel node biopsy in pediatric patients. J Pediatr Surg 2000;35:961.

74. Neville HL, et al: Preoperative staging, prognostic factors, and outcome for extremity rhabdomyosarcoma: A preliminary report from the Intergroup Rhabdomyosarcoma Study IV (1991-1997). J Pediatr Surg 2000;35:317.

75. Newton WA, et al: Pathology of rhabdomyosarcoma and related tumors. In Maurer HM, Ruyman FB, Pochedly C (eds): Rhabdomyosarcoma and Related Tumors in Children and Adolescents. Boca Raton, Fla, CRC Press, 1991.

76. Newton WA, et al: Classification of rhabdomyosarcomas and related sarcomas: Pathologic aspects and proposal for a new classification. An Intergroup Rhabdomyosarcoma Study. Cancer 1995;76:1073.

77. Olive D, et al: Paraaortic lymphadenectomy is not necessary in the treatment of localized paratesticular rhabdomyosarcoma. Cancer 1984;54:1283.

78. Ortega JA: A therapeutic approach to childhood pelvic rhabdomyosarcoma without pelvic exenteration. J Pediatr Surg 1979;94:205.

79. Pack GT, et al: Rhabdomyosarcoma of the skeletal muscle: Report of 100 cases. Surgery 1952;32:1023.

80. Pappo AS, et al: Biology and therapy of pediatric rhabdomyosarcoma. J Clin Oncol 1995;13:2123.

81. Pappo AS, et al: A phase II trial of high-dose methotrexate in previously untreated children and adolescents with high-risk unresectable or metastatic rhabdomyosarcoma. J Pediatr Hematol Oncol 1997;19:438.

82. Pappo AS, et al: Up-front window trial of topotecan in previously untreated children and adolescents with metastatic rhabdomyosarcoma: An Intergroup Rhabdomyosarcoma Study (IRSG). J Clin Oncol 2001;19:213.

83. Pinkel D, et al: Rhabdomyosarcoma in children. JAMA 1961;175:293.

84. Pollono DG, et al: Rhabdomyosarcoma of extrahepatic biliary tree: Initial treatment with chemotherapy and conservative surgery. Med Pediatr Oncol 1998;30:290.

85. Raney RB Jr: Rhabdomyosarcoma and related tumors of the head and neck in childhood. In Maurer HM, Ruymann FB, Pochedly C (eds): Rhabdomyosarcoma and Related Tumors in Children and Adolescents. Boca Raton, Fla, CRC Press, 1991.

86. Raney RB Jr, et al: Paratesticular rhabdomyosarcoma in children. Cancer 1978;42:729.

87. Raney RB Jr, et al (for the IRS Committee): Primary chemotherapy with or without radiation therapy and/or surgery for children with localized sarcoma of the bladder, prostate, vagina, uterus and cervix: A comparison of the results in Intergroup Rhabdomyosarcoma Studies I and II. Cancer 1980;66:2072.

88. Raney RB Jr, et al (for the IRS Committee): Soft-tissue sarcoma of the trunk in childhood: Results of the Intergroup Rhabdomyosarcoma Study (IRS), 1972-1976. Cancer 1982;49:2612.

89. Raney RB Jr, et al: Improved prognosis with intensive treatment of children with cranial soft tissue sarcomas arising in nonorbital parameningeal sites: A report from the Intergroup Rhabdomyosarcoma Study. Cancer 1987;59:147.

90. Raney RB Jr, et al: Sequelae of treatment in 109 patients followed from five to fifteen years after diagnosis of sarcoma of the bladder and prostate: A report from the Intergroup Rhabdomyosarcoma Study (IRS) Committee. Cancer 1993;71:2387.

91. Raney RB Jr, et al: Results of treating localized cranial parameningeal sarcoma on Intergroup Rhabdomyosarcoma (RMS) Studies (IRS)-II through IV. Med Pediatric Oncol 2000;35:178.

92. Raney RB Jr, et al: The Intergroup Rhabdomyosarcoma Study Group (IRSG): Major lessons from the IRS-I through IRS-IV studies as background for the current IRS-IV treatment protocols. Sarcoma 2001;5:9.

93. Raney RB Jr, et al: Results of treatment of 56 patients with localized retroperitoneal and pelvic rhabdomyosarcoma: A report from the Intergroup Rhabdomyosarcoma Study-IV, 1991-1997. Pediatr Blood Cancer 2004;42:618.

94. Rich DC, et al: Second malignant neoplasms in children after treatment of soft tissue sarcoma. J Pediatr Surg 1997;32:369.

95. Rodeberg DA, et al: Surgical principles for children/adolescents with newly diagnosed rhabdomyosarcoma: A report from the Soft Tissue Sarcoma Committee of the Children's Oncology Group. Sarcoma 2002;6:111.

96. Rodeberg DA, et al: Characteristics and outcomes of rhabdomyosarcoma patients with isolated lung metastases from IRS-IV. J Pediatr Surg 2005;40:256.

97. Ruymann FB: Rhabdomyosarcoma in children and adolescents: A review. Hematol Oncol Clin North Am 1987;1:621.

98. Ruymann FB, et al: Congenital anomalies associated with rhabdomyosarcoma: A report from the Intergroup Rhabdomyosarcoam Study. Med Pediatr Oncol 1988;16:13.

99. Ruymann FB, et al: Epidemiology of soft tissue sarcomas. In Maurer HM, Ruymann FB, Pochedly C (eds): Rhabdomyosarcoma and Related Tumors in Children and Adolescents. Boca Raton, Fla, CRC Press, 1991.

100. Ruymann FB, et al: Comparison of two double chemotherapy regimens and conventional radiotherapy in metastatic rhabdomyosarcoma: Improved overall survival using ifosfamide/etoposide compared to vincristine/melphalan in IRSG-IV. Proc Am Soc Clin Oncol 1997;16:521a.

101. Seymour-Dempsey K, et al: Neurofibromatosis: Implications for the general surgeon. J Am Coll Surg 2002;195:553.

102. Shapiro DN, et al: Relationship of tumor-cell ploidy to histologic subtype and treatment of outcome in children and adolescents with unresectable rhabdomyosarcoma. J Clin Oncol 1991;9:159.

103. Smith LM, et al: Which patients with rhabdomyosarcoma (RMS) and microscopic residual tumor (group II) fail therapy? A report from the Intergroup Rhabdomyosarcoma Study Group (IRSG). Proc Am Soc Clin Oncol 2000;19:577a.

104. Spunt SL, et al: Aggressive surgery is unwarranted for biliary tract rhabdomyosarcoma. J Pediatr Surg 2000;35:309.

105. Stobbe GC, et al: Embryonal rhabdomyosarcoma of the head and neck in children and adolescents. Cancer 1950;3:826.

106. Stout AP: Rhabdomyosarcoma of the skeletal muscle. Ann Surg 1946;123:447.

107. Strong LC, et al: The Li-Fraumeni syndrome: From clinical epidemiology to molecular genetics. Am J Epidemiol 1992;135:190.

108. Tapscott SJ, et al: Deficiency in rhabdomyosarcomas of a factor required for MyoD activity and myogenesis. Science 1993;259:1450.

109. Tefft M, et al: Radiation therapy combined with systemic chemotherapy of rhabdomyosarcoma in children: Local control in patients enrolled into the Intergroup Rhabdomyosarcoma Study. Natl Cancer Inst Monogr 1981;56:75.

110. Turc C: Consistent chromosomal translocation in alveolar rhabdomyosarcoma. Cancer Genet Cytogenet 1986;19:361.

111. Vietti T, et al: Topotecan window in patients with rhabdomyosarcoma (RMS): An IRSG study. Proc Am Soc Clin Oncol 1997;16:510a.

112. Weintraub H, et al: The MyoD gene family: Nodal point during specification of the muscle cell lineage. Science 1991;251:761.

113. Wexler LH, et al: Pediatric soft tissue sarcomas. CA Cancer J Clin 44:211,1994.

114. Wharam M, et al: Management of orbital rhabdomyosarcoma. In Jacob C (ed): Cancers of the Head and Neck, Boston, Martinus Niijhoff, 1987.

115. Wiener ES: Rhabdomyosarcoma: New dimensions in management. Semin Pediatr Surg 1993;2:47.

116. Wiener ES: Head and neck rhabdomyosarcoma. Semin Pediatr Surg 1994;3:203.

117. Wiener ES, et al (for the IRS Committee of CCSG, POG, UKCCSG): Second look operations in children in group III and IV rhabdomyosarcoma (RMS). SIOP XXII Meeting, October, 1990, Rome. Med Pediatr Oncol 1990;18:408.

118. Wiener ES, et al (for the IRS Committee of CCSG and POG): Complete response or not complete response? Second look operations are the answer in children with rhabdomyosarcoma. ASCO Annual Meeting, May 19-21, 1991, Houston, Texas. Proc Am Soc Clin Oncol 1991;10:316.

119. Wiener ES, et al: Rhabdomyosarcoma in extremity and trunk sites. In Maurer HM, Ruymann FB, Pochedly C (eds): Rhabdomyosarcoma and Related Tumors in Children and Adolescents. Boca Raton, Fla, CRC Press, 1991.

120. Wiener ES, et al: Retroperitoneal node biopsy in paratesticular rhabdomyosarcoma. J Pediatr Surg 1994;29:171.

121. Wiener ES, et al: Controversies in the management of paratesticular rhabdomyosarcoma: Is staging retroperitoneal lymph node dissection necessary for adolescents with resected paratesticular rhabdomyosarcoma? Semin Pediatr Surg 2001;10:146.

122. Wiener ES, et al: What is optimal management for children or adolescents with localized paratesticular rhabdomyosarcoma? Results in IRS-III and IRS-IV. J Pediatr Surg (in press).

123. Wolden SL, et al: Indications for radiotherapy and chemotherapy after complete resection in rhabdomyosarcoma: A report from the Intergroup Rhabdomyosarcoma Studies (IRS) I to III. J Clin Oncol 1999;17:3468.

124. Young JL, et al: Cancer incidence, survival, and mortality for children younger than 15 years. Cancer 1986;58:598.

Chapter 33

Other Soft Tissue Tumors

Thom E. Lobe

Soft tissue tumors, primarily sarcomas, are a complex group of childhood malignancies of varied histologic subtypes. The prognosis depends on the histology, age, site, extent of involvement, and a variety of other factors. This chapter focuses on those tumors classified as non-rhabdomyosarcoma soft tissue sarcomas and other soft tissue tumors of childhood. The discussion focuses on three areas: (1) classification and nomenclature, (2) current multimodal therapy, and (3) the surgical approach to problematic tumor types and sites.

Soft tissue tumors in children constitute a diverse group of pathologic entities whose phenotypic variations parallel the multipotential nature of mesenchymal tissues. As noted in Table 33-1,[86] the phenotypic diversity is expressed by benign and malignant variants of each cell type. However, the terms *benign* and *malignant* do not necessarily match the potential clinical aggressiveness of these tumors. Some tumors in the benign group can be

easily treated by simple excision, such as hemangioma; others can recur and require extensive resection, such as desmoid-type fibromatosis. Similarly, the malignant group includes low-grade sarcomas, such as infantile fibrosarcoma, that have little propensity for metastasis, as well as high-grade sarcomas that often present with disseminated bone marrow disease. Some of these tumors are better considered reactive rather than neoplastic in nature; examples include nodular fasciitis and inflammatory myofibroblastic tumor.

Pediatric sarcomas show striking differences in incidence compared with their adult counterparts. A prime example is malignant fibrous histiocytoma, which is often the most common sarcoma in adult series but is rare in children. Only the angiomatoid variant, a low-grade lesion of borderline malignant behavior, occurs with sufficient frequency to be seen by most pediatric pathologists. Similar differences in frequency exist for liposarcoma

TABLE 33-1 Soft Tissue Tumors in Children

Tissue Type	Benign	Sarcomatous
Fat	Lipoblastoma (relatively common)	Liposarcoma (rare)
Blood and lymphatic vessels	Hemangioma, lymphangioma, and variants (very common)	Angiosarcoma (rare); hemangiopericytoma, infantile and adult variants (relatively rare)
Fibrous	Post-traumatic scar (common); fibromatosis and variants (common); nodular fasciitis (relatively common)	Fibrosarcoma, infantile and adult type (relatively rare)
Fibrohistiocytic	Fibrous histiocytoma and variants (common)	Malignant fibrous histiocytoma (rare)
Skeletal muscle	Rhabdomyoma (rare)	Rhabdomyosarcoma (common)
Smooth muscle	Leiomyoma (rare)	Leiomyosarcoma (rare)
Peripheral nervous tissue	Neurofibroma (relatively common); neurilemmoma (relatively uncommon)	Malignant peripheral nerve sheath tumors and variants; peripheral primitive neuroectodermal tumors (relatively common)
Synovial-like	Pigmented villonodular synovitis and related lesions (relatively rare)	Synovial sarcoma (relatively common)
Osseous	Myositis ossificans (relatively common)	Extraosseous osteosarcoma (very rare?)
Chondrocytic	Chondromas of soft tissue (rare)	Extraskeletal chondrosarcoma, myxoid vs mesenchymal (relatively rare)
Epithelial	?	Epithelioid sarcoma (relatively rare)
Melanocytic	?	Clear cell sarcoma of tendons and aponeuroses
Myofibroblastic	Inflammatory myofibroblastic tumor (relatively rare)	Myofibrosarcoma (rare)

and leiomyosarcoma. Conversely, rhabdomyosarcoma is by far the most common soft tissue malignancy in children but is rare in adults. In adults, rhabdomyosarcoma typically occurs as the pleomorphic variety, but the very existence of this cell type in children has been questioned.[80] Synovial sarcoma and neural tumors have an increased occurrence in children.

Surgeons must also be aware of the borderline "malignant" nature of many pediatric soft tissue tumors, a situation similar to that noted with epithelial surface tumors of the ovary. An example is the aforementioned angiomatoid malignant fibrous histiocytoma; the infrequency of metastases has led to the omission of the "malignant" qualifier by some investigators.[35] Other borderline lesions include epithelioid hemangioendothelioma, spindle cell hemangioendothelioma, and dermatofibrosarcoma protuberans. Occasionally, however, these lesions present with metastases, and the histologic appearance is often not predictive of this capacity.

Several examples of pediatric soft tissue tumors are relatively benign when they occur in infants and children younger than 5 years old but behave in a more typically aggressive fashion in older children. Infantile fibrosarcoma may appear high grade on histologic examination and form large, expansile extremity lesions on clinical presentation, yet the rarity of metastatic disease in these lesions is well known, and conservative therapy is advised.[67] A similar lesion is infantile hemangiopericytoma, whose behavior is akin to a benign vascular lesion in infants but is potentially more malignant in older children and adolescents.

Because of the inconsistencies in predicted behavior, the grading scheme for pediatric soft tissue sarcomas takes into account cytohistologic features used for adult sarcomas but employs the caveats of the childhood lesions (Table 33-2).[86,88] For example, fibrosarcomas are

---

TABLE 33-2 Pediatric Oncology Group Scheme for Grading Nonrhabdomyosarcomatous Pediatric Sarcomas

Grade 1
  Myxoid and well-differentiated liposarcoma
  Deep-seated dermatofibrosarcoma protuberans
  Well-differeniated or infantile (age <5yr) fibrosarcoma
  Well-differentiated or infantile (age <5yr) hemangiopericytoma
  Well-differentiated malignant peripheral nerve sheath tumor
  Angiomatoid malignant fibrous histiocytoma

Grade 2
  Sarcomas not specifically include in grades 1 or 3; <15% of tumor shows geographic necrosis or the mitotic index is <5 per 10 high-power fields

Grade 3
  Pleomorphic or round cell liposarcoma
  Mesenchymal chondrosarcoma
  Extraskeletal osteosarcoma
  Malignant triton tumor
  Alveolar soft part sarcoma
  Other sarcomas not specifically induced in grades 1 or 2, in which >15% of tumor shows geographic necrosis or the mitotic index is >4 per 10 high-power fields

---

low grade (grade 1) when they occur in children younger than 5 years, regardless of features such as mitotic index, necrosis, or cytology. In older children, however, they are grade 2 or 3, depending on whether the mitotic index is low (<5 per 10 high-power fields) or high (>4 per 10 high-power fields) or whether there is little (<15%) or abundant (>15%) geographic necrosis. Cytologic features such as pleomorphism and cellularity are used to distinguish ambiguous cases. This system should not be used with rhabdomyosarcoma or peripheral primitive neuroectodermal tumors (PNETs), which are always considered high grade and are best treated with a systematic approach using surgical resection, combination chemotherapy, and radiation.

Fibromatoses are a heterogeneous group of lesions, some of which are potentially lethal entities requiring wide excision and careful follow-up for cure. These tumors all contain benign-appearing fibroblasts as major constituents, but they vary in their affected age range, histologic patterns, typical location, tendency toward multifocality or chondroid differentiation, and likelihood of recurrence with incomplete surgical margins. One entity, fibrous hamartoma of infancy, contains a mixture of fat, mature fibrous tissue, and immature fibrous tissue and is typically located in the subcutis of the back and shoulder; it usually does not recur. In contrast, infantile desmoid-type fibromatosis is a more homogeneous, diffusely infiltrating mass of mature fibroblasts and fat that may occur in locations not easily amenable to surgical excision; it leads to significant morbidity or mortality by invasion of adjacent anatomic structures. Infantile desmoid-type fibromatosis is distinguished from infantile fibrosarcoma by virtue of its lack of cellular pleomorphism or mitotic activity, and it does not metastasize. Older children and adolescents may also have desmoid-type musculoaponeurotic fibromatosis, with similar histology and behavior. Some pharmacologic agents have been found to be of therapeutic utility,[8,31] but large numbers of patients have not been tested in a prospective, randomized clinical trial. Another entity is infantile myofibromatosis, which may occur as solitary or multicentric lesions; visceral involvement with the latter may prove lethal.

Diagnosis of pediatric soft tissue tumors may be accomplished with routine histology or even fine-needle aspiration,[116] but it often requires a battery of special techniques that may include histochemistry, immunohistochemistry, electron microscopy, cytogenetics, flow cytometry, in situ hybridization, or reverse transcriptase polymerase chain reaction (RT-PCR). In general, because of their primitive, undifferentiated nature, round cell lesions require more extensive study, whereas spindle cell lesions are more likely to be diagnosed by routine histology if sufficient tissue is available. Paradoxically, round cell tumors usually yield better specimens on fine-needle aspiration cytology, whereas the more cohesive spindle cell lesions often give inadequate or insufficient samples by this technique. Close interaction among oncologists, surgeons, and pathologists is required to maximize diagnostic yield and utility. Occasional life-threatening situations may require an expedited diagnosis with less than adequate material. When time allows, however, a precise and accurate diagnosis is invaluable in clinical management.

The time required for the turnaround of ancillary data ranges from 1 day or less for immunohistochemistry and RT-PCR to several days for electron microscopy to 2 weeks for cytogenetics. The availability and reliability of these techniques depend on the nature and amount of material submitted; fresh tissue is required for cytogenetics and RT-PCR, and special fixation is required for electron microscopy and possibly for immunohistochemistry. RT-PCR has the advantage of extreme sensitivity, so only a small specimen is required. Cytogenetics may give misleading results if the specimen is contaminated by normal host tissues, or no results if there is poor sample viability.

Diagnostic features of the more common round and spindle cell sarcomas are listed in Table 33-3.[86] The initial pathologic evaluation generally attempts to determine first whether the lesion is benign or malignant and second whether it is a round or spindle cell tumor. Then a differential diagnosis is constructed, and special studies are acquired as necessary to eliminate or confirm the diagnostic possibilities. The differential diagnosis of a completely undifferentiated round cell tumor includes a variety of lesions, with the most likely candidates being rhabdomyosarcoma, lymphoma, neuroblastoma, PNET, or soft tissue Ewing's tumor. Immunohistochemical stains for desmin and muscle-specific actin (muscle markers), CD45 and other lymphoid markers, neuron-specific enolase and synaptophysin (neural markers), and vimentin and CD99 (Ewing's markers) are evaluated. The combination of results is usually of great utility in weighing the alternatives, but many caveats exist. For example, neuron-specific enolase is a sensitive neural marker but is often positive in rhabdomyosarcoma, so its presence is more helpful in the absence of muscle markers. Similarly, CD99 is a very sensitive and relatively specific marker of PNET, but it is also commonly found in T-cell lymphomas. Neural markers may be present in both PNET and neuroblastoma, but the latter are CD99 negative. Finally, some tumors such as primitive ectomesenchymoma commonly display multipotential differentiation patterns with positivity for diagnostically disparate markers. In these confusing situations, it is wise to consider results from alternative methods such as electron microscopy and cytogenetics.

NONRHABDOMYOSARCOMATOUS SOFT TISSUE SARCOMA

Malignant soft tissue sarcomas are derived from mesenchymal cells and account for 7% of all childhood tumors.[74,121] These tumors encompass two major histologic subgroups: rhabdomyosarcoma and nonrhabdomyosarcomatous soft tissue sarcomas. Rhabdomyosarcoma (see Chapter 32) is the most common soft tissue sarcoma in children and accounts for more than half of all cases of childhood soft tissue sarcomas, with 250 newly diagnosed patients encountered yearly in the United States.[87,121] Nonrhabdomyosarcomatous soft tissue sarcomas (NRSTSs) are a heterogeneous group of malignancies; they account for 47% of all pediatric soft tissue sarcomas and for 3% of all pediatric cancers.[74,75] The clinical behavior of these tumors has not been well defined.[75,99,121] Their rarity and histologic heterogeneity have precluded careful study of their natural history and response to therapy. Therefore, much of the information regarding treatment of these tumors in pediatric patients has been derived from adult studies. Further, despite their aggressive pathologic appearance, some subtypes of pediatric NRSTS (e.g., infantile fibrosarcoma) have a relatively benign clinical course after treatment with surgery alone.[23,75]

NRSTS, like rhabdomyosarcoma, can arise in any part of the body. Two series totaling 322 pediatric patients indicated that the most common sites were the extremities, trunk, and abdomen and pelvis.[79,99] Some sites such as the eye and orbit[18] and the breast[28] are extremely rare. In these series, synovial sarcoma, neurofibrosarcoma, malignant fibrous histiocytoma, and fibrosarcoma were the most frequent histologies.[97,99] NRSTSs have been associated with Li-Fraumeni syndrome, and some tumors (e.g., malignant fibrous histiocytoma) can develop in previously irradiated sites.[75] Approximately 4% of patients with neurofibromatosis type 1 (NF-1) develop malignant peripheral nerve sheath tumors; 40% of these rare malignancies are seen in patients with NF-1.[27] Leiomyosarcoma can occur in children infected with human immunodeficiency virus (HIV) and Epstein-Barr virus.[70]

Pediatric soft tissue sarcomas are increasingly being defined by both histologic appearance and underlying chromosomal abnormalities to determine their biologic behavior. Most sarcomas of this type have specific chromosomal translocations that create unique fusion genes. These fusion genes may have diagnostic, prognostic, and surveillance implications for the patient.[5]

Prognostic factors in children with NRSTS include whether the tumor can be resected, tumor size, histologic grade, tumor invasiveness, and the presence or absence of metastatic disease.[84,98] In a review of 37 children with synovial sarcoma, the 5-year probability of survival was $80 \pm 9\%$ for patients with completely resected lesions, compared with $17 \pm 15\%$ for those with unresected or metastatic lesions.[84] Of 154 children with NRSTS who were treated at a single institution, 31% with grade 1 or 2 lesions had treatment failure, and 73% with grade 3 disease developed recurrent disease. Similarly, 88% of those with large, invasive, grade 3 lesions failed therapy, compared with 2% of children with small, low-grade, noninvasive lesions.[99]

Unlike rhabdomyosarcoma, which is a highly chemosensitive tumor, the mainstay of treatment for NRSTS is complete surgical resection with or without adjuvant radiotherapy to prevent local recurrence. Several prospective adult trials of NRSTS failed to document a survival benefit of adjuvant chemotherapy.[72,127] The only prospective pediatric trial addressing the value of adjuvant chemotherapy was conducted by the Pediatric Oncology Group (POG). In this trial, 75 children with completely resected lesions were assigned either to receive adjuvant chemotherapy with vincristine, dactinomycin, cyclophosphamide, and doxorubicin or to be simply observed. The 3-year disease-free survival rates for these two groups did not differ (74% versus 76%). Subgroup analysis disclosed that patients with grade 3 lesions fared significantly worse than those with grade 1 or 2 disease (3-year event-free survival, 75% versus 91%; $P = 0.018$).[88] Distant relapse accounted for more than

TABLE 33-3 Differential Diagnosis of Relatively Common Pediatric Soft Tissue Sarcomas

Tumor	Immunohistochemistry	Electron Microscopy	Cytogenetics	RT-PCR or Other Molecular Technique	Other
Round Cell					
Rhabdomyosarcoma	Desmin, muscle actin, MyoD	Thick and thin filaments, Z bands, pools of glycogen, primitive cytoplasm, neurosecretory granules,	t(1;13); t(2;13) (alveolar only)	PAX7;FHKHR PAX3;FHKHR	PAS stain for glycogen
PNET, Ewing's tumor	CD99, synaptophysin, vimentin, NSE		t(11;22), t(21;22)	Fli-1;EWS ERG;EWS	PAS stain for glycogen; absent reticulin
Lymphoma	CD45, CD45RO, CD20, CD3, CD43, CD30	primitive cytoplasm, lack of inter-cellular junctions	Burkitt's: t(2;8), t(8;14), t(8;22) Anaplastic large cell: +(2;5)	Burkitt's: c-myc;IgH; c-myc; Igk: c-myc;Igλ ALK;ALM	Flow cytometry; consider extranodal
Desmoplastic small cell tumor	Vimentin, cytokeratin desmin, Synaptophysin, NSE, CD57	Not diagnostic	t(11;22)(p13;q12)	WT1;EWS	Characteristic desmoplastic stroma
Langerhans cell histiocytosis	S100, CD1a, peanut lectin	Birbeck granules	Not diagnostic	Not diagnostic	Eosinophils frequent
Neuroblastoma	NSE, synaptophysin, chromagranin (weak)	Processes with microtubules, neurosecretory granules, synaptic junctions	1p deletions, double minutes, homogeneous staining regions (nonspecific)	N-myc amplification (may be seen in alveolar rhabdomyosarcoma	Ganglionic differentiation; urinary catecholamines; CD99 negative
Spindle Cell					
Synovial sarcoma	Cytokeratin, EMA	Epithelial differentiation process, Luse bodies, basal lamina, pseudomesaxons	t(X;18)	SSX1;SYT SSX2;SYT	Beware confusion due to neural invasion
Malignant peripheral nerve sheath tumor	S100, CD57, GFAP		None	Deletion of NF-1?	History of neurofibromatosis; origin within major nerve; coexisting neurofibroma
Fibrosarcoma, myofibrosarcoma	Vimentin, smooth muscle actin	Lamellae of RER, terminal web, actin microfilaments, collagen granules, fibronexus junctions, pinocytotic vesicles	None	None	Inflammatory variants described; consider inflammatory myofibroblastic tumor

PNET, primitive neuroectodermal tumor; RT-PCR, reverse transcriptase-polymerase chain reaction; NF-1, neurofibromatosis type1; NSE, neuron-specific enolase

80% of the failures in the high-grade group. These data suggest that a prospective trial of adjuvant chemotherapy in children with high-grade, completely resected NRSTS may be warranted if prospective trials of children with unresectable or metastatic NRSTS identify active agents.

The outcome for children with metastatic NRSTSs continues to be poor, with less than 20% of patients disease free at 3 years.[84,95] Surgical resection is the treatment of choice for most NRSTSs. The role of chemotherapy and radiation therapy is poorly defined. Evaluation of the role of chemotherapy has been limited by the lack of randomized, controlled trials. The POG attempted to randomize patients after surgical resection of NRSTS (clinical groups I and II) to chemotherapy (vincristine, doxorubicin, cyclophosphamide, dactinomycin) or observation.[96] Of the 81 eligible patients, only 30 accepted randomization. The patients who received chemotherapy (both randomized and nonrandomized) did worse; however, this is likely due to a greater number of high-grade tumors among the treated patients. The most active drugs against NRSTS include ifosfamide and doxorubicin.[29] A prospective POG trial for children with unresectable or metastatic NRSTS compared VADRAC (vincristine, doxorubicin [Adriamycin], cytoxan) with VADRAC plus dacarbazine (DTIC). DTIC conferred no additional benefit: the 4-year overall and event-free survival estimates were 30.6 ± 8.5% and 18.4 ± 6.8%, respectively.[95] Identification of new agents in phase I and II trials, intensification of known active agents and concomitant growth factor support, and administration of preoperative chemotherapy are strategies that may help improve the outcome for children with NRSTS.

Children with metastatic disease, particularly those older than 10 years or those with bone or bone marrow involvement, tend to have a poor outcome and need new treatment options. The use of high-dose single, multiple, or combined chemotherapy-radiotherapy regimens with stem cell rescue has, for the most part, failed to improve the poor outcome, but this remains the cornerstone of today's clinical trials.[5]

Radiotherapy is generally administered for microscopic residual disease or histologic evidence of tumor extending close to the margin of resection and may be indicated for group I tumors larger than 5 cm. The efficacy of radiotherapy has not been proved, however, and the adverse effects of radiation exposure in children, including effects on body growth and secondary cancers, make its use in small, totally resected tumors questionable. Spunt et al.[114] described 121 patients with group I and II NRSTSs treated at St. Jude Children's Hospital. Radiation reduced the risk of local recurrence in group II patients but had no impact on event-free survival. Radiation did not impact local recurrence in patients with group I disease.

Pediatric soft tissue sarcomas arising as second malignancies can be cured using the same strategies used for de novo pediatric sarcomas.[11]

Synovial Sarcoma

Synovial sarcoma is one of the most common NRSTSs seen in pediatric patients; approximately 30% of synovial sarcomas occur in patients younger than 20 years. There are few reports concerning synovial sarcoma in pediatric patients.[38,63,82,84,107] As in adults, most of these sarcomas arise in the extremities, most commonly the lower extremity. Other common sites are the trunk and the head and neck. The 5-year event-free survival rate is approximately 70% for all pediatric patients; however, survival is approximately 80% for those with group I and II tumors and 0% to 58% for patients with group III and IV tumors. The outcome appears similar to that seen in adults. Because most reports include only adults or only children, and because different staging systems are used, direct comparison is difficult. Local recurrences are common, with metastases primarily to lung but also to lymph nodes.[38] Late relapses are common, and survival curves continue to fall off even at 10 and 15 years.

The primary treatment for synovial sarcoma is surgical resection. There are many reports of response to chemotherapy, but no study has clearly shown that chemotherapy improves survival. The CWS-81 study treated patients initially with chemotherapy using combinations of vincristine, doxorubicin, cyclophosphamide or ifosfamide, and actinomycin D. In five patients with group III and IV tumors, a complete response was seen in two and a partial response in three; complete resection and long-term survival were achieved in all five patients.[63] The use of high-dose ifosfamide (14 to 18 g/m^2) in 13 adult patients with metastatic disease resulted in a response in all patients treated. Most responses were partial or transient, but when combined with surgical resection of residual disease, disease-free status was noted in four patients at 3, 14, 21, and 42 months, respectively.[103] These data suggest that chemotherapy may have a role in shrinking tumors to permit subsequent surgical resection, but the use of chemotherapy in an adjuvant setting is unproved for synovial sarcoma. The optimal treatment strategy for synovial sarcoma is thus subject to debate, and different strategies have been used for pediatric and adult patients. One retrospective analysis examined a large group of patients of all ages treated at a single institution over a 30-year period. The study included 271 patients ranging in age from 5 to 87 years; 255 had localized disease that was macroscopically resected in 215 cases and was deemed unresectable at diagnosis in 40 cases. Chemotherapy was administered to 41% of patients, corresponding to 76% of patients aged 16 years of younger and less than 20% of older patients; 28% of patients with macroscopically resected disease received chemotherapy on an adjuvant basis. The overall 5-year event-free survival rate for the study cohort was 37%, although this rate varied with age (66% for patients aged 16 years or younger, 40% for those 17 to 30 years, and 31% for those older than 30 years). Among patients with surgically resected tumors, the 5-year metastasis-free survival rate was 60% for those treated with chemotherapy versus 48% for those who were not. The benefit associated with chemotherapy appeared greatest for patients aged 17 years or older who had tumors measuring greater than 5 cm (metastasis-free survival 47% with chemotherapy versus 27% without chemotherapy). In the subgroup of patients with measurable disease, the rate of tumor response to chemotherapy was approximately 48%.

Although the authors await more convincing proof of the efficacy of adjuvant chemotherapy in the treatment of adult soft tissue sarcoma, they recommend that patients with high-risk synovial sarcoma (tumor size >5 cm) be the first to be considered for this type of treatment.[40]

Radiotherapy for synovial sarcoma is often used for microscopic residual disease or histologic evidence of tumor close to the resected margin. As with other NRSTSs, its efficacy has not been proved, and radiation's negative effects on growth in children and the risk of secondary cancers and other late effects make its use in small, totally resected tumors questionable.[89]

Genetic evaluation of synovial sarcoma tumor tissue shows a poorer outcome for tumors associated with the SYT-SSX fusion type.[62] This fusion type is more common in patients presenting with metastases than is SYT-SSX2; in patients with localized disease, SYT-SSX1 is associated with a shorter overall survival time.

Certain primary sites, such as synovial sarcoma of the hand, are rare. No clear guidelines exist with regard to their management. A functional limb-saving approach, without compromising the principles of cancer management, should be individualized in each case.[51]

Primary renal synovial sarcomas are now an accepted entity and are likely a subset of what was previously considered an adult variant of Wilms' tumor.[3]

Infantile Fibrosarcoma

Infantile fibrosarcoma is the most common soft tissue sarcoma of infants, accounting for about half of fibrosarcomas in the pediatric population. These tumors usually present as a slowly enlarging mass that may have been present for months to years. Most occur on the extremities, but head and neck tumors are also common. The name *infantile* fibrosarcoma is a misnomer, because the improved prognosis it implies and the chromosomal changes associated with this tumor are also seen in children up to about 5 years of age. Younger children with fibrosarcoma also have a good prognosis, with a better than 90% long-term survival rate. Although childhood fibrosarcoma has a recurrence rate of about 50%, the metastatic potential is less than 10%.[24,113]

Infantile fibrosarcoma grows rapidly, infiltrates locally, but rarely metastasizes. Although complete surgical resection is curative, it is not always possible. Neoadjuvant chemotherapy causes many tumors to shrink sufficiently to allow resection. There does not seem to be a role for adjuvant chemotherapy or radiation after complete resection. Although recurrence is frequent, most cases can be managed with additional surgical excision. Overall survival is greater than 90%.[37]

Because of the typically benign course of infantile fibrosarcoma in children younger than 5 years, conservative surgical procedures are recommended to preserve function. Infantile fibrosarcoma is generally responsive to chemotherapy and in some instances can be successful as initial therapy.[60,110] Spontaneous regression has also been reported in infantile fibrosarcoma.[67] Pulmonary fibrosarcoma is a rare malignant tumor in childhood. In the absence of metastasis, complete resection appears to be curative.[91] Similar results can be expected with fibrosarcoma of the trachea.[93]

Hemangiopericytoma

Only 5% to 10% of hemangiopericytomas occur in children and adolescents,[34,57] and many of these are infantile hemangiopericytoma, an entity with a more benign course than that seen in older patients. The infantile form is more likely to occur in the head and neck and has a low metastatic potential.

Infants with incomplete removal of hemangiopericytoma often do well with no further therapy.[6] Responses to chemotherapy have been reported.[4,6] Congenital hemangiopericytoma generally does not metastasize and has a good prognosis, although some instances of metastases and death have been reported.[6] Spontaneous resolution has been reported after biopsy alone.[21]

This lesion can present in odd locations, such as a thyroglossal duct remnant,[50] on rare occasions. This tumor can mimic a benign arteriovenous malformation that is sometimes still referred to as an "angioma."[76] It has also been reported to occur in association with trisomy 15 as a sole anomaly.[117]

Neurogenic Sarcoma

Neurogenic tumors (malignant peripheral nerve sheath tumors, neurofibrosarcomas, neurosarcomas, and malignant schwannomas) often present with pain or neurologic symptoms that have been present for prolonged periods before diagnosis. Neurogenic sarcomas may arise de novo or from a preexisting fibroma. In pediatric series, NF-1 was present in 21% to 62% of patients.[17,32,71] Less than 5% of patients with NF-1 develop a sarcoma, however.[112]

Primary sarcomas of the central nervous system are rare in children. Their cell of origin is controversial, but the most widely accepted theory names the pluripotential primitive mesenchymal cells in the dura mater, the leptomeninges or their pial extensions into the brain and the spinal cord along the periadventitial spaces, the choroidea, and the stroma of the choroid plexus. The reported incidence of sarcomas at this site varies from 0.1% to 4.3%, owing to the inconsistent definitions from study to study. These tumors frequently arise in the supratentorial compartment in children. Dural attachment and central nervous system dissemination are often found. Metastasis outside the central nervous system is associated with a poor prognosis, although aggressive resection with postoperative radiation may offer a chance for long-term survival. Repeat craniotomy should be offered for recurrent local disease. Newer chemotherapy protocols may hold promise in the future.[1]

These are very aggressive tumors, and radical surgery is the primary treatment. In patients with NF-1, the tumors present at an earlier age and recur and metastasize more quickly and more frequently.[33,71,126] Malignant peripheral nerve sheath tumors are rare and usually fatal, with a high risk of local recurrence and distant metastasis.[115]

Complete excision is the most important prognostic factor, with a 5-year disease-free survival rate of 67%. With microscopic residual tumor, the 5-year disease-free survival rate is 43%; this falls to 22% when the tumor is not completely resected because recurrence is inevitable, with most tumors metastasizing to the lungs.[126] External beam radiation does not appear to impact survival, but brachytherapy (BRT) and intraoperative radiation are beneficial.[126]

Liposarcoma

Although liposarcoma is one of the more common soft tissue sarcomas in adults, it is rare in children.[19,39,64,111] Gross total resection is the indicated treatment. Tumor shrinkage to allow for complete excision has been achieved with radiation[19] and chemotherapy.[39] Adjuvant chemotherapy or radiation has been used in children with microscopic residual tumor, but its effectiveness has not been documented.[39,64] The 5-year survival rates in extremity liposarcoma in adults is dependent on histologic subtype and are as follows: for well-differentiated tumors, 100%; for myxoid tumors, 88%; for fibroblastic tumors, 58%; for pleomorphic tumors, 56%; and for lipoblastic tumors, 40%.[20] The better prognosis in children with liposarcoma compared with adults may be related to the higher incidence of myxoid and well-differentiated subtypes (70% to 85% of pediatric liposarcomas).

Desmoplastic Small Round Cell Tumor

Desmoplastic small round cell tumor occurs primarily in young men who present with pain, ascites, abdominal distention or mass, nausea and vomiting, or signs of bowel or bladder obstruction. Presentation with widely disseminated metastases to liver, lungs, and lymph nodes is common.[45] Although the precise tumor type may be difficult to determine, the RT-PCR method for formalin-fixed material has a 94% to 100% specificity for tumor type.[43]

Because of widespread dissemination at presentation, complete surgical resection is rarely possible. Response to chemotherapy, including high-dose chemotherapy and autologous stem cell rescue, has been documented.[10,36,46,61,104] Long-term survival remains dependent on the ability to resect all gross disease after neoadjuvant chemotherapy. Radiation therapy may be of benefit in treating microscopic residual disease. The use of radiofrequency for the ablation of unresectable hepatic metastasis in desmoplastic small round cell tumor may be effective.[30]

Malignant Melanoma of Soft Parts

Approximately 25% of these tumors occur in patients younger than 20 years. Most patients present with an enlarging mass in the extremities that has been present for a long time.[25,106] Local recurrence is common. Metastases occur to lung (59%), lymph nodes (53%), and bone (22%).

Treatment is surgical excision. The median overall survival duration is 49 months,[106] but patients with metastases at diagnosis generally survive less than 1 year. Local relapses and metastases can occur years after diagnosis and treatment. The role of adjuvant chemotherapy or radiation is uncertain for these tumors.[44]

Alveolar Soft Part Sarcoma

Approximately 25% of alveolar soft part sarcomas are seen in patients younger than 20 years. This tumor is predominant in women (61%), especially in younger patients.[66] Presentation consists of a painless enlarging mass of the extremity, with head and neck tumors also common in children.[16,85] It occurs in 0.8% to 1.8% of children. Mean length of survival is 20 years in patients age 0 to 9 years at diagnosis and 14 years in those age 10 to 19 years. Tumors greater than 5 cm in diameter have an increased risk of metastasis, which usually occurs early in the disease. Excision of metastasis can influence survival.[83] Approximately 20% of patients have metastases at diagnosis. Metastases can sometimes occur many years after the initial diagnosis and affect the lung, bone, and brain.

Treatment is primarily surgical, with complete excision being the best treatment. There is a low risk of local recurrence if adequate margins are obtained. In patients presenting with metastatic disease at diagnosis, the median survival duration is 3 years.[66] Younger patients have a longer survival time, but this is related primarily to a lower incidence of metastases at diagnosis.[66,85] According to the Soft-Tissue Sarcoma Italian Cooperative Group, pediatric alveolar soft part sarcoma has a more favorable prognosis than its adult counterpart.[16]

SPECIAL DIAGNOSTIC AND SURGICAL CONSIDERATIONS

New Imaging Modalities

Magnetic resonance spectroscopy appears to be effective in assessing tumor response in childhood cancer and could potentially be used to tailor chemotherapy to the individual child's needs.[118] The prognostic significance of magnetic resonance spectroscopy has been studied in sarcomas of the extremity, where the aim was to determine whether pretreatment spectra might be useful in defining good- versus poor-risk tumors and to determine whether changes that occur early during the course of therapy can be useful to predict tumor response.[59]

Fluorodeoxyglucose positron emission tomography scans have been assessed for their diagnostic and therapeutic role in childhood sarcomas through a systematic review of the relevant literature and a meta-analysis. There is no apparent indication for the use of this modality in the standard treatment of sarcomas at present, although it may be used for the detection, grading, treatment, and evaluation of locally advanced sarcomas.[7]

Biopsy and Surgery

The value of fine-needle aspiration is primarily to differentiate a solid mass from a fluid-containing mass or an abscess that may require drainage. In all other instances, at a minimum, a Tru-Cut needle biopsy is warranted.[12,52,65,94,99,100] Although needle tract recurrences have been documented, these are extremely rare events and are more common among patients with carcinoma.[108] When the tissue obtained is insufficient to obtain a specific diagnosis or a discrepancy exists, an open biopsy is indicated. For extremity lesions, the incision should be placed longitudinally or parallel to the neurovascular bundle. A transverse biopsy incision would contaminate multiple tissue compartments and thus preclude limb salvage surgery.[73,99,101] An excisional biopsy of a lesion is undertaken only if the tumor is small (< 2.5 cm) or situated such that an eventual wide local resection could be done without risk of functional deformity.[119] In all other instances, an incisional biopsy is obtained and should be carefully planned and placed, so that the tract can be *completely* excised at the time of definitive surgery.

It has been shown repeatedly that when resection is planned for a benign tumor or when resection of a malignant lesion is not carefully planned, the quality and amount of tumor resection are inadequate. In these instances, residual tumor can be identified following primary re-excision in 30% to 49% of patients.[12,14,47,99,102,122,124] If primary radical resection is not performed, local recurrence rates of 50% to 90% have been observed.[13,14,47,55,99,102,128] Therefore, whenever diagnostic imaging, the operative notes, or pathologic examination suggests that there is residual tumor or that the tumor is close to the specimen margin, it is recommended that the patient undergo primary re-excision of the operative site whenever possible.[12,14,58,99,101,119,125]

EXTREMITY TUMORS

Two major factors have contributed to reduced amputation rates in children with soft tissue sarcoma. First, although amputation results in a high rate of local control, it fails to improve overall survival.[14,55,99,102,122,124,125] Second, limb salvage procedures with or without adjuvant radiation therapy have effectively decreased local recurrence rates to less than 10%.[22,41,42,77,99,122,124] Although amputation may be logical in an elderly patient, it is not the best choice for a growing child. Amputation in adult patients obviates the musculoskeletal deformity or the risk of a second malignancy.[14,94,99,101,102]

The surgical principle is to obtain a wide local resection with adequate margins, generally considered to be about 2 cm.[101,119] Depending on the size and site of the tumor, wide local resection may be obtained by means of a radical compartmental resection, resection of a muscle from insertion to origin, or radical wide local resection.* Although wide margins are obtained in most directions,

---

*See references 12, 14, 53, 55, 92, 99, 102, 119, 122, 124.

in certain situations, especially in the vicinity of major nerves or vessels, the margins may be only a few millimeters. In this case, it is advisable to remove the adventitial sheath along with the specimen.[55,102] Although resection is the primary concern, dissection is often tailored to the individual patient, based on preoperative diagnostic imaging.

The skin from the previous biopsy site is completely ellipsed, and the flaps are raised. The deeper extent of the dissection is usually initiated on one side 2 to 3 cm from the tumor. Often the deep margins overlie the vessels or nerve. In this case, the adventitial sheath or perineural sheath adjacent to the tumor should be resected to acquire a little more margin. If the vessel is grossly involved, resection of the vessel with interposition of a vascular prosthesis can be considered. If the tumor abuts the bone, stripping of the periosteum, marginal resection of the bone, or resection of a segment of the bone can be performed. In these instances, the bony defect may be bridged by a vascularized fibula graft or allograft plus intramedullary nails.

In the popliteal fossa and the elbow, compartmental resection of a tumor with satisfactory margins is almost impossible because of the complex neurovascular anatomy, the loose connective tissue, and the close confines of adjacent structures.[90,105,109] These tumors are not confined by fascial boundaries and are considered extra-compartmental. It is my policy to maintain limb function whenever feasible with resection of these lesions, albeit with tenuous margins. Radiation therapy is added for local control in the form of interstitial brachytherapy, external beam radiation, or a combination of both. Major ablative procedures such as amputation should be considered when there is neurovascular involvement, for local recurrence, and in a skeletally immature child.

A similar situation arises in lesions of the hand or foot, which are relatively uncommon primary sites. The tight compartments interspersed with tendons and neurovascular bundles make resection with adequate margins difficult. Surgical procedures may include ray amputation of one or more digits, wide local excision of the area, and supplemental radiation or use of a neurovascular free transfer technique, especially in the case of resection of the thumb.[15,48,49,54] In the lower extremity, amputation still has a role in the management of large, high-grade invasive tumors or when combination therapy could result in a poor functional outcome. Amputation may also be appropriate for pain control, especially in a weight-bearing limb, and for recurrent local disease.

This combined-modality management has led to 90% to 95% limb salvage in NRSTS, with local recurrence rates in the vicinity of 10%.[12,99,101,122,124] In recent years, better understanding of tumor biology and improved techniques for the delivery of radiation have emerged. Radiation therapy may be administered preoperatively, intraoperatively, or postoperatively.[22,26,42,81,122,123]

MANAGEMENT OF EXTREMITY LYMPH NODE DRAINAGE

The role of regional node dissection in soft tissue sarcoma has become clearer in recent years. In a collective review of more than 2500 cases of NRSTS, the incidence of nodal involvement was around 3.9%. In the same series, the authors detected a slightly increasing incidence of lymph node metastasis with increasing tumor grade, ranging from 0% for grade 1 lesions to 12% for grade 3 lesions.[69] In a review of NRSTS at St. Jude Children's Hospital, a similar range was noted.[114] In another review, 76 of 204 patients underwent either lymph node dissection or biopsy of suspicious lesions; it was positive for tumor in nine, and in seven of the nine children the tumors were high-grade lesions.[48,99,101,102] It is my practice to biopsy only suspicious nodes of high-grade lesions that are more than 5 cm in size, or if the lymph nodes are present in the field of dissection of the primary tumor.

When lymph node involvement is suspected in extremity tumors, it can be assessed by injection with iso-sulfan blue dye into the lesion at the time of surgery. Uptake of the dye into the nodes draining the lesion can be determined in this fashion (Fig. 33-1).

Mandell et al.[68] evaluated 34 patients with extremity rhabdomyosarcoma, 27 of whom underwent evaluation of regional lymph node drainage. Thirteen patients (48%) demonstrated evidence of nodal involvement, only one of whom survived. In contrast, there were 12 survivors among the 14 patients without nodal involvement. Even when patients with distant metastasis were excluded, 11 of the 12 patients with no nodal

involvement survived. The need for nodal assessment in all patients with extremity rhabdomyosarcoma was confirmed in an analysis of Intergroup Rhabdomyosarcoma Study-III.[2]

FUNCTIONAL OUTCOME FOLLOWING LIMB SALVAGE SURGERY

Over the past two and a half decades, limb salvage surgery with adjuvant irradiation has emerged as the optimal treatment and has been performed on a substantial number of patients. Although the outcome of this combined modality addresses primarily cosmetic concerns, in young children and particularly the skeletally immature, attention should be given not only to quality of life but also to associated local complications, including a stiff, painful, shortened, or disfigured extremity or fractures associated with demineralization of bone.[9,54,56,120] Children should have active physical therapy to minimize contracture. Use of the Musculoskeletal Tumor Society functional outcome evaluation has been detailed mostly in the adult literature. Excellent to good results were obtained in 75% to 80% of patients, with more than 75% returning to full employment. A similar detailed study in the pediatric literature is lacking. Complications noted in my experience among long-term survivors after combined treatment include limb shortening requiring epiphysiodesis, flexion

A

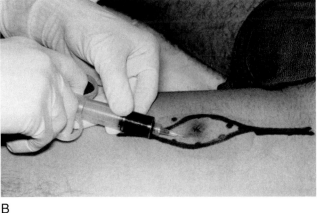

B

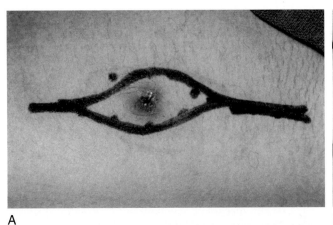

C

Figure 33–1 *A*, Epithelioid sarcoma of the left lower extremity. Note the longitudinal orientation of the proposed incision relative to the extremity, so that a wider excision can be carried out if required. *B*, Isosulfan blue is injected into the lesion before excision is carried out. *C*, A draining lymph node is identified containing the dye. (Courtesy of Dr. Bhaskar Rao, St. Jude Children's Research Hospital, Memphis, Tenn.)

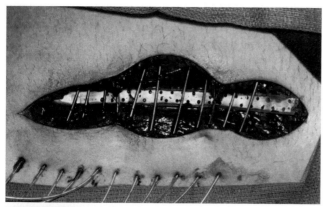

Figure 33–2 Afterloading catheters are placed for brachytherapy in the patient with epithelioid sarcoma depicted in Figure 33-1. (Courtesy of Dr. Bhaskar Rao, St. Jude Children's Research Hospital, Memphis, Tenn.)

deformity, fibrosis, chronic edema, fracture, and secondary osteosarcoma in 7 of 50 long-term survivors with extremity sarcoma. These patients have been followed for 12 to 104 months (median, 36 months).

SOFT TISSUE SARCOMA OF THE TRUNK

When a chest wall resection is indicated, a standard thoracotomy incision is appropriate. The investing layer of the serratus anterior or pectoralis is incised at an appropriate distance from the tumor. Careful palpation should be used to gauge the extent of resection, which may include resection of the periosteum with placement of afterloading catheters for brachytherapy. However, if imaging studies or visualization at the time of surgery indicates infiltration of the intercostal muscles or intrathoracic extension, a formal chest wall resection is indicated. The intercostal muscles are divided at an appropriate point, after ligation of the intercostal vessels. Careful palpation of the intrathoracic extension determines the extent of resection and the number of ribs to be removed. The anterior and posterior extent of resection should be 2.5 to 5 cm. The superior and posterior extent is generally a rib above or below the primary lesion. Any adhesions between the pulmonary parenchyma and tumor are excised using an endoscopic linear stapler, so that the specimen can be removed en bloc. The resultant defect is closed by a double layer of mesh and neighboring muscle flaps or myocutaneous flaps.

The abdominal wall is a rare primary tumor site. Accurate preoperative imaging can determine tumor resectability. The entire extent of the tumor is resected to obtain satisfactory margins. The deep margins should include resection of the peritoneum whenever possible. The peritoneal defect may be closed by an omental patch or absorbable mesh. Direct contact between the nonabsorbable mesh and the bowel should be avoided to reduce the risk of bowel fistula. It is my policy, especially in the case of lower abdominal wall lesions, to place the bowel loops away from the postoperative radiation field

by means of absorbable mesh and to deliver at least a portion of the radiation therapy dose as brachytherapy. Brachytherapy increases local control and reduces the probability of late complications (especially altered bone and organ growth) in comparison to external beam radiation (Fig. 33-2). Low-energy radionuclides and remote afterloading technology allow the treatment of infants and very young children while reducing radiation exposure to patients, family, and medical personnel.[78]

REFERENCES

1. Al-gahtany M, Shroft M, Bouffet E, et al: Primary central nervous system sarcomas in children: Clinical, radiological, and pathological features. Childs Nerv Syst 2003;19: 808-817.
2. Andrassy RJ, Corpron CA, Hays D, et al: Extremity sarcomas: An analysis of prognostic factors from the Intergroup Rhabdomyosarcoma Study III. J Pediatr Surg 1996;31: 191-196.
3. Argani P, Ladanyi M: Recent advances in pediatric renal neoplasia. Adv Anat Pathol 2003;10:243-260.
4. Atkinson JB, Mahour JB, Isaacs H, et al: Hemangiopericytoma in infants and children: A report of six patients. Am J Surg 1984;148:372-374.
5. Atra A, Pinkerton R: High-dose chemotherapy in soft tissue sarcoma in children. Crit Rev Oncol Hematol 2002;41: 191-196.
6. Bailey PV, Webber TR, Tracy TF, et al: Congenital hemangiopericytoma: An unusual vascular neoplasm of infancy. Surgery 1993;114:936-941.
7. Bastiaannet E, Groen H, Jager PL, et al: The value of FDG-PET in the detection, grading and response to therapy of soft tissue and bone sarcomas: A systematic review and meta-analysis. Cancer Treat Rev 2004;30:83-101.
8. Bauernhofer T, Stoger H, Schmid M, et al: Sequential treatment of recurrent mesenteric desmoid tumor. Cancer 1996;77:1061-1065.
9. Bell RS, O'Sullivan B, Davis A, et al: Functional outcome in patients treated with surgery and irradiation for soft tissue tumours. J Surg Oncol 1991;48:224-231.
10. Bisogno G, Roganovich J, Sotti G, et al: Desmoplastic small round cell tumour in children and adolescents. Med Pediatr Oncol 2000;34:338-342.
11. Bisogno G, Sotti G, Nowicki Y, et al: Soft tissue sarcoma as a second malignant neoplasm in the pediatric age group. Cancer 2004;100:1758-1765.
12. Brennan MF: Management of soft tissue sarcoma. Aust N Z J Surg 1990;60:419-428.
13. Brennan MF: The enigma of local recurrence. Ann Surg Oncol 1997;4:1-12.
14. Brennan MF, Casper ES, Harrison L, et al: The role of multimodality therapy in soft-tissue sarcoma. Ann Surg 1991; 214:328-338.
15. Brien EW, Terek RM, Geer RJ, et al: Treatment of soft-tissue sarcomas of the hand. J Bone Joint Surg Am 1995;77:564-571.
16. Casanova M, Ferrari A, Bisogno G, et al: Alveolar soft part sarcoma in children and adolescents: A report from the Soft-Tissue Italian Cooperative Group. Ann Oncol 2000;11:1445-1449.
17. Casanova M, Ferrari A, Spreafico F, et al: Malignant peripheral nerve sheath tumors in children: A single-institution twenty-year experience. J Pediatr Hematol Oncol 1999; 21:509-513.

18. Castillo BV, Kaufman L: Pediatric tumors of the eye and orbit. Pediatr Clin North Am 2003;50:1-20.

19. Castleberry RP, Kelly DR, Wilson ER, et al: Childhood liposarcoma: Report of a case and review of the literature. Cancer 1984;54:579-584.

20. Chang HR, Hajdu SI, Collin C, et al: The prognostic value of histologic subtypes in primary extremity liposarcoma. Cancer 1989;64:1514-1520.

21. Chen KT, Kassel SH, Medrano VA: Congenital hemangiopericytoma. J Surg Oncol 1986;31:127-129.

22. Cheng EY, Dusenbery KE, Winters MR, et al: Soft tissue sarcomas: Preoperative versus postoperative radiotherapy. J Surg Oncol 1996;61:90-99.

23. Chung EB, Enzinger FM: Infantile fibrosarcoma. Cancer 1976;38:729-739.

24. Chung EB, Enzinger FM: Infantile myofibromatosis. Cancer 1981;48:1807-1818.

25. Chung EB, Enzinger FM: Malignant melanoma of soft parts. Am J Surg Pathol 1983;7:405-413.

26. Cionini L, Marzano S, Olmi P: Soft tissue sarcomas: Experience with intraoperative brachytherapy in the conservative management. Ann Oncol 1992;3:S63-S66.

27. DeCou JM, Rao BN, Parham DM, et al: Malignant peripheral nerve sheath tumors: The St Jude Children's Research Hospital experience. Ann Surg Oncol 1995;2:524-529.

28. Dehner LP, Hill DA, Deschryver K: Pathology of the breast in children, adolescents and young adults. Semin Diagn Pathol 1999;16:235-247.

29. Demetri GD, Elias AD: Results of single agent and combination chemotherapy for advanced stage soft tissue sarcomas: Implications for decision making in the clinic. Hematol Oncol Clin North Am 1995;9:765-783.

30. de Oliveira-Filho AG, Miranda ML, Diz FL, et al: Use of radiofrequency for ablation of unresectable hepatic metastasis in desmoplastic small round cell tumor. Med Pediatr Oncol 2003;41:476-477.

31. Dominguez Malagon HR, Alfeiran Ruiz A, Chavarriaxicotencatl P, et al: Clinical and cellular effects of colchicine in fibromatosis. Cancer 1992;69:2478-2483.

32. Ducatman BS, Scheithouer BW, Peipgras DG, et al: Malignant peripheral nerve sheath tumors in childhood. J Neurooncol 1984;2:241-248.

33. Ducatman BS, Scheithouer BW, Peipgras DG, et al: Malignant peripheral nerve sheath tumors: A clinicopathologic study of 120 cases. Cancer 1986;57:2006-2021.

34. Enzinger FM: Hemangiopericytoma. In Weiss SW (ed): Soft Tissue Tumors, 2nd ed. St Louis, Mosby, 1988, pp 596-613.

35. Enzinger FM, Weiss SW: Soft Tissue Tumors, 3rd ed. St Louis, Mosby, 1995.

36. Farhat F, Culine S, Lhomme C, et al: Desmoplastic small round cell tumors: Results of a four-drug chemotherapy regimen in five adult patients. Cancer 1996;7:1363-1366.

37. Ferguson WS: Advances in the adjuvant treatment of infantile fibrosarcoma. Expert Rev Anticancer Ther 2003;3: 185-191.

38. Ferrari A, Casanova M, Massimino M, et al: Synovial sarcoma: Report of a series of 25 consecutive children from a single institution. Med Pediatr Oncol 1999;32:32-37.

39. Ferrari A, Casanova M, Spreafico F, et al: Childhood liposarcoma: A single-institution twenty year experience. Pediatr Hematol Oncol 1999;16:415-421.

40. Ferrari A, Gronchi A, Casanova M, et al: Synovial sarcoma: A retrospective analysis of 271 patients of all ages treated at a single institution. Cancer 2004;101:627-634.

41. Fontanesi J, Pappo AS, Parham DM, et al: Role of irradiation in management of synovial sarcoma: St Jude Children's Research Hospital experience. Med Pediatr Oncol 1996;26:264-267.

42. Frezza G, Barbieri E, Ammendolia I, et al: Surgery and radiation therapy in the treatment of soft tissue sarcomas of extremities. Ann Oncol 1992;3:S93-S95.

43. Fritsch MK, Bridge JA, Schuster AE, et al: Performance characteristics of a reverse transcriptase-polymerase chain reaction assay for the detection of tumor-specific fusion transcripts from archival tissue. Pediatr Dev Pathol 2003;6:43-53.

44. Gandolfo N, Marinoli C, Cafiero F, et al: Malignant melanoma of soft tissues (clear cell sarcoma) of the foot: Is MRI able to perform a specific diagnosis? Report of one case and review of the radiological literature. Anticancer Res 2000;20:3993-3998.

45. Gerald WL, Ladanyi M, de Alava E, et al: Clinical, pathological, and molecular spectrum of tumors associated with t(11;22)(p13;q12): Desmoplastic small round-cell tumor and its variants. J Clin Oncol 1998;16:3026-3036.

46. Gonzalez-Crussi F, Crawford SE, Sun CC: Intraabdominal desmoplastic small tumors with divergent differentiation: Observations on three cases of childhood. Am J Surg Pathol 1990;14:633-642.

47. Goodlad JR, Fletcher CD, Smith MA: Surgical resection of primary soft-tissue sarcoma: Incidence of residual tumour in 95 patients needing re-excision after local resection. J Bone Joint Surg Br 1996;78:658-661.

48. Gross E, Rao BN, Bowman L, et al: Outcome of treatment for pediatric sarcoma of the foot: A retrospective review over a 20-year period. J Pediatr Surg 1997;32:1181-1184.

49. Gross E, Rao BN, Pappo AS, et al: Soft tissue sarcoma of the hand in children: Clinical outcome and management. J Pediatr Surg 1997;32:698-702.

50. Gupta A, Maddalozzo J, Win Htin T, et al: Spindle cell rhabdomyosarcoma of the tongue in an infant: A case report with emphasis on differential diagnosis of childhood spindle cell lesions. Pathol Res Pract 2004;200:537-543.

51. Harjai MM, Bal RK, Hagpal BM, et al: Synovial sarcoma of the hand. Indian Pediatr 1999;36:194-197.

52. Heslin MJ, Lewis JJ, Woodruff JM, et al: Core needle biopsy for diagnosis of extremity soft tissue sarcoma. Ann Surg Oncol 1997;4:425-431.

53. Jaffe KA, Morris SG: Resection and reconstruction for soft-tissue sarcomas of the extremity. Orthop Clin North Am 1991;22:161-176.

54. Johnstone PA, Wexler LH, Venzon DJ, et al: Sarcomas of the hand and foot: Analysis of local control and functional result with combined modality therapy in extremity preservation. Int J Radiat Oncol Biol Phys 1994;29:735-745.

55. Karakousis CP, Proimakis C, Walsh DL: Primary soft tissue sarcoma of the extremities in adults. Br J Surg 1995;82: 1208-1212.

56. Karasek K, Constine LS, Rosier R: Sarcoma therapy: Functional outcome and relationship to treatment parameters. Int J Radiat Oncol Biol Phys 1992;24:651-656.

57. Kauffman SL, Stout AP: Hemangiopericytoma in children. Cancer 1960;13:695-710.

58. Keus RB, Rutgers EJ, Ho GH, et al: Limb-sparing therapy of extremity soft tissue sarcomas: Treatment outcome and long-term functional results. Eur J Cancer 1994;30A: 1459-1463.

59. Koutcher KA, Ballon D, Grahan M, et al: ^{31}P NMR spectra of extremity sarcomas: Diversity of metabolic profiles and changes in response to chemotherapy. Magn Reson Med 1990;16:19-34.

60. Kurkchubasche AG, Halvorson EG, Forman EN, et al: The role of preoperative chemotherapy in the treatment of infantile fibrosarcoma. J Pediatr Surg 2000;35:880-883.

61. Kushner BH, LaQuaglia MP, Wollner N, et al: Desmoplastic small round cell tumor: Prolonged progression-free

survival with aggressive multimodal therapy. J Clin Oncol 1996;14:1526-1531.

62. Ladanyi M, Antonescu CR, Leung DH, et al: Impact of SYT-SSX fusion type on the clinical behavior of synovial sarcoma: A multi-institutional retrospective study of 243 patients. Cancer Res 2002;62:135-140.

63. Ladenstein R, Treuner J, Koscielniak E, et al: Synovial sarcoma in childhood and adolescents: Report of the German CWS-81 study. Cancer 1993;71:3647-3655.

64. LaQuaglia MP, Spiro SA, Ghavimi F, et al: Liposarcoma in patients younger than or equal to 22 years of age. Cancer 1999;72:3114-3119.

65. Lawrence W, Neifield JP: Soft tissue sarcomas. Curr Probl Surg 1989;2:753-827.

66. Lieberman PH, Brennan MF, Kimmel M, et al: Alveolar soft-part sarcoma: A clinico-pathologic study of half a century. Cancer 1989;63:1-13.

67. Madden NP, Spicer RD, Allibone EB, et al: Spontaneous regression of neonatal fibrosarcoma. Br J Cancer Suppl 1992;18:S72-S75.

68. Mandell L, Ghavimi F, LaQuaglia M, et al: Prognostic significance of regional lymph node involvement in childhood extremity rhabdomyosarcoma. Med Pediatr Oncol 1990;18:466-471.

69. Mazeron JJ, Suit HD: Lymph nodes as sites of metastasis from sarcomas of soft tissue. Cancer 1987;60:1800-1808.

70. McClain KL, Leach CT, Jenson HB, et al: Association of Epstein-Barr virus with leiomyosarcomas in children with AIDS. N Engl J Med 1995;332:12.

71. Meis JM, Enzinger FM, Martz KL, et al: Malignant peripheral nerve sheath tumors (malignant schwannoma) in children. Am J Surg Pathol 1992;16:694-707.

72. Merens WC, Bramwell VH: Adjuvant chemotherapy for soft tissue sarcomas. Hematol Oncol Clin North Am 1995;9:801-815.

73. Meterissian SH, Reilly JA, Murphy A, et al: Soft-tissue sarcomas of the shoulder girdle: Factors influencing local recurrence, distant metastases, and survival. Ann Surg Oncol 1995;2:530-536.

74. Miller RW, Young JL, Novakovic B: Childhood cancer. Cancer 1995;75:395-405.

75. Miser JS, Triche TJ, Kinsella TJ, et al: Other soft tissue sarcomas of childhood. In Pizzo PA, Poplack DG (eds): Principles and Practice of Pediatric Oncology. Philadelphia, Lippincott-Raven, 1997, pp 865-888.

76. Mounayer C, Benndorf G, Bisdorff A, et al: Facial infantile hemangiopericytoma resembling an arteriovenous malformation. J Neuroradiol 2004;31:227-230.

77. Nag S, Olson T, Ruymann F, et al: High-dose-rate brachytherapy in childhood sarcomas: A local control strategy preserving bone growth and function. Med Pediatr Oncol 1995;25:463-469.

78. Nag S, Tippin DB: Brachytherapy for pediatric tumors. Brachytherapy 2003;2:131-138.

79. Neifeld J, Maurer H, Dillon P, et al: Non-rhabdomyosarcoma soft tissue sarcomas (NRSTS) in children. Society of Surgical Oncology, 1994.

80. Newton WA Jr, Soule EH, Hamoudi AB, et al: Histopathology of childhood sarcomas, Intergroup Rhabdomyosarcoma Studies I and II: Clinicopathologic correlation. J Clin Oncol 1988;6:67-75.

81. Nielsen OS, Cummings B, O'Sullivan B, et al: Preoperative and postoperative irradiation of soft tissue sarcomas: Effect of radiation field size. Int J Radiat Oncol Biol Phys 1991;21:1595-1599.

82. Okcu MF, Despa S, Choroszy M, et al: Synovial sarcoma in children and adolescents: Thirty three years of experience with multimodal therapy. Med Pediatr Oncol 2001;37:90-96.

83. Ordonez NG: Alveolor soft part sarcoma: A review and update. Adv Academ Pathol 1999;6:125-139.

84. Pappo AS, Fontanesi J, Luo X, et al: Synovial sarcoma in children and adolescents: The St Jude Children's Research Hospital experience. J Clin Oncol 1994;12:2360-2366.

85. Pappo AS, Parham D, Cain A, et al: Alveolar soft part sarcoma in children and adolescents: Clinical features and outcomes in 11 patients. Med Pediatr Oncol 1996;26:81-84.

86. Pappo AS, Parham D, Lobe TE: Soft tissue sarcomas in children. Semin Surg Oncol 1999;16:121-143.

87. Pappo AS, Shapiro DN, Crist WM, et al: Biology and therapy of pediatric rhabdomyosarcoma. J Clin Oncol 1995;13:2123-2139.

88. Parham DM, Webber BL, Jenkins JJ III, et al: Nonrhabdomyosarcomatous soft tissue sarcomas of childhood: Formulation of a simplified system for grading. Mod Pathol 1995;8:705-710.

89. Paulino AC: Late effects of radiotherapy for pediatric extremity sarcomas. Int J Radiat Oncol Biol Phys 2004;60:265-274.

90. Philippe PG, Rao BN, Rogers DA, et al: Sarcomas of the flexor fossae in children: Is amputation necessary? J Pediatr Surg 1992;27:964-967.

91. Picard E, Udassin R, Ramu N, et al: Pulmonary fibrosarcoma in childhood: Fiber-optic bronchoscopic diagnosis and review of the literature. Pediatr Pulmonol 1999;27:347-350.

92. Pitcher ME, Thomas JM: Functional compartmental resection for soft tissue sarcomas. Eur J Surg Oncol 1994;20:441-445.

93. Postovsky S, Peleg H, Ben-Itzhak O, et al: Fibrosarcoma of the trachea in a child: Case report and review of the literature. Am J Otolaryngol 1999;20:332-335.

94. Pratt CB, Kun LE: Soft Tissue Sarcomas of Children. Boston, Kluwer, 1993.

95. Pratt CB, Maurer HM, Salzberg A, et al: Treatment of unresectable or metastatic pediatric soft tissue sarcomas with surgery, irradiation and chemotherapy: A Pediatric Oncology Group study. Med Pediatr Oncol 1998;4:201-209.

96. Pratt CB, Pappo AS, Gieser P: Role of adjuvant chemotherapy in the treatment of surgically resected pediatric nonrhabdomyosarcomatous soft tissue sarcomas: A Pediatric Oncology Group Study. J Clin Oncol 1999;17:1219-1226.

97. Raney RB, Kollath J, Anderson J, et al: Late effects of therapy for patients with primary orbital rhabdomyosarcoma: A report from the Intergroup Rhabdomyosarcoma Study (IRS-III), 1984-1991. Med Pediatr Oncol 1997;29:425.

98. Rao BN: Malignant lesions of the chest and chest wall in childhood. Chest Surg Clin North Am 1993;3:461-475.

99. Rao BN: Nonrhabdomyosarcoma in children: Prognostic factors influencing survival. Semin Surg Oncol 1993;9:524-531.

100. Rao BN: Present day concepts of thoracoscopy as a modality in pediatric cancer management. Int Surg 1997;82:123-126.

101. Rao BN, Etcubanas EE, Green AA: Present-day concepts in the management of sarcomas in children. Cancer Invest 1989;7:349-356.

102. Rao BN, Santana VM, Parham D, et al: Pediatric nonrhabdomyosarcomas of the extremities: Influence of size, invasiveness, and grade on outcome. Arch Surg 1991;126:1490-1495.

103. Rosen G, Forscher C, Lowenbraun S, et al: Synovial sarcoma: Uniform response of metastasis to high dose ifosfamide. Cancer 1994;73:2506-2511.

104. Rosoff PM, Bayliff S: Successful clinical response to irinotecan in desmoplastic round blue cell tumor. Med Pediatr Oncol 1999;33:500-503.

105. Rydholm A, Gustafson P, Rooser B: Limb-sparing surgery without radiotherapy based on anatomic location of soft tissue sarcoma. J Clin Oncol 1991;9:1757-1765.

106. Sara AS, Evans HL, Benjamin RS: Malignant melanoma of soft parts (clear cell sarcoma): A study of 17 cases, with emphasis on prognostic factors. Cancer 1990;65:367-374.

107. Schmidt D, Thum P, Harms D, et al: Synovial sarcoma in children and adolescents: A report from the Kiel Pediatric Tumor Registry. Cancer 1991;67:1667-1672.

108. Schwartz HS, Spengler DM: Needle tract recurrences after closed biopsy for sarcoma: Three cases and review of the literature. Ann Surg Oncol 1997;4:228-236.

109. Serpell JW, Ball AB, Robinson MH, et al: Factors influencing local recurrence and survival in patients with soft tissue sarcoma of the upper limb. Br J Surg 1991;78:1368-1372.

110. Shetty AK, Yu LC, Gardner RV, et al: Role of chemotherapy in the treatment of infantile fibrosarcoma. Med Pediatr Oncol 1999;33:425-427.

111. Shmookler BM, Enzinger FM: Liposarcoma occurring in children: An analysis of 17 cases and review of the literature. Cancer 1983;52:567-574.

112. Sorensen SA, Mulvihill JJ, Nielsen A: Long-term follow-up of von Recklinghausen neurofibromatosis: Survival and malignant neoplasms. N Engl J Med 1986;314:1010-1015.

113. Soule EH, Pritchard DJ: Fibrosarcoma in infants and children. Cancer 1977;40:1711-1721.

114. Spunt SL, Poquette CA, Hurt YS, et al: Prognostic factors for children and adolescents with surgically resected non-rhabdomyosarcomatous soft-tissue sarcoma: An analysis of 121 patients treated at St Jude Children's Research Hospital. J Clin Oncol 1999;17:3697-3707.

115. Stark AM, Buhl R, Hugo HH, et al: Malignant peripheral nerve sheath tumors: Report of 8 cases and review of the literature. Acta Neurochir 2001;143:357-364.

116. Taylor SR, Nunez C: Fine-needle aspiration biopsy in a pediatric population: Report of 64 consecutive cases. Cancer 1984;54:1449-1453.

117. Vadlamani I, Ma E, Brink DS, et al: Trisomy 15 in a case of pediatric hemangiopericytoma and review of the literature. Cancer Genet Cytogenet 2002;138:116-119.

118. Vaiday SJ, Payne GS, Leach MO, et al: Potential role of magnetic resonance spectroscopy in assessment of tumour response in childhood cancer. Eur J Cancer 2003;39:728-735.

119. Valle AA, Kraybill WG: Management of soft tissue sarcomas of the extremity in adults. J Surg Oncol 1996;63: 271-279.

120. Wall JE, Kaste SC, Greenwald CA, et al: Fractures in children treated with radiotherapy for soft tissue sarcoma. Orthopedics 1996;19:657-664.

121. Wexler LH, Helman LJ: Rhabdomyosarcoma and the undifferentiated sarcomas. In Pizzo PA, Poplack DG (eds): Principles and Practice of Pediatric Oncology. Philadelphia, Lippincott-Raven, 1997, pp 799-829.

122. Wiklund T, Huuhtanen R, Blomqvist C, et al: The importance of a multidisciplinary group in the treatment of soft tissue sarcomas. Eur J Cancer 1996;32A:269-273.

123. Willett CG, Suit HD, Tepper JE, et al: Intraoperative electron beam radiation therapy for retroperitoneal soft tissue sarcoma. Cancer 1991;68:278-283.

124. Williard WC, Collin C, Casper ES, et al: The changing role of amputation for soft tissue sarcoma of the extremity in adults. Surg Gynecol Obstet 1992;175:389-396.

125. Wilson AN, Davis A, Bell RS, et al: Local control of soft tissue sarcoma of the extremity: The experience of a multidisciplinary sarcoma group with definitive surgery and radiotherapy. Eur J Cancer 1994;30A:746-751.

126. Wong WW, Hirose T, Scheithauer BW, et al: Malignant peripheral nerve sheath tumor: Analysis of treatment outcome. Int J Radiat Oncol Biol Phys 1998;42:351-360.

127. Zalupski MM, Baker LH: Systemic adjuvant chemotherapy for soft tissue sarcomas. Hematol Oncol Clin North Am 1995;9:787-800.

128. Zornig C, Peiper M, Schroder S: Re-excision of soft tissue sarcoma after inadequate initial operation. Br J Surg 1995;82:278-279.

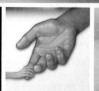

Chapter 34

Teratomas and Other Germ Cell Tumors

Richard G. Azizkhan

Pediatric germ cell tumors (GCTs) are a heterogeneous group of rare neoplasms. They occur at a rate of 2.4 cases per million children and account for approximately 1% of cancers diagnosed in children younger than 15 years.[195] These neoplasms occur in both gonadal and extragonadal sites, with extragonadal and testicular tumors predominating in children younger than 3 years and gonadal tumors predominating during and after puberty. GCTs exhibit a broad spectrum of clinical presentation and histopathologic features and carry varying risks for malignancy, depending on the type of lesion. Irrespective of such differences, lesions are presumed to originate from the primordial germ cell. Clinical and pathologic variations stem from differences in the stage of germ cell development at tumorigenesis, gender, and oncogenic influences.[36] Early in embryogenesis, germ cells begin to undergo a directed migration along the midline dorsal mesentery of the hindgut and are eventually incorporated into embryonic gonadal tissue. When this migratory process is perturbed, nests of germ cells may be deposited in abnormal locations. Thus, GCTs are found in the sacrococcygeal area, the mediastinum, the retroperitoneum, the pineal area of the brain, and the ovary and testis. Malignant transformation can occur at any of these sites. The broad spectrum of GCTs and tissue types in different anatomic locations reflects the totipotential nature of germ cells, with specific tumor types associated with the degree of cell differentiation.

Most GCTs are associated with a number of biologic markers that are useful in identifying and managing these tumors and assessing their recurrence. Treatment depends on multiple factors, including specific pathology, anatomic location, tumor stage, histology, and resectability. Optimal outcomes are achieved with complete surgical resection, accurate histologic examination, and the selective use of chemotherapy. Of particular importance, the introduction of cisplatinum chemotherapy in the late 1970s led to a dramatic improvement in both survival and salvage rates for recurrent and metastatic disease.[46] Current survival rates for low-stage extragonadal sites and for both low- and high-stage gonadal sites vary from 90% to 100%, depending on location. Survival for higher-stage extragonadal lesions approximates 75%.[148]

This chapter focuses on the most common extragonadal GCT, the teratoma, and on the malignant extragonadal GCTs typically seen by pediatric surgeons. Tumors of the ovaries and testes and intracranial tumors are discussed here only briefly but are covered in more detail in Chapters 36, 37, and 41, respectively.

EMBRYOLOGY

Primordial germ cells originate near the allantois of the embryonic yolk sac endoderm and become evident by the fourth week of gestation. By the fifth week, these cells migrate through the mesentery to the gonadal ridge[94] and eventually become the gonads. This migration appears to be mediated by the c-kit receptor and stem cell factor. The latter is expressed in an increasing gradient from the yolk sac to the gonadal ridge, along which germ cells appear to migrate.[108,171] Migration of cells cephalad to the gonadal ridges is complete by 6 weeks' gestation. At this stage, the ridges extend from the cervical to the lower lumbar levels on either side of the developing vertebral column.[67]

In animal models, the absence of c-kit receptor expression in primordial germ cells is associated with failure of migration and proliferation into the gonad.[36] The prevailing hypothesis is that extragonadal GCTs arise from aberrant migration or the deposition of germ cells along the path of migration.[65] Cells may migrate into areas that are not within the normal pathway (e.g., pineal and sacrococcygeal regions) or may remain outside the coalescence of gonadal tissue.

HISTOPATHOLOGIC CLASSIFICATION AND STAGING

Although there is slight variation among the published classifications, GCTs are generally considered to consist of seven main histologic types: dysgerminoma (or seminoma),

TABLE 34-1 Staging for Malignant Extragonadal Germ Cell Tumors
Stage I: Localized disease, with complete resection at any site (coccygectomy for sacrococcygeal site); negative tumor margins; tumor markers positive or negative
Stage II: Microscopic residual disease; capsular invasion; negative lymph nodes or microscopic lymph node involvement; tumor markers positive or negative
Stage III: Gross residual disease; gross lymph node involvement; cytologic evidence of tumor cells in ascites or pleural fluid; tumor markers positive or negative
Stage IV: Distant metastases involving lungs, liver, brain, bone, distant nodes, or other sites.

Adapted from staging systems of the Children's Oncology Group and the National Cancer Institute.

yolk sac (endodermal sinus) tumor, embryonal carcinoma, polyembryoma, choriocarcinoma, teratoma, and mixed GCT. Most malignant GCTs occur in pure form, but in 10% of cases, two or more tumor types are combined.[161] In order of frequency, the most common are teratoma, endodermal sinus tumor, germinoma, and mixed GCT. Choriocarcinoma, embryonal carcinoma, and polyembryoma are rarely seen.

The existence of multiple tumor types and sites of origin precludes the development of a homogeneous staging system comparable to that for other organ-specific malignancies. The Children's Oncology Group and the National Cancer Institute have, however, adopted a general staging system for malignant extragonadal GCTs (Table 34-1). (For staging systems for female and male gonadal tumors, see Chapters 36 and 37.)

MAJOR BIOLOGIC MARKERS

Alpha Fetoprotein

Over the past several decades, a number of biologic markers used in the diagnosis and management of GCTs have been the subject of intensive investigation,[25] and the clinical importance of these markers has become well established. Most GCTs secrete either alpha fetoprotein (AFP) or β-human chorionic gonadotropin (β-HCG); optimally, both markers should be measured before surgical excision of a suspected tumor to establish a baseline so that the impact of therapy can be determined.

AFP, which was first identified as a serum marker of liver tumors, is the predominant serum-binding fetal protein. The fetal and neonatal liver secretes AFP in large quantities, with newborn levels of 50,000 ng/mL being normal; higher levels are noted in premature infants. AFP reaches its peak concentration at 12 to 14 weeks' gestation and gradually drops to a normal adult level of 10 ng/dL by 8 months to 1 year of age.[62] Interpretation of AFP levels must thus be viewed within the context of the wide variability in normal levels during the first year of life. These levels become clinically relevant when they are significantly elevated over the normal range for any particular age (Fig. 34-1). Elevated serum AFP levels or positive immunohistochemical staining of GCTs for AFP indicates the presence of malignant components, specifically yolk sac or embryonal carcinoma.

Operative excision alone usually returns serum AFP levels to normal; its serum half-life is 5 to 7 days.[109] In most cases, treatment regimens are closely linked to the behavior of AFP, and postoperative monitoring is useful to detect tumor recurrence before it is clinically apparent. If metastasis or residual tumor is suspected because AFP levels do not fall as expected, an extensive search should be undertaken using diagnostic imaging and possibly surgery. Elevations of AFP are not, however, always indicative of tumor progression. Chemotherapy-induced tumor lysis can cause abrupt though transient AFP elevation.[187] Disorders associated with abnormal hepatic function, such as benign liver conditions, hepatic and gastrointestinal malignancies, viral hepatitis, cholestasis secondary to anesthesia, or drug-induced hepatic cholestasis, can also lead to persistently high AFP levels.[15,60,96] Other conditions associated with AFP elevation include hypothyroidism, ataxia telangiectasia, and hereditary tyrosinemia.[194] Although these disorders are readily distinguishable from

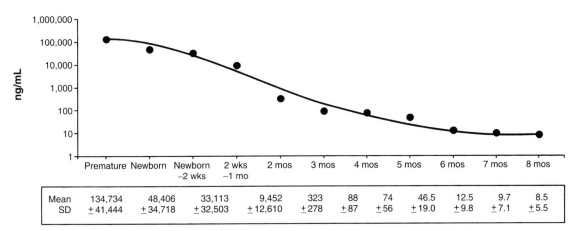

	Premature	Newborn	Newborn −2 wks	2 wks −1 mo	2 mos	3 mos	4 mos	5 mos	6 mos	7 mos	8 mos
Mean	134,734	48,406	33,113	9,452	323	88	74	46.5	12.5	9.7	8.5
SD	±41,444	±34,718	±32,503	±12,610	±278	±87	±56	±19.0	±9.8	±7.1	±5.5

Figure 34-1 Declining serum alpha fetoprotein levels in normal infants. (Adapted from Wu JT, Sudar K: Serum alpha fetoprotein (AFP) levels in normal infants. Pediatr Res 1981;15:50.)

GCTs, they should be considered when interpreting an elevated AFP level.

β-Human Chorionic Gonadotropin

β-HCG is a glycoprotein presumed to be produced by placental syncytiotrophoblasts. It is composed of α and β subunits, and the latter can be reliably assayed. β-HCG elevation suggests the presence of syncytiotrophoblasts as seen in choriocarcinoma, seminoma or dysgerminoma, and occasionally embryonal carcinoma.[73] In contrast to the long half-life of AFP, the β subunit of HCG has a half-life ranging from only 24 to 36 hours.[106] Its decline is rapid, and its sustained disappearance indicates complete tumor removal. Monitoring β-HCG levels helps assess the progress of patients with β-HCG-secreting tumors.

As with AFP, a sudden elevation of serum β-HCG can occur after cell lysis secondary to chemotherapy.[187] Also, rising levels of this marker may be associated with an increase in luteinizing hormone after bilateral orchiectomy or oophorectomy; this occurs because of immunologic cross-reactivity between the α subunit of luteinizing hormone and that of HCG.[60] Although a number of other neoplasms (e.g., multiple myeloma and malignancies of the pancreas, gastrointestinal tract, breast, lung, and bladder) are associated with modest serum β-HCG elevation, these disorders are seen primarily in adults.

Observations and Caveats

Over the past decade, investigators have made important observations that have stimulated debate regarding the interpretation of AFP and HCG serum levels. Of particular relevance, a study conducted by Trigo et al.[180] indicated that the lack of elevated tumor markers is not always a reliable indicator of the absence of recurrent disease. The authors suggested that although tumor marker assessment should be included in treatment follow-up, early detection of recurrence should not rely on this assessment alone.

The prognostic significance of the prolonged half-life clearance of AFP or HCG has been the focus of a number of studies, with findings reflecting a lack of consensus or, at the very least, a degree of confusion. Christensen et al.[34] questioned the concept of a fixed half-life for HCG, suggesting that a half-life delay following the later stages of chemotherapy may not always indicate persistent disease. This delay has been attributed to a biphasic pattern of half-life clearance, with a slower component occurring later in chemotherapy. Findings of other clinicians[125,131] suggest that the rate of marker decline early in chemotherapy is of prognostic value across risk groups. Bosl and Head[26] reported that pretreatment risk status and post-treatment marker clearance are independent and equal prognostic variables, with prolonged half-life clearance being an important variable in both previously untreated and treated patients. In contrast, Morris and Bosl[130] reported six cases in which stable, modest elevations in serum markers were present after treatment, even though there were no radiographic or clinical indications of persistent disease. Patients were closely monitored but did not require additional chemotherapy. Although it appears that tumor marker levels and the rate of half-life marker clearance are of prognostic importance, mild to moderate elevations during the later phases of chemotherapy may be less reliable indicators of persistent disease.

OTHER MARKERS

Elevated levels of serum lactate dehydrogenase (LDH), a glycolytic liver enzyme, have been observed in patients with GCTs and may be a prognostic indicator.[90] LDH is a nonspecific marker thought to correlate with tumor growth and regression, although it shows no particular association with any GCT type.[36,111] In patients with dysgerminoma, increased serum LDH isoenzyme 1 does, however, correlate with tumor burden and is useful in surgical management.[160] Spurious increases in LDH are seen with viral illnesses, liver diseases, and during and after chemotherapy.[111]

Placental alkaline phosphatase (PLAP) is a reliable marker of GCT differentiation,[93] and immunohistochemical staining for PLAP is useful for determining the origin of histologically undifferentiated GCTs.[106] PLAP is elevated in the sera of virtually all patients with advanced seminoma and in 30% of patients with stage I seminoma.[103,151] It may also be useful in the analysis of other tumors of uncertain histogenesis, particularly if the differential diagnosis lies between seminoma and lymphoma.[25]

Two recent studies indicate that the concentration of s-kit (the soluble isoform of c-kit) in cerebrospinal fluid may be a useful clinical marker for central nervous system germinomas, particularly for detecting recurrence or subarachnoid dissemination.[129,174] Another study indicates that combined CD117 (c-kit) and CD30 (Ki-1 antigen) immunohistochemistry may be a valuable tool for distinguishing seminoma from embryonal carcinoma.[113]

Vascular endothelial growth factor protein expression is higher in testicular GCTs than in normal testes and correlates with microvessel count and systemic metastases.[58] The epidermal growth factor receptor is a useful marker to identify the syncytiotrophoblastic cells in testicular GCTs.[81]

Investigators continue to look for biologic and immunohistochemical markers that will help differentiate GCT types and stratify patients.[5,59,96,114,124,188] Although many interesting observations have been made, further study in larger patient populations is required to validate the findings. Moreover, it is important to keep in mind that most studies have been conducted in adult populations rather than in children.

CYTOGENETICS

New cytogenetic technologies have improved our understanding of the genetics and molecular mechanisms involved in the development of GCTs. Genetic alterations may be associated with clinical outcome and are the subject of intense study. Flow cytometry has determined that pediatric GCTs have varied DNA ploidy and are thus unlike adult GCTs, which tend to have aneuploid DNA.[168] Most teratomas in children younger than 4 years are diploid, have normal karyotypes, and behave in a benign fashion regardless of site of origin.[28,85,98] Malignant GCTs in this age group are almost always yolk sac tumors and are generally diploid or tetraploid.[145,170] The most common cytogenetic abnormalities involve chromosomes 1, 3, and 6. Studies have demonstrated deletion of 1p36 in 80% to 100% of infantile malignant GCTs arising from testicular and extragonadal sites.[145,170] A small minority of these tumors show evidence of c-myc or n-myc amplification, proto-oncogenes that may have prognostic significance.[144]

In older children and adolescents, cytogenetic analysis of central nervous system teratomas has shown a high frequency of sex chromosome abnormalities, most commonly increased copies of the X chromosome.[32,197] Although isochromosome 12p or i(12p) is quite common in all types of adult GCTs, it is infrequently seen in childhood GCTs. Having three or more copies of this isochromosome has been associated with treatment failure and is considered to be of prognostic importance.[86] This abnormality has been described in pineal germinomas but has not been seen in pineal teratomas.[38,165,197] Isochromosome 12p has also been identified in ovarian tumors in both adolescents and adults.[4]

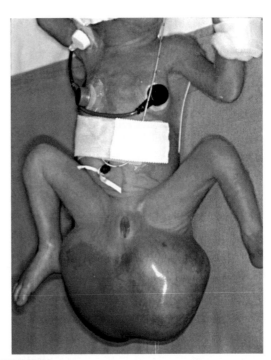

Figure 34–2 Sacrococcygeal teratoma in an infant at 30 weeks' gestation. The tumor was successfully resected, and the patient is now a young adult.

TERATOMAS

Teratomas are the most frequently occurring GCT. These neoplasms arise in both gonadal and extragonadal locations, and location is thought to correspond to the embryonic resting sites of primordial totipotential germ cells. Teratoma presentation correlates with both age and anatomic site. Teratomas occurring in infancy and early childhood are generally extragonadal, whereas those presenting in older children more commonly occur in the ovary or testis.[164] More than half of teratomas are observed at birth; they present in many locations but are most common in the sacrococcygeal area (Fig. 34-2). In prepubertal children, approximately 75% of teratomas occur in the sacrococcygeal area, and the diagnosis is generally made during the first year of life. Although more than one third of teratomas of the testis are recognized in the first year of life, these lesions are rarely diagnosed in the neonatal period.[99,176] The sacrococcyx is also the most common extragonadal location irrespective of age (45% to 65%) (Table 34-2). Cervicofacial tumors and tumors of the intracranial cavity are seen less frequently. Teratomas presenting in the mediastinum, heart, retroperitoneum, and liver are rare. Excluding testicular teratomas, 75% to 80% of teratomas occur in females. Approximately 20% of tumors contain malignant components, the most common being endodermal sinus tumor.

A spectrum of congenital anomalies is seen in association with teratomas,[8,87,142] with the type of anomaly often depending on the tumor site and size. Single or combined malformations of the genitourinary tract, rectum, anus, vertebrae, and caudal spinal cord are sometimes found in patients with extensive sacrococcygeal teratomas.[10,112,138,142]

Disfiguring cleft palate defects are found in newborns with massive cranial and nasopharyngeal teratomas.[65,146]

Teratomas can present as solid, cystic, or mixed solid and cystic lesions. By definition, these lesions are composed of representative tissues from each of the three germ layers of the embryonic disk (ectoderm, endoderm, and mesoderm) and usually contain tissues foreign to the anatomic site of origin.[40] One germ cell layer may predominate, and occasionally a teratoma can be monodermal. Most teratomas that are present at birth consist of ectodermal and mesodermal components. Epidermal and dermal structures such as hair and sebaceous and sweat glands are frequently present, as are fairly well-developed teeth. Pancreatic, adrenal, and thyroid tissue

TABLE 34–2 Site of Tumor Occurrence

Site	Incidence (%)
Sacrococcygeal region	45-65
Anterior mediastinum	10-12
Gonadal (ovary and testis)	10-35
Retroperitoneum	3-5
Cervical area	3-6
Presacral area	3-5
Central nervous system	2-4
Other rare sites (e.g., liver, kidney, vagina, stomach)	<1

From Shamberger RC: Teratomas and germ cell tumors. In O'Neill JA Jr, Grosfeld JL, Fonkalsrud EW, et al (eds): Principles of Pediatric Surgery, 2nd ed. St Louis, Mosby, 2004.

is also observed. Virtually all teratomas have mesodermal components, including fat, cartilage, bone, and muscle. Endodermal components commonly seen include intestinal epithelium and cystic structures lined by squamous, cuboidal, or flattened epithelium.[36] Mature and immature neuroepithelial and glial tissue is also frequently seen.

Tumor tissue shows varying levels of maturity, and tumors are classified histologically as either mature or immature (Fig. 34-3). Most pediatric teratomas are mature, exhibiting the absence of coexisting malignant cells with little or no tendency to undergo malignant degeneration. Mature teratomas of the gonads are encapsulated, multicystic, or solid tumors, whereas extragonadal teratomas do not have clearly defined external capsules.[41,77,78] Although a mature teratoma may be benign from a histologic standpoint, it is important to note that it may be fatal if the airway is compromised or if vital structures such as the brain or heart are involved. Moreover, depending on location and size, even benign tumors may be inoperable and incompatible with extrauterine life.

Immature teratomas are usually larger and more solid than mature lesions. They differ histologically in that various immature tissues, usually neuroepithelium, are present in lesions. A number of authors have devised and modified grading systems for immature teratomas.[137,153] Such systems generally consider the degree of immaturity of the tumor as well as the presence and quantity of its neuroepithelial components. Although grading has prognostic significance only for immature teratomas of the adult ovary,[36] in the management of adolescents, it provides clinicians with a useful indication of which tumors may have a propensity for malignant transformation and therefore require close surveillance. Grading systems are not as useful in the fetus or newborn because embryonic or immature elements may be appropriate for the stage of development.[92,184] Regardless of tumor grade in these patients, immature teratomas are associated with a favorable prognosis, and only in rare cases does immature neuroglial tissue metastasize to adjacent lymph nodes, lungs, and other distant organs from an immature primary site.[17,43,66,179]

The most important predictor of tumor recurrence in pediatric immature teratomas is the presence of microscopic foci of yolk sac tumor.[84] Because of their size, they may be missed by the pathologic sampling process. Such oversights may account for metachronous metastases after resection of the immature teratoma metastasis.

In general, prognosis depends on the patient's age, the resectability of the tumor, and the presence of metastases or metastatic potential.

Fetus in Fetu

The relationship between fetus in fetu and teratoma remains controversial and vague, with no clear distinction between the two.[2,48,65,83,134] Fetus in fetu is characterized by organized vertebral, musculoskeletal, and organ structures that may resemble a fetus (Fig. 34-4). It has been detected both pre- and postnatally, with an abdominal retroperitoneal mass being the most common clinical site.[48] Current thought is that fetus in fetu is a rare form of highly differentiated teratoma. According to the World Health Organization classification, it is presently categorized as a mature teratoma.[161]

Sacrococcygeal Teratoma

Clinical Presentation and Diagnosis

Sacrococcygeal teratoma (SCT) is the predominant teratoma as well as the most common neoplasm of the fetus and newborn. The tumor has an estimated incidence of 1 in 20,000 to 40,000 live births and a female predominance

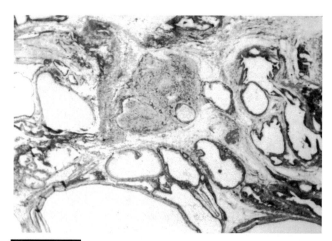

Figure 34–3   Histology of sacrococcygeal teratoma with hematoxylin-eosin stain demonstrating mature cystic epithelial elements, along with a dense central focus of immature neuroepithelial tissue.

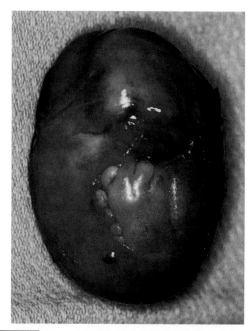

Figure 34–4   Retroperitoneal fetus in fetu removed from a 9-month-old female. This anencephalic tumor had extremities, a spine, and primitive facial structures.

ranging from 2:1 to 4:1.[10,39,117,158] Most SCTs are histologically benign; however, approximately 17% exhibit malignant histologic or clinical features.[3,20] Most cases of SCT occur sporadically, although 10% of patients have a family history of twinning.

Ten percent to 20% of patients with SCT have coexisting anomalies such as tracheoesophageal fistula, imperforate anus, anorectal stenosis, spina bifida, genitourinary malformations, meningomyelocele, and anencephaly.[10,68,142,150,191] Also, many patients have significant structural abnormalities of juxtaposed organs resulting from displacement by a large teratoma.

A classification system developed by Altman et al.[3] divides SCTs into four distinct anatomic types that differ in the degree of intra- and extrapelvic extension. Type I (46.7%) is predominantly external, with minimal presacral extension. Type II (34.7%) arises externally and has a significant intrapelvic component. Type III (8.8%) is primarily pelvic and abdominal but is apparent externally. Type IV (9.8%) is presacral and has no external manifestation (Fig. 34-5). These authors observed that the incidence of malignant components correlates not only with anatomic type (8% in type I versus 38% in type IV) but also with age at diagnosis and gender; however, the size of the tumor is unrelated.[3,79] The rate of malignancy of tumors found in older infants (older than 6 months) and in children is significantly higher than that of the visible exophytic tumors seen in neonates. Malignant change appears to be more frequent in males,[3,30,57] particularly those with solid versus complex or cystic tumors.[157] The most common malignant elements identified within sacrococcygeal lesions are yolk sac tumor and embryonal carcinoma.[80]

Many larger SCTs manifest in utero and can be diagnosed prenatally. To date, more than 60 such cases have been reported.[24,69] Although the diagnosis is usually made between 22 and 34 weeks' gestation, it has been made as early as 13 weeks. Uterine size larger than expected for gestational date (polyhydramnios or tumor enlargement) is the most common obstetric indication for performing a maternal-fetal ultrasound (US) examination.

US may reveal an external mass arising from the sacral area of the fetus (Fig. 34-6A). This mass is composed of solid and cystic areas, with foci of calcification sometimes apparent. Most prenatally diagnosed SCTs are extremely vascular and can be seen on color-flow Doppler studies.[21]

Lumbosacral myelomeningocele is the most likely entity to be confused with SCT. This type of myelomeningocele and cystic SCT have similar findings on sonography. Because both are associated with elevated maternal levels of AFP, these levels are not helpful in distinguishing the two entities. Other critical information gained from sonography includes the possible presence of abdominal or pelvic extension, evidence of bowel or urinary tract obstruction, assessment of the integrity of the fetal spine, and documentation of fetal lower extremity function.[163] Imaging of the fetal brain is helpful in establishing the diagnosis because most fetuses with lumbosacral myelomeningocele have cranial signs such as Arnold-Chiari malformation.[21] When there is doubt, fetal MRI can be extremely valuable in clarifying fetal anatomy and making a definitive diagnosis (Fig. 34-6B). Other soft tissue tumors that may mimic SCT include neuroblastoma, hemangioma, leiomyoma, and lipoma.[21]

Tumors can grow at an unpredictable rate to tremendous dimensions and may extend retroperitoneally, displacing pelvic or abdominal structures. Large tumors can cause placentomegaly, nonimmune fetal hydrops, and the mirror syndrome.[53,155] These conditions are thought to result from a hyperdynamic state induced by low-resistance vessels in the teratoma.[7] Without fetal intervention, high-output cardiac failure and hydrops resulting in fetal demise are almost certain. Thus, in a select subset of fetuses that meet stringent criteria, restoring more normal fetal physiology may be achieved by surgical debulking of the SCT in utero.[82]

Neonatal death may occur due to obstetric complications from tumor rupture, preterm labor, or dystocia.[24,54,71,132] Impending preterm labor from polyhydramnios or uterine distention from tumor mass may require treatment by amnioreduction or cyst aspiration. Dystocia and tumor

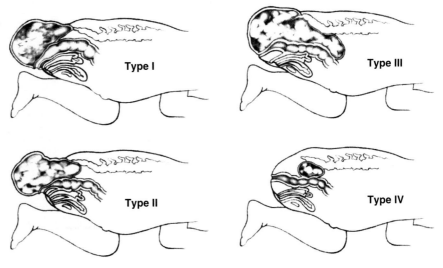

Figure 34–5 Sacrococcygeal teratoma classification scheme. (From Altman RP, Randolph JG, Lilly JR: Sacrococcygeal teratoma: American Academy of Pediatrics Surgical Section Survey—1973. J Pediatr Surg 1974;9:389.)

Type I

Type II

Type III

Type IV

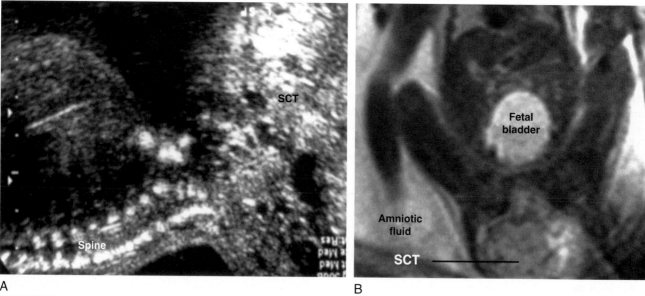

A   B

Figure 34–6 Fetal imaging of a fetus with a sacrococcygeal teratoma. *A,* Prenatal maternal-fetal ultrasonograpy depicting a fetus with a sacrococcygeal teratoma (SCT). *B,* Maternal-fetal magnetic resonance image depicting a sizable sacrococcygeal teratoma in a 20-week fetus. (Courtesy of Dr. Timothy Crombleholme.)

rupture can be avoided by planned cesarean section delivery for infants with tumors larger than 5 cm.[164]

Antenatal diagnosis carries a significantly less favorable prognosis than does diagnosis at birth, and prognostic factors outlined in the current SCT classification system are not applicable to fetal cases.[3,24] Whereas the mortality rate for SCT diagnosed in neonates is 5% at most, that for fetal SCT is close to 50%.[24,53,54] Results of most clinical series indicate that hydrops or polyhydramnios and placentomegaly portend a fatal outcome. The indication for maternal-fetal US is also a predictive factor.[24] If SCT is an incidental finding on routine prenatal sonography, the prognosis is favorable at any gestational age. Many of these lesions are predominantly cystic and relatively avascular and can be managed postnatally with surgical resection. If US is performed owing to maternal indications, the outcome is much less favorable. Additionally, prematurity from polyhydramnios or cesarean section performed before 30 to 32 weeks' gestation results in increased mortality.[164] In light of these factors, antenatal diagnosis requires referral to a high-risk obstetric center with immediately available neonatal intensive care and pediatric surgical and anesthesia expertise.

Postnatally, the diagnosis is determined by clinical findings on physical examination, serum AFP and β-HCG levels, and a number of radiographic imaging studies. Ninety percent of SCTs are noted at delivery, with a protruding caudal mass extending from the coccygeal region. Though uncommon, these tumors are easily recognized, and a reliable diagnosis can generally be made by physical examination alone. Intrapelvic components can be diagnosed by a rectal digital examination. SCTs seen at birth are predominantly benign, and many are functionally asymptomatic.

Intrapelvic variants may have a delayed postnatal presentation.[3,53,155] They are typically noted in infants and children between 4 months and 4 years of age. In contrast to the SCTs seen in neonates, these tumors are located in the pelvis and have no external component. More than one third are associated with malignancy. Clinical presentation may include constipation, anal stenosis, symptoms related to the tumor compressing the bladder or rectum, and a palpable mass. Presacral tumors are associated with sacral defects and anorectal malformations (Currarino's triad) (Fig. 34-7).

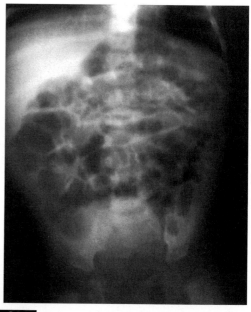

Figure 34–7 Abdominal radiograph in a 9-month-old female with Currarino's triad. A pelvic mass is seen displacing the intestine cephalad. A scimitar-shaped sacrum can also be visualized.

Radiographs of the pelvis identify any sacral defects or tumor calcifications. Computed tomography (CT) with intravenous and rectal contrast material defines the intrapelvic extent of the tumor, identifies any nodal or distant metastases, and demonstrates possible urinary tract displacement or obstruction. CT also identifies liver metastasis and periaortic lymph node enlargement. MRI is useful when spinal involvement is suspected or if the diagnosis is in doubt. A chest radiograph is useful for revealing obvious pulmonary metastases, but because chest CT is more reliable in picking up smaller metastatic lesions, it should be performed when there is a high index of suspicion.

The frequency of malignancy appears to correlate with age at diagnosis.[3] Approximately 8% of SCTs noted at birth are malignant. After 2 months of age, the frequency of malignant transformation rises sharply. By 6 months, 40% to 80% of SCTs are malignant, with the most common type of malignancy being yolk sac tumor. Because presacral (type IV) SCTs are often diagnosed at an older age, they have an increased rate of malignancy.

Operative Treatment

The treatment of choice for infants with SCT is complete surgical resection. With the exception of emergencies related to tumor rupture or hemorrhage that adversely affect the neonate's hemodynamic status, operative intervention can be undertaken on an elective basis early in the newborn period. The anatomic location of the tumor determines the operative approach. Tumors with extensive intrapelvic extension or a dominant abdominal component (type III or IV) are initially approached through the abdomen. A posterior sacral approach is sufficient for most type I and II tumors (Fig. 34-8).

Operative goals include (1) complete and prompt tumor excision, (2) resection of the coccyx to prevent tumor recurrence, (3) reconstruction of the muscles of anorectal continence, and (4) restoration of a normal perineal and gluteal appearance.[6,51] A significant delay in performing surgery may result in serious complications, including pressure necrosis, tumor hemorrhage, and malignant degeneration.

Initial control of the middle sacral and hypogastric arteries may be required to safely remove tumors in these fragile infants. Surgery is performed in a temperature-controlled environment, and infants are protected from heat loss with appropriate measures. The urinary bladder is catheterized, and the procedure is generally performed with the patient in a prone jackknife position, cushioned in a sterile foam ring (see Fig. 34-8A). After skin preparation and sterile draping, a frown-shaped

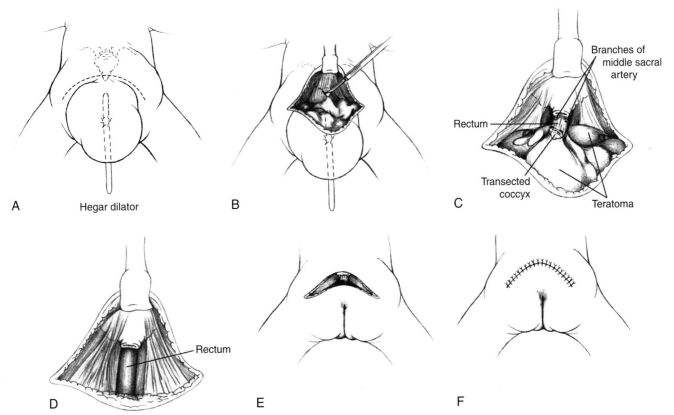

Figure 34-8 Operative treatment of sacrococcygeal teratoma. *A,* Prone positioning of the infant. It is helpful to place a Hegar dilator partially into the rectum to facilitate its identification during the tumor resection. *B,* A "frown" or inverted V posterior incision facilitates access to the tumor and the coccyx, which is being divided. *C,* Middle sacral vessels after division of the coccyx. Once these vessels are ligated and divided, the tumor can be dissected from the rectum and separated from the gluteal and levator muscles. *D,* Tumor has been removed, and underlying rectum and pelvic muscles can be visualized. *E,* Anatomic reconstruction of the anorectal muscles is performed. *F,* Final closure of the incision.

or inverted V incision is made superior to the tumor (see Fig. 34-8B). This incision provides excellent exposure and keeps the subsequent wound closure some distance from the anal orifice. To delineate the rectum, the surgeon's finger or a Hegar dilator may be inserted 3 cm into the anal canal. After raising skin flaps off the tumor, the attenuated retrorectal muscles are carefully identified and preserved. The mass is mobilized close to its capsule, and hemostasis is secured with electrocautery and suturing of vessels. To retard heat loss, warm gauze pads are placed over the exposed dissection and the tumor mass. The main blood supply to the tumor usually arises from a primitive middle sacral artery or from branches of the hypogastric artery. After division of the coccyx from the sacrum, the vessels can be observed exiting the presacral space ventral to the coccyx (see Fig. 34-8C). For patients with extremely large or vascular lesions in which excessive fluid shifts or hemorrhage may result in operative mortality, surgeons occasionally use extracorporeal membrane oxygenation in conjunction with hypothermia and hypoperfusion to facilitate better control of bleeding during resection.[116]

Because failure to remove the coccyx is associated with a recurrence rate as high as 37%,[70] the coccyx is excised in continuity with the tumor. The tumor is dissected free from the rectal wall, and the anorectal muscles are reconstructed (see Fig. 34-8D and E). The levator muscles are attached superiorly, providing support to the rectum and positioning the anus in the normal location. A closed suction drain may be placed below the subcutaneous flaps. The wound is then closed in layers with interrupted absorbable sutures (see Fig. 34-8F). A urinary catheter is left in position for several days. To maintain wound cleanliness, the patient is kept prone for several days postoperatively.

Premature newborns with large teratomas are challenging to manage. Owing to lung immaturity, increased tumor vascularity, and poor tolerance of blood loss, the surgical risks are high.[154] In these patients, devascularization and staged resection may be considered to avoid excessive blood loss. A fetus with a large SCT presents an even greater management challenge. As mentioned earlier, fetal hydrops and placentomegaly are associated with fetal demise.

The most serious complication of excision is intraoperative hemorrhage, and the major cause of mortality is hemorrhagic shock. One successful preoperative strategy for stabilizing patients with vascular tumors and significant bleeding is to tightly wrap the teratoma with an elastic bandage. As a salvage approach for acute life-threatening hemorrhage, Teitelbaum et al.[177] reported performing an emergent laparotomy and temporarily cross-clamping the distal abdominal aorta.

As with any surgical procedure, wound complications can occur. Resection of teratomas with significant intrapelvic and intraperitoneal extension may be associated with temporary or persistent urinary retention in the postoperative period, but these symptoms generally resolve. Although patients with small tumors invariably have normal anorectal continence, 30% to 40% of premature infants with large SCTs and in whom the levator and gluteal muscles are severely attenuated have fecal incontinence. Long-term bowel management strategies allow most patients to achieve socially acceptable bowel function.

Long-Term Outcome

Research over the past several decades indicates that age at diagnosis is the dominant prognostic factor for SCT. Fetuses diagnosed with SCT after 30 weeks' gestation tend to have better outcomes than those diagnosed earlier.[54,104,157] Postnatally, when the diagnosis is made before 2 months of age or excision is performed before 4 months of age, the malignancy rate is 5% to 10%.[44,189] Additionally, cystic tumors, which are generally mature, carry a better prognosis. Complications related to hemorrhage, vascular steal, and malignancy are seen more frequently in patients with solid tumors.

The long-term outcome in newborns with SCT is generally excellent. The Pediatric Onocology Group–Children's Cancer Group study reported 80% event-free survival and 100% survival with complete resection alone in immature teratomas, even when microscopic foci of yolk sac tumor were present.[120] Nevertheless, because all SCTs have a risk of local or distant recurrence, close follow-up at 3-month intervals for 3 to 4 years is essential. According to findings reported by Rescorla et al.,[150] a Children's Cancer Group study noted an 11% tumor recurrence rate with mature teratoma and a 4% recurrence rate with immature teratoma. Although 43% to 50% of these recurrences were malignant, the chemosensitivity of yolk sac (endodermal sinus) tumor resulted in a high survival rate. Serum AFP levels are monitored, and physical examinations are performed. Special attention is given to rectal examination because it may detect a presacral recurrence. When AFP levels do not fall appropriately, abdominal US is performed. When there is an index of suspicion, abdominopelvic CT or MRI is carried out, as well as lung CT. A recurrent tumor may be benign, but it should be re-excised to minimize the long-term risk of malignant transformation.

Adjuvant Therapy

Detection of malignant elements warrants adjuvant multiagent chemotherapy. The most active antineoplastic drugs include cisplatin, etoposide, and bleomycin. Current reports indicate impressive survival rates in patients with both locally advanced and metastatic disease after the administration of intensive chemotherapy.[63,64,149] Even with malignant transformation of SCT, Misra et al.[128] reported survival rates of 88% with local disease and 75% with distant metastases. Moreover, it appears that stage, extent of metastasis, and extension into bone have no prognostic significance when children are treated with platinum-based regimens.[29]

For patients in whom the primary malignant tumor is unresectable, a multiagent chemotherapy course is administered to facilitate subsequent resection. If a good tumor response is indicated by a diminishing serum AFP level and by CT and chest radiography, resection is undertaken after several cycles of chemotherapy.

In patients with localized malignant recurrence, complete resection remains the cornerstone of salvage treatment. This is done in conjunction with adjuvant chemotherapy.

Chemotherapy is also effective in the treatment of metastatic foci in the lungs and liver. However, to ensure the removal of any malignant elements, residual lesions must be excised. Though uncommon, radiation therapy may have a role in controlling unresectable disease in selected patients.

Head and Neck Teratoma

Head and neck teratomas account for 5% of all neonatal teratomas. These rare neoplasms may occur in the brain, orbit, oropharynx, nasopharynx, or cervical region.

Intracranial Teratoma

Intracranial teratomas (covered in depth in Chapter 41) present in a bimodal age pattern. They account for nearly 50% of all brain tumors in early infancy, and a high prevalence is seen in the teenage years (ages 12 to 16) as well. In neonates, intracranial teratomas have an equal sex predilection; in older children, they occur more commonly in boys (2:1). The pineal gland is the most common site of origin, although teratomas are also found in the hypothalamus, ventricles, and suprasellar and cerebellar regions. Whereas intracranial teratomas occurring in neonates are generally benign, those seen in older children and teenagers are almost always malignant. All histologic types have been observed, but intracranial teratomas are broadly classified into two groups: nearly 50% are classified as germinomas, and the remaining are considered nongerminoma GCTs. In many instances, however, the tumor shows a mixed histologic pattern. The most common presenting finding in infants is increased intracranial pressure related to obstructive hydrocephalus. Older children and teenagers present with severe headaches, seizures, lethargy, visual disturbances, and vomiting. Boys with tumors that produce β-HCG sometimes present with precocious puberty.

The diagnosis is supported by skull radiographs and CT or MRI revealing either midline or paraxial supratentorial lesions that are often calcified. Resection is the treatment of choice, but many neonatal intracranial teratomas are not resectable. Palliative shunting to alleviate intracranial pressure and relieve hydrocephalus clearly has a short-term benefit but does not necessarily prolong survival in patients with malignant teratomas. Moreover, in some infants, shunting is associated with the spread of tumor to extracranial sites.

Both chemotherapy and radiotherapy have been incorporated into contemporary treatment regimens. In children with germinoma, treatment with radiotherapy has yielded an excellent 5-year survival of 80% to 90%.[13,76,156] In patients with nongerminoma GCTs, however, treatment with surgery and radiotherapy has yielded a poor outcome, with 0% to 33% 5-year survival.[76,141] Although the role of chemotherapy in these patients has not yet been well established, it has been incorporated into contemporary research trials in an effort to reduce the long-term morbidity associated with radiotherapy, particularly in very young children. Additionally, both chemotherapy and radiotherapy have been used to salvage failures by these respective modalities.[11,12,127] Some authors maintain that adding chemotherapy to the treatment protocol of children with germinoma may not enhance the already high survival rates but may lead to less radiation-induced morbidity by allowing reduced radiation volumes and doses or by delaying radiation therapy in very young patients.[13,76,156] Optimally, future approaches for managing germinoma will combine minimal radiation doses and field sizes with less aggressive chemotherapeutic regimens. In contrast, high-risk patients with nongerminoma GCTs may benefit from a more aggressive approach including more intensive chemotherapy, radiation, and surgery. Considering the rarity of intracranial teratomas and the lengthy interval between treatment and the development of related side effects, evidence based on prospective randomized studies is a long-term goal.

Cervicofacial Teratoma

Cervical teratomas are extremely rare neoplasms. Although most of these tumors are histologically benign, they frequently cause significant airway and esophageal obstruction in the perinatal period and are thus potentially fatal. Primary tumor sites include the tongue, nasopharynx, palate, sinus, mandible, tonsil, anterior neck, and thyroid gland. As with SCTs, cervicofacial teratomas are predominantly congenital in origin. Males and females are equally affected.

Prenatal US is a reliable and essential diagnostic tool for detecting these lesions in utero, thereby allowing for careful arrangement of the time, mode, and place of delivery. When large cervical teratomas are detected prenatally, findings generally reveal multiloculated irregular masses with both solid and cystic components (Fig. 34-9).[72]

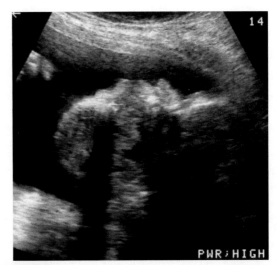

Figure 34–9 Prenatal ultrasonography depicting a large cervical teratoma.

To delineate anatomy more clearly, fetal MRI is the diagnostic study of choice. Among cases detected prenatally, lymphatic malformation (cystic hygroma) is the most likely entity to be mistaken for cervical teratoma. Similarities in size, sonographic findings, clinical characteristics, location, and gestational age at presentation can make this distinction difficult.[16] Other lesions to be considered in the differential diagnosis include large branchial cleft cyst and congenital thyroid goiter. Because less than 30% of cervical teratomas are associated with elevated serum AFP levels, this assay is not particularly helpful in the differential diagnosis of fetal cervical masses.[21] Approximately one third of prenatally diagnosed cases are complicated by maternal polyhydramnios, which is thought to be due to esophageal obstruction or interference with fetal swallowing. There is a high incidence of preterm labor and delivery that may be secondary to increased uterine size resulting from polyhydramnios or tumor.

Cervical teratomas are generally large and bulky, often measuring 5 to 12 cm in diameter (Fig. 34-10).[16,167] Tumor masses greater than the size of the fetal head have been reported,[16,95,140] as has involvement of the oral floor, protrusion into the oral cavity (epignathus), and extension into the superior mediastinum.[95] Massive lesions may cause dystocia, requiring a cesarean section to deliver the baby. Various anomalies occurring in association with cervical teratomas have been reported. These include craniofacial and central nervous system anomalies,[8] hypoplastic left ventricle, trisomy 13, and one case each of chondrodystrophia fetalis and imperforate anus. Mandibular hypoplasia has also been seen as a direct result of mass effect on the developing mandible.[21]

Up to 50% of cervicofacial teratomas contain calcifications,[72,100] and these are often seen best on postnatal plain radiographs.[74,172] When calcifications are present in a partially cystic and solid neck mass, they are virtually diagnostic of cervical teratoma.[72] A postnatal CT scan is particularly useful in delineating the anatomic extent and precise involvement of the neoplasm.

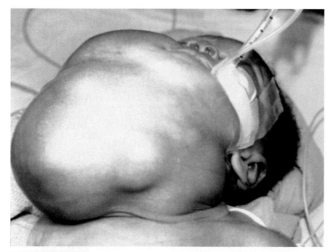

Figure 34–10 Large cervical teratoma in a 34-week premature baby. This infant had significant airway obstruction at birth and was successfully intubated in the delivery room.

As shown by Azizkhan et al.,[8] airway obstruction at birth is life threatening and is associated with a high mortality rate. In patients with massive fetal neck masses, this is generally associated with a delay in obtaining an airway and an inability to ventilate effectively. Delay can result in hypoxia and acidosis, and a delay longer than 5 minutes can result in anoxic injury. In light of these concerns, most cervicofacial teratomas are definitively treated after delivery, which should take place at a tertiary care center with an expert perinatal team that includes a pediatric surgeon. Optimally, if a cesarean section is performed, maternal-fetal placental circulation should be maintained while an airway is secured. This is done by employing an EXIT (ex utero intrapartum treatment) procedure. This method allows time to perform procedures such as direct laryngoscopy, bronchoscopy, tracheostomy, surfactant administration, and cyst decompression, which may be required to secure the airway.[21] Because precipitous airway obstruction may occur due to hemorrhage into the tumor,[16,72,89] orotracheal intubation is indicated in all patients, regardless of the presence or absence of symptoms.

In some series,[110,179] infants either had acute airway obstruction or lost a previously secure orotracheal airway within a few hours or days after delivery. Because early resection after stabilization is the most effective method of achieving total airway control, it is the treatment of choice. Delaying surgery can have other serious ramifications, including retention of secretions, atelectasis, or pneumonia due to interference with swallowing.[16,65] Resection also removes the risk of malignant degeneration, which occurs at much higher frequencies (>90%) in cases of cervical teratomas that are not diagnosed or treated until late adolescence or adulthood.[27]

To minimize operative morbidity, dissection of the teratoma should begin in areas distant to important regional nerves. Cervical teratomas often have a pseudocapsule, facilitating gentle elevation of the tumor out of the neck. If the tumor arises from the thyroid gland, the involved thyroid lobe is excised in continuity with the teratoma. Any enlarged lymph nodes should be excised with the tumor, because glial metastases may be present. After excision, a drain is left in place for 24 to 48 hours. Because these tumors are often large, envelopment of vital anatomic structures in the neck is common. In some cases, complete tumor excision with acceptable functional and cosmetic results may be achieved only by staged procedures.[8]

In contrast to the high incidence of malignancy (>60%) in adults, malignant cervicofacial teratomas with metastases are comparatively uncommon in neonates, with a 20% incidence reported by Azizkhan et al.[8] Despite the existence of poorly differentiated or undifferentiated tissue in the primary tumor, many infants remain free from recurrence following complete resection of a cervical teratoma. Such cases suggest that malignant biologic behavior is uncommon in this population.[16,45,72] Reported findings show a number of consistent histologic patterns.[8] Neuroectodermal elements and immature neural tissue are the most commonly observed tissues in metastatic foci. In approximately one third of cases, the metastases are more differentiated but are confined to regional nodes. Patients with isolated regional node metastases who are treated with excision of the primary tumor generally survive free of disease. This supports the concept that the presence of metastases containing only differentiated tumor usually correlates with a good prognosis.

There are currently no chemotherapy guidelines for neonates with malignant cervical teratomas. Based on results of their series, however, Azizkhan et al.[8] recommended that this modality be reserved for infants with disseminated disease (that has not differentiated) and those who have invasive tumors and residual disease after resection.

Although cervical teratoma is generally a benign tumor, the possibility of malignant transformation mandates close surveillance for tumor recurrence. Serum AFP levels should be monitored at 3-month intervals in infancy and annually thereafter, with a rising level alerting the clinician to the possibility of tumor recurrence. As discussed earlier in this chapter, serum AFP levels must be interpreted with caution and viewed within the framework of their natural half-life. Imaging studies twice a year for the first 3 years of life are also recommended for surveillance. Because the thyroid and parathyroid glands may be removed or affected by tumor excision, the risk of temporary or permanent hypothyroidism must be considered.[8] If encountered, these complications must be monitored and managed appropriately.

Mediastinal Teratoma

Mediastinal teratomas account for approximately 20% of all mediastinal pediatric neoplasms. They are the second most common extragonadal site of teratomas and affect boys and girls equally. Though uncommon, other malignant mediastinal GCTs with various histologic patterns also arise. Mediastinal teratomas more frequently arise in the anterior mediastinum but are also observed within the pericardium or heart and, rarely, in the posterior mediastinum. Less than 50% of childhood mediastinal teratomas occur in neonates. Although adolescents and young adults are frequently asymptomatic, infants and children usually have symptoms that are related to compression of the lung or bronchi; they may range from acute respiratory distress to a chronic cough, chest pain, or wheezing. Anterior mediastinal and pericardial tumors are associated with superior vena cava syndrome. Some boys with mediastinal teratomas may present with precocious puberty associated with a benign or malignant β-HCG-secreting neoplasm. Because such neoplasms are associated with Klinefelter's syndrome, chromosomal karyotyping should be performed.

More than 30 cases have been diagnosed prenatally. Accompanying polyhydramnios, fetal hydrops, and a number of other serious conditions have resulted in fatal outcomes. It is thought that open fetal surgery may have a role in a select subset of patients, although the two attempts to date have been unsuccessful. A postnatal chest radiograph may reveal a mediastinal mass; in approximately one third of cases, this mass is calcified. US of the chest shows a mass with cystic and solid components and may be useful in distinguishing the mass from the pericardium and heart. CT often clarifies the extent of the tumor and its relationship to surrounding anatomic structures. The differential diagnosis includes thymoma, thymic cyst, lymphatic malformation, mediastinal non-Hodgkin's lymphoma, esophageal duplication, and bronchogenic cyst. When there is an index of suspicion, bone scintigraphy may be performed to detect osseous metastases. Serum levels of AFP, β-HCG, LDH, and PLAP may be elevated.[52]

An overall malignancy rate of 15% has been reported in the pediatric age group.[40] A number of studies have shown that both mature and immature mediastinal teratomas occurring in newborns and infants behave in a benign fashion if resected.[31,107,176] Outcomes in these age groups have been shown to be more favorable than those in adolescents and adults.

Complete surgical removal is the treatment of choice for both benign and malignant lesions. Because anterior mediastinal masses frequently compress the airway, anesthesia management is critical. Once spontaneous respiration has been eliminated by intravenous paralytic agents, patients may lose their ability to be ventilated, even with a properly positioned endotracheal tube. A sternotomy or thoracotomy provides excellent operative exposure. Care should be taken to avoid injury to the phrenic nerves.

Histologic study reveals immature cellular elements in approximately 20% of mediastinal tumors in young children. Although this carries almost no increased risk of malignancy in these children, the presence of immature tissue is associated with high mortality from progressive tumor in older teenagers and young adults. Thus, they should be treated with adjuvant chemotherapy. In cases in which malignant tumor has infiltrated into vital structures, resection may not be possible, and chemotherapy may be required to make the teratoma amenable to subsequent resection. Because cure of malignancy is unusual with resection alone, all patients undergo adjuvant postoperative chemotherapy to prevent disease recurrence and progression.

Although results from cooperative multiagent chemotherapy trials have not been as impressive as those with sacrococcygeal lesions, they have been quite favorable. In a recent series,[22] 18 of 36 patients underwent biopsy followed by chemotherapy and then tumor resection. Tumor size remained stable or increased in 6 patients and decreased a mean of 57% in 12. The overall 4-year survival rate for children treated with a regimen of etoposide, bleomycin, and cisplatin was 71%; the event-free survival rate was 69%. The authors suggested that boys aged 15 years or older may be a high-risk subgroup for mortality from tumor progression.

Cardiac Teratoma

Although a teratoma may arise in the heart, this occurs only rarely and almost exclusively in girls. Cardiac teratomas typically present with signs and symptoms of congestive heart failure, confined to the right side of the heart. The diagnosis is suspected on echocardiography, which reveals the presence of a multicystic intracardiac mass.

Arrhythmias and an intraventricular block may be observed on an electrocardiogram. Associated congenital heart defects such as atrial septal defect and ventricular septal defect are frequently seen. To avoid the occurrence of complete outflow obstruction or a fatal arrhythmia, prompt resection is essential. Malignant teratomas (25%) require treatment with chemotherapy. For patients with benign, resectable cardiac teratomas, cardiac transplantation offers a reasonable therapeutic alternative.

Retroperitoneal Teratoma

The retroperitoneum is the third most common extragonadal site, accounting for 5% of all teratomas.[118] Most tumors are observed in early infancy, with 50% identified in the first year of life and 75% occurring by age 5. Girls are more commonly affected (2:1) than boys. Patients usually present with a large palpable abdominal mass that may cause symptoms of alimentary tract compression. The differential diagnosis includes a number of other tumors seen in early childhood (e.g., neuroblastoma and Wilms' tumor), as well as cystic retroperitoneal lymphatic malformations, omental cyst, and fetus in fetu. Plain abdominal radiographs may reveal displacement of bowel and calcification within the tumor. When calcification is present, the pattern is more distinct and noticeably different from the diffuse stippled calcification seen in neuroblastoma. CT or MRI of the abdomen helps differentiate this neoplasm from more common childhood tumors.

Laparotomy for complete tumor resection is the therapy of choice. Because most of these tumors are benign, this approach is usually successful. Approximately 20% of retroperitoneal teratomas are malignant at diagnosis, and 30% to 40% may have immature tissues. Benign glial implants have occasionally been observed, indicating a maturation process of these metastatic foci. Because malignant recurrence has been reported in patients with benign teratomas containing immature components, both malignant lesions and those containing high-grade immature elements should be treated with postoperative chemotherapy.[155]

Other Rare Extragonadal Teratomas

Gastric Teratoma

Gastric teratomas are exceedingly rare. These lesions may present as a palpable epigastric mass, with symptoms of gastric outlet obstruction or upper gastrointestinal bleeding occurring in infancy. These neoplasms are usually large and are often multicystic. Plain radiographs of the abdomen often show calcification. An upper gastrointestinal contrast study defines the stomach and tumor relationship. Upper endoscopy may reveal an extrinsic mass that compresses the gastric lumen or evidence of erosion by the tumor. Histologic examination reveals that these lesions are composed of mature tissues, frequently containing immature neuroglial elements. Resection of the tumor is the treatment of choice. The prognosis for this teratoma is generally favorable.[47,91,162]

Vaginal Teratoma

These rare lesions present in the first year of life, often in the neonatal period. Examination may reveal minor bleeding from an easily visible vaginal mass. Most lesions are yolk sac tumors. A chest radiograph is performed to rule out lung metastases, and CT delineates the extent of the lesion. If the tumor is localized, management entails local resection of the tumor by partial vaginectomy and low-dose multiagent chemotherapy. Involvement of the uterus requires a hysterectomy. Preliminary adjuvant chemotherapy may limit the extent of the required resection.[164]

Gonadal Teratomas

Ovarian Teratoma

Teratomas are the most common pediatric ovarian tumor, accounting for more than 50% of all ovarian neoplasms and 25% of all childhood teratomas. Most ovarian teratomas present between 5 and 16 years of age and are unusual in the first 2 to 3 years of life. Pain is the most common presenting symptom, observed in more than 50% of patients. Acute abdominal pain from torsion of the tumor is reported in 25% of patients. Because most tumors are large (10 to 15 cm), the identification of an asymptomatic abdominal mass is another common presentation. Intra-abdominal and pelvic calcifications resembling teeth are seen in approximately half of abdominal radiographs. Tumors occur equally on the right and left ovaries and are bilateral in 5% to 10% of cases. Although abdominopelvic US shows a mass composed of cystic and solid components as well as the structure of the contralateral ovary, CT is the optimal imaging study for preoperative staging. Serum AFP and HCG levels should be obtained. If elevated, they may be indicative of malignant potential.

Simple or salpingo-oophorectomy is the treatment of choice for benign tumors with an intact capsule and mature elements on histologic examination. At the time of surgery, any ascitic fluid is collected for cytologic analysis. If ascitic fluid is absent, peritoneal washings are obtained and evaluated for the presence of tumor cells. All peritoneal surfaces, including the underside of the diaphragm, are inspected for peritoneal implants. If they are observed, biopsy specimens are obtained. An infracolic omentectomy should be performed if the omentum has gross tumor. Gonad-sparing resection of benign cystic ovarian teratomas has been advocated by some surgeons. However, long-term follow-up is limited, and this approach remains controversial.[135]

The management of immature ovarian teratomas with extraovarian peritoneal involvement is complex. Fortunately, most patients have mature glial implants. They do not require chemotherapy and have an excellent prognosis.[155] Tumors with a higher histologic grade (grades II and III) have a risk of malignancy and require adjuvant multiagent chemotherapy. Treatment with current chemotherapeutic regimens has resulted in a survival rate approaching 90%.[97] (For a more detailed discussion, refer to Chapter 36.)

Testicular Teratoma

Testicular teratomas are the most common testicular neoplasms in childhood. They present bimodally in terms of age, with infants younger than 2 years and teenagers and young adults most commonly affected. Infants usually present with a nontender scrotal mass. In 15% of patients, a hydrocele may also be present. Preoperative serum AFP and HCG levels are obtained. A chest radiograph and an abdominal CT scan are obtained to evaluate for nodal and visceral metastases.

Tumors are staged by virtue of their resectability and the presence of nodal and distant metastases. In stage I disease (80% of cases), treatment consists of a transinguinal radical orchiectomy and includes excision of the spermatic cord at the internal ring. Radical orchiectomy alone in stage I disease in infants is associated with greater than 90% 5-year survival.

Most malignant tumors in infants are yolk sac tumors that rarely metastasize to retroperitoneal lymph nodes. Retroperitoneal lymph node dissection is thus not required for infants with stage I disease who are younger than 2 years and have a normal preoperative abdominal CT scan. If elevated serum tumor markers do not return to normal after resection (20% of cases), the teratoma is restaged, retroperitoneal lymph node dissection is subsequently performed, and adjuvant chemotherapy is administered. Retroperitoneal node dissection is usually performed unilaterally, using nerve-sparing techniques to prevent retrograde ejaculation. Suspicious contralateral lymph nodes should be biopsied. The frequency of relapse following lymphadenectomy is 10% to 15%, with disease usually recurring in the lungs or mediastinum. Most patients with metastatic disease benefit from multiagent chemotherapy. (For a more detailed discussion, refer to Chapter 37.)

YOLK SAC TUMOR

Yolk sac tumors are the most common malignant GCT affecting children from infancy to adolescence. In neonates and young children, these neoplasms are found primarily in extragonadal sites, particularly the sacrococcygeal area. However, they are also common in the testes of infants and young boys,[196] with yolk sac tumor being the predominant pediatric malignant GCT involving the testis. In older children and adolescents, the ovary is the most common location. Less common primary sites include the mediastinum, retroperitoneum, pineal area, and vagina. In adolescents, these tumors rarely occur in pure form in extragonadal sites but are seen as a component of mixed malignant GCTs.[42,49] Pediatric yolk sac tumor is cytogenetically and biologically distinct from its adult counterpart. Examination of pediatric tumor tissue has shown deletions in chromosomes 1 (1p) and 6 (6q), but no evidence of the i(12p) deletion observed in adult GCTs.[143]

Grossly, yolk sac tumors appear as pale gray to yellow friable, mucoid tissue with foci of cystic areas and necrosis.[36,73] One relatively recent and credible theory suggests that these neoplasms originate from the primary yolk sac,[136] a structure that develops early in embryogenesis. The yolk sac consists of multipotential primitive endoderm tissue capable of differentiating into the primitive gut and its derivatives, including the liver, thus leading to variable histologic patterns. The pseudopapillary (festoon) and microcystic (reticular) patterns are the most common and widely recognized. Both usually display perivascular sheaths of cells referred to as endodermal sinus structures or Schiller-Duval bodies. Most well-differentiated yolk sac tumors also contain intra- and extracellular hyaline deposits that are resistant to periodic acid–Schiff diastase staining and positive for AFP. However, in that the microcystic pattern is less differentiated, it is often associated with eosinophilic globules and strands that infrequently stain positively for AFP. Occasionally, endodermal sinus tumors are more solid and can be difficult to distinguish from embryonal carcinoma. Some tumors may have a hepatoid pattern that resembles fetal liver cells.[73] Variations in histologic pattern do not appear to correlate with outcome, which has improved considerably with multiagent chemotherapy. Nevertheless, as evidenced by the Pediatric Oncology Study (1971-1984),[79] neonatal SCTs may recur as yolk sac tumors, which are associated with a worse prognosis owing to their invasive nature.

EMBRYONAL CARCINOMA

Though far less common than yolk sac tumors, embryonal carcinoma also presents in the first year of life. It rarely occurs in pure form in children; more often, it is a component of a mixed malignant GCT. The major histologic pattern is epithelial, comprising large nests of cells with varying amounts of central necrosis. However, pseudotubular and papillary patterns, which may be confused with those of yolk sac tumors, are also common. Cells are AFP negative, and tumors generally lack the eosinophilic hyaline globules characteristic of some yolk sac tumors. In contrast to other GCTs, embryonal carcinoma is positive for cytokeratin by immunohistochemical staining.[36]

GERMINOMA

The term *germinoma* is currently used to refer to a group of neoplasms with common histologic characteristics. Formerly, a lesion was termed a *seminoma* if found in the testis, a *dysgerminoma* in the ovary, and a *germinoma* in an extragonadal site. These tumors are thought to arise from totipotential germ cells present at the undifferentiated stage of gonadal development. They are commonly seen in the ovary, anterior mediastinum, and pineal region and are the most common pure malignant GCT occurring in the ovary and central nervous system in children.[49,175] In children, germinomas account for 10% of all ovarian tumors and approximately 15% of GCTs in all locations. These tumors are rarely seen in infants and small children and occur most often in prepubertal girls and young women, with 44% of cases presenting before age 20 years.[73] Germinoma is the predominant malignancy found in dysgenetic gonads and undescended testes.

On gross examination, germinomas appear solid, encapsulated, gray-pink or tan in color, with occasional small foci of hemorrhage and necrosis and a rubbery consistency. Tumor cells are arranged in nests separated by bands of fibrous tissue associated with variable degrees of lymphocytic infiltration. The cells are large, with clear to slightly eosinophilic cytoplasm, distinct cell membranes, and large round nuclei having one or two prominent nucleoli.[36] Although granulomas with giant cells as well as syncytiotrophoblasts may be present, they alter tumor prognosis only when associated with cytotrophoblasts in foci of choriocarcinoma. Germinoma cells strongly stain for PLAP, whereas syncytiotrophoblasts stain for β-HCG. As noted by Scully et al.,[161] germinomas are also immunoreactive for vimentin and, in some cases, LDH, neuron-specific enolase, Leu-7, cytokeratin, desmin, and glial fibrillary acidic protein. In one study,[183] c-kit localization was found in 92% of germinomas.

CHORIOCARCINOMA

Choriocarcinoma is a rare, highly malignant tumor seen primarily in females. This tumor typically occurs as a component of a malignant mixed GCT. As with yolk sac tumors and embryonal carcinoma, this lesion can occur during the first year of life, either as a metastasis secondary to a placental choriocarcinoma[33,37] or as a primary tumor arising from locations such as the liver, lung, brain, kidney, or maxilla.[101,166] The most common site is the pineal region.[56,166] It presents in both prepubertal children and young adolescents, occurring primarily in the gonads and less frequently in the mediastinum. Pure choriocarcinoma in young infants almost always represents disseminated metastasis from maternal or placental gestational trophoblastic tumor.[19,55]

On gross examination, pure choriocarcinoma is characteristically solid, hemorrhagic, and friable. Microscopically, both cytotrophoblasts and syncytiotrophoblasts are present. Cytotrophoblasts typically appear as closely packed nests of relatively uniform, medium-sized cells with clear cytoplasm, distinct cell margins, and vesicular nuclei, whereas syncytiotrophoblasts represent giant multinucleated syncytial trophoblastic cells.[36] Both cell types are typically immunoreactive for cytokeratin. The syncytiotrophoblastic cells are also immunoreactive for HCG, human placental lactogen, and pregnancy-specific β₁-glycoprotein. In addition, immunoreactivity for PLAP, epithelial membrane antigen, neuron-specific enolase, alpha₁-antitrypsin, and carcinoembryonic antigen is seen in some tumors.[161]

POLYEMBRYOMA

Polyembryomas are exceedingly rare malignant tumors of the ovary, with fewer than 10 cases reported during the last 4 decades.[161] They are often reported in combination with other neoplastic components.[18,102] Patients are typically children or young women who present with clinical symptoms and signs indicative of the presence of a large pelvic mass. Rarely, patients have symptoms related to extraovarian spread of tumor at presentation.[182] The histologic tumor appearance is characterized by a preponderance of embryoid structures that resemble normal early embryos in various stages of development. These structures are composed of yolk sac, embryonal, and hepatic elements, as well as chorionic elements such as syncytiotrophoblastic giant cells. Mature and immature teratomatous elements, predominantly of endodermal derivation, are usually present as well.[161] In many cases, elevated serum levels of AFP and β-HCG have been noted. Histologically, both the yolk sac and the hepatic elements are immunoreactive for AFP and alpha₁-antitrypsin. Syncytiotrophoblastic elements are immunoreactive for HCG.[102,133,147,173]

GONADOBLASTOMA

Gonadoblastoma is a relatively rare tumor composed of germ cells intermixed with stromal cells.[139,185,186] It is considered a precursor to the development of a malignant GCT. Gonadoblastoma is most commonly found in dysgenetic gonads of phenotypic females who have at least a fragment of the Y chromosome.[181] Patients are generally older adolescents or in the third decade of life and have a history of primary amenorrhea. They may exhibit a lack of secondary sexual characteristics and the presence of elevated gonadotropin levels and streak gonads.[50,139,190] These tumors are often quite small, soft to firm, gray-tan to brown, and slightly lobulated. Microscopic features include the proliferation of both germ cells and gonadal sex cord cells. Germ cells show positivity for PLAP.[36]

Most gonadoblastomas behave in a benign fashion, although there is a 30% risk of overgrowth of a malignant germ cell element.[185] Varying malignant elements may be present; germinoma is the most common, occurring in approximately 50% of cases.[188,189] The malignant potential of this tumor is determined by the underlying malignant component. Gonadectomy is recommended for young patients with mixed gonadal dysgenesis because of the increased frequency of gonadoblastoma and germinoma and the virilizing effects of residual testicular tissue.[152]

MIXED GERM CELL TUMORS

GCTs often comprise two or more pure histologic types. Benign through possibly malignant GCTs such as immature teratomas may coexist with frankly malignant GCTs, and 10% to 40% of patients with malignant tumors have mixed histology.[1,61,105,121] Of these patients, 40% are diagnosed before puberty.[105] The most common histologic component of mixed GCTs is dysgerminoma (germinoma), although immature teratoma, endodermal sinus tumor, and embryonal carcinoma may be detected in varying proportions.[36] Also, mixed GCTs account for 8% to 10% of malignant primitive GCTs of the ovary.[105,159]

The occurrence of these tumors underscores the importance of careful gross examination and judicious tumor tissue sampling. The prognosis of patients with mixed GCTs is generally thought to depend on the tumor's most malignant element, but some investigators have reported that a minor component of a highly malignant element affects the prognosis less adversely than does a major component.[105]

TREATMENT OVERVIEW AND FUTURE PERSPECTIVES

Advances in surgical treatment, together with the use of platinum-containing multiagent chemotherapy regimens, have resulted in a dramatic improvement in the outcome for children with malignant GCTs. International studies using integrated multimodal treatment strategies are reporting impressive survival rates, ranging from 75% to 90%.[14,63,121,149,178,193] Although chemotherapy protocols in these studies differ somewhat, the standard chemotherapy regimen in the United States for children with malignant extragonadal GCTs includes a combination of cisplatin, etoposide, and bleomycin (PEB). This protocol has, however, been associated with a high risk of late effects, particularly the nephrotoxicity and ototoxicity of cisplatin.[35,75] Growing concern about these effects has spurred investigations into alternative protocols with less deleterious long-term effects. In the United Kingdom, the combination of carboplatin, etoposide, and bleomycin (JEB) has undergone clinical investigation in children younger than 16 years. Authors have reported comparable event-free survival with less ototoxicity and renal impairment than PEB.[119] Corroborating these findings, a recent prospective study conducted in the United States concluded that carboplatin could be substituted for cisplatin without sacrificing response or survival; overall survival and event-free survival were 91% and 87%, respectively.[169] In contrast, adult studies that substituted standard-dose carboplatin for cisplatin in combination with etoposide alone[9] or with etoposide and low-dose bleomycin[88] demonstrated inferior event-free and overall survival in patients with malignant GCTs. To date, no randomized comparison of PEB versus JEB has been conducted in children.

Because pediatric extragonadal GCTs are rare and treatment is effective, the number of relapsed patients is small, ranging from 20% to 30%. Children with recurrent malignancy following resection may be salvageable with the standard PEB regimen. For patients with cisplatin-refractory or poorly responding tumors, a further dose escalation of cisplatin under protection with amifostine is being evaluated in the United States, with results regarding toxicity still pending. Results from German protocols suggest that locoregional hyperthermia offers an attractive alternative, in that cisplatin is a good thermosensitizer and hyperthermia may thus overcome cisplatinum resistance.[192] Additionally, authors anticipate that locoregional hyperthermia will result in fewer systemic side effects than cisplatin dose escalation.

Although ifosfamide is not used as a first-line therapy, it has been incorporated into various treatment strategies for adults with relapsed or refractory disease[115,126] and, in combination with cisplatin and etoposide (ICE), has been used in a small number of pediatric patients.[122,123] There is, however, increasing concern about the nephrotoxicity of this drug combination in children. Another area of ongoing research, particularly for high-risk GCTs in older adolescents and young adults, is high-dose chemotherapy with peripheral blood stem cell transplant.[23] Outcomes of this approach have not yet been clearly established.

In a further effort to minimize the late toxic effects of treatment, the Pediatric Oncology Group and the Children's Cancer Group cooperatively developed a classification scheme that allows for less intense and more individualized treatment approaches. Based on the results of their studies, patients are stratified into three distinct risk groups:

> Low risk—patients with stage I malignant gonadal and extragonadal GCTs, including stage I immature teratomas
>
> Intermediate risk—patients with stage II to IV gonadal and stage II extragonadal GCTs
>
> High risk—patients with stage III and IV extragonadal GCTs

The Children's Oncology Group is currently developing risk-specific treatment strategies based on this new scheme. Under consideration is observation without adjuvant chemotherapy after surgical resection for all patients with stage I tumors.[63,119] To ensure that recurrent disease is detected early, strict guidelines for the evaluation and follow-up of these patients will be mandated. For patients with intermediate-risk tumors, consideration is being given to a modified standard PEB treatment that decreases the length of therapy. For children with high-risk extragonadal GCTs, the previously cited investigation using high-dose PEB in combination with amifostine is ongoing.

REFERENCES

1. Ablin A, Krailo M, Ramsey N, et al: Results of treatment of malignant germ cell tumors in 93 children: A report from the Children's Cancer Study Group. J Clin Oncol 1991;9:1782.
2. Alpers CE, Harrison MR: Fetus in fetu associated with an undescended testis. Pediatr Pathol 1985;4:37.
3. Altman RP, Randolph JG, Lilly JR: Sacrococcygeal teratoma: American Academy of Pediatrics Surgical Section Survey—1973. J Pediatr Surg 1974;9:389.
4. Atkin NB, Baker MC: Abnormal chromosomes including small metacentrics in 14 ovarian cancers. Cancer Genet Cytogenet 1987;26:355.
5. Aubry F, Satie AP, Rioux-Leclercq N, et al: MAGE-A4, a germ cell specific marker, is expressed differentially in testicular tumors. Cancer 2001;92:2778.
6. Azizkhan RG: Neonatal tumors. In Carachi R, Azmy A, Grosfeld JL (eds): The Surgery of Childhood Tumors. New York, Oxford University Press, 1999, ch 8.
7. Azizkhan RG, Caty MG: Teratomas in childhood. Curr Opin Pediatr 1996;8:287.
8. Azizkhan RG, Haase GM, Applebaum H, et al: Diagnosis, management, and outcome of cervicofacial teratomas in neonates: A Children's Cancer Group study. J Pediatr Surg 1995;30:312.
9. Bajorin DF, Sarosdy MF, Pfister DG, et al: Randomized trial of etoposide and cisplatin versus etoposide and carboplatin in patients with good-risk germ cell tumors: A multi-institutional study. J Clin Oncol 1993;11:598.

10. Bale PM: Sacrococcygeal developmental abnormalities and tumors in children. Perspect Pediatr Pathol 1984;8:9.

11. Balmaceda C, Diez B, Villablanca J, et al: Chemotherapy the only strategy in primary central nervous system germ cell tumours: Results of an international study. J Neurooncol 1993;15:S3.

12. Balmaceda C, Heller G, Rosenblum M, et al: Chemotherapy without irradiation: A novel approach for newly diagnosed CNS germ cell tumours: Results of an international cooperative trial. J Clin Oncol 1996;14:2908.

13. Balmaceda C, Modak S, Finlay J: Central nervous system germ cell tumours. Semin Oncol 1998;25:243.

14. Baranzelli MC, Patte C: The French experience in paediatric malignant germ cell tumours. In Jones WG, Appleyard I, Harnden T, et al (eds): Germ Cell Tumours, 4th ed. London, John Libbey & Co, 1998, p 219.

15. Bartlett NL, Freiha FS, Torti FM: Serum markers in germ cell neoplasms. Hematol Oncol Clin North Am 1991;5:1245.

16. Batsakis JG, Littler ER, Oberman HA: Teratomas of the neck. A clinicopathologic appraisal. Arch Otolaryngol 1964; 79:619.

17. Baumann FR, Nerlich A: Metastasizing cervical teratoma of the fetus. Pediatr Pathol 1993;13:21.

18. Beck JS, Fulmer HF, Lee ST: Solid malignant ovarian teratoma with "embryoid bodies" and trophoblastic differentiation. J Pathol 1969;99:67.

19. Belchis DA, Mowry J, Davis JH: Infantile choriocarcinoma: Re-examination of a potentially curable entity. Cancer 1993;72:2028.

20. Berry CL, Keeling J, Hilton C: Teratomata in infancy and childhood: A review of 91 cases. J Pathol 1969;98:241.

21. Bianchi DW, Crombleholme TM, D'Alton ME: Fetology: Diagnosis and Management of the Fetal Patient. New York, McGraw-Hill, 2000, chs 111, 116.

22. Billmire D, Vinocur C, Rescorla F, et al: Malignant mediastinal germ cell tumors: An intergroup study. J Pediatr Surg 2001;36:18.

23. Bokemeyer C, Kollmannsberger C, Meisner C, et al: First-line high-dose chemotherapy compared with standard-dose PEB/VIP chemotherapy in patients with advanced germ cell tumors: A multivariate and matched-pair analysis. J Clin Oncol 1999;17:3450.

24. Bond SJ, Harrison MR, Schmidt KG, et al: Death due to high-output cardiac failure in fetal sacrococcygeal teratoma. J Pediatr Surg 1990;25:1287.

25. Bosl GJ, Chaganti RS: The use of tumor markers in germ cell malignancies. Hematol Oncol Clin North Am 1994;8:573.

26. Bosl GJ, Head MD: Serum tumor marker half-life during chemotherapy in patients with germ cell tumors. Int J Biol Markers 1994;9:25.

27. Buckley NJ, Burch WM, Leight GS: Malignant teratoma in the thyroid gland of an adult: A case report and a review of the literature. Surgery 1986;100:932.

28. Bussey KJ, Lawce HJ, Olson SB, et al: Chromosome abnormalities of eighty-one pediatric germ cell tumors: Sex-, age-, site-, and histopathology-related differences—a Children's Cancer Group study. Genes Chromosomes Cancer 1999; 25:134.

29. Calaminus G, Schneider DT, Bokkerink JP, et al: Prognostic value of tumor size, metastases, extension into bone, and increased tumor marker in children with malignant sacrococcygeal germ cell tumors: A prospective evaluation of 71 patients treated in the German cooperative protocols Maligne Keimzelltumoren (MAKEI) 83/86 and MAKEI 89. J Clin Oncol 2003;21:781.

30. Carney JA, Thompson DP, Johnson CL, et al: Teratomas in children: Clinical and pathologic aspects. J Pediatr Surg 1972;7:271.

31. Carter D, Bibro MC, Touloukian RJ: Benign clinical behavior of immature mediastinal teratoma in infancy and childhood. Cancer 1982;49:398.

32. Casalone R, Righi R, Granata P, et al: Cerebral germ cell tumor and XXY karyotype. Cancer Genet Cytogenet 1994; 74:25.

33. Chandra SA, Gilbert EF, Viseskul C, et al: Neonatal intracranial choriocarcinoma. Arch Pathol Lab Med 1990; 114:1079.

34. Christensen TB, Engbaek F, Marqversen J, et al: ^{125}I-labelled human chorionic gonadotrophin (hCG) as an elimination marker in the evaluation of hCG decline during chemotherapy in patients with testicular cancer. Br J Cancer 1999; 80:1577.

35. Cushing B, Giller R, Lauer S, et al: Comparison of high dose or standard dose cisplatin with etoposide and bleomycin (HDPEB vs PEB) in children with stage I-IV extragonadal malignant germ cell tumors (MGCT): A Pediatric Intergroup report (POG9049/CCG8882) [abstract]. Proc Am Soc Clin Oncol 1998;17:525a.

36. Cushing B, Perlman E, Marina N, et al: Germ cell tumors. In Pizzo PA, Poplock DG (eds): Principles and Practice of Pediatric Oncology, 2nd ed. Philadelphia, JB Lippincott, 1993, ch 36.

37. Dautenhahn L, Babyn PS, Smith CR: Metastatic choriocarcinoma in an infant: Imaging appearance. Pediatr Radiol 1993;23:597.

38. deBruin TW, Slater RM, Defferari R, et al: Isochromosome 12p-positive pineal germ cell tumor. Cancer Res 1994; 54:1542.

39. Dehner LP: Neoplasms of the fetus and neonate. In Naeye RL, Kissane JM, Kaufman N (eds): Perinatal Diseases. International Academy of Pathology, Monograph No. 22. Baltimore, Williams & Wilkins, 1981, p 286.

40. Dehner LP: Gonadal and extragonadal germ cell neoplasia of childhood. Hum Pathol 1983;14:493.

41. Dehner LP: Gonadal and extragonadal germ cell neoplasms: Teratomas in childhood. In Finegold MJ, Bennington J (eds): Pathology of Neoplasia in Children and Adolescents. Philadelphia, WB Saunders, 1986, p 282.

42. Dehner LP: Germ cell tumors of the mediastinum. Semin Diagn Pathol 1990;7:266.

43. Dehner LP, Mills A, Talerman A, et al: Germ cell neoplasms of head and neck soft tissues: A pathologic spectrum of teratomatous and endodermal sinus tumors. Hum Pathol 1990;21:309.

44. Donnellan WA, Swenson O: Benign and malignant sacrococcygeal teratomas. Pediatr Surg 1988;64:834.

45. Dunn CJ, Nguyen DL, Leonard JC: Ultrasound diagnosis of immature cervical teratoma: A case report. Am J Perinatol 1992;9:445.

46. Einhorn LH, Donohue J: Cis-diamminedichloroplatinum, vinblastine, and bleomycin combination chemotherapy in disseminated testicular cancer. Ann Intern Med 1977;87:293.

47. Esposito G, Cigliano B, Paludetto R: Abdominothoracic gastric teratoma in a female newborn infant. J Pediatr Surg 1983;18:304.

48. Federici S, Ceccarelli PL, Ferrari M, et al: Fetus in fetu: Report of three cases and review of the literature. Pediatr Surg Int 1991;6:60.

49. Felix I, Becker LE: Intracranial germ cell tumors in children: An immunohistochemical and electron microscopic study. Pediatr Neurosurg 1990;16:156.

50. Fisher RA, Salm R, Spencer RW: Bilateral gonadoblastoma/dysgerminoma in a 46XY individual: Case report with hormonal studies. J Clin Pathol 1982;35:420.

51. Fishman SJ, Jennings RW, Johnson SM, et al: Contouring buttock reconstruction after sacrococcygeal teratoma resection. J Pediatr Surg 2004;39:439.

52. Fishman WH: Alkaline phosphatase isoenzymes: Recent progress. Clin Biochem 1990;23:94.
53. Flake AW: Fetal sacrococcygeal teratoma. Semin Pediatr Surg 1993;2:113.
54. Flake AW, Harrison MR, Adzick NS, et al: Fetal sacrococcygeal teratoma. J Pediatr Surg 1986;21:563.
55. Flam F, Lundstrom V, Silfversward C: Choriocarcinoma in mother and child: Case report. Br J Obstet Gynaecol 1989; 96:241.
56. Fraser GC, Blair GK, Hemming A, et al: The treatment of simultaneous choriocarcinoma in mother and baby. J Pediatr Surg 1992;27:1318.
57. Fraumeni JF Jr, Li FP, Dalager N: Teratomas in children: Epidemiologic features. J Natl Cancer Inst 1973; 51:1425.
58. Fukuda S, Shirahama T, Imazono Y, et al: Expression of vascular endothelial growth factor in patients with testicular germ cell tumors as an indicator of metastatic disease. Cancer 1999;85:1323.
59. Gels ME, Marrink J, Visser P, et al: Importance of a new tumor marker TRA-1-60 in the follow-up of patients with clinical stage 1 nonseminomatous testicular germ cell tumors. Ann Surg Oncol 1997;4:321.
60. Germa JR, Llanos M, Tabernero JM, et al: False elevations of alpha-fetoprotein associated with liver dysfunction in germ cell tumors. Cancer 1993;72:2491.
61. Gershenson DM, Del Junco G, Copeland LJ, et al: Mixed germ cell tumors of the ovary. Obstet Gynecol 1984; 64:200.
62. Gitlin D, Perricelli A, Gillin GM: Synthesis of fetoprotein by liver, yolk sac, and gastrointestinal tract of the human conceptus. Cancer Res 1972;32:979.
63. Göbel U, Calaminus G, Schneider DT, et al: Management of germ cell tumors in children: Approaches to cure. Onkologie 2002;25:14.
64. Göbel U, Schneider DT, Calaminus G, et al: Multimodal treatment of malignant sacrococcygeal germ cell tumors: A prospective analysis of 66 patients of the German cooperative protocols MAKEI 83/86 and 89. J Clin Oncol 2001;19:1943.
65. Gonzalez-Crussi F: Extragonadal teratomas. In Atlas of Tumor Pathology, 2nd ser, fascicle 18. Washington, DC, Armed Forces Institute of Pathology, 1982.
66. Gonzalez-Crussi F, Winkler RF, Mirkin DL: Sacrococcygeal teratomas in infants and children: Relationship of histology and prognosis in 40 cases. Arch Pathol Lab Med 1978; 102:420.
67. Gornall P: Malignant germ cell tumors. In Carachi R, Azmy A, Grosfeld JL (eds): The Surgery of Childhood Tumors. New York, Oxford University Press, 1999, ch 12.
68. Goto M, Makino Y, Tamura R, et al: Sacrococcygeal teratoma with hydrops fetalis and bilateral hydronephrosis. J Perinat Med 2000;28:414.
69. Grisoni ER, Gauderer MWL, Wolfson RN, et al: Antenatal diagnosis of sacrococcygeal teratomas: Prognostic features. Pediatr Surg Int 1988;3:173.
70. Gross RE, Clatworthy HW, Meeker IA: Sacrococcygeal teratoma in infants and children. Surg Gynecol Obstet 1951; 92:341.
71. Gross SJ, Benzie RJ, Sermer M, et al: Sacrococcygeal teratoma: Prenatal diagnosis and management. Am J Obstet Gynecol 1987;156:393.
72. Gundry SR, Wesley JR, Klein MD, et al: Cervical teratomas in the newborn. J Pediatr Surg 1983;18:382.
73. Haase GM, Vinocur CD: Ovarian tumors. In O'Neill JA Jr, Rowe MI, Grosfeld JL, et al (eds): Pediatric Surgery, vol 1, 5th ed. St Louis, Mosby, 1998, ch 33.
74. Hajdu SI, Faruque AA, Hajdu E, et al: Teratoma of the neck in infants. Am J Dis Child 1966;3:412.
75. Hale GA, Marina NM, Jones-Wallace D, et al: Late effects of treatment for germ cell tumors during childhood and adolescence. J Pediatr Hematol Oncol 1999;21:115.
76. Halperin EC, Constine LS, Tarbell NJ, Kun LE (eds): Supratentorial brain tumours. In Paediatric Radiation Oncology, 3rd ed. Philadelphia, Lippincott Williams & Wilkins, 1999, p 67.
77. Harms D, Janig U: Germ cell tumors of childhood: Report of 170 cases including 59 pure and partial yolk-sac tumors. Virchows Arch A Pathol Anat Histopathol 1986;409:223.
78. Hawkins EP: Pathology of germ cell tumors in children. Crit Rev Oncol Hematol 1990;10:165.
79. Hawkins EP, Finegold MJ, Hawkins HK, et al: Nongerminomatous malignant germ cell tumors in children: A review of 89 cases from the Pediatric Oncology Group, 1971-1984. Cancer 1986;58:2579.
80. Hawkins EP, Perlman EJ: Germ cell tumors in childhood: Morphology and biology. In Parham DM (ed): Pediatric Neoplasia: Morphology and Biology. New York, Raven Press, 1996, p 297.
81. Hechelhammer L, Storkel S, Odermatt B, et al: Epidermal growth factor receptor is a marker for syncytiotrophoblastic cells in testicular germ cell tumors. Virchows Arch 2003; 443:28.
82. Hedrick HL, Flake AW, Crombleholme TM, et al: Sacrococcygeal teratoma: Prenatal assessment, fetal intervention, and outcome. J Pediatr Surg 2004;39:430.
83. Heifetz SA, Alrabeeah A, Brown BS, et al: Fetus in fetu: A fetiform teratoma. Pediatr Pathol 1988;8:215.
84. Heifetz SA, Cushing B, Biller R, et al: Immature teratomas in children: Pathologic considerations. Am J Surg Pathol 1998;22:1115.
85. Hoffner L, Deka R, Chakravarti A: Cytogenetics and origins of pediatric germ cell tumors. Cancer Genet Cytogenet 1994;74:54.
86. Hoffner L, Shen-Schwarz S, Deka R, et al: Genetics and biology of human ovarian teratomas. III. Cytogenetics and origins of malignant ovarian germ cell tumors. Cancer Genet Cytogenet 1992;62:58.
87. Holzgreve W, Miny P, Anderson R, et al: Experience with 8 cases of prenatally diagnosed sacrococcygeal teratomas. Fetal Ther 1987;2:88.
88. Horwich A, Sleijfer DT, Fossa SD, et al: Randomized trial of bleomycin, etoposide, and cisplatin compared with bleomycin, etoposide, and carboplatin in good-prognosis metastatic nonseminomatous germ cell cancer: A multi-institutional Medical Research Council/European Organization for Research and Treatment of Cancer trial. J Clin Oncol 1997;15:1844.
89. Hurlbut HJ, Webb HW, Moseley T: Cervical teratoma in infant siblings. J Pediatr Surg 1967;2:424.
90. International Germ Cell Consensus Classification: A prognostic factor-based staging system for metastatic germ cell cancers. International Germ Cell Cancer Collaborative Group. J Clin Oncol 1997;15:594.
91. Isaacs H Jr: Tumors of the Newborn and Infant. St Louis, Mosby–Year Book, 1991.
92. Isaacs H Jr: Germ cell tumors. In Tumors of the Fetus and Newborn, vol 35 in Major Problems in Pathology. Philadelphia, WB Saunders, 1997, p 15.
93. Jacobsen GK, Norgaard-Pedersen B: Placental alkaline phosphatase in testicular germ cell tumours and in carcinoma in-situ of the testis: An immunohistochemical study. Acta Pathol Microbiol Immunol Scand (A) 1984;92:323.
94. Jirasek JE: Morphogenesis of the genital system in the human. Birth Defects Orig Artic Ser 1977;13:13.
95. Jordan RB, Gauderer MW: Cervical teratomas: An analysis, literature review and proposed classification. J Pediatr Surg 1988;23:583.

96. Kamoto T, Satomura S, Yoshiki T, et al: Lectin-reactive alpha-fetoprotein (AFP-L3%) curability and prediction of clinical course after treatment of non-seminomatous germ cell tumors. Jpn J Clin Oncol 2002;32:472.

97. Kapoor G, Advani SH, Nair CN, et al: Pediatric germ cell tumor: An experience with BEP. J Pediatr Hematol Oncol 1995;17:318.

98. Kashiwagi A, Nagamori S, Toyota K, et al: DNA ploidy of testicular germ cell tumors in childhood: Difference from adult testicular tumors. Nippon Hinyokika Gakkai Zasshi 1993;84:1655.

99. Kay R: Prepubertal testicular tumor registry. Urol Clin North Am 1993;20:1.

100. Kelly MF, Berenholz L, Rizzo KA, et al: Approach for oxygenation of the newborn with airway obstruction due to a cervical mass. Ann Otol Rhinol Laryngol 1990;99:179.

101. Kim SN, Chi JG, Kim YW, et al: Neonatal choriocarcinoma of the liver. Pediatr Pathol 1993;13:723.

102. King ME, Hubbell MJ, Talerman A: Mixed germ cell tumor of the ovary with a prominent polyembryoma component. Int J Gynecol Pathol 1991;10:88.

103. Koshida K, Nishino A, Yamamoto H, et al: The role of alkaline phosphatase isoenzymes as tumor markers for testicular germ cell tumors. J Urol 1991;146:57.

104. Kuhlmann RS, Warsof SL, Levy DL, et al: Fetal sacrococcygeal teratoma. Fetal Ther 1987;2:95.

105. Kurman RJ, Norris HJ: Malignant mixed germ cell tumors of the ovary: A clinical and pathologic analysis of 30 cases. Obstet Gynecol 1976;48:579.

106. Lachman MF, Kim K, Koo BC: Mediastinal teratoma associated with Klinefelter's syndrome. Arch Pathol Lab Med 1986;110:1067.

107. Lakhoo K, Boyle M, Drake DP: Mediastinal teratomas: Review of 15 pediatric cases. J Pediatr Surg 1993;28:1161.

108. Lamb DJ: Growth factors and testicular development. J Urol 1993;150:583.

109. Lange PH, Vogelzang NJ, Goldman A, et al: Marker half-life analysis as a prognostic tool in testicular cancer. J Urol 1982;128:708.

110. Langer JC, Tabb T, Thompson P, et al: Management of prenatally diagnosed tracheal obstruction: Access to the airway in utero prior to delivery. Fetal Diagn Ther 1992;7:12.

111. Lawton AJ, Mead GM: Staging and prognostic factors in testicular cancer. Semin Surg Oncol 1999;17:223.

112. Lemire RG, Beckwith JB: Pathogenesis of congenital tumors and malformations of the sacrococcygeal region. Teratology 1982;25:201.

113. Leroy X, Augusto D, Leteurtre E, et al: CD30 and CD117 (c-kit) used in combination are useful for distinguishing embryonal carcinoma from seminoma. J Histochem Cytochem 2002;50:283.

114. Lifschitz-Mercer B, Elliott DJ, Leider-Trejo L, et al: Absence of RBM expression as a marker of intratubular (in situ) germ cell neoplasia of the testis. Hum Pathol 2000;31:1116.

115. Loehrer PJ Sr, Gonin R, Nichols CR, et al: Vinblastine plus ifosfamide plus cisplatin as initial salvage therapy in recurrent germ cell tumor. J Clin Oncol 1998;16:2500.

116. Lund DP, Soriano SG, Fauza D, et al: Resection of a massive sacrococcygeal teratoma using hypothermic hypoperfusion: A novel use of extracorporeal membrane oxygenation. J Pediatr Surg 1995;30:1557.

117. Magee JF, McFadden DE, Pantzar JT: Congenital tumors. In Dimmick JE, Kalousek DK (eds): Developmental Pathology of the Embryo and Fetus. Philadelphia, JB Lippincott, 1992, p 235.

118. Mahour GH, Landing BH, Woolley MM: Teratomas in children: Clinicopathologic studies in 133 patients. Z Kinderchir 1978;23:365.

119. Mann JR, Raafat F, Robinson K, et al: The United Kingdom Children's Cancer Study Group's second germ cell tumor study: Carboplatin, etoposide, and bleomycin are effective treatment for children with malignant extracranial germ cell tumors, with acceptable toxicity. J Clin Oncol 2000;18:3809.

120. Marina NM, Cushing B, Giller R, et al: Complete surgical excision is effective treatment for children with immature teratomas with or without malignant elements: A Pediatric Oncology Group/Children's Cancer Group Intergroup Study. J Clin Oncol 1999;17:2137.

121. Marina NM, Fontanesi J, Kun L, et al: Treatment of childhood germ cell tumors: Review of the St Jude experience from 1979 to 1988. Cancer 1992;70:2568.

122. Marina NM, Rodman JH, Murry DJ, et al: Phase I study of escalating targeted doses of carboplatin combined with ifosfamide and etoposide in treatment of newly diagnosed pediatric solid tumors. J Natl Cancer Inst 1994;86:544.

123. Marina NM, Shema SJ, Bowman LC, et al: Failure of granulocyte-macrophage colony-stimulating factor to reduce febrile neutropenia in children with recurrent solid tumors treated with ifosfamide, carboplatin, and etoposide chemotherapy. Med Pediatr Oncol 1994;23:328.

124. Mazumdar M, Bacik J, Tickoo SK, et al: Cluster analysis of p53 and Ki67 expression, apoptosis, alpha-fetoprotein, and human chorionic gonadotrophin indicates a favorable prognostic subgroup within the embryonal carcinoma germ cell tumor. J Clin Oncol 2003;21:2679.

125. Mazumdar M, Bajorin DF, Bacik J, et al: Predicting outcome to chemotherapy in patients with germ cell tumors: The value of the rate of decline of human chorionic gonadotrophin and alpha-fetoprotein during therapy. J Clin Oncol 2001;19:2534.

126. McCaffrey JA, Mazumdar M, Bajorin DF, et al: Ifosfamide- and cisplatin-containing chemotherapy as first-line salvage therapy in germ cell tumors: Response and survival. J Clin Oncol 1997;15:2559.

127. Merchant TE, Davis BJ, Sheldon JM, et al: Radiation therapy for relapsed CNS germinoma after primary chemotherapy. J Clin Oncol 1998;16:204.

128. Misra D, Pritchard J, Drake DP, et al: Markedly improved survival in malignant sacrococcygeal teratomas—16 years' experience. Eur J Pediatr Surg 1997;7:152.

129. Miyanohara O, Takeshima H, Kaji M, et al: Diagnostic significance of soluble c-kit in the cerebrospinal fluid of patients with germ cell tumors. J Neurosurg 2002;97:177.

130. Morris MJ, Bosl GJ: Recognizing abnormal marker results that do not reflect disease in patients with germ cell tumors. J Urol 2000;163:796.

131. Murphy BA, Motzer RJ, Mazumdar M, et al: Serum tumor marker decline is an early predictor of treatment outcome in germ cell tumor patients treated with cisplatin and ifosfamide salvage chemotherapy. Cancer 1994;73:2520.

132. Musci MN Jr, Clark MJ, Ayres RE, et al: Management of dystocia caused by a large sacrococcygeal teratoma. Obstet Gynecol 1983;62(3 Suppl):10s.

133. Nakashima N, Fukatsu T, Nagasaka T, et al: The frequency and histology of hepatic tissue in germ cell tumors. Am J Surg Pathol 1987;11:682.

134. Naudin Ten Cate L, Vermeij-Keers C, Smit DA, et al: Intracranial teratoma with multiple fetuses: Pre- and postnatal appearance. Hum Pathol 1995;26:804.

135. Nirasawa Y, Ito Y: Reproduction-preserving technique for benign cystic teratoma of the ovary. Pediatr Surg Int 1995; 10:126.

136. Nogales FF: Embryologic clues to human yolk sac tumors: A review. Int J Gynecol Pathol 1993;12:101.

137. Norris HJ, Zirkin HJ, Benson WL: Immature (malignant) teratoma of the ovary: A clinical and pathologic study of 58 cases. Cancer 1976;37:2359.

138. Noseworthy J, Lack EE, Kozakewich HP, et al: Sacrococcygeal germ cell tumors in childhood: An updated experience with 118 patients. J Pediatr Surg 1981;16:358.

139. Olsen MM, Caldamone AA, Jackson CL, et al: Gonadoblastoma in infancy: Indications for early gonadectomy in 46XY gonadal dysgenesis. J Pediatr Surg 1988;23:270.

140. Owor R, Master SP: Cervical teratomas in the newborn. East Afr Med J 1974;51:376.

141. Packer RJ, Sutton LN, Rosenstock JG, et al: Pineal region tumors of childhood. Pediatrics 1984;74:97.

142. Parkes SE, Muir KR, Southern L, et al: Neonatal tumours: A thirty-year population based study. Med Pediatr Oncol 1994;22:309.

143. Perlman EJ, Cushing B, Hawkins E, et al: Cytogenetic analysis of childhood endodermal sinus tumors: A Pediatric Oncology Group study. Pediatr Pathol 1994;14:695.

144. Perlman EJ, Hu J, Ho D, et al: Genetic analysis of childhood endodermal sinus tumors by comparative genomic hybridization. J Pediatr Hematol Oncol 2000;22:100.

145. Perlman EJ, Valentine MB, Look AT, et al: Deletion of the short arm of chromosome 1 in childhood endodermal sinus tumor by two color fluorescence in situ hybridization. Lab Invest 1995;72:5.

146. Potter EL, Craig JM: Pathology of the Fetus and the Infant, 3rd ed. Chicago, Year Book Medical Publishers, 1975, p 177.

147. Prat J, Matias-Guiu X, Scully RE: Hepatic yolk sac differentiation in an ovarian polyembryoma. Surg Pathol 1989;2:147.

148. Rescorla FJ: Pediatric germ cell tumors. Semin Surg Oncol 1999;16:144.

149. Rescorla FJ, Billmire D, Stolar C, et al: The effect of cisplatin dose and surgical resection in children with malignant germ cell tumors at the sacrococcygeal region: A pediatric intergroup trial (POG 9049/CCG 8882). J Pediatr Surg 2001;36:12.

150. Rescorla FJ, Sawin RS, Coran AG, et al: Long-term outcome for infants and children with sacrococcygeal teratoma: A report from the Children's Cancer Group. J Pediatr Surg 1998;33:171.

151. Richie JP: Neoplasms of the testis. In Walsh PC, Retik AB, Stamey TA, et al (eds): Campbell's Urology, 6th ed. Philadelphia, WB Saunders, 1992, p 1222.

152. Robboy SJ, Miller T, Donahoe PK, et al: Dysgenesis of testicular and streak gonads in syndrome of mixed gonadal dysgenesis: Perspective derived from a clinicopathologic analysis of twenty one cases. Hum Pathol 1982; 13:700.

153. Robboy SJ, Scully RE: Ovarian teratoma with glial implants on the peritoneum: An analysis of 12 cases. Hum Pathol 1970;1:643.

154. Robertson FM, Crombleholme TM, Frantz ID, et al: Devascularization and staged resection of giant sacrococcygeal teratoma in the premature infant. J Pediatr Surg 1995;30:309.

155. Rowe MI, O'Neill JA, Grosfeld JL, et al: Teratomas and germ cell tumors. In Essentials of Pediatric Surgery. St Louis, Mosby, 1995, p 296.

156. Sawamura Y, Ikeda J, Shirato H, et al: Germ cell tumours of the central nervous system: Treatment considerations based on 111 cases and their long-term clinical outcomes. Eur J Cancer 1998;34:104.

157. Schey WL, Shkolnik A, White H: Clinical and radiographic considerations of sacrococcygeal teratomas: An analysis of 26 new cases and review of the literature. Radiology 1977;125:189.

158. Schropp KP, Lobe TE, Rao B, et al: Sacrococcygeal teratoma: The experience of four decades. J Pediatr Surg 1992;27:1075.

159. Schwartz PE, Chambers SK, Chambers JT, et al: Ovarian germ cell malignancies: The Yale University experience. Gynecol Oncol 1992;45:26.

160. Schwartz PE, Morris JM: Serum lactic dehydrogenase: A tumor marker for dysgerminoma. Obstet Gynecol 1988;72:511.

161. Scully RE, Young RH, Clement PB: Atlas of Tumor Pathology, 3rd ser, fascicle 23. Washington, DC, Armed Forces Institute of Pathology, 1998, ch 13.

162. Senocak ME, Kale G, Buyukpamukcu N, et al: Gastric teratoma in children including the third reported female case. J Pediatr Surg 1990;25:681.

163. Shaaban AF, Kim HB, Flake AW: Fetal surgery, diagnosis, and intervention. In Ziegler MM, Azizkhan RG, Weber TR (eds): Operative Pediatric Surgery. New York, McGraw-Hill, 2003, ch 3.

164. Shamberger RC: Teratomas and germ cell tumors. In O'Neill JA, Grosfeld JL, Fonkalsrud EW, et al (eds): Principles of Pediatric Surgery, 2nd ed. St Louis, Mosby, 2004, ch 24.

165. Shen V, Chaparro M, Choi BH, et al: Absence of isochromosome 12p in a pineal region malignant germ cell tumor. Cancer Genet Cytogenet 1990;50:153.

166. Shitara T, Oshima Y, Yugami S, et al: Choriocarcinoma in children. Am J Pediatr Hematol Oncol 1993;15:268.

167. Silberman R, Mendelson IR: Teratoma of the neck: Report of 2 cases and review of the literature. Arch Dis Child 1960;35:159.

168. Silver SA, Wiley JM, Perlman EJ: DNA ploidy analysis of pediatric germ cell tumors. Mod Pathol 1994;7:951.

169. Stern JW, Bunin N: Prospective study of carboplatin-based chemotherapy for pediatric germ cell tumors. Med Pediatr Oncol 2002;39:163.

170. Stock C, Ambros IM, Lion T, et al: Detection of numerical and structural chromosome abnormalities in pediatric germ cell tumors by means of interphase cytogenetics. Cancer 1994;11:40.

171. Strohmeyer T, Reese D, Press M, et al: Expression of the c-kit proto-oncogene and its ligand stem cell factor (SCF) in normal and malignant human testicular tissue. J Urol 1995;153:511.

172. Suita S, Ikeda K, Nakano H, et al: Teratoma of the neck in a newborn infant—a case report. Z Kinderchir 1982;35:9.

173. Takeda A, Ishizuka T, Goto T, et al: Polyembryoma of ovary producing alpha-fetoprotein and HCG: Immunoperoxidase and electron microscopic study. Cancer 1982;49:1878.

174. Takeshima H, Kuratsu J: A review of soluble c-kit (s-kit) as a novel tumor marker and possible molecular target for the treatment of CNS germinoma. Surg Neurol 2003; 60:321.

175. Talerman A: Germ cell tumors of the ovary. In Kurman RJ (ed): Blaustein's Pathology of the Female Genital Tract, 4th ed. New York, Springer-Verlag, 1994, p 849.

176. Tapper D, Lack EE: Teratomas in infancy and childhood: A 54-year experience at the Children's Hospital Medical Center. Ann Surg 1983;198:398.

177. Teitelbaum D, Teich S, Cassidy S, et al: Highly vascularized sacrococcygeal teratoma: Description of this atypical variant and its operative management. J Pediatr Surg 1994;29:98.

178. Toner GC, Stockler MR, Boyer MJ, et al: Comparison of two standard chemotherapy regimens for good prognosis germ cell tumors: A randomized trial. Lancet 2001;357:739.

179. Touran T, Applebaum H, Frost DB, et al: Congenital metastatic cervical teratoma: Diagnostic and management considerations. J Pediatr Surg 1989;24:21.

180. Trigo JM, Tabernero JM, Paz-Ares L, et al: Tumor markers at the time of recurrence in patients with germ cell tumors. Cancer 2000;88:162.

181. Troche V, Hernandez E: Neoplasia arising in dysgenetic gonads: A review. Obstet Gynecol Surv 1986;41:74.

182. Tsukahara Y, Fukuta T, Yamada T, et al: Retroperitoneal giant tumor formed by migrating polyembryoma with numerous embryoid bodies from an ovarian mixed germ cell tumor. Gynecol Obstet Invest 1991;31:58.

183. Tsuura Y, Hiraki H, Watanabe K, et al: Preferential localization of c-kit product in tissue mast cells, basal cells of skin, epithelial cells of breast, small cell lung carcinoma and seminoma/dysgerminoma in human: Immunohistochemical study on formalin-fixed, paraffin-embedded tissues. Virchows Arch 1994;424:135.

184. Valdiserri RO, Yunis EJ: Sacrococcygeal teratomas: A review of 68 cases. Cancer 1981;48:217.

185. Verp MS, Simpson JL: Abnormal sexual differentiation and neoplasia. Cancer Genet Cytogenet 1987; 25:191.

186. Vilain E, Jaubert F, Fellous M, et al: Pathology of 46,XY pure gonadal dysgenesis: Absence of testis differentiation associated with mutations in the testis-determining factor. Differentiation 1993;52:151.

187. Vogelzang NJ, Lange PH, Goldman A, et al: Acute changes of alpha-fetoprotein and human chorionic gonadotropin during induction chemotherapy of germ cell tumors. Cancer Res 1982;42:4855.

188. von Eyben FE, Madsen EL, Blaabjerg O, et al: Serum lactate dehydrogenase isoenzyme 1 and relapse in patients with nonseminomatous testicular germ cell tumors clinical stage I. Acta Oncol 2001;40:536.

189. Waldhausen JA, Kolman JW, Vellios F, et al: Sacrococcygeal teratoma. Pediatr Surg 1963;54:933.

190. Warner BA, Monsaert RP, Stumpf PG, et al: 46,XY gonadal dysgenesis: Is oncogenesis related to H-Y phenotype or breast development? Hum Genet 1985;69:79.

191. Werb P, Scurry J, Ostor A, et al: Survey of congenital tumors in perinatal necropsies. Pathology 1992;24:247.

192. Wessalowski R, Kruck H, Pape H, et al: Hyperthermia for the treatment of patients with malignant germ cell tumors: A phase I/II study in ten children and adolescents with recurrent or refractory tumors. Cancer 1998;82:793.

193. Wollner N, Ghavimi F, Wachtel A, et al: Germ cell tumors in children: Gonadal and extragonadal. Med Pediatr Oncol 1991;19:228.

194. Wu JT, Book L, Sudar K: Serum alpha fetoprotein (AFP) levels in normal infants. Pediatr Res 1981;15:50.

195. Young JL Jr, Ries LG, Silverberg E, et al: Cancer incidence, survival and mortality for children younger than age 15 years. Cancer 1986;58(2 Suppl):598.

196. Young R, Scully R: Germ cell tumors: Nonseminomatous Tumors, Occult Tumors, Effects of Chemotherapy in Testicular Tumors. Chicago: ASCP Press, 1990, p 37.

197. Yu IT, Griffin CA, Phillips PC, et al: Numerical sex chromosomal abnormalities in pineal teratomas by cytogenetic analysis and fluorescence in situ hybridization. Lab Invest 1995;72:419.

Chapter 35

Hodgkin's Disease and Non-Hodgkin's Lymphoma

Michael P. La Quaglia and Wendy T. Su

HODGKIN'S DISEASE

Hodgkin's disease was first described by Hodgkin in 1832, based on anatomic observation. The original paper was entitled "On Some Morbid Appearance of the Absorbent Glands and Spleen."[44] After the development of microscopic histology, Sternberg in 1898 and Reed in 1902 were the first to characterize the histopathology.[110,121] They emphasized the unique appearance of a multinucleated giant cell with prominent nucleoli, which distinguished it from tuberculosis. The first reports of radiotherapy for Hodgkin's disease were published in 1902 and 1903.[98] The radiotherapeutic principles required for curative treatment of Hodgkin's disease were reported by Gilbert.[33] Peters[94] in Toronto subsequently published a series of patients who survived disease-free 20 years after treatment. Staging laparotomy was developed in the late 1960s to map out patterns of metastatic spread and for research.[34] Kaplan et al.[13,51,103] at Stanford University laid the foundation for modern supervoltage treatment of Hodgkin's disease. Use of a derivative of nitrogen mustard to treat patients with lymphosarcoma and Hodgkin's disease was published in 1946,[36] and the results of multiagent treatment with MOPP (Mustargen [mechlorethamine], Oncovin [vincristine], procarbazine, prednisone) were reported in 1967.[22] As survival improved, it was noted that more patients developed adverse side effects, such as secondary malignancy and infertility. The non-cross-resistant ABVD regimen (Adriamycin [doxorubicin], bleomycin, vinblastine, dacarbazine) was developed in the 1970s, with less risk of secondary acute myelogenous leukemia and infertility. In the 1980s more investigators began to recognize the long-term sequelae of standard-dose radiotherapy and chemotherapy, especially in the pediatric population. A combined-modality regimen was applied to a subset of patients initially selected with staging laparotomy and later by diagnostic imaging in the 1990s. Risk-adaptive trials and tailored therapy were the main investigational efforts of that decade, with the aim of finding the optimal combination therapy with maximal efficacy and minimal toxicity.

Incidence and Epidemiology

Hodgkin's disease (HD) is characterized by a bimodal age distribution. The first peak is from 15 years to the late 20s, and the second peak occurs in those older than 50 years. Three forms of HD have been recognized by epidemiologic studies. The childhood form occurs in those younger than 14 years, the young adult form occurs in those 15 to 34 years old, and the older adult form occurs in those between 55 and 74 years. Children and adolescents account for 15% of all HD patients, and HD is twice as common in teenagers as it is in those younger than 10 years. HD accounts for 5% of all pediatric malignancies, with an incidence of about 6 cases per 1 million. Histologic subtypes also vary with age. Mixed cellularity HD is more common in young children, whereas nodular sclerosing HD is more frequently observed in adolescents.

The cause of HD is multifactorial, but there is an association with Epstein-Barr virus (EBV) exposure that is most frequently seen in children younger than 10 years. The viral infection appears to precede tumor cell expansion, and EBV may act alone or in conjunction with other carcinogens. Until recently, the origin of Reed-Sternberg cells was elusive. Advances in immunohistology and molecular biology have revealed the clonal nature of these cells. Reed-Sternberg, lymphocytic, and histiocytic cells seen in HD appear to derive from a single transformed B cell that has undergone monoclonal expansion. Immunophenotyping of HD cells has demonstrated B-cell antigens. HD is also characterized by many cytokine-producing and -responding cells, which are responsible for the nonspecific signs and symptoms seen with this tumor.

Clinical Presentation

Painless cervical or supraclavicular lymphadenopathy is the most common presenting symptom of HD (80%). Enlarged nodes primary to the axilla or groin are relatively

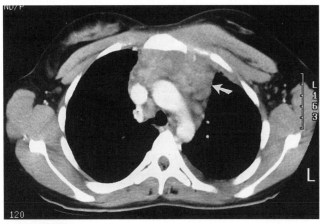

Figure 35-1 Thoracic computed tomography scan showing tumor in the mediastinum (*arrow*) in a patient with stage IIB Hodgkin's disease. These studies should be obtained before surgery to identify tracheobronchial obstruction.

uncommon (30%), and primary inguinal involvement is encountered in less than 5% of cases. The lymphadenopathy is usually firm, rubbery, and nontender. More than two thirds of patients have mediastinal involvement at presentation, and good posteroanterior chest radiographs are essential to evaluate the mediastinum and to rule out airway obstruction before any invasive procedures. When a mediastinal mass is identified by plain radiographs, it is also advisable to obtain a thoracic computed tomography (CT) scan with intravenous contrast material to evaluate the airway and obtain further anatomic information (Figs. 35-1 and 35-2). Clinicians should always assume that airway compression by tumor is a possibility before the institution of general anesthesia. The superior vena caval syndrome, with facial swelling, distended neck veins, and plethoric complexion above the neck, is highly suggestive of superior vena cava obstruction by mediastinal tumor.

Approximately one third of patients present with systemic symptoms (substage B symptoms; see later), which may include loss of more than 10% of body weight in the past 6 months, drenching night sweats, or fever greater

than 38°C (100.4°F). Pruritus is also commonly observed among HD patients but does not carry as much prognostic value. The immune profiles of HD patients are altered, and the disease is characterized by generalized immune deficiency, ineffective host autoimmune response, and cutaneous anergy.[123]

Diagnosis

The workup of patients with suspected HD should begin with a careful history and physical examination. All nodal groups should be evaluated, and enlarged lymph nodes measured. The lymphatic tissue composing Waldeyer's ring (adenoids and tonsils) should also be examined. The diagnosis of HD requires lymph node biopsy for histologic evaluation. The presence of Reed-Sternberg cells is pathognomonic of HD (Fig. 35-3). There are four histologic subtypes defined by the Rye classification—lymphocyte predominance, nodular sclerosing, mixed cellularity, and lymphocyte depletion—each with a unique immunophenotypic profile.[40] Nodular sclerosing is the most common subtype seen in children (>65%), followed by mixed cellularity and lymphocyte predominance. The lymphocyte-predominance subtype carries the best prognosis historically. However, since the development of highly effective multiagent and multidisciplinary treatment regimens, all histologic subtypes have become responsive to therapy.

Laboratory studies should include a complete blood cell count with differential, erythrocyte sedimentation rate, baseline hepatic and renal function tests, and electrolytes. The serum copper and lactate dehydrogenase (LDH) levels at diagnosis have been correlated with tumor burden, but there are no specific tumor markers.

Staging

Staging of HD can be either clinical or pathologic. Clinical staging is based on the well-established Ann Arbor

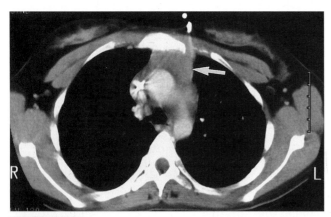

Figure 35-2 The same patient in Figure 35-1 after chemotherapy. The nodular mediastinal mass has resolved (*arrow*), but there is homogeneous thymic enlargement. This rebound thymic hyperplasia can be confused with disease persistence or recurrence.

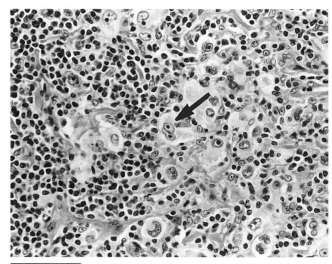

Figure 35-3 A histopathologic section from a patient with nodular sclerosing Hodgkin's disease. The *arrow* identifies a Reed-Sternberg cell.

TABLE 35-1 Ann Arbor Staging System for Hodgkin's Disease

Stage	Criteria
I	Involvement of a single lymph node region (I) or a single extralymphatic organ or site (IE)
II	Involvement of two or more lymph node regions on the same side of the diaphragm (II) or localized involvement of an extralymphatic organ or site and one or more lymph node regions on the same side of the diaphragm (IIE)
III	Involvement of lymph node regions on both sides of the diaphragm (III); this may include splenic involvement (IIIS) or localized involvement of an extralymphatic organ (IIIE) or site (IIIES)
IV	Disseminated involvement of one or more organs or sites with or without associated lymph node involvement

staging system (Table 35–1) and requires information obtained from the history, physical examination, and diagnostic imaging studies. The substage classifications A, B, and E are based on defined clinical features. Substage A indicates asymptomatic disease. Substage B symptoms are strictly defined as more than 10% weight loss over 6 months, drenching night sweats, and fever greater than 38°C for 3 days. Substage E denotes minimal extralymphatic disease.

Radiographic imaging is an integral component of clinical staging. Chest radiographs often reveal the presence of a mediastinal mass, and the ratio of its maximal diameter to that of the thoracic cavity on a posteroanterior view is prognostically important. A ratio greater than 1:3 places the patient in the subcategory of bulky mediastinal disease, which is associated with a worse prognosis and requires systemic chemotherapy for adequate treatment. CT of the chest and abdomen permits a more accurate assessment of disease extent. If high cervical nodes are involved, CT of the neck is also obtained to evalute Waldeyer's ring. CT of the chest provides the best information regarding the extent of mediastinal disease and also evaluates the pulmonary parenchyma, pleura, pericardium, and chest wall. Both intravenous and oral contrast agents should be administered for CT evaluation of infradiaphragmatic disease, to better distinguish lymphadenopathy from other structures. CT scanning is of limited usefulness in children because of the small quantity of retroperitoneal fat and the frequency of benign lymphadenopathy in this age group. Under these circumstances, CT scanning is inaccurate in detecting splenic or periaortic nodal involvement[14] and has a reported accuracy of 71% to 74% when compared with laparotomy. Magnetic resonance imaging (MRI) provides a more accurate evaluation of infradiaphragmatic disease compared with CT, with better visualization of fat-encased retroperitoneal nodes. Lymphangiography is technically difficult and is rarely performed in children.

Gallium 67 scans are less specific and do not differentiate inflammatory changes from malignancy, but persistent activity may indicate residual disease. Positron emission tomography has recently been shown to detect disease not identified on CT scans in adults, although data are limited in children.[30]

Pathologic staging theoretically requires surgical staging, including splenectomy, unless metastatic disease is found in bone, marrow, liver, or lung biopsies. However, modern HD therapy almost always includes systemic chemotherapy, so the results of pathologic staging do not affect treatment. Therefore, surgical staging with splenectomy is almost never done today. The only exception, which is very rare, is the treatment of localized HD in an adolescent male with radiotherapy alone.

Treatment

Surgery

All patients with HD require a biopsy, usually of involved lymph nodes, to establish the diagnosis and histologic subtype. Frozen sections are inadequate for diagnostic purposes, and permanent hematoxylin-eosin sections must always be obtained. In addition, it is important to procure tissue for more detailed studies, such as immunohistochemistry, immunophenotyping, and cytogenetics. Biopsies should be taken from the most easily accessible site. In patients with only mediastinal involvement, biopsy samples can be obtained via mediastinoscopy, Chamberlain procedure, or thoracoscopy.[35] Retroperitoneal lymphadenopathy is often accessible through laparoscopic biopsy. Fine-needle aspiration cytology is inadequate to detect sparse Reed-Sternberg cells, and 20% of interventional radiologic procedures for HD diagnosis were falsely negative in one study.[32] Excisional lymph node biopsy or incisional biopsy of massively enlarged or matted nodes is essential to make an accurate diagnosis. Every attempt should be made to provide a specimen that preserves cytoarchitecture without crush or cautery artifact.

The role of surgical staging has changed with the paradigm shifts in the treatment of HD. Staging laparotomy was initially devised by radiation oncologists to define the pathologic extent of disease and direct accurate supervoltage radiation fields, because all involved nodal sites required irradiation if cure was to be achieved. Low-stage HD presenting in the neck often followed a predictable route of progression that could be defined by sampling retroperitoneal lymph nodes and removing the spleen. If the disease had extended beyond reasonable radiation portals, chemotherapy would be necessary. The historical purpose of laparotomy-splenectomy in HD was to document the anatomic distribution of disease and thus determine nodal echelons requiring radiotherapy. It was not designed as a therapeutic maneuver. With the wide application of chemotherapy in all stages of HD,[25,62] surgical staging has become irrelevant because the additional information it provides does not alter treatment. As noted earlier, the exception is the rare male adolescent with localized disease who might be treated by radiation alone.

Traditionally, surgical staging requires laparotomy, splenectomy, bilobar liver needle and wedge biopsies, and thorough sampling of multiple lymph node sites (splenic hilum, porta hepatis, suprapancreatic, bilateral para-aortic, and mesenteric). Bilateral oophoropexies are also performed in girls. Staging performed laparoscopically may reduce postoperative morbidity,[110,116,117,129] including the risk of postoperative bowel obstruction.[27] However, the susceptibility to infection caused by splenectomy is not altered.

Chemotherapy

Effective chemotherapy regimens for HD contain drugs that are individually effective and that have different mechanisms of action so that multiple homeostatic functions in the tumor cell are attacked and drug resistance is minimized (Table 35–2). The agents should have nonoverlapping toxicities so that a full dose of each drug can be given. The MOPP regimen fulfills these requirements and was the first multidrug regimen found to be effective against HD. In a long-term study of 188 patients from the National Cancer Institute treated with MOPP, the complete remission rate was 89%, and 54% of patients remained disease free at 10 years.[67] The mean age at diagnosis for this group was 32 years and ranged from 12 to 69 years. In this study, 95% of patients had stage III or IV disease, and 89% had B symptoms. Maintenance therapy did not affect the remission rate and does not seem to be necessary in HD.

ABVD was the second regimen used in the treatment of HD.[11] It was developed for the treatment of patients failing MOPP therapy and contains individually effective drugs with nonoverlapping toxicities. In view of the effectiveness of both MOPP and ABVD and the fact that their toxicities do not overlap, trials combining the two regimens were done, with good preliminary results.[10] These regimens are given in an outpatient setting and have easily manageable acute toxicities. However, their significant long-term toxicity prompted the design of alternating regimens of MOPP-ABVD to avoid reaching cumulative doses associated with toxicity.

The current trend is the application of "tailored therapy" based on disease response. This approach aims to limit the cumulative dose, thus minimizing toxicity while maintaining efficacy. Results of response-based therapy were recently reported by the Pediatric Oncology Group.[114] For advanced-stage HD, early responders received only three cycles of ABVE-PC (Adriamycin, bleomycin, vincristine, etoposide, prednisone, cyclophosphamide) versus five cycles, followed by 25 Gy of radiation. The 2-year event-free survival was 90.8% for early responders and 87.7% for slow responders. Low-stage patients received either two or four cycles of ABVE (for early and slow responders, respectively), followed by radiotherapy, with no difference in outcome. New trials are under way to evaluate the use of dose- and time-intensive delivery.

Radiation Therapy

Historically, the application of radiation therapy was based on the concept of contiguous lymph node basin involvement. Ideally, a 4- to 8-MeV linear accelerator is used for treatment. Orthovoltage techniques are contraindicated, and cobalt 60 is associated with significant radiation scatter, which should be avoided in children. The risk of recurrence is 10% or less if doses of 3500 to 4400 cGy are used. Thus, clinically involved areas are usually given 4000 to 4400 cGy, whereas prophylactic treatment of subclinical areas can be accomplished with 3000 to 4000 cGy. The combination of chemotherapy and radiotherapy can be effective, with local control rates of 97%. However, the long-term toxicity prompted trials in the 1980s with protocols incorporating six cycles of chemotherapy and lower-dose (1500 to 2500 cGy), limited-field radiotherapy. This resulted in excellent disease control and decreased musculoskeletal deformity.[25,87]

The application of risk-adapted therapy using combination chemotherapy has achieved excellent disease-free survival and overall survival. Recent studies have shown that the addition of low-dose involved-field radiation improves event-free survival but does not affect overall survival in patients with a complete response to chemotherapy.[84] Currently, the standard of care for the majority of children and adolescents with HD is risk-adapted combined-modality therapy using low-dose, involved-field radiation in conjunction with multiagent chemotherapy.

Complications

Treatment Toxicity

Late effects of treatment include surgical complications, soft tissue and bone growth abnormalities, cardiopulmonary effects, endocrine sequelae, and secondary

---

TABLE 35–2 Chemotherapy Regimens for Hodgkin's Disease

Regimen	Agents
ABVD[9]	Doxorubicin (Adriamycin), bleomycin, vinblastine, dacarbazine
ABVE (DBVE)	Doxorubicin (Adriamycin), bleomycin, vincristine, etoposide
VAMP[23]	Vincristine, doxorubicin (Adriamycin), methotrexate, prednisone
OPPA ± COPP (females)[107]	Vincristine (Oncovin), prednisone, procarbazine, doxorubicin (Adriamycin), cyclophosphamide, vincristine (Oncovin), prednisone, procarbazine
OEPA ± COPP (males)[107]	Vincristine (Oncovin), etoposide, prednisone, doxorubicin (Adriamycin), cyclophosphamide, vincristine (Oncovin), prednisone, procarbazine
COPP/ABV[84]	Cyclophosphamide, vincristine (Oncovin), prednisone, procarbazine, doxorubicin (Adriamycin), bleomycin, vinblastine
BEACOPP (advanced stage)[54]	Bleomycin, etoposide, doxorubicin (Adriamycin), cyclophosphamide, vincristine (Oncovin), prednisone, procarbazine
COPP	Cyclophosphamide, vincristine (Oncovin), prednisone, procarbazine
CHOP	Cyclophosphamide, doxorubicin (Adriamycin), vincristine (Oncovin), prednisone
ABVE-PC (DBVE-PC)[12]	Doxorubicin (Adriamycin), bleomycin, vincristine, etoposide, prednisone, cyclophosphamide

malignancies. An alteration in the proportion of sitting to standing height has been noted in patients receiving radiation to the axial skeleton.[97] Boys seem to be more severely affected than girls. There is also shortening of the clavicles, reduced interclavicular distance, fibrosis of the soft tissues in the neck, and thinning of hair in the posterior cervical region. Growth disturbance is not significant in children with bone ages of 14 to 15 years at the time of treatment.

Significant radiation-induced pulmonary injury can occur, depending on the volume included in the radiation field, the dose, and the daily fraction size. Symptomatic pulmonary injury occurs in 3.6% of patients receiving high-dose mantle therapy. Bleomycin also may cause severe pulmonary dysfunction.

Radiation injury to the myocardium is also related to dose, fraction size, and volume irradiated. Approximately 13% of children receiving high-dose mantle therapy develop cardiac injury. The coronary arteries and great vessels can be affected as well. Doxorubicin is also known to cause cardiac injury, and Raynaud's syndrome has been reported in patients receiving vinblastine and bleomycin.

Endocrine effects include hypothyroidism, sterility, and other alterations in fertility. Using thyroid-stimulating hormone as a marker for hypothyroidism, between 4% and 79% of patients develop this complication.[19] Thyroid abnormalities depend on the dose given to the neck; 17% of patients receiving less than 26 Gy develop thyroid abnormalities, whereas 78% of those receiving 26 Gy or more become hypothyroid.

Gonadal dysfunction (both ovarian and testicular) has been documented after HD therapy.[111] Pelvic irradiation carries a high likelihood of ablating ovarian function. Ovarian transposition, whereby the ovaries are moved away from the radiation field, can preserve ovarian function and fertility.[31] The ovaries can be moved to the midline behind the uterus or to both flanks. A small clip should be placed on the peritoneum in the area where the ovaries were moved for identification by the radiotherapist. Sterility is a much greater problem in males, and gonadal dysfunction may exist at the time of diagnosis in 30% to 40% of patients.[15,88,127] Pretreatment storage of sperm in older patients should be considered.

Secondary Malignancies

Second malignancies include acute nonlymphocytic leukemia, non-Hodgkin's lymphoma, thyroid cancers (usually differentiated), breast cancer (in irradiated patients),[8,17,59,73,125] and bone or soft tissue sarcomas. Patients who underwent prior splenectomy also have a risk of developing leukemia. The MOPP regimen involves a higher risk of secondary malignancy compared with the ABVD regimen. Children who require retreatment also have higher risk of secondary malignancy as a direct dose effect.[49] The incidence of secondary leukemia in patients primarily treated with MOPP may be 5% to 7%; this increases to 10% if MOPP is given with radiotherapy. The risk of leukemia decreases after 10 years, whereas the risk of non-Hodgkin's lymphoma increases with time, underlying the importance of continual monitoring. Solid tumors may develop in as many as 4% of patients.

Complications of Laparotomy

Complications specific to staging laparotomy can be divided into three groups: (1) early postsurgical complications (<6 weeks after operation), (2) late complications (>6 months after surgery), and (3) septic complications related to splenectomy. Hays et al.[42,43] reviewed the experience of the Intergroup Hodgkin's Disease in Childhood Study, consisting of 234 staging laparotomies; in the initial report, 55% of children were followed for at least 2 years, and in the updated summary, the median follow-up was 5 years. In the first 6 weeks after laparotomy, three pulmonary and three abdominal complications were noted, for an overall incidence of 2.6%. These included one case of right ureteral obstruction secondary to scar, which required operative lysis; one intestinal obstruction from adhesions, requiring reoperation; one superficial wound infection; and three cases of atelectasis-pneumonia. There were no postoperative deaths. Five late surgical complications occurred (2.1%). There were four cases of bowel obstruction requiring adhesiolysis, and in one of these an intestinal perforation secondary to volvulus of a bowel segment around an adhesive band required repair. In the fifth patient, a right oophorectomy was necessary because of torsion and secondary necrosis. This ovary had been moved to the flank during staging laparotomy to avoid the major radiation portals. Thus, the combined incidence of early and late surgical complications specific for laparotomy was 4.7%, including clinically significant atelectasis.

Schneeberger and Girvan[112] reported on 39 children with HD who underwent staging laparotomy. No operative deaths were reported, and there were no minor complications such as atelectasis. There were five (12.8%) cases of small bowel obstruction, and four were managed nonoperatively with nasogastric suction. One patient required re-exploration 11 years after staging laparotomy because of a small bowel volvulus around adhesions. Donaldson and Kaplan[24] reported that the rate of significant, nonlethal complications in the immediate postoperative period after staging laparotomy in children was approximately 1%. Significant complications in this study included wound infection and dehiscence, subphrenic abscess, pulmonary infection, retroperitoneal hematoma, pancreatitis, and significant postoperative bleeding. Complications such as mild postoperative atelectasis were not included. Late complications such as adhesive bowel obstruction have been reported in 3% to 12% of patients in other series and may occur even if abdominal radiation is not given.[50]

Complications of Splenectomy

Increased susceptibility to infection after splenectomy was first noted by King and Shumacker[56] in 1952, and multiple confirmatory reports have been published since then.[29,119] The incidence of postsplenectomy sepsis is increased in younger children, especially those younger than 10 years. In interpreting data from patients undergoing splenectomy in the setting of HD, it should be remembered that the disease process itself and chemotherapeutic agents are immunosuppressive.

Serious questions about the use of splenectomy in children with HD were raised following the report of Chilcote et al.[16] in 1976. This was a retrospective study of 200 children aged 19 years or younger treated for HD at collaborating institutions of the Children's Cancer Study Group. In this study, 20 episodes of sepsis were noted in 18 patients, and the interval from splenectomy to infection varied from 8 days to 3 years. The median age of patients developing sepsis was 10 years. All but three of these patients had received or were receiving chemotherapy, and all but two had received radiation therapy. Organisms included pneumococci, *Haemophilus influenzae*, streptococci, and meningococci. Ten of the children who developed sepsis died, and most of them had a fulminant course. Significantly, only two contributing institutions used prophylactic antibiotics at the time, and neither reported serious infections. The overall follow-up interval was not stated.

Subsequent analysis of postsplenectomy sepsis rates by the Intergroup Hodgkin's Disease in Childhood Study showed that this was less of a problem with the use of vaccination and prophylactic antibiotics.[42] In the first report from this group, with 55% of patients followed 2 years or more, only two disease-free patients developed documented sepsis. An additional two children developed sepsis in the setting of chemotherapy given for relapse. There were also three cases of possible sepsis, but blood cultures were negative. Most important, no deaths were noted in this group. Significantly, 83% of these children received pneumococcal vaccination before splenectomy, and 74% were given prophylactic antibiotics. In an update of this series, with a median follow-up of 5.5 years, the total number of documented cases of sepsis had risen to five, but no deaths were reported. In two patients, pneumococcus was isolated from the blood, and in the remaining three, *H. influenzae* was found. Of the five children who developed sepsis, four had received pneumococcal vaccine, but only three had been vaccinated preoperatively. Four of the five children had antibiotics discontinued or interrupted before the development of sepsis. Age at diagnosis ranged from 4 to 14 years, with a median of 9 years in the group developing sepsis. An additional five patients became gravely ill and were thought to have sepsis because of a good response to antibiotics; blood cultures in these children were negative, and there was no mortality. With a mean follow-up of more than 5 years, there were five (2.1%) confirmed cases and five suspected cases of sepsis, and the lethality from this complication was zero.

The defect in humoral immunity caused by splenectomy is permanent, however, and additional cases of postsplenectomy infection can be expected in HD survivors undergoing staging laparotomy.[105] Using a sepsis incidence of 0.38% per year derived from the Intergroup Hodgkin's Disease in Childhood Study (2.1% incidence in 5.5 years), it was estimated that almost 20% of splenectomized HD patients would develop this complication over a 50-year period.[96] The incidence of sepsis is reduced in adults and falls with age, so this is probably an overestimate. The cumulative risk of sepsis over a lifetime is not known.

Treatment of Metastatic Disease and Relapse

The salvage therapy for patients with refractory or recurrent disease depends on the initial therapeutic regimen. Fifty percent to 80% of patients treated initially with radiation alone can be cured with chemotherapy or combined-modality therapy. With the use of combined-modality therapy for early-stage disease and a risk-adapted approach for advanced-stage disease, nearly 90% of patients with Hodgkin's lymphoma are cured with initial therapy. However, in patients who have primary refractory or relapsed disease, high-dose therapy and autologous stem cell transplantation constitute the best curative option. The use of peripheral blood progenitor cells has decreased transplant-related mortality to less than 3%, but long-term progression-free survival has shown minimal improvement.[77-79]

Prognostic Factors

The current treatment approach to HD is risk-adapted therapy. Risk features at the time of diagnosis include the presence of B symptoms, age, stage, nodal bulk, and number of involved nodal regions. Patients with localized nodal involvement and the absence of B symptoms have a favorable clinical presentation. Those with B symptoms, bulky mediastinal or peripheral lymphadenopathy, extranodal extension of disease, and advanced disease (stage IIIB to IV) have an unfavorable clinical presentation. Patients with an unfavorable clinical presentation are treated with standard non-cross-resistant chemotherapy on a conventional schedule, followed by consolidation therapy of low-dose, involved-field radiation. Alternatively, abbreviated, dose-intensive multiagent chemotherapy followed by consolidating radiation is being evaluated. Early response to therapy is correlated with better prognosis and reflects tumor bulk and biology.[12]

Outcome

The application of risk-adapted therapy consisting of chemotherapy alone has resulted in 5-year survival of greater than 90% and disease-free survival of greater than 85%. The goal of optimal therapy is to preserve the high survival rate, decrease the relapse rate, and minimize late adverse effects.

NON-HODGKIN'S LYMPHOMA

The non-Hodgkin's lymphomas are divided into Burkitt's and Burkitt's-like lymphomas, lymphoblastic lymphomas, diffuse large B-cell lymphomas, and anaplastic large cell lymphomas. The anatomic distribution of these neoplasms can be at least partially understood by reference to normal B-cell and T-cell ontogeny.

Incidence and Epidemiology

There are 750 to 800 new cases of non-Hodgkin's lymphoma each year in the United States.[93] Burkitt's and

Burkitt's-like lymphomas have a fivefold higher incidence in males than in females in patients younger than 20 years (3.2 versus 0.7 cases per million). The overall incidence of Burkitt's lymphoma rises after 5 years of age and falls again after age 15. In contrast, the incidence of diffuse large cell lymphoma rises steadily with age and has a male-female ratio of 1.4. Lymphoblastic lymphomas occur at similar frequencies in those younger than 20 years and have a male-female ratio of 2.5.

Biology

Lymphocyte Ontogeny and Differentiation

Although a detailed discussion of lymphoid cell development is beyond the scope of this chapter, a short review of this subject may help in understanding the various histologic subgroups and their unique clinical behavior. Basic to our current understanding of the normal and pathologic immune system is the idea that there are functionally separate B-cell and T-cell compartments.[68,76,130] A second important notion is that mature lymphocytes are not end-stage cells but can undergo transformation to an effector cell type in the presence of antigen. Lymphoid development can be conceptualized as progressing through a differentiation path from a stem cell to an activated cell. This is followed by transformation to an effector phenotype when the proper stimulus is provided. A simplified scheme for B-cell differentiation is illustrated in Figure 35-4. B cells originate in the bone marrow from totipotential stem cells that differentiate through many intermediate cell types to eventually become antibody-producing plasma cells. Malignant transformation can occur at any point along the differentiation path, thus producing some readily recognizable clinical syndromes or histopathologic subtypes. Of interest to the pediatric surgeon is that B cells, at the developmental stage when immunoglobulin M (IgM) surface immunoglobulin is detectable (see Fig. 35–4), can undergo malignant transformation into undifferentiated lymphoma. Because of their light microscopic appearance, these are also called small, noncleaved cell lymphomas. Burkitt's lymphoma is a subset of these undifferentiated lymphomas. Because B cells develop in the bone marrow and then migrate to secondary lymphoid organs (lymph nodes, spleen, Peyer's patches, liver), one would expect clinical localization of the developing neoplasm in those anatomic sites. As a corollary, B-cell lymphoma should not occur in the anterior mediastinum in the region of the thymus because normal B cells are not thymic dependent. Usually, but not always, this anatomic distribution is consistent with clinical observations. In the United States, Burkitt's lymphoma has a predilection for the abdomen (in western equatorial Africa, it usually arises in the mandible, but abdominal lymphoma is also noted in up to 20% of these patients). Burkitt's lymphoma of the tonsil and testis (as a site of relapse) has also been reported, but Burkitt's lymphoma of the anterior mediastinum is extremely rare.[53,57]

A simplified schema for the differentiation of T cells is depicted in Figure 35–5. Because thymic residence is a necessary part of T-cell development, most lymphomas presenting in the anterior mediastinum originate from the T-cell lineage. Fifty percent to 70% of patients with lymphoblastic lymphoma (T cell) present with an intrathoracic tumor, usually an anterior mediastinal mass; an abdominal presentation is uncommon. There is a general predilection for T-cell-dependent or B-cell-dependent anatomic areas of the lymphoid system to be involved by lymphomas that also express surface markers specific for their respective T or B lymphocytes. Of interest is the observation that removal of the thymus prevents T lymphomas in mice, whereas removal of the bursa of Fabricius prevents B lymphomas in chickens.[92,105]

Cytogenetic and Molecular Biologic Findings

In 1976, a characteristic chromosomal translocation involving chromosomes 8 and 14 was discovered in Burkitt's lymphoma.[135] It was subsequently shown that the *c-myc* proto-oncogene was translocated from chromosome 8 to the immunoglobulin heavy-chain locus on chromosome 14.[124] Finally, it was determined that in a minority of Burkitt's lymphomas, the 8;14 translocation was replaced by an 8;22 or 2;8 translocation.[99] This still involved the *c-myc* gene on chromosome 8. The difference in this minority of cases was that instead of an immunoglobulin heavy-chain locus, the κ light-chain locus on chromosome 2 or the λ light-chain locus on chromosome 22 was involved. Thus, a proto-oncogene was always juxtaposed to an immunoglobulin constant region coding sequence. Because Burkitt's lymphomas are of B-cell origin, it was thought that these cytogenetic abnormalities involving known proto-oncogene and immunoglobulin coding sequences were not coincidental and had pathophysiologic significance. It was subsequently shown that the translocated *c-myc* allele becomes activated by its proximity to the immunoglobulin coding region.[6] This may result in an inappropriate expression of c-myc RNA and protein in B lymphocytes at this stage of differentiation.[72]

In contrast to the extensive cytogenetic data in small, noncleaved cell tumors, most lymphoblastic lymphomas do not manifest specific, nonrandom mutations.[58] A small percentage of lymphoblastic tumors of T-cell origin have

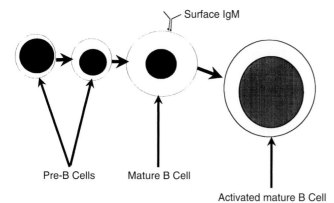

Surface IgM

Pre-B Cells   Mature B Cell

Activated mature B Cell

Figure 35–4 Simplified diagram of the B-cell differentiation pathway. Undifferentiated lymphoma develops just after cells express surface immunoglobulin M.

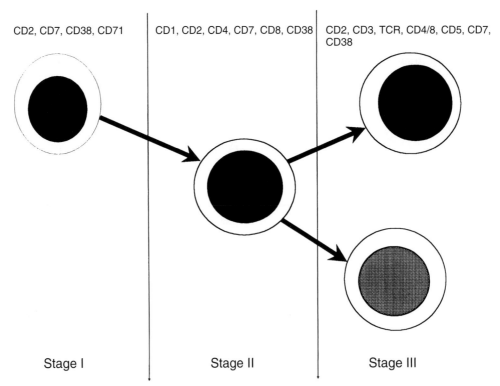

Figure 35–5 Simplified diagram of T-cell differentiation. Lymphoblastic lymphomas usually express the enzyme terminal deoxynucleotide transferase. T cells must traverse the thymus during differentiation.

translocations, most often involving chromosome 14 (14q11) in a region occupied by the T cc and 8 receptor gene (T-cell receptor) or chromosome 7 near Tβ.[21] This is analogous to the involvement of immunoglobulin gene coding regions in B-cell lymphomas. Information from cytogenetic and molecular biologic analysis has provided important insights into the molecular mechanisms of malignant degeneration of lymphoid cells.

Lymphoma Subtypes and Histopathology

This brief description of immune system ontogeny serves as a basis for understanding the three major subcategories of childhood non-Hodgkin's lymphoma: (1) undifferentiated, which are also called small, noncleaved cell lymphomas; (2) lymphoblastic; and (3) large cell (diffuse large B-cell and anaplastic large cell). All three are considered high grade in contrast to other subtypes observed in adult patients. The exceptions to this rule are certain large cell lymphomas with a follicular-center cell type, which are considered intermediate in grade but are rare in childhood and adolescence. The undifferentiated lymphomas are primarily abdominal in origin and develop from B-cell precursors. Malignant degeneration occurs before cleavage of the nucleus during differentiation. They can be divided into Burkitt's and non-Burkitt's categories based on their appearance under light microscopy. Burkitt's lymphoma is characterized by medium-sized nuclei that are approximately the same size as interspersed benign histiocytes, which provides a convenient method of measurement and confers a "starry-sky"

appearance (Fig. 35–6). There are usually two to five prominent basophilic nucleoli. A high nuclear-to-cytoplasmic ratio is observed. Non-Burkitt's varieties often show frequent, single, large nucleoli and more variation in nucleolar size and shape. A later age at presentation and an increased incidence of peripheral lymph node or bone marrow involvement have been associated with non-Burkitt's small, noncleaved cell lymphomas. No cytogenetic, immunohistochemical, or molecular biologic markers distinguish the two. Small, noncleaved cell lymphomas express surface immunoglobulin of the IgM class

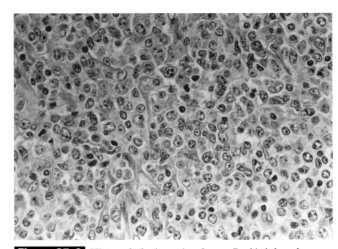

Figure 35–6 Histopathologic section from a Burkitt's lymphoma showing multiple prominent nucleoli.

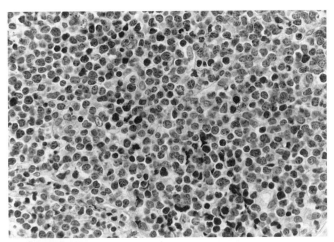

Figure 35–7 Representative section from a lymphoblastic lymphoma. The dark-staining cells are normal lymphocytes.

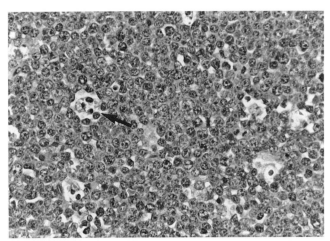

Figure 35–8 Representative section from a diffuse large cell lymphoma. Several macrophages *(arrow)* are seen ingesting tumor cells.

and surface antigens detected by the monoclonal antibodies CD19 and CD20.[109] They do not contain the enzyme terminal deoxynucleotide transferase, which is always found in lymphoblastic lymphomas. Small, noncleaved cell lymphoma must be distinguished from small cell nodular lymphomas that occur in adults and have a more indolent course.

Lymphoblastic lymphomas are located predominantly in the anterior mediastinum and are characterized by diffuse effacement of nodal architecture. A lobular appearance may be observed because of extension of tumor cells along normal tissue planes. Cytologically, the nuclei are smaller than those of the interspersed histiocytes, and the nucleoli are inconspicuous (Fig. 35–7). Again, the starry-sky pattern can be appreciated, and the nuclear-to-cytoplasmic ratio is higher than that seen in small, noncleaved cell lymphomas. In about half the cases, the nuclear membrane is convoluted or cleaved. The enzyme terminal deoxynucleotide transferase is invariably found, and most lymphoblastic lymphomas express T-cell markers, including CD7 or CD5.[65]

Large cell lymphomas (diffuse large cell lymphomas) are usually high grade. As noted previously, the follicular-center cell type is technically intermediate in grade but shows aggressive biologic behavior. The normal nodal architecture is effaced by cells with large nuclei and scant cytoplasm (Fig. 35–8). The nuclei are larger than those of invading histiocytes. These cells are large and cleaved and have cleaved nuclei, whereas nucleoli are inconspicuous. Another cell type consisting of large, cleaved cells with a narrow rim of cytoplasm and prominent, pyknotic nucleoli may also be present. The two cell types may coexist in the same tumor. A study done by the Pediatric Oncology Group categorized large cell lymphomas into two subtypes.[85] The first was a large cell, cleaved or uncleaved lymphoma arising in germinal centers of lymphoid follicles and of B-cell origin. The second type of large cell lymphoma was described as immunoblastic, and most of these originated from T-cell precursors. A plasmacytoid variant of the immunoblastic large cell lymphoma is thought to be of B-cell origin. A variant of large cell lymphoma expresses the Ki-1 antigen, which

is also found on Reed-Sternberg cells and is of T-cell origin.[4,104,113]

It should be emphasized that all childhood non-Hodgkin's lymphomas are diffuse and fast growing. This contrasts with the nodular and often indolent forms of lymphoma observed in adults. Thus, childhood lymphoma should be treated as a systemic disease from the time of diagnosis, with the early institution of multiagent chemotherapy. It is estimated that the growth fraction of childhood lymphoma approaches 100% in some cases and that uncorrected doubling times that do not take into account spontaneous cell death (apoptosis) are as low as 12 hours to several days. Measured doubling times that account for cell death have been reported to average approximately 3 days for small, noncleaved cell tumors injected subcutaneously into mice. It is estimated that the cell death rate for African Burkitt's lymphoma is 70% of all progeny cells. Undifferentiated B-cell tumors of childhood have the highest growth fractions, with up to 27% of cells in S phase by flow cytometry.[47,48]

Clinical Presentation

Undifferentiated Lymphoma

In the United States, children with non-Hodgkin's lymphoma present with a small number of defined syndromes that generally correlate with cell type. More than 90% of patients with small, noncleaved cell lymphoma present with a palpable abdominal tumor.[7,132] The tumor can cause abdominal pain, distention, change in bowel habits, nausea, vomiting, intestinal obstruction, intussusception, intestinal bleeding, ascites, or bowel perforation. Commonly, the lymphoma presents as a right iliac fossa mass and can be confused with appendicitis or an appendiceal abscess. These patients may have enlarged inguinal or iliac lymph nodes. Patients with extensive intra-abdominal involvement may have fatigue, malaise, and weight loss. An example of an extensive abdominal Burkitt's lymphoma almost totally replacing the liver is illustrated in Figure 35–9. Interestingly, Burkitt's lymphoma in equatorial Africa,

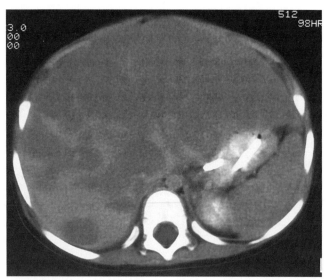

Figure 35–9 Abdominal computed tomography scan of a patient with Burkitt's lymphoma showing almost total hepatic replacement with tumor. The diagnosis was made by bone marrow aspiration.

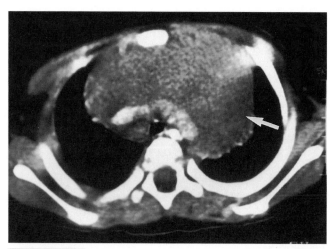

Figure 35–10 Thoracic computed tomography scan of a patient with lymphoblastic lymphoma and a large anterior mediastinal mass (*arrow*). The airway is displaced but not compressed.

although usually presenting as a diffuse jaw tumor, also involves the abdomen in more than 50% of patients. In the United States, other sites of involvement at presentation include bone marrow, pleural effusions, cerebrospinal fluid, central nervous system, peripheral nodes, kidneys, and pharynx.[57,132] The ovary is a common site of presentation in both the United States and Africa.[80]

For practical purposes, patients with abdominal non-Hodgkin's lymphomas can be divided into two groups. In the first group, the disease process is localized anatomically within the abdomen. In this case, the tumor often involves the bowel wall, and many of these children present with acute abdominal symptoms suggesting appendicitis or intussusception. The majority can undergo complete gross tumor resection, often with a simple bowel resection and reanastomosis, with little consequent morbidity. In the second group, there is extensive intra-abdominal tumor, and presentation with an abdominal mass without acute symptoms is more likely. The mesenteric root and retroperitoneum are heavily involved, and attempts at complete excision are associated with a higher complication rate.

Lymphoblastic Lymphoma

Fifty percent to 70% of patients with lymphoblastic lymphoma present with an anterior mediastinal mass or intrathoracic tumor (or both). Figure 35–10 shows a thoracic CT scan of a patient with mediastinal lymphoblastic lymphoma. These tumors may be distinguishable from the middle mediastinal mass associated with HD, but this is often not feasible, especially with extensive mediastinal masses. Fifty percent to 80% of patients have supra-diaphragmatic lymphadenopathy, including cervical, supraclavicular, and axillary regions. Abdominal involvement is uncommon and, when observed, usually includes hepatosplenomegaly. Bone marrow infiltration is common in this situation, making the distinction from acute

lymphoblastic leukemia difficult. In these cases, survival may be better after treatment with a lymphoblastic leukemia-type regimen. Pleural effusions are often observed, and patients may complain of dyspnea, chest pain, or dysphagia. Vena caval syndrome with facial, chest, and upper extremity edema and dilated cutaneous veins over the upper torso and shoulders, or airway compression with severe dyspnea or orthopnea (or both), may require the urgent institution of chemotherapy or radiation.[1,132] The central nervous system is rarely involved at diagnosis.

Large Cell Lymphoma

The anatomic distribution of primary sites in large cell lymphoma is similar to that observed for small, non-cleaved cell tumors. Unusual sites of presentation are possible, however, such as B-cell large cell lymphomas that arise in the anterior mediastinum. Ki-1-positive (anaplastic, usually derived from T cells) large cell lymphomas often involve the skin, central nervous system, lymph nodes, lung, testis, and muscle in addition to the gastrointestinal tract. Lung, facial, and intracerebral primary tumors are more likely to be large cell lymphomas.[86,106,108] A progressively enlarging mass is the most common mode of presentation.

Post-Transplant Lymphoproliferative Disease

Post-transplant lymphoproliferative disease (PTLD) occurs as a complication of allogeneic transplantation and can be progressive, with a fatal outcome. It can occur after both solid organ and bone marrow transplants. The probability of PTLD is increased after T-cell-depleted bone marrow grafts, after transplants from unrelated donors, in patients who develop graft-versus-host disease, and particularly in patients treated with aggressive immunosuppressive regimens, including those that contain antithymocyte globulin. PTLD that occurs after bone marrow transplantation arises from transformation of the donor B cells by EBV. These patients often present with gastrointestinal disturbance such as nausea and vomiting or derangement in hepatic function. For tumors arising in the gastrointestinal tract, endoscopic biopsy may establish the diagnosis. Multiple biopsies are usually required to identify the transformed cells. Liver lesions can be biopsied laparoscopically or percutaneously.[38,45,92,95,120,122]

Treatment of PTLD consists of stopping immunosuppression and administering an anti-CD20 monoclonal antibody (rituximab). In addition, various targeted cellular strategies directed against EBV-transformed cells have been developed, including reinfusion of donor lymphocytes at low dose. There is no role for surgical resection.

Diagnosis

The evaluation of a patient presenting with possible non-Hodgkin's lymphoma includes an extensive history and physical examination. This is followed by a complete blood count; liver function tests, including LDH, serum electrolytes, blood urea nitrogen, creatinine, and uric acid level; chest radiograph; bone marrow aspirations; and lumbar puncture with cytospin for cytology. A four-site bone marrow aspiration and two-site bone marrow biopsy frequently identify marrow involvement, which has serious implications for outcome. A gallium-67 scan and CT scan of the chest and abdomen with oral and intravenous contrast material can provide valuable information concerning tumor location and extent. Gallium is taken up by neoplastic lymphoid cells (in particular, small, noncleaved cells) and provides a good total-body screen for disease. Bone scans can identify suspected skeletal involvement. MRI may play a role, especially in the evaluation of epidural disease, but is probably not absolutely necessary. The role of positron emission tomography remains investigational.

Staging

Staging laparotomy is not performed in non-Hodgkin's lymphoma because all patients require systemic chemotherapy. Many patients also require surgical intervention because of abdominal complications such as intussusception or bleeding or to obtain diagnostic tissue. The pediatric surgeon must be aware that childhood lymphoma is a systemic disease, and the operative procedure should not delay the institution of chemotherapy. The Ann Arbor staging system for HD is not relevant to non-Hodgkin's lymphomas, and a number of groups have attempted to develop more appropriate classifications.[5,82] Presently, no clinical staging schema is entirely satisfactory, and it may be more important to assess the tumor volume at presentation rather than trying to fit a diffuse systemic process into a limited number of staging categories. The most widely used system for non-Hodgkin's lymphoma staging in childhood is that from St. Jude's Children's Research Hospital (Table 35–3). The Children's Oncology Group divides non-Hodgkin's lymphomas into two categories: limited and extensive. Limited disease corresponds to stages I and II in the St. Jude's system, and extensive correlates with stages III and IV.[81]

Treatment

Surgery

Magrath et al.,[70] basing their conclusions on an extensive experience with patients in Uganda with abdominal Burkitt's lymphoma, suggested that surgical reduction of tumor bulk has a favorable impact on survival. In retrospect, there are several problems with this conclusion. First, extent of disease at diagnosis was not evaluated for its predictive effect on outcome. Subsequent studies have shown that the most important predictor of survival is extent of disease. Second, only 9 of the 68 patients (13%) actually underwent total resection (defined as >90% resection). The vast majority had biopsy alone (63%) or subtotal resection (24%). This observation strongly suggests a biologic selection for the patients undergoing total resection. In addition, the patients received single-agent chemotherapy (cyclophosphamide), whereas the standard is currently a multiagent, histopathology-specific protocol. Finally, the reported surgical mortality rate in this

TABLE 35–3 St. Jude's Children's Research Hospital Staging System for Non-Hodgkin's Lymphoma*

Stage	Undifferentiated	Stage	Lymphoblastic
I	Single extra-abdominal tumor	I	Single extrathoracic tumor
IR	Resected intra-abdominal (>90%) tumor	II	Multiple extrathoracic tumors except BM and CNS
II	Multiple extra-abdominal sites except BM and CNS	IIIA	Single thymic tumor
IIIA	Unresected intra-abdominal tumor or non–stage IV epidural disease	IIIB	Mediastinal tumor with pleural effusion
IIIB	Intra-abdominal and extra-abdominal tumor except BM	IVA	Mediastinal tumor with extrathoracic extension except BM or CNS
IVA	BM without abdominal or CNS involvement	IVB	BM and intrathoracic tumor without CNS or other extrathoracic involvement
IVB	BM and abdominal tumor without CNS involvement	IVC	BM and extrathoracic tumor without CNS involvement
IVC	CNS disease (cells in cerebrospinal fluid, cranial nerve palsy)	IVD	Bone marrow and CNS disease

*Tumor burden is assessed at diagnosis, which is the main determinant of outcome.
BM, bone marrow; CNS, central nervous system.

series was 10%, which seems excessive under the present circumstances.

Kemeny et al.[55] evaluated the role of surgery for treatment of the primary tumor and for treatment of complications in patients with American Burkitt's lymphoma. They suggested that complete resection has an advantage but pointed out that extent of disease was not analyzed as an independent variable. A role for surgical intervention in the supportive therapy of non-Hodgkin's lymphoma was also suggested. As noted, small, noncleaved cell tumors in particular have high growth fractions. As a consequence, renal shutdown caused by urate nephropathy is a real danger and could be complicated by mechanical ureteral obstruction by a retroperitoneal mass. In addition, the tumor lysis syndrome may occur, especially during induction chemotherapy of small, noncleaved cell lymphomas.[18,126] Finally, multiple gastrointestinal complications, including bleeding, obstruction, or perforation, can occur. The authors pointed out that surgery can provide vascular access for dialysis or hydration, ureteral stenting in the face of obstruction, and definitive operations for intestinal complications.

Initial surgical management should include incisional biopsy for diagnosis, followed by intense, multiagent chemotherapy, except for small, easily resectable lesions.[52] Data regarding the role of surgery in abdominal Burkitt's lymphoma indicate that the extent of disease is a more significant predictive variable than is completeness of surgical resection.[115] Major surgical procedures in patients with extensive abdominal disease are unlikely to result in complete excision and may be associated with an increased complication rate, resulting in a delay in instituting chemotherapy.[115]

Similarly, the surgical committee of the Children's Cancer Group (CCG) evaluated the role of surgical therapy in 68 patients with non-Hodgkin's lymphoma in the CCG-551 study.[60] Variables analyzed included (1) extent of disease at diagnosis; (2) completeness of surgical resection (complete gross resection); (3) radiation therapy to the primary site; and (4) sex, age, and race. Laparotomy was performed in 67 children (99%), with complete gross resection accomplished in 28 (42%). Age at diagnosis, sex, and race had no effect on event-free survival. Tumor burden was the most important prognostic factor. Complete resection was also a significant predictor of event-free survival but was not as important as tumor burden. Of the 10 reported surgical complications, 8 occurred in the group with extensive disease and incomplete resection. These data support a role for complete surgical resection in the setting of localized disease, especially when confined to the bowel. Resections performed in these circumstances positively affect outcome by reducing tumor cell burden and preventing certain complications, such as bowel perforation.[75] Because extensive retroperitoneal dissection, with the possibility of significant hemorrhagic or septic complications, is avoided, chemotherapy can be initiated promptly.

Attempts at resection of massive retroperitoneal masses or large hepatic lymphomas are associated with an increased complication rate and serve to postpone essential chemotherapy. This is particularly deleterious because undifferentiated lymphomas grow so rapidly. In patients presenting with extensive abdominal disease, diagnosis can often be made by bone marrow aspiration because at least 20% of all patients have obvious marrow involvement (symptoms, positive bone scan), and an additional 20% have microscopic involvement that is unsuspected clinically. Additional sources of diagnostic tissue include ascites and pleural effusions, peripheral lymph nodes, or localized bone lesions, which can sometimes be biopsied by needle. Tumor may invade the bowel wall and undergo subsequent necrosis, resulting in free perforation and peritonitis or severe hemorrhage. Often, Burkitt's lymphoma is localized to the right lower quadrant in the region of Peyer's patches, and symptoms may mimic acute appendicitis. In this situation, resection of the ileocecal segment and adjacent mesentery often results in complete gross resection.

Patients with large mediastinal masses need careful preoperative evaluation; preoperative airway assessment by clinical and radiographic examination is crucial. Plain chest radiographs and CT scans indicate the degree of airway compression. Because cervical, supraclavicular, and axillary lymph node involvement approaches 50%, diagnostic biopsies performed at these sites under local anesthesia avoid the dangers associated with a general anesthetic and airway manipulation. Aspiration of malignant pleural effusions may also provide diagnostic material.

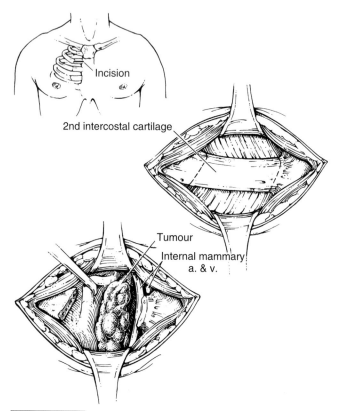

Figure 35–11 Technique of anterior mediastinotomy, or the Chamberlain procedure. This is a useful approach when the diagnosis of lymphoma cannot be made using less invasive techniques, such as lymph node biopsy, bone marrow aspiration, or thoracentesis.

If intrathoracic biopsy is required, the anesthetic technique may be modified so that patients can be safely intubated. Postoperative extubation is usually not feasible, however, until the tumor has been treated, and arrangements should be made for patient transfer to an intensive care environment.[29] Figure 35-11 depicts the technique for mediastinotomy, or the Chamberlain procedure. This approach can be useful in patients with large mediastinal masses but without more accessible nodal involvement. It can be performed on either side, depending on the CT findings, and thoracostomy drainage is almost never necessary. At present, there is no defined role for resection of mediastinal lymphomas, and operative removal is not indicated.

Rarely, patients with mediastinal lymphoblastic lymphoma present with a malignant pericardial effusion and incipient tamponade. If clinical signs are apparent, including tachycardia, tachypnea, neck vein distention, pulsus paradoxus, and muffled heart tones, an emergency echocardiogram must be done. A large pericardial effusion can almost always be drained by catheter pericardiocentesis.[74]

Minimally invasive techniques that allow much more thorough thoracic or abdominal exploration without the attendant morbidity of large incisions may have a role in the diagnosis, staging, and treatment of childhood non-Hodgkin's lymphomas. This role remains undefined by prospective or randomized studies; however, trials by both the Pediatric Oncology Group and the CCG are under way to determine their eventual role in this disease process. Laparoscopy may be the optimal method for managing lymphoproliferative disease in the following settings: for the differential diagnosis of hepatic or splenic focal lesions; when percutaneous needle biopsy fails or genetic analysis is needed for a therapeutic decision; for the primary diagnosis and abdominal staging of patients with diffuse retroperitoneal lymphadenopathy in the absence of peripheral lymphadenopathy; for cases of abdominal restaging after concurrent chemoradiotherapy, and in cases of suspected relapse when percutaneous biopsy is not technically possible; and for patients with lymphoproliferative disease when splenectomy is required.[110,116,117,129]

Significant bone marrow infiltration can cause severe thrombocytopenia; therefore, a complete blood count with platelet count should be available preoperatively. The production of serum clotting factors may also be affected by hepatic infiltration, and a full coagulation screen should be performed in preparation for surgery.

Surgical intervention in non-Hodgkin's lymphoma should obtain sufficient biopsy material when other sources are unavailable. If adequate diagnostic material can be obtained from bone marrow aspirates, a more invasive procedure may not be required. Laparotomy is indicated when acute abdominal symptoms are present or when sufficient diagnostic tissue cannot be obtained from other sources. Similarly, a thoracic or mediastinal procedure such as the Chamberlain procedure should be designed and carried out with minimal surgical trauma and prompt institution of systemic chemotherapy. An adequate workup to rule out life-threatening metabolic or hematologic problems and to establish airway integrity should be done before operation. The surgeon is obligated to verify that tissue samples are sent in an appropriate condition for immunohistochemistry, immunophenotyping, and cytogenetics. Children with localized abdominal disease, especially if it involves an intestinal segment, should undergo complete gross resection if this can be accomplished with speed and minimal morbidity. Patients with extensive infiltration of tumor throughout the small bowel mesentery or retroperitoneum or those with massive parenchymal involvement are best treated by adequate tissue biopsy through the smallest possible incision and prompt initiation of appropriate multiagent chemotherapy. Mediastinal or cervical primary tumors should undergo initial diagnostic biopsy, and complete tumor resection must be avoided. Laparoscopic and thoracoscopic approaches may prove useful in the diagnosis and treatment of non-Hodgkin's lymphomas. These techniques minimize tissue trauma, which may prove useful because systemic treatment can be initiated with little delay. Studies to evaluate the role of minimal-access surgery in patients with solid tumors are being undertaken by cooperative groups.

Chemotherapy

Non-Hodgkin's lymphomas in childhood are disseminated at diagnosis. This concept is supported by the finding that patients with completely excised, localized disease almost always relapse in distant sites (e.g., bone marrow, cerebrospinal fluid).[46,131] Effective therapy must therefore be systemic, and chemotherapy is the primary treatment modality. Historically, only 20% to 30% of patients with non-Hodgkin's lymphoma survived for 5 years until the pioneering work of Wollner et al.[28,133,134] in 1975, when the LSA2-L2 regimen, adapted from the treatment of acute lymphoblastic leukemia, resulted in a 73% salvage rate. At about the same time, Ziegler et al.[71,136] reported successful treatment of these patients using the COMP (cyclophosphamide, Oncovin [vincristine], methotrexate, prednisone) regimen. The Children's Cancer Study Group began a randomized trial comparing these two high-dose chemotherapy regimens for non-Hodgkin's lymphoma in 1977 (CCG-551),[3] with patients being randomized at diagnosis. The results suggested that therapy for non-Hodgkin's lymphoma in children should be modified to take into account the specific histopathologic subtype. A short summary of this trial is illustrative. Overall disease-free survival was 60% at 2 years for patients in CCG-551. Patients with nonlocalized disease and lymphoblastic histopathologic findings had a disease-free survival of 76% at 2 years if treated with LSA2-L2, whereas similar patients treated with COMP had only a 26% survival ($P = 0.00002$). Conversely, in patients with nonlocalized, undifferentiated (small, noncleaved cell) tumors, disease-free survival was 57% for COMP, compared to 28% for LSA2-L2 ($P = 0.02$). Lymphoblastic tumors did significantly better when treated with LSA2-L2, whereas COMP was more effective for undifferentiated lymphomas.

Chemotherapy is the primary treatment modality for all stages and histopathologic subtypes of non-Hodgkin's lymphoma. Given the high growth fractions encountered,

TABLE 35-4 Treatment Regimens for Non-Hodgkin's Lymphoma

Lymphoblastic Lymphoma		Small Noncleaved Lymphoma	
Stage I, II	Stage III, IV	Stage I, II	Stage III, IV
Vincristine, doxorubicin, cyclophosphamide, prednisone, mercaptopurine, methotrexate[64]	BFM-NHL 90: prednisone, dexamethasone, vincristine, daunorubicin, doxorubicin, L-asparaginase, cyclophosphamide, cytarabine, methotrexate, 6-mercaptopurine, 6-thioguanine, CNS irradiation[37]	COMP French LMB-89: high-dose cyclophosphamide, vincristine, prednisone, doxorubicin[89]	French LMB-89
CHOP + MTX (NCI-POB-7704): cyclophosphamide, doxorubicin, vincristine, and prednisone, alternating with infusional methotrexate[69] COMP: cyclophosphamide, vincristine, methotrexate, prednisone[3]	LMTB1: LSA2L2 regimen supplemented by 10 courses of high-dose methotrexate[90]	CHOP CHOP + MTX (NCI-POB-7704) NHL-BFM 90: prednisone, dexamethasone, vincristine, doxorubicin, cyclophospha-mide, ifosfamide, etoposide, cytarabine, methotrexate[102]	NHL-BFM 90 NCI-89-C-0041F: cyclophosphamide, vincristine, doxorubicin, and methotrexate (Codox-M), alternating with cytarabine, etoposide, and ifosfamide (IVAC)[2]

especially with undifferentiated non-Hodgkin's lymphoma, it is crucial that chemotherapy be initiated as expeditiously as possible.

Chemotherapeutic protocols for non-Hodgkin's lymphoma continue to evolve, and some of these regimens are listed in Table 35–4. Many lymphomas with localized gross disease still receive COMP chemotherapy. Mediastinal T-cell tumors are treated with regimens similar or identical to those used for lymphoblastic lymphoma, and LSA2-L2 is no longer widely used. Small, noncleaved cell lymphomas, including Burkitt's, are treated with regimens that are dose intense but shorter in duration. The use of supportive granulocyte-colony stimulating factor has been associated with a reduction in hospital readmission for febrile neutropenia.[61,66,91] An anti-CD20 monoclonal antibody has been used for refractory or recurrent B-cell lymphomas.[118] There are no reported trials in childhood lymphomas.

Radiation Therapy

In the treatment of localized non-Hodgkin's lymphoma, radiation therapy has been shown to add toxicity with no therapeutic benefit.[26,83] Conversely, external beam radiation cannot be used to treat diffuse involvement at multiple anatomic sites. At present, radiotherapy should be reserved for specific emergent situations, such as mediastinal involvement with airway obstruction or massive testicular involvement. Routine central nervous system prophylaxis is readily accomplished with intrathecal methotrexate and cytosine arabinoside.[69] A number of recent studies continue to show a favorable outcome for non-Hodgkin's lymphoma patients treated with chemotherapy without radiotherapy.[37,63,101]

Complications

As previously noted, childhood non-Hodgkin's lymphomas, especially the small, noncleaved cell subtype, have extremely high growth fractions and rapid cellular turnover rates. This results in a large turnover of tumor cells, either because they outgrow their blood supply or undergo cell death and lysis for other reasons. Depending on the size of the tumor, this places a tremendous metabolic load on the kidneys, composed of phosphates, potassium, purines, and protein. Patients may present with elevated serum uric acid, lactate, and potassium levels. This syndrome may be further aggravated during the initial massive cell lysis caused by chemotherapy. The result is the tumor lysis syndrome, which can result in hyperuricemic nephropathy and renal shutdown.[41] Obviously, the metabolic and hematologic status of the patient should be determined before surgery. A full serum electrolyte screen, as well as determinations of serum creatinine and blood urea nitrogen, is mandatory before surgical intervention, and preoperative hemodialysis may be required to control electrolyte disturbances. All patients should be treated with allopurinol and undergo alkaline diuresis before chemotherapy.

Ancillary roles for surgery include the establishment of vascular access for chemotherapy and, if necessary, hemodialysis. Decompression of the urinary tract may also be required in cases of ureteral obstruction by a large abdominal tumor. Cystoscopic placement of ureteral catheters (double-J) can result in marked improvement in urine output and renal function. This technique is preferable to percutaneous puncture both for patient comfort and to avoid infectious complications from percutaneous catheters when the granulocyte counts fall after chemotherapy.

Prognostic Factors

Clinical outcome depends on tumor burden at the time of diagnosis. This is reflected by the clinical stage, but no current staging system correlates linearly with tumor burden.[18,69] A number of serum parameters can be used to estimate tumor amount, as these substances are secreted or shed from malignant cells. These include LDH, interleukin-2 receptor, β_2-microglobulin, uric acid, lactic acid, and polyamines.[20,39,128] Determination of serum LDH levels is readily available and easy to obtain. LDH levels greater than 250 mg/U/L suggest significant tumor burden, whereas levels greater than 500 are associated with a significantly worse prognosis.

Summary

Non-Hodgkin's lymphoma is a heterogeneous group of lymphoid malignancies that can be systematized by reference to normal lymphoid ontogeny. Most abdominal tumors are of the undifferentiated histopathologic subtype (also called small, noncleaved cell), with Burkitt's lymphoma included in this group. Present data support complete resection of abdominal lymphomas only when this can be accomplished with minimal morbidity and without delaying the initiation of chemotherapy. Most mediastinal lymphomas are of T-cell orgin, and resection should not be performed. Surgical intervention may also be required to treat complications, such as massive tumor lysis, bowel perforation, gastrointestinal hemorrhage, or urinary tract obstruction.

REFERENCES

1. Abruzzo LV, Jaffe ES, Cotelingam JD, et al: T-cell lymphoblastic lymphoma with eosinophilia associated with subsequent myeloid malignancy. Am J Surg Pathol 1992;16:236-245.
2. Adde M, Shad A, Venzon D, et al: Additional chemotherapy agents improve treatment outcome for children and adults with advanced B-cell lymphomas. Semin Oncol 1998;25 (Suppl 4):33-39; discussion 45-48.
3. Anderson JR, Jenkin RD, Wilson JF, et al: Long-term follow-up of patients treated with COMP or LSA2l2 therapy for childhood non-Hodgkin's lymphoma: A report of CCG-551 from the Children's Cancer Group. J Clin Oncol 1993;11:1024-1032 (see comments).
4. Anderson MM, Ross CW, Singleton TP, et al: Ki-1 anaplastic large cell lymphoma with a prominent leukemic phase. Hum Pathol 1996;27:1093-1095.
5. Anderson T, Chabner BA, Young RC, et al: Malignant lymphoma. 1. The histology and staging of 473 patients at the National Cancer Institute: Validity of the Ann Arbor staging classification for the non-Hodgkin's lymphomas. Cancer 1982;50:2699-2707.
6. ar-Rushdi A, Nishikura K, Erikson J, et al: Differential expression of the translocated and the untranslocated c-myc oncogene in Burkitt lymphoma. Science 1983;222:390-393.
7. Arseneau JC, Canellos GP, Banks PM, et al: American Burkitt's lymphoma: A clinicopathologic study of 30 cases. I. Clinical factors relating to prolonged survival. Am J Med 1975;58:314-321.
8. Beaty O 3rd, Hudson MM, Greenwald C, et al: Subsequent malignancies in children and adolescents after treatment for Hodgkin's disease. J Clin Oncol 1995;13:603-609 (see comments).
9. Behrendt H, Brinkhuis M, Van Leeuwen EF: Treatment of childhood Hodgkin's disease with ABVD without radiotherapy. Med Pediatr Oncol 1996;26:244-248.
10. Bonadonna G, Valagussa P, Santoro A: Alternating non-cross-resistant combination chemotherapy or MOPP in stage IV Hodgkin's disease. A report of 8-year results. Ann Intern Med 1986;104:739-746.
11. Bonadonna G, Zucali R, Monfardini S, et al: Combination chemotherapy of Hodgkin's disease with Adriamycin, bleomycin, vinblastine, and imidazole carboxamide versus MOPP. Cancer 1975;36:252-259.
12. Carde P, Koscielny S, Franklin J, et al: Early response to chemotherapy: A surrogate for final outcome of Hodgkin's disease patients that should influence initial treatment length and intensity? Ann Oncol 2002;13(Suppl 1):86-91.
13. Castellino RA, Dunnick NR, Goffinet DR, et al: Predictive value of lymphography for sites of subdiaphragmatic disease encountered at staging laparotomy in newly diagnosed Hodgkin's disease and non-Hodgkin's lymphoma. J Clin Oncol 1993;1:532-536.
14. Castellino RA, Hoppe RT, Blank N, et al: Computed tomography, lymphography, and staging laparotomy: Correlations in initial staging of Hodgkin disease. AJR Am J Roentgenol 1984;143:37-41.
15. Chapman RM, Sutcliffe SB, Malpas JS: Male gonadal dysfunction in Hodgkin's disease: A prospective study. JAMA 1981;245:1323-1328.
16. Chilcote RR, Baehner RL, Hammond D: Septicemia and meningitis in children splenectomized for Hodgkin's disease. N Engl J Med 1976;295:798-800.
17. Chung CT, Bogart JA, Adams JF, et al: Increased risk of breast cancer in splenectomized patients undergoing radiation therapy for Hodgkin's disease. Int J Radiat Oncol Biol Phys 1997;37:405-409.
18. Cohen LF, Balow JE, Magrath IT, et al: Acute tumor lysis syndrome: A review of 37 patients with Burkitt's lymphoma. Am J Med 1980;68:486-491.
19. Constine LS, Donaldson SS, McDougall IR, et al: Thyroid dysfunction after radiotherapy in children with Hodgkin's disease. Cancer 1984;53:878-883.
20. Csako G, Magrath IT, Elin RJ: Serum total and isoenzyme lactate dehydrogenase activity in American Burkitt's lymphoma patients. Am J Clin Pathol 1982;78:712-717.
21. Denny CT, Yoshikai Y, Mak TW, et al: A chromosome 14 inversion in a T-cell lymphoma is caused by site-specific recombination between immunoglobulin and T-cell receptor loci. Nature 1986;320:549-551.
22. DeVita VTJ, Serpick A, Carbone PP: Combination chemotherapy in the treatment of advanced Hodgkin's disease. Ann Intern Med 1970;73:881-895.
23. Donaldson SS, Hudson MM, Lamborn KR, et al: VAMP and low-dose, involved-field radiation for children and adolescents with favorable, early-stage Hodgkin's disease: Results of a prospective clinical trial. J Clin Oncol 2002;20:3081-3087.
24. Donaldson SS, Kaplan HS: Complications of treatment of Hodgkin's disease in children. Cancer Treat Rep 1982;66:977-989.
25. Donaldson SS, Link MP: Combined modality treatment with low-dose radiation and MOPP chemotherapy for children with Hodgkin's disease. J Clin Oncol 1987;5:742-749.
26. Donaldson SS, Whitaker SJ, Plowman PN, et al: Stage I-II pediatric Hodgkin's disease: Long-term follow-up demonstrates equivalent survival rates following different management schemes. J Clin Oncol 1990;8:1128-1137 (see comments).
27. Duepree HJ, Senagore AJ, Delaney CP, Fazio VW: Does means of access affect the incidence of small bowel obstruction and ventral hernia after bowel resection?

Laparoscopy versus laparotomy. J Am Coll Surg 2003; 197:177-181.

28. Duque-Hammershaimb L, Wollner N, Miller DR: LSA2-l2 protocol treatment of stage IV non-Hodgkin's lymphoma in children with partial and extensive bone marrow involvement. Cancer 1983;52:39-43.

29. Eraklis AJ, Filler RM: Splenectomy in childhood: A review of 1413 cases. J Pediatr Surg 1972;7:382-388.

30. Franzius C, Schober O: Assessment of therapy response by FDG PET in pediatric patients. Q J Nucl Med 2003;47:41-45.

31. Gaetini A, De Simone M, Urgesi A, et al: Lateral high abdominal ovariopexy: An original surgical technique for protection of the ovaries during curative radiotherapy for Hodgkin's disease. J Surg Oncol 1988;39:22-28.

32. Garrett KM, Hoffer FA, Behm FG, et al: Interventional radiology techniques for the diagnosis of lymphoma or leukemia. Pediatr Radiol 2002;32:653-662.

33. Gilbert R: Radiotherapy in Hodgkin's disease (malignant granulomatosis): Anatomic and clinical foundations, governing principles, results. AJR Am J Roentgenol 1939;41: 198-241.

34. Glatstein E, Guernsey JM, Rosenberg SA, et al: The value of laparotomy and splenectomy in the staging of Hodgkin's disease. Cancer 1969;24:709-718.

35. Glick RD, La Quaglia MP: Lymphomas of the anterior mediastinum. Semin Pediatr Surg 1999;8:69-77.

36. Goodman LS, Wintrobe MM, Dameshek W, et al: Nitrogen mustard therapy: Use of methyl-bis(-chlorethyl)amine hydrochloride for Hodgkin's disease, lymphosarcoma, leukemia, and certain allied diseases and miscellaneous disorders. JAMA 1946;132:126-132.

37. Grenzebach J, Schrappe M, Ludwig WD, et al: Favorable outcome for children and adolescents with T-cell lymphoblastic lymphoma with an intensive ALL-type therapy without local radiotherapy. Ann Hematol 2001;80(Suppl 3): B73-B76.

38. Gross TG, Filipovich AH, Conley ME, et al: Cure of X-linked lymphoproliferative disease (XLP) with allogeneic hematopoietic stem cell transplantation (HSCT): Report from the XLP Registry. Bone Marrow Transplant 1996;17: 741-744.

39. Hagberg H, Killander A, Simonsson B: Serum beta 2-microglobulin in malignant lymphoma. Cancer 1983;51: 2220-2225.

40. Haluska FG, Brufsky AM, Canellos GP: The cellular biology of the Reed-Sternberg cell. Blood 1994;84:1005-1019.

41. Hande KR, Garrow GC: Acute tumor lysis syndrome in patients with high-grade non-Hodgkin's lymphoma. Am J Med 1993;94:133-139.

42. Hays DM: Malignant solid tumors of childhood. Curr Probl Surg 1986;23:161-242.

43. Hays DM, Ternberg JL, Chen TT, et al: Complications related to 234 staging laparotomies performed in the Intergroup Hodgkin's Disease in Childhood Study. Surgery 1984;96:471-478.

44. Hodgkin T: On some morbid appearances of the absorbent glands and spleen. Med Chir Trans Soc Lond 1832;17: 68-114.

45. Hurwitz M, Desai DM, Cox KL, et al: Complete immunosuppressive withdrawal as a uniform approach to posttransplant lymphoproliferative disease in pediatric liver transplantation. Pediatr Transplant 2004;8:267-272.

46. Hutter JJ Jr, Favara BE, Nelson M, Holton CP: Non-Hodgkin's lymphoma in children: Correlation of CNS disease with initial presentation. Cancer 1975;36:2132-2137.

47. Iversen OH, Bjerknes R, Iversen U, et al: Cell kinetics in Burkitt's lymphoma. In Drewinko B, Humphrey RM (eds): Growth Kinetics and Biochemical. 1997, pp 675-686.

48. Iversen OH, Iversen U, Ziegler JL, Bluming AZ: Cell kinetics in Burkitt lymphoma. Eur J Cancer 1974;10:155-163.

49. Jenkin D, Greenberg M, Fitzgerald A: Second malignant tumours in childhood Hodgkin's disease. Med Pediatr Oncol 1996;26:373-379.

50. Jenkin RD, Brown TC, Peters MV, Sonley MJ: Hodgkin's disease in children: A retrospective analysis: 1958-73. Cancer 1975;35:979-990.

51. Kaplan HS: Long-term results of palliative and radical radiotherapy of Hodgkin's disease. Cancer Res 1966;26: 1250-1252.

52. Kaufman BH, Burgert EO Jr, Banks PM: Abdominal Burkitt's lymphoma: Role of early aggressive surgery. J Pediatr Surg 1987;22:671-674.

53. Kellie SJ, Pui CH, Murphy SB: Childhood non-Hodgkin's lymphoma involving the testis: Clinical features and treatment outcome. J Clin Oncol 1989;7:1066-1070.

54. Kelly KM, Hutchinson RJ, Sposto R, et al: Feasibility of upfront dose-intensive chemotherapy in children with advanced-stage Hodgkin's lymphoma: Preliminary results from the Children's Cancer Group Study CCG-59704. Ann Oncol 2002;13(Suppl 1):107-111.

55. Kemeny MM, Magrath IT, Brennan MF: The role of surgery in the management of American Burkitt's lymphoma and its treatment. Ann Surg 1982;196:82-86.

56. King H, Shumacker HBJ: Splenic studies. I. Susceptibility to infection after splenectomy performed in infancy. Ann Surg 1952;136:239-242.

57. Kraus M, Fliss DM, Argov S, et al: Burkitt's lymphoma of the tonsil. J Laryngol Otol 1990;104:991-994.

58. Kristoffersson U, Heim S, Mandahl N, et al: Trisomy 5 and t(5;14)(q11;q32) as the sole abnormalities in two different clones from a centroblastic non-Hodgkin's lymphoma. Cancer Genet Cytogenet 1988;36:173-176.

59. Kushner BH, Zauber A, Tan CT: Second malignancies after childhood Hodgkin's disease: The Memorial Sloan-Kettering Cancer Center experience. Cancer 1988;62:1364-1370.

60. La Quaglia MP, Stolar CJ, Krailo M, et al: The role of surgery in abdominal non-Hodgkin's lymphoma: Experience from the Children's Cancer Study Group. J Pediatr Surg 1992;27: 230-235.

61. Laver J, Amylon M, Desai S, et al: Randomized trial of r-metHu granulocyte colony-stimulating factor in an intensive treatment for T-cell leukemia and advanced-stage lymphoblastic lymphoma of childhood: A Pediatric Oncology Group pilot study. J Clin Oncol 1998;16:522-526.

62. Leventhal BG, Kato GJ: Childhood Hodgkin and non-Hodgkin lymphomas. Pediatr Rev 1990;12:171-179.

63. Link MP, Donaldson SS, Berard CW, et al: Results of treatment of childhood localized non-Hodgkin's lymphoma with combination chemotherapy with or without radiotherapy. N Engl J Med 1990;322:1169-1174.

64. Link MP, Shuster JJ, Donaldson SS, et al: Treatment of children and young adults with early-stage non-Hodgkin's lymphoma. N Engl J Med 1997;337:1259-1266.

65. Link MP, Warnke R, Finlay J, et al: A single monoclonal antibody identifies T-cell lineage of childhood lymphoid malignancies. Blood 1983;62:722-728.

66. Little MA, Morland B, Chisholm J, et al: A randomised study of prophylactic G-CSF following MRC UKALL XI intensification regimen in childhood ALL and T-NHL. Med Pediatr Oncol 2002;38:98-103.

67. Longo DL, Young RC, Wesley M, et al: Twenty years of MOPP therapy for Hodgkin's disease. J Clin Oncol 1986; 4:1295-1306.

68. Magrath IT: Lymphocyte differentiation: An essential basis for the comprehension of lymphoid neoplasia. J Natl Cancer Inst 1981;67:501-514.

69. Magrath IT, Janus C, Edwards BK, et al: An effective therapy for both undifferentiated (including Burkitt's) lymphomas and lymphoblastic lymphomas in children and young adults. Blood 1984;63:1102-1111.

70. Magrath IT, Lwanga S, Carswell W, Harrison N: Surgical reduction of tumour bulk in management of abdominal Burkitt's lymphoma. BMJ 1974;2:308-312.

71. Magrath IT, Ziegler JL: Failure of BCG immunostimulation to affect the clinical course of Burkitt's lymphoma. BMJ 1976;1:615-618.

72. Maguire RT, Robins TS, Thorgeirsson SS, Heilman CA: Expression of cellular myc and mos genes in undifferentiated B cell lymphomas of Burkitt and non-Burkitt types. Proc Natl Acad Sci U S A 1983;80:1947-1950.

73. Mauch PM, Kalish LA, Marcus KC, et al: Second malignancies after treatment for laparotomy staged IA-IIIB Hodgkin's disease: Long-term analysis of risk factors and outcome. Blood 1996;87:3625-3632.

74. Medary I, Steinherz LJ, Aronson DC, La Quaglia MP: Cardiac tamponade in the pediatric oncology population: Treatment by percutaneous catheter drainage. J Pediatr Surg 1996;31: 197-199.

75. Meyers PA, Potter VP, Wollner N, Exelby P: Bowel perforation during initial treatment for childhood non-Hodgkin's lymphoma. Cancer 1985;56:259-261.

76. Miller JF: Immunologic functions of the thymus. Lancet 1961;2:748-749.

77. Moskowitz C: Risk-adapted therapy for relapsed and refractory lymphoma using ICE chemotherapy. Cancer Chemother Pharmacol 2002;49(Suppl 1):S9-S12.

78. Moskowitz C: An update on the management of relapsed and primary refractory Hodgkin's disease. Semin Oncol 2004;31(2 Suppl 4):54-59.

79. Moskowitz CH, Kewalramani T, Nimer SD, et al: Effectiveness of high dose chemoradiotherapy and autologous stem cell transplantation for patients with biopsy-proven primary refractory Hodgkin's disease. Br J Haematol 2004;124:645-652.

80. Mukhtar AU, Mugerwa B: Burkitt's lymphoma of the ovary. Cent Afr J Med 1999;45:104-105.

81. Murphy SB, Fairclough DL, Hutchison RE, Berard CW: Non-Hodgkin's lymphomas of childhood: An analysis of the histology, staging, and response to treatment of 338 cases at a single institution. J Clin Oncol 1989;7:186-193.

82. Murphy SB, Frizzera G, Evans AE: A study of childhood non-Hodgkin's lymphoma. Cancer 1975;36:2121-2131.

83. Murphy SB, Hustu HO: A randomized trial of combined modality therapy of childhood non-Hodgkin's lymphoma. Cancer 1980;45:630-637.

84. Nachman JB, Sposto R, Herzog P, et al: Randomized comparison of low-dose involved-field radiotherapy and no radiotherapy for children with Hodgkin's disease who achieve a complete response to chemotherapy. J Clin Oncol 2002;20:3765-3771.

85. Nathwani BN, Griffith RC, Kelly DR: A morphological study of childhood lymphoma of the diffuse histiocytic type: The Pediatric Oncology Group experience. Cancer 1976;38: 964-983.

86. Nathwani BN, Griffith RC, Kelly DR, et al: A morphologic study of childhood lymphoma of the diffuse "histiocytic" type: The Pediatric Oncology Group experience. Cancer 1987;59: 1138-1142.

87. Oberlin O, Leverger G, Pacquement H, et al: Low-dose radiation therapy and reduced chemotherapy in childhood Hodgkin's disease: The experience of the French Society of Pediatric Oncology. J Clin Oncol 1992;10:1602-1608.

88. Ortin TT, Shostak CA, Donaldson SS: Gonadal status and reproductive function following treatment for Hodgkin's disease in childhood: The Stanford experience. Int J Radiat Oncol Biol Phys 1990;19:873-880.

89. Patte C, Auperin A, Michon J, et al: The Societe Francaise d'Oncologie Pediatrique LMB89 protocol: Highly effective multiagent chemotherapy tailored to the tumor burden and initial response in 561 unselected children with B-cell lymphomas and L3 leukemia. Blood 2001;97: 3370-3379.

90. Patte C, Kalifa C, Flamant F, et al: Results of the LMT81 protocol, a modified LSA2L2 protocol with high dose methotrexate, on 84 children with non-B-cell (lymphoblastic) lymphoma. Med Pediatr Oncol 1992;20:105-113.

91. Patte C, Laplanche A, Bertozzi AI, et al: Granulocyte colony-stimulating factor in induction treatment of children with non-Hodgkin's lymphoma: A randomized study of the French Society of Pediatric Oncology. J Clin Oncol 2002;20:441-448.

92. Penn I: De novo malignances in pediatric organ transplant recipients. Pediatr Transplant 1998;2:56-63.

93. Percy CL, Smith MA, Linet M, et al: Lymphomas and reticuloendothelial neoplasms. In Ries LAG, Smith MA, Gurney JG, et al (eds): Cancer Incidence and Survival among Children and Adolescents: United States SEER Program 1975-1995. NIH Pub. No. 99-4649. Bethesda, Md, National Cancer Institute, SEER Program, 1999.

94. Peters MV: A study of survival in Hodgkin's disease treated radiologically. AJR Am J Roentgenol 1950;63: 299-311.

95. Pondarre C, Kebaili K, Dijoud F, et al: Epstein-Barr virus-related lymphoproliferative disease complicating childhood acute lymphoblastic leukemia: No recurrence after unrelated donor bone marrow transplantation. Bone Marrow Transplant 2001;27:93-95.

96. Pringle KC, Rowley D, Burrington JD: Immunologic response in splenectomized and partially splenectomized rats. J Pediatr Surg 1980;15:531-536.

97. Probert JC, Parker BR: The effects of radiation therapy on bone growth. Radiology 1975;114:155-162.

98. Pusey WA: Cases of sarcoma and Hodgkin's disease treated by exposure to x-rays: A preliminary report. JAMA 1902;38:166-169.

99. Rappold GA, Hameister H, Cremer T, et al: C-myc and immunoglobulin kappa light chain constant genes are on the 8q+ chromosome of three Burkitt lymphoma lines with t(2;8) translocations. EMBO J 1984;3:2951-2955.

100. Reed DM: On the pathological changes in Hodgkin's disease with especial reference to its relation to tuberculosis. Johns Hopkins Hosp Rep 1902;10:133-196.

101. Reiter A, Schrappe M, Ludwig WD, et al: Intensive ALL-type therapy without local radiotherapy provides a 90% event-free survival for children with T-cell lymphoblastic lymphoma: A BFM group report. Blood 2000; 92:416-421.

102. Reiter A, Schrappe M, Tiemann M, et al: Improved treatment results in childhood B-cell neoplasms with tailored intensification of therapy: A report of the Berlin-Frankfurt-Munster Group Trial NHL-BFM 90. Blood 1999;94:3294-3306.

103. Rosenberg SA, Kaplan HS: Evidence for an orderly progression in the spread of Hodgkin's disease. Cancer Res 1966;26:1225-1231.

104. Ross CW, Hanson CA, Schnitzer B: CD30 (Ki-1)-positive, anaplastic large cell lymphoma mimicking gastrointestinal carcinoma. Cancer 1992;70:2517-2523.

105. Rowley DA: The formation of circulating antibody in the splenectomized human being following intravenous injection of heterologous erythrocytes. J Immunol 1950;65: 515-521.

106. Rubie H, Gladieff L, Robert A, et al: Childhood anaplastic large cell lymphoma Ki-1/CD30: Clinicopathologic features of 19 cases. Med Pediatr Oncol 1994;22:155-161.

107. Ruhl U, Albrecht M, Dieckmann K, et al: Response-adapted radiotherapy in the treatment of pediatric Hodgkin's disease: An interim report at 5 years of the German GPOH-HD 95 trial. Int J Radiat Oncol Biol Phys 2001;51:1209-1218.

108. Samuelsson BO, Ridell B, Rockert L, et al: Non-Hodgkin lymphoma in children: A 20-year population-based epidemiologic study in western Sweden. J Pediatr Hematol Oncol 1999;21:103-110.

109. Sandlund JT, Downing JR, Crist WM: Non-Hodgkin's lymphoma in childhood. N Engl J Med 1996;334:1238-1248.

110. Sandoval C, Strom K, Stringel G: Laparoscopy in the management of pediatric intraabdominal tumors. JSLS 2004;8:115-118.

111. Schellong G, Bramswig JH, Hornig-Franz I, et al: Hodgkin's disease in children: Combined modality treatment for stages IA, IB, and IIA. Results in 356 patients of the German/Austrian Pediatric Study Group. Ann Oncol 1994;5(Suppl 2):113-115.

112. Schneeberger AL, Girvan DP: Staging laparotomy for Hodgkin's disease in children. J Pediatr Surg 1988;23:714-717.

113. Schnitzer B, Roth MS, Hyder DM, Ginsburg D: Ki-1 lymphomas in children. Cancer 1988;61:1213-1221.

114. Schwartz CL: Prognostic factors in pediatric Hodgkin disease. Curr Oncol Rep 2003;5:498-504.

115. Shamberger RC, Weinstein HJ: The role of surgery in abdominal Burkitt's lymphoma. J Pediatr Surg 1992;27:236-240.

116. Silecchia G, Fantini A, Raparelli L, et al: Management of abdominal lymphoproliferative diseases in the era of laparoscopy. Am J Surg 1999;177:325-330.

117. Silecchia G, Raparelli L, Perrotta N, et al: Accuracy of laparoscopy in the diagnosis and staging of lymphoproliferative diseases. World J Surg 2003;27:653-658.

118. Silverman DH, Delpassand ES, Torabi F, et al: Radiolabeled antibody therapy in non-Hodgkins lymphoma: Radiation protection, isotope comparisons and quality of life issues. Cancer Treat Rev 2004;30:165-172.

119. Singer DB: Postsplenectomy sepsis. Perspect Pediatr Pathol 1973;1:285-311.

120. Socie G, Curtis RE, Deeg HJ, et al: New malignant diseases after allogeneic marrow transplantation for childhood acute leukemia. J Clin Oncol 2000;18:348-357.

121. Sternberg C: Uber eine Eigenartige unter dem Bilde der Pseudoleukamie verlaufende Tuberculose des lymphatischen Apparates. Z Heilk 1898;19:21-90.

122. Su IJ, Wang CH, Cheng AL, Chen RL: Hemophagocytic syndrome in Epstein-Barr virus-associated T-lymphoproliferative disorders: Disease spectrum, pathogenesis, and management. Leuk Lymphoma 1995;19:401-406.

123. Tan CT, De Sousa M, Good RA: Distinguishing features of the immunology of Hodgkin's disease in children. Cancer Treat Rep 1982;66:969-975.

124. Taub R, Moulding C, Battey J, et al: Activation and somatic mutation of the translocated c-myc gene in Burkitt lymphoma cells. Cell 1984;36:339-348.

125. Thomson AB, Wallace WH: Treatment of paediatric Hodgkin's disease: A balance of risks. Eur J Cancer 2002;38:468-477.

126. Tsokos GC, Balow JE, Spiegel RJ, Magrath IT: Renal and metabolic complications of undifferentiated and lymphoblastic lymphomas. Medicine (Baltimore) 1981;60:218-229.

127. Vigersky RA, Chapman RM, Berenberg J, Glass AR: Testicular dysfunction in untreated Hodgkin's disease. Am J Med 1982;73:482-486.

128. Wagner DK, Kiwanuka J, Edwards BK, et al: Soluble interleukin-2 receptor levels in patients with undifferentiated and lymphoblastic lymphomas: Correlation with survival. J Clin Oncol 1987;5:1262-1274.

129. Walsh RM, Heniford BT: Role of laparoscopy for Hodgkin's and non-Hodgkin's lymphoma. Semin Surg Oncol 1999;16:284-292.

130. Warner NL, Szenberg A, Burnet FM: The immunological role of different lymphoid organs in the chicken. I. Dissociation of immunological responsiveness. Aust J Exp Biol Med Sci 1962;40:373-388.

131. Watanabe A, Sullivan MP, Sutow WW, Wilbur JR: Undifferentiated lymphoma, non-Burkitt's type: Meningeal and bone marrow involvement in children. Am J Dis Child 1973;125:57-61.

132. White L, Siegel SE, Quah TC: Non-Hodgkin's lymphomas in children. I. Patterns of disease and classification. Crit Rev Oncol Hematol 1992;13:55-71.

133. Wollner N: Non-Hodgkin's lymphoma in children. Pediatr Clin North Am 1976;23:371-378.

134. Wollner N, Burchenal JH, Lieberman PH, et al: Non-Hodgkin's lymphoma in children: A comparative study of two modalities of therapy. Cancer 1976;37:123-134.

135. Zech L, Haglund U, Nilsson K, Klein G: Characteristic chromosomal abnormalities in biopsies and lymphoid-cell lines from patients with Burkitt and non-Burkitt lymphomas. Int J Cancer 1976;17:47-56.

136. Ziegler JL: Treatment results of 54 American patients with Burkitt's lymphoma are similar to the African experience. N Engl J Med 1977;297:75-80.

Chapter 36

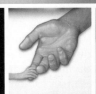
Ovarian Tumors

Claire L. Templeman and Mary E. Fallat

INCIDENCE

Primary cysts and tumors of the ovaries are uncommon in children. The majority of these masses are not malignant.[64] Gynecologic malignant conditions account for approximately 2% of all types of cancer in children, and 60% to 70% of these lesions arise in the ovary.[158] Recently the North American Association of Central Cancer Registries released data from 1992 to 1997 regarding more than 1.6 million women and children diagnosed with cancer.[233] This report revealed that 1.2% of ovarian cancer cases occurred in females between birth and age 19 years.[233] Lindfors[117] analyzed several large series of ovarian tumors in children and estimated that the annual incidence of combined benign and malignant lesions was 2.6 cases per 100,000 girls younger than 15 years.

Age distribution has an influence on the relative frequency of specific types of ovarian lesions. Lack et al.[112] reviewed 157 primary ovarian tumors from a 50-year experience at the Boston Children's Hospital. The incidence of mature cystic teratomas was relatively static beyond 5 years of age, the incidence of granulosa cell tumors dropped after 9 years of age, the peak incidence of yolk sac tumors occurred between 10 and 14 years of age and then dropped dramatically, and surface epithelial tumors were not seen in girls younger than 10 years.

The concept that the highest incidence of malignant conditions occurs in the youngest patients has been reassessed. Newer diagnostic imaging techniques have increased the detection of all gonadal masses, and the frequency of ovarian cancer has decreased. A 43-year review published in 1992 by Gribbon et al.[77] noted that malignant ovarian tumors are more frequent (70%) in the second decade of life.

Previous surveys reported a 55% to 67% incidence of malignant ovarian lesions.[78,142] An 11-year experience of 91 cases from the Children's Hospital of Philadelphia published in 1993 detected only a 21% incidence of malignant tumors.[26] Ninety-seven percent of the patients younger than 8 years had benign lesions, compared with 33% in older age groups. Imai et al.[96] reported a 20% incidence of malignancy among 114 ovarian tumors collected from a large hospital network in Japan. Several other series reported that the occurrence of malignant ovarian tumors in children and adolescents ranged from 10% to 40%.[48,53,190]

EPIDEMIOLOGY

A few syndromes or diseases have been associated with ovarian pathology. The Peutz-Jeghers syndrome has been associated with granulosa cell tumors, ovarian cystadenomas, and sex cord–stromal tumors with annular tubules.[161] Juvenile granulosa cell tumors have been detected with Ollier's disease (multiple enchondromatosis)[11] and Maffucci's syndrome (enchondromatosis and hemangiomas).[201] The Sertoli-Leydig cell tumor has been associated with Ollier's disease,[3] and fibrosarcoma has been linked with Maffucci's syndrome.[32] Sclerosing stromal tumors have been associated with the Chédiak-Higashi syndrome (oculocutaneous albinism, pyogenic infections, and leukocyte granule abnormalities that result in deficient phagocytosis).[97] The presence of ovarian cysts had been noted in various dysmorphic syndromes, including those with craniofacial, laryngeal, and digital malformations.[126] The McCune-Albright syndrome (triad of café au lait macules, polyostotic fibrous dysplasia, and autonomous endocrine hyperactivity) is generally characterized by gonadotropin-independent sexual precocity due to recurrent ovarian follicle formation and cyclic estradiol secretion.[224] Fibromas are often associated with the basal cell nevus syndrome.

Nulliparity is associated with a 1.5 to 3.2 times greater risk of the development of ovarian cancer than is parity. Women who have never used oral contraceptives have a risk 1.4 to 2.5 times greater than that of women who have used them. Other potential but more controversial risk factors include exposure to ovulation-inducing drugs without successful pregnancy and diets high in meat and animal fats, dairy products, and lactose. Prior tubal ligation and hysterectomy may reduce the risk of ovarian cancer.[130,184]

Approximately 5% to 10% of women with breast and ovarian cancer have a genetic predisposition. High percentages of hereditary breast and ovarian cancers arise from mutations in the tumor suppressor genes *BRCA1* and *BRCA2*. Approximately 70% of familial ovarian cancer cases are caused by *BRCA1* mutations and 20% by *BRCA2*. These mutations are inherited in an autosomal dominant fashion. If a woman is a carrier of one of these gene mutations, she has a lifetime risk of developing ovarian cancer as high as 60%.[51,130]

Genetic testing of adolescents is controversial.[185,222] Kodish[107] formulated the argument that physicians should respect the "rule of earliest onset" and defer testing until the age when the onset of disease becomes possible. Although it may seem premature to address these issues in adolescence, some mature young women at risk for breast or ovarian cancer may inquire about the efficacy of future surgical or medical interventions. In most cases, surgical intervention is not indicated until age 35 years or older or completion of childbearing. The use of oral contraceptives has been shown to reduce the risk of ovarian cancer in the general population. Whether the use of these agents in young women with *BRCA* mutations is beneficial remains to be determined.[130]

The American Society of Human Genetics and the American College of Medical Genetics issued a joint report on the genetic testing of children and adolescents in 1995.[10] If the primary goal of genetic testing is to promote the well-being of the child, testing is acceptable only if there are medical benefits, such as preventive measures and therapy. Currently, the benefits of prophylactic surgery or increased surveillance in adolescent patients have not been evaluated or tested, and there is no conclusive evidence that *BRCA* testing has a medical benefit in individuals younger than 18 years. An alternative view proposed by Elger and Harding[56] is that some mature adolescents may obtain significant psychological relief from knowing their mutation status and may be capable of using this information for reproductive and health decisions.

CLINICAL PRESENTATION

Ovarian lesions can present with variable signs and symptoms. Most often, the clinical presentation does not differentiate a benign tumor from a malignant one. Abdominal pain is the most common symptom.[26,96,190] With cysts and other non-neoplastic conditions, the pain can be acute in onset, with a crescendo pattern of severity because of torsion, rupture, or hemorrhage. The clinical picture may mimic appendicitis.[39]

A more chronic, insidious pattern of pain, increasing girth, and marked distention over several weeks to months may occur. Secondary symptoms include anorexia, nausea, vomiting, and urinary frequency and urgency. A palpable abdominal mass with or without tenderness is the most frequent finding on physical examination and is detected in more than 60% of patients with ovarian tumors.[26,190] These tumors are usually mobile and palpable above the pelvic brim. Bimanual palpation between the lower abdomen and rectum may be helpful in detecting smaller lesions. Vaginal examination is usually reserved for sexually active patients, although vaginal inspection is of value in all patients. An increasing number of ovarian lesions are discovered incidentally by abdominal radiographs or ultrasonography (US) done for other reasons.

Both neoplastic and non-neoplastic ovarian lesions demonstrate endocrine activity in approximately 10% of cases.[26,96,112] Ovarian cysts of the simple, follicular, or luteal type may secrete estrogen and can cause precocious isosexual development. The lesions usually function autonomously, and the girls have suppressed gonadotropin concentrations. As a result, they can be distinguished from patients with central precocious puberty (with accelerated skeletal maturation) or premature thelarche (isolated breast development) by estrogen withdrawal and vaginal bleeding after cyst involution or removal. Precocious pseudopuberty may occur due to the production of human chorionic gonadotropin in girls with germ cell tumors, including dysgerminomas, yolk sac tumors, and choriocarcinomas. Precocious puberty is most common with the sex cord–stromal tumors, such as juvenile granulosa cell tumors or some Sertoli-Leydig cell tumors, which cause elevated levels of circulating estrogen.

Virilization due to androgen excess can occur with Sertoli-Leydig cell tumors, and masculinization is occasionally seen in older girls with dysgerminomas that contain syncytial trophoblastic giant cells. Yolk sac tumors, steroid cell tumors, and polycystic ovaries can be associated with virilization.

DIAGNOSIS

Laboratory Tests

Many ovarian neoplasms are associated with the secretion of specific tumor markers or hormones. These are outlined in Tables 36-1 and 36-2 and are discussed further in the sections on individual tumors.

Tumor Markers

Germ cell tumors are associated with various biologic markers that are useful in identifying and managing this group

TABLE 36–1 Ovarian Tumors and Tumor Markers

Histologic Subtype	CA-125	CA-19.9	AFP	β-HCG	LDH
Endometrioma	+				
Epithelial					
Borderline	+				
Carcinoma	+				
Germ cell*					
Dysgerminoma				+	+
Yolk sac			+	+	
Immature teratoma					
Choriocarcinoma				+	
Embryonal			+	+	
Endodermal sinus			+		
Sertoli-Leydig				+	

*The markers indicated are elevated in pure tumors; mixed tumors may secrete several markers.

AFP, alpha fetoprotein; HCG, β-human chorionic gonadotropin; LDH, lactate dehydrogenase.

TABLE 36-2 Ovarian Tumors and Hormones

Histologic Subtype	Estradiol	Testosterone	Urinary 17-Ketosteroid	Gonadotropins
Ovarian cyst				
Simple	↑			
Follicular	↑			
Luteal	↑			
Sex cord–stromal				
Juvenile granulosa	↑	↑*		↓
Sertoli-Leydig	↑†	↑‡		↓
Luteinized thecoma	↑	↑*		
Sex cord tumor with annular tubules	↑			
Steroid cell tumor		↑	↑	
Gonadoblastoma	↑*	↑	↑	↓
Choriocarcinoma	↑			↑

*Indicates rarer variants of the tumor.
†Functioning Sertoli cells predominate.
‡Functioning Leydig cells predominate.

of tumors.[48] Protein markers, including alpha fetoprotein (AFP), β-human chorionic gonadotropin (β-HCG), and lactate dehydrogenase (LDH), are the most readily available. They are measured with serum assays or immunohistochemical staining of paraffin-fixed or frozen tumor.

Alpha Fetoprotein

The association of AFP with germ cell tumors was first described by Abelev et al.[1] Because the fetal yolk sac is the source of AFP early in human embryogenesis, elevations of the marker occur with yolk sac tumors.[207] This is also true with hepatoblastoma, hepatocellular carcinoma, and teratocarcinoma.[200] The elevation reflects the presence of fetal tissue from which normal progenitor cells arise.

There is wide variability in normal levels of AFP from birth through the first year of life,[230] and AFP is significantly elevated in premature and normal newborns (Table 36-3). Its usefulness in the diagnosis of yolk sac tumor or embryonal carcinoma in the first month of life is limited.[66,71] Its value in tumor identification begins when the AFP level is significantly elevated over the normal range at any particular age. The normal serum half-life of AFP is 5 to 7 days. Its decline after removal of an AFP-producing tumor signifies a response to treatment. The goal of any treatment is to return AFP to normal levels. Tumor recurrence is marked by a sudden elevation of the AFP level.

β-Human Chorionic Gonadotropin

β-HCG is a glycoprotein produced by placental syncytiotrophoblasts. It comprises two subunits, α and β; the latter can be reliably assayed.[214] β-HCG elevation in a patient with a germ cell tumor suggests the presence of syncytiotrophoblasts, as seen in seminoma, dysgerminoma, choriocarcinoma, and occasionally embryonal carcinoma.[152] Elevations above 100 ng/mL are unusual and suggest the diagnosis of choriocarcinoma.[154] Unlike the much longer half-life of AFP, the β subunit has a half-life of 20 to 30 hours.[154] Its rapid disappearance implies complete removal of a tumor.

Serum Lactate Dehydrogenase

Serum LDH is a nonspecific marker that is widely distributed in human tissues and is therefore of limited value in establishing tumor type or response to treatment. However, elevated LDH may indicate increased cell turnover and has been used as a nonspecific indicator of malignancy.[145] It is most useful as a prognostic marker for lymphoid tumors and neuroblastoma. The gene for this isoenzyme is located on 12p, and nonrandom structural changes in chromosome 12 have been seen in all histologic subtypes of germ cell tumors.

Cancer Genetics

Ovarian germ cell tumors are associated with sex chromosome abnormalities. Although a few case studies

TABLE 36-3 Average Normal Serum Alpha Fetoprotein Levels in Infants

Age	Number of Samples	Mean ± SD (ng/mL)
Premature	11	134,734 ± 41,444
Newborn	55	48,406 ± 34,718
Newborn-2 wk	16	33,113 ± 32,503
2 wk-1 mo	12	9452 ± 12,610
2 mo	40	323 ± 278
3 mo	5	88 ± 87
4 mo	31	74 ± 56
5 mo	6	46.5 ± 19
6 mo	9	12.5 ± 9.8
7 mo	5	9.7 ± 7.1
8 mo	3	8.5 ± 5.5

From Wu JT, Book L, Sudar K: Serum alpha-fetoprotein (AFP) levels in normal infants. Pediatr Res 1981;15:50.

suggest otherwise, a large study examining 456 first- or second-degree female relatives of 78 patients with ovarian germ cell tumors did not identify an increased risk for occurrence.[18,188,219]

The application of new cytogenetic technologies has increased our understanding of the genetics and molecular mechanisms involved in the development of germ cell tumors. Nonrandom changes in molecular structure have commonly been reported in chromosomes 1 and 12, as well as in others.[37,88,128] For example, the chromosomal aberration of trisomy 12 has been identified in many stromal tumors.[149] An isochromosome is a chromosome in which both arms are derived from one of the two arms by breakage at the centromere and subsequent duplication. Isochromosome 12p [i(12p)] has been identified in all types of germ cell tumors,[137,172,191] including testicular germ cell tumors in men.[21,172,196] The presence of three or more copies of i(12p) has been associated with treatment failure.[88] Nonrandom endodermal sinus tumors in children involve the deletion of segments of chromosome 1p and 6q. Deletion of the terminal portion of 1p has been identified in other tumors, indicating that it may be a locus of one or more tumor suppressor genes not yet characterized. Isochromosome 12p has been identified in ovarian tumors in adolescents and adults.[12] Endodermal sinus tumors in children may show cytogenetic differences from adults with no evidence of i(12p), but with deletions involving 1p, 3q, and 6q.[153] The *c-myc* oncogene has been found in a few endodermal sinus tumors, and the current Children's Oncology Group protocol will begin to correlate amplification with survival and response to therapy.[31] Further studies are required to determine the significance of these findings. Many germ cell tumors in children express P-glycoprotein, a membrane-bound protein that can decrease the response to chemotherapy; this may explain why these tumors are frequently resistant to treatment.[221]

Imaging Techniques

Various radiographic studies play an important role in the clinical evaluation of pediatric ovarian lesions. Prenatal US can usually differentiate ovarian lesions from intestinal duplication, hydronephrosis, duodenal atresia, choledochal cyst, urachal remnants, hydrometrocolpos, and intestinal obstruction (Fig. 36-1). Mesenteric and omental cysts are more difficult to distinguish from simple ovarian cysts, because the ovary is an abdominal rather than a pelvic organ in an infant.

US is the diagnostic study of choice for the initial evaluation of potential ovarian pathology in all age groups. Adequate urinary bladder distention is mandatory to displace gas-filled intestinal loops out of the pelvis and to ensure adequate sound wave transmission through the ovaries. Ovarian volume changes with age from less than 0.7 cm^3 in girls younger than 2 years to 1.8 to 5.7 cm^3 in postpubertal patients.[197] Morphologic characteristics also change. In children younger than 8 years, the ovaries are generally solid, ovoid structures with a homogeneous echogenic texture. During and after puberty, the ultrasonographic spectrum of the gonad undergoes cystic changes that parallel ovulatory follicle activity in the organ. Ovarian cysts are generally anechoic, thin-walled masses

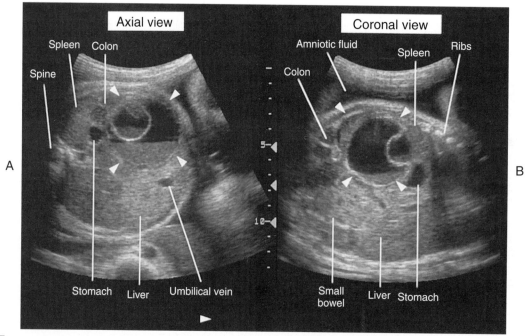

Figure 36–1 *A* and *B*, Two views of an ultrasonogram of a fetus in the third trimester. A large, complex ovarian cyst containing fluid debris, internal septation, and solid components can be seen. An ovarian neoplasm was identified during surgery after birth. (Courtesy of Gary A. Thieme, MD, Prenatal Diagnosis Center, University of Colorado School of Medicine.)

with through transmission. With torsion, fluid debris or septation may be present.[189] Most benign tumors are complex masses that are hypoechoic with peripheral echogenic mural nodules, which may exhibit acoustic shadowing. Malignant tumors are often larger than 10 cm in diameter and appear as complex soft tissue masses with ill-defined, irregular borders and central necrosis, thick septations, or papillary projections on US. Doppler color-flow imaging and transvaginal US are also valuable in postpubertal patients to determine morphologic characteristics of ovarian lesions.[22,169,215]

Computed tomography (CT) and magnetic resonance imaging (MRI) are useful when the origin of the pelvic mass cannot be established by US or when assessment of the full extent of a noncystic lesion is necessary. The characteristic finding of a benign tumor on CT is a fluid-filled mass with fat and calcifications.[99] Focal solid components arising from the tumor wall are common (Fig. 36-2). Malignant lesions are large and predominantly solid with occasional cystic areas as well as fine or coarse calcifications. Direct extension of tumors to adjacent pelvic structures or to the liver and lungs can also be demonstrated by CT, which provides more accurate staging of disease than US. Adnexal torsion in association with any tumor has a distinct appearance on CT, which is demonstrated by dynamic scanning after the administration of contrast medium. The appearance is generally characterized by lack of enhancement of mural nodules, which indicates interruption of blood flow, and demonstration of thick, engorged blood vessels that drape around the tumor and indicate markedly congested veins distal to the site of torsion.

MRI is well suited for imaging pelvic lesions because it is not influenced by extensive subcutaneous fat and offers superb soft tissue contrast resolution.[65] The technique is especially valuable in determining whether a mass is ovarian or uterine in origin, and it has a specific signal behavior and a distinct appearance that enable the detection of dermoid cysts, endometrioma, and endometrial implants.[106,194] The ability of MRI to delineate the extent of disease in endometriosis after laparoscopic biopsy may be useful for monitoring treatment response.[60] The character of cystic fluid, either simple hemorrhagic or complex, can be assessed by MRI.[65] The long imaging times required may cause peristalsis and respiratory motion to obscure peritoneal and intestinal surfaces, and sedation may be needed in small children. Ovarian torsion with hemorrhagic infarction can be detected on MRI by the finding of a high-intensity rim at the periphery of the mass on the T1-weighted image.[104]

DISEASE CLASSIFICATION AND STAGING

Ovarian lesions are generally divided into non-neoplastic and neoplastic entities; the former category includes several functioning cysts, and the latter includes benign and malignant tumors. The clinical system presented here is modified from the most recent version of the World Health Organization's proposal for the international histologic classification of diseases and its adaptation for oncology (Tables 36-4 and 36-5).[184] Non-neoplastic and neoplastic lesions may arise from surface epithelium, germ cell components, or support stroma. Neoplastic lesions are listed based on the tissue of origin.

Proper management of ovarian neoplasms requires accurate staging of the initial extent of disease. In malignant cases, recent advances in therapy have resulted in increased survival rates and preservation of fertility. Surgical staging with histologic confirmation must be done to supplement the clinical assessment of disease status. Precise staging is based on clinical examination, surgical exploration, tissue histology, and fluid cytology, as reaffirmed by the Cancer Committee of the International Federation of Gynecology and Obstetrics (FIGO) (Table 36-6).[62]

Because ovarian neoplasms are relatively uncommon, evaluation and treatment protocols developed from multi-institutional collaborative studies have been most valuable.

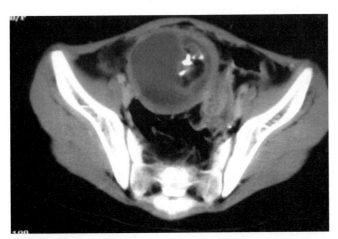

Figure 36–2 Computed tomography scan of a large, calcified abdominal mass. The mass has a large cystic component, with solid, thickened walls that are somewhat eccentric in appearance. The tumor was a thin-walled fibrous cyst with extensive hemorrhagic infarction throughout the entire cyst wall. Histology was consistent with a benign cystic teratoma.

TABLE 36–4 World Health Organization Histologic Classification of Non-neoplastic Ovarian Lesions

Solitary follicle cyst
Multiple follicle cysts (polycystic ovarian disease; sclerocystic ovaries)
Large solitary luteinized follicle cyst of pregnancy and puerperium
Hyperreactio luteinalis (multiple luteinized follicle cysts)
Corpus luteum cyst
Pregnancy luteoma
Ectopic pregnancy
Stromal hyperplasia
Stromal hyperthecosis
Massive edema
Fibromatosis
Endometriosis
Cyst, unclassified (simple cyst)
Inflammatory lesions

TABLE 36-5 World Health Organization Classification of Tumors of the Ovary

1. Surface epithelial–stromal tumors
    1.1. Serous tumors
    1.2. Mucinous tumors
    1.3. Endometrioid tumors
    1.4. Clear cell tumors
    1.5. Transitional cell tumors
    1.6. Squamous cell tumors
    1.7. Mixed epithelial tumors
    1.8. Undifferentiated and unclassified tumors
2. Sex cord–stromal tumors
    2.1. Granulosa–stromal cell tumors
        2.1.1. Granulosa cell tumor group
            2.1.1.1. Adult
            2.1.1.2. Juvenile
        2.1.2. Tumors in thecoma-fibroma group
    2.2. Sertoli–stromal cell tumors
    2.3. Sex cord–stromal tumors of mixed or unclassified cell types
        2.3.1. Sex cord tumor with annular tubules
        2.3.2. Gynandroblastoma
    2.4. Steroid cell tumors
3. Germ cell tumors
    3.1. Primitive germ cell tumors

    3.1.1. Dysgerminoma
    3.1.2. Yolk sac tumor (endodermal sinus tumor)
    3.1.3. Embryonal carcinoma
    3.1.4. Polyembryoma
    3.1.5. Nongestational choriocarcinoma
    3.1.6. Mixed germ cell tumors (specify components)
    3.2. Biphasic or triphasic teratomas
        3.2.1. Immature
        3.2.2. Mature
    3.3. Monodermal teratomas
4. Germ cell sex cord–stromal tumors
    4.1. Gonadoblastoma
    4.2. Mixed germ cell–sex cord–stromal tumor of nongonadoblastoma type
5. Tumors of rete ovarii
6. Miscellaneous tumors
    6.1. Small cell carcinomas, hypercalcemic type
    6.2. Gestational choriocarcinomas
    6.3. Soft tissue tumors not specific to ovary
7. Tumorlike conditions
8. Lymphoid and hematopoietic tumors
9. Secondary tumors

Stromal and germ cell tumors have been assessed in studies from the Children's Cancer Group (CCG), the Pediatric Oncology Group (POG), and the Gynecologic Oncology Group (GOG).[31,41,69,167] In children, the intergroup POG 9048/9049 and CCG 8882/8891 studies used a system that incorporated both surgical and pathologic findings. This concept has been preserved by the Children's Oncology Group (COG) (Table 36-7).[31]

Uniform surgical guidelines that incorporate standard approaches to these lesions have been formulated, although the approach to ovarian neoplasms has become more conservative with time.[208,209] Preoperative assessment should try to exclude obvious malignancy by the collection of serum tumor markers and carefully performed pelvic US to determine whether the ovarian mass is complex in nature.

TABLE 36-6 Staging of Carcinoma of the Ovary: International Federation of Gynecology and Obstetrics (FIGO)

Stage	Extent of Disease
	Primary tumor cannot be assessed
0	No evidence of primary tumor
I	Tumor confined to ovaries
IA	Tumor limited to one ovary, capsule intact
	No tumor on ovarian surface
	No malignant cells in ascites or peritoneal washings
IB	Tumor limited to both ovaries, capsule intact
	No tumor on ovarian surface
	No malignant cells in ascites or peritoneal washings
IC	Tumor limited to one or both ovaries, with any of the following:
	Capsule ruptured, tumor on ovarian surface, malignant cells in ascites or peritoneal washings
II	Tumor involves one or both ovaries with pelvic extension
IIA	Extension to or implants on uterus or tubes or both
	No malignant cells in ascites or peritoneal washings
IIB	Extension to other pelvic organs
	No malignant cells in ascites or peritoneal washings
IIC	IIA or IIB with positive malignant cells in ascites or peritoneal washings
III	Tumor involves one or both ovaries with microscopically confirmed peritoneal metastasis outside the pelvis or regional lymph nodes metastasis
IIIA	Microscopic peritoneal metastasis beyond the pelvis
IIIB	Macroscopic peritoneal metastasis beyond the pelvis 2 cm or less in greatest dimension
IIIC	Peritoneal metastasis beyond the pelvis more than 2 cm in greatest dimension or regional lymph nodes metastasis
IV	Distant metastasis beyond the peritoneal cavity

TABLE 36–7 Clinicopathologic Staging of Ovarian Germ Cell Tumors: Children's Oncology Group (COG)

Stage	Extent of Disease
I	Limited to ovary (peritoneal evaluation should be negative); no clinical, radiographic, or histologic evidence of disease beyond the ovaries (Note: The presence of gliomatosis peritonei does not change stage I disease to a higher stage)
II	Microscopic residual; peritoneal evaluation negative (Note: The presence of gliomatosis peritonei does not change stage II disease to a higher stage)
III	Lymph node involvement (metastatic nodule); gross residual or biopsy only; contiguous visceral involvement (omentum, intestine, bladder); peritoneal evaluation positive for malignancy
IV	Distant metastases, including liver

Elevated tumor markers and a complex mass on US strongly suggest a malignancy, and an abdominal and pelvic CT scan should be obtained. For potentially malignant lesions, an adequate abdominal incision is used, and violation of the tumor capsule is avoided. Alternatively, if tumor markers are negative and the mass is thought to be benign (e.g., a mature cystic teratoma) a laparoscopic approach can be considered (Fig. 36-3).

Initial resection in pediatric patients should virtually always be conservative. Pelvic washings, unilateral ovarian cystectomy, intraoperative frozen section, and careful visual inspection of the contralateral ovary are appropriate in the initial management of benign lesions or tumors of low malignant potential. Pelvic washings are part of the staging system for ovarian tumors and should be performed immediately on entry into the abdomen (via either laparoscopy or laparotomy) in an attempt to avoid contamination in the event of intraoperative tumor rupture. Because the final pathology will not be known until either frozen section or histologic evaluation of paraffin-embedded tissue, peritoneal washings should be performed in all patients with complex adnexal masses in case of an unsuspected malignancy. If there is no evidence of free fluid upon entering the abdomen, lactated Ringer's solution can be used to irrigate the pelvis and paracolic gutters, then aspirated and sent as washings.

Malignant germ cell and stromal tumors are almost never bilateral in early-stage disease, so unilateral salpingo-oophorectomy with a staging procedure is adequate first-line management. Excellent responses have been reported with chemotherapy, even in children with extensive tumors, and maintenance of childbearing capability is possible with this approach. In bilateral or more advanced disease, the current success of in vitro fertilization techniques has prompted the consideration of uterus-sparing procedures during the initial operation.[14,202] The expected biologic behavior of the tumor and its response to adjuvant therapy generally dictate the ultimate extent of surgery required.

The value of laparoscopic examination in the assessment of pelvic disease is well established (see Fig. 36-3). Elsheikh et al.[57] reported a series of 54 patients between 14 and 20 years of age with ovarian masses managed laparoscopically. Final pathology included mature cystic teratomas in 22 patients, 12 cases of endometriosis, 8 serous and 5 mucinous cystadenomas, 3 borderline tumors, and 3 cases of fibroma-thecoma. Héloury et al.[86] performed laparoscopy in 28 children with pathologic conditions of the adnexa. Several nonovarian lesions were detected among the 25 children who had laparoscopy for diagnostic purposes. In addition, the histologic nature of an ovarian tumor was confirmed in four children, and diagnostic aspiration was performed on nine functional cysts. Pelvic adhesions prevented successful laparoscopy in one case, and one postoperative complication necessitated secondary laparotomy.

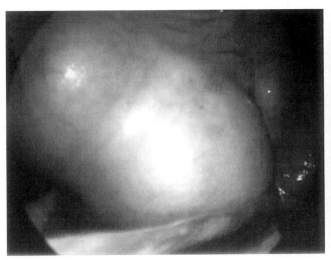
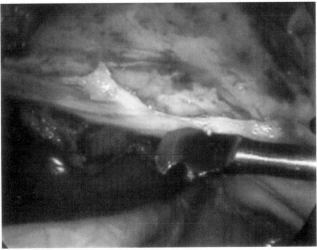

A   B

Figure 36–3 *A,* Laparoscopic view of an abdominal mass, originally palpated during a routine well-child examination. Workup included a computed tomography scan of the abdomen and pelvis, which disclosed a large cystic mass in the left ovary. *B,* The Harmonic Scalpel was used to make an incision over the central aspect or waist of the mass, enabling cyst dissection. The ovary was preserved.

The American Association of Gynecologic Laparoscopists reviewed more than 13,000 procedures performed for persistent ovarian masses.[93] Stage I ovarian cancer was detected in 0.4% of cases. Although these results are encouraging in adult women, there is concern about the difficulty of establishing the true nature of an ovarian tumor by gross examination in children, because experience with such an evaluation is so infrequent. Nevertheless, techniques are being established to avoid tumor spillage that may expand the use of this method. In addition, experienced surgeons are beginning to perform more extensive staging procedures and lymph node dissections using the laparoscope.[87]

TREATMENT

Non-neoplastic Ovarian Tumors

Ovarian cysts are known to arise from mature follicles. Autopsy studies of prepubertal girls have documented active follicular growth at all ages and normal oocytes, granulosa cells, and cysts in various stages of involution.[155,156] By convention, physiologic follicles are differentiated from pathologic ovarian cysts on the basis of size: any lesion larger than 2 cm in diameter is no longer considered a mature follicle.

Non-neoplastic cysts are benign and generally asymptomatic, although they represent approximately 35% of all surgically treated ovarian lesions in children and adolescents.[24] Although surgical intervention is rarely indicated, these lesions occasionally have clinical manifestations, based on size or associated functional activity, that warrant differentiation from true ovarian neoplasms. When an operation is necessary, a conservative approach should be undertaken. In most cases, it is possible to remove the cyst and preserve the adjacent normal ovarian tissue.

Follicular Cysts

Follicular cysts represent about 50% of the non-neoplastic ovarian lesions.[24] They are unilateral, unilocular, and histologically benign and often have a thin, yellowish, clear liquid content. These lesions are now known to be quite common in neonates and infants. Cohen et al.[35] detected cysts in 84% of all imaged ovaries in 77 patients from birth to 24 months of age. The prevalence was similar in each 3-month age bracket. Parallel findings were noted in premenarchal girls between 2 and 12 years of age.[34] Cysts were detected in 68% of patients; again, a generally equal distribution was noted across the age spectrum. The presence of cysts in the premenarchal ovary of an otherwise healthy child does not necessarily suggest endocrinologic or other disease. Occasionally, ovarian cysts persist and enlarge and are capable of secreting estrogen, thereby leading to precocious isosexual development.[118]

The size of an ovarian lesion has been a major factor in determining clinical management. Millar et al.[127] found 17 cysts larger than 2 cm in diameter in 99 prepubertal girls during a 5-year period. Seven were treated by observation alone, without adverse outcome. Benign follicular or luteinized cysts were excised in the other 10 girls;

two of these cysts (5 and 10 cm in diameter) had undergone adnexal torsion and left no identifiable ovarian tissue. In a series of 28 patients with early sexual development, 12 had isolated premature thelarche, 4 presented with vaginal bleeding, and 7 had true central precocious puberty. In these groups, no ovarian cysts were larger than 2 cm in diameter.[63] Girls with premature thelarche often had detectable ovarian microcysts. The remaining five patients with precocious pseudopuberty had larger ovarian cysts. Although two lesions regressed spontaneously, three others required surgical excision of luteinized follicular cysts.

Ovarian cysts have been recognized prenatally with some frequency with the increased use of maternal US.[23] The precise cause of fetal ovarian cysts remains unclear, but they may be due to either production of fetal follicle-stimulating hormone, maternal estrogen, or placental chorionic gonadotropin or stimulation of an immature hypothalamus-pituitary-ovarian axis. A postnatal decrease in hormonal stimulation often leads to a self-limited process.

Ovarian cysts noted in the prenatal and perinatal periods can be expected to spontaneously regress during the first year of life, and in utero therapy is not justified.[85,125] Cesarean section should be performed for obstetric indications only, even when a large cyst is suspected.[85,171] These lesions may occasionally be complicated by torsion, intestinal obstruction, or perforation and cyst rupture.[23,178] Bagolan et al.[15] and Giorlandino et al.[70] confirmed that patients with echogenic cysts with fluid debris, retracting clot, or septation should undergo surgical intervention because such findings were associated with torsion and hemorrhage.[195] In this age group, torsion is often a prenatal event, and viable ovarian tissue may not be identified, even with the most expeditious neonatal surgical intervention (Fig. 36-4).[6,23] Cysts that develop in utero are most often lined by luteinized cells, whereas those in older children are more often lined by granulosa cells.[154]

Most authors now advocate increasingly conservative measures for neonatal ovarian lesions. Small, asymptomatic

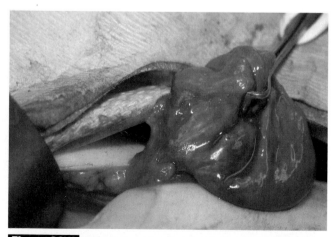

Figure 36-4 This newborn female infant had a prenatal diagnosis of an intra-abdominal cystic mass. Postnatal imaging showed a low-attenuation cystic structure with a curvilinear calcification along one wall. Laparotomy disclosed a torsed ovarian cyst and ovary, attached by only a small residual stalk. The fallopian tube was preserved. Pathology showed a thin-walled cyst containing dystrophic calcifications.

cysts are generally observed for regression with serial US. Cysts 5 cm in diameter or larger and those with a long adnexal pedicle are more likely to undergo torsion and should be excised with ovarian preservation[23] or aspirated.[6,129,171] US-guided cyst aspiration is associated with minimal recurrence and few complications.[43,52] Smaller simple cysts should be observed unless they become symptomatic, recur, or fail to regress after several months of observation.[30]

In prepubertal children, the occurrence of acute symptoms and endocrine activity are more problematic. Warner et al.[218] described the outcome of 92 patients with large ovarian cysts. Ninety percent of the cysts clinically regressed or completely resolved. Acute, severe abdominal pain was the indication for operative intervention in 17 of the 23 surgically treated patients. Cyst size and US characteristics did not accurately predict outcome. Laparotomy was recommended if symptoms did not resolve within 24 hours, a large mass was associated with intra-abdominal complications, or there was evidence of a neoplasm on imaging studies. Surgical intervention was also recommended for any cyst that increased in size or failed to regress on follow-up US.

As many as 75% of girls with juvenile hypothyroidism have multicystic ovaries and may show varying degrees of sexual precocity and galactorrhea due to increased secretion of pituitary gonadotropins and prolactin.[154] Multiple follicular cysts should also be distinguished from polycystic ovary syndrome, which is the most common cause of delayed puberty and heavy anovulatory bleeding in adolescent females.[170]

In one randomized study of postmenarchal patients, cysts 5 cm in diameter or larger and those with a complex appearance on imaging studies were followed for a short time with serial pelvic US. High regression rates were seen with those followed expectantly.[192] Exploratory laparotomy or laparoscopy was recommended for patients with cysts that had not resolved or had increased in size within 2 to 3 months[192] and for cysts associated with acute or severe chronic abdominal pain or intra-abdominal complications.

In non-neoplastic ovarian cysts, surgical preservation of as much normal ovarian tissue as possible is a high priority. A plane of dissection can usually be established between the normal gonadal tissue and the cyst after injecting saline with a fine-bore needle beneath the visceral peritoneum. If the surgical manipulation necessary to completely remove the lesion would threaten significant viable ovarian tissue, the cyst should be unroofed and debulked, and the cyst wall excised to the extent possible, while protecting the ovary. Unilateral oophorectomy is indicated only if there is a reasonable certainty that no viable gonadal tissue can be salvaged. The ipsilateral fallopian tube should be spared because fertilization is still possible from the contralateral normal ovary.

Corpus Luteum Cysts

True functioning corpus luteum cysts develop only in adolescents who are actively ovulating. Although these cysts may be bilateral and become quite large, they usually regress spontaneously with the cyclic decline in serum progesterone. The gross appearance of the external surface is often bright yellow, although it may take on a hemorrhagic appearance when filled with bloody fluid. The cyst lining is composed of luteinized granulosa and theca cells and is capable of actively producing estrogen and progesterone. These cysts may cause acute pelvic pain if they rupture or undergo torsion. Failure of the corpus luteum to involute may cause menstrual irregularity and dysfunctional uterine bleeding.

Surgical goals for corpus luteum cysts parallel those for other follicular lesions. Surgical intervention is indicated in the presence of cyst accident or persistence, demonstrated by repeat pelvic US performed 4 to 6 weeks after the initial assessment. Hasson[83] was able to treat 17 of 19 patients who had corpus luteum cysts with laparoscopic aspiration, fenestration, or cyst wall excision. Clinical symptoms resolved in all but one patient. Cyst recurrence was rare.

Parovarian Cysts

Parovarian cysts are usually small and rarely symptomatic. They do not arise from ovarian tissue but are usually considered with this group of lesions because of their proximity to the gonad. These cysts originate from the epoophoron and are located in the leaves of the mesosalpinx. Parovarian cysts cannot be distinguished from ovarian follicular cysts using any radiographic imaging technique. During an operation, their gross features are virtually identical to those of follicular lesions, but they can usually be accurately identified because of their anatomic position. When surgical treatment is required, both standard open and minimally invasive techniques have been used.[83,179] Large parovarian cysts (>3 cm) should be completely enucleated from the mesosalpinx in such a way that the fallopian tube and ovary are not damaged.[42] Those less than 3 cm may be treated with puncture and bipolar coagulation of the cyst wall.[42]

Endometriosis

Endometriosis is a disorder in which the endometrial glands and stroma are implanted on the peritoneal surfaces of extrauterine sites. The proposed mechanisms for the pathogenesis of this disease include menstrual flow obstruction with retrograde menstruation, mechanical transplantation and implantation of endometrial elements, and coelomic metaplasia.[81,105,144] The interval between the onset of menarche and the diagnosis of endometriosis may be as short as 1 month, and the incidence of disease in teenage girls may be far higher than previously anticipated or described.[165] Extensive disease is uncommon in young adolescents unless it is associated with an obstructive müllerian anomaly.[173]

The incidence of endometriosis reportedly ranges from 1% in younger girls to 47% in older girls.[73,89,124] Typical symptoms include a pattern of chronic cyclic or acyclic pelvic pain and dysmenorrhea.[13] Early diagnosis is critical so that treatment can preclude the development of extensive intraperitoneal inflammation, as indicated by extensive adhesions and endometriomas. Early lesions on the peritoneal surfaces appear as small petechiae that penetrate the surface less than 1 mm. More recently it has been recognized that endometriosis may have an atypical appearance, including vesicular lesions, white plaques, powder burns, and adhesions.[216]

The revised American Fertility Society classification of endometriosis is widely accepted as the staging system for the disease and was developed as a prognostic tool for patients with infertility.[7] However, the four stages do not correlate with pain symptoms; rather, they are associated with depth of disease.[108] For patients with pelvic pain and a suspected diagnosis of endometriosis, medical therapy with nonsteroidal anti-inflammatory drugs or oral contraceptives should be considered. Both medications act to suppress prostaglandins, which are known to be important in the pathophysiology of dysmenorrhea. These drugs along with gonadotropin hormone antagonists, used for a 6-month period, are the most commonly used medications.

Currently, laparoscopy with biopsy of any suspicious lesions is the accepted diagnostic procedure, although endometriomas are well visualized on US. A histologic diagnosis of endometriosis may be important, because minimal disease at a younger age has been shown in some cases to progress to more extensive disease with age.[109] If the surgeon is experienced with the management of endometriosis ablation, excision of all visible lesions is superior to placebo in the management of pelvic pain in patients with endometriosis.[198]

Simple Cysts

Most authors consider simple cysts to be follicular in origin. Anatomically, they are generally small, unilocular, thin walled, and similar to follicular lesions. They are always histologically benign and hormonally inactive. Large symptomatic lesions should be managed in a manner similar to that of follicular cysts. Laparoscopic inspection with fine-needle aspiration, fenestration, and biopsy with or without cyst lining excision was evaluated in 1990.[83] Only 1 of 56 functional simple or parovarian cysts recurred after laparoscopic management.

Neoplastic Ovarian Tumors

Most neoplastic ovarian tumors develop from cell lines derived from one of three sources: the germinal epithelium covering the urogenital ridge, the underlying stromal elements of the urogenital ridge, or the germ cells that arise from the yolk sac. Cells from each of these lineages may develop into an ovarian neoplasm by dedifferentiation, proliferation, and eventually malignant transformation.[190] Malignant ovarian tumors probably arise from their benign counterparts as a consequence of either direct or indirect hormonal stimulation. Histologically and biologically intermediate forms between benign and malignant epithelial lesions have been identified and designate tumors of low malignant potential.

Age influences the relative frequency of the various types of ovarian neoplasms. In adults, most tumors are derived from the epithelial line, and adenocarcinomas predominate. In children, germ cell tumors are most common and represent approximately 60% of cases.[47,190] Epithelial lesions account for only about 15% of tumors in the younger age group (Table 36-8).[36,47] Although germ cell tumors predominate in each age group, the peak incidence of sex cord–stromal tumors occurs in the first 4 years of life, and epithelial tumors are more common in older

TABLE 36-8 Age Distribution (%) of Various Types of Ovarian Tumors

Histologic Type	0-4 Yr	5-9 Yr	10-14 Yr	15-19 Yr	All Ages
Germ cell	48	59	68	47	62.2
Sex cord–stromal	40	17	5	12	9.7
Common epithelial	6	4	13	34	19.3
Miscellaneous	6	20	14	6	8.7

From Deprest J, Moerman P, Corneillie P, et al: Ovarian borderline mucinous tumor in a premenarchal girl: Review on ovarian epithelial cancer in young girls. Gynecol Oncol 1992;45:219.

teenagers. Neoplasms that are rare in children include endometrioid and clear cell tumors, which are usually malignant; Brenner tumors, which are usually benign; disseminated malignant lymphoma; and metastatic lesions to the ovary.

Surface Epithelial-Stromal Tumors

Epithelial tumors account for 70% of all ovarian neoplasms, but they are not common in children. In one recent series, they accounted for only 16% of all surgically resected ovarian masses.[134] Norris and Jensen[142] reported that 67 of 353 ovarian tumors (19%) in children were epithelial in origin, and 12% were malignant. The tumors are usually serous or mucinous.[112] Twenty percent of serous tumors are bilateral, and very few are malignant.[112,132] Mucinous tumors are usually unilateral, and 10% are malignant.[112] Deprest et al.[47] calculated a 16% malignancy rate for ovarian epithelial neoplasms derived from a collected series that reported more than 1700 pediatric patients with various types of ovarian tumors. Ovarian carcinoma is different in children than in adults. The proportion of mucinous tumors was 40% in children, compared with 12% in adults; in children, 30% were of borderline malignant potential, compared with the adult rate of less than 10% for these more favorable lesions.

Serum CA-125 is a useful tumor marker in malignant epithelial ovarian tumors. However, in premenopausal patients, CA-125 may also be raised in several benign gynecologic conditions, including endometriosis, pelvic inflammatory disease, fibroids, and pregnancy. Immunoscintigraphy, currently used in the research setting, may be useful in the future as a supplement to conventional diagnostic methods. This technique, which localizes CA-125 using a monoclonal antibody,[151] may also prove useful for localizing active disease after chemotherapy and monitoring for the presence of recurrent disease.[101]

Epithelial tumors are staged using the FIGO system.[62] Stage IA tumors may be treated with unilateral salpingo-oophorectomy. The opposite ovary should be examined externally and a biopsy taken of any surface abnormalities. Most young patients with stage IB tumors (tumors limited to both ovaries) may be adequately treated by bilateral gonadectomy; however, the uterus should be preserved to allow future in vitro fertilization.[14,146] In ovarian cancer of a more advanced stage, maximum cytoreduction is important and has been associated with an improved outcome.[217] Total abdominal hysterectomy and bilateral salpingo-oophorectomy are usually appropriate. Omentectomy and resection of as much gross intraperitoneal disease as possible should be accomplished. Adjuvant chemotherapy after appropriate surgical excision has been beneficial in cases of advanced ovarian carcinoma. Six cycles of carboplatin and cyclophosphamide has yielded 60% to 70% clinical response rates, with 5-year survival rates of 10% to 20%.[146] More recent trials using combined cisplatin and paclitaxel are promising. Radiation therapy, second-look surgery, and secondary cytoreduction may be useful in cases of advanced cancer, but their current role remains controversial.

Miscellaneous Tumors

Small cell carcinoma of the ovary is an extremely rare condition, with a very poor prognosis.[61] These tumors are very aggressive and are the most common undifferentiated ovarian carcinoma in young patients. They have been encountered in patients aged 9 to 44 years, with a mean age of 23 years.[163,183] Paraendocrine hypercalcemia occurs in two thirds of cases, but patients rarely have clinical manifestations of this abnormality. Serum parathormone levels are normal. Virtually all tumors are unilateral, although only 40% have been detected at stage IA. The gross appearance of the tumor is a fleshy white to pale tan color; extensive areas of hemorrhage or necrosis are common. Small cell carcinomas have an uncertain histogenesis, and electron microscopy is often needed to make the final diagnosis. Only one third of patients with stage IA tumors survive long term, and survival of patients with more widespread disease is rare.[112] Unilateral salpingo-oophorectomy has been associated with long-term survival in some patients with stage IA tumors. Metachronous appearance of tumor in a contralateral conserved ovary has been encountered, and bilateral adnexectomy may be a more appropriate surgical option. Despite various treatment modalities, including resection, radiation therapy, and intensive chemotherapy, the average life expectancy remains low, at 18 months.[163]

Tumors of Low Malignant Potential

Ovarian epithelial tumors of low malignant potential differ from epithelial cancer in two major ways: they occur in younger patients, and they have a better prognosis than ovarian cancer. They have been described for all subtypes of ovarian cancer.[47] The serous and mucinous tumors are by far the most common and resemble their benign counterparts. These borderline tumors are differentiated from standard adenocarcinoma in that they lack stromal invasion by neoplastic epithelial elements (Fig. 36-5). Up to

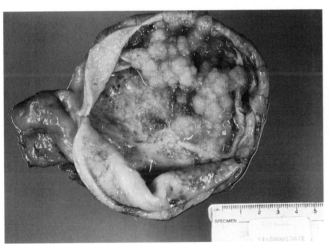

A

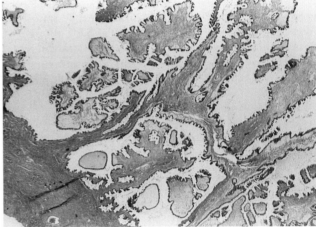

B

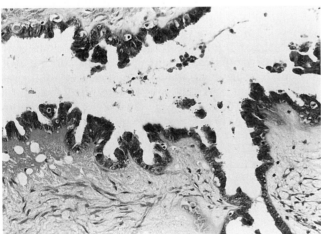

C

Figure 36–5 *A,* Ovarian tumor from a 17-year-old girl with massive bilateral ovarian lesions. The opened specimen shows a cavity filled with clear fluid, and the wall is lined by numerous nodules and papillary protuberances. *B,* Histologic section of the lesion shows serous papillary tumor of low malignant potential (hematoxylin-eosin stain, ×40). *C,* Higher-power photomicrograph of a section of the lesion shows that the papillae are fibrovascular cores lined by stratified epithelial cells without stromal invasion (hematoxylin-eosin stain, ×400).

50% of these tumors are bilateral, and they demonstrate a characteristic indolent clinical course. However, recurrences may occur as long as 10 to 15 years after surgery for the primary tumor, and they may take the form of invasive cancer.[38]

In a recent adult series, long-term survival among women with mucinous and serous borderline tumors was compared. Overall 10-year survival for women with serous ovarian borderline tumors and carcinomas was 96% and 30.4%, respectively. For patients with mucinous borderline tumors and carcinomas, it was 94% and 64%, respectively.[187] In adults, 91% of borderline mucinous tumors present as stage I disease, with a 5-year survival rate of 98%. Serous tumors have a similar outcome. The extensive review by Massad et al.[122] noted an overall survival of 98% for stage I tumors, 94% for stage II, and 79% for stages III and IV. In children, Morris et al.[135] noted that 75% of the patients presented with stage I disease, and overall survival was 100%. The combined 10-year survival rate for all stages was 73%.

Surgery is the primary method of therapy. Unilateral salpingo-oophorectomy is adequate for all low-stage tumors and has been standard treatment; however, recent studies have shown that ovarian cystectomy can be performed in young patients with careful follow-up.[133] These patients require close surveillance, with pelvic examinations, CA-125 serum samples, and US every 3 to 6 months, because patients managed with ovarian cystectomy have a higher risk of recurrence than those managed more aggressively.[239] Morice et al.[133] reported recurrence rates of 36.3%, 15.1%, and 5.7% after cystectomy, oophorectomy, and hysterectomy with bilateral oophorectomy, respectively. Despite the difference in recurrence risk, there was no demonstrated impact on overall survival; all patients were salvaged with further surgery. Conservative treatment should therefore be considered in young patients who wish to preserve their fertility and will comply with follow-up. Routine contralateral wedge biopsy is unnecessary[132] if the ovary appears normal on US.[16]

Bilateral tumors require bilateral oophorocystectomy or salpingo-oophorectomy. Uterus-sparing procedures are probably not appropriate for advanced-stage disease. The pathologic features that identify poor prognosis are still being elucidated,[38] and currently there are no clear candidates. At present, surgery remains the most effective therapy for these patients; the place of adjuvant therapy has yet to be established.[16,113] No individual treatment strategy has led to consistently superior outcomes, but the favorable biology of this tumor minimizes the importance of the limited clinical benefit achieved from adjuvant therapy.

Sex Cord–Stromal Tumors

Sex cord–stromal tumors probably arise from uncommitted mesenchymal stem cells that reside below the surface epithelium of the urogenital ridge.[164] This totipotential tissue may differentiate into several different cell lines, including granulosa-theca cells in the ovary and Leydig-Sertoli cells in the testicular interstitium. Sex cord–stromal tumors are referred to as functioning ovarian tumors because they result in systemic hormonal effects. They account for 13% of ovarian tumors encountered in the Boston Children's Hospital series[112] and 17% in another series of ovarian neoplasms in children.[190] Before 9 years of age, most sex cord–stromal tumors are feminizing; after 9 years of age, there is a predominance of virilizing neoplasms.[154]

Granulosa-Theca Cell Tumors

Granulosa-theca cell tumors are the most common type of sex cord–stromal neoplasms and the most common type of functioning ovarian neoplasm. The juvenile granulosa cell tumor is a specific subclassification of these lesions; 44% occur in the first decade of life, and 97% are seen by 30 years of age.[162] Isosexual pseudoprecocious puberty is the presenting sign in the majority of premenarchal girls who have this tumor (Fig. 36-6).[164] Most patients have elevated serum and urinary estrogen levels, whereas gonadotropin levels are low. This profile assists in differentiating children with these tumors from others with true sexual precocity, gonadotropin-secreting lesions, or feminizing adrenal tumors. Levels of serum inhibin, a glycoprotein produced by ovarian granulosa cells, may be a useful tumor marker.[114,140] Müllerian-inhibiting substance levels are elevated in some granulosa-theca cell tumors, which suggests a potential role as a prognostic marker.[80]

Clinical findings include premature thelarche, vaginal discharge or bleeding, labial enlargement, development of pubic or axillary hair, increased somatic growth, and advanced bone age. Clitoral enlargement is a rare manifestation of virilization and tumor androgen production. Postpubertal girls may present with an abdominal mass, relatively nonspecific symptoms of abdominal pain, or increased girth. Tumor rupture with hemoperitoneum, although rare, is a dramatic event that necessitates surgery. Amenorrhea and other menstrual irregularities may occur. Clinical emergencies can occur in young infants who have a rapid onset of pleural effusion and ascites that causes severe abdominal distention and respiratory distress.[95]

In addition to differences in clinical presentation, juvenile granulosa cell tumors demonstrate a pattern of histologic features and biologic behavior that are distinct from the adult counterpart. The juvenile variety is usually a relatively large lesion that averages 12.5 cm in diameter.[234] At laparotomy, it appears as a yellow-tan or gray solid neoplasm with cystic areas that often contain hemorrhagic fluid. In contrast to adult-type tumors, the juvenile type has abundant eosinophilic or luteinized cytoplasm, with atypical nuclei and a higher mitotic rate. DNA content and cell-cycle kinetics analyzed by flow cytometry do not necessarily correlate with the prognosis in children, as they often do in adults.[199]

Although the adult form is generally an indolent, slow-growing lesion of relatively low malignant potential, the biologic behavior of the juvenile tumor is more aggressive and correlates well with tumor size, disease stage, presence of rupture, and degree of nuclear atypia and mitotic activity. The lesion was unilateral in 122 of 125 cases reviewed by Young et al.[236] If the adult tumor recurs, it is usually more than 5 years after diagnosis. Malignant granulosa

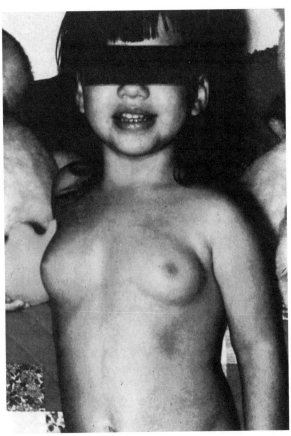

A

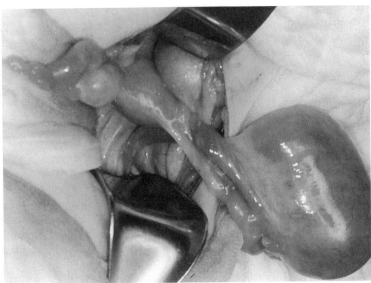

B

Figure 36-6 *A,* Three-year-old girl demonstrating isosexual pseudoprecocious puberty. *B,* Surgery revealed a benign juvenile granulosa cell tumor. Unilateral salpingo-oophorectomy was performed to remove the tumor.

cell tumors in young patients tend to recur much more quickly.

Granulosa cell tumors are staged similarly to other ovarian lesions (see Table 36-6). In children, these tumors are associated with a favorable prognosis because more than 90% of patients present with stage I disease. Overall survival is approximately 95% for stage IA patients and 80% for stage IC patients. Virtually all patients with stage II or greater disease die regardless of treatment. Plantaz et al.[159] analyzed a series of 39 juvenile granulosa cell tumors from several centers in France. Patients' median age was 6 years; 52% developed precocious pseudopuberty, and 10% had endocrine dysfunction after puberty. Tumor rupture caused a surgical emergency in three cases. Four of the five deaths within 6 months were in girls with stage III or IV disease.

Because of the low rate of bilateral occurrence and the favorable prognosis of stage I tumors, unilateral oophorectomy or salpingo-oophorectomy is adequate initial therapy when preservation of fertility is desired. Because of the poor prognosis for children with advanced-stage disease, aggressive multidisciplinary therapy is indicated, although the benefits remain unclear. Hysterectomy with bilateral salpingo-oophorectomy and 3000 cGy whole-abdominal radiation, with a boost to areas of residual disease, have been used in girls with stage III tumors that ruptured or had macroscopic tumor extension.[159] Multiple-drug chemotherapy, including methotrexate, actinomycin D, cyclophosphamide,

bleomycin, and the vinca alkaloids, has been used with some response. However, most patients subsequently relapsed and died. Currently, specific chemotherapeutic regimens must be considered investigational in those few patients with advanced malignant disease.

Fibromas and Thecomas

Fibromas and thecomas account for 14% of sex cord–stromal tumors in pediatric patients.[112] Although they are extremely uncommon in females younger than 20 years, fibromas are usually associated with the basal cell nevus syndrome and are frequently bilateral, multicentric, and calcified. Most ovarian thecomas occur in menopausal women; however, two variants of this lesion have been reported in the second decade of life. Calcified thecomas invariably cause amenorrhea or other menstrual irregularities and hirsutism.[235] If these tumors contain a substantial number of lutein cells, they are appropriately called luteinized thecomas, which can occur in younger girls and may be associated with androgenic manifestations.

On gross examination, fibromas are firm, solid masses with a whorled, trabeculated appearance on cross section. The lipid content of thecomas results in a pale yellow to orange color. These lesions are benign, and unilateral oophorectomy is adequate treatment. In the case of bilateral fibromas, all gross tumor tissue should be removed, with particular attention to sparing normal-appearing ovarian tissue.[90] Tumor recurrence is rare and is managed by reoperation. Virilizing symptoms usually resolve after resection of the tumor.

Sclerosing Stromal Tumors

Sclerosing stromal tumors have recently been recognized as entities distinct from fibromas and thecomas. These tumors occur in girls, with 30% of documented cases presenting in the first 2 decades of life. Estrogen secretion has occasionally been reported, whereas androgen manifestations are quite rare. The typical presentation includes the presence of a pelvic mass and pelvic pain in a young patient with a history of menstrual irregularity. This lesion has also been associated with the Chédiak-Higashi syndrome.[97]

Sclerosing stromal tumors are unilateral, usually larger than 5 cm in diameter, and benign. At laparotomy, these tumors are well-circumscribed, firm, whitish yellow masses with clearly demarcated areas of edema and cyst formation. Histologically, the tumor is characterized by a pseudolobulated pattern, with cellular foci clearly demarcated from the edematous and collagenized areas.[91] Gross tumor removal is generally adequate treatment.

Sertoli-Leydig Cell Tumors

Sertoli-Leydig cell tumors account for less than 0.5% of all ovarian tumors but constitute between 10% and 30% of the sex cord–stromal neoplasms.[112] Although most of these tumors are masculinizing, some are nonfunctional or even associated with estrogenic effects. Therefore, the older terms *arrhenoblastoma* and *androblastoma* are no longer favored. One third of cases occur in patients younger than 20 years. These tumors are almost always unilateral and present as stage IA at diagnosis. Survival is excellent, with tumor-related deaths in only 5% of affected individuals.[154] Similar to granulosa cell tumors, the gross appearance of Sertoli-Leydig cell tumors varies widely, but these lesions are less often filled with hemorrhagic fluid and rarely have a unilocular, thin-walled, cystic appearance.

Current classifications now recognize five histologic patterns based on the degree of differentiation and the presence of heterologous, endodermal, or mesenchymal elements. Tumor stage and histologic appearance are important prognostic factors. Sertoli-Leydig cell tumors with heterologous elements are more common in younger patients and may be difficult to distinguish from immature teratomas.[154] There are two phases of the masculinizing effects of androgen overproduction. Initially, defeminization takes place with amenorrhea, breast atrophy, and loss of female body habitus. This may be followed or overlapped by masculinization characterized by hirsutism, clitoral hypertrophy, and voice deepening. In prepubertal girls, masculinization and accelerated somatic growth predominate. Postpubertal girls usually have menstrual irregularities, acne, body habitus masculinization, and hirsutism. The virilizing effects are caused by testosterone accumulation resulting from a deficiency in catabolizing enzymes. Gonadotropin levels are low, and excretion of urinary 17-ketosteroid and pregnanetriol is normal. Because the testosterone level is often directly related to tumor tissue

volume, this hormone is a biologic marker for monitoring disease behavior.[49] Tumor markers most likely to be elevated are AFP and CA-125.[115] LDH may be elevated or normal. The hormonal profile of these lesions assists in differentiating them from exogenous androgen sources, adrenal tumors, true hermaphroditism, and polycystic ovaries. Similar to granulosa cell tumors, the Sertoli-Leydig cell lesions may be associated with multiple enchondromas caused by nonhereditary mesodermal dysplasia (Ollier's disease).[223]

Surgical therapy should be conservative for patients with low-stage disease. Unilateral oophorectomy or adnexectomy is adequate and preserves later childbearing capacity. If tumors are bilateral, are poorly differentiated, have ruptured, or demonstrate aggressive behavior, a more aggressive approach similar to that used for granulosa cell tumors is necessary.[50] Gershenson et al.[67] looked at the response of these tumors when treated with surgery and chemotherapy if poor prognostic indicators were present at initial diagnosis. Following completion of four cycles of bleomycin-etoposide-cisplatin chemotherapy, 50% of patients remained disease free at 28 months, with an overall response rate of 83%. Limited data are available regarding preserved ovarian function following chemotherapy. Oral contraceptives and gonadotropin-releasing hormone agonists may provide some ovarian protection both during and after chemotherapy.[28]

Sex Cord Tumors with Annular Tubules

Sex cord tumors with annular tubules are rare but distinct variants of sex cord–stromal tumors. They have the potential for bidirectional differentiation into granulosa or Sertoli cells.[112] These lesions are observed in patients with Peutz-Jeghers syndrome. When associated with this syndrome, the lesions are small, multifocal, and usually bilateral. The tumors are often calcified and are invariably noted incidentally during autopsy or in an ovary removed for reasons unrelated to neoplasia. Although patients with these tumors occasionally have menstrual irregularities suggesting hyperestrinism, surgical therapy is rarely indicated.

When these tumors occur in the absence of Peutz-Jeghers syndrome, the clinical difference is significant. Such lesions occur in older patients with a mean age of 34 years, although cases have been reported in patients from 6 to 76 years old. In younger patients, the tumor is unilateral and almost always larger than 5 cm in diameter; 20% are malignant. Even with aggressive therapy, 50% of patients with these tumors die.[234]

Steroid Cell Tumors

Steroid cell tumor is now the preferred name for lesions previously called lipid cell tumors. This term is more appropriate because of the morphologic features of the tumor and its propensity to secrete steroid hormones, and because many such lesions contain little or no lipids. The group is subclassified into three major categories according to the cells of origin: (1) Stromal luteoma is a small steroid cell tumor contained in the ovary arising from the stromal lutein cell. (2) Leydig cell tumor contains the classic intracytoplasmic Reinke's crystals and arises from histologically similar precursor cells found in the ovarian hilus. (3) Steroid cell tumors not otherwise specified account for approximately 60% of cases and typically occur in younger patients.

The first and second categories of lesion are usually encountered in postmenopausal women and are only rarely reported in patients in the first 3 decades of life. Most cases in the third category and in prepubertal children have been associated with androgenic, heterosexual pseudoprecocity.[82] The tumors are rarely estrogenic, but isosexual pseudoprecocious puberty has been reported.[45] The androgenic tumors show elevated testosterone and androstenedione levels, increased urinary 17-ketosteroid excretion, and decreased gonadotropin levels.

These lesions are well-demarcated, solid masses with a bright yellow to brownish appearance on gross examination; fossae of hemorrhage and necrosis may occasionally be observed. In older patients, malignant steroid cell tumors not otherwise specified may occur in 25% of patients and require aggressive surgery because adjuvant therapy is not effective.[84] In children, these lesions are virtually always benign and at a low stage. Unilateral salpingo-oophorectomy is adequate treatment, but close follow-up is essential. Most of the hormonal symptoms should progressively resolve after tumor removal, although younger children may develop true precocious puberty after tumor removal because chronic androgen exposure appears to induce an early maturation of the hypothalamus.[182]

Germ Cell Tumors

The path of descent of the primordial germ cells is imperfect; as a result, some of the cells occasionally miss their destination and can be deposited anywhere along this migration route. Germ cells have been found in the pineal area of the brain, mediastinum, retroperitoneum, sacrococcygeal area, and ovary and testis. If malignant transformation occurs at any of these sites, a gonadal or extragonadal neoplasm will develop. Because these nests of cells are totipotential in nature, a wide variety of tumors is seen. The specific type of tumor depends on the degree of differentiation that has occurred; this has been characterized by Telium.[205] If no differentiation occurs, a germinoma develops; with differentiation, embryonal carcinomas occur; and with extraembryonic differentiation, choriocarcinomas or endodermal sinus tumors develop. If embryonal differentiation occurs, the teratoma—the most mature of these tumor types—is seen.

Germ cell tumors are rare in children and adolescents, but when they occur, the gonad is the most frequent site. A summary of 13 reviews encompassing 1491 cases of benign and malignant germ cell tumors in children noted that 41% were gonadal in location,[2] and 71% of these were ovarian. Epithelial and stromal ovarian tumors prevail in adults; germ cell tumors predominate in children. Several large series of ovarian neoplasms report an incidence of germ cell tumors ranging from 48% to 62%.[92,96,142] This group of tumors develops from the same totipotential primordial germ cell, but each neoplasm has different behavioral characteristics, which are presented individually here; later they are discussed as a group with regard to overall management decisions.

Germinoma

The term *germinoma* encompasses a group of tumors with common histologic characteristics. It is the primary malignant tumor found in dysgenetic gonads. This tumor may be referred to as a seminoma if found in the testis, a dysgerminoma in the ovary, and a germinoma in an extragonadal site. Germinomas are believed to arise from the totipotential germ cells that were present at the undifferentiated stage of gonadal development.[220] Germinomas represent the most frequent ovarian malignant neoplasm seen in both children and adults.[154] They account for approximately 10% of all benign and malignant ovarian tumors.[44]

Germinomas are most often seen in prepubertal girls and young women, with 44% of cases occurring before 20 years of age and 87% by 30 years.[9] The typical patient is genotypically and phenotypically normal. These often bulky tumors may reach massive proportions and lead to abdominal pain and symptoms of pelvic pressure or symptoms related to obstruction of the gastrointestinal or urinary tract. Occasionally, girls with these tumors present with an acute abdomen as a result of torsion, rupture, or hemorrhage into the tumor (Fig. 36-7).[25] Ascites may be present. Because germinomas are endocrinologically inert, the presence of remote endocrine effects suggests that the tumor is a mixed germ cell tumor. In true germ cell tumors, LDH is elevated in 95% of patients, but other markers are negative.[102] In the mixed form of these tumors, markers may be positive or negative, depending on which germ cell component is present.

On gross examination, these tumors appear bulky, encapsulated, solid, and yellowish in color (see Fig. 36-7); they can be bilateral in 5% to 30% of cases.[25,46,220] Germinomas have a rather uniform microscopic appearance consisting of large, round cells that have vesicular nuclei and clear to eosinophilic cytoplasm. These cells resemble primordial germ cells. Lymphoid infiltrates may be present.

The management of germ cell tumors begins with surgical excision. Conservative surgery with a unilateral salpingo-oophorectomy, thorough inspection of the contralateral ovary with biopsy of suspicious lesions, and careful staging (as outlined in the section on surgical approach) is mandatory. Surgery alone is adequate for stage IA disease, although the older literature disputed this.[75] These tumors are very radiosensitive, but the cost of cure may be too high if fertility is compromised.[66] In children, other long-term effects such as growth abnormalities or secondary tumors must also be considered. Radiation has been abandoned in favor of effective multiagent chemotherapeutic programs that include platinum, etoposide, and bleomycin, which is now standard therapy.[31,76,225]

Endodermal Sinus Tumors

Endodermal sinus or yolk sac tumors are aggressively malignant neoplasms that, either alone or as a component of a mixed germ cell tumor, are the second most common

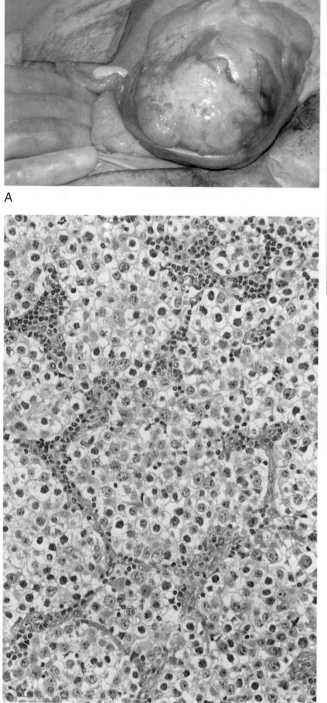

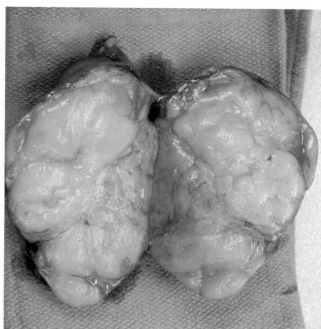

Figure 36–7 *A,* This encapsulated mass from a 5-year-old girl with acute abdominal pain proved to be a dysgerminoma. The child's contralateral tube and ovary are seen to the left of the tumor. A small portion of the ipsilateral tube and uterus were in the surgical specimen but uninvolved with tumor. *B,* The cut surface of the tumor is characterized by lobules divided by thin, fibrous septae. *C,* Micrograph of a dysgerminoma demonstrating polygonal, clear tumor cells divided into small lobules by fibrous septae that contain scattered lymphocytes. *(A, B see color plate.)*

histologic subtype of malignant ovarian germ cell tumors in children and adolescents.[154] In neonates and young children, the primary location of these tumors is the sacrococcygeal area. In older children and adolescents, it is found most frequently in the ovary. The origin of this particular tumor has been debated,[177,204,205] and many microscopic patterns of this tumor have been described. Nogales[141] suggested that this tumor originates from the primary yolk sac, a structure that develops very early in embryogenesis and consists of multipotential primitive endoderm. This tissue is capable of differentiating epithelial somatic tissues as well as secondary yolk sac tissue (a terminal, temporary structure with limited differentiating capacity) and mesenchyma. Yolk sac tumors with pure endodermal sinus subtypes are less mature than the differentiated glandular or hepatoid subtypes.[175]

These rapidly growing tumors are the second most common germ cell tumor in children.[59] Symptoms are generally present for less than a month and are related to the presence of an intra-abdominal mass. Seventy-five percent of patients present with abdominal pain and increased abdominal girth.[160] Elevation of the biologic marker AFP is the hallmark of this tumor.

The gross appearance of these tumors during surgery is pale yellow-tan and slimy, with foci of cystic areas and necrosis.[2] The tumors are soft and friable when handled. Most tumors show a distinct histologic subtype, with differentiation toward vitelline or yolk sac structures.[111] Microscopically, the most common papillary pattern has the so-called endodermal sinus structures (Schiller-Duval bodies) or perivascular sheaths of cells. Most well-differentiated yolk sac tumors also contain extracellular and intracellular droplets that are resistant to periodic acid–Sciff diastase staining and positive for AFP.

Embryonal Carcinomas

A relatively uncommon isolated germ cell tumor is embryonal carcinoma, which may resemble an anaplastic carcinoma with extensive necrosis. Embryonal carcinoma is more often found in association with other germ cell tumors and is referred to as a mixed germ cell tumor. One subtype of this tumor, the polyembryoma, is capable of producing both AFP and β-HCG, resulting in clinical endocrinopathies such as menstrual irregularities and isosexual precocious puberty. The histologic appearance is characterized by bodies that resemble tiny embryos.[206]

The workup and surgical approach to this tumor are similar to those for endodermal sinus tumor. Isolated, unilateral disease is managed by unilateral salpingo-oophorectomy. Advanced local disease necessitates panhysterectomy for local control; multiagent chemotherapy and radiation therapy are also indicated.

Choriocarcinomas

Choriocarcinomas are rare, endocrinologically active, highly malignant germ cell tumors that occur in girls and women. Estrogen is produced both by the tumor and by the ovary itself in response to the release of gonadotropin by the neoplastic chorionic tissue. The β-HCG level is elevated, and AFP is normal.

The clinical presentation is influenced by the age of the patient. Premenarchal girls present with signs of isosexual precocity and evidence of a rapidly growing neoplasm. These usually large, solid tumors generally adhere to surrounding tissues, and distant metastatic disease is associated with this tumor. The child may become cachectic and die quickly despite surgical excision and multidisciplinary therapy. In adolescents, the tumor also develops rapidly, but hormone production leads to menstrual disturbances and may initially simulate pregnancy. A gestational form of this tumor can arise in the placenta during pregnancy.[33]

Operative excision can be a formidable task because the tumor may be friable and quite vascular, and it often invades contiguous structures.[92] If the lesion is localized, surgery is limited to unilateral salpingo-oophorectomy; however, this is rarely the case. A more extensive extirpative procedure is usually required that involves removing the tumor, the opposite ovary, the uterus, and as much metastatic tissue as possible.

Grossly, these tumors appear nodular with a friable consistency. The tumor is purple with variegated areas of dark brown and yellow secondary to hemorrhage and necrosis. Microscopic evaluation of these tumors reveals cytotrophoblasts and syncytiotrophoblasts, with evidence of extensive necrosis and hemorrhage. Metastatic implants are friable and have a similar gross and microscopic appearance as the primary lesion. Multiagent chemotherapy is the treatment regimen of choice.

Teratomas

Teratomas are a group of neoplasms composed of tissue elements that are foreign to the organ or anatomic site where they are found.[74] Classically, these tumors are defined as being composed of tissue derived from the three germ layers: ectoderm, mesoderm, and endoderm. All three germ layers do *not* have to be present in each tumor, but some embryonic tissues must be found in an abnormal location. These tissues show elements of disorganization as well as various levels of maturation. As such, teratomas are histologically classified as mature and immature tumors and those with malignant components.[119] The development of a somatic malignancy within a teratoma is a rare event in childhood and is thought to occur within differentiated teratomatous elements rather than from totipotent embryonal cells.[154]

Mature Teratomas: Most teratomas in children are of the mature type. The majority of mature ovarian teratomas have entered but have not completed meiosis, suggesting that they arise from germ cells arrested in meiosis I.[154] There is little or no tendency for malignant degeneration of preexisting benign elements or the coexistence of malignant cells in a benign teratoma.[36] In neonates, mature teratomas are found most commonly in the sacrococcygeal area, followed by the head and neck.[98,119,203] The ovary becomes an important site later in childhood, especially during adolescence. Ovarian teratomas are predominantly cystic in nature.[36] Overall, benign cystic teratomas are the most common ovarian neoplasms in children[92] and can be bilateral in as many as 10% of patients.[36,193]

Symptoms of mature teratomas can be acute or chronic. Acute symptoms that mimic appendicitis are seen when torsion, hemorrhage, or rupture of the mass occurs. Gradual onset of symptoms may be related to the presence of an intra-abdominal adnexal mass, which may cause pressure on adjacent organs. Occasionally, a ruptured teratoma may lead to a chronic inflammatory response with the development of a mass of intestine and omentum adhering to the anterior abdominal wall; this condition is associated with pelvic adenopathy, which mimics a malignant tumor.[55]

On examination, findings are primarily related to the mass itself. These tumors are located in the abdomen in infants and young children. They are found in the

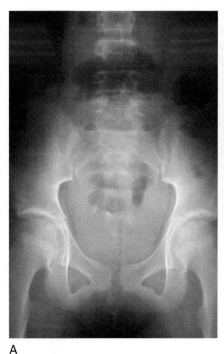

A

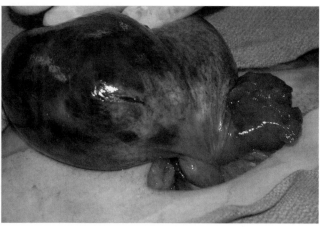

B

Figure 36–8 *A,* Plain abdominal radiograph of a 16-year-old girl with a unilateral ovarian teratoma; the pelvic mass contains toothlike calcifications. *B,* The patient presented to the emergency room with a several-day history of abdominal pain and was found to have a ruptured benign ovarian teratoma with torsion. Upon detorsion, the cyst was removed and the ovary preserved. Six months after surgery, the patient has evidence of two normal ovaries on ultrasonography.

pelvis of adolescents, although large tumors may be palpated in the abdomen, and there may be associated tenderness.

Plain abdominal radiographs demonstrate calcifications in up to 67% of cases (Fig. 36-8).[4] US is a commonly used diagnostic test. The positive predictive ability of US approaches 100% when two or more characteristic findings, such as shadowing echodensity and regionally bright echodensity, are present.[150] MRI may be more useful than CT in the diagnosis of mature cystic teratoma due to its ability to clearly define soft tissue components.[212]

Conservative ovarian surgery in childhood and adolescence is important for the development of normal puberty and future fertility. This must be balanced with complete removal of the mature cystic teratoma (Fig. 36-9). Traditional management of children with mature cystic teratomas has been oophorectomy via laparotomy. However, laparoscopic removal, either by cystectomy or oophorectomy, is a safe alternative when done by an experienced laparoscopist (see Fig. 36-3).[209] Campo and Garcea,[27] in a randomized, controlled trial, demonstrated that the use of an endobag when removing a mature cystic teratoma laparoscopically decreased the occurrence of spillage from 46% to 3.7% of cases.

Simple aspiration of a giant, predominantly cystic lesion as a means of "removal" should be avoided, because a malignant component may be present. Every effort should be made to spare the ovary, even when the mass is very large or bilateral, in an attempt to preserve hormonal and reproductive functions (see Figs. 36-8 and 36-9).[100] If this is not possible, the gonad and tumor alone should be removed, leaving the fallopian tube in place unless it is necrotic from torsion.

In adults, the reported incidence of recurrent mature cystic teratomas following cystectomy is 3% to 4%[8,29]

and usually occurs in patients younger than 40 years.[8] Also, in younger patients with multiple or bilateral mature cystic teratomas, there is a 2% to 3% incidence of the subsequent development of germ cell tumors.[8,20,232] In the absence of specific literature investigating recurrence in children, recommendations for postoperative surveillance are empirical. Given the sensitivity of US in the detection of mature cystic teratomas, annual imaging in prepubertal and young adolescents followed by annual pelvic examinations in older adolescents seems appropriate.

Miliary, intraperitoneal glial implants (i.e., grade 0), are occasionally encountered in association with mature teratomas.[58] These implants are never suspected before surgery. They appear as white or gray nodules, usually 1 to 3 mm in diameter, and are usually confined to the omentum, pelvic peritoneum, or adjacent or adherent to the tumor itself. Several explanations have been offered for the development of these implants.[166] The most widely accepted theory is that implantation occurs through a defect in the capsule of the primary tumor, permitting penetration by teratomatous elements under pressure. If the components near the defect are histologically mature, the metastatic implants will also be mature. In 11 of 12 cases reported by Robboy and Scully,[166] the capsule of the primary tumor was torn or had omentum or adnexal structures adhering to the mass. Implants can have a disturbing appearance, but no specific treatment is necessary when they are well differentiated, and their presence does not change management of the primary tumor. However, if adjacent components are immature, the lesions may progress and require adjuvant therapy.

Immature Teratomas: Immature teratomas are germ cell neoplasms composed of tissue derived from the three

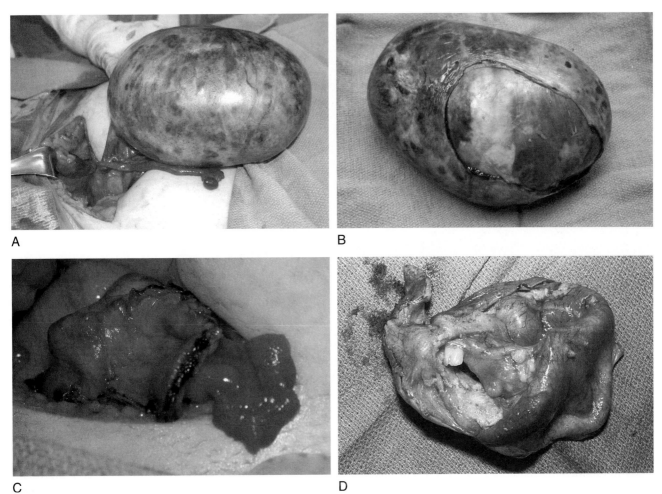

Figure 36–9 *A,* Large ovarian dermoid tumor in a 14-year-old girl with acute severe abdominal pain upon awakening. The fallopian tube is seen below the tumor. *B,* After tumor excision, the surface where the cyst was peeled away from the ovary can be seen. *C,* Ovarian tissue (*left*) and fallopian tube (*right*) remaining after cyst removal. *D,* Opened gross specimen of an ovarian dermoid showing multiple tooth- and jawlike calcifications. (*A, B, C, see color plate.*)

germ cell layers. These teratomas are clinically distinct from benign or malignant teratomas because they also contain immature, neuroepithelial elements (Fig. 36-10). Immature teratomas can coexist with the more mature solid or cystic benign teratomas or with malignant teratomas, in which case treatment is determined by the malignant component.[143]

Immature teratomas are graded by the degree of immaturity of the tumor and the presence and quantity of neuroepithelial components. The grade of the primary tumor is significant and is one of the major determinants of the likelihood of extraovarian metastasis. The current grading system was developed by Thurlbeck and Scully[211] and modified by Norris et al.[143] and Ihara et al.[94]

Grade I. Limited to ovary (peritoneal evaluation should be negative). No clinical, radiographic, or histologic evidence of disease beyond the ovaries. (The presence of gliomatosis peritonei does not change grade I disease to a higher grade.)

Grade II. Microscopic residual; peritoneal evaluation negative. (The presence of gliomatosis peritonei does not change grade II disease to a higher grade.)

Grade III. Lymph node involvement (metastatic nodule); gross residual or biopsy only; contiguous visceral involvement (omentum, intestine, bladder); peritoneal evaluation positive for malignancy.

Grade IV. Distant metastases, including liver.

Multidisciplinary therapy has improved the prognosis of immature teratomas. In a study published in 1976 by Norris et al.,[143] survival was 82% for patients with grade I tumors, 62% for grade II, and 30% for grade III with the use of combination therapy. The experience of the M. D. Anderson Cancer Center published in 1986 disclosed that 15 of 16 patients managed initially with surgery alone had recurrence of the tumor, but 10 of 11 who received subsequent chemotherapy were salvaged.[68] Eighteen of 21 patients who received combination vincristine, actinomycin D, cyclophosphamide (VAC) chemotherapy survived.

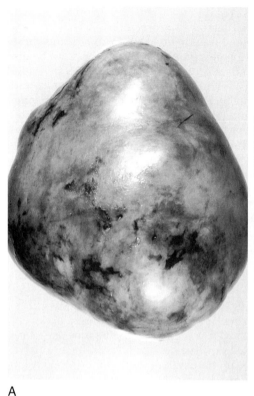

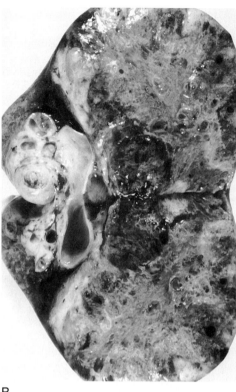

Figure 36-10 *A,* Characteristic gross appearance of an immature teratoma in a 5-year-old girl who presented with a left ovarian mass. The tumor is a solid and cystic globoid mass with a smooth, shiny surface. *B,* Cut section of an immature teratoma shows a variegated, solid, cystic appearance with focal areas of hemorrhage.

A   B

Based on improvement in survival, current management of immature teratomas must balance survival with the maintenance of childbearing capacity.[121] In 1989 Koulos et al.[110] reviewed 25 cases accrued from the Connecticut Tumor Registry and found that 18 of 23 patients with stage I disease were effectively treated with preservation of the opposite adnexa, with or without adjuvant chemotherapy. They concluded that it might be reasonable to withhold chemotherapy from patients with stage I, grade I and II immature teratomas who were initially treated with conservative surgery if the patient can be followed closely for possible recurrence. In cases of recurrence, rescue can be achieved with salvage therapy. Kawai et al.[103] agreed that unilateral salpingo-oophorectomy alone is adequate for stage I immature teratoma if the tumor has a histologic grade of I; however, chemotherapy with VAC or VAC with cisplatin is required for grade II or III tumors. In their study, 18 of 19 patients were disease free at a mean follow-up of 62 months. A similar conclusion was reached by Bonazzi et al.[19] based on a 10-year prospective study of 32 patients with ovarian immature teratoma. Patients with stage I or II, grade I or II tumors can be managed with fertility-sparing surgery without chemotherapy, whereas patients with stage III or grade III (regardless of stage) or with relapse are most effectively treated with platinum-based chemotherapy. In their study, all 32 patients were disease free with a median survival of 47 months.

Immature teratomas are rarely bilateral,[40] and biopsy of the unaffected ovary is unnecessary if it looks normal.[68] To preserve future childbearing potential in children,

unilateral salpingo-oophorectomy for stage I, grade I disease is adequate.[41,121] Platinum-based chemotherapy is required for grade II or III tumors. For tumors of stage II or higher, attempts should be made to preserve reproductive capability whenever possible, along with the addition of chemotherapy. It is also suggested that postinduction surgery should be used for grade II or III and stage II or higher tumors, with termination of chemotherapy if no tumors of grade I or higher are identified.[68]

Monodermal Teratomas: A monodermal teratoma is an ovarian tumor composed exclusively or almost exclusively of ectoderm or mesoderm or endoderm, for example, neuroectoderm.[5]

Gonadoblastomas

Gonadoblastoma, a tumor first described by Scully[180] in 1953, is relatively rare and occurs most commonly in patients with dysgenetic gonads. Most patients are virilized or nonvirilized phenotypic females. In the only large series reported, Scully[181] reviewed 74 cases and found that 89% were chromatin negative and the most common karyotype was 46XY or 45X/46XY. Troche and Hernandez,[213] in a literature review of 140 cases of neoplasms arising in dysgenetic gonads, found that 80% had these karyotypes. Patients are usually older adolescents or in the third decade of life with a history of primary amenorrhea. Androgen production by the tumor causes virilization. When a workup for amenorrhea or virilization is undertaken, an abnormal karyotype with a Y chromosome or chromosome fragment can be found in as many as 90% of patients.[213] These often small tumors may then be identified during examination or exploration. They may also be found incidentally during excision of gonadal streaks or dysgenetic gonads.[136,229] These tumors become invasive early, and gonadectomy is recommended as soon as 46XY gonadal dysgenesis is diagnosed.[139,181,213]

Gonadoblastomas are composed of germ cells and sex cord derivatives that are similar to granulosa and Sertoli cells, although immunohistochemical and ultrastructural findings are more supportive of Sertoli-like differentiation.[168] Lutein or Leydig-like stromal cells occur in two thirds of cases and probably reflect a stromal reaction to gonadotropin stimulation.[168] These tumors are considered precursors to germ cell tumors in dysgenetic or streak gonads because they may coexist with dysgerminomas and other germ cell tumors in more than half of patients.[213] The tumor may be difficult to identify on gross examination because of overgrowth by the malignant component and other changes, including calcification, fibrosis, or both. In fact, calcification may be the only remnant of the gonadoblastoma, and the presence of calcification in a dysgerminoma should raise the suspicion of an underlying gonadoblastoma. The malignant potential of this tumor is determined by the underlying malignant component and should be treated accordingly. The outcome for patients may be enhanced because abnormal sexual development prompts early evaluation and subsequent diagnosis of the tumor. The prognosis of nongerminomatous germ cell tumors has improved with the advent of bleomycin, etoposide, and cisplatin protocols, and survival rates of 70% to 90% have been reported.[154]

Mixed Germ Cell Tumors

Germ cell tumors in children are often composed of more than one pure histologic type. Benign but questionably malignant tumors (immature teratomas) and frankly malignant tumors (germinomas, choriocarcinomas, endodermal sinus tumors, embryonal carcinomas) may be present. Management of mixed tumors is geared toward the most malignant component.

SURGICAL GUIDELINES FOR OVARIAN GERM CELL TUMORS

The goal of surgery is to completely evaluate the extent of disease, safely and completely resect the tumor, and spare all uninvolved reproductive organs. Preservation of reproductive potential is a high priority during surgery for ovarian lesions in children. An increasinag number of laparoscopic procedures are being performed for the evaluation of pelvic masses, and data demonstrate that the benefits of a faster recovery time and a shorter hospital stay seen in adults are also applicable to children.[209,210] If a suspected ovarian malignancy is detected at the time of laparoscopy, complete surgical staging and resection by conventional laparotomy are currently recommended.

Benign lesions require only tumor resection via ovarian cystectomy or unilateral oophorectomy.

Benign tumors, frankly malignant tumors, and those with mixed histologic characteristics often cannot be distinguished based on gross appearance alone. If in doubt, staging is recommended, because the treatment and prognosis of malignancies depend on accurate staging. The current intergroup COG protocol includes thorough inspection, palpation, and biopsy of any suspicious peritoneal and liver nodules (including the subphrenic spaces).[31] Both ovaries are inspected. If a tumor is found in an ovary, it should be removed by unilateral oophorectomy. The opposite ovary should be inspected, and nodules or suspicious areas should be biopsied and removed. If a contralateral tumor is found, bilateral salpingo-oophorectomy is done.

Ascitic fluid is collected for cytologic evaluation. If no fluid is present, peritoneal washings using lactated Ringer's solution must be obtained. Biopsy of suspicious omental lesions should be done. Omentectomy is performed for tumors involving the omentum. Retroperitoneal lymph nodes are palpated, and suspicious or enlarged nodes are biopsied, including debulking of all obvious retroperitoneal lymphatic spread and removal of any large, bulky areas of metastatic tissue in the peritoneum. If tumor invasion has occurred to the extent that a safe, nonmutilating procedure cannot be done, attempts to surgically excise the tumor may be delayed until the effectiveness of chemotherapy can be determined. At week 12 of treatment, postinduction surgery is performed on patients with persistently elevated tumor markers or clinical evidence of gross residual intra-abdominal disease on physical examination or imaging studies. Postinduction surgery includes biopsy or resection of obvious disease, sampling of the lymph nodes, and biopsy of the kidney to assess cisplatin toxicity.

CHEMOTHERAPY FOR OVARIAN GERM CELL TUMORS

Forty years ago, no effective therapy for germ cell tumors existed. Based on the early success of managing testicular germ cell tumors using multiagent platinum-based chemotherapy, ovarian tumor treatment evolved along similar lines. The addition of chemotherapy reduced the risk of recurrent disease for adult patients with completely resected ovarian germ cell tumors.[226] Initially, adjuvant VAC was added to surgical excision.[226] Because it was effective on testicular germ cell tumors, cisplatin was added to more recent treatment protocols, and the regimen of cisplatin, etoposide, and bleomycin (PEB) became the preferred protocol. An 8-year study from the GOG that closed in 1992 evaluated PEB and found that 91 of 93 patients were free of recurrent germ cell tumors with a median follow-up of 38.6 months.[228]

Historically, several chemotherapeutic regimens were tried in children, and the best results were achieved with PEB.[116,120] In a pilot study, Pinkerton et al.[157] demonstrated the effectiveness of substituting cisplatin with carboplatin, a less toxic drug; carboplatin was then combined with bleomycin and etoposide. Eight of eight patients with ovarian germ cell tumors survived with this regimen. Using a platinum-based regimen, only 1 of 17 girls with resected ovarian nonseminomatous germ cell tumors in FIGO stage IA relapsed in an analysis of European trials by Göbel et al.[72]

In 1991 the CCG experience of 93 children with malignant germ cell tumors included 30 ovarian tumors.[3] By study design, immature teratomas and dysgerminomas were not included. Using a cisplatin-based regimen, the 4-year event-free survival rate was 63%. Tumor size affected prognosis. If the tumor was larger than 16 cm in diameter, the outcome was worse. Patients in whom complete tumor resection could not be done during the original procedure were more likely to have subsequent adverse events than were those in whom the tumor was completely removed ($P = 0.08$). In 1994 Nair et al.[138] reported their findings in 107 children with germ cell tumors, including 43 girls with ovarian tumors. Of these, 22 received multiagent chemotherapy. A complete response was seen in 6 of 11 patients treated with platinum, vinblastine, and bleomycin, compared with 10 of 11 patients who responded completely to treatment with PEB (with etoposide replacing vinblastine). The risk of chemotherapy-related complications is low relative to the effectiveness of the PEB regimen.[227]

There is currently a phase III study of reduced therapy in the treatment of children with low- and intermediate-risk extracranial germ cell tumors through the COG (COG-AGCT0132) that was activated November 3, 2003.[31] Based on data from the last POG-CCG intergroup study, patients with malignant germ cell tumors can be stratified into three risk groups (low, intermediate, and high) defined by stage and primary site. Based on preliminary data from POG 9048/CCG 8891, patients with stage I ovarian and extragonadal immature teratomas with malignant elements appear to do well following complete surgical resection.[41] In the current study, all patients with stage I tumors will be categorized in the low-risk category and treated with surgery followed by close observation and monitoring. The intermediate-risk group will consist of patients with stage II to III gonadal tumors. Such patients have been shown to have a 3-year event-free survival of about 90% with standard-dose PEB.[31,167] These patients will be treated with a modified PEB regimen consisting of three cycles of compressed PEB every 21 days. Saxman et al.[176] reported that long-term survival was equivalent for men with germ cell cancer who were treated with either three or four cycles of PEB. Patients who are partial responders may then have surgical resection of residual tumor. Therapy is discontinued upon pathologic complete response and normal markers, or it is continued for an additional three cycles in children who remain partial responders. Patients with recurring germ cell tumors may be salvaged with high-dose chemotherapy with autologous stem cell transplantation.

UNCLASSIFIED BENIGN TUMORS

Although the ovary is highly vascularized, hemangiomas are extremely rare; a review found only 40 published cases of these tumors.[79] Their occurrence is relatively evenly distributed between infancy and postmenopausal age groups. The lesions are usually quite small, asymptomatic, and discovered incidentally. Bilateral occurrence is rare, and the tumors are almost always cavernous. Benign-appearing ultrasonographic features have been described.[148] When the tumors are large, associated symptoms include abdominal pain, distention, and bloody ascites. Torsion or rupture may cause an acute surgical emergency. No malignant tumors of this type have been described, and oophorectomy or adnexectomy is curative if needed.

Primary ovarian leiomyomas are also extremely rare, although they have been reported in teenage girls.[174] Most reported cases are clinically silent; however, the lesion may be large enough to cause increased abdominal girth and pelvic pain. Tumor markers are normal, and imaging studies are generally unable to differentiate this benign solid tumor from a malignant process. Unilateral salpingo-oophorectomy is curative.

The ovarian myxoma is a rare benign tumor characterized by conspicuous vascularity and mesenchymal proliferation that requires only a conservative surgical procedure.[54]

UNCLASSIFIED MALIGNANT TUMORS

Primary ovarian sarcomas are a heterogeneous group of aggressive tumors associated with poor survival. Most cases occur in older women; however, a review of 151 cases described 10 of 29 patients with rhabdomyosarcoma who were younger than 20 years.[186] These patients presented with nonspecific symptoms of abdominal discomfort or swelling, with occasional urinary or gastrointestinal complaints secondary to mass effect. Accurate staging is critical. Hysterectomy with bilateral salpingo-oophorectomy and debulking of as much diseased intra-abdominal tissue as possible have been done. Radiation therapy is administered for residual pelvic disease, and several chemotherapeutic regimens have been used. In contrast to other rhabdomyosarcomas, the outcome for patients with ovarian lesions has generally been poor, perhaps because of the advanced stage of disease at diagnosis. Nevertheless, the most recent chemotherapeutic regimens used in cooperative group studies have been highly effective, and it is reasonable to assume that more conservative surgical resection will provide adequate treatment for these rare tumors.

Genuine stromal sarcomas and low-grade endometrial stromal sarcomas of the ovary have been occasionally reported in the second decade of life. These lesions are believed to arise from ovarian endometriosis, coelomic mesenchyma, or neometaplasia of stromal cells. Lesions are usually discovered because of nonspecific pelvic discomfort, although early infiltration into adjacent tissues may cause intestinal or ureteric obstruction. Tumor infiltration may not be grossly apparent, so initial surgical resection should be aggressive, with total hysterectomy and bilateral salpingo-oophorectomy. Progesterone administration may provide effective adjunctive therapy, although this has to be continued indefinitely because stromal sarcomas can reappear and spread dramatically when the medication is stopped. Radiation therapy has been used for local residual disease, although recurrence is common. The role of chemotherapy for these tumors has not been defined.

Cases of genuine ovarian fibrosarcoma in children are extremely rare. Patients present with pelvic pain and a palpable mass. Fibrosarcoma has been associated with Maffucci's syndrome.[32] Although the outcome is uniformly poor in older patients, survival of younger patients who have undergone aggressive surgical resection, including hysterectomy and bilateral salpingo-oophorectomy, has been reported. Success with subsequent radiation or chemotherapy has not been reported.

Primary leiomyosarcoma of the ovary is extremely rare in children. These tumors may arise de novo from any of the smooth muscle sites in the ovary or may represent malignant degeneration of leiomyoma, a benign counterpart.[131] As with most of these rare tumors, presenting symptoms are nonspecific, and discovery may occur in an advanced stage of disease. Aggressive surgical therapy is recommended because no adjuvant therapy has proved beneficial.

SECONDARY TUMORS

Although secondary ovarian malignancy is rare, the ovaries are a potential metastatic site for a wide variety of childhood malignancies (Table 36-9).[123,238] Distinguishing primary neoplasms from secondary neoplasms is important to prevent inappropriate therapy or adverse sequelae. Metastatic spread to the ovary occurs through four main pathways: (1) hematogenous spread, (2) lymphatic spread, (3) transcoelomic dissemination with surface implantation, and (4) direct spread.[123] Highly malignant tumors that have a predilection for the pelvic region are intra-abdominal desmoplastic small round cell tumors.[237]

Pais et al.[147] reviewed 23 cases of ovarian involvement in patients with relapsing leukemia. Abdominal pain was the most common symptom, and a mass could usually be palpated. Although most patients in whom leukemia treatment failed had systemic and not local disease, US

revealed a characteristic appearance and was effective in detecting ovarian involvement in these patients.[17] Survival was based on aggressive systemic multiagent chemotherapy and not on the degree of surgical resection of the ovarian lesion. Routine pelvic radiation therapy was of no benefit.

Reports have noted granulocytic sarcoma of the ovary occurring in patients with acute or relapsed acute myelogenous leukemia.[231] Although aggressive systemic chemotherapy is critical to survival, an ovarian mass should be investigated immediately to determine its nature (i.e., benign or malignant and exact cell type). In this instance, surgical resection of the ovary and any other involved gynecologic organs or pelvic tissue must be done. Radiation therapy has been used for residual disease in the pelvis. Although the ultimate outcome of granulocytic sarcomas is probably dependent on the effectiveness of chemotherapy, local measures of tumor control cannot be overlooked when this tumor is detected.

SUMMARY

The diagnosis and management of ovarian lesions in infants and children remain challenging because of the wide variety of possible pathologies, some of which are extremely rare. Non-neoplastic lesions are being detected more commonly as imaging techniques continue to improve. Neoplastic lesions are more readily diagnosed and completely characterized with advances in biochemical, immunohistologic, and cytogenetic technology.

Because of the relative rarity of ovarian tumors in children, clinical approaches may be based on experience with similar adult lesions. However, it is critical to recognize the differences exhibited by the juvenile forms of many of these entities, which often present at a less advanced stage and have a more favorable natural history and response to therapy. Preservation of reproductive and endocrine function is of paramount importance in the treatment of ovarian lesions in infants and children. Careful observation or nonoperative therapies may be appropriate for many non-neoplastic conditions. Most benign neoplasms are adequately managed with conservative surgical approaches. Even frankly malignant tumors increasingly yield to multidisciplinary therapy, which can include less radically ablative surgery and still result in long-term survival and possible fertility preservation for young patients. Radiation has been shown to be useful in specific cases to increase local control, but, given the paucity of cases, a survival advantage has not been demonstrated.

TABLE 36–9 Secondary (Metastatic) Tumors Occurring in the Ovary in Children
Colorectal
Breast
Gastric carcinoma
Carcinoid tumors (liver, lung)
Malignant melanoma
Burkitt's lymphoma
Rhabdomyosarcoma
Wilms' tumor
Neuroblastoma
Retinoblastoma
Ewing's sarcoma
Rhabdoid tumor of the kidney
Medulloblastoma
Osteogenic sarcoma
Chondrosarcoma
Leukemia

ACKNOWLEDGMENTS

The authors would like to thank Drs. Catheryn Yashar and Alexandra Cheerva for their kind review of the chapter.

REFERENCES

1. Abelev GI, Assecritova IV, Kraevsky NA, et al: Embryonal serum alpha-globulin in cancer patients: Diagnostic value. Int J Cancer 1967;2:551-558.

2. Ablin A, Isaacs H Jr: Germ cell tumors. In Pizzo PA, Poplack DG (eds): Principles and Practice of Pediatric Oncology, 2nd ed. Philadelphia, JB Lippincott, 1993, pp 867-887.

3. Ablin AR, Krailo MD, Ramsay NKC, et al: Results of treatment of malignant germ cell tumors in 93 children: A report from the Children's Cancer Study Group. J Clin Oncol 1991;9:1782-1792.

4. Adelman S, Benson CD, Hertzler JH: Surgical lesions of the ovary in infancy and childhood. Surg Gynecol Obstet 1975;141:219-222.

5. Aguirre P, Scully R: Malignant neuroectodermal tumor of the ovary, a distinctive form of monodermal teratoma: Report of five cases. Am J Surg Pathol 1982;6:283-292.

6. Alrabeeah A, Galliani CA, Giacomantonio M, et al: Neonatal ovarian torsion: Report of three cases and review of the literature. Pediatr Pathol 1988;8:143-149.

7. American Fertility Society: Revised American Fertility Society classification of endometriosis 1985. Fertil Steril 1985;43:351-352.

8. Anteby E, Ron M, Revel A, et al: Germ cell tumors of the ovary arising after dermoid cyst resection: A long term follow-up study. Obstet Gynecol 1994;83:605-608.

9. Asadourian LA, Taylor HB: Dysgerminoma, an analysis of 105 cases. Obstet Gynecol 1969;33:370-379.

10. ASHG/ACMG Report: Points to consider: Ethical, legal, and psychological implications of genetic testing in children and adolescents. Am J Hum Genet 1995;57:1233-1241.

11. Asirvatham R, Rooney RJ, Watts HG: Ollier's disease with secondary chondrosarcoma associated with ovarian tumour. Int Orthop (SICOT) 1991;15:393-395.

12. Atkin NB, Baker MC: Abnormal chromosomes including small metacentrics in 14 ovarian cancers. Cancer Genet Cytogenet 1987;26:355-361.

13. Attaran M, Gidwani GP: Adolescent endometriosis. Obstet Gynecol Clin North Am 2003;30:379-390.

14. Ayhan A, et al: Oncologic and reproductive outcome after fertility-saving surgery in ovarian cancer. Eur J Gynaecol Oncol 2003;24:223-232.

15. Bagolan P, Rivosecchi M, Giorlandino C, et al: Prenatal diagnosis and clinical outcome of ovarian cysts. J Pediatr Surg 1992;27:879-881.

16. Barakat RR: Borderline tumors of the ovary. Obstet Gynecol Clin North Am 1994;21:93-104.

17. Bickers GH, Siebert JJ, Anderson JC, et al: Sonography of ovarian involvement in childhood acute lymphocytic leukemia. Am J Res 1981;137:399-401.

18. Blake KI, Gerrard MR: Malignant germ cell tumours in two siblings. Med Pediatr Oncol 1993;21:299-300.

19. Bonazzi C, Pecctori F, Colombo N, et al: Pure ovarian immature teratoma, a unique and curable disease: 10 years' experience of 32 prospectively treated patients. Obstet Gynecol 1994;84:598-604.

20. Borenstein R, Czernobilsky B, Lancet M: Immature ovarian teratoma, an unusual case. Int J Obstet Gynecol 1982;20:159-162.

21. Bosl GJ, Dmitrovsky E, Reuter VE, et al: Isochromosome of chromosome 12: Clinically useful marker for male germ cell tumors. J Natl Cancer Inst 1989;81:1874-1878.

22. Bourne T, Campbell S, Steer C, et al: Transvaginal color flow imaging: A possible new screening technique for ovarian cancer. BMJ 1989;299:1367-1370.

23. Brandt ML, Luks FI, Filiatrault D, et al: Surgical indications in antenatally diagnosed ovarian cysts. J Pediatr Surg 1991;26:276-282.

24. Breen JL, Maxson WS: Ovarian tumors in children and adolescents. Clin Obstet Gynecol 1977;20:607-623.

25. Brody S: Clinical aspects of dysgerminoma of the ovary. Acta Radiol 1961;56:209-230.

26. Brown MF, Hebra A, McGeehin K, et al: Ovarian masses in children: A review of 91 cases of malignant and benign masses. J Pediatr Surg 1993;28:930-932.

27. Campo S, Garcea N: Laparoscopic conservative excision of ovarian dermoid cysts with and without an endobag. J Am Assoc Gynecol Laparosc 1998;5:165-170.

28. Chao H, Wang H: Gonadotropin-releasing hormone-agonist as a neoadjunctive therapy for Sertoli-Leydig cell tumors of the ovary. Int J Gynaecol Obstet 1999;66:189-190.

29. Chapron C, Dubuisson JB, Samouh N, et al: Treatment of ovarian dermoid cysts. Surg Endosc 1994;8:1092-1095.

30. Chiaramonte C, Piscopo A, Cataliotto F: Ovarian cysts in newborns. Pediatr Surg Int 2001;17:171-174.

31. Children's Oncology Group AGCT0132: A phase III study of reduced therapy in the treatment of children with low and intermediate risk extracranial germ cell tumors. (Activated November 3, 2003; version date, March 10, 2004.)

32. Christman JE, Ballon SC: Ovarian fibrosarcoma associated with Maffucci's syndrome. Gynecol Oncol 1990;37:290-291.

33. Christopherson WA, Kanbour A, Szulman A: Case report: Choriocarcinoma in a term placenta with maternal metastases. Gynecol Oncol 1992;46:239-245.

34. Cohen HL, Eisenberg P, Mandel FS, et al: Ovarian cysts are common in premenarchal girls: A sonographic study of 101 children 2-12 years old. Am J Res 1992;159:89-91.

35. Cohen HL, Shapiro MA, Manel FS, et al: Normal ovaries in neonates and infants: A sonographic study of 77 patients 1 day to 24 months old. Am J Res 1993;160:583-586.

36. Comerci JT, Licciardi F, Bergh PA et al: Mature cystic teratoma: A clinicopathologic evaluation of 517 cases and a review of the literature. Obstet Gynecol 1994;84:22-28.

37. Craig I, Rawlings C: Human gene mapping 10.5 Oxford conference. Cytogenet Cell Genet 1990;55:5-76.

38. Crispens MA: Borderline ovarian tumours: A review of the recent literature. Curr Opin Obstet Gynecol 2004;15:39-43.

39. Cronen PW, Nagaraj HS: Ovarian tumors in children. South Med J 1988;81:464-468.

40. Curry SL, Smite JP, Gallagher HS: Malignant teratoma of the ovary: Prognostic factors and treatment. Am J Obstet Gynecol 1978;131:845-849.

41. Cushing B, Giller R, Ablin A, et al: Surgical resection alone is effective treatment for ovarian immature teratoma in children and adolescents: A report of the Pediatric Oncology Group and the Children's Cancer Group. Am J Obstet Gynecol 1999;181:353-358.

42. Darwish AM, Amin AF, Mohamad SA: Laparoscopic management of paratubal and paraovarian cysts. JSLS 2003;7:101-106.

43. DeCrespigny LC, Robinson H, Davoren RA, et al: The "simple" ovarian cyst: Aspirate or operate? Br J Obstet Gynaecol 1989;96:1035-1039.

44. Dehner LP: Gonadal and extragonadal germ cell neoplasia in childhood. Hum Pathol 1983;14:493-511.

45. Dengg K, Fink FM, Heitger A, et al: Precocious puberty due to a lipid-cell tumour of the ovary. Eur J Pediatr 1993;152:12-14.

46. DePalo G, Pilotti S, Kenda R, et al: Natural history of dysgerminoma. Am J Obstet Gynecol 1982;143:799-807.

47. Deprest J, Moerman P, Corneillie P, et al: Ovarian borderline mucinous tumor in a premenarchal girl: Review on ovarian epithelial cancer in young girls. Gynecol Oncol 1992;45:219-224.

48. Diamond MP, Baxter JW, Peerman CG, et al: Occurrence of ovarian malignancy in childhood and adolescence: A community-wide evaluation. Obstet Gynecol 1988;71:858-860.

49. Dicker D, Dekel A, Feldberg D, et al: Bilateral Sertoli-Leydig cell tumor with heterologous elements: Report of

an unusual case and review of the literature. Eur J Obstet Gynecol Reprod Biol 1986;22:175-181.

50. Dietrich J, Kaplan A, Lopez H, et al: Clinical pathologic correlation: A case of poorly differentiated Sertoli-Leydig tumor of the ovary. J Pediatr Adolesc Gynecol 2004;17: 49-52.

51. Easton DF, Ford D, Bishop T, Breast Cancer Linkage Consortium: Breast and ovarian cancer incidence in BRCA1-mutation carriers. Am J Hum Genet 1995;56: 265-271.

52. Eggermont E, Lecoutere D, Devlieger H, et al: Ovarian cysts in newborn infants. Am J Dis Child 1988;142:702.

53. Ehren IM, Mahour GH, Isaacs H: Benign and malignant ovarian tumors in children and adolescents. Am J Surg 1984;147:339-344.

54. Eichhorn JH, Scully RE: Ovarian myxoma: Clinicopathologic and immunocytologic analysis of five cases and a review of the literature. Int J Gynecol Pathol 1991;10:156-169.

55. Ein SH, Darte JMM, Stephens CA: Cystic and solid ovarian tumors in children: A 44-year review. J Pediatr Surg 1970; 5:148-156.

56. Elger BS, Harding TW: Testing adolescents for a hereditary breast cancer gene (BRCA1): Respecting their autonomy is in their best interest. Arch Pediatr Adolesc Med 2000;154: 113-119.

57. Elsheikh A, Milingos S, Kallipolitis G, et al: Ovarian tumors in young females: A laparoscopic approach. Eur J Gynaecol Oncol 2001;22:243-244.

58. Fanning J, Bates J: Mature solid teratoma associated with gliomatosis peritonei. Am J Obstet Gynecol 1986;155: 661-662.

59. Farahmand SM, Marchetti DL, Asirwatham JE, et al: Ovarian endodermal sinus tumor associated with pregnancy: Case report and review of the literature. Gynecol Oncol 1991;41: 156-160.

60. Fedele L, Dorta M, Brioschi D, et al: Magnetic resonance evaluation of gynecologic masses in adolescents. Adolesc Pediatr Gynecol 1990;3:83-88.

61. Ferrera PC, Whitman MCW: Ovarian small cell carcinoma: A rare neoplasm in a 15-year-old female. Pediatr Emerg Care 2000;16:170-172.

62. FIGO Committee on Gynecologic Oncology: Staging classifications and clinical practice guidelines of gynaecologic cancers. Int J Gynecol Obstet 2000;70:207-312.

63. Freedman SM, Kreitzer PM, Elkowitz SS, et al: Ovarian microcysts in girls with isolated premature thelarche. J Pediatr Surg 1993;122:246-251.

64. Gallup DG, Talledo OE: Benign and malignant tumors. Clin Obstet Gynecol 1987;30:662-670.

65. Gedeit RG, Jay MS, Ross SP: The role of MRI in evaluation of an adolescent with a pelvic mass. J Adolesc Health Care 1990;11:516-518.

66. Gershenson DM, Del Junco G, Silva EG, et al: Immature teratoma of the ovary. Obstet Gynecol 1986;68:624-629.

67. Gershenson DM, Morris M, Burke T, et al: Treatment of poor-prognosis sex cord-stromal tumors of the ovary with a combination of bleomycin, etoposide and cisplatin. Obstet Gynecol 1996;87:527-531.

68. Gershenson DM, Morris M, Cangir A, et al: Treatment of malignant germ cell tumors of the ovary with bleomycin, etoposide and cisplatin. J Clin Oncol 1990;8: 715-720.

69. Giller R, Cushing B, Lauer S, et al: Comparison of high-dose or standard-dose cisplatin with etoposide and bleomycin (HDPEB vs PEB) in children with stage III or IV malignant germ cell tumors (MGCT) at gonadal primary site: A Pediatric Intergroup trial (POG 9049/CCG 8882). Proc Am Soc Clin Oncol 1998;17:525.

70. Giorlandino C, Bilancioni E, Bagolan P, et al: Antenatal ultrasonographic diagnosis and management of fetal ovarian cysts. Int J Gynecol Obstet 1993;44:27-31.

71. Gitlin D, Perricelli A, Gillin GM: Synthesis of fetoprotein by liver, yolk sac, and gastrointestinal tract of the human conceptus. Cancer Res 1972;32:979-982.

72. Göbel U, Haas RJ, Calaminus G, et al: Treatment of germ cell tumors in children: Results of European trials for testicular and non-testicular primary sites. Crit Rev Oncol Hematol 1990;10:89-98.

73. Goldstein D, deCholonoky C, Emans SJ: Adolescent endometriosis. J Adolesc Health 1980;1:37-41.

74. Gonzales-Crussi F: Extragonadal teratomas. In Atlas of Tumor Pathology, 2nd ser, fascicle 18. Washington, DC, Armed Forces Institute of Pathology, 1982, pp 1-43.

75. Gordon A, Lipton D, Woodruff D: Dysgerminoma: A review of 158 cases from the Emil Novak Ovarian Tumor Registry. Obstet Gynecol 1981;58:497-504.

76. Greist A, Roth B, Einhorn L, et al: Cisplatin-combination chemotherapy for disseminated germ cell tumors: Long-term follow-up. Proc Am Soc Clin Oncol 1985;4:100.

77. Gribbon M, Ein SH, Mancer K: Pediatric malignant ovarian tumors: A 43-year review. J Pediatr Surg 1992;27: 480-484.

78. Groeber WR: Ovarian tumors during infancy and childhood. Am J Obstet Gynecol 1963;86:1027-1035.

79. Gunes HA, Egilmez R, Dulger M: Ovarian haemangioma. Br J Clin Pract 1990;44:734-735.

80. Gustafson ML, Lee MM, Scully RE, et al: Mullerian inhibitory substance as a marker for ovarian sex cord tumor. N Engl J Med 1992;326:466-471.

81. Halme J, Hammond MG, Hulka JF, et al: Retrograde menstruation in healthy women and in patients with endometriosis. Obstet Gynecol 1984;64:151-154.

82. Harris AC, Wakely PE, Kaplowitz PB, et al: Steroid cell tumor of the ovary in a child. Arch Pathol Lab Med 1991;115:150-154.

83. Hasson HM: Laparoscopic management of ovarian cysts. J Reprod Med 1990;35:863-867.

84. Hayes MC, Scully RE: Ovarian steroid cell tumors (not otherwise specified): A clinicopathological analysis of 63 cases. Am J Surg Pathol 1987;11:835-845.

85. Heling K, Chaoui R, Kirchmair F, et al: Fetal ovarian cysts: Prenatal diagnosis, management and postnatal outcome. Ultrasound Obstet Gynecol 2002;20:47-50.

86. Héloury Y, Guiberteau V, Sagot P, et al: Laparoscopy in adnexal pathology in the child: A study of 28 cases. Eur J Pediatr Surg 1993;3:75-78.

87. Herd J, Fowler JM, Shenson D, et al: Laparoscopic para-aortic lymph node sampling: Development of a technique. Gynecol Oncol 1992;44:271-276.

88. Hoffner L, Shen-Schwarz S, Deka R, et al: Genetics and biology of human ovarian teratomas. III. Cytogenetics and origins of malignant ovarian germ cell tumors. Cancer Genet Cytogenet 1992;62:58-65.

89. Hoshiai H, Ishikawa M, Sawatari Y, et al: Laparoscopic evaluation of the onset and progression of endometriosis. Am J Obstet Gynecol 1993;169:714-719.

90. Howell CG Jr, Rogers DA, Gable DS, et al: Bilateral ovarian fibromas in children. J Pediatr Surg 1990;25: 690-691.

91. Hsu C, Ma L, Mak L: Sclerosing stromal tumor of the ovary: Case report and review of the literature. Int J Gynecol Pathol 1983;2:192-200.

92. Huffman JW: Ovarian tumors in children and adolescents. In Huffman JW, et al (eds): The Gynecology of Childhood and Adolescence, 2nd ed. Philadelphia, WB Saunders, 1981, pp 277-349.

93. Hulka JF, Parker WH, Surrey MW, et al: Management of ovarian masses: AAGL 1990 survey. J Reprod Med 1992; 37:599-602.

94. Ihara T, Ohama K, Satoh H: Histologic grade and karyotype of immature teratoma of the ovary. Cancer 1984;54: 2988-2994.

95. Imai A, Furui T, Shimokawa K, et al: Juvenile granulosa cell tumor in a 2-year-old infant: Report of a case complicated with ascites and acute respiratory distress. Gynecol Oncol 1992;46:397-400.

96. Imai A, Furui T, Tamaya T: Gynecologic tumors and symptoms in childhood and adolescence: 10-years' experience. Int J Gynecol Obstet 1994;5:227-234.

97. Inoue R, Kondo N, Motoyoshi F, et al: Chediak-Higashi syndrome: Report of a case with an ovarian tumor. Clin Genet 1991;39:316-318.

98. Issacs H Jr: Perinatal (congenital and neonatal) neoplasms: A report of 110 cases. Pediatr Pathol 1985;3:165-216.

99. Jabra AA, Fishman EK, Taylor GA: Primary ovarian tumors in the pediatric patient: CT evaluation. Clin Imaging 1993;17:199-203.

100. Jona JZ, Burchby K, Vitamvas G: Castration-sparing management of an adolescent with high bilateral cystic teratomas of the ovaries. J Pediatr Surg 1988;23:973-974.

101. Kalofonos HP, Karamouzis MV, Epenetos AA: Radio-immunoscintigraphy in patients with ovarian cancer. Acta Oncol 2001;40:549-557.

102. Kawai M, Kano T, Furuhashi Y, et al: Immature teratoma of the ovary. Gynecol Oncol 1991;40:133-137.

103. Kawai M, Kano T, Kikkawa F, et al: Seven tumor markers in benign and malignant germ cell tumors of the ovary. Gynecol Oncol 1992;45:248-253.

104. Kawakami K, Murata K, Kawaguchi N, et al: Hemorrhagic infarction of the diseased ovary: A common MR finding in two cases. Magn Reson Imaging 1993;11:595-597.

105. Kerner H, Gaton E, Czernobilsky B: Unusual ovarian, tubal and pelvic mesothelial inclusions in patients with endometriosis. Histopathology 1981;5:277-283.

106. Kier R, Smith RC, McCarthy SM: Value of lipid- and water-suppression MR images in distinguishing between blood and lipid within ovarian masses. Am J Res 1992;158:321-325.

107. Kodish ED: Testing children for cancer genes: The rule of earliest onset. J Pediatr 1999;135:390-395.

108. Koninckx PR, Meulman C, Demeyere S, et al: Suggestive evidence that pelvic endometriosis is a progressive disease, whereas deeply infiltrating endometriosis is associated with pelvic pain. Fertil Steril 1991;55:759-765.

109. Koninckx PR, Oosterlynck D, D'Hooghe T, et al: Deeply infiltrating endometriosis is a disease whereas mild endometriosis could be considered a non-disease. Ann N Y Acad Sci 1994;734:333-341.

110. Koulos JP, Hoffman JS, Steinhoff MM: Immature teratoma of the ovary. Gynecol Oncol 1989;34:46-49.

111. Kurman RJ, Norris HJ: Endodermal sinus tumor of the ovary: A clinical and pathologic analysis of 71 cases. Cancer 1976;38:2404-2419.

112. Lack EE, Young RH, Scully RE: Pathology of ovarian neoplasms in childhood and adolescence. Pathol Annu 1992; 27:281-356.

113. Lackman F, Carey MS, Kirk ME, et al: Surgery as sole treatment for serous borderline tumors of the ovary with non-invasive implants. Gynceol Oncol 2003;90:407-412.

114. Lappohn RE, Burger HG, Bouma J, et al: Inhibin as a marker for granulosa cell tumor. Acta Obstet Gynecol Scand 1992;71(Suppl 155):61-65.

115. Larsen WG, Felmar EA, Wallace ME, et al: Sertoli-Leydig cell tumor of the ovary: A rare cause of amenorrhea. Obstet Gynecol 1992;79:831-833.

116. LaVecchia C, Morris HB, Draper GJ: Malignant ovarian tumours in childhood in Britain, 1962-78. Br J Cancer 1983;48:363-374.

117. Lindfors O: Primary ovarian neoplasms in infants and children: A study of 81 cases diagnosed in Finland and Sweden. Ann Chir Gynaecol Fenn 1971;177(Suppl): 1-66.

118. Low LCK, Wang C, Leung A, et al: Undetectable levels of serum FSH immunoactivity and bioactivity in girls with sexual precocity due to ovarian cysts. Acta Paediatr 1994;83:623-626.

119. Mahour GH, Landing HB, Woolley MM: Teratomas in children: Clinicopathologic studies in 133 patients. Z Kinderchir 1978;23:365-380.

120. Mann JR, Pearson D, Barrett A, et al: Results of the United Kingdom Children's Cancer Study Group's germ cell tumor studies. Cancer 1989;63:1657-1667.

121. Marina NM, Cushing B, Giller R, et al: Complete surgical excision is effective treatment for children with immature teratomas with or without malignant elements: A Pediatric Oncology Group/Children's Cancer Group Intergroup Study. J Clin Oncol 1999;17:2137-2143.

122. Massad LS Jr, Hunter VJ, Szpak CA, et al: Epithelial ovarian tumors of low malignant potential. Obstet Gynecol 1991; 78:1027-1032.

123. McCarville MB, Hill DA, Miller BE, et al: Secondary ovarian neoplasms in children: Imaging features with histopathologic correlation. Pediatr Radiol 2001;31:358-364.

124. Meigs JV: Endometriosis. Ann Surg 1948;127:795-809.

125. Meizner I, Levy A, Katz M, et al: Fetal ovarian cysts: Prenatal ultrasonographic detection and postnatal evaluation and treatment. Am J Obstet Gynecol 1991;164:874-878.

126. Mena W, Krassikoff N, Philips JB III: Fused eyelids, airway anomalies, ovarian cysts, and digital abnormalities in siblings: A new autosomal recessive syndrome or a variant of Fraser syndrome? Am J Med Genet 1991;40:377-382.

127. Millar DM, Blake JM, Stringer DA, et al: Prepubertal ovarian cyst formation: 5 years' experience. Obstet Gynecol 1993; 81:434-438.

128. Mitelman F: Catalog of chromosomal aberrations. In Cancer, 4th ed. New York, Wiley-Liss, 1991.

129. Mittermayer C, Blaicher W, Grassauer D, et al: Fetal ovarian cysts: Development and neonatal outcome. Ultraschall Med 2003;24:21-26.

130. Modan B, Hartge P, Hirsh-Yechezkel G, et al: Parity, oral contraceptives, and the risk of ovarian cancer among carriers and noncarriers of a BRCA1 and BRCA2 mutation. N Engl J Med 2001;345:235-240.

131. Monk BJ, Nieberg R, Berek JS: Primary leiomyosarcoma of the ovary in a perimenarchal female. Gynecol Oncol 1993;48:389-393.

132. Moore DT: Ovarian epithelial tumor of low malignant potential in an adolescent. J Tenn Med Assoc 1992;85: 557-558.

133. Morice PCS, Camatte S, Hassan J, et al: Clinical outcomes and fertility after conservative treatment of borderline ovarian tumors. Fertil Steril 2001;75:92-96.

134. Morowitz M, Huff D, von Allmen D: Epithelial ovarian tumors in children: A retrospective analysis. J Pediatr Surg 2003;38:331-335.

135. Morris HB, LaVecchia C, Draper GJ: Malignant epithelial tumors of the ovary in childhood: A clinicopathological study of 13 cases in Great Britain 1962-1978. Gynecol Oncol 1984;19:290-297.

136. Müller J, Visfeldt J, Philip J, et al: Carcinoma in situ, gonadoblastoma, and early invasive neoplasia in a nine-year-old girl with 46,XY gonadal dysgenesis. APMIS 1992; 100:170-174.

137. Murty VV, Dmitrovsky E, Bosl GJ, et al: Nonrandom chromosome abnormalities in testicular and ovarian germ cell tumor lines. Cancer Genet Cytogenet 1990;50:67-73.

138. Nair R, Pai SK, Nair CN, et al: Malignant germ cell tumors in childhood. J Surg Oncol 1994;56:186-190.

139. Narod SA, Risch H, Moslehi R, et al: Oral contraceptives and the risk of hereditary ovarian cancer. N Engl J Med 1998;339:424-428.

140. Nishida M, Jimi S, Haji M, et al: Juvenile granulosa cell tumor in association with a high serum inhibin level. Gynecol Oncol 1991;40:90-94.

141. Nogales FF: Embryologic clues to human yolk sac tumors: A review. Int J Gynecol Pathol 1993;12:101-107.

142. Norris HJ, Jensen RD: Relative frequency of ovarian neoplasms in children and adolescents. Cancer 1972;30:713-719.

143. Norris HJ, Zirkin HJ, Benson WL: Immature (malignant) teratoma of the ovary: A clinical and pathologic study of 58 cases. Cancer 1976;37:2359-2372.

144. Olive DL, Hammond CB: Endometriosis: Pathogenesis and mechanisms of infertility. Postgrad Obstet Gynecol 1985;5:1-6.

145. Ortega JA, Siegel SE: Biologic markers in pediatric solid tumors. In Pizzo P, Poplack DG (eds): Principles and Practice of Pediatric Oncology, 2nd ed. Philadelphia, JB Lippincott, 1993, pp 179-194.

146. Ovarian cancer: Screening, treatment, and followup. NIH Consensus Statement 1994;12:1-30.

147. Pais RC, Kim TH, Zwiren GT, et al: Ovarian tumors in relapsing acute lymphoblastic leukemia: A review of 23 cases. J Pediatr Surg 1991;26:70-74.

148. Paladini D, Di Meglio A, Esposito A, et al: Ultrasonic features of an ovarian cystohemangioma: A case report. Eur J Obstet Gynecol Reprod Biol 1991;40:239-240.

149. Parham DM, Bugg FM, Pratt CB: Carcinomas, adenomas, precursor lesions, and second malignancies. In Parham DM (ed): Pediatric Neoplasia: Morphology and Biology. Philadelphia, Lippincott-Raven, 1996, pp 385-390.

150. Patel MD, Feldstein VA, Lipson SD, et al: Cystic teratomas of the ovary: Diagnostic value of sonography. AJR Am J Roentgenol 1998;171:1061-1065.

151. Perkins AC, Powell MC, Wastie ML, et al: A prospective evaluation of OC125 and magnetic resonance imaging in patients with ovarian carcinoma. Eur J Nucl Med 1990;16:311-316.

152. Perlin E, Engeler JE, Edson M, et al: The value of serial measurement of both human chorionic gonadotropin and alpha-fetoprotein for monitoring germ cell tumors. Cancer 1976;37:215-219.

153. Perlman EJ, Cushing B, Hawkins E, et al: Cytogenetic analysis of childhood endodermal sinus tumors: A Pediatric Oncology Group study. Pediatr Pathol 1994;14:695-708.

154. Perlman EJ, Fritsch MK: The female reproductive system. In Stocker JT, Dehner LP (eds): Pediatric Pathology, 2nd ed. Philadelphia, Lippincott Williams & Wilkins, 2001, pp 920-938.

155. Peters H, Byskov AG, Grinsted J: Follicular growth in fetal and prepubertal ovaries in humans and other primates. Clin Endocrinol Metab 1978;7:469-485.

156. Peters H, Himelstein-Braun R, Faber M: The normal development of the ovary in childhood. Acta Endocrinol 1976;82:617-630.

157. Pinkerton CR, Broadbent V, Horwich A, et al: "JEB"—a carboplatin based regimen for malignant germ cell tumours in children. Br J Cancer 1990;62:257-262.

158. Piver MS, Patton T: Ovarian cancer in children. Semin Surg Oncol 1986;2:163-169.

159. Plantaz D, Flamant F, Vassal G, et al: Juvenile granulosa cell tumor in children: A clinical study of 39 cases [abstract]. Med Pediatr Oncol 1991;19:396.

160. Pliskow S: Endodermal sinus tumor of the ovary: Review of 10 cases. South Med J 1993;86:187-189.

161. Podczaski E, Kaminski PF, Pees RC, et al: Peutz-Jeghers syndrome with ovarian sex cord tumor with annular tubules and cervical adenoma malignum. Gynecol Oncol 1991;42:74-78.

162. Powell JL, Johnson NA, Bailey CL, et al: Management of advanced juvenile granulosa cell tumor of the ovary. Gynecol Oncol 1993;48:119-123.

163. Powell JL, McAfee RD, McCoy RC, et al: Uterine and ovarian conservation in advanced small cell carcinoma of the ovary. Obstet Gynecol 1998;91:846-848.

164. Raafat F, Klys H, Rylance G: Juvenile granulosa cell tumor. Pediatr Pathol 1990;10:617-623.

165. Ranney B: Etiology, prevention and inhibition of endometriosis. Clin Obstet Gynecol 1980;23:875-883.

166. Robboy SJ, Scully RE: Ovarian teratoma with glial implants on the peritoneum: An analysis of 12 cases. Hum Pathol 1970;1:643-653.

167. Rogers PC, Olson TA, Cullen JW, et al: Treatment of children and adolescents with stage II testicular and stages I and II ovarian malignant germ cell tumors: A Pediatric Intergroup study—Pediatric Oncology Group 9048 and Children's Cancer Group 8891. J Clin Oncol 2004;22:3563-3569.

168. Roth LM, Eglen DE: Gonadoblastoma: Immunohistochemical and ultrastructural observations. Int J Gynecol Pathol 1989;8:72-81.

169. Rottem S, Levit N, Thaler I, et al: Classification of ovarian lesions by high frequency transvaginal sonography. J Clin Ultrasound 1990;18:359-363.

170. Rotterdam ESHRE/ASRM, Sponsored PCOS Consensus Workshop Group: Revised 2003 consensus on diagnosis criteria and long-term health risks related to polycystic ovary syndrome. Fertil Steril 2004;81:19-25.

171. Sakala EP, Leon ZA, Rouse GA: Management of antenatally diagnosed fetal ovarian cysts. Obstet Gynecol Surv 1991;46:407-414.

172. Samaniego F, Rodriquez E, Houldsworth J, et al: Cytogenetic and molecular analysis of human male germ cell tumors: Chromosome 12 abnormalities and gene amplification. Genes Chromosomes Cancer 1990;4:239-300.

173. Sanfilippo JS, Wakim NG, Schikler K, et al: Endometriosis in association with uterine anomaly. Am J Obstet Gynecol 1986;154:39-43.

174. SanMarco L, Londero F, Stefanutti V, et al: Ovarian leiomyoma. Clin Exp Obstet Gynecol 1991;18:145-148.

175. Sasaki H, Furusato M, Kiyokawa T, et al: Prognostic significance of histopathological subtypes in state I pure yolk sac tumors of the ovary. Br J Cancer 1994;69:529-536.

176. Saxman SB, Finch D, Gonin R, et al: Long term follow-up of a phase III study of three versus four cycles of bleomycin, etoposide, and cisplatin in favorable-prognosis germ-cell tumors: The Indiana University experience. J Clin Oncol 1998;16:702-706.

177. Schiller W: Mesonephroma ovarii. Am J Cancer 1939;35:1-21.

178. Scholz PM, Key L, Filston HC: Large ovarian cyst causing cecal perforation in a newborn infant. J Pediatr Surg 1982;17:91-92.

179. Schwobel MG, Stauffer UG: Surgical treatment of ovarian tumors in childhood. Prog Pediatr Surg 1991;26:112-123.

180. Scully RE: Gonadoblastoma: A gonadal tumor related to the dysgerminoma (seminoma) and capable of sex-hormone production. Cancer 1953;6:455-463.

181. Scully RE: Gonadoblastoma: A review of 74 cases. Cancer 1970;25:1340-1356.
182. Scully RE: Weekly clinicopathological exercises: Case 22-1982. N Engl J Med 1982;306:1348-1355.
183. Scully RE: Small cell carcinoma of hypercalcemic type. Int J Gynecol Pathol 1993;2:148-152.
184. Scully RE, Young RH, Clement PB: Atlas of Tumor Pathology, Tumors of the Ovary, Maldeveloped Gonads, Fallopian Tube and Broad Ligaments, 3rd ser, fascicle 23. Washington, DC, American Registry of Pathology, Armed Forces Institute of Pathology, 1998.
185. Seeber B, Driscoll D: Hereditary breast and ovarian cancer syndrome: Should we test adolescents? J Pediatr Adolesc Gynecol 2004;17:161-167.
186. Shakfeh SM, Woodruff JD: Primary ovarian sarcomas: Report of 46 cases and review of the literature. Obstet Gynecol Surv 1987;42:331-349.
187. Sherman ME, Mink PJ, Curtis R, et al: Survival among women with borderline ovarian tumors and ovarian carcinoma: A population-based analysis. Cancer 2004;100:1045-1052.
188. Shulman LP, Muram D, Marina N, et al: Lack of heritability in ovarian germ cell malignancies. Am J Obstet Gynecol 1994;170:1803-1808.
189. Siegel MJ, Surratt JT: Pediatric gynecologic imaging. Obstet Gynecol Clin North Am 1992;19:103-126.
190. Skinner MA, Schlatter MG, Heifetz SA, et al: Ovarian neoplasms in children. Arch Surg 1993;128:849-854.
191. Speleman F, DePotter C, Dal Cin P, et al: i(12p) in a malignant ovarian tumor. Cancer Genet Cytogenet 1990;45:49-53.
192. Steinkampf MP, Hammond KR, Blackwell RE: Hormonal treatment of functional ovarian cysts: A randomized, prospective study. Fertil Steril 1990;54:775-777.
193. Stern JK, Buscema J, Rosenshein NB, et al: Spontaneous rupture of benign cystic teratomas. Obstet Gynecol 1981;57:363-366.
194. Stevens SK, Hricak H, Stern JL: Ovarian lesions: Detection and characterization with gadolinium-enhanced MR imaging at 1.5T[1]. Radiology 1991;181:481-488.
195. Stickland JL: Ovarian cysts in neonates, children and adolescents. Curr Opin Obstet Gynecol 2002;14:459-465.
196. Suijkerbuijk RF, van de Veen Y, van Echten J, et al: Demonstration of the genuine i(12p) character of the standard marker chromosome of testicular germ cell tumors and identification of further chromosome 12 aberrations by competitive in situ hybridization. Am J Hum Genet 1991;489:269-401.
197. Surratt JT, Siegel MJ: Imaging of pediatric ovarian masses. Radiographics 1991;11:533-548.
198. Sutton CJ, Ewen SP, Whitelaw N, et al: Prospective, randomized, double-blind, controlled trial of laser laparoscopy in the treatment of pelvic pain associated with minimal, mild, and moderate endometriosis. Fertil Steril 1994;62:696-700.
199. Swanson SA, Norris HJ, Kelsten ML, et al: DNA content of juvenile granulosa tumors determined by flow cytometry. Int J Gynecol Pathol 1990;9:101-109.
200. Talerman A, Haije WG, Baggerman L: Serum alpha-feto protein (AFP) in patients with germ cell tumors of the gonads and extragonadal sites: Correlation between endodermal sinus (yolk sac) tumor and raised serum AFP. Cancer 1980;46:380-385.
201. Tanaka Y, Sasaki Y, Nishihira H, et al: Ovarian juvenile granulosa cell tumor associated with Maffucci's syndrome. Am J Clin Pathol 1992;97:523-527.
202. Tangir J, Zelterman D, Wenging M, et al: Reproductive function after conservative surgery and chemotherapy for malignant germ cell tumors of the ovary. Obstet Gynecol 2003;101:251-257.

203. Tapper D, Lack E: Teratomas in infancy and childhood, a 54 year experience at the Children's Hospital Medical Center. Ann Surg 1983;198:398-410.
204. Teilum G: Endodermal sinus tumor of the ovary and testis. Cancer 1959;12:1092-1105.
205. Teilum G: Classification of endodermal sinus tumor (meloblastoma vitellinum) and so-called embryonal carcinoma of the ovary. Acta Pathol Microbiol Scand 1965;64:407-429.
206. Teilum G: Special Tumors of Ovary and Testis, 2nd ed. Copenhagen, Munksgaard, 1976.
207. Teilum G, Albrechtsen R, Norgaard-Pedersen B: The histogenetic-embryologic basis for reappearance of AFP in endodermal sinus tumors (yolk sac tumors) and teratomas. Acta Pathol Microbiol Scand 1975;83:80-86.
208. Templeman C, Blenshevsky A, Fallat ME, et al: Noninflammatory ovarian masses in girls and young women. Obstet Gynecol 2000;96:229-233.
209. Templeman CL, Hertweck SP, Scheetz JP, et al: The management of mature cystic teratomas in children and adolescents: A retrospective analysis. Hum Reprod 2000;15:2669-2672.
210. Templeman CL, Reynolds AM, Hertweck SP, et al: Laparoscopic management of neonatal ovarian cysts. J Am Assoc Gynecol Laparosc 2000;7:401-404.
211. Thurlbeck W, Scully RE: Solid teratoma of the ovary: A clinico-pathologic analysis of 9 cases. Cancer 1960;13:801-811.
212. Togashi K: Ovarian cancer: The clinical role of US, CT, and MRI. Eur Radiol 2003;13(Suppl 4):L87-L104.
213. Troche V, Hernandez E: Neoplasia arising in dysgenetic gonads: A review. Obstet Gynecol Surv 1986;41:74-79.
214. Vaitukaitis JK, Braunstein GC, Ross GT: A radioimmunoassay which specifically measures human chorionic gonadotropin in the presence of human luteinizing hormone. Am J Obstet Gynecol 1972;113:751-758.
215. Van Voorhis BJ, Schwaiger J, Syrop CH, et al: Early diagnosis of ovarian torsion by color Doppler ultrasonography. Fertil Steril 1992;58:215-217.
216. Vercellini P, Bocciolone L, Vendola N, et al: Peritoneal endometriosis: Morphologic appearance in women with chronic pelvic pain. J Reprod Med 1991;36:533-536.
217. Vergote IB: Surgery for gynecologic malignancies. Curr Opin Oncol 1993;5:877-884.
218. Warner BW, Kuhn JC, Barr LL: Conservative management of large ovarian cysts in children: The value of serial pelvic ultrasonography. Surgery 1992;112:749-755.
219. Weinblatt M, Kochen J: An unusual family cancer syndrome manifested in young siblings. Cancer 1991;68:1068-1070.
220. Weinblatt ME, Ortega JA: Treatment of children with dysgerminoma of the ovary. Cancer 1982;49:2608-2611.
221. Weinstein RS, Kuszak JR, Kluskens LF: P-glycoproteins in pathology: The multidrug resistance gene family in humans. Hum Pathol 1990;21:34-48.
222. Wertz DC, Fanos JH, Reilly PR: Genetic testing for children and adolescents: Who decides? JAMA 1994;272:875-881.
223. Weyl-Ben Arush M, Oslander L: Ollier's disease associated with ovarian Sertoli-Leydig cell tumor and breast adenoma. Am J Pediatr Hematol Oncol 1991;13:49-51.
224. Wierman ME, Beardsworth DE, Mansfield MJ, et al: Puberty without gonadotropins: A unique mechanism of sexual development. N Engl J Med 1985;312:65-72.
225. Williams SD, Birch R, Einhorn LH, et al: Treatment of disseminated germ cell tumors with cisplatin, bleomycin, and either vinblastine or etoposide. N Engl J Med 1987;316:1435-1440.

226. Williams SD, Blessing JA, Liao SY, et al: Adjuvant therapy of ovarian germ cell tumors with cisplatin, etoposide, and bleomycin: A trial of the Gynecologic Oncology Group. J Clin Oncol 1994;12:701-706.

227. Williams SD, Blessing J, Slayton R, et al: Ovarian germ cell tumors: Adjuvant trials of the Gynecologic Oncology Group [abstract 584]. Proc Am Soc Clin Oncol 1989; 8:150.

228. Williams SD, Gershenson DM, Horowitz CJ, et al: Ovarian germ cell and stromal tumors. In Hoskins W, Perez CA, Young RC (eds): Principles and Practice of Gynecologic Oncology. Philadelphia, JB Lippincott, 1992, pp 715-730.

229. Wilson E, Vuitch F, Carr B: Laparoscopic removal of dysgenetic gonads containing a gonadoblastoma in a patient with Swyer syndrome. Obstet Gynecol 1992;79: 842-844.

230. Wu JT, Book L, Sudar K: Serum a-fetoprotein (AFP) levels in normal infants. Pediatr Res 1981;15:50-52.

231. Yamamoto K, Akiyama H, Maruyama T, et al: Granulocytic sarcoma of the ovary in patients with acute myelogenous leukemia. Am J Hematol 1991;38:223-225.

232. Yanai-Inbar ISR: Relation of ovarian dermoid cysts and immature teratomas: An analysis of 350 cases of immature teratoma and 10 cases of dermoid cyst with microscopic foci of immature tissue. Int J Gynecol Pathol 1987;6: 203-212.

233. Young JL Jr, Wu XC, Roffers SD, et al: Ovarian cancer in children and young adults in the United States 1992-1997. Cancer 2003;97(10 Suppl):2694-2700.

234. Young RH: Ovarian tumors other than those of surface epithelial-stromal type. Hum Pathol 1991;22: 763-775.

235. Young RH, Clement PB, Scully RE: Calcified thecomas in young women: A report of four cases. Int J Gynecol Pathol 1988;7:343-350.

236. Young RH, Dickersin GR, Scully RE: Juvenile granulosa cell tumor of the ovary: A clinicopathological analysis of 125 cases. Am J Surg Pathol 1984;8:575-596.

237. Young RH, Eichhorn JH, Dickersin GR, et al: Ovarian involvement by the intraabdominal desmoplastic small round cell tumor with divergent differentiation: A report of three cases. Hum Pathol 1992;23:454-464.

238. Young RH, Kozakewich HPW, Scully RE: Metastatic ovarian tumors in children: A report of 14 cases and review of the literature. Int J Gynecol Pathol 1993;12:8-19.

239. Zanetta GRS, Rota S, Chiari S, et al: Behaviour of borderline tumors with particular interest to persistence, recurrence, and progression to invasive carcinoma: A prospective study. J Clin Oncol 2001;19:2658-2664.

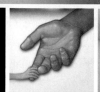

Chapter 37

Testicular Tumors

Hsi-Yang Wu and Eugene Wiener

Testicular tumors in prepubertal boys differ from those in postpubertal men in both pathology and tendency for metastasis. This difference allows testis-sparing procedures to be applied more liberally in younger patients but requires careful evaluation of pubertal development in older patients. The peak incidence for testicular tumors is 2 to 4 years of age.[13] These tumors represent 1% of all pediatric solid tumors and are rare in the African American and Asian populations. Testis tumors that arise later in life are associated with a history of cryptorchidism and mixed gonadal dysgenesis. The risk of malignancy arising from an undescended testis after puberty is 1% in inguinal testes and 5% in abdominal testes.[6] The most common pathology in a testis that remains undescended is seminoma, whereas a testis that has been surgically placed in the scrotum is more likely to have embryonal or teratocarcinoma pathology. Orchiopexy does not reduce the incidence of testicular cancer.[2] Because prepubertal testis biopsies rarely detect tumors in undescended testes, the pathologic finding of normal testicular parenchyma does not preclude the later development of tumor.

CLINICAL PRESENTATION

A nontender, solid scrotal mass is the usual presenting sign of a testicular tumor. Often a history of trauma is volunteered, but this likely alerted the boy or his parents to a previously unrecognized painless, enlarged testis, rather than being the cause. The differential diagnosis includes testicular torsion and epididymitis, but in the absence of pain, dysuria, and inflammation, tumor is more likely. However, it is not unusual for a patient with a tumor to be mistakenly operated on for suspected torsion. Physical examination should differentiate between epididymal swelling (spermatocele or epididymitis) and testicular swelling (orchitis or tumor). There may be an associated hydrocele. Transillumination does not rule out the presence of a tumor, because a tumor and a hydrocele can coexist. Stromal testicular tumors can present with precocious puberty (Leydig cell) or gynecomastia (Sertoli cell).

DIAGNOSIS

Imaging

If the testis cannot be palpated owing to a tense hydrocele or if the examination is unclear, scrotal ultrasonography is helpful in determining the architecture and echogenicity of the testis. The normal testis has a homogeneous texture, whereas a tumor has a heterogeneous texture in comparison to the normal testicular parenchyma next to it. If there are cystic areas in the involved testis, a teratoma or epidermoid cyst is the likely diagnosis, and testis-sparing surgery should be considered. The presence of multiple small calcifications (microlithiasis) is of unclear significance. It has been found in association with testis tumor in adult men. If microlithiasis is found in the contralateral (presumably normal) testis, follow-up imaging is warranted owing to the possibility of the later formation of a testis tumor.[11]

A metastatic evaluation is performed after the diagnosis of a malignant tumor is established. A chest computed tomography (CT) scan should be obtained because metastases from yolk sac tumors are more likely to occur in the lung than the retroperitoneum. A CT scan of the abdomen and pelvis to look for retroperitoneal nodal involvement is performed postoperatively.

Tumor Markers

Serum alpha fetoprotein (AFP) and β-human chorionic gonadotropin (β-HCG) levels should be obtained preoperatively in all patients with suspected testis tumor. Although elevated levels are occasionally useful in making the diagnosis, they are most beneficial in follow-up for recurrence. AFP (a marker for yolk sac tumors) is normally elevated in newborns until 8 months of age[27] and in patients with liver dysfunction, so serial determinations after orchiectomy are needed. The half-life of AFP is 5 days, so the level should be normal 25 days after orchiectomy if the entire tumor was removed. β-HCG is occasionally elevated in seminoma and more commonly in choriocarcinoma, both of which are rare

TABLE 37-1 American Academy of Pediatrics Testis Tumor Registry, 2002

Tumor Type	Percentage
Yolk sac	62
Teratoma	23
Gonadal stromal	4
Epidermoid cyst	3
Juvenile granulosa	3
Sertoli cell	3
Leydig cell	1
Gonadoblastoma	1

in the prepubertal population. Its half-life is 1 day, so it should return to normal by 1 week postoperatively.

STAGING AND CLASSIFICATION

Table 37-1 lists the distribution of pathologies in the 2002 American Academy of Pediatrics Testis Tumor Registry.[20] The predominance of yolk sac tumors may reflect a reporting bias; in many single-institution studies teratomas are more common, but they are often not reported to registries because they are benign.[1,14,23,26] Table 37-2 shows the staging system for testis tumor used by the Children's Oncology Group (COG).

TREATMENT BY TUMOR TYPE

Teratoma

Teratomas are derived from ectoderm, mesoderm, and endoderm and therefore can have solid and cystic components. Epidermoid cysts can be considered monophasic teratomas, in that they are derived only from ectoderm. Before puberty, teratoma can be managed with a testis-sparing approach[20,21,24] because it is always benign, even when the pathology shows immature elements.[8] In patients

TABLE 37-2 Children's Oncology Group Staging for Prepubertal Testis Tumor (from AGCT0132)

Stage	Description
I	Limited to testis, completely resected by high inguinal orchiectomy; no clinical, radiographic, or histologic evidence of disease beyond the testes; patients with normal or unknown tumor markers at diagnosis must have a negative ipsilateral retroperitoneal node sampling to confirm stage I disease if radiographic studies demonstrate lymph nodes >2 cm
II	Transscrotal biopsy, microscopic disease in scrotum or high in spermatic cord (≤5 cm from proximal end)
III	Retroperitoneal lymph node involvement, but no visceral or extra-abdominal involvement; lymph nodes >4 cm by computed tomography or >2 cm and <4 cm with biopsy proof
IV	Distant metastases, including liver

entering puberty, teratoma should be treated as it is in adult patients, with radical inguinal orchiectomy, owing to its more malignant behavior.

If the AFP level is elevated relative to age-adjusted levels, one should assume that yolk sac elements are present and not perform testis-sparing surgery. Scrotal ultrasonography showing internal calcifications and a heterogeneous mass in the testis, in association with a normal AFP level, suggests a teratoma. The testis is approached through an inguinal incision, and after vascular control has been obtained at the level of the internal inguinal ring, the teratoma can be shelled out from the testis; a frozen section can confirm the pathology.[21] Even when the teratoma significantly compresses normal testicular parenchyma, postoperative ultrasound studies usually show good recovery of testicular tissue, with presumably preserved function.[14]

There are two different approaches to the use of frozen sections. The classic approach is to obtain a frozen section to confirm teratoma pathology and that there are no maturation changes in the neighboring parenchyma.[20] Others have suggested that the combination of ultrasound findings and normal AFP level should be sufficient to make the diagnosis of teratoma preoperatively. They also recommend that any patient with pubertal development should be excluded from testis-sparing surgery.[14,23] Most prepubertal boys with teratomas have good gonadal preservation after testis-sparing surgery.

Germ Cell Tumor

Sixty percent of prepubertal testis tumors are germ cell tumors. The yolk sac tumor in children manifests a different pattern of metastasis than in adults. In children, hematogenous metastases to the lung occur in 20% of cases, whereas spread to the retroperitoneal nodes occurs in only 4% to 6% of cases; in adults, spread is usually to the retroperitoneal nodes. Most yolk sac tumors present during the first 2 years of life. The yolk sac tumor is managed with radical inguinal orchiectomy. The pathology reveals Schiller-Duval bodies. If the patient is stage I (no chest metastasis or retroperitoneal adenopathy, with appropriate drop in AFP), no chemotherapy is necessary.[20] The recommended surveillance program is shown in Figure 37-1. Patients with stage II disease (transscrotal orchiectomy, microscopic disease, or persistently elevated AFP) receive platinum-based chemotherapy (cisplatin, etoposide, bleomycin) and no radiation therapy.

Whether children who have undergone transscrotal orchiectomy also require hemiscrotectomy is controversial,[22] because it now appears that local therapy does not change the outcome if chemotherapy is given in adults, although no similar study has been performed in children.[7] The current COG protocol no longer requires hemiscrotectomy in this situation. Patients with stage II disease with persistent retroperitoneal mass or persistent elevated serum AFP levels after chemotherapy should have retroperitoneal lymph node dissection (RPLND). If viable tumor is found, the chemotherapy regimen is changed. Those with stage III (>2 cm retroperitoneal lymph node) and stage IV disease (metastasis) receive chemotherapy,

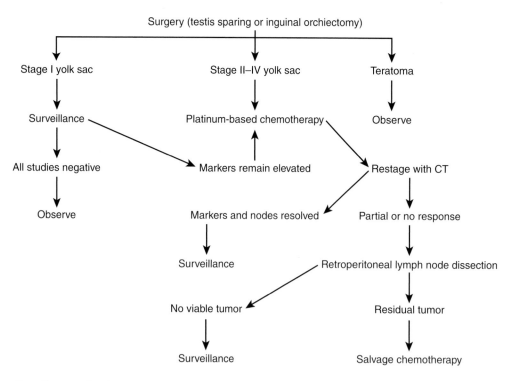

Figure 37–1 Algorithm for surveillance of germ cell tumors. CT, computed tomography. (Adapted from POG 9048/CCSG 8891.)

Surveillance protocol:
Markers every month x 1 year, then every 2 months x 1 year.
Chest radiograph every 2 months x 1 year, then every 3 months x 1 year.
CT every 3 months x 1 year, then every 6 months x 1 year.

followed by RPLND for any residual mass. The overall survival for all stages approaches 100%.

The rare extragonadal germ cell tumor (retroperitoneal and abdominal) is best treated with initial biopsy (complete resection if possible), chemotherapy, and re-resection of residual tumor. Event free-survival is 83% at 6 years.[4]

Gonadal Stromal Tumor

Leydig cell tumors are the most common gonadal stromal tumors of adults and children.[25] The classic triad of findings in Leydig cell tumors is precocious puberty (10%), unilateral testis mass (90%), and elevated 17-ketosteroid. Unlike precocious puberty induced by a pituitary lesion (high luteinizing hormone [LH], follicle-stimulating hormone [FSH], and testosterone levels), Leydig cell tumors have low LH and FSH and high testosterone levels. The precocious puberty may not resolve after resection, but this does not necessarily indicate the presence of residual tumor. Nodules induced by congenital adrenal hyperplasia tend to be bilateral (80%) and also have low LH and FSH and high testosterone. These nodules are suppressed with dexamethasone or adrenocorticotropic hormone administration and regress when treated with glucocorticoids. The Reinke crystal, which is pathognomonic for Leydig cell tumors in adults, is rarely found in children. Leydig cell tumors can also be managed using a testis-sparing approach, similar to teratoma, because they are benign in children.[12,24,25]

Sertoli cell tumors are rare in children, usually benign, and safely treated with testis-sparing procedures.[17,24,25]

They can present with gynecomastia. Follow-up CT scans of the retroperitoneum are necessary for at least 2 years because the pathology does not always predict outcome. Although these tumors are usually benign, the frequency of patients with retroperitoneal node involvement is not known, because the entire experience with malignant behavior in prepubertal patients is limited to a few case reports.[25]

Gonadoblastoma

Gonadoblastoma is classically encountered in patients with mixed gonadal dysgenesis (45,X/46,XY) or intersex with dysgenetic gonads in association with a Y chromosome in the karyotype. The tumors are small, bilateral in 33% of cases, malignant in 10%, and usually present after puberty. The pathology includes germ cells and stroma cells. Although it is a low-grade malignancy, the nonpalpable gonad is managed with early gonadectomy because it can degenerate into seminoma later in life.

Previously, it was recommended that both gonads be removed in patients with mixed gonadal dysgenesis.[9] The management of these tumors has become more complicated with the realization that neonatal testosterone imprints the brain; therefore, bilateral gonadectomy and rearing as a female may not correspond with the eventual gender role. If it is elected to leave a gonad in the scrotum, one suggestion is to perform annual scrotal examinations and ultrasonography until patients complete puberty, and to perform testis biopsies looking for testicular carcinoma in situ at the beginning and end of puberty.[15]

Secondary Tumor

Secondary tumors of the testis are usually due to lymphoma or leukemia and appear hypoechoic on ultrasonography. Although it was once common practice to biopsy the testes of patients who were completing chemotherapy for lymphoma and leukemia, no survival advantage has been shown, so this is no longer routinely performed.[16] If a patient has an enlarged testis after treatment for lymphoma or leukemia, a biopsy of the affected testis should be taken, and testicular radiation given. Additional chemotherapy should also be given, because the presence of tumor in a sanctuary site such as the testis suggests residual disease elsewhere.

Paratesticular rhabdomyosarcoma is discussed in detail in Chapter 32.

TECHNIQUE

Testis-sparing surgery is generally performed through an inguinal incision. The testis is delivered into the incision, and a Penrose drain is placed around the cord at the level of the internal inguinal ring to occlude the vessels. The tunica vaginalis of the testis is opened directly over the mass. Sometimes intraoperative ultrasonography is helpful in localizing the tumor if it is deep in the parenchyma. The edge of the knife blade is used to shell out the tumor; this preserves the neighboring parenchyma, which the pathologist needs to examine to ensure that pubertal maturation has not occurred. Hemostasis is accomplished with finely controlled bipolar cautery. The tunica vaginalis is closed with absorbable suture and replaced in the scrotum.

A radical orchiectomy is performed by high ligation of all cord structures at the level of the internal ring. If the mass is too large to mobilize from the scrotum, the inguinal incision should be lengthened to the superior aspect of the scrotum to avoid tumor rupture.

RPLND can be performed through a transabdominal, thoracoabdominal, or laparoscopic approach. The procedures are based on the dissections originally designed for adult testicular tumors.[10] The most common sites for lymph node metastases in instances of right-sided tumors are the interaortocaval and paracaval nodes, whereas left-sided tumors tend to spread to the para-aortic and interaortocaval nodes. The boundaries of the dissection depend on the initial stage of the tumor. If the tumor is stage II, a modified unilateral template may be used (Figs. 37-2 and 37-3). If the tumor is stage III or IV, a bilateral dissection is required (Fig. 37-4). The nodal packets

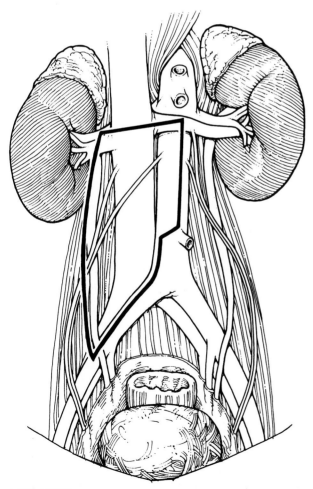

Figure 37-2 Right modified nerve-sparing retroperitoneal lymph node dissection template. (From Marshall FF [ed]: Textbook of Operative Urology. Philadelphia, WB Saunders, 1996, pp 368-369.)

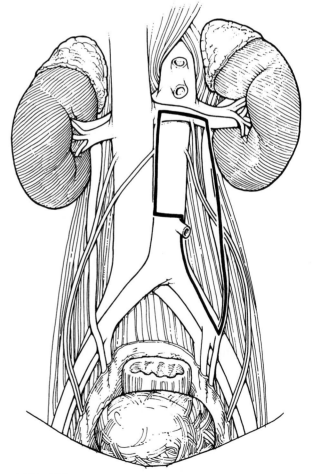

Figure 37-3 Left modified nerve-sparing retroperitoneal lymph node dissection template. (From Marshall FF [ed]: Textbook of Operative Urology. Philadelphia, WB Saunders, 1996, pp 368-369.)

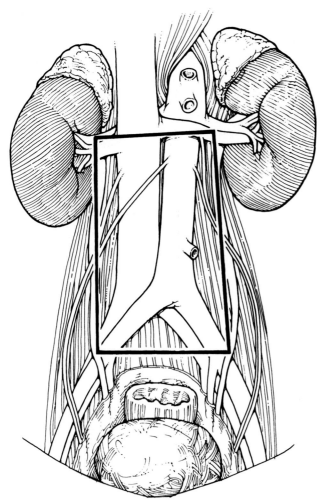

Figure 37–4 Template for full bilateral retroperitoneal lymph node dissection. (From Marshall FF [ed]: Textbook of Operative Urology. Philadelphia, WB Saunders, 1996, pp 368-369.)

are split over the great vessels, and the sympathetic ganglia are preserved as they course over the iliac veins to preserve ejaculation. Laparoscopic RPLND achieves a similar dissection using five transabdominal ports. Because the experience in adult patients has been limited to stage I and small residual masses in stage II tumors,[3,18] the use of laparoscopic RPLND in children should probably be limited to small stage II tumors.

COMPLICATIONS

Infertility and testicular failure are two long-term complications of treatment. Whereas adult patients with testis tumors have the option of pretreatment sperm banking, this is not possible for prepubertal boys. Survivors of childhood male genital tumors are only 0.45 times as likely as controls to be fertile.[5] If the sympathetic nerves are sacrificed during RPLND, loss of ejaculation will occur. Alkylating agents such as cyclophosphamide tend to affect sperm count the most but are not routinely used

for testis tumors. Leydig cells tend to be more resistant to chemotherapy, and androgen replacement is usually not necessary.[19]

SUMMARY

Testis-sparing surgery should be considered when the preoperative evaluation suggests that the pathology will be a non–germ cell tumor in a prepubertal boy. If yolk sac pathology is suspected based on an elevated AFP level, radical orchiectomy and treatment based on postoperative staging result in excellent survival outcomes.

REFERENCES

1. Andrassy RJ, Copron C, Ritchey M: Testicular tumors. In O'Neill JA, Rowe MI, Grosfeld JL, et al (eds): Pediatric Surgery, 5th ed. Philadelphia, WB Saunders, 1998, p 542.
2. Batata MA, Whitmore WF, Chu FCH, et al: Cryptorchidism and testicular cancer. J Urol 1980;124:382.
3. Bhayani SB, Ong A, Oh WK, et al: Laparoscopic retroperitoneal lymph node dissection for clinical stage I non-seminomatous germ cell testicular cancer: A long-term update. Urology 2003;62:324.
4. Billmire D, Vinocur C, Rescorla F, et al: Malignant retroperitoneal and abdominal germ cell tumors: An intergroup study. J Pediatr Surg 2003;38:315.
5. Byrne J, Fears TR, Gail MH, et al: Effects of treatment on fertility in long-term survivors of testicular cancer. N Engl J Med 1987;3178:1315.
6. Campbell HE: Incidence of malignant growth of the undescended testicle: A critical and statistical study. Arch Surg 1942;44:353.
7. Capelouto CC, Clark PE, Ransil BJ, et al: A review of scrotal violation in testicular cancer: Is adjuvant local therapy necessary? J Urol 1995;153:981.
8. Carney JA, Thompson DP, Johnson CL, et al: Teratomas in children: Clinical and pathologic aspects. J Pediatr Surg 1972;7:271.
9. Donahoe PK, Crawford JD, Hendren WH: Mixed gonadal dysgenesis, pathogenesis, and management. J Pediatr Surg 1979;14:287.
10. Donohue JP, Foster RS, Rowland RG, et al: Nerve-sparing retroperitoneal lymphadenectomy with preservation of ejaculation. J Urol 1990;144:287.
11. Furness PD III, Husmann DA, Brock JW III, et al: Multi-institutional study of testicular microlithiasis in childhood: A benign or premalignant condition? J Urol 1998;160:1151.
12. Konrad D, Schoenle EJ: Ten-year follow-up in a boy with Leydig cell tumor after selective surgery. Horm Res 1999;51:96.
13. Li FP, Fraumeni JF Jr: Testicular cancers in children: Epidemiologic characteristics. J Natl Cancer Inst 1972;48:1575.
14. Metcalfe PD, Farivar-Mosheni H, Farhat W, et al: Pediatric testicular tumors: Contemporary incidence and efficacy of testicular preserving surgery. J Urol 2003;170:2412.
15. Muller J, Ritzen EM, Ivarsson SA, et al: Management of males with 45,X/46,XY gonadal dysgenesis. Horm Res 1999;52:11.
16. Nachman J, Palmer NF, Sather HN, et al: Open-wedge testicular biopsy in childhood acute lymphoblastic leukemia after two years of maintenance therapy: Diagnostic accuracy and influence on outcome—a report from Children's Cancer Study Group. Blood 1990;75:1051.

17. Nonomura K, Koyama T, Kakizaki H, et al: Testicular-sparing surgery for the prepubertal testicular tumor: Experience of two cases with large cell calcifying Sertoli cell tumors. Eur Urol 2001;40:699.

18. Palese MA, Su LM, Kavoussi LR: Laparoscopic retroperitoneal lymph node dissection after chemotherapy. Urology 2002;60:130.

19. Relander T, Cavallin-Stahl E, Garwicz S, et al: Gonadal and sexual function in men treated for childhood cancer. Med Pediatr Oncol 2000;34:52.

20. Ross JH, Rybicki L, Kay R: Clinical behavior and a contemporary management algorithm for prepubertal testis tumors: A summary of the prepubertal testis tumor registry. J Urol 2002;168:1675.

21. Rushton HG, Belman AB, Sesterhenn I, et al: Testicular sparing surgery for prepubertal teratoma of the testis: A clinical and pathological study. J Urol 1990;144:726.

22. Schlatter M, Rescorla F, Giller R, et al: Excellent outcome in patients with stage I germ cell tumors of the testes: A study of the Children's Cancer Group/Pediatric Oncology Group. J Pediatr Surg 2003;38:319.

23. Shukla AR, Woodard C, Carr MC, et al: Experience with testis sparing surgery for testicular teratoma. J Urol 2004;171:161.

24. Sugita Y, Clarnette TD, Cooke-Yarborough C, et al: Testicular and paratesticular tumours in children: 30 years' experience. Aust N Z J Surg 1999;69:505.

25. Thomas JC, Ross JH, Kay R: Stromal testis tumors in children: A report from the Prepubertal Testis Tumor Registry. J Urol 2001;166:2338.

26. Walsh C, Rushton HG: Diagnosis and management of teratomas and epidermoid cysts. Urol Clin North Am 2000; 27:509.

27. Wu JT, Book L, Sudar K: Serum alpha fetoprotein (AFP) levels in normal infants. Pediatr Res 1981;15:50.

Chapter 38

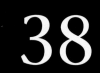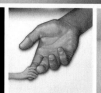

Adrenal Tumors

Stanley. T. Lau and Michael G. Caty

ANATOMY

Translated from its Latin root, *adrenal* means "near the kidney." The bilateral adrenal glands are found anteromedially in relation to the superior pole of the kidneys, covered by perirenal fat and enclosed by Gerota's fascia. In adults, the glands weigh approximately 5 g each. The right gland abuts the inferior vena cava and liver and lies on the posterior extension of the diaphragm, and the left gland lies next to the splenic vessels and the tail of the pancreas.

Although the blood supply to the adrenal glands is variable, it comes from three general sources: the inferior phrenic artery superiorly, the aorta medially, and the renal arteries inferiorly. The venous drainage does not parallel the arterial supply; instead, a single large adrenal vein provides the majority of the venous drainage for each gland. The right adrenal vein empties into the inferior vena cava, and the left adrenal vein joins the left renal vein.

The adrenal lymphatics arise from one plexus beneath the capsule and from a second plexus in the medulla. The right adrenal lymph vessels drain into the periaortic lymph nodes near the diaphragmatic crus, and the left adrenal lymphatics empty into lymph nodes near the take-off of the left renal artery.

The innervation of the adrenal glands arises from the celiac plexus and the greater thoracic splanchnic nerves. The preganglionic sympathetic fibers enter the hilum and end in ganglia within the medulla.

The two distinct regions of the adrenal gland are the cortex and the medulla. These regions not only are distinct on gross examination but also are different embryologically, structurally, and functionally. The adrenal medulla is derived from ectodermal cells from the neural crest. These early cells form the chromocell system and the neuronal system, which accounts for the possible development of two distinct medullary neoplasms: pheochromocytoma and neuroblastoma. The preganglionic sympathetic neural cells innervate the secretory chromaffin cells, which synthesize norepinephrine and epinephrine.

The cortex comprises the outer portion of the adrenal gland and secretes sex hormones, mineralocorticoids, and glucocorticoids. It is divided into three separate zones with separate synthetic functions. The zona glomerulosa is the outermost cortical zone and produces aldosterone and related mineralocorticoids. The zona fasciculata lies beneath the zona glomerulosa and secretes cortisol and the adrenal sex hormones. The inner zona reticularis maintains cholesterol stores as a precursor for steroidogenesis and secretes cortisol, androgens, and estrogens.

EMBRYOLOGY

The primordium of the adrenal cortex becomes visible as early as the fourth week of gestation and is clearly seen by the sixth week. On prenatal ultrasonography (US), the adrenal glands may be visible as early as 20 weeks' gestation and are identifiable in the majority of fetuses by 30 weeks' gestation.[30] During the fourth to sixth weeks of gestation, the mesodermal cells of the posterior abdominal wall at the adrenogenital ridge become more columnar and invade the mesenchyma beneath the epithelial surface, ultimately forming the fetal adrenal cortex. Another proliferation of epithelial cells subsequently forms a cap over these primitive cortical cells, becoming the zona glomerulosa of the definitive cortex. The ectodermal chromaffin cells of the adrenal medulla arise from the neural crest as early as the fifth week, with primitive cells from the thoracic ganglia from the 6th to 12th segments invading the gland and forming the medulla. Differentiation of these primitive medullary cells into chromaffin cells begins at the third month of gestation, ultimately leading to the cells' production of epinephrine and norepinephrine.

The fetal zone of the adrenal cortex begins to appear around the sixth week of gestation. This zone continues to enlarge and occupy the majority of the gland. In fact, because of the large size of the fetal cortical zone, the fetal adrenal gland is four times the size of the kidney during the fourth month of gestation. This fetal cortex subsequently decreases in size, disappearing in the first year of life.

During fetal development, ectopic rests of medullary and cortical tissue may remain and persist after birth. Extra-adrenal medullary rests are usually found along the aorta and its branches. The organ of Zuckerkandl is an example of a chromaffin mass at the origin of the inferior mesenteric artery. Most extra-adrenal chromaffin rests involute after birth; the chromaffin cells in the medulla differentiate.

Extra-adrenal cortical rests are common in children and are found in the kidney or liver or along the migratory path of the gonads, in hernia sacs, or in the gonads themselves. Approximately 50% of newborns have adrenocortical rests, but these rests typically atrophy and disappear within a few weeks after birth.[30]

PHYSIOLOGY

Adrenal Medullary Function

The adrenal medulla synthesizes and releases catecholamines—dopamine, epinephrine, and norepinephrine. Catecholamine synthesis begins with tyrosine, a nonessential amino acid. Tyrosine hydroxylase converts tyrosine into dihydroxyphenylalanine (DOPA) and is the rate-limiting step in the synthetic pathway. DOPA decarboxylase converts DOPA into dopamine. Phenylamine ß-hydroxylase converts dopamine into norepinephrine. Finally, phenylethylamine *N*-methyltransferase converts norepinephrine into epinephrine.

The chromaffin cells within the medulla contain cytoplasmic granules that store the catecholamines. Preganglionic sympathetic nerve endings release acetylcholine, which causes calcium-dependent exocytosis of these cytoplasmic storage granules and release of the catecholamines. Regulation of adrenal medullary catecholamine release is accomplished through inhibitory feedback mechanisms involving norepinephrine. Norepinephrine inhibits acetylcholine release from the presynaptic α_2 receptors and also inhibits tyrosine hydroxylase activity when present in high concentrations.

Adrenal Cortical Function

The adrenal cortex synthesizes three types of hormones: glucocorticoids, mineralocorticoids, and sex hormones. Regulation of these hormones is accomplished by the hypothalamic-pituitary-adrenal axis. The hypothalamus produces corticotropin-releasing hormone (CRH); this is transported to the anterior pituitary gland, where it stimulates the release of adrenocorticotropic hormone (ACTH). ACTH then stimulates the production of adrenal hormones from the adrenal cortex.

The physiologic diurnal variation in CRH release leads to a cyclic variation in ACTH and the hormones regulated by it. Serum concentrations peak shortly before or at the time of awakening and decline throughout the remainder of the day. Both cortisol and ACTH inhibit CRH release, creating a negative feedback loop.

Adrenocortical production of glucocorticoids begins with a cholesterol substrate and is regulated by ACTH. The majority of serum cortisol is bound by cortisol-binding protein (90%) and albumin (6%), leaving only a small percentage (4%) free and physiologically active. As with most steroids, the unbound cortisol fraction is lipophilic and therefore readily crosses the plasma membrane of target cells. Specific receptors then bind with cortisol and act in the cell nucleus to regulate messenger RNA synthesis.

Cortisol affects metabolism primarily by opposing insulin. It causes hyperglycemia by increasing the proteolysis necessary for gluconeogenesis and inducing hepatic gluconeogenic enzymes. Cortisol also decreases the use of glucose by peripheral tissues; it inhibits glucose uptake into fat cells and decreases the amount of insulin bound by insulin-sensitive tissues.

Cortisol also decreases inflammation and immune function, affecting wound healing. Cortisol lowers both the lymphocytic and the granulocytic cellular immune response by decreasing the lymphocyte response to antigenic stimulation and impairing chemotaxis and phagocytosis of leukocytes. These two immune functions are an important part of early wound healing; thus, wounds have decreased tensile strength and impaired healing in the setting of excess cortisol.

Aldosterone, a mineralocorticoid, is synthesized in the zona glomerulosa and metabolized primarily by the liver. The renin-angiotensin system controls the majority of aldosterone regulation, with ACTH playing only a small role. The macula densa of the renal juxtaglomerular apparatus releases renin in response to a drop in renal perfusion or hyponatremia. Renin converts angiotensinogen, which is produced by the liver, to angiotensin I. Angiotensin-converting enzyme, found in the lung, converts angiotensin I to angiotensin II. Angiotensin II stimulates the synthesis of aldosterone by directly acting on the cells of the adrenal zona glomerulosa; it also acts as a vasoconstrictor. By increasing the renal retention of sodium, aldosterone increases blood pressure and corrects hyponatremia, thus reducing the release of renin.

The serum potassium concentration also provides a small amount of aldosterone regulation. Hyperkalemia leads to increased aldosterone production by directly acting on the zona glomerulosa cells, as well as increasing renin release from the juxtaglomerular cells. Aldosterone promotes an increased renal excretion of potassium, thus lowering aldosterone production and providing another feedback mechanism.

Adrenal androgens are synthesized in the zona reticularis and are regulated primarily by ACTH. These hormones are released in a cyclic manner, correlating with the release of cortisol and ACTH. The adrenal androgens are only weakly active but are converted by peripheral tissues into more active forms such as testosterone and dihydrotestosterone. Metabolism of these hormones occurs in the liver.

IMAGING OF THE ADRENAL GLAND

In children, imaging of the adrenal glands is necessary when an intra-abdominal mass is detected or when there are secondary signs of a hyperfunctioning adrenal gland. Imaging of the abdomen and retroperitoneum identifies the organ of origin, detects metastatic disease, and demonstrates bilaterality. Nuclear medicine studies can be used to localize tumors to their adrenal origin and demonstrate extra-adrenal tumors. The use of specific radiopharmaceuticals allows one to predict the cell type of an adrenal tumor.

Plain abdominal radiographs have minimal clinical utility in the assessment of an adrenal mass. Small functional adrenal masses will not be visualized, and although large masses, such as neuroblastoma, will demonstrate calcifications and mass effect, they are often palpable and more readily diagnosed by physical examination.

The initial screening examination to evaluate an abdominal mass is often abdominal US. US offers the advantages of correlating imaging with physical examination findings and avoiding ionizing radiation. The goals of abdominal US are to identify the organ of origin, define the character and size of the mass, and determine its vascularity. It may be difficult to identify the adrenal gland as the organ of origin for large masses, owing to compression from adjacent organs such as the kidney.

The normal adrenal gland is easily visualized by US during the first week of life. The adrenal soon involutes, and the distinction between the cortex and the medulla is lost. Adrenal hemorrhage may manifest as an adrenal mass in newborns. Affected newborns may have predisposing factors such as asphyxia or a difficult delivery. The appearance of the adrenal gland following adrenal hemorrhage is varied. The adrenal gland may be echogenic, hypoechoic, or a mixture of the two.[41] Adrenal hemorrhage may be confused with neuroblastoma. Patients with normal urinary catecholamine levels and the appropriate risk factors for adrenal hemorrhage can be observed and undergo repeat US. Differentiation of adrenal adenoma and carcinoma by US is difficult; in addition, both resemble an adrenal pheochromocytoma. An ultrasonographic characteristic that suggests malignancy is central necrosis from rapid growth. Biochemical testing and the use of computed tomography (CT), magnetic resonance imaging (MRI), and nuclear medicine studies narrow the diagnostic possibilities.

When US identifies a solid mass in the retroperitoneum, planar imaging is performed to identify the organ of origin and define resectability. The two immediate choices in children are CT and MRI. Although CT is an accurate method of diagnosing adrenal lesions, it is less accurate in younger children owing to the absence of retroperitoneal fat. Other disadvantages of CT are the need for intravenous contrast material and exposure to ionizing radiation. Simultaneous scanning of the chest to rule out pulmonary metastases in patients suspected of having adrenal carcinoma is a benefit of CT. Imaging of adrenal lesions with MRI offers the advantage of multiplanar imaging. Coronal imaging is a useful modality to distinguish adrenal masses from the adjacent kidney and vice versa.[27,33,38] Pheochromocytomas demonstrate low or intermediate signal intensity on T1-weighted images and enhance with gadolinium–diethylenetriaminepentaacetic acid (DTPA).[20]

The unique cellular properties of tumors of the adrenal gland allow imaging with radiopharmaceuticals. The selective uptake of specific compounds allows the identification of adrenal and extra-adrenal locations of pheochromocytoma and the location of adrenal adenomas.

The adrenal gland and pheochromocytoma cells contain transporter systems for norepinephrine. Metaiodobenzylguanidine (MIBG), which is structurally similar to norepinephrine, is taken up by the norepinephrine transporter system into intracytoplasmic vesicles. Radionuclide imaging is achieved by labeling MIBG with one of two iodine isotopes at the meta position of the benzoic ring. The iodine isotope ^{131}I has a half-life of 8.2 days and emits high-energy radiation. The iodine isotope ^{123}I has a shorter half-life and emits lower-energy radiation.[15] Patients undergoing MIBG scanning should be given a saturated solution of potassium iodide to block thyroid uptake of the free iodine isotope. Scintigraphy is performed at 24 and 48 hours. MIBG scanning is valuable for the detection of extra-adrenal and metastatic pheochromocytoma. It also confirms the adrenal location of a pheochromocytoma in patients with positive urine or serum catecholamine tests.

Positron emission tomography (PET) may be a useful imaging study for pheochromocytoma in the near future. PET scanning uses short-lived positron-emitting agents to identify specific areas of uptake in the body. Because of the increased metabolism of tumors, labeled glucose can be used to identify malignant tissue. The most common form of labeled glucose in use for PET scanning is [18F]-fluorodeoxyglucose (FDG). Resolution of pheochromocytoma and distinction between benign and malignant pheochromocytoma are not optimal with FDG PET, however. A more useful agent may be 6-[18F]-fluorodopamine (DA). The similarity between norepinephrine and DA allows selective uptake by sympathoadrenal tissue.[32] One study found that FDG PET demonstrated metastases better than MIBG scanning did.[37] PET scanning results in lower radioactivity exposure than standard scintigraphy. When specific agents such as DA become generally available, it may prove to be the imaging method of choice.

Another useful radiopharmaceutical is ^{131}I-iodomethyl-1-19-norcholesterol (NP-59). This cholesterol analogue is taken up as cholesterol into the steroid pathways of the adrenal cortex. It is used to identify the adrenal cortex and can differentiate adenomas from adrenocortical hyperplasia.

LESIONS OF THE ADRENAL MEDULLA

Pheochromocytoma

In 1886 Frankel of Freiburg, Germany, published the first description of bilateral pheochromocytomas found during the postmortem examination of an 18-year-old woman who had presented with symptoms of anxiety, palpitations, and headache.[44] In 1912 Pick named the tumor for its predominant cell type, the pheochromocyte, but it was not until 1922 that Labbe et al. first described a clear relationship between pheochromocytoma and paroxysmal hypertension. In 1927 Mayo performed the first successful removal of a pheochromocytoma in a patient with paroxysmal hypertension who underwent surgical exploration without a preoperative diagnosis. In 1929 Pincoffs made the first correct preoperative diagnosis, and the successful operation was performed by Shipley.[14] Since that time, the behavior of pheochromocytomas has become better understood, particularly with respect to children.

Pheochromocytoma is an uncommon tumor of childhood, and there are several characteristics that distinguish

TABLE 38–1 Comparison of Pheochromocytoma in Children and Adults		
	Pediatric	**Adult**
Incidence	1:500,000	1:50,000
Familial pattern (%)	10	2-3
Bilateral (%)	24-70	10
Extra-adrenal site (%)	30	10
Malignant (%)	3	10

it from its adult counterpart. The incidence of pheochromocytoma in childhood is 10% of the adult incidence, occurring in approximately 1 in 500,000 children compared with 1 in 50,000 adults.[34] Approximately 10% of childhood pheochromocytomas are familial, which is about four times the frequency in adults. Whereas only 7% of pheochromocytomas are bilateral in adults, the reported incidence of bilateral pheochromocytomas in children ranges from 24% to as high as 70%. Extra-adrenal pheochromocytomas are approximately twice as prevalent in children compared with adults[11,36] (Table 38-1).

Pheochromocytomas originate from medullary chromaffin cells, which produce the catecholamines that cause the symptoms of the tumor. These cells migrate along the aorta, usually remaining near the branches off the aorta.

Symptoms

In children with pheochromocytoma, the average age at presentation is 11 years, although the tumor can occur at any age. Over half the children present with headaches, fever, palpitations, thirst, polyuria, sweating, nausea, and weight loss, but the most common presentation is sustained hypertension.[4,34,36] In children, most causes of hypertension are secondary, with renal abnormalities being most common (78%), followed by renal artery disease (12%), and coarctation of the aorta (2%).[23] Pheochromocytoma accounts for 0.5% of children with hypertension and must be considered once other causes are eliminated. In children with pheochromocytoma, hypertension is sustained in up to 70% to 90% of cases, with only a small minority presenting with paroxysmal hypertension. In contrast, up to 50% of adults with pheochromocytoma have paroxysmal hypertension.[36]

Diagnosis

The diagnosis of pheochromocytoma relies on elevated levels of blood and urinary catecholamines and their metabolites. A 24-hour urine measurement of catecholamines, metanephrine, and vanillylmandelic acid is the best diagnostic test.[18,43] Urinary metanephrine levels are increased in about 95% of patients, and urinary vanillylmandelic acid and catecholamine levels are increased in approximately 90% of patients.[43] There is also a linear relationship between the amount of vanillylmandelic acid and the size of the pheochromocytoma.[10] The normal 24-hour urinary secretion is less than 100 mg for free catecholamines, less than 7 mg for vanillylmandelic acid, and less than 1.3 mg for metanephrine. Plasma catecholamines

can also be measured by radioenzyme assay. However, patients must remain supine and calm during the blood draws, which can be difficult in children. Patients with normal plasma catecholamine levels during a hypertensive episode probably do not have pheochromocytoma, but levels greater than 2000 pg/mL are diagnostic of pheochromocytoma. Plasma catecholamine levels between 500 and 1000 pg/mL are suspicious for a pheochromocytoma, and further testing is indicated.[36]

After obtaining the chemical diagnosis of pheochromocytoma, the tumor must be localized. Although large masses such as a neuroblastoma can be seen on plain abdominal films, most adrenal masses cannot be visualized without the use of other imaging methods. Almost all pheochromocytomas occur in the abdomen or pelvis, and although the adrenal gland is the most common site, up to 43% of children may have multifocal disease.[36] The initial study in infants and children is often US, which can be useful in distinguishing between solid and cystic masses but may not visualize small adrenal lesions. CT and MRI offer the advantage of much better resolution and sensitivity, particularly MRI (Fig. 38-1). Another useful

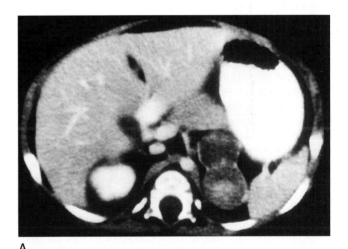

A

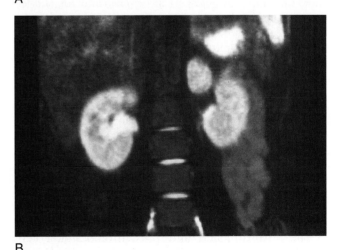

B

Figure 38–1 *A,* Computed tomography of the abdomen in a 10-year-old girl with a left adrenal mass associated with hypertension. *B,* Magnetic resonance image demonstrates a left adrenal pheochromocytoma. No other masses were noted. No contrast agent was required.

imaging technique is ^{131}I-labeled MIBG scanning; this radioisotope accumulates where norepinephrine is taken up and allows detection of the tumor. This can be particularly useful in localizing extra-adrenal pheochromocytomas, but this location is rare in the pediatric population. The head and neck may be a more common site of these tumors in children compared with adults, followed by the retroperitoneum.[42]

Treatment

The treatment of pheochromocytoma is surgical excision, but medical management is an essential part of the preoperative preparation. The high levels of catecholamines increase the risk of sudden and severe intraoperative hypertension, as well as profound hypotension once the tumor is removed and catecholamine release has ceased. In fact, these complications accounted for the high mortality rate associated with surgical resection in the past.[36] Improvements in preoperative and intraoperative management have reduced the operative mortality from 24% to 45% in the past to less than 10% today.[9] Preoperative use of α-adrenergic blockers such as phenoxybenzamine and phentolamine minimizes the effects of epinephrine and norepinephrine by blocking the α-adrenergic receptors. These agents should be used at least 3 to 7 days before the procedure to minimize the intraoperative risks.

β-Adrenergic blockade with agents such as propranolol and labetalol may be used once an α-adrenergic blockade is achieved, particularly if a resting tachycardia develops. If these agents are used, it is crucial that α-blockade be established first.

Patients with pheochromocytomas tend to be slightly hypovolemic at baseline, with an average 15% reduction in plasma volume. As the pharmacologic blockade is established preoperatively, it may be necessary to administer intravenous fluid replacement. This volume re-expansion also helps minimize intraoperative blood pressure fluctuations and cardiac arrhythmias.

Despite good preoperative normalization of blood pressure, the anesthesiologist must be prepared for sudden fluctuations. The times of significant intraoperative risk are during anesthetic induction and intubation, during surgical manipulation of the tumor, and immediately following ligation of the tumor's venous drainage.[7] An arterial catheter and a central venous line are crucial for monitoring intraoperative blood pressure and fluid status. The anesthesiologist must also be prepared to use fast-acting agents to raise or lower blood pressure as needed. Sodium nitroprusside and nitroglycerin are useful agents, as are vasopressors and intravenous fluids. Cardiac arrhythmias can be managed with the use of propranolol, esmolol, and lidocaine.

The traditional operative approach uses a transabdominal incision, usually subcostal. Through this incision, both adrenal glands can be visualized, as well as the periaortic sympathetic ganglia, the small bowel mesentery, and the pelvis. More than 95% of pediatric pheochromocytomas are located in the abdomen, and this approach reveals the majority of tumors. The surgeon must make a conscious effort to minimize direct manipulation of the tumor during dissection. Early control and ligation of

the adrenal vein limit the release of catecholamines as the tumor is removed.

The surgeon can expose the right adrenal gland by reflecting the transverse colon inferiorly and mobilizing the duodenum medially. This exposes the upper portion of the right kidney as well as the right adrenal gland. Reflecting the liver superiorly and rolling the lateral border of the inferior vena cava medially expose the adrenal gland further. There is a greater risk of hemorrhage on the right side than on the left, owing to the shorter length of the right adrenal vein and the greater risk of tearing this vessel.

The surgeon can expose the left adrenal gland by incising the peritoneum lateral to the splenic flexure and mobilizing the colon in a medial direction. The perirenal fascia can then be incised, exposing the left adrenal gland. Alternatively, the surgeon can divide the gastrocolic ligament, mobilizing the stomach superiorly and the transverse colon inferiorly. The posterior peritoneum along the inferior pancreatic border can then be incised, allowing mobilization of the pancreatic tail and exposure of the adrenal vein.

An adrenal pheochromocytoma is typically encapsulated, and although there may be small amounts of normal adrenal tissue, the entire adrenal gland should be removed. It is rarely necessary to perform a nephrectomy because the tumor is usually not adherent to the kidney.

As previously mentioned, once the adrenal vein is ligated and the tumor is removed, the patient may become hypotensive due to the removal of the catecholamine excess. In fact, it may be several days before the blood pressure normalizes. If hypertension returns postoperatively, one should suspect a second pheochromocytoma. All patients should undergo follow-up to confirm normalization of catecholamine levels. Long-term follow-up is indicated because of the possibility of a metachronous occurrence of a multifocal pheochromocytoma.[7,36]

Associated Disorders

Familial pheochromocytomas may occur in the setting of several syndromes. The most common syndromes are multiple endocrine neoplasia type 2 (MEN-2) and von Hippel-Lindau disease. There is a smaller incidence of familial pheochromocytomas in patients with neurofibromatosis type 1 and in patients without any other abnormalities.

MEN-2 is an autosomal dominant disorder caused by a mutation of the *RET* proto-oncogene on chromosome 10. These patients are at risk for medullary thyroid carcinoma, and up to 50% will develop adrenal pheochromocytoma. These tumors are almost always bilateral and are almost never malignant. Patients with MEN-2A are also at risk for hyperparathyroidism, and patients with MEN-2B may have a marfanoid habitus or mucosal ganglioneuromas.

A mutation of the von Hippel-Lindau gene on chromosome 3 leads to von Hippel-Lindau disease. This condition is characterized by retinal angiomas, hemangioblastomas of the central nervous system, renal cysts, renal cell carcinoma, pancreatic cysts, and pheochromocytomas. These pheochromocytomas are often multifocal and are frequently extra-adrenal (Fig. 38-2).

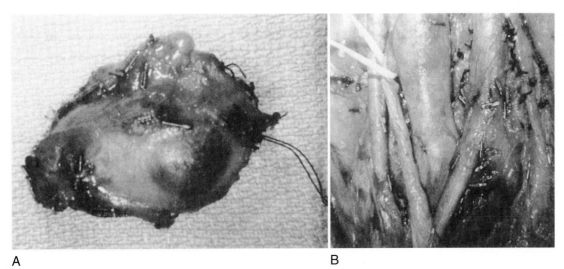

Figure 38–2 *A*, Relatively small extra-adrenal pheochromocytoma that arose from a paraspinal sympathetic ganglion in a 13-year-old girl who experienced paroxysmal hypertension and severe headache while horseback riding. *B*, The operative field after tumor excision shows the vena cava and aortic bifurcation. A vessel loop is around the ureter.

Malignancy

Histologic examination of a pheochromocytoma cannot accurately determine malignancy, which has been reported to occur in up to 10% of children with this tumor.[4] The diagnosis of a malignant pheochromocytoma often relates to the tumor's clinical behavior. A malignant pheochromocytoma may have local infiltration or distant metastasis, which most commonly occurs in bone, liver, lymph nodes, lung, and central nervous system. Synchronous or metachronous pheochromocytomas may present anywhere along the sympathetic chain. Although surgical resection remains the treatment of choice, long-term palliation may be obtained through a multimodal approach including local excision, radiation, and chemotherapy.[8]

LESIONS OF THE ADRENAL CORTEX

Adrenocortical neoplasms are rare in the pediatric population, accounting for less than 0.2% of all pediatric tumors and 6% of all adrenal tumors in children.[6] The incidence of these neoplasms has been reported to be approximately 25 cases per year in the United States, of which about 75% are adrenocortical carcinomas.[35,45] Adrenocortical tumors occur more frequently in girls, with a male-female ratio of approximately 1:2 to 1:3.[26] Like pheochromocytomas, adrenocortical neoplasms behave differently in children than in adults. Approximately 85% to 95% of these tumors are hormonally active in children, compared with less than 50% in adults.[5,28] Further, whereas there are clear pathologic criteria for malignancy in the adult population, these guidelines do not always hold true in the pediatric population. Because the clinical behavior of these tumors does not always correlate with the pathologic appearance, the diagnosis of malignancy should be based on clinical behavior.

Age less than 3.5 years at the time of diagnosis and symptom duration of less than 6 months before diagnosis are favorable prognostic indicators in adrenocortical carcinoma. Early detection is essential in these children, because a delay in diagnosis adversely affects clinical outcome.[30]

Adrenocortical tumors are associated with several congenital anomalies, including hemihypertrophy; other tumors associated with hemihypertrophy include nephroblastoma and hepatoblastoma. Patients with Beckwith-Wiedemann syndrome (exomphalos, macroglossia, and gigantism) also have a higher than expected incidence of adrenocortical carcinoma.[21] Most adrenocortical tumors, however, occur sporadically.[30]

Cushing's Syndrome

In 1932 Cushing first described the syndrome that bears his name in a patient with a pituitary adenoma. Since that time, the understanding of the pathophysiology and cause has expanded considerably.

Endogenous Cushing's syndrome is a rare condition in the pediatric population. In general, the incidence of spontaneous Cushing's syndrome is approximately 5 per million population; it occurs primarily in young adult women, with a female-male ratio of 9:1. Ten percent of cases occur in children and adolescents.[24]

The typical manifestation of Cushing's syndrome in children is generalized obesity and long bone growth retardation.[24] Other symptoms include hypertension, weakness, thin skin with striae and easy bruising, acne, menstrual irregularity, osteoporosis, and glucose intolerance. Unlike in adults with Cushing's syndrome, muscle weakness, sleep disturbances, and mental changes such as emotional lability, irritability, or depression are rare in children.[24]

CRH is secreted by the hypothalamus and is the most potent stimulator of ACTH release from the anterior pituitary. ACTH then stimulates the production of glucocorticoids, mineralocorticoids, and sex hormones from the adrenal cortex. Cushing's syndrome can be divided into ACTH-dependent and ACTH-independent types. In the former condition, the inappropriately high ACTH levels stimulate the adrenal cortex to produce excessive cortisol. In the ACTH-independent type, abnormal adrenal tissue produces excessive cortisol irrespective of ACTH levels.

Cushing's disease refers to Cushing's syndrome caused by pituitary tumors that lead to excessive ACTH production. Typically, these tumors are microadenomas and are less than 1 cm in diameter; however, large, invasive pituitary adenomas may develop. These tumors lead to bilateral adrenocortical hyperplasia, with a corresponding glucocorticoid excess. As the age of the patient increases, there is a greater likelihood of a pituitary cause of the syndrome.

In patients younger than 6 years, the most likely cause of endogenous Cushing's syndrome is an adrenal tumor.

Although adrenocortical carcinomas represent only 0.2% of all childhood malignancies and 6% of adrenal cancers, approximately 60% to 80% of pediatric Cushing's syndrome cases are caused by adrenocortical carcinomas.[5]

The clinical diagnosis of hypercortisolism must be confirmed biochemically to diagnose Cushing's syndrome. In addition, the specific source of the syndrome must be localized (Fig. 38-3). Because the normal circadian rhythm of cortisol secretion is lost in Cushing's syndrome, random serum cortisol levels are of limited value. Screening with morning and evening serum cortisol levels to assess diurnal variation has a low sensitivity. Instead, the 24-hour urinary free cortisol level is the best way to diagnose hypercortisolism, with a sensitivity of approximately 98%.[16] In children, this value must be corrected for size. A normal value is less than 70 µg/m² per day; this is elevated with Cushing's syndrome. Another useful test is the 24-hour urinary 17-hydroxysteroid excretion; this is an indirect measure of cortisol secretion and

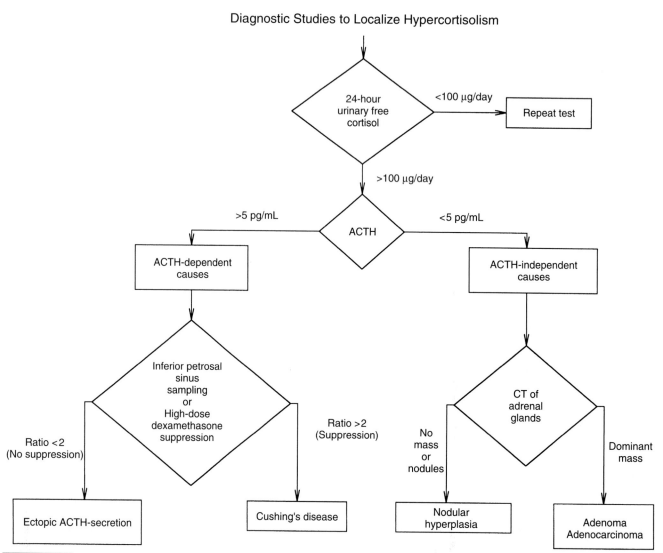

Diagnostic Studies to Localize Hypercortisolism

Figure 38-3 Algorithm to localize the cause of hypercortisolism in children with suspected Cushing's syndrome. ACTH, adrenocorticotropic hormone; CT, computed tomography.

is elevated with hypercortisolism. Once it is corrected for creatinine excretion, the normal value is between 2 and 7 mg per gram of creatinine per day. Another useful screening test is the overnight 1-mg dexamethasone suppression test (or 0.3 mg/m² in children). After the administration of dexamethasone, a morning cortisol level above 5 μg/dL indicates unsuppressed cortisol secretion consistent with Cushing's syndrome.

Once the diagnosis of Cushing's syndrome has been established, the next step is to determine the underlying cause of the hypercortisolism. As shown in Figure 38-3, measurement of the ACTH level can distinguish between ACTH-dependent and ACTH-independent causes. If the ACTH level is greater than 5 pg/mL, the source is ACTH dependent; if the level is less than 5 pg/mL, it is ACTH independent.

ACTH-dependent causes of hypercortisolism include both pituitary and ectopic ACTH-secreting neoplasms. Although ectopic production of ACTH is rare in children, Wilms' tumors and tumors of the thymus, pancreas, or neural tissue can produce ACTH. Most patients with ACTH-secreting tumors have Cushing's disease (Cushing's syndrome caused by a pituitary tumor). Although a high-dose dexamethasone suppression test or an inferior petrosal sinus sampling can distinguish a pituitary source from an ectopic source, MRI can also show a pituitary tumor. An ectopic tumor producing CRH is another ACTH-dependent source of Cushing's syndrome, but this condition has not been reported in children.[3,16]

In both adults and children, the treatment of choice for Cushing's disease is a transsphenoidal resection of the pituitary adenoma. In patients with no postoperative improvement or with recurrence, some response may be obtained with pituitary irradiation using cobalt 60.

If an ectopic ACTH-secreting tumor is indicated by the workup, the patient must undergo screening for medullary carcinoma of the thyroid (serum calcitonin levels) and screening for pheochromocytoma (24-hour urine measurement of catecholamines, metanephrine, and vanillylmandelic acid). Other ectopic locations such as a bronchial, thymic, or intestinal carcinoid tumor may be seen on CT of the chest and abdomen. Ectopic ACTH-producing tumors should be resected if possible. If resection is not possible, bilateral adrenalectomy can offer an effective treatment of Cushing's syndrome.

ACTH-independent causes of Cushing's syndrome include adrenal neoplasms and nodular adrenal hyperplasia. ACTH-independent Cushing's syndrome is relatively more frequent in children than in adults.[16] In children, an adrenocortical tumor most frequently occurs in the setting of a virilizing syndrome, and the majority of children present with virilizing symptoms. Approximately 33% of these patients have Cushing's syndrome; less than 10% present with isolated Cushing's syndrome without any virilizing signs.[28,35]

Nodular adrenal hyperplasia is a rare condition that occurs in children and young adults. This disease usually presents in the first 2 decades of life, predominantly in girls. Although this entity can occur sporadically, many cases are familial and appear in an autosomal dominant fashion.[16] The adrenal glands contain multiple nodules approximately 3 to 5 mm in size. Histologic examination

reveals lymphocytic infiltration of the cortex, suggesting an autoimmune cause of the disorder. The treatment of this cause of Cushing's syndrome is bilateral adrenalectomy.[16] This procedure is associated with significant morbidity rates and requires permanent postoperative mineralocorticoid and glucocorticoid replacement.

Sex Hormone-Producing Tumors

An adrenocortical lesion may lead to either a virilizing or a feminizing tumor. As previously mentioned, most adrenocortical tumors in children are hormonally active. Virilization with or without hypercortisolism is the most common presentation.[22,28,40,45] These virilizing tumors may be more difficult to recognize in boys than in girls. Boys may present with precocious puberty, including penile enlargement, acne, and premature development of pubic, axillary, and facial hair. Girls may develop clitoral hypertrophy, hirsutism, and acne (Fig. 38-4). The treatment of choice is adrenalectomy.

Although feminizing adrenocortical tumors are rare in children, they are usually malignant. In the normal adrenal gland, very small amounts of estrogens may be secreted. With adrenocortical tumors, however, overproduction of estrogens, particularly estradiol, may occur. In girls, these tumors present with precocious isosexual development, including early breast enlargement, accelerated growth, and advanced bone age. In boys, these tumors cause bilateral gynecomastia, accelerated growth rate, and delayed pubertal development; there is also an absence of spermatogenesis.

Treatment of Adrenocortical Tumors

Surgical resection is the mainstay of treatment for adrenocortical tumors. The treatment of choice for a benign adrenal adenoma is adrenalectomy. Adrenocortical carcinomas, however, require a wide excision with adequate abdominal exploration for metastatic disease. In either case, postoperative steroid replacement is typically required until the contralateral gland can recover from its suppression.

CT or MRI can help distinguish between adrenal hyperplasia and an adrenal tumor. An NP-59 scintiscan may aid in the evaluation of an adrenal lesion. Adrenal adenomas usually have an increased uptake of NP-59, whereas adrenocortical carcinomas typically do not take up the isotope. Bilateral uptake of NP-59 indicates bilateral adrenal hyperplasia, which can be the result of ACTH oversecretion.

The most common sites of metastatic adrenocortical carcinomas are the lung, liver, lymph nodes, contralateral adrenal gland, bones, kidneys, and brain. If complete resection is not possible, tumor debulking may be of some benefit. Medical therapy with mitotane may also play a role in treating patients with unresectable disease. Mitotane acts as an adrenolytic agent by altering mitochondrial function, blocking adrenal steroid hydroxylation, and altering the extra-adrenal metabolism of cortisol and androgens. The success of chemotherapy

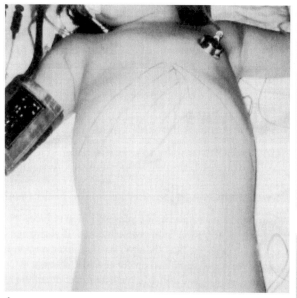

A

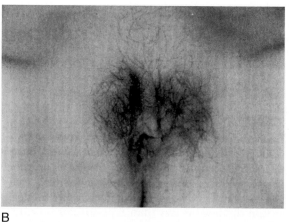

B

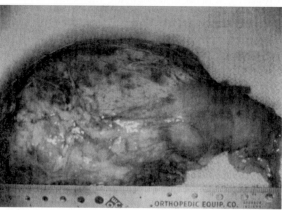

C

Figure 38–4 *A,* This 3-year-old girl presented with a large right upper quadrant mass. *B,* She was noted to have pubic hair. *C,* The mass was a virilizing adrenocortical carcinoma. Despite complete excision and treatment with chemotherapy, the child developed metastases and eventually succumbed.

has not been clearly shown, however, and complete surgical resection is the only treatment that makes a significant difference in terms of survival.[31]

HYPERALDOSTERONISM

Overproduction of aldosterone, or hyperaldosteronism, may be due to either adrenal dysfunction or overproduction of renin. Primary hyperaldosteronism refers to adrenal dysfunction, such as an aldosterone-secreting tumor or bilateral adrenal hyperplasia. Secondary hyperaldosteronism refers to an overproduction of renin, which can be caused by cirrhosis, congestive heart failure, a renin-producing juxtaglomerular cell tumor, or renovascular abnormalities such as renal artery stenosis.

The symptoms of hyperaldosteronism include headaches, fatigue, weakness, lethargy, poor weight gain, polyuria, polydipsia, and nocturia. Hypertension develops as a result of increased sodium and water reabsorption. Weakness occurs due to hypokalemia, which is the most common laboratory finding, although metabolic alkalosis may be observed from the loss of hydrogen ions in the urine. The biochemical diagnosis of hyperaldosteronism is demonstrated by excessive aldosterone secretion in the setting of suppressed renin secretion. Once the diagnosis of primary hyperaldosteronism has been established,

patients with aldosterone-secreting adrenal tumors must be distinguished from those with the more common condition of bilateral adrenocortical hyperplasia. In patients with bilateral adrenocortical hyperplasia, dexamethasone administration normalizes the abnormally high aldosterone level and low renin level.[43]

In the pediatric population, the incidence of aldosteronoma, or an adrenal adenoma causing primary hyperaldosteronism, is extremely low. There are only a handful of reported cases in the literature. As previously mentioned, the more common cause of primary hyperaldosteronism is bilateral cortical hyperplasia.[1] An aldosteronoma is best treated by unilateral adrenalectomy. Patients with bilateral adrenocortical hyperplasia do not respond well to surgical treatment and are best managed with medical therapy using spironolactone and amiloride.[43] Adrenal insufficiency resulting from bilateral adrenalectomy is more difficult to manage than hyperaldosteronism.

ADDISON'S DISEASE

Insufficient production of steroid hormones (either glucocorticoids or mineralocorticoids) can lead to Addison's disease. Children with Addison's disease present with a variety of symptoms, including weakness, anorexia, weight loss, fatigue, nausea, vomiting, and diarrhea.

If the child has an elevated ACTH level, hyperpigmentation will develop, because melanocytes are stimulated by ACTH. Seizures may also occur in the setting of the hypoglycemia, which occurs with adrenal crisis.

There are many causes of adrenal insufficiency in children. Congenital adrenal hypoplasia can result from either an autosomal recessive disorder or an X-linked disorder that occurs in boys. Errors in steroid metabolism can also lead to adrenal insufficiency. The most common group of inborn errors involves defects in glucocorticoid synthesis and is collectively known as congenital adrenal hyperplasia. Acquired lesions involving the hypothalamus or pituitary can also lead to adrenal insufficiency through a reduction in CRH or ACTH secretion.

Destruction of the adrenal glands can also lead to adrenal insufficiency. Conditions causing adrenal demise include hemorrhage, infection, adrenoleukodystrophy, and autoimmune diseases. In older patients, overwhelming infection can lead to adrenal hemorrhage. Tuberculosis used to be a common cause of infectious adrenal destruction; however, the incidence of this condition has fallen in modern times. One of the more common causes of acute adrenal insufficiency is cessation of chronic exogenous glucocorticoid administration.

In newborns, adrenal hemorrhage is not an uncommon event. In fact, the adrenal gland is the second most common source of hemoperitoneum in the newborn period.[39] The pathogenesis of adrenal hemorrhage in newborns is not fully understood. Associated factors include traumatic delivery, asphyxia, maternal hypotension, overwhelming infection, or hemorrhagic disorders.[19,30] The incidence of adrenal hemorrhage is almost 2 cases per 1000 live births,[30] but as the sensitivity of imaging technology improves, this number may increase. Adrenal hemorrhage occurs three to four times more frequently in the right adrenal gland than the left and is bilateral in 8% to 10% of patients.[19] This bias toward the right side may be due to the direct drainage of the right adrenal gland into the inferior vena cava, making the right gland more susceptible to changes in venous pressure. The left gland remains somewhat protected by its drainage into the left renal vein. The fetal cortex contributes to fetal and neonatal adrenal hemorrhage due to both its size and its later involution. The large size of the fetal cortex makes the adrenal glands relatively large, increasing the vulnerability to trauma. The physiologic involution of the fetal cortex may occur quite rapidly, tearing the unsupported central adrenal gland vessels.[39]

On prenatal US, adrenal hemorrhage appears as an echogenic mass. This mass becomes increasingly hypoechoic and usually involutes on subsequent sonograms. The lesion may completely resolve, leaving only residual calcifications. However, the lesion may not resolve, and surgical resection may be necessary to differentiate the mass from a cystic neuroblastoma.

The treatment of Addison's disease is replacement of the deficient steroid hormone. This may be accomplished with a mineralocorticoid such as fludrocortisone or a glucocorticoid such as hydrocortisone or prednisone. During periods of acute stress, such as infection or operation, increased doses of glucocorticoids are needed.

INCIDENTAL ADRENAL MASS

The incidental discovery of adrenal lesions on imaging studies performed for other reasons has been increasing in both children and adults, perhaps due to the increased frequency of imaging studies being performed and the increased sensitivity of those imaging modalities. In adults, the current recommendation is to remove all hormonally active tumors regardless of size. In the case of nonfunctional adrenal masses, it is considered safe to observe a mass less than 4 cm in size.[2,13,25] In the pediatric population, however, there are no clear guidelines about incidental, nonfunctional adrenal masses. Owing to the higher incidence of both functional tumors and malignant tumors in the pediatric adrenal gland, many surgeons recommend adrenalectomy in this setting.[25]

ADRENALECTOMY

The objective of adrenal surgery is to attain complete tumor resection, resulting in normalization of endocrine function and cure of malignancy. Perioperative planning includes correction of potential electrolyte abnormalities, establishing alpha and beta blockade in the case of pheochromocytoma, and performing localizing studies to guide the surgical approach. The surgical approach is based on the probable histology of the adrenal mass, the presence of bilaterality, and the surgeon's preference. The introduction of laparoscopic adrenal resection has provided an attractive alternative for the resection of many adrenal masses in children.

Traditional approaches to adrenal resection have included anterior, posterior, and thoracoabdominal approaches. The anterior approach to adrenalectomy permits resection of either the left or the right adrenal gland. It also allows bilateral resection through a single incision. During the anterior approach to right adrenalectomy, the duodenum is mobilized by the Kocher maneuver (Fig. 38-5). Gerota's fascia is opened, and the right lobe of the liver is retracted in a cephalad direction. The most important element of the procedure is the dissection between the medial border of the adrenal mass and the lateral wall of the inferior vena cava. This plane is developed in a cephalad direction until the relatively short right adrenal vein is identified entering the vena cava. Multiple veins may be present and should be identified to prevent accidental avulsion. During the anterior approach to the left adrenal gland, the initial maneuver is to mobilize the splenic flexure of the colon. The pancreas and spleen are retracted superiorly, and Gerota's fascia is opened. The left adrenal vein enters the renal vein superiorly and can be ligated in this plane. Several arteries enter the medial surface of the adrenal gland from the lateral side of the aorta; these arteries need to be divided before adrenal removal. The posterior approach to the adrenal gland is accomplished most commonly through the bed of the 11th rib. This strategy avoids intraperitoneal dissection, eliminates postoperative adhesions, and decreases postoperative ileus. The posterior approach is not useful for bilateral adrenal lesions,

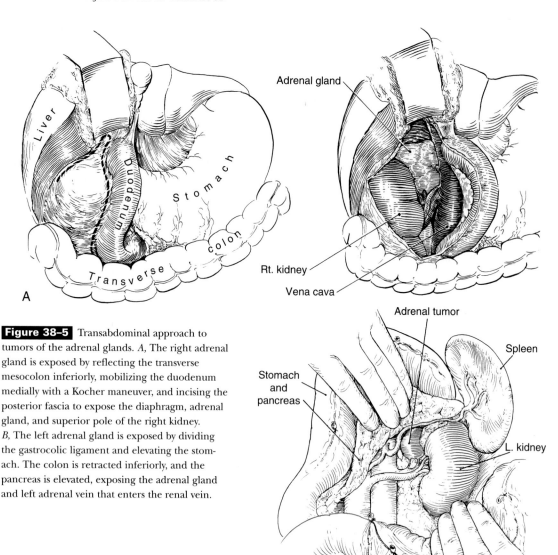

Figure 38–5 Transabdominal approach to tumors of the adrenal glands. *A,* The right adrenal gland is exposed by reflecting the transverse mesocolon inferiorly, mobilizing the duodenum medially with a Kocher maneuver, and incising the posterior fascia to expose the diaphragm, adrenal gland, and superior pole of the right kidney. *B,* The left adrenal gland is exposed by dividing the gastrocolic ligament and elevating the stomach. The colon is retracted inferiorly, and the pancreas is elevated, exposing the adrenal gland and left adrenal vein that enters the renal vein.

malignancies, or large vascular tumors. The thoracoabdominal approach to adrenalectomy is best applied to very large unilateral lesions. Although this approach provides optimal exposure of large vascular tumors, postoperative pain and impairment of ventilation limit its application.

The first laparoscopic adrenalectomy was reported in an adult in 1991.[12] Since then, a number of studies involving laparoscopic adrenalectomy in children have been published,[17,29] demonstrating the feasibility and safety of this approach. Most commonly, laparoscopic adrenalectomy is performed with the patient in the lateral position. A kidney rest elevates the flank opposite the adrenal lesion. Four or five trocars are placed in a subcostal position on the side of the adrenal gland to be resected. Exposure is improved on the right side by dividing the right triangular ligament of the liver. Division of the lienocolic ligament on the left improves exposure of the left adrenal gland. When possible, the adrenal vein is

ligated with clips at the initial point of dissection. The adrenal specimen should be removed in a specimen bag because of the potential for malignancy. Most adrenal lesions in children are small and benign, making laparoscopic resection an appropriate choice in the majority of cases. Although no absolute contraindications to laparoscopic resection exist, an open approach should be considered in patients with large tumors, malignancies with potential lymph node involvement, and highly vascular pheochromocytomas.

REFERENCES

1. Agarwala S, Mitra DK, Bhatnagar V, et al: Aldosteronoma in childhood: A review of clinical features and management. J Pediatr Surg 1994;29:1388-1391.
2. Arnaldi G, Masini AM, Giachetti G, et al: Adrenal incidentaloma. Braz J Med Biol Res 2000;33:1177-1189.

3. Bickler SW, McMahon TJ, Campbell JR, et al: Preoperative diagnostic evaluation of children with Cushing's syndrome. J Pediatr Surg 1994;29:671-676.

4. Caty MG, Coran AG, Geagan M, Thompson NW: Current diagnosis and treatment of pheochromocytoma in children: Experience with 22 consecutive tumors in 14 patients. Arch Surg 1990;125:978-981.

5. Chudler RM, Kay R: Adrenocortical carcinoma in children. Urol Clin North Am 1989;16:469-479.

6. Ciftci AO, Senocak ME, Tanyel FC, et al: Adrenocortical tumors in children. J Pediatr Surg 2001;36:549-554.

7. Ein SH, Pullerits J, Creighton R, Balfe JW: Pediatric pheochromocytoma: A 36-year review. Pediatr Surg Int 1997; 2:595-598.

8. Ein SH, Weitzman S, Thorner P, et al: Pediatric malignant pheochromocytoma. J Pediatr Surg 1994;29:1197-1201.

9. Ellis D, Gartner JC: The intraoperative medical management of childhood pheochromocytoma. J Pediatr Surg 1980;15:655-659.

10. Farndon JR, Davidson HA, Johnston ID, Well SA Jr: VMA excretion in patients with pheochromocytoma. Ann Surg 1980;191:259-263.

11. Fonkalsrud EW: Pheochromocytoma in childhood. Prog Pediatr Surg 1991;26:103-111.

12. Gagner M, LaCroix A, Bolte E: Laparoscopic adrenalectomy in Cushing's syndrome and pheochromocytoma. N Engl J Med 1992;327:1033.

13. Grumbach MM, Biller BM, Braunstein GD, et al: Management of the clinically inapparent adrenal mass ("incidentaloma"). Ann Intern Med 2003;138:424-429.

14. Hume DM: Pheochromocytoma in the adult and in the child. Am J Surg 1960;99:458-496.

15. Ilias I, Pacak K: Current approaches and recommended algorithm for the diagnostic localization of pheochromocytoma. J Clin Endocrinol Metab 2004;89:479-491.

16. Jones KL: The Cushing syndromes. Pediatr Clin North Am 1990;37:1313-1332.

17. Kadamba P, Habib Z, Rossi L: Experience with laparoscopic adrenalectomy in children. J Pediatr Surg 2004;39:764-767.

18. Kaufman BH, Telander RL, vanHeerden JA, et al: Pheochromocytoma in the pediatric age group: Current status. J Pediatr Surg 1983;18:879-884.

19. Khuri FJ, Alton DJ, Hardy BE, et al: Adrenal hemorrhage in neonates: Report of 5 cases and review of the literature. J Urol 1980;124:684-687.

20. Krestin GP, Steinbrich W, Friedmann G, et al: Adrenal masses: Evaluation with fast gradient-echo MR imaging and Gd-DTPA-enhanced dynamic studies. Radiology 1989; 171:675-680.

21. Lack EE, Mulvihill JJ, Travis WD, Kozakewich HP: Adrenal cortical neoplasms in the pediatric and adolescent age group: Clinicopathologic study of 30 cases with emphasis on epidemiological and prognostic factors. Pathol Annu 1992; 27(Pt 1):1-53.

22. Lee PD, Winter RJ, Green OC: Virilizing adrenocortical tumors in childhood: Eight cases and a review of the literature. Pediatrics 1985;76:437-444.

23. Londe S: Causes of hypertension in the young. Pediatr Clin North Am 1978;25:55-65.

24. Magiakou MA, Mastorakos G, Oldfield EH, et al: Cushing's syndrome in children and adolescents: Presentation, diagnosis, and therapy. N Engl J Med 1994;331:629-636.

25. Masiakos PT, Gerstle JT, Cheang T, et al: Is surgery necessary for incidentally discovered adrenal masses in children? J Pediatr Surg 2004;39:754-758.

26. Mayer SK, Oligny LL, Deal C, et al: Childhood adrenocortical tumors: Case series and reevaluation of prognosis—a 24-year experience. J Pediatr Surg 1997;32:911-915.

27. Meyer JS: Retroperitoneal MR imaging in children. Magn Reson Imaging Clin North Am 1996;4:657-678.

28. Michalkiewicz E, Sandrini R, Figueiredo B, et al: Clinical and outcome characteristics of children with adrenocortical tumors: A report from the International Pediatric Adrenocortical Tumor Registry. J Clin Oncol 2004;22: 838-845.

29. Miller KA, Albanese C, Harrison M, et al: Experience with laparoscopic adrenalectomy in pediatric patients. J Pediatr Surg 2002;37:979-982.

30. Nadler EP, Barksdale EM: Adrenal masses in the newborn. Semin Pediatr Surg 2000;9:156-164.

31. Ng L, Libertino JM: Adrenocortical carcinoma: Diagnosis, evaluation and treatment. J Urol 2003;169:5-11.

32. Pacak K, Eisenhofer G, Carrasquillo JA, et al: Diagnostic localization of pheochromocytoma: The coming of age of positron emission tomography. Ann N Y Acad Sci 2002; 970:170-176.

33. Petrus LV, Hall TR, Boechat MI, et al: The pediatric patient with suspected adrenal neoplasm: Which radiological test to use? Med Pediatr Oncol 1992;20:53-57.

34. Reddy VS, O'Neill JA Jr, Holcomb GW III, et al: Twenty-five-year surgical experience with pheochromocytoma in children. Am Surg 2000;66:1085-1091.

35. Ribeiro RC, Michalkiewicz EL, Figueiredo BC, et al: Adrenocortical tumors in children. Braz J Med Biol Res 2000;33:1225-1234.

36. Ross JH: Pheochromocytoma: Special considerations in children. Urol Clin North Am 2000;27:393-402.

37. Shulkin BL, Thompson NW, Shapiro B, et al: Pheochromocytomas: Imaging with 2-[fluorine-18]fluoro-2-deoxy-D-glucose PET. Radiology 1999;212:35-41.

38. Siegel MJ: MR imaging of the pediatric abdomen. Magn Reson Imaging Clin North Am 1995;3:161-182.

39. Skandalakis J, et al: The suprarenal glands. In Skandalakis J, Gray S: Embryology for Surgeons, 2nd ed. Baltimore, Williams & Wilkins, 1994.

40. Stewart JN, Flageole H, Kavan P: A surgical approach to adrenocortical tumors in children: The mainstay of treatment. J Pediatr Surg 2004;39:759-763.

41. Teele R: Abdominal masses. In Share J, Teele R: Ultrasonography of Infants and Children. Philadelphia, WB Saunders, 1991.

42. Tekautz TM, Pratt CB, Jenkins JJ, Spunt SL: Pediatric extraadrenal paraganglioma. J Pediatr Surg 2003;38: 1317-1321.

43. Telander RL, Zimmerman D, Kaufman BH, vanHeerden JA: Pediatric endocrine surgery. Surg Clin North Am 1985;65:1551-1587.

44. Welbourn RB: Early surgical history of phaeochromocytoma. Br J Surg 1987;4:594-596.

45. Wieneke JA, Thompson LD, Heffess CS: Adrenal cortical neoplasms in the pediatric population: A clinicopathologic and immunophenotypic analysis of 83 patients. Am J Surg Pathol 2003;27:867-881.

Chapter 39

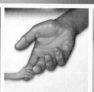

Tumors of the Lung

Stephen J. Shochat

The majority of pulmonary neoplasms in children are due to metastatic disease; however, primary pulmonary tumors of the lung do occur in the pediatric age group. The approximate ratio of primary pulmonary tumors to metastatic neoplasms and non-neoplastic lesions of the lung is 1:5:60.[13,15] Although primary pulmonary tumors are rare in children, the majority of these tumors are malignant. In a review of 383 primary pulmonary neoplasms in children by Hancock et al.,[29] 76% were malignant and 24% were benign. This incidence is similar to that previously reported by Hartman and Shochat.[31] Table 39-1 demonstrates the variety of primary pulmonary neoplasms seen in children. This chapter addresses the more common benign and malignant primary pulmonary tumors in children and discusses the treatment of pulmonary metastatic disease in the pediatric population.

BENIGN TUMORS

Plasma Cell Granuloma (Inflammatory Pseudotumor)

Plasma cell granuloma has also been called inflammatory myofibroblastic tumor, fibroxanthoma, histiocytoma, and fibrohistiocytoma. This lesion, which is seen frequently in adults, occurs rarely in children younger than 10 years (approximately 8% of cases). However, plasma cell granuloma is the most common benign tumor in children and accounts for slightly more than 50% of all benign lesions and approximately 20% of all primary lung tumors.[31] These tumors usually present as peripheral pulmonary masses but occasionally present as polypoid endobronchial tumors.[3,5] The pathogenesis of plasma cell granuloma is not well understood, but an antecedent pulmonary infection has been reported in approximately 30% of cases. The mean age at presentation in children is 7 years, and 35% of the children are between 1 and 15 years of age.[2,5,81] Many children are asymptomatic at the time of presentation, but fever, cough, pain, hemoptysis, pneumonitis, and dysphagia may be present. The natural history is that of a slow-growing

mass starting as a focus of organized pneumonia with a tendency for local invasion. Extension of the tumor beyond the confines of the lung is common. At least four deaths have been reported due to tracheal obstruction or involvement of the mediastinum by massive lesions.

Treatment consists of a conservative pulmonary resection with removal of all gross disease if possible. Primary hilar adenopathy may be present, and local invasion with disregard for tissue planes mimics malignancy. A frequent problem is identifying the benign nature of these masses.

TABLE 39–1 Primary Pulmonary Neoplasms in Children

Type of Tumor	No. of Patients (%)*
Benign (n = 92)	
Plasma cell granuloma	48 (52.2)
Hamartoma	22 (23.9)
Neurogenic tumor	9 (9.8)
Leiomyoma	6 (6.5)
Mucous gland adenoma	3 (3.3)
Myoblastoma	3 (3.3)
Benign teratoma	1 (1.1)
Malignant (n = 291)	
Bronchial "adenoma"	118 (40.5)
Bronchioalveolar carcinoma	49 (16.8)
Pulmonary blastoma	45 (15.5)
Fibrosarcoma	28 (9.6)
Rhabdomyosarcoma	17 (5.8)
Leiomyosarcoma	11 (3.8)
Sarcoma	6 (2.1)
Hemangiopericytoma	4 (1.4)
Plasmacytoma	4 (1.4)
Lymphoma	3 (1.0)
Teratoma	3 (1.0)
Mesenchymoma	2 (1.7)
Myxosarcoma	1 (0.3)

*Percent of benign or malignant tumors.
Modified from Hancock BJ, DiLorenzo M, Youssef S, et al: Childhood primary pulmonary neoplasms. J Pediatr Surg 1993;28:1133.

However, the diagnosis can usually be confirmed by frozen section. Malignant fibrous histiocytoma of the lung, an extremely rare tumor in children, can mimic plasma cell granuloma and must be considered in the differential diagnosis.[53] Recurrences following resection are rare but have been reported. Nonsteroidal anti-inflammatory drugs have been used to treat large inoperable lesions, with encouraging results.[72]

Hamartoma

Pulmonary hamartoma is the second most frequent benign lesion seen in children. These lesions usually present as parenchymal lesions and can be quite large. Approximately one quarter are calcified, and "popcorn-like" calcification is pathognomonic.[21] Two endobronchial lesions have been reported. Four tumors occurring in the neonatal period were quite large and were associated with significant respiratory distress; all were fatal. An interesting triad is the combination of pulmonary hamartoma, extra-adrenal paraganglioma, and gastric smooth muscle tumors; the majority of these patients are young women. Conservative pulmonary resection is the treatment of choice; however, lobectomy or even pneumonectomy may be required, especially for large lesions and endobronchial lesions when sleeve resection is not possible.

MALIGNANT TUMORS

Bronchial Adenoma

The most frequently encountered malignant primary pulmonary tumor is bronchial adenoma. These tumors are a heterogeneous group of primary endobronchial lesions. Although *adenoma* implies a benign process, all varieties of bronchial adenomas occasionally display malignant behavior. There are three histologic types: carcinoid tumor (most common), mucoepidermoid carcinoma, and adenoid cystic carcinoma. Carcinoid tumors account for 80% to 85% of all bronchial adenomas in children. The presenting symptoms are usually due to incomplete bronchial obstruction, with cough, recurrent pneumonitis, and hemoptysis. Owing to diagnostic difficulties, symptoms are often present for months; occasionally, children with wheezing have been treated for asthma, delaying diagnosis as long as 4 to 5 years. Metastatic lesions are reported in approximately 6% of cases, and recurrences occur in 2%. There is a single report of a child with a carcinoid tumor and metastatic disease who developed the classic carcinoid syndrome.[43] Bronchial adenomas of all histologic types are associated with an excellent prognosis in children, even in the presence of local invasion.[68]

The management of bronchial adenomas is somewhat controversial because most are visible endoscopically. Biopsy in these lesions may be hazardous because of the risk of hemorrhage, and endoscopic resection is not recommended. Bronchography or computed tomography

(CT) may be helpful to determine the degree of bronchiectasis distal to the obstruction, because the degree of pulmonary destruction may influence surgical therapy.[3] However, Tagge et al.[76] described a technique for pulmonary salvage despite significant distal atelectasis. Conservative pulmonary resection with removal of the involved lymphatics is the treatment of choice. Sleeve segmental bronchial resection is possible in children and is the treatment of choice when feasible.[24,38] Adenoid cystic carcinomas (cylindroma) have a tendency to spread submucosally, and late local recurrence or dissemination has been reported. In addition to en bloc resection with hilar lymphadenectomy, a frozen section examination of the bronchial margins should be carried out in children with this lesion.

Bronchogenic Carcinoma

Although bronchogenic carcinoma is rare in children, this tumor was the second most common malignant lesion reported by Hancock et al.[29] Interestingly, squamous cell carcinoma was rare, with the majority of tumors being either undifferentiated or adenocarcinomas. The term *bronchioalveolar carcinoma* has been used in most cases.[45] These tumors are associated with both cystic adenomatoid malformations and intrapulmonary bronchogenic cysts (Table 39-2).* Only rare survivors have been reported, and mortality exceeds 90%. The majority of children present with disseminated disease, and the average survival is only 7 months. Localized lesions can be treated by complete resection, followed by adjuvant therapy. Mucoepidermoid carcinoma of the bronchus has also been described in children as young as 4 years (Fig. 39-1).[66]

Pulmonary Blastoma

Pulmonary blastoma is a rare malignant tumor that occurs primarily in adults and arises from mesenchymal blastema. This tumor is an aggressive lesion, with metastatic disease at presentation in approximately 20% of cases.[17,29] They may arise from the lung, pleura, and mediastinum.[56] Occasionally, these tumors may arise in an extralobar sequestration or in a previous lung cyst (Table 39-3).† The majority of cases occur in the right hemithorax (Fig. 39-2). Frequent sites of metastases are the liver, brain, and spinal cord. Local recurrences are frequent, and the mortality rate is approximately 40%.[6,29] The majority of children present before 4 years of age, and symptoms include persistent cough, chest pain, episodes of pneumonia that are refractory to antibiotics, and hemoptysis. Diagnosis is achieved by CT of the chest, bronchoscopy, and biopsy. Because most of these tumors are located peripherally, resection is usually possible by segmental or lobar resection. The use of multimodal

---

* See references 7, 19, 22, 27, 37, 40, 45, 51, 58, 59, 73.
† See references 1, 11, 23, 36, 47, 57, 64, 65, 71, 74, 80, 84.

TABLE 39–2 Bronchioalveolar Carcinoma Associated with Congenital Cystic Lung Malformations

Author	Year of Publication	Type of Lung Cyst	Age at Diagnosis (yr)	Comments
Prichard[58]	1984	CCAM type 1	30	Died of metastatic disease
Hurley[37]	1985	CCAM type 1		
Benjamin[7]	1991	CCAM type 1	19	BAC diagnosed in same lobe with segmental resection 19 yr earlier; died at 23 yr
Morresi[51]	1995	CCAM type 1	20	
Ribet[59]	1995	CCAM type 1	42	
Kaslovsky[40]	1997	CCAM type 1	11	Incomplete resection of CCAM in neonatal period
Granata[27]	1998	CCAM type 1	11	Lobectomy for recurrent infection; BAC was finding
Endo[22]	1982	Bronchogenic (intrapulmonary)	37	Abnormal CXR noted 10 yr earlier; presented with dyspnea, BAC was incidental finding, 3×1 mm
De Perrot[19]	2001	Bronchogenic (intrapulmonary)	79	Long-standing history of cyst infections
MacSweeney[45]	2003	CCAM type 1 0.5, 13, 18 30, 36		1 BAC in a recurrent cyst; 1 other patient with a typical adenomatous hyperplasia (both patients underwent segmental resection)
Sudou[73]	2003	CCAM type 1	17	Abnormality seen on CXR from 10 yr earlier

BAC, bronchioalveolar carcinoma; CCAM, congenital cystic adenomatoid malformation; CXR, chest radiograph.
Adapted from LaBerge JM, Puligandla P, Flageole H: Asymptomatic congenital lung malformations. Semin Pediatr Surg 2005;14:16.

neoadjuvant chemotherapy and radiation following surgical resection has shown promising results in a few patients with extensive disease and dissemination.[56,67] Chemotherapeutic agents that have been used include actinomycin D, vincristine, cyclophosphamide alternating with courses of doxorubicin, and cisplatin. Histologic evaluation of the tumor shows an exclusive mesenchymal composition, including primitive tubules, immature blastema, and spindle cell stroma. Some demonstrate elements of embryonal rhabdomyosarcoma arising within a multicyctic lesion.

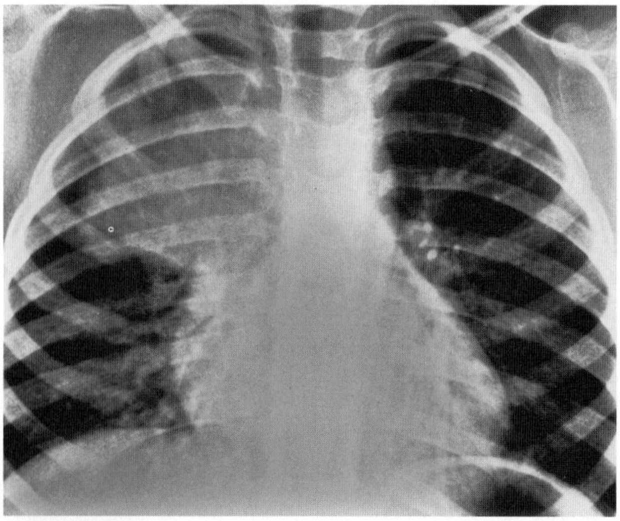

Rhabdomyosarcoma

Rhabdomyosarcomas of the lung are rare and account for only 0.5% of all childhood rhabdomyosarcomas (see Chapter 32).[9] Many of the lesions are endobronchial in origin (Fig. 39-3); however, several cases apparently originated in congenital cystic anomalies. (see Table 39-3).* This is an important issue because 4% of benign tumors and 8.6% of malignant tumors enumerated in Table 39-1 were associated with previously documented cystic malformations.[29] Tumors that developed in these malformations included 11 sarcomas, 9 pulmonary blastomas, 3 bronchogenic carcinomas, and 2 mesenchymomas.

Comments

Although children with primary lung tumors represent a heterogeneous group of patients, analysis of the reported cases suggests that evaluation and treatment are similar in the majority of patients. Many children are asymptomatic, especially those with benign tumors; however, cough, recurrent pneumonitis, and symptoms of atypical bronchial asthma may be the initial presentation. Radiographic findings usually indicate a solitary mass

Figure 39–1 Anteroposterior view of a right upper lobe lesion in a 4-year-old girl. The tumor was resected by right upper lobectomy and was shown to be a mucoepidermoid carcinoma. (Courtesy of Jay L. Grosfeld, MD.)

* See references 4, 8, 10, 16, 33, 41, 49, 52, 54, 67, 79, 86.

TABLE 39-3 Mesenchymal Malignancy and Cystic Lung Malformations

Author	Year	Type of Lung Cyst	Type of Malignancy	Age at Diagnosis (mo)
Stephanopoulos[70]	1963	"Cystic hamartoma"	Myxosarcoma	
Ueda[79]	1977	CCAM	RMS	18
Martinez[47]	1978	"Polycystic disease"	Pulmonary blastoma	24
Valderrama[80]	1978	Extralobar sequestration	Pulmonary blastoma	
Sumner[74]	1979	Peripheral cyst	Pulmonary blastoma	48
Weinbera[83]	1980	Congenital lung cyst	Mixed mesenchymal sarcoma	108
Krous[41]	1980	Bronchogenic cyst (intrapulmonary)	Embryonal RMS	30
Weinblatt[84]	1982	"Cystic lung disease"	Pulmonary blastoma	30
Holland-Moritz[36]	1984	"Pneumatocele"	PPB	48
Morales[50]	1986	Congenital cyst	Pulmonary blastoma	
Williams[86]	1986	CCAM	Embryonal RMS	21
Allan[4]	1987	"Congenital origin of cysts not confirmed"	RMS	21, 30
Shariff[67]	1988	CCAM type 1	RMS	15
Hedlund[33]	1989	"Cystic hamartoma"	RMS	18, 22
Cairoli[10]	1990	CCAM	RMS	36
Domizio[20]	1990	"Congenital cyst"	Malignant mesenchymoma	48
Senac[65]	1991		PPB	
Murphy[52]	1992	Bronchogenic cyst, CCAM (2)	Embryonal RMS	24, 36, 42
Bogers[8]	1993	Lobar emphysema	RMS	18
Calabria[11]	1993	"Pneumatoceles"	Pulmonary blastoma	
McDermott[49]	1993	Congenital cyst	Embryonal RMS	36
Paupe[57]	1994	Cystic lung lesion	Pulmonary blastoma	
Seballos[64]	1994	CCAM	Pulmonary blastoma	22
Tagge[75]	1996	Bilateral pneumatocele	PPB	45
Adirim[1]	1997	CCAM type 1	Pulmonary blastoma	
D'Agostino[16]	1997	CCAM type 2	Embryonal RMS	22
Federici[23]	2001	CCAM type 1	PPB	36
Ozcan[54]	2001	CCAM	Embryonal RMS	13
Papagiannopoulos[55]	2001	CCAM type 4	PPB	30
Stocker[71]	2002	CCAM type 4	PPB	48

CCAM, congenital cystic adenomatoid malformation; CPAM congenital pulmonary airway malformation; PPB, pleuropulmonary blastoma; RMS, rhabdomyosarcoma.
Adapted from LaBerge JM, Puligandla P, Flageole H: Asymptomatic congenital lung malformations. Semin Pediatr Surg 2005;14:16.

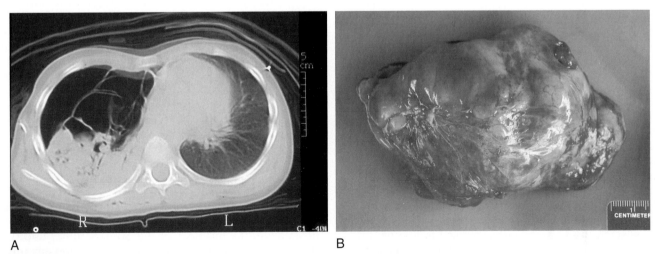

A B

Figure 39-2 *A,* Computed tomography scan of the chest shows a cystic lesion in the right hemithorax. *B,* The tumor was resected (lobectomy), and the histology showed findings consistent with a pleuropulmonary blastoma. (Courtesy of Jay L. Grosfeld, MD.)

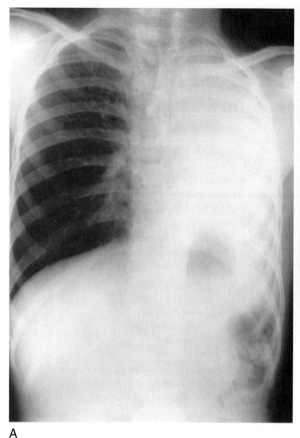

A

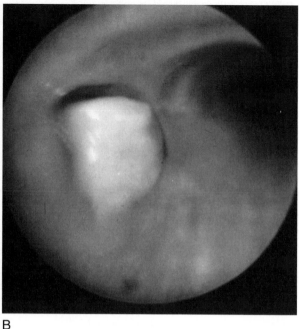

B

Figure 39–3   Patient with complete atelectasis of the left lung and obstruction of the left main bronchus secondary to rhabdomyosarcoma.

lesion or evidence of airway obstruction with resultant atelectasis and pneumonitis. Because many of these tumors can be visualized by bronchoscopy, a bronchoscopic examination should be performed. Flexible bronchoscopic techniques may be helpful for diagnosis, but the use of rigid bronchoscopy with modern magnification, along with general anesthesia, is necessary if endoscopic biopsy is contemplated. Preparation for emergency thoracotomy should be made at the time of bronchoscopy in the event of life-threatening hemorrhage.

Bronchoscopic removal of some isolated lesions may be attempted, but owing to the high incidence of recurrence and the possibility of severe hemorrhage, this technique should be used selectively. Conservative surgical resection is the procedure of choice for benign pulmonary tumors to achieve histologic diagnosis and preserve maximum functioning lung tissue. Thoracoscopic resection is an option in these children.[35] CT and magnetic resonance imaging should be performed in children with large space-occupying lesions to determine resectability. Fine-needle aspiration for cytology or core needle biopsy may be performed as the initial procedure for diagnosis in selected cases. Treatment of malignant lesions varies, depending on location and histology. Sleeve resections should be considered for bronchial adenomas. Resection of involved lymphatics should be considered with malignant lesions. Combined-modality therapy with adjuvant chemotherapy and possibly radiation therapy may be helpful in children with large primary malignancies or dissemination.

An important consideration is the association of primary lung tumors with congenital cystic pulmonary malformations. These lesions may be asymptomatic and be discovered incidentally. In some instances, the natural history of the lung cyst is unknown, and a few may regress.[42] Although some authors recommend simple observation, most pediatric surgeons argue against prolonged observation of cystic lesions because of an increased risk of infection, pneumothorax, sudden cyst enlargement with potential respiratory compromise, and associated malignancy.[1,11,42,47,55,57,65,75] If patients with asymptomatic cystic malformations are observed without resection, they should be followed closely and evaluated frequently.

TREATMENT OF METASTATIC DISEASE

Pulmonary metastases occur much more frequently than primary tumors in children, and the surgical approach depends on the histology of the primary tumor and the response of the primary site to combined-modality therapy. Pulmonary metastases should not be considered for resection until the primary tumor is eradicated without evidence of recurrence and other sites of metastatic disease are ruled out. Tumors most frequently considered

TABLE 39-4 Pulmonary Metastasectomy for Osteogenic Sarcoma

Author	No. of Patients	Average Interval to Relapse (mo) (Range)	No. of Procedures (No. of Lesions)	Disease-Free Survival, No. (%)	Median Follow-up for Survivors/ (mo) (Range)
Martini[48]	22	10 (2-25)	59 (113)	7 (32)	33 (15-234)
Spanos[69]	29	15.7 (4-30)	52 (124)	11 (37)	36 (9-234)
Telander[77]	28	9/6 (2-34)	60 (173)	13 (46)	25 (6-48)
Giritsky[25]	12	9 (1-21)	19	6 (50)	17 (9-39)
Rosenberg[60]	18	—	—	7 (39)	—
Burgers[9]	12	13 (2-20)	9	5 (42)	(36-72)
Schaller[63]	17	—	34	7 (41)	(12-192)
Goorin[26]	32	12.5 (4-59)	26 (>63)	9 (28)	55 (19-101)
Carter[12]	43	13 (1-83)	—	4 (10)	69 (59-80)

From LaQuaglia MP: The surgical management of metastases in pediatric cancer. Semin Pediatr Surg 1993;2:75.

for pulmonary metastasectomy are osteosarcoma, soft tissue sarcoma, and Wilms' tumor.[39]

Osteosarcoma

Children with osteosarcoma should be considered for resection of pulmonary metastases once the primary lesion is controlled. The overall disease-free survival is approximately 40% in children who develop metachronous pulmonary metastases. Multiple factors, such as number of pulmonary nodules and time of recurrence, play an important role in children with osteosarcoma and pulmonary metastases.[32,78] Roth et al.[61] showed that patients with fewer than four pulmonary nodules had an improved survival over those with more than four lesions. According to Goorin et al.,[26] a complete resection of all pulmonary lesions is an important determinant of outcome, and penetration through the parietal pleura is associated with an adverse outcome. Although somewhat controversial, the outlook seems to be somewhat improved, even in patients presenting with pulmonary metastases, if complete resection of all metastatic lesions can be accomplished.[46] Harris et al.[30] reported a 68% survival rate in 17 patients with fewer than eight pulmonary nodules at presentation following chemotherapy, resection of the primary tumor, and pulmonary metastasectomy. The data in Table 39-4 suggest that an aggressive attempt at surgical resection of pulmonary metastases is indicated in osteosarcoma, possibly irrespective of the number of lesions or the interval to the development of metastases.

Soft Tissue Sarcoma

The usefulness of resecting pulmonary metastases in patients with soft tissue sarcoma depends on the histologic subtype. Rarely is pulmonary resection of metastatic lesions required in rhabdomyosarcoma, and resection of pulmonary metastasis in Ewing's sarcoma has not been found to be efficacious.[34] The remaining sarcomas should be considered for resection if complete excision is possible and the patient's primary tumor is under control. The time to development of pulmonary metastases, number of lesions, and tumor doubling time are all significant prognostic factors in soft tissue sarcomas. Historically, approximately 10% to 20% of these patients can be salvaged by resection of pulmonary metastases.[44]

Wilms' Tumor

Rarely is pulmonary resection of metastatic disease required in children with Wilms' tumor. In a review of the National Wilms' Tumor Study by Green et al.,[28] no advantage of pulmonary resection was found compared with chemotherapy and radiation therapy alone. In an attempt to avoid pulmonary radiation, deKraker et al.[18] suggested a protocol using primary pulmonary resection after chemotherapy for pulmonary metastases. The overall results were not encouraging, and few patients ultimately required resection of pulmonary metastases following chemotherapy. Because the results of chemotherapy and whole-lung irradiation are excellent for children with Wilms' tumor and pulmonary metastases, pulmonary resection of metastases should be reserved for only selected cases (see Chapter 27).

Comments

Operation for pulmonary metastases in children depends on the histology of the primary tumor, the extent of the metastatic disease, and whether the metastatic disease is responsive to chemotherapy. The surgical approach varies, depending on the disease process and the age of the patient. No difference in survival has been demonstrated with sequential lateral thoracotomy versus sternotomy, but the latter is preferable in older patients with osteosarcoma. Complete resection of all metastatic disease is an important consideration, and the use of automatic stapling devices can be helpful. Wedge resection is usually possible in children with osteosarcoma. However, formal lobectomy or segmentectomy may be required to remove all tumor completely, especially when the primary tumor is not responsive to chemotherapy or radiation.[6] Muscle-sparing techniques are available in those children requiring posterolateral thoracotomies, and thoracoscopy may be appropriate in certain cases.[55] However, port site recurrences have been reported following thoracoscopic resection of pulmonary metastatic disease.[62,85]

REFERENCES

1. Adirim AD, King R, Klein BL: Radiologic case of the month: Congenital cystic adenomatoid malformation of the lung and pulmonary blastoma. Arch Pediatr Adolesc Med 1997;151:1053.
2. Agrons GA, Rosado-de-Christenson ML, Kirejczyk WM, et al: Pulmonary inflammatory pseudotumor: Radiologic features. Radiology 1998;206:51.
3. Ahel V, Zubovic I, Rozmanic V: Bronchial adenoid cystic carcinoma with saccular bronchiectasis as a cause of recurrent pneumonia in children. Pediatr Pulmonol 1992: 12:160.
4. Allan BT, Day DL, Dehner LP: Primary pulmonary rhabdomyosarcoma of the lung in children: Report of two cases presenting with spontaneous pneumothorax. Cancer 1987;59:1005.
5. Bahadoni M, Liebow AA: Plasma cell granulomas of the lung. Cancer 1973;31:191.
6. Ballantine TVN, Wiseman NE, Filler RM: Assessment of pulmonary wedge resection for the treatment of lung metastases. J Pediatr Surg 1975;10:671.
7. Benjamin DR, Cahill JL: Bronchioalveolar carcinoma of the lung and congenital cystic adenomatoid malformation. Am J Clin Pathol 1991;95:889.
8. Bogers AJ, Hazebroek FW, Molenaar J, et al: Surgical treatment of congenital bronchopulmonary disease in children. Eur J Cardiothorac Surg 1993;7:117.
9. Burgers JM, Brear K, van Dobbenburgh OA, et al: Role of metastasectomy without chemotherapy in the management of osteosarcoma in children. Cancer 1980; 45:1664.
10. Cairoli G, Bertana S, Giuntoli M, et al: Cystic adenomatoid malformation of the lung: Experience in four operated cases. Pediatr Med Chir 1990;12:681.
11. Calabria R, Srikanth MS, Chamberlin K, et al: Management of pulmonary blastoma in children. Am Surg 1993; 59:192.
12. Carter SR, Grimer RJ, Sneath RS, et al: Results of thoracotomy in osteogenic sarcoma with pulmonary metastases. Thorax 1991;46:727.
13. Crisei KL, Greenberg SB, Wolfson BJ: Cardiopulmonary and thoracic tumors of childhood. Radiol Clin North Am 1997;35:1341.
14. Crist WM, Raney RB, Newton W, et al: Intrathoracic soft tissue sarcomas in children. Cancer 1982;50:598.
15. Cohen MC, Kaschula ROC: Primary pulmonary tumors in childhood: A review of 31 years' experience and the literature. Pediatr Pulmonol 1992;40:222.
16. D'Agostino S, Bonoldi E, Dante S, et al: Embryonal rhabdomyosarcoma of the lung arising in cystic adenomatoid malformation: Case report and review of the literature. J Pediatr Surg 1997;32:1381.
17. Dehner LP: Pleuropulmonary blastoma is the pulmonary blastoma of childhood. Semin Diagn Pathol 1994; 11:144.
18. deKraker J, Lemerle J, Voute PA, et al: Wilms' tumor with pulmonary metastases at diagnosis: The significance of primary chemotherapy. J Clin Oncol 1990;8:1187.
19. De Perrot M, Pache JC, Spiliopoulous A: Carcinoma arising in congenital lung cysts. Thorac Cardiovasc Surg 2001;49:184.
20. Domizio P, Liesner RL, Dicks-Mireaux C, et al: Malignant mesenchymoma associated with a congenital lung cyst in a child: Case report and review of the literature. Pediatr Pathol 1990;10:785.
21. Eggli KD, Newman B: Nodules, masses and pseudomasses in the pediatric lung. Radiol Clin North Am 1993; 31:651.
22. Endo T, Inoue M, Waatanabe N, et al: Two operative cases of pulmonary blastoma. Kyobu Geka 1982;35:219.
23. Federici S, Domenichelli V, Tani G: Pleuropulmonary blastoma in congenital cystic adenomatoid malformation: Report of a case. Eur J Pediatr Surg 2001;11:196.
24. Gaissert HA, Mathisen DJ, Grillo HC, et al: Tracheobronchial sleeve resection in children and adolescents. J Pediatr Surg 1994;29:192.
25. Giritsky AS, Etcubawas E, Mark JBD: Pulmonary resection in children with metastatic osteogenic sarcoma. J Thorac Cardiovas Surg 1978;75:354.
26. Goorin AM, DeCorey MJ, Lack EE, et al: Prognostic significance of complete surgical resection of pulmonary metastases in patients with osteogenic sarcoma: Analyses of 32 patients. J Clin Oncol 1984;2:425.
27. Granata C, Gambini C, Balducci T, et al: Bronchioalveolar carcinoma arising in a cystic adenomatoid malformation in a child: A case report and review on malignancies originating in congenital adenomatoid malformations. Pediatr Pulmonol 1998;25:62.
28. Green DM, Breslow N, Ii Y, et al: The role of surgical excision in the management of relapsed Wilms' tumor patients with pulmonary metastases: A report from the National Wilms' Tumor Study. J Pediatr Surg 1991;26:728.
29. Hancock BJ, DiLorenzo M, Youssef S, et al: Childhood primary pulmonary neoplasms. J Pediatr Surg 1993; 28:1133.
30. Harris M, Gieser P, Goorin AM, et al: Treatment of metastatic osteosarcoma at diagnosis: A Pediatric Oncology Group study. J Clin Oncol 1998;11:3641.
31. Hartman GE, Shochat SJ: Primary pulmonary neoplasms of childhood: A review. Ann Thorac Surg 1983;36:108.
32. Hawkins DS, Arndt CA: Pattern of disease recurrence and prognostic factors in patients with osteosarcoma treated with contemporary chemotherapy. Cancer 2003; 98:2447.
33. Hedlund GL, Bisset GS III, Bove KE: Malignant neoplasms arising in cystic hamartomas of the lung in childhood. Radiology 1989;173:77.
34. Heij HA, Vos A, deKraker J, et al: Prognostic factors in surgery for pulmonary metastases in children. Surgery 1994; 115:687.
35. Holcomb GW III, Tomita SS, Haase GM, et al: Minimally invasive surgery in children with cancer. Cancer 1995; 76:121.
36. Holland-Moritz RM, Heyn RM: Pulmonary blastoma associated with cystic lesions in children. Med Pediatr Oncol 1984;12:85.
37. Hurley P, Corbishsley C, Pepper J: Bronchoalveolar carcinoma arising in longstanding lung cysts. Thorax 1985; 40:960.

38. Jalal A, Jeyasingham K: Bronchoplasty for malignant and benign conditions: A retrospective study of 44 cases. Eur J Cardiothorac Surg 2000;17:370.

39. Karnak I, Senocak ME, Kutluk T, et al: Pulmonary metastases in children: An analysis of surgical spectrum. Eur J Pediatr Surg 2002;12:15.

40. Kaslovsky RA, Purdy S, Dangman BC, et al: Bronchioalveolar carcinoma in a child with congenital cystic adenomatoid malformation. Chest 1997;112:548.

41. Krous HF, Harper PE, Perlman M: Congenital cystic adenomatoid malformation in bilateral renal agenesis: Its mitigation of Potter's syndrome. Arch Pathol Lab Med 1980;104:368.

42. LaBerge JM, Puligandla P, Flageole H: Asymptomatic congenital lung malformations. Semin Pediatr Surg 2005; 14:16.

43. Lack EE, Harris GBC, Eraklis AJ, et al: Primary bronchial tumors in childhood: A clinicopathologic study of six cases. Cancer 1983;51:492.

44. LaQuaglia MP: The surgical management of metastases in pediatric cancer. Semin Pediatr Surg 1993;2:75.

45. MacSweeney F, Papagiannopoulos K, Goldstraw P, et al: Assessment of the expanded classification of congenital cystic adenomatoid malformations and their relationship to malignant transformation. Am J Surg Pathol 2003; 27:1139.

46. Marina NM, Pratt CB, Rao BN, et al: Improved prognosis of children with osteosarcoma metastatic to the lung(s) at the time of diagnosis. Cancer 1992;70:2722.

47. Martinez JC, Pecero FC, Gutierrez de la Pena C, et al: Pulmonary blastoma: Report of a case. J Pediatr Surg 1978;13:93.

48. Martini N, Havos AG, Mike V, et al: Multiple pulmonary resections in the treatment of osteogenic sarcoma. Ann Thorac Surg 1971;12:271.

49. McDermott VG, MacKenzie S, Hendry GM: Case report: Primary intrathoracic rhabdomyosarcoma: A rare childhood malignancy. Br J Radiol 1993;66:937.

50. Morales L, Julia V, Tardio E, et al: Pulmonary blastoma at the site of a congenital pulmonary cyst. Chir Pediatr 1986; 27:53.

51. Morresi A, Wockel W, Karg O: Adenomatoid cystic lung abnormality in adults with associated bronchioalveolar carcinoma. Pathologe 1995;16:292.

52. Murphy JJ, Blair GK, Fraser GC, et al: Rhabdomyosarcoma arising within congenital pulmonary cysts: Report of three cases. J Pediatr Surg 1992;27:1364.

53. Nistal M, Jimenez-Hefferman JA, Hardisson D, et al: Malignant fibrous histiocytoma of the lung in a child. Eur J Pediatr 1997;156:107.

54. Ozcan C, Celik A, Ural Z, et al: Primary pulmonary rhabdomyosarcoma arising within cystic adenomatoid malformation: A case report and review of the literature. J Pediatr Surg 2001;36:1062.

55. Papagiannopolous KA, Sheppard M, Bush AP, et al: Pleuropulmonary blastoma: Is prophylactic resection of congenital lung cysts effective? Ann Thorac Surg 2001; 72:604.

56. Parsons SK, Fishman SJ, Hoorntje LE, et al: Aggressive multimodal treatment of pleuropulmonary blastoma. Ann Thorac Surg 2001:72:939.

57. Paupe A, Martelli H, Lenclen R, et al: Pneumothorax revealing pneumoblastoma in an infant. Arch Pediatr 1994;1:919.

58. Prichard MG, Brown PJ, Sterrett GF: Bronchioalveolar carcinoma arising in longstanding lung cysts. Thorax 1984;39:545.

59. Ribet ME, Copin MC, Soots JG, et al: Bronchalveolar carcinoma and cystic adenomatoid malformation. Ann Thorac Surg 1995;60:1126.

60. Rosenberg SA, Flye MW, Conkle D, et al: Treatment of osteogenic sarcoma. II. Aggressive resection of pulmonary metastases. Cancer Treat Rep 1979;63:753.

61. Roth JA, Putnam JB, Wesley MN, et al: Differing determinants of prognosis following resection of pulmonary metastases from osteogenic and soft tissue sarcoma patients. Cancer 1985;55:1361.

62. Sartorelli KH, Patrick D, Meagher DP Jr: Port-site recurrence after thoracoscopic resection of pulmonary metastasis owing to osteogenic sarcoma. J Pediatr Surg 1996;31:1443.

63. Schaller RT Jr, Haas J, Schaller J, et al: Improved survival in children with osteosarcoma following resection of pulmonary metastases. J Pediatr Surg 1982;17:546.

64. Seballos RM, Klein RL: Pulmonary blastoma in children: Report of two cases and review of the literature. J Pediatr Surg 1994;29:1553.

65. Senac MO Jr, Wood BP, Isaacs H, et al: Pulmonary blastoma, a rare childhood malignancy. Radiology 1991;179:743.

66. Seo IS, Warren M, Mirkin LD, et al: Mucoepidermoid carcinoma of the bronchus in a four year old child. Cancer 1984;53:1600.

67. Shariff S, Thomas JA, Shetty N, et al: Primary pulmonary rhabdomyosarcoma in a child with a review of the literature. J Surg Oncol 1988;38:261.

68. Soga J, Yakuwa Y: Bronchopulmonary carcinoids: An analysis of 1875 reported cases with special reference to a comparison between typical carcinoids and atypical varieties. Ann Thorac Cardiovasc Surg 1999;5:211.

69. Spanos PK, Payne WS, Ivins JC, Pritchard DJ: Pulmonary resection for metastatic osteogenic sarcoma. J Bone Joint Surg Am 1976;58:624.

70. Stephanopoulos C, Catsaras H: Myxosarcoma complicating a cystic hamartoma of the lung. Thorax 1963;18:144.

71. Stocker JT: Congenital pulmonary airway malformations— a new name for and an expanded classification of congenital cystic adenomatoid malformation of the lung. Histopathology 2002;41(Suppl):S424.

72. Su W, Ko A, O'Connell TX, et al: Treatment of pseudotumors with nonsteroidal anti-inflammatory drugs. J Pediatr Surg 2000;35:1635.

73. Sudou M, Sugi K, Murakami T: Bronchioalveolar carcinoma arising from a congenital cystic adenomatoid malformation in an adolescent: The first case in the Orient. J Thorac Cardiovasc Surg 2003;126:902.

74. Sumner TE, Phelps CR, Crowe JE, et al: Pulmonary blastoma in a child. AJR Am J Roentgenol 1979; 133:147.

75. Tagge EP, Mulvihill D, Chandler JC, et al: Childhood pleuropulmonary blastoma: Caution against nonoperative management of congenital lung cysts. J Pediatr Surg 1996; 31:187.

76. Tagge EP, Yanis E, Chopy KJ, et al: Obstructing endobronchial fibrous histiocytoma: Potential for lung salvage. J Pediatr Surg 1991;26:1067.

77. Telander RL, Pairolero PC, Pritchard DJ, et al: Resection of pulmonary metastatic osteogenic sarcoma in children. Surgery 1978;84:335H.

78. Thompson RC Jr, Cheng EY, Clohisy DR, et al: Results of treatment for metastatic osteosarcoma with neoadjuvant chemotherapy and surgery. Clin Orthop 2002;397:240.

79. Ueda K, Gruppo R, Unger F, et al: Rhabdomyosarcoma of lung arising in congenital cystic adenomatoid malformation. Cancer 1977;40:383.

80. Valderrama E, Salija G, Shende A, et al: Pulmonary blastoma: Report of two cases in children. Am J Surg Pathol 1978;2:415.

81. Verbeke JIML, Verberne AAPH, Den Hollander JC, Robben SGF: Inflammatory myofibroblastic tumor of the lung manifesting as progressive atelectasis. Pediatr Radiol 1999;29:816.

82. Vujanic GM, Dojcinov D: Inflammatory pseudotumor of the lung in children. Pediatr Hematol Oncol 1991;8:121.

83. Weinberg AG, Currarino G, Moore GC, Votteler TP: Mesenchymal neoplasia and congenital pulmonary cysts. Pediatr Radiol 1980;9:179.

84. Weinblatt ME, Siegel SE, Isaacs H: Pulmonary blastoma associated with cystic lung disease. Cancer 1982; 49:669.

85. Wille GA, Gregory R, Guernsey JM: Tumor implantation at port site of video-assisted thoracoscopic resection of pulmonary metastasis. West J Med 1997;166:65.

86. Williams RA: Embryonal rhabdomysosarcoma occurring in cystic adenomatoid malformation. Pediatr Pathol 1986; 5:118.

87. Zaidi A, Zamvar V, Macbeth F, et al: Pulmonary blastoma: Medium-term results from a regional center. Ann Thorac Surg 2002;73:1572.

Chapter 40

Bone Tumors

Saminathan S. Nathan and John H. Healey

Bone tumors are rare. In the United States there were 166,487 cases of breast cancer and 164,753 cases[28] of prostate cancer in 2000. By comparison, there were only 2,051 of all types of bone sarcomas that year. A large proportion of these tumors occur in the pediatric population. In one published database 26.8% of all bone sarcomas occurred in the pediatric age group. There are no population-based benign bone registries so it would be impossible to guess at the true incidence of benign bone tumors. Most databases of this nature derive from tertiary referral institutions, and so benign conditions, which are often asymptomatic, would be grossly underrepresented. Nevertheless, one study has shown that up to 43% of children have a bone lesion during skeletal development.[18] This implies that the overwhelming majority of lesions are benign.

The pediatric surgeon will often be called into the management of the patient with bone tumors for a number of reasons. The very young child on follow-up for an unrelated condition may manifest with a bone lesion secondary to osteomyelitis or leukemia. The older child with a metastatic osteogenic sarcoma may require the expertise of the pediatric thoracic surgeon for the resection of pulmonary nodules. The teenager with a pathologic fracture through a unicameral bone cyst or nonossifying fibroma may present first to the pediatric surgeon on call in the pediatric emergency department.

The diagnosis of these rare groups of conditions is readily attained through a careful clinical evaluation. In that regard, the utility of plain radiographs can never be overstated. They facilitate the initial workup of these patients and allow them to be referred to specialized centers with multidisciplinary expertise. Although the subsequent imaging modalities are important, the radiographs form a key part of surgical planning.

It is with the pediatric surgeon in mind that this chapter is written. Lengthy discourse on the pathology is avoided, and several excellent references exist.[62,67,128,135] Instead, the format adopted is a practical approach to the management of these conditions. Where prudent, insights and controversies are highlighted to spur interest into specific areas.

GENERAL CONSIDERATIONS

Pathophysiology

The main aim of this section is to illustrate the specific issues of the pathophysiology of bone tumors that distinguish them from tumors of soft tissue.

Bone tumors should be approached initially from the standpoint of being benign or malignant. Whereas traditional approaches regarding the treatment of most nonskeletal benign lesions have been one of benign neglect if these lesions are not perceived to be causing problems, the management of benign bone lesions is complicated by a potential compromise of skeletal structural integrity. Cortical deficiency weakens bones and can mandate treatment to prevent fracture. The prudent, if rare, consideration is one of syndromic presentation and malignant transformation. Many of these principles are applicable to malignant lesions as well. However, malignant lesions have at their cornerstone of consideration their implication on survival, which will be elaborated. Metastatic lesions to bone are not common in the pediatric age group. Their pathophysiologic implications tend to be structural or diagnostic.

In the pediatric age group benign lesions far outnumber primary malignant lesions, which in turn outnumber metastatic lesions. Owing to the protean manner in which benign lesions behave, some are not evident in the physician's office. Conclusions about their natural history and malignant potential are therefore difficult to ascertain.[67] This is obviously not the problem with malignant and metastatic lesions. In this section we discuss pathologic conditions of the bone that occur most commonly in the pediatric age group. In the pediatric population the commonly occurring benign lesions are the unicameral bone cyst, aneurysmal bone cyst, enchondroma, osteochondroma, nonossifying fibroma, and osteoid osteoma. The common malignant bone tumors are osteogenic sarcoma and Ewing's family tumor (Table 40-1). Here we highlight specific features of each tumor. For a more thorough understanding of pathology the reader is directed to any one of a number of fine books on the subject.[62,67,128,135]

TABLE 40-1 Commonly Occurring Tumors by Age Group

Age	Benign Tumors	Malignant Tumors	Tumor-like Conditions
Birth to 5 years	Eosinophilic granuloma	Leukemia Metastatic neuroblastoma	Osteomyelitis Nonaccidental injury
5 to 15 years	Unicameral bone cyst Osteochondroma Aneurysmal bone cyst Osteoid osteoma Enchondroma Nonossifying fibroma Chondromyxoid fibroma Chondroblastoma	Ewing's sarcoma Osteogenic sarcoma	Fibrous dysplasia Osteomyelitis Osteofibrous dysplasia Stress fracture
15 to 20 years	Unicameral bone cyst Osteochondroma Osteoid osteoma Aneurysmal bone cyst Nonossifying fibroma Giant cell tumor Enchondroma Chondroblastoma Chondromyxoid fibroma	Osteogenic sarcoma Ewing's sarcoma	Fibrous dysplasia Stress fracture

By considering the factors age, frequency, and location in the long bones (see Fig. 40-3), a diagnosis can be arrived in the majority of cases. The possibility of trauma should always be borne in mind and in the noncommunicative child younger than 5 years old, nonaccidental injury may be the cause.

Benign Lesions

The typical benign lesion in the pediatric age group (Table 40-2) is determined incidentally. These lesions rarely cause any symptoms and are often diagnosed when a parent notices a lump or deformity (e.g., osteochondroma) or a radiograph is obtained for an unrelated

TABLE 40-2 Incidence of the More Commonly Diagnosed Bone Tumors

Tumors	All Bone Tumors (%)	Bone Tumors in the First Two Decades (%)
Benign		
Osteochondroma	7.86	4.69
Aneurysmal bone cyst	2.60	1.96
Osteoid osteoma	2.99	1.94
Nonossifying fibroma	1.13	0.99
Enchondroma	3.02	0.98
Giant cell tumor	5.10	0.80
Chondroblastoma	1.07	0.66
Chondromyxoid fibroma	0.41	0.14
Unicameral bone cyst	Unknown	Unknown
Malignant		
Osteogenic sarcoma	14.9	7.53
Ewing's sarcoma	4.6	3.50

In using this table a number of caveats need to be remembered. Most benign lesions are often asymptomatic, and only symptomatic ones will present. Of these, most will be managed at the primary care setting. Malignant lesions will, however, usually present to a referral center. Hence in terms of population incidence these figures are unreliable. In relative terms, however, they have some utility in indicating their prevalence. Unicameral bone cysts are left in this list as a reminder of their frequency.

condition (e.g., nonossifying fibroma). In these cases there are two main surgical indications: diagnosis through a biopsy and surgical stabilization of bones that have fractured or are likely to fracture, especially through a precarious location. For example, a bone cyst in the neck of a femur should be seriously considered for surgical stabilization because a fracture through this area may result in avascular necrosis of the femoral head. The biopsy itself cannot be undertaken lightly because it can weaken the bone, mandating surgical or external splinting. This is pertinent because benign lesions are often asymptomatic whereas the biopsy itself incurs morbidity. The challenge is in improving the yield from biopsy in terms of distinguishing malignant from benign disease.

Size of the Tumor

Size is an important consideration. For example, cartilaginous tumors larger than 4 cm in a heterogeneous group of patients with cartilaginous rib lesions were found to have increased likelihood of malignant behavior.[62] Because of their aggressive malignant potential large cartilaginous tumors should be resected widely despite their relatively bland histologic appearance (Fig. 40-1). Large tumors can also grow into neighboring compartments and cause mechanical compromise to joints. Although this is less critical in joints of the upper limb, it is more important in the spine and in the lower limbs, where they cause mechanical impingement and pain. The disruption of a tubular bone that results from the growth of a lesion results in weakening of the bone. Thus, lesions that involve more than 50% of the cross-section of a bone should be treated from a mechanical standpoint.[45,46,58] These lesions are at increased risk of fracture and, on the

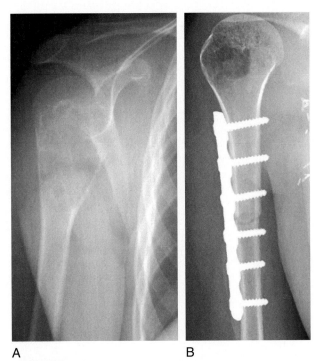

A   B

Figure 40–1 *A,* Chondrosarcoma in the proximal humerus of a 13-year-old boy. This is an exceedingly rare diagnosis in this age group. *B,* A proximal humeral resection with allograft reconstruction was performed. In children, the available prostheses may be too large and hence bulk allografts may be the only choice.

of the growth plate, caused disordered linear growth of the long bone.[135] These cases are often familial and rarely compromised by their condition. Joints of the upper limb often have high tolerance for the resultant deformity. In the occasional case, however, especially in the lower limb, degenerative arthritis develops necessitating premature surgery.

Multiplicity of Bone Tumors

Multiple bone lesions are often syndromic and may confer a higher incidence of malignant degeneration.[67,128,135] Multiple osteochondromas occur in multiple hereditary exostoses—an autosomal dominant condition caused by abnormalities of the *EXT1, EXT2,* and *EXT3* genes on chromosomes 8, 11 and 19.[30,74,142] Patients with this condition have an increased incidence of malignant degeneration into chondrosarcomas of 10% to 27.6%. By comparison, isolated osteochondromas have a malignant degeneration rate of about 1%.[62,67,128] Because only symptomatic lesions will present to the physician, the true incidence of malignant degeneration in isolated lesions is probably impossible to ascertain with certainty. Multiple enchondromatoses is a sporadic condition that confers an increased incidence of malignant transformation of up to 50% in the involved bones.[67] Limb-length inequality and malalignment are also common. *Ollier's disease,* as this condition is termed, has another counterpart

chance that they may be malignant, could result in a potential limb-sparing operation being deferred for an amputation.

Fracture Through a Benign Lesion

The fractured benign lesion is typified by the unicameral bone cyst. These lesions may appear aggressive, but a careful history and physical examination with appropriate imaging modalities will usually establish their benign nature (Fig. 40-2). Unicameral bone cysts that fracture have been known to resolve spontaneously. However, the vast majority of them will continue to fracture through a child's lifetime and prove to be disabling.[98] In general, they should be treated surgically, especially if they are symptomatic.

The timing of surgery is critical. An early biopsy would show callus formation that would be difficult to distinguish from a malignant process. Therefore, these lesions should be observed during fracture healing for about a month, following which a biopsy and a definitive procedure are performed.

Location in Relation to the Physis

Location in relation to the physes is an important consideration distinguishing tumor assessment and management of children versus adults (Fig. 40-3). The term *diaphyseal aclasis* was coined to highlight a condition in which multiple osteochondromas, a condition primarily

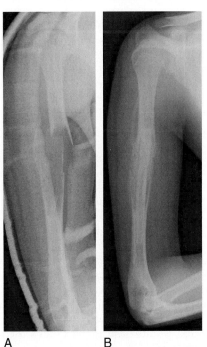

A   B

Figure 40–2 *A,* Large unicameral bone cyst of the proximal humerus that had fractured. The aggressive appearance may lead one to suspect a malignant process, but a careful evaluation of the margins of this lesion and absence of periosteal reaction reaffirms the management decision of observation before surgery. *B,* This cyst was curetted and packed with an allograft 1 month after the fracture. Treatment with an intramedullary fibular graft provided stabilization, and supplemental bone graft healed the lesion.

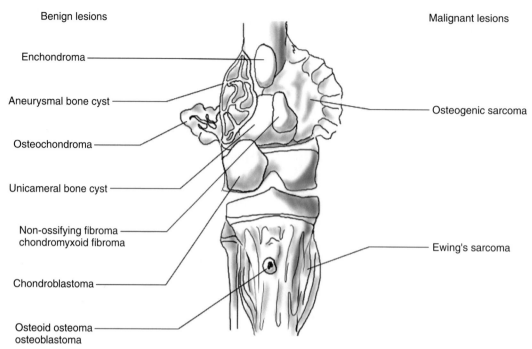

Benign lesions

Enchondroma

Aneurysmal bone cyst

Osteochondroma

Unicameral bone cyst

Non-ossifying fibroma
chondromyxoid fibroma

Chondroblastoma

Osteoid osteoma
osteoblastoma

Malignant lesions

Osteogenic sarcoma

Ewing's sarcoma

Figure 40-3 The location of lesions in relation to the physis gives a clue to the diagnosis. In most cases the diagnosis can be made on radiographs, leaving further imaging to plan for surgery.

classically affecting one limb anlage. A variant, *Maffucci's syndrome,* describes widespread enchondromas associated with hemangiomas of the hand. The occurrence of multiple nonossifying fibromas, associated with mental retardation, café-au-lait spots, endocrine disorders, cardiovascular malformations, and ocular abnormalities has been termed *Jaffe-Campanacci syndrome* but has no malignant implications.[67,94]

Site of Involvement

The site of benign cartilaginous lesions has important implications on malignant potential. Peripheral lesions in the hand rarely turn malignant, whereas those toward the axial skeleton have important malignant potential even if they appear benign histologically.[62,67,86,94,128,135] Lesions in bones about weight-bearing joints should be regarded with special care. In the pediatric group these lesions are usually chondroblastomas. They grow epiphyseally and in so doing can cause weakening of the subchondral bone and ultimately an intra-articular extension or fracture that may even mimic osteochondral defects. In the case of sarcomas, a relatively conservative resection in this context would have to be deferred to an extra-articular resection.

Metastatic Potential

A unique feature of benign bone tumors is that there is a small incidence of metastasis in these lesions. Accordingly 1.7% of chondroblastomas and 3% of giant cell tumors[56,61,72,128] do metastasize. It is controversial if some of these lesions were, in fact, malignant from

the outset.[73] However, of the truly benign lesions that do metastasize, they tend to be in atypical lesions and have had surgical manipulation that may have embolized tumor cells. When followed, some of these metastatic lesions, primarily in the lung, may remain dormant and not progress. The possibility, therefore, is that they represent a transport phenomenon more akin to a mechanical embolism and not true metastasis, which would require a number of mutations before finally seeding.[62,73]

Malignant Lesions

Epidemiology

The main histologic types of bone tumors are osteogenic sarcoma, Ewing's family tumor, chondrosarcoma, and other sarcomas. They affect children at a rate of 6:3:2:1.[28,128]

Osteogenic sarcomas (also known as osteosarcomas) are malignant bone-forming tumors of the bone. They occur at any age but most frequently present in middle teenage years in the extremity. There are various subtypes with varying implications on survival. In general, the subtypes perform similarly except perhaps for telangiectatic osteogenic sarcomas, which bear special mention. In the pre-chemotherapy era this was regarded as the tumor with the poorest prognosis.[91] Presently, however, it has the best prognosis.[63] The lytic nature of these sarcomas weakens bone, resulting in the highest rate of pathologic fracture. Increasingly, rarer forms of osteogenic sarcoma are described. Two variants of note are the small cell sarcoma and giant cell rich osteogenic sarcoma. The former can be confused with Ewing's family tumor and as such is often treated by similar chemotherapy protocols.[90,116] The latter can be confused in the appropriate setting with giant cell tumors of the bone, which is a benign condition.[12,13,41]

Ewing's sarcoma occurs at a younger age (see Table 40-1) and may affect any bone, particularly the femur, pelvis, and humerus. It is the most common cancer in the pelvis, ribs, foot, and fibula. It was once considered to be distinct from peripheral neuroectodermal tumors but has been shown to be genetically identical to this entity. It is presently considered to be in the same family of neoplasms also known as Ewing's family tumors.[62,135]

Chondrosarcoma is less prevalent in the pediatric age group. It is more widely distributed in the body compared with its occurrence in adults.

Genetics

There have been few consistent genetic or syndromic associations with osteogenic sarcoma. Patients with the Li-Fraumeni syndrome[77] have a *TP53* germline mutation[78,81] on 9p21 and are predisposed to osteogenic sarcoma, breast cancer, and leukemia (Fig. 40-4). Two to 3 percent of patients with osteogenic sarcoma will be the proband for Li-Fraumeni families.[124] Another germline mutation of 13q14, hereditary retinoblastoma, predisposes to osteogenic sarcomas.[11] Children who received radiation therapy for retinoblastoma, Hodgkin's and non-Hodgkin's lymphoma, Ewing's family tumor, and other cancers are at 5% to 10% risk of developing osteogenic sarcoma. Patients with an *RB* gene deletion and a history of alkylating agent exposure from a prior malignancy are predisposed to this complication as well.[127] About 5% of all osteogenic sarcomas occur as postradiation sarcomas.[65]

Ewing's family tumor is a malignancy associated with a number of translocations. The 11 to 22 translocation resulting in an EWS-FLI1 fusion transcript is the most common variant, and type 1 is associated with the best prognosis.[15] Other translocations include type 2 EWS-FLI1, EWS-ERG from a 21,22 translocation, and EWS-ETV1 from a 7,22 translocation. These rarer variants have not been as well studied but appear to confer a poorer prognosis.[15] Further additive mutations involving cell-cycle genes reduce the prognosis of these tumors further. Ewing's family tumor is the most common solid tumor to metastasize to the brain.[32]

Diagnosis and Staging

Bone tumors are diagnosed based on the well-recognized triad of history, physical examination, and investigation. After a clinical diagnosis it is imperative that imaging and staging procedures are done before biopsy. Preoperative imaging allows for planning of the definitive procedure and hence placement of the biopsy incision. In addition, changes that would occur in the lesion after biopsy would be difficult to distinguish from changes due to tumor growth on imaging. Furthermore, changes in the lung after general anesthesia (e.g., atelectasis) are difficult to distinguish from metastatic deposits.

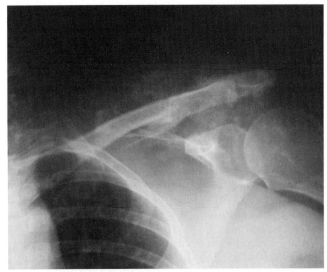

A

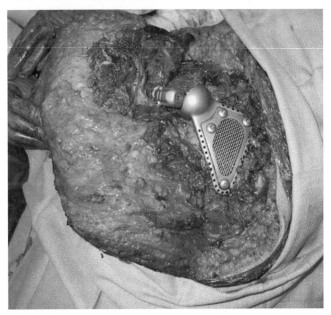

B

Figure 40–4 *A,* Osteogenic sarcoma in the left scapula of a female patient with Li-Fraumeni syndrome. This patient had a family history of osteogenic sarcoma in a first-degree relative. At the time of staging for the osteogenic sarcoma in the scapula a lesion in the breast was discovered on CT of the chest. This was subsequently found to be an adenocarcinoma. *B,* The patient underwent a scapular replacement. A latissimus dorsi flap was used for skin cover.

Clinical Evaluation

Although it is not possible to be comprehensive in this section, the history and physical examination are important parts of the assessment of a patient with a bone tumor. Patient demographics and tumor location narrow the differential diagnosis and focus the workup efficiently.

The patient's age is important (see Table 40-2). Most malignancies occur in the second decade of life.[62,67,128,135] Among children, subtle variation occurs in the prevalence of disease with respect to age (see Table 40-1).

Demographically, it is exceedingly rare for patients of African descent to have Ewing's family tumor.[135]

Pain at rest is an important sign that occurs in tumors and in other organic conditions such as infection and bone infarction. It distinguishes these conditions from mechanical pain, which occurs with activity. Most malignant tumors will present as pain. Pain relieved by nonsteroidal anti-inflammatory drugs (NSAIDs) is pathognomonic of osteoid osteoma.[59] This can occur at any age and is characterized by painful scoliosis when it occurs in the spine.

A family history of malignancy should be discerned especially in possible sentinel cases of the Li-Fraumeni syndrome.[77,78,81] Such patients should have systemic workups to rule out other sites of involvement in the form of radioisotope bone scans or positron emission tomographic scans.

As described earlier, the surgeon should be alert to any dysmorphism that the patient may have. Cutaneous stigmata are evident in patients with neurofibromatosis, fibrous dysplasia, and Jaffe-Campanacci syndrome.[94] Limb discrepancies are seen in patients with multiple enchondromatoses and multiple hereditary exostoses.[119]

Infection should be a differential diagnosis in almost every case seen. Tumor epidemiology is very telling. For example, childhood leukemia is nearly 10 times as common as Ewing's family tumor and so rare manifestations of leukemia are more common than routine presentations of Ewing's family tumor.

The nature of bony reconstruction also requires that the method chosen be matched with the demands of the patient. As such, an idea of the patient's expectation should be sought at this time.

Radiology

The minimal radiologic assessment at the first visit should be two orthogonal radiographic views of the area in question. Radiographs remain the most specific diagnostic imaging tests and are the only ones that give the "gestalt" of overall assessment of skeletal biology and mechanics. By analyzing the location of the tumor (see Fig. 40-3) as well as whether it is benign or malignant, the diagnosis can be arrived at in the majority of cases.[62,67,128,135]

Benign lesions are well circumscribed, with a good sclerotic border, and have no soft tissue edema. Malignant lesions have lucent or variegated matrices and permeative borders. Edema is often apparent as the presence of fat lines.

The often-quoted eponymous phrases are not specific to specific malignancies. *Codman's triangle* refers to the lifting and ossification of periosteum at the periphery of an osteogenic sarcoma. The *sunburst appearance* is due to the ossification of fibers and vessels subperiosteally as the tumor expands out of the cortex. *Onion skinning* refers to the periodic ossification and expansion of periosteum from the cortex. Any of these conditions can be seen in tumors or infections that are sufficiently fast growing.

In the diagram, epiphyseal lesions are typical of chondroblastoma or giant cell tumors; physeal lesions are typical of osteochondromas; metaphyseal lesions are typical of osteogenic sarcomas, unicameral bone cysts, aneurysmal bone cysts, and nonossifying fibromas; and diaphyseal lesions are typical of Ewing's family tumor, fibrous dysplasia, or enchondromas.

Laboratory Evaluation

The main blood parameters of importance are lactate dehydrogenase and alkaline phosphatase.[50,76,123] Lactate dehydrogenase levels have been used as a surrogate for tumor load and have been correlated with survival in the case of Ewing's family tumor.[50] Serum alkaline phosphatase elevation is characteristic of osteogenic sarcoma and is correlated with poor survival in this condition.[76,123] Glucose intolerance is associated with chondrosarcoma of the bone.[48,85] Erythrocyte sedimentation rates, C-reactive protein, and white blood cell and differential counts should be sought to rule out infection.

Preoperative Planning

Magnetic resonance imaging (MRI) of the lesion offers an assessment of compartmentalization of the tumor. A compartment is an abstract concept and refers to any plane that offers a fascial or cortical bone barrier to contiguous spread. It has implications on the extent of surgery, which by definition must be outside the compartment to be radical (see later).[37] Also by forming a baseline assessment one is able to make an assessment of response to chemotherapy in the case of neoadjuvant treatment.[60] It has secondary importance in providing the actual diagnosis. In specific examples it is useful in histologic diagnosis. The aneurysmal bone cyst shows fluid-fluid levels on an MR image. Pigmented villonodular synovitis is hypointense (dark) on T1- and T2-weighted imaging owing to hemosiderin deposition. Cartilaginous lesions are hyperintense (light) on T2-weighted imaging. Mineralized and dense fibrous tissue are dark on T1- and T2-weighted imaging.[4,96]

Staging

Staging studies are meant to assess the degree of spread of the disease. In the case of bone tumors two systems are used: the Enneking system or Surgical Staging System (SSS)[39] as adopted by the Musculoskeletal Tumor Society and the American Joint Committee on Cancer (AJCC) system, which at the time of writing is in its sixth revision.[53] In the case of Ewing's family tumor a different classification from Enneking is used.[36]

In the SSS, tumors are designated G0, G1, and G2 for benign, low-grade, and high-grade lesions. Benign lesions (G0) are classified as latent, active, or aggressive designated by Arabic numerals 1, 2, and 3, respectively. Malignant lesions are designated I if low grade and II if high grade. The further designation A or B denotes intracompartmental or extracompartmental disease. Stage III disease is metastatic disease. Therefore, in this classification, grade, compartmentalization, and metastases are the fundamental prognostic factors.

In the AJCC system, I and II similarly designate low- and high-grade lesions. A and B designate tumors smaller or larger than 8 cm, respectively. III denotes multicentric disease, and IV denotes metastatic disease. IVA denotes pulmonary metastases, and IVB denotes extrapulmonary metastases. Therefore, this classification considers grade, size, multicentricity, and metastases as prognostic factors.

In the Enneking staging system of Ewing's family tumor, stage I tumors are solitary intraosseous lesions, stage II are solitary lesions with extraosseous extension, stage III are multicentric lesions, and stage IV are metastatic. It is unclear how to stage patients who have independent sites of bone marrow involvement versus those who have circulating tumor cells identified by light microscopy (i.e., Enneking stage III or IV). Modern pathology analysis extends these concepts to include immunohistochemistry or reverse transcriptase polymerase chain reaction (RT-PCR) of recombinant gene products.

The modalities used for staging are bone scans and computed tomography (CT) of the chest.[39] Positron emission tomographic scans are presently being evaluated but have fundamental utility in the management of recurrent or metastatic disease.[16] In the case of Ewing's family tumor, bone marrow biopsies are done in an attempt to capture cases that are multicentric at presentation. The utility of this approach is being evaluated.[40]

Biopsy

The biopsy is a critical procedure that can complicate management severely if not performed appropriately. Misplaced incisions continue to be important causes of resectable tumors being rendered nonamenable to limb salvage surgery.[37,84] A good pathologist comfortable in handling bony tissue is critical to this process. In the appropriate case, extra tissue may be needed for cytogenetic studies. Ewing's family tumors are particularly fragile, and biopsy specimens should be handled carefully to allow for processing.

Presurgical Considerations

As a general rule, all imaging and staging should be completed before biopsy. The lesion that warrants biopsy should be given consideration for a primary wide excision. This approach is typically applicable to small lesions less than 3 cm, lesions in expendable bones (e.g., distal phalanx), distal ulna lesions, and proximal fibula lesions, where there is a risk of common peroneal nerve contamination (Fig. 40-5).

Figure 40–5 *A* and *B*, An aneurysmal bone cyst of the right proximal fibula in a 17-year-old boy. *C*, In this instance a primary wide resection was done because the bone was expendable and it prevented contamination of the common peroneal nerve *(arrow).*

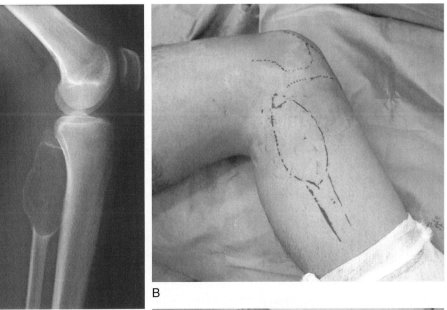

A

B

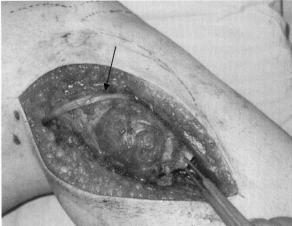

C

The lesion should preferably be sampled in the institution where the definitive procedure is to be done by the definitive surgeon. It has been shown repeatedly that when this was not adhered to the results were compromised.[83,84]

Consideration should be given to needle biopsies in the case of lesions in the pelvis or about the spine where the exposure necessary for an open biopsy may be extensive and oblige the commitment to a definitive procedure.

A pathologist familiar with processing bone tissue should be on hand to evaluate the biopsy. If tumor tissue can be cut with a knife, then it can be cut with a microtome. Frozen-section analysis is required primarily to ascertain the adequacy and representativeness of the specimen and secondarily for the definitive diagnosis.

Antibiotics should be withheld before the biopsy to improve the yield of microbiologic assessment. The biopsy may be done with use of a tourniquet to prevent bleeding and dissemination of the tumor locally. When the tourniquet is applied, simple elevation should be used for exsanguination. Compressive exsanguination should be avoided because this could rupture the tumor. At all times the limb should be protected from fracturing because this would cause extensive local dissemination of disease.

Surgical Considerations

The planned incision for the definitive surgery should be marked. This should generally follow extensile exposures and be longitudinal along the line of the definitive incision. The incision should be placed directly over the lesion. Flaps and dissection should be avoided.

The incision is developed directly into the tumor. If there is a soft tissue component of the tumor, then this alone needs be sampled. If a bone biopsy is necessary, then the edges of the biopsy specimen should be rounded to minimize a stress riser. Frozen section analysis will confirm the adequacy of the biopsy. In the meantime, a culture is taken, the tourniquet is released, and antibiotics are given. Absolute hemostasis is needed at the conclusion of the procedure to minimize spread of tumor cells in the hematoma.

The wound is closed in layers. If a drain is necessary, this should be brought out in the line of the incision so that it can be excised at the time of definitive surgery.

Postsurgical Considerations

The patient should be limited to protected weight bearing at least until some healing of the biopsy or ossification of the tumor as a response to neoadjuvant chemotherapy occurs. This typically takes up to 6 weeks.

Fractures through osteogenic sarcomas have traditionally precluded limb salvage surgery. Recent studies have shown that limb salvage may still be possible in selected cases.[2,7,113,114] Special surgical consideration is needed in these cases.

Adjuvant Therapy

This section concentrates on the use of radiation and chemotherapy. In general, these modalities are not used in the treatment of benign conditions. Up to 10% risk of malignant transformation occurs when benign lesions are irradiated.[19,62,65,67,127,128,135]

Both chemotherapy and radiation therapy can be used in the neoadjuvant (preoperative) or adjuvant (postoperative) setting in the treatment of malignant conditions. The neoadjuvant approach has the advantage of "shrinking" the tumor and provides a more discernible margin, theoretically improving local control of the disease. In the case of chemotherapy, before the era of modular prosthesis, the neoadjuvant route was necessary while the custom prostheses were manufactured. This technique has been shown to be as efficacious as primary surgery. Even so, the one randomized trial of preoperative and postoperative chemotherapy versus only postoperative chemotherapy failed to show any difference in survival. Therefore, in selected cases it is reasonable and may be prudent to perform surgery first.[92]

Chemotherapy

Historically, before the era of chemotherapy, survival in osteogenic sarcomas was less than 20%. Between 1972 and 1981 the development of chemotherapy protocols for osteogenic sarcoma revolutionized treatment and the present 5-year disease free survival rates are 60% to 76%.[6,55,64,87,92,106]

At present the standard approach to the treatment of osteogenic sarcoma has been neoadjuvant therapy to treat unrecognized microscopic disease, followed by definitive resection and then adjuvant chemotherapy. This approach has been more traditional than empirical. Still the availability of comparison tissue at the time of definitive resection has been an important tool in prognostication.

Chemotherapy-associated necrosis in resected specimens has been graded. Grade I necrosis is necrosis amounting to less than 50% of a tumor. Grade II necrosis amounts to necrosis of 50% to 90% of a tumor. Grade III necrosis is necrosis in more than 90% of a tumor, and grade IV necrosis is necrosis in virtually the entire tumor. This has further been grouped with grades I and II necrosis being referred to as standard response and grades III and IV necrosis being designated good response. Good response in post-resection specimens is an important indicator of good prognosis in osteogenic sarcoma as well as Ewing's family tumor patients.[92,143]

It should be remembered that historically 20% of patients had been cured by surgery alone and even now up to 24% to 40% are not cured of their disease. This means that 44% to 64% of patients have no change in cure. Nevertheless, even they benefit from chemotherapy by enjoying longer survival, better local disease control, and higher limb salvage rates.[92]

The typical agents used can be classified as cell cycle–specific and cell cycle–nonspecific agents. Cell cycle–specific agents include methotrexate and doxorubicin. These interfere with cell division and hence affect cells that are actively proliferating. In any cell population there are quiescent cells. These cells would not be affected by cell cycle–specific agents. For this purpose the cell cycle–nonspecific agents are used. Cisplatin and alkylating agents (e.g., cyclophosphamide and ifosfamide) directly damage the DNA of a cell and so even quiescent cells are affected. This Goldie-Coldman model of chemotherapeutic administration is the most commonly used in the treatment of osteogenic sarcomas and Ewing's family tumors.[51]

Multiple-agent chemotherapy has been adopted by a number of working groups in the treatment of osteogenic sarcoma. In Europe the Cooperative Osteosarcoma Study group (COSS) reports an actuarial 10-year survival of 64%.[14] The Rizzoli Institute reports an 8-year disease-free survival rate of 59%.[43] Hence, it appears that in its present form multimodality treatment with multiple-agent chemotherapy and surgical resection appears to have stagnated in the past 20 years. Novel approaches and agents are continually being developed.

The traditional agents cisplatin, doxorubicin, and high doses of methotrexate have been combined with ifosfamide in a number of centers. Preliminary results are promising. The Rizzoli Institute, as part of the Italian Sarcoma Group/Scandinavian Sarcoma Group, reports that the combination is associated with a 5-year overall survival of 87% and a 5-year disease-free survival of 73%, improving on their earlier results.[8,43] Ifosfamide has been used in this manner at our center with variable results. Chemotherapy-associated necrosis has not been dramatic, nor has this been associated with an increased survival benefit in our patients.

Chemotherapy as the sole agent in the treatment of osteogenic sarcoma has been reported to have inferior results.[68] The complications with this approach include increased local recurrence and metastases. Cure was convincingly achieved in only 10% of patients.

Recently, it has been discovered that bisphosphonates may have important anticancer properties and these agents are being investigated clinically in some centers.[70]

The optimal route of delivery for chemotherapeutic agents continues to be developed. In a recent study, the use of neoadjuvant intra-arterial cisplatin and intravenous doxorubicin, followed by surgical resection of the tumor and completion of chemotherapy, conferred an 84% 10-year event-free survival rate. Necrosis was monitored preoperatively by angiography, and surgery was performed only after 90% or greater reduction in neovascularity was achieved. After resection and assessment of necrosis, adjuvant chemotherapy was tailored according to the chemotherapeutic response seen in the resection specimen. This state of the art represents a culmination of a number of techniques that have been developed in the field and represents the necessary multidisciplinary approach in these conditions.[137]

Radiation Therapy

Radiation therapy has been used in both the neoadjuvant and adjuvant setting in the treatment of Ewing's family tumor. Osteogenic sarcoma does not respond well to radiation therapy, and its use in this tumor has been limited to only very select situations.[34,75]

Regimens for treatment of Ewing's family tumor differ according to site and center. Radiation is generally effective but has been reported to have a higher rate of local recurrence than surgery alone. When used alone, doses up to 6600 cGy may be necessary to produce local control.[122] In contrast, 3000 to 4000 cGy in divided doses is given in this condition when surgery is combined with radiation therapy.[89] Because of its propensity to cause premature physeal closure and bone necrosis[52,97] and the additional concern of radiation sarcoma developing in these genetically altered patients in whom alkylating agents have been used,[19,34,52,65,127] the role of radiation therapy in local control in some institutions has been limited to the treatment of spine and pelvic lesions. In these settings the treatment may be used solely or intraoperatively in conjunction with surgery (Fig. 40-6). In the treatment of extremity lesions a purely surgical approach may be desirable, reserving irradiation for when margins of resection are compromised or when the response to preoperative chemotherapy has been incomplete.[89,108,143]

Although not studied specifically in the pediatric age group, radiation therapy has been shown to increase wound complications in the perioperative period, which is another factor to consider if the patient is to have chemotherapy.[102] Thus, in general this modality is best used judiciously.

In Langerhans histiocytosis, low-dose radiation therapy amounting to less than 1000 rads effects good local control of disease while avoiding the skeletal side effects of radiation therapy.[115]

Surgery

In bone tumors, resection and reconstruction are two aspects of management that have largely complementary but occasionally conflicting goals (e.g., cryotherapy is good for extending the margins of resection of a tumor

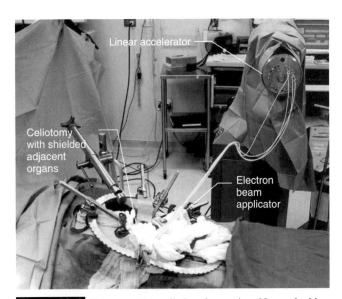

Figure 40–6 Intraoperative radiation therapy in a 19-month-old girl who underwent a wide resection with nodal clearance for a rhabdomyosarcoma of the pelvis.

but results in weakening of the bone). Therefore, while the goals of resection are generally quite clear (i.e., cure), the goals of reconstruction are often compromised, especially in malignant conditions. In benign conditions, reconstruction tends to have to be more restorative of function. In this section we present a general list of considerations that will be elaborated on in the section on specific considerations.

Minimally Invasive Options

The minimally invasive option is reserved for benign conditions. It is born of two management philosophies—the desire to effect local control and the hesitation to cause more morbidity than the primary lesion. Whichever modality is chosen, it is imperative that a histologic diagnosis be obtained a priori.

Radiofrequency Ablation

Radiofrequency ablation employs high-intensity heat in proximity to a lesion to effect thermal necrosis. It has wide utility in the ablation of various solid tumors. In bone tumors it has principally been used in the ablation of osteoid osteomas. This condition is a painful condition marked by increased night pain and is promptly relieved by the use of NSAIDs. Otherwise it is relatively benign. It can be found most commonly in the proximal femur. In these locations, surgical ablation in the form of a resection can incur high morbidity. Hence an option such as radiofrequency ablation is ideal, although it incurs a 10% to 15% recurrence rate[33,107] compared with surgery, which has a near 0% recurrence rate.[23] It has limited utility in the spine owing to the indiscriminate high heat generated.

Injection

This technique is principally used in the treatment of unicameral bone cysts. Clinically apparent bone cysts have a tendency to recurrent fracture and need to be treated.[98] However, they have no malignant potential and have been known to regress.[67,98] It is controversial if corticosteroid injection is a necessary element of treatment—it has been shown that simple decompression of a cyst is sufficient to induce a regression.[126] Cure rates of up to 50% are reported, with a median injection rate of three and a range of one to up to nine injections.[22,110] Each of these sessions requires the child to be under anesthesia. Therefore, it has not been widely received.

As alluded to earlier, various forms of decompression have been advocated in the literature with varying success. One approach involves the injection of bone marrow.[35,71,79,109,144] Cure rates of up to 50% to 70% may be achieved. However, with this technique repeated injections may be necessary, incurring multiple inductions of anesthesia and donor site morbidity.

Curettage, widely regarded to be the gold standard, has a recurrence rate of 5% to 50%.[98] Thus there is no clearly superior modality in the treatment of this condition.

NSAID Treatment

Although not a surgical modality, NSAID treatment has been used in the treatment of osteoid osteomas in selected individuals. In patients who have lesions in the spine or in the acetabular area, surgical or radiofrequency ablation could result in disordered growth, necessitating spinal fusions or corrective hip surgery. In these instances, NSAID treatment associated with a predictable amelioration of symptoms may be attempted. This can be continued as long as there are no gastric or renal side effects. Cure rates of up to 45% are possible but require protracted ingestion of NSAIDs for about 30 months.[66]

Resection

Surgical decisions are based on the concept of compartments in relation to a tumor (Fig. 40-7). The compartment is bound by a barrier, which naturally limits the expansion of a tumor. When first described it was useful in teaching the principles of wide resection or a resection with a margin of healthy tissue: if a resection was performed outside a compartment it resulted in a margin that was free of malignant involvement.[39] This idea was useful in drawing parallels to conventional cancer surgery of the time. We realize now that this theory is flawed at many levels. For example, most osteogenic sarcomas present with tumors that have breached the cortex and so their distinction from a "contained" osteogenic sarcoma is moot. In the lower limb a tumor that has involved the rectus femoris has involved a compartment extending from the anterior inferior iliac spine of the pelvis to the tibial tubercle. Clearly it would not be practical in this setting to perform a hindquarter amputation. Finally, especially in the region of the linea aspera, there are numerous perforating vessels, which go through the lateral intermuscular septum—clearly these do not form a continuous barrier to tumor spread.

Still, the concept of compartmentalization is useful when one describes the surgical procedures as intralesional, marginal, wide, and radical.[37] Although not often used in the context of amputations, these principles are applicable as well. Intralesional procedures, as the name implies, are procedures that leave macroscopic residual tissue. A biopsy or injection of a lesion is an intralesional procedure. A marginal procedure stops at the level of the extent of maximal expansion of a tumor. Curettage is a marginal procedure. A wide procedure goes beyond the reactive zone of the tumor. When first described, the "reactive zone" referred to the zone of reaction around the tumor marked by inflammatory change (i.e., hyperemia and edema).[36,37] This assessment was made predominantly at the time of surgery. With the advent of more sophisticated imaging modalities it can now be demonstrated that this "zone" may extend further than previously appreciated. Therefore, it appears that the description of a reactive zone is rather more abstract than real. As a general rule, resecting a tumor beyond its capsule where vessel tortuosity and edema is seen is a wide resection and hence this appreciation, while strongly influenced by newer imaging, remains largely surgical. Most malignant tumors are resected widely. A radical resection is an excision of the compartment in

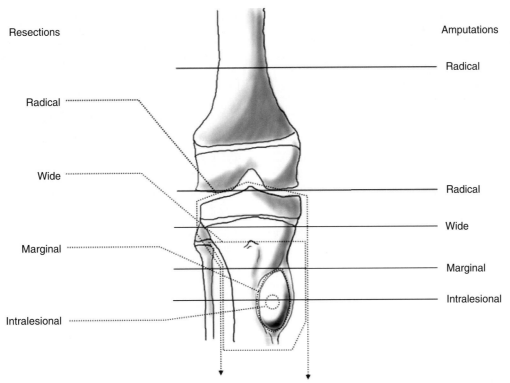

Resections

Amputations

Radical

Radical

Wide

Radical

Wide

Marginal

Marginal

Intralesional

Intralesional

Figure 40-7   Surgical margins in relation to the compartments involved. At left are the resections, and at right are the amputations. These classifications are largely academic because in the strictest terms most of the resections except radical resections and only wide or radical amputations are performed. Radical resections involve the compartment bearing the tumor and hence in this case would amount to removing the tibia *(arrows)*. Marginal amputations may be resorted to in the spine and pelvis whereupon local adjuvants assume significant roles in disease control (see Fig. 40-6). Intralesional amputations are obviously not therapeutic applications in tumor surgery but are included here for completeness. Of interest, intercalary amputations in the pediatric population can be problematic when the remnant stump elongates through appositional growth. To avoid this complication it may be necessary to resort to a through-joint (e.g., through-knee) amputation.

which a tumor resides. An above-knee amputation for a tibial lesion is a radical resection.

There are a number of surgical adjuvants that may be employed. This can be in the form of heat (e.g., argon beam coagulator) or cold (e.g., liquid nitrogen cryotherapy).[80,88] In addition, chemical measures may be employed (e.g., phenol, polymethylmethacrylate cement).[25,103] In the occasional case, specialized forms of radiation (e.g., brachytherapy, intraoperative radiation therapy) may be used especially in the pelvis (see Fig. 40-6). The purpose of these surgical adjuvants is to extend the margins of resection beyond what can be mechanically removed by the surgeon. These improve local control of the tumor.

Benign Lesions

It is useful at this juncture to recall the staging system for benign lesions. This is classified as benign, active, and aggressive. It is evident in these entities that even within this group specific nuances of the condition warrant special considerations. In benign bony conditions the procedures available are curettage, high-speed burring of lesional walls, adjuvant procedures, and wide resection.[25,80] It is helpful to describe these procedures from most to least aggressive.

In benign conditions, *wide resection* may occasionally be resorted to when the involved bone is expendable (e.g., rib or terminal phalanx of the little toe) or at the

end of a bone (e.g., distal ulna or proximal fibula). In these situations, reconstruction provides little value and can, in fact, be the source of considerable morbidity. Additionally, it may be resorted to in the context of a recalcitrant recurrent benign or aggressive lesion. Typical lesions that are resected in this manner are giant cell tumors, aneurysmal bone cysts, or fibrous dysplasia.

Marginal excision is typified conceptually by the technique used to excise a soft tissue lipoma. Such a procedure is not technically feasible in most bony lesions. Osteochondromas and periosteal chondromas may be removed in such a fashion.

Intralesional procedures are more commonly performed in benign tumors. This typically involves curettage of a lesion with high-speed burring of the wall. By and large this is the typical procedure for most latent or active benign bony conditions (e.g., unicameral bone cyst). The use of heat, cold (Fig. 40-8), or chemical modalities serves to extend this margin of clearance further and is typically used in active or aggressive tumors (e.g., giant cell tumor, chondroblastoma).

Malignant Lesions

The sine qua non of the resection of malignant bone lesion is that at minimum a *wide resection* must be performed. In certain situations, however, this may not be possible

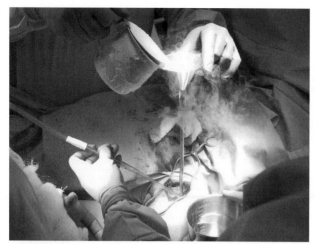

Figure 40-8 Cryosurgery in a patient with chondrosarcoma. Liquid nitrogen is poured into a funnel that directs the agent into the lesion while avoiding contact with the surrounding skin. The effect of freezing extends the margins of necrosis beyond that which can be felt by the surgeon, effectively extending the surgical margins from an intralesional or marginal excision to a wide resection.

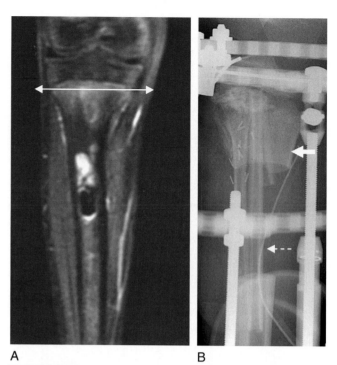

A   B

Figure 40-9 *A,* Ewing's sarcoma of the tibia in an 11-year-old boy. The lesion extended to 1 cm from the growth plate. It responded well to chemotherapy with virtually no remaining soft tissue involvement. A physeal-sparing resection was done along a resection plane *(double-headed arrow)* carefully performed under image intensifier guidance. *B,* The use of a pin fixator in this regard is extremely advantageous because it allows stabilization of the small proximal tibial segment that precludes routine pin fixation. The remaining gap was reconstructed with a proximal tibial allograft *(thick arrow)* and vascularized fibular graft *(broken arrow)* harvested with a paddle of skin, which provided skin cover of the construct.

(e.g., a tumor that has expanded into the spinal canal or a tumor that has invaded into the pelvic cavity). In these instances, the results tend to be suboptimal.

With newer imaging modalities it is now often possible to perform a physeal-sparing procedure in growing children (Fig. 40-9). Although it used to be believed that the physis is an effective barrier to tumor spread, it has been shown that up to 80% of tumors abutting the physis have in fact breached it.[38,69,99,118] Physeal-sparing procedures must therefore be carefully balanced with the response to chemotherapy to determine if this is feasible.

As a variation on this theme it is occasionally possible to save the epiphysis and hence the neighboring joint by performing a distraction procedure through the growth plate. This effectively increases the margin of normal tissue proximal to a tumor. A resection may then be performed through this now-lengthened segment.[24]

Another approach to retaining a joint would be to perform a Van Nes rotationplasty (Fig. 40-10).[133] This procedure, generally undertaken for high-grade tumors about the knee, involves wide extra-articular resections whereupon the distal leg and foot are joined to the proximal remaining femur. In the process, the sciatic nerve is retained and a segmental resection of the femoral artery with a true femoral-popliteal arterial anastomosis is performed. The foot is rotated with the heel pointing anteriorly. Of practical interest the distal segment is rotated externally, bringing the sciatic nerve and vessels anteromedially. This should be documented in the surgical note to facilitate further surgical procedures as may be necessary. The ankle, therefore, functions as a knee joint. This procedure has poor acceptance among patients owing to their cosmetic abhorrence but is highly functional and durable.[20] A similar Winkelmann procedure may be performed where the proximal tibia is brought to the hip. In children it is remarkable to note the plasticity and remodeling of these disparate bones, which in time will accommodate each other in a stable fashion.[139,140]

Radical procedures and amputations have received poor support because they are regarded as being disfiguring. Studies have shown that patients with limb salvage procedures do better in terms of function and cost savings.[54,104] Although this appears true at face value, in-depth analysis shows that these studies are too heterogeneous to allow any firm conclusions. With the aid of modern prosthesis, patients with amputations are able to achieve very high levels of activity. Furthermore, complications are three to four times higher in limb salvage compared with limb ablative surgery. Although most series have not shown a significant survival benefit between amputation and limb-sparing surgery, these studies are underpowered or include cases of amputation being salvage procedures.[47,92,117] The primary question that needs to be answered is whether there is any survival and functional benefit in two-site and stage-controlled groups with respect to amputation or wide resection. This would require a case-controlled study with amputation and wide resection arms, and it is a safe assumption that this will never be done.

There is still a role for amputations, especially when the tumor is in the distal extremity, adjuvant therapies are ineffective, or reconstruction is too problematic because of nerve, vessel, or soft tissue problems.

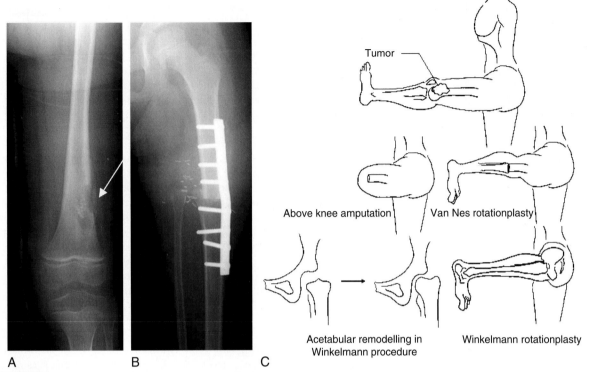

Above knee amputation

Van Nes rotationplasty

Acetabular remodelling in
Winkelmann procedure

Winkelmann rotationplasty

Figure 40–10 *A,* Osteogenic sarcoma *(arrow)* with large soft tissue extension in an 8-year-old child. The small size of the child and high level of activity precluded endoprosthetic reconstruction. *B,* A Van Nes rotationplasty was performed. *C,* Variants of the rotationplasty are compared with the above-knee amputation. The bottom panel illustrates how the proximal tibia remodels and accommodates the acetabulum in the Winkelmann procedure.

Local recurrence in malignant lesions is a poor prognostic factor and is associated with a 90% fatality rate. It is generally a reflection of compromised local control, although in one study good chemotherapy response was associated with a low local recurrence rate.[47] Specifically, in this series when intralesional procedures had been performed for osteogenic sarcoma, standard responders were three times as likely to get a local recurrence as good responders. However, even among good responders, local recurrence was 14 times more likely if a intralesional procedure had been done as opposed to a wide resection. This underscores the need both for good surgical margins *and* effective chemotherapy.

Reconstruction

In most instances after the resection of benign lesions, small defects arise. These are easily dealt with through the use of various gap fillers. With malignant lesions, large creative solutions are needed. It becomes difficult to determine which lesions are best treated by which technique because of the relative paucity of cases and the high-risk nature of these procedures. In this section we will highlight the various modalities available and the pertinent qualifiers for each modality.

Benign Lesions

Following the resection of these lesions one is usually left with a small defect. In latent and perhaps active

conditions there is a low rate of local recurrence. Thus the aim here is the reconstitution of bone. The modalities that have been tried are bone graft and bone graft substitutes. In general, autografts tend to have better incorporation rates but incur the risk of donor site morbidity or—worse—donor site tumor implantation. Allografts have a low risk of disease transmission and immunologic response.[10,125] Synthetic grafts tend not to incorporate as well.[31,132]

In the more aggressive lesions the risk of recurrence increases. In these situations bone substitutes could be resorbed by the disease process and increase the delay before subsequent radiologic imaging is able to distinguish between postoperative change and recurrence. In this setting, bone cement becomes a good alternative.[80,103] Furthermore, radiopaque cement acts as a contrast agent. Recurrence at the margin of the cemented defect can readily be identified and treated.

Malignant Lesions

The solutions that have been tried to solve the complex bone, joint, and soft tissue defects left after tumor resections form a veritable cornucopia of techniques, spanning all of orthopedic and plastic surgery. It is impossible to reiterate all these solutions here. Instead, we present a list of principal solutions pertinent to the specific reconstructive option.

The paramount requirement of all solutions is as a *space filler* and *skin closure.* Without these two requirements chemotherapy cannot resume and the patient will not survive. Most solutions will provide space-filling ability if there is adequate skin for closure. If skin closure is not possible a local flap or vascularized pedicular graft may be necessary. In some instances, especially with intercalary resections, the ability to provide intercalary stability with overlying skin closure can be provided by a vascularized fibular graft with a skin paddle. The skin paddle affords the additional advantage of monitoring the viability of the flap. Rotationplasties and their variants are remarkably functional solutions to the problem but have poor acceptance among patients because of their appearance. Similarly, amputations are often an instant solution to the problem, although even here the occasional exception exists.[104]

Joint reconstruction is a challenging endeavor. Biologic solutions include the use of bulk allograft (Fig. 40-11). They have the advantage of becoming incorporated by the body. The disadvantages[82] are high fracture rates of 19%, nonunion rates of 17%, and infection rates of 11%.

Osteoarticular allografts also become arthritic (16%) with time. Theoretically, however, with good incorporation of the allograft one would be able to perform a conventional less constrained joint replacement (Fig. 40-12). The endoprosthetic solution tends to be easier but is less resilient, suffering from wear and loosening with time.[57,130,145] With advancements in technology, better designs will allow for longer-lasting implants (Fig. 40-13). The allograft prosthetic composite is another approach that appears to capitalize on the lasting nature of allografts and their soft tissue capsular attachments and the simplicity of prosthetics (Fig. 40-14). In very young children the available endoprostheses may be too large, and this may be a relative indication for the use of bulk allografts instead (see Fig. 40-1). Downsized pediatric implants are incapable of holding up in adults and are destined for failure and revision (Fig. 40-15). Prosthetic reconstruction has the distinct advantage of allowing immediate weight bearing, which is very important in patients who may have a reduced life expectancy. In truth, the various modalities are complementary rather than independent.

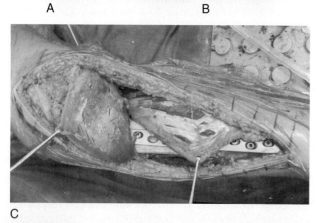

C

Figure 40–11 *A*, Ewing's sarcoma of the proximal tibia in an 11-year-old. *B* and *C*, This was widely resected and reconstructed with an osteoarticular tibial allograft. A gastrocnemius flap was raised to provide soft tissue cover to the construct.

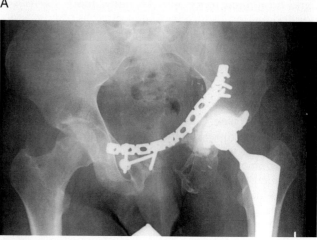

B

Figure 40–12 *A*, Resection and reconstruction of Ewing's sarcoma of the pelvis. *B*, Degenerative changes developed in his hip 2 years later and required hip replacement surgery.

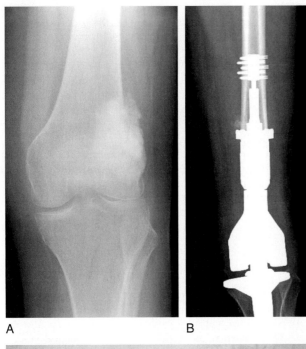

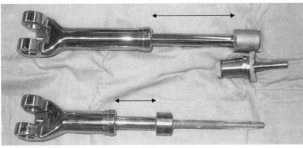

Figure 40-13 *A,* Osteogenic sarcoma in a 16-year-old girl. *B,* An endoprosthetic device was placed in the patient after resection of the lesion. *C,* With growth of the child, it becomes occasionally necessary to swap implants with devices that can provide further extensibility.

Figure 40-14 *A,* Osteogenic sarcoma in proximal humerus of a 16-year-old boy. *B,* A proximal humeral resection with allograft and prosthetic composite was used to reconstruct the defect.

Growth is a complex problem in the management of these patients. In the year that patients receive chemotherapy growth is often stunted. After this, however, the child resumes growth. There are various means to predict this growth.[3,95] As a rule of thumb, the distal femur grows 1 cm a year and the proximal tibia grows 7 mm a year. Girls generally stop growing at 14 years and boys at 16 years. Therefore, a 10-year-old boy who had an extra-articular resection would have potentially 10 cm of growth to accommodate. In general, a 2-cm length discrepancy is considered compensable and does not require treatment. Thus, in this example an additional 8-cm correction is needed.

The modalities available include contralateral epiphysiodeses. This method ablates the growth plate of the contralateral knee. The procedure needs to be timed accurately and tends to be really only practical in the older child approaching the last few centimeters of growth.

Bone transport is another option. This yields good results but the child must remain in the apparatus for long periods of time. At an elongation rate of 1 mm/day, the child with an 8-cm defect must remain in the apparatus at minimum for 3 months for the elongation and a further 3 months for consolidation of the regenerate (Fig. 40-16). This duration is commonly doubled when distraction osteogenesis is done during chemotherapy. Even in healthy individuals the risk of pin tract infection during the procedure is greater than 90%.[17] In the patient with malignant disease who is to receive chemotherapy this would be an important consideration.[105] In addition, the regenerate tends to be weak and is prone to fracture (Fig. 40-17). Patients on chemotherapy are prone to osteoporosis and are already at risk for fracture.

The extensible prosthesis is a marvel of modern science that is presently undergoing "teething" issues.[111,112,130,134] The manual designs require repeated surgical procedures to periodically lengthen the limb to keep pace with

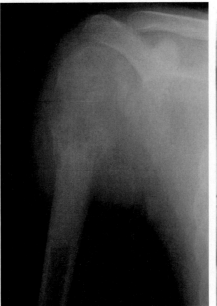

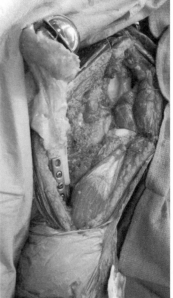

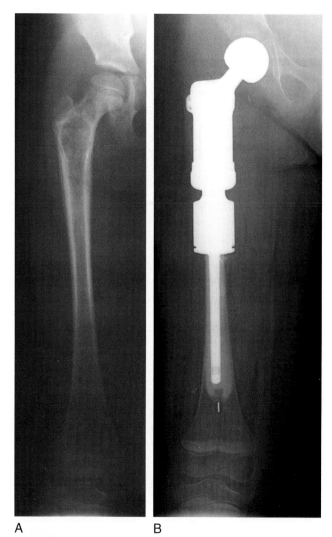

Figure 40-15 *A,* Osteogenic sarcoma of the proximal femur in a 14-year-old girl. *B,* A wide resection and bipolar hemiarthroplasty with proximal femoral replacement was performed. Of note, the femoral head matched the acetabulum so an additional bipolar component was not added.

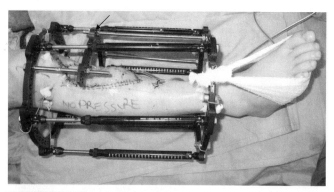

Figure 40-16 Ewing's sarcoma of the tibia. The patient underwent wide resection and a planned bone transport procedure. The middle ring *(arrow)* is secured to a segment of bone that has been osteotomized. This segment of bone is allowed 5 days for a provisional callus to form. By progressively advancing the ring distally at a rate of 1 mm/day, the segment of bone is transported to fill the defect while at the same time remaining connected to the proximal tibia. This regenerate is weak and requires an equivalent amount of time to consolidate. For example, an 80-mm defect would require 5 days to form provisional callus, 80 days to lengthen, and 80 days to consolidate before removal of the frame. This ungainly device needs to be tolerated by the patient for the duration of the limb-lengthening procedure.

As such there are many solutions to the problem but no perfect one. Therefore, it is apparent that the surgeon dealing with this condition must be able to perform or at least facilitate all of these procedures. Any one of these procedures is applicable to the individual case, and they remain complementary to each other.

SPECIFIC CONSIDERATIONS

In this section specific issues are highlighted that pertain to characteristics of the individual case and the way they may affect management. A discussive rather than a didactic style is used to facilitate familiarity with the problems and to unify the concepts as presented in the section on general considerations. Features specific to respective diagnoses are covered in the section on pathophysiology.

Age

Diagnosis

In the very young child, below 5 years of age, the patient who presents with a lesion in the bone is likely to have one of only a few diagnoses (see Table 40-1). The main considerations in this group are infection and localized manifestations of systemic malignancies (i.e., leukemias). Consideration should be given to metastatic disease, which in this group is often neuroblastoma. In the group between 5 and 10 years of age, Ewing's family tumor needs to be considered. In the second decade, with increased activity of the child and increased use of radiographs in assessing incidental trauma, many of the benign conditions are diagnosed. In addition, osteogenic sarcoma and Ewing's family tumor become prevalent.

normal growth (see Fig. 40-13C). The Stanmore implants have been used for nearly 20 years and have a 23% revision rate.[130] Survivorship analysis, however, shows a near-zero survivorship at 10 years.[129] Self-extending designs work through electromagnetic couplers or heating coils that allow motors or heat release springs to extend the implant. The Phenix device is presently undergoing evaluation in the United States.[138] Preliminary results show a complication rate of up to 44%, necessitating revision. The Repiphysis system uses an external electromagnetic field to provide controlled released of a spring held in place by a locking mechanism. This device is associated with a implant revision rate of 44%.[49] In general, the stems in these devices are too narrow and mechanically insufficient and fixation techniques remain inadequate. As such, all these designs have poor longevity but reduce immediate surgical complications (e.g., infection). They are well tolerated by patients and families.

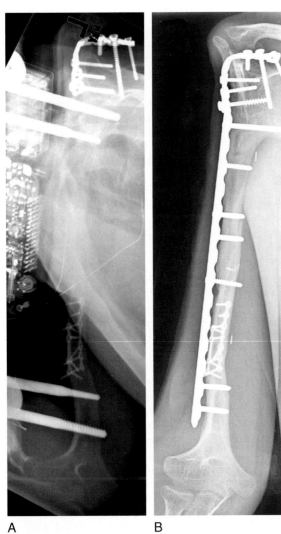

A　　　　　B

Figure 40–17 *A,* A patient presented with osteogenic sarcoma of the proximal humerus that was resected and reconstructed with a vascularized fibular graft shoulder arthrodesis at 6 years of age. He developed a shortened humerus at maturity, which was lengthened. *B,* Post lengthening, the regenerate was protected with a plate and hypertrophied with time.

Growth

Issues of linear growth have been touched on earlier. In the treatment of conditions of the bone adjacent to a physis the potential for future growth should be considered. This is more prudent in the benign case when conceivably nonsurgical management can be offered without dire consequences. Thus in the typical case of the unicameral bone cyst adjacent to the growth plate it may be prudent not to subject the physis to curettage, accepting that this may increase recurrence rates. In the case of a chondroblastoma, which tends to be more aggressive, however, growth plate damage may be unavoidable and a local adjuvant may be indicated (e.g., cryosurgery). By contrast in malignant conditions, sacrificing the growth plate with the aim of achieving good surgical margins is an acceptable concession (see Fig. 40-13).

Site

The implications of site of disease in relation to pathology and pathophysiology have been alluded to earlier. Here the focus is on the implications of site of involvement to the reconstruction of a defect.

Upper Limbs

In general terms, load-bearing requirements in the upper limbs differ considerably from those in the lower limb. In the upper limb the prehensile functions of feeding and personal hygiene are considered fundamental in terms of goals of surgery. In the lower limb, weight bearing is paramount. With that in mind the upper limb tends to be more forgiving in terms of reconstructive durability but more demanding in terms of mobility. The following discussion is more applicable to large segmental bony defects. Cavitary lesions are managed with appropriate bone fillers (see bone graft and bone graft substitutes, earlier).

In the *shoulder,* good function can be achieved by periscapular resections and reconstructions.[26,101,141] The options for reconstruction here involve suspensory arthroplasties or scapular replacements (see Fig. 40-4). Abduction is limited, but otherwise prehensile function remains good. Humeral resections generally perform well but, owing to the indicated pathologic processes, tend to be applicable only to lower grade lesions. Replacements with osteoarticular allografts (see Fig. 40-1) or allograft prosthetic composites (see Fig. 40-13) afford good replacement of function. In lower-grade lesions, in which the deltoid and rotator cuff may be retained, abduction is often acceptable.

The *elbow* has limited options because of the poor soft tissue coverage in this area.[120,131,136] Osteoarticular allografts and endoprosthesis provide reasonable flexion and extension and pronation and supination. *Forearm* bone resections are highly specialized affairs involving intercalary bone resections and replacement with vascularized fibular grafts. In the event of wrist disruption, this may have to be fused. Involvement of various nerves in the forearm may necessitate tendon transfers. Cross circulation in the palm is an important sign to document in the event of the need to sacrifice the radial or ulnar artery.

Lesions occurring distally in the *hand* rarely require treatment if benign and often require varying forms of amputation if malignant.

Lower Limbs

In the lower limb, *pelvic resections* are classified into type I resections above the acetabulum, type II resections in the periacetabular area, and type III resections below the acetabulum.[1,21,100] Complications in this type of surgery are very high, mainly because the internal iliac supply to the posterior gluteal flap is often disrupted in the process of resection and because the duration of the procedures is long. In addition, because of the limited bone available afterward, reconstructive options become challenging.

In type I resections, the need is for a strut to span the remaining hemipelvis to the sacrum. Allografts or autogenous fibular grafts are usually used in this context. This is occasionally not possible and a defect is left. In these cases patients are able to function reasonably well. In type II resections, replacement of the joint becomes necessary. This can be achieved through a custom prosthesis, an allograft-prosthetic composite (see Fig. 40-12), or an arthrodesis. Type III resections are usually stable and can be left with a defect. Combination defects especially after type I-II resections are especially challenging. The options include allograft prosthetic composites and saddle prostheses. Occasionally, hindquarter amputations are still necessary.

In *proximal femoral* lesions, articular involvement may necessitate type II–like extra-articular pelvic resections and reconstructions. Contained proximal femoral lesions are treated with prostheses or allograft prosthetic composites. Intercalary femoral and tibial resections are generally managed with allografts or vascularized fibular autografts or combinations of these. Bone transport is another viable option but, as mentioned, takes a protracted course and has a high complication rate. Recent work suggests that pin fixators are safe even if the patient is to undergo chemotherapy.

Resections about the *knee* are generally treated with endoprosthetic reconstruction.[111,130,145] Bulk osteoarticular allografts have been used and provide reasonable function (see Fig. 40-11). These invariably become arthritic with time.[82] But at that point a more traditional joint replacement may be performed. Arthrodeses have generally fallen out of favor, although they remain good alternatives with reasonable function in the appropriate setting.[104]

In the *ankle*, variable resections of the fibula may be performed with reasonable expectation of function. In general, with tibial resections, arthrodesis needs to be performed.[27,29,104] In the *foot*, as with the hand, various types of amputations are generally recommended.

Metastatic Disease

The implications of aggressiveness in the case of benign lesions and compartmentalization in the case of malignancies have been touched on previously. Here the discussion is confined to metastatic osteogenic sarcoma and Ewing's family tumor.

Patients with metastatic osteogenic sarcoma may present in two settings: the patient with metastasis at the outset and the patient who has developed metastasis despite having had a remission. It has been shown that patients who present with early unilateral pulmonary metastasis within 2 years of diagnosis have a high incidence of contralateral disease and should undergo staged bilateral thoracotomies.[121] Late unilateral pulmonary metastasis tends not to be associated with contralateral disease.

Patients with metastasis at the outset have been shown to have a survival of 11% to 36%.[9,93] Management of this group requires the aggressive implementation of chemotherapy to treat unrecognized microscopic disease and surgical induction of remission by removal of all macroscopic disease. These are multidisciplinary efforts that should be reserved for specialized centers. Patients may have to undergo segmental pulmonary resections together with resections of their tumors and reconstructions thereof.

The patient who develops metastases after a remission has a very variable prognosis, ranging from 0% to 26% in various series.[42,44] In these patients, although the principles of management are similar, the expectation is different. Surgical induction of remission is still a very effective method in these patients and the main determinant of survival.[44] This entails bilateral thoracotomies and segmental resections of solitary bony metastases as needed.[5,121]

Ironically, owing to the poor prognosis, limb salvage surgery is relatively indicated. This, however, needs to be balanced with the duration of recuperation from surgery during which the child will not be on chemotherapy. The surgeon should select the operation with the fastest most predictable recovery. For example, this would drive the decision to use a cemented prosthesis rather than the uncemented implant that would be used in localized disease in children.

Timing of surgery can be complex. Pulmonary metastasis occurring at presentation of the primary lesion should be resected in a staged manner during recovery from the primary resection. A lesion that develops during consolidation chemotherapy should be resected after completion of a round of chemotherapy. Metastasis that develops after chemotherapy should be aggressively resected, with consideration given to staged bilateral thoracotomies if this occurs early.

In these patients the issues of management may not necessarily be curative. The surgeon needs to be able to balance the procedures that may be offered with the expected prognosis of the child. Two actual cases illustrate this point.

Case 1

A patient with advanced osteogenic sarcoma of the tibia fungating through the skin presents for the first time with multiple metastases to the lungs and regional lymph nodes. Note that in the AJCC staging system this patient has stage IVB disease. This patient underwent an amputation before chemotherapy.

A few questions arise, the foremost being why a limb salvage procedure was not performed in this case. Limb salvage in this case would have required either an allograft or vascularized fibular graft and hardware to be placed into the defect. This would have incurred a significant risk of skin breakdown and infection, requiring a free muscle flap. In the meantime the metastatic disease would have progressed and the patient might have died. When a thoracotomy for this patient is done to resect the pulmonary metastases, it should be planned with consideration that a free latissimus flap may be needed and so the muscle should not be compromised.

A second question may be posed as to the use of neoadjuvant therapy in this setting. Here, the patient would have been immunocompromised in the presence of an infected wound. Hence in this situation the most prudent approach was an amputation.

Case 2

A patient with a history of osteogenic sarcoma of the left distal femur that has been resected and reconstructed and is 2 years out from chemotherapy now presents with metastasis in the right distal femur and proximal tibia. This patient underwent resection and reconstruction with an endoprosthesis.

An amputation would not have been curative in this case because it is assumed that other sites of metastases must exist. Yet a surgical induction of remission was necessary because the patient developed metastases soon after chemotherapy and thus may have developed resistance to the chemotherapeutic agents.

These two cases illustrate the many levels of complexity that underlie the management of these patients. Only through a careful consideration of all factors can the most appropriate line of management be offered.

REFERENCES

1. Aboulafia AJ, Buch R, Mathews J, et al: Reconstruction using the saddle prosthesis following excision of primary and metastatic periacetabular tumors. Clin Orthop Relat Res 1995;(314):203-213.
2. Abudu A, Sferopoulos NK, Tillman RM, et al: The surgical treatment and outcome of pathological fractures in localised osteosarcoma. J Bone Joint Surg Br 1996;78:694-698.
3. Anderson M, Green WT, Messner MB: Growth and predictions of growth in the lower extremities. Am J Orthop 1963;45A:1-14.
4. Araki Y, Tanaka H, Yamamoto H, et al: MR imaging of pigmented villonodular synovitis of the knee. Radiat Med 1994;12:11-15.
5. Aung L, Gorlick R, Healey JH, et al: Metachronous skeletal osteosarcoma in patients treated with adjuvant and neoadjuvant chemotherapy for nonmetastatic osteosarcoma. J Clin Oncol 2003;21:342-348.
6. Bacci G, Briccoli A, Ferrari S, et al: Neoadjuvant chemotherapy for osteosarcoma of the extremity: Long-term results of the Rizzoli's 4th protocol. Eur J Cancer 2001;37:2030-2039.
7. Bacci G, Ferrari S, Longhi A, et al: Nonmetastatic osteosarcoma of the extremity with pathologic fracture at presentation: Local and systemic control by amputation or limb salvage after preoperative chemotherapy. Acta Orthop Scand 2003;74:449-454.
8. Bacci G, Ferrari S, Longhi A, et al: High dose ifosfamide in combination with high dose methotrexate, Adriamycin and cisplatin in the neoadjuvant treatment of extremity osteosarcoma: Preliminary results of an Italian Sarcoma Group/Scandinavian Sarcoma Group pilot study. J Chemother 2002;14:198-206.
9. Bacci G, Picci P, Briccoli A, et al: Osteosarcoma of the extremity metastatic at presentation: Results achieved in 26 patients treated with combined therapy (primary chemotherapy followed by simultaneous resection of the primary and metastatic lesions). Tumori 1992;78:200-206.
10. Bauer TW, Muschler GF: Bone graft materials: An overview of the basic science. Clin Orthop Relat Res 2000;(371):10-27.
11. Berg HL, Weiland AJ: Multiple osteogenic sarcoma following bilateral retinoblastoma: A case report. J Bone Joint Surg Am 1978;60:251-253.
12. Bertoni F, Bacchini P, Staals EL: Malignancy in giant cell tumor. Skeletal Radiol 2003;32:143-146.
13. Bertoni F, Bacchini P, Staals EL: Malignancy in giant cell tumor of bone. Cancer 2003;97:2520-2529.
14. Bielack SS, Kempf-Bielack B, Delling G, et al: Prognostic factors in high-grade osteosarcoma of the extremities or trunk: An analysis of 1,702 patients treated on neoadjuvant cooperative osteosarcoma study group protocols. J Clin Oncol 2002;20:776-790.
15. Bonin G, Scamps C, Turc-Carel C, Lipinski M: Chimeric EWS-FLI1 transcript in a Ewing cell line with a complex t(11;22;14) translocation. Cancer Res 1993;53:3655-3657.
16. Brenner W, Bohuslavizki KH, Eary JF: PET imaging of osteosarcoma. J Nucl Med 2003;44:930-942.
17. Brownlow HC, Simpson AH: Complications of distraction osteogenesis: A changing pattern. Am J Orthop 2002;31:31-36.
18. Caffey J: On fibrous defects in cortical walls of growing tubular bones: Their radiologic appearance, structure, prevalence, natural course, and diagnostic significance. Adv Pediatr 1955;7:13-51.
19. Cahan WG, Woodard HQ, Higinbotham NL, et al: Sarcoma arising in irradiated bone: Report of eleven cases: 1948. Cancer 1998;82:8-34.
20. Cammisa FP Jr, Glasser DB, Otis JC, et al: The Van Nes tibial rotationplasty: A functionally viable reconstructive procedure in children who have a tumor of the distal end of the femur. J Bone Joint Surg Am 1990;72:1541-1547.
21. Campanacci M, Capanna R: Pelvic resections: The Rizzoli Institute experience. Orthop Clin North Am 1991;22:65-86.
22. Campanacci M, De Sessa L, Trentani C: Scaglietti's method for conservative treatment of simple bone cysts with local injections of methylprednisolone acetate. Ital J Orthop Traumatol 1977;3:27-36.
23. Campanacci M, Ruggieri P, Gasbarrini A, et al: Osteoid osteoma: Direct visual identification and intralesional excision of the nidus with minimal removal of bone. J Bone Joint Surg Br 1999;81:814-820.
24. Canadell J, Forriol F, Cara JA: Removal of metaphyseal bone tumours with preservation of the epiphysis: Physeal distraction before excision. J Bone Joint Surg Br 1994;76:127-132.
25. Capanna R, Sudanese A, Baldini N, Campanacci M: Phenol as an adjuvant in the control of local recurrence of benign neoplasms of bone treated by curettage. Ital J Orthop Traumatol 1985;11:381-388.
26. Capanna R, van Horn JR, Biagini R, et al: The Tikhoff-Linberg procedure for bone tumors of the proximal humerus: The classical "extensive" technique versus a modified "transglenoid" resection. Arch Orthop Trauma Surg 1990;109:63-67.
27. Casadei R, Ruggieri P, Giuseppe T, et al: Ankle resection arthrodesis in patients with bone tumors. Foot Ankle Int 1994;15:242-249.
28. Centers for Disease Control and Prevention, National Cancer Institute, and North American Association of Central Cancer Registries: United States Cancer Statistics: 2000 Incidence. 2000.
29. Chou LB, Malawer MM: Analysis of surgical treatment of 33 foot and ankle tumors. Foot Ankle Int 1994;15:175-181.
30. Cook A, Raskind W, Blanton SH, et al: Genetic heterogeneity in families with hereditary multiple exostoses. Am J Hum Genet 1993;53:71-79.

31. Damien CJ, Parsons JR: Bone graft and bone graft substitutes: A review of current technology and applications. J Appl Biomater 1991;2:187-208.

32. de Alava E, Antonescu CR, Panizo A, et al: Prognostic impact of P53 status in Ewing sarcoma. Cancer 2000;89:783-792.

33. de Berg JC, Pattynama PM, Obermann WR, et al: Percutaneous computed-tomography-guided thermocoagulation for osteoid osteomas. Lancet 1995;346:350-351.

34. de Moor NG: Osteosarcoma: A review of 72 cases treated by megavoltage radiation therapy, with or without surgery. S Afr J Surg 1975;13:137-146.

35. Docquier PL, Delloye C: Treatment of simple bone cysts with aspiration and a single bone marrow injection. J Pediatr Orthop 2003;23:766-773.

36. Enneking WF: Musculoskeletal Tumor Surgery. New York: Churchill Livingstone, 1983, vol 2, p 1351.

37. Enneking, WF. Musculoskeletal Tumor Surgery. New York: Churchill Livingstone, 1983, vol 1, pp 89–122.

38. Enneking WF, Kagan A: Transepiphyseal extension of osteosarcoma: Incidence, mechanism, and implications. Cancer 1978;41:1526-1537.

39. Enneking WF, Spanier SS, Goodman MA: A system for the surgical staging of musculoskeletal sarcoma. Clin Orthop Relat Res 1980;(153):106-120.

40. Fagnou C, Michon J, Peter M, et al: Presence of tumor cells in bone marrow but not in blood is associated with adverse prognosis in patients with Ewing's tumor. Société Française d'Oncologie Pediatrique. J Clin Oncol 1998; 16:1707-1711.

41. Fain JS, Unni KK, Beabout JW, Rock MG: Nonepiphyseal giant cell tumor of the long bones: Clinical, radiologic, and pathologic study. Cancer 1993;71:3514-3519.

42. Ferrari S, Bacci G, Picci P, et al: Long-term follow-up and post-relapse survival in patients with non-metastatic osteosarcoma of the extremity treated with neoadjuvant chemotherapy. Ann Oncol 1997;8:765-771.

43. Ferrari S, Bertoni F, Mercuri M, et al: Predictive factors of disease-free survival for non-metastatic osteosarcoma of the extremity: An analysis of 300 patients treated at the Rizzoli Institute. Ann Oncol 2001;12:1145-1150.

44. Ferrari S, Briccoli A, Mercuri M, et al: Postrelapse survival in osteosarcoma of the extremities: Prognostic factors for long-term survival. J Clin Oncol 2003;21:710-715.

45. Fidler M: Prophylactic internal fixation of secondary neoplastic deposits in long bones. BMJ 1973;1:341-343.

46. Fidler M: Incidence of fracture through metastases in long bones. Acta Orthop Scand 1981;52:623-627.

47. Gherlinzoni F, Picci P, Bacci G, Campanacci D: Limb sparing versus amputation in osteosarcoma: Correlation between local control, surgical margins and tumor necrosis: Istituto Rizzoli experience. Ann Oncol 1992;3(Suppl 2): S23-S27.

48. Ghosh L, Huvos AG, Mike V: The pancreatic islets in chondrosarcoma: A qualitative and quantitative study in humans. Am J Pathol 1973;71:23-32.

49. Gitelis S, Neel MD, Wilkins RM, et al: The use of a closed expandable prosthesis for pediatric sarcomas. Chir Organi Mov 2003;88:327-333.

50. Glaubiger DL, Makuch R, Schwarz J, et al: Determination of prognostic factors and their influence on therapeutic results in patients with Ewing's sarcoma. Cancer 1980;45:2213-2219.

51. Goldie JH, Coldman AJ, Gudauskas GA: Rationale for the use of alternating non-cross-resistant chemotherapy. Cancer Treat Rep 1982;66:439-449.

52. Goldwein JW: Effects of radiation therapy on skeletal growth in childhood. Clin Orthop Relat Res 1991;(262):101-107.

53. Greene FL: AJCC Cancer Staging Manual, 6th ed. New York, Springer-Verlag, 2002.

54. Grimer RJ, Carter SR, Pynsent PB: The cost-effectiveness of limb salvage for bone tumours. J Bone Joint Surg Br 1997; 79:558-561.

55. Grimer RJ, Taminiau AM, Cannon SR: Surgical outcomes in osteosarcoma. J Bone Joint Surg Br 2002;84:395-400.

56. Haas A, Ritter SA: Benign giant-cell tumor of femur with embolic metastasis in prepuce of penis. Am J Surg 1955; 89:573-578.

57. Ham SJ, Schraffordt KH, Veth RP, et al: Limb salvage surgery for primary bone sarcoma of the lower extremities: Long-term consequences of endoprosthetic reconstructions. Ann Surg Oncol 1998;5:423-436.

58. Harrington KD: The role of surgery in the management of pathologic fractures. Orthop Clin North Am 1977; 8:841.

59. Hasegawa T, Hirose T, Sakamoto R, et al: Mechanism of pain in osteoid osteomas: An immunohistochemical study. Histopathology 1993;22:487-491.

60. Hogeboom WR, Hoekstra HJ, Mooyaart EL, et al: Magnetic resonance imaging (MRI) in evaluating in vivo response to neoadjuvant chemotherapy for osteosarcomas of the extremities. Eur J Surg Oncol 1989;15:424-430.

61. Huvos AG: "Benign" metastasis in giant cell tumor of bone. Hum Pathol 1981;12:1151.

62. Huvos AG: Bone Tumors—Diagnosis, Treatment & Prognosis, 2nd ed. Philadelphia, WB Saunders, 1991.

63. Huvos AG, Rosen G, Bretsky SS, Butler A: Telangiectatic osteogenic sarcoma: A clinicopathologic study of 124 patients. Cancer 1982;49:1679-1689.

64. Huvos AG, Rosen G, Marcove RC: Primary osteogenic sarcoma: Pathologic aspects in 20 patients after treatment with chemotherapy en bloc resection, and prosthetic bone replacement. Arch Pathol Lab Med 1977;101:14-18.

65. Huvos AG, Woodard HQ, Cahan WG, et al: Postradiation osteogenic sarcoma of bone and soft tissues: A clinicopathologic study of 66 patients. Cancer 1985;55:1244-1255.

66. Ilyas I, Younge DA: Medical management of osteoid osteoma. Can J Surg 2002;45:435-437.

67. Jaffe HL: Tumors and Tumorous Conditions of the Bones and Joints. Philadelphia, Lea & Febiger, 1958.

68. Jaffe N, Carrasco H, Raymond K, et al: Can cure in patients with osteosarcoma be achieved exclusively with chemotherapy and abrogation of surgery? Cancer 2002;95:2202-2210.

69. Jesus-Garcia R, Seixas MT, Costa SR, et al: Epiphyseal plate involvement in osteosarcoma. Clin Orthop Relat Res 2000;(373):32-38.

70. Klenner T, Wingen F, Keppler BK, et al: Anticancer-agent-linked phosphonates with antiosteolytic and antineoplastic properties: A promising perspective in the treatment of bone-related malignancies? J Cancer Res Clin Oncol 1990;116:341-350.

71. Kose N, Gokturk E, Turgut A, et al: Percutaneous autologous bone marrow grafting for simple bone cysts. Bull Hosp Jt Dis 1999;58:105-110.

72. Kyriakos M, Land VJ, Penning HL, Parker SG: Metastatic chondroblastoma: Report of a fatal case with a review of the literature on atypical, aggressive, and malignant chondroblastoma. Cancer 1985;55:1770-1789.

73. Ladanyi M, Traganos F, Huvos AG: Benign metastasizing giant cell tumors of bone: A DNA flow cytometric study. Cancer 1989;64:1521-1526.

74. Le Merrer M, Legeai-Mallet L, Jeannin PM, et al: A gene for hereditary multiple exostoses maps to chromosome 19p. Hum Mol Genet 1994;3:717-722.

75. Lee ES: Osteosarcoma: A reconnaissance. Clin Radiol 1975; 26:5-25.

76. Levine AM, Rosenberg SA: Alkaline phosphatase levels in osteosarcoma tissue are related to prognosis. Cancer 1979;44:2291-2293.

77. Li FP, Fraumeni JF Jr: Soft-tissue sarcomas, breast cancer, and other neoplasms: A familial syndrome? Ann Intern Med 1969;71:747-752.

78. Li FP, Garber JE, Friend SH, et al: Recommendations on predictive testing for germ line p53 mutations among cancer-prone individuals. J Natl Cancer Inst 1992;84:1156-1160.

79. Lokiec F, Ezra E, Khermosh O, Wientroub S: Simple bone cysts treated by percutaneous autologous marrow grafting: A preliminary report. J Bone Joint Surg Br 1996;78:934-937.

80. Malawer MM, Dunham W: Cryosurgery and acrylic cementation as surgical adjuncts in the treatment of aggressive (benign) bone tumors: Analysis of 25 patients below the age of 21. Clin Orthop Relat Res 1991;(262):42-57.

81. Malkin D, Jolly KW, Barbier N, et al: Germline mutations of the p53 tumor-suppressor gene in children and young adults with second malignant neoplasms. N Engl J Med 1992;326:1309-1315.

82. Mankin HJ, Gebhardt MC, Jennings LC, et al: Long-term results of allograft replacement in the management of bone tumors. Clin Orthop Relat Res 1996;(324):86-97.

83. Mankin HJ, Lange TA, Spanier SS: The hazards of biopsy in patients with malignant primary bone and soft-tissue tumors. J Bone Joint Surg Am 1982;64:1121-1127.

84. Mankin HJ, Mankin CJ, Simon MA: The hazards of the biopsy, revisited. Members of the Musculoskeletal Tumor Society. J Bone Joint Surg Am 1996;78:656-663.

85. Marcove RC, Francis KC: Chondrosarcoma and altered carbohydrate metabolism. N Engl J Med 1963;268:1399-1400.

86. Marcove RC, Huvos AG: Cartilaginous tumors of the ribs. Cancer 1971;27:794-801.

87. Marcove RC, Mike V, Hajek JV, et al: Osteogenic sarcoma under the age of twenty-one: A review of one hundred and forty-five operative cases. J Bone Joint Surg Am 1970;52:411-423.

88. Marcove RC, Miller TR: Treatment of primary and metastatic bone tumors by cryosurgery. JAMA 1969;207:1890-1894.

89. Marcove RC, Rosen G: Radical en bloc excision of Ewing's sarcoma. Clin Orthop Relat Res 1980;(153):86-91.

90. Martin SE, Dwyer A, Kissane JM, Costa J: Small-cell osteosarcoma. Cancer 1982;50:990-996.

91. Matsuno T, Unni KK, McLeod RA, Dahlin DC: Telangiectatic osteogenic sarcoma. Cancer 1976;38:2538-2547.

92. Meyers PA, Heller G, Healey J, et al: Chemotherapy for nonmetastatic osteogenic sarcoma: The Memorial Sloan-Kettering experience. J Clin Oncol 1992;10:5-15.

93. Meyers PA, Heller G, Healey JH, et al: Osteogenic sarcoma with clinically detectable metastasis at initial presentation. J Clin Oncol 1993;11:449-453.

94. Mirra JM, Gold RH, Rand F: Disseminated nonossifying fibromas in association with cafe-au-lait spots (Jaffe-Campanacci syndrome). Clin Orthop 1982;(168):192-205.

95. Moseley CF: A straight-line graph for leg-length discrepancies. J Bone Joint Surg Am 1977;59:174-179.

96. Moser RP Jr, Madewell JE: An approach to primary bone tumors. Radiol Clin North Am 1987;25:1049-1093.

97. Mould JJ, Adam NM: The problem of avascular necrosis of bone in patients treated for Hodgkin's disease. Clin Radiol 1983;34:231-236.

98. Neer CS, Francis KC, Johnston AD, Kiernan HA Jr: Current concepts on the treatment of solitary unicameral bone cyst. Clin Orthop Relat Res 1973;(97):40-51.

99. Norton KI, Hermann G, Abdelwahab IF, et al: Epiphyseal involvement in osteosarcoma. Radiology 1991;180:813-816.

100. O'Connor MI, Sim FH: Salvage of the limb in the treatment of malignant pelvic tumors. J Bone Joint Surg Am 1989;71:481-494.

101. O'Connor MI, Sim FH, Chao EY: Limb salvage for neoplasms of the shoulder girdle: Intermediate reconstructive and functional results. J Bone Joint Surg Am 1996;78:1872-1888.

102. Peat BG, Bell RS, Davis A, et al: Wound-healing complications after soft-tissue sarcoma surgery. Plast Reconstr Surg 1994;93:980-987.

103. Persson BM, Wouters HW: Curettage and acrylic cementation in surgery of giant cell tumors of bone. Clin Orthop Relat Res 1976;(120):125-133.

104. Renard AJ, Veth RP, Schreuder HW, et al: Function and complications after ablative and limb-salvage therapy in lower extremity sarcoma of bone. J Surg Oncol 2000;73:198-205.

105. Rodl R, Gosheger G, Leidinger B, et al: Correction of leg-length discrepancy after hip transposition. Clin Orthop Relat Res 2003;(416):271-277.

106. Rosen G, Nirenberg A, Caparros B, et al: Osteogenic sarcoma: Eight-percent, three-year, disease-free survival with combination chemotherapy (T-7). Natl Cancer Inst Monogr 1981;(56):213-220.

107. Rosenthal DI, Hornicek FJ, Wolfe MW, et al: Percutaneous radiofrequency coagulation of osteoid osteoma compared with operative treatment. J Bone Joint Surg Am 1998;80:815-821.

108. Rosito P, Mancini AF, Rondelli R, et al: Italian Cooperative Study for the treatment of children and young adults with localized Ewing sarcoma of bone: A preliminary report of 6 years of experience. Cancer 1999;86:421-428.

109. Rougraff BT, Kling TJ: Treatment of active unicameral bone cysts with percutaneous injection of demineralized bone matrix and autogenous bone marrow. J Bone Joint Surg Am 2002;84:921-929.

110. Scaglietti O, Marchetti PG, Bartolozzi P: The effects of methylprednisolone acetate in the treatment of bone cysts: Results of three years follow-up. J Bone Joint Surg Br 1979;61:200-204.

111. Schiller C, Windhager R, Fellinger EJ, et al: Extendable tumour endoprostheses for the leg in children. J Bone Joint Surg Br 1995;77:608-614.

112. Schindler OS, Cannon SR, Briggs TW, et al: Use of extendable total femoral replacements in children with malignant bone tumors. Clin Orthop Relat Res 1998;(357):157-170.

113. Scully SP, Ghert MA, Zurakowski D, et al: Pathologic fracture in osteosarcoma: Prognostic importance and treatment implications. J Bone Joint Surg Am 2002;84:49-57.

114. Scully SP, Temple HT, O'Keefe RJ, et al: The surgical treatment of patients with osteosarcoma who sustain a pathologic fracture. Clin Orthop Relat Res 1996;(324):227-232.

115. Selch MT, Parker RG: Radiation therapy in the management of Langerhans cell histiocytosis. Med Pediatr Oncol 1990;18:97-102.

116. Sim FH, Unni KK, Beabout JW, Dahlin DC: Osteosarcoma with small cells simulating Ewing's tumor. J Bone Joint Surg Am 1979;61:207-215.

117. Simon MA, Aschliman MA, Thomas N, Mankin HJ: Limb-salvage treatment versus amputation for osteosarcoma of the distal end of the femur. J Bone Joint Surg Am 1986;68:1331-1337.

118. Simon MA, Bos GD: Epiphyseal extension of metaphyseal osteosarcoma in skeletally immature individuals. J Bone Joint Surg Am 1980;62:195-204.

119. Solomon L: Bone growth in diaphysial aclasis. J Bone Joint Surg Br 1961;43:700-716.

120. Sperling JW, Pritchard DJ, Morrey BF: Total elbow arthroplasty after resection of tumors at the elbow. Clin Orthop Relat Res 1999;(367):256-261.

121. Su WT, Chewning J, Abramson S, et al: Surgical management and outcome of osteosarcoma patients with unilateral pulmonary metastases. J Pediatr Surg 2004;39:418-423.

122. Suit HD: Role of therapeutic radiology in cancer of bone. Cancer 1975;35:930-935.

123. Thorpe WP, Reilly JJ, Rosenberg SA: Prognostic significance of alkaline phosphatase measurements in patients with osteogenic sarcoma receiving chemotherapy. Cancer 1979;43:2178-2181.

124. Toguchida J, Yamaguchi T, Dayton SH, et al: Prevalence and spectrum of germline mutations of the p53 gene among patients with sarcoma. N Engl J Med 1992;326:1301-1308.

125. Tomford WW: Bone allografts: Past, present and future. Cell Tissue Bank 2000;1:105-109.

126. Tsuchiya H, Abdel-Wanis ME, Uehara K, et al: Cannulation of simple bone cysts. J Bone Joint Surg Br 2002;84:245-248.

127. Tucker MA, D'Angio GJ, Boice JD Jr, et al: Bone sarcomas linked to radiotherapy and chemotherapy in children. N Engl J Med 1987;317:588-593.

128. Unni KK: Dahlin's Bone Tumors—General Aspects and Data on 11,087 Cases, 5th ed. Philadelphia, Lippincott-Raven, 1996.

129. Unwin PS, Blunn GW: Advances in the design of extendible replacements: An analysis of 597 replacements. In: Proceedings of the Musculoskeletal Tumor Society, Long Beach, CA: Musculosketal Tumor Society, 2004, p 51.

130. Unwin PS, Walker PS: Extendible endoprostheses for the skeletally immature. Clin Orthop Relat Res 1996;(322):179-193.

131. Urbaniak JR, Aitken M: Clinical use of bone allografts in the elbow. Orthop Clin North Am 1987;18:311-321.

132. Vaccaro AR, Chiba K, Heller JG, et al: Bone grafting alternatives in spinal surgery. Spine J 2002;2:206-215.

133. Van Nes CP: Rotation-plasty for congenital defects of the femur: Making use of the shortened limb to control the knee joint of a prosthesis. J Bone Joint Surg Br 1950;32:12-16.

134. Verkerke GJ, Schraffordt KH, Veth RP, et al: An extendable modular endoprosthetic system for bone tumour management in the leg. J Biomed Eng 1990;12:91-96.

135. Vigorita VJ: Orthopaedic Pathology. Philadelphia, Lippincott Williams & Wilkins, 1999.

136. Weber KL, Lin PP, Yasko AW: Complex segmental elbow reconstruction after tumor resection. Clin Orthop Relat Res 2003;(415):31-44.

137. Wilkins RM, Cullen JW, Odom L, et al: Superior survival in treatment of primary nonmetastatic pediatric osteosarcoma of the extremity. Ann Surg Oncol 2003;10:498-507.

138. Wilkins RM, Soubeiran A: The Phenix expandable prosthesis: Early American experience. Clin Orthop Relat Res 2001;(382):51-58.

139. Winkelmann WW: Hip rotationplasty for malignant tumors of the proximal part of the femur. J Bone Joint Surg Am 1986;68:362-369.

140. Winkelmann WW: Type-B-IIIa hip rotationplasty: An alternative operation for the treatment of malignant tumors of the femur in early childhood. J Bone Joint Surg Am 2000;82:814-828.

141. Wittig JC, Bickels J, Kellar-Graney KL, et al: Osteosarcoma of the proximal humerus: Long-term results with limb-sparing surgery. Clin Orthop Relat Res 2002;397:156-176.

142. Wu YQ, Heutink P, de Vries BB, et al: Assignment of a second locus for multiple exostoses to the pericentromeric region of chromosome 11. Hum Mol Genet 1994;3:167-171.

143. Wunder JS, Paulian G, Huvos AG, et al: The histological response to chemotherapy as a predictor of the oncological outcome of operative treatment of Ewing sarcoma. J Bone Joint Surg Am 1998;80:1020-1033.

144. Yandow SM, Lundeen GA, Scott SM, Coffin C: Autogenic bone marrow injections as a treatment for simple bone cyst. J Pediatr Orthop 1998;18:616-620.

145. Zeegen EN, Aponte-Tinao LA, Hornicek FJ, et al: Survivorship analysis of 141 modular metallic endoprostheses at early followup. Clin Orthop Relat Res 2004;420:239-250.

Chapter 41

Brain Tumors

Phillip B. Storm and Leslie N. Sutton

Except for injuries, neoplasms are the most common cause of death in children younger than the age of 15 years. Tumors of the central nervous system are the most common solid neoplasms found in children, account for 20% of cancer deaths, and are second only to leukemia in overall cancer frequency.[20,22,70] Approximately 1700 pediatric brain tumors are diagnosed each year, for an incidence of 3.1/100,000 children at risk.[10]

Important factors in diagnosing brain tumors are location, age, and cell type. Location is probably the most important factor radiographically, with age being the second most important. The brain is divided into two compartments by the tentorium. Above the tentorium (supratentorial) are the cerebral hemispheres, the basal ganglia, and the thalamus. Below the tentorium (infratentorial) are the pineal gland, the tectum, the pons, the medulla, and the cerebellum. Unlike adult tumors, which tend to be supratentorial, pediatric tumors are evenly split between supratentorial and infratentorial. There is an interesting division of location based on age. In children younger than 2 years of age, the tumors are typically supratentorial, whereas children between the ages of 3 and 15 predominately have infratentorial tumors (Table 41-1).[15,20] The prognosis is usually poor in children who present with brain tumors when younger than the age of 1 year,[8] with choroid plexus papilloma being the exception.

The development of immunohistochemical techniques has allowed pediatric tumors to be classified by histology. Tumors can arise from any of a number of cell types in the brain. The brain is composed of neurons and glial cells. The glial cells far outnumber the neurons and provide a nourishing and supportive role. The three main glial cells are astrocytes, oligodendrocytes, and ependymal cells, and the neoplasms they give rise to are gliomas. More specifically they form astrocytomas, oligodendrogliomas, and ependymomas, respectively. Tumors involving both neuronal and glial cells are called ganglion cell tumors and consist of gangliogliomas, desmoplastic infantile gangliogliomas, and gangliocytomas. Another mixed neuronal and glial tumor is a dysembryoplastic neuroepithelial tumor (DNET). Lastly are the embryonal tumors or primitive neuroectodermal tumors (PNETs). Embryonal tumors include medulloblastoma, medulloepithelioma,

neuroblastomas, melanotic neuroectodermal tumors in infancy, and atypical teratoid/rhabdoid tumors (ATRT).

CLINICAL FEATURES

The signs and symptoms of brain tumors in children vary considerably based on tumor type and location and on the age of the child. In the absence of a seizure or a focal neurologic deficit, such as a sixth nerve paresis causing double vision, the vast majority of the symptoms are nonspecific and easily attributable to many more common and less serious causes. Common symptoms are headache, nausea, vomiting, lethargy, subtle changes in personality, and worsening school performance. This constellation of symptoms is often attributed to gastrointestinal problems, depression, school anxiety, migraines, sinusitis, or a prescription for glasses. Even a long-standing seizure disorder ultimately may be caused by a supratentorial brain tumor. Infants typically present with a failure to thrive, decreased intake, macrocephaly, or lethargy.

TABLE 41-1 Brain Tumors in Children

Age	Tumor Histology
0-2	Teratoma
	Primitive neuroectodermal tumor
	Astrocytoma (high grade)
	Choroid plexus papilloma
2-15	Supratentorial tumors (50%)
	Astrocytoma (low grade)
	Craniopharyngioma
	Hypothalamic glioma
	Primitive neuroectodermal tumor
	Ependymoma
	Choroid plexus papilloma
	Infratentorial tumors (50%)
	Primitive neuroectodermal tumor: medulloblastoma
	Cerebellar astrocytoma
	Ependymoma
	Brainstem glioma

Pediatric patients with brain tumors are typically between the ages of 2 and 14 years with a few days to weeks of *headache, nausea/vomiting, gait ataxia,* and/or *diplopia,* who have an enhancing midline posterior fossa tumor on magnetic resonance imaging (MRI) with associated hydrocephalus. In fact, it is the resultant hydrocephalus that is responsible for this constellation of symptoms rather than the tumor itself. Headaches are common in children with viral infections, but frequent, daily, morning headaches should raise the clinical suspicion for a mass lesion, especially in the absence of fever or other sequela of a viral infection. Patients with elevated intracranial pressure often have an exacerbation of their symptoms in the morning because lying in the recumbent position overnight raises intracranial pressure compared with being upright. Furthermore, sleeping results in hypoventilation, which results in an increase in P_{CO_2}, causing an even greater increase in the intracranial pressure. The elevated intracranial pressure can also cause the cerebellar tonsils to herniate into the foramen of magnum and result in occipital headaches and neck pain.

There are two instances in which tumors cause nausea and vomiting. One is the elevation of intracranial pressure, and the other is direct irritation/infiltration of the vomiting center. The vomiting center (area postrema) is located on the floor of the fourth ventricle and is vulnerable from compression from large posterior fossa tumors or from direct invasion of intrinsic brainstem tumors causing vomiting. Because an intrinsic tumor in the medulla can cause vomiting in the absence of other neurologic findings, persistent vomiting should raise the possibility of a posterior fossa tumor and not be attributed to gastrointestinal diseases such as reflux without a detailed history and neurologic examination. Ataxia is often described by the parents as clumsiness, "walking like he is drunk," walking with the head tilted to one side, or falling to one side.

The visual complaints resulting from posterior fossa tumors are most frequently diplopia, difficulty looking up (sunsetting eyes—Parinaud's syndrome), and occasionally decreased visual acuity. Again, these findings are a result of the hydrocephalus. Decreased visual acuity can occur because of papilledema. Loss of vision is more common in supratentorial tumors because of optic nerve atrophy from direct compression. Patients with posterior fossa tumors are usually diagnosed by MRI because their other symptoms occur long before they develop visual loss; thus, a lack of visual signs or symptoms does not exclude a tumor. Visual loss is still seen in some patients with posterior fossa tumors because of poor access to medical care.

Even though the "typical" pediatric brain tumor is in the posterior fossa there are many supratentorial tumors, especially in patients younger than 2 years old. Children younger than 2 years of age often present with a failure to thrive, hemiparesis, seizures, or a full bulging anterior fontanelle with an enlarged head circumference.[18,35,43] Children who are older than age 2 years with supratentorial tumors present similarly to adult patients with brain tumors, with headaches and/or seizures. Patients who present with sudden onset of severe headache and/or rapidly declining mental status usually have hemorrhaged into their lesion. Occasionally, obstructive hydrocephalus can cause a rapid decline, but because of the relative slow rate of growth of the tumor they present before the cerebrospinal fluid (CSF) pathways are completely obstructed.

Less common signs and symptoms arise from endocrine abnormalities such as weight gain, weight loss, diabetes insipidus, short stature, truncal obesity, and delayed puberty; and galactorrhea is from tumors affecting the hypothalamic-pituitary axis. Because of the proximity of these tumors to the optic nerves and chiasm they often cause decreased vision as well as visual field cuts, most of which are asymptomatic.

RADIOGRAPHIC EVALUATION

Patients suspected of having a brain tumor need to be evaluated with MRI with and without gadolinium enhancement. Even though MRI is the gold standard for evaluating tumors, patients presenting to an emergency department with clinical signs and symptoms of a brain tumor need head computed tomography (CT) without instillation of a contrast medium. CT is excellent in evaluating hydrocephalus and hemorrhage, the two main causes of a rapid neurologic decline. Furthermore, CT can be done in minutes and frequently does not require sedation, gives excellent detail and information, and is considerably less expensive. If the patient's condition is rapidly deteriorating, a contrast agent–enhanced head CT needs to be performed to better characterize the lesion for the radiologist and the neurosurgeon if the patient requires emergent surgical intervention. If the patient's condition is stable, the contrast agent can be omitted and MRI with and without gadolinium can be done, the timing of which is dictated by the clinical signs and symptoms.

MRI provides much better brain resolution and provides images in the sagittal, axial, and coronal planes and, with newer imaging sequences and spectroscopy, may even point to a specific histologic diagnosis.[62] This is far superior to the axial-only images that are obtained with CT. Furthermore, it is difficult to evaluate the lower brainstem with CT because of the bony artifact from the skull base. A limitation of MRI is that it does not show intratumoral calcifications very well and occasionally patients require both studies to aid in the proper diagnosis.

The addition of gadolinium provides more information about the tumor. The blood-brain barrier is made up of tight junctions in the endothelial cells lining the brain capillaries, which prevent most blood contents from entering the brain, including gadolinium. Certain brain tumors cause breakdown of the blood-brain barrier and permit the gadolinium to enter the tumor and then appear bright on an enhanced T1-weighted image. In general, especially in the adult population, contrast medium enhancement in an intra-axial lesion means a more aggressive brain tumor and a poorer prognosis. This is not as consistent in pediatric tumors. There are enhancing pediatric brain tumors that are not aggressive and are curable with a total resection. In general, tumors that do not enhance are less aggressive.

When looking at MRIs the important factors to consider are (1) the location of the tumor (e.g., supratentorial, infratentorial, pineal region, suprasellar), (2) whether it is intra-axial (within the brain tissue) or extra-axial (outside brain tissue), (3) the age of the patient, (4) whether it enhances, and (5) if it is single or multiple. By systematically looking at the scans and considering these factors, the differential diagnosis can be narrowed considerably and can be extremely helpful in preoperative planning.

If there are multiple lesions in the brain, or the location and enhancement suggest a tumor type that metastasizes or tends to cause "drop mets" to the spine, then a spinal MRI with and without enhancement is performed. It is preferable to obtain the spinal MRI preoperatively but this is often dictated by the patient's clinical examination.

All patients with brain tumors receive a postoperative MRI within 48 hours to evaluate the extent of resection and rule out hydrocephalus, bleeding, or ischemia. The timing is important because after 48 hours expected postoperative changes/"scarring" can enhance and make it difficult to distinguish scarring from residual tumor. If the patient did not get a preoperative MRI evaluation of the spine and the histologic diagnosis is consistent with tumors that produce "drop mets," then the study should be done 2 weeks after surgery for staging of the tumor.

SURGICAL INTERVENTION

The goal of surgical intervention is to safely debulk as much tumor as possible, to obtain a histologic diagnosis, and to reestablish normal CSF pathways or divert CSF. The location of the tumor often determines how aggressively the tumor is debulked. In fact, some tumors because of their location and their ability to be diagnosed with MRI are not sampled. For example, a pontine glioma, which is an intrinsic astrocytoma of the brainstem, cannot be debulked safely and has a characteristic finding on MRI. These patients are referred to the neuro-oncologist for management without needing a tissue diagnosis. Pineal region tumors are another example of a lesion that may be diagnosed without surgical intervention. Patients with a pineal lesion need to have serum beta–human chorionic gonadotropin (β-hCG), alpha-fetoprotein (AFP), and placental alkaline phosphate (PLAP) levels obtained. If these are negative, then CSF markers are needed. If the markers are positive, then a diagnosis of pineal germ cell tumor is made. The treatment is stereotactic radiation without the need for a tissue diagnosis, and the cure rate approaches 100% for a germinoma.

Most tumors, however, require surgical intervention consisting of either a stereotactic biopsy or an open craniotomy. The most important tool for preoperative planning is MRI. Tumors that are diffuse, intrinsic tumors of the thalamus or basal ganglia typically undergo stereotactic biopsy. This procedure involves rigidly fixing an MRI-compatible frame to the patient's skull. The patient then has an MRI, and the X, Y, and Z coordinates are determined. These coordinates are used to position the frame and arc so that the tip of the needle is exactly where these three points intersect in the brain. The advantages of a stereotactic biopsy are that the surgical procedure is done quickly, diagnosis is possible in areas of the brain that carry an unacceptable morbidity and mortality with an open craniotomy, and the patient is discharged on

postoperative day 1. The disadvantages are that the pathologist is only given a small amount of tissue; if bleeding is encountered at the time of surgery it may not be recognized until the patient deteriorates neurologically after the procedure; and if the diagnosis requires the neurosurgeon to operate, the patient needs a second operative procedure and the tissue in that area may not be representative of the true grade of the tumor.

The majority of pediatric tumors are treated with a craniotomy/craniectomy for open biopsy with an attempt at maximal microsurgical tumor resection, because prognosis of many tumors is strongly influenced by the amount of postsurgical residual tumor.[59] Cerebral hemispheric tumors are approached by craniotomy. Preoperative planning consists of an MRI coupled with a frameless stereotactic navigation study. The navigation study allows the neurosurgeon to view the tumor in the operating room in the sagittal, axial, and coronal planes and can be used to plan the incision and find the tumor. The limitation of this technology is that it is not a real time study and as the brain is retracted, cysts or CSF spaces are drained, the brain shifts position, and the accuracy is compromised. Intraoperative ultrasound is extremely helpful in finding lesions when brain shifting has decreased the accuracy of the intraoperative navigation system. Intraoperative MRI aims at correcting the limitation of the navigation systems by providing a real-time image; however, intraoperative MRI is severely limited by the resolution because the magnet is considerably weaker than those used for conventional MRI. This is exciting technology and as the resolution improves it will be used on all tumor cases and be an invaluable tool to the tumor surgeon. Functional MRI techniques can localize speech and motor cortex in relation to the tumor and aid in selecting the safest site to incise the cortex if these areas of eloquent cortex are involved by the tumor.[48] Functional MRI requires a cooperative, nonsedated patient, which in the pediatric population can be challenging. Electrophysiologic recording and stimulation are sometimes helpful in locating the motor strip.

Even though these advances have substantially aided the neurosurgeon there is still no substitute for an outstanding understanding of the three-dimensional anatomy of the brain. When choosing a route, anatomic planes such as the interhemispheric fissure, the Sylvian fissure, and the cranial base are used if possible to avoid resecting normal brain. If there is no plane, the approach is usually through the least amount of brain tissue, with the obvious exception of areas of eloquent cortex such as language and motor.

Tumors of the midline (hypothalamus, thalamus, basal ganglia, and brainstem) were once considered inoperable. Microsurgical techniques and innovative instrumentation, however, now make these tumors approachable. At the same time, advances in chemotherapy and single-dose and fractionated radiosurgery offer alternatives, and it is unclear at this time which strategy or combination of strategies is best for a particular tumor. Pineal region tumors may be approached via a posterior fossa route, retracting the cerebellum from the underside of the tentorium, or by a supratentorial route between the hemispheres and through the posterior corpus callosum, or through the tentorium itself. The relationship of the pineal tumor to the tentorium dictates the approach.

Tumors of the cerebellum and lower brainstem are approached by a posterior fossa craniotomy or craniectomy. Midline tumors of the fourth ventricle usually present as obstructive hydrocephalus. Although some neurosurgeons prefer to place a shunt before tumor resection, most now favor giving the child corticosteroids and placing a ventriculostomy at the time of the craniectomy, which is either removed or converted to a shunt if needed in the postoperative period. Between 20% to 40% of children will ultimately require a shunt.[33] The patient is placed in the prone position, and the bone overlying the cerebellum is removed, occasionally including the posterior ring of C1. After opening the dura, the cerebellar vermis is vertically incised, providing access to the cavity of the fourth ventricle. The tumor is removed with bipolar cautery, suction, or the ultrasonic aspirator. Laterally placed tumors of the cerebellopontine angle are reached by retracting the cerebellum medially, and working around the cranial nerves, using electrophysiologic monitoring of cranial nerves V, VII, VIII, IX, X, XI, and XII as required. Tumors of the brainstem may be debulked, if they are dorsally exophytic and have low-grade histology. The dura is closed and covered with DuraGen, a collagen product that augments dura, but replacement of bone is not required. Postoperative problems include acute hydrocephalus and pseudomeningoceles, aseptic meningitis, mutism, pseudobulbar palsy,[69] cranial nerve or brainstem dysfunction, gastrointestinal hemorrhage,[50] and spinal instability.[58] Patients with swallowing dysfunction and aspiration may require tracheostomy and feeding gastrostomy.

TUMOR TYPES

Cerebellar Astrocytomas

These tumors are usually histologically benign and curable with total surgical resection. The average age at presentation is 9 years, and patients present with pernicious vomiting, intermittent morning headache, and disturbances of balance, often over a period of months. The classic CT appearance[71] is of a low-intensity cystic cerebellar mass in proximity to the vermis with a brilliantly enhancing "mural nodule." About one fourth will be entirely solid, however. MRI is helpful in defining the surgical anatomy, particularly the relationship of the tumor to the brainstem, and the nature of the cyst wall. Cerebellar astrocytomas are typically of low signal intensity on T1-weighted MRI sequences, are of increased intensity on T2-weighted sequences, and show enhancement of the solid component with intravenous gadolinium (Fig. 41-1). Obstructive hydrocephalus is common.

Histologically, the tumors are composed of benign-appearing astrocytes. Subtypes are the juvenile pilocytic form (60%) and the fibrillary form (30%). A "diffuse" form has also been described, which may carry a poorer prognosis.[21] Detailed examination may reveal cellular pleomorphism and tumor extension to the subarachnoid space, but these tumors rarely disseminate. Malignant tumors

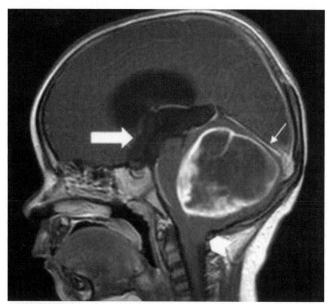

Figure 41–1 A 2-year-old girl presented after several days of vomiting and lethargy. A sagittal T1-weighted MR image with gadolinium shows a large posterior fossa tumor based in the cerebellum (*small arrow*). The patient has hydrocephalus (*large arrow* showing a dilated third ventricle). She also has herniation of the cerebellar tonsils through the foramen magnum (*arrowhead*). At surgery a diagnosis of cerebellar astrocytoma was made.

are rare and usually follow radiation therapy given for a previously benign tumor.[57]

Treatment is complete surgical excision. This may be accomplished in a high percentage of cases in which there is no brainstem involvement. These tumors rarely recur after radiographically confirmed complete excision, and no adjuvant therapy is indicated.[1] Therefore, if there is residual tumor on the postoperative scan, reoperation for total excision is recommended. Radiation therapy may be considered for multiply recurrent lesions or in cases in which brainstem involvement precludes complete removal, but even in these cases residual tumor may remain indolent for years without specific therapy. Regular postoperative surveillance scanning is appropriate when there is suspicion for residual tumor. Recurrence is treated with reoperation if this is feasible.

Primitive Neuroectodermal Tumor and Medulloblastoma

A posterior fossa PNET is termed a *medulloblastoma*. Medulloblastoma is the most common malignant brain tumor of childhood. Histologically, the classic medulloblastoma is composed of densely packed cells with hyperchromatic nuclei and little cytoplasm, giving the histologic slides a blue color when stained with hematoxylin and eosin. When the lesion is located in the posterior fossa, the tumor is termed *medulloblastoma* or *posterior fossa PNET*. Tumors with identical histology can occur in the cerebral hemispheres and are termed *supratentorial PNETs*. Children with medulloblastomas typically present with headache, vomiting, and lethargy of relatively short duration, and the mean age at diagnosis is younger than that for cerebellar astrocytomas. Infants may present with failure to thrive. Supratentorial PNETs present with increased intracranial pressure and focal neurologic signs depending on location.

On a CT scan, medulloblastomas typically appear as well-marginated homogeneously dense masses filling the fourth ventricle causing obstructive hydrocephalus; however, unlike ependymomas, they lack calcifications. They usually enhance brilliantly with contrast medium instillation. MRI shows variable signal characteristics. The images are often slightly hypointense on T1 weighting, becoming brighter on fluid-attenuated inversion recovery (FLAIR) sequences, and may be bright or dark on T2-weighted studies. They usually enhance on MRI (Fig. 41-2). MRI of the spine is indicated either preoperatively or postoperatively to evaluate for spinal metastases ("drop mets").

Treatment begins with biopsy and surgical excision. These tumors are not curable with surgery alone; and in cases with metastases at diagnosis or extensive brainstem involvement, the major mass should be debulked but no attempt should be made to resect tumor from vital areas. After the operation, radiation therapy is usually administered to the entire brain and spinal canal, with a boost to the tumor bed. Younger children suffer significant cognitive problems as a result of whole-brain irradiation in an age- and dose-dependent fashion.[38] Because chemotherapy has proven effective in both newly diagnosed and recurrent medulloblastomas,[14,30,40,63] recent trials have attempted to reduce, eliminate, or delay radiation and replace it with chemotherapy, particularly in the younger age groups.[12] In determining the best treatment, staging

criteria are important to define risk groups. In the past, the Chang system was used, which used the surgeon's estimate of the tumor size at operation and the extent of metastatic disease based on postoperative imaging.[9] In most centers today, patients are assigned to a high-risk group based on younger age, postoperative residual disease, and presence of disseminated disease.[31,39,40]

The rate of progression-free survival ranges from more than 70% at 5 years in groups with favorable risk factors[7] to less than 30% in certain high-risk groups.[14] Recent reports suggest that intensive adjuvant chemotherapy results in improved survival in high-risk patients comparable to low-risk patients treated with radiation alone.[40]

Patients require long-term supportive care, which is best done in the setting of a multidisciplinary pediatric neuro-oncology clinic. Surveillance scanning is of unproven value, because patients with tumors that recur after primary therapy almost invariably die of their disease.[64] Late sequelae of therapy include pituitary dysfunction,[11] growth retardation,[47] cardiomyopathy,[28] cognitive delay,[49] psychosocial adjustment and family problems, and radiation-induced meningiomas, astrocytomas, and sarcomas.[25]

Ependymomas

Ependymomas occur in the region of the fourth ventricle or cerebellopontine angle (Fig. 41-3), spinal cord, or supratentorial compartment. Most are histologically

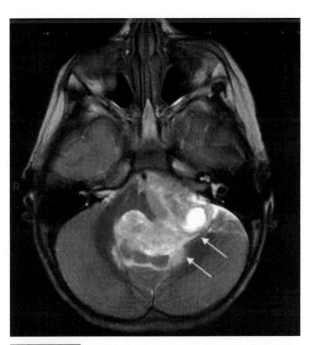

Figure 41–3 An 18-month-old boy presented after 3 days of headaches and vomiting and 2 days of gait ataxia. On the day of admission he was unresponsive at home. Emergent MRI revealed a large posterior fossa tumor. An axial T2-weighted MR image shows a tumor occupying the fourth ventricle and "oozing" out of the foramen of Luschka into the cerebellar pontine angle and encasing all of the posterior fossa cranial nerves *(arrows)*. The patient was found to have an ependymoma.

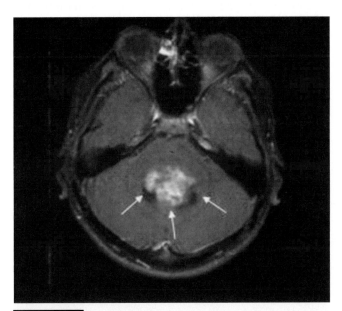

Figure 41–2 An 8-year-old boy presented after several weeks of morning headaches and vomiting. An axial T1-weighted MR image with gadolinium shows a heterogeneously enhancing lesion occupying the fourth ventricle *(arrows)*. The lesion does not "ooze" out of the lateral CSF pathways (foramen of Luschka) like an ependymoma. The pathologic diagnosis was medulloblastoma.

benign, but, despite this, they rank among the worst of all pediatric brain tumors. They have a tendency to recur in the local tumor bed but may also disseminate throughout the neuraxis. The median age at diagnosis is between 3 and 5 years,[23] but tumors in infants and adults are not uncommon. When they arise in the posterior fossa (75% of cases), symptoms are similar to those of other tumors in this location. Cranial nerve and brainstem dysfunction suggest involvement of these structures. Vomiting may arise without hydrocephalus, which suggests infiltration of the region of the obex, which is characteristic of ependymomas. When they arise in the supratentorial compartment in children, they are often extremely large and, despite their presumed ependymal origin, may demonstrate no connection with the ventricle.

CT typically shows an isodense mass with flecks of calcification and an inhomogeneous pattern of enhancement. Posterior fossa lesions may extend through the foramina of Luschka into the cerebellopontine angle. On T1-weighted MRI, ependymomas are usually isointense to hypointense and are hyperintense on T2/proton-weighted images.[55] They often enhance inhomogeneously.

Treatment is primarily surgical. Prognosis is strongly dependent on extent of surgical resection as determined by postoperative imaging. The 5-year progression-free survival after complete resection is 60% to 80%, compared with less than 30% after incomplete resection.[26] Radical surgical resection may result in permanent neurologic damage and may not be possible in some cases. Unless the tumor has disseminated at diagnosis, postoperative radiation is usually confined to the operative bed with a generous margin. Adjuvant chemotherapy was thought to be of little or no benefit,[36] but recent studies show improved outcomes with chemotherapy.[19,52] Trials of radiosurgery for unresectable tumors are under way in several centers.

Brainstem Gliomas

It is now recognized that there are several types of brainstem gliomas, with very different outcomes.[13] The most common variety is the *diffuse intrinsic pontine glioma*, which is not amenable to surgical resection. These tumors typically present as cranial neuropathies rather than hydrocephalus. Patients are young children with bilateral sixth nerve palsies, facial weakness, and ataxia. The diagnosis is established by MRI, which shows a swollen pons with diffuse signal abnormality (see Fig. 41-3). Surgery is not indicated. Radiation therapy provides symptomatic relief, but most children die within a year.[37] *Cervicomedullary astrocytomas* are considered to be rostral extensions of intrinsic spinal cord tumors and carry a favorable prognosis. Signs and symptoms may include vomiting, torticollis, slowly evolving motor weakness, or symptoms of hydrocephalus. MRI shows an enlarged upper cervical spinal cord, with a rostral extension presenting in the cisterna magna. These tumors are often amenable to aggressive surgical resection; and if the histology is benign, adjuvant radiation therapy is deferred. *Tectal gliomas* are now recognized to be a not infrequent cause of hydrocephalus.[46] They typically present as symptoms referable

to ventricular obstruction and are usually treated with either a ventriculoperitoneal shunt or endoscopic third ventriculostomy. These are usually extremely indolent, and treatment of the tumor itself is required only if it progressively enlarges.

Hypothalamic/Chiasmatic Astrocytomas

Suprasellar astrocytomas are usually low-grade neoplasms, which may occur in association with neurofibromatosis type 1 or as isolated tumors. The etiology of these tumors is not well understood, but the association with neurofibromatosis type 1, which is localized to chromosome 17q, suggests a molecular genetics basis. These tumors may present as primarily visual abnormalities (visual field cuts or asymmetrical loss of visual acuity in association with optic atrophy) or as hypothalamic dysfunction (precocious puberty, growth failure, obesity, or the *diencephalic syndrome,* which consists of failure of weight gain and loss of subcutaneous tissue). Often visual and hypothalamic complaints coexist.

Imaging studies usually cannot distinguish hypothalamic tumors from those arising from the visual apparatus. The tumors typically do not calcify, which helps distinguish them from craniopharyngiomas, and appear as solid hypodense lesions on CT or T1-weighted MRI sequences with contrast agent enhancement. Extension to the intraorbital optic nerves or along the optic radiations is diagnostic and rules out craniopharyngiomas, germinomas, or other tumors (Fig. 41-4).

Treatment is controversial. Traditionally, treatment has been surgical biopsy, followed by radiation therapy. Recently, chemotherapy with dactinomycin and vincristine,

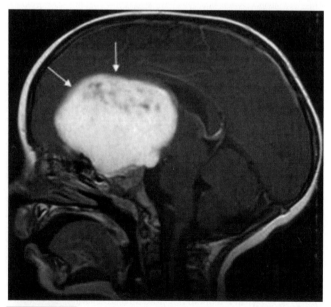

Figure 41–4 A 14-month-old boy presented with a 1-week history of lethargy and a 2-day history of vomiting. Sagittal T1-weighted MR image with gadolinium shows a large enhancing suprasellar and frontal tumor arising from the optic chiasm and hypothalamus *(arrows).* The diagnosis of a hypothalamic astrocytoma was confirmed at surgery.

or other combinations, has shown promise, especially in infants and young children in whom radiation therapy is damaging to the brain.[45] Radical surgical resection as primary therapy has also been reported.[68]

Craniopharyngioma

Craniopharyngiomas are histologically benign masses believed to arise from embryonic rests derived from the hypophyseal-pharyngeal duct. Symptoms arise from optic chiasm or nerve compression, hypopituitarism, hypothalamic dysfunction, or increased intracranial pressure in association with hydrocephalus. They also occur in adults, but the childhood form represents a distinct entity, characterized by large size and extensive calcification. There are two varieties of craniopharyngioma, the adamantinomatous and the papillary types. The most common variety in children is the adamantinomatous type. Histologically, they typically are composed of a squamous epithelial cyst wall, with cystic fluid composed of cholesterol crystals, and calcifications. They are usually inseparable from the pituitary gland and may have an interdigitating gliotic interface with the hypothalamus above. This makes complete surgical removal uncertain, because small rests of tumor may reside in the brain, and is also the explanation for hypothalamic dysfunction that may be seen after surgical excision.

Radiographically, CT reveals either a rim-enhancing cystic mass with basal calcifications or an entirely solid tumor. MRI shows the sagittal anatomy well but may miss the calcifications (Fig. 41-5).[24] In some instances, imaging

cannot distinguish a craniopharyngioma from a hypothalamic glioma.

Treatment is complete surgical excision via craniotomy, which is possible in a high percentage of cases.[27] In cases in which complete resection is not possible, or when tumor recurs, radiation therapy is a useful adjunct.[66] Post-treatment problems include panhypopituitarism, obesity, visual problems, emotional lability,[54] and pseudo-aneurysms of the carotid artery.[60] Long-term survival is in the range of 90% at 10 years,[53] but local recurrences are not uncommon. Recurrences are treated by reoperation,[67] instillation of colloidal ^{32}P into cysts, or radiosurgery.

Low-Grade Supratentorial Astrocytomas

Low-grade astrocytomas and gangliogliomas of the cortical regions and temporal lobes often present as intractable seizures. CT may show masses of low density, which may or may not enhance with contrast medium instillation. MRI usually shows a mass of decreased signal on T1-weighted images and increased signal on T2 weighting.

Complete resection is the goal of surgery, but this may be difficult owing to problems in defining the tumor margins and proximity to eloquent areas. Adjuncts to aid in this include language and motor mapping using implantable grids or intraoperative electrophysiologic monitoring techniques,[2] functional MRI techniques, and image-directed tumor resection.[29] Tumors of the temporal lobe are often treated by formal temporal lobectomy to decrease the likelihood of seizures. Seizure mapping techniques have also been employed with cortical tumors, but simple removal of the tumor usually provides good seizure control,[41] and the value of these strategies is uncertain.

The outcome of low-grade astrocytomas,[59] gangliogliomas[61] (Fig. 41-6), and DNETs (Fig. 41-7) that are

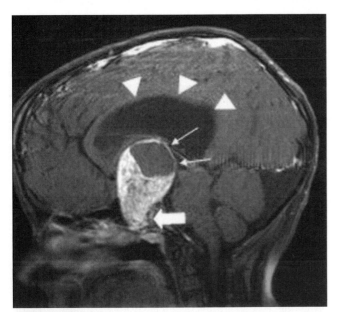

Figure 41-5 An 11-year-old boy presented with a several-month history of headaches and lethargy and extreme thirst and high urine output. Sagittal T1-weighted MR image with gadolinium shows an enhancing intrasellar lesion enlarging the sella turcica (*large arrow*). The tumor occupies the third ventricle and has a cystic component (*small arrows*). The patient also has obstructive hydrocephalus with dilated lateral ventricles and a thinned corpus callosum (*arrowheads*).

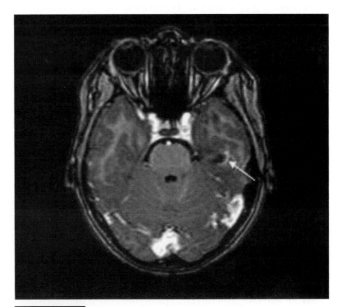

Figure 41-6 A 9-year-old boy presented with intractable seizures. Axial T1-weighted MR image with gadolinium shows a minimally enhancing lesion in the left temporal lobe (*arrow*). A ganglioglioma was completely resected, and the patient is seizure free.

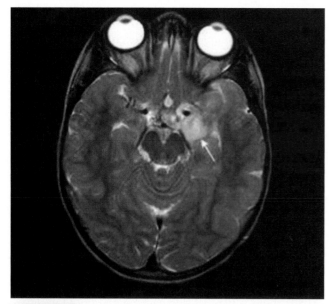

Figure 41-7 A 14-year-old boy presented with left-sided headaches for months and a seizure. Axial T2-weighted image shows a hyperintense mesial temporal lobe lesion involving the cortex *(arrow)*. The lesion was hypointense on T1-weighted images and did not enhance. The diagnosis was dysembryoplastic neuroepithelial tumor (DNET).

completely resected is favorable, although surveillance scanning is warranted. About 70% of children will be long-term survivors. Recurrent tumors can be treated by reoperation or reoperation followed by radiation therapy.[32]

Pineal Region Tumors

Tumors of the pineal region encompass a wide variety of histologic types. They can be divided into *germ cell tumors* (teratoma, germinoma, choriocarcinoma, embryonal cell carcinoma, yolk sac tumor), *pineal parenchymal tumors* (pineocytoma, pineoblastoma), *tumors of surrounding structures* (astrocytomas, meningiomas), and *other benign conditions* (cysts, vascular malformations). The older term *pinealoma* is no longer used.

Patients present with signs and symptoms of hydrocephalus, upgaze paresis, and rarely precocious puberty. MRI confirms the presence of a tumor and excludes other possibilities but is nonspecific regarding the histologic type. Specific germ cell tumors may secrete "tumor markers," which may be measured in CSF obtained from lumbar puncture or ventriculostomy or blood. Elevated β-hCG (>50.0 IU/L) is seen in choriocarcinomas, elevated AFP (>25.0 IU/L) is seen in endodermal sinus tumors and embryonal cell carcinomas, and PLAP is elevated in germinomas.

In the past, surgery in the pineal region was considered prohibitively dangerous and tumors were often treated without histologic confirmation. This region is now readily approachable using the supracerebellar/infratentorial or interhemispheric-transcallosal routes with minimal morbidity, and in most centers biopsy is performed. As in the suprasellar region, pure germinomas of

the pineal carry a good prognosis after irradiation, although in cases with disseminated disease whole-brain and spinal irradiation will be required.[34] Treatment with chemotherapy alone is advocated in some centers. The other malignant germ cell tumors are usually fatal.[42] Pineoblastomas are treated like PNETs in other locations. Pineocytomas may be simply observed if totally resected or given focal radiation for residual tumor.

Rhabdoid/Atypical Teratoid Tumors

These tumors have only recently been defined. They are highly malignant tumors with histologic resemblance to rhabdoid tumors of the kidney. They typically occur in the posterior fossa in young children and infants but may be located in the spine or supratentorial space. In the past, many of these were probably misclassified as PNETs but are distinguished by larger cells with pink cytoplasm that show immunohistochemical staining for smooth muscle actin, vimentin, and epithelial membrane antigen. Chromosomal analysis reveals monosomy 22 in a high percentage of cases.[5] Treatment is surgical excision, chemotherapy, and irradiation in older children, but virtually all the patients in reported cases have died.

Malignant Supratentorial Astrocytomas

Anaplastic astrocytomas and glioblastoma multiforme account for only about 6% of childhood tumors, which is a smaller incidence than that in adults. Clinical signs and symptoms reflect location. Imaging features are similar to those seen in adults, and the masses are often large, with enhancing rings and necrotic centers. Dissemination occurs in about 10%.[65]

Treatment is maximal resection followed by radiation therapy, but the prognosis remains poor. Although more extensive resection confers better outcome, this may reflect the fact that more favorable tumors are more amenable to aggressive surgery. Chemotherapy prolongs life in children with high-grade astrocytomas, but overall 5-year progression-free survival is only 33%.[17] Trials of high-dose chemotherapy with autologous marrow rescue are ongoing.[16]

Choroid Plexus Tumors

Tumors of the choroid plexus are divided into the benign choroid plexus papilloma and the malignant choroid plexus carcinoma. In children, they tend to arise in the trigone of the lateral ventricle, and they often present in infancy by producing hydrocephalus. The radiographic appearance is an intraventricular, homogeneously enhancing, lobulated mass. Carcinomas are typically larger and may disseminate. The vascular supply is the choroidal arteries, which may be seen with high-resolution MRI.

Treatment is surgical excision, which is curative for papillomas. The procedure is hazardous, because these tumors may be extremely vascular and the patients are typically small. Carcinomas are particularly difficult to remove because of extreme vascularity. This has prompted some to recommend biopsy, followed by chemotherapy, and later resection.[56] Prolonged survival and even cure are possible after complete removal of malignant choroid plexus tumors.

Meningiomas

Meningeal tumors are uncommon in childhood, accounting for about 2% of tumors. They may be associated with neurofibromatosis. Meningiomas occur in the orbit, sphenoid wing, or virtually any portion of the intracranial compartment and need not have a dural attachment. Radiographically, they typically enhance and may be extremely large. Treatment is surgical resection, which is curative if complete removal can be accomplished. Irradiation is of benefit in recurrences or when complete removal is not possible.[44]

Metastases

Metastatic brain tumors are uncommon in children. Primary tumors that may metastasize to brain include Wilms' tumor, osteogenic sarcoma, and embryonal rhabdomyosarcoma. Presentation is often abrupt, often with catastrophic neurologic symptoms due to hemorrhage.

TUMOR GENETICS

Despite rapid developments in imaging, navigational systems, and surgical instruments and techniques, many tumors, especially high-grade lesions, are still incurable with surgery alone and in conjunction with chemotherapy and radiation therapy. The future in treating brain tumors lies in better biologic and molecular understanding of the tumors. Such techniques have given us better understanding of neurofibromatosis type 2, which is associated with the development of meningiomas and acoustic neuromas in children. The gene locus was identified on chromosome 22,[51] the same chromosome that has been identified in pediatric meningiomas in patients without neurofibromatosis type 2.[4] The genetic abnormalities result in a loss of a tumor-suppressor gene. Monosomy 22 has been associated with rhabdoid and atypical teratoid tumors.[5] Neurofibromatosis type 1 is associated with childhood gliomas, particularly of the hypothalamus, brainstem, and optic chiasm. The gene locus is at 17q11.2, which encodes for the protein neurofibromin. Neurofibromin is an "off switch" for the *RAS* oncogene. Tissue from astrocytomas frequently has abnormalities of chromosome 17, which are primarily in the short arm (p). The short arm of chromosome 17 is where the *TP53* tumor suppressor gene is located. The possibility exists that mutation of a "control gene" leads to development of the brain tumor, and if one copy of the gene is already dysfunctional, as in neurofibromatosis type 1, the likelihood of a tumor arising is increased. Abnormalities of chromosome 17 are also found in medulloblastoma,[6] but some work suggests that the locus is distinct from

the *TP53* suppressor gene.[3] In neuroblastoma, amplification of N-*MYC* correlates with tumor growth and aggressiveness.

The continued collaboration between neurosurgeons, oncologists, radiologists, and molecular biologists is imperative to improving the fight against pediatric brain tumors.

REFERENCES

1. Abdollahzadeh M, Hoffman HJ, Blazer SI, et al: Benign cerebellar astrocytoma in childhood: Experience at the Hospital for Sick Children 1980-1992. Childs Nerv Syst 1994;10:380.
2. Berger MS, Ojemann GA, Lettich E: Neurophysiological monitoring during astrocytoma surgery. Neurosurg Clin N Am 1990;1:65.
3. Biegel JA, Burk CD, Barr FG, Emmanuel BS: Evidence for a 17p tumor related locus distinct from p53 in pediatric primitive neuroectodermal tumors. Cancer Res 1992;52:3391.
4. Biegel JA, Parmiter AH, Sutton LN, et al: Abnormalities of chromosome 22 in pediatric meningiomas. Genes Chromosomes Cancer 1994;9:81.
5. Biegel JA, Rorke LB, Packer RJ, Emanuel BS: Monosomy 22 in rhabdoid or atypical tumors of the brain. J Neurosurg 1990;73:710.
6. Biegel JA, Rorke LB, Packer RJ, et al: Isochromosome 17q in primitive neuroectodermal tumors of the central nervous system. Genes Chromosomes Cancer 1989;1:139.
7. Bourne JP, Geyer R, Berger M, et al: The prognostic significance of postoperative residual contrast enhancement on CT scan in pediatric patients with medulloblastoma. J Neurooncol 1992;14:263.
8. Buetow PC, Smirniotopoulos JG, Done S: Congenital brain tumors: A review of 45 cases, AJNR Am J Neuroradiol 1990;11:793.
9. Chang CH, Housepian EM, Herbert C Jr: An operative staging system and a megavoltage radiotherapeutic technic for cerebellar medulloblastomas. Radiology 1969;93:1351.
10. Crist WM, Kun LE: Common solid tumors of childhood. N Engl J Med 1991;324:461.
11. Duffner PK, Cohen ME, Voorhess ML, et al: Long-term effects of cranial irradiation on endocrine function in children with brain tumors: A prospective study. Cancer 1985;56:2189.
12. Duffner PK, Horowitz ME, Krischer JP, et al: Postoperative chemotherapy and delayed radiation in children less than three years of age with malignant brain tumors. N Engl J Med 1993;328:1725.
13. Epstein FJ, Farmer JP: Brain-stem glioma growth patterns. J Neurosurg 1993;78:408.
14. Evans AE, Jenkin RD, Sposto R, et al: The treatment of medulloblastoma: Results of a prospective randomized trial of radiation therapy with and without CCNU, vincristine, and prednisone. J Neurosurg 1990;72:572.
15. Farwell JR, Dohrmann GJ, Flannery JT: Central nervous system tumors in children. Cancer 1977;40:3123.
16. Finlay JL, August C, Packer R, et al: High-dose multi-agent chemotherapy followed by bone marrow 'rescue' for malignant astrocytomas of childhood and adolescence. J Neurooncol 1990;9:239.
17. Finlay JL, Boyett JM, Yates AJ, et al: Randomized phase III trial in childhood high-grade astrocytoma comparing vincristine, lomustine, and prednisone with the eight-drugs-in-1-day regimen. Children's Cancer Group. J Clin Oncol 1995;13:112.

18. Freeman CR, Farmer JP, Montes J: Low-grade astrocytomas in children: Evolving management strategies. Int J Radiat Oncol Biol Phys 1998;41:979.

19. Geyer JR, Sposto R, Jennings M, et al: Children's Cancer Group. Multiagent chemotherapy and deferred radiotherapy in infants with malignant brain tumors: a report from the Children's Cancer Group. J Clin Oncol 2005;23:7621.

20. Giuffre R: Biological aspects of brain tumors in infancy and childhood. Childs Nerv Syst 1989;5:55.

21. Gjerris F, Klinken L: Long-term prognosis in children with benign cerebellar astrocytoma. J Neurosurg 1978; 49:179.

22. Gold EB, Leviton A, Lopez R, et al: Parental smoking and risk of childhood brain tumors. Am J Epidemiol 1993; 137:620.

23. Goldwein JW, Leahy JM, Packer RJ, et al: Intracranial ependymomas in children. Int J Radiat Oncol Biol Phys 1990;19:1497.

24. Harwood-Nash DC: Neuroimaging of childhood craniopharyngioma. Pediatr Neurosurg 1994;21(Suppl 1):2.

25. Hawkins MM, Draper GJ, Kingston JE: Incidence of second primary tumours among childhood cancer survivors. Br J Cancer 1987;56:339.

26. Healey EA, Barnes PD, Kupsky WJ, et al: The prognostic significance of postoperative residual tumor in ependymoma. Neurosurgery 1991;28:666.

27. Hoffman HJ, De Silva M, Humphreys RP, et al: Aggressive surgical management of craniopharyngiomas in children. J Neurosurg 1992;76:47.

28. Jakacki RI, Goldwein JW, Larsen RL, et al: Cardiac dysfunction following spinal irradiation during childhood. J Clin Oncol 1993;11:1033.

29. Kelly PJ: Image-directed tumor resection. Neurosurg Clin North Am 1990;1:81.

30. Krischer JP, Ragab AH, Kun L, et al: Nitrogen mustard, vincristine, procarbazine, and prednisone as adjuvant chemotherapy in the treatment of medulloblastoma. A Pediatric Oncology Group study. J Neurosurg 1991; 74:905.

31. Laurent JP, Chang CH, Cohen ME: A classification system for primitive neuroectodermal tumors (medulloblastoma) of the posterior fossa. Cancer 1985;56:1807.

32. Laws ER Jr, Taylor WF, Clifton MB, Okazaki H: Neurosurgical management of low-grade astrocytoma of the cerebral hemispheres. J Neurosurg 1984;61:665.

33. Lee M, Wisoff JH, Abbott R, et al: Management of hydrocephalus in children with medulloblastoma: Prognostic factors for shunting. Pediatr Neurosurg 1994;20:240.

34. Legido A, Packer RJ, Sutton LN, et al: Suprasellar germinomas in childhood: A reappraisal. Cancer 1989;63:340.

35. Loftus CM, Copeland BR, Carmel PW: Cystic supratentorial gliomas: Natural history and evaluation of modes of surgical therapy. Neurosurgery 1985;17:19.

36. Nazar GB, Hoffman HJ, Becker LE, et al: Infratentorial ependymomas in childhood: Prognostic factors and treatment. J Neurosurg 1990;72:408.

37. Packer RJ, Allen JC, Goldwein JL, et al: Hyperfractionated radiotherapy for children with brainstem gliomas: A pilot study using 7,200 cGy. Ann Neurol 1990;27:167.

38. Packer RJ, Sutton LN, Atkins TE, et al: A prospective study of cognitive function in children receiving whole-brain radiotherapy and chemotherapy: 2-year results. J Neurosurg 1989;70:707.

39. Packer RJ, Sutton LN, D'Angio G, et al: Management of children with primitive neuroectodermal tumors of the posterior fossa/medulloblastoma. Pediatr Neurosci 1985;12:272.

40. Packer RJ, Sutton LN, Elterman R, et al: Outcome for children with medulloblastoma treated with radiation and cisplatin, CCNU, and vincristine chemotherapy. J Neurosurg 1994;81:690.

41. Packer RJ, Sutton LN, Patel KM, et al: Seizure control following tumor surgery for childhood cortical low-grade gliomas. J Neurosurg 1994;80:998.

42. Packer RJ, Sutton LN, Rorke LB, et al: Intracranial embryonal cell carcinoma. Cancer 1984;54:520.

43. Palma L, Russo A, Mercuri S: Cystic cerebral astrocytomas in infancy and childhood: Long-term results. Childs Brain 1983;10:79.

44. Perilongo G, Sutton LN, Goldwein JW, et al: Childhood meningiomas: Experience in the modern imaging era. Pediatr Neurosurg 1992;18:16.

45. Petronio J, Edwards MS, Prados M, et al: Management of chiasmal and hypothalamic gliomas of infancy and childhood with chemotherapy. J Neurosurg 1991;74:701.

46. Pollack IF, Pang D, Albright AL: The long-term outcome in children with late-onset aqueductal stenosis resulting from benign intrinsic tectal tumors. J Neurosurg 1994;80:681.

47. Probert JC, Parker BR, Kaplan HS: Growth retardation in children after megavoltage irradiation of the spine. Cancer 1973;32:634.

48. Puce A, Constable RT, Luby ML, et al: Functional magnetic resonance imaging of sensory and motor cortex: Comparison with electrophysiological localization. J Neurosurg 1995; 83:262.

49. Radcliffe J, Bunin GR, Sutton LN, et al: Cognitive deficits in long-term survivors of childhood medulloblastoma and other noncortical tumors: Age-dependent effects of whole brain radiation. Int J Dev Neurosci 1994;12:327.

50. Ross AJ 3rd, Siegel KR, Bell W, et al: Massive gastrointestinal hemorrhage in children with posterior fossa tumors. J Pediatr Surg 1987;22:633.

51. Rouleau GA, Wertelecki W, Haines JL, et al: Genetic linkage of bilateral acoustic neurofibromatosis to a DNA marker on chromosome 22. Nature 1987;329:246.

52. Sandri A, Massimino M, Mastrodicasa L, et al: Treatment with oral etoposide for childhood recurrent ependymomas. J Pediatr Hematol Oncol 2005;27:486.

53. Scott RM, Hetelekidis S, Barnes PD, et al: Surgery, radiation, and combination therapy in the treatment of childhood craniopharyngioma—a 20-year experience. Pediatr Neurosurg 1994;21(Suppl 1):75.

54. Shiminski-Maher T: Patient/family preparation and education for complications and late sequelae of craniopharyngiomas. Pediatr Neurosurg 1994;21(Suppl 1):114.

55. Spoto GP, Press GA, Hesselink JR, Solomon M: Intracranial ependymoma and subependymoma: MR manifestations. AJR Am J Roentgenol 1990;154:837.

56. St. Clair SK, Humphreys RP, Pillary RK, et al: Current management of choroid plexus carcinoma in children. Pediatr Neurosurg 1991;17:225.

57. Steinberg GK, Shuer LM, Conley FK, Hanbery JW: Evolution and outcome in malignant astroglial neoplasms of the cerebellum. J Neurosurg 1985;62:9.

58. Steinbok P, Boyd M, Cochrane D: Cervical spinal deformity following craniotomy and upper cervical laminectomy for posterior fossa tumors in children. Childs Nerv Syst 1989;5:25.

59. Sutton LN: Current management of low-grade astrocytomas of childhood. Pediatr Neurosci 1987;13:98.

60. Sutton LN, Gusnard D, Bruce DA, et al: Fusiform dilatations of the carotid artery following radical surgery of childhood craniopharyngiomas. J Neurosurg 1991;74:695.

61. Sutton LN, Packer RJ, Rorke LB, et al: Cerebral gangliogliomas during childhood. Neurosurgery 1983;13:124.

62. Sutton LN, Wang Z, Gusnard D, et al: Proton magnetic resonance spectroscopy of pediatric brain tumors. Neurosurgery 1992;31:195.

63. Tait DM, Thomton-Jones H, Bloom HJ, et al: Adjuvant chemotherapy for medulloblastoma: The first multi-centre control trial of the International Society of Paediatric Oncology (SIOP I). Eur J Cancer 1990;26:464.

64. Torres CF, Rebsamen S, Silber JH, et al: Surveillance scanning of children with medulloblastoma. N Engl J Med 1994; 330:892.

65. Vertosick FT Jr, Selker RG: Brain stem and spinal metastases of supratentorial glioblastoma multiforme: A clinical series. Neurosurgery 1990;27:516.

66. Weiss M, Sutton L, Marcial V, et al: The role of radiation therapy in the management of childhood craniopharyngioma. Int J Radiat Oncol Biol Phys 1989;17:1313.

67. Wisoff JH: Surgical management of recurrent craniopharyngiomas. Pediatr Neurosurg 1994;21(Suppl 1):108.

68. Wisoff JH, Abbott R, Epstein F: Surgical management of exophytic chiasmatic-hypothalamic tumors of childhood. J Neurosurg 1990;73:661.

69. Wisoff JH, Epstein FJ: Pseudobulbar palsy after posterior fossa operation in children. Neurosurgery 1984;15:707.

70. Young JL Jr, Percy CL, Asire AJ, et al: Cancer incidence and mortality in the United States, 1973-77. Natl Cancer Inst Monogr 1981;(57):1.

71. Zimmerman RA, Bilaniuk LT, Bruno L, Rosenstock J: Computed tomography of cerebellar astrocytoma. AJR Am J Roentgenol 1978;130:929.

Part IV

TRANSPLANTATION

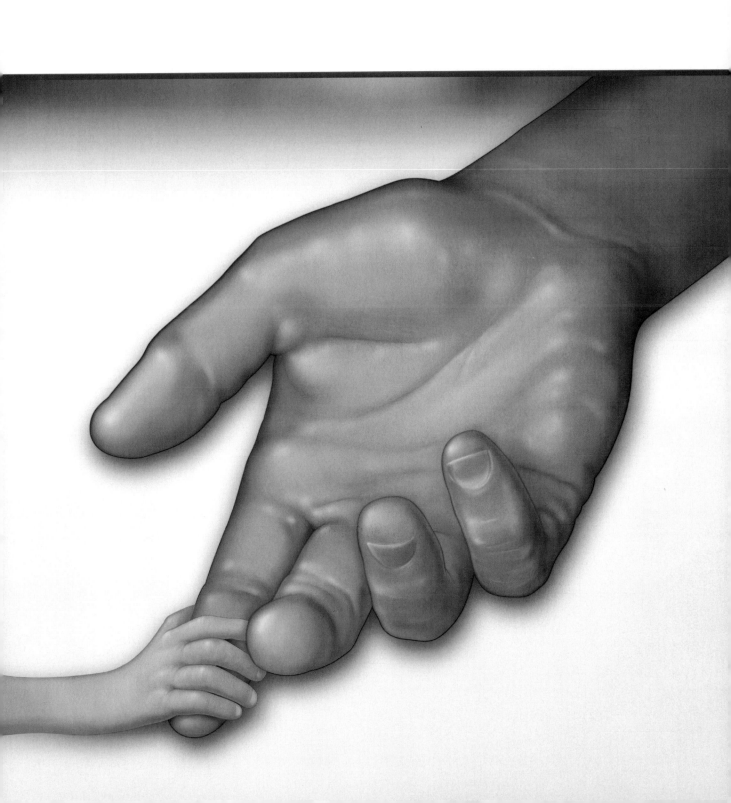

Chapter 42

Principles of Transplantation

Jorge Reyes, Noriko Murase, and Thomas E. Starzl

Histocompatibility matching, immunosuppression, tissue preservation, and techniques of implantation have been considered to be the generic struts of both organ and bone marrow cell transplantation. However, neither kind of transplantation could have emerged as a clinical service were it not for the induction by the graft itself of various degrees on donor-specific nonreactivity (tolerance). Without this fifth factor, no transplant recipient could survive for long if the amount of immunosuppression given to obtain initial engraftment had to be continued.

THE ENIGMA OF ACQUIRED TOLERANCE

The variable acquired tolerance on which transplantation depends has been one of the most enigmatic and controversial issues in all of biology. This was caused, in part, by the unexpected achievement of organ engraftment at an early time—a decade before successful bone marrow transplantation and in ostensible violation of the very principles that would shape the impending revolution in general immunology. As a consequence, clinical organ transplantation was developed empirically rather than as a branch of classic immunology. This occurred in four distinct phases, each lasting more than a decade. Only at the end was it possible to explain organ engraftment and thereby eliminate the mystique of transplantation.

Phase 1: 1953-1968

Phase 1 began between 1953-1956 with the demonstration that neonatal mice[8,9] and irradiated adult mice[36] develop donor-specific tolerance after successful engraftment of donor hematolymphopoietic cells. The key observation was that the mice bearing donor cells (donor leukocyte chimerism) could now accept skin grafts from the original donor strain but from no other strain (Fig. 42-1). The chimeric neonatal mice and the irradiated adult mice were analogues of today's bone marrow transplantation into immune deficient and cytoablated humans, respectively. But because a good histocompatibility match was required for avoidance of graft-versus-host disease (GVHD) and of rejection,[39] clinical application

of bone marrow transplantation had to await discovery of the human leukocyte antigens (HLA). When this was accomplished,[3,21,99] the successfully treated human bone marrow recipients of 1968 were oversized versions of the tolerant chimeric mice.

By the time of the clinical bone marrow transplant breakthrough of 1968, kidney transplantation[22,23,29,42,48,49,64] already was an established clinical service, albeit a flawed one.[65] In addition, the first long survivals had been recorded after liver[72] and heart transplantation[5]; these were followed in 1968-1969 by the first prolonged survival of a lung[18] and a pancreas recipient[34] (Table 42-1). All of the organ transplant successes had been accomplished in the ostensible absence of leukocyte chimerism, without HLA matching and with no evidence of GVHD. By going

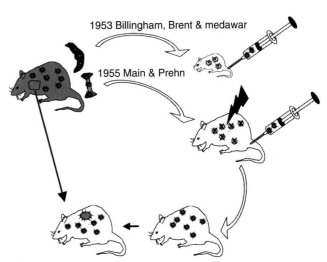

Figure 42-1 The mouse models of acquired tolerance described between 1953 and 1956. White cells (leukocytes) were isolated from the spleen or bone marrow of adult donor mice *(upper left)* and injected into the bloodstream of newborn mice *(upper right)* or of irradiated adult mice *(middle right)*. Under both circumstances, the recipient immune system was too weak to reject the foreign cells *(dark shaded)*. With engraftment of the injected cells (i.e., donor leukocyte chimerism), the recipient mice now could freely accept tissues and organs from the leukocyte donor but from no other donor *(bottom left)*.

TABLE 42–1 First Successful Transplantation of Human Allografts (Survival > 1 Year)

Organ	City	Date	Physician/ Surgeon	Reference
Kidney	Boston	Jan. 24, 1959	Merrill/ Murray	42, 48
Liver	Denver	July 23, 1967	Starzl	72
Heart	Cape Town	Jan. 2, 1968	Barnard	5
Lung	Ghent	Nov. 14, 1968	Derom	18
Pancreas	Minneapolis	June 3, 1969	Lillehei	34

beyond the leukocyte chimerism boundaries established by the mouse tolerance models, organ transplantation had entered unmapped territory.

"Pseudotolerant" Organ Recipients

Two unexplained features of the alloimmune response had made it feasible to forge ahead precociously with organ transplantation.[64] The first was that organ rejection is highly reversible. The second was that an organ allograft, if protected by nonspecific immunosuppression, could induce its own acceptance. "Self-induced engraftment" was observed for the first time in 1959 in two fraternal twin kidney recipients, first in Boston by Joseph Murray[48] and then in Paris by Jean Hamburger.[22] These were the first successful transplantations in the world of an organ allograft, in any species. Both patients had been conditioned with 450 R sublethal total-body irradiation before transplantation. The renal allografts functioned for more than 2 decades without a need for maintenance drug therapy, which was, in fact, not yet available.

A similar drug-free state was next occasionally observed after kidney transplantation (and more frequently after liver replacement) in mongrel dogs who were treated with a single immunosuppressive agent: 6-mercaptopurine (6-MP),[55,112] azathioprine,[50,66] prednisone,[113] or antilymphocyte globulin (ALG).[70] After treatment was stopped, rejection in some animals never developed (Fig. 42-2A). Such results were exceedingly rare; less than 1% of the canine kidney experiments done under 6-MP and azathioprine up to the summer of 1962. However, the possibility that an organ could be inherently tolerogenic was crystallized by the human experience summarized in the title of a report in 1963 of a series of live donor kidney recipients treated in Denver: "The Reversal of Rejection in Human Renal Homografts with Subsequent Development of Homograft Tolerance."[64] The recipients had been given azathioprine *before* as well as after renal transplantation, adding large doses of prednisone to treat rejections that were monitored by serial testing of serum creatinine (Fig. 42-3A). Rejection occurred in almost every case, and 25% of the grafts were lost to uncontrolled acute rejection. However, the 1-year survival of 46 allografts obtained from familial donors over a 16-month period in 1962-1963 was an unprecedented 75%.

The development of partial tolerance in many of the survivors was inferred from the rapidly declining need

for treatment after rejection reversal (see Fig. 42-3A). Nine (19%) of the 46 allografts functioned for the next 4 decades, each depicted in Figure 42-4 as a horizontal bar. Moreover, all immunosuppression eventually was stopped in seven of the nine patients without rejection for periods ranging from 6 to 40 years (the solid portion of the bars). Eight of the nine patients are still alive and bear the longest surviving organ allografts in the world.[92]

What was the connection between the tolerant mouse models, the irradiated fraternal twin kidney recipients in Boston and Paris, the ultimate drug-free canine organ recipients (see Fig. 42-2A), and the unique cluster of "pseudotolerant" human kidney recipients in Denver (Fig. 42-4)? The mystery deepened with the demonstration in 1966 in France,[16] England,[11,12,53] and the United States[74] that the liver can be transplanted in about 20% of outbred pigs without any treatment at all (see Fig. 42-2B). None of the animal or human organ recipients, whether off or on maintenance immunosuppression, was thought to have donor leukocyte chimerism.

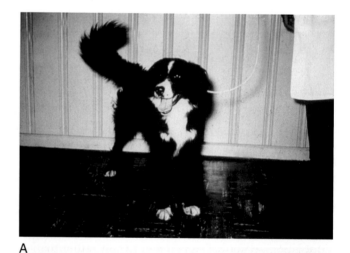

A

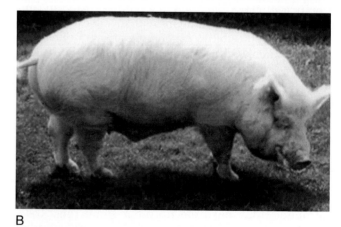

B

Figure 42–2 *A,* Caine recipient of an orthotopic liver homograft, 5 years later. The operation was on March 23, 1964. The dog was treated for only 120 days with azathioprine and died of old age after 13 years. *B,* A spontaneously tolerant pig recipient described by Calne.[12]

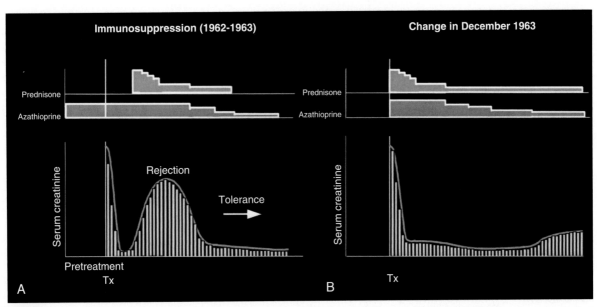

Figure 42–3 *A,* Empirically developed immunosuppression used for kidney transplant recipients in 1962-1963. Note the reversal of rejection with the addition of prednisone to azathioprine. More than a third of a century later it was realized that the timing of drug administration had been in accord with the tolerogenic principles of immunosuppression (see text). *B,* Treatment revisions in immunosuppression made at the University of Colorado in December, 1963, that unwittingly violated principles of tolerogenic immunosuppression. Pretreatment was de-emphasized or eliminated, and high doses of prednisone were given prophylactically instead of as needed. Although the frequency of acute rejection was reduced, the drug-free tolerance shown in Figure 42-4 was no longer seen.

False Premises of Phase 1

Thus, organ transplantation became disconnected at a very early time from the scientific anchor of leukocyte chimerism that had been established by the mouse models and was soon to be exemplified by human bone marrow transplantation. The resulting intellectual separation of the two kinds of transplantation (Fig. 42-5) was an unchallenged legacy of phase 1, passed on from generation to generation ever since.

There was another dark legacy of phase 1. This was a modified version of the treatment strategy that had been developed with azathioprine and prednisone (see Fig. 42-3B). The principal change was the use of large prophylactic doses of prednisone from the time of operation, instead of the administration of corticosteroids only when needed. In a second modification, the pretreatment was de-emphasized (see Fig. 42-3B). The incidence of acute rejection was greatly reduced after these changes. However, no cluster of drug-free kidney recipients like that shown in Figure 42-4 was ever seen again, anywhere in the world. More than 35 years passed before the long-term immunologic consequences of the modifications were realized.

Figure 42–4 Nine (19%) of the 46 live donor kidney recipients treated at the University of Colorado over an 18-month period beginning in the autumn of 1962. The solid portion of the horizontal bars depicts the time off immunosuppression. Note that the current serum creatinine concentration (CR) is normal in all but one patient. *Murdered: kidney allograft normal at autopsy.

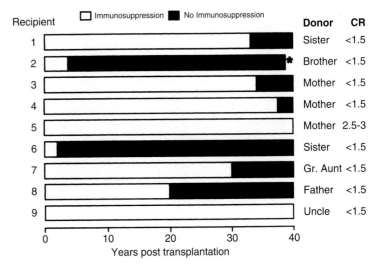

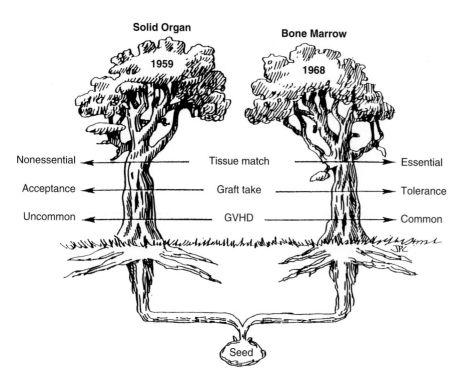

Solid Organ — 1959

Bone Marrow — 1968

Nonessential ←	Tissue match	→ Essential
Acceptance ←	Graft take	→ Tolerance
Uncommon ←	GVHD	→ Common

Seed

Figure 42–5 The developmental tree of bone marrow *(right)* and organ transplantation *(left)* after it was demonstrated that rejection is an immunologic response. GVHD, graft-versus-host disease.

Phase 2: 1969-1979

Throughout the succeeding phase 2 that began in 1969, immunosuppression for organ transplantation was based on azathioprine and prophylactic high-dose prednisone to which ALG was added after 1966[70,71] in about 15% of centers. Phase 2 was a bleak period. In the view of critics, the heavy mortality, and particularly the devastating morbidity caused by corticosteroid dependence, made organ transplantation (even of kidneys) as much a disease as a treatment. Most of the liver and heart transplant programs that had been established in an initial burst of optimism after the first successful cases closed down.

But in the few remaining centers, patients like the one shown in Figure 42-6 bore witness to what some day would be accomplished on a grand scale. Four years old at the time of her liver replacement for biliary atresia and a hepatoma in 1969, she is the longest surviving recipient of an extrarenal organ.

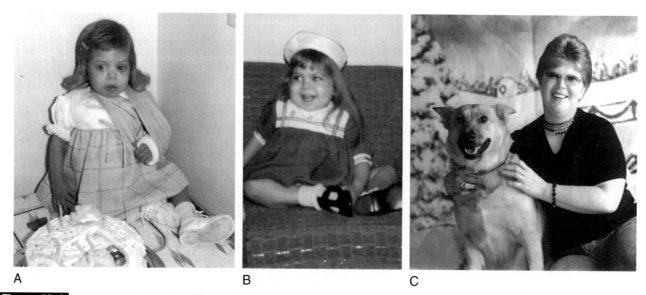

A B C

Figure 42–6 Four-year-old at the time of liver replacement for biliary atresia and a hepatoma but now in her 35th post-transplant year. She is the longest surviving recipient of an extrarenal organ.

Phase 3: 1980-1991

In fact, what had appeared to be the sunset of extrarenal organ transplantation was only the dawn of phase 3, which began with the clinical introduction of cyclosporine,[13,14,77,78] followed a decade later by that of tacrolimus.[20,81,82,102] The use of these drugs was associated with stepwise improvements with all organs, but their impact was most conclusively demonstrated with liver and heart transplantation. The results with liver transplantation shown in Figure 42-7 using azathioprine-, cyclosporine-, and tacrolimus-based immunosuppression were presented at the meeting of the American Surgical Association in April 1994.[103] By then, intestinal transplantation under tacrolimus-based immunosuppression had become a service.[104,105]

As the new agents became available, they were simply incorporated into the modified formula of heavy prophylactic immunosuppression that had been inherited from phases 1 and 2. Used in a variety of multiple-agent combinations from the time of surgery, the better drugs fueled the golden age of transplantation of the 1980s and early 1990s. Acute rejection had become almost a "non" problem. However, the unresolved issues now were chronic rejection, risks of long-term immunosuppression (e.g., infections and de novo malignancies), and drug toxicity (e.g., the nephrotoxicity of cyclosporine and tacrolimus).

Phase 4: 1992-Present

It was clear that relief from the burden of lifetime immunosuppression would require elucidation of the mechanisms of alloengraftment and of acquired tolerance. An intensified search for the engraftment mechanisms has dominated the current phase 4, which began in the early 1990s.

The Historical Dogma

Until this time, organ engraftment had been attributed to mechanisms that did not involve either the presence or a role of leukocyte chimerism. Although it was known that organs contain large numbers of passenger leukocytes, these donor cells were largely replaced in the successfully transplanted allograft by recipient leukocytes as shown in Figure 42-8A. The missing donor cells were thought to have undergone immune destruction with selective sparing of the specialized parenchymal cells. As for bone marrow transplantation (see Fig. 42-8B), the ideal result had been perceived as complete replacement of recipient immune cells (i.e., total hematolymphopoietic chimerism).

The Discovery of Microchimerism

A flaw in this historical dogma began to be exposed in the early 1990s. The first puzzling observation in Seattle[56] and Helsinki[107] was the invariable presence of a small residual population of recipient hematolymphopoietic cells in patients previously thought to have complete bone marrow replacement (see Fig. 42-8D). This was followed in 1992 by the discovery of donor leukocyte microchimerism in long-surviving human organ recipients. Now it was evident that organ engraftment (see Fig. 42-8C) and bone marrow cell engraftment (see Fig. 42-8D) were mirror-image versions of leukocyte chimerism, differing in the reversed proportion of donor and recipient cells.

The discovery of microchimerism in organ recipients was made with a very simple clinical study.[83-87] With the use of sensitive detection techniques, donor hematolymphopoietic cells of different lineages (including dendritic cells) were found in the blood, lymph nodes, skin, or other tissues of 30 of 30 liver or kidney recipients who had borne functioning allografts for up to 30 years. The donor leukocytes obviously were progeny of donor precursor or pluripotent hematolymphopoietic stem cells that had migrated from the graft into the recipient after surviving a double immune reaction that presumably had occurred just after transplantation, years or decades earlier.[35,45,57,94]

It was concluded that organ engraftment had been the result of "responses of co-existing donor and recipient cells, each to the other, causing reciprocal clonal exhaustion, followed by peripheral clonal deletion."[83,85] The host response (the upright curve in Fig. 42-9) was the dominant one in most cases of organ transplantation but with the occasional exception of GVHD. In the conventionally treated bone marrow recipient, host cytoablation simply transferred immune dominance from the host to the graft (the inverted curve in Fig. 42-9), explaining the high risk of GVHD. All of the major differences between the two kinds of transplantation were caused by the recipient cytoablation. After an estrangement of more than a third of a century, the intellectual separation of bone marrow and organ transplantation was ended (Fig. 42-10).

Immune Regulation by Antigen Migration and Localization

But how was the exhaustion-deletion of the double immune reaction shown in Figure 42-9 maintained after its

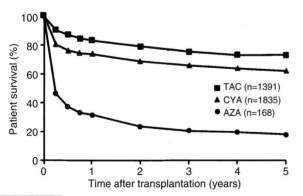

Figure 42–7 Patient survival: results with orthotopic liver transplantation at the Universities of Colorado (1963-1980) and Pittsburgh (1981-1993), in periods defined by azathioprine (AZA)-, cyclosporine (CYA)-, and tacrolimus (TAC)-based immune suppression. Stepwise improvements associated with the advent of these drugs also were made with other kinds of organs.

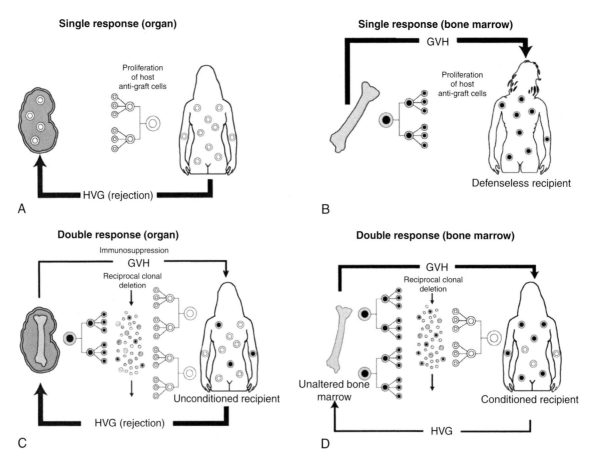

Figure 42–8 Old (*A* and *B*) and new views (*C* and *D*) of transplantation recipients. *A,* The early conceptualization of immune mechanisms in organ transplantation in terms of a unidirectional host-versus-graft (HVG) response. Although this readily explained organ rejection, it limited possible explanations of organ engraftment. *B,* Mirror image of *A* depicting the early understanding of successful bone marrow transplantation as a complete replacement of the recipient immune system by that of the donor, with the potential complication of an unopposed lethal unidirectional graft-versus-host (GVH) response, that is, rejection of the recipient by the graft. *C,* Our current view of bidirectional and reciprocally modulating immune responses of coexisting immune competent cell populations. Because of variable reciprocal induction of deletional tolerance, organ engraftment was feasible despite a usually dominant HVG reaction. The bone silhouette in the graft represents passenger leukocytes of bone marrow origin. *D,* Our currently conceived mirror image of *C* after successful bone marrow transplantation. Recipient's cytoablation has caused a reversal of the size proportions of the donor and recipient populations of immune cells.

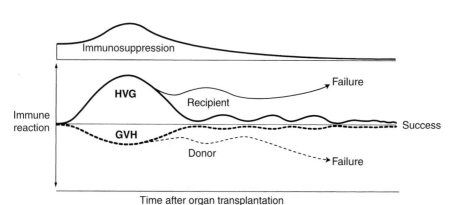

Figure 42–9 Contemporaneous HVG (*upright curves*) and GVH (*inverted curves*) responses after transplantation. In contrast to the usually dominant HVG reaction of organ transplantation, the GVH reaction usually is dominant after bone marrow cell transplantation to the irradiated or otherwise immunodepressed recipient. Therapeutic failure with either type of transplantation implies the inability to control one, the other, or both of the contemporaneous responses with a protective umbrella of immunosuppression. (Starzl TE, Zinkernagel R: Antigen localization and migration in immunity and tolerance. N Engl J Med 1998;339:1905-1913.)

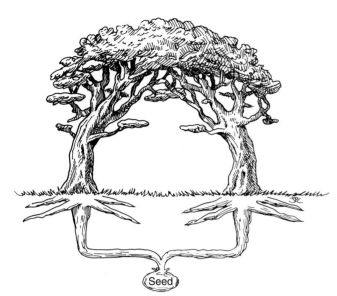

Figure 42–10 Unification of organ and bone marrow transplantation (See text).

acute induction by the first wave of migratory leukocytes? Rolf Zinkernagel, in Zurich (Fig. 42-11), had addressed this question during the 1990s in experimental studies of the nonresponsiveness that may develop to intracellular microorganisms such as tubercle bacillus and noncytopathic viruses.[43,109-111] The analogies between the syndromes caused by such infectious agents and the events following transplantation were described in 1998 in a joint review with Zinkernagel in the *New England Journal of Medicine*.[89]

The analogies between transplantation and infection had been obscured by the characteristic double immune reaction of transplantation and by the complicating factor of immunosuppression. Now, these analogies were obvious. The antidonor response induced by the initially selective migration of the graft's leukocytes to host lymphoid organs (Fig. 42-12, left)[17,32,44,51] is comparable to the response induced by a spreading intracellular pathogen. The migration patterns of the donor leukocytes were the same whether these cells emigrated from an organ or were delivered as a bone marrow cell infusion. Cells that survived the antidonor response that they had induced begin within a few days to move on (see Fig. 42-12, right) to protected nonlymphoid niches where their presence may be detected no longer by the immune system (immune ignorance[4,27,30,31,89]). This was a survival tactic of noncytopathic microorganisms.

The migration of donor leukocytes is shown schematically in Figure 42-13, left by centrifugal arrows: first by hematogenous routes to lymphoid organs and, after a few weeks, on to nonlymphoid sites (outer circle). A subsequent reverse migration of donor cells from protected nonlymphoid niches back to host lymphoid organs is depicted by the inwardly directed dashed arrows in Figure 42-13, right. The retrograde migration is a two-edged sword. On one hand, these cells may sustain the clonal exhaustion-deletion induced at the outset, usually requiring an umbrella of maintenance immunosuppression. But on the other hand, these cells can perpetuate alloimmunity in the same way as surviving residual microorganisms perpetuate protective immunity. Not surprisingly, therefore, an alternative consequence of microchimerism may be the high panel reactive antibody (connoting sensitization to HLA antigens) that commonly develops after unsuccessful transplantation.[25,61]

Therapeutic Implications

How could the new insight be exploited clinically? The window of opportunity for the donor leukocyte-induced clonal deletion that corresponds with collapse of the antigraft response (Fig. 42-14, left) is open only for the first few post-transplant weeks.[46,47,57,95] It was apparent that the window could be closed by excessive postoperative immunosuppression (see Fig. 42-14, middle). With later reduction of the initial overimmunosuppression, recovery of the inefficiently deleted clone would be expected, leading to the delayed acute rejection, or the chronic rejection, that was being seen in the transplant clinics. Even in the best-case scenario, the patients would be predestined to lifetime dependence on immunosuppression. However, too little immunosuppression would result in uncontrolled rejection (see Fig. 42-14, right).

The problem faced by clinicians was how to find just the right amount of post-transplant immunosuppression. In 2001, it was suggested that this dilemma could be addressed by successively applying two historically rooted therapeutic principles: recipient pretreatment, followed by minimalistic post-transplant immunosuppression.[90] With pretreatment, the recipients, immune responsiveness would be reduced

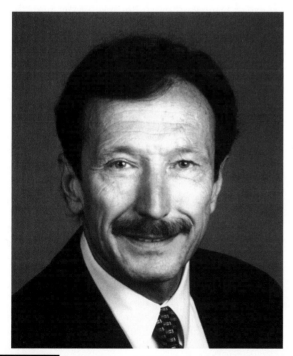

Figure 42–11 Rolf Zinkernagel (1944-). Swiss physician-immunologist whose discovery (with Peter Doherty) of the mechanisms of the adaptive immune response to noncytopathic microorganisms earned the Nobel prize in 1996.

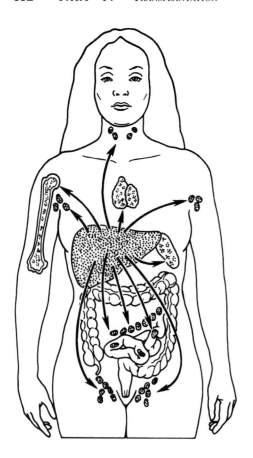
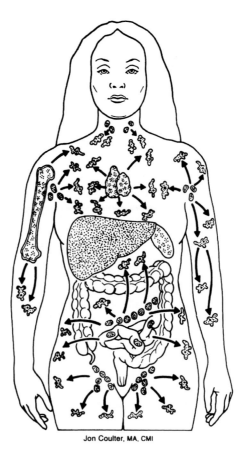

Jon Coulter, MA, CMI

Figure 42–12 Initial preferential migration of passenger leukocytes from organ allografts (here a liver) to host lymphoid organs *(left),* where they induce a donor-specific immune response. After about 30 days, many of the surviving cells move on to nonlymphoid sites *(right).*

before exposure to donor antigen, thereby lowering the anticipated donor-specific response into a more readily deletable range (Fig. 42-15). Clonal deletion by the kidneys' passenger leukocytes undoubtedly is what had been accomplished after sublethal irradiation alone in the ground-breaking fraternal twin (i.e., sublethal total body irradiation or myelotoxic drugs) cases of 1959.[22,48] In fact, radical pretreatment by recipient cytoablation ultimately

became the essential therapeutic step for conventional bone marrow transplantation. Because of the high risk of GVHD, this approach was too dangerous and too restrictive to be practical for organ transplantation.

However, less drastic lymphoid depletion by ALG or other measures (so-called nonmyeloablative conditioning) had been repeatedly shown since the 1960s to be effective without causing GVHD[71] (see Fig. 42-15).

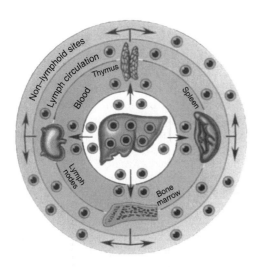
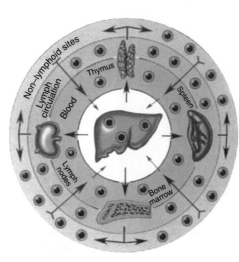

Figure 42–13 The migration routes of passenger leukocytes of transplanted organs are similar to those of infused bone marrow cells. *Left,* Selective migration at first to host lymphoid organs. After 15 to 30 days, surviving leukocytes begin to secondarily move to nonlymphoid sites. *Right,* Establishment of reverse traffic by which the exhaustion-deletion induced at the outset can be maintained.

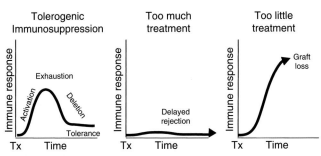

Figure 42–14 The effect of post-transplant immunosuppression on the seminal mechanism of clonal exhaustion deletion. *Left,* Just the right amount. *Middle,* Too much. *Right,* Too little. See text.

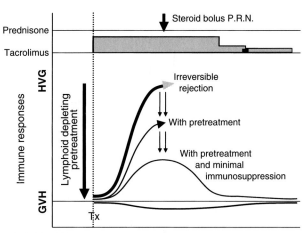

Figure 42–16 Conversion of rejection *(thick dark arrow)* to an immune response that can be exhausted and deleted by combination of pretreatment and minimalistic post-transplant immunosuppression.

After pretreatment with one of today's potent antilymphoid antibody preparations, the preemptively weakened clonal activation could proceed efficiently to clonal deletion under minimalistic short- and long-term maintenance therapy (Fig. 42-16). In July 2001, we instituted the double-principle strategy in adult organ recipients. The pretreatment was with a single infusion of 5 mg/kg of thymoglobulin. Beginning in 2002, a single Campath dose of 30 mg was substituted for thymoglobulin in most adult cases. After either kind of lymphoid depletion, treatment after transplantation was given with a conservative daily dose of a single drug (usually tacrolimus), adding other agents only in the event of breakthrough rejection and for as brief a period as possible. The strategy was extended to infants and children for intestinal transplantation in 2002 and for all kidney transplantations after April 2003.

After 4 to 8 months, weaning from monotherapy to less than daily doses was begun in adults whose graft function was stable: every other day, then three times per week, twice a week, and in many cases to once a week by 1 year (Fig. 42-17). The strategy has been used for the treatment of more than 1000 adult kidney, liver, intestine, pancreas, and lung recipients.[40,59,91] This experience has demonstrated that the quality of life of transplant recipients can be improved. For the first time, children are being considered for spaced weaning.

ORGAN PRESERVATION

Procurement

The breakthroughs of the early 1960s that made transplantation clinically practical were so unexpected that almost no formal preparation had been made to preserve the transplanted organs. Cardiac surgeons had used hypothermia for open-heart operations from 1950 onward and knew that ischemic damage below the level of aortic cross-clamping could be reduced by cooling the subdiaphagmatic organs.[58] In an early report, Lillehei and colleagues[33] immersed intestines in iced saline before autotransplantation. In Boston, Sicular and Moore[60] reported greatly slowed enzyme degradation in cold slices of liver.

Despite this awareness, kidneys were routinely transplanted until 1963 with no protection from warm ischemia during organ transfer. The only attempt to cool kidney allografts until then was by the potentially dangerous practice

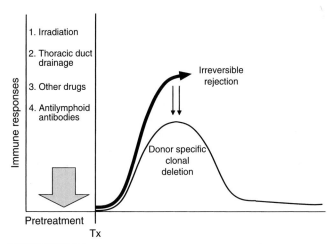

Figure 42–15 Rather than producing rejection *(thick dark arrow),* the donor-specific immune response to allografts may be exhausted and deleted, *as depicted by the fall of the initially ascending continuous thin line,* when recipient immune responsiveness is weakened in advance of transplantation (the pretreatment principle).

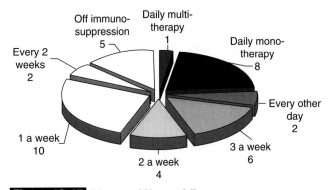

Figure 42–17 Diagram of 2½-year follow-up.

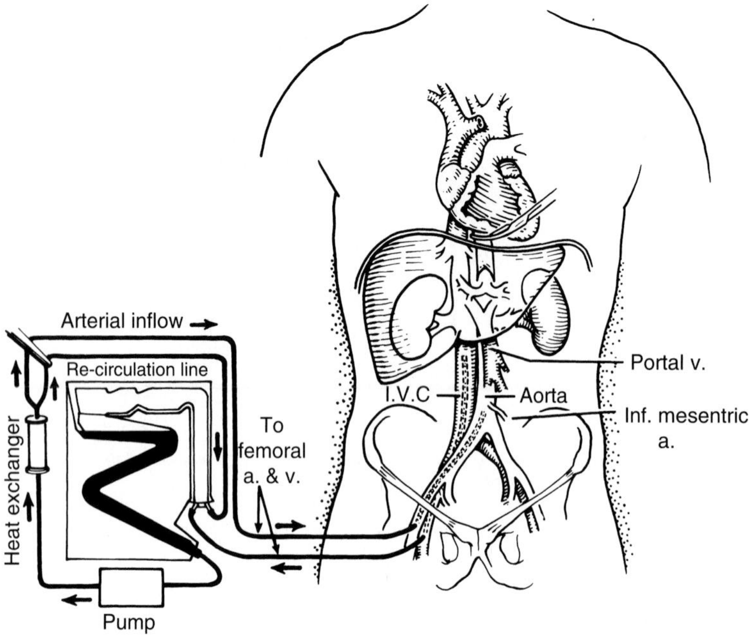

Figure 42–18 First technique of in situ cooling by extracorporeal hypothermic perfusion. The catheters were inserted into the aorta and vena cava by way of the femoral vessels as soon as possible after death. Temperature control was provided with a heat exchanger. Cross-clamping of the thoracic aorta limited perfusion to the lower part of the body. This method of cadaveric organ procurement was used from 1962 to 1969, before the acceptance of brain death criteria. The preliminary stages of this approach provided the basis for subsequent in situ infusion techniques.

(used by thoracic surgeons for open-heart surgery) of immersing the live donor in a bathtub of ice water (total-body hypothermia).[63] This cumbersome method of cooling was quickly replaced by infusion of chilled solutions into the renal artery after donor nephrectomy,[67] exploiting a principle of core (transvascular) cooling that had been standardized several years earlier for experimental liver transplantation.[62]

Core cooling in situ, the first critical step in the preservation of all cadaveric whole organs, is done today with variations of the technique described in 1963 by Marchioro and coworkers,[37] which permits in situ cooling to be undertaken[68] (Fig. 42-18). Ackerman and Snell[1] and Merkel and associates[41] popularized in situ cooling of cadaveric kidneys with simple infusion of cold electrolyte solutions into the donor femoral artery or distal aorta. Procurement techniques were eventually perfected that allowed removal of all thoracic and abdominal organs, including the liver, without jeopardizing any of the individual organs (Fig. 42-19).[79] Modifications of this flexible procedure have been made for unstable donors and even for donors whose hearts have stopped beating.[80] During the 5 years between 1980 and 1985, such techniques had become interchangeable in all parts of the world, setting the stage for reliable organ sharing. After the chilled organs are removed, subsequent preservation is possible with prototype strategies: simple refrigeration or continuous perfusion (see later).

Extended Preservation

Continuous Vascular Perfusion

Efforts to continuously perfuse isolated organs have proved to be difficult. For renal allografts, Ackerman and Barnard[2] used a normothermic perfusate primed with

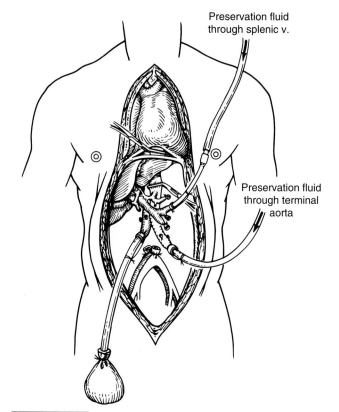

Figure 42–19 Principle of in situ cooling used for multiple organ procurement. With limited preliminary dissection of the aorta and of the great splanchnic veins (in this case the splenic vein), cold infusates can be used to chill organs in situ. In this case, the kidneys and liver were being removed. Note the aortic cross-clamp above the celiac axis.

blood that was oxygenated within a hyperbaric chamber. Brettschneider and colleagues[10] modified the apparatus and were able to preserve canine livers for 2 days, an unprecedented feat at the time. When Belzer and associates[6] eliminated the hemoglobin and hyperbaric chamber components, their asanguinous hypothermic perfusion technique was immediately accepted for clinical renal transplantation but then slowly abandoned in most centers when it was learned that the quality of 2-day preservation was not markedly better than that of simpler and less expensive infusion and slush methods (see later). However, refinement of perfusion techniques may someday permit true organ banking.

Static Preservation

With these "slush techniques," special solutions, such as those described by Collins and coworkers,[15] were instilled into the renal vascular system of kidneys or the vascular system of other organs after their preliminary chilling and separation. The original Collins solution or modifications of it were used for nearly 2 decades before they were replaced with the University of Wisconsin (UW) solution that was developed by the team of Folkert Belzer. Although it was first used for the liver,[7,26,101] the UW solution provides superior preservation of kidneys and other organs.[24,106] The UW preservation permitted longer and safer preservation of kidneys (2 days) and livers (18 hours), a higher rate of graft survival, and a lower rate of primary nonfunction. With the UW solution, national organ sharing was made economical and practical.

TISSUE TYPING

Antigen Matching

The first prospective antigen matching trials were begun in 1964 by Terasaki and associates[97] in collaboration with the University of Colorado kidney transplantation team. Although the value of this serologic technology was demonstrable when the kidney donor was a highly compatible family member (the "perfect match"),[75] lesser degrees of matching correlated poorly with renal transplantation outcome.[88] The reasons for this paradox were inexplicable until the discovery of recipient chimerism (Fig. 42-20). However, the belief that matching should be a prime determinant of success resulted in its use as an overriding factor for the allocation of cadaver kidneys in the United States.

The propriety of this kidney allocation policy has been repeatedly challenged on ethical as well as scientific grounds for nearly a third of a century. Those in favor of perpetuating the role of graded HLA matches cite multicenter case compilations in the United States and Europe showing a small gain in allograft survival with histocompatible kidneys, whereas many of the individual contributing centers see no such trend in their own experience.[19,38,58,93] In a compelling study, Terasaki and associates[98] reported that early survival and the subsequent half-life of kidneys from randomly matched, living unrelated donors was

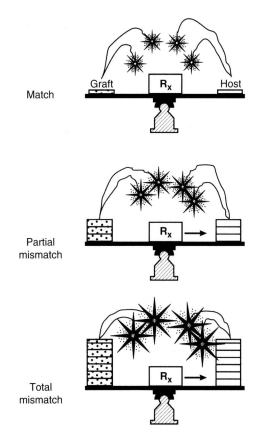

Figure 42–20 The nullification effect of simultaneous host-versus-graft (HVG) and graft-versus-host (GVH) reactions when organs are transplanted to recipients whose immune system has not been cytoablated. The reciprocal induction of tolerance, each to the other, of the coexisting cell populations is the explanation for the poor correlation of HLA matching with outcome after organ transplantation.

identical to that of parent-offspring (one haplotype matched) grafts. The inescapable conclusion is that more effective timing and dosage of immunosuppressive therapy rather than refinements in tissue matching and organ sharing will be the primary method of improving the results of whole-organ transplantation.

Crossmatching

None of the immunosuppressive measures available today can prevent immediate destruction of kidneys and other kinds of organ grafts in what has been called hyperacute rejection. This complication was first seen with the transplantation of kidneys from ABO-incompatible donors when they were placed in recipients with antidonor isoagglutinins.[69] After the description by Terasaki and associates[96] of hyperacute kidney rejection by a recipient with antidonor lymphocytotoxic antibodies, Kissmeyer-Nielsen and colleagues[28] and others[73,76,100,108] confirmed the association of hyperacute rejection with these antigraft antibodies. Although hyperacute rejection can usually be avoided with the lymphocytotoxic crossmatch originally recommended by Terasaki and associates, the precise pathogenesis of such rejection remains poorly understood more than 30 years after its recognition as a complement activation syndrome.[73,76]

FUTURE PROSPECTS

The revisions in timing and dose control that encourage the seminal mechanisms of clonal exhaustion-deletion and immune ignorance should make it possible to systematically reduce exposure to the risks of chronic immunosuppression. Our prediction is that completely drug free tolerance will be largely, but not exclusively, limited to recipients of HLA-matched organs. But variable partial tolerance will be more regularly attainable in most of the others, not so much by developing better drugs as by the mechanism-based use of drugs we already have in hand. Xenotransplantation will have to be developed within the same immunologic framework. Here, the problem in principle is to create a better interspecies tissue match by transgenic modification. Although the α-1,3GT gene responsible for hyperacute rejection of pig organs by higher primates has been knocked out in pigs,[54] it is not yet known what further changes have to be made before porcine organs can be used clinically. Where stem cell biology will fit remains unknown. But it also will have to conform to the same immunologic rules.

REFERENCES

1. Ackermann JR, Snell MR: Cadaveric renal transplantation. Br J Urol 1963;40:515.
2. Ackermann JR, Barnard CN: Successful storage of kidneys. Br J Surg 1966;53:525-532.
3. Bach FH: Bone-marrow transplantation in a patient with the Wiskott-Aldrich syndrome. Lancet 1968;2:1364-1366.
4. Barker CF, Billingham RE: The role of afferent lymphatics in the rejection of skin homografts. J Exp Med 1968;128:197-221.
5. Barnard CN: What we have learned about heart transplants. J Thorac Cardiovasc Surg 1968;56:457-468.
6. Belzer FO, Ashby BS, Dunphy JE: 24-hour and 72-hour preservation of canine kidneys. Lancet 1967;2:536-538.
7. Belzer FO, Southard JH: Principles of solid-organ preservation by cold storage. Transplantation 1988;45:673-676.
8. Billingham RE, Brent L, Medawar PB: "Actively acquired tolerance" of foreign cells. Nature 1953;172:603-606.
9. Billingham R, Brent L, Medawar P: Quantitative studies on tissue transplantation immunity: III. Actively acquired tolerance. Philos Trans R Soc Lond (Biol) 1956;239:357-412.
10. Brettschneider L, Daloze PM, Huguet C, et al: The use of combined preservation techniques for extended storage of orthotopic liver homografts. Surg Gynecol Obstet 1968;126:263-274.
11. Calne RY, White HJO, Yoffa DE, et al: Prolonged survival of liver transplants in the pig. BMJ 1967;4:645-648.
12. Calne RY, Sells RA, Pena JR, et al: Induction of immunological tolerance by porcine liver allografts. Nature 1969;223:472-474.
13. Calne RY, White DJG, Thiru S, et al: Cyclosporin A in patients receiving renal allografts from cadaver donors. Lancet 1978;2:1323-1327.
14. Calne RY, Rolles K, White DJG, et al: Cyclosporin A initially as the only immunosuppressant in 34 recipients of cadaveric organs; 32 kidneys, 2 pancreases, and 2 livers. Lancet 1979;2:1033-1036.
15. Collins GM, Bravo-Shugarman M, Terasaki PI: Kidney preservation for transportation: Initial perfusion and 30 hours ice storage. Lancet 1969;2:1219-1224.
16. Cordier G, Garnier H, Clot JP, et al: La greffe de foie orthotopique chez le porc. Mem Acad Chir (Paris) 1966;92:799-807.
17. Demetris AJ, Qian S, Sun H, et al: Early events in liver allograft rejection. Am J Pathol 1991;138:609-618.
18. Derom F, Barbier F, Ringoir S, et al: Ten-month survival after lung homotransplantation in man. J Thorac Cardiovasc Surg 1971;61:835-846.
19. Ferguson R: For the Transplant Information Share Group (TISG): A multicenter experience with sequential ALG/cyclosporine therapy in renal transplantation. Clin Transpl 1988;2:285.
20. Fung JJ, Todo S, Tzakis A, et al: Conversion of liver allograft recipients from cyclosporine to FK506-based immunosuppression: Benefits and pitfalls. Transplant Proc 1991;23:14-21.
21. Gatti RA, Meuwissen HJ, Allen HD, et al: Immunological reconstitution of sex-linked lymphopenic immunological deficiency. Lancet 1968;2:1366-1369.
22. Hamburger J, Vaysse J, Crosnier J, et al: Transplantation of a kidney between nonmonozygotic twins after irradiation of the receiver: Good function at the fourth month. Presse Med 1959;67:1771-1775.
23. Hamburger J, Vaysse J, Crosnier J, et al: Renal homotransplantation in man after radiation of the recipient. Am J Med 1962;32:854-871.
24. Hoffman B, Sollinger H, Kalayoglu M, Belzer FO: Use of UW solution for kidney transplantation. Transplantation 1988;46:338-339.
25. Inman B, Halloran B, Melk A, et al: Microchimerism in sensitized renal patients. Transplantation 1999;67:1381-1383.
26. Kalayoglu M, Sollinger HW, Stratta RJ, et al: Extended preservation of the liver for clinical transplantation. Lancet 1988;1:617-619.
27. Karrer U, Althage A, Odermatt B, et al: On the key role of secondary lymphoid organs in antiviral immune responses studied in alymphoplastic (aly/aly) and spleenless (Hox11(-)/-) mutant mice. J Exp Med 1997;185:2157-2170.
28. Kissmeyer-Nielsen F, Olsen S, Peterson VP, Fjeldborg O: Hyperacute rejection of kidney allografts, associated with preexisting humoral antibodies against donor cells. Lancet 1966;2:622.
29. Kuss R, Legrain M, Mathe G, et al: Homologous human kidney transplantation: Experience with six patients. Postgrad Med J 1962;38:528-531.
30. Lafferty KJ, Prowse SJ, Simeonovic CJ: Immunobiology of tissue transplantation: A return to the passenger leukocyte concept. Ann Rev Immunol 1983;1:143-173.
31. Lakkis FG, Arakelov A, Konieczny BT, Inoue Y: Immunologic ignorance of vascularized organ transplants in the absence of secondary lymphoid tissue. Nature Med 2000;6:686-688.
32. Larsen CP, Morris PJ, Austyn JM: Migration of dendritic leukocytes from cardiac allografts into host spleens: A novel route for initiation of rejection. J Exp Med 1990;171:307-314.
33. Lillehei RC, Goott B, Miller FA: The physiological response of the small bowel of the dog to ischemia including prolonged in vitro preservation of the bowel with successful replacement and survival. Ann Surg 1959;150:543-560.
34. Lillehei RC, Simmons RL, Najarian JS, et al: Pancreaticoduodenal allotransplantation: Experimental and clinical observations. Ann Surg 1970;172:405-436.

35. Lu L, Rudert WA, Qian S, et al: Growth of donor-derived dendritic cells from the bone marrow of murine liver allograft recipients in response to granulocyte/macrophage colony-stimulating factor. J Exp Med 1995;182:379-387.

36. Main JM, Prehn RT: Successful skin homografts after the administration of high dosage X radiation and homologous bone marrow. J Natl Cancer Inst 1955;15:1023-1029.

37. Marchioro TL, Waddell WR, Starzl TE: Use of extracorporeal cadaver perfusion for preparation of organ homografts. Surg Forum 1963;14:174-176.

38. Matas AJ, Sutherland DER, Najarian JS: The impact of HLA matching on graft survival. Transplantation 1992;54: 568-569.

39. Mathe G, Amiel JL, Schwarzenberg L, et al: Haematopoietic chimera in man after allogeneic (homologous) bone-marrow transplantation. BMJ 1963;2:1633-1635.

40. McCurry K, Iacono A, Zeevi A, et al: Early outcomes in human lung transplantation utilizing thymoglobulin or campath 1H for recipient pretreatment followed by post-transplant tacrolimus near-monotherapy. J Thorac Cardiovasc Surg, 2005;2:528-537.

41. Merkel FK, Jonasson O, Bergan JJ: Procurement of cadaver donor organs: Evisceration technique. Transplant Proc 1972;4:585-589.

42. Merrill JP, Murray JE, Harrison JH, et al: Successful homotransplantation of the kidney between non-identical twins. N Engl J Med 1960;262:1251-1260.

43. Moskophidis D, Lechner F, Pircher H, Zinkernagel RM: Virus persistence in acutely infected immunocompetent mice by exhaustion of antiviral cytotoxic effector T cells. Nature 1993;362:758-761.

44. Murase N, Demetris AJ, Woo J, et al: Lymphocyte traffic and graft-versus-host disease after fully allogeneic small bowel transplantation. Transplant Proc 1991;23:3246-3247.

45. Murase N, Starzl TE, Ye Q, et al: Multilineage hematopoietic reconstitution of supralethally irradiated rats by syngeneic whole organ transplantation: with particular reference to the liver. Transplantation 1996;61:1-4.

46. Murase N, Demetris A, Woo J, et al: Graft versus host disease (GVHD) after BN to LEW compared to LEW to BN rat intestinal transplantation under FK 506. Transplantation 1993;55:1-7.

47. Murase N, Starzl TE, Tanabe M, et al: Variable chimerism, graft versus host disease, and tolerance after different kinds of cell and whole organ transplantation from Lewis to Brown-Norway rats. Transplantation 1995;60:158-171.

48. Murray JE, Merrill JP, Dammin GJ, et al: Study of transplantation immunity after total body irradiation: Clinical and experimental investigation. Surgery 1960;48:272-284.

49. Murray JE, Merrill JP, Harrison JH, et al: Prolonged survival of human-kidney homografts by immunosuppressive drug therapy. N Engl J Med 1963;268:1315-1323.

50. Murray JE, Sheil AGR, Moseley R, et al: Analysis of mechanism of immunosuppressive drugs in renal homotransplantation. Ann Surg 1964;160:449-473.

51. Nemlander A, Soots A, von Willebrand E, et al: Redistribution of renal allograft-responding leukocytes during rejection: II. Kinetics and specificity. J Exp Med 1982;156:1087-1100.

52. Peacock JH, Terblanche J: Orthotopic homotransplantation of the liver in the pig. In Read AE (ed): The Liver. London, Butterworth, 1967, p 333.

53. Phelps CJ, Koike C, Vaught TD, et al: Production of α1,3-galactosyltransferase-deficient pigs. Science 2003;299: 411-414.

54. Pierce JC, Varco RL: Induction of tolerance to a canine renal homotransplant with 6-mercaptopurine. Lancet 1962;1:781-782.

55. Przepiorka D, Thomas ED, Durham DM, Fisher L: Use of a probe to repeat sequence of the Y chromosome for detection of host cells in peripheral blood of bone marrow transplant recipients. Am J Clin Pathol 1991;95:201-206.

56. Sakamoto T, Ye Q, Lu L, et al: Donor hematopoietic progenitor cells in non-myeloablated rat recipients of allogeneic bone marrow and liver grafts. Transplantation 1999; 67:833-840.

57. Owens JC, Prevedel AE, Swan H: Prolonged experimental occlusion of thoracic aorta during hypothermia. Arch Surg 1955;70:95-97.

58. Salvatierra O Jr: Optimal use of organs for transplantation. N Engl J Med 1988;318:1329-1331.

59. Shapiro R, Jordan M, Basu A, et al: Kidney transplantation under a tolerogenic regimen of recipient pre-treatment and low-dose postoperative immunosuppression, with subsequent weaning. Ann Surg 2003;238:520-527.

60. Sicular A, Moore FD: The postmortem survival of tissues. J Surg Res 1961;1:16.

61. SivaSai KS, Jendrisak M, Duffy BF, et al: Chimerism in peripheral blood of sensitized patients waiting for renal transplantation: Clinical implications. Transplantation 2000;69:538-544.

62. Starzl TE, Kaupp HA Jr, Brock DR, et al: Reconstructive problems in canine liver homotransplantation with special reference to the postoperative role of hepatic venous flow. Surg Gynecol Obstet 1960;111:733-743.

63. Starzl TE, Brittain RS, Stonnington OG, et al: Renal transplantation in identical twins. Arch Surg 1963;86:600-607.

64. Starzl TE, Marchioro TL, Waddell WR: The reversal of rejection in human renal homografts with subsequent development of homograft tolerance. Surg Gynecol Obstet 1963;117:385-395.

65. Starzl TE: Experience in Renal Transplantation. Philadelphia, WB Saunders, 1964.

66. Starzl TE: Host-graft adaptation. In Starzl TE: Experience in Renal Transplantation. Philadelphia, WB Saunders, 1964, pp 164-170.

67. Starzl TE: Donor nephrectomy. In Starzl TE: Experience in Renal Transplantation. Philadelphia, WB Saunders, 1964, pp 68-82.

68. Starzl TE: The role of cadaveric donors in homotransplantation. In Starzl TE: Experience in Renal Transplantation. Philadelphia, WB Saunders, 1964, pp 54-58.

69. Starzl TE: Patterns of permissible donor-recipient tissue transfer in relation to ABO blood groups. In Starzl TE: Experience in Renal Transplantation. Philadelphia, WB Saunders, 1964, pp 37-46.

70. Starzl TE, Marchioro TL, Porter KA, et al: The use of heterologous antilymphoid agents in canine renal and liver homotransplantation and in human renal homotransplantation. Surg Gynecol Obstet 1967;124:301-318.

71. Starzl TE, Porter KA, Iwasaki Y, et al: The use of antilymphocyte globulin in human renal homotransplantation. In Wolstenholme GEW, O'Connor M (eds): Antilymphocytic Serum. London, J & A Churchill, 1967, pp 4-34.

72. Starzl TE, Groth CG, Brettschneider L, et al: Orthotopic homotransplantation of the human liver. Ann Surg 1968; 168:392-415.

73. Starzl TE, Lerner RA, Dixon FJ, et al: Shwartzman reaction after human renal transplantation. N Engl J Med 1968;278: 642-648.

74. Starzl TE: Rejection in unmodified animals. In Starzl TE: Experience in Renal Transplantation. Philadelphia, WB Saunders, 1964, p 184.

75. Starzl TE, Porter KA, Andres G, et al: Long-term survival after renal transplantation in humans: With special reference to histocompatibility matching, thymectomy, homograft

glomerulonephritis, heterologous ALG, and recipient malignancy. Ann Surg 1970;172:437-472.

76. Starzl TE, Boehmig HJ, Amemiya H, et al: Clotting changes, including disseminated intravascular coagulation, during rapid renal-homograft rejection. N Engl J Med 1970;283:383-390.

77. Starzl TE, Weil R III, Iwatsuki S, et al: The use of cyclosporin A and prednisone in cadaver kidney transplantation. Surg Gynecol Obstet 1980;151:17-26.

78. Starzl TE, Klintmalm GBG, Porter KA, et al: Liver transplantation with use of cyclosporin A and prednisone. N Engl J Med 1981;305:266-269.

79. Starzl TE, Hakala TR, Shaw BW Jr, et al: A flexible procedure for multiple cadaveric organ procurement. Surg Gynecol Obstet 1984;158:223-230.

80. Starzl TE, Miller C, Broznick B, Makowka L: An improved technique for multiple organ harvesting. Surg Gynecol Obstet 1987;165:343-348.

81. Starzl TE, Todo S, Fung J, et al: FK 506 for human liver, kidney and pancreas transplantation. Lancet 1989;2:1000-1004.

82. Starzl TE, Fung J, Jordan M, et al: Kidney transplantation under FK 506. JAMA 1990;264:63-67.

83. Starzl TE, Demetris AJ, Murase N, et al: Cell migration, chimerism, and graft acceptance. Lancet 1992;339:1579-1582.

84. Starzl TE, Demetris AJ, Trucco M, et al: Systemic chimerism in human female recipients of male livers. Lancet 1992;340:876-877.

85. Starzl TE, Demetris AJ, Trucco M, et al: Cell migration and chimerism after whole-organ transplantation: The basis of graft acceptance. Hepatology 1993;17:1127-1152.

86. Starzl TE, Demetris AJ, Trucco M, et al: Chimerism after liver transplantation for type IV glycogen storage disease and type I Gaucher's disease. N Engl J Med 1993;328:745-749.

87. Starzl TE, Demetris AJ, Trucco M, et al: Chimerism and donor-specific nonreactivity 27 to 29 years after kidney allotransplantation. Transplantation 1993;55:1272-1277.

88. Starzl TE, Eliasziw M, Gjertson M, et al: HLA and cross reactive antigen group (CREG) matching for cadaver kidney allocation. Transplantation 1997;64:983-991.

89. Starzl TE, Zinkernagel R: Antigen localization and migration in immunity and tolerance. N Engl J Med 1998;339:1905-1913.

90. Starzl TE, Zinkernagel R: Transplantation tolerance from a historical perspective. Nature Rev Immunol 2001;1:233-239.

91. Starzl TE, Murase N, Abu-Elmagd K, et al: Tolerogenic immunosuppression for organ transplantation. Lancet 2003;361:1502-1510.

92. Starzl TE, Murase N, Demetris AJ, et al: Lessons of organ-induced tolerance learned from historical clinical experience. Transplantation 2004;77:926-929.

93. Takemoto S Terasaki PI, Cecka JM, et al: Survival of nationally shared HLA-matched kidney transplants from cadaveric donors. N Engl J Med 1992;327:834-839.

94. Taniguchi H, Toyoshima T, Fukao K, Nakauchi H: Presence of hematopoietic stem cells in the adult liver. Nat Med 1996;2:198-203.

95. Terakura M, Murase N, Demetris AJ, et al: Lymphoid/non-lymphoid compartmentalization of donor leukocyte chimerism in rat recipients of heart allografts, with or without adjunct bone marrow. Transplantation 1998;66: 350-357.

96. Terasaki PI, Marchioro TL, Starzl TE: Sero-typing of human lymphocyte antigens: Preliminary trials on long-term kidney homograft survivors. In Russel PS, Winn HJ, Amos DB (eds): Histocompatibility Testing. Washington, DC, National Academy of Science—National Research Council, 1965.

97. Terasaki PI, Vredevoe DL, Mickey MR, et al: Serotyping for homotransplantation: VII. Selection of kidney donors for thirty-two recipients. Ann N Y Acad Sci 1966;129:500.

98. Terasaki PI, Cecka JM, Gjertson DW, Takemoto S: High survival rates of kidney transplants from spousal and living unrelated donors. N Engl J Med 1995;333:333-336.

99. Thomas ED, Storb R, Clift RA, et al: Bone marrow transplantation. N Engl J Med 1975;292:832, 895-902 (2 parts).

100. Ting A: The lymphocytotoxic crossmatch test in clinical renal transplantation. Transplantation 1983;35:403-407.

101. Todo S, Nery J, Yanaga K, et al: Extended preservation of human liver grafts with UW solution. JAMA 1989;261:711-714.

102. Todo S, Fung JJ, Starzl TE, et al: Liver, kidney, and thoracic organ transplantation under FK 506. Ann Surg 1990;212:295-305.

103. Todo S, Fung JJ, Starzl TE, et al: Single center experience with primary orthotopic liver transplantation under FK506 immunosuppression. Ann Surg 1994;220:297-309.

104. Todo S, Tzakis A, Reyes J, et al: Small intestinal transplantation in humans with or without colon. Transplantation 1994;57:840-848.

105. Todo S, Reyes J, Furukawa H, et al: Outcome analysis of 71 clinical intestinal transplantations. Ann Surg 1995;222:270-282.

106. Ueda Y, Todo S, Imventarza O, et al: The UW solution for canine kidney preservation: Its specific effect on renal hemodynamics and microvasculature. Transplantation 1989;48:913-918.

107. Wessman M, Popp S, Ruutu T, et al: Detection of residual host cells after bone marrow transplantation using non-isotopic in situ hybridization and karyotype analysis. Bone Marrow Transplant 1993;11:279-284.

108. Williams GM, et al: Studies in hyperacute and chronic renal homograft rejection in man. Surgery 1967;62:204.

109. Zinkernagel RM, Ehl S, Aichele P, et al: Antigen localization regulates immune responses in a dose- and time-dependent fashion: A geographical view of immune reactivity. Immunol Rev 1997;156:199-209.

110. Zinkernagel RM, Hengartner H: Antiviral immunity. Immunol Today 1997;18:258-260.

111. Zinkernagel RM, Bachmann MF, Kundig TM, et al: On immunologic memory. Annu Rev Immunol 1996;14:333-367.

112. Zukoski CF, Callaway JM: Adult tolerance induced by 6-methyl mercaptopurine to canine renal homografts. Nature (London) 1963;198:706-707.

113. Zukoski CF, Callaway JM, Rhea WG Jr: Tolerance to a canine renal homograft induced by prednisolone. Surg Forum 1963;14:208-210.

Chapter 43

Renal Transplantation

John C. Magee and Darrell A. Campbell, Jr.

Transplantation is the preferred treatment option for children with end-stage renal disease (ESRD) because it provides the best opportunity for health, growth, and development. Progress continues in pediatric transplantation, and currently patient and graft survival for pediatric renal recipients is excellent. The improvement in outcomes reflects better pretransplant care, a growing understanding of immunosuppression management in pediatric recipients, improvements in donor selection, and refinements in surgical technique and perioperative management. Several single-center experiences have documented the excellent results possible, even in small children.[34,42,47,57]

Although single-center expertise provides great insight into many issues in transplantation, it is generally agreed that larger registry type data provide the most meaningful reflection of the state of transplantation as practiced across the country. One leading source of such information is the North American Pediatric Renal Transplant Cooperative Study (NAPRTCS), which was initiated in 1987.[6,59,80] Additionally, national data in the United States are collected through the Organ Procurement Transplant Network (OPTN) and regularly analyzed by the Scientific Registry of Transplant Recipients (SRTR).[14,46]

END-STAGE RENAL DISEASE IN CHILDREN

According to the United States Renal Data System (USRDS), 1216 individuals aged 19 or younger began treatment for ESRD in 2002.[96] The incidence of ESRD in this age group is 14.5 per million individuals per year. Because ESRD is much more uncommon in children than adults, this rate is well below the overall national incidence of ESRD of 333 per million per year.

The etiology of renal disease in the pediatric transplant population is summarized in Table 43-1. According to these NAPRTCS data, the five most common diagnoses are obstructive uropathy, renal aplasia/hypoplasia/dysplasia, focal segmental glomerulo sclerosis (FSGS), reflux nephropathy, and chronic glomerulonephritis. These diagnoses account for just over half the transplants performed. The causes of renal failure in children are distinctly different from those in the adult population;

specifically, congenital abnormalities and obstructive uropathy are some of the leading causes for renal transplantation in children. Additionally, FSGS is the most common acquired renal disease and is much more common in the pediatric age range compared with the adult population.

TABLE 43–1 Primary Diagnosis for Renal Transplant Recipients (N = 7939) Age 20 Years and Younger

Disease	%
Obstructive uropathy	16.1
Aplasia/hypoplasia/dysplasia	16.0
Focal segmental glomerulosclerosis	11.4
Reflux nephropathy	5.2
Chronic glomerulonephritis	3.5
Medullary cystic disease	2.8
Hemolytic-uremic syndrome	2.8
Polycystic disease	2.7
Prune belly syndrome	2.6
Congenital nephrotic syndrome	2.5
Familial nephritis	2.3
Cystinosis	2.1
Idiopathic crescentic glomerulonephritis	1.9
Membranoproliferative glomerulonephritis type I	1.9
Pyelo/interstitial nephritis	1.9
Systemic lupus erythematosus nephritis	1.7
Renal infarct	1.5
Henoch-Schönlein nephritis	1.3
Berger's (IgA) nephritis	1.3
Membranoproliferative glomerulonephritis type II	0.9
Wilms' tumor	0.6
Denys-Drash syndrome	0.6
Oxalosis	0.5
Wegener's granulomatosis	0.5
Membranous nephropathy	0.5
Other systemic immunologic disease	0.4
Sickle cell nephropathy	0.2
Diabetic glomerulonephritis	0.1
Other	8.0
Unknown	6.2

From North American Pediatric Renal Transplant Cooperative Study (NAPRTCS) 2004 annual report. Available at www.naprtcs.org.

Within the pediatric population, the prevalence of causes varies by age, sex, and race. Congenital causes are more prevalent in younger children, whereas acquired diseases tend to become manifest in older children. Overall, 60% of the recipients are male, and males represent the majority of the recipients with obstructive uropathy (86%), aplasia/hypoplasia/dysplasia (62%), and FSGS (58%). Reflux nephropathy, chronic glomerulonephritis, and lupus nephritis are more prevalent in female recipients, with females accounting for 55%, 59%, and 81%, respectively. With regard to recipient race, for black children, FSGS was the most prevalent diagnosis (23%), followed by obstructive uropathy (16%), aplasia/hypoplasia/dysplasia (14%), chronic glomerulonephritis (4%), and lupus nephritis (4%). In white recipients, obstructive uropathy was the most prevalent etiology (17%), followed by aplasia/hypoplasia/dysplasia (17%), FSGS (9%), reflux nephropathy (6%), and medullary cystic disease (4%).

RECIPIENT EVALUATION

Any child with ESRD should be considered a candidate for renal transplantation. Absolute contraindications are rare and include untreated malignancy or systemic sepsis. Relative contraindications include severe systemic disease that would severely shorten the patient's lifespan or a social situation that makes follow-up with post-transplant care and immunosuppression regimen absolutely impossible. At times the decision whether to perform a transplant in a given child with a poor quality of life or significant impairment can be extremely difficult for all involved. There is often no readily apparent correct answer. In such situations, a thorough discussion considering what are the expectations and goals for that particular child is helpful.

All children with progressive chronic renal insufficiency should be evaluated by a multidisciplinary pediatric transplant team, including a pediatric nephrologist, a transplant surgeon, social worker, and nutritionist. In addition, many teams include pediatric urologists and clinical psychologists, with other experts included as indicated. It is optimal if a child can be fully evaluated before initiating dialysis. This can facilitate evaluation of any potential living donor and prepare all involved for transplant. Ideally, this early evaluation can allow preemptive transplantation, obviating the need for dialysis. With respect to infant size, renal transplantation can be performed successfully in infants as small as 6.0 kg, although we and others[57] believe 10.0 kg is ideal if this can be accomplished without compromising the health of the child.

Our standard evaluation of process is summarized in Table 43-2. Every effort should be made to optimize the medical management of the child with ESRD, including management of bone disease, optimization of nutrition, and completing childhood immunizations. Several aspects of the evaluation of the pediatric recipient are unique from adult patients and deserve special attention. One is the evaluation and management of bladder function. Many patients will have lower-pole anomalies and may or may not have a bladder suitable for transplantation. Many children will have also undergone previous urologic procedures. Expertise in such issues, or a close working

TABLE 43-2 Evaluation of Pediatric Kidney Transplant Candidate
History and physical examination
Laboratory tests:
Hematologic (complete blood cell count with platelets; prothrombin time/partial thromboplastin time)
Biochemistry (renal function, electrolytes, liver function)
Serologic studies (hepatitis B and C, herpesvirus, cytomegalovirus, Epstein-Barr virus, varicella-zoster, human immunodeficiency virus)
ABO blood typing
Tissue typing (human leukocyte antigen typing; alloantibody screening)
Urinalysis
Chest radiograph
Electrocardiogram
Psychosocial assessment
As needed evaluations:
Voiding cystourethrogram
Vascular imaging

collaboration with pediatric urology, is essential. Nutrition is also of paramount importance in the pediatric population to optimize growth and development. Finally, it is important to evaluate and optimize issues related to the psychologic state of the child and caregivers. Adequate social support is vital for all involved. The stress of a chronically ill child undergoing a complex procedure places a great strain on all, and the need for ongoing education and reassurance is significant. In older children it is important to ensure they are actively involved in the process. Issues in the adolescent population can be particularly challenging, because the risk of noncompliance is held to be greatest in this group, both before and after transplantation.

In addition to these factors, several other issues require special attention. One is the potential need to evaluate the patient's vasculature. As renal replacement therapy has improved, it is now possible to hemodialyze smaller and smaller children, including neonates. Unfortunately, these therapies require the use of indwelling catheters, which has been linked to increased rates of iliac vein and vena cava thrombosis. The lack of adequate venous outflow can make transplantation difficult and limit the standard surgical options. Thomas and coworkers summarized their experience with these venous thromboses and suggested a screening algorithm utilizing radiographic imaging for patients at risk, focusing on young children with a history of femoral vein catheterization or history of any intra-abdominal process associated with inflammation.[92]

The potential need for native nephrectomy is often an issue addressed during the evaluation process. Native nephrectomy is much more common in the pediatric population compared with the adult transplant population. Nationally, 23% of pediatric recipients have had all native renal tissue removed before transplantation.[72] Potential indications for native nephrectomy include recurrent severe infections due to reflux nephropathy, uncontrolled hypertension, and congenital nephrotic syndrome. The indication for patients with nephrotic syndrome arises from the fact that frequently these children are prothrombotic due to the significant proteinuria. Children with polycystic kidney disease may require native nephrectomies owing to issues related to bleeding, recurrent infections, or pain. Occasionally, native nephrectomy can be warranted if the native kidneys are so enlarged that the transplanted kidney would be compromised. Some contend that massive polyuria in small infants is an indication for nephrectomy, arguing that postoperative fluid management is made easier, thus decreasing the risk of graft hypoperfusion. Although this has appeal on a superficial level, careful attention to postoperative management can often avoid this as the sole indication for nephrectomy. Additionally, there are those who believe that children with FSGS should undergo native nephrectomy, suggesting it simplifies the diagnosis of recurrent disease, because any proteinuria reflects disease in the graft rather than persistent proteinuria from the native kidneys. In such situations, an initial attempt at "medical nephrectomy" with nonsteroidal therapy is worth consideration.

In addition to a rational consideration of the indications for native nephrectomy, the timing of the nephrectomy is important. In children already on renal replacement therapy, if bilateral native nephrectomies are indicated, it may be safer and easier to accomplish this weeks before transplantation. In children not on renal replacement therapy, the issue is more complex. We prefer not to perform bilateral nephrectomies at the time of transplantation because this is a major procedure to combine with renal transplantation. Additionally, even in small infants, we perform the transplant via a retroperitoneal approach, which does not provide access to the contralateral native kidney. For children requiring bilateral native nephrectomy, and who are not yet on renal replacement therapy, many will have sufficient renal reserve to tolerate a unilateral left nephrectomy before transplantation and still not require dialysis. In this situation, at the time of the transplantation procedure we proceed with a standard retroperitoneal incision and extend the incision slightly cephalad, allowing us to perform a right native nephrectomy. In cases where unilateral native nephrectomy would require initiation of renal replacement therapy before transplantation, we have typically removed the ipsilateral native kidney at the time of the transplant procedure. The remaining contralateral native kidney can be removed several months after transplantation if still indicated.

In considering when to perform the transplant, any child currently on renal replacement therapy should undergo transplantation as soon as a suitable living donor is identified or a deceased donor organ becomes available. In children not yet on dialysis, transplantation should be done before the onset of symptoms of uremia. It is important to be aware of the impact of ESRD on growth and development. In patients with FSGS or lupus nephritis, transplantation is typically delayed until the disease is quiescent, which may preclude preemptive transplantation. In most other situations, preemptive transplantation allows the children to avoid the need for dialysis with no real disadvantage.[24] Unfortunately, at present only 33% of children who receive a living donor transplant receive preemptive transplant and only 13% of deceased donor recipients are transplanted before initiation of dialysis.[6]

UROLOGIC ISSUES

The high incidence of urologic issues in the pediatric ESRD population requires careful evaluation of bladder function before transplantation. In addition to dysplasia and bladder outlet obstruction, bladder function may be abnormal due to neuropathy, acquired voiding dysfunction, or acquired bladder pathology. Any previous surgical bladder augmentation will impair normal bladder function. A history of urinary incontinence, frequent urinary tract infections, previous urologic procedures, and the need for bladder catheterization should prompt further investigation. In patients with suspected bladder dysfunction, a voiding cystourethrogram (VCUG) should be obtained with urodynamic measurements. A pressure of less than 30 cm H_2O during the filling portion of the VCUG generally indicates the bladder will be suitable.

The timing of any surgical intervention warrants careful consideration. In some patients with anuria/oliguria, the bladder may not be functional, although it is often too early to tell if it will eventually become suitable. Once bladder augmentation is performed, the patient will need to continue catheterizing long term because the bladder will not be functional. Urologic procedures that preserve native renal function for many years are clearly prudent, but interventions before transplantation should be planned by carefully considering the risks and benefits of the procedure and being mindful of the impact on subsequent transplantation and the long-term management.

DIALYSIS ACCESS

For children who do not undergo preemptive transplantation or who initially present with ESRD, establishment of adequate dialysis access is of paramount importance. Proper dialysis access is necessary for adequate dialysis, which is directly linked to the quality of life and health of the patient. Both hemodialysis and peritoneal dialysis are suitable options. According to USRDS data, at the end of 2002, 61% of patients aged 19 years and younger were on hemodialysis, whereas 39% were on peritoneal dialysis.[96] The choice of hemodialysis or peritoneal dialysis is best made on an individual basis, considering the patient and family's preferences and skill levels, as well as the treatment options available at the local site.

With respect to hemodialysis, all attempts should be made to create a primary arterial venous fistula. For patients without adequate veins, a polytetra fluoroethylene graft is required. A native fistula is clearly preferred because of superior patency rates, although this option does require the presence of suitable veins. Additionally, a native fistula requires several weeks to mature following the procedure before it can be accessed. For patients in need of urgent hemodialysis with no access, the only option is a temporary catheter. Approximately three fourths of all pediatric patients have a temporary catheter as their access at time of initiation of dialysis.[61] The use of these catheters is associated with increased risks of infection and poor clearance with dialysis. Additionally, these catheters can lead to central venous stenosis and thrombosis, which can make future permanent upper extremity vascular access more difficult to achieve. Accordingly, the jugular vein is preferred over the subclavian vein for catheter placement.

Peritoneal dialysis is performed after placement of a Tenckhoff catheter. A double-cuffed peritoneal dialysis catheter is inserted via an open surgical procedure under general anesthesia. The loop of the catheter is placed in the pelvis. During the procedure it is important to ascertain that fluid can run freely through the catheter into the abdomen and drain freely as well. The use of double-cuffed catheters and orienting the catheter so that the exit site is oriented with the catheter pointing downward are associated with a lower incidence of infection.[61]

DONOR SELECTION

Living donor transplantation is the preferred option for all patients with ESRD. Living donor transplantation offers the best outcomes after transplantation, compared with deceased donor transplantation. In addition, living donor transplantation can be performed as soon as a suitable donor is identified, avoiding the need for waiting on the transplant list for a deceased donor. Living donors may be either genetically related or unrelated to the potential recipient. The results from both types of living donors are equivalent, and both are superior to outcomes from deceased donors. Although there is no need for the living donor to be genetically related, nearly all donors share a significant relationship with the intended recipient. Potential living donors should undergo a full evaluation by a transplant center experienced in this process. The donor must be willing, be in good health, and have two normal kidneys. In addition, the donor and recipient must be ABO compatible. Although there is a growing interest in strategies to cross this barrier, such efforts are still in their early stages and the experience in the pediatric population is limited.[66,83] In addition, the recipient should have a negative lymphocytotoxic crossmatch with the potential donor. Crossmatching is done to determine that the recipient does not have preformed antibodies directed against the recipient's human leukocyte antigens (HLA), which would likely cause hyperacute rejection and rapid graft loss. The onset of this process is immediate and nearly impossible to reverse. Strategies to manipulate anti–donor antibody activity are being investigated and include intravenous immunoglobulin and plasmapheresis. The most common causes of anti-HLA antibodies in the recipient are blood transfusions, previous transplantation, and pregnancy.

Evaluation of the Potential Living Donor

Evaluation of potential living kidney donors should proceed independent of the recipient's evaluation, placing donor safety as the highest priority. Our standard evaluation of process is summarized in Table 43-3. Although HLA matching has traditionally played an important role in choosing which living donor to evaluate, current immunosuppression has minimized the impact of matching, and we believe the best potential living donor is the

TABLE 43-3 Evaluation of Living Kidney Donor

History and physical examination
Laboratory tests:
    Hematologic (complete blood cell count with platelets; prothrombin time/partial thromboplastin time)
    Biochemistry (renal function, electrolytes, liver function)
    Serologic studies (hepatitis B and C, herpesvirus, cytomegalovirus, Epstein-Barr virus, human immunodeficiency virus)
    ABO blood typing
    Tissue typing (human leukocyte antigen typing)
Urinalysis
Chest radiograph
Electrocardiogram
Psychosocial assessment
Helical CT scan

individual who is most motivated. Lacking that distinction, and all else equal, we would choose the donor with the best HLA match. It is also important to consider other issues unique to each donor, including psychosocial concerns such as the need to care for other children, the need to care for the recipient, and what options would be least disruptive to the family unit. When discussing the situation with the family, it is important to consider other siblings who may also need renal transplantation in the future because this can play a role in deciding which donor donates to which recipient. The use of live donors younger than 18 years of age is very rare, and this practice is not encouraged.[16,44]

Living kidney donation appears to be safe and has now been in practice for 50 years. The risk of operative mortality appears to be 3 in 10,000.[50] After the procedure, living kidney donors appear to do well over the long term as well. The introduction of laparoscopic donor nephrectomy has been a significant step forward for the individuals who consider kidney donation. The laparoscopic procedure is associated with quicker recovery and appears as safe as open donor nephrectomy.[93,100] Although there was some concern that laparoscopic donation might result in inferior outcomes compared with open donor nephrectomy, particularly in small infants, this concern has not been substantiated at centers that have examined this issue.[41,95] Regardless of the approach utilized, however, the surgical team performing the donor nephrectomy should be experts at that approach.

Evaluation of the Deceased Donor

For children who do not have a suitable living donor, deceased donor transplantation is the only option. Deceased donors can be individuals who have either suffered brain death or whose heart has irreversibly stopped beating. The latter group has often been referred to as "non-heartbeating donors." In the United States, organ allocation is governed by policies established by the OPTN. These policies undergo constant refinement as data support more rational and fair allocation strategies. At present, deceased donor kidneys are allocated both on a national and a local level. After a potential deceased donor is identified, the blood type, HLA type, and other relevant donor factors are entered into the national database maintained by the United Network for Organ Sharing (UNOS). If an ABO-compatible, HLA-identical recipient is identified, that individual would be offered this kidney. These zero antigen mismatch kidneys are shared on a national level. Although there is some benefit to this strategy, such an approach is also often associated with an increase in the cold ischemic time owing to the need to transport the kidney to the recipient's center. In cases in which no zero antigen mismatch recipient is identified, the kidneys are usually transplanted locally. Allocation of these kidneys is guided by a point system that factors in the degree of the HLA match at the DR locus and recipient waiting time. Additional points are given to recipients with a high level of anti-HLA antibodies because these individuals face considerable difficulty in finding a suitable kidney donor. Based on data that pediatric patients do poorly while on dialysis, the allocation strategy was adjusted to give additional points to pediatric patients based on their age. Further priority with respect to allocation is given to pediatric candidates who have not been transplanted within age-specific time goals after listing: candidates birth to 5 years old listed for 6 months; candidates 6 to 10 years old listed for 12 months; and candidates 11 to 17 years old listed for 18 months. In total, these allocation policies result in pediatric candidates waiting for shorter times on transplant lists than adult candidates. Nonetheless, many children wait longer than intended. In late 2004, a further revision to the allocation policy was adopted whereby kidneys from all deceased donors younger than 35 years of age will be preferentially offered to pediatric candidates.

The overall number of deceased donors each year has remained relatively stable. The criteria for donor acceptability, however, have expanded. Donors are now much older than those previously utilized, and a significant percentage of donors have a history of hypertension or other medical comorbidities, which may impact the quality of the organs donated. In attempts to improve utilization of kidney donors in the higher risk groups, a subset of such donors have been defined as extended criteria donors (ECD), and the kidneys are allocated based on principles designed to facilitate utilization of such organs.[55,69] The ECD criteria include any deceased donor older than the age of 60 years or older than the age of 50 years with two of the following: a history of hypertension, a terminal pre-donation serum creatinine value greater than or equal to 1.5 mg/dL, or death resulting from a cerebrovascular accident (stroke). The relative risk of graft failure for such kidneys is greater than 1.7 times the risk of a reference group of ideal deceased donors. Whereas accepting ECD kidneys will benefit many adult transplant candidates, the allocation priorities already provided to pediatric candidates obviate the need for utilizing such kidneys in children. Consequently, most children should not be listed for ECD kidneys.

Driven by the severe shortage of donor organs, interest in Donation after Cardiac Death (DCD) has had a resurgence. DCD, formerly known as "non-heartbeating organ donation," has the potential to significantly increase the number of available organs. Patients meeting the strict criteria for brain death make up a relatively small fraction of all patients who die in hospitals. Most patients who die never progress to brain death before cardiac arrest. Patients who sustain a severe and unrecoverable neurologic injury but do not meet the criteria for brain death may be eligible for organ donation if a determination to withdraw intensive care unit (ICU) support is made jointly by the legal next-of-kin and the physicians caring for the patient. DCD is an option that can allow such patients and their families to pursue organ donation. DCD accounted for only 3.3% of all deceased donor kidneys transplanted in 2002, a slight increase from 1.2% in 1994.[67] Although the initial results using DCD kidneys have been good, there is often a higher risk of delayed graft function.[12,15]

In considering which organ to accept for a given pediatric recipient, the transplant surgeon must balance the desire to obtain the "perfect kidney" (e.g., quality of the donor, degree of HLA matching) with the benefit of rendering the patient free of dialysis. Refinements in organ allocation have made this process more straightforward. The pediatric recipient will, hopefully, require many years of function from the graft and, consequently, this limits enthusiasm for accepting older or marginal donors. Generally, ECD or DCD donors should not be used in the pediatric population. Additionally, the use of kidneys from smaller pediatric deceased donors is associated with poorer outcomes and kidneys from such donors are rarely appropriate for pediatric candidates. An important exception might be the highly sensitized recipient who has waited for a long period of time and has had no suitable offers. In such a situation, the decision needs to be made on a case-by-case basis, weighing the various risks and benefits of the options available.

TRANSPLANTATION

Preoperative Preparation

Deceased donor transplant recipients are admitted to the hospital once a suitable kidney is accepted. We currently still admit our pediatric living donor recipients, although these patients could be potentially admitted on the day of their procedure if their dialysis regimen was stable or if they were not on dialysis. On admission, the need for a dialysis is assessed. It is also important to ask about any intervening health issues since the patient's last office visit, as well as examining for any evidence of ongoing infection.

Anesthesia

Close coordination with the anesthesia team is vital to the conduct of any operation, although this is particularly important in kidney transplantation in small infants. Maintaining adequate volume status is critical. Because a kidney from an adult donor is typically used, blood flow to the graft often equals the entire cardiac output in the recipient, and thus hypotension can be particularly problematic. Many children have an obligate polyuria that can cause hypovolemia if not carefully monitored. After reperfusion, the new kidney can also sequester several hundred milliliters of blood, further aggravating hypovolemia.

Operative Procedure

The child is taken to the operating room and general anesthesia induced. Adequate intravenous access is established. In children larger than 20.0 kg we typically do not place a central venous line if adequate peripheral access can be established. For smaller children we find central venous access useful, both for fluid administration as well as for monitoring central venous pressure. In these smaller children we also place an arterial line as well to permit constant blood pressure monitoring. The child is placed in the supine position and a Foley catheter is inserted into the bladder. We connect the urinary catheter to a three-way irrigation system using dilute povidone-iodine (Betadine) in saline. In other centers an antibiotic solution may be preferred. This arrangement allows the bladder to be filled and drained outside of the operative field as necessary. The abdomen is then prepped and draped. The child's temperature should be monitored closely, especially with small children who may become hypothermic with either fluid resuscitation or the perfusion of the cold kidney. The operating room temperature should be maintained and warming blankets used. In addition to routine anesthetic monitoring, a constant focus of attention must be the volume status of the recipient. It is vital that the arterial blood pressure and central venous pressure are adequate when the kidney is reperfused. For infants and small children, the central venous pressure is usually maintained in the range of 12.0 to 18.0 cm H_2O by administration of either crystalloid and/or colloid as necessary. Near completion of the vascular anastomoses, we typically give 0.5 mg/kg of mannitol intravenously. We do not routinely employ a loop diuretic.

Operative Techniques

Small Children (<20.0 kg)

In years past many have performed kidney transplants intra-abdominally in infants and small children via a midline incision. Since 1998 we have used a retroperitoneal approach similar to that used in adults. In small children, placing the kidney on the right side is preferable, because this gives the easiest access to the vena cava. A curvilinear skin incision is made in the right lower quadrant. The abdominal wall musculature is divided, and the preperitoneal space is entered. Attempts are made to stay outside the peritoneum during the course of the dissection. We use a fixed retractor for exposure. The spermatic cord is mobilized and preserved in males, whereas the round ligament is routinely divided in females. The dissection is carried medially until the common iliac vessels, the distal aorta, and vena cava are visualized. If a native nephrectomy is necessary on the right side, this can be performed at this point as well, tracing the ureter up to the kidney.

The exact site of the vascular anastomosis depends on the size of the kidney as well as the size of the child. Generally in small children the renal vein is anastomosed to the vena cava and the renal artery is anastomosed to either the distal aorta or the common iliac artery. The lymphatics overlying these vessels are divided between silk ties to hopefully minimize the risk of a lymphocele developing postoperatively. When an aortic anastomosis is planned, it is mobilized from below the inferior mesenteric artery to the bifurcation. Lumbar branches are controlled with Pott's ties rather than ligated. In the case of an aortic anastomosis, both the right and left common iliac arteries are controlled just distal to the aortic bifurcation. The vena cava is mobilized to allow placement of a side-biting vascular clamp, which can require ligation of some lumbar veins. Vessel loops are frequently used to help gently control the vessels during the dissection. Once the recipient's vessels have been exposed, the donor kidney is brought into the operative field. The kidney should be inspected for any evidence of unsuspected pathology, and the renal vessels are examined. After preparing the kidney, thoughtful consideration needs to be given for the fit of the kidney in the recipient's body cavity. Particular attention needs to be focused on the length of the renal vessels as well as their orientation. It is important to consider the final resting position of the kidney after it is perfused, the retractor is removed, and the wound closed.

The venous anastomosis is performed first. The vena cava or iliac vein is controlled with a side-biting clamp. A longitudinal venotomy is made along the anterolateral or lateral aspect of the vein. The renal vein is cut to length, again after considering the lie of the kidney, and mindful that a redundant renal vein may predispose to thrombosis. We place and tie two corner sutures of 5-0 Prolene. The anastomosis is then performed in a running manner, making sure it is widely patent. An end-to-side arterial anastomosis is then performed, between the donor artery and the recipient's distal aorta or common iliac artery. The recipient vessels are controlled using gentle spring clips or occasionally a small vascular clamp. A longitudinal arteriotomy is made, mindful of the final orientation of the renal artery. We enlarge the arteriotomy using a 4.0 mm aortic punch. The renal artery is then sewn end-to-side using a running 6-0 Prolene suture. We typically perform the procedure with loupe magnification, which allows for more precise suture placement.

If two renal arteries are present, they can either be implanted separately or they can be syndactylized before reimplantation. When the vessels are syndactylized, it is important to consider if this will allow the vessels to lie in good position at the end of the procedure, since syndactylization will fix both vessels relatively firmly in two dimensions. This can limit the options of where the anastomosis can be suitably performed or lead to kinking of one or both of the donor arteries if the final resting position of the kidney is not properly anticipated.

Before completion of the arterial anastomosis it is worthwhile to discuss the hemodynamic state of the patient with the anesthesia team. Intraoperative assessment of the vascular volume by direct assessment of the vena cava is possible. Mannitol is also given at this time. Because of the size of the adult kidney volume, and given the normal pediatric blood volume, the kidney can be both slow to perfuse as well as sequester a significant volume of blood. The anesthesiologist must be ready to give volume replacement promptly as indicated. At this point the clamp is removed from the vein and any bleeding assessed. Next, during gentle occlusion of the renal artery with vascular pickups, the clamps are removed from the recipient's vessel, restoring distal blood flow. After a few seconds, flow is established to the kidney. In small children we occasionally will briefly re-clamp the recipient's vessels distal to the arterial anastomosis to provide preferential blood flow to the kidney. The operative field is carefully examined for any bleeding sites that should be controlled. The color and turgor of the graft are assessed. The renal artery should have a good pulse, and a thrill can usually be appreciated as well. Both the lower and upper poles should be assessed for perfusion. The renal vein should be full but not tense, with a turgor similar to the vena cava. The lie of the kidney is again examined.

Attention is then directed to performance of the ureteroneocystostomy. We generally perform the ureteral anastomosis as an extravesical ureteroneocystostomy,[47,64] although others prefer the transvesical Politano-Leadbetter approach.[42,57] The Foley catheter is clamped, and the bladder is filled. A site on the dome of the bladder is selected where the ureter will sit without any angulation. The muscle coat of the bladder is divided, exposing the bladder mucosa. An opening is then made in the mucosa. The donor ureter should be trimmed to length. Care should be taken to make sure it is sufficient to allow a tension-free anastomosis to the bladder, but excessive length should be minimized because of the risk of ureteral obstruction or stricture due to inadequate perfusion of the distal ureter. The end of the ureter is spatulated, and a mucosa to mucosa anastomosis is performed using running 5-0 PDS suture. Running suture is adequate in this situation, but great care must be taken to avoid cinching on the suture when the knot is tied because this results in a pursestring effect causing stenosis of the anastomosis. To prevent vesicoureteral reflux, the bladder muscle wall is approximated over the ureteral anastomosis using the interrupted 4-0 PDS suture. This allows the ureter to take a tangential course under the bladder wall so that during micturition, the transvesical portion of the ureter is compressed by the overlying bladder wall. In patients with a normal bladder and a good blood supply to the distal ureter, we do not routinely place a stent. If there is any concern regarding the ureteral anastomosis, either due to the donor ureter or the quality of the recipient's bladder, we place a double-J ureteral stent. The stent can be removed several weeks after transplantation as an outpatient procedure.

After completing the ureteral anastomosis, the kidney is again inspected with attention to the renal vessels and the lie of the kidney once the retractor is removed. Careful planning and attention to detail before performing the anastomosis is usually well rewarded at this point.

The retractor is removed, and the fascia is closed in one or two layers with a running suture. The skin is closed using a running absorbable suture. The urinary catheter is flushed with saline to remove any clots that might obstruct the catheter, and the catheter is then connected to a urimeter. For small infants, the volume resuscitation required to ensure excellent renal perfusion, combined with the size of the kidney contributing to a decrease in respiratory excursion, may make ventilatory support in the immediate postoperative period necessary. If the patient's oxygen saturation and pulmonary mechanics are satisfactory, the patient can be extubated in the operating room.

Larger Children (>20.0 kg)

The technique for renal transplantation in larger children is similar to that in the adults. We prefer to put the kidney on the right side when possible. An incision is made in the right lower quadrant, extending up from a fingerbreadth or two above the pubis to just lateral of the rectus sheath. The preperitoneal space is again developed, and the iliac vessels are mobilized. Again we divide the lymphatics over these vessels between silk ties in hopes of minimizing the risk of postoperative development of lymphocele. As in smaller children, the placement of the arterial and venous anastomoses depends on the size of the child and the renal vessels. The venous anastomosis can be done to the vena cava, the common iliac, or the external iliac vein. The arterial anastomosis is performed to the distal aorta, the common iliac, or the external iliac artery. We have not used the internal iliac artery for well over a decade. After revascularizing the kidney, the ureteroneocystostomy is performed using an extravesicular technique. At the completion of the operation these larger children are extubated.

Ureteral Reconstruction in Patients with Previous Urologic Procedures

The ideal urinary reservoir stores a reasonable volume at a low pressure, does not leak, and empties nearly completely with voiding.[24] In the majority of cases, the ideal reservoir is the patient's bladder. If the bladder functioned normally before development of oliguria, it is likely to function adequately after transplantation. Nonetheless, up to 30% of pediatric recipients will not have normal bladder function, and frequently a surgical augmentation or other urologic procedure has been performed before referral for transplantation.

Drainage of transplanted kidneys into an augmented bladder or urinary conduit is an appropriate management strategy when the native bladder is unsuitable or absent.[10,26] When indicated, we prefer to have the intended urinary reservoir created and suitable for use before the transplant procedure. Intraoperatively, when planning the ureteroneocystostomy to an augmented bladder, it is important to consider the blood supply to the augmented section so as not to compromise it during the transplant. It is preferable to perform the ureteroneocystostomy to the native bladder, and this can be accomplished in most situations. We strongly believe that an antireflux ureteroneocystostomy is mandatory for all patients, and it is most readily performed when the bladder wall is used.

Patients with kidney transplants drained into an augmented bladder or urinary conduit are at increased risk for urine infection, but compared with historical controls, graft survival is not adversely affected.[32] The rate of surgical complications related to the ureteral anastomosis is higher in these patients, approximately 20%.[25,32,43] Regardless of the etiology of the bladder dysfunction, such patients require regular clean intermittent straight catheterization after transplantation.

Children with obstructive uropathy from posterior urethral valves will not have normal bladder function, and this can contribute to renal dysfunction after transplantation.[26] Awareness of these issues is vital, and evaluation with follow-up urodynamic studies is frequently indicated in children with voiding disorders. Bladder dysfunction, such as hypocompliance and/or hyperreflexia, requires medical or surgical treatment.[76]

POSTOPERATIVE CARE

Careful attention to detail in the postoperative period is essential. Special care must be directed to the fluid and electrolyte status. Many children are polyuric before transplant, and this obligate urine loss will continue in the immediate postoperative period. Intravenous fluids are administered, taking into account urine output as well as insensible losses. The composition of these solutions is adjusted as needed, depending on regular measurement of serum electrolytes. Serum sodium, potassium, and calcium levels are followed closely and replaced as necessary. Heart rate, blood pressure, and central venous pressure are carefully monitored. No single factor alone is entirely reliable in assessing intravascular volume, and some readings may not reflect the true status of the patient.

For patients who were oliguric or who had native nephrectomies before transplantation, if the graft functions immediately, monitoring urine output is an excellent measurement of graft function. For patients who made significant urine before transplantation, or who have delayed graft function, evaluation of graft function is more difficult. In situations in which the patient made urine before transplantation, the volume of urine production is often suggestive of graft function. In addition, the serum creatinine concentration should fall over time. Recipients with oliguria should be carefully evaluated. The urinary catheter should be flushed with small volumes of sterile saline. The volume status of the patient should be carefully assessed. A fluid bolus is usually warranted, both as a diagnostic test and as therapeutic intervention. An ultrasound with Doppler study will be helpful at confirming adequate arterial flow to the graft and adequate venous outflow. In addition, the ultrasound will show if there is any evidence of fluid or blood around the kidney, as well as assess for possible ureteral obstruction. In patients who appear to be adequately volume loaded and hemodynamically stable, a dose of diuretic can be given to monitor response. It is important to do this carefully because sudden massive urine output can

cause significant intravascular volume depletion, which can then lead to problems with renal perfusion. In situations in which the patient is massively volume overloaded or has significant electrolyte abnormalities, dialysis may be indicated.

If ventilated postoperatively, the smaller children are weaned from the ventilator generally within the first 24 hours. Enteral feedings can be started at a slow rate almost immediately after the extraperitoneal approach. Infants who were on tube feedings before transplantation should resume these tube feedings because they usually will not be fed per os in the immediate post-transplantation period. Hypertension can be problematic. The volume loading associated with the procedure, as well as the use of calcineurin inhibitors for immunosuppression, can result in significant hypertension, which can be severe and require aggressive therapy to prevent seizures and other sequelae.

In order to monitor and replace urine output on an hourly basis we usually admit our patients to the ICU. If this can be accomplished on a surgical floor unit, larger children could be admitted to an area specializing in the care of renal transplant patients. Children who are admitted into the ICU are typically transferred to the floor unit within 1 to 2 days. Most children can leave the hospital in 5 to 7 days after transplantation assuming they are able to eat and the family is familiar with the immunosuppression regimen.

EVALUATION OF EARLY ALLOGRAFT DYSFUNCTION

Ideally, the donor kidney should begin to make urine shortly after revascularization. The likelihood of this occurring depends on multiple factors, beginning with the quality of the donor organ. Living donor kidneys will generally function immediately because of the healthy state of the donor as well as the shorter cold ischemic time. For deceased donor kidneys the cold ischemic time is generally longer. In addition and more importantly, there are multiple factors associated with the donor death, including hypotension, the potential need for high doses of vasopressors, and other issues related to the overall health of the donor.

Regardless of the donor source, the assessment of the graft begins in the operating room, evaluating the graft for color and turgor as well as inspecting the arterial and venous anastomoses. Particular attention should be directed to considering how the kidney is positioned once the abdomen is closed and how this could impact the vasculature. The renal artery will often have a thrill suggestive of excellent flow and low intrarenal resistance. Assuming the technical aspects of the procedure appear satisfactory, additional volume for the kidney not making urine is the best option. Once the patient is adequately volume loaded, loop diuretics may be used to gently encourage a diuresis. In patients who are aneuric before the procedure, continued failure to make urine in the postoperative period should prompt a bedside Doppler ultrasound examination. For patients who made urine before the transplantation, determining whether the transplanted kidney is making urine is more difficult, although sometimes the amount of volume being produced will give a sign that the kidney is working. Over the next 24 hours the serum creatinine level should fall as well. If there is still concern about function, a Doppler ultrasound study should be obtained and any suggestion of problems with the arteriovenous signal should initiate a prompt return to the operating room. Generally the ultrasound will be fine, or occasionally there will be a modest reduction in flow suggestive of increased intrarenal resistance, most commonly due to acute tubular necrosis. This condition resolves without any specific intervention. Other diagnostic studies are less frequently required. Renal arteriography is rarely indicated. Radionucleotide scans are used by some centers, but we find them less helpful than ultrasonography. A radionucleotide scan may be helpful in documenting a suspected urinary leak before proceeding with percutaneous nephrostomy.

Complications related to the ureteral anastomosis include leaks and obstruction. The risk of ureteral complications is approximately 9%.[57] A leak at the ureteral anastomosis generally becomes manifest in the first few days after the transplant. Leaks can generally be managed nonoperatively by placing a percutaneous nephrostomy tube. This tube is subsequently advanced across the anastomosis into the bladder and converted to a universal stent. The stent is usually left open to external dependent drainage for several days, at which time it can be capped until healing occurs. If a large urinoma is present, separate drainage of the perinephric fluid collection may be required.

Obstruction of the urinary system can occur at any time. Obstructions that occur earlier are usually related to technical problems with the anastomosis of the donor ureter or other mechanical issues such as torsion of the ureter, if the ureter was twisted before anastomosis. Because the ureter relies on small arterial feeding vessels from the lower pole of the kidney for its vascular supply, it is prudent to avoid leaving it excessively long. Ureteral stenoses occurring late after transplant generally require operative intervention, with resection of the stenotic segment and a urologic reconstruction.

Another complication after retroperitoneal kidney transplantation is lymphocele. Lymphoceles may produce discomfort or allograft dysfunction. The diagnosis is established when ultrasound-guided percutaneous aspiration reveals clear fluid with a creatinine concentration equivalent to serum. Percutaneous drainage is associated with a very high incidence of recurrence, and generally the preferred approach is creation of a peritoneal window. This can be accomplished either via a laparoscopic approach or through a small open incision with drainage of the lymphocele into the peritoneal cavity.

In instances of renal vein thrombosis, the graft is usually not salvageable. The cause of renal vein thrombosis is uncertain, but it may more likely be due to immunologic factors and recipient hypercoagulable state rather than any technical issue.

IMMUNOSUPPRESSION

Over the past several decades, significant advances have been made in our understanding of the immune response and several new immunosuppressive agents have been introduced into clinical care. There are now several regimens available, but all require a balance between prevention of rejection and unwanted side effects associated with immunosuppression.[87] Some centers use a standard protocol for all recipients, whereas other centers individualize the regimen for each patient. Immunosuppressive agents are used for induction, maintenance, and treatment of rejection episodes.

ANTIBODY PREPARATIONS

Both polyclonal and monoclonal antibody preparations are utilized. Antibody preparations have a role in induction regimens and for the treatment of rejection.

Antilymphocyte Antibodies

Antilymphocyte antibodies include polyclonal preparations, such as equine antithymocyte globulin (ATGAM) and rabbit antithymocyte globulin (Thymoglobulin), and the monoclonal antibody muromonab-CD3 (OKT3). These agents act by lymphodepletion, as well as by interactions with cellular receptors. The use of antilymphocyte preparations in induction regimens was routine, but their use has declined precipitously over time.[6] We currently restrict the use of these agents to recipients at higher risk for immunologic graft loss, such as patients requiring retransplantation, highly sensitized patients, or black recipients.

Anti–Interleukin-2 Receptor Monoclonal Antibodies

Two monoclonal antibodies have been developed that bind to the alpha subunit of interleukin (IL)-2 receptor (CD25) and inhibit IL-2–mediated lymphocyte proliferation. Both received approval by the U.S. Food and Drug Administration (FDA) in 1998. Basiliximab (Simulect) is a chimeric human/mouse monoclonal antibody.[39] Daclizumab (Zenapax) is a humanized murine monoclonal antibody.[99] Both agents are effective in reducing the incidence of acute cellular rejection, with good long-term results and no evidence of increased risk of infection or malignancy.[8,63,88] The IL-2 receptor antibodies are used in induction regimens but are not effective in treating rejection.

Calcineurin Inhibitors

The introduction of cyclosporine after its FDA approval in 1983 is widely accepted as one of the most significant advances in transplantation. Its efficacy in pediatric renal transplantation is established.[31] Tacrolimus received FDA approval in 1994. Both cyclosporine and tacrolimus act through inhibition of calcineurin activity.

The agents first enter the cell and bind to specific cytoplasmic proteins; cyclosporine binds to cyclophilin, and tacrolimus binds to tacrolimus binding protein (also known as FK-binding protein). Both drug-protein complexes then bind to calcineurin, a phosphatase that controls the transport of transcriptional regulator factors across the nuclear membrane. By inhibiting the translocation of these factors into the nucleus, both drugs inhibit transcription of several early T-cell activation genes, most significantly IL-2.

Both cyclosporine and tacrolimus are effective at preventing rejection.[40] A recent randomized prospective open label trial performed in Europe in pediatric renal recipients compared tacrolimus to cyclosporine, along with azathioprine and steroids. There was a significantly lower incidence of acute rejection in the tacrolimus group (36.9%) compared with cyclosporine therapy (59.1%).[94] In contrast to this observation, a retrospective analysis of NAPRTCS data comparing cyclosporine to tacrolimus, along with mycophenolate mofetil and corticosteroids, showed equal rates of rejection and graft survival. Although rejection rates were similar, tacrolimus therapy was associated with improved graft function at 1 and 2 years after transplant.[60] According to a recent analysis of OPTN data, most pediatric recipients were reported as being discharged on tacrolimus compared with cyclosporine (71.4% versus 22.5%).[46]

The side effects of cyclosporine include hirsutism and gingival hyperplasia, whereas tacrolimus is associated with increased incidence of post-transplant diabetes and neurotoxicity. Both cyclosporine and tacrolimus share significant nephrotoxicity, and appreciation of the role of calcineurin inhibitor–induced nephrotoxicity in both renal and nonrenal transplantation is growing. It is important to balance the side effects of either agent and risk/benefit for each child.[40] In children who develop a problematic side effect from one agent, conversion to the other agent is appropriate.

Mycophenolate Mofetil

Mycophenolate mofetil (MMF, CellCept) inhibits purine synthesis and has essentially replaced azathioprine (Imuran) as the primary antiproliferative agent.[6,46] MMF is converted in vivo to mycophenolic acid, a noncompetitive inhibitor of inosine monophosphate dehydrogenase (IMPDH), which is a key enzyme in de novo purine biosynthesis. Although most cells can synthesize purines by either the de novo or the salvage pathway, B and T lymphocytes lack the salvage pathway. MMF is thus a selective inhibitor of lymphocyte proliferation. It has been demonstrated to be safe and effective in pediatric patients.[9,37] The primary side effects are related to leukopenia and gastrointestinal intolerance. An enteric-coated mycophenolate (Myfortic) has been developed with similar efficacy and side effect profile.

Prednisone

Glucocorticoids have played an integral role in most immunosuppression regimens since the earliest days of transplantation. They act primarily through transcriptional regulation. They first diffuse across the plasma membrane and bind to cytoplasmic steroid receptors. This complex is translocated to the nucleus, where it binds to specific gene promoters and other regulatory regions, inhibiting cytokine synthesis. Corticosteroids are also lymphocytotoxic and possess significant anti-inflammatory activity. They inhibit macrophage function and other nonspecific aspects of the inflammatory response.

Long-term corticosteroid therapy is associated with increased risk of hypertension, hyperlipidemia, diabetes, bone loss, cosmetic disfigurement, and cataracts. Attempts at minimizing corticosteroids have not had a significant effect on these side effects, and new efforts are being directed to corticosteroid avoidance. Although it is appealing to consider withdrawal of corticosteroids over time, corticosteroid withdrawal appears associated with increased risk of acute and chronic rejection.[73] Some investigators believe that not introducing corticosteroids would prevent subsequent corticosteroid dependence. Corticosteroid-free regimens have been introduced and show promise in retrospective studies.[7] Sarwal and associates have shown excellent initial results in a corticosteroid-free protocol using an extended induction with daclizumab, tacrolimus, and mycophenolate mofetil.[78] With a mean follow-up of 20 months, overall graft and patient survival was 98%, and the rate of acute rejection was 8% at 1 year. This preliminary study has led to a prospective, multicenter randomized study that is currently underway.

Sirolimus

Sirolimus, or rapamycin, is a macrolide antibiotic with immunosuppressive properties. Sirolimus inhibits a protein, target of rapamycin (TOR), a key regulatory kinase controlling cytokine-mediated cellular proliferation. A potential role for sirolimus in renal transplantation has been established.[30,38] There is interest in using sirolimus in protocols to avoid calcineurin inhibitors or corticosteroids. Additionally, there is a role for conversion to sirolimus for complications due to other agents. Sirolimus interacts with calcineurin inhibitors, particularly cyclosporine, and careful monitoring is essential. Like many other immunosuppressive agents, there is evidence to suggest more rapid metabolism of sirolimus in children compared with adults.[79] Another agent in this class, everolimus, is under development.[36] Experience with sirolimus is limited, and care is warranted given concerns for long-term risks that may be associated with the drug.

Treatment of Rejection

Suspected rejection episodes should be confirmed by biopsy. The first-line therapy for acute cellular rejection is pulse corticosteroid therapy. Typically, intravenous methylprednisolone is administered for 3 days, with doses ranging from 5.0 to 25.0 mg/kg/day (maximum dose, 1.0 g) depending on local protocols. We utilize 10.0 mg/kg for children younger than age 6 and 5.0 mg/kg for children aged 6 years and older, with a maximum dose of 500 mg/day. Severe rejection, or rejection episodes refractory to pulse corticosteroid therapy, are treated with polyclonal antilymphocyte globulin or monoclonal OKT3 antibody; we prefer the former. There is no role for the use of IL-2 receptor antibodies in treating rejection. Treatment of acute rejection episodes is nearly always successful, although late episodes of rejection are more unlikely to respond appropriately. After successful treatment, many centers consider altering the maintenance immunosuppression, including changing to the other calcineurin inhibitor, or substituting sirolimus for MMF; however, there is little evidence to support this approach. An assessment of adherence to the immunosuppression regimen should also be initiated. If after treatment the patient's creatinine level does not fall to the baseline value, a follow-up biopsy should be strongly considered.

OUTCOMES

Graft and Patient Survival

There are approximately 800 pediatric kidney transplants performed annually in the United States. In 2002, there were 769 transplants, with 57% living donor and 43% deceased donor kidneys.[46] Over the past decade there has been continued improvement in graft survival (Fig. 43-1). For all pediatric recipients, 1-year deceased donor kidney graft survival has increased from 83% in 1993 to 91% for transplants performed in 2002. Similarly, graft survival after living donor transplantation increased from 90% to 97% over the same period. Current graft and patient survival after renal transplantation is excellent. At our center, for the 38 pediatric transplants performed between January 1, 2001, and June 30, 2003, graft and patient survival was 100%. Nationally, graft and patient survival during the same time period was 94.5% and 98.9%, respectively. Current graft survival for pediatric recipients of living donor and deceased donor kidney transplants are shown in Figure 43-2. Recipient survival stratified by age range is summarized in Figure 43-3. While patient survival is good, it is important to realize that even with transplantation, these children face a significantly increased risk of mortality compared with the general population.[54]

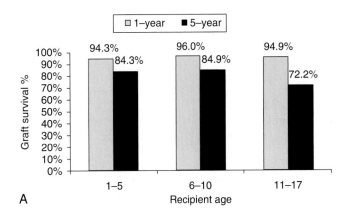

A

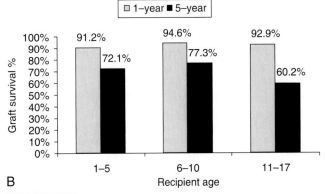

B

Figure 43–2 *A,* Adjusted 1- and 5-year graft survival of living donor kidney transplants by recipient age. *B,* Adjusted 1- and 5-year graft survival of deceased donor kidney transplants by recipient age. (From OPTN/SRTR: 2003 OPTN/SRTR Annual Report: Transplant Data 1993-2002. HHS/HRSA/SPB/DOT; UNOS; URREA. Available online at: www.ustransplant.org.)

The past decade has seen improvement in all pediatric age ranges. This improvement is particularly noteworthy in children younger than 2 years of age who had previously had the worse outcomes; these children now have outcomes that equal the outcomes of any age group.[6,46] Recent reports demonstrate that the longest transplant

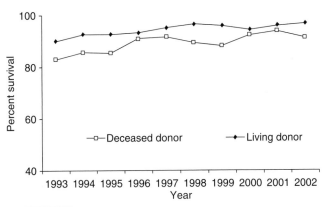

Figure 43–1 Adjusted 1-year graft survival for pediatric kidney recipients, 1993-2002. (From SRTR analysis, August 2004.)

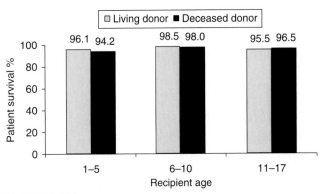

Figure 43–3 Adjusted 5-year patient survival of living and deceased donor kidney transplants by recipient age. (From OPTN/SRTR: 2003 OPTN/SRTR Annual Report: Transplant Data 1993-2002. HHS/HRSA/SPB/DOT; UNOS; URREA. Available online at: www.ustransplant.org.)

half-lives of all recipients are now the youngest recipients, especially if the pediatric recipient receives an adult kidney that functions immediately.[11,77] These improvements likely reflect better donor selection, improvement in surgical techniques, better immunosuppression agents, and a better understanding of immunosuppression management in children.

Although the current short-term success in the pediatric population is encouraging, it is also important to realize that long-term graft survival in the adolescent group (ages 11 to 17) is poor (see Fig. 43-2). The graft survival is lower than all age groups except adults older than 65 years.[46] The reasons behind this significant rate of graft loss are speculative, but noncompliance likely plays a significant role.[85] The higher incidence of recurrent FSGS in this age group may also contribute to graft loss.[5] Regardless of the cause, improving the long-term outcomes in this patient population represents one of the largest challenges in pediatric transplantation.

Post-Transplant Outcomes and Risk Factors Associated with Graft Loss

Benfield and coworkers reported that the most common causes responsible for 1605 primary allograft failures reported to NAPRTCS are chronic rejection (32.4%), acute rejection (15.2%), vascular thrombosis (11.6%), death of the recipient with a functioning graft (10.1%), and recurrence of the primary disease (5.9%).[6] Analysis of large single-center experiences and registry data has revealed risk factors associated with specific post-transplantation outcomes. For a given child, some of these risk factors are not modifiable—such as their race, age, or primary disease. Other factors are potentially modifiable, and efforts should be made to improve the risk ratio when possible.

The type and timing of the transplant affect outcomes. Living donor transplantation is associated with better graft survival compared with deceased donor transplantation,[28] although the difference appears to be becoming smaller in more recent cohorts of recipients.[6] Preemptive transplantation is associated with better graft survival compared with patients on dialysis at time of transplantation.[98] For children on dialysis, the choice of dialysis therapy does not impact on graft survival, although graft loss from vascular thrombosis is more common in children on peritoneal dialysis compared with hemodialysis.

Delayed Graft Function

Delayed graft function (DGF) is defined as the need for dialysis during the first week after transplantation and is a manifestation of significant acute tubular necrosis (ATN). DGF is more common in recipients of deceased donor kidneys compared with living donor transplants. In pediatric recipients, analysis of over 5000 transplants has demonstrated that DGF is an independent risk factor for subsequent graft loss.[91] DGF is also associated with increased risk for acute and chronic rejection. It is believed that this association reflects the impact of renal injury on the subsequent immune response. DGF also limits the ability to use renal dysfunction as a sign of acute rejection, and diagnosis of rejection could be delayed. We believe that all allografts with DGF lasting longer than 5 to 7 days should be sampled, and biopsies should be performed even earlier in patients with increased risk of rejection.

Because of the impact of DGF on graft survival, all efforts should be made to decrease the risk for ATN. Over the past decade, the incidence of DGF after deceased donor renal transplantation has decreased from 16% to 12.5% in 2002.[46] This observation likely represents improvements in recipient management and donor selection. The rate of DGF in these pediatric recipients is half that observed in adult patients (23.4%), reflecting the differential donor selection made possible by the allocation system.

Vascular Thrombosis

Vascular thrombosis is the third most common reported cause of graft loss.[6] Risk factors that appear associated with thrombosis include donor age younger than 6 years, cold ischemic time greater than 24 hours, prior transplant, and peritoneal dialysis below transplantation.[53] Careful consideration of donor quality, along with efforts to ensure adequate perfusion to the graft, are strategies to minimize the risk of thrombosis. Patients with ESRD have a higher incidence of hypercoagulable conditions and any history of thrombosis, including recurrent or unexplained thrombosis of hemodialysis access, should prompt further evaluation.

Acute Rejection

Acute rejection typically occurs between 1 week and 3 months after transplantation, although it can happen at any time. A rise in the serum creatinine level is frequently the first sign of rejection. Other findings such as low-grade fever, graft tenderness, hypertension, or decreased urine output may or may not be present. Any evidence of renal dysfunction should be promptly investigated. A percutaneous renal biopsy should be obtained to confirm the diagnosis because many other processes can lead to allograft dysfunction, including calcineurin toxicity, ureteral obstruction, infection, renal artery stenosis, and recurrence of original disease. Acute rejection episodes are treated by either pulse corticosteroids or antilymphocyte antibodies as detailed previously.

Acute rejection, and, in particular, late acute rejection episodes occurring more than 1 year after transplant, are independent risk factors for graft loss due to chronic rejection.[90] One episode of acute rejection increases the risk of graft loss from chronic rejection graft failure 3-fold, and two episodes of acute rejection increase the risk 12-fold. The incidence of acute rejection is decreasing over time and is likely the major factor for the observed improvement in graft survival.[6] An analysis of NAPRTCS cohort from 1997-1999 yielded an acute rejection rate of 40% in the first year after transplant compared with 71% for transplants performed in 1987-1989.[52] Currently, rejection rates are 20% to 30%.

Acute rejection, even successfully treated, profoundly impacts graft survival and all efforts to minimize this risk are important. Unfortunately, merely intensifying the immunosuppression regimen is limited by the consequences of nonspecific systemic immunosuppression. Ensuring the patient remains on therapeutic immunosuppression is vital and noncompliance can have disastrous implications. Prompt recognition and treatment of rejection is another important principle. Because serum creatinine is a relatively insensitive indicator of renal dysfunction, particularly in small children with an adult kidney, some advocate protocol renal biopsies to detect subclinical rejection that may benefit from treatment.

Chronic Allograft Nephropathy

Whereas short-term results are excellent, continued graft failure becomes a progressive renal dysfunction due to chronic allograft nephropathy, the most common cause of graft failure. Chronic allograft nephropathy, often called "chronic rejection," involves both immunologic and nonimmunologic factors. Although acute rejection episodes are the major risk factor for chronic allograft nephropathy, it is clear other processes can contribute as well.[49] Efforts to reduce chronic allograft nephropathy are limited by our understanding of the process. In addition to eventually causing graft loss, renal dysfunction associated with chronic allograft nephropathy also adversely impacts the recipient's general health and development.

Noncompliance

Compliance with the medical regimen is essential for the success of transplantation. Noncompliance is believed to contribute to significant graft loss in all patients and be largely responsible for the poorer long-term graft survival seen in adolescent recipients. Shaw and coworkers reviewed 112 pediatric renal transplant recipients and found one third had clinically significant periods of medication nonadherence.[82] Nonadherence was significantly more common in adolescents compared with younger recipients. Nonadherence was associated with both acute and chronic rejection, as well as graft loss. Improved parental involvement and discussion of the child-parent relationship may improve adherence.

Recurrent Disease

The recurrence of the patient's primary disease is variable, and recurrence may or may not lead to graft loss. Recurrent disease is a more significant issue in the pediatric population, because of the nature of the diagnoses leading to ESRD, and their association with higher rates of graft loss after recurrence.[81]

FSGS is the most prevalent and clinically significant disease to recur after renal transplantation.[4] In children, the recurrence rate can be as high as 40%.[3] It can recur almost immediately after transplant, and most recurrences are within the first month. Patients with FSGS should be followed closely after transplantation with urine protein measurements. Graft survival is often worse in adolescents with recurrent FSGS, with up to a 38% risk of graft loss.[62] A circulating permeability factor is believed to play a critical role in the pathogenesis of FSGS. Plasmapheresis is the most frequently used therapy for recurrence, although evidence-based controlled trials supporting its efficacy are lacking.[62] Early institution of pheresis is associated with better outcomes,[70] and some have proposed a role for preoperative plasmapheresis to decrease the risk of recurrence.[65] Others have suggested a role for intensifying the immunosuppression.[13] In addition to FSGS, other primary renal causes associated with recurrent disease and potential graft loss include membranoproliferative glomerulonephritis types 1 and 2 and IgA nephropathy.[81] Again, the risk of graft loss is variable, and none constitute an absolute contraindication to transplantation.

In addition to these primary glomerulopathies, there are other recurrent diseases that disproportionately affect the pediatric population. Hemolytic-uremic syndrome can recur after transplantation. The patients at greatest risk of recurrence and subsequent graft loss are those with atypical nondiarrhea–associated hemolytic-uremic syndrome.[45,71] Henoch-Schönlein purpura can also recur after transplantation.[56] The 5-year risk of renal recurrence after transplantation for Henoch-Schönlein purpura is 35%, and the risk for subsequent graft loss is 11%.[56] Aggressive initial progression to ESRD is associated with a higher risk of recurrence, and recurrence can occur greater than a year after disappearance of the purpura.

Oxalosis (primary hyperoxaluria type 1) is a metabolic disease caused by a defect in hepatic peroxisomal alanine:glyoxlate aminotransferase, which leads to increased synthesis and excretion of oxalate. The excessive oxalate load leads to urolithiasis, medullary calcinosis, and eventual ESRD. There is also significant extrarenal oxalate deposition as well. The primary metabolic defect is not corrected by kidney transplantation, and after transplantation the persistent oxalate load causes subsequent renal graft loss. The morbidity associated with the persistent extrarenal oxalate deposition is responsible for early patient death. Given this natural history, simultaneous liver-kidney transplantation has been advocated as the primary treatment in these individuals.[21,27,35] The risk of this approach is substantial as well, and kidney transplantation alone can be appropriate in selected patients, most notably those who are pyridoxine sensitive or those with lower oxalate burdens.[74]

Medical Complications

Infection

Infection is a constant risk of immunosuppression and is one clinical representation of the precarious balance between over and under immunosuppression. Great vigilance should be maintained during periods of heaviest immunosuppression, as occurs immediately after transplant or during treatment of rejection. Additional prophylaxis is warranted during these periods of greatest risk.

Currently, post-transplant infection accounts for more hospitalizations than acute rejection, even in the first 6 months after transplantation.[18] Post-transplantation infections are predominantly bacterial and viral. Fungal infections, although accounting for 0.2% to 2.7% of infection-related hospitalizations, can be particularly dangerous. Several viral pathogens are worthy of discussion. Pediatric recipients are often at higher risk, because the likelihood that they will be more naïve to a particular pathogen is greater than the majority of the population.

Cytomegalovirus (CMV)

CMV represents the most common viral infection after transplantation. CMV infection can occur in any recipient, although the risk is highest when a seronegative recipient is transplanted with a kidney from a seropositive donor. Infection occurs in the seropositive recipient as well owing to activation of latent virus. The incidence and the severity of CMV have declined with more effective prophylaxis. The severity of CMV infection may range from asymptomatic to organ involvement and death. The typical presentation occurs 1 to 3 months after transplantation, with the patient feeling relatively well but having fevers or sometimes with flu-like symptoms. Leukopenia is a common laboratory finding. Patients with tissue-invasive CMV disease will appear toxic and there will be evidence of end-organ dysfunction. Currently, the diagnosis is confirmed using either a CMV pp65 antigenemia assay or the CMV polymerase chain reaction (PCR) assay. Both methods allow monitoring of the response to therapy. Treatment of CMV disease includes ganciclovir or valganciclovir. In more severe cases, treatment with CMV hyperimmune globulin may be helpful. Unfortunately, ganciclovir-resistant CMV strains are emerging.

Varicella-Zoster Virus (VZV)

In pediatric recipients, there is high risk of a primary chickenpox infection. Treatment is with intravenous acyclovir until the lesions crust over, then conversion to oral acyclovir. Primary infections can be quite severe. We immunize our VZV seronegative candidates before transplantation. For seronegative recipients who have a defined exposure, we administer VZV immune globulin.

BK Virus

BK virus is a ubiquitous polyomavirus that has recently been identified as a significant concern in renal transplantation.[97] There is a high incidence of seroconversion (60% to 100%) by late childhood, and the virus is dormant in the renal epithelium until reactivated. The recent growing awareness of this pathogen may reflect the impact of more potent immunosuppression protocols. Early reports, primarily in the adult literature, suggested BK virus was an important cause of renal allograft dysfunction, and BK interstitial nephritis resulted in a loss of up to 45% to 70% of infected grafts.

BK nephropathy should be considered in the evaluation of renal allograft dysfunction. BK nephropathy can be definitively diagnosed on biopsy using immunohistochemistry, but the histology can be confused at times with acute rejection. Treatment with additional immunosuppression does not improve renal function, and it often will cause further deterioration. The initial treatment for BK nephropathy consists of lowering maintenance immunosuppression. Treatment with low doses of cidofovir or intravenous immunoglobulin has also been utilized. Measurement of BK virus by PCR is becoming more widespread, both for diagnosis and monitoring response to treatment.

There has been concern that children, who may be less likely to be seropositive, will be at an increased risk of BK infection. In one study involving 18 pediatric recipients, the incidence of BK seropositivity was 56% and that of BK viruria was 33%.[33] These figures are comparable to incidence of seropositivity and viral activation observed in adult transplant recipients. The incidence of BK virus–associated transplant nephropathy is estimated to be 4% to 7%.[97] In the largest examination of the issue in the pediatric population, Smith and coworkers evaluated a single-center cohort of 173 renal transplant recipients and identified BK nephropathy in 6 children (3.5%).[86] The diagnosis was made on biopsy at a median of 15 months after transplantation. Treatment consisted of lowering the baseline immunosuppression; and with a median of 25 months' follow-up, all grafts are functioning with stable function. In addition, Smith and coworkers demonstrated a strong association between BK nephropathy and recipient seronegativity.[86] It is likely that improved awareness, prompt diagnosis, and treatment may reduce the risk of graft loss initially associated with this disease process.

Malignancy

Transplant recipients face an increased risk of de novo malignancy related to their immunosuppression. Lymphomas, specifically post-transplant lymphoproliferative disorder (PTLD), are the most common. The incidence is approximately 1% in renal transplantation.[19,20] PTLD actually represents a spectrum of pathology. Epstein-Barr virus (EBV) is believed to be causative in much of the progression to PTLD, especially in the B-cell lymphomas.[2] The treatment and prognosis of PTLD depend on the histology.[29] A wide variety of factors have been proposed to be associated with an increased risk, including the use of antilymphocyte induction therapy, EBV-seronegative recipient, era of transplant, and EBV infection though these associations are not always consistently demonstrated within the pediatric population. PTLD does appear to be related to the overall intensity of immunosuppression.[17,19] More recent analysis suggests the incidence of PTLD is increasing, and young white males appear to be at greatest risk.[20]

The second most common cancer in pediatric recipients is skin cancer. Squamous cell carcinoma accounts for the majority of cutaneous neoplasms, followed by malignant melanoma and basal cell carcinoma. The best strategy combines sun block and sun avoidance. All transplant recipients should undergo regular skin follow-up, specifically focusing on this risk. Long-term immunosuppression is also associated with increased risks of cervical, vulvar, and anal carcinoma.

Other Medical Issues

In addition to the risks of infection and malignancy, transplant recipients face many other risks owing to their history of ESRD, their underlying renal disease, and the individual risks associated with all their medications.

Renal transplant recipients are at higher risk for cardiovascular disease. The preexisting renal insufficiency, the time on dialysis, and the immunosuppressive medications after transplantation all contribute to this risk. Additionally, the prevalence of hypertension in pediatric kidney recipients is 50% to 80%.[58] Many recipients will have additional cardiovascular risk factors, including hyperlipidemia, hyperhomocysteinemia, anemia, malnutrition, and chronic inflammation.[84] Matteucci and colleagues evaluated 28 pediatric renal transplant patients and demonstrated that 82% had evidence of left ventricular hypertrophy.[51] Although there are little data examining the magnitude of the risk in pediatric patients, young adult patients with ESRD have a 1000-fold higher risk of cardiovascular death compared with the general population. Although the risk of cardiovascular death decreases after successful transplantation compared with dialysis, it does not become normal.[68] In addition to contributing to cardiovascular risk, hypertension after transplantation is associated with a higher risk of graft dysfunction and graft loss.[89] Every effort should be made to modify these cardiovascular risk factors to promote health and prolong life.

Transplant recipients also face significant problems with bone metabolism and growth.[22] This is in part owing to the chronic renal insufficiency, malnutrition, graft dysfunction after transplantation, and immunosuppressive medications. Renal osteodystrophy is a substantial problem, but proper management with calcium supplementation, vitamin D supplementation, and the use of other agents has improved overall bone health. The risk of osseous complications seems to be improving over time, and the risk decreases after transplantation when compared with dialysis therapy.[75] The introduction of recombinant human growth hormone has proved to be safe and effective. Although recombinant human growth hormone was a large step forward in promoting linear growth in these patients, many still will not obtain optimal final adult height.[1]

Cognitive and Psychosocial Development

The negative impact of ESRD on cognitive development in children has diminished over the years, owing to significant improvements in medical management and renal replacement therapy.[23] It is believed that children with ESRD who undergo transplants may now reach a level of cognitive function close to or at the level of healthy children. Psychosocial development remains below the healthy population, although renal transplantation offers a better outlook compared with the dialysis population. Overall quality of life for the child and the family appears to be better after transplantation compared with dialysis, although again, when compared with the normative population, there are disparities.[23,48,72]

REFERENCES

1. Acott PD, Pernica JM: Growth hormone therapy before and after pediatric renal transplant. Pediatr Transplant 2003;7:426-440.
2. ASTS/AST: Epstein-Barr virus and lymphoproliferative disorders after transplantation. Am J Transplant 2004;4:59-65.
3. Baqi N, Tejani A: Recurrence of the original disease in pediatric renal transplantation. J Nephrol 1997;10:85-92.
4. Baum MA: Outcomes after renal transplantation for FSGS in children. Pediatr Transplant 2004;8:329-333.
5. Baum MA, Ho M, Stablein D, et al: Outcome of renal transplantation in adolescents with focal segmental glomerulosclerosis. Pediatr Transplant 2002;6:488-492.
6. Benfield MR, McDonald RA, Bartosh S, et al: Changing trends in pediatric transplantation: 2001 Annual Report of the North American Pediatric Renal Transplant Cooperative Study. Pediatr Transplant 2003;7:321-335.
7. Birkeland SA: Steroid-free immunosuppression in renal transplantation: A long-term follow-up of 100 consecutive patients. Transplantation 2001;71:1089-1090.
8. Bumgardner GL, Hardie I, Johnson RW, et al: Results of 3-year phase III clinical trials with daclizumab prophylaxis for prevention of acute rejection after renal transplantation. Transplantation 2001;72:839-845.
9. Bunchman T, Navarro M, Broyer M, et al: The use of mycophenolate mofetil suspension in pediatric renal allograft recipients. Pediatr Nephrol 2001;16:978-984.
10. Capizzi A, Zanon GF, Zacchello G, Rigamonti W: Kidney transplantation in children with reconstructed bladder. Transplantation 2004;77:1113-1116.
11. Cecka JM, Gjertson DW, Terasaki PI: Pediatric renal transplantation: A review of the UNOS data. United Network for Organ Sharing. Pediatr Transplant 1997;1:55-64.
12. Cho YW, Terasaki PI, Cecka JM, Gjertson DW: Transplantation of kidneys from donors whose hearts have stopped beating. N Engl J Med 1998;338:221-225.
13. Cochat P, Schell M, Ranchin B, et al: Management of recurrent nephrotic syndrome after kidney transplantation in children. Clin Nephrol 1996;46:17-20.
14. Colombani PM, Dunn SP, Harmon WE, et al: Pediatric transplantation. Am J Transplant 2003;3(Suppl 4):S53-S63.
15. Cooper JT, Chin LT, Krieger NR, et al: Donation after cardiac death: The University of Wisconsin experience with renal transplantation. Am J Transplant 2004;4:1490-1494.
16. Delmonico FL, Harmon WE: The use of a minor as a live kidney donor. Am J Transplant 2002;2:333-336.
17. Dharnidharka VR, Ho PL, Stablein DM, et al: Mycophenolate, tacrolimus and post-transplant lymphoproliferative disorder: A report of the North American Pediatric Renal Transplant Cooperative Study. Pediatr Transplant 2002;6:396-399.
18. Dharnidharka VR, Stablein DM, Harmon WE: Post-transplant infections now exceed acute rejection as cause for hospitalization: A report of the NAPRTCS. Am J Transplant 2004;4:384-389.
19. Dharnidharka VR, Sullivan EK, Stablein DM, et al: Risk factors for posttransplant lymphoproliferative disorder (PTLD) in

pediatric kidney transplantation: A report of the North American Pediatric Renal Transplant Cooperative Study (NAPRTCS). Transplantation 2001;71:1065-1068.

20. Dharnidharka VR, Tejani AH, Ho PL, Harmon WE: Post-transplant lymphoproliferative disorder in the United States: Young Caucasian males are at highest risk. Am J Transplant 2002;2:993-998.

21. Ellis SR, Hulton SA, McKiernan PJ, et al: Combined liver-kidney transplantation for primary hyperoxaluria type 1 in young children. Nephrol Dial Transplant 2001;16:348-354.

22. Fine RN: Growth following solid-organ transplantation. Pediatr Transplant 2002;6:47-52.

23. Fine RN, Alonso EM, Fischel JE, et al: Pediatric transplantation of the kidney, liver and heart: Summary report. Pediatr Transplant 2004;8:75-86.

24. Fine RN, Tejani A, Sullivan EK: Pre-emptive renal transplantation in children: Report of the North American Pediatric Renal Transplant Cooperative Study (NAPRTCS). Clin Transplant 1994;8:474-478.

25. Fontaine E, Gagnadoux MF, Niaudet P, et al: Renal transplantation in children with augmentation cystoplasty: Long-term results. J Urol 1998;159:2110-2113.

26. Franc-Guimond J, Gonzalez R: Renal transplantation in children with reconstructed bladders. Transplantation 2004;77:1116-1120.

27. Gagnadoux MF, Lacaille F, Niaudet P, et al: Long term results of liver-kidney transplantation in children with primary hyperoxaluria. Pediatr Nephrol 2001;16:946-950.

28. Gjertson DW, Cecka JM: Determinants of long-term survival of pediatric kidney grafts reported to the United Network for Organ Sharing kidney transplant registry. Pediatr Transplant 2001;5:5-15.

29. Green M, Webber S: Posttransplantation lymphoproliferative disorders. Pediatr Clin North Am 2003;50:1471-1491.

30. Groth CG, Backman L, Morales JM, et al: Sirolimus (rapamycin)-based therapy in human renal transplantation: Similar efficacy and different toxicity compared with cyclosporine. Sirolimus European Renal Transplant Study Group. Transplantation 1999;67:1036-1042.

31. Harmon WE, Sullivan EK: Cyclosporine dosing and its relationship to outcome in pediatric renal transplantation. Kidney Int Suppl 1993;43:S50-S55.

32. Hatch DA, Koyle MA, Baskin LS, et al: Kidney transplantation in children with urinary diversion or bladder augmentation. J Urol 2001;165 (Suppl):2265-2268.

33. Haysom L, Rosenberg AR, Kainer G, et al: BK viral infection in an Australian pediatric renal transplant population. Pediatr Transplant 2004;8:480-484.

34. Healey PJ, McDonald R, Waldhausen JH, et al: Transplantation of adult living donor kidneys into infants and small children. Arch Surg 2000;135:1035-1041.

35. Hoppe B, Langman CB: A United States survey on diagnosis, treatment, and outcome of primary hyperoxaluria. Pediatr Nephrol 2003;18:986-991.

36. Hoyer PF, Ettenger R, Kovarik JM, et al: Everolimus in pediatric de nova renal transplant patients. Transplantation 2003;75:2082-2085.

37. Jungraithmayr T, Staskewitz A, Kirste G, et al: Pediatric renal transplantation with mycophenolate mofetil-based immunosuppression without induction: Results after three years. Transplantation 2003;75:454-461.

38. Kahan BD, Julian BA, Pescovitz MD, et al: Sirolimus reduces the incidence of acute rejection episodes despite lower cyclosporine doses in Caucasian recipients of mismatched primary renal allografts: A phase II trial. Rapamune Study Group. Transplantation 1999;68:1526-1532.

39. Kahan BD, Rajagopalan PR, Hall M: Reduction of the occurrence of acute cellular rejection among renal allograft recipients treated with basiliximab, a chimeric anti-interleukin-2-receptor monoclonal antibody. United States Simulect Renal Study Group. Transplantation 1999;67:276-284.

40. Kari JA, Trompeter RS: What is the calcineurin inhibitor of choice for pediatric renal transplantation? Pediatr Transplant 2004;8:437-444.

41. Kayler LK, Merion RM, Maraschio MA, et al: Outcomes of pediatric living donor renal transplant after laparoscopic versus open donor nephrectomy. Transplant Proc 2002;34:3097-3098.

42. Khwaja K, Humar A, Najarian JS: Kidney transplants for children under 1 year of age—a single-center experience. Pediatr Transplant 2003;7:163-167.

43. Koo HP, Bunchman TE, Flynn JT, et al: Renal transplantation in children with severe lower urinary tract dysfunction. J Urol 1999;161:240-245.

44. Live Organ Donor Consensus Group. Consensus statement on the live organ donor. JAMA 2000;284:2919-2926.

45. Loirat C, Niaudet P: The risk of recurrence of hemolytic uremic syndrome after renal transplantation in children. Pediatr Nephrol 2003;18:1095-1101.

46. Magee JC, Bucuvalas JC, Farmer DG, et al: Pediatric transplantation. Am J Transplant 2004;4(Suppl 9):S54-S71.

47. Magee JC, Sung RS, Turcotte JG, et al: Renal transplantation at the University of Michigan 1964 to 1999. In Cecka JM, Terasaki PI, eds: Clinical Transplants 1999, Los Angeles: UCLA Tissue Typing Laboratory, 2000, pp 139-148.

48. Manificat S, Dazord A, Cochat P, et al: Quality of life of children and adolescents after kidney or liver transplantation: Child, parents and caregiver's point of view. Pediatr Transplant 2003;7:228-235.

49. Matas AJ: Impact of acute rejection on development of chronic rejection in pediatric renal transplant recipients. Pediatr Transplant 2000;4:92-99.

50. Matas AJ, Bartlett ST, Leichtman AB, Delmonico FL: Morbidity and mortality after living kidney donation, 1999-2001: Survey of United States transplant centers. Am J Transplant 2003;3:830-834.

51. Matteucci MC, Giordano U, Calzolari A, et al: Left ventricular hypertrophy, treadmill tests, and 24-hour blood pressure in pediatric transplant patients. Kidney Int 1999;56:1566-1570.

52. McDonald R, Ho PL, Stablein DM, et al: Rejection profile of recent pediatric renal transplant recipients compared with historical controls: A report of the North American Pediatric Renal Transplant Cooperative Study (NAPRTCS). Am J Transplant 2001;1:55-60.

53. McDonald RA, Smith JM, Stablein D, Harmon WE: Pretransplant peritoneal dialysis and graft thrombosis following pediatric kidney transplantation: A NAPRTCS report. Pediatr Transplant 2003;7:204-208.

54. McDonald SP, Craig JC, Australian and New Zealand Paediatric Nephrology A: Long-term survival of children with end-stage renal disease. N Engl J Med 2004;350:2654-2662.

55. Metzger RA, Delmonico FL, Feng S, et al: Expanded criteria donors for kidney transplantation. Am J Transplant 2003;3(Suppl 4):S114-S125.

56. Meulders Q, Pirson Y, Cosyns JP, et al: Course of Henoch-Schönlein nephritis after renal transplantation: Report on ten patients and review of the literature. Transplantation 1994;58:1179-1186.

57. Millan MT, Sarwal MM, Lemley KV, et al: A 100% 2-year graft survival can be attained in high-risk 15-kg or smaller infant recipients of kidney allografts. Arch Surg 2000;135:1063-1068; discussion 1068-1069.

58. Mitsnefes MM: Hypertension and end-organ damage in pediatric renal transplantation. Pediatr Transplant 2004;8:394-399.

59. NAPRTCS: North American Pediatric Renal Transplant Cooperative Study (NAPRTCS) 2004 Annual Report. Available online at www.naprtcs.org.

60. Neu AM, Ho PL, Fine RN, et al: Tacrolimus vs. cyclosporine A as primary immunosuppression in pediatric renal transplantation: A NAPRTCS study. Pediatr Transplant 2003; 7:217-222.

61. Neu AM, Ho PL, McDonald RA, Warady BA: Chronic dialysis in children and adolescents. The 2001 NAPRTCS Annual Report. Pediatr Nephrol 2002;17:656-663.

62. Newstead CG: Recurrent disease in renal transplants. Nephrol Dial Transplant 2003;18(Suppl 6):vi68-74.

63. Offner G, Broyer M, Niaudet P, et al: A multicenter, open-label, pharmacokinetic/pharmacodynamic safety, and tolerability study of basiliximab (Simulect) in pediatric de novo renal transplant recipients. Transplantation 2002; 74:961-966.

64. Ohl DA, Konnak JW, Campbell DA, et al: Extravesical ureteroneocystostomy in renal transplantation. J Urol 1988;139: 499-502.

65. Ohta T, Kawaguchi H, Hattori M, et al: Effect of pre- and postoperative plasmapheresis on posttransplant recurrence of focal segmental glomerulosclerosis in children. Transplantation 2001;71:628-633.

66. Ohta T, Kawaguchi H, Hattori M, et al: ABO-incompatible pediatric kidney transplantation in a single-center trial. Pediatr Nephrol 2000;14:1-5.

67. OPTN/SRTR: 2003 OPTN/SRTR Annual Report: Transplant Data 1993-2002. HHS/HRSA/SPB/DOT; UNOS; URREA. Available online at: www.ustransplant.org.

68. Parekh RS, Carroll CE, Wolfe RA, Port FK: Cardiovascular mortality in children and young adults with end-stage kidney disease. J Pediatr 2002;141:191-197.

69. Port FK, Bragg-Gresham JL, Metzger RA, et al: Donor characteristics associated with reduced graft survival: An approach to expanding the pool of kidney donors. Transplantation 2002;74:1281-1286.

70. Pradhan M, Petro J, Palmer J, et al: Early use of plasmapheresis for recurrent post-transplant FSGS. Pediatr Nephrol 2003; 18:934-938.

71. Quan A, Sullivan EK, Alexander SR: Recurrence of hemolytic uremic syndrome after renal transplantation in children: A report of the North American Pediatric Renal Transplant Cooperative Study. Transplantation 2001;72: 742-745.

72. Qvist E, Narhi V, Apajasalo M, et al: Psychosocial adjustment and quality of life after renal transplantation in early childhood. Pediatr Transplant 2004;8:120-125.

73. Roberti I, Reisman L, Lieberman KV, Burrows L: Risk of steroid withdrawal in pediatric renal allograft recipients (a 5-year follow-up). Clin Transplant 1994;8:405-408.

74. Saborio P, Scheinman JI: Transplantation for primary hyperoxaluria in the United States. Kidney Int 1999; 56:1094-1100.

75. Saland JM: Osseous complications of pediatric transplantation. Pediatr Transplant 2004;8:400-415.

76. Salomon L, Fontaine E, Guest G, et al: Role of the bladder in delayed failure of kidney transplants in boys with posterior urethral valves. J Urol 2000;163:1282-1285.

77. Sarwal MM, Cecka JM, Millan MT, Salvatierra O Jr: Adult-size kidneys without acute tubular necrosis provide exceedingly superior long-term graft outcomes for infants and small children: A single center and UNOS analysis. United Network for Organ Sharing. Transplantation 2000;70: 1728-1736.

78. Sarwal MM, Vidhun JR, Alexander SR, et al: Continued superior outcomes with modification and lengthened follow-up of a steroid-avoidance pilot with extended daclizumab

79. Schachter AD, Meyers KE, Spaneas LD, et al: Short sirolimus half-life in pediatric renal transplant recipients on a calcineurin inhibitor-free protocol. Pediatr Transplant 2004;8:171-177.

80. Seikaly MG: Recurrence of primary disease in children after renal transplantation: An evidence-based update. Pediatr Transplant 2004;8:113-119.

81. Seikaly M, Ho PL, Emmett L, Tejani A: The 12th Annual Report of the North American Pediatric Renal Transplant Cooperative Study: Renal transplantation from 1987 through 1998. Pediatr Transplant 2001;5:215-231.

82. Shaw RJ, Palmer L, Blasey C, Sarwal M: A typology of nonadherence in pediatric renal transplant recipients. Pediatr Transplant 2003;7:489-493.

83. Shishido S, Asanuma H, Tajima E, et al: ABO-incompatible living-donor kidney transplantation in children. Transplantation 2001;72:1037-1042.

84. Silverstein DM: Risk factors for cardiovascular disease in pediatric renal transplant recipients. Pediatr Transplant 2004;8:386-393.

85. Smith JM, Ho PL, McDonald RA, et al: Renal transplant outcomes in adolescents: A report of the North American Pediatric Renal Transplant Cooperative Study. Pediatr Transplant 2002;6:493-499.

86. Smith JM, McDonald RA, Finn LS, et al: Polyomavirus nephropathy in pediatric kidney transplant recipients. Am J Transplant 2004;4:2109-2117.

87. Smith JM, McDonald RA, Nemeth TL: Current immunosuppressive agents in pediatric renal transplantation: Efficacy, side-effects and utilization. Pediatr Transplant 2004;8:445-453.

88. Sollinger H, Kaplan B, Pescovitz MD, et al: Basiliximab versus antithymocyte globulin for prevention of acute renal allograft rejection. Transplantation 2001;72:1915-1919.

89. Sorof JM, Sullivan EK, Tejani A, Portman RJ: Antihypertensive medication and renal allograft failure: A North American Pediatric Renal Transplant Cooperative Study report. J Am Soc Nephrol 1999;10:1324-1330.

90. Tejani A, Sullivan EK: The impact of acute rejection on chronic rejection: A report of the North American Pediatric Renal Transplant Cooperative Study. Pediatr Transplant 2000;4:107-111.

91. Tejani AH, Sullivan EK, Alexander SR, et al: Predictive factors for delayed graft function (DGF) and its impact on renal graft survival in children: A report of the North American Pediatric Renal Transplant Cooperative Study (NAPRTCS). Pediatr Transplant 1999;3:293-300.

92. Thomas SE, Hickman RO, Tapper D, et al: Asymptomatic inferior vena cava abnormalities in three children with end-stage renal disease: Risk factors and screening guidelines for pretransplant diagnosis. Pediatr Transplant 2000; 4:28-34.

93. Tooher RL, Rao MM, Scott DF, et al: A systematic review of laparoscopic live-donor nephrectomy. Transplantation 2004;78:404-414.

94. Trompeter R, Filler G, Webb NJ, et al: Randomized trial of tacrolimus versus cyclosporin microemulsion in renal transplantation. Pediatr Nephrol 2002;17:141-149.

95. Troppmann C, Pierce JL, Wiesmann KM, et al: Early and late recipient graft function and donor outcome after laparoscopic vs open adult live donor nephrectomy for pediatric renal transplantation. Arch Surg 2002;137: 908-915; discussion 915-916.

96. U.S. Renal Data System: USRDS 2004 Annual Data Report: Atlas of End-Stage Renal Disease in the United States, National Institutes of Health, National Institute of Diabetes and Digestive and Kidney Diseases, Bethesda, MD, 2004. Available at www.usrds.org.

97. Vats A: BK virus-associated transplant nephropathy: Need for increased awareness in children. Pediatr Transplant 2004;8:421-425.

98. Vats AN, Donaldson L, Fine RN, Chavers BM: Pretransplant dialysis status and outcome of renal transplantation in North American children: A NAPRTCS Study. North American Pediatric Renal Transplant Cooperative Study. Transplantation 2000;69:1414-1419.

99. Vincenti F, Kirkman R, Light S, et al: Interleukin-2-receptor blockade with daclizumab to prevent acute rejection in renal transplantation. Daclizumab Triple Therapy Study Group. N Engl J Med 1998;338:161-165.

100. Wolf JS Jr, Merion RM, Leichtman AB, et al: Randomized controlled trial of hand-assisted laparoscopic versus open surgical live donor nephrectomy. Transplantation 2001;72:284-290.

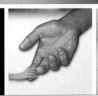

Chapter 44

Pancreas and Islet Cell Transplantation

David E. R. Sutherland, Angelika C. Gruessner, Bernhard J. Hering,

and Rainer W. G. Gruessner

Type 1 diabetes, most commonly presenting in childhood, continues to represent a therapeutic challenge. Secondary diabetes complications, observed in 30% to 50% of patients who live more than 20 years after onset of the disease, result in poor quality of life, premature death, and considerable health care costs.[54] The principal determinant of the risk of devastating diabetes complications is the total lifetime exposure to elevated blood glucose levels.[1] Therefore, establishing safe and effective methods of achieving and maintaining normoglycemia will have substantial implications for the health and the quality of life of individuals with diabetes.

The Diabetes Control and Complications Trial (DCCT) demonstrated that, given a qualified diabetes care team and intensive insulin treatment control, near-normalization of glycemia could be achieved and sustained for several years. However, such a near-perfect level of treatment would increase a patient's burden of day-to-day diabetes management, be difficult to implement for many patients, require more attention and medical services than are routinely available in clinical practice,[6] and be accompanied by an increased frequency of severe hypoglycemia.[1] Currently, the only way to restore sustained normoglycemia without the associated risk of hypoglycemia is to replace the patient's glucose-sensing and insulin-secreting pancreatic islet beta cells, either by the transplantation of a vascularized pancreas[81] or by the infusion of isolated pancreatic islets.[75] The tradeoff is the need for immunosuppression to prevent rejection of allogenic tissue, and for this reason most pancreas or islet transplant recipients have been adults. However, the potential for application earlier in the course of the disease exists, particularly in diabetic children already on immunosuppression for other indications.[3]

PANCREAS TRANSPLANTATION

History

The first clinical pancreas transplant was performed in 1966 by Drs. William Kelly and Richard Lillehei, simultaneous with a kidney transplant, in a uremic diabetic patient at the University of Minnesota.[46] Shortly thereafter a few institutions around the world began to perform pancreas transplants, as detailed in a comprehensive history in another book.[84]

The success rate (long-term insulin independence) with pancreas transplantation was initially low but increased considerably in the 1980s, leading to increased application (Fig. 44-1). Innovations in both surgical techniques and immunosuppression were responsible for the improvements.

The first pancreas transplant was a duct-ligated segmental (body and tail) graft,[46] but this approach was associated with multiple complications. In a series of 13 more

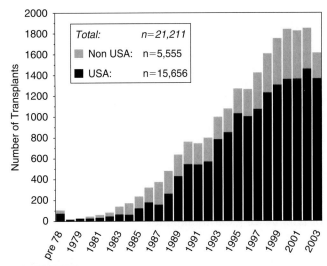

Pancreas Transplants Worldwide

Total: n=21,211
Non USA: n=5,555
USA: n=15,656

Figure 44–1 Annual number of U.S. and non-U.S. pancreas transplants reported to the International Pancreas Transplant Registry (IPTR), 1978-2003.

pancreas transplants between 1966 and 1973 at the University of Minnesota,[48,49] Lillehei devised the whole pancreas-duodenal transplant technique to the iliac vessels with enteric drainage via a duodenoenterostomy to native small bowel that is now routine at most centers. The initial results, however, were not as good as today, and several surgeons devised alternative techniques during the 1970s and early 1980s.[84] Dubernard, in Lyon, France, introduced duct injection of a synthetic polymer as a method to block secretions and cause fibrosis in the exocrine pancreas of a segmental graft with sparing of the endocrine component,[19] and many pioneering centers adopted this technique, although it is little used today. Gliedman introduced urinary drainage via a ureteroductostomy for segmental grafts,[23] and Sollinger later modified this approach with direct anastomosis of a duodenal patch of a whole pancreas graft to the recipient bladder.[70] Drs. Dai Nghiem and Robert Corry did further modification of urinary drainage,[57] retaining a bubble of duodenum for duodenocystostomy as Lillehei had done for duodenoenterostomy.[49] From the early 1980s until the mid-1990s, the bladder-drainage technique with duodenocystostomy was the predominant technique for pancreas transplants. The bladder-drainage technique had a low acute complication rate and was helpful in monitoring for rejection by detection of a decline in urine amylase activity, but chronic complications, such as recurrent urinary tract infections or dehydration from fluid loss via the exocrine secretions, were common. Thus, in the mid-1990s, a change occurred and enteric drainage, as described by Lillehei and colleagues[49] and never totally out of fashion,[72,79] overtook bladder drainage as the predominant drainage procedure. In addition, portal rather than systemic venous drainage was used by some groups for enteric-drained whole pancreas duodenal transplants.[65] Portal venous drainage was originally introduced by Calne in 1984 for segmental pancreas grafts as a more physiologic technique[12] and was applied by several groups sporadically over the years.[84]

With advances in immunosuppression, including the introduction of cyclosporine by Calne and coworkers in 1979,[13] tacrolimus by Starzl and associates in 1989,[73] and mycophenolate mofetil by Sollinger and coworkers in 1995,[61] bladder drainage had become less important for monitoring rejection. Furthermore, in recipients of simultaneous pancreas and kidney transplants from the same donor, the kidney could be monitored for rejection episodes (elevation of serum creatinine) as a surrogate marker for pancreas rejection before there was sufficient pancreas damage to cause hyperglycemia. However, in solitary pancreas transplants, serum creatinine could not be used as a marker for rejection, and in such cases bladder drainage is useful and continues to be employed.[84]

Details of Surgical Techniques

As mentioned in the history section, a variety of techniques have been used for management of the exocrine secretions and venous drainage of pancreas transplants. The majority of pancreas grafts are procured from multiorgan deceased donors; and because the liver and pancreas share the origins of their arterial blood supply, a whole-organ pancreas graft usually requires reconstruction.[8,52] The blood supply to the tail of the pancreas is supplied by the splenic artery originating from the celiac axis, and the head of the pancreas is supplied by the pancreaticoduodenal arcades originating from the superior mesenteric artery and the hepatic artery. Because the latter goes with the liver, along with the celiac axis, the usual approach is to attach an arterial Y-graft of the donor iliac vessels, with anastomosis of the hypogastric artery to the graft splenic artery and the external iliac artery to the graft superior mesenteric artery, leaving the common iliac artery segment of the Y-graft for anastomosis to the recipient arterial system, usually the right common iliac artery. The portal vein of the pancreas graft can be anastomosed and divided to bring it into the field or vena cava or to the recipient's superior mesenteric vein.

When venous drainage is to the recipient's iliac vein, the whole pancreas graft can be oriented with the head directed into either the pelvis or the upper abdomen. When directed cephalad, enteric drainage is the only option. When directed caudad, the duodenum can be anastomosed to either the bladder (Fig. 44-2) or bowel (Fig. 44-3). Figure 44-2 shows the bladder-drainage technique and also depicts a kidney transplant to the left iliac vessels, but, as mentioned, with a kidney transplant, enteric drainage is more common than bladder drainage.

With the bladder drainage technique, the anastomosis may be handsewn or performed with an EEA stapler brought through the distal duodenum (which is subsequently stapled closed) for connection to the post of the anvil projected through the posterior bladder via an anterior cystotomy (see Fig. 44-2). The inner layer is then reinforced with a running absorbable suture for hemostasis and for burying the staples under the mucosa.

With enteric drainage/systemic venous drainage, the anastomosis may be handsewn in an end-to-side fashion (Fig. 44-3), or it can be done in a side-to-side fashion by handsewing or by using an EEA stapler.[22a] The barrel of the EEA stapler is inserted into the end of the graft duodenum, and the post is projected through the side wall. The anvil is inserted into the recipient bowel through an enterotomy secured around the connecting post by a pursestring suture. The two posts are connected and the stapler is fired, creating the anastomosis. The end of the duodenum is then closed with a simple stapler. The enteric anastomosis can be done directly to the most convenient proximal small bowel loop of the recipient or to a Roux-en-Y segment of recipient bowel that is created at the time. Outcome analyses do not show any statistical advantage of a Roux-en-Y loop.

For portal drainage of the pancreas graft venous effluent (Fig. 44-4), the head and duodenum of the graft is oriented cephalad, and the graft portal vein is anastomosed directly to the recipient superior mesenteric vein. In the illustration, the pancreas graft is ventral to the recipient small bowel mesentery so the venous anastomosis is to the ventral side of the vein, and the arterial Y-graft must be brought through a window of mesentery for anastomosis to the recipient's aorta or common iliac artery. The graft duodenum is anastomosed to recipient small bowel by the same techniques described for systemic

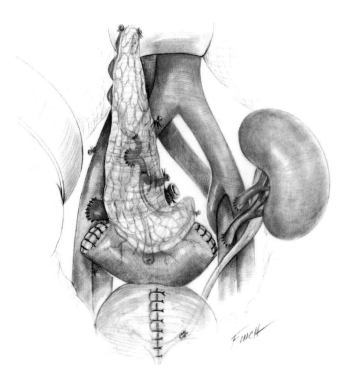

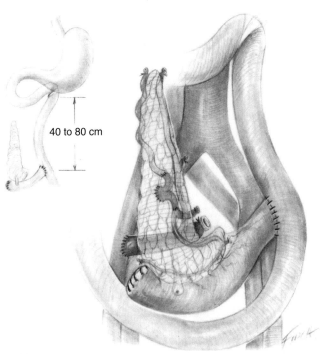

40 to 80 cm

Figure 44–3 Pancreas-duodenal transplant using a deceased donor with systemic venous drainage and enteric drainage of graft exocrine secretions to a proximal loop of recipient jejunum. In this particular case, an end-to-side two-layer duodenojejunostomy using the distal end of the graft duodenum is illustrated and the anastomosis is located 40 to 80 cm distal to the ligament of Treitz *(inset)*. Alternatively, a side-to-side stapled or handsewn duodenojejunostomy, with or without a Roux-en-Y loop, can be done. (Reproduced from Gruessner RWG, Sutherland DER [eds]: Transplantation of the Pancreas. New York, Springer-Verlag, 2004.)

Figure 44–2 Simultaneous pancreas and kidney (SPK) transplant using a whole pancreas/duodenal graft from a deceased donor with systemic venous drainage to the right iliac vein and bladder drainage of the pancreas exocrine secretions via a duodenocystostomy. Both the pancreas and kidney are placed in the peritoneum through a midline incision. The donor splenic artery, supplying the pancreatic tail, and the donor superior mesenteric artery, supplying the pancreatic head, have been joined by a Y-graft constructed from the donor common external/internal iliac artery complex during a bench procedure, and the base of the Y-graft is anastomosed to the recipient common iliac artery. The mid-duodenum is anastomosed to the posterior dome of the bladder, and the duodenal stumps are oversewn. The kidney graft could be from a living donor or the same deceased donor as the pancreas graft, but in either case is preferentially placed to the left iliac vessels so the right side, with its more superficial vessels, can be used for the pancreas transplant. In this particular illustration, the donor ureter was implanted into the bladder using the Politano-Leadbetter technique via an anterior cystotomy, a technique that also allows the duodenocystostomy to be performed with an EEA stapler, with internal oversewing of the anastomotic line using an absorbable suture to cover the staples, followed by closure of the cystotomy. However, when enteric drainage is used for an SPK transplant, an external ureteroneocystostomy is usually performed. (Reproduced from Gruessner RWG, Sutherland DER [eds]: Transplantation of the Pancreas. New York, Springer-Verlag, 2004.)

venous drainage, with or without (as depicted) a Roux-en-Y loop of recipient bowel.

An alternative approach for portal venous drainage of the pancreas graft effluent is to place the pancreas retroperitoneally by reflecting the right colon to the left and exposing the dorsal surface of the superior mesenteric vein, as described by Boggi and associates.[7,9] The arterial Y-graft can then be anastomosed directly to the right common iliac artery, but this approach does mandate creation of a Roux-en-Y limb of recipient bowel to bring

through the small bowel or transverse colon mesentery for a graft duodenoenterostomy.

Other techniques can be used, including duct injection for a segmental graft. Segmental grafts are rarely used except in the few cases of living donor pancreas transplants,[4,33,82] and most of these have the exocrine secretions managed by either a ductoenterostomy to a Roux-en-Y limb of recipient bowel or a ductocystostomy to the recipient's bladder (Fig. 44-5). Segmental pancreas transplants from living donors, with or without a kidney transplant, are particularly useful in candidates who would otherwise have a long wait for a deceased donor organ, such as those with a high level of human leukocyte antigen (HLA) antibodies but with a negative crossmatch to a living volunteer. For more details concerning the variety of surgical techniques in pancreas donors (deceased and living) and recipients, the reader is referred to work by Benedetti and colleagues.[5]

General Information, Pancreas Transplant Categories, and Immunosuppression

By the mid-1990s, more than 1500 pancreas transplants were being done annually worldwide (see Fig. 44-1), as reported

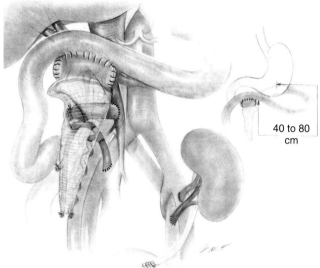

Figure 44–4 Whole pancreas/duodenum transplant using a deceased donor with portal venous drainage via an end-to-side anastomosis to the recipient superior mesenteric vein accessed below its confluence with the splenic vein. Drainage of exocrine secretions is via a side-to-side duodenojejunostomy, 40 to 80 cm distal to the ligament of Treitz. Note that the cephalad position of the pancreatic head when portal venous drainage is employed, as opposed to the caudal orientation possible with systemic venous drainage, is no different than that needed when bladder drainage is done. In this particular illustration, the pancreas graft overlies the root of the small bowel mesentery, with the duodenal segment below the transverse colon, and the arterial Y-graft is anastomosed to the recipient common iliac artery through a mesenteric tunnel. However, a retroperitoneal approach under the right colon is also possible, in which case the arterial Y-graft can be anastomosed directly to the recipient iliac artery but the enteric anastomosis must be via a Roux-en-Y limb of recipient bowel brought through the mesentery. If a kidney is simultaneously transplanted to the left iliac vessels, the ureter can be implanted into the bladder using the extravesical ureteroneocystostomy (Lich) technique, as illustrated. (Reproduced from Gruessner RWG, Sutherland DER [eds]: Transplantation of the Pancreas. New York, Springer-Verlag, 2004.)

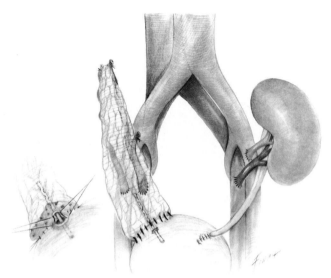

Figure 44–5 Living donor segmental (body and tail) pancreas transplant to right iliac vessels (systemic venous drainage) and bladder drainage of exocrine secretions via a ductocystostomy by means of an intraperitoneal approach. The donor splenic artery and splenic vein are anastomosed end to side to the recipient external iliac artery and vein after ligation and division of all hypogastric veins to bring the main vein as superficial as possible. The splenic artery anastomosis is lateral and proximal to the splenic vein anastomosis. A two-layer ductocystostomy is constructed: the pancreatic duct is approximated to the urothelial layer (inner layer) using interrupted 7-0 absorbable sutures over a stent *(inset)*. If the kidney is transplanted simultaneously, the donor ureter is implanted into the bladder using the extravesical ureteroneocystostomy (Lich) technique. (Reproduced from Gruessner RWG, Sutherland DER [eds]: Transplantation of the Pancreas. New York, Springer-Verlag, 2004.)

to the International Pancreas Transplant Registry (IPTR).[29] By 2003, more than 21,000 vascularized pancreas transplants had been performed, approximately three-fourths in the United States, with very large series at some centers.[79] The vast majority were done to establish insulin independence in patients with de novo type 1 diabetes mellitus, but enteric-drained pancreas transplants have been used to correct both endocrine and exocrine deficiency after total pancreatectomy in some patients[31,34] and to treat diseases such as cystic fibrosis in others.[74]

Specialists in more than 120 institutions in the United States and nearly the same number elsewhere have performed pancreas transplants.[29] The IPTR was founded in 1980 to analyze the cases.[80] In 1987, reporting of U.S. cases became obligatory through the United Network for Organ Sharing (UNOS), and annual reports have been made thereafter.[28-30]

There are three categories of pancreas transplant recipients: (1) uremic diabetic patients who undergo a simultaneous pancreas and kidney (SPK) transplant from either a deceased or living donor[33]; (2) nephropathic patients who already have had renal insufficiency corrected, usually by a living donor kidney transplant, and then undergo a pancreas after kidney (PAK) transplant; and (3) nonuremic diabetic patients who undergo a pancreas transplant alone (PTA). The Pancreas Transplant Registry has compared outcomes in the three categories over several eras of data collection.[28-30]

The majority of pancreas transplants have been in the SPK category, but in recent years there has been an increased emphasis in performing living donor kidney transplants to preempt the need for dialysis in diabetics with nephropathy. Thus, the number of PAK transplants has increased as the number of SPK transplants has declined (Fig. 44-6). Concomitantly, there has also been an increase in the number of PTA cases to treat diabetics without advanced nephropathy who have diabetic management problems justifying immunosuppression and to treat patients who would also be candidates for islet transplantation given the conditions discussed later.

Immunosuppression management of pancreas transplant recipients is similar to that of recipients of other solid organs, including kidneys, which the majority of pancreas recipients also receive. Thus, induction immunosuppression with anti–T-cell monoclonal or polyclonal depleting

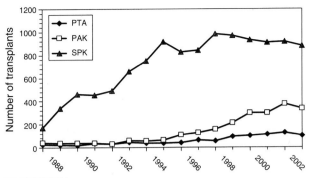

Figure 44–6 Number of pancreas transplants performed annually in the United States from 1988 through 2003 by recipient category. PTA, pancreas transplant alone; SPK, simultaneous pancreas-kidney; PAK, pancreas after kidney transplant.

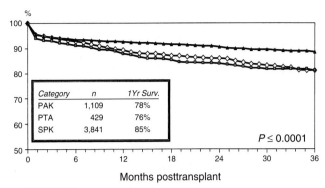

Figure 44–8 Pancreas graft functional survival rates (insulin independence) for 2000-2004 U.S. deceased donor primary transplants by recipient category. PTA, pancreas transplant alone; SPK, simultaneous pancreas-kidney; PAK, pancreas after kidney transplant.

or nondepleting agents may be used or reserved for rejection episodes. Maintenance immunosuppression usually consists of a combination of a calcineurin inhibitor (cyclosporine or tacrolimus), with the dose and blood levels adjusted to minimize nephrotoxicity, and an antiproliferative agent (mycophenolate mofetil or sirolimus), with or without prednisone. Corticosteroid-free regimens are now quite common for all organ transplants, including the pancreas.[45]

Pancreas Transplant Outcomes

Current outcomes with deceased donor pancreas transplants according to recipient categories, surgical technique, and immunosuppression protocol, for U.S. cases as reported to UNOS from January 2000 to June 2004, are summarized here. During this period, more than 5,800 pancreas transplants were reported to UNOS, including more than 3,800 SPK transplants, more than 1,300 PAK transplants, and more than 400 PTAs.

The primary transplant patient survival rates in the three recipient categories are shown in Figure 44-7. At 1 year,

95% of the SPK, 95% of the PAK, and 98% of the PTA recipients were alive; at 3 years, 90%, 88%, and 95%, respectively, were alive ($P = 0.05$). The highest patient survival rate was in the PTA category, presumably because this group had less advanced complications before transplantation.

The primary pancreas graft survival rates in the three recipient categories are shown in Figure 44-8. At 1 year, 85% of the SPK, 78% of the PAK, and 76% of the PTA recipients were insulin-independent; at 3 years, 77%, 62% and 62%, respectively, were insulin-independent ($P < 0.001$). The highest pancreas graft survival rates are in the SPK category, presumably because the kidney graft (usually from the same donor as the pancreas) can be used to detect rejection episodes earlier than in the other categories where only the pancreas can be monitored. Support for this hypothesis comes from Registry data showing no significant differences in graft technical failure rates between categories but large differences in rejection loss rates.

Of the 2000-2004 primary pancreas grafts, 8% failed for technical reasons, with thrombosis being the highest risk for technical loss (5%); infection, pancreatitis, and anastomotic leak made up the rest. There were no significant differences between categories in regard to technical losses.

The primary pancreas graft failure rates from rejection are shown in Figure 44-9. At 1 year, 2% of the SPK, 8% of the PAK, and 10% of the PTA recipients of technically successful grafts had to resume exogenous insulin (significantly lower in the SPK category; $P = 0.0001$).

In regard to management of pancreatic duct exocrine secretions for 2000-2004 cases, enteric drainage predominated for SPK transplants (81%); for PAK and PTA, the proportion that were enteric-drained was slightly lower (67% and 56%, respectively). Overall, the technical failure rate was slightly higher with enteric drainage than with bladder drainage (8% versus 6%). Pancreas graft survival rates, however, were not significantly different for enteric-drained versus bladder-drained transplants in any of the categories: at 1 year they were 85% (n = 3047) versus 87% (n = 707) for SPK; 77% (n = 733) versus 80% (n = 364) for PAK; and 72% (n = 238) versus 79% (n = 184) for PTA cases. For PTA, the failure rate from rejection

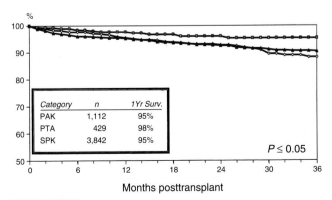

Figure 44–7 Patient survival rates for 2000-2004 U.S. deceased donor primary transplants by recipient category. PTA, pancreas transplant alone; SPK, simultaneous pancreas-kidney; PAK, pancreas after kidney transplant.

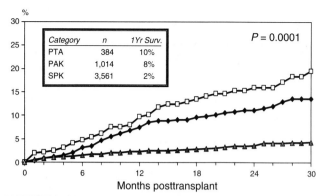

Figure 44–9 Technically successful pancreas graft immunologic failure rates (return to exogenous insulin) for 2000-2004 U.S. deceased donor primary transplants by recipient category. PTA, pancreas transplant alone; SPK, simultaneous pancreas-kidney; PAK, pancreas after kidney transplant.

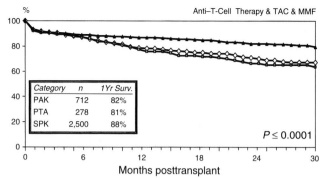

Figure 44–10 Pancreas graft functional survival rates (insulin independence) for 2000-2004 U.S. deceased donor primary transplants by category in diabetic recipients given anti–T-cell agents for induction and tacrolimus (TAC) and mycophenolate mofetil (MMF) for maintenance immunosuppression. PTA, pancreas transplant alone; SPK, simultaneous pancreas-kidney; PAK, pancreas after kidney transplant.

for technically successful grafts was significantly lower with bladder drainage than enteric drainage: 5% (n = 161) versus 15% (n = 216) at 1 year (P = 0.03).

In the SPK category, bladder drainage and enteric drainage would be expected to give similar results: in most cases both grafts come from the same donor, and monitoring of serum creatinine serves as a surrogate marker for rejection in the pancreas transplant, allowing easy detection and reversal by treatment. In contrast, for solitary pancreas transplants (PAK and PTA), serum creatinine cannot be used as a marker of pancreas rejection; hyperglycemia is a late manifestation of rejection and exocrine markers must be used. Although serum amylase and lipase may elevate during a rejection episode, this does not occur in all cases; but for bladder-drained grafts, a decrease in urine amylase eventually always accompanies rejection (100% sensitive, even though it is not specific) and nearly always precedes hyperglycemia, so a rejection episode is more likely to be diagnosed in a bladder-drained graft and lead to treatment and reversal.

Of note, for enteric-drained grafts in all categories, the pancreas graft survival rates were slightly lower when a Roux-en-Y loop of recipient bowel was used for the enteric anastomosis.[29] Approximately one-third of enteric-drained pancreas grafts reported to UNOS were done with a Roux-en-Y loop, but the outcomes are not improved by this procedural addition; and at least in PTA recipients the technical failure rate was higher when a Roux-en-Y loop was used.[29]

Another variation in surgical technique is portal drainage of the venous effluent for enteric-drained grafts.[64] It establishes normal physiology and a theoretic metabolic advantage over systemic venous drainage, and some groups have reported that portal venous enteric-drainage grafts are less prone to rejection than systemic venous enteric-drainage grafts.[58,78] The latest Registry analysis shows that portal venous drainage was used for one-fifth of enteric-drainage transplants, but there were no significant differences in pancreas graft survival versus systemic venous enteric-drainage transplants in any of the categories: at 1 year, 85% (n = 610) versus 85% (n = 2437)

for SPK; 78% (n = 168) versus 77% (n = 564) for PAK; and 71% (n = 85) versus 72% (n = 153) for PTA cases.

In regard to immunosuppression, according to the latest Registry analysis, anti–T-cell agents were used for induction therapy in about three-fourths of 2000-2004 U.S. pancreas recipients in each category.[30] The most frequently used regimen for maintenance immunosuppression (two-thirds of the recipients in each category) was tacrolimus and mycophenolate mofetil in combination, with or without prednisone. In recipients of primary deceased donor pancreas grafts given anti–T-cell agents for induction and tacrolimus and mycophenolate mofetil for maintenance immunosuppression (Fig. 44-10), the 1-year graft survival rates in the SPK, PAK, and PTA categories were 88% (n = 2500), 82% (n = 712), and 81% (n = 278), respectively. Sirolimus was used as a maintenance immunosuppressive drug in about one-sixth of recipients in each category (Fig. 44-11), with comparable outcomes: the 1-year pancreas graft survival rates in the SPK, PAK, and PTA categories were 87% (n = 675), 82% (n = 184),

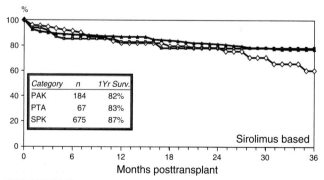

Figure 44–11 Pancreas graft functional survival rates (insulin independence) for 2000-2004 U.S. deceased donor primary transplants by category in diabetic recipients given sirolimus-based maintenance immunosuppression. PTA, pancreas transplant alone; SPK, simultaneous pancreas-kidney; PAK, pancreas after kidney transplant.

and 83% (n = 67), respectively. In contrast, the remaining one-sixth of recipients given alternative immunosuppressive regimens had distinctly lower pancreas graft survival rates in each category: at 1 year, 63% in SPK (n = 666), 61% in PAK (n = 213), and 54% in PTA (n = 84) cases. A center effect may play a role in the outcomes of the Registry analysis according to immunosuppressive regimens.

In regard to the logistics of pancreas transplantation, the recent Registry data[30] showed a slight increase in technical failure rates and a slight decrease in graft survival rates with increasing preservation time. For example, in the SPK category, 1-year pancreas graft survival rates were 86% with 4 to 7 hours of preservation versus 81% with 28 to 31 hours of preservation. HLA matching had virtually no impact on SPK graft survival rates, but matching at least at the class I loci had a beneficial effect in the PAK and the PTA categories.

In regard to pancreas recipient age, the recent Registry analysis of 2000-2004 cases showed an effect on outcome mainly in PTA recipients, with rejection more likely in the youngest patients. In the PAK category, all recipients were older than 20 years; per an analysis of rejection rates by decade of age, at 1 year the rates varied from 4% to 7%. In the SPK category, the rejection rate at 1 year was 2% to 4% in the various age groups older than 20 years but 0% for those younger than 20 years (n = 4). In contrast, in the PTA category the rejection rate at 1 year was 50% for those younger than 20 (n = 14) and 13% for those 20 to 29 (n = 39); for PTA recipients older than 30 the 1-year rejection loss rates were 4% to 6%, similar to the other two recipient categories. Thus, the young nonuremic diabetic is highly immunocompetent and more prone to reject a pancreas graft, consistent with an earlier analysis of outcomes in U.S. pediatric pancreas transplant recipients from 1988 to 1999.[27] In that analysis, out of slightly more than 8,000 pancreas transplants, only 49 were in recipients younger than 21 (<1%), 34 in the SPK, 2 in the PAK, and 13 in the PTA category; all were deceased donor pancreas transplants except for two PTA segmental grafts from living donors. Less than half of the pediatric pancreas recipients were younger than 19. In the PTA recipients, the 1-year graft survival rate was only 15%, with all but one loss being from rejection in less than 1 year. The Registry data do not include the indications for a PTA in the pediatric recipients, but presumably they had extremely labile diabetes, justifying placement on immunosuppression in an attempt to gain control. In the pediatric SPK recipients, however, the 1-year patient, pancreas, and kidney graft survival rates were 96%, 78%, and 71%, respectively, which were outcomes comparable to those of adult SPK recipients for the entire period. Of the pediatric SPK recipients, most had a renal disease other than diabetic nephropathy.

Thus, pancreas transplants in the pediatric age group are uncommon, and most are in diabetic children who also have renal failure and thus need a kidney transplant, obligating them to immunosuppression. At least in this group, the outcomes are such that it seems reasonable to recommend the addition of the pancreas so the child can become insulin-independent as well as dialysis-free for the price of immunosuppression. For nonuremic diabetic children with extreme lability in whom a successful pancreas transplant would be appropriate treatment, the antirejection strategies need to be optimized to improve the graft survival rates over what has been achieved in the past.

With respect to outcome measures other than insulin independence, prevention and reversal of secondary complications, improvement in quality of life, expansion of life span, and reduction of health care costs per quality-adjusted life year have all been positively demonstrated in type 1 diabetic pancreas transplant recipients.[18,20,26,56,76,88,97] In patients with labile diabetes and hypoglycemic unawareness, a pancreas transplant can resolve an otherwise intractable and life-threatening course.[47,55,63]

Whether a pancreas transplant has an effect on survival probabilities for the diabetic population selected for the procedure is controversial. Two separate analyses of U.S. data from UNOS and the Organ Procurement Transplant Network (OPTN) for pancreas transplant candidates and recipients between 1995 and 2000 compared the survival probabilities for patients who remained on the waiting list versus those receiving a transplant by category.[32,90] In the first analysis,[90] SPK recipients had a significantly higher probability of survival than those remaining on the waiting list for the procedure, but for solitary (PAK or PTA) recipients just the opposite was the case. In the second analysis,[32] the higher survival probability for SPK recipients was confirmed, and, in addition, the overall survival probabilities of solitary pancreas transplant recipients compared with those waiting and even after 1 year were favorable for transplantation. In the second analysis, patients who listed at multiple centers were identified and were counted only once, corrections were made for patients who changed categories, and longer follow-up was available. Thus, pancreas transplantation does not entail a higher risk than staying on exogenous insulin for those on the waiting list and may improve survival probabilities for solitary as well as SPK recipients.

ISLET TRANSPLANTATION

The less invasive alternative to transplantation of the pancreas or an immediately vascularized graft solely for beta cell replacement is transplantation of isolated islets as a free graft.[39,41,59,94] The first clinical islet allograft was in 1974 in a diabetic recipient of a previous kidney transplant[53]; and more than 700 islet allotransplants have since been performed. The success rate with islet allotransplants was low until recently (beginning in 2000). However, islet autotransplants have had a relatively high success rate in preventing diabetes after total pancreatectomy for more than 2 decades, so they are briefly described before reviewing the current status of islet allografts for type 1 as well as for surgical diabetes.

Islet Autotransplants at Pancreatectomy for Benign Disease

Islet autotransplants to prevent diabetes after a total pancreatectomy for benign disease, such as chronic pancreatitis,

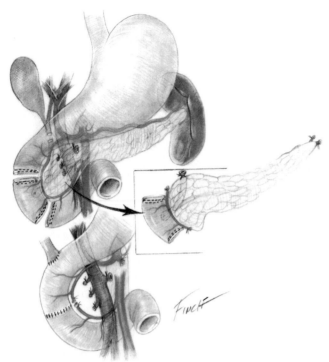

Figure 44–12 Pylorus-sparing total pancreatectomy and partial duodenectomy technique for patients with chronic pancreatitis undergoing islet autotransplants. The bile duct is transected and reimplanted into the duodenum, shown here proximal to a duodenoduodenostomy or duodenojejunostomy, but more commonly it is placed distal to the enteric anastomosis, with the site depending on the individual anatomy. When possible, only the second portion of the duodenum is resected and an end-to-end duodenoduodenostomy is created; but if viability is not maintained, the entire distal duodenum must be resected and an end-to-end or end-to-side duodenojejunostomy performed. The short gastric vessels are preserved, as well as the gastroepiploic artery if possible, and the spleen is not removed if its viability is maintained. (Reproduced from Gruessner RWG, Sutherland DER [eds]: Transplantation of the Pancreas. New York, Springer-Verlag, 2004.)

have been successful since the first case was performed in the 1970s, but depend on the number of islets transplanted.[83,85,92] Children with chronic pancreatitis and intractable pain who required pancreatectomy for resolution of narcotic dependence have had diabetes prevented by islet autotransplants.[83,91] The surgical technique of pylorus-sparing total pancreatectomy and duodenectomy is shown in Figure 44-12. The procedure can be staged, but when the body and tail of the pancreas are removed they should always be processed for islet isolation for an intraportal autotransplant (Fig. 44-13A).

If a distal pancreatectomy is the primary procedure and a Whipple (completion) pancreatectomy becomes necessary, diabetes will have been prophylactically prevented by the initial islet autograft. If a Whipple procedure was the primary procedure but pain persists and a distal (body and tail) completion pancreatectomy is required, it should be done in an institution capable of isolating islets from the excised gland for an autotransplant.

Islet Allotransplants

Islet allografts in patients with surgical diabetes have also been associated with a very high success rate.[62,89] Islet allograft transplants in patients with autoimmune type 1 diabetes have been more challenging; insulin independence in this recipient group, even on an anecdotal basis, was not achieved until the early 1990s.[11,24,67,68,93]

Islet allotransplants, as with autotransplants, are usually done with embolization of the islets to the liver via the portal vein, where at least some islets will survive by nutrient diffusion until revascularization occurs (see Fig. 44-13B). A drawback of islet allotransplants, as compared with pancreas transplants, is the reduced beta cell mass; much attention has been given to compensating for the attrition that occurs.

Recently, increasing the mass of transplanted islet cells and choosing combinations of antirejection agents to reduce the diabetogenic side effects of immunosuppressive drugs have markedly improved the success rate of islet allografts. Shapiro and associates reported achieving insulin independence after repeated islet transplants (sequential multiple donors) in 7 of 7 type 1 diabetic patients given glucocorticoid-free immunosuppression with daclizumab, sirolimus, and relatively low-dose tacrolimus.[69]

Corticosteroids are highly diabetogenic and are a known risk factor for posttransplant diabetes in recipients of organ allografts of all types. Although the incidence of drug-induced diabetes is low in pancreas allograft recipients, this is because an intact normal pancreas has a high beta cell mass but with islet isolation there is a substantial reduction. Thus, in the presence of diabetogenic immunosuppression, a single islet donor may not suffice. By eliminating one agent that is diabetogenic (corticosteroids) and by reducing the dose of another diabetogenic but potent immunosuppressant, tacrolimus, and adding sirolimus (a less diabetogenic but perhaps as potent an immunosuppressant as tacrolimus), the beta cell mass transplanted was sufficient to eliminate the need for exogenous insulin in an expanding series.[66] The results of the Edmonton group suggested that if a totally nondiabetogenic immunosuppressive regimen potent enough to prevent rejection could be devised, even a single islet donor could suffice.[66] Alternatively, improving the efficiency of islet cell isolation in terms of viable beta cell mass might allow a single donor to suffice even if the immunosuppressive regimen was not completely free of diabetogenicity, as is the case for the Edmonton protocol.

The diabetogenic side effects of prior conventional immunosuppressive therapy certainly is one reason for the historically poor success rate of human islet allografts. Less than 50% of the islets are usually isolated, and less than 50% of transplanted islet beta cells engraft.[17] That immunosuppressive drugs are diabetogenic (not only glucocorticoids but also the calcineurin inhibitors tacrolimus and cyclosporine) particularly at high doses, increasing insulin need while inhibiting insulin secretion, is well documented.[15] The full islet mass of an immediately vascularized pancreas graft is able to overcome drug-induced insulin resistance whereas achieving

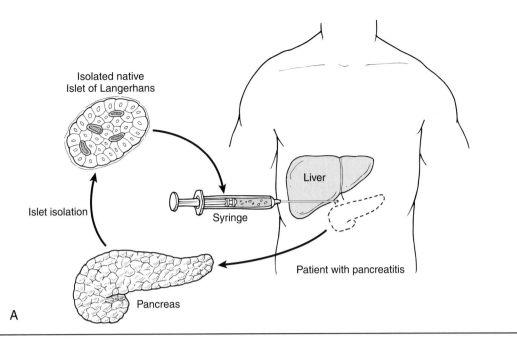

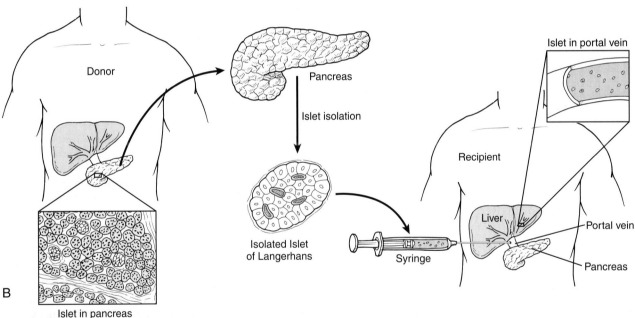

Figure 44–13 Islet transplantation using the portal vein for embolization to the liver where revascularization will occur, either as an autograft of islets isolated from the excised specimen after pancreatectomy for benign disease (*A*) or as an allograft of cells isolated from a donor for treatment of a patient with type 1 diabetes (*B*).

the critical beta cell mass necessary to do so with an islet graft is more difficult, at least at the moment. Fortunately, the new generation of immunosuppressive drugs has made the use of prednisone unnecessary for the majority of recipients in clinical transplantation and also has allowed calcineurin inhibitors to be used in lower, less diabetogenic doses.[21,22]

The ability to consistently achieve insulin independence in diabetic patients by islet allotransplants, first reported by the Edmonton group,[69] has been confirmed at other institutions.[25,36,37,44,51] In most series, however, the recipients

required islets from two or more donor pancreases.[25,44,51,69] For islet allotransplantation to replace pancreas transplantation, or to become a clinically significant treatment option on a large scale for the diabetic population, will require additional advances, including maximization of the islet cell yield and potency as well as minimization of immunosuppressive failures and risks.

Several strategies designed to promote the potency, engraftment, and functional survival of transplanted islet cells were evaluated in two recent islet transplant trials at the University of Minnesota: (1) excluding pancreases from donors older than 50 years, (2) limiting ischemic injury of islets during pancreas storage, (3) avoiding islet-toxic reagents during islet processing, (4) culturing islets to allow pretransplant initiation of immunosuppression, (5) providing potent prophylactic anticoagulation and aggressive insulin therapy peritransplant, (6) increasing the immunosuppressive and anti-inflammatory potency of induction immunosuppression, and (7) avoiding glucocorticoids and minimizing calcineurin inhibitors in maintenance immunosuppression.[36,37] In two pilot islet transplant trials in type 1 diabetic patients with hypoglycemia unawareness, 12 of 14 recipients with type 1 diabetes achieved insulin independence after single-donor islet transplants, with normal HbA_{1c} levels. The outcome suggests that some or all of the seven strategies facilitate consistent reversal of type 1 diabetes with islets prepared from one pancreas. Three of the strategies are of particular importance:

First, pancreas preservation methods that are adequate for prolonged cold storage before vascularized pancreas transplants are inadequate for even a short period of cold storage before islet isolation and transplants. The cellular stress encountered during islet isolation is compounded by any preceding cold ischemic injury of the donor pancreas; moreover, such stress exceeds the cellular stress associated with reperfusion injury that islets are subjected to after a vascularized pancreas transplant.[38] Experimental evidence indicates that the two-layer (perfluorodecalin/University of Wisconsin [UW] solution) pancreas preservation method both increases the yield of the islet isolation process and preserves the ability of isolated islets to reverse diabetes.[42,87]

Second, the intravascular location of intraportally transplanted islets immediately exposes the graft to primed autoreactive, islet beta cell–directed T cells. This location may also hasten the mounting of alloimmune responses. Pretransplant islet culture permits achievement of an immunosuppressed state well before islet infusion; it may also limit the diminution of islet mass, immediately post-transplant, because of autoimmunity, alloimmunity, and innate immunity.[35] The allogeneic islet mass needed to achieve insulin independence is higher in type 1 diabetic patients, as compared with surgically diabetic patients. This difference suggests that engraftment and survival of allogeneic islets is compromised in an autoimmune environment.[39] The need for more than one donor pancreas in the Edmonton experience[69] may reflect the inability of anti–IL-2R monoclonal antibodies (mAbs) to abrogate early effector responses mediated by persisting autoimmunity. Consequently, we targeted autoreactive T cells in the peritransplant period with anti-CD3 antibodies or polyclonal T cell antibodies, two of the very few strategies proven effective in inhibiting activated autoreactive T cells.[14,50,96]

Finally, pretransplant islet culture was a critical component of our study protocols. It allows achievement of T cell–directed immunosuppression in the recipient well before islet infusion, which is likely important in reducing islet-directed immune responses mediated by autoreactive, primed T cells to which the intravascularly transplanted islets are immediately exposed.

Delaying transplantation until 2 days after the initiation of therapy with T cell–depleting antibodies prevents exposure of transplanted islets to the cytokine release associated, to varying degrees, with the first and second antibody infusions. Pretransplant culture also allows quality control studies to be performed before the infusion of tissue, thereby avoiding transplantation of tissue not meeting more thorough release criteria. Studies in animals indicate improved metabolic efficacy of cultured (as opposed to freshly isolated) islets.[43] The results of our recent clinical trials are consistent with those of experimental studies, suggesting that pretransplant islet culture does not have deleterious, and may have beneficial, metabolic effects beyond the immunologic advantages.

Thus, incorporation of several advances into revised islet transplant protocols appears to facilitate outcomes in selected islet recipients. Novel, glucocorticoid-free and calcineurin inhibitor-free, nondiabetogenic immunosuppressive regimens have proven safe and effective in the relevant preclinical nonhuman primate islet allotransplant model[2,95] and are expected to lead to further significant improvements in islet transplant outcomes.

Nonetheless, until the logistical and islet yield problems have been solved, pancreas transplants will remain the most efficient use of the majority of donor organs. Obviously, for correction of diabetes, a simple cell transplant is preferable to the major surgery of a pancreas transplant, but islet isolation requires a specialized facility whereas pancreas transplants can be done at virtually any hospital with a transplant program and appropriately trained surgeons. Demonstration of control and consistency of human islet processing techniques, predictability of posttransplant islet function by islet product potency assays, and documentation of clinical safety and efficacy of islet transplants are needed for licensure of isolated human islets as a biologic product. Such a license will be critical to securing third-party reimbursement, which may provide a strong incentive for maximizing donor pancreas utilization. Progress in pancreas preservation techniques and the creation of regional islet processing centers may lead to adjustments in donor pancreas allocation algorithms and overcome logistical and technical impediments, resulting in increased availability of islet transplants.

At the moment, generalized immunosuppression is needed to prevent rejection of either an immediately vascularized pancreas or a neovascularized islet allograft. However, protocols designed to induce immunologic tolerance specific to the donor can be tested more readily in islet than in solid organ recipients: the magnitude of the surgical procedure and the consequences of rejection failure are less.[40] Thus, it is critical to continue islet allotransplants with novel immune monitoring and antirejection strategies even if at the moment pancreas transplants predominate as the clinical mode of beta cell replacement for type 1 diabetes mellitus.

Although a transition from pancreas to islet transplants as the dominant form of beta cell replacement therapy may occur over the next few years, pancreas transplants will not disappear entirely. Patients with high pretransplant insulin requirements in whom diabetes reversal with islet transplants is less likely would best be served with a vascularized pancreas transplant. Furthermore, diabetic patients with exocrine deficiency would best be served by an enteric-drained pancreas transplant. In addition, in patients who have very high insulin requirements or insulin resistance (type 2 diabetes), an intact organ may be needed to obtain a sufficient islet mass to restore insulin independence from a single donor in the presence of insulin resistance.

Tissue availability will be the limiting factor in determining the magnitude of the impact of beta cell replacement therapy. Six thousand deceased donors are available each year in the United States, but it is estimated that only half have a pancreas suitable for transplantation. Thus, the maximal number of pancreas transplants that could be done in the United States is 12,000 per year, assuming that each deceased pancreas could be split for use in two recipients,[86] and that living donors would be used for segmental pancreas transplants[33] to the extent that they have been for kidney transplants (currently about 6000 per year in the United States). This scenario has not yet materialized, but the potential is there to transplant at a rate approaching half of the annual incidence of new-onset cases of type 1 diabetes (30,000/year in the United States). The numbers could be increased further if enough islets could be isolated from one donor for transplants into more than two recipients. Although the efficacy of islet transplant protocols will continue to improve and the procedural and immunosuppressive risks now associated with islet transplants will continue to diminish, islet transplants will not be the ultimate approach to diabetes care. Just as pancreas transplants set the stage for islet transplants, the real value of islet transplants will be to create and build momentum for the development of xenogeneic and stem/precursor cell–derived islet beta cell therapy[10,60,71] that will then make cell replacement therapy routine and commonplace in diabetes care.

Pancreas transplants, and eventually islet transplants, should be in the armamentarium of every transplant center for the treatment of diabetic patients. Likewise, every endocrinologist should consider beta cell replacement in the treatment of patients in whom type 1 diabetes is complicated by hypoglycemia-associated autonomic failure[16] and/or progressive microvascular complications. Continued clinical research on pancreas and islet transplants is needed to identify the most appropriate recipient population, the optimal timing in the course of diabetes, and the most suitable donor tissue and transplant protocol for a given patient. Both pancreas and islet transplants need to be made as economical as possible.[77] Studies such as those done in pancreas-kidney transplant recipients showing the efficiency in the treatment of complicated diabetes[18] are needed in islet recipients as well. Currently, beta cell replacement has a well-defined clinical role for adult patients with incapacitating hypoglycemic unawareness and is also appropriate in children and adults who otherwise need immunosuppression, such as for a kidney transplant. As antirejection strategies become safer with fewer side effects, the indications for pediatric beta cell replacement therapy can be liberalized.

ACKNOWLEDGMENT

We are indebted to Heather Nelson for assistance in preparing the manuscript.

REFERENCES

1. The effect of intensive treatment of diabetes on the development and progression of long-term complications in insulin-dependent diabetes mellitus. The Diabetes Control and Complications Trial Research Group. N Engl J Med 1993;329:977-986.
2. Adams AB, Shirasugi N, Durham MM, et al: Calcineurin inhibitor-free CD28 blockade-based protocol protects allogeneic islets in nonhuman primates. Diabetes 2002;51:265-270.
3. Bendel-Stenzel MR, Kashtan CE, Sutherland DER, Chavers BM: Simultaneous pancreas-kidney transplant in two children with hemolytic-uremic symptoms. Pediatr Nephrol 1997;11:485-487.
4. Benedetti E, Dunn T, Massad MG, et al: Successful living related simultaneous pancreas-kidney transplant between identical twins. Transplantation 1999;67:915-918.
5. Benedetti E, Sileri P, Kandaswamy R, et al: Surgical aspects of pancreas transplantation. In Gruessner RW, Sutherland DER (eds): Transplantation of the Pancreas. New York, Springer-Verlag, 2004, pp 111-178.
6. Bloomgarden ZT: American Diabetes Association Postgraduate Course, 1996: treatment and prevention of diabetes. Diabetes Care 1996;19:784-786.
7. Boggi U, Vistoli F, Del Chiaro M, et al: Portal enteric-drained solitary pancreas transplantation without surveillance biopsy: Is it safe? Transplant Proc 2004;36:1090-1092.
8. Boggi U, Vistoli F, Del Chiaro M, et al: A simplified technique for the en bloc procurement of abdominal organs that is suitable for pancreas and small-bowel transplantation. Surgery 2004;135:629-641.
9. Boggi U, Vistoli F, Signori S, et al: A new technique for retroperitoneal pancreas transplantation with portal-enteric drainage. Transplantation 2005;79:1137-1142.
10. Bonner-Weir S, Sharma A: Pancreatic stem cells. J Pathol 2002;197:519-526.
11. Bretzel RG, Hering BJ, Federlin KF: Islet cell transplantation in diabetes mellitus—from bench to bedside. Exp Clin Endocrinol Diabetes 2004;103(Suppl 2):143-159.
12. Calne RY: Paratopic segmental pancreas grafting: A technique with portal venous drainage. Lancet 1984;1:595-597.
13. Calne RY, Rolles K, White DJ, et al: Cyclosporin A initially as the only immunosuppressant in 34 recipients of cadaveric organs: 32 kidneys, 2 pancreases, and 2 livers. Lancet 1979;2:1033-1036.
14. Chatenoud L, Thervet E, Primo J, Bach JF: Anti-CD3 antibody induces long-term remission of overt autoimmunity in nonobese diabetic mice. Proc Natl Acad Sci U S A 1994;91:123-127.
15. Christiansen E, Andersen HB, Rasmussen K, et al: Pancreatic beta-cell function and glucose metabolism in human segmental pancreas and kidney transplantation. Am J Physiol 1993;264(3 Pt 1):E441-E449.
16. Cryer PE: Banting lecture. Hypoglycemia: The limiting factor in the management of IDDM. Diabetes 1994;43:1378-1389.
17. Davalli AM, Ogawa Y, Scaglia L, et al: Function, mass, and replication of porcine and rat islets transplanted into diabetic nude mice. Diabetes 1995;44:104-111.

18. Douzdjian V, Ferrara D, Silvestri G: Treatment strategies for insulin-dependent diabetics with ESRD: A cost-effectiveness decision analysis model. Am J Kidney Dis 1998;31:794-802.

19. Dubernard JM, Traeger J, Neyra P, et al: A new method of preparation of segmental pancreatic grafts for transplantation: Trials in dogs and in man. Surgery 1978;84:633-640.

20. Fioretto P, Steffes MW, Sutherland DER, et al: Reversal of lesions of diabetic nephropathy after pancreas transplantation. N Engl J Med 1998;339:69-75.

21. First MR: Immunosuppressive agents and their actions. Transplant Proc 2002;34:1369-1371.

22. First MR, Gerber DA, Hariharan S, et al: Posttransplant diabetes mellitus in kidney allograft recipients: Incidence, risk factors, and management. Transplantation 2002;73: 379-386.

22a. Fridell JA, Milgrom M, Henson S, et al: Use of the end-to-end anastomotic circular stapler for creation of the duodenoenterostomy for enteric drainage of the pancreas allograft. J Am Coll Surg 2004;198:495-497.

23. Gliedman ML, Gold M, Whittaker J, et al: Clinical segmental pancreatic transplantation with ureter-pancreatic duct anastomosis for exocrine drainage. Surgery 1973;74: 171-180.

24. Gores PF, Najarian JS, Stephanian E, et al: Insulin independence in type I diabetes after transplantation of unpurified islets from a single donor using 15-deoxyspergualin. Lancet 1993;341:19-21.

25. Goss JA, Schock AP, Brunicardi FC, et al: Achievement of insulin independence in three consecutive type-1 diabetic patients via pancreatic islet transplantation using islets isolated at a remote islet isolation center. Transplantation 2002;74:1761-1766.

26. Gross CR, Limwattananon C, Matthees BJ: Quality of life after pancreas transplantation: A review. Clin Transplant 1998;12:351-361.

27. Gruessner AC: Pediatric pancreas transplants in the USA 1988-2000. Pediatr Transplant 2000;4:100.

28. Gruessner AC, Sutherland DER: Pancreas transplant outcomes for United States and non-US cases as reported to the United Network for Organ Sharing and the International Pancreas Transplant Registry as of October 2002. In Cecka JM, Terasaki PI (eds): Clinical Transplants 2002. Los Angeles, UCLA Immunogenetics Center, 2003.

29. Gruessner AC, Sutherland DER: Pancreas transplant outcomes for United States (US) and non-US cases as reported to the United Network for Organ Sharing (UNOS) and the International Pancreas Transplant Registry (IPTR) as of May 2003. In Cecka JM, Terasaki PI (eds): Clinical Transplants 2003. Los Angeles, UCLA Immunogenetics Center, 2004.

30. Gruessner AC, Sutherland DER: Pancreas Transplantation Analyses of United States (US) and non-US cases as reported to the United Network for Organ Sharing (UNOS) and the International Pancreas Transplant Registry (IPTR) as of June 2004. In Cecka JM, Terasaki PI (eds): Clinical Transplants 2004. Los Angeles, UCLA Immunogenetics Center, 2005.

31. Gruessner RW, Sutherland DE, Dunn DL, et al: Transplant options for patients undergoing total pancreatectomy for chronic pancreatitis. J Am Coll Surg 2004;198:559-567.

32. Gruessner RW, Sutherland DE, Gruessner AC: Mortality assessment for pancreas transplants. Am J Transplant 2004; 4:2018-2026.

33. Gruessner RWG, Kendall DM, Drangstveit MB, et al: Simultaneous pancreas-kidney transplantation from live donors. Ann Surg 1997;226:471-482.

34. Gruessner RWG, Manivel DC, Dunn DL, Sutherland DER: Pancreaticoduodenal transplantation with enteric drainage following native total pancreatectomy for chronic pancreatitis: A case report. Pancreas 1991;6:479-488.

35. Hering BJ, Bretzel RG, Hopt UT, et al: New protocol toward prevention of early human islet allograft failure. Transplant Proc 1994;26:570-571.

36. Hering BJ, Kandaswamy R, Ansite JD, et al: Successful single donor islet transplantation in type 1 diabetes. Am J Transplant 2003;3(Suppl 5):296.

37. Hering BJ, Kandaswamy R, Harmon JV, et al: Transplantation of cultured islets from two-layer preserved pancreases in type 1 diabetes with anti-CD3 antibody. Am J Transplant 2004;4:390-401.

38. Hering BJ, Matsumoto I, Sawada T, et al: Impact of two-layer pancreas preservation on islet isolation and transplantation. Transplantation 2002;74:1813-1816.

39. Hering BJ, Ricordi C: Islet transplantation for patients with type I diabetes. Graft 1999;2:12-27.

40. Hering BJ, Ricordi C, Sutherland DER, Bluestone JA: Islet transplantation: At the forefront of clinical research on immune tolerance. In Norman DJ, Suki WN (eds): Primer on Transplantation. Thorofare, NJ, American Society of Transplant Physicians, 2000.

41. Hering BJ, Wijkstrom M, Eckman PM: Islet transplantation. In Gruessner RW, Sutherland DER (eds): Transplantation of the Pancreas. New York, Springer-Verlag, 2004.

42. Hiraoka K, Trexler A, Fujioka B, et al: Optimal temperature in pancreas preservation by the two-layer cold storage method before islet isolation. Transplant Proc 2001;33(1-2): 891-892.

43. Jahr H, Hussmann B, Eckhardt T, Bretzel RG: Successful single donor islet allotransplantation in the streptozotocin diabetes rat model. Cell Transplant 2002;11:513-518.

44. Kaufman DB, Baker MS, Chen X, et al: Sequential kidney/islet transplantation using prednisone-free immunosuppression. Am J Transplant 2002;2:674-677.

45. Kaufman DB, Leventhal JR, Koffron AJ, et al: A prospective study of rapid corticosteroid elimination in simultaneous pancreas-kidney transplantation: Comparison of two maintenance immunosuppression protocols: Tacrolimus/mycophenolate mofetil versus tacrolimus/sirolimus. Transplantation 2002;73:169-177.

46. Kelly WD, Lillehei RC, Merkel FK: Allotransplantation of the pancreas and duodenum along with the kidney in diabetic nephropathy. Surgery 1967;61:827-835.

47. Kendall DM, Rooney DP, Smets YF, et al: Pancreas transplantation restores epinephrine response and symptom recognition during hypoglycemia in patients with long-standing type I diabetes and autonomic neuropathy. Diabetes 2000;46:249-257.

48. Lillehei RC, Ruiz JO, Aquino C, Goetz FC: Transplantation of the pancreas. Acta Endocrinol 1976;83(Suppl 205): 303-320.

49. Lillehei RC, Simmons RL, Najarian JS, et al: Pancreaticoduodenal allotransplantation: Experimental and clinical experience. Ann Surg 1970;172:405-436.

50. Maki T, Ichikawa T, Blanco R, Porter J: Long-term abrogation of autoimmune diabetes in nonobese diabetic mice by immunotherapy with anti-lymphocyte serum. Proc Natl Acad Sci U S A 1992;89:3434-3438.

51. Markmann JF, Deng S, Huang X, et al: Insulin independence following isolated islet transplantation and single islet infusions. Ann Surg 2003;237:741-749.

52. Marsh CL, Perkins JD, Sutherland DER, et al: Combined hepatic and pancreaticoduodenal procurement for transplantation. Surg Gynecol Obstet 1989;168:254-258.

53. Najarian JS, Sutherland DER, Matas AJ, et al: Human islet transplantation: A preliminary experience. Transplant Proc 1977;9:233-236.

54. Nathan DM: Long-term complications of diabetes mellitus. N Engl J Med 1993;328:1676-1685.

55. Navarro X, Kennedy WR, Aeppli D, Sutherland DER: Neuropathy and mortality in diabetes: Influence of pancreas transplantation. Muscle Nerve 1996;19:1009-1016.

56. Navarro X, Sutherland DER, Kennedy WR: Long-term effects of pancreatic transplantation on diabetic neuropathy. Ann Neurol 1997;42:727-736.

57. Nghiem DD, Corry RJ: Technique of simultaneous pancreaticoduodenal transplantation with urinary drainage of pancreatic secretion. Am J Surg 1987;153:405-406.

58. Philosophe B, Farney AC, Schweitzer EJ, et al: Superiority of portal venous drainage over systemic venous drainage in pancreas transplantation: A retrospective study. Ann Surg 2001;234:689-696.

59. Pileggi A, Ricordi C, Alessiani M, Inverardi L: Factors influencing islet of Langerhans graft function and monitoring. Clin Chim Acta 2001;310:3-16.

60. Poggioli R, Inverardi L, Ricordi C: Islet xenotransplantation. Cell Transplant 2002;11:89-94.

61. Rayhill SC, Kirk AD, Odorico JS, et al: Simultaneous pancreas-kidney transplantation at the University of Wisconsin. In Cecka JM, Terasaki PI (eds): Clinical Transplants 1995. Los Angeles, UCLA Tissue Typing Laboratory, 1996.

62. Ricordi C, Tzakis A, Carroll PB, et al: Human islet isolation and allotransplantation in 22 consecutive cases. Transplantation 1992;53:407-414.

63. Robertson RP, Sutherland DE, Kendall DM, et al: Metabolic characterization of long-term successful pancreas transplants in type I diabetes. J Investig Med 1996;44:549-555.

64. Rosenlof LK, Earnhardt RC, Pruett TL, et al: Pancreas transplantation: An initial experience with systemic and portal drainage of pancreatic allografts. Ann Surg 1992;215:586-595.

65. Rosenlof LK, Earnhardt RC, Pruett TL, et al: Pancreas transplantation: An initial experience with systemic and portal drainage of pancreatic allografts. Ann Surg 1992;215:586-595.

66. Ryan EA, Lakey JR, Paty BW, et al: Successful islet transplantation: Continued insulin reserve provides long-term glycemic control. Diabetes 2002;51:2148-2157.

67. Scharp DW, Lacy PE, Santiago JV, et al: Insulin independence after islet transplantation into type I diabetic patient. Diabetes 1990;39:515-518.

68. Secchi A, Socci C, Maffi P, et al: Islet transplantation in IDDM patients. Diabetologia 1997;40:225-231.

69. Shapiro AM, Lakey JR, Ryan EA, et al: Islet transplantation in seven patients with type 1 diabetes mellitus using a glucocorticoid-free immunosuppressive regimen [see comments]. N Engl J Med 2000;343:230-238.

70. Sollinger HW, Cook K, Kamps D: Clinical and experimental experience with pancreaticocystostomy for exocrine pancreatic drainage in pancreas transplantation. Transplant Proc 1984;16:749-751.

71. Soria B, Roche E, Berna G, et al: Insulin-secreting cells derived from embryonic stem cells normalize glycemia in streptozotocin-induced diabetic mice. Diabetes 2000;49:157-162.

72. Starzl TE, Iwatsuki S, Shaw BW Jr, et al: Pancreaticoduodenal transplantation in humans. Surg Gynecol Obstet 1984;159:265-272.

73. Starzl TE, Todo S, Fung J, et al: FK 506 for liver, kidney, and pancreas transplantation. Lancet 1989;2:1000-1004.

74. Stern RC, Mayes JT, Weber FL Jr, et al: Restoration of exocrine pancreatic function following pancreas-liver-kidney transplantation in a cystic fibrosis patient. Clin Transplant 1994;8:1-4.

75. Stock PG, Bluestone JA: Beta-cell replacement for type I diabetes. Annu Rev Med 2004;55:133-156.

76. Stratta RJ: The economics of pancreas transplantation. Graft 2000;3:19.

77. Stratta RJ, Cushing KA, Frisbie K, Miller SA: Analysis of hospital charges after simultaneous pancreas-kidney transplantation in the era of managed care. Transplantation 1997;64:287-292.

78. Stratta RJ, Shokouh-Amiri MH, Egidi MF, et al: A prospective comparison of simultaneous kidney-pancreas transplantation with systemic-enteric versus portal-enteric drainage. Ann Surg 2001;233:740-751.

79. Sutherland DE, Gruessner RW, Dunn DL, et al: Lessons learned from more than 1,000 pancreas transplants at a single institution. Ann Surg 2001;233:463-501.

80. Sutherland DER: International human pancreas and islet transplant registry. Transplant Proc 1980;12(No 4, Suppl 2):229-236.

81. Sutherland DER: Pancreas and islet transplant population. In Gruessner RWG, Sutherland DER (eds): Transplantation of the Pancreas. New York, Springer-Verlag, 2004.

82. Sutherland DER, Goetz FC, Najarian JS: Pancreas transplants from living related donors. Transplantation 1984;38:625-633.

83. Sutherland DER, Gruessner RG, Jie T, et al: Pancreatic islet auto-transplantation for chronic pancreatitis. Clin Transplant 2004;18(Suppl 13):17-18.

84. Sutherland DER, Gruessner RWG: History of pancreas transplantation. In Gruessner RWG, Sutherland DER (eds): Transplantation of the Pancreas. New York, Springer-Verlag, 2004.

85. Sutherland DER, Matas AJ, Najarian JS: Pancreatic islet cell transplantation. Surg Clin North Am 1978;58:365-382.

86. Sutherland DER, Morel P, Gruessner RWG: Transplantation of two diabetic patients with one divided cadaver donor pancreas. Transplant Proc 1990;22:585.

87. Tanioka Y, Sutherland DER, Kuroda Y, et al: Excellence of the two-layer method (University of Wisconsin solution/perfluorochemical) in pancreas preservation before islet isolation. Surgery 1997;122:435-442.

88. Tyden G, Bolinder J, Solders G, et al: Improved survival in patients with insulin-dependent diabetes mellitus and end-stage diabetic nephropathy 10 years after combined pancreas and kidney transplantation. Transplantation 1999;67:645-648.

89. Tzakis A, Ricordi C, Alejandro R, et al: Pancreatic islet transplantation after upper abdominal exenteration and liver replacement. Lancet 1990;336:402-405.

90. Venstrom JM, McBride MA, Rother KI, et al: Survival after pancreas transplantation in patients with diabetes and preserved kidney function. JAMA 2003;290:2817-2823.

91. Wahoff DC, Papalois B, Najarian JS, et al: Islet autotransplantation after total pancreatectomy in a child. J Pediatr Surg 1996;31:1-6.

92. Wahoff DC, Papalois B, Najarian JS, et al: Autologous islet transplantation to prevent diabetes after pancreatic resection. Ann Surg 1995;222:562-579.

93. Warnock GL, Kneteman NM, Ryan E, et al: Normoglycaemia after transplantation of freshly isolated and cryopreserved pancreatic islets in type 1 (insulin-dependent) diabetes mellitus. Diabetologia 1991;34:55-58.

94. White SA, James RF, Swift SM, et al: Human islet cell transplantation—future prospects. Diabet Med 2001;18:78-103.

95. Wijkstrom M, Kenyon NS, Kirchhof N, et al: Islet allograft survival in nonhuman primates immunosuppressed with basiliximab, RAD, and FTY720.Transplantation 2004;77: 827-835.

96. Woodle ES, Xu D, Zivin RA, et al: Phase I trial of a humanized, Fc receptor nonbinding OKT3 antibody, huOKT3gamma1(Ala-Ala), in the treatment of acute renal allograft rejection. Transplantation 1999;68:608-616.

97. Zehrer CL, Gross CR: Quality of life of pancreas transplant recipients. Diabetologia 1991;34 (Suppl 1):S145-S149.

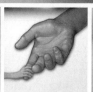

Chapter 45

Liver Transplantation

Bob H. Saggi, Douglas G. Farmer, and Ronald W. Busuttil

The treatment of liver disease in children with transplantation has its roots in the origin of liver transplantation itself, with the initial cases performed by Thomas E. Starzl on two children in 1963 and 1968.[19] Although the initial results were disappointing, over the ensuing 2 decades, liver transplantation developed into the standard therapy for end-stage liver disease (ESLD), certain malignancies of the liver and biliary tract, acute liver failure, and many metabolic derangements. The National Institutes of Health Development Conference designated it as such in 1983, and the National Organ Transplantation Act created a nationally regulated system of organ allocation in 1987. The United Network for Organ Sharing (UNOS) was thus created and currently regulates the field by a peer review process. In 2003, more than 5600 liver transplant procedures were performed, including 546 in pediatric patients.[21] This number of transplant procedures performed has been relatively stable since the mid 1990s, but there has been a shift to utilization of an increasing number of "partial" liver grafts from cadaveric and living donors. The pediatric population offers unique challenges due to size, perhaps enhanced immune responsiveness, and a relative organ scarcity. Although nearly two thirds of the pediatric recipients of liver transplants are younger than 5 years of age, donors younger than the age of 5 comprise only 26% of the pediatric cadaveric donors (Fig. 45-1).[21] As a consequence, achieving success in this patient population requires technical perfection, both from the standpoint of obtaining a suitable graft and performing a meticulous transplant operation. With reduction in transplant waiting time and improvements in immunosuppression, surgical technique, and long-term posttransplantation care, survival has been significantly improved and now approaches 90% at 1 year and 80% at 5 years, with many children surviving into adolescence and adulthood with a good quality of life.[3] In this chapter, we review the major indications for liver transplantation in children, the basic pathophysiology and clinical presentation of liver failure, operative strategies with emphasis on the unique surgical options available to children, postoperative management with emphasis on management of surgical complications, and outcome analysis.

Figure 45–1 Distribution of pediatric liver transplants by age. (Data from www.unos.org)

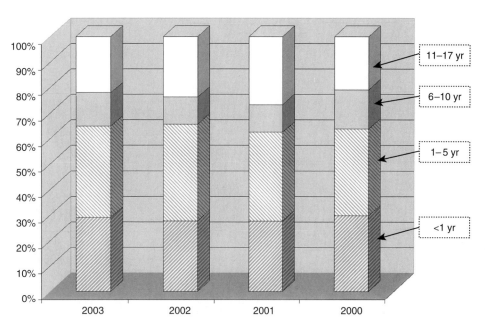

INDICATIONS

Liver transplantation is currently indicated for children with ESLD due to cholestatic and noncholestatic causes of cirrhosis, acute hepatic failure, some metabolic liver diseases, select tumors, and a variety of miscellaneous indications (Fig. 45-2). The general indication for liver transplantation in children is liver disease that limits long-term survival or quality of life or markedly impairs normal growth and development. Cirrhosis alone is not an indication for transplantation because many of these patients can be medically managed for a prolonged period before decompensation. In acute liver failure, the development of clear symptoms such as refractory coagulopathy, acidosis, and cerebral edema that correlate with a poor prognosis for spontaneous recovery of liver function is an indication for transplantation. Otherwise, medical support in those patients with a better prognosis is provided until liver function returns to normal.[5]

With long-standing cirrhosis, the development of a constellation of symptoms and signs that represent decompensation of hepatocellular function or portal hypertension heralds a need for transplantation. These include progressive jaundice, coagulopathy, protein-calorie malnutrition and growth retardation, impaired cognitive development, encephalopathy, hypersplenism, variceal hemorrhage, and advanced or refractory ascites. The majority of patients undergoing transplantation in this population are deeply jaundiced owing to secondary or primary biliary cirrhosis from long-standing intrahepatic and/or extrahepatic biliary obstruction. On physical examination, these patients often have muscle wasting, an enlarged spleen, a hard, palpable liver, abdominal distention from ascites, and peripheral edema. With decompensation, long-term survival without liver transplantation is limited, and referral for transplantation must be made before decompensation.[3,12]

Cholestatic Liver Disorders

The most common indications for liver transplantation are the cholestatic liver disorders, with the most common being biliary atresia. This group accounts for roughly 50% of the transplants performed on children in 2003, and biliary atresia accounts for 70% of this cholestatic group (see Fig. 45-2).[21] The management of biliary atresia rests on early diagnosis, using surgical exploration with biopsy as the central confirmatory test in most cases. The diagnostic workup is detailed elsewhere in this textbook. Portoenterostomy is the preferred treatment if diagnosis precedes the development of cirrhosis, usually before 3 months of age, although long-term results from portoenterostomy are optimal if it is done before 8 weeks.[22] This procedure is essential for slowing, and in some cases arresting, the progression of liver disease to cirrhosis and portal hypertension. Unfortunately, despite effective biliary drainage, more than 70% of patients will go on to develop ESLD by the age of 5 years and require transplantation.[4,22] However, in many cases, portoenterostomy allows reasonable growth and development so that transplantation is forestalled until the child is older and larger. Primary portoenterostomy performed late in the course of biliary atresia and re-exploration for failing biliary drainage are usually unsuccessful and only complicate transplantation outcomes. Instead, once a portoenterostomy has failed, patients should be evaluated for liver transplantation. Liver transplantation is indicated when the diagnosis is made in infants older than 3 months of age, when ESLD is clearly present at any age, or after a portoenterostomy failure. Patients with biliary atresia should be managed by a pediatric hepatologist experienced in the nuances of liver transplantation to ensure early transplantation is pursued when signs of liver decompensation are observed.

Other uncommon causes of cholestatic liver injury and cirrhosis include familial paucity of intrahepatic bile ducts, which exists in syndromic (Alagille's syndrome) and nonsyndromic forms; familial cholestatic syndromes; primary or secondary sclerosing cholangitis; and uncorrectable choledochal cyst disease, including Caroli's disease. The cystic diseases have a component of uncorrectable extrahepatic obstruction whereas the others are the result of malformation or destruction of intrahepatic bile ducts and/or arterial systems. All of these conditions have in common a variable and unpredictable progression to

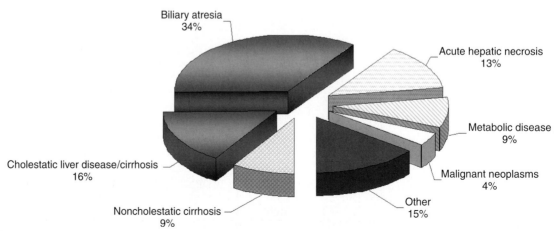

Figure 45-2 Indications for pediatric liver transplantation. (Data obtained from www.unos.org, based on 2003 transplants.)

advanced fibrosis, cirrhosis, and portal hypertension. These patients typically present with progressive jaundice at an older age than patients with biliary atresia. Although their management does not entail a portoenterostomy, the indications for transplantation in these patients follow the same rationale as that for biliary atresia.

Noncholestatic Cirrhosis

This is an uncommon indication for liver replacement in children, accounting for less than 10% of all procedures performed in 2003 (see Fig. 45-2).[21] These children usually present later in life than the cholestatic disorders. Causes of cirrhosis and ESLD in these patients include chronic autoimmune hepatitis, neonatal hepatitis, chronic viral (B or C) hepatitis, and cryptogenic cirrhosis.

Acute Liver Failure

Fulminant hepatic failure is usually defined as the onset of encephalopathy within 28 days after the onset of jaundice in a patient with acute liver failure without evidence of chronic liver disease. The hallmarks of acute liver failure include profound coagulopathy, acidosis, hypoglycemia, and progressive hyperbilirubinemia. These patients can develop acute renal failure, multiorgan failure syndrome, or cerebral edema progressing to herniation. Early referral is essential to avoid progression to a condition that contraindicates transplantation. A number of criteria to determine the need for transplantation have been devised in European centers, where these patients are managed in a highly structured and centralized manner.[15] The most common known cause in children is viral hepatitis, followed by acetaminophen and other drug toxicities and Wilson's disease. However, in nearly two thirds of patients a cause cannot be identified. Liver transplantation is the only acceptable therapy in patients who meet the criteria of fulminant hepatic failure, and early referral of all patients with acute liver failure is essential.[5]

Metabolic Liver Disease

These disorders have in common an enzyme deficiency or some other defect in hepatocellular function. This impairment can result in progressive fibrosis or cirrhosis (e.g., cystic fibrosis, chronic Wilson's disease, and neonatal iron storage disease) with a typical presentation of ESLD. In other cases the liver is structurally normal but harmful byproducts of metabolism accumulate to cause neurologic injury (e.g., Crigler-Najjar syndrome, ornithine transcarbamylase deficiency, and Wilson's disease), cardiovascular disease (e.g., familial hypercholesterolemia), or renal injury (familial hyperoxaluria). Some disorders are associated with the development of malignancies (e.g., tyrosinemia), and transplantation should be considered preemptively. Transplant evaluation of all patients with known metabolic disorders of the liver involves a thorough evaluation of extrahepatic organ function. This will ensure transplantation of only those patients who can benefit from liver transplantation and prevents progression of extrahepatic disease. In some patients, simultaneous or sequential dual-organ transplantation may be necessary (e.g., lung, kidney, heart).

Tumors

The most common liver malignancy in children is hepatoblastoma.[16] Although sporadic cases have been reported, hepatocellular carcinoma is primarily seen in older children with viral hepatitis, tyrosinemia, or in association with cirrhosis from other causes. Nonmetastatic malignancies in pediatric patients are managed by surgical resection unless tumor size and/or location preclude resection. The benefit of neoadjuvant and/or adjuvant chemotherapy and rarely irradiation for hepatoblastoma has been well documented, but there is no well-established role for it in hepatocellular carcinoma.[17,20] Benefit may be derived from preoperative transarterial chemoembolization and/or radiofrequency ablation.[1] If the lesion is unresectable, transplantation can be considered after excluding extrahepatic disease.[14] The long-term survival after liver transplantation for hepatoblastoma is approximately 50%, whereas outcomes from hepatocellular carcinoma are not nearly as good.[14,17] The major issue that remains to be resolved is whether transplantation should be attempted for large hepatoblastomas primarily or as a salvage after recurrence after resection. Data from Europe suggest a worse outcome when liver transplantation is performed as a salvage procedure. The most common benign tumor of the liver is hemangioendothelioma; and although the vast majority regress with growth and medical therapy, occasionally progression of heart failure or mass effect warrants transplantation.[16]

Miscellaneous Conditions

Other conditions include diagnoses such as Budd-Chiari syndrome, trauma, and biliary cirrhosis secondary to intestinal failure and long-term use of total parenteral nutrition, which is detailed in Chapter 46.

ORGAN ALLOCATION AND PRETRANSPLANT CARE

Patients who have evidence of ESLD are candidates for liver transplantation. However, the small size of the pediatric patient combined with a nationwide shortage of organs relative to patients on a waiting list makes achieving transplantation in a timely fashion problematic. In 2003, there were 546 pediatric liver transplants performed. In that same year, there were 800 pediatric-aged cadaveric donors. The problem and discrepancy is particularly evident in the younger-than-age-6-year category in which there were 354 liver recipients but only 207 donors. Another problem is of course timing: at the time a pediatric donor is available, there is not necessarily a size-matched pediatric recipient available. Compounding this problem is the fact that adults older than age 18 years can be offered pediatric donors and therefore contribute to the pediatric donor problem (see Fig. 45-1).[21] This creates a relative shortage of organs that necessitates a system that allocates these scarce organs to those who will derive the most benefit. Since 2002, the Pediatric End-stage Liver Disease (PELD) score was implemented to allocate organs based on this "sickest first" paradigm.[12] The PELD score consists of five variables: International Normalized Ratio, total serum bilirubin concentration, serum albumin level, growth retardation (= 2 standard deviations below the median height or weight for age), and young age (< 1 or 1 to 2 years). Status I is used to designate patients with fulminant hepatic failure, primary graft nonfunction after transplantation, early hepatic artery thrombosis, and miscellaneous acute conditions. Unlike adults, pediatric ESLD patients requiring care in an intensive care unit for any reason are listed as status I because their mortality is high despite minimal change in PELD score. In an effort to ameliorate the shortage of potential organs, the liver of all donors 18 years of age and younger is preferentially allocated to pediatric recipients. This combined with the widespread use of split-liver transplantation (see later) has markedly reduced waiting times and positively impacted waiting list mortality.[7,25]

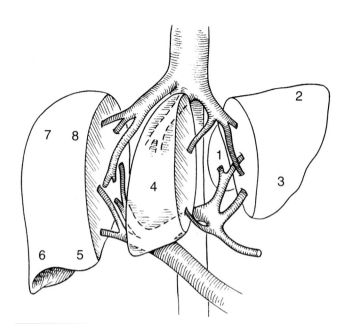

Figure 45-3 Segmental liver anatomy. The division of the liver into independently vascularized and drained segments is based on the parallel bifurcation of the portal vein and hepatic artery.

DONOR PROCUREMENT AND HEPATOBILIARY ANATOMY

Hepatobiliary Anatomy

The performance of a donor hepatectomy or transplant operation requires a thorough understanding of foregut anatomy. In addition, a very detailed understanding of this anatomy is essential to the field of segmental liver transplantation and has impacted hepatobiliary surgery. The blood supply to the liver is based on a highly variable hepatic arterial and portal venous system. Venous drainage is via the right, mid, and left hepatic veins that join the inferior vena cava, which traverses the dorsal surface of the liver (the retrohepatic vena cava). The liver is composed of the major right and left lobes, which are separated by external landmarks and further subdivided into the right anterior and posterior and left medial and lateral segments. This nomenclature is still used to describe major anatomic liver resections. However, through the elegant anatomic techniques of the pioneering surgical anatomist Couinaud, hepatic anatomy was found to be much more intricate (Fig. 45-3). The "Couinaud nomenclature" describes nine hepatic segments based on portal vein branching in relationship to the *transverse plane* (a cross-sectional plane located at "midpoints" of the hepatic veins) and the *longitudinal planes* of the individual hepatic veins (see Fig. 45-3). Each of the segments is supplied by an independent portal venous and hepatic arterial branch and drained by an independent biliary radicle. The biliary tree is second only to the arterial system in its variability. The hepatic venous drainage is intersegmental. A more detailed review of the anatomy of the liver is available elsewhere and its discussion is beyond the scope of this chapter.

THE DONOR OPERATION

The use of organs from cadaveric donors in pediatric liver transplantation involves selecting an appropriate quality and size-matched donor, organizing an experienced transplant harvest team, and performing a precise technical operation that recognizes arterial anatomic variants and allows for multiorgan procurement. The advent of segmental liver transplantation has expanded the acceptable donor age to approximately 40 years. Preharvest donor management should focus on maintenance of hemodynamic stability with adequate but not excessive volume loading, minimizing the use of vasopressors, optimizing oxygenation without excessive use of positive end-expiratory pressure (PEEP), and correcting hypernatremia that results from diabetes insipidus. In the stable donor, once these goals are achieved, the procurement operation can be performed. In the properly selected unstable donor, unnecessary delays are to be avoided because expedient hypothermic perfusion and cold storage only help minimize the ongoing organ ischemia.

The donor operation begins with midline laparotomy and median sternotomy for wide exposure. The abdominal great vessels are exposed by a medial visceral rotation of the right colon and small intestine, and the aorta and inferior mesenteric vein are cannulated. The liver quality is assessed, and the biliary tree is flushed via the gallbladder. After full systemic heparinization, the supraceliac aorta is cross-clamped and the intrapericardial inferior vena cava is incised to exsanguinate the donor. Then cold-organ perfusion is initiated through the previously placed cannulas and the abdominal cavity is immersed in ice in an attempt to achieve a liver core temperature of 4°C. University of Wisconsin (UW) solution has been used as the standard solution in the United States since 1987 when it was developed by Belzer and Southhard. This solution extended the limit of preservation to as long as 12 to 18 hours, after which the incidence of primary graft failure increases substantially. However, the acceptable preservation time depends on numerous donor and recipient variables and should still be minimized when possible. This is especially important in instances of reduced size or split-liver transplantation. The UW solution is a hyperkalemic, hyperosmolar solution that prevents cellular swelling, maintains stable transmembrane electrical gradients upon reperfusion by preventing efflux of intracellular potassium during storage, and contains a variety of oxygen- free radical scavengers. Recently, some centers have employed histidine-tryptophan-ketoglutarate solution because of its low potassium content and viscosity.[2] However, this solution has not been thoroughly evaluated using long-term, randomized controlled trials. Until these data are available, UW solution remains the gold standard for organ preservation. Once the donor organ is procured, the harvest team typically transports the liver graft to the transplant center and prepares it for engraftment by a separate recipient team.

SEGMENTAL LIVER TRANSPLANTATION: LIVING DONOR, REDUCED SIZE AND SPLIT

The shortage of pediatric organs coupled with a significant wait-list death rate has driven the development of alternative organ sources. Three alternatives to use of a whole-organ graft are available: living donor, reduced size, and split liver grafts.[6,7,24,25] Living donor transplantation was developed as an alternative to scarce whole-organ grafts and typically utilizes a segment 2 and 3 (left-lateral segment [LLS]) graft. Because of the small but real risk of safety in a healthy donor, reduced size transplantation was simultaneously developed as an alternative and involves resecting the LLS graft before or after cold-organ perfusion and discarding the remaining liver. Obviously, this benefits the pediatric recipient but wastes an organ that could be utilized by an adult recipient. Splitting the whole organ into a right trisegment and LLS graft to utilize in an adult and pediatric recipient, respectively, was first described by Pichlmayr in Hanover, Germany, in 1988. This can be done either before cold-organ perfusion (in-situ technique) (Fig. 45-4) or after cold-organ perfusion and removal of the liver from the donor (ex-vivo technique).[24] This technique provides a suitable graft for the pediatric population without worsening the already severe organ shortage in the adult population. Although the initial results were discouraging, with increased experience the survival rates of patients and grafts are nearly equal to whole-organ and living-donor transplantation, although the risk of vascular and biliary complications is somewhat higher.[8,25] At the University of California in Los Angeles (UCLA), we are only performing living donor transplantation when a whole or split graft is not available in a timely fashion or for special indications. There has been a marked reduction in transplant wait time since the routine use of segmental grafts following this strategy.[7,25]

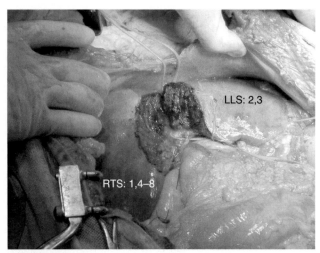

Figure 45–4   Cadaveric in-situ split liver procedure. The liver is separated just to the left of the umbilical fissure into a right trisegment (RTS) graft and a left-lateral segment (LLS) graft.

THE LIVER TRANSPLANTATION OPERATION

The performance of the whole-organ cadaveric liver transplantation procedure has changed little over the past 2 decades. Whereas there are tremendous individual and institutional differences in the subtleties of using certain techniques, the basic steps in the procedure remain the same. What follows is a description of how a liver transplantation procedure is generally performed at UCLA today and has been applied in over 800 pediatric cases.[13] The procedure can be roughly divided into four major phases, each with its own anatomic and physiologic challenges: hepatectomy phase, anhepatic phase with engraftment, reperfusion with arterialization, and biliary reconstruction. Perhaps the most challenging step during liver transplantation is the hepatectomy. Coagulopathy, portal hypertension, and poor liver and renal function create a surgical environment in which continuous bleeding is possible. During this phase, the anesthesiologist plays a key role in maintaining volume, rapid transfusion, correcting coagulopathy and fibrinolysis, and maintaining body temperature. The goal of this phase is to devascularize the liver by ligating and dividing the hepatic artery and portal vein as well as to mobilize the suprahepatic and infrahepatic vena cava to enable removal. These goals are achieved while leaving in the recipient adequate lengths of each vessel for later implantation of the donor graft. In the majority of pediatric liver transplant operations, the retrohepatic vena cava is retained as the liver is dissected off the vena cava by dividing the tributaries from the right and caudate lobes, and often only partial occlusion of the vena cava is necessary. Meticulous but expedient surgical technique is essential during the hepatectomy in ensuring optimal patient outcome. During the anhepatic phase, the anesthesiologist must support certain aspects of hepatic function to prevent or treat acidemia, hypothermia, coagulopathy, and, occasionally, fibrinolysis. In addition, they must ensure adequate

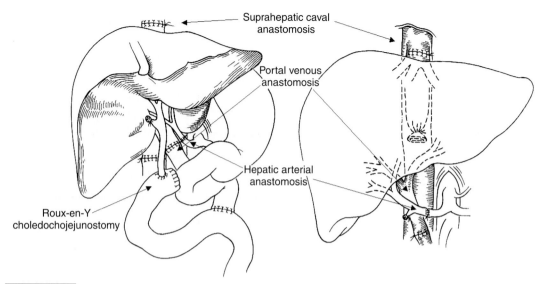

Figure 45–5   Whole-organ engraftment. Both the standard orthotopic and the "piggyback" techniques are depicted.

circulating volume and maintain hemodynamic stability. In children, veno-venous bypass is rarely used.

While the patient is anhepatic the liver graft is removed from hypothermic storage and engrafted. The insertion of the graft begins with the suprahepatic vena caval, followed by the infrahepatic vena caval and the portal anastomoses. If the retrohepatic cava was retained, the "piggyback" technique is used, in which the suprahepatic vena cava of the graft is sewn to the cloacae created from the confluence of the recipient hepatic veins and the donor infrahepatic vena cava is ligated (Fig. 45-5). Before reperfusion, the liver is flushed with a cold colloid and albumin solution via the donor portal vein to reduce the risk of potential reperfusion-associated complications.

Reperfusion is then undertaken in a controlled manner. Communication between the surgical and anesthesia teams is essential to allow the anesthesiologist time to institute preparative and preventive measures. Reperfusion is undertaken by first removing the suprahepatic vena cava clamp, then the infrahepatic vena cava clamp, and lastly the portal venous clamp. As blood is reintroduced into the liver allograft and allowed to drain into the right atria, many serious and potentially life-threatening complications can develop. The major challenges encountered by the anesthesiologist at this point are life-threatening hyperkalemia, acidosis, arrhythmias, and hemodynamic instability with or without surgical or coagulopathic bleeding. A factor that contributes is the return of cold, acidotic, and hyperkalemic blood directly into the right atrium. It is at this point that maintenance of physiologic stability by the surgeon and anesthesiologist in the preceding phases, the preoperative state of the recipient, and the intrinsic quality of the graft converge to determine early graft function as well as the course of the remainder of the operation. Without a doubt, this is one of the most hazardous portions of the liver transplant procedure.

The hepatic arterial anastomosis is then performed. In general arterial inflow is obtained from one of the branches of the celiac trunk. However, in some instances, inflow from these vessels is not adequate, necessitating the use of aortic conduits. A conduit can be placed either on the supraceliac or infrarenal aorta. In some cases, when the arteries are of very small caliber (<3 mm), the arterial anastomosis is performed before reperfusion. The biliary tree is then reconstructed by choledocho-choledochostomy or by Roux-en-Y choledochojejunostomy, the latter being more common in small children and used exclusively in partial liver grafts because of the size of the donor duct (see Fig. 45-5). After ensuring sufficient hemostasis, drains are placed and the abdominal cavity is closed. The patient is then transferred directly to the intensive care unit. Segmental transplantation, using split, reduced-sized, or living donor grafts, involves variations in the manner in which the anastomoses are performed, but the general steps are similar (Fig. 45-6).

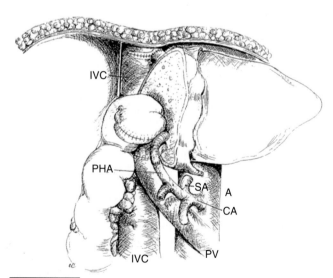

Figure 45–6   Left-lateral segment engraftment. IVC, inferior vena cava; PHA, proper hepatic artery; SA, splenic artery; CA, celiac artery; A, aorta; PV, portal vein. (Reprinted with permission from Goss J, Yersiz H, Shackleton CR, et al: In situ splitting of the cadaveric liver for transplantation. Transplantation 1997;64:871-877.)

POST-TRANSPLANTATION CARE

The early and long-term postoperative care of the liver transplant recipient is almost as important as the performance of the operation in ensuring optimal outcomes. The immediate postoperative care is aimed at assessing graft function, providing supportive care for the recipient, and early detection of complications. Graft function can be assessed in many ways. Physiologic and clinical assessment can be done almost immediately, with a warm, arousable, and hemodynamically stable patient with a liver producing "golden-brown" bile (in the infrequent case in which a biliary drainage tube is placed) being the hallmark of a functional graft. Graft function is then confirmed biochemically by evidence of synthetic and metabolic function (e.g., correcting prothrombin time, reversal of acidemia). Although the degree of preservation injury, as measured by liver enzyme levels, does not linearly correlate with graft function, grafts with severe injury are more likely to exhibit delayed function or nonfunction. Failure of a graft without vascular compromise (primary nonfunction) requires retransplantation in almost all cases, with the outcome directly related to the time to retransplantation. The incidence of primary nonfunction in pediatric patients is 5% to 10%.[6,10,25]

TECHNICAL COMPLICATIONS

Technical complications can be divided into vascular, biliary, and general surgical complications. In the early postoperative period, infectious and general surgical complications of liver transplantation today are similar to those that occur after any major abdominal operation. However, the incidence of fungal infection is higher and the incidence of bowel perforation in pediatric recipients is as high as 19% in some series.[23]

Vascular Complications

Major vascular complications include hepatic artery thrombosis, portal vein thrombosis, and vena caval thrombosis or stenosis. Intravenous low-dose unfractionated heparin with or without low-molecular-weight dextran is routinely used for prophylaxis to prevent vascular thromboses. Duplex ultrasonography and computed tomography or conventional angiography are accepted means of diagnosis. Hepatic artery thrombosis is the most common vascular complication, with an incidence that varies from 5% to 18% depending on patient age and type of graft.[6,10,23,25] Early vascular complications are usually technical in nature, whereas immunologic and infectious (e.g., cytomegalovirus) causes have been ascribed to those occurring months after transplantation. Hepatic artery thrombosis occurring in the first week after liver transplantation is commonly associated with graft nonfunction and biliary necrosis or leak, whereas those instances occurring later do not necessarily affect graft function immediately but can produce biliary complications. These include intrahepatic biliary abscesses, biliary anastomotic stricture, and sclerosing cholangitis with

sepsis, all of which lead to significant morbidity. If diagnosed early, some patients can be managed by thrombectomy and surgical revision. However, most patients with early hepatic artery thrombosis require urgent retransplantation. Late hepatic artery thrombosis with preserved graft function can be managed by radiologic interventional techniques, and the patient can undergo retransplantation remote from the time of the initial transplant procedure. Thrombosis of the portal vein occurs in 2% to 4% of pediatric liver transplant procedures and is usually associated with loss of the graft. Prompt retransplantation is required for patient salvage. Late portal vein thrombosis usually presents as recurrent variceal bleeding or ascites and can be managed medically, endoscopically, or surgically with either shunting or retransplantation. Vena caval or hepatic vein thrombosis or stenosis occurs in 3% to 6% of pediatric liver transplant patients and is usually best managed with balloon dilation in an interventional radiology unit.[6,10,23,25]

Biliary Complications

Biliary complications that are not associated with hepatic artery thrombosis occur in 3% to 20% of patients depending on the type of graft and whether a choledochojejunostomy was employed. These usually result from technical errors, but occasionally warm ischemia or immunologic and infectious factors can be implicated (e.g., cytomegalovirus). Diagnosis is achieved by cholangiography, and treatment can be by endoscopic or radiologic intervention or by surgical revision.[6,10,23,25]

IMMUNOSUPPRESSIVE THERAPY AND REJECTION

Immunosuppression for liver transplantation in the modern era rests on a class of drugs known as calcineurin inhibitors (CNI), the prototype of which is cyclosporine (Table 45-1). Cyclosporine, especially its microemulsion formulation that allows better bioavailability and more consistent therapeutic levels, revolutionized organ transplantation by reducing the incidence of rejection in all solid organs. The second-generation CNI tacrolimus was first used clinically in 1990. The greater potency of tacrolimus allowed for a further reduction in the early incidence of rejection after liver transplantation while also allowing the earlier weaning of corticosteroid therapy. Initial reports of a higher incidence of opportunistic infections and post-transplant lymphoproliferative disorder have been refuted by modern data. Currently, most liver transplantation centers utilize a tacrolimus-based regimen, combined with corticosteroid therapy with or without adjunctive agents. Cyclosporine and tacrolimus share certain acute and long-term side effects while having some that are unique to each agent. The most important of these is nephrotoxicity, which occurs in an acute variety from vasoconstriction of the afferent renal arterioles and is reversible, as well as a more chronic variety marked by tubular atrophy, interstitial fibrosis, and glomerulosclerosis. The chronic variety is variably reversible depending on the degree of disease. To minimize acute toxicity and to

TABLE 45-1 Modern Immunosuppressants Used in Liver Transplantation

Name	Mechanism of Action	Principal Use	Common Toxicities
Calcineurin inhibitors (CNI) Cyclosporine Tacrolimus	Exact and complete mechanism unknown. Inhibits IL-2 and other cytokine gene transcription, thus preventing T-helper cell expansion.	Induction and maintenance of immunosuppression long-term. Tacrolimus is the only agent approved for monotherapy, whereas cyclosporine must generally be used with another agent long term.	Shared: nephrotoxicity, hypertension, hyperglycemia, neurotoxicity (seizures, myoclonus, essential tremors) Cyclosporine: hirsutism, gingival hyperplasia, more diabetes Tacrolimus: diarrhea, anorexia, more neurotoxicity, more hypertension
Glucocorticoids Methylprednisolone Prednisone	Diffuse action on immune system by its anti-inflammatory properties, especially inhibition of IL-1	Induction of immunosuppression and maintenance. May be weaned off long-term in some patients.	Hyperlipidemia, osteopenia, hypertension, diabetes, impaired wound healing, growth retardation, cushingoid features, striae, acne
Mycophenolate mofetil	Purine antimetabolite, semi-selective for salvage pathway present, primarily used in lymphocytes	Used as an adjunctive agent to reduce the dose of CNI or corticosteroid	Myelosuppression, diarrhea, anorexia, nausea, vomiting, gastrointestinal mucosal ulceration?
Mammalian target of rapamycin inhibitors Rapamycin RAD	Inhibits cell cycle progression in stimulated cells, thus preventing clonal expansion of stimulated B and T cells	Unclear; use in pediatric patients preliminary. May be useful in minimizing CNI dose when toxicity exists or in refractory or chronic allograft rejection	Hyperlipidemia, impaired wound healing, pneumonitis, oral ulceration
OKT-3 monoclonal antibody	Clonal deletion of (CD-3+) T cells	Severe or refractory acute allograft rejection	Systemic inflammatory response syndrome (SIRS) and other infusional reactions, increased risk of viral infections and post-transplant lymphoproliferative disorder
Antilymphocyte globulin (Thymoglobulin)	Exact and complete mechanism unknown but produces central and peripheral deletion of lymphoid cells	Severe or refractory acute allograft rejection	Increased risk of viral infections and post-transplant lymphoproliferative disorder, lower incidence of infusional reactions than OKT-3, thrombocytopenia
IL-2 receptor antagonists Basiliximab Daclizumab	Competitive inhibition of IL-2 receptors	Induction of immunosuppression as an adjunct to CNI. Used to minimize other immunosuppression (CNI, corticosteroids)	Increased risk of viral infections, possible post-transplant lymphoproliferative disorder, rare infusional reactions

allow lower early CNI levels, especially with pre-transplant renal insufficiency, a purine antimetabolite mycophenolate mofetil is sometimes used as an adjunctive agent (see Table 45-1). The newest class of immunosuppressive agents are the inhibitors of the mammalian target of rapamycin, the prototype of which is sirolimus. This agent has been used sparingly in pediatric liver transplantation, and only preliminary data regarding its efficacy are available. Although this drug has no nephrotoxicity, it is associated with other long-term sequelae, such as hypercholesterolemia. At present there are no perfect immunosuppressive agents available (i.e., one with minimal side effects).

Acute rejection is common in pediatric liver transplantation, with the peak incidence being within the first 6 months, and 30% to 50% of patients experience at least one episode.[6,10,25] It is less common after the first post-transplantation year, occurring in less than 10% of cases. Diagnosis of acute rejection is suspected when elevated aspartate or alanine transaminase levels or elevated alkaline phosphatase levels and gamma-glutamyl transferase levels are observed. Acute rejection is an alloantigen specific, T cell–mediated inflammatory process that targets vascular endothelium and biliary epithelium but not hepatocytes. This is related to the greater expression of donor human leukocyte antigens on the former cell types. The histologic hallmark of acute rejection is a mixed inflammatory cell infiltrate (polymorphonuclear cells, lymphocytes, and eosinophils) in the portal triad with evidence of endothelitis and/or biliary epithelial injury. Rejection is graded as mild, moderate, or severe depending on the proportion of involved portal triads, the degree of infiltrate and injury, and the presence of central vein endothelitis, which is a sign of severe acute rejection. Treatment of acute rejection is centered on a high-dose methylprednisolone bolus, but unresponsive cases may require use of antibody therapy (OKT-3, ATG; see Table 45-1). Acute rejection does not influence long-term graft survival in adults or children unless it occurs in multiple or corticosteroid refractory episodes.[6,9] Acute rejection accounts for less than 3% of overall patient and graft loss. However, treatment of acute rejection is an important risk factor for the development of cytomegalovirus and Epstein-Barr virus infections in children. The latter is a risk factor for the development of post-transplant lymphoproliferative disorder. Therefore, a balance between adequate immunosuppression to prevent acute rejection and overimmunosuppression to avoid toxicity is necessary. Currently, long-term morbidity from immunosuppressive drug therapy is the major challenge facing long-term survival and quality of life in the pediatric solid organ transplantation population.

Chronic rejection is a common cause of late graft loss in children, whereas disease recurrence is uncommon. Chronic rejection is not entirely alloantigen driven and may be due to a number of factors that share a final common pathway of graft injury. Its hallmark is the intrahepatic loss of bile ducts, which has been termed *vanishing bile duct syndrome* owing to this histologic finding noted on biopsy. Rejection is suspected by the presence of progressive jaundice and a rising serum alkaline phosphatase level. Currently, there is no prophylactic or therapeutic agent available to treat chronic rejection, although progression of graft fibrosis may be forestalled by sirolimus, based on animal data.[11] The only accepted treatment when decompensated graft failure occurs is retransplantation.

INFECTIOUS COMPLICATIONS

Post-transplant infections are the most common cause of morbidity and mortality after liver transplantation. The highest incidence of bacterial and fungal infections is in the first month after transplantation. Fungal infections occurring months to years after transplantation are unusual and are more commonly the atypical or endemic organisms such as *Cryptococcus, Mucor, Blastomyces,* or *Coccidioides* species. Viral infections are the most common infections after the early post-transplant period. Cytomegalovirus and Epstein-Barr virus infections account for the vast majority of opportunistic viral infections. Overall reduction and more selective immunosuppression and prophylaxis with ganciclovir have reduced the incidence and morbidity of these infections. The other agents responsible for infectious morbidity, their presentation, diagnosis, and treatment are included in Table 45-2. Of particular importance in children is the prophylaxis and effective treatment of Epstein-Barr virus. This is associated with the development of numerous malignant consequences. The most common of these is a diffuse proliferation of lymphoid tissue known as post-transplant lymphoproliferative disorder, which can present as a mononucleosis-like syndrome with diffuse lymphadenopathy or as lymphoma involving any organ. A variety of other tumors are also associated with Epstein-Barr virus infections.[9] The general therapy for post-transplant lymphoproliferative disorder is reduction or elimination of immunosuppression and, occasionally, surgical intervention and/or chemotherapy. The complete discussion of these disorders is beyond this chapter's scope but is extensively covered in a report by Holmes and Sokol.[9]

OUTCOME

Numerous factors are known to impact patient and graft survival in children after liver transplantation.[3,6,10,23,25] Overall, survival has improved, with 1-year and 5-year patient survival approaching 90% and 80%, respectively, in patients younger than 18 years of age.[3] Age, nutritional status, urgency of transplantation, the indication for transplantation, and presence of renal dysfunction are all major factors that determine outcome. Whereas early data suggested that patients with biliary atresia have worse outcomes owing to their often-malnourished state, young age, and previous surgical intervention, more recent data suggest that this difference is not significant.[4] Patients with metabolic disease do exceedingly well because they often are older, do not have liver failure and its sequelae, and have not previously undergone an abdominal operation. Finally, transplantation for malignancy in children is associated with survival that is substantially below average but much better than the natural

TABLE 45-2 Infectious Complications After Liver Transplantation

Organism	Presentation	Diagnosis	Antimicrobials
Cytomegalovirus (CMV)	Infection results from: reactivation of virus; blood transfusion; infected transplanted organ. Mild viral, "flu-like" syndrome Invasive tissue infection (retinitis, pneumonitis, myocarditis, enterocolitis, hepatitis, central nervous system)	Quantitative CMV-DNA PCR PP-65 Antigen Tissue cultures Blood or fluid cultures Biopsy with immunostains	Prophylaxis: intravenous ganciclovir, oral valganciclovir Therapy: intravenous ganciclovir with or without CMV immunoglobulin
Epstein-Barr virus (EBV)	Spectrum: infectious mononucleosis to lymphoproliferative disease to lymphoma to EBV-associated soft tissue tumors Occurs with EBV and immunosuppression, 10% to 15% infant liver transplantation Gastrointestinal tract, neck, thorax, central nervous system	Quantitative EBV-DNA PCR Blood smear Biopsy with immunostains CT scans of suspected sites	Prophylaxis: intravenous ganciclovir, oral valganciclovir Therapy: acyclovir, reduction or withdrawal of immunosuppression. Possible use of systemic chemotherapy for lymphoproliferative disorders or lymphoma
Herpes simplex virus (HSV)	Skin lesions, gastrointestinal tract disseminated herpes: fever, fatigue, abnormal liver functions, hepatitis, pneumonia	HSV-1 and HSV-2 antibodies Biopsy with viral cultures	Acyclovir
Pneumocystis	Atypical pneumonia, can progress to life-threatening pneumonitis	Bronchoalveolar lavage, lung biopsy	Prophylaxis: Low-dose oral trimethoprim/sulfamethoxazole, dapsone, or pentamidine Therapy: High-dose intravenous trimethoprim/sulfamethoxazole
Candida	Local mucous membrane, invasive tissue infection, fungemia	Blood, fluid, and tissue cultures, fundoscopic examination	Prophylaxis: Fluconazole, in very-high-risk patients possibly lipid formulation of amphotericin B Therapy: Fluconazole (for sensitive candidal species) or lipid formulation of amphotericin B, caspofungin, or voriconazole (insensitive Candida or Aspergillus)
Aspergillus	Entry via upper or lower respiratory tract with metastatic spread (central nervous system, intra-abdominal, solid organ)	Blood, fluid, and tissue cultures, Bronchoalveolar lavage, CT scans	
Bacteria	Gram-negative: Enterobacteriaceae, Escherichia coli, Pseudomonas Gram-positive: Enterococcus, Staphylococcus	Blood, fluid, and tissue cultures, Bronchoalveolar lavage, CT scans, surgical exploration	Varies

history of the disease. Numerous large series exist in the literature detailing the improvement in outcome with experience.[6,10]

Although outcomes have improved, many issues still remain to be resolved. The first and foremost is the organ shortage. The number of listed patients is increasing steadily, while the number of suitable donors, even with segmental liver transplantation, has plateaued. Strategies aimed at expanding the donor pool and allocating organs to those patients who have not only the greatest survival benefit compared with pretransplant survival but also the greatest chance of optimal posttransplant outcome are essential. National policies aimed at effectively identifying donors amenable for organ splitting and development of local, regional, and national sharing of split grafts still await refinement.

Finally, the development of gene therapy or optimization of hepatocyte transplantation as alternatives to whole-organ transplantation for metabolic diseases may alleviate some of the current organ shortage.

Another important challenge for the liver transplantation community is the perfection of immunosuppression. Currently, all immunosuppressive agents have long-term side effects that result in impaired growth and development, infectious morbidity, malignancies, and numerous medical complications, including renal failure. The development of drug therapy that minimizes or eliminates these complications is essential. Furthermore, a better understanding of the immunology of peripheral T-cell tolerance and chronic rejection is important. Although in the past decade we witnessed improvements in many technical and immunosuppressive aspects of liver transplantation, improvements in survival and quality of life in the next decade will rest firmly on a better understanding of our immune system on a cellular and molecular level. The quest to achieve immunotolerance has been elusive.

REFERENCES

1. Arcement CM, Towbin RB, Meza MP, et al: Intrahepatic chemoembolization in unresectable pediatric liver malignancies. Pediatr Radiol 2000;30:779-785.
2. Canelo R, Hakim NS, Ringe B: Experience with histidine tryptophan ketoglutarate versus University Wisconsin preservation solutions in transplantation. Int Surg 2003; 88:145-151.
3. Colombani PM, Dunn SP, Harmon WE, et al: Pediatric transplantation. Am J Transplant 2003;3(Suppl 4):53-63.
4. Diem HV, Evrard V, Vinh HT, et al: Pediatric liver transplantation for biliary atresia: Results of primary grafts in 328 recipients. Transplantation 2003;75:1692-1697.
5. Farmer DG, Anselmo DM, Ghobrial RM, et al: Liver transplantation for fulminant hepatic failure: Experience with more than 200 patients over a 17-year period. Ann Surg 2003;237:666-675.
6. Goss JA, Shackleton CR, McDiarmid SV, et al: Long-term results of pediatric liver transplantation: An analysis of 569 transplants. Ann Surg 1998;228:411-420.
7. Gridelli B, Spada M, Petz W, et al: Split-liver transplantation eliminates the need for living-donor liver transplantation in children with end-stage cholestatic liver disease. Transplantation 2003;75:1197-1203.
8. Heffron TG, Pillen T, Welch D, et al: Biliary complications after pediatric liver transplantation revisited. Transplant Proc 2003;35:1461-1462.
9. Holmes RD, Sokol RJ: Epstein-Barr virus and post-transplant lymphoproliferative disease. Pediatr Transplant 2002;6:456-464.
10. Jain A, Mazariegos G, Kashyap R, et al: Pediatric liver transplantation in 808 consecutive children: 20-years experience from a single center. Transplant Proc 2002;34:1955-1957.
11. Markiewicz M, Kalicinski J, Teisseyre J, et al: Rapamycin in children after liver transplantation. Transplant Proc 2003;35:2284-2286.
12. McDiarmid SV, Anand R, Lindblad AS; Principal investigators and Institutions of the Studies of Pediatric Liver Transplantation (SPLIT) Research Group. Development of a pediatric end-stage liver disease score to predict poor outcome in children awaiting liver transplantation. Transplantation 2002;74:173-181.
13. Klintmalm GB, Busuttil RW: The recipient hepatectomy and grafting. In Busuttil RW, Klintmalm GB (eds): Transplantation of the Liver. Philadelphia, WB Saunders, 1996, pp 405-418.
14. Molmenti EP, Wilkinson K, Molmenti H, et al: Treatment of unresectable hepatoblastoma with liver transplantation in the pediatric population. Am J Transplant 2002;2:535-538.
15. O'Grady JG, Alexander GJ, Hayllar KM, et al: Early indicators of prognosis in fulminant hepatic failure. Gastroenterology 1989;97:439-445.
16. Reynolds M: Pediatric liver tumors. Semin Surg Oncol 1999;16:159-172.
17. Schnater JM, Aronson DC, Plaschkes J, et al: Surgical view of the treatment of patients with hepatoblastoma: Results from the first prospective trial of the International Society of Pediatric Oncology Liver Tumor Study Group. Cancer 2002;94:1111-1120.
18. Sieders E, Peeters PM, TenVergert EM, et al: Early vascular complications after pediatric liver transplantation. Liver Transpl 2000;6:326-332.
19. Starzl TE, Groth CG, Brettschneider L, et al: Orthotopic homotransplantation of the human liver. Ann Surg 1968;168:392-415.
20. Suita S, Tajiri T, Takamatsu H, et al: Improved survival outcome for hepatoblastoma based on an optimal chemotherapeutic regimen—a report from the study group for pediatric solid malignant tumors in the Kyushu area. J Pediatr Surg 2004;39:195-198.
21. United Network for Organ Sharing: http://www.unos.org/data/about/viewDataReports.asp
22. Wildhaber BE, Coran AG, Drongowski RA, et al: The Kasai portoenterostomy for biliary atresia: A review of a 27-year experience with 81 patients. Transplantation 2003;75: 1692-1697.
23. Yamanaka J, Lynch SV, Ong TH, et al: Surgical complications and long-term outcome in pediatric liver transplantation. Hepatogastroenterology 2000;47:1371-1374.
24. Yersiz H, Renz JF, Hisatake GM, et al: The conventional technique in in-situ split-liver transplantation. J Hepatobiliary Pancreat Surg 2003;10:11-15.
25. Yersiz H, Renz JF, Farmer DG, et al: One hundred in situ split-liver transplantations: A single-center experience. Ann Surg 2003;238:496-505; discussion 506-507.

Chapter 46

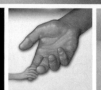

Intestinal Transplantation

Douglas G. Farmer and Sherilyn A. Gordon

The field of intestinal transplantation (ITx) has undergone significant advances over the past 10 to 15 years. From the unsuccessful attempts in the 1960s, patient survival rates approaching 80% to 90% can now be offered to selected recipients of ITx. Advances in surgical techniques have undoubtedly played a significant role. However, true leaps forward have been associated with the development of novel, more powerful immunomodulatory agents. In this chapter we review these developments and discuss the indications and techniques used in this field. Outcomes and obstacles to more widespread success of the procedure are also reviewed.

HISTORY

In the late 1950s, the experimental era of ITx was initiated by the pioneering work of two independent investigators, Lillehei[34] and Starzl,[46] who developed technically successful canine models of ITx. These models, coupled with the successful transplantation of human kidneys, led to nine published attempts at human ITx in the 1960s and 1970s (Table 46-1).[35] The outcomes of these clinical attempts performed under the standard immunosuppression of that era (steroids, azathioprine, antilymphocyte globulin, or any combination of these agents) were disheartening because of severe and uncontrollable rejection or technical failure. It was apparent that long-term survival of the lymphoid-rich intestinal allograft

would require more specific immunosuppression and more technical advances before clinical application. Nearly simultaneously, the development of total parenteral nutrition (TPN) by Wilmore and Dudrick[16] and long-term intravascular central lines by Broviac[6] in 1968 and 1972, respectively, enabled the short- and long-term administration of fluids, electrolytes, and nutrients to patients with insufficient intestinal function, thus dramatically changing the prognosis of this patient population. These clinical developments relegated ITx to a purely research entity for the next 15 years.

The subsequent discovery and successful clinical application of cyclosporine to other solid organ transplants[5,10] led to renewed interest in human ITx. Importantly, several landmark clinical case reports emerged, including the first successful human multivisceral transplantation by Starzl and associates in 1987,[49] isolated intestinal transplantation by Deltz and associates[13] in 1987, and combined liver-intestinal transplantation by Grant and colleagues in 1988 (Table 46-2).[35] However, success was limited to case reports and rejection remained the primary obstacle to long-term graft survival.

The modern era of transplantation was ushered forth in the 1990s by the discovery and clinical application of the powerful immunosuppressant FK-506 (tacrolimus, Prograf; off-label use).[31] With use of this agent, for the first time, reports of series of patients undergoing successful ITx were published[35] (personal communication, W. Burns, 2003). Today, tacrolimus remains the mainstay of most

TABLE 46-1 Early Attempts at Human Intestinal Transplantation

Year	Center	Graft	Graft Survival	Cause of Graft Loss
1964	Boston Floating Hospital	Living related isolated intestine	12 hours	Intestinal necrosis
1964	Boston Floating Hospital	Isolated intestine	2 days	Intestinal necrosis
1967	Univ of Minnesota	Intestine + colon	12 hours	Patient died of pulmonary embolism
1968	Univ of São Paulo	Isolated intestine	12 days	Rejection
1969	Univ of Paris	Intestine + colon	23 days	Rejection
1969	Univ of Mississippi	Living related isolated intestine	32 days	Rejection
1969	Univ of São Paulo	Isolated intestine	5 days	Rejection
1969	Albert Einstein Hospital	Isolated intestine	18 hours	Patient died of hypovolemic shock
1970	Cornell Univ Hospital	Living related isolated intestine	79 days	Rejection

TABLE 46–2 Outcomes of Initial Experience in Clinical Intestinal Transplantation with Cyclosporine Immunosuppression

Year	Author	Graft	Graft Survival	Cause of Graft Loss
1985	Cohen	Isolated intestine	12 days	Rejection
1987	Goulet	Isolated intestine	3 hours	Thrombosis
1987	Goulet	Isolated intestine	211 days	Rejection
1987	Deltz	Isolated intestine (living related)	12 days	Rejection
1987	Starzl	Multivisceral	192 days	Patient died of multisytem organ failure
1988	Grant	Combined liver/small bowel	5 years	Unknown

immunotherapeutic regimens for recipients of ITx and has been one of the crucial developments leading to the establishment of ITx as the standard of care for the treatment of children and adults with intestinal failure and life-threatening TPN-related morbidity.

RECIPIENT SELECTION

Selection of children with intestinal failure for ITx is based on the presence of TPN-related complications, the potential for gut adaptation, and medical and surgical suitability. To better understand candidates for ITx, a brief description of short-bowel/gut syndrome, intestinal failure, and intestinal adaptation is required. In general, short-gut syndrome is a clinical entity in which patients have insufficient gastrointestinal absorptive capacity to meet their daily fluid, electrolyte, and nutritional requirements. There are a variety of congenital, surgical, and functional causes of short-gut syndrome that may potentially lead to intestinal failure and ITx (Table 46-3).[25] Before the availability of TPN, the diagnosis of short-gut syndrome carried an extremely poor prognosis because most patients suffered premature mortality as a result of some degree of dehydration, catabolism, or starvation (Fig. 46-1).[23]

Not only is TPN lifesaving because it provides complete nutritional, fluid, and electrolyte support, but it also facilitates the process of intestinal adaptation. Adaptation is a complex process in which the remnant bowel undergoes hypertrophy, dilation, and motility changes that effectively increase the net absorption of nutrients per unit of length of bowel. This process is initiated within 24 hours of the onset of intestinal resection and is probably maximal at 2 to 3 years from onset, although isolated case reports of complete intestinal adaptation much later have been published.[14] Several keys to adaptation as outlined in other chapters include the presence of adequate calories and nutrients provided by TPN and the presence of intestinal luminal nutrients. The prognosis for complete adaptation from TPN is dependent on a number of factors, including the length of remnant bowel, the presence or absence of an ileocecal valve, the length of remaining colon, the age of the patient, the length of time since the onset of short-gut syndrome, and the presence of residual disease in the remnant bowel.[43] Patients who carry a poor prognosis for adaptation or who fail to adapt are considered to have intestinal failure and are thus relegated to lifelong TPN support. It is estimated that in Western countries, intestinal failure will eventually be diagnosed in two infants per million live births.[2]

Efforts to enhance the adaptive process have included medical interventions such as the administration of intraluminal glutamine, glutathione, and short-chain fatty acids, as well as systemic growth hormone. Unfortunately, these protocols are offered only at specialized centers of bowel rehabilitation and success has been limited to select patients.[7,43] Surgical procedures such as tapering

TABLE 46–3 Indications for Intestinal Transplantation in Pediatric Patients

Indication	% of Pediatric ITx Performed
Gastroschisis	21%
Volvulus	18%
Necrotizing enterocolitis	12%
Pseudo-obstruction	9%
Intestinal atresia	7%
Failed primary transplant	7%
Aganglionosis/Hirschprungs's disease	7%
Microvillus inclusion disease	6%
Short gut/other	6%
Malabsorption	4%
Dysmotility	2%
Tumor	1%

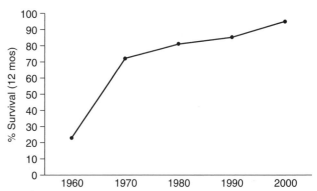

Figure 46–1 Mortality associated with short-gut syndrome before and after the clinical use of total parenteral nutrition.[11,15,50,59]

enteroplasties, artificial valves, and antiperistaltic and isoperistaltic colonic interposition have also been cited as putative methods of enhancing adaptation.[12] However, like medical therapies, widespread application does not seem possible because only select patients appear to benefit from these interventions.[7] Recently, the serial transverse enteroplasty procedure has been advocated as a surgical method for bowel lengthening.[56] Unfortunately, too few patients with short follow-up limit conclusions at this time. Ultimately, approximately 50% of all children with intestinal failure will fail attempts at adaptation.[29]

Analysis of patients maintained on long-term home TPN therapy reveals that in general, these patients do quite well with few serious complications. Unfortunately, not all patients tolerate TPN well and instead suffer from any of a number of life-threatening complications, in addition to the lifestyle-limiting issues. The most frequent life-threatening complications include the development of TPN-associated liver disease, loss of central vascular access sites, recurrent central line infections, difficult fluid and electrolyte management, osteopenia, vertical growth limitation, and death.[29] In fact, many TPN series report 5-year survival rates of only 80%,[59] which is well below that expected for age-matched healthy cohorts.

Indications

Simplistically speaking, the indication for ITx is intestinal failure in patients in whom one or more TPN-associated life-threatening complications have developed or are at high risk for developing. Statistically, this strategy is successful because when these types of complications develop in patients with intestinal failure, their prognosis for survival on long-term TPN is worse than after ITx. Kaufman and associates from the American Society of Transplantation published the first definitive manuscript on the indications for pediatric ITx, and these indications are summarized herein.[27]

The first group of indications is very discretely defined and includes patients with intestinal failure and impending or existing life-threatening TPN-associated complications, including hepatic failure, recurrent central line sepsis, and loss of central access sites. Advanced liver disease secondary to TPN is perhaps the most straightforward because death from liver disease is the inevitable outcome without transplantation.[29,59] However, early liver dysfunction is not as straightforward inasmuch as the rate of progression to advanced disease cannot be predicted.[30] Certainly, the ability to reverse early hepatic dysfunction with isolated ITx has been reported and must be a strong consideration for such patients because the critical shortage of donor liver organs increases the mortality in patients awaiting combined liver-intestinal transplantation.

Recurrent line sepsis in patients with intestinal failure is also an indication for ITx. In general, this indication does not include patients with the occasional infection, but instead those with multiple, recurring infections, infections associated with metastatic foci such as endocarditis, infections associated with multiorgan failure syndromes, and infections caused by multiple-antibiotic–resistant microbes.

Finally, a patient with intestinal failure and limited vascular access should also be considered for ITx. Limited access is appropriately defined as loss of approximately half the standard jugular, subclavian, or iliac vein access sites and not the extreme cases in which intrahepatic, intra-atrial, or intrathoracic access lines are the only available options.

The second group in whom ITx should be considered is the subset of patients at high risk for early death or TPN failure. This group includes young infants, patients with very short lengths of remnant bowel (<10 cm of intestine, absence of the colon, proximal jejunostomies, etc.), patients with gastrocolonic discontinuity (absence of the entire jejunoileal segment with separate drainage of foregut and hindgut secretions required), and patients with congenital epithelial disorders that carry no realistic prognosis for adaptation, such as microvillus inclusion disease, tufting enteropathy, and congenital villus atrophy.

Finally, patients with intestinal failure as a result of disorders associated with high morbidity and poor quality of life should be considered for ITx. This group typically includes patients with difficult fluid and electrolyte management situations that render them hospital bound. Patients with motility disorders such as chronic intestinal pseudo-obstruction, wherein severe dysmotility is associated with severe pain, are also included in this subset.

Evaluation/Listing

Early referral to a center offering both intestinal rehabilitation and ITx is critical for optimizing both pre-ITx care and post-ITx outcome. In particular, children who by virtue of their underlying disease are not candidates for rehabilitation therapy, such as those with gastrocolonic discontinuity and microvillus inclusion disease, warrant immediate referral so that they can be monitored closely by the transplant team for early evaluation and listing. Additionally, patients with risk factors known to be associated with decreased wait list survival, including age younger than 1 year, bridging fibrosis or cirrhosis, bilirubin levels higher than 3 mg/dL, and thrombocytopenia,[9] require prompt evaluation.

Children who are candidates for intestinal rehabilitation may undergo a cursory evaluation by the transplant team with a full workup for ITx only if criteria are met later. Otherwise, initial attempts at intestinal rehabilitation are warranted. Before listing any patient for ITx, a comprehensive evaluation of all major organ systems must be undertaken. The protocol at our center is noted in Table 46-4. Of note, this protocol includes many details that assist with operative planning, such as the type of transplant to be performed, the target vascular access sites, the target inflow and outflow vessels for the graft, the diseased organs to be removed, and the potential sites of gastrointestinal reconstruction. Contraindications to ITx include profound neurologic impairment, uncontrolled systemic sepsis, uncorrectable systemic illnesses not directly related to the digestive system, severe immunologic deficiencies, and the presence of unresectable malignancies.

Once deemed a suitable candidate for ITx, the child is listed with the United Network for Organ Sharing (UNOS)

TABLE 46–4 Prelisting Evaluation of Pediatric Intestinal Transplant Recipients at the University of California, Los Angeles, Intestinal Transplantation Program	
Laboratory Tests	**Studies**
Type and screen, HLA typing, cytotoxic antibody screen	Upper/lower gastrointestinal contrast studies
Serum chemistries, liver function panel, albumin, prealbumin, transferrin, cholesterol	Abdominal imaging via computed tomography or magnetic resonance imaging
Zinc, ferritin, copper, selenium, chromium, folate, vitamin B_{12}, A, D, E levels	Duplex Doppler or magnetic resonance imaging of central veins
Complete blood count/platelets, PT/APTT, fibrinogen	Nuclear medicine glomerular filtration rate
Urinalysis	Nuclear medicine gastric emptying study
Viral serology:	Echocardiography (history of chemotherapy, known congenital defects, endocarditis)
Epstein-Barr virus	
Cytomegalovirus	
Human immunodeficiency virus	
Hepatitis B, C virus	

APTT, activated partial thromboplastin time; PT, prothrombin time.

separately for each organ required and the urgency needed. For the intestine, the current categories include status 1 (urgent), status 2 (nonurgent), or status 7 (temporarily inactive, usually because of active infection). If concomitant liver transplantation is required, separate listing according to the Pediatric End Stage Liver Disease scoring system is performed.[36] Finally, if concomitant pancreas transplantation is required, a third separate listing is initiated.

A comment regarding listing and waiting for liver-inclusive allografts is warranted. ITx recipients are allocated the liver portion of the grafts based solely on their Pediatric End Stage Liver Disease score. Unfortunately, this scoring system was developed for pediatric candidates with biliary atresia, the most common type of pediatric liver disease, to the exclusion of those with parenteral nutrition–associated liver disease. After implementation of this system, alarmingly high mortality rates were reported in the UNOS annual reviews. Fryer et al. expanded on these statistics in a 2003 report[19] and reviewed the outcome of candidates with hepatic failure who were awaiting multiorgan transplants. In retrospect, these high mortality rates were due to the fact that the natural history and progression of TPN-associated liver disease differ significantly from that of other forms of pediatric liver disease and that many of the measured variables used to calculate liver disease scores, such as the prothrombin time and international normalized ratio, do not become abnormal until late in the progression of hepatic failure. As a consequence, UNOS has now adopted measures to ensure that multiorgan recipients with liver disease are more competitive for the liver portions of their allografts. Because these measures were recently instituted, it is too early to determine their impact on ITx candidate wait-list mortality.

GRAFT SELECTION

Five general graft options are available to ITx candidates, depending on the integrity of the remnant gastrointestinal tract and the status of the other visceral organs: (1) isolated bowel consisting of all or part of the jejunoileum (Fig. 46-2A); (2) combined liver and intestine graft (Fig. 46-2B); (3) multivisceral graft consisting of the liver, stomach, pancreas, duodenum, or jejunoileum (Fig. 46-2C); (4) modified multivisceral graft to include option 3 without the liver; and (5) isolated liver graft.[18]

Isolated intestinal transplantation is indicated for patients with intestinal failure and reversible or no disease in other viscera such as the stomach, liver, and pancreas. Combined liver and intestinal grafts are offered to children who have intestinal failure with irreversible liver disease (congenital or acquired). Multivisceral grafts are reserved for children with extensive disease involving the entire gastrointestinal tract/viscera and irreversible liver disease. Pan-gastrointestinal motility disorders are common indications for this type of graft. In addition, children with low-grade malignancies such as desmoid tumors involving the root of the mesentery and requiring sacrifice of the superior mesenteric and celiac arteries may also be candidates for multivisceral grafts. A modified multivisceral graft is used in candidates who have criteria similar to those for a multivisceral graft except that the degree of liver disease is deemed reversible. Finally, the use of an isolated liver graft is an option in select candidates for ITx. Isolated liver grafts are used only when a transplant candidate has advanced liver disease but carries a good prognosis for intestinal adaptation. This situation is most common in infants with a suitable length of remnant bowel but in whom end-stage liver disease develops rapidly. It is not an appropriate option for patients with intestinal failure and evolving liver dysfunction. In appropriate cases, isolated liver transplantation cures the liver disease and allows the recipient to later adapt off TPN. Appropriate selection is absolutely critical because isolated liver transplantation in a candidate with intestinal failure in whom adaptation does not occur and the need for TPN persists carries a very poor prognosis.

DONOR SELECTION

In addition to the standard criteria for selection of deceased donor liver grafts, including the absence of recent systemic

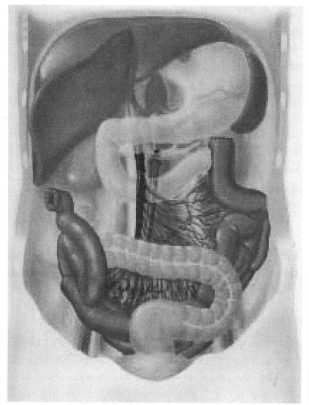

A

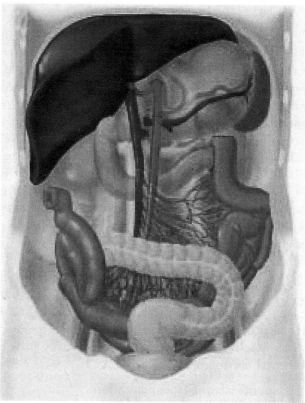

B

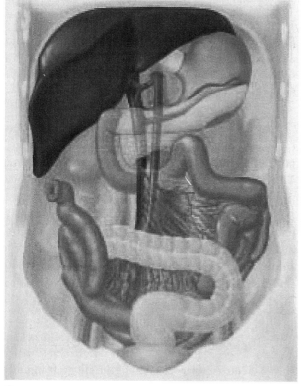

C

Figure 46–2   *A,* Isolated intestinal graft. *B,* Combined liver-intestinal graft. *C,* Multivisceral graft. (*See color plate.*) (From Fishbein TM, Gondolesi GE, Kaufman SS: Intestinal transplantation for gut failure. Gastroenterology 2003;126:1615.)

viral, bacterial, or fungal infection or malignancy, donor selection for ITx is based on size. Frequently, an ITx candidate has had multiple abdominal procedures, loss of bowel, and scarring that result in a "loss of domain" effect manifested by less intra-abdominal space for donor organs from patients of similar age and size. To circumvent this problem, targeting a donor size that is 25% to 30% smaller than the intended recipient is optimal. Furthermore, because of the sensitivity of allograft mucosa to ischemia, the donor mechanism of death, including downtime, prolonged resuscitative efforts, and the use of high-dose vasopressors that shunt blood away from the bowel, should be critically evaluated. The donor and recipient should be blood group identical/compatible. Some authors discourage the use of cytomegalovirus (CMV)-positive donors[39]; however, donor availability can be significantly impaired with this policy, particularly for infants who are likely to be seronegative. Human leukocyte antigen (HLA) and cytotoxic crossmatching is generally performed by most centers but is not a factor in donor selection because prolongation of cold ischemia times while awaiting results can have a great impact on graft function. In addition, the geographic location of the donor can be a factor related to cold ischemia time inasmuch as most ITx teams desire times less than 8 to 12 hours.

Living donation for isolated ITx has been performed, with theoretical benefits including improved graft function because of minimal ischemia time and decreased immunologic complications because of HLA similarity in living related donors.[41,57] Unfortunately, although single-center reports are quite promising, Intestinal Transplant Registry data have shown no difference in graft survival to date (Fig. 46-3).[25] These data, coupled with the current favorable discrepancy between ITx donors and recipients (5500 cadaveric donors versus 120 ITx recipients in the United States in 2003), limit the applicability of living donor ITx until further data regarding benefit are available.

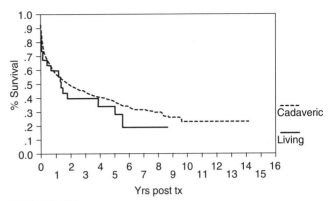

Figure 46–3 Graft survival by donor type. (From International Transplant Registry. Available at http://www/intestinaltransplant.org. Accessed 2004.)

OPERATIVE PROCEDURES

Donor

All multivisceral procurement techniques represent modifications of those originally described by Starzl et al.[45] Later modifications have been published by Grant,[22] Starzl,[47,51,52] Bueno,[9] and Abu-Elmagd[1] and their colleagues. Common to all these techniques is that procurement of thoracic and renal organs is not precluded and that minor modifications enable procurement of all of the various visceral grafts described earlier. The general principles as outlined in a previous report[61] include the use of a midline incision, obtaining vascular control of the donor aorta in the supraceliac and infrarenal locations, mobilization of the target graft organ or organs, and coordinated donor perfusion (Fig. 46-4A and B).

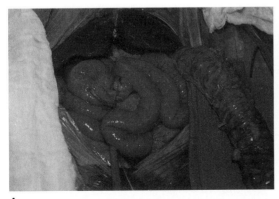 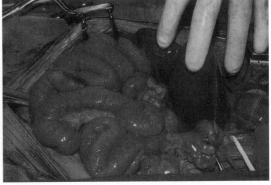

A   B

Figure 46–4 Operative approach to a multivisceral donor. *A,* The round and falciform ligaments have been divided and the liver completely mobilized. In addition, the left colon has been mobilized to the splenic flexure, the terminal ileum has been stapled (*left lower corner*), and the aortic cannula has been positioned. *B,* The aortic cannula is in position with the supraceliac aorta encircled with umbilical tape (*lower right*). The donor is prepared for systemic heparin, cross-clamping, and organ perfusion. (*See color plate.*) (From Yersiz H, Renz J, Histaki G, et al: Multivisceral and isolated intestinal procurement techniques. Liver Transpl 2003;9:881.)

After removal of the thoracic grafts, the target abdominal viscera are removed en bloc. In the case of an isolated intestinal graft, the liver, pancreas, and intestine can all be procured separately for transplantation into different recipients.[1] The entire jejunoileum is usually procured with vascular inflow from the celiac and superior mesenteric arteries and outflow via the suprahepatic vena cava. Of note, use of the duodenal-sparing variation for procurement of the liver-intestinal allograft (the "Omaha technique")[55] represents a modification in which the donor duodenum and the head of the pancreas are retained with the liver-intestinal graft, thus eliminating the need for recipient biliary reconstruction. Many centers now commonly use this technique. Finally, multivisceral grafts incorporate all the viscera en bloc with vascular inflow again from the celiac and superior mesenteric arteries and outflow via the suprahepatic vena cava. Ex vivo multivisceral allograft preparation, minimized through increased dissection and organ separation in situ, consists of preparation of a donor thoracic aorta conduit and oversewing of the transected pancreas and distal vena cava. Thus, total cold ischemia time is reduced and inadvertent rewarming is avoided.

Recipient

The surgical approach to the recipient is challenging, and accurate preoperative assessment and operative planning are essential. Identification of an established surgical plan to include the target organs to be removed, vascular inflow and outflow targets, organ or organs to implant, and target remnant viscera for gastrointestinal continuity is crucial. In general, this operative plan is individualized for the disease and anatomy of each recipient. Multiple previous surgeries, dense adhesions, and coagulopathy/portal hypertension are the norm, especially for patients with advanced liver disease.

The recipient operation can be considered in five phases, depending on the type of transplant required. Stage 1 consists of ensuring that adequate multilumen access has been obtained for intraoperative management and postoperative administration of TPN and intravenous medications. Special note should be made of preoperative vascular imaging studies to avoid complications associated with attempted access in occluded sites. Our standard is magnetic resonance venography performed during transplant evaluation to establish vascular access targets.

Stage 2 is abdominal dissection and removal of diseased organs. For the recipient of an isolated intestinal graft, this can safely be performed through a midline incision with lysis of adhesions below the mesocolon and resection of the diseased remnant jejunoileum. For a liver-intestinal recipient, we prefer a bilateral subcostal incision with the initial dissection confined to the perihepatic region. Total hepatectomy is undertaken, usually with retention of the inferior vena cava and without the use of venovenous bypass. Finally, for recipients of multivisceral grafts, an en bloc foregut resection to include a partial gastrectomy, total hepatectomy, total pancreaticoduodenosplenectomy, and remnant enterectomy is performed.

After this dissection phase is complete and before implantation, vascular inflow and outflow targets are sought and vascular conduits used liberally as needed. Conduit placement allows for a much more technically facile anastomosis. It should also be noted that the preferred outflow for an isolated intestinal graft is either a branch of the recipient portal venous system or the inferior vena cava. For liver-intestinal recipients, the native foregut viscera drained by the portal venous system must also be addressed. In our experience, performing a native portacaval shunt is probably the easiest, but the use of an end-to-side donor portal–to–recipient portal anastomosis is an option as well.

The third phase, consisting of implantation, then ensues (Fig. 46-5). In cases of isolated ITx, intestinal revascularization is achieved via anastomosis of the donor superior mesenteric artery with the recipient infrarenal aorta. In liver-containing multiorgan grafts, arterial inflow is obtained from the supraceliac aorta. We prefer to piggyback the liver, thus eliminating the need for an infrahepatic inferior vena cava anastomosis. Modified multivisceral grafts can be implanted via the same principles as for isolated intestinal grafts in some cases, but others require more extensive resection of diseased organs such as the stomach and duodenum/pancreas.

The fourth phase is devoted to restoration of gastrointestinal continuity. For an isolated intestinal graft recipient, the target proximal anastomosis is usually the remnant jejunum, but direct anastomosis to the stomach is sometimes required. A distal ileostomy is almost always created with various techniques to facilitate allograft monitoring after transplantation. In cases in which suitable remnant colon exists, anastomosis of the graft ileum to the native colon is also performed. In the case of a multivisceral recipient, the entire foregut of the recipient has been removed, with only a small remnant of proximal stomach and colon left. Therefore, the graft stomach or jejunum is anastomosed to the recipient stomach/esophagus, and the distal anastomoses are similar to those described earlier. Pyloroplasty is required if the stomach is included.

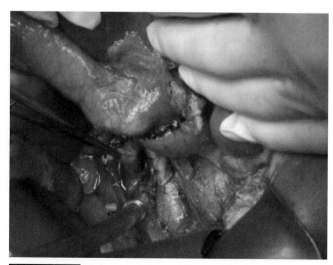

Figure 46–5   Operative photo, graft implantation demonstrating complete vascular anastomoses below the graft pancreas.

For the recipient of a liver-intestinal allograft, our technique necessitates dissection and removal of diseased remnant gut after reperfusion of the graft. We use this technique to avoid extensive dissection in the presence of portal hypertension and coagulopathy before removal of the native liver. Furthermore, we have been successfully able to "stage" this type of transplant in difficult cases.[44] Specifically, rather than proceed with the latter stages of the transplant operation in a coagulopathic patient with significant transfusion requirements, we terminate the procedure at this stage, drain the distal end of the bowel, and pack and close the abdomen. A second-stage operation conducted after the patient has stabilized in the intensive care unit then completes the procedure. Regardless of the method used, a liver-intestine recipient will require dissection and removal of diseased bowel with restoration of intestinal continuity as described earlier.

The final phase of the operation consists of establishment of enteral access. The major centers use differing techniques. Irrespective of the technique used, having access to the transplanted bowel for administration of enteral nutrients and medications is essential for a successful outcome. We prefer to use a 2-in-1 gastrojejunostomy tube. With this method, one ostomy (gastrostomy) is created, and the jejunal portion of the gastrojejunostomy is manually fed down into the transplanted jejunum. Others report performing separate tube gastrostomies and jejunostomies.

For closure, spatial constraints and lack of abdominal domain may require splenectomy, liver resection, or partial allograft enterectomy. Alternatives such as the use of split-liver donor grafts have been advocated. Compressive closure can lead to ischemic allograft necrosis or vascular thrombosis, or both, and is thus to be avoided. In this case, prosthetic-assisted or skin-only closures with delayed reconstruction may be indicated. The University of Miami has reported good results with transplantation of the abdominal wall after ITx.[33]

POSTOPERATIVE MANAGEMENT

Medical

Patients are monitored in the pediatric intensive care unit with invasive lines and regular assessment of volume status, gastrointestinal loss, renal function, and indicators of graft perfusion, including serial serum lactate, chemistry panels, liver function studies, and arterial blood gas analysis for the first several days postoperatively. Because of their smaller plasma volume, children are subject to greater shifts in hemoconcentration and procoagulant factor concentration than are adults.[24] This response is augmented in recipients of liver grafts as a result of initial fluctuating hepatic function. Agents such as prostaglandin, dopamine, dextran, and low-dose heparin are used at our center to promote splanchnic perfusion and prevent thrombosis. In addition, it is anticipated that the patient will require TPN until the absorptive capacity of the graft is demonstrated by tolerance of increasing volumes of dilute and then full-strength enteral feeding.

Immunosuppression

Contemporary immunosuppression for ITx is predicated on the observation that graft and patient survival rates have improved as immunosuppression has become more potent and specific. Although various protocols vary, many centers use an induction agent for the purpose of depleting T cells or T-cell products and encouraging microchimerism or tolerance. Drugs/mechanisms used to achieve induction include antithymocyte globulin,[48] alemtuzumab (off-label),[58] infusion of donor bone marrow–derived cells,[32] and interleukin-2 receptor blockade.[17,53] Tacrolimus in addition to steroids is usually the mainstay of maintenance therapies. Our protocol consists of induction of daclizumab (Zenapax, Roche Laboratories, Nutley, NJ; off-label use) preoperatively and postoperatively with initiation of enterically administered maintenance tacrolimus within 24 hours of ITx. We also administer secondary and tertiary immunosuppression consisting of intravenous steroid pulse and taper and mycophenolate mofetil (CellCept, Roche Laboratories; off-label use), with enteric conversion only after allograft absorptive capacity has been demonstrated. With this regimen we have seen a marked increase in patient and graft survival along with a decrease in rejection and infection. In cases of tacrolimus intolerance or increased risk of rejection (or both), we have demonstrated graft salvage in a subset of both adults and children who have converted to sirolimus (Rapamune, Wyeth; off-label use) rescue therapy.[21]

The primary cause of morbidity and mortality after ITx is sepsis. Based on registry data, Beath et al. report sepsis as the leading cause of death (50%) of transplant recipients reviewed.[4] Therefore, intermediate and long-term immunosuppressive goals for most centers include steroid weaning and a reduction in trough serum levels of tacrolimus to avoid cumulative morbidity. In addition to the universal risk for infection with immunosuppression, the well-known adverse effects of prolonged steroid use, such as osteoporosis, adrenal insufficiency, peptic ulcer disease, psychosis, cataracts, growth failure, and glucose intolerance, are augmented by the toxicities associated with other immunosuppressants used in ITx. For tacrolimus, neurotoxicity, nephrotoxicity, glucose intolerance, and hypertension predominate; with mycophenolate, bone marrow depression, mucosal ulcerations, and gastrointestinal disturbances are problematic; and the use of sirolimus has been shown to result in bone marrow depression, stomatitis, and hyperlipidemia. Weaning of immunosuppression to avoid these complications must be tempered by the long-term risk for rejection, a significant problem in ITx recipients.

COMPLICATIONS

Rejection

After sepsis, rejection is the second most common cause of death following ITx, but the primary reason for graft loss.[4] Compounding this problem is the fact that detection of rejection can be difficult when relying on nonspecific clinical signs and symptoms. Symptoms vary from fever to high-output gastrointestinal loss, abdominal pain, and hematochezia. Rarely, obstructive symptoms may predominate. In addition, the liver portion of the composite graft is usually late to reject, and therefore the use of liver function tests to alert the clinician to rejection often proves unreliable. Serum markers such as intestinal fatty acid binding protein,[28] citrulline,[20] and granzyme B[37] have been championed as markers of rejection, but because of lack of bowel specificity, as well as changes that can occur in other inflammatory bowel conditions, none have demonstrated clinical utility.

Endoscopy and biopsy are used as the gold standard for the early diagnosis of acute rejection after ITx. Endoscopic features of rejection include edema, hyperemia, mucosal granularity, loss of the fine mucosal vascular pattern, diminished peristalsis, and mucosal ulceration. Histologic features of acute rejection include mononuclear infiltration, crypt injury with nuclear enlargement and hyperchromasia, decreased cell height, mucin depletion, crypt apoptosis, and distortion of villous and crypt architecture (Fig. 46-6).[60] Recently, use of the zoom video endoscope has been advocated as a method to more accurately visualize the mucosa and diagnose rejection.[26] Widespread application has not been achieved to date.

The frequency with which surveillance endoscopy is performed depends on the center. In general, most centers initiate regular surveillance endoscopy within 1 to 2 weeks after ITx and continue these procedures at least weekly for the first 6 to 8 weeks thereafter. When clinical signs and symptoms suspicious for rejection are noted, diagnostic endoscopy and biopsy are quickly performed, regardless of timing.

Treatment of rejection is based on clinical and histologic severity. Severe episodes warrant monoclonal antilymphocyte antibody therapy and are generally indicative of a high risk for graft loss. Antilymphocyte therapies require empirical antiviral therapy and carry a cumulative risk for post-transplant lymphoproliferative disorder (PTLD).

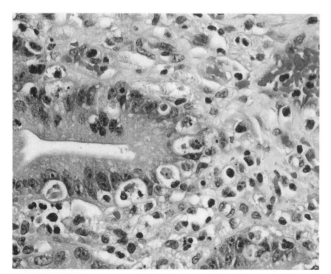

Figure 46–6 Histologic features of intestinal allograft acute cellular rejection, including crypt distortion with apoptosis and an extensive inflammatory infiltrate. (*See color plate.*)

Mild to moderate episodes can be treated with an increased level of maintenance immunosuppression or a steroid bolus, or both. In patients refractory to immunotherapy, it is critical to proceed swiftly to enterectomy and cessation of immunosuppression to avoid sepsis and death.

Infection

As mentioned previously, infection is the primary cause of mortality in ITx recipients. In general, the prevalence of infection/sepsis varies directly with the amount of immunosuppression used. Recipients of ITx are undoubtedly some of the most heavily immunosuppressed transplant recipients. Furthermore, the necessity of a long and complex abdominal procedure renders ITx recipients more susceptible to infection. Common foci of infection are intra-abdominal and pulmonary sites. Aggressive evaluation and treatment must be undertaken when clinical signs or symptoms of infection arise.

Although standard intra-abdominal and pulmonary post-transplant infections occur and are serious, these types of infections are not unique to recipients of ITx. Other infections unique to this population occur and are worthy of discussion. Infectious enteritides are an increasingly recognized complication after ITx.[62] Not only do these infections mimic rejection (and many times are incorrectly treated as such), but they can also precipitate a subsequent rejection episode and graft loss. In our experience, the major infections have been viral, primarily adenovirus and rotavirus, but other agents, including *Cryptosporidium*, *Giardia lamblia*, and *Clostridium difficile*, have been encountered as well.

CMV and Epstein-Barr virus (EBV) also present unique problems after ITx. In fact, rates of infection with these viruses can be as high as 40% after ITx[62]—a rate much higher than that seen after any other solid organ transplant. Both viruses can directly infect the bowel and represent a major source of morbidity and mortality. Several protocols are used to control their replication after ITx. At the University of California, Los Angeles, we have used a standard prophylaxis protocol consisting of intravenous ganciclovir for the first 100 days after ITx, followed by conversion to oral acyclovir. In addition, we use a preemptive monitoring and therapeutic protocol consisting of frequent testing for the presence of EBV or CMV viral DNA in blood with polymerase chain reaction. Detection of CMV or EBV viral DNA prompts preemptive therapy that includes intravenous ganciclovir or CMV immune globulin (or both). With this protocol we have significantly reduced the incidence of CMV and EBV viremia and infection after ITx.[62]

Post-Transplant Lymphoproliferative Disorder

PTLD is a B-cell malignancy caused in many instances by EBV infection. Intestinal Transplant Registry data reveal that PTLD is the cause of graft loss in 1.6% and patient death in 6.1% of pediatric ITx patients.[4] Prompt diagnosis and treatment are necessary to improve these outcomes. A thorough evaluation of the patient should be performed, including physical examination and complete radiologic imaging. Suspicious adenopathy should prompt biopsy and bone marrow sampling. Treatment consists of ganciclovir, CMV immune globulin, and reduction in immunosuppression. Early data regarding graft and patient salvage with the use of humanized anti-CD20 monoclonal antibody (rituximab) as treatment of PTLD instead of chemotherapy are convincing.[38] Severe refractory or EBV-negative patients may require chemotherapy. Prevention with a preemptive monitoring protocol such as that just outlined allows for maximal treatment success. In our experience, the incidence of PTLD has been less than 2%.

OUTCOMES

To evaluate outcomes, several data sources are now available. Large, single-center series have been reported from the Universities of Pittsburgh, Miami, Nebraska, California (Los Angeles), and Mount Sinai. Additionally, pooled center data are available from two sources. The Intestinal Transplant Registry is a worldwide, voluntary registry that is believed to contain data regarding all human intestinal transplant attempts ever performed. From this standpoint, it is a unique and useful source of data analysis. Additionally, in the United States, mandatory data collection though UNOS is made available in the Scientific Registry of Transplant Recipients Annual Report. Outcome data will reflect these major sources.

As previously noted, outcomes after ITx have been demonstrated to be dependent on the era of immunosuppression. From the Intestinal Transplant Registry, overall patient and graft survival rates at 1 year now exceed 75% and 65%, respectively, in select recipients (Fig. 46-7A and B).[25] Further observations include differential prognoses based on the type of ITx, location of the recipient before ITx, and the type of induction therapy used (Fig. 46-8A to C).[25] Of particular note is the fact that successful ITx is associated with a 90% rate of freedom from TPN.[25]

An underassessed outcome variable after transplantation of any kind has been quality of life. Sudan et al. report that pediatric ITx recipients rate their quality of

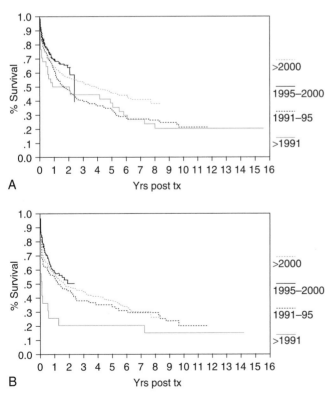

Figure 46–7 Patient (*A*) and graft (*B*) survival after intestinal transplantation by era. (From International Transplant Registry. Available at http://www.intestinaltransplant.org. Accessed 2004.)

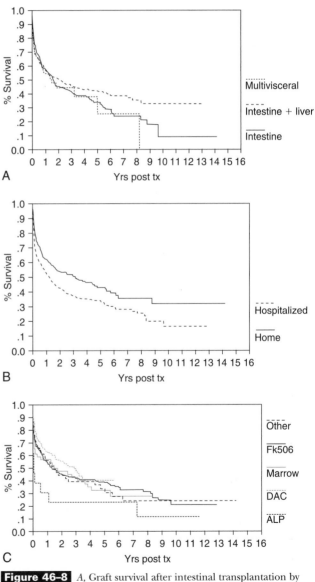

Figure 46–8 *A*, Graft survival after intestinal transplantation by graft type (multivisceral versus intestine plus liver versus isolated intestine). *B*, Graft survival after intestinal transplantation by pretransplant location. *C*, Graft survival by induction agent. ALP, antilymphocyte product; DAC, daclizumab; marrow, bone marrow. (From International Transplant Registry. Available at http://www.intestinaltransplant.org. Accessed 2004.)

life as not significantly different from that of their healthy peers,[54] thus indicating that successful ITx truly restores a patient to a better lifestyle than that preceding the transplant. However, these data must be interpreted with caution because patients undergoing long-term home TPN without complications have similar quality-of-life assessments.

CONCLUSION

The field of ITx has changed dramatically since the experimental eras of the 1950s, 1960s, and 1970s. Today, ITx is a common procedure performed at a few specialized transplant centers worldwide. Recipients enjoy unprecedented success rates not seen previously after ITx. Advances in surgical techniques, immunotherapy, and experience in management have contributed significantly to these improvements. Unfortunately, the field remains limited to specialized centers and only to patients with intestinal failure and life-threatening TPN-associated complications. More widespread application will require a reduction in post-transplant surgical morbidity, infections, immunosuppression-related complications, length of hospitalization, and cost. However, as the field grows, these goals are realistically obtainable in the near future.

REFERENCES

1. Abu-Elmagd K, Fung J, Bueno J, et al: Logistics and technique for procurement of intestinal, pancreatic, and hepatic grafts from the same donor. Ann Surg 2000;232:680.
2. American Gastroenterological Association Clinical Practice Committee: AGA technical review on short bowel syndrome and intestinal transplantation. Gastroenterology 2003; 125:1111.
3. Asfar S, Atkinson P, Ghent C, et al: Small bowel transplantation, a life-saving option for selected patients with intestinal failure. Dig Dis Sci 1996;441:875.
4. Beath S, deVille Goyet J, Kelly D: Risk factors for death and graft loss after small bowel transplantation. Curr Opin Organ Transplant 2003;8:195.
5. Borel J, Feurer C, Magnee C, et al: Effects of the new antilymphocytic peptide cyclosporine A in animals. Immunology 1977;32:1017.
6. Broviac J, Cole J, Scribner B: A silicone rubber atrial catheter for prolonged parenteral nutrition. Surg Gynecol Obstet 1974;139:24.
7. Byrne T, Cox S, Karimbakas M, et al: Bowel rehabilitation: An alternative to long-term parenteral nutrition and intestinal transplantation for some patients with short bowel syndrome. Transplant Proc 2002;34:887.
8. Bueno J, Abu-Elmagd K, Mazariegos G, et al: Composite liver–small bowel allografts with preservation of donor duodenum and hepatic biliary system in children. J Pediatr Surg 2000;35:291.
9. Bueno J, Ohwada S, Kocoshis S, et al: Factors impacting the survival of children with intestinal failure referred for intestinal transplantation. J Pediatr Surg 1999;34:27.
10. Calne R, Rolles K, White D, et al: Cyclosporin-A in clinical organ grafting. Transplant Proc 1981;13:349.
11. Caniano D, Starr J, Ginn-Pease M, et al: Extensive short-bowel syndrome in neonates: Outcome in the 1980's. Surgery 1989;105:119.
12. Carlson G: Surgical management of intestinal failure. Proc Nutr Soc 2003;62:711.
13. Deltz E, Schroeder P, Gebhard H, et al: Successful clinical small bowel transplantation: A report of a case. Clin Transpl 1989;21:89.
14. DiBaise J, Young R, Vanderhoof J: Intestinal rehabilitation and the short bowel syndrome: Part 2. Am J Gastroenterol 2004;99:1823.
15. Dorney S, Ament M, Berquist W, et al: Improved survival in very short small bowel of infancy with use of long-term parenteral nutrition. J Pediatr 1985;107:521.
16. Dudrick S, Wilmore D, Rhoads J: Long-term total parenteral nutrition with growth, development and positive nitrogen balance. Surgery 1968;64:138.
17. Farmer D, McDiarmid S, Edelstein S, et al: Induction therapy with interleukin-2 receptor antagonist after intestinal transplantation is associated with reduced acute cellular rejection and improved renal function. Transplant Proc 2004;36:331.
18. Fishbein TM, Gondolesi GE, Kaufman SS: Intestinal transplantation for gut failure. Gastroenterology 2003;126:1615.
19. Fryer J, Pellar S, Osmond D, et al: Mortality in candidates waiting for combined liver-intestine transplants exceeds that for other candidates waiting for liver transplants. Liver Transpl 2003;9:748.
20. Gondolesi G, Fishbein T, Chehade M, et al: Serum citrulline is a potential marker for rejection of intestinal allografts. Transplant Proc 2002;34:918.
21. Gordon S, Yersiz H, McDiarmid S, et al: Rescue immunotherapy using sirolimus after small bowel transplantation. Presented at the IXth International Small Bowel Transplantation symposium, 2005.
22. Grant D, Wall W, Mineualt R, et al: Successful small bowel/liver transplantation. Lancet 1990;335:181.
23. Hancock B, Wiseman N: Lethal short-bowel syndrome. J Pediatr Surg 1990;25:1131.
24. Harper P, Luddington R, Carrell R, et al: Protein C deficiency and portal thrombosis in liver transplantation in children. Lancet 1988;2:924.
25. International Transplant Registry. Available at http: www.intestinaltransplants.org. Accessed 2004.
26. Kato T, O'Brien CB, Nishida S, et al: The first case report of the use of a zoom videoendoscope for the evaluation of small bowel graft mucosa in a human after intestinal transplantation. Gastrointest Endosc 1999;50:257.
27. Kaufman S, Atkinson J, Bianchi A, et al: Indications for pediatric intestinal transplantation: A position paper of the American Society of Transplantation. Pediatr Transplant 2001;5:80.
28. Kaufman S, Lyden E, Marks W, et al: Lack of utility of intestinal fatty acid binding protein levels in predicting intestinal allograft rejection. Transplantation 2001; 71:1058.
29. Kaufman SS: Prevention of parenteral nutrition–associated liver disease in children. Pediatr Transplant 2002;6:37.
30. Kelly D: Liver complications of pediatric parenteral nutrition—epidemiology. Nutrition 1998;14:153.
31. Kino T, Hatanaka H, Miyata S, et al: FK-506, a novel immunosuppressant isolated from a *Streptomyces*. II. Immunosuppressive effect of FK-506 in vitro. J Antibiot (Tokyo) 40:1256, 1987.
32. Levi D, Tzakis A, Kato T, et al: Immune responses and their regulation by donor bone marrow cells in clinical organ transplantation. Transpl Immunol 2003;11:307.

33. Levi D, Tzakis A, Madariaga J, et al: Transplantation of the abdominal wall. Lancet 2003;361:2173.

34. Lillehei R, Goot B, Miller F: The physiologic response of the small bowel of the dog to ischemia including prolonged in vitro preservation of the bowel with successful replacement and survival. Ann Surg 1959;150:543.

35. McAllister V, Grant DR: Clinical small bowel transplantation. In Grant DR, Rim (eds): Small Bowel Transplantation. London, Edward Arnold, 1994, pp 121-132.

36. McDiarmid SV, Anand R, Lindblad AS: Principal Investigators and Institutions of the Studies of Pediatric Liver Transplantation (SPLIT) Research Group. Development of a pediatric end-stage liver disease score to predict poor outcome in children awaiting liver transplantation. Transplantation 2002;74:173.

37. McDiarmid S, Farmer D, Kuniyoshi J, et al: Perforin and granzyme B. Cytolytic proteins up-regulated during rejection of rat small intestine allografts. Transplantation 1995; 69:762.

38. McGhee W, Mazariegos G, Sindhi R, et al: Rituximab in the treatment of pediatric small bowel transplant patients with post transplant lymphoproliferative disorder unresponsive to standard treatment. Transplant Proc 2002; 34:955.

39. Manez R, Kusne S, Green M, et al: Incidence and risk factors associated with the development of cytomegalovirus disease after intestinal transplantation. Transplantation 1995;59:1010.

40. The Organ Procurement and Transplantation Network: Available at http://www.optn.org. Accessed 2004.

41. Pollard S: Intestinal transplantation: Living related. Br Med Bull 1997;53:868.

42. Potts W: Pediatric surgery. JAMA 1955;157:627.

43. Quiros-Tejeira R, Ament M, Reyen L: Long-term parenteral nutritional support and intestinal adaptation in children with short bowel syndrome: A 25-year experience. J Pediatr 2004;145:157.

44. Renz J, McDiarmid S, Edelstein S, et al: Application of combined liver-intestinal transplantation as a staged procedure. Transpant Proc 2004;36:314.

45. Starzl T, Hakala T, Shaw B, et al: A flexible procedure for multiple cadaveric organ procurement. Surg Gynecol Obstet 1984;158:228.

46. Starzl T, Kaupp H: Mass homotransplantations of abdominal organs in dogs. Surg Forum 1960;11:28.

47. Starzl T, Miller C, Bronznick B, et al: An improved technique for multiple organ harvesting. Surg Gynecol Obstet 1987;165:343.

48. Starzl T, Murase N, Abu-Elmagd K, et al: Tolerogenic immunosuppression for organ transplantation. Lancet 2003; 361:1502.

49. Starzl T, Rowe M, Todo S, et al: Transplantation of multiple abdominal viscera. JAMA 1989;261:1449.

50. Starzl T, Todo S, Fung J, et al: FK 506 for liver, kidney, and pancreas transplantation. Lancet 1989;2:1000.

51. Starzl T, Todo S, Tzakis A, et al: Abdominal organ cluster transplantation for the treatment of upper abdominal malignancies. Ann Surg 1989;210:374.

52. Starzl T, Todo S, Tzakis A, et al: The many faces of multivisceral transplantation. Surg Gynecol Obstet 1991;172:335.

53. Sudan D, Chinnakotla S, Horslen S, et al: Basiliximab decreases the incidence of acute rejection after intestinal transplantation. Transplant Proc 2002;34:940.

54. Sudan D, Horslen S, Botha J, et al: Quality of life after pediatric intestinal transplantation: The perception of pediatric recipients and their parents. Am J Transplant 2004;4:407.

55. Sudan D, Iyer K, Deroover A, et al: A new technique for combined liver-intestinal transplantation. Transplantation 2001;72:1846.

56. Tannuri U: Serial transverse tapering enteroplasty (STEP): A novel bowel lengthening procedure, and serial transverse enteroplasty for short bowel syndrome. J Pediatr Surg 2003;38:1845.

57. Tesi R, Beck R, Lambiase L, et al: Living-related small bowel transplantation: Donor evaluation and outcome. Transplant Proc 1997;29:686.

58. Tzakis A, Dato T, Nishida S, et al: Alemtuzumab (Campath 1-H) combined with tacrolimus in intestinal and multivisceral transplantation. Transplantation 2001;75:1512.

59. Vantini I, Benini L, Bonfante F, et al: Survival rate and prognostic factors in patients with intestinal failure. Dig Liver Dis 2004;36:46.

60. Wu T, Abu-Elmagd K, Bond G, et al: A schema for histologic grading of small intestine allograft acute rejection. Transplantation 2002;75:1241.

61. Yersiz H, Renz J, Hisatake G, et al: Multivisceral and isolated intestinal procurement techniques. Liver Transpl 2003;9:881.

62. Ziring D, Tran R, Edelstein S, et al: Infectious enteritis after intestinal transplantation: Incidence, timing, and outcome. Transplantation 2005;79:702.

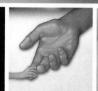

Chapter 47

Heart Transplantation

Thomas L. Spray and Stephanie M. P. Fuller

Thoracic organ transplantation has been successfully performed in pediatric patients since the mid-1980s and now serves as an important option in the treatment of both congenital and end-stage heart and lung disease in children. Approximately 350 pediatric heart transplants are performed annually in the Unites States, or roughly 10% of all thoracic organ transplants.[4,15] Despite the clinical success of heart and lung transplantation in children, limited donor availability has prevented more widespread application of this therapy. Complications such as acute and chronic rejection, graft coronary artery disease (CAD), and bronchiolitis obliterans, as well as the infectious and neoplastic complications of current methods of immunosuppression, threaten cardiac transplant longevity. This chapter focuses on the clinical aspects of heart transplantation in infants and children, including indications, preoperative evaluation, operative techniques, postoperative management, complications, and outcome.

HISTORICAL NOTES

Kantrowitz et al. performed the first pediatric heart transplant in 1967 when they transplanted the heart of an infant with anencephaly into a 3-week-old infant with tricuspid atresia. The next year, Cooley transplanted the heart and lungs of a newborn with anencephaly into a 3-month-old with an atrioventricular septal defect and pulmonary hypertension. Although neither of the infants survived for more than a few hours because of allograft rejection, these pioneering procedures emphasized the technical feasibility of thoracic organ transplantation in children. It was only in 1980 with the introduction of cyclosporine as an immunosuppressive agent that meaningful clinical success became possible. In November 1985, Bailey performed the first successful cardiac transplantation on a 4-day-old neonate with hypoplastic left heart syndrome (HLHS) at Loma Linda.[1] Throughout the last 2 decades, outcomes have been improved by technical advances, better immunosuppression, including reduced steroid use and the advent of induction therapy, a decreased incidence of rejection, increased attention to viral prophylaxis, and aggressive treatment of post-transplant lymphoma and other post-transplant complications.

INDICATIONS

As published by the Registry for the International Society for Heart and Lung Transplantation in the Seventh Official Pediatric Report in May 2004, the number of pediatric heart transplants has remained relatively constant over the last 10 years (Fig. 47-1).[4] The most common indications for cardiac transplantation in the pediatric population remain congenital cardiac disease and cardiomyopathy, as demonstrated in Figures 47-2 to 47-4. According to age distribution, congenital heart disease is seen more commonly in infants, most of whom are younger than 2 months, whereas cardiomyopathy is more prevalent in older children. As expected, the incidence of retransplantation increases with increasing patient age.

The primary indication for heart transplantation in infancy remains complex congenital heart disease without a reasonable corrective or palliative surgical option. Of such conditions, the most common anomaly treated by transplantation is HLHS, a group of defects characterized by aortic or mitral atresia/stenosis with a diminutive

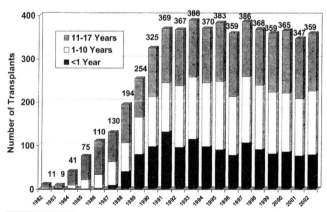

Figure 47-1 Age distribution of pediatric heart recipients by year of transplantation performed from January 1996 to June 2003. (Reprinted from Journal of Heart and Lung Transplantation, August 2004, with permission from International Society of Heart and Lung Transplantation.)

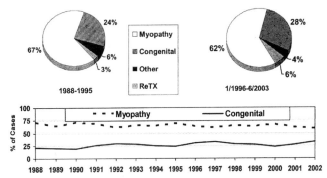

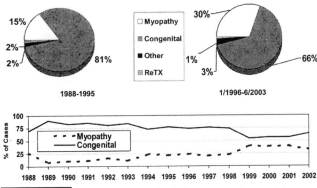

Figure 47–2 Diagnoses for pediatric heart transplant recipients (age <1 year). ReTX, retransplantation. (Reprinted from Journal of Heart and Lung Transplantation, August 2004, with permission from International Society of Heart and Lung Transplantation.)

Figure 47–4 Diagnoses for pediatric heart transplant recipients (age 11 to 17 years). ReTX, retransplantation. (Reprinted from Journal of Heart and Lung Transplantation, August 2004, with permission from International Society of Heart and Lung Transplantation.)

left ventricle. Initial poor results with a staged palliative approach to HLHS led some centers to consider orthotopic heart transplantation as the primary treatment of this anomaly. Long transplant waiting lists have led other institutions to advocate performing a stage I palliation (Norwood or Sano procedure) to help stabilize the patient and then list the patient for transplantation.[5] However, with improvement in early survival from the Norwood procedure followed by a Fontan repair, the majority of cardiac centers have abandoned primary transplantation as initial therapy for HLHS. Instead, transplantation is an option now reserved for patients with unusually high risk, including aortic atresia with a diminutive ascending aorta and severe tricuspid regurgitation.[6]

Other forms of congenital heart disease that have been treated by cardiac transplantation during infancy include an unbalanced atrioventricular canal, single ventricle, complex truncus arteriosus, double-outlet right ventricle, Ebstein's anomaly, L-transposition of the great arteries, and pulmonary atresia with an intact ventricular septum.[3] Even the most complex forms of congenital heart disease, such as heterotaxy syndromes with anomalies of systemic and venous drainage, are amenable to cardiac

transplantation with suitable reconstruction.[14] Other pediatric candidates include infants with congenital heart disease who have undergone previous corrective or palliative procedures yet who exhibit residual or progressive cardiac dysfunction manifested by left ventricular failure that ultimately requires transplantation. In these cases, postoperative cardiac dysfunction is often related to atrioventricular or semilunar valvar insufficiency that eventually results in dilated cardiomyopathy. Of note, multiple previous palliative procedures do not preclude successful transplantation.[12]

Cardiomyopathy is the other most common indication for heart transplantation in infancy and childhood. Most pediatric heart transplantations outside infancy are performed for idiopathic cardiomyopathy. Other causes of cardiomyopathy include viral, familial, and hypertrophic. Despite the diverse causes of cardiomyopathy, several variables have been associated with poor outcome, including very high left ventricular end-diastolic pressure, a left ventricular ejection fraction less than 20%, ventricular arrhythmia, and a family history of cardiomyopathy.[18,30] Cardiomyopathy attributable to inflammation or arrhythmia tends to have a more favorable outcome, and these patients should be supported as long as possible before transplantation to allow for the possibility of spontaneous recovery. Other less common indications for cardiac transplantation are doxorubicin-induced cardiotoxicity from chemotherapy for malignancy and obstructive cardiac tumors such as fibromas and rhabdomyomas that are not amenable to surgical resection.

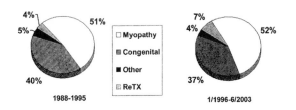

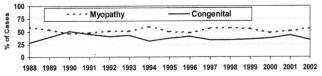

Figure 47–3 Diagnoses for pediatric heart transplant recipients (age 1 to 10 years). ReTX, retransplantation. (Reprinted from Journal of Heart and Lung Transplantation, August 2004, with permission from International Society of Heart and Lung Transplantation.)

PREOPERATIVE EVALUATION

The pretransplant evaluation is a multidisciplinary screening process that serves as the key to successful organ transplantation (Table 47-1). Potential recipients undergo a thorough physical and psychosocial evaluation with careful examination of the cardiac, pulmonary, neurologic, renal, infectious, and socioeconomic systems. The presence of an adequate family support system is of paramount importance to survival postoperatively. Parents must demonstrate the ability and resources to

TABLE 47-1 Evaluation of Candidates for Heart Transplantation

History and physical examination
Blood type
Panel-reactive antibody
Complete blood count with differential
Chemistry panel with electrolytes
Liver function tests
Lipid profile
Serologic examination for antibodies to varicella, CMV, EBV, herpes simplex, measles, hepatitis A to D, HIV, toxoplasmosis
Chest radiograph
Chest computed tomography
Pulmonary function tests
Cardiology evaluation with electrocardiogram, echocardiogram, MUGA scan—ventricular ejection fraction, cardiac catheterization, exercise stress test
Consultation with pediatric cardiologist, transplant coordinator, infectious disease specialist, pulmonologist, nutritionist, psychiatrist, social worker, dentist

CMV, cytomegalovirus; EBV, Epstein-Barr virus; HIV, human immunodeficiency virus; MUGA, multiple uptake gated acquisition.

comply with the complex medical regimens required and to cope with the potential for long or frequent hospitalizations even years after transplantation. As part of this multidisciplinary evaluation, patients undergo screening laboratory tests, including a viral serology panel (e.g., human immunodeficiency virus [HIV], cytomegalovirus [CMV], human Epstein-Barr virus [EBV], hepatitis).

Cardiac evaluation is performed mainly by echocardiography and cardiac catheterization in which the anatomy of the systemic and pulmonary venous connections of the heart and lungs are precisely identified. Important hemodynamic data, including systemic cardiac output and pulmonary vascular resistance (PVR), both indexed to the patient's body area, are obtained at cardiac catheterization and used to screen candidates. These numbers become significant because the major contraindication to transplantation is fixed pulmonary hypertension unresponsive to pulmonary vasodilators. Patients with elevated PVR (>4 to 6 Wood units) are tested with pulmonary vasodilators, including sodium nitroprusside, oxygen (FIO_2 100%), and inhaled nitric oxide, to establish whether the pulmonary vascular bed is reactive. In general, the presence of a fixed PVR in excess of 6 to 8 Wood units is a contraindication to orthotopic heart transplantation because the donor heart is unable to tolerate right-sided dilation caused by high pulmonary resistance. Patients who demonstrate improvement with vasodilators may undergo transplantation with a survival rate comparable to that in patients with normal resistance.[12] Although patients with fixed pulmonary hypertension have successfully undergone transplantation, they have a much higher mortality rate, usually because of postoperative right ventricular failure. Other contraindications to cardiac transplantation include multiple noncardiac congenital anomalies, active malignancy, infection, severe metabolic disease (i.e., diabetes mellitus), multiple organ failure, multiple congenital anomalies, and the lack of an adequate family support

system, in addition to socioeconomic factors that lead to noncompliance with drug regimens and follow-up care.

Children suffering from cardiomyopathy and manifesting symptoms of chronic congestive heart failure that limit activity or uncontrollable arrhythmias are often referred for transplantation, particularly if these patients are unresponsive to medications. The timing for transplantation in these children, especially those with hypertrophic cardiomyopathy, is less clear because some patients may improve with medication and conservative therapy.

As previously stated, the mortality for idiopathic dilated cardiomyopathy in children is highest in the first year after diagnosis and is mainly determined by the degree of left ventricular failure.

Children listed for heart transplantation should be closely monitored until their transplantation, either as outpatients if their condition permits or while hospitalized. Good nutritional status should be maintained and supplementation such as tube feedings or total parenteral nutrition used as needed. A close watch for infectious complications is important, and any subtle indications of infection should be thoroughly investigated. Major infections require patients to have their transplantation status put on hold until they are treated adequately. Anticongestive therapy should be optimized with digoxin, diuretics, and afterload reduction with captopril or other angiotensin-converting enzyme inhibitors. If heart failure worsens, hospitalization may be required for inotropic support with dobutamine or phosphodiesterase inhibitors such as milrinone. Long-term therapy may require the placement of an intravenous access device such as a Broviac catheter. The use of extracorporeal membrane oxygenation (ECMO) as a bridge to cardiac transplantation in critically ill children has been limited mostly to those with postcardiotomy ventricular failure. In general, the results have been poor, although several studies show survival rates ranging from 45% to 73% when ECMO is used as a bridge to cardiac transplantation.[13,16] Older children and adolescents have excellent survival with the use of long-term ventricular assist devices as a bridge to transplantation, although size restrictions limit their application in the infant population.

A neonate referred for cardiac transplantation requires several other unique considerations. Infants with complex congenital heart disease such as HLHS are commonly confined to a neonatal intensive care unit and are usually maintained on a continuous infusion of prostaglandin E_1 to prevent closure of the ductus arteriosus if there is duct-dependent physiology. Implantation of expansile stents in the ductus may allow discontinuation of prostaglandin during waiting. Balloon atrial septostomy with or without stenting to improve mixing of saturated and desaturated blood and to decompress the left atrium may be helpful if there is a restrictive patent foramen ovale. Other important issues are the maintenance of adequate nutritional support, avoidance of renal and metabolic complications, and prompt and thorough treatment of any infectious complications, especially line sepsis, in these fragile infants. Common neonatal problems such as seizures, necrotizing enterocolitis, and intraventricular hemorrhage are also seen in these patients. At the minimum, 10% to 20% of infants die while awaiting a donor heart.

As mentioned earlier, initial palliative procedures such as the Norwood procedure for HLHS or a Blalock-Taussig shunt for lesions with ductal-dependent pulmonary blood flow can be performed in the face of a prolonged wait for a donor.

The United Network for Organ Sharing determines organ allocation and in 2002 revised their classification for pediatric patients awaiting heart transplantation. Status 1A applies to patients requiring ventilatory or mechanical circulatory support (i.e., left ventricular assist device, ECMO, or a balloon pump) or multiple- or high-dose inotropes, infants younger than 6 months with pulmonary pressure greater than 50% of systemic levels, or any patient with a life expectancy of less than 14 days without a heart transplant. Status 1B applies to patients requiring single-dose inotropic support or infants younger than 6 months who have significant failure to thrive (less than the 5th percentile for weight or height or loss of 1.5 SD of expected growth). All other patients with less acuity are classified as status 2. A patient's status may change depending on changes in clinical condition, or the patient may be placed on hold (status 7) because of an infectious, malignant, or other complication and then later be reactivated.

DONOR EVALUATION AND ORGAN PROCUREMENT

The criteria for an ideal organ donor are as follows: meets requirements for brain death, consent from next of kin, ABO compatibility in older children, weight compatibility (one to three times that of the recipient), normal echocardiogram, age younger than 35 years, and normal heart by visual inspection at the time of harvest. A history of cardiopulmonary resuscitation is not an absolute contraindication to cardiac donation for pediatric recipients. All potential donors are evaluated carefully for the cause of death, including the presence of chest trauma, need for cardiopulmonary resuscitation, and cardiac function before death. For neonates, most donors have suffered sudden infant death syndrome or birth asphyxia, whereas older donors are victims of violence and car accidents.

The shortage of suitable organ donors, especially for neonatal recipients, has led to many attempts at expanding the donor pool. Hearts from donors with moderately impaired ventricular function by echocardiography (left ventricular shortening fraction greater than 25% without major wall motion abnormalities) have been successfully transplanted into infant recipients.[14] Donor-to-recipient weight ratios of up to 4:1 have been used in infants. Tamisier and colleagues demonstrated that the higher the PVR, the larger the donor heart needed for successful transplantation and that hearts with PVR values thought to be in excess of normal can also be used.[28] Although ideal donor ischemia time is from 2 to 4 hours, ischemic times have been successfully extended beyond 9 hours. Deviations from the "ideal" donor criteria should be individualized, and even though the use of a marginal donor for a dying infant maintained on ECMO may be justified, use of the same heart for a child who is stable as an outpatient might not.

ABO-incompatible transplantation has been introduced as a method to decrease recipient waiting times and associated waiting list mortality.[29] Because neonates do not have the ability to produce antibodies to T-cell antigens, including major blood group antigens, ABO incompatibility becomes a negligible complication. ABO-incompatible transplantation has been infrequently used in the United States, and the age at which it is no longer feasible is still not clearly defined.

Good donor management is a vital part of successful organ transplantation. The main goals are maintenance of normothermia, euvolemia, and adequate tissue perfusion and prevention of infection. Often, donors with poor cardiac function on initial evaluation will respond to volume loading and low-dose inotropic support with a significant improvement in function after heart retrieval, usually as part of a multiorgan retrieval procedure. All donors are screened for agents that might cause serious infection in an immunocompromised host, such as CMV, EBV, HIV, hepatitis, and *Toxoplasma*. The presence of antibodies to CMV, EBV, and *Toxoplasma* is not a contraindication to transplantation but helps guide post-transplant therapy.

The four major goals in procurement of a donor heart are to (1) work effectively with the other teams to ensure optimal condition of each recovered organ, (2) evaluate the hemodynamic status of the patient and the gross function of the heart by inspection, (3) use an effective cardioplegia and venting procedure that maximizes preservation of the heart, and (4) expertly remove the heart and adjoining vascular connections to ensure optimal anatomy for implantation. Procurement is performed via a median sternotomy. Donor blood is obtained for viral titers and retrospective HLA typing. The initial dissection involves separating the aorta from the main pulmonary artery to allow cross-clamping. Careful inspection of the heart is performed, and the patient is systemically heparinized. Procurement commences when the aorta is cross-clamped. Cardioplegia solution is infused through the aortic root, and the heart is vented via the right atrial appendage or superior vena cava for the right side and the superior pulmonary vein or left atrial appendage for the left side. The superior vena cava is dissected free of its pericardial attachments up to the innominate vein, and the azygos vein is ligated and divided. The pericardial reflections around the right superior pulmonary vein and the inferior vena cava are sharply divided. The cardiectomy begins with inferior vena cava transection, followed by right and left pulmonary vein transection at the pericardial reflection. The main pulmonary artery is divided and then the posterior pericardial attachments and the superior vena cava. Last of all, the aorta is transected at the level of the innominate artery or more distally if the aorta is needed for the recipient. The donor heart is immersed in cold (4° C), sterile saline and then triple-bagged in a sterile manner for transport. In general, the cold ischemia time should be limited to a maximum of 4 to 5 hours.

RECIPIENT PREPARATION AND TECHNIQUES OF IMPLANTATION

The standard technique for orthotopic heart transplantation was first described by Lower and Shumway in 1960 and consists of biatrial anastomoses, thus avoiding

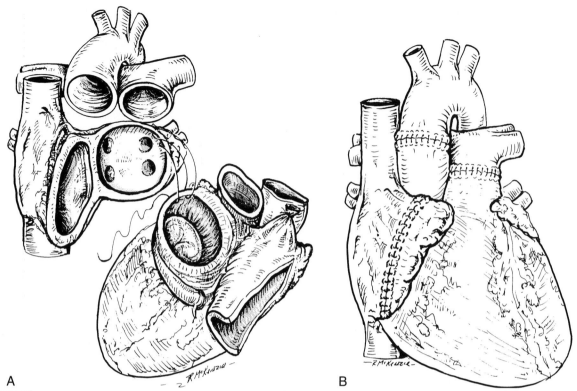

A

B

Figure 47–5 Standard heart transplantation using biatrial anastomosis. *A*, A recipient ventricular mass has been removed, and the left atrial anastomosis has been started. *B*, Final appearance after all anastomoses are complete.

individual caval and pulmonary vein connections (Fig. 47-5).[19] Currently, however, the majority of cardiac transplant centers now use the bicaval technique because it preserves atrial morphology and kinesis and is simpler when reconstruction after previous congenital heart repair is necessary. Once adequate hemodynamic monitoring is in place and the recipient is properly anesthetized, a median sternotomy is performed and the heart is suspended in a pericardial cradle. If previous sternotomies have been performed, appropriate precautions should be taken, including exposing the groins in the sterile field for access for femoral bypass. Once in the chest, the main pulmonary artery is dissected off the aorta past the bifurcation, and the pericardial reflection is mobilized off the aortic arch. Normally, aortic and bicaval cannulation is used.

In the case of a recipient with HLHS, the aortic arch vessels are mobilized proximally and controlled with snares, and the descending thoracic aorta is dissected to a level 2 to 3 cm below the insertion of the ductus arteriosus. The right and left pulmonary arteries are mobilized and controlled with snares in preparation for cardiopulmonary bypass. After heparinization, the main pulmonary artery is cannulated for arterial inflow, and a single venous cannula is placed in the right atrium because circulatory arrest will be used. Immediately on instituting cardiopulmonary bypass, the pulmonary arteries are snared tight and the body perfused through a patent ductus arteriosus. The recipient is cooled to 18° C for circulatory arrest.

Once the donor organ is available in the operating room and the patient has been adequately cooled, circulatory arrest is established, the arch vessels are snared

tightly, and the patient is exsanguinated into the venous reservoir. The aorta is divided just above the valve and incised longitudinally along the lesser curve of the aortic arch to a level 1 to 2 cm below the ductal insertion site on the descending aorta. The ductus is ligated next to the pulmonary artery and divided, and then the main pulmonary artery is transected just below the bifurcation. The right atrial incision is started superiorly at the base of the appendage. This incision is then carried down into the coronary sinus and across the atrial septum into the left atrium. The superior aspect of the right atrial incision is next carried across the septum to open the roof of the left atrium. The lateral wall of the left atrium is incised above the left pulmonary veins, with the left atrial appendage included with the specimen.

The donor organ is prepared on the back table in cold saline solution. The right atrium is incised from the inferior vena cava laterally to the base of the appendage; the area of the sinoatrial node is avoided if atrial anastomoses rather than caval anastomoses are to be performed. The pulmonary vein confluence is excised off the back of the left atrium, leaving an opening comparable in size to the recipient left atrial cuff. The pulmonary artery is transected just below the bifurcation to provide a wide anastomosis. The aorta is trimmed, depending on the level required in the recipient. Care must be taken to check for and adequately close a patent foramen ovale, which is frequently present, especially in infant hearts. Failure to do so may result in significant postoperative right-to-left shunting in the face of pulmonary hypertension.

The implantation is begun by anastomosing the lateral wall of the left atrium from the level of the left atrial appendage inferiorly. A left ventricular vent is placed through the right superior pulmonary vein, and the left atrial anastomosis is completed by reconstructing the intra-atrial septum. The arch of the aorta is then reconstructed. The right atrial anastomosis is begun at the inferior vena cava orifice and then taken superiorly along the intra-atrial septum. Once the right atrial anastomosis is completed, the ligature is removed from the donor superior vena cava and the venous cannula is placed through the vena caval stump. The ascending aorta

is then cannulated by a new purse-string suture, air is evacuated, and cardiopulmonary bypass is resumed. The snares are released from the head vessels and warming is commenced. The pulmonary anastomosis is then performed in an end-to-end fashion. If time permits, this step may be done during circulatory arrest in a drier field. After adequate warming, the patient is weaned from cardiopulmonary bypass and the cannulas removed (Fig. 47-6).[19] Right atrial, left atrial, and occasionally pulmonary artery pressure catheters are placed before

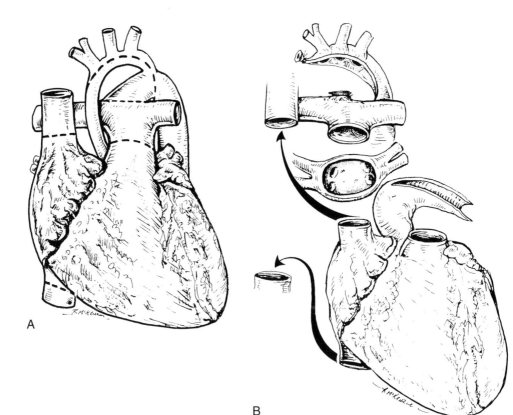

Figure 47–6 Technique for transplantation in hypoplastic left heart syndrome (with the use of bicaval anastomosis). *A,* Recipient anatomy before cardiectomy. *B,* Appearance of the recipient after cardiectomy. Note that the aortic incision must be extended into the descending aorta beyond the level of the arterial duct. *C,* Final appearance after all anastomoses are complete.

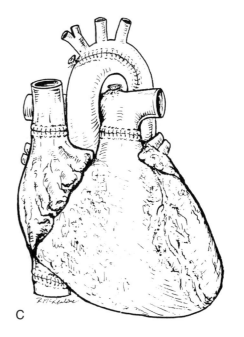

discontinuing bypass and brought out through the skin below the incision.

In older children with cardiomyopathy or infants without aortic arch abnormalities, the recipient procedure is similar to that performed in adults. The ascending aorta is mobilized to the pericardial reflection and used for arterial cannulation. The child is cooled to 28° C to 34° C because the implantation is performed under aortic cross-clamp rather than circulatory arrest. After the left atrial anastomosis has been completed, the right atrial connection can be sewn either directly or by using a bicaval technique if a previous cavopulmonary connection has been performed. This may decrease the incidence of tricuspid regurgitation in certain patients. The aortic anastomosis is then completed in an end-to-end fashion in the mid-ascending aorta. The pulmonary artery anastomosis may or may not be performed during aortic cross-clamp, depending on how long the implant procedure takes.

Numerous other variations of the implantation procedure can be used, depending on the recipient anatomy present. Modifications accounting for a persistent left superior vena cava, previous cavopulmonary shunt or Fontan procedure, corrected transposition of the great arteries, and situs inversus totalis have all been described.

POSTOPERATIVE MANAGEMENT

The recipient is returned from the operating room to an isolation room in the intensive care unit. Mechanical ventilation is required initially but is weaned as rapidly as possible. Antibiotics are continued until all monitoring lines and chest tubes have been removed.

Some level of inotropic support is required in virtually all heart transplant recipients. Isoproterenol is often an ideal choice owing to its pulmonary vasodilatory effects, as well as its inotropic and chronotropic effects because many patients have a slower than optimal heart rate initially. This transient sinus node dysfunction is rarely permanent. Dobutamine and dopamine, especially at "renal doses," are also frequently used to augment ventricular contractility. Epinephrine and norepinephrine are usually reserved for poor graft function. Sodium nitroprusside infusion or phosphodiesterase inhibitors are used for afterload reduction in the early postoperative period. Right ventricular dysfunction secondary to pulmonary hypertension may respond to phosphodiesterase inhibitors such as milrinone. Inhaled nitric oxide has been shown to be an effective selective pulmonary vasodilator with few systemic side effects and is useful in cardiac transplant recipients with pulmonary hypertension.

TRANSPLANT IMMUNOSUPPRESSION

A combination of immunosuppressive agents are used for the prevention and treatment of rejection. Standard triple-drug immunosuppression therapy consisting of prednisone, cyclosporine, and azathioprine has been successfully used in pediatric cardiac transplant recipients and remains the most common regimen.[11] The induction and maintenance doses of medications used for immunosuppression at the Children's Hospital of Philadelphia are listed in Table 47-2. Because of the adverse effects of corticosteroids, withdrawal from prednisone is usually attempted 6 months after transplantation. Up to 80% of recipients may be successfully weaned from steroids; only a quarter of these patients have an episode of rejection in the first 6 months.[10] Tacrolimus (formerly called FK-506) has been shown[27] to be an effective immunosuppressive agent in children, and its use has increased over the last 5 years, with approximately 40% of all pediatric cardiac transplant patients receiving it for maintenance immunosuppression 1 year after transplantation in the place of cyclosporine.[4] Overall, patients taking tacrolimus appear to have a lower incidence of rejection. Side effects of

TABLE 47–2 Heart Transplantation Immunosuppression Regimen at the Children's Hospital of Philadelphia

Drug	Dosage
Azathioprine/ mycophenolate mofetil (MMF)	2 mg/kg IV given in the operating room, before transplantation
	Then 2 mg/kg IV given once daily for 5 days (neonates), 7 days (infants), or 9 days (adolescents)
	Change to MMF, 120 mg/kg/day IV given twice daily (target level, 2.5-3.0), after the azathioprine course is completed
	Change to MMF orally as intestinal function returns
Cyclosporine	0.02 mg/kg/hr IV infusion beginning in the operating room, before transplantation
	Then 0.02 mg/kg/hr IV infusion for 24 hr (target level, 100)
	Change to ATG on postoperative day 3 and give 1.5 mg/kg IV once daily for 3 days (neonates), 5 days (infants), or 7 days (adolescents)
	Change back to cyclosporine orally after ATG course is completed to maintain target levels of approximately 125 in neonates and 150-175 in older children by discharge
	Dosing should be carefully adjusted over the next 2 months to achieve levels of 125-150 in neonates, 175-200 in infants, 250 in 6- to 12-year-olds, and 250-300 in adolescents
Solu-Medrol	10-15 mg/kg IV given in the operating room, before transplantation
	Then 3 mg/kg IV twice daily for 3 doses

ATG, rabbit antithymocyte globulin; IV, Intravenous.

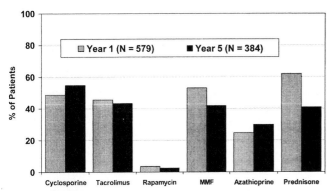

Figure 47-7 Pediatric heart recipients: maintenance immuno-suppression at the time of follow-up between January 2000 and June 2003. Different patients were analyzed at years 1 and 5. MMF, mycophenolate mofetil. (Reprinted from Journal of Heart and Lung Transplantation, August 2004, with permission from International Society of Heart and Lung Transplantation.)

azathioprine therapy, such as bone marrow depression, have precipitated the use of mycophenolate mofetil in its place. It is well tolerated with few side effects and has been shown in large clinical trials to have benefits in survival and treated rejection episodes[17] (Fig. 47-7). An increasing number of centers recommend the use of induction immunosuppression in pediatric cardiac recipients, with close to 40% of patients now receiving either a polyclonal anti–T-cell preparation, OKT3 (a murine monoclonal CD3 antibody), or an interleukin-2 receptor antibody immediately after transplantation (Fig. 47-8). However, there have been no significant differences in the average number of rejection episodes in patients treated for rejection regardless of the type of induction agent used.[4]

Infectious prophylaxis includes oral nystatin for fungal prophylaxis and oral trimethoprim-sulfamethoxazole three times per week. Pentamidine inhalation treatment is an effective alternative to trimethoprim-sulfamethoxazole for *Pneumocystis carinii* prophylaxis if bone marrow

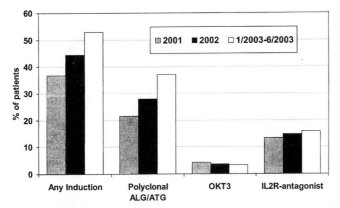

Figure 47-8 Pediatric heart recipients: induction immunosup-pression (follow-up from January 2001 to June 2003). ALG, antilym-phocyte globulin; ATG, antithymocyte globulin; IL-2R, interleukin-2 receptor. (Reprinted from Journal of Heart and Lung Transplantation, August 2004, with permission from International Society of Heart and Lung Transplantation.)

suppression is a problem. Routine CMV prophylaxis is not used in cardiac transplant recipients at our institution.

EARLY COMPLICATIONS

Acute rejection and infection are the most common early complications after cardiac transplantation. Nearly 60% to 75% of patients have at least one episode of rejection, and it should be expected that about a third will have an episode in the first 3 months and 50% within the first year after transplantation.[7] Some studies suggest that infants may be less prone to rejection than older children. Rejection surveillance is based on clinical evaluation, echocardiography, and endomyocardial biopsy. Clinical assessment includes observation of changes in a patient's activity or appetite. Atrial or ventricular ectopy, including tachycardia, is suspicious for rejection and mandates evaluation. Echocardiography is particularly useful in neonates, in whom biopsy is technically difficult and carries significant risk because of patient size. Echocardiographic evaluation is typically performed weekly for the first month and then monthly for the first year after transplantation. Echocardiography-guided transjugular endomyocardial biopsy has been shown to be an effective means of monitoring pediatric transplant recipients for rejection and remains the gold standard for detection of rejection.[9] An aggressive approach consisting of routine endomyocardial biopsy weekly for the first month after transplantation, every second week for the second month, and then once monthly for the remainder of the first year has been adopted at the Children's Hospital of Philadelphia for rejection surveillance. Subsequent biopsies are obtained twice annually or whenever rejection is clinically suspected. Most biopsies are performed on an outpatient basis. The international grading system for cardiac transplant rejection is shown in Table 47-3.

Episodes of acute rejection are usually treated with a 3-day course of intravenous methylprednisolone (10 mg/kg). OKT3 and antithymocyte globulin are reserved for an incomplete response or rejection refractory to steroids. Response is confirmed by follow-up biopsy 1 to 2 weeks after treatment.

TABLE 47-3 International Society for Heart and Lung Transplantation Categories of Acute Rejection

Grade 0	No evidence of cellular rejection
Grade 1A	Focal perivascular or interstitial infiltrate without myocyte injury
Grade 1B	Multifocal or diffuse sparse infiltrate without myocyte injury
Grade 2	Single focus of dense infiltrate with myocyte injury
Grade 3A	Multifocal dense infiltrate with myocyte injury
Grade 3B	Diffuse, dense infiltrate with myocyte injury
Grade 4	Diffuse and extensive polymorphous infiltrate with myocyte injury—may have hemorrhage, edema, and microvascular invasion

From Rodriguez ER: The pathology of heart transplant biopsy specimens: Revisiting the 1990 ISHLT working formulation. J Heart Lung Transplant 2003;22:3.

Although infectious complications are common in cardiac transplant recipients, infection-related deaths do not appear to be. Bacterial infections are most frequent in the early post-transplant period but can occur late after transplantation and usually respond to proper antibiotic therapy. Of viral infections, CMV appears to be the most common and is treated with intravenous ganciclovir. Viral respiratory infections usually occur at a frequency similar to that in normal children and appear to be well tolerated by the recipient.

Aside from rejection and infection, the immediate postoperative complications after heart transplantation are hypertension, seizures, renal dysfunction, and diabetes. Nearly 10% of infant heart transplant recipients require perioperative peritoneal dialysis. Among neonates, 10% to 15% require phenobarbital therapy for postoperative seizures, which may result from the use of circulatory arrest in these patients.[2]

LATE COMPLICATIONS

The primary late complications in pediatric cardiac transplant recipients are chronic rejection, PTLD, and transplant CAD. Rejection may account for up to 40% of deaths after cardiac transplantation.[4] Lymphoproliferative disease is currently treated by a reduction in immunosuppressants, acyclovir, and chemotherapy.

The onset of transplant CAD has a prevalence of 10% to 15% and may be suggested by symptoms of congestive heart failure in recipients. Echocardiograms are performed routinely during follow-up visits of heart transplant recipients, and worsening ventricular function is a sign of graft CAD. A new onset of arrhythmias after transplantation, especially ventricular arrhythmias, may also be an indication of underlying CAD.[23] Additionally, CAD may be found on routine follow-up catheterization or intracoronary ultrasound, without any previous suggestion of disease. A number of causes have been implicated in the development of graft CAD, including chronic cellular rejection, hyperlipidemia, vascular rejection, and CMV infection. Unlike adult cardiac transplant recipients, CAD appears to develop in pediatric patients relatively early after transplantation, with one series demonstrating an incidence of 35% by 2 years after transplantation.[8] A review of 815 pediatric transplant patients found nearly 8% to have significant CAD by angiogram or autopsy findings.[22] The mean time after transplantation to diagnosis was 2.2 years, with one patient having significant CAD 2 months after transplantation. Only 20% of patients in whom graft CAD was diagnosed were still alive, and most of the deaths were sudden or unexpected. Retransplantation appears to be the only viable option for these patients, although the results in general are not encouraging, with 1- and 3-year survival rates of 71% and 47%, respectively, and CAD developing in the second grafts in 20% of retransplantation patients.[20] However, the Loma Linda group has reported a significantly better retransplantation experience in infants who were first transplanted when younger than 6 months.[14] In this group, a 10-year actuarial survival rate of 91% was observed after retransplantation, potentially related to this center's early adoption of

a steroid-free immunosuppressive regimen. In addition, medical treatment targeted at cholesterol and lipid-lowering therapies are currently under investigation.[25]

RESULTS

The largest group of infant cardiac transplant recipients reported in the literature is from Loma Linda, where 233 heart transplantations in infants younger than 6 months have been performed.[14] Nearly 65% were for HLHS, and the rest were for other complex congenital anomalies (29%) or cardiomyopathy or tumor (8%). The operative (30-day) survival rate was 89%, with the primary causes of mortality being primary graft failure, technical problems, pneumonia, or acute rejection. The overall 1-year survival rate was 84%, with a 5- and 10-year actuarial survival rate of 73% and 68%, respectively. In addition, patients undergoing transplantation when younger than 30 days had a significantly better outcome than did older infants, with an actuarial survival rate of 80% and 77% at 5 and 10 years, potentially related to improved immune tolerance in the younger subgroup.

Stanford University[24] reported its series of 72 patients younger than 18 years who have undergone heart transplantation since 1977. Only 25% were younger than 1 year (mean of 9 years), and nearly two thirds had cardiomyopathy unrelated to congenital heart disease. The operative survival rate was 87.5%, with deaths mainly caused by pulmonary hypertension/right ventricular failure and acute rejection. There were 20 late deaths; 24% were due to rejection and 17% were due to graft CAD. Actuarial survival rates at 1, 5, and 10 years were 75%, 60%, and 50%, respectively.

At St. Louis Children's Hospital, 45 heart transplantations were performed from 1983 to 1993, more than half in infants with HLHS.[26] The infant group had a survival rate (92%) similar to that of the Loma Linda series, whereas the pediatric group (older than 1 year) had an 80% early survival rate.

Results from the Registry of the International Society for Heart and Lung Transplantation reveal a perioperative mortality rate higher for infants than for older children (Fig. 47-9).[4] Despite the much greater early mortality,

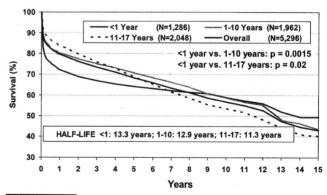

Figure 47–9 Pediatric heart transplantation: Kaplan-Meier survival (January 1982 to June 2002). (Reprinted from Journal of Heart and Lung Transplantation, August 2004, with permission from International Society of Heart and Lung Transplantation.)

however, the half-life of 13.3 years is longer than that of the childhood or adolescent survivors. For the childhood age group of 1 to 10 years, the half-life was 17.5 years versus 13.7 years for the adolescent age group, thus conferring the younger patients a significant survival advantage. Averaged over 15 years, an infant recipient would have an approximate 2% per year risk of mortality, whereas for older children it remains approximately 4%, again indicating a long-term survival advantage for younger cardiac transplant recipients. The most predictive risk factors for 1-year mortality in the pediatric population remain congenital heart disease, retransplantation, donor age, pulmonary artery systolic pressure greater than 35 mm Hg, and need for mechanical ventilation and hospitalization while awaiting transplantation. Among the most significant risk factors for 5-year mortality are dialysis, congenital heart disease, and female gender. Causes of death include CAD, acute rejection, lymphoma, graft failure, and infection. Prevalent post-transplant morbidities for survivors include hypertension (45%), renal dysfunction (5.4%), hyperlipidemia (9.9%), and diabetes (3.2%).[4]

Aside from survival, it has been demonstrated that transplanted hearts in children appear to grow normally and the left ventricle increases muscle mass to maintain the normal left ventricular mass-volume ratio over time.[31] Exercise testing in older children has shown peak heart rate and oxygen consumption to be consistently two thirds of that predicted in heart transplant recipients.[21] Somatic growth appears to be normal in infants after heart transplantation, and neurologic development is generally preserved, although some neurologic abnormalities may be seen in up to 20% of neonatal recipients on long-term follow-up.[4]

CONCLUSION

Despite further improvements in surgical technique, immunosuppression, perioperative management, and rejection surveillance, long-term results of pediatric heart transplantation have shown little change, with a 15-year survival rate of approximately 50% (see Fig. 47-9). Chronic rejection, graft CAD, and the long-term effects of steroids on growth continue to cloud the development of cardiac transplantation as the primary treatment of complex congenital heart disease. However, for many children with end-stage cardiomyopathy and structural heart disease not amenable to corrective surgery, transplantation is the only option. Future areas of research interest include the use of xenografts, ABO incompatibility, permanent mechanical support, and widening the bridge to transplantation with smaller and more adaptable assist devices.

REFERENCES

1. Bailey LL: Role of cardiac replacement in the neonate. J Heart Lung Transplant 1985;4:506.
2. Bailey LL, Gundry SR, Razzouk AJ, et al: Bless the babies: One hundred fifteen late survivors of heart transplantation during the first year of life. J Thorac Cardiovasc Surg 1993;105:805.
3. Boucek MM, Bernstein D: Heart transplantation in infancy. Prog Pediatr Cardiol 1993;2(4):20.
4. Boucek MM, Edwards LB, Keck BM, et al: The Registry of the International Society for Heart and Lung Transplantation: Seventh Official Pediatric Report—2004. J Heart Lung Transplant 2004;23:933.
5. Bove EL: Transplantation after first-stage reconstruction for hypoplastic left heart syndrome. Ann Thorac Surg 1991; 52:701.
6. Bove EL: Surgical treatment for hypoplastic left heart syndrome. Jpn J Thorac Cardiovasc Surg 1999;47(2):47.
7. Braunlin EA, Canter CE, Olivari MT, et al: Rejection and infection after pediatric cardiac transplantation. Ann Thorac Surg 1990;49:385.
8. Braunlin EA, Hunter DW, Canter CE, et al: Coronary artery disease in pediatric cardiac transplant recipients receiving triple-drug immunosuppression. Circulation 1991;84(Suppl):III303.
9. Canter CE, Appleton RS, Soffitz JE, et al: Surveillance for rejection by echocardiographically guided endomyocardial biopsy in the infant heart transplant recipient. Circulation 1991;84(Suppl III)III-310.
10. Canter CE, Moorehead S, Soffitz JE, et al: Steroid withdrawal in the pediatric heart transplant recipient initially treated with triple immunosuppression. J Heart Lung Transplant 1994;13:74.
11. Canter CE, Soffitz JE, Moorehead S, et al: Early results after pediatric cardiac transplantation with triple immunosuppression therapy. Am J Cardiol 1993;71:971.
12. Cooper MM, Fuzesi L, Addonizio LI, et al: Pediatric heart transplantation after operations involving the pulmonary arteries. J Thorac Cardiovascular Surg 1991;102:386.
13. del Nido PJ, Armitage JM, Fricker FJ, et al: Extracorporeal membrane oxygenation support as a bridge to pediatric heart transplantation. Circulation 1994;90(5 Pt 2, Suppl):II66.
14. Fortuna KS, Chinnock RE, Bailey LL, et al: Heart transplantation among 233 infants during the first six months of life: The Loma Linda experience. Loma Linda Pediatric Heart Transplant Group. Clin Transpl 1999;263.
15. Hosenpud JD, Bennen LE, Keck BM, et al: The Registry of the International Society for Heart and Lung Transplantation: Eighteenth Official Report—2001. J Heart Lung Transplant 2001;20:805.
16. Kirshborn PM, Bridges ND, Myung RJ, et al: Use of extracorporeal membrane oxygenation in pediatric thoracic organ transplantation. J Thorac Cardiovasc Surg 2002;123:130.
17. Kobashigawa JA: Mycophenolate mofetil in cardiac transplantation. Curr Opin Cardiol 1998;13:117.
18. Lewis AB: Prognostic value of echocardiography in children with idiopathic dilated cardiomyopathy. Am Heart J 1994;128:133.
19. Lower RR, Shumway NE: Studies on orthotopic homotransplantations of the canine heart. Surg Forum 1960;11:18.
20. Michler RE, Edward NM, Hsu D, et al: Pediatric retransplantation. J Heart Lung Transplant 1993;12:5319.
21. Nixon PA, Fricker FJ, Noyes BE, et al: Exercise testing in pediatric heart, heart-lung and lung recipients. Chest 1995; 107:1328.
22. Pahl E, Zalos VR, Ficker FI, et al: Posttransplant coronary artery disease in children: A multicenter national survey. Circulation 1994;9(5 Pt 2, Suppl):II56.
23. Park JK, Hus DT, Hordof AI, et al: Arrhythmias in pediatric heart transplant recipients: Prevalence and association with death, coronary artery disease, and rejection. J Heart Lung Transplant 1993;12:596.
24. Sarris CE, Smith JA, Bernstin D, et al: Pediatric cardiac transplantation: The Stanford experience. Circulation 1994;90(5 Pt 2, Suppl):II51.

25. Seipelt IM, Crawford SE, Rodgers S, et al: Hypercholesterolemia is common after pediatric heart transplantation: Initial experience with pravastatin. J Heart Lung Transplant 2004;23:317.

26. Spray TL: Transplantation of the heart and lungs in children. Annu Rev Med 1994;45:139.

27. Swenson JM, Fricker FJ, Armitage JM: Immunosuppression switch in pediatric heart transplant recipients: Cyclosporine to FK506. J Am Coll Cardiol 1995;25:1183.

28. Tamisier D, Vouhe P, Le Bidois J, et al: Donor-recipient size matching in pediatric heart transplantation; a word of caution about small grafts. J Heart Lung Transplant 1996; 15:190.

29. West LJ, Pollock-Barziv SM, Dipchand AI, et al: ABO-incompatible heart transplantation in infants. N Engl J Med 2001;344:793.

30. Wiles HB: Prognostic features of children with idiopathic dilated cardiomyopathy. Am J Cardiol 1991;68:1372.

31. Zales VR, Wright KL, Pahl E, et al: Normal left ventricular muscle mass and mass/volume ratio after pediatric cardiac transplantation. Circulation 1994;90(5 Pt 2, Suppl):II61.

Chapter 48

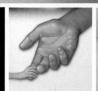

Lung Transplantation

Charles B. Huddleston and Joel Cooper

The first reported attempt at lung transplantation occurred in 1963 and was performed by Dr. James Hardy at the University of Mississippi Medical Center.[27] The patient did not survive the hospitalization, dying 18 days after the transplant. There were a number of additional attempts at this over the next few years, with most failures related to poor healing in the airway anastomosis. Approximately 20 years after Dr. Hardy's ill-fated effort, the first truly successful lung transplant was performed in Toronto, Canada, by a team led by Dr. Joel Cooper. This patient had a single-lung transplant for pulmonary fibrosis and survived for more than 6 years, ultimately dying of renal failure.[8] Over the years since, and particularly in the late 1990s, pediatric lung transplantation has emerged as a viable treatment option for children with end-stage pulmonary parenchymal and vascular diseases. However, the number of children undergoing transplants throughout the world since 1989 remains relatively small, representing only 4% of all lung transplants performed.[67] In this chapter, pediatric lung transplantation is described as an isolated procedure and heart-lung transplantation is not included.

INDICATIONS

Isolated lung transplantation is applicable to any child with life-threatening and progressive disability due to pulmonary parenchymal or vascular disease. In general, this treatment modality is indicated for increasing the duration of life, not solely for improvement of the quality of life. The current long-term survival after lung transplantation is approximately 50% at 5 years. Thus, the selection of patients for transplantation and the timing of the procedure are critically important. One would like to be able to predict when a child would be within 2 years of dying without any form of medical treatment. Obviously this may be very difficult. The major diagnostic groups for pediatric lung transplantation are cystic fibrosis, interstitial lung disease with pulmonary fibrosis, primary pulmonary hypertension, pulmonary hypertension associated with congenital heart disease, retransplantation, and a "miscellaneous" category (Table 48-1).

Chronic obstructive lung disease, the most common indication for transplantation in adults, is remarkably absent from this list.[67]

Cystic Fibrosis

This disease, the most common lethal hereditary disease in North America, comprises the largest diagnostic group of children younger than age 18 years undergoing lung transplantation. Although the median survival now exceeds 29 years, one third of the deaths from cystic fibrosis occurs in the pediatric age group. Without question, the most common cause of death is respiratory. About 100 transplants are performed annually in the United States for cystic fibrosis,[13] and although this number is growing slowly each year, donor availability still remains a major limiting factor.

As with other diagnostic groups, timing of transplantation in the course of a chronic disease is a crucial issue. Kerem, in the early 1990s, demonstrated that an FEV_1 less than 30% of predicted, PaO_2 less than 55 mm Hg, and/or a PCO_2 greater than 50 mm Hg was associated with a survival beyond 2 years of less than 50%.[39] The impact of these factors is magnified in the pediatric age group, particularly in girls. However, more recent studies on the natural history of cystic fibrosis patients once they have severely compromised lung function show that an isolated measure of the FEV_1 alone may not be sufficiently predictive.

TABLE 48-1 Indications for Lung Transplantation in Children

Cystic fibrosis
Pulmonary fibrosis
Pulmonary vascular disease
    Primary pulmonary hypertension
    Eisenmenger's syndrome
Bronchiolitis obliterans
Retransplant
Other

The rate of decline in the FEV_1 may be a more accurate determinant of survival.[47,58] Other factors that may serve as relative indicators in deciding to proceed toward transplantation include the need for continuous supplemental oxygen, increased frequency for hospitalizations, and diminished weight for height (below the 80th percentile).[39]

The presence of antibiotic-resistant organisms in the sputum is a relative contraindication to lung transplant. The synergistic effectiveness of antibiotic combinations is certainly an important evaluation of any resistant organism, whether consideration for transplantation is underway or not. It is reasonable to proceed with transplantation in the presence of most organisms with a highly resistant antibiotic profile as long as there are synergistic combinations available. However, *Burkholderia cepacia* colonization is associated with a particularly poor prognosis and therefore is of particular concern.[24,61] Portal hypertension with hepatic cirrhosis occurs in 5% to 10% of patients with cystic fibrosis. These children are at risk for variceal bleeding as well as derangements of synthetic function. In general, if the synthetic function is preserved, decompression of the portal venous system with percutaneous procedures will lower the risk to a level satisfactory for lung transplantation.[44] However, when there is also synthetic dysfunction of the liver, combined liver-lung transplantation may be the only appropriate option.[11] Diabetes mellitus is generally not considered a contraindication to transplantation unless there is evidence of vasculopathy, bearing in mind that control of serum glucose will be more difficult after transplantation.[19] As many as 10% to 15% of CF lung transplant candidates will have had prior thoracotomies for either pneumothorax or pulmonary resection. Most centers do not consider this a contraindication to transplantation, although the resultant adhesions from these prior operations do increase the difficulty and the risk of bleeding.[18] Mechanical ventilation or presence of a tracheostomy are not in and of themselves contraindications to transplantation, but the overall medical condition of patients requiring this level of support must be carefully considered.

Pulmonary Vascular Disease

This rather broad classification of patients includes those with primary pulmonary hypertension (PPH) and those with pulmonary hypertension associated with congenital heart disease (PH/CHD). The latter category includes patients with Eisenmenger's syndrome but is not limited to this. These patients die of either progressive right-sided heart failure, arrhythmias, or a lethal episode of hemoptysis. It is difficult to predict when a patient might have a fatal arrhythmia or hemoptysis episode. However, most patients with pulmonary vascular disease will die of progressive right-sided heart failure over a protracted period of time.[15] In the past several years a number of somewhat selective pulmonary vasodilators have become available for use in these patients. These include intravenous prostacyclin,[1] prostacyclin analogues iloprost (inhaled)[29] and betaprost (oral),[50] and bosentan,[5] an endothelin receptor antagonist. These drugs have enabled patients to put off the need for transplantation

for years. In fact, the number of patients undergoing transplantation for pulmonary vascular disease has significantly dropped in recent years.

The timing of transplantation for patients with pulmonary vascular disease is influenced significantly by the response to medical therapy and the underlying cause of the pulmonary vascular disease. While primary pulmonary hypertension and Eisenmenger's syndrome result in identical histologic changes in the pulmonary vascular bed, the latter of these two is associated with a much more favorable long-term prognosis. A retrospective analysis by Hopkins of 100 adults with severe pulmonary hypertension due to either Eisenmenger's syndrome or PPH revealed that, in the former group, actuarial survival without transplantation was 97% at 1 year, 89% at 2 years, and 77% at 3 years. In contrast, survival was 77%, 69%, and 35% over the same respective time intervals in the PPH cohort.[30] It is presumed that the intracardiac defect allows the right ventricle to "decompress" via the defect when the afterload in the pulmonary vascular bed becomes prohibitively high. On the basis of this and other observations, atrial septostomy performed in the cardiac catheterization suite has been demonstrated to provide clinical benefit in patients with PPH.[41] Results from a multicenter study of patients with PPH performed before the advent of long-term intravenous prostacyclin therapy demonstrated a median survival from time of diagnosis of 2.8 years. In that study, a formula was developed incorporating hemodynamic variables to assist in predicting the 2-year mortality[15] and it was recommended that patients should be listed when this figure is less than or equal to 50%. Studies regarding natural history in adults have been applied to children, but it is unclear whether this disease behaves the same in a younger population. Clabby and coworkers reviewed 50 patients from many centers to provide a means of estimating survival in children with PPH.[6] There was a direct correlation of mortality with the product of the mean right atrial pressure and the pulmonary vascular resistance.[6] With progress in the medical therapy of PPH to identify selective pulmonary vasodilators as well as the underlying mechanisms of this disease, these formulas predicting survival may be obsolete. The durability of medical therapy is unclear. How this therapy might be applied to secondary pulmonary hypertension, such as Eisenmenger's syndrome, is speculative.

The two main issues in considering patients with Eisenmenger's syndrome or PH/CHD for lung transplantation are the timing of listing and the complexity of the cardiac lesion to be repaired. As noted earlier, it is clear that, once the diagnosis is made, these patients can live much longer than those with PPH.[30] The mode of death in these patients is by progressive heart failure, pulmonary hemorrhage, stroke, or sudden death presumably due to arrhythmias.[6] Patients should be listed when symptoms develop, when there has been a single pulmonary hemorrhage, or perhaps arbitrarily when they reach their late 30s. Most patients with PH/CHD have an atrial septal defect, ventricular septal defect, or patent ductus arteriosus. All of these require relatively simple cardiac repairs. However, there are patients with unrepaired atrioventricular canal defects, transposition of the great arteries, and truncus arteriosus who would require more complex procedures. An alternative for these patients would be a heart-lung transplant. The likelihood of obtaining a donor heart-lung block for anyone over 40 kg is low because of the distribution policy for thoracic donor organs. In addition, the long-term survival after heart-lung transplantation is particularly poor (approximately 40% at 5 years post transplant).[67] These two issues must be factored into the decision as to whether one should perform the higher-risk procedure of lung transplantation in combination with repair of a complex cardiac lesion or a heart-lung transplantation.

Some patients with congenital heart disease who have undergone repair may not experience the expected decline in pulmonary vascular resistance after appropriate correction. Occasionally the repair has been performed relatively late in life, but there are children who have undergone timely repair and still present later on with severe pulmonary hypertension. It is not clear how to classify these patients. In general, this is a less uniform group than either the patients with PPH or those with Eisenmenger's syndrome. They seem to follow a clinical course similar to that seen in patients with PPH and should be treated in a similar fashion.[30]

Another diagnostic group with pulmonary vascular disease are patients with an inadequate pulmonary vascular bed. Examples of this include pulmonary atresia, ventricular septal defect and multiple aortopulmonary collaterals, and congenital diaphragmatic hernia, where there is primarily a general deficiency of pulmonary parenchyma. In the former group, complete correction (repair of the ventricular septal defect combined with reconstruction of the right ventricular outflow tract with a conduit to the unifocalized aortopulmonary collaterals) represents a high-risk but viable option for the majority of these patients. However, when the anatomy of the aortopulmonary collaterals is not amenable to unifocalization or when unifocalization has not produced satisfactory growth of the pulmonary vascular tree, the result is progressive cyanosis or progressive pulmonary hypertension or both. Lung transplantation with repair of the residual cardiac defect may be the only feasible option for survival. Children with congenital diaphragmatic hernias, despite having undergone a successful hernia repair, may still be left with inadequate pulmonary parenchyma and vascular bed to handle the full cardiac output. The resultant severe pulmonary hypertension is the usual cause of death in these infants and is an indication for transplantation. The problem here is that these infants often will require extracorporeal membrane oxygenator support during the perioperative period. This reduces the time that patients such as this can wait for a donor offer once listed for lung transplantation. It is possible that a single-lung transplant on the affected side would be sufficient in this circumstance. In this scenario, once the patient has grown it may be possible to remove the transplanted lung altogether, leaving the patient with a presumably normal contralateral lung to maintain normal respiratory function. In reality, those patients with insufficient pulmonary reserve will have to be identified very early in the course for lung transplantation to be a realistic option. The mortality is quite high even when donor organs are identified.

In all the previous situations, isolated lung transplantation is appropriate only when left ventricular function is normal. Poor left ventricular function will result in elevated left ventricular end-diastolic pressure post transplant, which will add significantly to problems with pulmonary edema and early graft failure. Right ventricular function is frequently poor, particularly in the patient group with PPH. That should not be a deterrent to isolated lung transplantation because the right ventricular function always returns to normal within a relatively short period of time.[53]

Although a prior thoracotomy is generally not a contraindication to lung transplantation in patients with pulmonary parenchymal disease, this is not true for those with pulmonary vascular disease, especially when secondary to congenital heart disease and associated with cyanosis. The adhesions that develop after a thoracotomy for palliation of cyanotic congenital heart disease are extremely vascular. Intercostal and internal mammary arteries will form direct connections through the pleura into the parenchyma of the lung in a compensatory attempt to enhance pulmonary blood flow. The bleeding that results during the recipient pneumonectomy portion of the transplant procedure is often horrendous and life threatening.

Pulmonary Fibrosis

These patients account for 5% to 10% of pediatric patients undergoing lung transplantation.[67] Placed in this category are those patients with "usual" interstitial fibrosis, radiation-induced fibrosis, bronchopulmonary dysplasia, and pulmonary fibrosis secondary to chronic aspiration. The progression of these disease processes is quite variable. Generally, patients should be listed when normal activities are markedly limited and minor viral illnesses lead to significant deterioration. Most patients will be oxygen dependent and may well have evidence of coexistent pulmonary hypertension. For those in whom aspiration is the underlying problem, the source of the aspiration must be eliminated.

The prognosis of children with idiopathic pulmonary fibrosis is not altogether clear. This may be because there is not a "usual interstitial pulmonary fibrosis" disease in children—the underlying causes are frequently unique and unusual. Decisions regarding listing for transplantation are somewhat difficult because of this. Pulmonary fibrosis presenting during infancy was once believed to have a poor prognosis; however, recent studies have demonstrated much improved survival with high doses of corticosteroid therapy.[51] The prognosis for adults with total lung capacity less than 60% predicted is still poor; nearly all are dead within 2 years.[37] It is difficult to translate this information into the pediatric experience. Pulmonary hypertension frequently accompanies this disease as it progresses. These patients should be evaluated and listed for transplantation when they become symptomatic. If there is a favorable response to corticosteroids they can be followed with standard (age > 5 years) or infant (age < 5 years) pulmonary function tests. One problem with this disease is that patients with progression of their disease tend to remain on relatively high doses of corticosteroids and come to transplantation in a rather cushingoid state. This should not exclude them from transplantation.

Bronchiolitis Obliterans and Retransplantation

Bronchiolitis obliterans is not a specific disease but rather a histologic description characterized by the obstruction and destruction of the distal airways. It may occur as a consequence of any severe lung injury, including viral pneumonia, graft-versus-host disease after bone marrow transplant, autoimmune diseases, chemical injury, Stevens-Johnson syndrome, and others. Of course, it is a relatively common late complication of lung transplantation (see later). The underlying etiology is unknown. "Primary" bronchiolitis obliterans (not related to a prior lung transplant) is a perfectly legitimate indication for lung transplantation: it is a slowly progressive disease in virtually all cases with no known effective treatment. When this disorder occurs as a consequence of an isolated lung injury, transplantation is a fairly straightforward decision process. However, those patients with prior bone marrow transplants (usually for leukemia) offer special considerations.[54] Although the standard definition of "cure" is remission of the malignancy for more than 5 years, most of these patients present within 2 or 3 years. Another problem is the deranged immune competency seen after bone marrow transplant and how the immunosuppressant agents used after lung transplantation might further affect this. We have found that these patients have less acute rejection than most other lung transplant recipients but may be more prone to opportunistic infections.[54] However, the number of patients transplanted in this setting is low. For patients who acquire bronchiolitis obliterans through other immunologic injuries, such as autoimmune disorders, there are concerns about the likelihood of recurrence in transplanted lungs. One would have to ascertain that the primary process has completely abated before transplantation.

Retransplantation for acute graft failure after transplantation has an extremely poor prognosis[49] and is not an option from a practical standpoint because of the long waiting times. Rarely, consideration may be given to this option in infants who generally have significantly shorter waiting times. Retransplantation for bronchiolitis obliterans is a controversial issue. Bronchiolitis obliterans accounts for the majority of deaths occurring more than 90 days post transplant.[67] This figure is borne out in our pediatric series.[65] Although early mortality after retransplantation is higher than for "first-time" lung transplants, those who do survive this early phase have long-term survival similar to the non-redo transplants.[49] Risk factors for poor early outcome include nonambulatory status, short period of time since the first transplant, transplantation at a center with limited experience, and dependence on mechanical ventilation. We have further noted that a low glomerular filtration rate is an independent risk factor. Because patients continue to die on the waiting list, one could argue that no patient should ever be retransplanted because this might deprive an otherwise lower-risk patient from receiving organs in a timely fashion. At present this

issue is unresolved. One can only advise use of proper judgment in selecting only the best candidates when the issue of retransplantation arises.

Miscellaneous

A variety of diagnoses fall into this group. Congenitally based pulmonary parenchymal diseases constitute one of the more interesting broad categories. Typically, these full-term newborns present with severe respiratory distress and no obvious cause such as meconium aspiration, sepsis, or persistent fetal circulation. The diagnoses falling into this category include surfactant protein B deficiency, other forms of pulmonary alveolar proteinosis, alveolar-capillary dysplasia, pulmonary dysmaturity, congenital interstitial pneumonitis, and others. These infants usually have severe respiratory failure and require a high level of ventilatory support. Often extracorporeal membrane oxygenation (ECMO) has been or is currently being used. An open-lung biopsy is often necessary to either make the diagnosis or to exclude other diagnoses. Surfactant protein B deficiency can now be diagnosed by looking for the specific genetic mutation in peripheral blood and assaying tracheal effluent for the presence of this surfactant protein.[25] All children with this diagnosis survive less than 3 months even with aggressive therapy. Additionally, because the surfactant proteins are expressed only in the lungs, extrapulmonary organ dysfunction is rare. Until other therapies become available, lung transplantation is the only viable therapeutic option. Abnormalities in the gene coding surfactant protein C have also been identified as a cause for interstitial lung disease in infants, which may progress to the point of requiring lung transplantation.[26] In general, the waiting time for an organ offer is relatively short in infants. Therefore, one might realistically believe that an infant with a 3-month life expectancy could undergo a transplant and survive. When an infant is on ECMO every effort should be made to wean from it using whatever means possible, including high-frequency oscillating ventilator and/or nitric oxide. Although ECMO is not an absolute contraindication to transplantation, one should be very cautious in this setting because of the relatively high incidence of other organ dysfunction.

CONTRAINDICATIONS

Contraindications to transplantation in children are also based on experience obtained in adults (Table 48-2). Absolute contraindications include systemic disease with major extrapulmonary manifestations or severe dysfunction of other organ systems. Thus, widespread malignancy, collagen vascular disease, human immunodeficiency virus infection, and severe neuromuscular disease are absolute contraindications. The acceptable degree of renal insufficiency is open to some interpretation. Given the nephrotoxicity of cyclosporine and tacrolimus, the drugs that form the basis of nearly all immunosuppressant regimens, a serum creatinine value greater than 2.0 mg/dL and a probable need for post-transplant dialysis are clinical parameters that would mitigate strongly against proceeding with transplantation. A glomerular filtration rate

TABLE 48-2 Contraindications to Lung Transplantation

Absolute
Malignancy
Human immunodeficiency virus infection
Multisystem organ failure
Left ventricular dysfunction
Active collagen vascular disease
Severe neuromuscular disease

Relative
Renal insufficiency
Liver function impairment
Malnutrition
Resistant organisms in the sputum
Poorly controlled diabetes mellitus
Osteopenia
Prior thoracotomies in the presence of pulmonary vascular disease
Prior pneumonectomy with mediastinal shift
Extreme prematurity
Poor compliance
Inadequate psychosocial support system

less than 50 mL/min has been associated with a poor outcome in some patients. Significantly deranged hepatic synthetic function precludes transplantation unless concomitant liver transplantation is also being undertaken. More complex issues include severe malnutrition, poorly controlled diabetes mellitus, osteopenia, vertebral compression fractures, and the need for mechanical ventilation. None of these factors in and of themselves serves as an absolute contraindication. Nonetheless, all such concerning aspects of the clinical presentation must be evaluated and carefully considered in the scope of the patient's overall state of health to assess the likelihood for successful recovery after the transplant. Chronic administration of corticosteroids before the transplant is considered to be undesirable; and, when possible, one should reduce the total daily dose or change to an every-other-day dosage schedule. Previously, corticosteroids were believed to have a significant negative impact on airway healing, particularly in the case of double-lung transplant with a tracheal anastomosis. Bilateral sequential lung transplantation with bronchial anastomoses has obviated this problem to a large degree. Severe psychiatric disorder in either the patient or, in the case of a young child, the care provider is a strong relative contraindication. Finally, a history of poor compliance with either a medical regimen or in keeping follow-up appointments is considered by most to be a strong relative contraindication to transplantation. Graft failure due to lack of proper care not only results in death to the recipient involved but also results in either a delayed or denied transplant for a more appropriate candidate.[26]

Special Circumstances

Some infants born extremely prematurely survive the early days of their lives only to develop severe bronchopulmonary dysplasia with respiratory failure within the first year of life. The incidence of significant cerebral injury in this group is high; approximately 50% of those surviving have some disability.[45] We can only assume that the incidence is higher in those with severe residual lung disease requiring transplantation. It is often difficult to assess the neurologic status in these infants because of their small size and often the need for sedation and neuromuscular paralysis for maintenance of satisfactory ventilation. It is probably unwise to submit an infant born at 25 to 28 weeks' estimated gestational age to lung transplantation unless there has been an opportunity for an accurate neurologic examination. Imaging studies may offer some reassurance but are inconclusive. Another unusual situation that arises where lung transplantation may be considered appropriate is the child with severe acute respiratory distress syndrome. Those children still in the acute phase of this illness often have other organ dysfunction and their condition is too unstable for them to wait the obligatory time once listed for transplantation given the current organ allocation system. Those who survive the early phase of acute respiratory distress syndrome and are left with fibrotic lungs and stable ventilatory requirements should be evaluated. Finally, occasionally a patient with a history of prior pneumonectomy will be referred for lung transplantation. After pneumonectomy in children, the mediastinum shifts to the affected side. This distorts the hilar structures to the point that bilateral or single lung transplant is virtually impossible. When possible, a patient undergoing pneumonectomy who might require lung transplant in the future should have a prosthetic spacer placed in that side of the chest to maintain normal mediastinal geometry.

DONOR EVALUATION AND ORGAN PROCUREMENT

Donor availability remains a major limitation to the applicability of transplantation for end-stage lung disease. Donors must be matched by ABO blood type compatibility and within a reasonable size range of the recipient. Height is used as the most accurate correlate to lung size. Height that falls within 25% of the recipient height is probably suitable. Extending this range upward is certainly feasible, because it is not difficult to reduce the size of the lungs by trimming off the edge or even using only the lower lobes. However, extending the lower limit should be done with great caution—the transplanted lungs may not fill the chest and may be more prone to pulmonary edema. Donors are excluded in the presence of positive HIV serology, active hepatitis, history of asthma, tuberculosis, or other significant pulmonary disease. A history of limited cigarette smoking is probably acceptable if other parameters of the evaluation fall within the guidelines. In general, the upper limit of donor age is approximately 55 years. The chest radiograph should be free of infiltrates and the arterial oxygen tension should be more than 300 mm Hg on an inspired oxygen fraction of 1.0 with an appropriate tidal volume and 5 cm H_2O positive end-expiratory pressure. Mild pulmonary contusions and subsegmental atelectasis would not necessarily exclude a donor as long as these criteria are met. When the procurement team arrives at the donor institution, flexible bronchoscopy should be performed to examine the airways for erythema suggestive of aspiration of gastric contents. In addition, this provides an opportunity to assess the nature and quantity of pulmonary secretions. The presence of purulent secretions that do not clear well with suctioning should exclude the donor even if the chest radiograph is clear and the oxygenation is adequate.

The surgical part of the procurement process is performed via a median sternotomy. Both pleural spaces are opened widely to allow visual inspection of the lungs and also the topical application of cold saline and slush. The trachea is dissected out between the superior vena cava and aorta. It may be helpful to develop the interatrial groove also to allow a more accurate division of the left atrial tissue that must be shared with the cardiac donor team in most situations. The principles of the procurement process beyond this are (1) anticoagulation with high dose (300 units/kg) heparin; (2) bolus injection of prostaglandin E_1 (50 to 70 µg/kg) directly into the main pulmonary artery; (3) decompressing the right side of the heart by incising the inferior vena cava; (4) decompressing the left side of the heart by amputating the left atrial appendage; (5) high volume (50 mL/kg), low pressure flush of cold (4°C) pulmonary preservation solution of choice; (6) topical application of cold saline and slush to the lungs; and (7) continued ventilation of the lungs with low volumes and low pressures using an FiO_2 of 0.4. When all the preservation solution has been administered, the lungs are excised en bloc with the posterior mediastinal tissue, including the esophagus and descending aorta. The esophagus is isolated with a stapling device to avoid contamination. The trachea is divided while the lungs are held in gentle inflation (pressure of ~ 20 cm H_2O) with the FiO_2 at 0.4. The lungs are then extracted, placed in a bag containing the preservation solution used for the flush, and then placed in cold storage for transport.

Much research has been devoted to finding the "ideal" preservation solution to extend potential ischemic times and avoid reperfusion injury.[35] A full discussion of this complex topic goes beyond the scope of this chapter. The most commonly employed preservation solutions at this time are modified Euro-Collins solution, University of Wisconsin solution, Perfadex, and Celsior. None of these is clearly superior to the others, and all work reasonably well. However, none reliably allows for preservation times greater than 8 hours and none completely avoids reperfusion injury.

TECHNIQUE OF TRANSPLANTATION

The surgical technique used for children is like that for adults with the exception that virtually all children will require cardiopulmonary bypass, whereas that is not always necessary in adults. Transplantation without cardiopulmonary bypass would require single-lung ventilation during the procedure. Maintaining single-lung ventilation in these small children is extremely difficult because the airways are too small to accommodate double-lumen endobronchial tubes. Bilateral lung transplant is performed for nearly all children because of concerns over the growth potential of the transplanted lungs. Trans-sternal bilateral anterior thoracotomy incision (the so-called "clamshell incision") via the fourth intercostal space provides excellent exposure of the heart and hilar regions. Absorbable suture is used for all anastomoses to provide the greatest potential for growth.[20] We recommend a simple end-to-end rather than a telescoping anastomosis for the airway because of the high incidence of stenosis in the latter.[17,32] If the patient requires concomitant repair of an intracardiac lesion (e.g., with Eisenmenger's syndrome), that is best performed after the recipient pneumonectomies and before implanting the donor lungs. Many of these patients have significant aortopulmonary collaterals resulting in significant pulmonary venous return to the heart while on cardiopulmonary bypass. After the recipient lungs have been removed, the absence of pulmonary venous return to the heart from bronchial arteries and other collateral vessels will allow for a bloodless operative field for the intracardiac repair. The subsequent period during which allograft implantation is performed provides sufficient time for cardiac reperfusion before weaning from cardiopulmonary bypass.

Living donor lobar transplantation, and the use of cadaveric lobes, has become more commonplace as an alternative to standard cadaveric "whole lung" transplantation.[62] This has been driven primarily by donor shortage. Although the upper lobes have been used, lower lobes seem better suited anatomically, with each lobe serving as an entire lung. When lobes come from a living donor there is less bronchial and vascular tissue with which to work and thus longer cuffs of the bronchus, pulmonary artery, and pulmonary vein of the recipient will facilitate the procedure. A technique has been devised whereby a single left lung can be partitioned such that the upper lobe is used on the right and the lower lobe on the left.[12] The circumstances under which one might employ this technique would be quite unusual—a single left lung from a large donor being made available to a desperately ill child. Nonetheless, it is another attempt at solving the ongoing problem of inadequate donor organ supply.

IMMUNOSUPPRESSION

Although the precise protocols differ from one center to another, most employ the so-called triple-drug immunosuppression approach (Table 48-3). Combinations of these immunosuppressant drugs allow for a better overall effect with a relatively less toxic dose of any one agent. Drug regimens generally include cyclosporine or tacrolimus in combination with azathioprine and prednisone. There is no clear advantage of cyclosporine over tacrolimus or vice versa in terms of efficacy or side effect profile. The use of induction cytolytic therapy using antithymocyte globulin or OKT3 is somewhat controversial but is generally not recommended because of infectious complications associated with their use. Daclizumab and basiliximab, specific monoclonal antibodies to interleukin 2, have been introduced as an alternative to cytolytic

TABLE 48–3 Immunosuppressant Agents

Class of Drug	Side Effects
Interleukin-2 Synthesis inhibitors	
Cyclosporine	Hypertension, seizures, nephrotoxicity, hirsutism, gingival hyperplasia
Tacrolimus	Hyperglycemia, seizures, nephrotoxic
Lymphocyte Proliferation Inhibitors	
Azathioprine	Leukopenia, nausea
Mycophenolate mofetil	Leukopenia, nausea, diarrhea, elevated liver enzymes
Sirolimus	Hypertriglyceridemia, delayed wound healing
Corticosteroids	Hypertension, hyperglycemia, cushingoid appearance
Induction Agents	
Antithymocyte globulin	Fever, chills, leukopenia, cytomegalovirus infections, post-transplant lymphoproliferative disorder
OKT3	Fever, chills, cytomegalovirus infections, post-transplant lymphoproliferative disorder
Daclizumab, basiliximab	Nausea, diarrhea

agents to "induce" tolerance.[4] Rather than cytolytic, these drugs work by blocking a critical pathway in the activation of lymphocytes involved in cellular rejection. The low infection rate using these monoclonal antibodies has stimulated the reemergence of induction therapy early after lung transplant.[3]

The initial target trough cyclosporine blood level is 300 to 400 ng/mL by whole blood monoclonal assay. When tacrolimus is used, that target trough level is 10 to 15 ng/mL. The initial corticosteroid dose is 0.5 mg/kg daily of prednisone or methylprednisolone. Azathioprine is given in a dose of 2.5 to 3.0 mg/kg daily. Acute rejection is treated with 3 consecutive days of intravenous methylprednisolone at a dose of 10 mg/kg. Rejection refractory to methylprednisolone is treated with antithymocyte globulin for 7 to 10 days. Recurrent (>2) bouts of acute rejection prompt a change of the baseline immunosuppression from cyclosporine and azathioprine to tacrolimus and mycophenolate mofetil. Although the corticosteroid dose is gradually tapered over time, we do not believe it is appropriate to stop this drug altogether. The side effects of immunosuppressive drugs in children are similar to those seen in adults, although the hirsutism associated with cyclosporine is clearly a more significant problem in young, female children. This adverse effect may be of sufficient magnitude to occasionally warrant a switch to tacrolimus. Sirolimus (rapamycin) is chemically similar to tacrolimus but inhibits the proliferative response of lymphocytes to interleukin-2.[63] It does not share the nephrotoxic potential of tacrolimus. It is currently reserved for situations of failure of other immunosuppressant drugs. Some caution should be exercised in using sirolimus as initial immunosuppression early after

transplantation because there has been evidence of impaired wound and airway healing resulting in serious complications.[43]

All patients receive prophylaxis against *Pneumocystis carinii* pneumonia with either sulfamethoxazole-trimethoprim orally three times per week or monthly treatment with aerosolized pentamidine when sulfa allergy or intolerance is present. Prophylaxis against mucocutaneous *Candida* infections is also employed.

POST-TRANSPLANT SURVEILLANCE

Surveillance after transplantation is based on periodic spirometry and bronchoscopy with biopsies and bronchoalveolar lavage. Before discharge from the hospital, patients are provided with a home spirometer and are asked to perform spirometry at least once daily. A decrease in FEV_1 of greater than 10% from baseline is considered an indication for evaluation. All patients, regardless of size, undergo regularly scheduled surveillance bronchoscopy to diagnose lower respiratory infections, subclinical graft rejection, and airway anastomotic complications. Virtually all episodes of suspected rejection should be confirmed with transbronchial biopsies. The main challenge occurs in small infants in whom a flexible fiberoptic bronchoscope large enough to provide a lumen for biopsy forceps may obstruct the airway. A technique of nonbronchoscopic "blind" transbronchial biopsy using a suction catheter for guiding the biopsy forceps into the proper position has been devised.[48] More recently, a mini-forceps has been developed for use in the 3.5-mm pediatric flexible fiberoptic bronchoscope. Bronchoscopy with biopsy is performed at 10 to 14 days, 6 weeks, and then 3, 6, 9, 12, 18, and 24 months after transplant as a surveillance procedure. Worsening pulmonary function, infiltrates on a chest radiograph, or deterioration in clinical status, such as fever or an oxygen requirement, also prompt bronchoscopy and biopsy. Bronchoalveolar lavage is performed at these procedures for quantitative bacterial, routine viral, and fungal cultures.

POST-TRANSPLANT COMPLICATIONS

Surgical Complications

Anastomotic Complications

Anastomotic complications can involve either the airway or the vascular anastomoses. Airway dehiscence was the major source of early morbidity and mortality in the early days of lung transplantation when tracheal anastomoses were performed. Not until this problem was solved by using an omental wrap for the airway anastomosis could clinical lung transplantation progress.[9] Currently, dehiscence is rare in spite of the fact that most do not use the omental wrap any longer but rather approximate donor and recipient peribronchial tissue over the anastomosis. Dehiscence of the airway may be either partial or total. Partial dehiscence can usually be treated expectantly but puts the airway at increased risk of late stenosis.[56] Complete dehiscence requires emergent therapy and is generally a lethal complication. Although reanastomosis should be attempted when possible, it is associated with a high failure rate and transplant pneumonectomy is required. Smaller airway size in children prompted concerns about whether the incidence of bronchial anastomotic stenosis would be higher and also whether the anastomoses would grow. Current evidence suggests that the airways at the anastomoses grow and that the incidence of bronchial stenosis is not affected by age or size at the time of transplant.[31,57] Bronchial stenosis is usually treated with dilatation initially with either progressively larger rigid bronchoscopes or with an angioplasty balloon. Balloon dilatation of a stricture may be preferable because it is less likely than a rigid bronchoscope to traumatize the distal airway. Repeat bronchoscopy 10 to 14 days after initial dilatation of a bronchial stenosis is necessary to judge the overall effectiveness and to assess the likelihood of recurrence. Depending on the severity of the initial stricture or the rapidity with which it recurs, one might consider placing a stent. There are two basic types of stents applicable to this situation: Silastic and wire mesh. In general, wire mesh stents are easier to insert but much more difficult to remove and Silastic stents are harder to place and easier to remove. Alternatives to stent placement include sleeve resection (of the bronchus or upper lobe) or retransplantation. Resection has been performed with good results in adults but would be a very difficult procedure in children.[59] Retransplantation should be reserved for situations in which the stricture extends beyond the bronchial bifurcation on either side and cannot be managed with either endobronchial techniques or local resection.

Vascular Anastomotic Complications

Problems with either the arterial or venous anastomoses are rare. In most instances, a stenosis in either of these is secondary to excessive length on the donor pulmonary artery or left atrial cuff or torsion of either of these structures when undertaking the anastomosis. Stenosis in one of the pulmonary artery anastomoses may or may not be manifest by right ventricular hypertension. Because pulmonary artery catheters are not often placed in children, one should check the right ventricular pressure by direct puncture once off cardiopulmonary bypass. If elevated, the pressure distal to each anastomosis should be checked also by direct puncture. Unilateral mild to moderate pulmonary arterial anastomotic stenosis may not result in significant elevation of right ventricular pressure. A perfusion lung scan is routinely performed within 24 hours of the transplant to screen for technical problems with the vascular anastomoses. Any significant discrepancy between right- and left-sided perfusion should be immediately evaluated with either direct visualization in the operating room or angiography. Stenosis in either or both pulmonary venous anastomoses is manifest by pulmonary hypertension, profuse pink frothy sputum, and diffuse infiltrates on a chest radiograph. These findings may also be present with a severe reperfusion injury or diffuse alveolar damage. However, the pulmonary capillary wedge pressure is generally normal in the latter two instances and elevated with a stenosis in the pulmonary venous anastomosis. Transesophageal echocardiography is particularly helpful in the diagnosis of pulmonary venous anastomotic problems. Confirmation of the diagnosis usually requires direct measurement of the pulmonary venous and left atrial pressures, particularly in small children. Early correction is mandatory.

Bleeding

A number of factors place these patients at increased risk for bleeding after transplantation. Nearly all transplants in children require prolonged cardiopulmonary bypass for recipient pneumonectomies and implantation of donor organs. Additionally, many of these patients have undergone prior thoracotomies or sternotomies. Aprotinin is an important adjunct in the prevention of bleeding complications in these patients.[38] Patients with cyanotic heart disease and a prior thoracotomy have the greatest risk of serious bleeding, as mentioned earlier.

Phrenic Nerve Injury

This complication occurs in about 20% of lung transplants and is secondary to trauma due to stretch while retracting to expose the hilar regions; it is more common on the right side.[60] Recovery of diaphragmatic function within 6 months of transplantation is the general rule. The reason for the right side being injured more commonly probably relates to the proximity of the nerve to the pulmonary artery and the superior vena cava on that side. The superior vena cava (and thus the phrenic nerve) must be retracted to expose the proximal right pulmonary artery. Prior thoracotomy puts the nerve at greater risk for injury because it may be obscured by adhesions.

Hoarseness

Vocal cord paralysis caused by recurrent laryngeal nerve injury has an incidence of approximately 10%. This diagnosis is made at the time of flexible fiberoptic bronchoscopy with direct examination of the cords. In most cases, anatomic asymmetry improves without directed therapy within 6 months of transplantation. The left vocal cord is nearly always the one involved, and the injury presumably occurs as a result of dissection of the left pulmonary artery in the region of the ligamentum arteriosum.

Gastrointestinal Complications

Gastroesophageal reflux has occurred almost exclusively in the very young infants undergoing lung transplantation. Fifty percent of infants surviving more than 30 days in our series suffered this complication, as documented by upper gastrointestinal series, 24-hour esophageal pH probe, or evidence of aspiration by the presence of lipid-laden macrophages on bronchoalveolar lavage.[34] The etiology of this high incidence of gastroesophageal reflux is not clear but may be due to injury to the vagus nerves bilaterally in the process of performing the recipient pneumonectomies. Decreased intestinal motility is also a common problem in all age groups. A relatively high incidence of gastroesophageal reflux has been noted in adults undergoing lung transplantation. A link to bronchiolitis obliterans has been proposed by some.[16] Patients with cystic fibrosis are at risk for distal intestinal obstruction syndrome. This can be avoided by aggressively treating with osmotic cathartics after transplant. Gastrografin enemas may be necessary if there is no response to oral cathartics.

Atrial Flutter

Atrial arrhythmias are relatively common with significant episodes of atrial flutter occurring in 10% of transplant recipients. Many require long-term treatment.[21] Recent investigation into this entity using a model of lung transplantation has shown that the suture lines for the left atrial anastomoses provide sufficient substrate for the maintenance of atrial flutter when initiated by programmed extrastimulus.[22]

Graft Complications

Reperfusion injury manifesting as graft failure with diffuse infiltrates on chest radiography, frothy sputum, and poor oxygenation is the most common graft complication early after lung transplantation, occurring in 20% to 30% of transplant recipients.[42] It is the most common cause of death within the first 30 days after transplant.[67] The underlying cause is probably multifactorial, with both donor and recipient conditions contributing to this problem. The best preventive measures include careful evaluation and procurement of the donor organs as well as having a recipient free of active infection or other acute problems. A well-conducted transplant procedure is also of utmost importance. The treatment of reperfusion injury is mostly supportive, although nitric oxide[14] and prostaglandin E_1[46] may be of some primary benefit.

Rejection is a common occurrence after lung transplantation, perhaps more so than in other solid organ transplants (Fig. 48-1). The lung has a much larger endothelial surface than other organs. Because the major histocompatibility antigen expression on endothelial surfaces is the primary signal for local immune recognition, the lung would seem to be the least easily camouflaged organ in the body. In addition, the lung graft comes with its own parenchymal bronchial lymphocytes and macrophages. Gradually, these are replaced by the recipient lymphocytes and macrophages. This rather intense immunologic activity adds to the risk of rejection. Acute graft rejection early after transplant presents in such a nonspecific fashion that each suspected episode should be documented with histologic evidence obtained via either transbronchial biopsy or open-lung biopsy. The great majority of episodes of acute rejection occur in the first 6 months after the transplant. Although the incidence of acute rejection in all children is about the same as that seen in adults, it appears that infants have a much lower incidence.[36] The precise reason for this is unclear but may have to do with the relative immaturity of the immunologic system in infants.

Bronchiolitis obliterans is viewed by most clinicians to be a manifestation of chronic rejection and occurs in nearly 50% of all long-term survivors.[64] The precise cause is unknown, although donor ischemic time and episodes of early acute rejection have been identified as risk factors.[33] Bronchiolitis obliterans presents as a significant fall in FEV_1 without other obvious cause. The chest radiograph is generally clear, and the computed tomographic examination of the chest is usually without infiltrates. Ventilation/perfusion lung scanning demonstrates a mosaic pattern of perfusion with air trapping. Bronchoscopy with transbronchial biopsy and bronchoalveolar lavage should be

Figure 48–1 Acute rejection. Present are multiple lymphocytes in a perivascular position involving many blood vessels, which can be seen better on higher power. This was interpreted as grade A2 acute rejection.

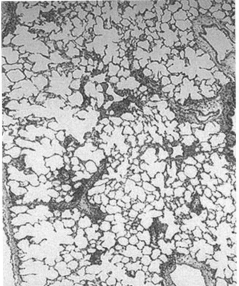
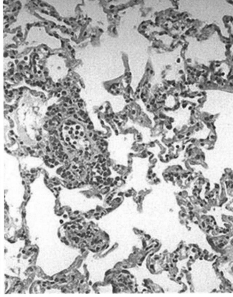

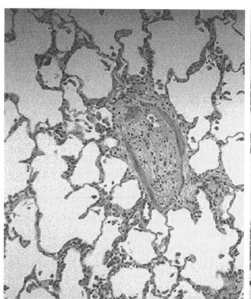
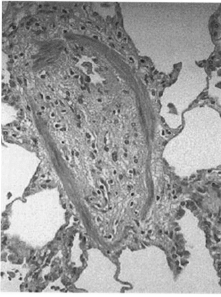

Figure 48–2 Histologic slide taken from the lung of a patient undergoing retransplantation for bronchiolitis obliterans. Small airways are obliterated by fibrous tissue.

done as part of the evaluation to rule out other potential causes such as acute rejection or infection and to assess the degree of active lymphocytic infiltration of the airways. The histologic picture of bronchiolitis obliterans is one of dense scarring of the membranous and respiratory bronchioles (Fig. 48-2). It may be inferred by the absence of identifiable bronchioles on biopsy material. Diagnosis of bronchiolitis obliterans by histologic examination of transbronchial biopsy material may be very difficult, however, and many do not consider it necessary to establish the diagnosis. A staging system has been established based on the degree of decline of FEV_1 from the peak value: post-transplant stage 1 = 20% to 35%, stage 2 = 35% to 50% decline, and stage 3 = more than 50% decline.[10] The current recommended treatment for bronchiolitis obliterans is to augment immunosuppression beginning usually with antithymocyte globulin daily for 7 to 10 days; the clinical response has been variable. A change in the maintenance immunosuppression is also appropriate. Antiproliferative agents may provide a more effective approach but that has yet to be proved. Total lymphoid irradiation and photopheresis are other modalities that have been proposed. Patients not responding to these measures may be suitable candidates for retransplantation. As mentioned earlier, this is a somewhat controversial topic because there is a shortage of donor organs and the results with retransplantation overall are not quite as good as first-time transplants. However, if the candidates are ambulatory, not ventilator dependent, and at an experienced lung transplant center, the survival results are not significantly different from first-time transplants.[49]

Post-transplant lymphoproliferative disease (PTLD) occurs in 5% to 10% of patients undergoing lung transplantation. PTLD occurs more frequently in association with a primary Epstein-Barr virus (EBV) infection.[68] Children may be somewhat more prone to this complication because they are frequently seronegative for EBV infection at the time of transplant and therefore likely to acquire a primary EBV infection during their post-transplant life. Reduction in immunosuppression is the mainstay of early therapy, although this may be insufficient and not uncommonly leads to the subsequent development of bronchiolitis obliterans. Rituximab, an anti-CD20 monoclonal antibody, has been used effectively in the treatment of PTLD.[64] Other treatment modalities include conventional chemotherapy,[66] irradiation,[20] and infusion of human leukocyte antigen–matched T lymphocytes.[52]

Infection

Although infection is generally common after any solid organ transplant, lung transplant recipients are at greater risk. Donors are all on mechanical ventilation, resulting in colonization of the airway with bacteria from an intensive care unit. With the exception of the small bowel, the lung is the only solid organ constantly in contact with the nonsterile outside world. An endotracheal tube necessary early after the transplant bypasses some of the natural defenses available to the respiratory tract. Obligate denervation of the lung that occurs with transplantation results in the cough reflex being markedly diminished or absent altogether. These and numerous other factors demand that the caregivers maintain constant vigilance in the diagnosis and treatment of respiratory infections and also emphasize to the recipient the importance of pulmonary toilet.

All potential candidates are screened for the presence of organisms in the airway and evidence of previous infections. Evidence of prior viral infections is evaluated by serologic testing for antibodies to cytomegalovirus, herpes simplex virus, varicella, EBV, hepatitis A, B, and C, and human immunodeficiency virus. Viral serologic screening is less informative in young infants whose immunoglobulin pool reflects passively transferred maternal antibodies. The initial antimicrobial therapy given in the early post-transplant period is directed in part by the results of pretransplant studies. Ganciclovir is given at a dose of 5 mg/kg/day for 6 weeks for any positive donor or recipient serology for cytomegalovirus. If patients have evidence of present or past *Aspergillus* infection, intravenous amphotericin B (3.0 mg/kg/day) is given for 5 to 10 days, followed by aerosolized amphotericin B (10 mg three times a day) depending on the clinical situation.

A number of viral respiratory infections are quite common in pediatric patients. Adenovirus and parainfluenza viruses are particularly bothersome in these children. As for cytomegalovirus, primary disease is generally more likely to be severe than reactivation disease.[10] As mentioned earlier, primary infection with EBV is an important risk factor for the development of PTLD.

Fungal infections are uncommon but potentially devastating. Nystatin oral suspension is employed to reduce the risk of infection from *Candida* species. Virtually all infections caused by *Candida* species can be successfully treated with oral or intravenous triazole antifungal agents. Invasive *Aspergillus* infections, however, are much more difficult to treat and may result in widespread dissemination if appropriate antifungal therapy is delayed.

Bacterial infections are the most common serious infection after lung transplantation. Bacterial lower respiratory tract infections, which include both purulent bronchitis and pneumonia, occur in most patients at some point after transplantation. Patients with cystic fibrosis are more likely to experience this complication, with the organism usually the same as that colonizing the airway before the transplant. Prophylaxis against lower respiratory tract infections in cystic fibrosis lung transplant recipients may be accomplished by administering aerosolized antibiotics (tobramycin or colistin) just as one might for end-stage cystic fibrosis.

Other Complications

Hypertension is a common problem after transplantation and is presumably due to treatment with the calcineurin inhibitors cyclosporine and tacrolimus as well as prednisone. Renal insufficiency occurs with increasing time after transplantation and is also related to treatment with cyclosporine and tacrolimus. Diabetes mellitus occurs in approximately 15% of patients after transplant, primarily in patients with cystic fibrosis.[8] Tacrolimus predictably increases the likelihood for the development of hyperglycemia.

SURVIVAL

The 3- and 5-year actuarial survival for children undergoing lung transplantation is approximately 54% and 45%, respectively, according to the International Society for Heart and Lung Transplantation registry (Fig. 48-3).[67] Acute graft failure accounts for the majority of deaths in the first 30 days. Infection is the cause of death in approximately 50% of those dying in the first year beyond the transplant hospitalization. Bronchiolitis obliterans is the cause of death in 50% of patients beyond 1 year after transplant and is clearly the major impediment to longterm survival.[49]

PULMONARY FUNCTION AND GROWTH

It is unclear whether transplanted lungs grow in terms of number and size of alveoli, and experimental data are inconclusive.[28,40] Measurement of lung growth is fraught with a number of complicating factors. One cannot use pulmonary function tests and lung volume size as measured by either chest radiograph or computed tomography because there are a number of elements that affect these studies that would not accurately reflect the number or size of alveoli. The impact of lung growth is particularly critical in small infants because their transplanted lungs will have to grow substantially over the rest of their lives to handle the physiologic load presented to them. Those children in our series too young to undergo standard pulmonary function testing underwent infant pulmonary function tests that provide a measurement of functional residual capacity, a reasonable surrogate for

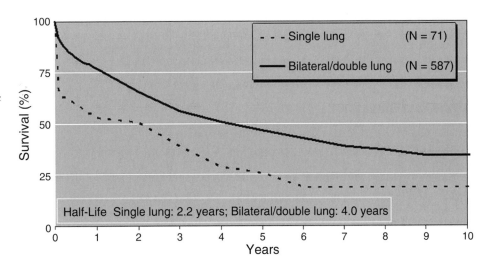

Figure 48–3 Kaplan-Meier survival curve for pediatric lung transplantation. (From Boucek MM, Faro A, Novick RJ, et al: The Registry of the International Society for Heart and Lung Transplantation: Fourth official pediatric report—2000. J Heart Lung Transplant 2001;20:39-52.)

Half-Life Single lung: 2.2 years; Bilateral/double lung: 4.0 years

- - - Single lung   (N = 71)
—— Bilateral/double lung   (N = 587)

lung volume. The average functional residual capacity per centimeter in height at 3 months after transplant was 2.3 mL/cm and remained between 2.1 and 2.8 mL/cm through 15 months after transplant. During this time substantial somatic growth occurred in these infants.[7] Thus, in the absence of central or peripheral airway obstruction, these data suggest that lung growth appropriate for size is occurring. We do not know whether this represents an increase in the number of alveoli and/or an increase in the size of existing alveoli, however.

LIVING DONOR LUNG TRANSPLANTATION

The use of living donors for lung transplantation (LDLTx) follows the same path proposed for kidney and liver transplantation in which successes (especially with the kidney) had already been experienced. The principle with this is that a normal, healthy adult should be able to donate a lower lobe from either the right or left lung to a child (or small adult) and have it serve as a "whole lung."[62] The donor presumably would have sufficient reserve so that the 20% to 25% loss of lung volume would not result in any loss of functional capacity for day-to-day living. The differences between LDLTx and living donor transplants for the kidney or liver is that two donors are required for LDLTx and the procurement is performed via a thoracotomy, which is generally perceived to be a higher risk procedure than laparotomy. Thus, two normal individuals are risking their lives for one. There are obviously significant ethical issues involved in this, particularly given the survival statistics for lung transplantation. However, there are clearly some advantages over cadaveric lung transplantation: short ischemic times for the donor lungs, extensive evaluation to ensure that the donors have normal lungs, a scheduled transplant at a time optimal for all concerned, and the potential for better human leukocyte antigen matching. It is a more challenging procedure technically, however. LDLTx is reserved for situations in which the recipient will not survive long enough to receive donor lungs from a cadaveric source. The survival in these patients after LDLTx has been similar to that seen in patients transplanted with lungs from a cadaveric source. One fascinating finding in this group has been the very low incidence of bronchiolitis obliterans.[69] This may be related to the very short ischemic times in the LDLTx donor organs, which are harvested in an adjoining hospital. Another possible explanation is an immunologic advantage in the case of the donors being close relatives.

FUTURE CONSIDERATIONS

Factors that limit the success of lung transplantation in children are similar to those in adults: donor shortage, balance of immunosuppression and prevention of infection, and development of bronchiolitis obliterans. As part of the solution to the donor shortage issue, it is likely that living donor lung transplantation will be used more commonly over the next several years but will likely not have a major impact overall on the donor pool and waiting times. Xenotransplantation may eventually offer another solution, but realistically this is many years from application. Newer immunosuppressive agents aimed at more specific areas of the immune response involved with organ recognition are necessary. Bronchiolitis obliterans remains the "Achilles heel" of long-term survival after lung transplantation. Although still not completely characterized as to its precise cause, most investigators ascribe this development to chronic rejection. To that end, clinical and basic research aimed at understanding the vectors of injury and disease progression in bronchiolitis obliterans are of paramount importance to the field of lung transplantation. Because the airway as the site of injury is accessible for assessment and therapy, bronchiolitis obliterans may provide a model system whereby chronic rejection, which also affects long-term success in heart, kidney, and liver transplantation, can be understood and overcome.

REFERENCES

1. Barst RJ, Rubin LJ, Long WA, et al: A comparison of continuous intravenous epoprostenol (prostacyclin) with conventional therapy for primary pulmonary hypertension. N Engl J Med 1996;334:296-302.
2. Boucek MM, Faro A, Novick RJ, et al: The Registry of the International Society for Heart and Lung Transplantation: Fourth official pediatric report—2000. J Heart Lung Transplant 2001;20:39-52.
3. Brock MV, Borja MC, Ferber L, et al: Induction therapy in lung transplantation: A prospective, controlled clinical trial comparing OKT3, anti-thymocyte globulin, and daclizumab. J Heart Lung Transplant 2001;20:1282-1290.
4. Bumgardner GL, Hardie I, Johnson RW, et al: Phase III Daclizumab Study Group: Results of 3-year phase III clinical trials with daclizumab prophylaxis for prevention of acute rejection after renal transplantation. Transplantation 2001;72:839-845.
5. Channick RN, Simonneau G, Sitbon O, et al: Effects of the dual endothelin-receptor antagonist bosentan in patients with pulmonary hypertension: A randomised placebo-controlled study. Lancet 2001;358:1119-1123.
6. Clabby ML, Canter CE, Moller JH, Bridges ND: Hemodynamic data and survival in children with pulmonary hypertension. J Am Coll Cardiol 1997;30:554-560.
7. Cohen AH, Mallory GB, Ross K, et al: Growth of lungs after transplantation in infants and in children younger than 3 years of age. Am J Respir Crit Care Med 1999;159:1747-1751.
8. Cooper JD, Ginsberg RJ, Goldberg M, the Toronto Lung Transplant Group: Unilateral transplantation for pulmonary fibrosis. N Engl J Med 1986;314:1140-1145.
9. Cooper JD, Pearson FG, Patterson GA, et al: Technique of successful lung transplantation in humans. J Thorac Cardiovasc Surg 1987;93:173-181.
10. Cooper JD, Billlingham M, Egan T, et al: A working formulation for the standardization of nomenclature and for clinical staging of chronic dysfunction in lung allografts. J Heart Lung Transplant 1993;12:713-716.
11. Couetil JP, Houssin DP, Soubrane O, et al:. Combined lung and liver transplantation in patients with cystic fibrosis: A 4½-year experience. J Thorac Cardiovasc Surg 1995;110:1415-1422.
12. Couetil J-P, Achkar A, Chevalier P, et al: Split lung with bilateral lobar transplantation: A two-year experience. J Heart Lung Transplant 1995;14(Suppl):S60.

13. Cystic Fibrosis Foundation: Patient Registry 1999 Annual Report. Bethesda, MD, September 2000.

14. Date H, Triantafillou AN, Trulock EP, et al: Inhaled nitric oxide reduces human lung allograft dysfunction. J Thorac Cardiovasc Surg 1996;111:913-919.

15. D'Alonzo GE, Barst RJ, Ayres SM, et al: Survival in patients with primary pulmonary hypertension: Results from a national prospective registry. Ann Intern Med 1991;115: 343-349.

16. Davis RD, Lau CL, Eubanks S, et al: Improved lung allograft function after fundoplication in patients with gastroesophageal reflux disease undergoing lung transplantation. J Thorac Cardiovasc Surg 2003;125:533-542.

17. Egan TM, Westerman JH, Lambert CJ, et al: Isolated lung transplantation for end-stage lung disease: A viable therapy. Ann Thorac Surg 1992;53:590-596.

18. Egan TM, Detterbeck FC, Mill MR, et al: Improved results of lung transplantation for patients with cystic fibrosis. J Thorac Cardiovasc Surg 1995;109:224-235.

19. Finkelstein SM, Wielinski CL, Elliott GR, et al: Diabetes mellitus associated with cystic fibrosis. J Pediatr 1988;112: 373-377.

20. Friedman E, Perez-Atayde AR, Silvera M, Jonas RA: Growth of tracheal anastomoses in lambs. J Thorac Cardiovasc Surg 1990;100:188-193.

21. Gandhi SK, Bromberg BI, Mallory GB, Huddleston CB: Atrial flutter—a newly recognized complication of pediatric lung transplantation. J Thorac Cardiovasc Surg 1996;112: 984-991.

22. Gandhi SK, Bromberg BI, Schuessler RB, et al: Left sided atrial flutter—characterization of a novel complication of pediatric lung transplantation in an acute canine model. J Thorac Cardiovasc Surg 1996;112:992-1001.

23. Ganne V, Siddiqi N, Kamaplath B, et al: Humanized anti-CD20 monoclonal antibody (Rituximab) treatment for post-transplant lymphoproliferative disorder. Clin Transplant 2003;17:417-422.

24. Gilligan PH, Neuringer IP, Gott KK, et al: The effects of panresistant bacteria in cystic fibrosis patients on lung transplant outcome. Am J Respir Crit Care Med 1997; 155:1699-1704.

25. Hamvas A, Mallory GB, Spray TL, et al: Lung transplantation for treatment of infants with surfactant protein B deficiency. J Pediatr 1997;130:231-239.

26. Hamvas A, Nogee LM, White FV, et al: Progressive lung disease and surfactant dysfunction with a deletion in surfactant protein C gene. Am J Respir Cell Mol Biol 2004; 30:771-776.

27. Hardy JD, Webb WR, Dalton ML, et al: Lung homotransplantation in man. JAMA 1963;186:1065-1074.

28. Hislop AA, Odom NJ, McGregor CGA, Haworth SG: Growth potential of the immature transplanted lung: An experimental study. J Thorac Cardiovasc Surg 1990;100: 360-370.

29. Hoeper MM, Schwarze M, Ehlerding S, et al: Long-term treatment of primary pulmonary hypertension with aerosolized iloprost, a prostacyclin analogue. N Engl J Med 2000;342:1866-1870.

30. Hopkins WE, Ochoe LL, Richardson GW, Trulock EP: Comparison of the hemodynamics and survival of adults with severe primary pulmonary hypertension or Eisenmenger syndrome. J Heart Lung Transplant 1996;15:100-105.

31. Huddleston CB, Spray TL, Mallory GB: Airway complications following pediatric lung transplant. J Heart Lung Transplant 1995;14 (Suppl):S60.

32. Huddleston CB: Airway complications in children following lung transplantation. In Cooper DKC, Miller L,

Patterson GA (eds): The Transplantation and Replacement of Thoracic Organs. Lancaster, UK, Kluwer, 1996, pp 581-588.

33. Huddleston CB, Sweet SC, Cohen AH, et al: Bronchiolitis obliterans after pediatric lung transplantation. J Heart Lung Transplant 1998;17:65.

34. Huddleston CB, Sweet SC, Mallory GB, et al: Lung transplantation in very young infants. J Thorac Cardiovasc Surg 1999;118:796-804.

35. Huddleston CB, Mendeloff EN: Heart and lung preservation for transplantation. J Cardiac Surg 2000;15:108-121.

36. Ibrahim JE, Sweet SC, Flippin MC, et al: Rejection is reduced in thoracic organ recipients when transplanted in the first year of life. J Heart Lung Transplant 2002;21: 311-318.

37. Jackson LK: Idiopathic pulmonary fibrosis. Clin Chest Med 1982;3:579.

38. Jaquiss RDB, Huddleston CB, Spray TL: Use of aprotinin in pediatric lung transplantation. J Heart Lung Transplant 1995;14:302-307.

39. Kerem E, Reisman J, Corey M, et al: Prediction of mortality in patients with cystic fibrosis. N Engl J Med 1992;326: 1187-1191.

40. Kern JA, Tribble CG, Flanagan TL, et al: Growth potential of porcine reduced-size mature pulmonary lobar transplants. J Thorac Cardiovasc Surg 1992;104:1329-1332.

41. Kerstein D, Levy PS, Hsu DT, et al: Blade balloon atrial septostomy in patients with severe primary pulmonary hypertension. Circulation 1995;91:2028-2035.

42. King RC, Binns OAR, Rodriguz F, et al: Reperfusion injury significantly impacts clinical outcome after pulmonary transplantation. Ann Thorac Surg 2000;69:1681-1685.

43. King-Biggs MB, Dunitz JM, Park SJ, et al: Airway anastomotic dehiscence associated with use of sirolimus immediately after lung transplantation. Transplantation 2003;75:1437-1443.

44. Klima LD, Kowdley KV, Lewis SL, et al: Successful lung transplantation in spite of cystic fibrosis-associated liver disease: A case series. J Heart Lung Transplant 1997;16:934-938.

45. Kurland G: Pediatric lung transplantation: Indications and contraindications. Semin Thorac Cardiovasc Surg 1996;8: 277-285.

46. Matsuzaki Y, Waddell TK, Puskas JD, et al: Amelioration of post-ischemic lung reperfusion injury by prostaglandin E_1. Am Rev Respir Dis 1993;148:882-889.

47. Milla CE, Warwick WJ: Risk of death in cystic fibrosis patients with severely compromised lung function. Chest 1998;113:1230-1234.

48. Mullins D, Livne M, Mallory GB, Kemp JS: A new technique for transbronchial biopsy in infants and small children. Pediatr Pulmonol 1995;20:253-257.

49. Novick RJ, Stitt LW, Al-Kattan K, et al: Pulmonary retransplantation: Predictors of graft function and survival in 230 patients. Ann Thorac Surg 1998;65:227-234.

50. Okano Y, Yoshioka T, Shimouchi A, et al: Orally active prostacyclin analogue in primary pulmonary hypertension. Lancet 1997;349:1365.

51. Osika E, Muller MH, Boccon-Gibod L, et al: Idiopathic pulmonary fibrosis in infants. Pediatr Pulmonol 1997;23:49-54.

52. Papadopoulos EB, Ladanyi M, Emanuel D, et al: Infusions of donor leukocytes to treat Epstein-Barr virus-associated lymphoproliferative disorders after allogeneic bone marrow transplantation. N Engl J Med 1994;330:1185-1191.

53. Pasque MK, Trulock EP, Cooper JD, et al: Single lung transplantation of pulmonary hypertension: Single institution experience in 34 patients. Circulation 1995;92:2252-2258.

54. Pechet TV, de la Morena MT, Mendeloff EN, et al: Lung transplantation in children following treatment for malignancy. J Heart Lung Transplant 2003;22:154-160.

55. Ramirez J, Patterson GA: Airway complications after lung transplantation. Semin Thorac Cardiovasc Surg 1992;4:147-153.
56. Rand KH, Pollard RB, Merigan TC: Increased pulmonary superinfections—cardiac transplant recipients undergoing primary cytomegalovirus infection. N Engl J Med 1987;298:951-953.
57. Ro PS, Bush DM, Kramer SS, et al: Airway growth after pediatric lung transplantation. J Heart Lung Transplant 2001;20:619-624.
58. Robinson W, Waltz DA: FEV$_1$ as a guide to lung transplant referral in young patients with cystic fibrosis. Pediatr Pulmonol 2000;30:198-202.
59. Schafers HJ, Schafer CM, Zink C, et al: Surgical treatment of airway complications after lung transplantation. J Thorac Cardiovasc Surg 1994;107:1476-1480.
60. Sheridan PH, Cheriyan A, Doud J, et al: Incidence of phrenic neuropathy after isolated lung transplantation. J Heart Lung Transplant 1995;14:684-691.
61. Snell GI, de Hoyos A, Krajden M, et al: *Pseudomonas cepacia* in lung transplant recipients with cystic fibrosis. Chest 1993;103:466-471.
62. Starnes VA, Barr ML, Cohen RG: Lobar transplantation: Indications, technique, and outcome. J Thorac Cardiovasc Surg 1994;108:403-411.
63. Stepkowski SM, Chen H, Daloze P, Kahan BD: Rapamycin, a potent immunosuppressive drug for vascularized heart, kidney and small bowel transplantation in the rat. Transplantation 1991;51:22-26.
64. Sundaresan S, Trulock EP, Mohanakumar T, et al: Prevalence and outcome of bronchiolitis syndrome after lung transplantation. Ann Thorac Surg 1995;60:1341-1346.
65. Sweet SC, Spray TL, Huddleston CB, et al: Pediatric lung transplantation at St. Louis Children's Hospital 1990-1995. Am J Respir Crit Care Med 1997;155:1027-1035.
66. Swinnen LJ, Mullen GM, Carr TJ, et al: Aggressive treatment for postcardiac transplant lymphoproliferation. Blood 1995;86:3333-3340.
67. Trulock EP, Edwards LB, Taylor DO, et al: The Registry of the International Society for Heart and Lung Transplantation: Twentieth official adult lung and heart-lung transplant report—2003. J Heart Lung Transplant 2003;22:625-635.
68. Walker RC, Paya CV, Marshall WF, et al: Pretransplantation sero-negative Epstein-Barr virus status is the primary risk factor for post-transplantation lymphoproliferative disease in adult heart, lung and other solid organ transplantation. J Heart Lung Transplant 1995;14:214-221.
69. Woo MS, MacLaughlin EF, Horn MV, et al: Bronchiolitis obliterans is not the primary cause of death in pediatric living donor lobar lung transplant recipients. J Heart Lung Transplant 2001;20:491-496.
70. Wood NS, Marlow N, Costeloe K, et al: Neurologic and developmental disability after extremely preterm birth. N Engl J Med 2000;343:378-384.
71. Wood P: The Eisenmenger syndrome or pulmonary hypertension with reversed central shunt. BMJ 1958;2:701-762.

Chapter 49

Surgical Implications Associated with Bone Marrow Transplantation

Paul M. Colombani and Mark L. Kayton

Bone marrow transplantation (BMT) is now being used to treat children with a variety of disorders, including hematologic malignancies, solid tumors, and immunologic disorders. Pediatric surgeons are called on regularly to provide vascular access and to address complications that occur in BMT patients. Understanding the process, indications, and problems associated with BMT can position pediatric surgeons to become important contributors to the patient care effort in this growing patient population.

The term *bone marrow transplantation* is often used as a catch phrase to subsume all prevalent methods of reconstituting hematopoietic stem cells, but in practice the stem cells may be provided from umbilical cord blood, peripheral blood stem cells, or bone marrow itself.[25] The cells may be autologous (collected when the patient is in remission) or allogeneic (from, for instance, a relative who is a close human leukocyte antigen [HLA] match). The recipient of the transplant receives a preparative regimen of chemotherapy with or without total-body irradiation, and this regimen is geared toward ablation of the underlying hematologic malignancy as well as ablation of the hematopoietic progenitor cells, thus paving the way for reconstitution of the blood with donor cells. An immunosuppressive regimen, as well as a prophylactic regimen designed to eliminate graft-versus-host disease (GVHD), is administered. As expected, complications at any phase of this process, whether involving cell harvest, immune system ablation, immunosuppression, or GVHD, routinely require involvement by a pediatric surgeon.

STEM CELL HARVEST AND VASCULAR ACCESS ISSUES

At our institutions we use a variety of temporary catheters in the groin or neck when one-time venous access is desired for blood cell harvest, but, increasingly, we have been placing tunneled, cuffed, dual-lumen subclavian vein lines (8 French Medcomp catheter for small children or 13.5 French Hickman catheter for older adolescents) that can function for pheresis and then remain in place to serve the long-term central venous access needs of the child.

BMT patients may require temporary access for dialysis or hemofiltration. For example, at the University of Minnesota, 5% of pediatric BMT patients needed dialysis for acute renal failure over a 12-year period.[13] Some have implicated the use of cyclosporine and amphotericin B, and the use of total-body irradiation, in the development of renal insufficiency in pediatric recipients of BMT.[33]

Acute access needs may arise in the intensive care unit (ICU) setting. To try to improve outcome among children with acute respiratory distress syndrome (ARDS), a group at Stanford University instituted early continuous venovenous hemofiltration (CVVH) at the time of intubation in a cohort of 10 pediatric oncology patients with respiratory failure and ARDS.[4] Six of the 10 children had undergone BMT. Eight (80%) survived; although there was no control group, this survival rate contrasts notably to that reported in the literature. For instance, a retrospective study of BMT patients from the Great Ormond Street Hospital found only a 40% rate of survival to ICU discharge among BMT patients with respiratory failure.[10] If this practice of early CVVH becomes more widespread, the need for surgeons to address vascular access will only escalate.

Even more dramatic needs for vascular access can arise. Leahey and colleagues at the Children's Hospital of Philadelphia have provided a case report on the use of extracorporeal membrane oxygenation (ECMO) 3 days after BMT.[15] The patient, an 8-month-old girl with severe combined immunodeficiency syndrome (SCID) and bronchiolitis from respiratory syncytial virus and influenza A virus, survived 15 days of ECMO and suffered a stroke but succeeded in engraftment of her transplant from an HLA-identical sibling, recovering adequate lymphocyte counts to resist infection. She survived and was discharged from the hospital.

COMPLICATIONS OF IMMUNE SYSTEM ABLATION AND IMMUNOSUPPRESSION

Intestinal Complications

The differential diagnosis of abdominal pain with diarrhea in the pediatric BMT recipient should include GVHD, mucositis secondary to medications, bacterial gastroenteritis, viral gastroenteritis (including adenovirus, rotavirus, and cytomegalovirus), *Clostridium difficile* infection, and amebiasis. Some of these causes are elaborated on because they are not common considerations in pediatric surgery.

In particular, considerations of intestinal GVHD will often prompt consultation with a pediatric surgeon to obtain, or else to manage the complications that may follow, upper or lower gastrointestinal biopsies. Upper gastrointestinal biopsies may be taken during endoscopy of the esophagus, stomach, or duodenum. A report by Ramakrishna and Treem recommends caution in biopsy of the duodenum in thrombocytopenic patients, with duodenal hematomas arising in two pediatric bone marrow transplant patients with platelet counts of 55,000/mm³ and 65,000/mm³, respectively.[23] Whereas the stomach and duodenum remain important sites to consider a biopsy, we have had success in diagnosing GVHD in specimens taken from the rectum using a rectal suction biopsy gun, which can be performed with little or no sedation of the patient on the ward unit and obviates the need for general anesthesia in the operating room.

In an intestinal tract already compromised by GVHD, unexpected pathologic processes may be noted. For instance, trophozoites of *Entamoeba histolytica* were recovered from the stool of two patients in Chile who had incomplete improvement after corticosteroid administration for concurrent GVHD.[21] Adenovirus enterocolitis has been described in a similar setting of intestinal GVHD.[27]

Clostridium difficile colitis can develop with striking manifestations in this population. One case report described *C. difficile* colitis in a 13-year-old BMT recipient who progressed to an obstructing post-colitis stricture of the descending colon requiring a transverse colostomy.[12]

Although rare, typhlitis (neutropenic enteropathy) does occur in BMT recipients (Fig. 49-1). Clinically, typhlitis presents as fever, abdominal pain or tenderness, and neutropenia. Hobson and colleagues noted that diarrhea was often observed in patients with typhlitis.[9] In a retrospective from Alberta, Canada, 5 of 142 pediatric BMT patients developed typhlitis. All were treated with bowel rest, total parenteral nutrition, and broad-spectrum antimicrobial medications, including systemic antifungal agents, and all survived and were discharged. This is in striking contrast to classic surgical teaching concerning typhlitis in adults in whom a 50% mortality is observed. Improvements in outcome after typhlitis may be a reflection of earlier diagnosis, aggressive use of granulocyte colony-stimulating factor, better antimicrobial agents, or all of these factors. Surprisingly, not all patients required computed tomography (CT) to make the diagnosis of typhlitis. One patient had the diagnosis made by plain abdominal radiography, and two of the five had an ultrasound study without CT.[1] On CT in children with typhlitis,

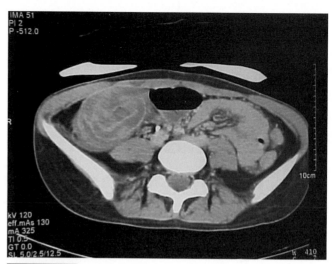

Figure 49-1 Typhlitis in a teenager with acute myelocytic leukemia who had undergone BMT. Note the thickened, onionskin appearance of the cecal wall and the pinpoint lumen. This patient underwent right hemicolectomy with ileostomy and mucous fistula; 1 year later, still in clinical remission from her leukemia, her condition was successfully reversed. Most cases of typhlitis are handled nonoperatively.

abnormal thickening of the cecal wall associated with surrounding inflammatory changes is observed.

Hepatobiliary Problems

Abnormal results of liver function tests are common among BMT patients, and surgeons will frequently be called on to differentiate obstructive biliary conditions from hepatocellular processes. Safford and colleagues have provided retrospective data regarding the incidence and natural history of gallstones among pediatric BMT patients.[24] Of 235 patients undergoing post-transplant ultrasound, 20 (8.5%) had gallstones. After stratifying these children based on the underlying diagnosis prompting transplant, Safford and colleagues found that among patients who received their transplant for neoplasia, inherited metabolic disorders, or immunologic disorders, about 7% had gallstones, whereas among patients receiving transplantation for various anemias and primary bone marrow disorders, 27% had gallstones, which suggests that factors such as hemolysis were more prevalent in the latter group. Nonetheless, of the 20 BMT recipients with gallstones, only 3 required surgical intervention (at a mean interval of 1.9 years after diagnosis of cholelithiasis), whereas 5 showed sonographic resolution of their gallstones (at an average of 150 days after diagnosis of cholelithiasis). Although this was not a prospective study, this observation should give surgeons some pause before being tempted to incidentally remove a stone-laden but asymptomatic gallbladder.

Another vexing problem affecting the liver in BMT patients is veno-occlusive disease. This refers to a syndrome usually seen within the first month after BMT, which may be a toxic response to the ablative and conditioning regimens used at the time of transplant.

This condition is characterized by congestion and fibrotic obliteration of the liver sinusoids and hepatic venules. Injury to zone 3 hepatocytes and endothelial cells is postulated as the inciting event. Hypercoagulable states and release of cytokines such as tumor necrosis factor-α may also play a role.[29]

The clinical diagnosis, summarized by the McDonald criteria,[18] is made when any two of the following three signs are present shortly after BMT: (1) ascites with a weight gain over 2% of baseline; (2) hepatomegaly or right upper quadrant tenderness; and (3) a total serum bilirubin level above 2 mg/dL. Prophylactic treatment with heparin has not been convincingly shown to improve outcome in this disease. Other strategies that have been described, although not validated in controlled studies, include the use of tissue plasminogen activator administered with heparin[14] and, in one pediatric case report, performance of a liver transplantation.[3]

Veno-occlusive disease has also been described in the lungs, may present as pulmonary hypertension, and has been fatal in nearly all instances.[32] Echocardiography can contribute to the diagnosis, but unfortunately most cases have been diagnosed at autopsy and some by open-lung biopsy.

Pulmonary Complications

A number of conditions, most far more common than veno-occlusive disease, can be diagnosed by lung biopsy. Infectious conditions include those caused by bacteria, viruses, fungi, *Legionella*, mycobacteria, and *Pneumocystis*. Among viral infections, cytomegalovirus, respiratory syncytial virus, adenovirus, and herpesviruses figure prominently. Noninfectious causes include hemorrhage, malignancy, drug toxicity, and interstitial pneumonitis, the last referring to an observed inflammatory response in the presence of negative cultures.[30] Finally, bronchiolitis obliterans organizing pneumonia (BOOP), a corticosteroid-responsive restrictive disease in which granulation tissue is deposited in terminal airways, also may be observed.[16]

Requests for lung biopsies are common in BMT centers. There is active debate about their impact on outcome. Shorter and coworkers, recounting the experience from 1976 to 1986 at Children's Hospital of Philadelphia, observed that 13 of 21 patients continued to deteriorate and died within 11 weeks despite the procedure, and only two patients required a significant change in therapy leading to survival.[28] Dunn and associates[5] described 15 stem cell transplant recipients. Eight of nine patients who required mechanical ventilation at the time of biopsy died. Therapy was changed by the results of biopsy in only 1 of the 15 patients. A more recent retrospective series by Hayes-Jordan and colleagues recapitulates these findings: a large proportion (7 of 19 [37%]) died within 30 days after lung biopsy, and only 3 of the 19 patients had a change in treatment leading to long-term survival.[8]

One subgroup that may benefit more from open-lung biopsy, if the entire involved area can be excised, are the patients with aspergillosis. The St. Jude group reported that 27 of 43 patients with aspergillosis had BMT.[6] Those patients who had all involved lung parenchyma resected had a significant survival benefit compared with those who did not have their lung that was involved with *Aspergillus* resected. This was not a randomized or prospective study, and all four survivors (with follow-up ranging from 1.7 to 43 months) had disease amenable to wedge resection, with one lobectomy. However, pulmonary aspergillosis is a disease process associated with a nearly 100% mortality in immunocompromised children. This implies it is reasonable to consider surgical resection in these cases.

Soft Tissue Complications

Skin and deep soft tissue infections including necrotizing fasciitis, necrotizing myositis, and cutaneous infection with *Mucor* may occur in BMT patients, especially during periods of neutropenia. Several case series exist describing soft tissue infections among neutropenic pediatric oncology patients, with some transplant recipients included in these groups.[11,19] Notably, enteric organisms—including *Escherichia coli*, *Pseudomonas*, and *Enterococcus*—are recovered from the cultures of BMT recipients. It is postulated that bacterial translocation from the gastrointestinal tract is a factor, resulting in hematogenous dissemination. This contrasts to standard assumptions that soft tissue infections originate when gram-positive bacteria or anaerobes colonize soft tissues after breaks in the skin. In the BMT population, broad-spectrum antibiotic coverage is required, including agents that target gram-negative organisms. Surgical débridement is every bit as much of an emergency as it is in other patient populations and can be even more challenging if bone marrow ablation has depleted the platelet count. Granulocyte colony-stimulating factor and granulocyte infusions should be considered in neutropenic patients. Johnston and associates[11] described fever, tachycardia, and localized pain out of proportion to findings on examination as helpful diagnostic signs and symptoms. If uncertainty exists, magnetic resonance imaging (MRI) may be useful, provided that time and the patient's clinical condition permit.

Cutaneous infection with *Mucor* (mucormycosis) should be considered in the differential diagnosis of any skin and soft tissue infection. This fungal infection, like bacterial soft tissue infections, usually mandates early débridement. In young BMT recipients, cutaneous infection with *Mucor* may present as tender induration that can progress to necrosis. Hyphae are demonstrable on microscopic examination of the involved tissue and blood vessels.[20,31]

Hemorrhagic Cystitis

Bleeding from the bladder epithelium can become a clinically devastating problem in BMT recipients. Hemorrhagic cystitis may be associated with toxicity from conditioning chemotherapies such as cyclophosphamide or busulfan,[26] or it may result from viral infections. Presentation may range from microscopic hematuria to gross hematuria with clots causing bladder outlet obstruction. Ultrasound shows thickening of the bladder wall; addition of color Doppler imaging may identify the focal areas of hypervascularity or active bleeding, which often leads to diagnostic cystoscopy.[17] Depending on the clinical severity of hemorrhagic cystitis, patients may be treated by intravenous hydration with forced diuresis, by Foley catheter drainage using continuous bladder irrigation, or by cystoscopy with removal of clot and fulguration of the bladder epithelium. The urethra in small children may not permit passage of a large enough Foley catheter to prevent recurrent obstruction by clot. In these patients, operative placement of large suprapubic catheters may be necessary.[34]

Thrombocytopenia

Refractory thrombocytopenia can be seen after BMT and often prompts the consideration of splenectomy. Thrombocytopenia may be related to medications, decreased marrow production of megakaryocytes, or platelet sequestration. However, platelets may be sequestered at other sites, and splenectomy does not prove curative in all patients with platelet sequestration. Hammersmith and associates have described a nuclear medicine technique for documenting splenic sequestration of platelets that can contribute to the decision whether to perform splenectomy.[7] Platelets are labeled with indium-111 and infused; platelet sequestration in the spleen is confirmed by observing the ratio of labeling density in the spleen to labeling density in the liver at various time points after infusion. A spleen-to-liver ratio of greater than 1.9 is consistent with abnormal splenic sequestration. However, this technique is not widely available and there are no data as to whether a positive scan predicts a good outcome after splenectomy. Thus, clinicians caring for patients with refractory thrombocytopenia must still make an empirical decision as to whether to perform splenectomy.

Unusual Problems

Acute suppurative thyroiditis has been described in a case report, in a 3-year-old undergoing a second BMT for chronic myelomonocytic leukemia.[22] Although the patient received total-body irradiation, which has been implicated as causing thyroid dysfunction, he developed swelling of the thyroid gland and hypothyroidism shortly after transplantation. In this instance, the authors considered the problem unrelated to radiation. Ultrasound showed "translucent" zones in the thyroid gland, and surgical drainage of purulent material was required.

COMPLICATIONS OF TRANSFUSIONS

Because surgeons and surgical house staff are often involved in ordering blood products for perioperative usage, it is important to remember that transfused blood itself can cause GVHD. Passenger T lymphocytes, which

can contaminate preparations of red cells, plasma, or platelets, mediate an immune response against the immunocompromised recipient. Manifestations of transfusion-associated GVHD include rash, abnormal liver function test results, pancytopenia, and, in 84% of affected patients, death.[2] Two techniques—leukocyte filtration and irradiation—are used respectively to reduce the load of, and to inactivate, leukocytes in banked blood products. Thus, blood products for BMT patients should be both leukocyte filtered and irradiated.

Chronic GVHD

Chronic GVHD is characterized by generalized sclerosis of skin and soft tissue structures and sometimes cholestatic jaundice. Even acquired phimosis has been observed in an advanced case, requiring circumcision in a 13-year-old boy.

CONCLUSION

Whereas the development of BMT has traditionally been in the realm of medical, pediatric, and oncologic specialists, this discussion highlights the multitude of organ systems that can manifest surgical pathologic processes after BMT. The lungs, intestinal tract, liver, spleen, bladder, soft tissue, and hematologic system are all subject to various surgical complications. Moreover, virtually every patient subjected to BMT will require vascular access for medications, alimentation, dialysis, or cell harvest. These expected implications of BMT mandate that every hospital with a pediatric BMT program have access to a general pediatric surgeon. In return, pediatric surgeons should educate and position themselves to advise their medical colleagues, manage these problems with expertise, and contribute to the development of this expanding aspect of transplantation.

REFERENCES

1. Al Otaibi A, Barker C, Anderson R, et al: Neutropenic enterocolitis (typhlitis) after pediatric bone marrow transplant. J Pediatr Surg 2002;37:770-772.
2. Anderson KC, Weinstein HJ: Transfusion-associated graft-versus-host disease. N Engl J Med 1990;323:315-321.
3. Bunin N, Leahey A, Dunn S: Related donor liver transplant for veno-occlusive disease following T-depleted unrelated donor bone marrow transplantation. Transplantation 1996; 61:664-666.
4. DiCarlo JV, Alexander SR, Agarwal R, et al: Continuous veno-venous hemofiltration may improve survival from acute respiratory distress syndrome after bone marrow transplantation or chemotherapy. J Pediatr Hematol Oncol 2003;25:801-805.
5. Dunn JC, West KW, Resurla FJ, et al: The utility of lung biopsy in recipients of stem-cell transplantation. J Pediatr Surg 2001;36:1302-1303.
6. Gow KW, Hayes-Jordan AA, Billups CA, et al: Benefit of surgical resection of invasive pulmonary aspergillosis in pediatric patients undergoing treatment for malignancies and

immunodeficiency syndromes. J Pediatr Surg 2003;38: 1354-1360.

7. Hammersmith SM, Jacobson AF, Mankoff DA: Scintigraphy with indium-111 labeled homologous (donor) platelets in the platelet transfusion refractory bone marrow transplant patient. J Nucl Med 1997;38:1135-1138.

8. Hayes-Jordan A, Benaim E, Richardson S, et al: Open lung biopsy in pediatric bone marrow transplant patients. J Pediatr Surg 2002;37:446-452.

9. Hobson MJ, Carney DE, Molik KA, et al: Appendicitis in childhood hematological malignancies: Analysis and comparison with typhlitis. J Pediatr Surg 2005;40:214-219; discussion 219-220.

10. Jacobe SJ, Hassan A, Veys P, et al: Outcome of children requiring admission to an intensive care unit after bone marrow transplantation. Crit Care Med 2003;31:1299-1305.

11. Johnston DL, Waldhausen JHT, Park JR: Deep soft tissue infections in the neutropenic pediatric oncology patient. J Pediatr Hematol Oncol 2001;23:443-447.

12. Kavan P, Sochor M, Nyc O, et al: Pseudomembranous *Clostridium* after autologous bone marrow transplantation. Bone Marrow Transplant 1998;21:521-523.

13. Lane PH, Mauer SM, Blazar BR, et al: Outcome of dialysis for acute renal failure in pediatric bone marrow transplant patients. Bone Marrow Transplant 1994;13:613-617.

14. Leahey AM, Bunin NJ: Recombinant human tissue plasminogen activator for the treatment of severe hepatic veno-occlusive disease in pediatric bone marrow transplant patients. Bone Marrow Transplant 1996;17:1101-1104.

15. Leahey AM, Bunin NJ, Schears GJ, et al: Successful use of extracorporeal membrane oxygenation (ECMO) during BMT for SCID. Bone Marrow Transplant 1998;21:839-840.

16. Mathew P, Bozeman P, Krance RA, et al: Bronchiolitis obliterans organizing pneumonia (BOOP) in children after allogeneic bone marrow transplantation. Bone Marrow Transplant 1994;13:221-223.

17. McCarville MB, Hoffer FA, Gingrich JR, et al: Imaging findings of hemorrhagic cystitis in pediatric oncology patients. Pediatr Radiol 2000;30:131-138.

18. McDonald GB, Sharma P, Matthews DE, et al: Veno-occlusive disease of the liver after bone marrow transplantation: Diagnosis, incidence, and predisposing factors. Hepatology 1984;4:116-122.

19. Murphy JJ, Granger R, Blair GK, et al: Necrotizing fasciitis in childhood. J Pediatr Surg 1995;30:1131-1134.

20. Nomura J, Ruskin J, Sahebi F, et al: Mucormycosis of the vulva following bone marrow transplantation. Bone Marrow Transplant 1997;19:859-860.

21. Perret C, Harris PR, Rivera M, et al: Refractory enteric amebiasis in pediatric patients with acute graft-versus-host disease after allogeneic bone marrow transplantation. J Pediatr Gastroenterol Nutr 2000;31:86-90.

22. Poelman M, Benoit Y, Laureys G, et al: Acute suppurative thyroiditis complicating second allogeneic transplant for juvenile CMML. Bone Marrow Transplant 1992;10: 547-548.

23. Ramakrishna J, Treem WR: Duodenal hematoma as a complication of endoscopic biopsy in pediatric bone marrow transplant recipients. J Pediatr Gastroenterol Nutr 1997; 25:426-429.

24. Safford SD, Safford KM, Martin P, et al: Management of cholelithiasis in pediatric patients who undergo bone marrow transplantation. J Pediatr Surg 2001;36:86-90.

25. Sanders JE: Bone marrow transplantation for pediatric malignancies. Pediatr Clin North Am 1997;44:1005-1020.

26. Seber A, Shu XO, Defor T, et al: Risk factors for hemorrhagic cystitis following BMT. Bone Marrow Transplant 1999;23:35-40.

27. Shayan K, Saunders F, Roberts E, et al: Adenovirus enterocolitis in pediatric patients following bone marrow transplantation. Arch Pathol Lab Med 2003;127: 1615-1618.

28. Shorter NA, Ross AJ III, August C, et al: The usefulness of open-lung biopsy in the pediatric bone marrow transplant population. J Pediatr Surg 1988;23:533-537.

29. Shulman HM, Hinterberger W: Hepatic veno-occlusive disease—liver toxicity syndrome after bone marrow transplantation. Bone Marrow Transplant 1992;10:197-214.

30. Stokes DC: Pulmonary complications of tissue transplantation in children. Curr Opin Pediatr 1994;6:272-279.

31. Trigg ME, Comito MA, Rumelhart SL: Cutaneous *Mucor* infection treated with wide excision in two children who underwent marrow transplantation. J Pediatr Surg 1996; 31:976-977.

32. Trobaugh-Lotrario AD, Greffe B, Deterding R, et al: Pulmonary veno-occlusive disease after autologous bone marrow transplant in a child with stage IV neuroblastoma: Case report and literature review. J Pediatr Hematol Oncol 2003;25:405-409.

33. Van Why SK, Friedman AL, Wei LJ, et al: Renal insufficiency after bone marrow transplantation in children. Bone Marrow Transplant 1991;7:383-388.

34. Vogeli TA, Peinemann F, Burdach S, et al: Urological treatment and clinical course of BK polyomavirus-associated hemorrhagic cystitis in children after bone marrow transplantation. Eur Urol 1999;36:252-257.

Part V

HEAD AND NECK

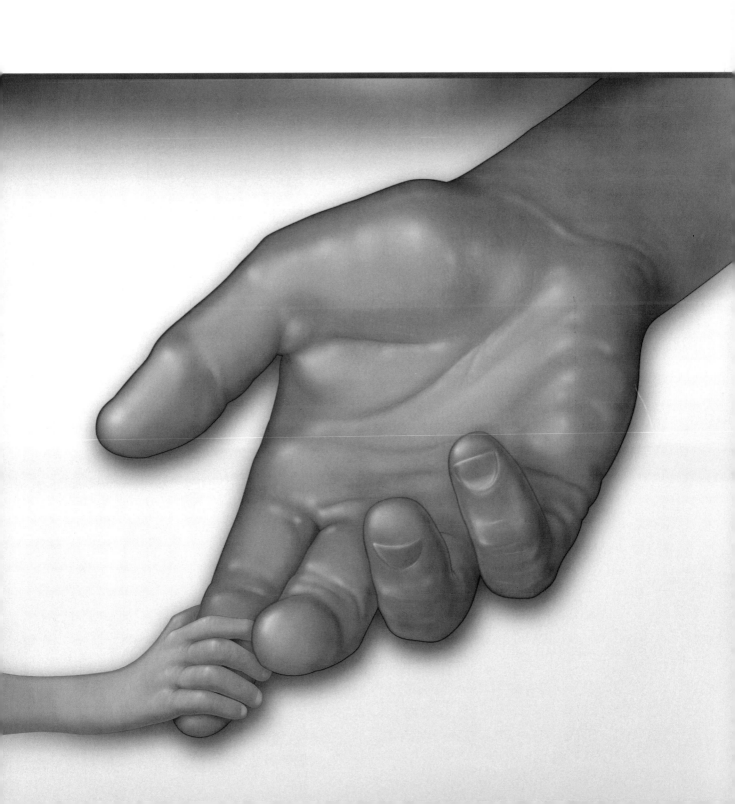

Chapter 50

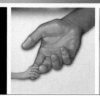

Craniofacial Anomalies

Henry K. Kawamoto, Jr.

Craniofacial anomalies are devastating when they occur. A lasting impression is made on initial encounter, and confusion may reign as to care. Some of these malformations are relatively common, such as a cleft of the lip or palate. Others are rare to the point that they may never be witnessed during a clinician's professional life. Yet, gathered together, the total number of children disfigured by craniofacial malformations is vast.

The term *craniofacial surgery* is automatically associated with the name of its founder Paul L. Tessier. Until the late 1960s, when word of his seminal work spread, only what now seems like a Band-Aid approach was available to correct these malformations.[54] Tessier and his coworkers showed that anatomic correction could be achieved by widely exposing the twisted craniofacial skeleton, restoring anatomic alignment with osteotomies, replacing missing parts with autogenous tissues, providing stable fixation, and adding an intracranial approach when indicated. The classic teaching of avoiding purposeful contamination (i.e., exposing the sterile intracranial environment to the filth of the nasal and oral cavities) was challenged directly under the cover of antibiotics. The concern about infection and other morbid events was shown to be unfounded as a new subspecialty was born.

Over the next 25 years, visiting Paris to observe Dr. Tessier's work became obligatory for surgeons who wished to gain proficiency in the field. Knowledge disseminated and expanded quickly. Now, throughout the world, most major medical centers have craniofacial anomalies teams composed of an anesthesiologist, audiologist, geneticist, neurosurgeon, ophthalmologist, oral surgeon, orthodontist, otolaryngologist, pediatrician, plastic surgeon, radiologist, social worker, and speech pathologist to care for patients with these complex anomalies.

Although the variety of craniofacial anomalies is enormous, they can be conveniently divided into two large groups: (1) craniofacial clefts and (2) craniosynostosis. The latter can be further subdivided into nonsyndromic and syndromic malformations. Entire texts are devoted to describing these entities. Additional books detail their surgical treatment, but centers differ in terms of timing and techniques. What follows is an overview that highlights the more common anomalies and their correction. Acquired disfigurement owing to neoplasm and trauma is also part of the field, but its discussion lies beyond the scope of this chapter.

BASIC CRANIOFACIAL SURGICAL PRINCIPLES

Immediately beneath the thin veneer and variety of expression of a child's face lies the complex end organs that produce sight, olfaction, hearing, speech, and mastication. Children with a craniofacial malformation are seriously handicapped in their social interactions. They deserve the coordinated long-term care of a dedicated team of specialists to look after their complicated needs. Surgeons who undertake such repairs must have special training and experience. A moment of carelessness can destroy the chance for normalcy forever.

The primary concern in the timing of surgical intervention is the preservation and restoration of function. Once these demands are satisfied, attention is focused on coordinating the operation with facial growth and development and the psychosocial needs of the child. Normal individual anatomic differences as well as inherent disparate growth of a malformed part must be considered. Surgical treatment generally is directed toward the end of the growth curve of each regional component. Access to the deformed area is gained through concealed incisions. Wide exposure of the pathologic process is required to relocate the affected craniofacial skeleton through socially invisible coronal, palpebral, and intraoral incisions (Fig. 50-1). If a visible scar is unavoidable, the incisions should so be designed as to mimic normal anatomic features or fall within aesthetic facial junctions or units.

The distorted facial skeleton must be restored as close to normal as possible. Similar to any project, establishing a sound foundation should precede the details. Thus, reconstructing the integrity of the facial skeleton receives priority. Anatomic relocation of maligned sections is basic. Missing parts should be replaced with autogenous material whenever possible. For osseous reconstruction,

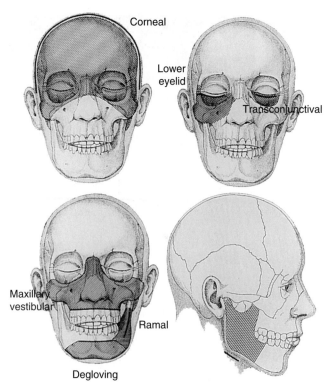

Corneal

Lower eyelid

Transconjunctival

Maxillary vestibular

Ramal

Degloving

Figure 50–1 Incision and exposure of craniofacial skeleton. *Shaded areas* represent areas of exposure provided by each incision.

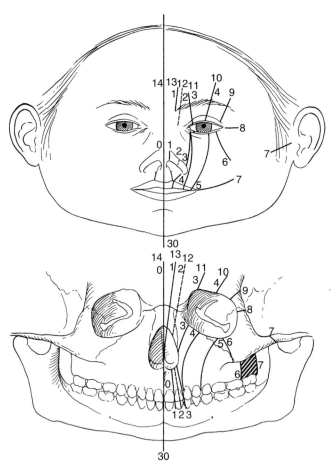

Figure 50–2 Tessier classification. Meridian represents the pathology of craniofacial clefts and their relationship to anatomic facial features. When both are present, *facial clefts* (0 to 7) usually follow their *cranial* (9 to 14) counterparts along the same meridian.

split calvarial bone is the popular choice because of its proximity to the main surgical field, a low percent of resorption, minimal associated morbidity, and an embryonic origin that is similar to the bone that it replaces. Alloplastic building blocks are poor substitutes for the real thing, and their use should especially be avoided on the growing skeleton.

CRANIOFACIAL CLEFTS

The kaleidoscopic world of craniofacial clefts is bewildering on first glance. Similar to a kaleidoscope, a slight turn can convert a forme fruste expression into a complete representation of the malformation. A further twist can produce more bizarre alterations or an entirely new entity.

Various classification systems have been proposed in an attempt to bring some order to the seeming chaos. The Tessier classification[26,53] enjoys the widest acceptance (Fig. 50-2). The categorization is founded on Tessier's personal observations and is clinically oriented. The topographic meridians prompt a search for any underlying faults in the facial skeleton. On the map of clefts, cleft 8 occupies the equator, clefts 0 to 7 depict the facial clefts, and clefts 9 to 14 delineate their cranial prolongations. Although a cleft may appear to be confined to either the facial or cranial hemisphere, careful inspection made along the entire meridian often will reveal subtle yet important findings.

Some craniofacial clefts are extremely rare and are noted only by surgeons who see a large number of these

patients. Therefore, this discussion is focused on those more commonly observed examples.

Cleft Lip and Palate

These clefts are described in detail in Chapter 51.

Craniofacial Microsomia

Other common names for craniofacial microsomia are the *first and second branchial arch syndrome, hemifacial microsomia,* and *otomandibular dysostosis.* In the Tessier classification, it is represented as cleft 7 (see Fig. 50-2). Earliest recording of this malformation is said to be about 2000 BC in the teratologic tables scribed by Chaldeans of Mesopotamia.[4] The first contemporary language report was by Reissman in 1869.[46] The incidence of craniofacial microsomia is estimated to be between 1 in 3000[42] and 1 in 5642[19] live births.

Unilateral expression is the rule. Nevertheless, approximately 10% show bilateral involvement and features that are asymmetrical.[10,48] The affected structures are all

Figure 50–3 Craniofacial microsomia (Tessier cleft 7). Note macrostomia, ear tags, and also the groove running toward a microtic ear.

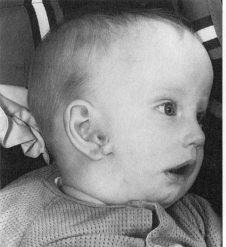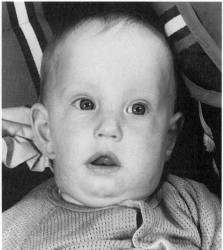

derived from the embryonic first and second branchial arches. Beginning at an enlarged oral commissure (macrostomia), a groove is commonly seen that is directed toward the ear with ear tags scattered along the route (Fig. 50-3). Partial absence of the external ear (microtia) is frequent and accompanied by a conductive hearing loss. Portions of the mandible, zygoma, and maxilla are deficient (Fig. 50-4). The ascending mandible shows the greatest range of hypoplasia by being entirely absent to displaying minor discrepancies of the condyle and ramus.

Being derivatives of the first and second branchial arches, the muscles of facial expression (Möbius syndrome) and mastication also can be involved in varying degrees. Hypoplasia or absence of the parotid gland is also seen.

Treatment varies with the degree of severity. Usually, greater disruptions demand earlier intervention. The correction of the macrostomia with local flaps and the removal of ear tags are performed generally within the first year of life. When the entire ramus is absent, it can

be replaced with a costochondral bone graft.[32] At the University of California at Los Angeles, we prefer to perform this surgery when the patient is about 6 years old. This is the same age that the construction of the external ear with a costochondral graft is initiated. When more of the ramus is present, distraction osteogenesis, using the Ilizarov principle, is used to lengthen the existing mandible or a previously inserted costal bone graft.[33] When most of the ramus is present, correction of the maxillofacial skeletal deformities can be deferred until late adolescence and the cessation of facial growth. As a necessary preliminary step, the teeth are orthodontically aligned within each jaw. The maxilla and the mandible are repositioned using a LeFort I osteotomy and intraoral bilateral ramal sagittal splitting procedure, respectively. An osseous genioplasty centers and elongates the deviated and retruded chin (Fig. 50-5). All the bony segments are rigidly held with biocompatible miniature plates and screw, thus eliminating the need to wire the jaws together and greatly simplifying the postoperative course.

Treacher Collins Syndrome

A confluence of clefts 6, 7, and 8 in the Tessier classification represents the Treacher Collins malformation (see Fig. 50-2). The earliest report of this entity was by Thompson in 1847.[43] However, Berry[6] is credited with the first description of the eyelid malformation, followed by Treacher Collins recording two cases with hypoplastic malar bones.[56] The syndrome is also known as *mandibulofacial dysostosis*. A comprehensive narrative of a series of 200 patients is recounted by Rogers.[49]

The incidence of the malformation is estimated at 1 in 10,000 live births. Inheritance is in an autosomal dominant manner with high but variable penetrance and expressivity.[17] Mutations in the *TCOF1* gene have been identified in family members with the malformation.[12,13]

Clinically, symmetrical bilateral involvement is seen of the eyelids, ears, zygomas, maxilla, and mandible (Fig. 50-6). The palpebral fissures are oriented with an

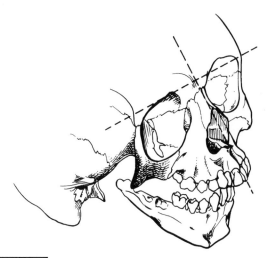

Figure 50–4 Line drawing of skeletal malformation of craniofacial microsomia. The ramus is partially absent, as is the zygomatic arch. The maxilla is also hypoplastic.

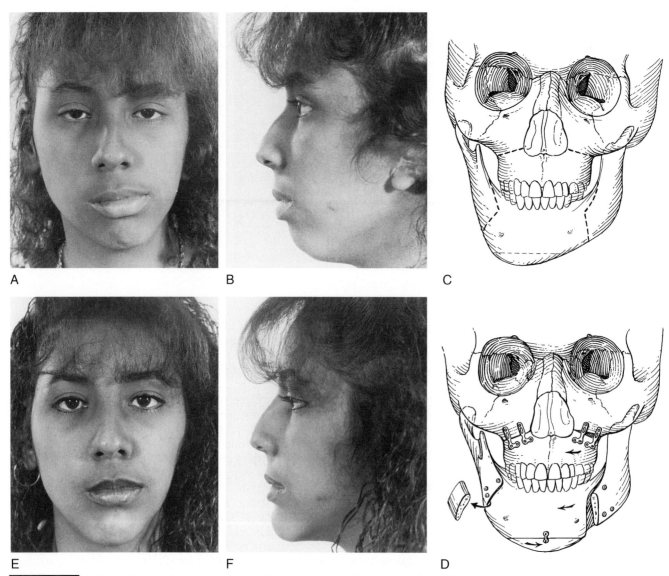

Figure 50–5 Patient with craniofacial microsomia. *A,* Preoperative frontal appearance. *B,* Profile view showing retrogenia. *C,* Line drawing of LeFort I (maxillary), sagittal splitting ramal osteotomies, and osseous genioplasty. *D,* Appearance after relocations of segments and fixation. *E* and *F,* Postoperative views.

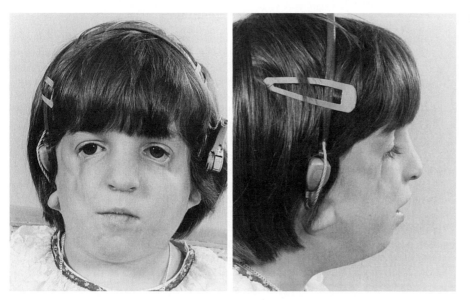

Figure 50–6 Patient with Treacher Collins syndrome. Note bilateral involvement of antimongoloid slant of palpebral fissures, absence of malar prominence, microtia, and retruded mandible and chin.

antimongoloid slant, and a coloboma occupies the lower eyelid, which lacks eyelashes in its medial two thirds. The zygomatic bones are hypoplastic and absent in the full expression of the malformation. Microtia of varying degrees is associated with conductive hearing loss. The preauricular hair is swept forward onto the cheek. The shortened posterior maxillary height restricts the size of the posterior choana and the passage of air. The mandible is also deficient in ramal height and body length. The intervening antegonial notch is acutely accentuated, and the chin is severely retruded.

The severity of the malformation dictates the timing of surgical intervention. Mandibular retrusion can be so profound as to compromise the airway and create a need for a tracheostomy. Early distraction osteogenesis can be used to increase the size of the airway and avoid a tracheostomy or allow its early removal.

Construction of the external ears with costal chondral grafts usually begins around the age of 6 years when the auricle is approximately 95% of adult size. Less popular means of fabricating an auricle are the use of alloplastic implants or external prosthesis. In the same period, the zygomas and orbits are built using calvarial bone grafts and simultaneously the lower eyelid colobomas and antimongoloid slant of the palpebral fissures are corrected with local flaps. At the end of the adolescent period, definitive management is directed to the maxillary and mandibular deformities using techniques that are similar to those applied to craniofacial microsomia (Fig. 50-7).

Cranial Clefts

The laterally placed types of the cranial clefts 9 to 14 are rare. As the midline is approached, their numbers increase in frequency. Nevertheless, the true incidence of each of these clefts is unknown because of their small numbers.

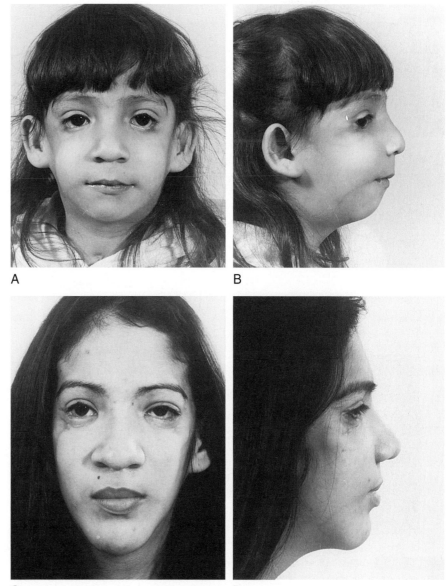

Figure 50–7 Patient with Treacher Collins syndrome. *A* and *B,* Preoperative appearance. *C* and *D,* Appearance after construction of zygomas, lateral orbital rim, lateral canthopexies, and upper to lower laterally based skin flaps.

A

B

C

D

Those clefts located medially to the orbit (clefts 11 to 14) disturb the position of the orbit by increasing the interorbital distance. Hypertelorbitism is thus produced. It is a sign and not a syndrome per se. Birth defects and orbital encroaching neoplasms can cause similar deformation. The medial orbital wall (interdacryon interval) is used to measure the interorbital distance. The normal measurement for a woman is 25 mm and is achieved by 13 years of age. Men reach their maximum of 28 mm by age 21 years.[21]

Tessier classified the hypertelorbitism into three grades: (1) 30 to 34 mm, (2) greater than 34 mm with normal shape and orientation of the orbits, and (3) greater than 40 mm.[52] Depending on the magnitude of separation, an extracranial approach alone or combined with an intracranial one is used, with the former being reserved for the lesser displacements.

Surgical correction is elective. No evidence exists that shows early intervention prevents amblyopia or alternating vision. Thus, surgical management is mainly directed at restoring normal facial features. In most centers the 5- to 7-year period is used as an appropriate age for correction. These children are starting to attend school, and this is a time when the upper face has attained most of its growth. In other centers operation is done as early as the second year of life. In any case, treatment of these complex malformations is best reserved for teams that routinely care for these children. These procedures are not for the occasional surgeon.

By and large, a combined intracranial and extracranial approach is required. The neurosurgeon provides the exposure of the orbital roof via a frontal craniotomy. The classic periorbital box osteotomies originally described by Tessier[52,54] largely have been replaced by a midline bipartition of the face (Fig. 50-8).[50]

The basic steps include unmasking the craniofacial skeleton through coronal and maxillary vestibular incisions (see Fig. 50-1), performing a frontal craniotomy, freeing the bony orbits using the classic box or facial bipartition technique, removing the excess bone from the nasal midline, closing the space by bringing the orbits together, securing rigid fixation of the segments, and closing of the wounds. If all goes well, the child spends a few days in the intensive care unit and is usually discharged after approximately a week's stay.

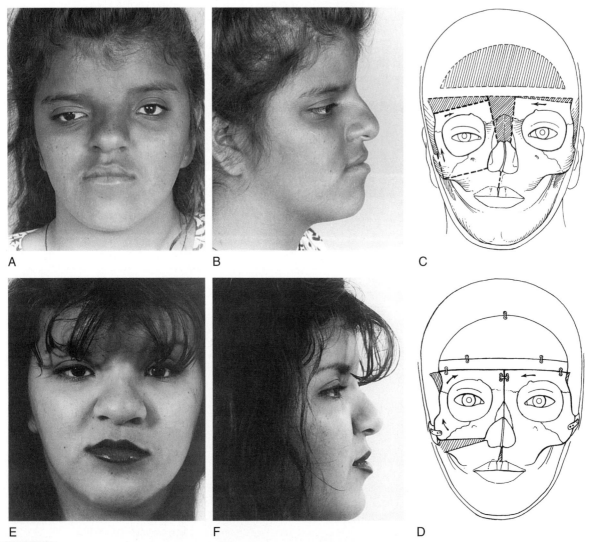

A   B   C

E   F   D

Figure 50–8 Patient with asymmetrical hypertelorbitism due to frontonasal dysplasia and left unilateral coronal synostosis. *A* and *B,* Preoperative view showing increased interorbital distance, orbital dystopia, greater left facial height, and flattened left forehead. *C,* Line drawing of skeletal deformity and osteotomies. *D,* Skeletal reconstruction and fixation of segments. *E* and *F,* Postoperative view.

CRANIOSYNOSTOSIS

During the first year the brain more than doubles its size and attains 60% of its adult weight.[8] Except for the uniqueness of the cranial vault sutures, the brain would be intolerably imprisoned and irreversibly damaged by mounting intracranial pressure. In the past the sutures were believed to be sites of active growth that push the plates apart, but further investigation has shown their role to be passive. In response to the rapidly enlarging brain, bone is deposited along their edges and the epicranium while resorption occurs along the dural surface.[14,36]

Normally, the cranial sutures are patent at birth and progress in early infancy to a yielding fibrous union that allows continuation of appositional bony growth. By 6 years of age the cranium has attained 90% of its adult size,[8] but complete solid bony union of the sutures must await at least the 50s.[31,32] Should a suture close prematurely, however, growth is arrested in a direction perpendicular to the fused suture, whereas compensatory expansion occurs in a parallel plane to the affected suture (Virchow's law). The resulting distortion of the skull depends on the suture or sutures that are closed.

The two subdivisions of craniosynostosis have important genetic and long-term growth implications. In general, the malformations of the nonsyndromic subset occur sporadically, whereas the syndromic ones have a hereditary component. Furthermore, after surgical correction, normal craniofacial development is the rule for the nonsyndromic patients, whereas those with syndromic attributes fare poorly.

Nonsyndromic Craniosynostosis

The overall incidence of nonsyndromic premature stenosis of cranial sutures has been stated to be 1 in 1000 live births.[7] This includes all forms of single suture fusion, with the sagittal suture being most commonly affected and unilateral coronal, metopic, and lambdoidal areas following in frequency. Bilateral fusion of the coronal as well as multiple suture involvement also occurs.

There would be less confusion if the specific name of the closed suture were used to describe the deformation of the calvarial cap. The following descriptive terms are widely acknowledged: *scaphocephaly* (boat shaped)—sagittal; *plagiocephaly* (oblique)—unilateral coronal; *brachycephaly* (short)—bilateral coronal; *trigonocephaly* (triangular)—metopic; and *acrocephaly* (topmost) or *turricephaly* (tower) or *oxycephaly* (sharp)—multiple sutures (Fig. 50-9).

Diagnosis can be established in most cases on clinical examination alone because of the characteristic deformation of the skull cap and on palpation of a ridge formed by the fused suture. Plain radiographic skull views can be taken to help confirm the clinical impression. A radiographic linear opacity replaces the wormian lucency of a patent suture. For unilateral coronal synostosis, a

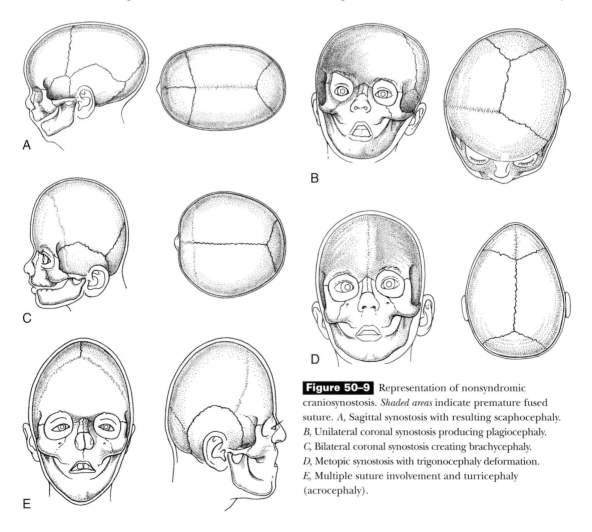

Figure 50–9 Representation of nonsyndromic craniosynostosis. *Shaded areas* indicate premature fused suture. *A,* Sagittal synostosis with resulting scaphocephaly. *B,* Unilateral coronal synostosis producing plagiocephaly. *C,* Bilateral coronal synostosis creating brachycephaly. *D,* Metopic synostosis with trigonocephaly deformation. *E,* Multiple suture involvement and turricephaly (acrocephaly).

classic *harlequin eye* sign formed by the elevated ipsilateral lesser wing of the sphenoid can be seen on a posteroanterior skull radiograph. Computed tomography (CT) usually is not needed nor is it diagnostically very helpfully unless reformatted in a three-dimensional manner.

The importance of establishing a clear diagnosis cannot be overstressed. The deformation of the craniofacial skeleton can be secondary. Muscular torticollis, cervical spinal abnormalities, and favored sleeping positions can produce *positional* distortions. The sutures are patent in these conditions. Treatment should be focused primarily on the cause of positional deformations rather than on the physical warping of the skull. When the sutures are open, early infant institution of molding helmets can restore normal contours but they are ill advised as primary therapy for true craniosynostosis contortions.

To lessen the possibility of sudden infant death syndrome, the American Academy of Pediatrics promoted a "Back to Sleep" program in June of 1992.[1] A substantial rise in the number of infants with unilateral or bilateral occipital deformations was experienced by all craniofacial anomalies centers.[3,57] These positional deformations were sometimes misdiagnosed, and blame fell on a "sticky" lambdoid suture when radiographs failed to verify opacification of the suture. Unnecessary posterior calvarial vault reconstructions were performed, which should have been avoided if differentiating clinical signs had been observed. Positional posterior plagiocephaly, when viewed from the vertex, has an oblique orientation of the skull cap, and the ear on the affected side is pushed anteriorly and away from the flattened posterior side. In contrast, true unilateral lambdoidal synostosis produces a trapezoid deformation with the ipsilateral ear being drawn toward the defective suture.[20] Fortunately, heightened awareness of deformation has dramatically reduced the number of operations for *positional* deformations to practically zero.

Nonsyndromic craniostenosis should be corrected because of the severe distortions that can be reflected onto the face. Other reasons address possible functional problems that the condition might cause, all of which are

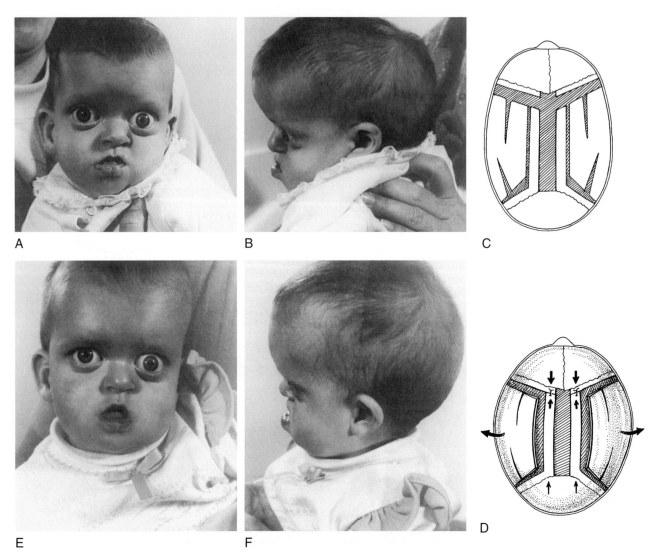

Figure 50–10 Patient with premature closure of sagittal suture (scaphocephaly). *A* and *B*, Preoperative appearance showing anteroposterior elongation of skull cap, decreased biparietal width, and anterior location of ears with greater posterior length. *C,* Illustration of π (pi) osteotomy with *shaded area* representing areas of resection. *D,* After decreasing anteroposterior dimension and lateral displacement of temporoparietal bone segments. *E* and *F,* Postoperative views.

related to increased intracranial pressure. Renier and associates found 13% of infants with single suture synostosis have elevated pressures and that this occurred in 42% of those with multiple suture involvement.[47] Visual impairment can occur but is rare when only one suture prematurely fused.[35] Whether higher intracranial pressure is associated with developmental retardation is debated. One study showed an association,[47] and another did not.[29]

Before the era of craniofacial surgery, the classically accepted method of treatment was a linear strip craniectomy of the pathologic suture. The incidence of refusion and continued deformation, however, was disappointingly high. In a review of 519 cases, Shillito and Matson[50] found that satisfactory appearance was achieved in only 52%, with the best results seen in infants with isolated sagittal synostosis. An unusual technique of total removal of the calvarial vault and orbital roofs was published by Powiertowsky and Matlosz in 1965.[44] Because of unpredictable reossification resulting in full-thickness defects and irregular contours, the method has fallen into disuse.

To take advantage of the rapidly expanding infant brain, early operative intervention is advised. Most centers favor the period of 3 to 6 months of age; others wait longer. All would agree that an operation should be performed before passage of the first year. Early correction produced better results in a long-term study of patients treated for metopic synostosis.[15]

Because of disappointment with the strip craniectomy techniques, the principles of treatment changed. Regardless of the type of craniosynostosis, emphasis was directed toward releasing the affected suture and immediately restoring normal architecture by repositioning and recontouring the deformed bones (Figs. 50-10 and 50-11). Hoffman and Mohr[22] applied these measures in their treatment of unilateral coronal synostosis. Marchac and Renier[31,32] refined the approach, and

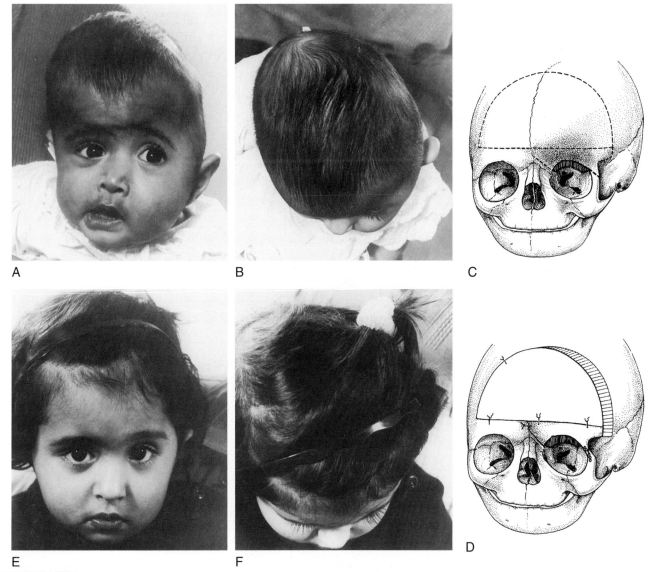

A   B   C
E   F   D

Figure 50–11 Example of unilateral coronal synostosis. *A* and *B,* Preoperative view. Note asymmetry of facial height of left and right side with ipsilateral side being taller, curvature of facial midline with contralateral deviation of chin and ipsilateral flattening, and contralateral bossing of forehead. *C,* Line drawing of deformity and osteotomies. *D,* Restoration of contour and fixation of mobilized segments. *E* and *F,* Postoperative appearance.

numerous geometric designs and fixation methods followed. Surgeons were attracted to the benefits offered by rigid fixation provided by using biocompatible metallic plates and screws. Subsequently, their use on a growing skull cap found the devices being translocated from the epicranium onto the dura.[16] Although initial reaction was one of alarm, detrimental consequences have not been observed.[27] Nevertheless, the metallic fixation hardware has been replaced by biodegradable plates and screws.

The strip craniectomy has been revived with the addition of endoscopic surgical techniques plus the use of a cranial molding helmet.[5,25] The involved suture is removed with the aid of the endoscope, and additional osteotomies of the cranial vault are made depending on the involved suture(s). A molding helmet is then used to obtain the desired contour. The benefits of this approach are a less invasive procedure, less blood loss, and a shorter hospital stay. The disadvantages are the additional cost of the molding helmet and increased postoperative visits for adjustment. Furthermore, to obtain satisfactory results, use of this method is limited to the first 5 months of life.

Syndromic Craniosynostosis

In contrast to nonsyndromic fusion, syndromic craniosynostosis behaves differently and has genetic implications. Early release of fused sutures does not lead to subsequent normal growth of the craniofacial skeleton. Therefore, additional operations will be required as the child matures. In contrast to the sporadic occurring nonsyndromic group, patterns of inheritance have been established for these malformations.

Crouzon Syndrome

It is somewhat ironic that a French surgeon, Paul Tessier, launched a subspecialty on a craniofacial malformation

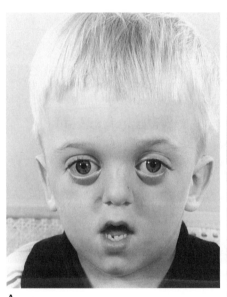
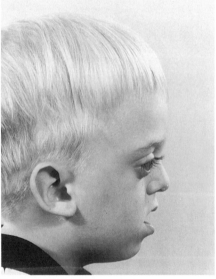
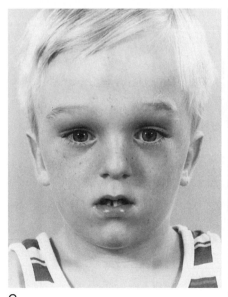
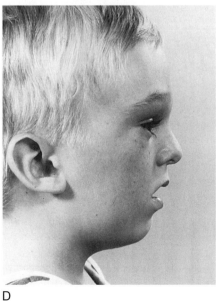

A

B

C

D

Figure 50–12 Patient with Crouzon syndrome. *A* and *B,* Preoperative view of child with exorbitism, midfacial retrusion, and pseudomandibular prognathism. *C* and *D,* Appearance after monobloc frontofacial advancement with advancement of forehead, normal globe position, and overcorrection of midfacial retrusion.

originally described over a half century before by a French neurologist.[11] Crouzon syndrome is the most commonly seen syndromic craniosynostosis anomaly, and its incidence has been estimated as being as high as 1 in 100,000 births.[17] The inheritance pattern is autosomal dominant with almost complete penetrance. Mutations in the *FGFR2* gene have been established in patients with the syndrome.[18,24,28,38,45]

Although any or all of the cranial sutures can be involved, bilateral coronal synostosis is most commonly observed. Cardinal features of the face include exorbitism (normal ocular contents housed in a hypoplastic orbit), midfacial retrusion with a collapsed maxilla, pseudomandibular prognathism, and a *parrot beak* appearance of the nose (Fig. 50-12). Mild hypertelorbitism can also be seen. Intelligence falls within the normal range. Features of the rest of body are normal, in contrast to the digital anomalies found in individuals with other malformations of this series.

Apert Syndrome

Originally described by Wheaton in 1894,[59] this malformation is known by the name of another French neurologist who described four cases 12 years later and applied the term *acrocephalosyndactyly*.[2] Its incidence has been estimated to be 1:160,000 live births.[17] The inheritance mode is that of autosomal dominant, although occurrence tends to be sporadic. As with Crouzon syndrome, a defect in the *FGFR2* gene has been identified.[30,41,60]

The exorbitism, midfacial retrusion with maxillary constriction, and pseudomandibular prognathism,

Figure 50–13   Child with Apert syndrome. *A* and *B,* Appearance before correction with flattened facies, retruded forehead and midface, and moderate exorbitism and hypertelorbitism. *C* and *D,* Appearance after monobloc frontofacial advancement to correct facial retrusion and facial bending to restore curvature to face and reduction of interorbital distance.

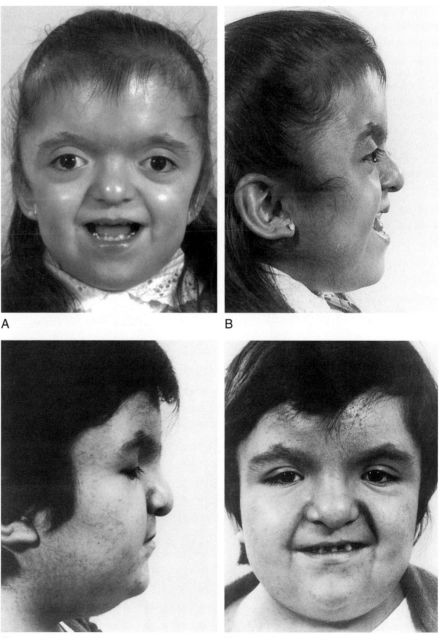

A

B

C

D

as in Crouzon syndrome, are present (Fig. 50-13). The exorbitism is more moderate and asymmetrical. The distance between the orbits is greater. The face also is flattened transversely. A major distinguishing feature is the symmetrical syndactyly of the hands and feet, with fusion of the interphalangeal joints that can be severe enough to produce a mitten deformity. In addition, an acne-like rash distributed over the face, trunks, and extremities appears in adolescence. Also unique is the presence of mild mental retardation.

Other Syndromes

Over 50 syndromes associated with craniosynostosis have been described in addition to the most common ones of Crouzon and Apert syndromes.[9] Because they are few in number, their frequency is not well established. Pfeiffer, Carpenter, and Saethre-Chotzen syndromes belong to this group and are distinguished respectively by broad toes and thumbs (Pfeiffer), preaxial polysyndactyly with soft tissue syndactyly of shortened fingers (Carpenter), and soft tissue webs between the second and third digits (Saethre-Chotzen). Pfeiffer and Saethre-Chotzen syndromes are transmitted in an autosomal dominant manner, and Carpenter syndrome is autosomal recessive.

Once seen, the rare kleeblattschädel (cloverleaf skull) anomaly is not easily forgotten. The skull cap assumes a trilobular configuration with a protruding vertex and bulging temporal regions (Fig. 50-14).

Treatment

The surgical management of all the syndromic craniosynostosis malformations generally falls into three chronologic stages. In contrast to the nonsyndromic variety, in this group normalization of facial growth is not realized after surgical intervention. Treatment is directed at the immediate problem; thus, a staged approach is used. Elements that must be addressed are release of elevated intracranial pressure caused by the premature suture closure, compromise of the airway by severe midfacial retrusion, and protection of the corneas because of the exorbitism. During the first year of life, the synostotic suture is released and a fronto-orbital advancement is performed (Fig. 50-15). This frees the rapidly expanding brain, more normal calvarial contours are achieved, and the corneas are offered more protection.

Treatment schemes and timing will then vary according to experience and preference of the surgeon. The management protocol at the University of California at Los Angeles is one that is popular. A second operation is performed around the sixth year of life when the orbits and skull cap have attained 90% of their adult size.[8] If the forehead is of normal shape, the classic LeFort III midfacial advancement is used to bring the entire midface forward. The maxilla is placed deliberately in an overcorrected anterior position, knowing that future midfacial growth will be limited (Fig. 50-16). This will open the crowded nasopharynx and correct the exorbitism.

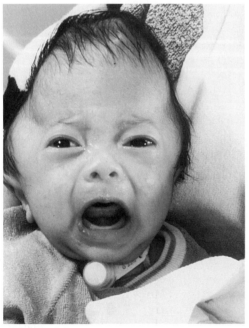

A

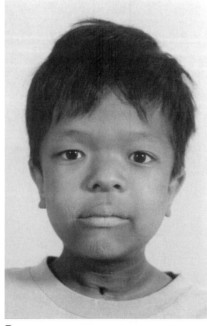

B

Figure 50–14 Example of kleeblattschädel (cloverleaf) malformation produced by premature closure of multiple sutures. *A,* Note trilobular configuration of skull cap and retrusion of forehead and midface. *B,* Appearance 8 years after fronto-orbital advancement in infancy and after monobloc advancement at 6 years of age.

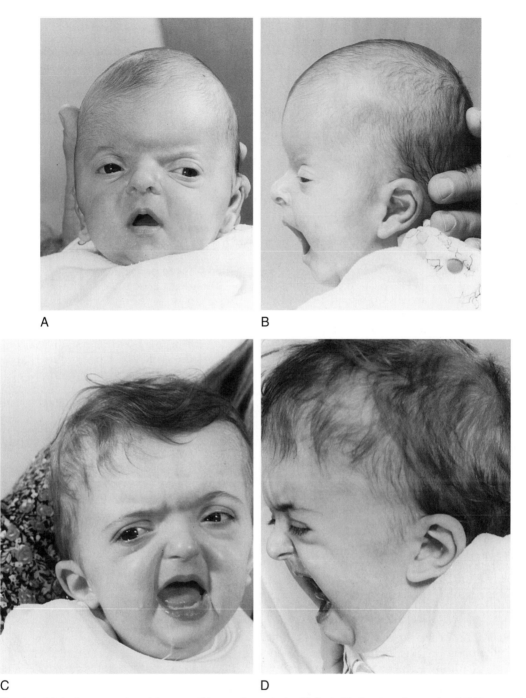

Figure 50–15 Fronto-orbital advancement used to correct bicoronal synostosis of infant with Apert syndrome. *A* and *B*, Preoperative views showing recession of superior orbital rims and forehead and exorbitism. *C* and *D*, Appearance after operation with normalization of forehead contours and orbital relationships.

If the forehead is found to be recessed, as is often the case, two alternative paths can be followed. As a preliminary operation, a second fronto-orbital advancement is performed. Approximately 6 months later, a LeFort III procedure is added. This approach is safer because sterility is maintained by separating a clean intracranial procedure from the contamination introduced by the subsequent

extracranial midfacial advancement. The dura expands slowly in a child of this age as compared with during infancy. Thus, a longer period must pass as the brain enlarges to obliterate the epidural dead space created by the fronto-orbital advancement.

The other approach is the monobloc frontofacial advancement.[40] The advantage of this technique is that

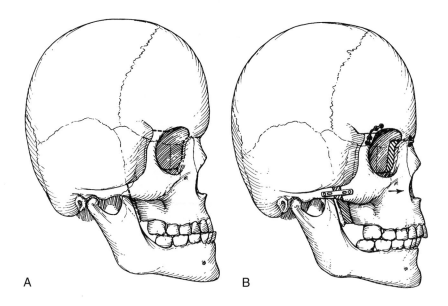

Figure 50-16 Illustration of LeFort III midface advancement. *A,* Line drawing depicting midfacial retrusion, pseudomandibular prognathism, and design of osteotomies. *B,* After mobilization to overcorrected anterior position and fixation.

only one operation is required to reposition the forehead and midfacial mass. The best cosmetic results are often achieved.[61] The risk of infection is increased, however, and the procedure is best avoided when a shunt is present that will inhibit the expansion of the brain and prolong the existence of the dead space.[28] Many of the hazards of the monobloc acute advancements have been reduced by applying distraction osteogenesis with its gradual frontofacial advancement rate of 1 mm/day.[51]

When hypertelorbitism is present, a facial bipartition (see Fig. 50-8) procedure can be added to either the LeFort III or frontofacial monobloc advancement. This procedure is particularly indicated in correcting the flattened forehead and midface that is typically seen in patients with Apert syndrome.[54] The final stage must await the completion of facial growth. After presurgical orthodontic alignment of the dentition, the pseudomandibular prognathism is corrected with a LeFort I (maxillary) advancement. A simultaneous advancement osseous genioplasty is frequently required to correct the retruded chin.

REFERENCES

1. American Academy of Pediatrics Task Force on Infant Positioning and SIDS: Positioning and SIDS. Pediatrics 1992;89:1120-1126.
2. Apert E: De l'acrocephalosyndactylie. Bull Soc Med Hôp Paris 1906;23:1310.
3. Argenta LC, David LR, Wilson JA, et al: An increase in infant cranial deformity with supine sleeping position. J Craniofac Surg 1996;7:5-11.
4. Ballatyne JW: The teratological records of Chaldea. Teratologia 1894;1:127.
5. Barone CM, Jimenez EF: Endoscopic craniectomy for early correction of craniosynostosis. Plast Reconstr Surg 1999; 104:1965-1973.
6. Berry GA: Note on a congenital defect (? coloboma) of the lower lid. Roy Lond Ophth Hosp Rep 1889;12:255.
7. Bertelson TL: The premature synostosis of the cranial sutures. Acta Ophthalmol Suppl 1958;51:47.
8. Blinkov SM, Glezer II: The Human Brain in Figures and Tables: A Quantitative Handbook. New York, Plenum Press, 1968.
9. Cohen MM Jr: Craniosynostosis and syndromes with craniosynostosis: Incidence, genetics, penetrance, variability, and new syndrome updating. Birth Defects 1979; 15:13-63.
10. Converse JM, Coccaro PJ, Becker M, Wood-Smith D: On hemifacial microsomia: The first and second branchial arch syndrome. Plast Reconstr Surg 1973;51: 268-279.
11. Crouzon O: Dysotose, cranio-faciale héréditaire. Bull Soc Med Hôp Paris 1912;33:545.
12. Dixon MJ, Hann E, Baker E, et al: Association of Treacher Collins syndrome and translocation 6p21.31/16p13.11: Exclusion of the locus from these candidate regions. J Hum Genet 1991;48:274-280.
13. Dixon MJ: Treacher Collins syndrome. Hum Mol Genet 1996;5(Spec):1391-1396.
14. Enlow DH, Azuma M: Functional growth boundaries in the human and mammalian face. Birth Defects 1975;11: 217-230.
15. Fearon JA, Kolar JC, Munro IR: Trigonocephaly—associated hypotelorbitism: Is treatment necessary? Plast Reconstr Surg 1996;97:503-509.
16. Fearon JA, Munro IA, Bruce DA: Observations on the use of rigid fixation for craniofacial deformities in infants and young children. Plast Reconstr Surg 1995;95: 634-637.

17. Gorlin RJ, Pindborg JH, Cohen MM Jr: Syndromes of the Head and Neck, 2nd ed. New York, McGraw-Hill, 1976, pp 220-224.
18. Gorry MC, Preston RA, White GJ, et al: Crouzon syndrome: Mutations in two spliceoforms of FGFR2 and a common point mutation shared with Jackson-Weiss syndrome. Hum Mol Genet 1995;4:1387-1390.
19. Grabb WC: The first and second branchial arch syndrome. Plast Reconstr Surg 1965;36:485-508.
20. Gruss JS: The diagnosis of plagiocephaly due to lambdoid suture synostosis: Clinical, radiological and operative findings. Craniofacial Surgery: State of the Art Symposium. New York, March 20, 1996.
21. Hangman CB: Growth of interorbital distance and skull thickness as observed in roentgenographic measurements. Radiology 1966;86:87.
22. Hoffman HJ, Mohr G: Lateral canthal advancement of the supraorbital margin. J Neurosurg 1976;45:376-381.
23. Hollway GE, Phillip HA, Ades LC, et al: Localization of craniosynostosis Adelaide type to 4p16. Hum Mol Genet 1995;4:681-683.
24. Jabs EW, Li X, Scott AF, et al: Jackson-Weiss and Crouzon syndromes are allelic with mutations in fibroblast growth factor receptor. Nat Genet 1994;8:275-279.
25. Jimenez DF, Barone CM, McGee ME, et al: Endoscopy-assisted wide-vertex craniectomy, barrel stave osteotomies, and post-operative helmet molding therapy in the management of sagittal suture craniosynostosis. J Neurosurg Spine 2004;100:407-417.
26. Kawamoto HK: The kaleidoscopic world of rare craniofacial clefts: Order out of chaos (Tessier classification). Clin Plast Surg 1976;3:529-572.
27. Kawamoto HK, McCarthy JG: Discussion of Fearon JR, et al: Observation on the use of rigid fixation for craniofacial deformities in infants and young children. Plast Reconstr Surg 1995;95:638.
28. Kawamoto HK Jr, Stuzin JM: Complication associated with the monobloc-frontofacial advancement. Presented before the American Association of Plastic Surgeons meeting, Palm Beach, May 3, 1988.
29. Kapp-Simon KA, Figueroa A, Jocher A, Schafer M: Longitudinal assessment of mental development in infants with nonsyndromic craniosynostosis with and without cranial release and reconstruction. Plast Reconstr Surg 1993;92:831-839.
30. Lewanda AF, Cohen MM Jr, Hood J, et al: Cytogenetic survey of Apert syndrome: Reevaluation of translocation (2;9)(p11.2;q34.2) in patient suggests the breakpoints are not related to the disorder. Am J Dis Child 1993;147:1306-1308.
31. Marchac D: Radical forehead remodeling for craniostenosis. Plast Reconstr Surg 1978;61:823-835.
32. Marchac D, Renier D: Craniofacial Surgery for Craniosynostosis. Boston, Little Brown, 1982.
33. McCarthy JG: The role of distraction osteogenesis in the reconstruction of the mandible in unilateral craniofacial microsomia. Clin Plast Surg 1994;21:625-631.
34. Molina F, Ortiz-Monasterio F: Mandibular elongation and remodeling by distraction: A farewell to major osteotomies. Plast Reconstr Surg 1995;96:825-840.
35. Montaut J, Stricker M: Dysmorphies Craniofaciales: Les Synostoses Prematures (Craniostenosis et Faciostenosis). Paris, Masson, 1977.
36. Moss ML: New studies of cranial growth. Birth Defects 1975;11:283-295.
37. Murray DJ, Kaban LP, Mulliken JB: Analysis and treatment of hemifacial microsomia. Plast Reconstr Surg 1984;74:186-199.
38. Neilson KM, Friesel RE: Constitutive activation of fibroblast growth factor receptor-2 by a point mutation associated with Crouzon syndrome. J Biol Chem 1995;270:26037-26040.
39. Oldridge M, Wilkie AO, Slaney SF, et al: Mutations in the third immunoglobulin domain of the fibroblast growth factor receptor-2 gene in Crouzon syndrome. Hum Mol Genet 1995;4:1077-1082.
40. Ortiz-Monasterio F, Fuente del Campo A, Carrillo A: Advancement of the orbits and the midface in one piece, combined with frontal repositioning for the correction of Crouzon's deformities. Plast Reconstr Surg 1978;61:507-516.
41. Park W-J, Theda C, Maestri NE, et al: Analysis of phenotypic features and FGFR2 mutations in Apert syndrome. Am J Hum Genet 1995;57:321-328.
42. Poswillo D: Orofacial malformations. Proc R Soc Med 1974;67:343-349.
43. Poswillo D: The pathogenesis of the Treacher Collins syndrome (mandibulofacial dysostosis). Br J Oral Surg 1975;13:1-26.
44. Powiertowsky H, Matlosz Z: The treatment of craniostenosis by a method of extensive resection of the vault of the skull. In: Proceedings of the Third International Congress on Neurosurgery. Excerpta Med Int Cong Ser 1965;110:834.
45. Readon W, Winter RM, Rutland P, et al: Mutations in the fibroblast growth factor receptor 2 gene cause Crouzon syndrome. Nat Genet 1994;8:98-103.
46. Reissmann H: Ein Fall von Makrostoma. Arch Minerva Chir 1869;6:858.
47. Renier D, Sainte-Rose C, Marchac D, Hirsh JF: Intracranial pressure in craniosynostosis. J Neurosurg 1982;57:370-377.
48. Renier D, Marchac D.: Craniofacial surgery for craniosynostosis: Functional and morphologic results. Ann Acad Med Singapore 1988;17:415.
49. Rogers BO: Berry–Treacher Collins syndrome: A review of 200 cases. Br J Plast Surg 1964;17:109-137.
50. Shillito J, Matson DD: Craniosynostosis: A review of 519 surgical patients. Pediatrics 1968;41:829-853.
51. Taub PJ, Bradley JP, Stuzin JM, Kawamoto HK: Decreased morbidity in monobloc advancement with distraction osteogenesis. Presented before the 71st annual meeting of the American Society of Plastic Surgery, San Antonio, TX, November 4, 2002.
52. Tessier P: Orbital hypertelorism: I. Successive surgical attempts, materials and methods, causes and mechanisms. Scand J Plast Reconstr Surg 1972;6:133-155.
53. Tessier P: Anatomical classification of facial, craniofacial and laterofacial clefts. J Maxillofac Surg 1976;4:69-92.
54. Tessier PL: Apert's syndrome: Acrocephalosyndactyly type I. In Caronni E (ed): Craniofacial Surgery. Boston, Little Brown, 1985, p 280.
55. Tessier P, Guiot B, Rougerie J, et al: Ostéotomies cranio-naso-orbito-faciales hypertélorisme. Ann Chir Plast 1967;12:103-118.
56. Treacher Collins E: Case with symmetrical congenital notches in the outer part of each lower lid and defective development of the malar bones. Trans Ophthalmol Soc UK 1900;20:190.
57. Turk AE, McCarthy JG, Thorne CHM, et al: The "Back to Sleep" campaign and deformational plagiocephaly: Is there cause for concern? J Craniofac Surg 1996;7:12-18.

58. van der Meulen JC: Medial faciotomy. Br J Plast Surg 1979;32:339.

59. Wheaton SW: Two specimens of congenital cranial deformities in infants in association with fusion of the fingers and toes. In Smith DW (ed): Major Problems in Clinical Pediatrics, Vol 7, Recognizable Patterns of Human Malformation. Philadelphia, WB Saunders, 1982, p 308.

60. Wilkie AOM, Slaney SF, Oldridge M, et al: Apert syndrome results from localized mutations of FGFR2 and is allelic with Crouzon syndrome. Nat Genet 1995;9: 165-172.

61. Wolfe SA, Morrison G, Page LK, et al: The monobloc fronto-facial advancement: Do the pluses outweigh the minuses? Plast Reconstr Surg 1993;91:977-987.

Chapter 51

 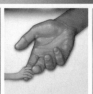

Cleft Lip and Palate

A. Michael Sadove and Barry L. Eppley

Clefting anomalies of the lip and palate are the most frequently encountered congenital facial defects. They constitute most of major congenital facial malformations and the majority of all orofacial cleft types. Clefts of the lip may be associated with dentoalveolar defects anterior to the incisive foramen and are classified as clefts of the *primary palate*. Clefts that disrupt the hard and soft portions of the palate posterior to the incisive foramen are called clefts of the *secondary palate*. Clefts can occur in many different forms and combinations from the most minor, incomplete isolated lip clefts to the most severe, complete bilateral cleft lip and palate.

The differences in racial occurrence are well known and are the result of ethnic variations in the timing and coordination of the facial merging process in utero. This may be due to the differences in facial tissue thickness between differing races. As a result of these differences, the frequency of occurrence of cleft lip may range from an incidence of 1 in 500 live births in Asians and Native Americans to 1 in 1500 to 2000 live births in African-American populations. Susceptibility of whites is intermediate at 1 in 750 to 900 live births.[18] The left side of the lip, for reasons as yet unclear, is more often cleft than the right. In contrast, the frequency of isolated cleft palate is much more similar among the races (approximately 0.50 in 1000 live births).

DEVELOPMENT OF CLEFT LIP

Facial processes arise as a result of migration and later proliferation of neural crest mesenchyme. Coalescence of these facial processes, around day 30 in the human embryo, results in the formation of the primary lip or palate, which creates the initial separation between the oral and nasal cavities. This eventually gives rise to portions of the upper lip and maxilla. Virtually all cases of cleft lip are due to the failure of the median nasal (globular) process either to contact or to maintain contact with the lateral nasal and maxillary processes. A failure to merge or to adhere after contact (failure of contact maintenance) in any one component of this midfacial convergence of processes can result in the presentation of a facial cleft (Fig. 51-1).

DEVELOPMENT OF CLEFT PALATE

The development of the hard and soft palate requires a consideration of both the primary palate (prepalate) and the secondary palate (palate proper). The primary palate is related to the development of structures anterior to the incisive foramen (i.e., the face, lips, premaxilla, and upper four incisor teeth). It is closely related to the facial merging process that has been described for cleft lip, and it commences during the fourth week of gestation and is completed by the seventh week. For this reason, cleft lip and palate implies a complete deformity extending from the lip through the alveolus back through the soft palate (Fig. 51-2A).

The secondary palate relates to structures posterior to the incisive foramen (i.e., hard palate, soft palate, and maxillary teeth). This region develops bilaterally from the palatal processes or plates of the maxillary bones, which become prominent during the sixth to seventh weeks. They extend from the primary palate to the tonsillar pillars and hang vertically beside the tongue. Between the eighth and ninth weeks, the palatal processes commence a positional change from the vertical to a horizontal plane. For a time, the palatal shelves are kept apart by the tongue, but as the tongue lowers in the floor of the mouth and moves forward, the two palatal plates fuse. Failure of the tongue to lower produces palatal clefts (see Fig. 51-2B). The best clinical example of this interrelated process is found in the Pierre Robin sequence, in which a soft palatal cleft, glossoptosis, and mandibular hypoplasia are present, which predisposes to a potential airway obstruction.

UNUSUAL FACIAL CLEFTS

Whereas cleft lip and palate as described earlier is the traditional type of facial cleft, other more unusual patterns may occur radiating out from the orofacial region.[8] They may be midline through the upper lip (Tessier 0), obliquely skirting around the nose toward the eye (Tessier 4, 5, and 6), or out from the corner of the mouth (Tessier 7). These types of facial clefts occur more

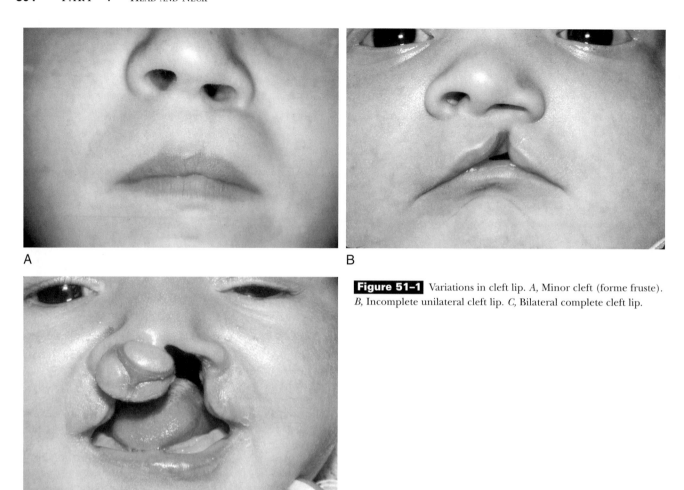

A

B

C

Figure 51-1 Variations in cleft lip. *A*, Minor cleft (forme fruste). *B*, Incomplete unilateral cleft lip. *C*, Bilateral complete cleft lip.

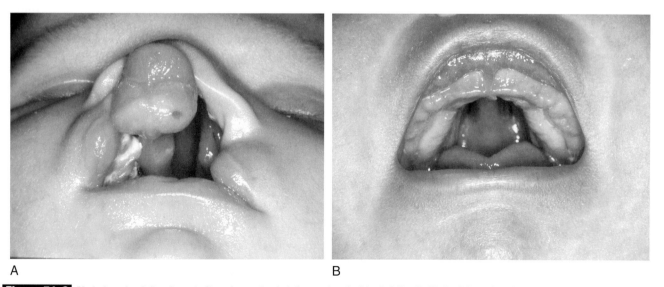

A

B

Figure 51-2 Variations in cleft palate. *A*, Complete palatal cleft associated with cleft lip. *B*, Cleft of the soft palate only.

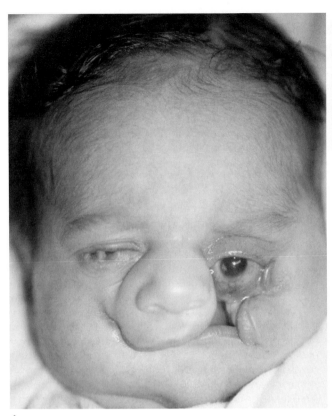

A

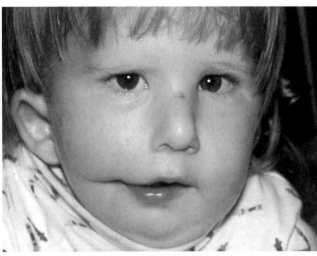

B

Figure 51-3 Atypical facial clefts. *A,* Oblique Tessier 4 cleft. *B,* Lateral Tessier 7 cleft.

rarely, involve different anatomic structures, and require innovative repair techniques. They usually are associated with more global facial defects and/or deficiencies. When present, they merit close evaluation of the face and brain because median lip clefts should be evaluated for frontonasal and brain deformities, whereas oblique and lateral oral clefts may involve eye, ear, and jaw deformities (Fig. 51-3).

ETIOLOGY OF CLEFTS

The cause of cleft lip and palate is multifactorial, involving both genetic and environmental factors. Although facial clefts occur in a variety of genetic syndromes (about 15% of cleft cases are syndromic; more than 170 syndromes have it as a feature), identification of a single gene controlling lip and palatal clefts has not yet been found.[18,24] Clefting loci have been identified on chromosomes 1, 2, 4, 6, 11, 14, 17, and 19. Certain specific chromosomal aberrations are consistently seen (e.g., trisomy D syndrome with medial cleft lip) or cleft lip associated with lower lip pits (van der Woude's syndrome). Because of their frequent syndromic association, it is important to search for other congenital defects, which occur most commonly on other parts of the head and neck, heart, and extremities. Only a few environmental factors are known, including certain drugs taken during gestation (phenytoin, retinoic acid, folic acid antagonists). Maternal smoking is now well known to increase the

incidence of clefting.[3] Multivitamin supplementation, particularly the folates, during the first 4 months of pregnancy, is currently thought to have a protective effect.[17]

SURGICAL CLEFT CORRECTION

Team Management

The anatomic complexity of the cleft deformity and its effects on multiple orofacial functions (facial growth, dental eruption and hygiene, jaw development, hearing, speech) as well as its effect on orofacial growth and development make a team approach to the cleft patient mandatory. Cleft teams consisting of specialists in plastic surgery, dentistry (pedodontics, orthodontics, and oral surgery), audiology, speech pathology, otolaryngology, and genetics can best provide the many needs of the cleft patient over time. Such a team approach offers the combined expertise to blend treatment intervention with growth and development, providing more efficient and cost-effective services.[1]

Neonatal Management

Parents

The presence of a facial cleft at birth may be historically unexpected, but the contemporary use of prenatal

TABLE 51–1 Genetic Risks of Cleft		
	Cleft Lip With or Without Cleft Palate (%)	**Cleft Palate (%)**
Frequency in general population	0.08	0.02
Risk of second affected child		
(a) If both parents are normal	3.7	2.5
(b) If one parent has cleft similar to patient's	19.4	14.3
Risk of third affected child (a and b)	9.0	0.90
Risk of first affected child if parent has a cleft	4.04	5.82

ultrasound allows for early detection of facial deformities.[13] This allows parents today an opportunity to seek prenatal counseling and consult with the cleft team before the birth of the child to lay the foundations of subsequent surgical reconstruction. Parents often feel guilty with the unfounded assumption that the cleft deformity could have been prevented. Reassurance to the parents can be done by arranging for genetic counseling to discuss the risk to future offspring (Table 51-1).

Child

Besides the obvious facial deformity from an external cleft lip, immediate functional concerns are for airway patency and the ability to feed. Certain cleft deformities isolated to the palate (e.g., Pierre Robin sequence) involve airway obstruction and may require differing forms of management. The disruption of the lip and hard palate makes suckling difficult because of the inability to create negative pressure by compression of the tongue against an open palate. Therefore, nasal regurgitation of liquids is common, and altered feeding regimens, including the use of a cross-cut nipple and a palatal obturator, may be needed to create effective feeding.

Neonatal Maxillary Orthopedics

In complete cleft lip and palate deformities in which the maxilla and hard palate are disrupted, repositioning of the displaced dentoalveolar segments before lip repair with various forms of intraoral and extraoral orthodontic appliances has been advocated. These methods may include simple methods such as adhesive taping across the cleft lip and circumferential elastic traction. Nasoalveolar molding orthopedic devices, however, are becoming popular because they are the most effective method of molding the nose, lip, and alveolus into the best possible presurgical position.[9] This makes the lip repair easier by decreasing the distance between the lip segments. This is of particular value in bilateral cases, in which the prolabial segment containing the premaxilla and central lip is anteriorly positioned. More involved mechanical methods such as fixed intraoral appliances have been used in some patients but increase the risk of injury to developing teeth by pinning into the bone, which is full of developing teeth.

Surgical Timing

The cleft lip is always repaired first at 3 to 4 months of age. Although it can technically be repaired within the first few weeks of life, a more traditional repair is obtained when the infant is older. The historic *rule of 10s* is a good guideline: 10 weeks of age, 10 grams of hemoglobin, and 10 pounds of weight. These conditions favor adequate wound healing and safe anesthesia. Associated anomalies, such as congenital heart disease, may alter the timing of repair until a later age.

The cleft palate is traditionally repaired after the lip and may be done between 9 and 15 months of age depending on the surgeon's philosophy. Early surgical efforts are purported to result in better speech function. Although this is controversial, delaying the repair until after 18 months of age is clearly associated with poorer speech outcomes. An exception to this would be the child with a history of early respiratory difficulties (e.g., Pierre Robin sequence). Delaying repair up until the age of 18 months may be necessary in such a child to decrease the risk of postoperative airway obstruction from decreasing the size of the nasopharyngeal airway.

The cleft alveolus (tooth-bearing portion of upper jaw) is usually repaired with an autogenous bone graft between 5 and 8 years of age. This not only establishes maxillary arch continuity but also permits subsequent tooth eruption and provides improved support for the cleft nasal base. A few centers favor early bone grafting before palate repair, around 9 to 12 months of age provided there is end-to-end maxillary segment alignment, in an effort to provide an earlier stabilization of the maxilla and closure of the oronasal fistula.

Cleft Lip Repair

The many types of cleft lip repairs attest to the fact that not all clefts are the same. They differ in both amount and extent of contiguous anatomic disruption. Therefore, it is difficult to find one operation that is the ideal solution for all cleft cases. The Millard rotation-advancement cleft lip repair, however, has become the most commonly performed procedure for repair of the unilateral cleft lip.[21] It effectively returns displaced lip and nasal structures into their normal position, allows the resultant scars to be less discernible because they lie along anatomic boundaries, and minimizes the amount of tissue discarded. The concept involves an inferior rotation of the medial lip segment with an advancement of the lateral lip segment into the subcolumellar space to join with the medial lip segment (Fig. 51-4). This procedure achieves a lengthening of the lip along the philtral line, reconstruction of the orbicularis muscle across the cleft, rotation of the

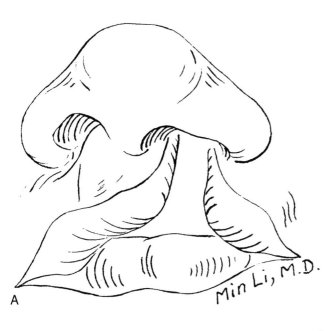

A

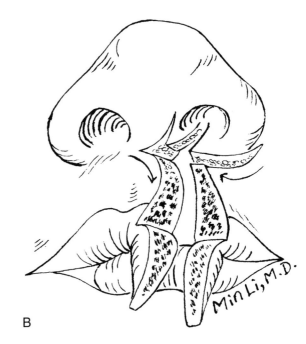

B

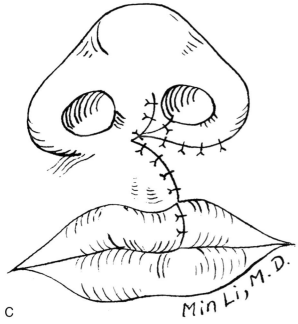

C

Figure 51–4 Rotation-advancement unilateral cleft lip repair. *A,* Original deformity with widened nasal base, lip cleft, and shortened medial and lateral lip elements. *B,* Cuts and separation of the lip elements around the nasal base and lateral lip, across the base of the columella to the opposite philtral ridge as well as the raising of bilateral vermilion flaps. The *arrows* indicate the downward rotation of the medial lip element and the advancement of the lateral lip element toward the columella. *C,* Completed skin closure after joining the orbicularis muscle across the defect.

displaced nasal base medially, a slight lengthening of the columella, and establishment of a labial sulcus. The conceptual simplicity and the ability to tailor and make adjustment as the repair proceeds is one of the major strengths of this type of lip repair. In addition, the minimal sacrifice of tissue and the location of the scar lines favor secondary revisions of the repair, which are almost always needed. Additions to the technique revolve around concurrent manipulation of the nose, mobilizing and translocating the ipsilateral lower alar cartilage and nasal base.[29]

The bilateral cleft lip represents more than just a doubling of the problem of the unilateral cleft lip. The lack of a columella, splaying of the alar cartilages and nasal bases, and protrusion of the underlying premaxilla not only make the initial lip repair different from a unilateral cleft but also ensure that subsequent operations will be needed. Decisions regarding repair of the bilateral cleft include whether to repair both lip clefts simultaneously or in stages, whether to adhese the lip elements before a definitive lip repair, and how to manage the protrusive premaxilla. All of these issues are controversial, and approaches may vary widely among cleft teams. Our approach is to do synchronous lip repair if the width of the clefts and the premaxilla permit closure without excessive tension on the orbicularis muscle coaptation and skin suture lines.[22] The technique of Millard's rotation-advancement is effective in creating a Cupid's bow and bilateral straight philtral lines (Fig. 51-5). When the premaxilla is too protrusive and concern exists regarding

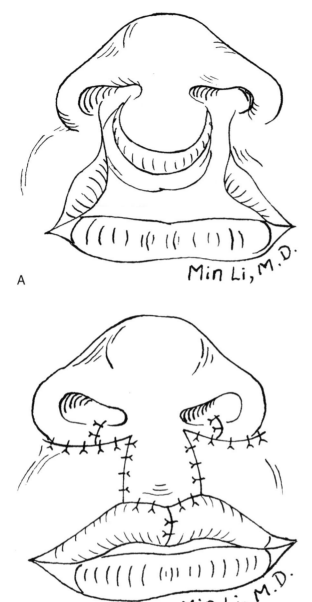

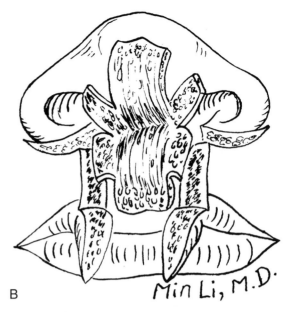

Figure 51-5 Bilateral cleft lip repair. *A,* Original deformity with protruding premaxilla and prolabium. Note the absence of a columella. *B,* The raising of a central prolabial skin flap, lateral lip flaps, and bilateral vermilion tissue converge to form the bilateral repair after the orbicularis muscle is joined over the protruding premaxilla. *C,* Completed lip repair.

the potential integrity of the lip repair, a more simplified lip adhesion may be performed first at 8 to 10 weeks of age. The definitive lip repair is then performed 2 to 3 months later after the premaxilla is retropositioned.

Cleft Palate Repair

Despite a long history, the surgical treatment of the cleft palate is controversial owing to conflicting opinions about how the type of surgical repair influences subsequent speech and facial skeletal development.[25] As such, cleft palate operations differ in regard to timing of intervention, staged versus complete hard and soft palatal repairs, and the arrangement of the tissue flaps to create palatal closure. The fundamental goals of the procedure are a soft palatal muscular reconstruction, a two-layer

(nasal and oral) lining closure of both hard and soft palatal defects, and adequate palatal length. Although there remains no uniform palatal repair technique or approach, the operation may be conceived as three basic types: straight-line closure, V-Y lengthening, or Z-plasty rearrangement.

Opening the mucosa along the cleft edges, mobilizing tissue at the subperiosteal level, and mobilizing of the palatal flaps medially enables a straight-line repair to be completed in two layers. This technique, known as the von Langenbeck repair, is straightforward but may not provide adequate soft palatal length. To achieve this goal, the straight-line repair has been modified by the creation of oblique incisions anteriorly to connect with the incision along the posterior alveolar ridge. Once the palatal flaps are mobilized, they are moved posteriorly and medially, which results in a V-Y rearrangement (Fig. 51-6).

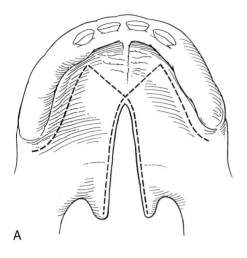

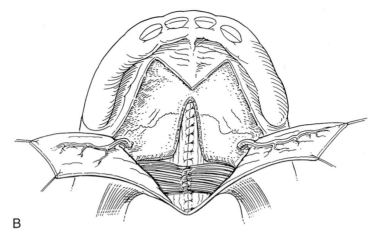

A

B

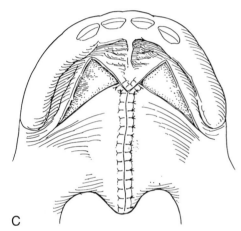

C

Figure 51–6 V-Y pushback cleft palate repair. *A*, Outline of incision placement. *B*, Raising of full-thickness mucoperiosteal flaps based on the greater palatine vessels, mucosal nasal lining closure, and soft palatal muscle apposition. *C*, Oral closure obtained by lengthening of the palate by a posterior repositioning of the palatal mucosal tissues, leaving an open area of anterior palatal bone.

As such, this technique has become known as a *push-back* palatal procedure or a Veau-Wardill-Kilner repair. With either approach, the aberrant attachments of the levator and tensor palatini muscles are detached from the posterior and medial edges of the palatal shelves and sutured together in the midline of the soft palatal closure (intravelar veloplasty). A more recent addition to palatal repair techniques has been the clever application of the Z-plasty principle with double-reversing musculomucosal flaps of oral and nasal tissue, often referred to as the Furlow palate repair.[4,7] This not only effectively reorients the soft palatal muscular fibers but also increases palatal length (Fig. 51-7). Mounting clinical evidence indicates that long-term speech outcomes may be improved with this type of muscular repair.[15] In addition, the risk of postoperative fistula formation is decreased because the suture lines between the oral and nasal linings do not lie directly over each other.

Alveolar Bone Grafting

Bone grafting of the tooth-bearing portion of the maxilla (alveolus) completes the primary repair sequence of the original cleft deformities. This procedure not only unifies the maxilla into a single unit and eliminates any residual oronasal fistulas but also provides the proper tissue to support subsequent tooth eruption. The use of autogenous bone is generally accepted as the graft material of choice, and most centers undertake graft placement when the child is between 5 and 8 years of age.[6,11] At this time, the canine teeth have sufficient root development so that the graft may provide support for the path of subsequent tooth eruption into the proper position in the dental arch. A few centers favor earlier alveolar bone graft placement within the first year of life in an effort to prevent maxillary collapse and decrease the need for extended orthodontic care later in life.[27] Long-term assessment of this technique shows favorable facial growth, improved maxillary arch forms, and decreased need for maxillary osteotomies and bone grafting at a later age.[28] *Boneless* alveolar bone grafts, in which a periosteal closure is obtained across the cleft defect by tibial periosteal grafts (periosteoplasty), have also been tried, but significant regenerated bone has not been consistently shown.

Secondary Cleft Management

Lip and Nasal Revision

Despite optimal execution of primary facial repair, most clefts require secondary revision of the lip, nose, or both. These revisions may entail a variety of procedures,

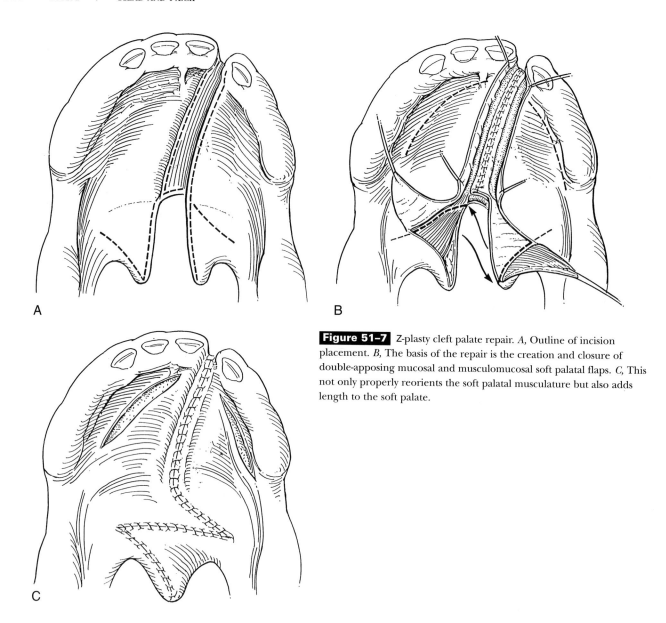

Figure 51-7 Z-plasty cleft palate repair. *A*, Outline of incision placement. *B*, The basis of the repair is the creation and closure of double-apposing mucosal and musculomucosal soft palatal flaps. *C*, This not only properly reorients the soft palatal musculature but also adds length to the soft palate.

including scar revision, vermilion realignment, philtral lengthening, nasal base rotation, or the correction of nasal tip cartilages.[31] In particular, the secondary creation of a columella in the bilateral cleft patient is necessary because this nasal element is congenitally absent in this cleft deformity.[23] Many of these lip and nasal revisions are done in the 2- to 4-year age range to allow scar maturation to occur before the child enters the public scrutiny of the school environment. Further cleft lip revisions in adolescence are also likely as the psychosocial demands of the teenage years escalate.[14] Most patients will eventually require a complete septorhinoplasty reconstruction to treat the entire nose once the pubertal growth phase has been passed.[5]

Palatal Revisions

The incidence of postoperative fistula formation after primary repair of the cleft palate is relatively high, averaging 10% to 20% even in experienced hands. These usually occur at the junction of the hard and soft palate posteriorly or at the premaxillary-maxillary junction anteriorly. Palatal fistula closure using local tissue may be necessary depending on the magnitude of its associated symptoms, such as nasal liquid regurgitation and nasal air escape affecting speech. In large fistulas or those occurring anteriorly behind the upper incisor teeth, the need for regional tissue coverage from the tongue through pedicled reconstructive techniques may be needed.

If the soft palate fails to contact the posterior pharyngeal wall properly during speech, excessive air escape through the nose occurs, resulting in hypernasal speech. This occurs in about 15% of all patients who have had clefts involving the secondary palate. This velopharyngeal dysfunction may require surgical management based on a nasoendoscopic assessment of palate and pharyngeal wall movement.[12] Competent velopharyngeal function may be attained by either rearranging tissues of the lateral

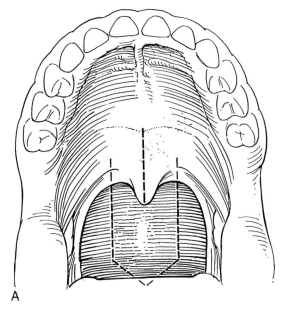

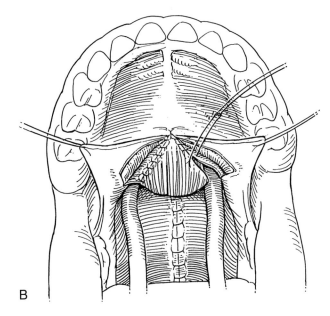

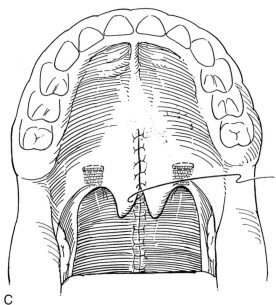

Figure 51-8 Pharyngeal flap for velopharyngeal dysfunction. *A,* Outline of incisions, including a split of the soft palate for access and flap inset and a superiorly based musculomucosal flap of the posterior pharyngeal wall. *B,* Raising of the pharyngeal flap and inset into the soft palate using small catheters to size the lateral ports and closure of the pharyngeal wall donor site. *C,* Closure of the soft palate. The flap effectively separates the velopharyngeal orifice into two small lateral orifices, thus decreasing nasal air loss during speech.

and posterior pharyngeal walls to create a *tightening* of the velopharyngeal sphincter[16] or attaching a musculomucosal flap from the posterior pharyngeal wall to the soft palate pharyngeal flap,[2] which decreases the cross-sectional dimensions of the velopharyngeal airway (Fig. 51-8). The success of these operations is dependent on matching the type of operation to the decision made at the pre-operative assessment of velopharyngeal dysfunction as determined by nasoendoscopy.

Orthognathic Surgery

The negative growth affect of clefting on the maxilla is typically manifest by restrictive anterior and transverse bone development. This creates a midfacial deficiency by appearance and a cross-bite/underbite type of occlusion. As a result, orthodontic alignment of the teeth and bony

osteotomies may be needed to properly place the maxilla into a correct skeletal and occlusal relationship with the mandible. The need for LeFort I advancements is estimated to be 20% to 30% in all cleft patients.[10] In cases of severe midfacial retrusion, as may occur in the bilateral cleft patient, the midfacial skeleton may need to be moved by osteotomies combined with postoperative distraction devices to obtain a significant movement that is postoperatively stable.[20]

ASSOCIATED CONGENITAL ANOMALIES

Lip Fistulas (Pits)

This condition, often inherited, may or may not be associated with cleft lip and palate. Symmetrical blind-ended fistulas or pits occur on the central segment of the lower lip vermilion. Known as van der Woude's syndrome, treatment consists of excision with removal of the mucosal tract and adjacent glandular tissue between 1 and 3 years of age.[26]

Submucous Cleft Palate

This seemingly least serious form of cleft palate often escapes detection until speech development occurs. Careful intraoral examination must demonstrate three physical findings: median depression or notch in the hard palate, a bifid uvula, and failure of the soft palatal muscles to join in the midline even though the overlying mucous membrane is intact. It may cause velopharyngeal dysfunction and require surgical therapy.[30]

Pierre Robin Sequence

The classic triad of cleft of the soft palate, posterior positioning of the tongue (glossoptosis), and mandibular hypoplasia is well known as the Pierre Robin sequence. It is not rare and should be excluded when clefts of the soft palate only are discovered. The significant mandibular retropositioning frequently causes airway issues immediately after birth that may require differing forms of management, including surgery, depending on its severity.[19] Palate repair is frequently delayed beyond 1 year of age in these patients to decrease the risk of secondary airway problems. By this time, growth of the mandible helps to bring the tongue forward.

REFERENCES

1. American Cleft Palate/Craniofacial Association: Parameters for the evaluation and treatment of patients with cleft lip/palate or other craniofacial anomalies. Cleft Palate Craniofac J 1993;30(suppl 1):4.
2. Cable BB, Canady JW, Karnell MP, et al: Pharyngeal flap surgery: Long-term outcomes at the University of Iowa. Plast Reconstr Surg 2004;113:475.
3. Chung KC, Kowalski CP, Kim HM, Buchman SR: Maternal cigarette smoking during pregnancy and the risk of having a child with cleft lip/palate. Plast Reconstr Surg 2000; 105:485.
4. Cohen M: Cleft lip and palate. Clin Plast Surg 2004;31:57.
5. Cutting C: Secondary cleft lip nasal reconstruction: State of the art. Cleft Palate Craniofac J 2000;37:538.
6. Dempf R, Telzrow T, Kramer FJ, Hausamen JE: Alveolar bone grafting in patients with complete clefts: A comparative study between secondary and tertiary bone grafting. Cleft Palate Craniofac J 2002;39:18.
7. Eppley BL: Pediatric plastic surgery revisited. Clin Plast Surg 2001;28:731.
8. Eppley BL, van Aalst J, Robey A: The spectrum of orofacial clefting. Plast Reconstr Surg 2005;115:101e-114e.
9. Grayson BH, Cutting CB: Presurgical nasoalveolar orthopedic molding in primary correction of the nose, lip, and alveolus of infants born with unilateral and bilateral clefts. Cleft Palate Craniofac J 2001;38:193.
10. Heliovaara A, Ranta R, Hukki J, Rintala A: Skeletal stability of LeFort I osteotomy in patients with isolated cleft palate and bilateral cleft lip and palate. Int J Oral Maxillofac Surg 2002;31:358.
11. Horswell BB, Henderson JM: Secondary osteoplasty of the alveolar cleft defect. J Oral Maxillofac Surg 2003;61:1082.
12. Johns DF, Rohrich RJ, Awada M: Velopharyngeal incompetence: A guide for clinical evaluation. Plast Reconstr Surg 2003;112:1890.
13. Johnson N, Sandy J: Prenatal diagnosis of cleft lip and palate. Cleft Palate Craniofac J 2003;40:186.
14. Kane AA, Pilgram TK, Moshiri M, Marsh JL: Long-term outcome of cleft lip nasal reconstruction in childhood. Plast Reconstr Surg 2000;105:1600.
15. LaRossa D, Jackson OH, Kirschner RE, et al: The Children's Hospital of Philadelphia modification of the Furlow double-opposing Z-palatoplasty: Long-term speech and growth results. Clin Plast Surg 2004;31:243.
16. Losken A, Williams JK, Burstein FD, et al: An outcome evaluation of sphincter pharyngoplasty for the management of velopharyngeal insufficiency. Plast Reconstr Surg 2003; 112:1755.
17. Loffredo LC, Souza JM, Freitas JA, Mossey PA: Oral clefts and vitamin supplementation. Cleft Palate Craniofac J 2001; 38:76.
18. Marazita ML, Mooney MP: Current concepts in the embryology and genetics of cleft lip and palate. Clin Plast Surg 2004;31:125.
19. Matsas R, Thomson A, Goodacre T: Management of infants with Pierre Robin sequence. Cleft Palate Craniofac J 2004; 41:219.
20. Molina F: Distraction osteogenesis for the cleft lip and palate patient. Clin Plast Surg 2004;31:291.
21. Mulliken JB, Martinez-Perez D: The principle of rotation advancement for repair of unilateral complete cleft lip and nasal deformity: Technical variations and analysis of results. Plast Reconstr Surg 1999;104:1247.
22. Mulliken JB: Primary repair of bilateral cleft lip and nasal deformity. Plast Reconstr Surg 2001;108:181.
23. Mulliken JB, Wu JK, Padwa BL: Repair of bilateral cleft lip: Review, revisions, and reflections. J Craniofac Surg 2003; 14:609.
24. Murray JC: Gene/environment causes of cleft lip and/or palate. Clin Genet 2002;61:248.
25. Pigott RW, Albery EH, Hathorn IS, et al: A comparison of three methods of repairing the hard palate. Cleft Palate Craniofac J 2002;39:383.
26. Rizos M, Spyropoulos MN: Van der Woude syndrome: A review. Cardinal signs, epidemiology, associated features, differential diagnosis, expressivity, genetic counseling and treatment. Eur J Orthod 2004;26:17.
27. Rosenstein SW: Early bone grafting of alveolar cleft deformities. J Oral Maxillofac Surg 2003;61:1078.
28. Rosenstein SW, Grasseschi M, Dado DV: A long-term retrospective outcome assessment of facial growth, secondary surgical need, and maxillary lateral incisor status is a surgical-orthodontic protocol for complete clefts. Plast Reconstr Surg 2003;111:1.
29. Salyer KE, Genecov ER, Genecov DG: Unilateral cleft lip-nose repair: A 33-year experience. J Craniofac Surg 2003; 14:549.
30. Sommerlad BC, Fenn C, Harland K, et al: Submucous cleft palate: A grading system and review of 40 consecutive submucous cleft palate repairs. Cleft Palate Craniofac J 2004; 41:114.
31. Stal S, Hollier L: Correction of secondary cleft lip deformities. Plast Reconstr Surg 2002;109:1672.

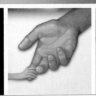

Chapter 52

Otolaryngologic Disorders

William P. Potsic and Ralph F. Wetmore

EAR

Anatomy

The ear is divided into three anatomic and functional areas: the external ear, the middle ear, and the inner ear. The external ear consists of the auricle, external auditory canal, and the lateral surface of the tympanic membrane. The auricle is a complex fibroelastic skeleton that is covered by skin and subcutaneous tissue that directs sound into the external ear canal.

The external auditory canal is oval with the long axis in the superior to inferior direction. In neonates, the external canal is almost entirely supported by soft, collapsible cartilage. As the temporal bone grows over several years, the bony portion of the canal enlarges to comprise the inner one third, leaving the outer two thirds supported by firm cartilage. Hair and cerumen glands are present in the outer two thirds of the external canal. The ear canal is lined by skin that is continuous with the lateral surface of the tympanic membrane, and it is innervated by cranial nerves V, VII, and X and cervical nerve III.

The tympanic membrane separates the external ear canal from the middle ear. It has three layers: an outer layer of skin; a middle layer of fibrous tissue that is attached to the malleus, the most lateral middle ear ossicle; and an inner layer of mucosa that is continuous with the mucosa lining the middle ear. The fibrous layer is also attached to a thick fibrous annulus that anchors it to the temporal bone.

The middle ear is an air-filled space within the temporal bone of the skull that is lined by ciliated, columnar respiratory epithelium. The middle ear communicates with the mastoid air cell system posteriorly and is lined by the same mucosa. It also communicates with the nasopharynx anteriorly through the eustachian tube. The mucociliary transport system of the middle ear moves mucus and debris into the nasopharynx, where it is swallowed. Secretory cells are not evenly distributed throughout the middle ear and mastoid complex and are more numerous anteriorly near the eustachian tube.

Three ossicles are present in the middle ear—the malleus, incus, and stapes—that transmit sound from the vibrating tympanic membrane to the stapes footplate. Stapes movement creates a fluid wave in the inner ear that travels to the round window membrane and is dissipated by reciprocal motion to the stapes.

There are two striated muscles in the middle ear. The tensor tympani muscle lies along the side of the eustachian tube, and its tendon attaches to the medial surface of the malleus. The stapedius muscle lies along the vertical portion of the facial nerve in the posterosuperior part of the middle ear. Its tendon attaches to the head of the stapes. These muscles stiffen the ossicular chain in the presence of sustained loud noise.

The facial nerve traverses the middle ear with its horizontal portion lying superior to the stapes. Posterior to the stapes, the facial nerve turns inferiorly in a vertical fashion to exit the stylomastoid foramen deep to the tip of the mastoid. The chorda tympani nerve is a branch of the facial nerve that innervates taste to the anterior two thirds of the tongue. It exits the facial nerve in the vertical segment and passes under the posterosuperior surface of the tympanic membrane, crossing the middle ear lateral to the long process of the incus and medial to the malleus. The facial nerve lies within a protective bony canal throughout its course in the middle ear. However, the bony canal may be absent (in the horizontal portion) in as many as 30% of patients. Cranial nerve IX supplies sensation to the floor of the middle ear.

The inner ear consists of the cochlea, semicircular canals, and vestibule. The cochlea is a coiled fluid-filled tube consisting of $2\frac{3}{4}$ turns surrounded by dense bone. It contains the membranes that support the organ of Corti and has hair cells that detect the fluid wave from vibration of the stapes footplate. The hair cells create the neural impulses that are transmitted from the auditory nerve (cranial nerve VIII) to the brain, providing the sensation of hearing.

The three paired semicircular canals (horizontal, superior, and inferior) are also fluid-filled tubes surrounded by dense bone. The semicircular canals each have a hair cell–containing structure (the ampulla) that detects motion. The utricle and saccule of the vestibule also have hair cell structures that detect acceleration.[26]

Embryology

The external ear develops during the sixth week of gestation and is completely developed by the 20th week. Six hillocks fuse to form the basic units of the pinna. Defects in the fusion of the hillocks lead to preauricular tags and sinuses. The external auditory canal develops from the first pharyngeal cleft. A solid epithelial plug forms during the beginning of the third month of gestation and canalizes in the seventh month to form the external auditory canal.

The middle ear canal develops from the first pharyngeal pouch. The ossicles develop from the first and second pharyngeal arches. The inner ear arises from neuroectodermal tissue within the otic placode that forms the otic pit.[26]

Any combination of anomalies may occur. Abnormalities of the development of the ear may create anomalies of the pinna, external auditory canal, middle ear structures, and inner ear. One of the anomalies that involves the external and middle ear is aural atresia (absence of the external auditory canal). Absence of the external canal may occur with a deformed or normal external ear. The ossicles may be deformed and are usually fused to each other as well as the bony plate representing the undeveloped tympanic membrane. The facial nerve may also be altered in its course through the temporal bone. Reconstruction of the atretic canal, removal of the bony tympanic plate, release of the fused ossicles, and reconstruction of a new eardrum is a complex surgical procedure that may improve hearing. Rarely there is incomplete development of the inner ear structures. The most common of these is dysplasia of the cochlea, and it may vary in severity. Dysplasia causes sensorineural hearing loss.[6,14]

Examination

The examination of the ear should always start with inspection of the outer ear and surrounding structures. Deformities of the outer ear structure may suggest the presence of other anomalies, such as a first branchial cleft sinus. A first branchial cleft sinus usually presents below the ear lobe near the angle of the jaw. The sinus tract may connect to the ear canal or, rarely, the middle ear.

The external auditory canal and tympanic membrane are best examined with a hand-held otoscope with a bright fiberoptic light source. The largest speculum that comfortably fits in the external canal should be used to maximize visualization and minimize pain. A very small speculum may be inserted deeply, but it might lacerate the ear canal as well as limit visibility of the tympanic membrane. The otoscope permits visualization of the ear canal and tympanic membrane. A translucent tympanic membrane will also permit visualization of the contents of the middle ear.

Cerumen may be encountered in the ear canal that obstructs the view of the tympanic membrane. Removal of cerumen may be performed by using an operating otoscope head and an ear curet. However, the use of a headlight such as the Lumiview (Welch Allyn, Skaneateles, NY) or operating microscope permits the use of both hands and superior visualization. Care

should be taken to secure the child to prevent sudden movement, and the ear curet should be used gently to avoid causing pain and a laceration of the ear canal.

Examination of a child with an apparent or suspected ear condition often requires objective assessment of hearing by audiometry. Current technology and expertise makes it possible to test a child at any age.

Behavioral audiometry can usually be accurately performed for a child who is older than 6 months of age by sound-field testing. Older children are presented with a tone through insert earphones and a range of frequencies between 250 and 8000 Hz for ear-specific testing. The hearing thresholds are recorded at each presented frequency; and this represents the air conduction threshold. The sound has to traverse the ear canal, tympanic membrane, and middle ear. The inner ear must respond by creating electrical impulses that are transmitted to the brain. Normal thresholds are less than 20 dB for children.

Bone conduction thresholds test the sensorineural component of hearing. A bone oscillator is used to test a range of frequencies by vibrating the skull, which stimulates the inner ear, directly bypassing the external and middle ear. Normally, air conduction thresholds require less energy than bone conduction thresholds. If bone conduction thresholds require less sound intensity than air conduction to be heard, the child has a conductive hearing loss. If air conduction and bone conduction thresholds are elevated but the same, the child has a sensorineural hearing loss. Most sensorineural hearing loss in children is a result of hair cell dysfunction in the organ of Corti. Hearing loss may be conductive, sensorineural, or mixed. Electrophysical tests such as brainstem auditory evoked response and sound emission tests that measure the intrinsic sounds from the inner ear (otoacoustic emissions) may be employed in young infants and children who cannot participate in behavioral audiometry. A mechanical test of tympanic membrane compliance (tympanometry) may also be used for audiometric assessment. All of these tools are employed by pediatric audiologists.[23]

For purposes of describing hearing loss, a threshold between 20 and 40 dB is considered mild, 40 to 65 dB is moderate, 55 to 70 dB is moderately severe, 70 to 90 dB is severe, and greater than 90 dB is profound. Four of 1000 children are born with a hearing loss, and 1 of those children is born with a severe to profound hearing loss.

Conductive hearing loss may be corrected with otologic surgery. Hearing aids and FM systems may be helpful to children with both conductive and sensorineural hearing loss. Assistance may be needed through auditory training, speech language therapy, and education to maximally develop communication skills. When a child has a sensorineural hearing loss that is too severe to be helped with hearing aids, a cochlear implant may be considered.

A cochlear implant is an electrical device that is implanted under the scalp behind the ear. Its processor converts sound to electrical impulses. A cable travels through the mastoid and facial recess to reach the middle ear, and the electrode array is inserted into the scala tympani of the cochlea through an opening that is made in the cochlea.

Cochlear implants stimulate the neural elements of the cochlea directly and bypass the hair cells. Because the vast majority of sensorineural hearing loss in children is due to hair cell dysfunction, nearly all children get sound perception from a cochlear implant. Rare conditions such as an absent auditory nerve or an absent cochlea preclude the use of a cochlear implant.

A multidisciplinary evaluation by a cochlear implant team is required to evaluate a child and determine family expectations before performing a cochlear implant. A temporal bone computed tomographic (CT) scan and/or magnetic resonance imaging (MRI) is performed to assess the cochlea and auditory nerves.

Children who are born deaf and are younger than the age of 3 years, as well as children who have already developed communication skills, language, and speech before losing their hearing, derive the greatest benefit from cochlear implants. Cochlear implantation is approved for children 12 months of age or older by the U.S. Food and Drug Administration. After a cochlear implant is performed, considerable auditory oral training is required to maximize a child's benefit to develop skills of audition, speech, and language. A child who has been deaf and without sound perception for several years is expected to benefit to a lesser degree.[33]

Otitis Media with Effusion and Inflammatory Disorders

Otitis media with effusion is the most common chronic condition of the ear during childhood. All children are born with small eustachian tubes that may at times be unable to clear mucus that is secreted in the mastoid and middle ear.

Fluid may develop in the middle ear during an upper respiratory infection. It usually clears within a few weeks as the upper respiratory tract infection resolves. Children with craniofacial anomalies such as cleft palate and Down syndrome are also prone to middle ear effusions; there is no medication that is consistently effective in resolving such effusions.

Persistent effusion may cause a conductive hearing loss in the range of 20 to 40 dB. A middle ear effusion may also function as a culture medium and predispose children to recurrent acute suppurative otitis media (ASOM).

When fluid persists in the middle ear for 3 to 4 months, causing a hearing loss or is associated with ASOM, myringotomy and tympanostomy tube placement is helpful to resolve the hearing loss and reduce the frequency and severity of infection.

Myringotomy and placement of a tube is performed under general anesthesia using an operating microscope. A small incision is made in any quadrant of the tympanic membrane except the posterosuperior quadrant, where there would be risk of injuring the ossicles. The mucus is suctioned from the ear, and a Silastic tube is placed in the myringotomy to provide prolonged ventilation of the middle ear. The tube will usually be extruded and the tympanostomy will heal in 6 months to 1 year. When the ear is no longer ventilated by a tube, the eustachian tube must ventilate the middle ear. If fluid recurs and persists, a repeat procedure may be needed. Most children outgrow this problem as their eustachian tube grows. Occasionally, adenoid tissue in the nasopharynx may contribute to the persistence of middle ear effusion and may also be removed at the time that a tube is placed. Children who have had multiple sets of tubes are candidates for adenoidectomy.

Acute Suppurative Otitis Media

Acute suppurative otitis media is the most common infection of childhood except for acute upper respiratory tract infections. It is the most common condition for which children seek medical care from their primary care physician. Usual pathogens causing ASOM include *Streptococcus pneumoniae, Haemophilus influenzae,* and *Moraxella catarrhalis.*[25]

Acute suppurative otitis media usually causes severe deep ear pain, fever, and a conductive hearing loss in the affected ear. The purulence in the middle ear is also present in the mastoid air cells because they are connected.

ASOM is treated with broad-spectrum oral antibiotics; however, there is growing concern that indiscriminant use of antibiotics may result in antibiotic resistance. For this reason, accurate diagnosis by otoscopy should be made before initiating a course of antibiotics.

Occasionally, ASOM does not respond as expected to standard antibiotic therapy. When this occurs, culture and sensitivity testing can be obtained by tympanocentesis. After sterilizing the ear canal with alcohol, a 22-gauge spinal needle can be placed through the posterior or anterior inferior quadrant of the tympanic membrane and fluid can be aspirated with a small syringe.

Complications of ASOM are uncommon if appropriate antibiotic therapy is used. The conductive hearing loss resolves as the middle ear effusion clears. However, infection may necrose the tympanic membrane, causing a spontaneous perforation. Small perforations usually heal in less than 7 days, but larger perforations may persist, cause a conductive hearing loss, and require a tympanoplasty for closure. The ossicular chain may also be disrupted by necrosis of the long process of the incus requiring ossicular reconstruction to restore hearing.

Acute coalescent mastoiditis occurs when infection erodes the bony mastoid cortex and destroys bony septa within the mastoid. A subperiosteal abscess may also be present. There is usually postauricular erythema and edema over the mastoid area. The auricle is displaced laterally and forward (Fig. 52-1). Otoscopy reveals forward displacement of the posterior superior skin of the ear canal.

In addition to antibiotics, treatment should include a wide field myringotomy from the anterior inferior quadrant to the posterior inferior quadrant, a tympanostomy tube placement for middle ear drainage, and a postauricular mastoidectomy to drain the subperiosteal abscess and the mastoid.

Facial nerve paralysis may occur from inflammation of that portion of the facial nerve that is exposed in the

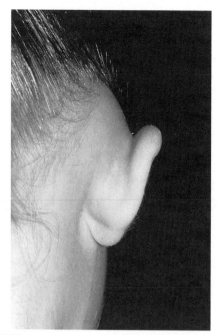

Figure 52-1 Acute mastoiditis. Extension of the acute inflammatory process from the middle ear and mastoid air cell systems to the overlying soft tissues displaces the auricle in an inferior and lateral direction from the side of the head. Fluctuance may be palpated over the mastoid cortex, and a defect in the cortical bone can frequently be appreciated. Surgical drainage with mastoidectomy is required.

middle ear during ASOM. Treatment with parenteral antibiotics, ototopical antibiotic drops applied in the ear canal, and a wide field myringotomy and tympanostomy tube placement almost always result in complete recovery of facial function. Facial nerve recovery may take a few weeks to several months.

Intracranial complications of ASOM may include meningitis, epidural abscess, brain abscess, otitic hydrocephalus, and lateral sinus thrombosis. Meningitis is the most common intracranial complication of ASOM and may be associated with profound sensorineural hearing loss and loss of vestibular function. Treatment of the intracranial complications of ASOM is focused on appropriate treatment of the intracranial process, in addition to a wide field myringotomy and tympanostomy tube placement in the affected ear.[2]

Chronic Otitis Media

Chronic otitis media is a descriptive term that refers to a persistent perforation of the tympanic membrane or the presence of a cholesteatoma of the middle ear. A cholesteatoma is a squamous epithelial-lined cyst that may be congenital or acquired. Congenital cholesteatomas are caused by epithelial rests that persist in the middle ear during temporal bone development. They present behind an intact tympanic membrane and appear as a white, smooth mass in the middle ear. They expand over time and are filled with squamous debris and may erode the ossicular chain and extend into the mastoid.

Acquired cholesteatoma develops from skin entering the middle ear after a tympanic membrane perforation or a retraction pocket from eustachian tube dysfunction.

Cholesteatomas are usually painless, cause a conductive hearing loss, and, in acquired cases, often present as otorrhea. The otorrhea should be treated with ototopical antibiotic eardrops, but the only treatment of cholesteatomas is complete surgical excision by tympanomastoid surgery and ossicular reconstruction.[27][pp 18-59] The potential complications of cholesteatomas are the same as those for ASOM.

Trauma

Objects stuck deeply into the ear canal such as a cotton-tipped applicator may perforate the tympanic membrane. This usually causes acute pain, bleeding, and a conductive hearing loss. If the ossicular chain is not disrupted, the vast majority of these perforations will heal spontaneously in about 2 weeks. If the tympanic membrane is perforated and the middle ear is contaminated with water, oral antibiotics should be given.

Lacerations of the auricle should be cleaned to prevent tattooing and repaired by careful approximation of the skin and soft tissue to restore the contours of the ear. The cartilage itself does not usually need to be sutured. Partially or totally avulsed tissue should be replaced. If necrosis of tissue occurs, it can be débrided as needed. In severe injuries of the auricle, oral antibiotic treatment is helpful to prevent chondritis and loss of the cartilage framework.

Blunt trauma to the ear is commonly seen in wrestlers, in children with poor neuromuscular tone, or in children with self-injurious behaviors. Blood or serum collects between the periosteum and the auricular cartilage. If the cartilage is fractured, the collection may occur on both sides of the ear. Evacuation of the collection is required to restore the contours of the ear, prevent infection, and prevent scarring with formation of a "cauliflower ear." Aspiration of the fluid and placement of a mastoid dressing for compression may be tried but is most often unsuccessful. Incision and drainage provides for complete evacuation of the blood or serum. Cotton dental rolls placed in each side of the auricle and held in place with bolster mattress sutures is the most effective management. The dental rolls should be left in place for 7 to 10 days while the patient also continues with a course of oral antibiotics. No outer dressing is required.[27][pp 106-109]

Blunt head trauma may disrupt the inner ear membranes causing sensorineural hearing loss and vertigo. No treatment is required, and the injury and symptoms may resolve spontaneously, but the sensorineural hearing loss may persist. Severe head trauma may cause fracture of the temporal bone of the skull. Temporal bone fractures can be classified as longitudinal, transverse, or mixed (Fig. 52-2) but are often complex and do not neatly fit into one category or another. A high-resolution, thin section CT scan of the temporal bone will define the extent of the fracture. The middle ear and mastoid are filled with blood when a fracture is present. The blood causes a conductive hearing loss that resolves when the ear clears.

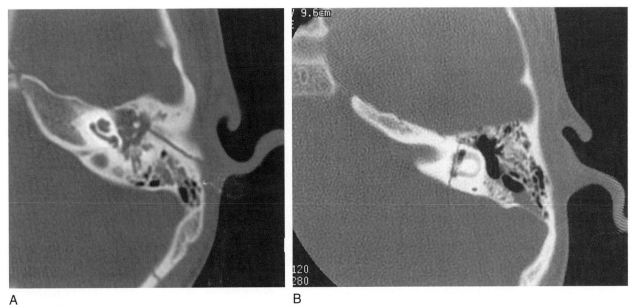

A   B

Figure 52-2   *A,* Longitudinal temporal bone fracture. These fractures run parallel to the petrous pyramid. The otic capsule is generally not affected by the fracture lines. Balance, hearing, and facial function are generally preserved. *B,* Transverse temporal bone fracture. These fractures generally extend through the cochlea and facial canal and result in deafness, vertigo, and facial nerve paralysis of immediate onset. Facial nerve exploration with repair should always be considered in these cases.

Otoscopic evaluation of a child with a temporal bone fracture may reveal a laceration of the ear canal and tympanic membrane. Blood is usually present in the ear canal, and the tympanic membrane appears to be dark blue because the middle ear is filled with blood. There is often ecchymosis of the mastoid area (Battle's sign).

It is important during evaluation of a skull and temporal bone fracture to note and record the function of the facial nerve if the patient is not unconscious. Facial nerve paralysis may be immediate or delayed in onset. Delayed facial nerve paralysis has a good prognosis for spontaneous recovery. Immediate facial paralysis may indicate disruption of the nerve or compression by bone fragments. Immediate facial nerve paralysis requires exploration and repair once the patient is stable and sufficiently recovered from any associated trauma. The facial nerve should be decompressed in the mastoid, middle ear, and middle cranial fossa. Bone chips impinging on the nerve should be removed, and the nerve should be sutured or grafted if needed. All patients with temporal bone fractures should have an audiogram once their condition has stabilized. If the fracture disarticulates the ossicles, a conductive hearing loss will persist after the blood has cleared from the middle ear and mastoid.

Fractures of the temporal bone may transverse the cochlea and vestibular apparatus. These fractures usually cause a severe sensorineural hearing loss and loss of vestibular function on the affected side. A concussive injury of the cochlea may also simultaneously be present in the opposite ear in severe head trauma.

Temporal bone fractures may permit leakage of cerebrospinal fluid (CSF) into the middle ear and mastoid. CSF may also drain through the lacerated tympanic membrane, causing CSF otorrhea. These leaks usually stop spontaneously, but persistent CSF otorrhea may require a lumbar drain to reduce the pressure and permit healing. Rarely, tympanomastoid exploration is required to close the leak. Persistent CSF leaks in the ear are associated with meningitis.

Tumors

Benign and malignant tumors of the ear are rare. Glomus tympanicum tumors and neuromas of the facial nerve may present in the middle ear. Also, eosinophilic granuloma and rhabdomyosarcoma may involve the structures of the temporal bone.[5,13]

NOSE

Anatomy

The nose can be divided into three anatomic sections. The bony vault is the immobile portion of the nose. It consists of the paired nasal bones, the frontal process of the maxillary bone, and the nasal process of the frontal bone. The cartilaginous vault is supported by the upper lateral cartilages and the cartilaginous nasal septum. The nasal lobule is supported by the lower lateral cartilages and the cartilaginous septum. The nasal septum is formed by the quadrilateral cartilage anteriorly. The posterior septum is composed of bone from the vomer, perpendicular plate of the ethmoid, nasal crest of the maxillary bone, and palatine bone.

Both the internal and external carotid artery systems supply blood to the nose. The roof and lateral wall of the internal nasal cavity are supplied by the anterior and posterior ethmoidal arteries, sphenopalatine artery, and greater palatine artery. The septum is supplied by the anterior and posterior ethmoidal arteries, palatine artery, and the superior labial artery. The convergence of these vessels in the anterior segment of the nose is referred to as Kiesselbach's plexus or Little's area. Venous drainage is accomplished mainly by the ophthalmic, anterior facial, and sphenopalatine veins.

The olfactory bulb is positioned high in the roof of the nasal cavity and is responsible for the sense of smell. Sensory information is transported by nerves that penetrate the cribriform plate and traverse cranial nerve I (the olfactory nerve) to the brain. Smell is also an important component of what is perceived as taste.

Bony projections, turbinates, form the lateral nasal wall and significantly increase the surface area of the nose, allowing for more efficient humidification and warming of the air to 36°C. Three turbinates are usually present (i.e., inferior, middle, and superior). A supreme turbinate, which is essentially a flap of mucosa, is occasionally present. The turbinates contribute to the turbulent airflow that creates approximately 50% of the total airflow resistance to the lungs.

Cleaning of air is accomplished through the nasal hairs (vibrissae) and the mucosal surface. Anteriorly, the nose is lined with stratified squamous epithelium, which changes to respiratory epithelium immediately anterior to the turbinates. Trapped debris is transported in a posterior direction into the nasopharynx by a mucociliary transport mechanism.

Speech is affected by nasal anatomy and pathologic conditions. Hyponasality from nasal obstruction or hypernasality from an excessive air leak can affect voice quality and intelligibility of speech.

Embryology

The nose serves as a drainage port for the paranasal sinuses. The meati are spaces between the lateral aspect of the nasal turbinates and the medial aspects of the lateral nasal wall. Each meatus is named for the turbinate that surrounds it. The maxillary, frontal, and anterior ethmoidal sinuses drain into the middle meatus. The posterior ethmoidal sinuses drain into the superior meatus. The sphenoidal sinus drains into an area known as the sphenoethmoidal recess that is located posterior and superior to the superior turbinate. The nasolacrimal duct drains into the inferior meatus.

The nasal cavities develop from the nasal pits in the 4-week embryo. These pits deepen and move medially to form the nasal cavity. The oronasal membrane that separates the nose from the mouth resolves in the seventh week to permit communication between the nose and nasopharynx.

The paranasal sinuses develop from an outpouching of the lateral nasal walls during the third and fourth months of development. The maxillary and ethmoidal sinuses are present at birth. The frontal and sphenoidal sinuses begin to develop several years after birth. The frontal sinus begins to develop at 7 years of age but is not fully aerated until adulthood.[1]

Inflammatory Conditions

Viral rhinosinusitis (the common cold) accounts for the majority of nose and sinus infections. It is caused by many strains of viruses and is a self-limited infection. Symptoms of fever, nasal congestion, headache, and clear rhinorrhea usually resolve over 5 to 7 days. Treatment is symptomatic.

Bacterial Rhinosinusitis

Acute bacterial rhinosinusitis may often follow an acute viral upper respiratory tract infection. The most common bacteria causing rhinosinusitis are *Streptococcus pneumoniae*, *Haemophilus influenzae*, and *Moraxella catarrhalis*. Acute rhinosinusitis causes malaise, headache, and nasal congestion. There may also be pain localized to the sinus region or pain on palpation over the maxillary or frontal sinuses. Chronic sinus infection may persist after the acute phase and symptoms often last longer than 30 days.

The "gold standard" for diagnosing sinusitis is a CT of the sinuses, but a thorough history and nasal examination is usually sufficient to diagnose acute rhinosinusitis. The nasal cavity can be visualized by using a large speculum on an otoscopic head. The posterior nasal cavity can be visualized with either a straight rod endoscope or a flexible fiberoptic nasopharyngoscope.

The treatment of rhinosinusitis includes oral antibiotics, short-term use of topical nasal decongestants (e.g., oxymethazoline), and saline nasal sprays. Topical nasal corticosteroid sprays may be helpful for the treatment of chronic sinusitis.

Chronic sinusitis in a child may be exacerbated by gastroesophageal reflux disease, immunodeficiencies, mucociliary dysfunction, and, more commonly, upper respiratory allergy. These predisposing conditions should be managed while treating the sinus infection. If the signs and symptoms of chronic sinus infection persist, a sinus CT is required to evaluate the condition of the sinus mucosa and the drainage pathways. Endoscopic sinus surgery may be necessary to open the involved sinuses to provide drainage.

Chronic inflammation of the nasal and sinus mucosa may lead to nasal and sinus polyp formation that chronically obstructs the nose and sinuses. Antrochoanal polyps are large polyps that originate from the walls of the maxillary sinus and extend through the nasal cavity into the nasopharynx. Nasal polyps may be removed endoscopically, but a large antrochoanal polyp may require removal through an open maxillary sinus procedure. Nasal polyps in a child should always prompt an evaluation for cystic fibrosis.

Complications of Sinusitis

The sinuses surround the orbit so a common complication of acute rhinosinusitis in children is orbital cellulitis with erythema and edema of the eyelids. Chemosis (edema of the ocular conjunctiva) is usually absent. However, if a periorbital subperiosteal abscess forms adjacent to an infected sinus, there may be proptosis, chemosis, ophthalmoplegia, and loss of vision. Infection in the ethmoidal sinuses most commonly results in this complication. Subperiosteal periorbital abscess is demonstrated best by sinus CT. Initial treatment should include intravenous antibiotics. Endoscopic or external drainage may be required in some cases.

Intracranial complications of sinusitis include cerebritis, cavernous sinus thrombosis, as well as epidural, subdural, and brain abscess. Treatment of intracranial complications or impending intracranial complications requires surgical drainage of the involved sinus and concurrent treatment of the intracranial lesion by a neurosurgeon.[30]

Fungal Sinusitis

Fungal sinusitis may occur in immunocompromised children, specifically severe diabetics, children undergoing chemotherapy, and bone marrow transplant recipients. The treatment of fungal sinusitis involves surgical drainage and intravenous antifungal agents.

However, a chronic form of fungal sinusitis is allergic fungal sinusitis. These patients usually have other signs of allergy, such as asthma. The treatment of this condition is corticosteroids and débridement of the involved sinuses. The diagnosis is made by sinus CT findings and the presence of eosinophils as well as fungi in the sinus secretions that are removed at the time of surgery.[11]

Congenital Malformations

Pyriform Aperture Stenosis

Congenital stenosis of the anterior bony aperture causes partial nasal obstruction that may be severe enough to cause difficulty feeding, respiratory distress, and failure to thrive. Anterior rhinoscopy demonstrates a very constricted nasal opening bilaterally. CT of the nose shows marked narrowing of the pyriform aperture.

Neonates are obligate nasal breathers, and severe stenosis must be surgically corrected. Because the stenotic segment is very anterior and the remainder of the nasal cavity is normal, removal of the constricting bone with drills is done through a sublabial approach. The nasal openings are stented with 3.0-mm endotracheal tube stents that are sutured in place and removed after a few days.

Choanal Atresia

Choanal atresia may be unilateral or bilateral. The obstructing tissue is usually a bony plate, but a few cases will have only membranous atresia. Unilateral choanal atresia presents as chronic unilateral rhinorrhea. There is no significant respiratory distress. Because neonates are obligate nose breathers, bilateral choanal atresia is associated with severe respiratory distress, difficulty feeding, and failure to thrive. The diagnosis is suspected if catheters cannot be passed through the nose and into the pharynx.

The obstruction may be visualized with a narrow flexible nasopharyngoscope after the nasal cavity has been suctioned of mucus and the nasal mucosa has been constricted with a nasal decongestant (e.g., oxymetazoline). The diagnosis is best made with CT of the nasal cavity. CT will demonstrate the atresia, define the tissue (bony or membranous), and show the configuration of the entire nasal cavity.

Choanal atresia may be successfully treated by removing the obstructing tissue transnasally. Curets, bone punches, and drills may all be effective to remove the atresia plate. However, when the bony plate is very thick and there is an extremely narrow posterior nasal cavity, a transpalatal repair is more direct. A transpalatal repair provides better access for more effective removal of the bony plate and posterior septum (Fig. 52-3). Stents fashioned from endotracheal tubes are placed and secured with sutures to the septum. They are removed in several weeks. The stents must be moistened with saline and suctioned several times daily to prevent mucus plugging and acute respiratory distress. Transpalatal repair of choanal atresia has a lower incidence of restenosis.[27[pp 196-205]]

Nasal Dermoid

Nasal dermoid cysts or sinuses present in the midline of the nasal dorsum (Fig. 52-4). They usually appear as a round bump or a pit with hair present in the pit (Fig. 52-5). They also may become infected. Nasal dermoid sinuses may extend through the nasal bones into the nasofrontal area and have an intracranial component. Both CT and MRI may be necessary to demonstrate the extent of the dermoid. Surgical removal is required to prevent infection and recurrence. This may be done between ages 3 and 5 years if prior infection has not occurred. Dermoids confined to the nose are resected completely using a midline incision with an ellipse around the sinus tract.

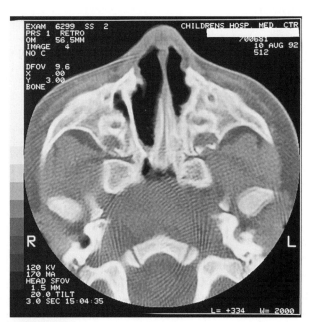

Figure 52–3 Choanal atresia. This disorder frequently presents at birth with respiratory distress.

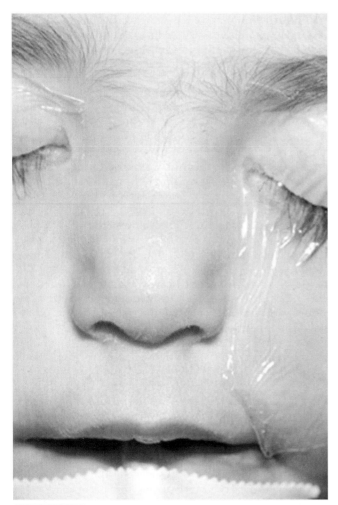

Figure 52–4 Nasal dermoid presenting in the midline as a pit.

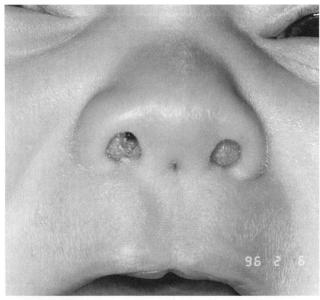

Figure 52–5 Nasal dermoid. These lesions typically present on the nasal dorsum as a single midline pit, often with a hair extruding from the depths of the pit. The pits may also be found on the columella. The dermoid will then tract through the septum toward the cranial base.

The tract is followed to its termination, and the nasal bones may need to be separated to reach the end of the tract.[27[pp 188-191]] If an intracranial component is present, a combined craniotomy and nasal approach with a neurosurgeon is recommended.

Nasal Glioma and Encephalocele

A nasal glioma presents as an intranasal mass and may be confused with a nasal polyp. The mass contains dysplastic brain tissue and may have an intracranial connection. CT and MRI are important to define the extent of the glioma and intracranial component as well as to plan the surgical approach.

An encephalocele presents as a soft compressible mass and may also be confused with a nasal polyp. Intranasal encephaloceles extend through a defect in the skull at the cribriform plate. CT and MRI define the extent of the encephalocele and are necessary to design the surgical approach. Surgical removal often includes a frontal craniotomy. Nasal encephaloceles may be associated with CSF rhinorrhea and meningitis.

Trauma

Nasal Fracture

An infant may be born with the soft nasal bones and the septum deviated to one side either as a result of a difficult delivery or from persistent intrauterine compression of the nose. The nasal structures can most often be returned to the midline with digital manipulation. If the nasal deformity is partially reduced, the nose usually straightens with growth during the first year to 18 months of age.

Nasal bone and nasal septal fractures in older children usually occur from a blow to the face during sports. There is usually a brief period of epistaxis and deviation of the nasal dorsum to one side. Swelling occurs rapidly, and the degree of the cosmetic deformity or the need for fracture reduction may not be easily determined. At the fourth to sixth day after injury, the edema subsides and the need for reduction can be determined. Nasal bone radiographs are of little help in making this judgment, so the need for nasal fracture reduction is usually based solely on clinical examination. Effective nasal fracture reduction may be done up to 2 weeks after the injury. Closed reduction under general anesthesia is the method of choice. Oral antibiotics prevent infection and are essential if nasal packing is used to support the nasal bone.

Although nasal fracture reduction is not urgent, a septal hematoma from a fractured septum should be excluded by the initial physician seeing the child. A septal hematoma that remains untreated may cause cartilage necrosis and loss of nasal support, with a resulting saddle-nose deformity. Treatment of a septal hematoma is with incision and evacuation of the clot. The mucoperichondral flap should then be sutured in place by bolster sutures through the septum. A small rubber band drain should remain in place for 12 to 24 hours, and antibiotics should be given.

Epistaxis in children usually occurs in Little's area of the anterior septum and frequently results from digital trauma (nose picking). The bleeding usually stops with pressure by squeezing the nasal ala. Infrequently, cauterization of the vessels under general anesthesia is needed.

Nasal Foreign Bodies

Children may be observed inserting a foreign body into their nose, or they may inform their parents of the event. Most children, however, present with a foul-smelling unilateral purulent nasal discharge and deny putting anything into their nose.

Most nasal foreign bodies are painless and do no harm to the nose except cause a foul nasal discharge. Disc batteries, on the other hand, cause very rapid alkali burns of the nasal cavity and pain. Batteries must be removed from the nose quickly because the chemical burn occurs in minutes to hours. If extensive tissue necrosis occurs, it may cause a nasal stenosis.

Removal of a nasal foreign body is aided by decongesting the nasal mucosa and using a headlamp to visualize the foreign body. A variety of forceps or hooks may be used. If the object is deep in the nose, the removal is best performed under general anesthesia. The endotracheal tube prevents aspiration of the object into the tracheobronchial tree if it is pushed back into the nasopharynx. One must remember that multiple foreign bodies may be present.

Nasal Lacerations

Nasal lacerations should be closed with care to match edges and restore the contours of the nose. Standard wound closure technique is employed. The nasal mucosa does not need to be sutured unless a large flap is displaced.

Nasal Tumors

Rhabdomyosarcoma, lymphoma, squamous cell carcinoma, and esthesioneuroblastoma may occur in the nose and sinuses of children. Fortunately, these malignant tumors are very rare in children. The treatment of children with malignant tumors of the nose and sinuses usually involves a multidisciplinary, multimodal approach.

Juvenile nasopharyngeal angiofibroma is a benign tumor of adolescent males that originates from the lateral wall of the nose and nasopharynx. The tumor may completely obstruct the nose and fill the nasopharynx. This type of angiofibroma may also extend intracranially through the base of the skull. Patients with these tumors present with nasal obstruction, recurrent epistaxis, and rhinorrhea.

The tumor may be seen with a flexible fiberoptic nasopharyngoscope or a rod lens telescope after decongesting the nasal mucosa. It appears as a smooth reddish mass. Biopsy of the mass should be avoided because of the potential for severe bleeding. CT and MRI define the extent and location of the tumor. MR angiography helps to delineate the blood supply, which may originate from both the internal and external carotid arteries. Contrast angiography may be reserved for presurgical planning and embolization of the copious blood supply that is often present.

The treatment of juvenile nasopharyngeal angiofibroma is complete surgical resection after preoperative embolization. Depending on the material used, the embolization may be effective for days to weeks. A variety of surgical approaches may be used, including endoscopic resection of small tumors. Extensive tumors may require a combined midfacial and craniotomy approach.[29]

Some authors have proposed radiation therapy as the primary treatment of juvenile nasopharyngeal angiofibroma, but many surgeons are concerned about the long-term effects of radiation in children, including the induction of malignant tumors.

ORAL CAVITY/PHARYNX

Anatomy

The boundaries of the oral cavity include the lips anteriorly, the cheeks laterally, and the palate superiorly. The posterior boundary is a plane that extends from the soft palate to the junction of the anterior two thirds and posterior one third of the tongue. The oral cavity is composed of the vestibule, the space between the lips and cheeks and alveolar ridges, and the oral cavity proper. The vestibule and oral cavity proper are separated by the alveolar ridge and teeth. The vestibule is divided in the midline by the labial frenula of the upper and lower lips. The alveolar ridge is contiguous superiorly with the hard palate. The parotid ducts (Stensen's ducts) enter the vestibule opposite the second maxillary molars. The submandibular ducts (Wharton's ducts) enter the floor of mouth near the lingual frenulum.

The palate is formed by a fusion of the primary palate anteriorly and medial growth of the palatal processes that form the secondary palate. The hard palate divides the nasal and oral cavities and is formed by the premaxilla and the horizontal plates of the palatine bones. The soft palate is formed by a muscular aponeurosis of the tensor veli palatini tendon. Five muscles insert into this aponeurosis and include the tensor veli palatini, levator veli palatini, palatoglossus, palatopharyngeus, and the musculus uvulae. Defects in formation of the hard and/or soft palate result in clefting. The sensory and motor innervation of the palate is through the trigeminal nerve and pharyngeal plexus.

The circumvallate papillae divide the tongue into the anterior two thirds that lies in the oral cavity and the posterior one third lying in the oropharynx. The innervation and vascular supply to the two major divisions of the tongue reflect their differences in origin—the anterior two thirds of the tongue being a first branchial arch derivative (trigeminal) whereas the posterior one third being a combination of third and fourth arch derivatives (pharyngeal plexus). The hypoglossal nerve supplies motor innervation to the intrinsic musculature. In addition to the intrinsic tongue musculature, the action of four extrinsic muscles combine to provide mobility. The genioglossus protrudes and depresses, the hyoglossus retracts and depresses, the styloglossus retracts, and the palatoglossus elevates. In addition to the circumvallate papilla, other taste buds on the tongue surface include conical, filiform, fungiform, and foliate papillae.

The pharynx is a fibromuscular tube that extends from the skull base to the level of the cricoid cartilage of the larynx and can be divided into three levels. The nasopharynx extends from the skull base to the level of the soft palate, the oropharynx extends from the soft palate to the tongue base, and the hypopharynx extends from the tongue base to the cricoid cartilage. Three muscular constrictors combine to form the muscular portion of the pharynx: superior, middle, and inferior constrictors. Passavant's ridge is a muscular segment of the superior constrictor that is involved in velopharyngeal closure. Lower fibers of the inferior constrictor help to form the upper esophageal sphincter. The motor and sensory innervation of the pharynx is from the glossopharyngeal and vagus nerves via the pharyngeal plexus.

A collection of lymphoid tissue within the pharynx forms Waldeyer's ring that includes the palatine tonsils, the adenoid (pharyngeal tonsil), and lymphoid follicles lining the lateral and posterior pharyngeal walls.

Acute Pharyngotonsillitis

In addition to the acute onset of sore throat, viral pharyngitis typically presents with fever and malaise. Signs include erythema of the pharynx and cervical lymphadenopathy. Depending on the viral agent, associated symptoms of nasal obstruction and rhinorrhea may also be present. Rhinovirus, coronavirus, parainfluenza virus, respiratory syncytial virus, adenovirus, and influenza virus are agents responsible for viral pharyngitis.

Primary herpetic gingivostomatitis, caused by herpes simplex types 1 or 2, presents as fever, adenopathy, and vesicles and ulcers on the lips, tongue, buccal mucosa, soft palate, and pharyngeal mucosa. Herpangina and hand-foot-and-mouth disease are viral infections that involve the oropharynx. Epstein-Barr virus (EBV) infection (infectious mononucleosis) presents as acute pharyngotonsillitis, fever, generalized adenopathy, malaise, and splenomegaly. Although EBV infection is suspected by the appearance of 10% or more atypical lymphocytes on a complete blood cell count and the presence of a positive Monospot test, the definitive diagnosis is confirmed by elevated titers of EBV.

Group A β-hemolytic *Streptococcus* (GABHS, i.e., *S. pyogenes*) commonly infects the pharynx. In addition to sore throat, associated symptoms include fever, headache, and abdominal pain. Associated signs include pharyngeal erythema, halitosis, tonsillar exudates, and tender adenopathy. Diagnosis may be confirmed initially with a rapid streptococcal antigen test. Because rapid antigen testing is more sensitive than formal plating on blood agar, a negative test does not need confirmation, but positive rapid streptococcal tests should be confirmed with formal plating. Other bacterial pathogens that cause acute pharyngitis include *Haemophilus influenzae* and groups C and G β-hemolytic streptococci. Occasionally, concurrent infection with penicillin-resistant *Staphylococcus aureus* may interfere with treatment of a GABHS infection.[28] Although many cases of GABHS infections respond to treatment with penicillin V or amoxicillin, emerging resistance to oropharyngeal pathogens mandates treatment of recalcitrant cases with an antibiotic having known effectiveness against β-lactamase–producing organisms. In cases in which a lack of compliance is suspected, intramuscular benzathine penicillin or ceftriaxone may be used.

Acute pharyngitis may also be associated with acute bacterial infections of the nose, nasopharynx, and sinuses. These infections may be caused by a variety of viral and bacterial pathogens; and in addition to sore throat, symptoms include fever, mucopurulent nasal drainage, nasal obstruction, and facial pain.

Recurrent Pharyngotonsillitis

Recurrent infection of the pharynx may be either viral or bacterial. GABHS are the most worrisome bacterial organisms because recurrent infection may lead to complications such as scarlet fever, acute rheumatic fever, septic arthritis, and acute glomerulonephritis. In addition to a history of multiple positive cultures for *S. pyogenes*, elevated antistreptolysin-O (ASO) titers may identify patients with chronic infection who are at risk for developing complications. Some asymptomatic children may be chronic carriers of GABHS, and elevated ASO titers may not be a reliable indicator for distinguishing between an active infection and the carrier state.

Treatment of recurrent streptococcal infection or the child who is a carrier should include a trial course of an antibiotic shown to reduce carriage (e.g., clindamycin, vancomycin, or rifampin). Children with recurrent pharyngotonsillitis unresponsive to medical therapy or those who suffer a complication should be considered for surgical management. Whereas treatment of each child should be individualized, suggested guidelines for surgical candidates include seven infections in 1 year, five or more infections per year for 2 years, or three or more infections per year for 3 years.[24] Other factors to be considered in employing a surgical option include severity of infection, response to antibiotic therapy, loss of time from school, and need for hospitalization.

Chronic Pharyngotonsillitis

The pharynx and specifically the tonsils may be the target of chronic infection. Affected children complain of chronic throat pain, halitosis, and production of white particles or tonsilliths. Signs include erythema of the tonsils, cryptic debris, and chronically enlarged cervical adenopathy. A variety of viral and bacterial agents can be blamed for chronic infection of the pharynx. Cultures may or may not be positive in these patients, because surface cultures may be negative while core tissue is positive. Antibiotic therapy directed at anaerobes or *S. aureus* may be helpful in resistant cases. Children with infections unresponsive to medical management are candidates for tonsillectomy.

Peritonsillar Cellulitis/Abscess

Localized extension of tonsillar infection may result in peritonsillar cellulitis. The same pathogens that cause acute pharyngotonsillitis are responsible for peritonsillar cellulitis. In addition to severe sore throat, symptoms and signs include drooling, trismus, muffled voice, ipsilateral referred otalgia, and tender lymphadenopathy. The affected tonsil is usually displaced in a medial and inferior position. Peritonsillar cellulitis may progress to frank abscess formation (quinsy).

Early cases of peritonsillar cellulitis may respond to oral antibiotics, such as the penicillins, cephalosporins, erythromycins, or clindamycin. Unresponsive cases of cellulitis or abscess should be treated with intravenous antibiotics. In children with suspected abscess formation, a variety of surgical drainage procedures can be performed. Needle aspiration or incision and drainage have been shown to be equally effective.[15] In persistent cases or in those children who will require general anesthesia for drainage, consideration should be given to performing a tonsillectomy (quinsy tonsillectomy).

Retropharyngeal/Parapharyngeal Space Infections

Signs and symptoms of deep neck space (retropharyngeal/ parapharyngeal) infections that involve the pharynx typically present as fever, drooling, irritability, decreased oral intake, torticollis, and/or trismus. Often there is a history of a preceding viral illness. Stridor or symptoms of upper airway obstruction may be seen in half of patients.[32] A neck mass or enlarged cervical nodes may be present depending on the location of the infection. Usual pathogens include coagulase-positive staphylococci and GABHS. Anaerobic bacteria have been found in as many as 50% of cases.[32] Complications of deep neck space infections include airway obstruction, bacteremia, rupture of the abscess into the pharynx with aspiration, mediastinal extension of infection, jugular thrombosis, and carotid artery rupture.

In suspected cases, the diagnosis of a retropharyngeal/parapharyngeal space infection is confirmed with either contrast medium–enhanced CT or MRI. Widening of the retropharynx on a lateral neck radiograph suggests a retropharyngeal infection. While ultrasound can detect the presence of an abscess cavity, CT or MRI are most helpful in demonstrating the extent of infection and the location of surrounding structures of importance, specifically the great vessels. Contrast medium–enhanced CT is particularly useful in distinguishing a phlegmon (cellulitis) from cases of frank suppuration. Demonstration of a hypodense region with surrounding rim enhancement has been shown to correlate with an abscess in 92% of cases (Fig. 52-6).

The initial management of a deep neck infection should begin with intravenous antibiotics, including oxacillin, clindamycin, cefazolin, β-lactamase penicillins, or a combination thereof. Surgical drainage should be reserved for those children who fail to show clinical improvement or progress to frank abscess formation on CT. The usual approach to surgical drainage is intraoral if the abscess points medial to the great vessels or extraoral if the infection points lateral to the great vessels.

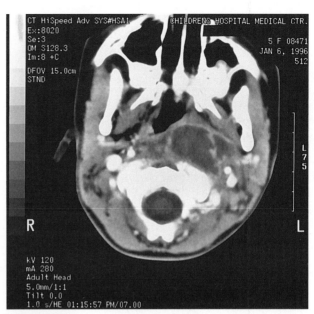

Figure 52–6   Retropharyngeal abscess. Computed tomography of the cervical area demonstrates fluid loculated in the retropharyngeal space. The abscess is typically unilateral and frequently extends into the medial aspect of the peripharyngeal space. In the absence of associated complications, drainage can be done intraorally.

Complications of deep neck infections should be treated aggressively. Mediastinal spread requires prompt surgical drainage in most cases. An infected jugular thrombosis (Lemierre's syndrome) can be a source of metastatic spread of infection as septic emboli. Signs and symptoms include spiking chills and fever (picket-fence fevers) and a neck mass in spite of appropriate antibiotic therapy. Ligature or excision of the infected thrombus may be required to eradicate the infection.

Sleep-Disordered Breathing

In the past decade, the impact of sleep-disordered breathing (SDB) on the health of children has been well described, beginning with the report of normative sleep data by Marcus and colleagues.[20] Children appear to have briefer but more frequent episodes of partial (hypopnea) and complete (apnea) obstruction. Because an apnea of less than 10 seconds may represent several missed breaths in a child, an apnea of any duration is abnormal. In most cases the site of obstruction during sleep is in the pharynx. In contrast to adults with this disorder in whom the pharyngeal impingement is due to adipose tissue surrounding the pharyngeal musculature, the major cause of airway obstruction in children results from adenotonsillar hypertrophy.

The apnea index represents the number of apneas in an hour, with a normal value being less than 1 in children. Because most children have an increased frequency of partial obstructions compared with adults, a measure of hypopneas may be more significant. A hypopnea is variably described as a reduction in airflow or respiratory

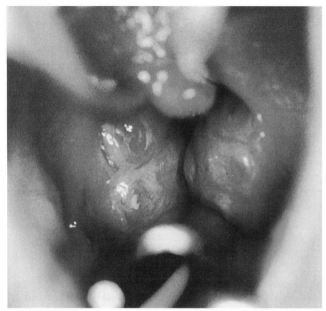

Figure 52–7 Tonsillar hypertrophy. Tonsillar hypertrophy is rated on a scale of 1 to 4. Grade 1+ tonsils are hypertrophic, grade 2+ tonsils extend slightly beyond the tonsillar pillars, grade 3+ tonsils extend in a medial direction beyond the anterior tonsillar pillars, and grade 4+ tonsils touch in the midline.

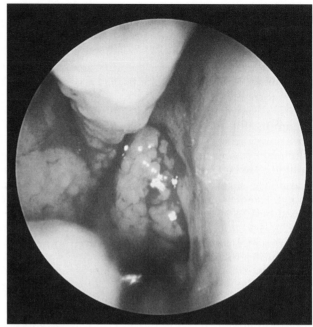

Figure 52–8 Adenoid hypertrophy. Hypertrophy of the adenoids may cause the nasopharynx to be obstructed with tissue. Smaller amounts of tissue are also able to obstruct nasal respiration by growing into the posterior choana as shown in this photograph.

effort or oxygen desaturation or combination thereof. Respiratory disturbance index is a measure of both apneas and hypopneas in an hour and may be a better reflection of SDB in children. A respiratory disturbance index greater than 5 is abnormal. Upper airway resistance syndrome represents obstructed breathing with normal respiratory indices but with sleep fragmentation and electroencephalographic arousals that indicate disordered sleep.

The major group at risk for SDB includes children with adenotonsillar hypertrophy secondary to lymphoid hyperplasia (Figs. 52-7 and 52-8). Whereas the age of affected children ranges from 2 years through adolescence, the prevalence mirrors the age of greatest lymphoid hyperplasia, 2 to 6 years, the age the tonsils and adenoids are largest in size. Other at-risk groups include syndromic children with Down syndrome, children with craniofacial disorders, and patients with cleft palate or storage diseases (Hunter's, Hurler's syndromes). Adverse effects of obstructive sleep apnea on children include poor school performance, failure to thrive, facial and dental maldevelopment, and, rarely, severe cardiac impairment, including systemic hypertension, cardiac arrhythmias, and cor pulmonale.

Daytime symptoms include noisy mouth-breathing, nasal obstruction and congestion, hyponasal speech, and dyspnea on exertion. In contrast to adults, hypersomnolence is uncommon in children because of the lower incidence of gas exchange abnormalities, specifically hypercarbia. Children may complain of headaches, seem irritable, and perform poorly in school. Nighttime symptoms are more obvious and include snoring, gasping and choking respirations, apnea, coughing, and a variety of other behaviors including sleepwalking, sleeptalking, rocking, head banging, and bruxism. Enuresis may appear in children with airway obstruction and then resolve after surgical treatment. In addition to enlarged tonsils, signs include the presence of a posterior pharyngeal flap in cleft palate patients, a craniofacial disorder, adenoid facies, and, rarely, evidence of right-sided heart failure.

The diagnosis of SDB is suggested by history and physical examination. Confirmation of obstruction and apnea may be made with overnight pulse oximetry and video or audio monitoring of sleep. The "gold standard" in the diagnosis of obstructive sleep apnea remains formal polysomnography, including measures of nasal and oral airflow, chest wall movements, electrocardiography, extraocular muscle movements, and gastric pH monitoring in selected cases. Depending on the suspected site of obstruction, adjuvant studies such as a lateral neck radiograph, MRI of the head and neck, and flexible upper airway endoscopy might be helpful.

The nonsurgical management of SDB consists of weight loss in obese patients and treatment of underlying allergies and gastroesophageal reflux. Nasal and dental appliances to maintain airway patency that may be useful in adults are usually poorly tolerated in children. Nasal continuous positive airway pressure, the mainstay of treatment in adults, is tolerated in many children and should be considered as a treatment option, especially in patients in whom other therapies have been exhausted or proven ineffective.

The initial surgical treatment for most children with SDB remains a tonsillectomy and adenoidectomy, a therapy that is usually curative. In patients with documented sleep apnea or a sleep disorder, both procedures should be utilized even if the tonsils appear small. Tonsillectomy and adenoidectomy techniques that have been standard for decades have been supplanted in some institutions by new technology including use of Coblation, Harmonic Scalpel, and the microdebrider. Efficacy of these newer techniques over established methods remains unproven.

Complications after tonsillectomy and adenoidectomy usually consist of respiratory compromise and acute or delayed bleeding. Since the advent of modern pediatric anesthesia, respiratory complications such as aspiration with resultant pneumonia and lung abscess are rare. Humidification, corticosteroids, and antibiotics have all been shown to improve the postoperative course after tonsil and adenoid surgery. Young children are most vulnerable to complications, and in most institutions children younger than 4 years of age are observed overnight for signs of dehydration and respiratory compromise.

Adjuvant surgery in the management of SDB includes craniofacial repair or posterior flap revision surgery in appropriate patients. Midface, mandibular, and hyoid advancement have proved useful in selected patients, along with nasal surgery such as septoplasty, partial inferior turbinectomy, or nasal polypectomy. Tracheostomy remains the treatment of last resort in patients who fail to respond to other forms of therapy.

Ankyloglossia

Ankyloglossia or tongue-tie is a common congenital disorder involving the lingual frenulum (Fig. 52-9). Neonates with diminished tongue mobility due to a foreshortened frenulum may have problems in sucking and feeding. Because the frenulum is thin and relatively avascular in neonates and young infants, it can often be incised as an office procedure. In older children the greatest effect of ankyloglossia is on speech. Because the tip of the tongue curls under on extrusion and has limited lateral and superior movement, speech articulation may be affected. Surgical treatment in these patients may require a short general anesthetic as the frenulum is thicker and more vascular, requiring surgical correction that includes either simple division with or without a Z-plasty repair.

Macroglossia

Macroglossia is uncommon. Generalized macroglossia, as seen in association with omphalocele, visceromegaly, and adrenal and renal disorders (Beckwith-Wiedemann syndrome), with glycogen storage diseases (Hunter's and Hurler's syndromes) or hypothyroidism, is rare. Relative macroglossia can be seen normally on occasion but is most common in Down syndrome. The most serious complication of this condition is airway obstruction. In infants, macroglossia should be distinguished from focal enlargement of the tongue seen in patients with a lymphatic malformation or hemangioma. Glossoptosis, posterior displacement of a normal-sized tongue, is seen in association with cleft palate and micrognathia in infants afflicted with the Pierre Robin sequence. Infants with airway obstruction secondary to an enlarged or displaced tongue may require a tracheostomy. Macroglossia in older children that affects cosmesis, interferes with speech, or causes drooling may be treated with a variety of tongue reduction techniques.

Benign Lesions

Epulis is a congenital granular cell tumor that typically presents as a soft, pink submucosal mass on the anterior alveolar ridge of the maxilla (Fig. 52-10). Females are

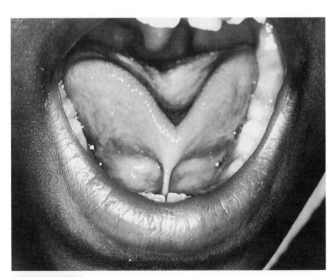

Figure 52–9 Ankyloglossia. Abnormal development of the lingual frenulum that limits extension of the tongue tip beyond the mandibular incisors frequently causes articulation disorders and should be corrected.

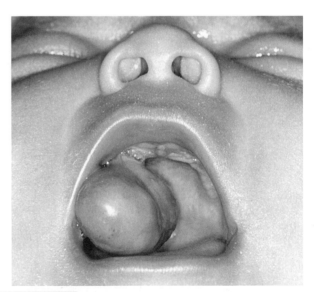

Figure 52–10 Congenital epulis. The congenital epulis is an unusual benign lesion that frequently arises from the anterior maxillary alveolar ridge. Airway and feeding difficulties may develop secondary to large lesions. Surgical excision is required.

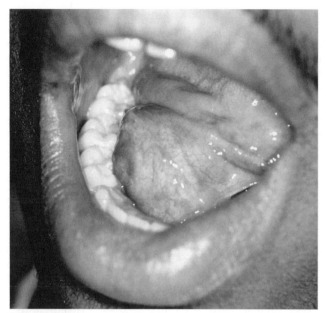

Figure 52–11 A ranula is a pseudocyst caused by obstruction of a sublingual gland. It generally presents as a unilateral, painless swelling in the floor of the mouth.

more commonly affected, and symptoms are usually confined to feeding problems. Surgical excision is curative.

Ranula is a pseudocyst located in the floor of the mouth that may occur congenitally or result from intraoral trauma (Fig. 52-11). Large ranulas may extend through the mylohyoid musculature and present in the neck as a "plunging ranula." Treatment of ranulas is by excision or marsupialization of the pseudocyst, often in conjunction with excision of the sublingual gland. *Mucoceles* are also pseudocysts of minor salivary gland origin and frequently rupture spontaneously. Recurrent or symptomatic mucoceles respond to surgical excision.

Hemangioma is a proliferative endothelial lesion found commonly in the head and neck. Their growth characteristics include enlargement during the first year of life, followed by spontaneous resolution. Surgical excision or treatment with corticosteroids may be necessary in lesions that cause ulceration and bleeding, airway obstruction, cardiovascular compromise, or platelet-trapping coagulopathy (Kasabach-Merritt syndrome). *Vascular malformations,* including venous, arterial, or arteriovenous malformations, rarely occur in the oral cavity and pharynx and necessitate intervention only if they cause pain, bleeding, ulceration, or heart failure. Management of complicated cases is by surgical excision or sclerotherapy for low-flow lesions (venous) and angiographic embolization for high-flow lesions.

Lymphatic malformation, formerly known as lymphangioma or cystic hygroma, is congenital and usually presents before 2 years of age. Histologically, lymphatic malformations consist of multiple dilated lymphatic channels or may contain either capillary or venous elements (venolymphatic malformations). Lymphatic malformations can occur anywhere in the neck and may cause extensive cosmetic deformity and functional problems in

cases with involvement of the tongue, floor of mouth, mandible, or larynx. Surgical resection of lymphatic malformations may be fraught with difficulty because they lack a capsule and are infiltrative. During surgical excision, care should be taken to avoid damaging nearby vital structures, and debulking is an acceptable option to total radical excision in many cases. Postoperative suction drains can be helpful in preventing the recurrence of lymphatic drainage under skin flaps. Carbon dioxide laser therapy has been employed in superficial lymphatic malformations of the tongue, and sclerotherapy of large cystic lesions may be an option.

Foregut cysts are true cysts, lined with respiratory epithelium, that present in the floor of mouth and should be distinguished from *dermoid cysts,* lined with stratified squamous epithelium and skin appendages, which may also be found in this location. A *thyroglossal duct cyst* may rarely present in the base of the tongue. Likewise, aberrant thyroid tissue, *lingual thyroid,* presents as a purple mass in the tongue base. Thyroid tissue in this location is usually hypofunctioning, and affected children require thyroid supplementation. Other aberrant rests of tissue, *choristomas,* consist of gastric, enteric, or neural tissue of normal histology in an abnormal location.

Second branchial cleft derivatives will rarely present as a cystic mass near the superior pole of the tonsil. Their extent and associated tracts can be demonstrated on MRI. *Tornwaldt's cyst* is a blind pouch in the nasopharynx that represents a persistence of an embryonic connection between the primitive notochord and the pharynx. Other benign nasopharyngeal masses include *nasopharyngeal teratomas, dermoid lesions (hairy polyp),* and *nasopharyngeal encephaloceles.* Most of these lesions are best evaluated by CT and/or MRI to determine their extent and the presence of an intracranial connection. Surgical excision is curative in most cases.

Squamous papillomas are benign slow-growing lesions typically found on the soft palate, uvula, and tonsillar pillars and are the result of infection with serotypes 6, 14, or 22 of the human papillomavirus (HPV). Because of concern that these lesions could spread to the larynx or trachea, complete surgical excision is usually recommended. *Pleomorphic adenoma* (mixed tumor) is a benign neoplasm of minor salivary glands with a predilection for the palate, although it may also be found in the lip and buccal mucosa. Treatment is with surgical excision.

Malignant Lesions

Rhabdomyosarcoma, the most frequent soft tissue malignancy of childhood, typically occurs in the 2- to 6-year age group and is derived from embryonic skeletal muscle.[4,18] In the oral cavity and oropharynx it presents as a rapidly growing mass in the tongue, palate, and uvula or cheek. These tumors metastasize early to local nodes, lung, and bone. Surgical therapy is limited to biopsy, excision of small lesions, or surgical salvage of treatment failures. The usual therapy includes a combination of chemotherapy and radiation therapy.

Lymphoma of the oral cavity and oropharynx typically involves the lymphoid tissue of Waldeyer's ring and presents as a mass of the tonsil or in the nasopharynx.[8] The diagnosis may be suspected by evidence of involved adenopathy in the neck but is confirmed by surgical biopsy. Treatment is with a combination of chemotherapy and radiation therapy.

Other rare malignant neoplasms of the oral cavity and pharynx include malignant salivary gland tumors (*mucoepidermoid carcinoma*) and *epidermoid* or *squamous cell carcinoma*. This latter tumor has been reported in organ transplant patients and adolescents who use snuff or chewing tobacco.[19] Treatment is usually surgical depending on the site and extent of involvement.

LARYNX

Anatomy

With the exception of the hyoid bone, the major structural framework of the larynx consists of cartilage and soft tissue. The hyoid bone lies superior to the larynx and is attached to it by the thyrohyoid membrane and strap muscles. The hyoid bone is derived from the second and third branchial arches. The cartilaginous structures of the larynx are composed of hyaline cartilage, with the exception of the epiglottis, which is composed of elastic cartilage. The cartilaginous structures of the larynx develop from the fourth, fifth, and sixth branchial arches. There are nine laryngeal cartilages, three that are single (thyroid, cricoid, and epiglottis) and six that are paired (arytenoid, cuneiform, and corniculate). The thyroid cartilage consists of two quadrilateral cartilages that form the anterior framework of the larynx. The cricoid cartilage is the only complete cartilaginous structure in the airway and provides posterior stability and a base of support for the cricoarytenoid and cricothyroid joints.

The cricothyroid muscles are paired extrinsic laryngeal muscles that serve to tilt the larynx down and forward, tensing the vocal folds. Paired intrinsic muscles—the thyroarytenoid, thyroepiglottic, and aryepiglottic muscles—act as a sphincter to close the larynx. The vocalis muscle comprises the internal fibers of the thyroarytenoid muscle and attaches to the vocal ligament. Action of this muscle serves to regulate the pitch of the vocal ligament. The other set of paired muscles includes the posterior cricoarytenoid, lateral cricoarytenoid, and interarytenoid muscles. The posterior cricoarytenoid muscles serve to abduct the vocal folds, whereas the cricoarytenoid and interarytenoid muscles adduct the vocal folds.

The quadrangular membrane is a connective tissue covering of the superior larynx that ends in a free margin along the vestibular ligament of the false cord. The conus elasticus is a membrane of elastic tissue that extends superiorly from the cricoid cartilage to form the paired vocal ligaments, the supporting structures of the vocal folds.

The blood supply of the larynx arises from the superior and inferior laryngeal arteries. The former is a branch of the superior thyroid artery, whereas the latter is a branch from the thyrocervical trunk. The intrinsic muscles of the larynx are innervated by the recurrent laryngeal nerve, which also supplies sensory branches to the inferior larynx. The superior laryngeal nerve has two branches: the external branch innervates the cricothyroid muscle, while the internal branch supplies sensation to the superior larynx.

The larynx has multiple functions within the upper airway. During respiration, it regulates airflow by opening during inspiration. The posterior cricoarytenoid muscle contracts with each inspiration to abduct the cords just before activation of the diaphragm. The protective function of the larynx produces two reflexes: cough and closure. Cough is important to expel mucus and foreign objects. The closure reflex serves to prevent aspiration of foreign matter. In addition to closure, the larynx elevates during swallowing. Both closure and elevation occur simultaneously along with relaxation of the cricopharyngeus muscle during the swallow of a bolus. Finally, the larynx plays an important role in speech production by generating sound. Vibration of the mucosa covering the vocalis structures produces sound whose pitch and register is altered by changes in tension, length, and mass of the underlying vocalis muscle and ligament.

The larynx of an infant sits much higher than that of an adult. The cricoid is located at the level of C4, whereas the tip of the epiglottis is at C1. The close approximation of the epiglottis to the soft palate makes the infant an obligate nose breather. By 2 years of age, the larynx has descended to the level of C5 and reaches the adult level of C6 to C7 by puberty. The glottis of the newborn is 7 mm in the anteroposterior dimension and 4 mm in the lateral dimension. The narrowest area of the infant airway, the subglottis, is approximately 4 mm in diameter.

Upper Airway Assessment

Symptoms of acute airway obstruction include dyspnea, cough, vocal changes, dysphagia, and sore throat. Dyspnea and rapid or labored breathing are indications of inadequate ventilation and may be triggered by changes in P_{CO_2} and P_{O_2}. A stimulus anywhere in the airway may produce cough. It is difficult to localize the site of the stimulus from the quality of the cough. Changes in the child's vocal character such as hoarseness or a muffled or weak cry may help in localizing the area of obstruction. Dysphagia for solids and/or liquids is often associated with airway obstruction. Depending on the cause of airway obstruction, affected patients may complain of sore throat.

The child's overall appearance is the first sign to be assessed in airway obstruction, because airway status often dictates how quickly further evaluation and intervention need to be performed. The level of consciousness should be determined because the unconscious or obtunded patient may need immediate airway management. Along with cyanosis in a patient without cyanotic heart disease, the presence of anxiety, restlessness, and diaphoresis are all ominous signs of impending airway compromise. Other symptoms of airway obstruction include tachypnea and substernal retractions. The child with airway obstruction is often tachycardic. The presence of bradycardia is a late indicator of severe hypoxia. The presence of a muffled cry often suggests obstruction at the level of the pharynx, whereas a barking cough is associated with laryngeal inflammation and edema. Stertor is a snorting sound whose origin is often in the pharynx. Stridor is noise produced by turbulent airflow in the laryngeal or tracheal airway. Inspiratory stridor suggests turbulence at or above the glottis. Expiratory stridor results from turbulent airflow in the distal trachea or bronchi. Biphasic stridor suggests a tracheal source. The degree and loudness of the sound is not always indicative of the severity of obstruction, because stridor can become softer just before complete obstruction. Other important signs of airway obstruction include drooling and use of accessory respiratory muscles.

In addition to determination of the child's physical status, assessment of the degree of airway obstruction should include an evaluation of the ventilatory status. Pulse oximetry provides an immediate record of arterial oxygenation while transcutaneous monitoring of CO_2 is a good indicator of ventilation. The lateral neck radiograph remains the best study for the initial evaluation of a child with airway obstruction because it demonstrates the anatomy from the tip of the nose to the thoracic inlet. The anteroposterior view of the neck is also helpful, specifically in defining areas of narrowing, such as a steeple sign associated with subglottic edema. A chest radiograph is also important in the initial assessment to identify foreign bodies or other conditions such as unilateral emphysema, atelectasis, or pneumonia that may account for the child's respiratory compromise. If time permits, a barium swallow or airway fluoroscopy may provide additional information.

Additional airway evaluation may include a brief flexible endoscopic examination. The nose is first sprayed with a combination of 2% lidocaine and oxymetazoline, and the child is gently restrained. The airway can be examined from the nares to the glottis. Attempts to pass a flexible scope through the glottis in a child with airway obstruction should be avoided. Likewise, flexible endoscopy should be avoided in a child with supraglottitis because of the possibility of precipitating complete obstruction. Children with suspected airway pathology distal to the glottis or those in whom the possibility that flexible endoscopy could compromise the airway should undergo any airway examination in the operating room where rigid endoscopes and other airway equipment is immediately available to secure the airway if necessary.

Nonsurgical intervention in the child with acute airway obstruction may begin with just observation alone in a high surveillance unit. Humidified oxygen administered by face mask will improve Po_2 and clearance of secretions. Racemic epinephrine administered by nebulizer acts to reduce mucosal edema and is useful in conditions such as laryngotracheobronchitis (infectious croup). Because its length of action lasts 30 to 60 minutes, treated patients should be observed for signs of rebound for 4 to 6 hours after administration. Corticosteroids have been shown to have value in the management of postintubation croup, adenotonsillar hypertrophy that results from EBV infection, allergic edema, and spasmodic croup. Use of corticosteroids in infectious croup and in infants with a subglottic hemangioma remains controversial.[10,16]

Other adjuvant therapies include antibiotics and inhalation of helium/oxygen mixture (heliox). Although viral agents are often responsible for inflammation in the larynx and trachea, bacterial superinfection is also common. Because of the prevalence of penicillin-resistant organisms, broad-spectrum antibiotics, including a higher-generation cephalosporin, penicillinase-resistant penicillin, or β-lactamase penicillin, are useful in preventing or eradicating infection. Heliox is a mixture of gas in which helium is used to replace nitrogen. The advantage of the helium-oxygen mixture is that its low density reduces air turbulence and gas resistance, allowing improved delivery of oxygen in patients with airway obstruction.

Nonsurgical airway management may include use of nasal or oral airways, endotracheal intubation, and, rarely, transtracheal ventilation. Nasal airways of rubber or other synthetic material can be easily inserted into the nose of most children after adequate lubrication with a water-soluble lubricant. Their best use is in cases where the pharynx is the site of obstruction. Oral airways are not as readily tolerated by children and only serve as a brief solution to an airway problem. During the 1970s, endotracheal intubation with polyvinyl chloride tubes revolutionized the management of supraglottitis, and even today intubation remains the mainstay of initial airway therapy in most children with severe airway obstruction. The size of the endotracheal tube used correlates with the age of the child. The subglottis, the narrowest part of the infant airway, typically admits a 3.5- or 4.0-mm inner diameter tube. The tube used in children older than a year can be roughly estimated by using the following formula: tube size = (16 + age in years) ÷ 4. Once the airway has been established, the tube should be carefully secured and the child appropriately sedated and/or restrained if necessary to avoid accidental self-extubation. Another method of airway management should be considered in children with an unstable cervical spine or in whom oral or neck trauma makes visualization difficult. Transtracheal ventilation, insertion of a 16-gauge needle through the cricothyroid membrane for the delivery of oxygen, should be reserved for emergencies and used only until a more stable airway can be obtained.

The surgical management of the child with acute airway obstruction should begin with endoscopy. The larynx can be visualized with one of a variety of pediatric laryngoscopes and the airway secured with a rigid pediatric ventilating bronchoscope of appropriate size. Once the airway is secured, a more stable form of airway management can be utilized. Rarely, in a child with acute airway obstruction, an airway cannot be established, and a cricothyrotomy may need to be performed. As in adults, this procedure avoids some of the risks of bleeding and pneumothorax inherent in a formal emergency tracheostomy. A small endotracheal or tracheostomy tube can be inserted through the incision in the cricothyroid membrane, but conversion should be made to a more stable airway as soon as possible. Tracheostomy remains the preferred airway in cases of acute obstruction in which a translaryngeal approach is unsuccessful or must be avoided. The emergent tracheostomy should be avoided if at all possible to lessen complications of bleeding, pneumothorax, pneumomediastinum, subcutaneous

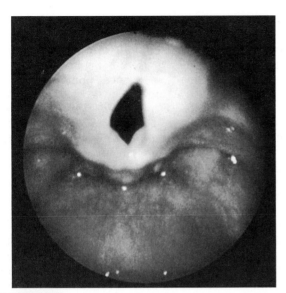

Figure 52–12 Laryngomalacia. This disorder classically presents as an omega-shaped epiglottis. The arytenoid mucosa is redundant, and the aryepiglottic folds are foreshortened. The result is a hooding of tissue over the glottic inlet that leads to airway obstruction on inspiration.

emphysema, or damage to surrounding structures. The incidence of these complications can be reduced by careful attention to surgical technique, good lighting, and adequate assistance.

Congenital Laryngeal Anomalies

Laryngomalacia is the most common cause of newborn stridor and is caused by prolapse of the supraglottic structures (arytenoid cartilages, aryepiglottic folds) during inspiration (Fig. 52-12). Symptoms typically appear at birth or soon thereafter and include inspiratory stridor, feeding difficulties, and, rarely, apnea or signs of severe airway obstruction. Gastroesophageal reflux disease tends to worsen symptoms of laryngomalacia. The diagnosis is confirmed by flexible endoscopy of the larynx, and other airway pathology can be excluded with lateral neck, chest, and barium swallow radiography. In most cases, laryngomalacia is self-limited and resolves by 18 months of age. Changes in positioning and feeding, treatment of reflux, and, in some neonates, use of monitoring may be necessary. In severe cases, surgical intervention with either a supraglottoplasy (surgical division of the aryepiglottic folds) or a tracheostomy may be necessary.

Tracheobronchomalacia is defined as collapse of the tracheobronchial airway. It may be congenital or acquired (from long-standing intubation and infection) and may be segmental or involve the entire tracheobronchial tree. Depending on the extent and location, symptoms include low-pitched biphasic stridor and signs of respiratory compromise. The diagnosis is usually made with endoscopy, although fluoroscopy of the airway may often demonstrate it. Treatment ranges from observation in most cases to airway management with a tracheostomy tube and positive-pressure ventilation in severe cases.

Vocal fold paralysis is the second most common congenital laryngeal anomaly (after laryngomalacia) and may be unilateral or bilateral. Congenital vocal fold paralysis may be caused by neurologic abnormalities (hydrocephalus, Arnold-Chiari malformation), birth trauma, or rarely in association with neoplasms of the larynx or neck. Neonates with bilateral involvement typically present with high-pitched inspiratory or biphasic stridor but a good cry. Respiratory compromise and feeding difficulties may accompany the stridor. In infants with unilateral involvement, the airway may be adequate although a few infants will show evidence of compromise, especially during feeding. The cry is often hoarse or breathy. Acquired vocal fold paralysis may result from trauma or from neoplasms of the chest or neck or may be iatrogenic, typically after surgery of the neck or arch of the aorta. The diagnosis of unilateral or bilateral vocal fold paralysis is confirmed with endoscopy. Additional studies in the evaluation of patients with vocal fold paralysis include lateral neck and chest radiography, barium swallow, and CT or MRI of the head and neck. Most cases of unilateral involvement can be observed, but infants with bilateral vocal fold paralysis often require a tracheostomy. In addition, infants with associated feeding difficulties may necessitate a gastrostomy. In older children (> 4 or 5 years of age) a more permanent solution such as a cordotomy or arytenoidectomy can be considered to improve the glottic airway.

Congenital subglottic stenosis is the third most common congenital laryngeal anomaly and is defined as a neonatal larynx that fails to admit a 3.5-mm endotracheal tube without a history of prior instrumentation or intubation (Fig. 52-13). The underlying abnormality is a cricoid cartilage that is either small or deformed. Infants with congenital subglottic stenosis present with inspiratory or biphasic stridor, barking cough, and other symptoms of airway obstruction. The diagnosis is often suggested by narrowing of the subglottis on a lateral neck radiograph and confirmed by endoscopy. Treatment depends on the severity of symptoms and ranges from observation to laryngeal reconstruction to tracheostomy.

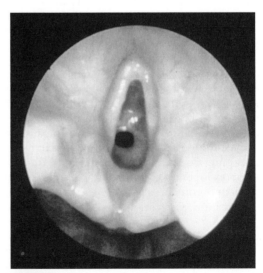

Figure 52–13 Subglottic stenosis. Congenital and acquired stenosis create airway obstruction, depending on the severity and type of stenosis. Various forms of reconstruction are available (see Chapter 63).

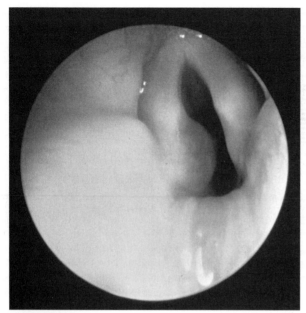

Figure 52–14   Subglottic hemangiomas typically arise from the posterior lateral aspect of the larynx. Small lesions may be managed conservatively, whereas lesions with aggressive growth patterns require tracheotomy to bypass the laryngeal obstruction.

A child with a *subglottic hemangioma* presents with the onset of progressive stridor during the first few months of life (Fig 52-14). Hemangiomas are proliferative endothelial lesions that can form in the submucosa of the posterior subglottis. Occasionally, they may involve the subglottis in a circumferential pattern. Associated cutaneous hemangiomas may be found in approximately 50% of patients. Symptoms are dependent on the amount of airway compromise and include biphasic stridor, barking cough, difficulty feeding, and other symptoms and signs of airway obstruction. The diagnosis may be suggested on a lateral neck radiograph but is confirmed with endoscopy. Nonsurgical management of infants with a subglottic hemangioma includes observation or treatment with systemic corticosteroids. Surgical therapy includes laser excision, open excision through a laryngofissure, or a tracheostomy.

A *laryngocele* is an air-filled dilatation of the saccule of the larynx that communicates with the laryngeal airway. It may present internally into the posterior superior false cord region or externally through the thyrohyoid membrane. A *saccular cyst* is fluid filled and protrudes between the true and false vocal folds. The diagnosis of this lesion is confirmed endoscopically, and CT of the larynx is helpful in assessing its extent and if it is fluid or air filled. Treatment is with endoscopic marsupialization or excision through a laryngofissure.

Inflammatory Disease of the Upper Airway

Laryngotracheobronchitis (viral croup) is an inflammation of the subglottic airway caused by a variety of parainfluenza and influenza viral agents. The infection may involve the entire glottis and extend into the trachea and bronchi. Affected children fall typically into the 1- to 3-year age group; males are more commonly affected than females. Symptoms and signs of viral croup include biphasic stridor, barking cough, and hoarseness, often in association with a prodromal viral upper respiratory tract infection. The diagnosis of croup is made clinically, but endoscopic examination may help to exclude other pathologic processes. Care should be taken not to instrument the subglottis, causing more swelling and inflammation and precipitating acute obstruction. Lateral neck radiography demonstrates subglottic narrowing, whereas anteroposterior neck films show a "steeple sign," the result of subglottic edema. Treatment of viral croup is typically supportive with humidification. Use of corticosteroids remains controversial. Treatment with nebulized racemic epinephrine in the emergency department or hospital setting often relieves symptoms; however, rebound of signs may occur several hours later and children should be monitored accordingly. Severely affected children may require intubation for respiratory failure. A smaller than normal tube should be employed. In rare cases, a tracheostomy may be required if the inflammation fails to resolve.

A child younger than 1 year of age with recurrent bouts of "croup" should be suspected of having either congenital subglottic stenosis or a hemangioma. Spasmodic croup is the recurrence of croup-like symptoms in a child who is otherwise well. Fever is rarely present, and the attacks frequently occur at night. Gastroesophageal reflux disease has been suggested as a possible inciting process. Treatment of spasmodic croup is usually observant, although corticosteroids or reflux medications may prove beneficial.

Supraglottitis (epiglottitis) is an infectious disease that involves the supraglottic larynx. In children the typical pathogen is type B *Haemophilus influenzae* (HIB). Other pathogens have been implicated in adolescent and adult cases. The incidence of supraglottitis in children has diminished markedly since the introduction of the conjugated HIB vaccine in the early 1990s.[17] Affected children are somewhat older than those seen with croup—in the 3- to 6-year age group. Symptoms and signs have a rapid onset, progress quickly to frank airway obstruction, and include stridor, dysphagia, fever, muffled voice, and signs of systemic toxicity. Affected children frequently sit and assume the "sniffing" position in an attempt to maximize their airway. Intraoral or endoscopic examination should be avoided in suspected patients because of concern for precipitating complete obstruction. Lateral neck radiography demonstrates a classic "thumbprinting" of the epiglottis but should only be obtained if facilities are present in close proximity to secure the airway.

Prompt airway management is essential in children with supraglottitis. The child's airway should be secured in either the emergency department or operating room with team members who include a pediatrician, anesthesiologist, critical care physician, otolaryngologist, or pediatric surgeon or others familiar with the pediatric airway. After inducing the child with general anesthesia, the airway should be intubated. Examination of the supraglottis may be made, and cultures of the larynx and blood are obtained. Equipment to perform a tracheostomy should be readily available. The child should remain intubated for 24 to 72 hours and should be supported with intravenous fluids and antibiotics that treat antibiotic-resistant *Haemophilus* (third-generation cephalosporins, chloramphenicol).

Bacterial tracheitis (membranous croup) often occurs as a complication of another infection, such as measles, varicella, or other viral agents. The most common organisms include *S. aureus*, GABHS, *M. catarrhalis*, or *H. influenzae*. It can occur in any age child and present with stridor, barking cough, and low-grade fever. Symptoms and signs then progress to include high fever and increasing obstruction and toxicity. The diagnosis may be suspected by diffuse narrowing of the tracheal air shadow on chest radiograph but is confirmed by endoscopic examination in the operating room. Purulent debris and crusts can be removed at this time. Cultures of secretions and crusts may be helpful in guiding intravenous antibiotic therapy that should be aimed initially at the usual pathogens. The airway should be secured with an endotracheal tube or, rarely, a tracheostomy. Repeat endoscopic examination of the airway may be warranted to continue débridement and to determine the feasibility of extubation.

Chronic Airway Obstruction

The chronic management of subglottic stenosis and other prolonged airway disorders is discussed in Chapter 63.

Benign Laryngeal Neoplasms

Recurrent respiratory papillomatosis is the most common benign neoplasm of the larynx in children. Squamous papillomas involve the larynx and occasionally the trachea and lower respiratory tract as exophytic lesions. Because of its recurrent nature, recurrent respiratory papillomatosis causes morbidity and, rarely, mortality due to malignant degeneration. Patients may be almost any age, but the disease is more aggressive in children. Human papillomavirus subtypes 6, 11, 16, and 18 have all been identified within papilloma tissue. The first two subtypes have been associated with genital warts, whereas the latter two have been associated with cervical and laryngeal cancers. The exact mechanism of human papillomavirus infection in the larynx remains unknown. Transmission of virus to the child from a mother with genital warts is suspected in many cases, but there is no concrete evidence to support this route of infection.

Children afflicted with recurrent respiratory papillomatosis present initially with hoarseness but may also have symptoms and signs of airway obstruction, including stridor. Lateral neck radiography may suggest laryngeal involvement, but the diagnosis is confirmed by direct laryngoscopy and biopsy (Fig. 52-15). In addition to the trachea and bronchi, squamous papillomas may also be found in the oral cavity.

Surgical excision is the mainstay of therapy in patients with recurrent respiratory papillomatosis. In the past, papillomas were excised using the carbon dioxide laser. More recently, the laryngeal microdebrider has become

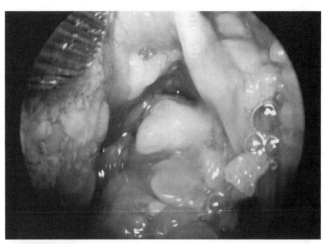

Figure 52-15 Recurrent respiratory papillomatosis. Severe papillomatosis may completely obstruct the larynx. Papillomas are characterized by malignant degeneration and aggressive growth patterns.

the preferred method of excision in many centers. In aggressive cases with swift recurrence and accompanying airway obstruction, tracheostomy may be necessary for airway management, although tracheostomy has been implicated in the spread of disease to the trachea and lower respiratory tract. Medical adjuvant therapy that has been employed with mixed results includes interferon, photodynamic therapy with dihematoporphyrin ether, indole-3-carbinol, or antiviral agents such as cidofovir.

Other benign laryngeal neoplasms are rare and include connective tissue tumors such as chondromas or fibromas, neurogenic tumors such as neurofibromas, or granular cell tumors and other cell types such as hamartomas or fibrous histiocytomas. Malignant tumors of the larynx are also rare and include squamous cell carcinoma and a variety of epithelial and connective tissue malignancies such as spindle cell carcinoma, rhabdomyosarcoma, muco-epidermoid carcinoma, and chondrosarcoma. Metastatic tumors and lymphoma may also rarely involve the larynx in children. Diagnosis is suspected by the sudden appearance of stridor, hoarseness, and airway obstruction and confirmed by biopsy. Treatment is dependent on cell type and may include surgical excision, radiation therapy, and/or chemotherapy.

NECK

Anatomy

The surgical anatomy and embryology of the neck is discussed in Chapter 56.

Clinical Evaluation

The initial examination of a disease or disorder of the neck begins with a thorough history. A detailed history can often serve to focus the differential diagnosis of a neck disorder. The age of the child is an important first consideration. The appearance of a neck mass in an infant often suggests a congenital disorder, whereas the sudden appearance of a mass in an adolescent might suggest a malignant process. Inflammatory diseases of the neck may occur in any age group but typically mirror the incidence of upper respiratory tract infections in children. Growth and temporal relationships are often important clues to a diagnosis. Neck masses that grow rapidly suggest either an inflammatory or malignant process, whereas slow-growing masses are typically benign. A history of systemic infection elsewhere in the body or recent travel or exposure to farm animals often points to an infectious origin. A history of trauma to the neck may explain the sudden appearance of a neck mass. Likewise, changes in the size of a neck mass with eating may suggest a salivary gland origin. Vascular lesions enlarge with straining or crying. Finally, systemic symptoms of fever, weight loss, night sweats, or fatigue in association with the sudden development of a neck mass may indicate a malignant process.

The physical examination of a child with a neck mass should begin with a comprehensive examination of the entire head and neck. Because the vascular, neural, and lymphatic patterns of the head drain into the neck, the source of neck disorders may be found in the head. Depending on the differential diagnosis, a physical examination of the entire body, including an assessment of lymph nodes in the groin and axillae and the presence of an enlarged spleen or liver, is essential. Palpable lymph nodes in the neck of children are a common finding, but lymph nodes larger than 2 cm fall outside the range of normal hyperplastic nodes and should be either monitored or investigated. The sudden appearance of large nodes in either the posterior cervical or supraclavicular regions may suggest a malignancy.[31] The consistency of a neck mass is also important in narrowing the differential diagnosis. Hard masses tend to be associated with either infection or malignancy. Fixation of a neck mass to skin or nearby structures is also suggestive of a malignancy. Cysts or abscesses tend to have a characteristic feel on palpation.

Depending on the differential diagnosis after a history and physical examination, radiologic studies may be useful. A lateral neck radiograph may demonstrate an abnormality of the nasopharynx, retropharynx, or cervical spine. Likewise, a chest radiograph may identify a malignancy, sarcoidosis, or tuberculosis. Infection or a neoplastic process in the sinuses may appear on a sinus series. CT and MRI are useful in the evaluation of a neck mass. Demonstration of hypodensity on CT suggests an inflammatory or necrotic process. Ring enhancement of a hypodense region on a contrast CT scan is indicative of an abscess. MRI is excellent for distinguishing fine detail within soft tissue and in the evaluation of vascular lesions of the neck. Finally, ultrasound is helpful in distinguishing solid and cystic masses. Use of ultrasound preoperatively in patients with a thyroglossal duct cyst is also a simple and economic way to assess the presence of normal thyroid tissue when it is not easily felt. Ultrasound and thyroid scanning should be employed in the assessment of any thyroid mass.

Selected laboratory studies may be helpful in the evaluation of a child with a neck disorder. A complete blood cell count with differential may identify patients with either a malignancy or systemic infection. Serologic testing for EBV or cytomegalovirus infection, toxoplasmosis, or cat-scratch disease may be diagnostic. Thyroid function testing is essential in any child with a suspected thyroid disorder. Finally, collection of urine for catecholamine metabolites (vanillylmandelic acid) may assist in the diagnosis of neuroblastoma.

If the diagnosis remains in doubt at this point, incisional or excisional biopsy may be indicated. Biopsy provides material for pathologic examination, culture, and other more sophisticated testing if necessary. Fine-needle aspiration of a neck mass in children for suspected malignancy is not as reliable as in adults.

Congenital Tracts and Cysts

Congenital sinuses and cysts are discussed in Chapter 56.

Inflammatory and Infectious Masses

Viral adenitis is the most common infectious disorder to involve the neck in children. Enlarged or hyperplastic lymph nodes are frequently the result of viral upper respiratory tract illnesses. Common pathogens include rhinovirus, adenovirus, and enterovirus, but measles, mumps, rubella, varicella, EBV, and cytomegalovirus may also cause lymphadenopathy. The diagnosis is often suspected by other findings in the history or physical examination and can be confirmed by serologic testing. Acute human immunodeficiency virus infection may present, as do other viral syndromes, with fever, headache, malaise, gastrointestinal symptoms, and a neck mass.

The usual source of *bacterial cervical adenitis* is the pharynx. Causative organisms are often streptococcal or staphylococcal species. Patients present with systemic symptoms of fever and malaise in addition to a neck mass that is diffusely swollen, erythematous, and tender. In contrast to viral adenitis, which is frequently bilateral, bacterial infections of the neck are usually unilateral. CT with contrast medium enhancement may be helpful in the evaluation of large infectious neck masses that may contain an abscess cavity. Needle aspiration of suspected infectious masses may provide material for culture and decompress the mass. Broad-spectrum antibiotic therapy, administered either orally or intravenously, may be curative, although surgical drainage is usually necessary in extensive cases.

Cat-scratch disease is caused by *Bartonella henselae* infection. The clinical picture includes the sudden appearance of unilateral lymphadenopathy after a scratch from a cat. Fever and malaise may be accompanying symptoms in many cases. Serologic testing for antibodies to *Bartonella* is diagnostic. Cat-scratch disease is usually self-limited, although some benefit has been described with the use of erythromycins and other antibiotics.[21]

In the past most mycobacterial infections have been caused by atypical organisms such as *Mycobacterium avium-intracellulare, M. scrofulaceum, M. bovis,* or *M. kansasii.* In the past decade or so, mycobacterial tuberculosis has made a resurgence as the pathogen responsible for a neck infection. Atypical mycobacterial infections present as nontender nodes in the preauricular, intraparotid, or posterior triangle regions. The skin overlying the node typically assumes a violet color, and systemic symptoms are rare. A chest radiograph should be obtained if *M. tuberculosis* is suspected. The diagnosis is made by obtaining material for acid-fast stain and culture with needle aspiration, surgical drainage, or excision of involved nodes. Surgical curettage or total excision is curative for atypical lesions. Tuberculosis should be treated with appropriate antituberculin chemotherapy.

Rarely, the neck may be involved with infections such as tularemia, brucellosis, actinomycosis, plague, histoplasmosis, or toxoplasmosis. Inflammatory disorders that may affect the neck include Kawasaki syndrome, sarcoidosis, sinus histiocytosis (Rosai-Dorfman disease), Kikuchi-Fujimoto disease, and PFAPA syndrome (periodic recurrent fever).

Malignant Neoplasms

Thyroid malignancies are not uncommon in the adolescent age group, with 10% of thyroid carcinomas occurring in patients younger than 21 years of age.[3] Well-differentiated tumors, usually *papillary carcinoma*, make up the majority of tumors. *Follicular, mixed,* and *medullary* tumors occur less commonly. Most patients present with a painless midline neck mass. On presentation, cervical adenopathy can be palpated in a majority of patients, a finding that reflects the high incidence of papillary disease that metastasizes via the lymphatics.[9] Other important symptoms and signs include a rapid rate of growth, pain, hoarseness, and dysphagia. Children who have received prior radiation are at greater risk of thyroid malignancy. The occurrence of thyroid malignancy may be associated with iodine deficiency, Hashimoto's thyroiditis, and Graves' disease.[9,22] Preoperative assessment should include thyroid nucleotide scanning to distinguish between cold (hypofunctioning) and hot (hyperfunctioning) nodules. Up to a third of cold nodules can be malignant, whereas hot nodules are rarely malignant.[12] Ultrasonography can distinguish between solid and cystic lesions, and fine-needle aspiration is an alternative to surgical biopsy for diagnosis. Surgical management includes near-total or total thyroidectomy, neck dissection if indicated, and postoperative ^{131}I ablation.

Lymphoma is a common pediatric malignancy and can present in the neck as painless lymphadenopathy. *Hodgkin's disease* occurs most often in late adolescence and has four histologic subtypes: lymphocyte predominance, nodular sclerosing, mixed cellularity, and lymphocyte depletion. Lymphocyte predominance and nodular sclerosing types make up most cases. Staging of Hodgkin's disease depends on the amount and location of nodal involvement and the presence or absence of systemic or B symptoms (fever, night sweats, weight loss). Treatment is with multiple-agent chemotherapy and localized radiation therapy. Non-Hodgkin's lymphoma can be divided into low-, intermediate-, or high-grade subtypes.

High-grade tumors may be further divided into large cell, lymphoblastic, and small cell types. Staging of non-Hodgkin's lymphoma is by location and extent. Treatment is with multiple-agent chemotherapy.

Langerhans' cell histiocytosis (previously histiocytosis X) includes the disease entities known as eosinophilic granuloma, Hand-Schüller-Christian syndrome, and Letterer-Siwe disease. The exact nature of this entity remains an enigma: it may represent a neoplasm or a hyperimmune response.[7] Symptoms and signs include lymphadenopathy, rashes, otorrhea, oral lesions, and hepatosplenomegaly. Diagnosis is dependent on the identification of Langerhan's cells on pathologic specimens. Treatment ranges from curettage or excision to intralesional or systemic corticosteroids to chemotherapy and radiation therapy.

Two major categories of neural tumors may be found in the neck. *Neurofibromatosis* is a benign disorder that in some forms (plexiform) may infiltrate surrounding tissues. For this reason, CT and/or MRI are vital in the preoperative evaluation of these lesions. Surgical resection is the mainstay of treatment. *Neuroblastoma* is a malignancy that develops from neural crest cells and may present as a solitary tumor or as lymphadenopathy. Clinical staging determines the mode of therapy that includes surgery, chemotherapy, and radiation therapy.

Rhabdomyosarcoma rarely presents as a primary tumor in the neck, more often being found as a primary tumor in the orbit, temporal bone, or nasopharynx. The diagnosis is made by biopsy, and patients are staged according to involvement. Treatment includes surgery, chemotherapy, and radiation therapy.

Malignancies of almost any type and location in the body can metastasize to the neck. The most common are thyroid malignancies. In adolescents, carcinomas, especially those arising in the nasopharynx, may spread to the neck lymphatics.

REFERENCES

1. Anon JB, Rontal M, Zinreich SJ: Anatomy and Embryology of the Paranasal Sinuses. New York, Thieme, 1996.
2. Bluestone CD, Klein JO: Otitis media and eustachian tube dysfunction. In Bluestone CD, Stool SE, Alper CM, et al (eds): Pediatric Otolaryngology, 4th ed. Philadelphia, WB Saunders, 2003, pp 474-686.
3. Buckwalter JA, Guril NJ, Thomas CG Jr: Cancer of the thyroid in youth. World J Surg 1981;5:15-25.
4. Cole RR, Cotton RT: Pediatric malignancies. In Bailey BJ, Johnson JT, Kohut RI, et al (eds): Head and Neck Surgery—Otolaryngology. Philadelphia, JB Lippincott, 1993, p 1388.
5. Cunningham MJ: Neoplasms of the ear and temporal bone. In Wetmore RF, Muntz HR, McGill TJ, et al (eds): Pediatric Otolaryngology: Principles and Practice Pathways. New York, Thieme, 2000, pp 385-408.
6. De la Cruz A, Chandrasekhar SS: Congenital malformations of the temporal bone. In Brackman DE, Shelton C, Arriaga MA (eds): Otologic Surgery. Philadelphia, WB Saunders, 1994, pp 69-84.
7. Devaney KO, Putzi MJ, Ferlito A, et al: Head and neck Langerhans' cell histiocytosis. Ann Otol Rhinol Laryngol 1997;106:526-532.

8. Fierstein J, Thawley S: Lymphomas of the head and neck. Laryngoscope 1978;88:582-593.

9. Geiger JD, Thompson NW: Thyroid tumors in children. Otolaryngol Clin North Am 1996;4:711-719.

10. Hawkins DB, Crockett DM, Shum TK: Corticosteroids in airway management. Otolaryngol Head Neck Surg 1983; 91:593-596.

11. Houser SM, Corey JP: Allergic fungal sinusitis: Pathophysiology, epidemiology and diagnosis. Otolaryngol Clin North Am 2000;33:399.

12. Hung W, Anderson KD, Chandra R: Solitary thyroid nodules in 71 children and adolescents. J Pediatr Surg 1992;27: 1407-1409.

13. Jacobs IN, Potsic WP: Glomus tympanicum in infancy. Arch Otolaryngol Head Neck Surg 1994;120:203-205.

14. Jahrsdoerfer RA, Yeakley JW, Aguilar EA, et al: Grading system for the selection of patients with congenital aural atresia. Am J Otol 1992;13:6-12.

15. Johnson RF, Stewart MG, Wright CC: An evidence-based review of the treatment of peritonsillar abscess. Otolaryngol Head Neck Surg 2003;128:332-343.

16. Kairys SW, Olmstead EM, O'Connor GT: Steroid treatment of laryngotracheitis: A meta-analysis of the evidence from randomized trials. Pediatrics 1989;83:683-693.

17. Kessler A, Wetmore RF, Marsh RR: Childhood epiglottitis in recent years. Int J Pediatr Otorhinolaryngol 1993;25:155-162.

18. Kodet R, Fajstavr J, Kabelka Z, et al: Is fetal cellular rhabdomyoma an entity or a differentiated rhabdomyosarcoma? A study of patients with rhabdomyoma of the tongue and sarcoma of the tongue enrolled in the intergroup rhabdomyosarcoma studies I, II and III. Cancer 1991;67: 2907-2913.

19. Lee YW, Gisser SD: Squamous cell carcinoma of the tongue in a nine-year renal transplant survivor: A case report with a discussion of the risk of development of epithelial carcinoma in renal transplant survivors. Cancer 1978;41:1-6.

20. Marcus CL, Omlin KJ, Basinki DJ, et al: Normal polysomnographic values for children and adolescents. Am Rev Respir Dis 1992;146:1235-1239.

21. Maurin M, Birtles R, Raoult D: Current knowledge of *Bartonella* species. Eur J Clin Microbiol Infect Dis 1997; 16:487-506.

22. Millman B, Pellitteri PK: Thyroid carcinoma in children and adolescents. Arch Otolaryngol Head Neck Surg 1995; 121:1261-1264.

23. Neault MW: Pediatric audiology. In Wetmore RF, Muntz HR, McGill TJ, et al (eds): Pediatric Otolaryngology: Principles and Practice Pathways. New York, Thieme, 2000, pp 183-202.

24. Paradise JL, Bluestone CD, Bachman RZ, et al: Efficacy of tonsillectomy for recurrent throat infection in severely affected children: Results of parallel randomized and non-randomized clinical trials. N Engl J Med 1984;310: 674-683.

25. Pichichero ME: First-line treatment of otitis media. In Alper CM, Bluestone CD, Casselbrant ML, et al (eds): Advanced Therapy of Otitis Media. Hamilton, ON, BC Decker, 2004, p 32.

26. Poje CP, Rechtweg JS: Structure and function of the temporal bone. In Wetmore RF, Muntz HR, McGill TJ, et al (eds): Pediatric Otolaryngology: Principles and Practice Pathways. New York, Thieme, 2000, pp 127-146.

27. Potsic WP, Cotton RT, Handler SD (eds): Surgical Pediatric Otolaryngology. New York, Thieme, 1997, pp 18-59, 106-109, 188-191, 196-205.

28. Quie PG, Pierce HC, Wannamaker LW: Influence of penicillin-producing staphylococci and the eradication of group A streptococci from the upper respiratory tract by penicillin treatments. Pediatrics 1966;37:467-476.

29. Radkowski D, McGill TJ, Healhy GB, et al: Angiofibroma: Changes in staging and treatment. Arch Otolaryngol Head Neck Surg 1996;122:122-129.

30. Richardson MA: Regional and intracranial complications of sinuses. In Wetmore RF, Muntz HR, McGill TJ, et al (eds): Pediatric Otolaryngology: Principles and Practice Pathways. New York, Thieme, 2000, pp 487-496.

31. Torsiglieri AJ, Tom LWC, Ross A, et al: Pediatric neck masses: Guidelines for evaluation. Int J Pediatr Otorhinolaryngol 1988;16:199-210.

32. Wetmore RF, Mahboubi S, Soyupak SK: Computed tomography in the evaluation of pediatric neck infections. Otolaryngol Head Neck Surg 1998;119:624-627.

33. Woolley AL, Lusk RP: Pediatric cochlear implantation. In Wetmore RF, Muntz HR, McGill TJ, et al (eds): Pediatric Otolaryngology: Principles and Practice Pathways. New York, Thieme, 2000, pp 359-370.

Chapter 53

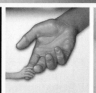

Salivary Glands

Nina L. Shapiro, MD

Salivary gland disorders are rare in children. They often present as a painful or, less commonly, a painless swelling in the affected gland. Disease processes may be of infectious, inflammatory, systemic, autoimmune, congenital, neoplastic, or traumatic origin.[6] Treatment is guided by the medical or surgical nature of the specific disease process.

CLASSIFICATION

Salivary glands may be divided into major and minor categories. The former category includes the parotid, submandibular, and sublingual glands, all of which are paired structures with their own well-defined anatomy, including blood supply and ductal drainage. Their function is augmented and facilitated by the minor salivary glands, which include the mucus-secreting tissues in the buccal mucosa, palate, mucosal surfaces of the lips, and floor of the mouth.

EMBRYOLOGY

In the sixth week of gestation, solid epithelial buds of ectoderm from the developing mouth invaginate into the surrounding mesenchyme. A groove from this invagination develops into a tunnel, which subsequently forms branches of salivary ductal tissue. The mesenchymal tissue forms the capsule and connective tissue of the salivary glands. The ends of the solid ducts form secretory acini, which become hollow. This process is similar for all of the major salivary gland embryogenesis.[9] During early gestation, the parotid ductules begin to grow around the facial nerve and its branches. This is of great clinical and surgical significance, because the facial nerve may be compressed or invaded by parotid gland lesions or its branches may be injured during parotid gland surgery.[28]

ANATOMY AND PHYSIOLOGY

The parotid gland is located in the space between the external auditory canal and the mandible. Its main duct (Stensen's duct) crosses the masseter muscle and opens in the buccal mucosa at the level of the second maxillary molar. The deep lobe of the parotid gland lies medial to the facial nerve branches and the mandible. Deep lobe parotid gland masses may extend to the parapharyngeal space and present as intraoral growths. The submandibular gland is located in the submandibular triangle of the neck. The main submandibular duct (Wharton's duct) exits the gland at a right angle and enters the mouth just lateral to the midline lingual frenulum. The sublingual gland is located at the lateral aspect of the floor of the mouth.[6]

Physiologic function of the salivary glands may be initiated by various stimuli, including cerebral, visual, olfactory, or gustatory. These stimuli promote the flow of saliva, which acts to lubricate the mouth for hygiene, speech, and deglutition; to moisten food for taste and mastication; and to initiate early starch digestion with α-amylase.[6]

PATHOLOGY

The response of a salivary gland to any pathologic process is swelling, which may be accompanied by symptoms such as pain, tenderness, erythema, or abnormal ductal discharge. Lesions may be congenital or acquired.[62] Congenital lesions include hemangiomas and lymphatic malformations. The majority of salivary masses in children are congenital vascular lesions, with hemangiomas seen in 50% to 60% of salivary gland masses and lymphatic malformations in approximately 25%.[3] Acquired lesions are of inflammatory, infectious, autoimmune, traumatic, or neoplastic origin. Major salivary gland disease initially presents as swelling of the gland and its surrounding structures. Advanced stages of disease may lead to cranial nerve involvement with resultant paresis or paralysis.

DIAGNOSIS

History

A careful history should be taken, with specific focus on duration of the lesion, its bilateral or unilateral presentation, and whether there is any symptom fluctuation associated with eating. A complete medical history is essential because the salivary glands may be involved in several systemic conditions.

Physical Examination

The physical examination should include careful inspection of the overlying skin, both local and distant, to evaluate for any cutaneous hemangiomas, as well as of the intraoral mucosa to evaluate for intraoral extension of the mass. Bimanual examination of the parotid glands and submandibular glands is crucial to fully evaluate the nature of the lesion. Longitudinal duct massage will assess for duct obstruction or purulent material in the saliva. Benign salivary lesions tend to be mobile, soft, and spongy, whereas malignant lesions are more often fixed and firm on palpation.

Radiographic Imaging

Plain radiographs of the salivary glands are helpful in detecting salivary duct calculi or diffuse glandular calcification.[6] Sialography is performed by injecting radiographic contrast medium through a small polyethylene tube into the salivary duct (Stensen's duct or Wharton's duct) in question. This technique is useful in identifying strictures, sialectasis, calculi, or saccular dilatation (Fig. 53-1).[33] The major limitation of this study is that it may cause pain; and in younger children, sedation or general anesthesia may be necessary.

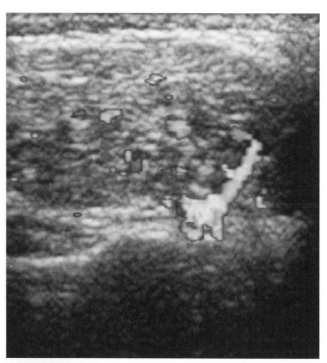

Figure 53-2 Doppler ultrasound study shows vascular pooling in a parotid hemangioma.

High-resolution ultrasonography is a useful, noninvasive technique in the diagnosis of sialectasis and salivary gland calculi.[19] The addition of color-flow Doppler imaging can provide accurate information regarding the consistency of the lesion and its vascular pattern and blood flow (Fig. 53-2).[66]

Computed Tomography

Computed tomography (CT) is an excellent diagnostic modality to assess both pathology and anatomy of the salivary glands. It can aid in distinguishing intrinsic or extrinsic lesions and can identify abscess formation by ring enhancement surrounding inflamed tissue. Instillation of an intravenous contrast agent is necessary to evaluate the presence of an abscess or to delineate vascularity of congenital and acquired vascular lesions.[6] These features aid in both medical and surgery planning.[10,16]

Magnetic Resonance Imaging

Magnetic resonance imaging (MRI) provides the best soft tissue detail of the salivary glands, and it is the only imaging technique that can delineate the facial nerve anatomy within the parotid glands. Signal intensity variations (T1- and T2-weighted images) provide additional valuable information regarding the nature of the mass.[24,58] For instance, hemangiomas, which are the most commonly seen parotid masses, have a characteristic appearance of high flow with intermediate intensity on T1-weighted images and high intensity on T2-weighted images.[6]

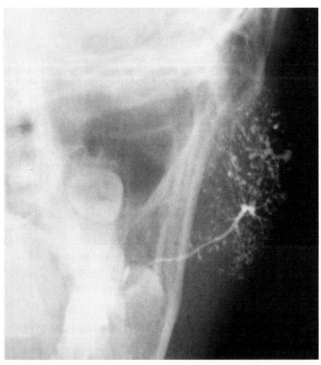

Figure 53-1 Sialogram shows saccular sialolithiasis of the parotid gland.

Biopsy

Fine-needle aspiration biopsy is an excellent tool in the diagnostic evaluation of salivary gland masses.[8,21] It can often be performed using local anesthesia in an outpatient setting with a cooperative child. The overall diagnostic accuracy is 84%.[1,40] Obtaining an adequate needle biopsy specimen may preclude the necessity for surgical therapy or, more often, aid in surgical planning. For deeper salivary gland tumors, fine-needle aspiration may be performed under ultrasound, CT, or MRI guidance. Open excisional biopsy is the definitive tool for investigation and may be curative. If the lesion is amenable to excision, an intraoral or extraoral approach may be used. When a biopsy specimen is obtained, it should be sent to the pathologist with a complete clinical description and proper markers to provide a precise orientation of the lesion. In many instances, a definitive diagnosis cannot be obtained on the frozen section and it is therefore desirable to wait until the permanent histologic report is received before further extensive and potentially disfiguring surgery is done. If the size and location of the lesion are favorable, the entire tumor may be resected intact with a clear surrounding cuff of normal tissue. The diagnosis of Sjögren's syndrome may be obtained by incisional biopsy of the minor salivary glands of the labial mucosa, or, alternatively, of the parotid gland.[39]

INFLAMMATORY DISEASE

Viral Sialadenitis

Acute inflammation of the salivary glands may be viral in up to 85% of cases, and the majority of viral sialadenitis involves the parotid glands. Viral infections are characterized by a benign self-limiting course over a 2- to 3-week period. Antipyretics, analgesics, and anti-inflammatory agents may be given for relief of symptoms. Causative organisms include coxsackievirus A and echovirus. Before the development of the mumps vaccine, mumps virus (paramyxovirus) was the most common cause of acute parotid inflammation in children.[13] As a result of nearly universal mumps immunization in the United States, which began in 1967, mumps parotitis is exceedingly rare.[12,43,50] Other potential causes of viral sialadenitis include cytomegalovirus, which is most commonly seen as a component of disseminated cytomegaloviral infection in infants and young children,[59] and Epstein-Barr virus (EBV), which in healthy children is associated with infectious mononucleosis and in chronically ill children may be associated with human immunodeficiency virus (HIV) infection.[14,60]

Bacterial Suppurative Sialadenitis

Acute suppurative sialadenitis most often presents as rapidly developing pain and swelling, with associated fever and poor oral intake. There may be associated purulent drainage from the duct of the affected gland. It is primarily seen in the parotid glands and less commonly in the submandibular or sublingual glands. The causative organisms are usually *Staphylococcus aureus* and *Streptococcus viridans*.[49] Acute sialadenitis often occurs in dehydrated patients because of decrease in salivary flow and dry oral mucosa. Most cases will respond to antistaphylococcal antibiotics, with careful attention to hydration, oral hygiene with mouthwashes, warm local compresses, and sialogogues such as sour lemon drop candies to stimulate salivary flow. Rarely, acute sialadenitis will not respond to medical therapy and the infected tissue will coalesce to form an abscess. Treatment of a salivary gland abscess includes intravenous antibiotics and surgical drainage.[52] If an abscess develops in the parotid gland, surgical drainage is carried out via a parotidectomy incision, with skin flap elevation. Multiple fascial incisions parallel to the course of the facial nerve are made to drain the abscess. If the facial nerve is paretic preoperatively, abscess drainage will usually facilitate resolution of nerve function.[6]

Chronic Sialadenitis

Chronic sialadenitis is the most common cause of inflammatory salivary gland disease in children (Fig. 53-3). Repeated episodes of infection may lead to a progressive sequence of structural changes in the gland, including sialectasis with stasis and resultant acinar destruction. It is important to distinguish between obstructive and nonobstructive causes of this condition. Obstruction is caused by ductal stenosis, which may be congenital or caused by a stone. Endogenous injury may result from chewing or biting the ductal opening. In such cases, the duct should be probed with a small-diameter lacrimal probe and laid open for continuous drainage. Nonobstructive chronic sialadenitis may occur in conjunction with metabolic disorders such as Sjögren's syndrome or chronic granulomatous disease such as sarcoidosis, tuberculosis, or atypical mycobacterial disease.

The treatment of obstructive sialadenitis is initially conservative, with warm compresses and anti-inflammatory medications. Ductal dilatation or marsupialization may be necessary for recalcitrant disease. Gland excision is rarely required.

Sialolithiasis (salivary gland or duct calculi) is rare in children. When present, it occurs in the submandibular gland in 80% of cases. When the stone is at the distal salivary duct and is visible or palpable intraorally, it may be excised by a simple incision at the orifice of Wharton's or Stensen's duct. Temporary stent placement through the duct may be necessary to avoid duct scarring and stricture. Rarely, a large calculus will be located in the proximal salivary duct or salivary gland parenchyma. If this results in chronic inflammation, complete gland excision with the stone-containing duct may be required.

CYSTIC DISEASE

Cystic disease may be acquired, congenital, or traumatic. It occurs most often in the minor salivary glands or in the parotid glands.[64] Congenital cystic disease may occur in the salivary glands, but it is not of salivary gland origin. Work type I and type II first branchial cleft cysts may present as

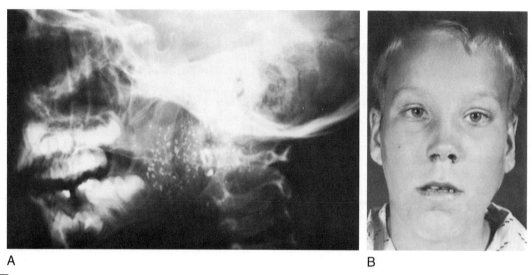

A   B

Figure 53–3 *A,* Sialogram of patient with history of recurrent parotid swelling. Note normal ductal system with early diffuse punctate sialectasis. *B,* Parotid gland swelling between acute attacks of inflammation.

parotid gland masses.[65] Congenital lymphatic malformations may also present in the parotid, submandibular, or sublingual glands. Large, bilateral intraparotid lymphoepithelial cysts are characteristic of HIV infection.[6]

Small mucous retention cysts may present in the minor salivary glands of the labial or buccal mucosa; these cysts usually result from single or repeated local trauma to the minor salivary glands and may lead to recurrent local mucosal swellings. If they do not resolve spontaneously, they will require complete excision. Local drainage or marsupialization will result in recurrence.

Ranula

A ranula is a mucus extravasation cyst of the sublingual gland. Initial presentation is that of a bluish, cystic mass at the floor of mouth, which may lead to lingual elevation and difficulty with deglutition (Fig. 53-4).

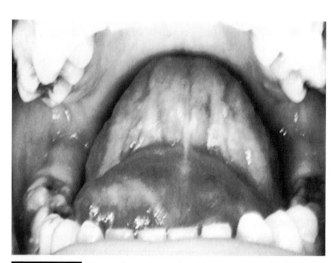

Figure 53–4 Floor of mouth ranula with posterosuperior lingual elevation.

Surgical management of ranulas is an area of much debate. Although some groups recommend marsupialization as definitive therapy,[31,44] others have described high incidence of cyst recurrence and subsequent extension to the neck via the mylohyoid (plunging ranula) and advocate complete sublingual gland excision as the definitive therapy.[35,48] During sublingual gland excision, care must be taken to avoid Wharton's duct injury. This can be avoided by placing a lacrimal probe in the duct intraoperatively to avoid duct entry. The lingual nerve must also be meticulously dissected just deep to the sublingual gland.

NEOPLASMS

Salivary gland neoplasms are extremely rare in children.[3,51] Less than 5% of salivary gland neoplasms occur in patients younger than 16 years of age.[4,34] However, when present, a pediatric salivary tumor must be assessed to rule out malignancy.[7,47,54]

Benign Neoplasms and Malformations

Benign neoplasms account for 60% of salivary tumors in children and are most commonly vascular in origin.[3] Vascular lesions include hemangiomas and lymphatic malformations, which are both congenital lesions (Fig. 53-5).

Hemangiomas

Hemangiomas are one of the most common salivary (primarily intraparotid) neoplasms in children. They usually present in infancy as a soft, nontender parotid swelling, with or without associated pigmented cutaneous lesions.[45] Diagnosis is usually confirmed by ultrasound with color-flow Doppler studies or MRI.[38] Biopsy of a suspected salivary gland hemangioma is rarely performed.[15] Parotid hemangiomas often resolve spontaneously and do not require medical or surgical therapy. If they are

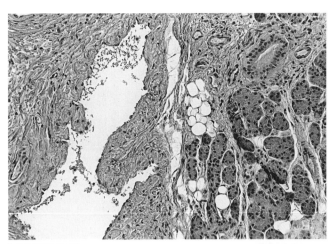

Figure 53-5 Vascular malformation of the parotid gland, showing large, irregular vascular spaces. (Hematoxylin-eosin stain, ×50.)

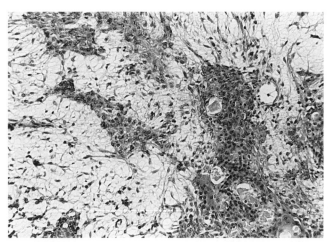

Figure 53-6 Pleomorphic adenoma (mixed tumor) of the parotid gland. Epithelial areas are mixed with myxomatoid and chondroid stroma. (Hematoxylin-eosin stain, ×50.)

rapidly growing or are causing functional impairments such as facial nerve weakness, external auditory canal obstruction, or cutaneous breakdown, systemic therapy such as corticosteroids or interferon alfa-2a or -2b are viable options to inhibit vascular growth and promote involution of the tumor.[5,30]

A less common vascular tumor is the kaposiform hemangioendothelioma. This is a benign, although locally aggressive, tumor that is firm to palpation with a nodular growth pattern and violaceous pigmentation. Therapy is controversial and may include systemic corticosteroids, interferon alfa, or surgical resection.[42]

Lymphatic Malformations

Lymphatic malformations are less common than hemangiomas, and the biology of these congenital vascular malformations results in a clinical course that differs from that of hemangiomas.[45] They do not undergo spontaneous involution, are usually present at or soon after birth, and grow with the growth of the child. They are not actual salivary lesions, but they are most commonly seen in the submandibular and parotid region in infants and young children.[46] Because they are lesions of the lymphatic system, they are susceptible to infection, with potential for cellulitis, intralesional bleeding, abscess formation, or lymphatic fluid extension to the floor of mouth or trachea with airway compromise. Treatment modalities have been an area of much investigation. Surgical resection must be complete to obviate recurrence. This is often difficult, owing to the fragility of the tumor lining and its proximity to major vessels and branches of the facial nerve.[23,29] In an effort to avoid surgical morbidity, success with intralesional sclerotherapy has been demonstrated, resulting in reduction in tumor size and minimal scarring or recurrence.[57]

Pleomorphic Adenomas

Pleomorphic adenomas (benign mixed tumors) are the most common nonvascular benign salivary tumors in children (Fig. 53-6).[51,54] They present as firm, rubbery masses, most often in the parotid gland, with an average age at presentation of 9.5 years within the pediatric population.[26,51] The tumor presents as a painless, slowly growing mass and is rarely infiltrative.[22] Treatment of superficial lobe tumors includes superficial parotidectomy with facial nerve dissection and preservation. Recurrence rates have been reported to be up to 40%, so long-term follow-up is recommended.[36,55] Rarely, recurrent pleomorphic adenomas may undergo malignant degeneration.[11]

The submandibular glands, minor salivary glands, tongue, and soft palate may also develop pleomorphic adenomas, although these are rare.[3]

Monomorphic Adenomas

Monomorphic adenomas are rare in children. Histologically, they may resemble adenoid cystic carcinoma, a highly aggressive malignant salivary tumor.[37] Treatment includes complete surgical resection and close long-term follow-up.

Papillary Cystadenoma Lymphomatosum (Warthin's Tumor)

These tumors are most commonly seen in men and are often bilateral parotid lesions. They may rarely present as benign parotid tumors in children.[6] Treatment is similar to that for pleomorphic adenomas.

Malignant Neoplasms

Malignant salivary neoplasms are rare in children. When present, they are often low-grade lesions, located most commonly in the parotid gland, and have a female preponderance.[51] Diagnostic evaluation should include CT or MRI and fine-needle aspiration biopsy. Treatment is surgical, with complete tumor excision with clear margins. Invasive malignancies may require sacrifice of the facial nerve branches, with subsequent nerve grafting to restore facial muscle function. Postoperative radiation therapy is recommended for high-grade lesions.[27,41]

Mucoepidermoid Carcinoma

Mucoepidermoid carcinoma is the most common pediatric salivary malignancy and is most commonly low grade and located in the parotid gland. Surgery with superficial or total parotidectomy, depending on tumor extent, is usually curative.[32,34] For high-grade mucoepidermoid carcinomas, or those involving the submandibular or minor salivary glands, concomitant neck dissection and adjuvant radiation therapy is recommended by many institutions.[17,25,53]

Acinic Cell Carcinoma

Acinic cell carcinomas present in a similar fashion as mucoepidermoid carcinomas. They tend to be low grade, and treatment is similar to that of mucoepidermoid carcinoma (Fig. 53-7).

Adenoid Cystic Carcinoma

Adenoid cystic carcinoma is a rare, high-grade salivary gland tumor. Perineural invasion may result in facial paralysis or, for submandibular gland tumors, in lingual nerve, hypoglossal nerve, and marginal mandibular branch deficits. There is a high incidence of regional nodal metastases, as well as distant metastases to the lungs, liver, and bone. Treatment includes wide surgical resection, neck dissection, and adjuvant radiation therapy.[27]

Rhabdomyosarcoma

Rhabdomyosarcoma may present as a parotid mass. Histologic variants include undifferentiated and embryonal types (Fig. 53-8). Treatment and outcomes depend on tumor stage and may include wide local surgical resection, with radiation and chemotherapy.

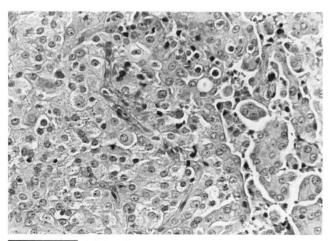

Figure 53-7 Acinic cell carcinoma of the parotid gland showing invasive proliferation. (Hematoxylin-eosin stain, ×100.)

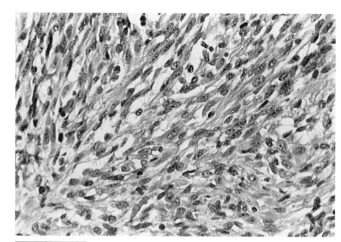

Figure 53-8 Rhabdomyosarcoma of the parotid gland showing spindle cell sarcoma with myogenous differentiation. (Hematoxylin-eosin stain, ×100.)

SURGICAL CONSIDERATIONS

The anatomic studies by Davis and colleagues[20] and the contribution by Beahrs and Chong[2] have laid the foundations for parotid surgery. Careful facial nerve dissection and preservation intraoperatively is enhanced by routine use of the facial nerve monitor.[63] Collaboration with anesthesia colleagues regarding reversal of muscle paralysis at the onset of surgery is crucial.

Parotid Gland

An S-shaped incision is made, beginning in the preauricular crease and extending in a curvilinear fashion to the postauricular region, followed by an inferior extension to 2 fingerbreadths below the angle of the mandible (Fig. 53-9). Skin flaps are elevated in a plane deep to the subcutaneous tissue and superficial to the investing fascia of the parotid gland. Posteriorly, skin flaps are elevated in the subplatysmal plane until the anterior border of the sternocleidomastoid is visualized. The greater auricular nerve and posterior facial vein will be identified and may need to be sacrificed to expose the posterior border of the parotid gland. To identify the main trunk of the facial nerve, which will divide the superficial and deep lobes of the gland, the earlobe must be retracted superiorly and the parotid gland is retracted anteriorly. Blunt dissection along the tragal pointer and mastoid process will allow visualization of the main trunk of the facial nerve as it emerges from the stylomastoid foramen. Meticulous dissection along the facial nerve branches in an anterior direction will elevate the superficial lobe of the parotid gland. If deep lobe dissection is required, the nerve branches must be gently retracted to gain access to the deep extent of the tumor. Careful blunt dissection, with utilization of the bipolar cautery and facial nerve monitor, will maximize excellent surgical results with minimal morbidity.[18]

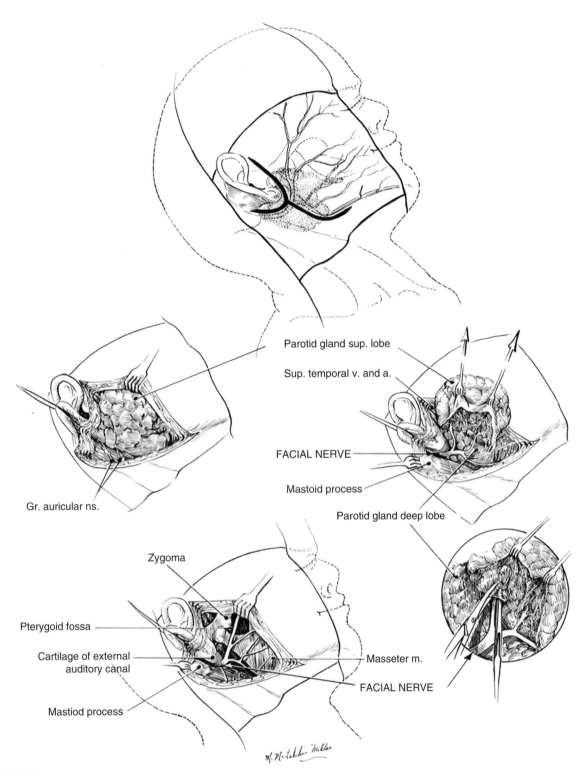

Parotid gland sup. lobe

Sup. temporal v. and a.

FACIAL NERVE

Mastoid process

Parotid gland deep lobe

Gr. auricular ns.

Zygoma

Pterygoid fossa

Cartilage of external auditory canal

Mastiod process

Masseter m.

FACIAL NERVE

Figure 53–9   Technique for parotidectomy.

Submandibular Gland

For submandibular gland resection, a horizontal skin incision is made in a natural skin crease approximately 2 fingerbreadths inferior to the body of the mandible. The dissection plane is carried out below the subcutaneous tissue and platysma, to the investing fascia of the submandibular gland. Exposure should reveal the mylohyoid muscle anteriorly, the sternocleidomastoid muscle posteriorly, and the digastric muscle inferiorly. The submandibular gland fascia is entered sharply. Identification and division of the anterior facial vein, just deep to this fascia, will facilitate protection and elevation of the marginal mandibular branch of the facial nerve. The hypoglossal nerve will be visualized deep to the digastric muscle. Anterior retraction of the mylohyoid muscle and downward retraction on the submandibular gland will enable identification of the lingual nerve and Wharton's duct. Division of the duct will free the lingual nerve from the gland and allow for complete blunt dissection of the gland.[18]

COMPLICATIONS AND RESULTS

Although salivary gland disorders are rare in childhood, the surgeon's knowledge of the anatomy of the major salivary glands and understanding of both systemic and neoplastic physiology is critical in performing appropriate evaluation and therapy. Neoplasms of the salivary glands are very rare in children and are commonly benign.[56] Evaluation and management should be tailored to the specific entity, whether it be of systemic or neoplastic origin. A multitude of diagnostic tools are available and may include radiologic or pathologic studies.

Inflammatory and infectious disorders are often treated medically, whereas neoplastic disorders require surgical intervention. The surgeon must have experience with facial nerve dissection and must have an understanding of the variations of facial nerve anatomy in infants, young children, and adolescents. Patients and families must be counseled regarding potential short- and long-term complications of facial nerve injury, whether temporary from nerve traction or permanent from nerve transection or sacrifice.

Despite the rigorous demands of parotid and submandibular gland surgery, in experienced hands, with adequate monitoring and meticulous dissection and hemostasis, surgical results are excellent.[61]

REFERENCES

1. Al-Khafaiji BM, Nestok BR, Katz RL: Fine needle aspiration of 154 parotid masses with histologic correlation: Ten year experience at the University of Texas MD Anderson Cancer Center. Cancer 1998;84:153.
2. Beahrs OH, Chong GC: Management of the facial nerve in parotidectomy. Am J Surg 1972;124:473.
3. Bentz BG, Hughes A, Ludemann JP, Maddalozzo J: Masses of the salivary gland region in children. Arch Otolaryngol Head Neck Surg 2000;126:1435-1439.
4. Bianchi A, Cudmore RE: Salivary gland tumors in childhood. J Pediatr Surg 1978;13:512.
5. Blei F, Isakoff M, Deb G: The response of parotid hemangiomas to the use of systemic interferon alfa-2a or corticosteroids. Arch Otolaryngol Head Neck Surg 1997;123:841-844.
6. Bower CM, Dyleski RA: Diseases of the salivary glands. In Bluestone CD, Stool SE, Kenna M (eds): Textbook of Pediatric Otolaryngology. Philadelphia, WB Saunders, 2004, pp 1251-1267.
7. Camacho AE, Goodman ML, Eavey RD: Pathologic correlation of the unknown solid parotid mass in children. Otolaryngol Head Neck Surg 1989;101:566-571.
8. Candel A, Gattuso P, Reddy V, et al: Is fine needle aspiration biopsy of salivary gland masses really necessary? Ear Nose Throat J 1993;72:485.
9. Carlson GW: The salivary glands: Embryology, anatomy, and surgical applications. Surg Clin North Am 2000;80:261-273.
10. Casselman JW, Mancuso AA: Major salivary gland masses: comparison of MR imaging and CT. Radiology 1987;165:183.
11. Castro EB, Huvos AG, Atrong EW, Foote FW Jr: Tumors of the major salivary glands in children. Cancer 1972;29:312.
12. Centers for Disease Control: Mumps prevention. MMWR Morb Mortal Wkly Rep 1989;38:338-392, 397-400.
13. Cherry JD: Mumps virus. In Feigen RD, Cherry JD, Demmler GJ, Kaplan SL (eds): Textbook of Pediatric Infectious Diseases, 5th ed. Philadelphia, WB Saunders, 2004, pp 2305-2314.
14. Chetty R, Vaithilingum M, Thejpal R: Epstein-Barr virus status and the histopathological changes of parotid gland lymphoid infiltrates in HIV-positive children. Pathology 1999;31:413-417.
15. Childers EL, Furlong MA, Fanburg-Smith JC: Hemangioma of the salivary gland: A study of ten cases of a rarely biopsied/excised lesion. Ann Diagn Pathol 2002;6:339-344.
16. Corr P, Cheng P, Metrweli C: The role of ultrasound and computed tomography in the evaluation of parotid masses. Aust Radiol 1993;37:195.
17. Conley J, Tinsley PP Jr: Treatment and prognosis of mucoepidermoid carcinoma in the pediatric age group. Arch Otolaryngol 1985;111:322-324.
18. Cunningham MJ: Tumors of the head and neck. In Bluestone CD, Stool SE (eds): Atlas of Pediatric Otolaryngology. Philadelphia, WB Saunders, 1995, pp 530-570.
19. Cvetinovic M, Jovic N, Mijatovic D: Evaluation of ultrasound in the diagnosis of pathologic processes in the parotid gland. J Oral Maxillofac Surg 1991;49;147.
20. Davis RA, Anson BJ, Budinger JM, Kurth LR: Surgical anatomy of the facial nerve and parotid gland based on 350 cervicofacial halves. Surg Gynecol Obstet 1956;102:358.
21. Dean GT, Briggs K, Spence RAG: An audit of surgery of the parotid gland. Ann R Coll Surg Engl 1995;77:188.
22. Ethunandan M, Ethunandan A, Macpherson D, et al: Parotid neoplasms in children: Experience of diagnosis and management in a district general hospital. Int J Oral Maxillofac Surg 2003;32:373-377.
23. Fageeh N, Manoukian J, Tewfik T, et al: Management of head and neck lymphatic malformations in children. J Otolaryngol 1997;26:253-258.
24. Freling NJ, Molenaar WM, Verney A: Malignant parotid tumors: Clinical use of MR imaging and histological correlation. Radiology 1992;185:691.
25. Friedman M, Levin B, Grybauskas V, et al: Malignant tumors of the major salivary glands. Otolaryngol Clin North Am 1986;19:625-636.
26. Galick R: Salivary gland neoplasms in children. Arch Otolaryngol 1969;89:878.
27. Garden AS, el-Naggar AK, Morrison WH, et al: Postoperative radiotherapy for malignant tumors of the parotid gland. Int J Radiat Oncol Biol Phys 1997;37:79.
28. Gasser RF: The early development of the parotid gland around the facial nerve branches. Anat Rec 1992;15:244.
29. Giguere CM, Bauman NM, Smith RJ: New treatment options for lymphangioma in infants and children. Ann Otol Rhinol Laryngol 2002;111:1066-1075.
30. Greene AK, Rogers GF, Mulliken JB: Management of parotid hemangioma in 100 children. Plast Reconstr Surg 2004;113:53-60.
31. Haberal I, Gocmen H, Samim E: Surgical management of pediatric ranula. Int J Pediatr Otorhinolaryngol 2004;68:161-163.

32. Hicks J, Flaitz C: Mucoepidermoid carcinoma of the salivary glands in children and adolescents: Assessment and proliferation of markers. Oral Oncol 2000;36:454-460.

33. Ilgit ET, et al: Digital subtraction sialography techniques: Advantages and results in 107 cases. Eur J Radiol 1992;15:44.

34. Jaques DA, Krolls SO, Chambers RG: Parotid tumors in children. Am J Surg 1976;132:469-471.

35. Kobayashi T, Ochi K, Komatsuzaki Y, et al: Blanket removal of the sublingual gland for treatment of plunging ranula. Laryngoscope 2003;113:386-388.

36. Koral K, Sayre J, Bhuta S, et al: Recurrent pleomorphic adenoma of the parotid gland in pediatric and adult patients: Value of multiple lesions as a diagnostic indicator. AJR Am J Roentgenol 2003;180:1171-1174.

37. Krolls SO, Trodahl JN, Boyers R: Salivary gland lesions in children. Cancer 1972;30:459.

38. Lowe LH, Stokes LS, Johnson JE, et al: Swelling at the angle of the mandible: Imaging of the pediatric parotid gland and periparotid region. Radiographics 2001;21:1211-1227.

39. McGuirt WF, Whang C, Moreland W: The role of parotid biopsy in the diagnosis of pediatric Sjögren syndrome. Arch Otolaryngol Head Neck Surg 2002;128:1279-1281.

40. Megerian CA, Maniglia AJ: Parotidectomy: A ten-year experience with fine needle aspiration and frozen section biopsy correlation. Ear Nose Throat J 1994;73:377.

41. Mendenhall WM, Morris CG, Amdur RJ, et al: Radiotherapy alone or combined with carbogen breathing for squamous cell carcinoma of the head and neck: A prospective, randomized trial. Cancer 2005;104:332-337.

42. Metry DW, Hebert AA: Benign cutaneous vascular tumors of infancy: When to worry, what to do. Arch Dermatol 2000;136:905-914.

43. Modlin JF: Current status of mumps in the United States. Infection 1975;132:106.

44. Morita Y, Sato K, Kawana M, et al: Treatment of ranula—excision of the sublingual gland versus marsupialization. Auris Nasus Larynx 2003;30:311-314.

45. Mulliken JB, Glowacki J: Hemangiomas and vascular malformations in infants and children: A classification based on endothelial characteristics. Plast Reconstr Surg 1982;69:412-420.

46. Orvidas LJ, Kasperbauer JL: Pediatric lymphangiomas of the head and neck. Ann Otol Rhinol Laryngol 2000;109:411-421.

47. Orvidas LJ, Kasperbauer JL, Lewis JE, et al: Pediatric parotid masses. Arch Otolaryngol Head Neck Surg 2000;126:177-184.

48. Pandit RT, Park AH: Management of pediatric ranula. Otolaryngol Head Neck Surg 2002;127:115-118.

49. Pershall KE, Koopman CF, Coultard SW: Sialadenitis in children. J Pediatr Otolaryngol 1986;11:199.

50. Peter G (ed): 1997 Red Book: Report of the Committee on Infectious Diseases, 24th ed. Elk Grove Village, IL, American Academy of Pediatrics, 1997, pp 366-369.

51. Ribeiro Kde C, Kowalski LP, Saba LM, de Camargo B: Epithelial salivary gland neoplasms in children and adolescents: A forty-four year experience. Med Pediatr Oncol 2002;39:504-600.

52. Rice DH: Non-neoplastic diseases of the salivary glands. In Paparella MM, et al (eds): Otolaryngology. Philadelphia, WB Saunders, 1991.

53. Rogers DA, Rao BN, Bowman L, et al: Primary malignancy of the salivary gland in children. J Pediatr Surg 1994;29:44-47.

54. Schuller DE, McCabe BF: Salivary gland neoplasms in childhood. Otolaryngol Clin North Am 1977;10:39.

55. Shikani AH, Johns ME: Tumors of the major salivary glands in children. Head Neck Surg 1998;10:257.

56. Siefert G, Sobin LH: The World Health Organization's Histological classification of salivary gland tumours: A commentary on the second edition. Cancer 1992;70:379.

57. Sung MW, Lee DW, Kim DY, et al: Sclerotherapy with picibanil (OK-432) for congenital lymphatic malformation in the head and neck. Laryngoscope 2001;111:1430-1433.

58. Tabor EK, Curtin HD: MR of the salivary glands. Radiol Clin North Am 1989;379:27.

59. Variend S, O'Neill D, Arnold P: The possible significance of cytomegaloviral parotitis in infant and early childhood deaths. Arch Pathol Lab Med 1997;121:1272.

60. Venkateswaran L, Gan YJ, Sixbey JW, Santana VM: Epstein-Barr virus infection in salivary gland tumors in children and young adults. Cancer 2000;89:463-466.

61. Watanabe Y, et al: Facial nerve palsy as a complication of parotid surgery and its prevention. Acta Otolaryngol Suppl (Stockh) 1993;504:137.

62. White AK: Salivary gland diseases in infancy and childhood. J Otorhinolaryngol 1992;21:422.

63. Woods JE: Parotidectomy: Points of technique for a brief and safe operation. Am J Surg 1983;145:678.

64. Work WP: Cysts and congenital lesions of the parotid gland. Otorhinolaryngol Clin North Am 1977;10:339.

65. Work WP: Newer concepts of first branchial cleft defects. Laryngoscope 1972;82:1581.

66. Yang WT, Ahuja A, Metreweli C: Sonographic features of head and neck hemangiomas and vascular malformations: Review of 23 patients. J Ultrasound Med 1997;16:39.

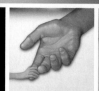

Chapter 54

Lymph Node Disorders

Kurt D. Newman and Andrea A. Hayes-Jordan

GENERAL APPROACH TO ADENOPATHY

An enlarging or persistent neck mass in a child is a common source of concern for parents and pediatricians and is a frequent reason for referral to a surgeon. Most cervical masses in children are either congenital lesions (i.e., thyroglossal duct or branchial cleft origin) or enlarged lymph nodes. Clinically palpable cervical lymphadenopathy is extremely common during childhood, with a reported prevalence of 28% to 55% in otherwise normal infants and children.[23,32] Although reactive hyperplasia caused by presumptive or proven infection accounts for most cases of cervical lymphadenopathy, the possibility of a malignant condition must be considered in all clinically suspicious lesions that become chronic or persist despite antibiotic therapy.[19] Surgical intervention is indicated in specific infectious conditions, such as atypical mycobacterial adenitis, and may be required in inflammatory lymphadenitis that is complicated by suppuration or fistula formation or is recalcitrant to appropriate medical management. Persistent lymphadenopathy despite 2 weeks of antibiotic therapy, unilateral adenopathy involving the supraclavicular or posterior triangle of the neck, and adenopathy in the presence of an unclear diagnosis are best treated by expedient excisional biopsy to exclude the possibility of malignancy. Diagnostic imaging may be helpful in distinguishing a solid versus cystic or mixed lesion.[16]

ANATOMY

The regional lymph node groups of the head and neck are shown in Figure 54-1. Drainage to lymphatic basins follows predictable, anatomic routes, with the nomenclature reflecting the site of the lymph nodes. The face and oropharynx drain predominantly to the preauricular, submandibular, and submental nodes; the posterior scalp drains to the occipital nodal group; and the mouth, tongue, tonsils, oropharynx, and nasopharynx drain to superficial and deep chains of the anterior cervical nodes. Significant lymphatic collateralization exists. A classification system for grouping cervical lymph nodes has been described by Shah and associates (Fig. 54-2).[49]

This scheme describes nodal groups as follows: level I—submental triangle nodes; levels II, III, and IV—upper, middle, and lower thirds of the internal jugular chain, respectively; level V—posterior cervical triangle nodes; level VI—tracheoesophageal groove nodes; and level VII—superior mediastinal nodes.

ACUTE LYMPHADENITIS

The most common cause of self-limiting, acute, inflammatory lymph node enlargement is a viral infection.[5] Acute bilateral cervical adenopathy is most often caused by a viral respiratory tract infection or streptococcal pharyngitis, whereas unilateral cervical lymphadenitis is usually caused by a streptococcal or staphylococcal infection in 40% to 80% of cases.[29] Bilateral lymphadenopathy secondary to viral infections usually resolves spontaneously. Acute suppurative lymphadenitis is typically caused by

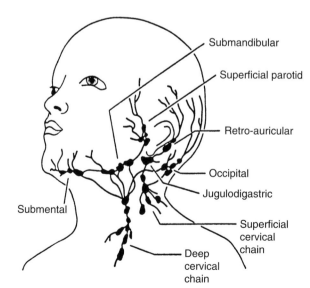

Figure 54–1 Regional lymph node groups of the head and neck. (From Bodenstein L, Altman RP: Cervical lymphadenitis in infants and children. Semin Pediatr Surg 1994;3:134. Used with permission.)

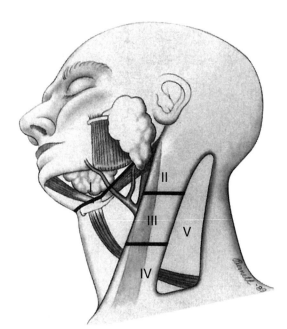

Figure 54–2 Lymphatic node levels of the neck. Level VI (tracheoesophageal) and level VII (superior mediastinum) groups are not shown. (From Shah JP, Medina JE, Shaha AR, et al: Cervical lymph node metastasis. Curr Prob Surg 1993;30:273. Used with permission.)

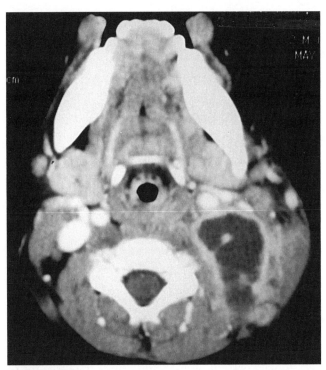

Figure 54–3 Although not necessary in the vast majority of cases, this CT scan demonstrates a deep cervical abscess from suppurative lymphadenitis. This 2-year-old child presented with diffuse unilateral cervical edema secondary to abscess, located posterior to the left carotid sheath.

bacterial infection from penicillin-resistant staphylococci, group A streptococci, or both.[3] *Staphylococcus* infection leading to lymphadenitis seems to occur more commonly in infants.[25] Anaerobic bacteria, group B streptococci, and *Haemophilus influenzae* type B are less frequent causal organisms.[8,20,47] Recently, a new pattern of resistance has been identified. Community-acquired methicillin-resistant, clindamycin-sensitive *Staphylococcus aureus* (MRSA) has been isolated from superficial abscesses and suppurative lymphadenitis in children.[29,41] Regardless of the causative bacterial agent, the local inflammatory signs of suppurative lymphadenitis strongly suggest the diagnosis. Children typically present with unilateral, tender adenopathy that involves the submandibular or deep cervical nodes (or both) draining the oropharynx. Erythema of the overlying skin may be present. Fever, malaise, and signs of systemic illness occur to varying extents. A careful search for a primary infection in the head and neck region, including the oropharynx and middle ear, should be conducted and treated appropriately.

Initial therapy for uncomplicated cervical lymphadenitis should begin with an empirical 5- to 10-day course of an oral, β-lactamase–resistant antibiotic. Most patients can be treated safely and effectively on an outpatient basis. If systemic signs of infection, including associated cellulitis, are present or if infection occurs in very young infants, intravenous antibiotics may be more clinically appropriate. Response of the infectious process should be observable within the first 72 hours of therapy. Failure to note clinical signs of improvement indicates the need for further diagnostic testing, including ultrasonography or fine-needle aspiration (FNA) of the involved mass.[6] The determination of the causative organism or organisms by aspirate culture allows for appropriate,

organism-specific antimicrobial therapy; however, FNA may require sedation or anesthesia to be performed safely in children. The aspirate should be sent for aerobic, anaerobic, and acid-fast bacterial stain and culture. Treatment should be based on aspirate results. If the aspirate reveals MRSA, clindamycin treatment should be used.[29,41]

Ultrasonography may help to differentiate between solid and cystic masses in the neck. In addition, identification of fluid associated with enlarged, inflammatory nodes may assist in determining the necessity for operative drainage. Other diagnostic methods such as computed tomography (CT) and magnetic resonance imaging (MRI) for suspected adenitis are unnecessary in most cases (Fig. 54-3). The enlarged lymph node will generally respond to appropriate antimicrobial therapy with prompt resolution of the lymphadenitis. The development of fluctuance caused by suppuration of the involved nodes can be effectively treated with repeated aspiration and antibiotics[7] or more definitively with open incision and drainage. In a retrospective study of 110 children, 95 had 107 cervical infectious sites drained surgically. The remaining 15 improved with medical therapy. CT accurately predicted operative findings in only 81 (76%) of cases. Of the 26 cases with a discrepancy between CT and operative findings, 18 showed false-positive findings in which the CT scan showed an abscess but only cellulitis was found at operation.[16]

ATYPICAL MYCOBACTERIAL ADENITIS

The genus *Mycobacterium* is characterized on light microscopy to be bacilli distinguished by their dense lipid capsules. The lipid capsules resist decolorization by acid alcohol after staining and thus are termed *acid-fast bacilli*.[1] Atypical mycobacteria are now the most common causative agents in mycobacterial lymphadenitis. The more common atypical mycobacteria include *M. avium-intracellulare, M. scrofulaceum, M. fortuitum,* and *M. chelonei*.[1] In contrast to tuberculous adenitis, atypical (or nontuberculous) mycobacterial adenitis is generally considered a local infectious process, without systemic involvement in immunocompetent hosts.[35] Disseminated disease is more commonly observed in patients with underlying acquired or congenital immunodeficiency states. Atypical mycobacterial adenitis is not contagious, and the portal of entry in otherwise healthy children is presumed to be the oropharynx.[2]

Atypical mycobacterial adenitis usually occurs in young children between 1 and 5 years of age. The common clinical presentation is focal, unilateral involvement of the jugulodigastric, preauricular, or submandibular nodal group. In contrast to acute suppurative lymphadenitis, the involved nodal group with atypical mycobacterial disease is minimally tender, firm, and rubbery to palpation, is well circumscribed, and may adhere to underlying structures. Although remarkably nontender, these lesions occasionally present as a draining sinus tract.[36] Signs of systemic illness or inflammation are usually minimal or nonexistent. Chest radiographs are typically normal.

Skin testing with tuberculin purified protein derivative (PPD) or old tuberculin (tine) in patients with atypical mycobacterial adenitis may yield an intermediate reaction resulting from cross-reactivity.[58] Specific, atypical mycobacterial antigens for skin testing have been developed[5,26] but are not widely available for clinical use. An in-vitro whole-blood assay measuring increased lymphocyte production of interferon-γ in patients with atypical mycobacterial adenitis has also been described.[15] FNA may yield acid-fast bacteria and provide a definitive diagnosis by aspirate culture. However, the preoperative clinical distinction between tuberculous and nontuberculous adenitis often remains difficult. Cervical lymphadenitis arising from infection with tuberculous and atypical mycobacteria has been reported but is extremely infrequent.[35] Unlike tuberculous adenitis, atypical mycobacterial adenitis generally does not respond to chemotherapy. The treatment of choice is complete surgical excision with primary wound closure.

In a literature review of the surgical treatment of atypical mycobacterial cervicofacial adenitis in children, excision, incision and drainage, curettage, and needle aspiration were compared among 16 studies. The cure rates were 92%, 10%, 86%, and 41%, respectively. Also, of 510 patients who underwent surgical excision, 11 transient and 1 permanent seventh nerve palsies were observed. Thirteen patients had persistent drainage after excision, and there were seven recurrences beneath the incision site.[18] At least 15 of 70 patients who underwent incision and drainage suffered draining sinuses. Of the 35 patients from four different studies who underwent curettage as treatment of atypical mycobacterial adenitis, 2 experienced delayed healing, in 1 a second curettage was necessary, and there was 1 recurrence.[18]

Incision and drainage alone should be avoided. Elliptical excision of the overlying skin, subcutaneous tissue, and the involved node is required; formal lymph node dissection is not necessary. Curettage is recommended only if surgical excision is not possible. A nerve stimulator may be helpful for lesions at the angle of the mandible to avoid injury to branches of the facial nerve. Antituberculous chemotherapy or patient isolation is not required for confirmed cases of atypical mycobacterial adenitis treated with adequate local excision.

MYCOBACTERIAL ADENITIS

Tuberculous lymphadenitis, or scrofula, is almost exclusively caused by *M. tuberculosis* in developed countries (Fig. 54-4). Before control of bovine tuberculosis, the predominant cause of tuberculous adenitis was *M. bovis*. Occasional cases of *M. bovis* are observed in patients from underdeveloped regions in which consumption of contaminated raw milk occurs. Patients proven to have human tuberculous adenitis often report previous exposure to a known carrier of tuberculosis,[48] but most patients have no evidence of active disease on a chest radiograph.[44] Tuberculous adenopathy is generally associated with other clinical symptoms and signs, including a strongly positive tuberculin PPD skin test and hilar adenopathy or apical calcification on a chest radiograph.[56] One study found a 92% sensitivity when two of three of the following criteria were fulfilled: positive PPD skin test, abnormal chest radiograph, or contact with someone with known infectious tuberculosis.[44] Tuberculous adenitis is therefore currently considered to be a local manifestation of a systemic disease and not an initial, primary focus of tuberculous infection.[5,10] Clinically, patients

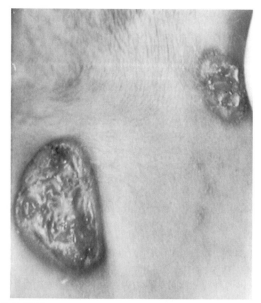

Figure 54–4 Cervical tuberculous adenitis (ear at right of photograph). Posterior cervical lymph nodes in a 7-year-old boy with a family history of contact and a positive PPD skin test. Medical management of tuberculosis with two-drug therapy for 7 months led to complete resolution. (From Jones PG: Glands of the neck. In Welch KJ, et al (eds): Pediatric Surgery, 4th ed. St. Louis, Mosby-Year Book, 1986. Used with permission.)

with tuberculous adenitis are usually older children and adolescents who present with nonsuppurative lymphadenitis,[31] which may be bilateral. A retrospective review of 24 immunocompetent children with tuberculous lymphadenitis showed that no patient had bilateral disease and the submandibular (29%) and the anterior cervical (71%) sites were the only areas of lymph node involvement.[44] However, posterior triangle nodal involvement does occur.[34]

The diagnosis of tuberculous adenitis can be made in the setting of an appropriate history, suspicious adenopathy associated with a strongly positive tuberculin PPD skin test, and positive acid-fast bacteria on stain or culture of nodal tissue. Diagnostic confirmation may be aided by FNA with aspirate culture and cytologic examination.[14,33] Rapid diagnosis of tuberculous adenitis by DNA amplification of nodal material using polymerase chain reaction (PCR) has been reported.[42] In contrast, a negative tuberculin PPD test essentially excludes the diagnosis of tuberculous adenitis. If a diagnostic dilemma persists, excisional biopsy in the operating room with the patient under general anesthesia is warranted. Incisional biopsy or incision and drainage should be avoided to prevent development of chronic, draining sinus tracts.[5,51,56] Fistula and cheloid formation can be seen in up to 100% of patients who underwent incision and drainage of tuberculous infected lymph nodes.[44]

Tuberculous adenitis generally responds to medical management that consists of multiple-agent chemotherapy. If tuberculous infection is directly observed, the World Health Organization recommends directly observed short-course therapy, which includes isoniazid, rifampin, and pyrazinamide for the first 2 months, followed by isoniazid and rifampin for an additional 4 months.[60] Although antituberculous chemotherapy remains essential, the role of complete surgical excision of involved nodes is more controversial.[6,12] Complete excision of involved nodes is prudent when biopsy is required for diagnosis; when a chronic, draining sinus tract evolves during medical treatment; or when optimal medical management fails.

CAT-SCRATCH DISEASE

Cat-scratch disease is a common cause of lymphadenitis in children, with an estimated incidence in the United States of 9.3 per 100,000 ambulatory pediatric and adult patients per year.[27] The highest age-specific incidence is among children younger than 10 years of age.[32] Current microbiologic and PCR-directed DNA analysis demonstrates that the pleomorphic, gram-negative bacillus *Bartonella henselae* (formerly *Rochalimaea*) is the causative organism of cat-scratch disease.[4,13,22] Most cases can be directly related to contact with a cat, and the usual site of inoculation is a limb. Subsequent adenitis occurs at regional lymphatic drainage basins (inguinal, axillary, epitrochlear nodes).[11] Similarly, cervical lymphadenopathy is observed with scratches in the head and neck region (Fig. 54-5). Although the primary manifestation of *B. henselae* infection is lymphadenopathy, some series report up to 25% of cases result in severe systemic illnesses.[30]

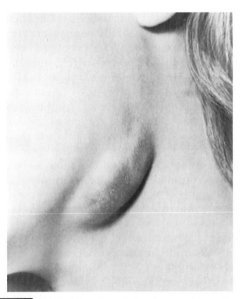

Figure 54-5 Cervical lymph node involvement in a patient with cat-scratch disease. The organism responsible for this infection is the pleomorphic, gram-negative bacillus *Bartonella henselae* (formerly *Rochalimaea*). (From Jones PG: Glands of the neck. In Welch KJ, et al [eds]: Pediatric Surgery, 4th ed. St. Louis, Mosby-Year Book, 1986. Used with permission.)

Initial infection occurs at a portal of entry in the skin, such as a scratch or bite. Papule formation may be observed at the site of inoculation in 3 to 5 days, with development of subacute lymphadenopathy at regional nodal drainage basins within 1 to 2 weeks. Early systemic symptoms of fever, malaise, myalgia, and anorexia are commonly reported. Although most cases involve the lymph node of the limbs, approximately 25% of cases involve the cervical lymph nodes.[11] Diagnosis based on a history of exposure to cats, presence of a site of inoculation (which may be healed by the time lymphadenopathy develops), and regional lymphadenopathy. Identification of *Bartonella* organisms from involved lymph nodes by Warthin-Starry silver impregnation stain has traditionally been used, but recently this stain has been found to be unreliable and found to lack species specificity.[40] PCR for *B. henselae* using paraffin sections from lymph nodes or other tissue is more reliable and accurate.[40] Because of its usual benign, self-limiting course, lymphadenopathy resolves in most cases within 6 to 8 weeks without specific treatment.[39] Suppuration is unusual. Excisional biopsy is generally unnecessary but may be warranted if a draining sinus tract develops or if the diagnosis is uncertain and the potential for malignancy cannot be excluded.

MISCELLANEOUS LESIONS

Various other infectious and inflammatory conditions can produce lymphadenopathy in infants and children. Most patients with these disorders do not require surgical management or, in particular, excisional biopsy of the lesions. A systematic approach to evaluation of these patients, including a thorough history, physical examination, and directed diagnostic tests, generally leads to the correct diagnosis. Surgical management of these lesions should be directed to patients who present diagnostic dilemmas, have nodal disease in suspicious areas (supraclavicular or posterior cervical triangle), or have persistent adenopathy despite adequate medical therapy.

Lymphadenopathies caused by infectious agents include toxoplasmosis (caused by *Toxoplasmosis gondii*), tularemia (caused by *Francisella tularensis*), and infectious mononucleosis (caused by Epstein-Barr virus).[28,53,57] Infection with *Actinomyces israelii* in the head and neck may lead to cervicofacial actinomycosis that is characterized by a woody, indurated cervical mass and development of chronic, draining fistulas. Direct involvement of the lymph nodes is uncommon, but the induration can make clinical differentiation difficult.[9] Infection with human immunodeficiency virus can produce generalized lymphadenopathy in infants and children.[17]

Other less frequent disorders that present as lymphadenopathies include Kawasaki disease or mucocutaneous lymph node syndrome. Kawasaki disease is a febrile disorder of childhood that is characterized in part by the abrupt onset of erythematous changes in the oropharyngeal mucosa; acute vasculitis; and extensive, nonsuppurative, nontender cervical adenopathy.[24] Histiocytic necrotizing lymphadenitis, or Kikuchi's disease, may present as cervical lymphadenopathy that resolves spontaneously. This disease can be clinically confused with malignant lymphadenopathy, and the patients often appropriately undergo diagnostic excisional lymph node biopsy for definitive diagnosis.[21] Castleman's disease, or giant lymph node hyperplasia, may also occasionally present as a solitary, enlarged cervical node.[45] These disorders do not require lymph node biopsy or excision.

Lymphomas are one of the more common malignant conditions in children. They may present as primary neck adenopathy that does not resolve with antibiotics or is enlarging. Patients with congenital or acquired immunodeficiency states, including human immunodeficiency virus infection, are at greater risk for developing malignant lymphoproliferative conditions.[17] The surgical management of Hodgkin's disease and non-Hodgkin's lymphoma is discussed in detail in Chapter 35. It is important to reiterate that although most neck masses in children are benign, a high index of suspicion regarding any neck mass that persists despite otherwise appropriate therapy must be maintained. Such masses must be assumed to be malignant until proven otherwise by excisional biopsy.

Although lymphoma is the most common malignant disorder manifested by cervical adenopathy, neuroblastoma and thyroid carcinoma are other childhood cancers that can also present as enlarged cervical lymph nodes. In neuroblastoma, cervical adenopathy is often bilateral. These patients have stage 4 disease, and the abdominal adrenal primary may not be palpable. After imaging of the chest, abdomen, and pelvis, if an abdominal primary tumor is detected, excisional biopsy of cervical lymph nodes may be done for initial diagnosis of stage 4 neuroblastoma (see Chapter 28). A child with metastatic thyroid carcinoma may present with unilateral cervical lymph node enlargement that should not be mistaken for ectopic thyroid gland. If thorough neck examination does not reveal a thyroid nodule, and a history of neck irradiation or other high-risk factors is obtained, thyroid ultrasound should be included in the evaluation of neck adenopathy.

REFERENCES

1. Albright JT, Pransky SM: Nontuberculous mycobacterial infections of the head and neck. Pediatr Clin North Am 2003;50:503-514.
2. Altman RP, Margileth AM: Cervical lymphadenopathy from atypical mycobacteria: Diagnosis and surgical treatment. J Pediatr Surg 1975;10:419.
3. Barton LL, Feigin RD: Childhood cervical lymphadenitis: A reappraisal. J Pediatr 1974;84:846.
4. Bergmans AM, Groothedde JW, Schellekens JF, et al: Etiology of cat-scratch disease: Comparison of polymerase chain reaction detection of *Bartonella* (formerly *Rochalimaea*) and *Afipia felis* DNA with serology and skin tests. J Infect Dis 1995;171:916.
5. Bodenstein L, Altman RP: Cervical lymphadenitis in infants and children. Semin Pediatr Surg 1994;3:134.
6. British Thoracic Society Research Committee: Short course chemotherapy for tuberculosis of lymph nodes: A controlled trial. BMJ 1985;290:1106.
7. Brodsky L, Belles W, Broday A, et al: Needle aspiration of neck masses in infants and children. Clin Pediatr 1992; 31:71.
8. Brook I: Aerobic and anaerobic bacteriology of cervical adenitis in children. Clin Pediatr 1980;19:693.
9. Burden P: Actinomycosis. J Infect 1989;19:95.
10. Cantrell RW, Jensen JH, Reid D: Diagnosis and management of tuberculous cervical adenitis. Arch Otolaryngol 1975;101:53.
11. Carithers HA: Cat-scratch disease: An overview based on the study of 1,200 patients. Am J Dis Child 1985;139:1124.
12. Castro DJ, Hoover L, Zuckerbraun L: Cervical mycobacterial lymphadenitis: Medical vs. surgical management. Arch Otolaryngol 1985;111:816.
13. Dalton MJ, Robinson LE, Cooper J, et al: Use of *Bartonella* antigens for serologic diagnosis of cat-scratch disease at a national referral center. Arch Intern Med 1995;155:1670.
14. Dasgupta A, Ghosh RN, Poddar AK, et al: Fine needle aspiration of cervical lymphadenopathy with special reference to tuberculosis. J Indian Med Assoc 1994;92:44.
15. Davidson PM, Creati K, Wood PR, et al: Lymphocyte production of gamma-interferon as a test for non-tuberculous mycobacterial lymphadenitis in childhood. Eur J Pediatr 1993;152:31.
16. Elden LM, Grundfast KM, Vezina G: Accuracy and usefulness of radiographic assessment of cervical neck infections in children. J Otolaryngol 2001;30:82.
17. Falloon J, Eddy J, Weinter K, Pizzo PA: Human immunodeficiency virus infection in children. J Pediatr 1989; 114:1.
18. Fergusson JAE, Simpson E: Surgical treatment of atypical mycobacterial cervicofacial adenitis in children. Aust NZ J Surg 1999;69:426.
19. Filston HC: Common lumps and bumps of the head and neck in infants and children. Pediatr Ann 1989;18:180.
20. Fishaut JM, Mokrohisky ST: Cervical lymphadenitis caused by *Haemophilus influenzae* type B. Am J Dis Child 1977; 131:925.
21. Fulcher AS: Cervical lymphadenopathy due to Kikuchi disease: US and CT appearance. J Comput Assist Tomogr 1993;17:131.

22. Goral S, Anderson B, Hager C, et al: Detection of *Rochalimaea henselae* DNA by polymerase chain reaction from suppurative nodes of children with cat-scratch disease. Pediatr Infect Dis J 1994;13:994.

23. Hartzog LW: Prevalence of lymphadenopathy of the head and neck in infants and children. Clin Pediatr 1983;22:485.

24. Hicks RV, Melish ME: Kawasaki syndrome. Pediatr Clin North Am 1986;33:1151.

25. Hieber JP, Davis AT: Staphylococcal cervical adenitis in young infants. Pediatrics 1976;57:424.

26. Huebner RE, Schein MF, Cauthern GM, et al: Usefulness of skin testing with mycobacterial antigens in children with cervical lymphadenopathy. Pediatr Infect Dis J 1992;11:450.

27. Jackson LA, Perkins BA, Wenger JD: Cat-scratch disease in the United States: An analysis of three national databases. Am J Public Health 1993;83:1707.

28. Jacobs RF, Condrey YM, Yamauchi T: Tularemia in adults and children: A changing presentation. Pediatrics 1985;76:818.

29. Johnigan RH, Periera KD, Poole MD: Community-acquired methicillin-resistant *Staphylococcus aureus* in children and adolescents: Changing trends. Arch Otolaryngol Head Neck Surg 2003;129:1049.

30. Kaplan S, Rawlings J, Paddock C, et al: Cat-scratch disease in children. MMWR 2002;51:212.

31. Lai KK, Stottmeier KD, Sherman IH, McCabe WR: Mycobacterial cervical lymphadenopathy: Relation of etiologic agents to age. JAMA 1984;251:1286.

32. Larsson LO, Bentzon MW, BergKelly K, Mellander L: Palpable lymph nodes of the neck in Swedish school children. Acta Paediatr 1994;83:1091.

33. Lau SK, Wei WI, Kwan S, Yew WW: Combined use of fine-needle aspiration cytologic examination and tuberculin skin test in the diagnosis of cervical tuberculous lymphadenitis. Arch Otolaryngol Head Neck Surg 1991;117:87.

34. Leung AK, Robson WL: Childhood cervical lymphadenopathy. J Pediatr Health Care 2004;18:3.

35. Lincoln EM, Gilbert LA: Disease in children due to mycobacteria other than *Mycobacterium tuberculosis*. Am Rev Respir Dis 1972;105:683.

36. Mair IWS, Elverland HH: Cervical mycobacterial infection. J Laryngol 1975;89:933.

37. Margileth AW: Management of nontuberculous (atypical) mycobacterial infections in children and adolescents. Pediatr Infect Dis 1985;4:119.

38. Margileth AM: Cat-scratch disease: No longer a diagnostic dilemma. Semin Vet Med Surg 1991;6:199.

39. Margileth AM: Antibiotic therapy for cat-scratch disease: Clinical study of therapeutic outcome in 268 patients and a review of the literature. Pediatr Infect Dis J 1992;11:474.

40. Margolis B, Kuzu I, Herrmann M, et al: Rapid polymerase chain reaction–based confirmation of cat-scratch disease and *Bartonella henselae* infection. Arch Pathol Lab Med 2003;127:706-710.

41. Martinez-Aguilar G, Hammerman WA, Mason EO Jr, Kaplan SL: Clindamycin treatment of invasive infections caused by community-acquired methicillin-resistant and methicillin-susceptible *Staphylococcus aureus* in children. Pediatr Infect Dis J 2003;22:593.

42. Narita M, Shibata M, Togashi T, Kobayashi H: Polymerase chain reaction for detection of *Mycobacterium tuberculosis*. Acta Pediatr 1992;81:141.

43. Ord RJ, Matz GJ: Tuberculosis cervical lymphadenitis. Arch Otolaryngol 1974;99:327.

44. Panagiotis S, Maltezou HC, Hantzakos A, et al: Mycobacterial cervical lymphadenitis in children: Clinical and laboratory factors of importance for differential diagnosis. Scand J Infect Dis 2001;33:362.

45. Penfold CN, Cottrell BJ, Talbot R: Neonatal giant lymph node hyperplasia (Castleman's disease) presenting in the head and neck. Br J Oral Maxillofac Surg 1991;29:110.

46. Piersimoni C, Felici L, Giorgi P, et al: Mixed mycobacterial infection of the cervical lymph nodes. Pediatr Infect Dis 1991;10:544.

47. Rathmore MH: Group B streptococcal cellulitis and adenitis concurrent with meningitis. Clin Pediatr 1989;28:411.

48. Schuit KE, Powell DA: Mycobacterial lymphadenitis in childhood. Am J Dis Child 1978;132:675.

49. Shah JP, Mdina JE, Shaha AR, et al: Cervical lymph node metastasis. Curr Prob Surg 1993;30:273.

50. Sigalet D, Lees G, Fanning A: Atypical tuberculosis in the pediatric patient: Implications for the pediatric surgeon. J Pediatr Surg 1992;27:1381.

51. Siu KF, Ng A, Wong J: Tuberculous lymphadenopathy: A review of results of surgical treatment. Aust NZ J Surg 1983;53:253.

52. Speck WT: Tuberculosis. In Behrman RE, et al (eds): Nelson Textbook of Pediatrics, 14th ed. Philadelphia, WB Saunders, 1992.

53. Sumaya CV, Ench Y: Epstein-Barr virus infectious mononucleosis in children: I. Clinical and laboratory findings. Pediatrics 1985;75:1003.

54. Taha AM, Davidson PT, Bailey WC: Surgical treatment of atypical mycobacterial lymphadenitis in children. Pediatr Infect Dis 1985;4:664.

55. Talmi YP, Cohen AH, Finkelstein Y, et al: *Mycobacterium tuberculosis* cervical adenitis: Diagnosis and management. Clin Pediatr 1989;28:408.

56. Telander RL, Filston HC: Review of head and neck lesions in infancy and childhood. Surg Clin North Am 1992;72:1429.

57. Thomaidis T, Anastassea-Vlachou K, Mandalenaki-Lambrou C, et al: Chronic lymphoglandular enlargement and toxoplasmosis in children. Arch Dis Child 1977;52:403.

58. Tomblin JL, Roberts FJ: Tuberculous cervical lymphadenitis. Can Med Assoc J 1979;121:324.

59. Wear DJ, Margileth AM, Hadfield TL, et al: Cat-scratch disease: A bacterial infection. Science 1983;221:1403.

60. World Health Organization: Global Tuberculosis Program: Global Tuberculosis Control. WHO report 1997, publication WHO/TB/225. Geneva, World Health Organization, 1997.

Chapter 55

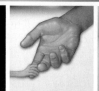

Surgical Diseases of the Thyroid and Parathyroid Glands

Michael A. Skinner

Diseases of the thyroid or parathyroid gland are uncommon in the pediatric age group. In one population-based study of school-aged children in the United States, thyroid disease prevalence was 36.7 per 1000 individuals.[36] Diffuse gland hypertrophy (goiter) was the most common diagnosis, occurring in about half of cases, and thyroiditis was the second most common abnormality. Thyroid nodules and thyroid hormone level disorders were less common, and malignant neoplasms were exceedingly rare; only two cases of papillary thyroid carcinoma were found in this population of nearly 5000 children observed clinically for 3 years.

Surgical evaluation or treatment of thyroid disease may be necessary in patients with benign or malignant neoplasia or in children exhibiting a physiologic abnormality, such as increased hormone secretion.

EMBRYOLOGY

The thyroid gland is the first endocrine organ to mature in embryologic development, arising at about 24 days' gestation as an outpouching of the embryonic alimentary tract at the primitive pharyngeal floor. As the embryo enlarges, the developing thyroid gland descends into the neck from the base of the tongue, passing ventrally to the hyoid bone and the laryngeal cartilages, and maintaining a tubular connection to the tongue known as the thyroglossal duct. The opening of this duct into the base of the tongue is called the foramen cecum. Typically, the thyroglossal duct changes from a hollow structure to a solid diverticulum; the original opening into the oropharynx usually remains as a blind pit at the base of the tongue. The thyroid gland has usually reached its final location in the neck by 7 weeks' gestation. Accessory thyroid tissue originating from remnants of the thyroglossal duct may appear in the tongue or anywhere along the course of caudal migration during development. Of occasional surgical importance, the gland fails to descend altogether, resulting in a lingual thyroid. Incomplete descent results in the gland appearing high in the neck or near the hyoid bone.

Histologically, in about the tenth week of gestation, the primordial thyroid cells begin to form discrete cords that further differentiate to form small cellular groups. Colloid begins to form, and thyroxine can be demonstrated in the embryo in about the 11th week. Early in the development of the thyroid gland, the ventral portions of the fourth pharyngeal pouches develop into the ultimobranchial bodies. These structures contain neural crest cells that fuse with the embryonic thyroid gland to form the parafollicular cells or C cells.

The parathyroid glands derive from the third and fourth pharyngeal pouches beginning in about the fifth week of gestation. During the sixth week of development, the parathyroid glands associated with the third pair of pharyngeal pouches migrate caudally with the thymic primordium, finally coming to rest on the dorsal surface of the thyroid gland low in the neck. The parathyroid glands arising from the fourth pharyngeal pouches also descend in the neck, ultimately coming to rest at a position superior to the glands derived from the third pouches. Functioning chief cells are active during fetal development to assist in regulating calcium metabolism.

PHYSIOLOGY

Production of thyroid hormone occurs in the thyroid gland at the interface between the follicular cell and the thyroglobulin or colloid. The initial step in thyroid synthesis is the iodination of tyrosine molecules to form either monoiodotyrosine, if there is one iodine molecule attached, or diiodotyrosine, if two iodine molecules are bound. These iodinated tyrosine molecules are then coupled to form the definitive thyroid hormones triiodothyronine (T_3) and thyroxine (T_4). If monoiodotyrosine is attached to diiodotyrosine, then T_3 results; two diiodotyrosines bound together constitute a T_4 molecule.

The thyroid gland secretes primarily T_4; approximately 80% of the T_3 in the circulation represents metabolized T_4, which has been partially deiodinated in the liver, kidney, or other peripheral tissues. In the circulation, most of the thyroid hormones are protein bound to increase their solubility. The most abundant hormone carrier is thyroid-binding globulin (TBG); other carriers include prealbumin and albumin. Because the protein-bound thyroid hormone is physiologically inactive, the plasma levels of these proteins must be considered when evaluating patients for abnormalities of thyroid function. Whereas T_4 is nearly 50-fold more concentrated in the plasma than T_3, the latter moiety binds much more avidly to the thyroid receptor and therefore accounts for most of the physiologic effect of thyroid hormone.

The production and secretion of T_3 and T_4 by the thyroid gland is chiefly controlled by thyroid-stimulating hormone (TSH). This protein is secreted by the anterior pituitary gland, principally in response to thyrotropin-releasing hormone (TRH), which is secreted by the hypothalamus. Under the influence of TSH, thyroid follicular cells extend pseudopods into the colloid to encircle the thyroglobulin and form vesicles that then fuse with protease-containing lysosomes. The thyroglobulin is then subjected to hydrolysis and proteolysis to release free thyroxine into the circulation.

NON-NEOPLASTIC THYROID CONDITIONS

The evaluation of a child with thyroid disease should begin with a physical examination of the neck to assess the size and consistency of the gland. Diffuse enlargement makes the diagnosis of simple colloid goiter more likely; or if the child is hyperthyroid, Graves' disease should be suspected. Chronic lymphocytic (Hashimoto's) thyroiditis is classically associated with a gland that feels granular or pebbly. Firmness in the gland suggests an infiltrative process, whereas a very hard gland is more suggestive of neoplasia. Tenderness in the thyroid gland is most commonly associated with an acute inflammatory process. Finally, the presence of enlarged neck lymph nodes should be noted; thyroid carcinoma may be associated with local metastases before the primary tumor can be palpated.

Laboratory tests are essential to assess for altered thyroid function. The TSH is elevated in hypothyroid states. The plasma free T_4 level is an accurate measure of the biologically active hormone, because it is generally unaffected by the amount of protein binding in the circulation. Conversely, when plasma total T_3 and T_4 are measured, an evaluation of TBG may be necessary to gauge the level of biologically active (unbound) hormone. Plasma levels of TBG are altered in a number of conditions, affecting the level of total thyroxine. In particular, TBG is increased in the neonatal period and decreased in the presence of exogenous glucocorticoids, androgens, and anabolic corticosteroids. Other medications that affect thyroxine metabolism include phenytoin and phenobarbital, which induce hepatic degradation of T_4 and decrease hormone binding to TBG. Finally, there exist rare conditions in which the TBG level is congenitally altered.

Several radiologic modalities are available to assist in imaging the thyroid gland. Ultrasonography is increasingly used to assess for thyroid cysts and in the evaluation of multinodular glands. This modality is especially useful in the serial evaluation of nodules managed nonoperatively. Radionuclide scintigraphy is another commonly used test. The three nuclides usually available for diagnostic imaging include iodine-123 (^{123}I), iodine-131 (^{131}I), and technetium-99m (^{99m}Tc). The radioiodines are most effective in detecting ectopic thyroid tissue or metastatic thyroid carcinoma, whereas ^{99m}Tc-pertechnetate is thought by some radiologists to enable superior imaging of thyroid gland nodules or tumors.

Hypothyroidism

Disorders of hypothyroidism are rarely treated surgically and may result from a defect anywhere in the hypothalamic-pituitary-thyroid axis. In rare cases, a hypothyroid state may be seen in conditions of thyroid hormone unresponsiveness, such as when there is a defect in the thyroid receptor gene; in such cases, the plasma thyroxine level is often elevated.

The most common cause of hypothyroidism diagnosed in neonatal screening programs is thyroid gland dysgenesis, accounting for approximately 90% of these patients. In about a third of these infants, no thyroid tissue is seen on radionuclide scanning; in the rest of the patients, a rudimentary gland may be found in an ectopic location, such as at the base of the tongue. Children with complete thyroid agenesis are often asymptomatic at birth, owing to the transplacental passage of maternal thyroid hormone through development. In some cases, ectopically located thyroid tissue may supply a sufficient amount of thyroxine for years or the diminutive gland may fail in childhood. Such conditions may come to clinical attention with the discovery of a sublingual or midline neck mass, and surgeons should be mindful of this possibility when evaluating children with neck masses. Consideration should be given to performing radionuclide thyroid scanning before removing any unusual neck mass to ensure that the functioning thyroid tissue is not accidentally resected.

Goiter and Thyroiditis

A goiter is found in about 3% of the population when children are specifically surveyed for abnormalities of the thyroid gland.[36] Goiters may be classified as either diffusely enlarged or nodular, and they may be associated with normal hormone secretion or thyrotoxicosis. The differential diagnosis of diffuse thyroid enlargement is listed in Table 55-1. Physiologically, diffuse goiters may be related to autoimmune diseases or as a response to a nonautoimmune inflammatory condition, or the enlargement may be a compensation for some defect in hormone production. Most children with goiters are euthyroid, and surgical resection is rarely indicated.

In a population-based study of over 5000 Croatian schoolchildren, thyromegaly was found in 2.78% of the subjects.[19] The causes of thyroid enlargement in this population are presented in Table 55-2. As in other populations with adequate dietary iodine intake, most of these patients had simple colloid goiter, also frequently called

TABLE 55-1 Differential Diagnosis of Goiter in Children

Autoimmune Mediated
Chronic lymphocytic (Hashimoto's) thyroiditis
Graves' disease
Simple colloid goiter

Compensatory
Iodine deficiency
Medications
Goitrogens
Hormone or receptor defect

Inflammatory Conditions
Acute suppurative thyroiditis
Subacute thyroiditis

adolescent goiter or nontoxic goiter. The diagnosis is established after normal levels of TSH and thyroid hormone are documented and when the diffuse nature of the goiter is documented scintigraphically or by ultrasound. The natural history of colloid goiter is not well known, but in one study in which adolescents with the condition were reevaluated some 20 years later, nearly 60% of the glands were found to be normal in size.[36] The spontaneous rate of colloid goiter resolution was not significantly different than the response rate in children treated with exogenous thyroid hormone. Thus, simple colloid goiters should generally not undergo any specific treatment. In rare cases, surgical resection of the gland may be indicated if there are symptoms related to the size of the goiter, if there is a suspicion of neoplasia, or for cosmetic reasons.

Chronic lymphocytic thyroiditis, also known as Hashimoto's thyroiditis, is another common cause of diffusely enlarged thyroid glands in children. This condition occurs most commonly in adolescent females and is part of the spectrum of autoimmune thyroid disorders. Indeed, the condition is associated with the presence of other autoimmune disorders such as juvenile rheumatoid arthritis, Addison's disease, and type 1 diabetes mellitus. Patients are usually euthyroid and slowly progress to become hypothyroid. Approximately 10% of these patients are

TABLE 55-2 Etiology of Thyroid Gland Enlargement in 5462 Croatian Schoolchildren

Diagnosis	Frequency (%)
Simple goiter	2.3
Chronic lymphocytic thyroiditis	0.35
Graves' disease	0.07
Benign adenoma	0.04
Cyst	0.02
Total	2.78

Adapted from Jaksic J, Dumic M, Filipovic B, et al: Thyroid disease in a school population with thyromegaly. Arch Dis Child 1994;70:103-103.

hyperthyroid; this condition has been termed *hashitoxicosis*. Patients with chronic lymphocytic thyroiditis are characterized by high titers of the circulating antithyroglobulin and antimicrosomal autoantibodies, which are presumably responsible for the B-lymphocytic infiltrate found in the thyroid gland on histologic evaluation.

Children with chronic lymphocytic thyroiditis generally come to clinical evaluation because of thyroid gland enlargement. The gland is generally pebbly or granular and may be mildly tender, and the diagnosis may be established by the discovery of high-titer antithyroid antibodies in association with the proper clinical and laboratory circumstances. Plasma thyroid hormone levels are generally not very useful, but the TSH level may be elevated in 70% of patients. Thyroid ultrasound demonstrates diffuse hypoechogenicity, and scintigraphy shows a patchy uptake of the tracer. In rare cases, fine-needle aspiration (FNA) of the gland may be needed to confirm the diagnosis if autoantibodies cannot be detected. The management of chronic lymphocytic thyroiditis is usually expectant; as many as a third of adolescent patients with the condition will resolve spontaneously, with normalization of gland size and disappearance of the antithyroid antibodies. Administration of thyroid hormone to euthyroid patients has not been shown to be useful in reducing the size of the goiter and is thus probably not indicated.[39] Thyroid function studies should be obtained every 6 months, and exogenous hormone should be administered if hypothyroidism develops.

Subacute (de Quervain's) thyroiditis is caused by a viral infection and is very rarely seen in children. Physical findings include tender, painful swelling of the thyroid gland. Usually, there is mild thyrotoxicosis owing to injury to the thyroid follicles with leakage of thyroid hormone into the circulation. Radioactive iodine uptake is decreased, as a result of thyroid follicular cell dysfunction; this finding distinguishes subacute thyroiditis from Graves' disease. Histologically, granulomas and epithelioid cells may be seen. Treatment is symptomatic and generally consists of nonsteroidal anti-inflammatory agents or corticosteroids. The disease usually lasts 2 to 9 months, and complete recovery may be expected.

Acute suppurative thyroiditis is caused by a bacterial infection of the gland, and the patient may have evidence of sepsis, with an acutely inflamed thyroid gland. Patients are usually euthyroid. The offending organisms are usually staphylococci or mixed aerobic and anaerobic flora. There may be a congenital pharyngeal sinus tract predisposing to infection. Treatment consists of antibiotics; if an abscess develops, incision and drainage may be necessary. The thyroid gland may be expected to recover completely.

Hyperthyroidism

With rare exceptions, hyperthyroidism of childhood is caused by Graves' disease, which is also termed *diffuse toxic goiter*. Other possible causes of this condition are listed in Table 55-3. In these patients, the onset of the condition may be delayed until 2 to 3 weeks after birth.

TABLE 55-3 Causes of Hyperthyroidism in Children

Graves' disease (toxic diffuse goiter)
Toxic nodular goiter
Subacute thyroiditis
Chronic lymphocytic thyroiditis
Neonatal thyroiditis
Thyroid-secreting hormone–secreting pituitary tumor
McCune-Albright syndrome
Thyrotropin receptor mutation

Graves' disease occurs in girls about five times more often than in boys, and the incidence steadily increases throughout childhood, peaking in the adolescent years. The condition usually develops insidiously over several months, and initial symptoms include nervousness, emotional lability, and declining school performance. Later in the course of the disease there will be weight loss and increased sweating, palpitations, heat intolerance, and malaise. True exophthalmos is an unusual finding in children, but a conspicuous stare is common. The thyroid gland is smooth, firm, and nontender, and a goiter is evident on physical examination in over 95% of cases. A bruit may be heard on auscultation. Laboratory evaluation usually demonstrates elevated free T_4 and a decreased TSH. In 10% to 20% of patients there is only elevation of T_3, a condition known as T_3 toxicosis. The diagnosis of Graves' disease is further supported by the presence of TSH-stimulating immunoglobulins.

Graves' disease is an autoimmune disease caused by TSH receptor antibodies, which stimulate the thyroid follicles to increase iodide uptake and induce increased production and secretion of thyroid hormone. It has been suggested that the TSH-binding proteins are present in a number of gram-positive and gram-negative bacteria, and it is possible that infection with such organisms may elicit production of antibodies that cross-react with the TSH receptor.[47] An infectious cause of Graves' disease is further supported by some epidemiologic reports of disease clustering.[33]

Graves' disease is currently managed by antithyroid medications, or the thyroid gland is ablated using either radioactive ^{131}I or surgical resection.[11] Most pediatric endocrinologists initiate therapy with antithyroid medications, although there is increasing use of radioablation as the first line of treatment.[26] The most commonly used antithyroid medications are methimazole or propylthiouracil (PTU), which reduce thyroid hormone production by inhibiting follicle cell organification of iodide and coupling of iodotyrosines. Methimazole is usually the preferred antithyroid medication because of its longer half-life and increased potency. The initial dose is 30 mg once daily, which should be reduced if the patient is younger than the usual adolescent. The TSH should be monitored carefully; rising levels signal overtreatment and may cause further increase in the goiter size. When the patient is euthyroid, as determined by normal T_3 and T_4 levels, the dose of methimazole should be reduced to 10 mg and maintained at a level to ensure normal thyroid hormone levels.

The most serious side effect of methimazole is an idiosyncratic agranulocytosis. This can occur at any time during the course of treatment or even during a second course of the drug. The onset of a sore throat with fevers should raise concern, and a neutrophil count should be obtained. Typically, the granulocyte count will rise 2 to 3 weeks after stopping the drug, but in rare cases, fatal opportunistic infections have been reported. Treatment with parenteral antibiotics during the recovery period has been recommended. Other adverse reactions to methimazole include nausea, minor skin reactions, urticaria, arthralgias, arthritis, and fevers.

The length of medical treatment is controversial. Usually, treatment is continued for 3 to 4 years. Remission of Graves' disease is approximately 25% if medication is discontinued after 2 years of treatment, and the continuing remission rate is about 25% every 2 years. In most children, the remission of Graves' disease will occur within 6 months of discontinuing antithyroid therapy. The resolution rate is decreased in children who have persistent detection of TSH receptor antibodies during and after treatment. In patients with Graves' disease who do not respond to treatment with antithyroid medications, or if there is a severe reaction to the medication, then the thyroid gland must undergo definitive ablation. Current methods of definitively treating Graves' disease include either surgical resection or ablation with radioactive ^{131}I. Neither of these modalities is without complications. Whereas ^{131}I therapy is effective, and the disease remission rate is low, patients have a 50% to 80% incidence of long-term hypothyroidism after treatment.[3] In some cases, larger doses of radioiodine have been administered to intentionally destroy the entire gland and to induce an easily managed state of permanent hypothyroidism.[26] Recent studies demonstrate there is no scientific merit to concerns over the possibility of teratogenic or carcinogenic effects of ^{131}I therapy in these younger patients.[9,22]

Surgical treatment may be occasionally recommended for pediatric patients with Graves' disease refractory to medical treatment. Subtotal thyroidectomy is the surgical procedure of choice for the treatment of Graves' disease and is appropriate treatment for patients who refuse radioiodine treatment or who fail medical management or if the thyroid is so large that there are symptoms related to compression. Patients should be rendered euthyroid with methimazole before undergoing surgery. Moreover, β-adrenergic blocking agents such as propranolol may be used to ameliorate the adrenergic symptoms of hyperthyroidism. Finally, iodine in the form of Lugol's solution, 5 to 10 drops/day, should be administered for 4 to 7 days before surgery to reduce the vascularity of the gland. In large studies of adults treated with a subtotal thyroidectomy for Graves' disease, the rate of recurrent hyperthyroidism is 6% to 10% at 10 years' follow-up.[3] Patients continue to relapse even later, and 30% of patients will exhibit recurrent hyperthyroidism 25 years after their subtotal thyroidectomy.[11] There is also a significant risk of permanent hypothyroidism in these patients, affecting approximately 5% of patients 1 year after surgery, increasing to as high as 50% of patients who are observed for 25 years. These findings demonstrate the importance of carefully observing such patients postoperatively to monitor thyroid status.

NEOPLASTIC THYROID CONDITIONS

Thyroid Nodules

Thyroid nodules are uncommon in children but can be the presenting finding in cases of thyroid cancer. In recent pediatric studies, the incidence of malignancy in thyroid nodules has been 20% or less.[2,8,16,53] This is a much lower incidence of cancer than was reported in previous decades and probably reflects the decreased number of children who have been exposed to neck irradiation for trivial reasons. It is important to properly evaluate and manage these lesions, because the cancer may be at an easily curable stage. A summary of pathologic results from recent studies of children who underwent surgery for thyroid nodules is presented in Table 55-4.

The differential diagnosis of solitary thyroid nodules is listed in Table 55-5. In most large pediatric series, females having nodules outnumber males approximately 2 to 1.[53] The majority of patients will come to clinical attention because of the mass in their neck. A careful neck examination should be performed, with special attention directed to determine if there are enlarged cervical lymph nodes suspicious for locally advanced carcinoma. The serum TSH level should be measured to identify patients with unsuspected thyrotoxicosis resulting from an autonomously functioning nodule. Imaging studies are

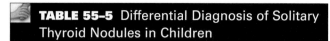

TABLE 55-5 Differential Diagnosis of Solitary Thyroid Nodules in Children

Adenoma
Carcinoma
Thyroid cyst
Ectopic thyroid gland
Cystic hygroma
Thyroglossal duct remnant
Germ cell tumor

unreliable at distinguishing benign from malignant nodules. For example, malignant nodules may be either functioning or nonfunctioning on thyroid scintiscan. Ultrasonography is also nondiagnostic because malignant nodules may be either solid or cystic. Thus, such imaging studies should be interpreted carefully in the evaluation of thyroid nodules in pediatric patients. A therapeutic trial of exogenous thyroid hormone to induce nodule regression is not recommended.

The use of FNA cytology to evaluate thyroid nodules is well established in adults, but the effectiveness of this technique is still being defined in children. Children are usually more difficult to evaluate than adults, owing to the smaller size of the nodules and the frequent need to sedate the child to allow safe and accurate aspiration. Moreover, the effectiveness of any diagnostic test is in part dependent on the pretest probability of a positive result. Because in young children there is a higher incidence of cancer in any thyroid nodule (when compared with adults), there is a slightly increased probability of a negative cytologic result that in fact may be associated with cancer. Such a false-negative cytologic result would delay the diagnosis and treatment of thyroid cancer. However, in light of the overall good clinical outcome in children with differentiated thyroid neoplasia, it must be acknowledged that such a delay will probably not result in any negative impact on survival.

In adolescent patients, thyroid nodules may be safely evaluated with FNA. The pattern of thyroid disease in the adolescent age group is similar to that of adults, in whom the safety of FNA has been established. In one large series, the incidence of malignancy in thyroid nodules in patients from 13 to 18 years old was only 11%.[53] In another study of 57 children with thyroid nodules evaluated by FNA, the incidence of malignancy was 18%.[34] There was one papillary carcinoma initially misdiagnosed as a benign lesion, which was eventually recognized as a malignancy with clinical follow-up. In another study of 57 children subjected to FNA for the evaluation of thyroid nodules, there was a similar incidence of cancer and 1 child initially had a false-negative FNA. In this case, the nodule was noted to increase in size over the ensuing 6 months, and excisional biopsy demonstrated the presence of Hürthle cell carcinoma.[20] Thus, these studies in mostly adolescent patients support the safety and effectiveness of FNA in this population.

The results of FNA cytology either will indicate unequivocal cancer or a benign lesion or the diagnosis will be indeterminant for carcinoma. If the nodule is

TABLE 55-4 Diagnoses in Pediatric Patients Who Had Surgical Resection for Thyroid Nodules

	Yip et al., 1994	Lafferty and Batch, 1997
No. of patients	122	52
No. malignant (%)	16* (13)	17 (33)
Histologic subtype		
Papillary	12	7
Follicular	3	7
Mixed	0	0
Anaplastic	0	0
Medullary	0	3
No. benign (%)	106 (87)	35 (67)
Diagnosis		
Thyroiditis	17	1
Thyroglossal cyst	0	2
Follicular adenoma	26	16
Colloid nodule	57	2
Branchial cyst	0	0
Other	6	14

*One patient in this series had lymphoma of the thyroid gland.
Data from Yip FWK, Reeve TS, Poole AG, Delbridge L: Thyroid nodules in childhood and adolescence. Aust NZ J Surg 1994;64:676-678; and Lafferty AR, Batch JA: Thyroid nodules in childhood and adolescence—thirty years of experience. J Pediatr Endocrinol Metab 1997;10:479-486.

judged to be benign, then it can be followed with serial physical examinations and with ultrasound studies. Surgical resection should be performed if the nodule is malignant or indeterminant or if a benign nodule is shown to increase in size. Some endocrinologists suppress benign thyroid nodules with exogenous thyroid hormone, but this has not been shown to alter the natural history of such nodules. If a cystic lesion disappears after aspiration, then surgery may be deferred. The lesion should be removed if it recurs. Whereas cyst fluid may be sent for cytologic analysis, the sensitivity of this test is probably low for detecting the presence of cancer.[25]

In prepubertal children, there is increased difficulty in obtaining aspiration cytology and the pattern of benign disease is different than adults; thus, the natural history of these lesions is unknown and the safety of nonoperative treatment has not been demonstrated. Therefore, it is recommended that all thyroid nodules be removed in children younger than 13 years. Some surgeons obtain preoperative ultrasound examination and thyroid scintigraphy as an aid in determining the anatomy.[16,27] It cannot be overstated that if there is any question about the reliability of the cytologic evaluation, then excisional biopsy of all thyroid nodules irrespective of patient age should be performed.

Thyroid Carcinoma

Carcinoma of the thyroid gland is relatively unusual in children, and population-based studies in Wales and Los Angeles demonstrate that the yearly incidence of thyroid carcinoma is between 1 and 2 cases per million individuals younger than 20 years of age.[14,32] This represents only about 3% of all pediatric malignancies. The peak incidence of thyroid cancer in children occurs between 10 and 18 years of age, and girls usually outnumber boys 2 to 1. Approximately 10% of all malignant thyroid tumors occur in children. The incidence of thyroid tumors in children has decreased over the past 2 decades owing to the reduced use of radiation to treat benign diseases. The importance of radiation as a cause of thyroid cancer was recently reemphasized by the marked increase of such tumors noted in the Republic of Belarus following the 1986 Chernobyl nuclear power plant catastrophe.[29,31] The latency period for the development of thyroid cancer after radiation exposure is 4 to 6 years, and in the Belarus population there was a 62-fold increase in thyroid tumor incidence after the Chernobyl accident.

Thyroid carcinoma also occurs at an increased incidence after treatment for a previous childhood malignancy. In one study, thyroid cancers constituted about 9% of second malignancies occurring after treatment for childhood tumors.[45] Hodgkin's lymphoma is the most common first malignancy associated with the subsequent development of thyroid cancer, and most thyroid neoplasms follow the previous use of radiation to the neck, but alkylating agents alone also predispose to thyroid cancer. The median interval from radiation therapy to the recognition of thyroid disease is about 12 years,[1] underscoring the importance of careful surveillance for second tumors in children who have been successfully treated for cancer.

Recent research has elucidated some of the genetic events responsible for the neoplastic process in thyroid tumors. The *RET* proto-oncogene, a receptor tyrosine kinase molecule located on the 10th chromosome, is frequently rearranged in papillary cancers so that the intracellular portion of the gene is juxtaposed to one of several ubiquitously expressed genes. The fusion genes are termed *RET/PTC* and exhibit increased expression of the tyrosine kinase activity of the molecule. These genetic rearrangements involving RET are especially frequent in radiation-induced thyroid tumors. After the Chernobyl accident, children from Belarus with thyroid cancer were found to exhibit *RET* fusion genes in over 62% of cases.[35] In some studies, the particular *RET* fusion gene combination has been correlated with particular histologic subtypes.[41]

The *RET* proto-oncogene is also important in the development of medullary thyroid carcinoma (MTC), and various mutations in *RET* are associated with the multiple endocrine neoplasia type 2 syndromes (MEN 2A, MEN 2B) and familial medullary thyroid carcinoma (FMTC). MTC is usually the first tumor to develop in these patients. Moreover, as many as 40% of patients with sporadic nonfamilial MTCs possess *RET* mutations.[10] The *RET* mutations in the susceptible tissues perturb the intracellular signaling pathways to alter the proliferation or differentiation of the neural crest–derived tissues involved in the MEN 2 syndromes.

Carcinoma of the thyroid gland typically presents clinically as a thyroid mass, as enlarged cervical lymph nodes, or with both of these findings. In one large clinical study of thyroid carcinoma in children, the more recently diagnosed patients were somewhat less likely to have enlarged regional lymph nodes at their initial presentation.[13] A compilation of the clinical aspects of several recent, large clinical series of pediatric patients with differentiated thyroid carcinoma is presented in Table 55-6. The pathologic diagnosis can be established either using FNA cytology or by frozen-section analysis of a biopsy specimen at the time of surgery. Recent studies have suggested that frozen-section analysis is less accurate in evaluating follicular lesions. As shown in Table 55-6, most of these patients will have papillary thyroid carcinoma. Before surgery, most children should have a thyroid scan, to determine if the thyroid mass contains functioning thyroid tissue. Some investigators also recommend an ultrasound study to determine if the lesion is cystic and to serve as a guide during the surgical procedure.[27] Because of the relatively high incidence of pulmonary metastasis in children having thyroid carcinoma, preoperative chest radiography or computed tomography should be performed.

The surgical management of thyroid cancer in children is controversial, because there have been no prospective clinical trials comparing more aggressive to less extensive surgical management options. As shown in Table 55-6, the long-term outcome is usually excellent, irrespective of the particular surgical procedure employed. Surgeons arguing in favor of aggressive thyroid resections hold that total thyroidectomy, with lymph node dissection if the regional nodes are involved with cancer, is the most successful method of obtaining local control of the tumor.[5,13,28,42]

TABLE 55-6 Clinical Aspects of Differentiated Thyroid Cancer in Children from a Large Pediatric Series

Total number of patients	329
Mean age	15.2
Percent female	76
Histology	
Papillary	297
Follicular	32
Medullary	0
Other	0
% With metastasis	74
Surgical procedure	
Total thyroidectomy	178
Subtotal thyroidectomy	55
Lobectomy or other	96
Lymph node procedure	255
% Receiving radiotherapy	43
Median follow-up (yr)	11.3
Cancer mortality (%)	0.7

Data from Newman KD, Black T, Heller G, et al: Differentiated thyroid cancer: Determinants of disease progression in patients <21 years of age at diagnosis: A report of the Surgical Discipline Committee of the Children's Cancer Group. Ann Surg 1998;227:533-541.

Moreover, removing the entire thyroid gland makes adjuvant radioiodine ablative therapy more effective, because there is less functioning normal thyroid tissue to compete with remaining tumor for the uptake of radionuclide. Finally, if all of the thyroid gland has been removed or ablated, then the serum thyroglobulin levels can be used to assess for tumor recurrence.

Surgeons favoring lesser thyroid gland resection argue that differentiated thyroid carcinoma in children is a relatively indolent disease and that survival is apparently not related to the extent of gland removal.[24,54] Moreover, there is an increased incidence of major surgical complications associated with total thyroidectomy in children. For example, the reported incidence of recurrent laryngeal nerve injury is 0% to 24%[13] and the reported frequency of permanent hypocalcemia is 6% to 27%.[7,13,24] Such complications are reported to occur less commonly in the more recent clinical series.[13]

In one retrospective study of 329 children treated for differentiated thyroid cancer there was multivariate analysis of the factors predicting early disease recurrence.[28] The only disease or treatment features significantly predictive of early recurrence were a lower age at diagnosis and the presence of residual neck disease after surgery. Children older than 15 years of age at diagnosis were less likely to experience tumor recurrence than younger children. After a median follow-up of 11.3 years, the tumor recurrence rate after treatment was 32% and there were only two cancer-related deaths. The overall progression-free survival of patients with differentiated thyroid cancer in this series was 67% at 10 years and 60% at 20 years after diagnosis. Factors not affecting progression-free survival included extent of thyroid surgery or node dissection, primary tumor size, extrathyroidal extension of tumor, regional lymph node involvement, distant metastases, use of ^{131}I radiotherapy in the initial management, or the antecedent exposure to radiation.[28] On balance, it appears that tumor factors may be more important than treatment factors in determining the clinical outcome in children having differentiated thyroid cancer.

Therefore, in the absence of controlled prospective trials, it is difficult to make firm recommendations regarding the surgical management of differentiated thyroid cancer in children. However, a consensus is emerging that more aggressive resections are preferred.[17] Surgeons and pediatric endocrinologists increasingly recommend either total or near-total thyroidectomy, followed by ^{131}I remnant ablation in conjunction with long-term suppressive thyroxine therapy. A modified neck dissection should be performed to remove as much gross disease as possible if there are large lymph nodes suggestive of the presence of regional metastasis. In patients with locally advanced disease, it is especially important to remove as much of the thyroid gland as possible to allow subsequent scanning and re-treatment with radioiodine as necessitated by tumor recurrence. Tumors involving the recurrent laryngeal nerve should not be aggressively resected to sacrifice the nerve, because residual tumor on the nerve can be adequately treated with radioiodine.

The risk of major surgical complications increases with the extent of the surgical procedure,[24] and complications occur significantly more frequently in younger children than older patients. The most common severe complications of thyroid resection include recurrent laryngeal nerve injury and permanent hypoparathyroidism. To reduce the likelihood of hypoparathyroidism, the inferior thyroid artery should be ligated near the thyroid capsule.[46] One method of preserving parathyroid gland function is to identify and autotransplant one or two of the glands into the sternocleidomastoid muscle or into the nondominant forearm.[44,52] If parathyroid gland perfusion is compromised during the dissection, then one should immediately autotransplant the gland into the nearby sternocleidomastoid muscle. To aid in the identification and protection of the recurrent laryngeal nerve, intraoperative nerve stimulation has been employed; the usefulness of this technique in children has been demonstrated in one report.[4]

The incidence of pulmonary metastases at diagnosis of thyroid cancer in childhood is about 6%.[50,54] In such cases there is nearly always significant cervical lymph node metastasis. Postoperative radioiodine treatment is required. Plain chest radiographs may demonstrate the pulmonary disease in only about 60% of cases.[50] Thus, scanning with radioiodine is necessary to detect these metastatic deposits. It should be recalled that radionuclide scans may be falsely negative if there is significant residual thyroid gland remaining in the neck, supporting the current recommendations for aggressive thyroid resection in children with differentiated thyroid cancer.[17]

The recurrence rate of thyroid cancer in patients followed for 20 years is about 30%,[24,28,42] emphasizing the importance of aggressive, early treatment and relatively frequent, long-term followup. An ^{131}I whole-body scan and chest CT scan performed approximately 6 weeks after the thyroid resection will detect residual tumor remaining in the neck and in the lungs.[17] In most cases, therapeutic doses of the radionuclide should then be administered to ablate residual thyroid tissue. This treatment should be repeated as necessary to manage residual metastatic disease.[13] To assay for recurrence of the neoplasm, diagnostic radioiodine scans should be repeated yearly. Recently, thyroglobulin has been shown to be a useful marker of residual or metastatic thyroid cancer; the plasma level of this protein should be measured yearly, and an elevated value should raise the suspicion for recurrent disease.[21] The diagnostic accuracy of this test is significantly decreased in children having residual thyroid tissue and in those who are taking thyroid hormone supplementation. To increase the sensitivity of thyroglobulin measurements for residual or recurrent thyroid cancer, the TSH can be raised by inducing a short period of iatrogenic hypothyroidism or by the administration of recombinant human TSH.[17]

Approximately 5% of thyroid neoplasms in children are medullary carcinomas that arise from the parafollicular C cells. MTC may occur sporadically, and familial tumors develop in patients having MEN type 2A or MEN 2B or the FMTC syndrome. MTC is usually the first tumor to develop in MEN patients. The neoplasm is particularly virulent in patients with MEN 2B and has been reported to occur in infancy.[30,40] As with other thyroid neoplasms, the clinical diagnosis of MTC is usually made after there is significant spread of the tumor to the adjacent cervical lymph nodes or to distant sites.[12]

Surgical resection is the only effective treatment for MTC, underscoring the importance of early diagnosis and therapy before metastasis occurs. Therefore, current management of MTC in children from families having the MEN 2 syndrome relies on the presymptomatic detection of the *RET* proto-oncogene mutation responsible for the disease, followed by prophylactic total thyroidectomy by about the age of 5 years, before the cancer spreads beyond the thyroid gland.[51] Approximately 80% of children who have thyroidectomy based solely on the presence of the RET mutation will already have foci of MTC within the thyroid gland.[43] Owing to the increased virulence of the MTC in children having MEN 2B, it may be preferable for them to have their thyroid glands removed in infancy.

THE PARATHYROID GLANDS

The parathyroid glands regulate calcium and phosphate homeostasis. Parathyroid hormone (PTH) is secreted as an 84-amino acid protein that is cleaved in the liver and kidney into the carboxy-terminal, amino-terminal, and midregion fragments. In the kidney, PTH interacts with its receptor to stimulate the production of the active vitamin D metabolite 1,25-dihydroxycholecalciferol, which then acts on the intestinal mucosa to increase calcium absorption. In the bones, PTH directly stimulates the mobilization of calcium through a process that also requires vitamin D.

The biologic activity of PTH resides in the amino-terminal segment, but the plasma level of this moiety is quite low, owing to its very short half-life in the circulation.

Most clinical assays of plasma PTH measure carboxy-terminal levels of the hormone, whose concentration is 50- to 500-fold those amino-terminal fragment. These assays are usually quite effective for the evaluation of hyperparathyroidism, but it should be noted that the carboxy-terminal fragment is cleared in the kidney and that plasma levels of the protein may therefore be elevated if there is impaired renal function. The laboratory hallmark of hyperparathyroidism is the finding of an elevated plasma PTH level with hypercalcemia. Radiographic evaluation is useful in patients who have had chronically elevated PTH levels, but the characteristic bone findings are not seen acutely.

The first step in the evaluation of hypercalcemia is to obtain a 24-hour measurement of urinary calcium to rule out familial hypocalciuric hypercalcemia. This condition, also known as familial benign hypercalcemia, usually comes to clinical attention in an asymptomatic child with an elevated serum calcium level. Serum levels of magnesium may also be elevated, and other family members may be affected. The condition is caused by an inherited mutation in the gene coding for the calcium sensing receptor, resulting in an insensitivity to calcium ion at the cellular level. There is an autosomal dominant inheritance pattern. The PTH level and parathyroid glands are normal, and there is usually no benefit to parathyroidectomy. In rare cases, a newborn born to affected parents may present with severe and life-threatening hypercalcemia owing to mutations in both alleles of the gene. These infants often have hyperplasia of the parathyroid glands and benefit from parathyroidectomy.

The differential diagnosis of hypercalcemia in childhood is presented in Table 55-7. Children, unlike adults, very rarely develop abnormal serum calcium levels related to neoplasms. However, some pediatric neoplasms may secrete a parathyroid-related polypeptide that will elevate the calcium level; this has been reported in malignant rhabdoid tumor, mesoblastic nephroma, rhabdomyosarcoma, neuroblastoma, and lymphoma. In these cases, the PTH level is generally normal or decreased.

TABLE 55-7 Differential Diagnosis of Hypercalcemia in Childhood

Elevated parathyroid hormone level
  Primary hyperparathyroidism
  Secondary hyperparathyroidism
  Tertiary hyperparathyroidism
  Ectopic parathyroid hormone production
Hypervitaminosis D
Sarcoidosis
Subcutaneous fat necrosis
Familial hypocalciuric hypercalcemia
Idiopathic hypercalcemia of infancy
Thyrotoxicosis
Hypervitaminosis A
Hypophosphatasia
Prolonged immobilization
Thiazide diuretics

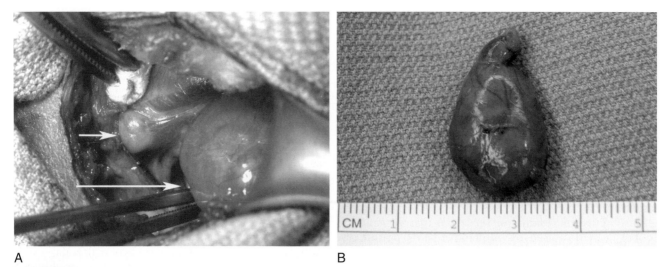

Figure 55-1 *A*, Parathyroid adenoma responsible for hypercalcemia. The *large arrow* identifies the enlarged upper gland, and the *small arrow* identifies the normal-sized lower gland. *B*, Resected parathyroid adenoma.

Primary hyperparathyroidism in childhood most commonly results from a solitary hyperfunctioning adenoma, as demonstrated in Figure 55-1. More rarely there is diffuse hyperplasia of all four glands.[37] Hyperparathyroidism resulting from hyperplasia in all four glands is a feature of MEN syndrome. Moreover, parathyroid hyperplasia is a feature in approximately 30% of patients having MEN 2A, but hypercalcemia in this syndrome rarely occurs in childhood.[15] Primary hyperparathyroidism of infancy is a rare disorder that is often fatal[23,38] and demonstrates a familial component in about half of cases. The condition usually develops within the first 3 months of life, and presenting signs include hypotonicity, respiratory distress, failure to thrive, lethargy, and polyuria. Early recognition and treatment of primary hyperparathyroidism of infancy is essential to allow normal growth and development of the baby. Pathologically, there is usually diffuse parathyroid gland hyperplasia.

There is no place for medical management of primary hyperparathyroidism in children; and once the diagnosis of hyperparathyroidism is established, the offending parathyroid tissue should be resected. Recent advances in imaging and real-time PTH measurements have allowed the use of minimally invasive techniques.[18,49] Currently, it is recommended that patients with primary hyperparathyroidism undergo preoperative localization with ^{99m}Tc-sestamibi scan.[6] If the scan demonstrates a single parathyroid lesion, a less invasive procedure can be considered. A small incision can be made over the offending gland, which can often be localized using a hand-held gamma probe. To confirm that the offending gland has been removed, a rapid parathyroid hormone analysis can be performed while the child remains asleep.[48] These modalities have not been widely used in children, but their use in adults has demonstrated a reduction in morbidity, hospital stay, and costs.[49]

The preferred surgical management of parathyroid gland hyperplasia involving all of the glands remains controversial. Some surgeons recommend removing three and one-half glands, whereas others prefer to remove all of the glands and heterotopically transplant some tissue into the nondominant forearm.[38] The latter approach has the advantage of avoiding repeated neck exploration if hyperparathyroidism should recur and has been shown to be safe in infants and children.[43] Moreover, there is evidence that total parathyroidectomy with heterotopic autotransplantation results in improved survival in infants with severe hypercalcemia.[38]

Secondary hyperparathyroidism occurs when the parathyroid glands are stimulated to increase PTH secretion in response to a decreased serum calcium level. This is most commonly associated with renal insufficiency but may also be associated with malabsorption syndromes. Patients with secondary hyperparathyroidism usually respond to medications that decrease intestinal phosphorus absorption. In rare cases, children will develop severe renal osteodystrophy manifested by skeletal fractures and metastatic calcifications; these children are candidates for either three and one-half gland parathyroidectomy or total parathyroidectomy with autotransplantation.[37] In some patients with chronic renal failure and secondary hyperparathyroidism who undergo renal transplantation, there is persistent hyperfunction of the glands even after the inciting stimulus (hypocalcemia from renal failure) is removed. This is termed *tertiary hyperparathyroidism* and results from four-gland hyperplasia; children with this condition are also candidates for total parathyroidectomy with autotransplantation.

REFERENCES

1. Acharya S, Sarafoglou K, LaQuaglia MP, et al: Thyroid neoplasms after therapeutic radiation for malignancies during childhood or adolescence. Cancer 2003;97:2397-2403.
2. Al-Shaikh A, Ngan B, Daneman A, et al: Fine-needle aspiration biopsy in the management of thyroid nodules in children and adolescents. J Pediatr 2001;138:140-142.

3. Berglund J, Christensen SB, Dymling JF, et al: The incidence of recurrence and hypothyroidism following treatment with antithyroid drugs, surgery, or radioiodine in all patients with thyrotoxicosis in Malmo during the period 1970-1974. J Intern Med 1991;229:435-442.

4. Brauckhoff M, Gimm O, Thanh PN, et al: First experience in intraoperative neurostimulation of the recurrent laryngeal nerve during thyroid surgery in children and adolescents. J Pediatr Surg 2002;37:1414-1418.

5. Ceccarelli C, Pacini F, Lippi F, et al: Thyroid cancer in children and adolescents. Surgery 1988;104:1143-1148.

6. Chen H: Surgery for primary hyperparathyroidism: What is the best approach? Ann Surg 2002;236:552-553.

7. de Roy van Zuidewijn DBW, Songun I, Kievit J, et al: Complications of thyroid surgery. Ann Surg Oncol 1995;2: 56-60.

8. Desjardins JG, Khan AH, Montupet P, et al: Management of thyroid nodules in children: A 20-year experience. J Pediatr Surg 1987;22:736-739.

9. Dickman PW, Holm L-E, Lundell G, et al: Thyroid cancer risk after thyroid examination with ^{131}I: A population-based cohort study in Sweden. Int J Cancer 2003;106:580-587.

10. Eng C, Smith DP, Mulligan LM, et al: Point mutation within the tyrosine kinase domain of the RET proto-oncogene in multiple endocrine neoplasia type 2B and related sporadic tumours. Hum Mol Genet 1994;3:237-241.

11. Franklyn JA: The management of hyperthyroidism. N Engl J Med 1994;330:1731-1738.

12. Gorlin JB, Sallan SE: Thyroid cancer in childhood. Endocrinol Metab Clin North Am 1990;19:649-662.

13. Harness JA, Thompson NW, McLeod MK, et al: Differentiated thyroid carcinoma in children and adolescents. World J Surg 1992;16:547-554.

14. Haselkorn T, Bernstein L, Preston-Martin S, et al: Descriptive epidemiology of thyroid cancer in Los Angeles County, 1972-1995. Cancer Causes Control 2000;11:163-170.

15. Howe JR, Norton JA, Wells SA Jr: Prevalence of pheochromocytoma and hyperparathyroidism in multiple endocrine neoplasia type 2A: Results of long-term follow-up. Surgery 1993;114:1070-1077.

16. Hung W, Anderson KD, Chandra RS, et al: Solitary thyroid nodules in 71 children and adolescents. J Pediatr Surg 1992;27:1407-1409.

17. Hung W, Sarlis NJ: Current controversies in the management of pediatric patients with well-differentiated nonmedullary thyroid cancer: A review. Thyroid 2002;12:683-702.

18. Irvin GL III, Molinari AS, Figueroa C, et al: Improved success rate in reoperative parathyroidectomy with intraoperative PTH assay. Ann Surg 1999;229:874-879.

19. Jaksic J, Dumic M, Filipovic B, et al: Thyroid disease in a school population with thyromegaly. Arch Dis Child 1994;70: 103-106.

20. Khurana KK, Labrador E, Izquierdo R, et al: The role of fine-needle aspiration biopsy in the management of thyroid nodules in children, adolescents, and young adults: A multi-institutional study. Thyroid 1999;9:383-386.

21. Kirk JM, Mort C, Grant DB, et al: The usefulness of serum thyroglobulin in the follow-up of differentiated thyroid carcinoma in children. Med Pediatr Oncol 1992;20: 201-208.

22. Klein I, Becker DV, Levey GS: Treatment of hyperthyroid disease. Ann Intern Med 1994;121:281-288.

23. Kulczycka H, Kaminski W, Wozniewicz B, et al: Primary hyperparathyroidism in infancy: Diagnostic and therapeutic difficulties. Klin Padiatr 1991;203:116-118.

24. La Quaglia MP, Corbally MT, Heller G, et al: Recurrence and morbidity in differentiated thyroid carcinoma in children. Surgery 1988;104:1149-1156.

25. Mazzaferri EL: Management of a solitary thyroid nodule. N Engl J Med 1993;328:553-559.

26. Nebesio TD, Siddiqui AR, Pescovitz OH, et al: Time course to hypothyroidism after fixed-dose radioablation therapy of Graves' disease in children. J Pediatr 2002;141: 99-103.

27. Newman KD: The current management of thyroid tumors in childhood. Semin Pediatr Surg 1993;2:69-74.

28. Newman KD, Black T, Heller G, et al: Differentiated thyroid cancer: Determinants of disease progression in patients < 21 years of age at diagnosis. Ann Surg 1998;227:533-541.

29. Nikiforov Y, Gnepp DR: Pediatric thyroid cancer after the Chernobyl disaster: Pathomorphologic study of 84 cases (1991-1992) from the Republic of Belarus. Cancer 1994;74: 748-765.

30. Norton JA, Froome LC, Farrell RE, et al: Multiple endocrine neoplasia type IIb: The most aggressive form of medullary thyroid carcinoma. Surg Clin North Am 1979;59:109-118.

31. Pacini F, Vorontsova T, Molinaro E, et al: Thyroid consequences of the Chernobyl nuclear accident. Acta Paediatr Suppl 1999;433:23-27.

32. Paterson ICM, Greenlee R, Adams Jones D: Thyroid cancer in Wales 1985-1996: A cancer registry-based study. Clin Oncol 1999;11:245-251.

33. Phillips DI, Barker DJ, Rees Smith B, et al: The geographical distribution of thyrotoxicosis in England according to the presence or absence of TSH-receptor antibodies. Clin Endocrinol 1985;23:283-287.

34. Raab SS, Silverman JF, Elsheikh TM, et al: Pediatric thyroid nodules: Disease demographics and clinical management by fine needle aspiration biopsy. Pediatrics 1995;95:46-49.

35. Rabes HM, Demidchik EP, Siderow JD, et al: Pattern of radiation-induced RET and NTRK1 rearrangement in 191 post-Chernobyl papillary thyroid carcinomas: Biological, phenotypic, and clinical implications. Clin Cancer Res 2000; 6:1093-1103.

36. Rallison ML, Dobyns BM, Meikle AW, et al: Natural history of thyroid abnormalities: Prevalence, incidence, and regression of thyroid diseases in adolescents and young adults. Am J Med 1991;91:363-370.

37. Ross AJ III: Parathyroid surgery in children. Prog Pediatr Surg 1991;26:48-59.

38. Ross AJ III, Cooper A, Attie MF, et al: Primary hyperparathyroidism in infancy. J Pediatr Surg 1986;21:493-499.

39. Rother KI, Zimmerman D, Schwenk WF: Effect of thyroid hormone treatment on thyromegaly in children and adolescents with Hashimoto disease. J Pediatr 1994;124: 599-601.

40. Samaan NA, Draznin MB, Halpin RE, et al: Multiple endocrine syndrome type IIb in early childhood. Cancer 1991;68:1832-1834.

41. Santoro M, Thomas GA, Vecchio G, et al: Gene rearrangement and Chernobyl related thyroid cancers. Br J Cancer 2000;82:315-322.

42. Schlumberger M, De Vathaire F, Travagli JP, et al: Differentiated thyroid carcinoma in childhood: Long term follow-up in 72 patients. J Clin Endocrinol Metab 1987;65:1088-1094.

43. Skinner MA, DeBenedetti MK, Moley JF, et al: Medullary thyroid carcinoma in children with multiple endocrine neoplasia types 2A and 2B. J Pediatr Surg 1996;31:177-182.

44. Skinner MA, Norton JA, Moley JF, et al: Heterotopic autotransplantation of parathyroid tissue in children undergoing total thyroidectomy. J Pediatr Surg 1997;32:510-513.

45. Smith MB, Xue H, Strong L, et al: Forty-year experience with second malignancies after treatment of childhood cancer: Analysis of outcome following the development of the second malignancy. J Pediatr Surg 1993;28:1342-1349.

46. Thomusch O, Machens A, Sekulla C, et al: The impact of surgical technique on postoperative hypoparathyroidism in bilateral thyroid surgery: A multivariate analysis of 5846 consecutive patients. Surgery 2003;133:180-185.

47. Tomer Y, Davies TF: Infection, thyroid disease, and autoimmunity. Endocrine Rev 1993;14:107-120.

48. Udelsman R, Aruny JE, Donovan PI, et al: Rapid parathyroid hormone analysis during venous localization. Ann Surg 2003;237:714-721.

49. Udelsman R, Donovan PI, Sokoll LJ: One hundred consecutive minimally invasive parathyroid explorations. Ann Surg 2000;232:331-339.

50. Vassilopoulou-Sellin R, Klein MJ, Smith TH, et al: Pulmonary metastases in children and young adults with differentiated thyroid cancer. Cancer 1993;71:1348-1352.

51. Wells SA Jr, Chi DD, Toshima K, et al: Predictive DNA testing and prophylactic thyroidectomy in patients at risk for multiple endocrine neoplasia type 2A. Ann Surg 1994;220: 237-250.

52. Wells SA Jr, Farndon JR, Dale JK, et al: Long term evaluation of patients with primary parathyroid hyperplasia managed by total parathyroidectomy and heterotopic autotransplantation. Ann Surg 1980;192:451-458.

53. Yip FWK, Reeve TS, Poole AG, et al: Thyroid nodules in childhood and adolescence. Aust NZ J Surg 1994;64: 676-678.

54. Zimmerman D, Hay ID, Gough IR, et al: Papillary thyroid carcinoma in children and adults: Long-term follow-up of 1039 patients conservatively treated at one institution during three decades. Surgery 1988;104:1157-1163.

Chapter 56

Cysts and Sinuses of the Neck

C. D. Smith

Cysts and sinuses of the neck constitute one of the most intriguing areas of pediatric pathology. Although congenital in origin, they may not be recognized or cause clinical problems until well into adulthood. In adulthood, they may masquerade as carcinoma.[5,8] In childhood, even though normally benign, they may, in rare cases, harbor malignancy.[7,29] The most common lesions, thyroglossal duct cysts and second branchial anomalies, are usually easily diagnosed on physical examination, do not necessarily require additional workup, and can often be excised safely in a day surgery unit. There are many pitfalls, however, for the surgeon, who through ignorance of anatomic variants or of well-established surgical techniques, may predispose the patient to the morbidity of multiple, painful recurrences or nerve deficits. A working knowledge of the embryologic origin of these cysts and sinuses and their relationship to normal neck structures is a prerequisite for successful management, as is the knowledge that total excision is required for a successful outcome. In addition, a familiarity with a number of unusual presentations, such as acute suppurative thyroiditis (piriform sinus arising from third or fourth branchial anomaly), otorrhea (first branchial anomaly), severe respiratory distress or sudden death in an infant (thyroglossal duct cyst, branchial anomaly), or an ectopic thyroid mimicking a thyroglossal duct cyst prevents delay in proper treatment. This chapter focuses on pertinent features of the embryology of the neck. Usual and unusual presentations of each entity are described, and surgical strategies for primary and recurrent lesions are discussed. New approaches that challenge conventional management principles and initial forays into the application of minimally invasive approaches to these congenital neck lesions are highlighted.

EMBRYOLOGY

There are potentially six branchial arches supplied by six aortic arches connecting the paired dorsal and ventral aortas in the primitive embryo (Fig. 56-1). The fifth arch is present transiently, if at all, and disappears without a trace. Each branchial arch is covered externally with ectoderm, lined internally with endoderm, and filled with mesoderm, containing an artery, a nerve, a cartilage rod, and muscle. The depressions between the arches are called *clefts* externally and *pouches* internally. The clefts are lined with ectoderm and the pouches endoderm (Fig. 56-2). The point at which they oppose each other is called the *closing membrane*. In the human, obliteration of these membranes does not normally occur to form a true gill as it does in the fish.

The contribution that each arch, cleft, and pouch makes to the formation of the neck and jaw is summarized in Table 56-1. Theories about the origin of cysts and sinuses of the neck are based on the relationship of these anomalies to adjacent arteries, muscles, and nerves; on known pathways taken by the thyroid, parathyroid, and thymus glands in their embryonic migrations; and, to a lesser extent, on the type of epithelial lining of the various anomalies.

Figure 56-1 shows the transformation of the aortic arches and aortas into the definitive vascular pattern. Three examples illustrate how knowledge of this process has been used to deduce the origin of branchial anomalies. First, one can predict that a piriform sinus tract (third or fourth branchial arch lesion) will course posterior to the internal carotid artery, a third arch structure, rather than between the internal and external carotid arteries, as is the case with second branchial cleft anomalies (Fig. 56-3). Second, an external sinus opening anterior to the sternocleidomastoid muscle in the lower neck does not distinguish between second, third, and fourth branchial cleft remnants. In the embryo, these clefts have a common exit site in the neck, the cervical sinus of His, which forms when the second branchial arch overgrows the openings of these clefts (Fig. 56-4A). The relationship of a cyst, sinus, or fistula to internal neck structures, such as the carotid bifurcation, the hypoglossal nerve, or the stylohyoid and digastric muscles, therefore, determines the site of origin of one of these particular anomalies, not the location of an external opening.[76] Third, although a complete fourth branchial cleft fistula has yet to be identified clinically, its

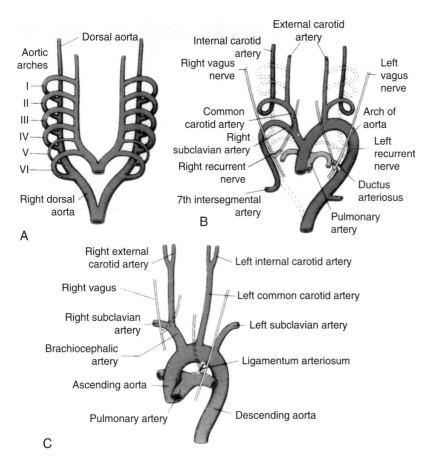

A

B

C

Figure 56–1 *A*, Diagram of the aortic arches and dorsal aortas before transformation into the definitive vascular pattern. *B*, Diagram of the aortic arches and dorsal aortas after the transformation. Obliterated components are indicated by *broken lines*. Note the patent ductus arteriosus and position of the seventh intersegmental artery on the left. *C*, The great arteries in the adult. Compare the distance between the place of origin of the left common carotid artery and the left subclavian in *B* and *C*. After the disappearance of the distal part of the sixth aortic arch (the fifth arches never form completely), the right recurrent laryngeal nerve hooks around the right subclavian artery. On the left, the nerve remains in place and hooks around the ligamentum arteriosum. (From Sadler TW: Head and neck. In Langman's Medical Embryology, 7th ed. Baltimore, Williams & Wilkins, 1995.)

course has been predicted to differ on the two sides of the neck. On the left side, this fistula would dive into the superior mediastinum beneath the arch of the aorta, the successor of the left fourth embryonic aortic arch. Because the right fourth embryonic aortic arch becomes the subclavian artery, the fistula would pass beneath that structure on the right side (see Figs. 56-1 and 56-5).

The nerves of the arches are important landmarks not only for deducing the origin of the various branchial anomalies but also for being at risk during excision of each one of them. In first branchial anomalies the tract may pass below, between, or above the branches of the facial nerve.[46] This is the reason identification of the branches of this nerve is a cardinal principle in the excision

of one of these lesions. The danger of injuring an adjacent nerve is much less of a clinical problem with uncomplicated lesions of the lower clefts but can become more of an issue when previous inflammation or operative procedures result in distortion of the normal anatomy. Figures 56-3 and 56-5 illustrate the paths of second, third, and fourth branchial fistulas vis-á-vis the glossopharyngeal (IX), the superior laryngeal and recurrent branches of the vagus (X), and the hypoglossal (XII) nerves.

Knowledge of the location of the internal openings of branchial cleft tracts can be helpful in both diagnosis and operative management. A first branchial anomaly often enters the external auditory canal (or rarely the middle ear). A second branchial anomaly enters the

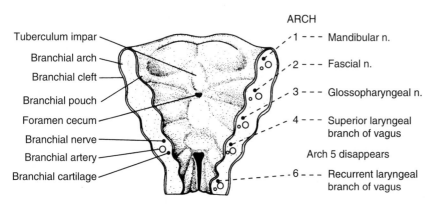

ARCH

Tuberculum impar
Branchial arch
Branchial cleft
Branchial pouch
Foramen cecum
Branchial nerve
Branchial artery
Branchial cartilage

1 – – – Mandibular n.
2 – – – Fascial n.
3 – – – Glossopharyngeal n.
4 – – – Superior laryngeal branch of vagus
Arch 5 disappears
6 – – – Recurrent laryngeal branch of vagus

Figure 56–2 Early development of branchial apparatus. (From Donegan JO: Congenital neck masses. In Cummings CW, et al [eds]: Otolaryngology—Head and Neck Surgery, 2nd ed. St Louis, Mosby–Year Book, 1993.)

TABLE 56-1 Derivatives of Branchial Arches, Clefts, and Pouches

	Dorsal	Ventral	Midline Floor of Pharynx
I			
Arch	Incus body	Meckel's cartilage	Body of tongue
External maxillary artery	Malleus head	Malleus	
Nerve V	Pinna		
Cleft	External auditory canal		
Pouch	Eustachian tube		
	Middle ear cavity		
	Mastoid air cells		
II			
Arch	Stapes	Styloid process	Root of tongue
Stapedial artery		Hyoid (lesser horn and part of body)	Foramen cecum
Nerves VII and VIII			Thyroid gland's median anlage
Pouch	Palatine tonsil		
	Supratonsillar fossa		
III			
Arch		Hyoid (greater horn and part of body)	
Internal carotid artery		Part of epiglottis	
Nerve IX		Thymus	
Pouch	Inferior parathyroid		
	Piriform fossa		
IV			
Arch		Thyroid cartilage	
Arch of aorta (L)		Cuneiform cartilage	
Part of subclavian artery (R)		Part of epiglottis	
Nerve X			
Pouch	Superior parathyroid (lateral anlage of thyroid gland)	Thymus (inconstant)	
V			
Arch			
Pouch	Ultimobranchial body (lateral anlage of thyroid gland)		
VI			
Arch		Cricoid	
Pulmonary artery		Arytenoid	
Ductus arteriosus (L)		Corniculate cartilage	
Nerve X (recurrent laryngeal)			

From Skandalakis JE, Gray SW, Todd NW: The pharynx and its derivatives. In Skandalakis JE, Gray SW (eds): Embryology for Surgeons, 2nd ed. Baltimore, Williams & Wilkins, 1994.

supratonsillar fossa. Third and fourth pouch sinuses and fistulas enter the pharynx through the piriform sinus but in different extremes of the sinus. Franciosi and associates have emphasized that third branchial cleft anomalies enter the base (superior portion) of the piriform sinus and ascend over the superior laryngeal nerve, whereas fourth anomalies enter the apex (inferior portion) and descend below that nerve.[24]

The only pouch, closing membrane/cleft complex to persist is the first one, which becomes the eustachian tube/middle ear, tympanic membrane, and external auditory canal (see Fig. 56-4A). The remainder of the branchial pouches normally give rise to the tonsils, the thymus, the parathyroids, and the C cells of the thyroid gland. The outer cleft components regress (see Figs. 56-4B and 56-6). Of these glands, only the tonsils remain at their pouch of origin. The third branchial pouch becomes elongated and

eventually loses its communication with the pharynx. It differentiates dorsally into the future inferior parathyroid (III), coming to rest close to the inferior pole of the thyroid and ventrally into the ipsilateral lobe of the thymus in the superior mediastinum. Embryologists agree that the future superior parathyroid gland arises from the fourth branchial pouch. They disagree as to whether the ultimobranchial body (lateral anlage of the thyroid gland and source of the calcitonin-producing C cells) arises from the fourth branchial or a vestigial fifth pouch (see Fig. 56-4). Based on immunohistochemical studies of resected specimens of the thyroid glands and fistulas from 15 patients, Miyauchi and colleagues have argued convincingly that these fistulas are in fact remnants related to the ultimobranchial body.[52] Himi and Kataura's work on the distribution of C cells in the thyroid gland with piriform sinus fistula supports this interpretation.[34]

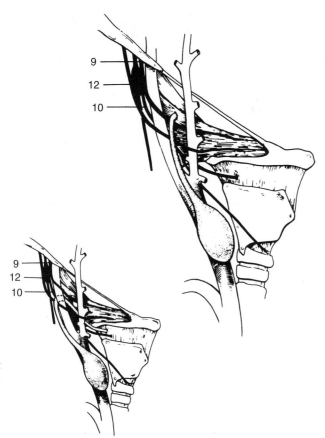

Figure 56–3 Second branchial cleft cyst and sinus tract (*right*); third branchial cleft cyst and sinus tract (*left*). (From Donegan JO: Congenital neck masses. In Cummings CW, et al [eds]: Otolaryngology—Head and Neck Surgery, 2nd ed. St Louis, Mosby–Year Book, 1993.)

The migration of fourth pouch structures is much less extensive than that of the third pouch derivatives: the parathyroid tissue normally is found on the dorsal surface of the superior thyroid, and the C cells find their way into the thyroid gland itself. Lateral cysts and sinuses of the neck can result from persistence of the second, third, or fourth pouches themselves or from rests of thymic or parathyroid tissue, which may be left anywhere along the route of their migrations. Demonstration of thymic tissue within a cyst wall does not reliably indicate origin because both third and fourth pouches may normally contain thymic tissue.

The thyroid gland develops from a bilobate diverticulum in between the muscular forerunners of the anterior and posterior portions of the tongue at a site that persists as the foramen cecum (Fig. 56-6). The gland descends in the midline of the neck anterior to the hyoid bone and comes to rest in the lower neck. Its transient connection to its point of origin is a cord of cells known as the thyroglossal duct. The lower end of this duct often persists as the pyramidal lobe. When the thyroglossal duct itself persists, the most important features to remember from a surgical point of view are the relation of this duct to the hyoid bone and the structure of the ductal remnants between the hyoid bone and the foramen cecum. The demonstration by three-dimensional reconstructions of thyroglossal duct surgical specimens by Horisawa elegantly shows why the central portion of the hyoid bone as well as a core of tissue from the hyoid to the foramen cecum must be removed with the cyst to prevent recurrence (Fig. 56-7).[35]

Rarely the thyroid gland may not complete its descent. It most commonly remains in the base of the tongue but

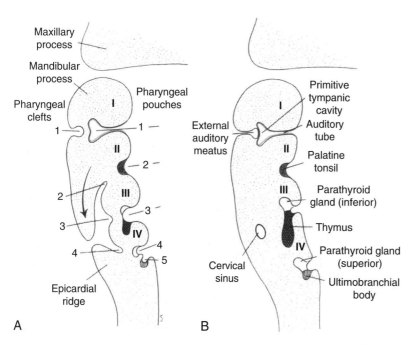

Maxillary process

Mandibular process

Pharyngeal clefts

Pharyngeal pouches

I

1 — — 1

II

— 2 —

2

III

— 3

3

IV

— 4

4

— 5

Epicardial ridge

A

Primitive tympanic cavity

Auditory tube

External auditory meatus

I

II

Palatine tonsil

III

Parathyroid gland (inferior)

Thymus

IV

Parathyroid gland (superior)

Cervical sinus

Ultimobranchial body

B

Figure 56–4 *A,* Schematic representation of the development of the pharyngeal clefts and pouches. Note that the second arch grows over the third and fourth arches, thereby burying the second, third, and fourth pharyngeal clefts. *B,* Remnants of the second, third, and fourth pharyngeal clefts form the cervical sinus, which is normally obliterated. Note the structures formed by the various pharyngeal pouches. (From Sadler TW: Head and neck. In Langman's Medical Embryology, 7th ed. Baltimore, Williams & Wilkins, 1995.)

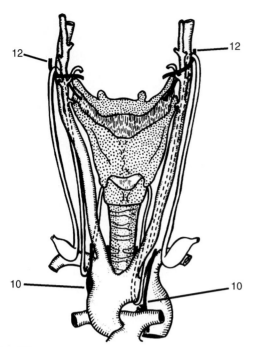

Figure 56–5 Anatomic relationships of probable course of fourth branchial fistula. (From Liston SL: Fourth branchial fistula. Otolaryngol Head Neck Surg 1981;89:520.)

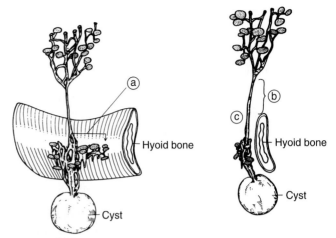

Figure 56–7 Diagram of the common running pattern of the thyroglossal duct based on anatomic reconstruction. a, Horizontal distance from midline to the most distant thyroglossal duct; b, length of the single duct above the hyoid bone; c, point where the diameter of the duct is measured. (From Horisawa M, Niinomi N, Ito T: What is the optimal depth for core-out toward the foramen cecum in a thyroglossal duct cyst operation? J Pediatr Surg 1992;27:710.)

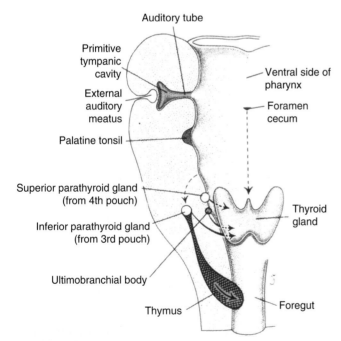

Figure 56–6 Schematic representation of migration of the thymus, parathyroid glands, and ultimobranchial body. The thyroid gland originates in the midline at the level of the foramen cecum and descends to the level of the first tracheal ring. (From Sadler TW: Head and neck. In Langman's Medical Embryology, 7th ed. Baltimore, Williams & Wilkins, 1995.)

at times can come to rest at a more distal site along the route to the base of the neck. This anomaly now has not only surgical, but also medicolegal implications related to informed consent, preoperative workup, and intraoperative management.[62]

INCIDENCE

In a review of 481 procedures in 445 pediatric patients 18 years and younger whose neck masses were excised at Children's Hospital of Philadelphia during a 5-year period, congenital neck masses were diagnosed in 244 patients (55%). Of these, 78 (32%) were branchial cleft anomalies, 73 (30%) were thyroglossal duct cysts, and 43 (18%) were dermoids.[78] Thyroglossal duct cysts were somewhat more common than branchial anomalies in the Mayo Clinic series of 612 adults and children: 55% versus 45%.[72] In a 15-year French series of 191 children, defects of midline closure outnumbered those of branchial migration: 53% had thyroglossal duct cysts, 11% had dermoid cysts, 19% had second cleft anomalies, 10% had first cleft anomalies, 4% had fourth pouch anomalies, and 2% had thymic cysts.[57]

SECOND BRANCHIAL ANOMALIES

More than 90% of branchial cleft anomalies are estimated to arise from the second branchial system. Approximately 8% are attributed to first branchial malformations, whereas those of the third and fourth systems rarely occur.[11] The male:female ratio is generally reported to be equal. When a sinus is present, most branchial anomalies are diagnosed in the first decade of life; when there is no external sinus, the diagnosis may not be made until well into adulthood. Seventy-four percent of the branchial anomalies in the Mayo Clinic series were cysts, 25% were fistulas, and 1% were skin tags or cartilages.[72] Surprisingly, in the review from the Hospital for Sick Children, London, 92 of 98 second branchial cleft/pouch anomalies over a 32-year period had sinus openings in the neck, which may be partially explained by the fact that all but two of the patients were diagnosed by the age of 10 and 78% by the age of 5 years.[23] Six patients had cartilaginous remnants in the neck without a sinus opening (Fig. 56-8). Six (6%) anomalies were bilateral. Other reports of bilaterality range from 2% to 10%.[26]

Typically, drainage from a tiny pit in the skin anterior to the lower third of the sternocleidomastoid muscle draws attention to the presence of a second branchial cleft sinus or fistula (Fig. 56-9). A cord may be palpable running upward in the neck from the ostium. Milking or stripping the tract provides a mucoid discharge. A cyst presents as a soft mass deep to the upper third of the same muscle. The sudden appearance of a painful mass in this location may be the first sign of one of these lesions.

Unusual presentations include stridor, pharyngeal cyst causing sore throat, feeling of fullness in the throat, hyponasal speech, dysphagia or odynophagia, a cold nodule on thyroid scan,[70] a hot nodule on thyroid scan,[70] an isolated hypoglossal nerve palsy,[25] or multiple cranial nerve palsies.[18] Branchial anomalies may occur as part of the branchio-oculofacial syndrome.[44] Branchiogenic carcinoma has been diagnosed in adults but not in children.[27]

Because of the likelihood of infection developing in any of the branchial cleft anomalies, excision is generally recommended at the time of diagnosis in a noninfected lesion. Surgery in infants is delayed until 3 to 6 months. Excision is delayed in any patient in the presence of infection. Antibiotics and possibly needle aspiration are advised to eradicate the infection. Incision and drainage are avoided when possible because this results in distortion

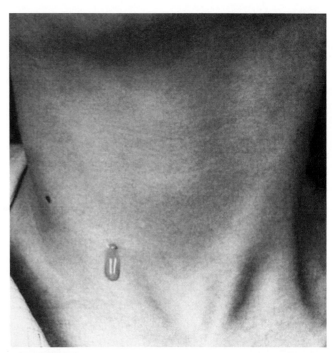

Figure 56–9 Unilateral discharging second cleft sinus. (From Ford GR, et al: Branchial cleft and pouch anomalies. J Laryngol Otol 1992;106:137.)

of normal tissue planes, which may contribute to the higher recurrence rate after excision in this group of patients. Two thirds of the patients in the Mayo Clinic series who had recurrences after surgery for branchial cleft anomalies had had previous surgery or infection (or both).[72]

In a child, a second branchial anomaly with an external opening can usually be excised through a single incision incorporating the sinus opening, whereas in adolescents and adults two stepladder incisions may be required. In contrast to thyroglossal duct cysts, these tracts are single and relatively well defined, which allows one to stay close to the tract wall in the dissection. Placement of a catheter, Prolene suture, or metal probe in the tract may be helpful. Injection of methylene blue into the tract can complicate the dissection if there is any spillage. Preoperative fistulography can be helpful but is not generally employed.[10] The primary objective in the excision of all of these lesions is to do a complete excision without injuring important adjacent structures, which, in a second branchial anomaly, includes the external and internal carotid arteries and the hypoglossal and glossopharyngeal nerves (see Fig. 56-3). The excision of a second branchial cyst varies only in that the incision is made over the cyst and adjacent to the carotid artery bifurcation.

Techniques for minimally invasive surgery on the neck are in the process of development using porcine and cadaver models.[73,74] A telescope and two dissecting ports placed in three incisions located at the base of the neck are employed. Use of a hernia balloon designed for laparoscopic herniorrhaphy to create a surgical pocket that can be maintained with compressed carbon dioxide pressures as low as 4 mm Hg has been demonstrated in

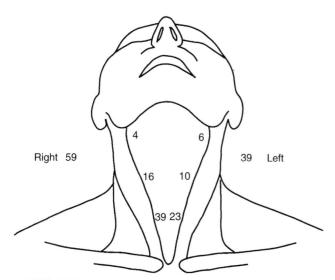

Right 59
4   6
16   10
39 23
39 Left

Figure 56–8 Site of branchial cleft sinuses. (From Ford GR, et al: Branchial cleft and pouch anomalies. J Laryngol Otol 1992;106:137.)

these models to be free of complications noted in earlier techniques, namely, subcutaneous emphysema, pneumothorax, pneumomediastinum, and air embolism. "Compelling" advantages in further porcine experiments by these same researchers using endorobotic technology (the DaVinci system) were noted: increased surgical precision and dexterity and decreased impact of tremor with the three-dimensional imaging, EndoWrist articulation, and motion scaling.[32] The technique has been used successfully only once in this country as of this writing to remove a lymph node, but broader application, including use in excision of congenital neck lesions, may be on the horizon as the technique is refined and instrumentation is improved.[1]

FIRST BRANCHIAL CLEFT ANOMALIES

First branchial cleft anomalies can be hard to diagnose. They are rare, yet when inflamed they may present in the same areas where infected submandibular or sebaceous glands typically manifest themselves (Fig. 56-10). Several hints may serve to alert the clinician that a first branchial anomaly is the underlying cause: a history of drainage below the angle of the mandible before infection, lack of deep induration, relatively nonpurulent drainage from the ear, or a cystic lesion of the tympanic membrane or middle ear coexisting with a sinus or abscess above the hyoid bone.[16,77] Obviously a careful otologic examination is an important part of the evaluation of such patients. As with second cleft anomalies, cysts outnumber sinuses and fistulas in all age groups and tend to present later. Of 460 patients with branchial cleft anomalies treated at the Mayo Clinic from 1950 to 1978, 38 (8%) were defects of the first branchial cleft. Twenty-six of the 38 (68%) were cysts, and 17 (65%) occurred in females. The mean age of patients with cysts was 15 years with a range of 13 to 18 years. In contrast, patients with sinuses and fistulas are diagnosed or first treated at a younger age when sex distribution tends to be equal.[59] Infection, which commonly occurs before the correct diagnosis is made, leads to scar formation and distortion of normal landmarks.

Two types of anomalies have been distinguished by Arnot[6] and Work.[83] The rarer of the two, type I, is considered a duplication of the membranous external auditory canal. It presents at a later age, is located lateral to the facial nerve, has an ectodermal (squamous epithelial) lining, and tends to parallel the external canal presenting just in front or just behind the ear. Type II lesions are duplication anomalies of the membranous external auditory canal and pinna and consist of both ectodermal and mesodermal (cartilage) elements (Fig. 56-11). Olsen and coworkers maintain that a classification dividing the lesions into isolated cysts, sinuses, or fistulas more accurately depicts the anatomic findings and achieves a better understanding of the appropriate diagnosis and management.[59] When a first branchial anomaly is suspected, it may be helpful to obtain a sonogram or computed tomographic (CT) scan to demonstrate the course of the tract and its relationship to the facial nerve and middle ear.

First branchial anomalies are hazardous to repair, particularly in younger age groups. The most important point in this operation is to expose the main trunk of the facial nerve at the beginning of the operation and to expose all branches of the nerve to the periphery.[40] It is important to emphasize the fact that injury to the facial nerve during parotid surgery is one of the most common causes of facial paralysis in children.[2,42] On the basis of dissections in infant cadavers, Farrior and Santini point out why: in children, the facial nerve is smaller, more superficial, and more difficult to identify because of the underdevelopment of surrounding structures.[22] They and others[55]

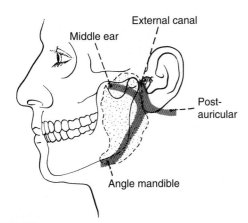

Figure 56-10 General location of first branchial cleft anomalies. (From Olsen KD, Maragos NE, Weiland LH: First branchial cleft anomalies. Laryngoscope 1980;90:423.)

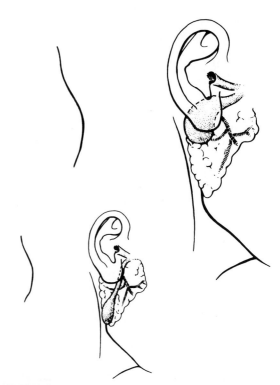

Figure 56-11 Type I branchial cleft abnormality (*right*); type II branchial cleft abnormality (*left*). (From Donegan JO: Congenital neck masses. In Cummings CW, et al [eds]: Otolaryngology—Head and Neck Surgery, 2nd ed. St Louis, Mosby–Year Book, 1993.)

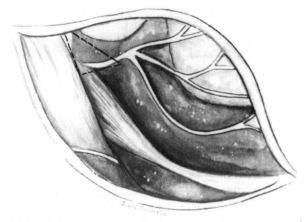

Figure 56–12 Facial nerve trunk exits stylomastoid foramen through triangle formed by cartilaginous ear canal, sternocleidomastoid muscle, and digastric muscle *(dotted lines)*. In infants, pes anserinus is located posterior to ramus of the mandible. (From Farrior JB, Santini H: Facial nerve identification in children. Otolaryngol Head Neck Surg 1985;93:173.)

recommend initial exposure of the nerve as it exits the stylomastoid foramen by making a retroauricular, rather than preauricular, incision and identifying it in the triangle formed by the sternocleidomastoid muscle, posterior belly of the digastric muscle, and cartilaginous ear canal (Fig. 56-12). In cases in which previous infection makes identification of the facial nerve outside the temporal bone difficult, Todd alternatively recommends finding the nerve within the mastoid, then following it to the stylomastoid foramen.[76] After the main trunk of the nerve is exposed, its branches are dissected peripherally and the superficial lobe of the parotid gland is removed. When the tract is located deep to the nerve, a total parotidectomy is carried out. The tract is then separated from the branches of the nerve and followed to its junction with the ear canal. Even when the tract does not enter the canal, a portion of the adjacent cartilage and skin lining of the ear canal should be excised to prevent recurrence. The resulting defect in the canal is allowed to close by secondary intention and rarely results in stenosis. It is uncommon for the tract to involve the tympanic membrane or middle ear, but when it does, partial tympanic membrane excision, tympanoplasty, and curettage of the small portion of the tract that traverses the temporal bone is required.[77] Ikarashi and colleagues state that in excising one of these lesions the surgeon should recognize the possibility that the tract may extend parallel to the eustachian tube as far as the nasopharynx.[37] When the tract is closely adherent to the submandibular gland, this gland should be removed with the tract.[59]

Electrophysiologic facial nerve localization has been used in type I branchial cleft cyst excision to allow safe total excision through a smaller surgical approach than generally advocated, obviating facial nerve trunk localization. In a report on 11 children operated on over a 9-year period, Isaacson and Martin emphasize that this technique is appropriate when the lesion is superior to the stylomastoid foramen and not previously infected or surgically violated.[38]

PIRIFORM SINUS FISTULAS

The rarest anomalies of the branchial apparatus, those attributed to remnants of the third and fourth pouch/cleft complexes, have the potential for causing two difficult clinical scenarios: life-threatening respiratory compromise in the neonatal period[12,24,45,51,54] and acute thyroiditis.[51,53] Because both presentations are rare, delay in diagnosis often occurs, with the result that landmark-distorting incision and drainage procedures are done, which complicate definitive management. More commonly, children with a piriform sinus give a history of repeated upper respiratory tract infections and sore throats and often pain and tenderness of the thyroid with or without suppuration. Adults with the condition often recall their initial episodes from childhood. Hoarseness is frequent. Swallowing is often painful, and the head may be held preferentially in extension.[51]

The keys to correct diagnosis are a high index of suspicion and the demonstration of the mouth of a fistula in the piriform sinus. As noted previously it is now believed that third branchial anomalies enter the base of the piriform sinus (superior portion) and fourth branchial anomalies enter the apex (inferior portion).[24] Most of these anomalies—and all of them in neonates reported to date—occur on the left side of the neck. In utero diagnosis has now been made.[65] In this report the possibility of the development of congenital high airway obstruction syndrome (CHAOS) was entertained and a multidisciplinary team was assembled at delivery for management of possible life-threatening airway obstruction, which fortunately did not occur.[65] A prenatally diagnosed cyst may be absent at birth only to become evident with feedings.[12]

Beyond the newborn period, delay in diagnosis occurs when patients present with evidence of infection associated with a swelling usually in the left neck adjacent to the upper pole of the thyroid gland. This may be diagnosed as unilateral thyroiditis or as suppurative lymphadenitis. Because incision and drainage can complicate definitive management, it is important to recognize the possibility of an underlying piriform sinus fistula as the source of the infection. Upper endoscopy or imaging can be used to make the diagnosis. In one retrospective study comparing the effectiveness of barium esophagography, CT, magnetic resonance imaging (MRI), and sonography, CT was the most reliable study for visualizing the sinus or fistulous tract and for evaluating the extent of the lesion.[60] In the presence of acute infection a barium esophagogram may fail to show the fistula, which is then able to be demonstrated when the infection resolves.

At the time of definitive surgery, cannulation with a Fogarty catheter, guidewire, or lacrimal duct probe, most easily performed by direct, rather than flexible, endoscopy, has been reported to be an aid in the dissection during surgery, as has placing an esophageal bougie to aid in the palpation of the catheter.[20,43,58,79] Nonomura and associates advocate a horizontal incision of the thyroid cartilage ala followed by medial retraction of the strap muscles, vertical incision of the inferior pharyngeal constrictor muscle, disarticulation of the cricothyroid joint, and anterior retraction of the thyroid ala.[58] Others favor exposing the thyroid gland near its upper pole and then

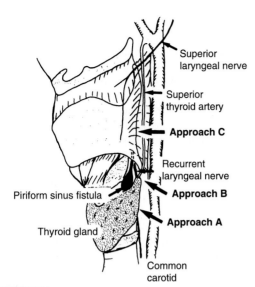

Figure 56–13 Schema of surgical approaches to a piriform sinus fistula. Approach C is approach recommended by Nonomura and colleagues. (From Nonomura N, et al: Surgical approach to piriform sinus fistula. Am J Otolaryngol 1993;14:111.)

dissecting superiorly[51] or identifying the fistula at the inferior border of the thyroid cartilage after incising the skin over the cricoid cartilage, retracting the thyroid gland laterally, and then exposing the cricothyroid and cricopharyngeal muscles (Fig. 56-13).[53] Enepekides stresses that the recurrent laryngeal nerve, which runs deep and medial to these lesions, must be identified and protected and notes that partial resection of the thyroid cartilage may be required for adequate exposure.[20] The external branch of the superior laryngeal nerve is also at risk in these dissections (Fig. 56-14). Resection of the

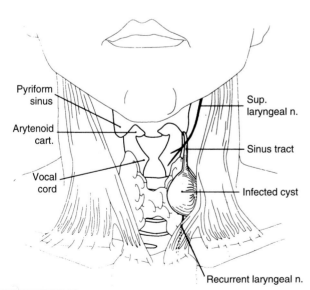

Figure 56–14 Thyroid abscess with piriform sinus tract. The tract passed up to the superior laryngeal nerve and superficial to the recurrent laryngeal nerve. *Note:* this would correspond to the course of a fourth branchial cleft sinus opening at the apex of the piriform sinus and descending deep to the superficial laryngeal nerve.

tract, adjacent scar tissue, and a portion of the thyroid gland or even hemithyroidectomy, when adherent to the tract, as well as ligation of the fistula opening in the piriform sinus, are regarded as essential steps in totally eradicating these lesions and reducing the chance of recurrence to a minimum.

There are possible exceptions to the rule of complete excision to prevent recurrence in the piriform sinus fistulas. The course of fourth branchial anomalies remains theoretical, a complete tract as illustrated in Figure 56-5 looping around the subclavian artery on the right and around the aorta on the left never having been demonstrated. Shugar and Healy advise against an overly aggressive attempt to remove a mediastinal tract.[67] To date, dissections of suspected fourth cleft tracts descending deep to the clavicle have been performed from the neck with no attempt to expose the aorta without reported recurrence.[28,67,71] Furthermore, there are now reports of obliteration of the piriform sinus tracts endoscopically with either electrocautery[39] or trichloroacetic acid.[60] Follow-up in the limited number of patients so treated has been short with the longest follow-up only 6 years. Additional experience with these techniques may support their use in patients in whom repeated infection and previous surgery make further attempts at complete excision hazardous.

THYROGLOSSAL DUCT CYSTS

Surgeons may rarely be in doubt preoperatively about the diagnosis of a midline neck mass, but they are often wrong. Knight and coworkers found specific preoperative diagnosis made by 28 surgeons over a 10-year period to be correct in only 61% of 146 cases.[41] The surgeon's postoperative diagnosis was the same as the final diagnosis in only 83% of the cases. Slightly more than 50% of their cases were thyroglossal duct cysts, 25% were epidermoid cysts, 15% were enlarged lymph nodes, 1.4% were median ectopic thyroid, and the remaining 5% were inflammation of unknown cause. Similarly, Torsiglieri and colleagues found only 70% of 97 children with thyroglossal duct cysts were diagnosed correctly before surgery.[72] In the Mayo Clinic series, the presentation was that of a cyst in 78% of 263 cases and a draining sinus— always the result of spontaneous or surgical drainage—in the remainder; 40% were located slightly lateral to the midline.[72] In a collected series of 381 patients, 60% were adjacent to the hyoid, 24% above the hyoid, 13% below the hyoid, and 8% intralingual.[4] A third had history of prior infection, and a fourth had prior surgical intervention. A variety of aerobic and anaerobic organisms have been isolated. *Haemophilus influenzae* and *Staphylococcus aureus* were the most commonly identified bacteria in one large series.[69] Males and females are equally affected in most series.

Most cases have a relatively benign presentation as a painless swelling, a draining sinus, or a tender mass. Occasionally, a patient complains of a bad taste in the mouth associated with spontaneous decompression of a cyst. Movement of the cyst with swallowing is often cited as a reliable diagnostic sign but can be difficult to evaluate in young children and is often present with other lesions when located near the hyoid bone. Unusual pediatric presentations include severe respiratory distress or even sudden infant death when these lesions are located at the base of the tongue,[9,66] a solitary cold thyroid nodule,[48,70] lingual thyroid presenting after previous thyroglossal cyst excision,[3] a lateral neck mass,[70] anterior tongue fistula,[56] actinomycosis in a persistent thyroglossal duct,[13] sublingual contiguous thyroglossal and dermoid cysts,[17] Hodgkin's disease,[29] and coexistence of thyroglossal and branchial cleft cysts.[72]

It is ideal to be as accurate as possible preoperatively about the diagnosis of a suspected thyroglossal duct cyst; however, more important is determining when not to operate and when to alter a planned procedure intraoperatively.

The question of what preoperative tests are needed for suspected thyroglossal duct cysts is a complex and controversial one. Many authorities state categorically that a thyroid scan should be done in all such cases to rule out an ectopic thyroid gland. Hypothyroidism as a result of removing a patient's only functioning thyroid tissue could thereby be avoided, although as Enepekides points out, most patients with cervical ectopic thyroid are hypothyroid.[20] Treatment with exogenous thyroid in such patients might result in reduction in the size of an ectopic gland that has hypertrophied in response to increased metabolic needs. In such cases, surgery could be avoided altogether. Furthermore, it has been reported anecdotally that physicians have been successfully sued for excising an ectopic thyroid.[62]

The financial implications of scanning all patients with midline masses in the neck, however, are significant, and alternate strategies for dealing with this issue have been proposed. The incidence of ectopic thyroid misdiagnosed as a thyroglossal duct cyst is reported to be between 1% and 2%.[4] The incidence is lower if one considers that the denominator should include dermoid cysts and anterior cervical lymph nodes, which are also frequently misdiagnosed as thyroglossal duct cysts. It would therefore theoretically require performing more than 100 negative scans to identify one ectopic thyroid, a substantial expense, not to mention the unnecessary radiation exposure to hundreds of patients. Basing their recommendations on a retrospective study of children undergoing thyroid scans at Boston Children's Hospital, Cleveland's Rainbow Babies, and Children's Hospital between 1978 and 1987, Radkowski and colleagues advise obtaining scans only when a careful history and physical examination or abnormal thyroid function studies suggest hypothyroidism (i.e., chronic constipation, developmental and growth delay, excessive somnolence, weight gain despite poor feeding habits, and elevated thyroid-stimulating hormone).[64] Others recommend obtaining a scan when preoperative ultrasound indicates the neck mass to be solid or thyroid tissue cannot be demonstrated in the normal location.[78,81] When a solid lesion is discovered unexpectedly at surgery, it is reasonable to obtain a frozen section to confirm the diagnosis. A decision then has to be made whether to preserve the gland by autotransplantation or

to excise the possibly dysgenetic gland. In both cases, lifetime treatment with exogenous thyroid is generally recommended, although in some cases with residual thyroid tissue supplementation has not been necessary.[30] Ideally, parents should be informed preoperatively about these possibilities.

CT,[21] MRI,[21] fistulography,[47] and fine-needle aspiration[63] in addition to thyroid hormone levels, ultrasound, and thyroid scans have all been described or advocated for preoperative workup of midline cervical masses. Their use in children in the absence of associated pathologic adenopathy, suspicion of impingement on laryngeal structures, or multiple recurrences is rarely needed; however, with appropriate indications, they can be helpful (Figs. 56-15 and 56-16).

An infected thyroglossal duct cyst should be treated initially with antibiotics and, if necessary, needle aspiration. Incision and drainage, which may result in seeding of ductal epithelium, is to be avoided when possible to reduce the chance of recurrence after subsequent excision. Perioperative antibiotics are recommended at the time of a Sistrunk procedure for a previously infected cyst. Overnight admission after excision is not required in the absence of difficulty with breathing or swallowing or an unreliable family situation.[33]

Management of recurrent thyroglossal duct cysts has been addressed in a number of reports.[19,36,50,61,75] Although most recurrences are identified early, intervals of up to 39 years have been reported.[36] Young patient age, skin involvement, previous or concurrent infection, lobulation of the cyst, rupture of the cyst at operation, and failure to remove the central portion of the hyoid and a core of tissue above it are all factors that predispose to recurrence. Principles in reoperations include a wider dissection extending inferiorly to remove a pyramidal lobe if present, removal of the central 3 to 4 cm of strap muscles down to the level of the pretracheal fascia, and a wider re-excision of the mid-hyoid bone and core of tissue to the foramen cecum.[50] Adherence to these guidelines should reduce the 25% to 35% recurrence rates reported after re-excision.[50,69]

It is estimated that less than 1% of thyroglossal duct cysts develop carcinoma.[4] Most of the 158 cases cited through 1994 have occurred in adults, but a child as young as 6 years old has been reported[4,80]; 80% are papillary carcinoma, but all types of thyroid malignancy are represented except for medullary carcinoma.[80] A Sistrunk procedure is considered adequate treatment when invasion of the capsule and regional or distant metastases are not present. Cure rate of 95% is expected for papillary carcinoma with this procedure. More radical surgery and postoperative radiation are indicated for other types of carcinoma.[80]

DERMOID CYSTS

The diagnosis of a cervical dermoid cyst is based on the histologic findings of epidermis with epidermal appendages, such as hair follicles, hair, and sebaceous glands, within the cyst wall.[14] These cysts form along the

Figure 56–15 Lateral (*A*) and anteroposterior (*B*) views of the two anterior neck masses in a clinically euthyroid 14-year-old girl. The superior one had been present for a year. The lower one had been present for 2 to 3 months and was increasing in size.

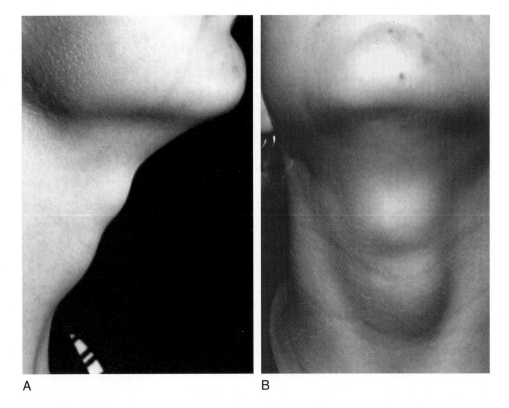

A   B

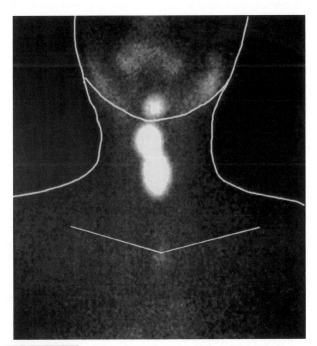

Figure 56–16 Anterior view of a ^{99m}Tc sodium pertechnetate thyroid scan performed after ultrasound showed the masses to be solid. The thyroid-stimulating hormone level was found to be at the upper limits of normal. Activity in the two clinically obvious masses, a previously unrecognized lingual mass at the base of the tongue, and no activity in the lower neck are evident. These findings were consistent with ectopic thyroid tissue at the three sites. The patient received ^{131}I for ablation of this tissue at the recommendation of a pediatric endocrinologist. The masses resolved. Now 9 years later as a pharmacy student she continues to do well on thyroid replacement therapy.

lines of embryonic fusion in the anterior neck. They are frequently confused preoperatively with thyroglossal duct cysts because they have the same distribution and may become inflamed. Similarly, there may also be confusion intraoperatively when these lesions are closely approximated to the hyoid bone. It is now recommended that a Sistrunk procedure be performed when there is doubt.[15,76] Aspirating or opening these cysts may result in spillage of cyst contents, which, in turn, may lead to infection or recurrence.

PREAURICULAR CYSTS

Preauricular cysts are included in this discussion not because they truly represent cysts or sinuses of the neck but because they need to be distinguished from first branchial cleft cysts. The former are common; are often bilateral; tend to be inherited; and only in rare cases are complicated by infection, involve the facial nerve, or enter into the external auditory canal.[49] They are believed to arise as a result of anomalies in the formation of the external ear from the two sets of three hillocks located on the dorsal end of the first two branchial arches. Singer stressed the fact that typically a series of cysts are found in continuity with the cutaneous sinus.[68] Successful excision through an inverted L-shaped incision requires removal of all ductal epithelium, which can be quite difficult when there is scarring from prior infection. It is generally agreed that surgery is indicated for symptomatic lesions, but it is not clear when or if asymptomatic ones should be removed. Many never cause a problem.

THYMIC CYSTS

Parenchymal cysts of the lower neck in children are rare. Wagner and coworkers collected 75 cases of thymic cysts in patients younger than 20 years of age up to 1988 and added 10 additional cases.[82] Diagnosis was based on the presence of spindle-shaped, spiral, or columnar cells; cholesterol crystals; Hassall's corpuscles; and giant cell reaction, all of which may occur in lower branchial cleft anomalies. They present as mobile, cystic masses, located anterior to but extending beneath the lower third of the sternocleidomastoid muscle. Although usually asymptomatic, they may cause significant respiratory problems as well as dysphagia, cervical pain, or hoarseness in 10% of cases.[31] They are most likely remnants of the third or fourth branchial pouches.

REFERENCES

1. Adams A: First endoscopic neck surgery deemed a success. Stanford Hosp Clin Med Staff Update Online 2002;26:1.
2. Alberti PW, Biagioni E: Facial paralysis in children: A review of 150 cases. Laryngoscope 1972;82:1013.
3. Alderson DJ, Lannigan FJ: Lingual thyroid presenting after previous thyroglossal cyst excision. J Laryngol Otol 1994; 108:341.
4. Allard RH: The thyroglossal cyst. Head Neck Surg 1982; 5:134.
5. Androulakis M, Johnson JT, Wagner RL: Thyroglossal duct and second branchial cleft anomalies in adults. Ear Nose Throat J 1990;69:318.
6. Arnot RS: Defects of the first branchial cleft. S Afr J Surg 1971;9:93.
7. Borger JA, Bercu BB: Papillary-follicular carcinoma arising in a thyroglossal duct cyst in a 12-year-old child. J Pediatr Surg 1988;23:362.
8. Burgess KL, Hartwick RW, Bedard YC: Metastatic squamous carcinoma presenting as a neck cyst: Differential diagnosis from inflamed branchial cleft cyst in fine needle aspirates. Acta Cytol 1993;37:494.
9. Byard RW, Bourne AJ, Silver MM: The association of lingual thyroglossal duct remnants with sudden death in infancy. Int J Pediatr Otorhinolaryngol 1990;20:107.
10. Celis I, Bijnens E, Peene P, Cleeren P: The use of preoperative fistulography in patients with a second branchial cleft anomaly. Eur Radiol 1998;8:1179.
11. Chandler JR, Mitchell B: Branchial cleft cysts, sinuses, and fistulas. Otolaryngol Clin North Am 1981;14:175.
12. Chin AC, Radhakrishnan J, Slatton D, Geissler G: Congenital cysts of the third and fourth pharyngeal pouches or pyriform sinus cysts. J Pediatr Surg 2000;35:1252.
13. Cobb RA, Ross HB: Actinomycosis in a persistent thyroglossal duct. Br J Surg 1986;73:751.
14. Cunningham MJ: The management of congenital neck masses. Am J Otolaryngol 1992;13:78.
15. deMello DE, Lima JA, Liapis H: Midline cervical cysts in children: Thyroglossal anomalies. Arch Otolaryngol Head Neck Surg 1987;113:418.
16. Dougall AJ: Anomalies of the first branchial cleft. J Pediatr Surg 1974;9:203.
17. Drucker C, Gerson CR: Sublingual contiguous thyroglossal and dermoid cysts in a neonate. Int J Pediatr Otorhinolaryngol 1992;23:181.
18. Durrant TJ, Sevick RJ, Lauryssen C, MacRae ME: Parapharyngeal branchial cleft cyst presenting with cranial nerve palsies. Can Assoc Radiol J 1994;45:134.
19. Ein SH, Shandling B, Stephens CA, Mancer K: The problem of recurrent thyroglossal duct remnants. J Pediatr Surg 1984;19:437.
20. Enepekides DJ: Management of congenital anomalies of the neck. Facial Plast Surg Clin North Am 2001;9:131.
21. Faerber EN, Swartz JD: Imaging of neck masses in infants and children. Crit Rev Diagn Imaging 1991;31:283.
22. Farrior JB, Santini H: Facial nerve identification in children. Otolaryngol Head Neck Surg 1985;93:173.
23. Ford GR, Balakrishnan A, Evans JN, Bailey CM: Branchial cleft and pouch anomalies. J Laryngol Otol 1992;106:137.
24. Franciosi JP, Sell LL, Conley SF, Bolender DL: Pyriform sinus malformations: A cadaveric representation. J Pediatr Surg 2002;37:533.
25. Gatot A, Tovi F, Fliss DM, Yanai-Inbar I: Branchial cleft cyst manifesting as hypoglossal nerve palsy. Head Neck 1991; 13:249.
26. Gatti WM, Zimm J: Bilateral branchial cleft fistulas: Diagnosis and management of two cases. Ear Nose Throat J 1988;67:256.
27. Girvigian MR, Rechdouni AK, Zeger GD, et al: Squamous cell carcinoma arising in a second branchial cleft cyst. Am J Clin Oncol 2004;27:96.
28. Godin MS, Kearns DB, Pransky SM, et al: Fourth branchial pouch sinus: Principles of diagnosis and management. Laryngoscope 1990;100:174.
29. Good GM, Isaacson G: Hodgkin's disease simulating a pediatric thyroglossal duct cyst. Am J Otolaryngol 2000; 21:277.
30. Grant DB, Hulse JA, Jackson DB, et al: Ectopic thyroid: Residual function after withdrawal of treatment in infancy and later childhood. Acta Paediatr Scand 1989;78:889.
31. Guba AM Jr, Adam AE, Jaques DA, Chambers RG: Cervical presentation of thymic cysts. Am J Surg 1978;136:430.
32. Haus BM, Kambham N, Le D, et al: Surgical robotic applications in otolaryngology. Laryngoscope 2003;113:1139.
33. Helmus C, Grin M, Westfall R: Same-day-stay head and neck surgery. Laryngoscope 1992;102:1331.
34. Himi T, Kataura A: Distribution of C cells in the thyroid gland with pyriform sinus fistula. Otolaryngol Head Neck Surg 1995;112:268.
35. Horisawa M, Niinomi N, Ito T: Anatomical reconstruction of the thyroglossal duct. J Pediatr Surg 1991;26:766.
36. Howard DJ, Lund VJ: Thyroglossal ducts, cysts and sinuses: A recurrent problem. Ann R Coll Surg Engl 1986;68:137.
37. Ikarashi F, Nakano Y, Nonomura N, et al: Clinical features of first branchial cleft anomalies. Am J Otolaryngol 1996; 17:233.
38. Isaacson G, Martin WH: First branchial cleft cyst excision with electrophysiological facial nerve localization. Arch Otolaryngol Head Neck Surg 2000;126:513.
39. Jordan JA, Graves JE, Manning SC, et al: Endoscopic cauterization for treatment of fourth branchial cleft sinuses. Arch Otolaryngol Head Neck Surg 1998;124:1021.
40. Kaneko T, Kitamura T, Asano H: Anomalies of the first branchial cleft (fistula and cyst). J Laryngol Otol 1974;88:1213.
41. Knight PJ, Hamoudi AB, Vassy LE: The diagnosis and treatment of midline neck masses in children. Surgery 1983;93:603.
42. Kornblut AD: Traumatic facial nerve injuries in children. Adv Otorhinolaryngol 1977;22:171.
43. Kubota M, Suita S, Kamimura T, Zaizen Y: Surgical strategy for the treatment of pyriform sinus fistula. J Pediatr Surg 1997;32:34.

44. Lin AE, Losken HW, Jaffe R, Biglan AW: The branchio-oculo-facial syndrome. Cleft Palate Craniofac J 1991;28:96.
45. Lin JN, Wang KL: Persistent third branchial apparatus. J Pediatr Surg 1991;26:663.
46. Liston SL: The relationship of the facial nerve and first branchial cleft anomalies—embryologic considerations. Laryngoscope 1982;92:1308.
47. Massoud TF, Schnetler JF: Case report: Taste of success in thyroglossal fistulography. Clin Radiol 1992;45:281.
48. McHenry CR, Danish R, Murphy T, Marty JJ: Atypical thyroglossal duct cyst: A rare cause for a solitary cold thyroid nodule in childhood. Am Surg 1993;59:223.
49. Melnick M, Myrianthopoulos NC, Paul NW: External ear malformations: Epidemiology, genetics, and natural history. Birth Defects Orig Artic Ser 1979;15:i.
50. Mickel RA, Calcaterra TC: Management of recurrent thyroglossal duct cysts. Arch Otolaryngol 1983;109:34.
51. Miller D, Hill JL, Sun CC, et al: The diagnosis and management of pyriform sinus fistulae in infants and young children. J Pediatr Surg 1983;18:377.
52. Miyauchi A, Matsuzuka F, Kuma K, Katayama S: Piriform sinus fistula and the ultimobranchial body. Histopathology 1992;20:221.
53. Miyauchi A, Matsuzuka F, Kuma K, Takai S: Piriform sinus fistula: An underlying abnormality common in patients with acute suppurative thyroiditis. World J Surg 1990;14:400.
54. Mouri N, Muraji T, Nishijima E, Tsugawa C: Reappraisal of lateral cervical cysts in neonates: Pyriform sinus cysts as an anatomy-based nomenclature. J Pediatr Surg 1998; 33:1141.
55. Murthy P, Shenoy P, Khan NA: First cleft branchial fistula in a child—a modified surgical technique. J Laryngol Otol 1994;108:1078.
56. Ngo HH, Frenkiel S, Satin R: Thyroglossal duct cyst presenting as an anterior tongue fistula, J Otolaryngol 1988; 17:227.
57. Nicollas R, Guelfucci B, Roman S, Triglia JM: Congenital cysts and fistulas of the neck. Int J Pediatr Otorhinolaryngol 2000;55:117.
58. Nonomura N, Ikarashi F, Fujisaki T, Nakano Y: Surgical approach to pyriform sinus fistula. Am J Otolaryngol 1993;14:111.
59. Olsen KD, Maragos NE, Weiland LH: First branchial cleft anomalies. Laryngoscope 1980;90:423.
60. Park SW, Han MH, Sung MH et al: Neck infection associated with pyriform sinus fistula: Imaging findings. AJNR Am J Neuroradiol 2000;21:817.
61. Pelausa ME, Forte V: Sistrunk revisited: A 10-year review of revision thyroglossal duct surgery at Toronto's Hospital for Sick Children. J Otolaryngol 1989;18:325.
62. Pinczower E, Crockett DM, Atkinson JB, Kun S: Preoperative thyroid scanning in presumed thyroglossal duct cysts. Arch Otolaryngol Head Neck Surg 1992;118:985.
63. Pitts WC, Tani EM, Skoog L: Papillary carcinoma in fine needle aspiration smears of a thyroglossal duct lesion. Acta Cytol 1988;32:599.
64. Radkowski D, Arnold J, Healy GB, et al: Thyroglossal duct remnants: Preoperative evaluation and management. Arch Otolaryngol Head Neck Surg 1991;117:1378.
65. Robichaud J, Papsin BC, Forte V: Third branchial cleft anomaly detected in utero. J Otolaryngol 2000;29:185.
66. Samuel M, Freeman NV, Sajwany MJ: Lingual thyroglossal duct cyst presenting in infancy. J Pediatr Surg 1993;28:891.
67. Shugar MA, Healy GB: The fourth branchial cleft anomaly. Head Neck Surg 1980;3:72.
68. Singer R: A new technic for extirpation of preauricular cysts. Am J Surg 1966;111:291.
69. Solomon JR, Rangecroft L: Thyroglossal-duct lesions in childhood. J Pediatr Surg 1984;19:555.
70. Sonnino RE, Spigland N, Laberge JM, et al: Unusual patterns of congenital neck masses in children. J Pediatr Surg 1989;24:966.
71. Takimoto T, Yoshizaki T, Ohoka H, Sakashita H: Fourth branchial pouch anomaly. J Laryngol Otol 1990;104:905.
72. Telander RL, Deane SA: Thyroglossal and branchial cleft cysts and sinuses. Surg Clin North Am 1977;57:779.
73. Terris DJ, Haus BM, Gourin CG: Endoscopic neck surgery: Resection of the submandibular gland in a cadaver model. Laryngoscope 2004;114:407.
74. Terris DJ, Monfared A, Thomas A, et al: Endoscopic selective neck dissection in a porcine model. Arch Otolaryngol Head Neck Surg 2003;129:613.
75. Tetteroo GW, Snellen JP, Knegt P, Jeekel J: Operative treatment of median cervical cysts. Br J Surg 1988;75:382.
76. Todd NW: Common congenital anomalies of the neck: Embryology and surgical anatomy, Surg Clin North Am 1993;73:599.
77. Tom LW, Kenealy JF, Torsiglieri AJ Jr: First branchial cleft anomalies involving the tympanic membrane and middle ear. Otolaryngol Head Neck Surg 1991;105:473.
78. Torsiglieri AJ Jr, Tom LW, Ross AJ 3rd, et al: Pediatric neck masses: Guidelines for evaluation. Int J Pediatr Otorhinolaryngol 1988;16:199.
79. Tyler D, Effmann E, Shorter N: Pyriform sinus cyst and fistula in the newborn: The value of endoscopic cannulation. J Pediatr Surg 1992;27:1500.
80. Van Vuuren PA, Balm AJ, Gregor RT, et al: Carcinoma arising in thyroglossal remnants. Clin Otolaryngol 1994;19:509.
81. Wadsworth DT, Siegel MJ: Thyroglossal duct cysts: Variability of sonographic findings. AJR Am J Roentgenol 1994;163:1475.
82. Wagner CW, Vinocur CD, Weintraub WH, Golladay ES: Respiratory complications in cervical thymic cysts. J Pediatr Surg 1988;23:657.
83. Work WP: Newer concepts of first branchial cleft defects. Laryngoscope 1972;82:1581.

Chapter 57

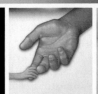

Torticollis

Spencer Beasley

There are many causes of torticollis in childhood (Table 57-1), but most of these causes are rare. The most common cause of torticollis is tightness and shortening of one sternomastoid muscle, a condition that occurs in about 0.4% of all births. Typically, at about 3 weeks of age, a visible or palpable swelling develops in part or all of the muscle; this swelling is called a sternomastoid tumor. It affects the right side in about 60%,[31] is bilateral in 2% to 8%,[43,45] and often persists for up to 1 year. Older children may have a fibrotic, shortened sternomastoid muscle, which is presumed in many to be the legacy of a previously unrecognized sternomastoid tumor.

HISTORY

Alexander the Great may have had torticollis, according to Plutarch.[38] Antyllus is said to have performed tenotomies in 350 AD, but the first authenticated division of the sternocleidomastoid was by Minnus in Amsterdam in 1641.[44]

A sternocleidomastoid tumor was described by Heusinger in 1826.[23] Torticollis was also a subject of interest to Dupuytren.[18]

ETIOLOGY

Little is known about the etiology of sternomastoid fibrosis, although several theories have been put forward to explain the condition. It may be due to an idiopathic intrauterine embryopathy[29] or could be the manifestation of an intrauterine positional disorder with development of the sternocleidomastoid compartment syndrome.[25] The high incidence of obstetric difficulties, such as breech presentation and the need for assisted delivery,[10,11] may be the result rather than the cause of the shortened sternomastoid muscle. There is no report of a sternomastoid tumor detected by antenatal ultrasound.[49] Concomitant hip dysplasia is common.[10]

PATHOLOGY

The basic abnormality on histology is fibrous replacement of muscle bundles.[34] Jones[29] has described endomysial fibrosis involving the deposition of collagen and fibroblasts around individual muscle fibers that undergo atrophy. The sarcoplasmic nuclei are compacted to form giant cells that appear to be multinucleated. The maturity of the fibrous tissue in neonates suggests that the disease may begin before birth[17,29,32] and may therefore contribute to the frequency of obstetric difficulties during delivery. The reported incidence of breech deliveries is about 20% to 30%[14]—much higher than the normal incidence. About 60% of affected infants are involved in a complicated birth,[14] which suggests that the fibrosis may affect the position of the fetus in utero and perhaps prevent normal engagement of the head in the maternal pelvis.

The natural history of untreated sternomastoid fibrosis is complete resolution in 50% to 70% of patients at 6 months of age. In about 10%, the tumor and sternomastoid shortening persist beyond 12 months of age.[15,43] The severity and distribution of the fibrosis vary and have led

TABLE 57–1 Causes of Torticollis in Infants and Children	
Cause	**Comment**
Sternomastoid tumor	Common; appears at 3 weeks of age
Abnormal position in utero	Tends to improve with age
Cervical hemivertebrae	Structural; confirmed on plain radiograph
Cervical lymphadenitis/ abscess	Acute; usually occurs in first 2 years of life
Retropharyngeal abscess[21]	Acute; signs of toxicity
Posterior fossa tumors[46]	A rare cause; other neurologic signs present
Acute atlantoaxial subluxation	May occur after tonsillectomy[2]
Atlantoaxial rotatory subluxation	Significance disputed[25]; diagnosed on dynamic CT
Spasmodic with gastroesophageal reflux	Sandifer's syndrome
Postural	Familial

to a variety of classifications based either on a palpable localized sternomastoid tumor or thickening and shortening of the whole muscle or on ultrasonographic findings.[27,42] The systems of classification have some prognostic significance in that localized lesions within the sternomastoid (clinically or ultrasonographically) are more likely to resolve spontaneously than those involving the whole muscle. In older children with torticollis, the appearance of degenerating fibers is more consistent with disuse atrophy produced by limitation of movement caused by the fibrosis.

CLINICAL FEATURES

Sternomastoid Torticollis

The tumor is a hard, spindle-shaped, painless discrete swelling usually about 1 to 3 cm in diameter within the substance of the sternomastoid muscle. Over 90% develop before the age of 3 months.[10] However, it usually first becomes evident at about 3 weeks after birth. Obvious head tilt or torticollis tends to develop later.[49] In infants, the head is rotated to the side opposite the tumor, with only slight flexion of the head to the affected side (Fig. 57-1).

In other patients, the sternomastoid tumor is less discrete, and the sternomastoid appears to be thickened and tightened along its whole length. These changes restrict rotation and lateral flexion of the head (Fig. 57-2). The rotational component of the action of the sternomastoid is easy to measure. It is assessed by standing behind the child's head and passively rotating the head while it is held between both hands. The sternomastoid muscle is stretched to its maximum length by rotation to the side of the affected muscle. Where the muscle is fibrotic, it cannot be stretched to its full length, and rotation to the ipsilateral side is restricted.

Older children with torticollis compensate for the more pronounced tilt by elevating one shoulder to enable the eyes to keep as level as possible (Fig. 57-3). Such compensation is not seen in infants because there is no need for them to maintain their eyes in a horizontal plane until they stand up.[28] Moreover, older children do not turn their heads to the contralateral side as much because

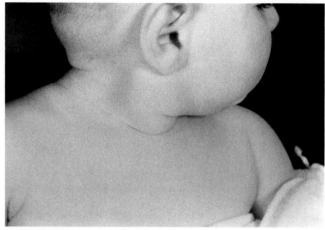

Figure 57–1 Appearance of a right sternomastoid tumor in infancy; the head is turned to the contralateral side.

they tend to compensate by twisting the neck and back to keep their eyes pointing forward.

Differential Diagnosis

Initial clinical assessment must establish whether the wry neck is caused by shortness of one sternomastoid muscle or by some other condition. In sternomastoid fibrosis, the anterior border of the muscle stands out as a tight band, although in some small infants in whom the neck is relatively short, the muscle may be difficult to see readily. For this reason, the full length of the muscle must be palpated to determine whether there is an area of thickening or fibrosis along part or all of its length. In about two thirds, there is a definite localized swelling (tumor) in the muscle; in the remainder, the whole muscle appears to be affected. Though not required for diagnosis, it has a characteristic appearance on ultrasonography that may help predict (to a degree) the likelihood of spontaneous resolution.[19,31,42] It can also be diagnosed on magnetic resonance imaging (MRI)[19] and computed tomography (CT).[33] In cases in which the muscle is neither prominent nor shortened, the torticollis is not caused by an abnormality

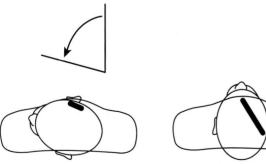

Normal range   Neutral position

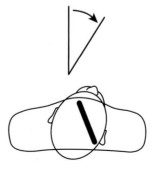

Limited range

Figure 57–2 Restriction of rotation of the head secondary to shortening of the sternomastoid muscle as viewed from above the head. The *black bars* represent the right sternomastoid muscle and show that its inability to lengthen limits rotation to that side.

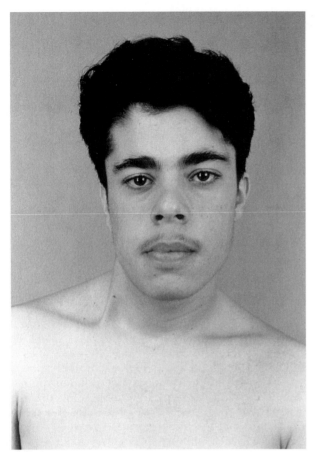

Figure 57-3 Appearance of torticollis as a result of sternomastoid fibrosis in an older child. The eyes are kept horizontal, but the shortened sternomastoid muscle causes compensatory elevation of the shoulder. (From Beasley SW: Pediatric Diagnosis. London, Chapman & Hall, 1994.)

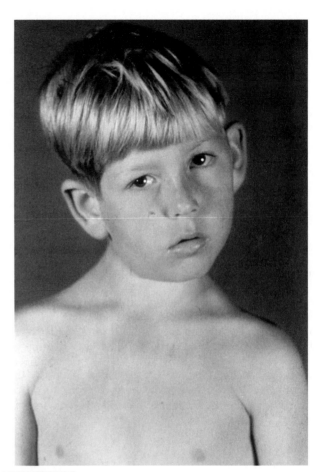

Figure 57-4 Torticollis caused by atlanto-occipital subluxation after tonsillectomy. Notice that there is no tightness of the sternomastoid muscle on either side. (From Beasley SW: Pediatric Diagnosis. London, Chapman & Hall, 1994.)

of the sternomastoid muscle, and alternative diagnoses must be sought (see Table 57-1 and Fig. 57-4).[3,28]

A squint may cause head tilt from imbalance in rotation of the eyes. The squint may not be obvious at first because the tilt compensates for the abnormal position of the eyes. When the head is straightened passively, the squint becomes apparent. Occasionally, sternomastoid fibrosis may occur coincidentally with ocular torticollis.

Posterior fossa tumors may compress the brainstem at the foramen magnum and produce acute stiffness of the neck that causes it to be held to one side. The neck is frozen in this position and is difficult to move actively or passively. The presence of a central nervous system tumor may be known already, but occasionally, acute torticollis is the first manifestation. Careful neurologic examination may show abnormalities of the lower cranial nerves and cerebellar function, and the causative lesion is demonstrated on CT or MRI.

Hemivertebrae involving the cervical spine may produce a tilt of the head that is evident from birth and does not progress. Vertebral lesions can be identified clinically by inspection and palpation of the dorsal cervical spines and confirmed on plain radiographs of the neck.

Acute torticollis has been attributed to atlantoaxial rotatory subluxation as determined on dynamic CT,[36,37] but others doubt the existence or significance of these findings and suggest that CT scans are not necessary at the initial examination.[24] Atlantoaxial subluxation has been reported after tonsillectomy.[2] Acute torticollis can also result from inflammatory conditions of the neck, including retropharyngeal abscess,[21] and can be a symptom of acute lymphoblastic leukemia.[39]

SECONDARY EFFECTS OF TORTICOLLIS

Table 57-2 lists the secondary effects of torticollis.

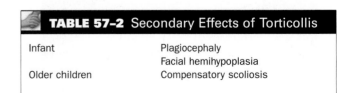

TABLE 57-2 Secondary Effects of Torticollis

Infant	Plagiocephaly
	Facial hemihypoplasia
Older children	Compensatory scoliosis

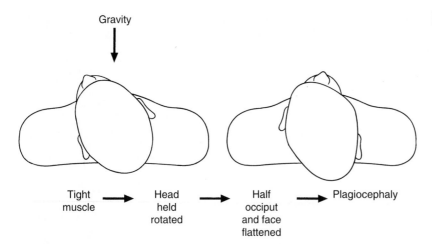

Gravity

Tight muscle → Head held rotated → Half occiput and face flattened → Plagiocephaly

Figure 57–5 Plagiocephaly.

Plagiocephaly

In small infants with torticollis and fixed rotation of the head, gravity deforms the relatively soft head as it lies in the same position for a prolonged period. Flattening of one occiput leads to secondary flattening of the contralateral forehead (Fig. 57-5). This asymmetric skull deformity is called *plagiocephaly* and develops in the first few months of life.[26] It is best observed from above the head. Once the child begins to sit up or the torticollis resolves, the plagiocephaly tends to resolve as well.[35] It may take several years to disappear, and a few children have a slight permanent deformity.

Facial Hypoplasia

Progressive facial deformity is seen when one sternomastoid muscle immobilizes the face for a long time. The malar eminence on the side of the face limited by the fibrotic muscle grows more slowly than the normal side does[25] and causes progressive asymmetry (Fig. 57-6). This inhibition of growth

of the mandible and maxilla embodies an important principle of pediatrics: normal growth of bones depends on normal muscular movement.

The degree of hemihypoplasia of the face can be determined by the angle between the plane of the eyes and the plane of the mouth. Normally these lines are parallel, but they form an angle to each other when the face is asymmetric. The development of hemihypoplasia is one indication for surgery; division of the tight sternomastoid muscle allows resolution of the skeletal abnormality and subsequent normal growth.[25]

Significant facial hemihypoplasia takes about 8 months to develop[29] but is more often recognized at about 3 to 4 years of age.[15] It becomes less obvious with ongoing growth once the torticollis has resolved.

Postural Compensation

When children are old enough to walk, the eyes are kept horizontal to facilitate balance and horizontal eye movement. The child compensates for the short fibrous sternomastoid by elevating the ipsilateral shoulder (see Fig. 57-3). In addition, there may be compensatory cervical and thoracic scoliosis. Adjacent muscles, such as the trapezius, may be wasted because of inactivity.[29]

CONSERVATIVE MANAGEMENT

Sternomastoid fibrosis resolves spontaneously in the vast majority of infants. Therefore, surgery is required only rarely. The value of manipulation of the head and neck has not been proved,[49] although it is widely used and may have some benefit in the first year of life.[12] Physiotherapy and regular neck exercises appear to be safe[12] and may make the parents feel that "something is being done" for their infant. Unintentional snapping during manipulation has been reported with no apparent deleterious effect on outcome.[8] Some clinicians advocate early institution of intensive passive neck range-of-motion stretching exercises and have reported high rates of resolution,[5,6,25,41] but no convincing evidence has shown that these measures alter the natural history of the condition.

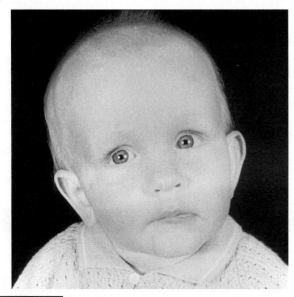

Figure 57-6 Facial hemihypoplasia on the right side.

Others consider it important to encourage parents to place toys and other desirable objects on the ipsilateral side to encourage the infant to turn toward the affected side.[29] Again, this strategy probably helps the parent more than the infant but is unlikely to do any harm. Attempts to put the infant to sleep with the head facing toward the affected side tend to fail, particularly if the muscle is tight. In most cases, reassurance is all that is required.

OPERATIVE TREATMENT

Indications for Surgery

Indications for surgery include

1. Persistent sternomastoid tightness limiting head rotation beyond 12 to 15 months of age[47]
2. Persistent sternomastoid tightness with progressive facial hemihypoplasia
3. Diagnosis in children older than 1 year[16]

Operative Technique

The procedure is performed under general anesthesia with laryngeal or endotracheal intubation, according to the expertise and preference of the pediatric anesthetist. The child is placed supine with the shoulders elevated and the neck rotated to the contralateral side. The muscle is best divided at its lower end,[25,38] although division at its upper end,[30] at both ends,[1,7,22] or in its midportion[20,29] have all been described. Endoscopic tenotomy of the muscle is also feasible.[4,13,40]

A 3- to 4-cm transverse incision is made in a skin crease about 1 cm above the sternal and clavicular heads of the affected sternomastoid (Fig. 57-7). The platysma is divided in the line of the incision. The external jugular vein can be retracted if it is within the field of view.

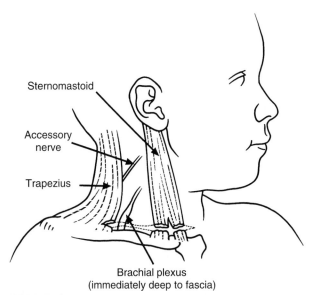

Figure 57-8 Division of the sternomastoid and investing cervical fascia to the anterior border of the trapezius.

The two heads of the sternomastoid muscle are dissected free, and the muscle is divided via diathermy so that no bleeding occurs. The investing cervical fascia anterior and posterior to the muscle must also be divided and the division continued posteriorly across the lower part of the posterior triangle of the neck (Fig. 57-8). Tightness of the cervical fascia between the sternomastoid and trapezius is usually palpable, and the fascia should be divided under direct vision to avoid damage to other structures, particularly the accessory nerve and branchial plexus.

The wound is infiltrated with bupivacaine or other local anesthetic agent. The platysma is closed with continuous 4-0 absorbable suture and the skin with subcuticular 5-0 Monocryl absorbable suture. No drains are required.

The procedure can be performed as a day case, and no postoperative restriction of movement is necessary. Full range of the neck is normally achieved within 1 week of surgery. Physiotherapy is usually unnecessary, although some advocate an extended period of physiotherapy postoperatively.[1] In older children, however, it may take longer, and the final cosmetic appearance is less certain.[9]

Complications

A hematoma may develop if hemostasis was inadequate at the time of surgery. Diathermy dissection keeps blood loss to a minimum. Larger superficial veins may require ligation and division if they cannot be retracted.

Incomplete division of both heads of the sternocleidomastoid muscle or failure to divide the cervical fascia over the posterior triangle of the neck may produce persistent torticollis. Careful inspection and palpation of the neck for residual tightness and bands at the time of surgery should prevent this complication from occurring. Recurrent torticollis is rare after surgical treatment and is seen in less than 3% of patients.[48]

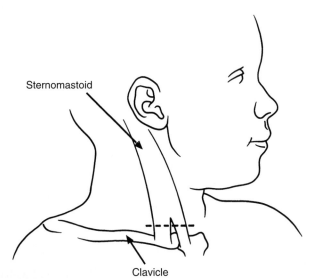

Figure 57-7 Skin incision for low division of the sternomastoid muscle.

Follow-up

Patients should be monitored until (1) the torticollis has resolved completely, (2) there is full range of movement of the head and neck, and (3) the sternomastoid muscle feels normal. In an older child with secondary scoliosis, follow-up, including radiologic studies if required, should continue until the scoliosis has resolved.

REFERENCES

1. Arslan H, Gunduz S, Subasy M, et al: Frontal cephalometric analysis in the evaluation of facial asymmetry in torticollis, and outcomes of bipolar release in patients over six years of age. Arch Orthop Trauma Surg 2002;122:489.
2. Bedi HS, Angliss RD, Williams SA, Connelly DP: Torticollis following adenotonsillectomy. Aust N Z J Surg 1999;69:63.
3. Bredenkamp JK, Hoover LA, Berke GS, Shaw A: Congenital muscular torticollis. A spectrum of disease. Arch Otolaryngol Head Neck Surg 1990;116:212.
4. Burstein FD, Cohen SR: Endoscopic surgical treatment for congenital muscular torticollis. Plast Reconstr Surg 1998;101:20.
5. Cameron BH, Langer JC, Cameron GS: Success of non-operative treatment for congenital muscular torticollis is dependent on early therapy. Pediatr Surg Int 1994;9:391.
6. Celayir AC: Congenital muscular torticollis: Early and intensive treatment is critical. A prospective study. Pediatr Int 2000;42:504.
7. Chen CE, Ko JY: Surgical treatment of muscular torticollis for patients above six years of age. Arch Orthop Trauma Surg 2000;120:149.
8. Cheng JC, Chen TM, Tang SP, et al: Snapping during manual stretching in congenital muscular torticollis. Clin Orthop 2001;384:237.
9. Cheng JC, Tang SP: Outcome of surgical treatment of congenital muscular torticollis. Clin Orthop 1999;362:190.
10. Cheng JC, Tang SP, Chen TM: Sternocleidomastoid pseudotumor and congenital muscular torticollis in infants: A prospective study of 510 cases. J Pediatr 1999;134:712.
11. Cheng JC, Tang SP, Chen TM, et al: The clinical presentation and outcome of treatment of congenital muscular torticollis in infants—a study of 1,086 cases. J Pediatr Surg 2000;35:1091.
12. Cheng JC, Wong MW, Tang SP, et al: Clinical determinants of the outcome of manual stretching in the treatment of congenital muscular torticollis in infants. A prospective study of 821 cases. J Bone Joint Surg Am 2001;83:679.
13. Cole R: Endoscopic surgical treatment for congenital muscular torticollis. Plast Reconstr Surg 1998;102:579.
14. Davids JR, Wenger DR, Mubarak SJ: Congenital muscular torticollis: Sequela of intrauterine or perinatal compartment syndrome. J Pediatr Orthop 1993;13:141.
15. de Chalain TM, Katz A: Idiopathic muscular torticollis in children: The Cape Town experience. Br J Plast Surg 1992;45:297.
16. Demirbilek S, Atayurt HF: Congenital muscular torticollis and sternomastoid tumour: Results of non-operative treatment. J Pediatr Surg 1999;34:549.
17. Dunn PM: Congenital sternomastoid torticollis: An intrauterine postural deformity. J Bone Joint Surg Br 1973;55:877.
18. Dupuytren G: Lecons Orales de Clinique Chirurgicale. Paris, JB Bailliere et Fils, 1839.

19. Entel RJ, Carolan FJ: Congenital muscular torticollis: Magnetic resonance imaging and ultrasound diagnosis. J Neuroimaging 1997;7:128.
20. Gurpinar A, Kiristioglu I, Balkan E, Dogruyol H: Surgical correction of muscular torticollis in older children with Peter G. Jones technique. J Pediatr Orthop 1998;18:98.
21. Harries PG: Retropharyngeal abscess and acute torticollis. J Laryngol Otol 1997;111:1183.
22. Hellstadius A: Torticollis congenita. Acta Chir Scand 1972;62:586.
23. Heusinger KP: Berichte von konighlichen, anthropanatomischen Anstalt zur Wurtzburg, Ber F D Schuljahr 1824/25, Etlinger, Wurtzburg 1826;4:43.
24. Hicazi A, Acaroglu E, Alanay A, et al: Atlantoaxial rotatory fixation-subluxation revisited: A computed tomographic analysis of acute torticollis in pediatric patients. Spine 2002;27:2771.
25. Hirschl RB: Sternocleidomastoid torticollis. In Spitz L, Coran A (eds): Rob & Smith's Operative Surgery: Pediatric Surgery, 5th ed. London, Chapman & Hall, 1995.
26. Hollier L, Kim J, Grayson BH, McCarthy JG: Congenital muscular torticollis and the associated craniofacial changes. Plast Reconstr Surg 2000;105:827.
27. Hsu TC, Wang CL, Wong MK, et al: Correlation of clinical and ultrasonographic features in congenital muscular torticollis. Arch Phys Med Rehabil 1999;80:637.
28. Hutson JM, Beasley SW: The Surgical Examination of Children. London, Heinemann, 1988.
29. Jones PG: Torticollis in Infancy and Childhood. Springfield IL, Charles C Thomas, 1967.
30. Lange C: Zur Behandlung des Schiefhalses. Wochenschr Orthop Chir 1910;27:440.
31. Lin JN, Chou ML: Ultrasonographic study of the sternocleidomastoid muscle in the management of congenital muscular torticollis. J Pediatr Surg 1997;32:1648.
32. MacDonald D: Sternomastoid tumour and muscular torticollis. J Bone Joint Surg Br 1969;41:432.
33. McGuire KJ, Silber J, Flynn JM, et al: Torticollis in children: Can dynamic computed tomography help determine severity and treatment? J Pediatr Orthop 2002;22:766.
34. Middleton DS: The pathology of congenital torticollis, Br J Surg 1930;18:188.
35. Morrison DL, Macewen GD: Congenital muscular torticollis: Observations regarding clinical findings, associated conditions and results of treatment. J Pediatr Orthop 1982;2:500.
36. Muniz AE, Belfer RA: Atlantoaxial rotary subluxation in children. Pediatr Emerg Care 1999;15:25.
37. Nicholson P, Higgins T, Fogarty E, et al: Three-dimensional spiral CT scanning in children with acute torticollis. Int Orthop 1999;23:47.
38. Peterson F: Zur Frage des Kopfnickerhamatoms bei Neugeborenen. Zentralbl Gynzkol 1886;10:777.
39. Rauch R, Jungert J, Rupprecht T, Greil J: Torticollis revealing as a symptom of acute lymphoblastic leukaemia in a 14 month old girl. Acta Paediatr 2002;90:587.
40. Sasaki S, Yamamoto Y, Sugihara T, et al: Endoscopic tenotomy of the sternocleidomastoid muscle: New method for surgical correction of muscular torticollis. Plast Reconstr Surg 2000;105:1764.
41. Stassen LF, Kerawala CJ: New surgical technique for the correction of congenital muscular torticollis (wry neck). Br J Oral Maxillofac Surg 2000;38:142.
42. Tang SF, Hsu KH, Wong AM, et al: Longitudinal followup study of ultrasonography in congenital muscular torticollis. Clin Orthop 2002;403:179.
43. Thomsen JR, Koltai PJ: Sternomastoid tumour of infancy. Ann Otol Rhinol Laryngol 1989;98:955.
44. Tubby AH: Deformities, 2nd ed. London, Macmillan, 1912.

45. Tufano RP, Tom LW, Austin MB: Bilateral sternocleidomastoid tumors of infancy. Int J Pediatr Otorhinolaryngol 1999;51:41.
46. Turgut M: Torticollis secondary to posterior fossa tumors. J Pediatr Orthop 1998;18:415.
47. Wei JL, Schwartz KM, Weaver AL, Orvidas LJ: Pseudotumor of infancy and congenital muscular torticollis: 170 cases. Laryngoscope 2001;111:688.

48. Wirth CJ, Hagena FW, Wuelker N, Siebert WE: Biterminal tenotomy for the treatment of congenital muscular torticollis. Long-term results. J Bone Joint Surg Am 1992;74:427.
49. Wright JE: Sternomastoid tumour and torticollis in infancy and childhood. Paediatr Surg Int 1994;9:172.

Part VI

THORAX

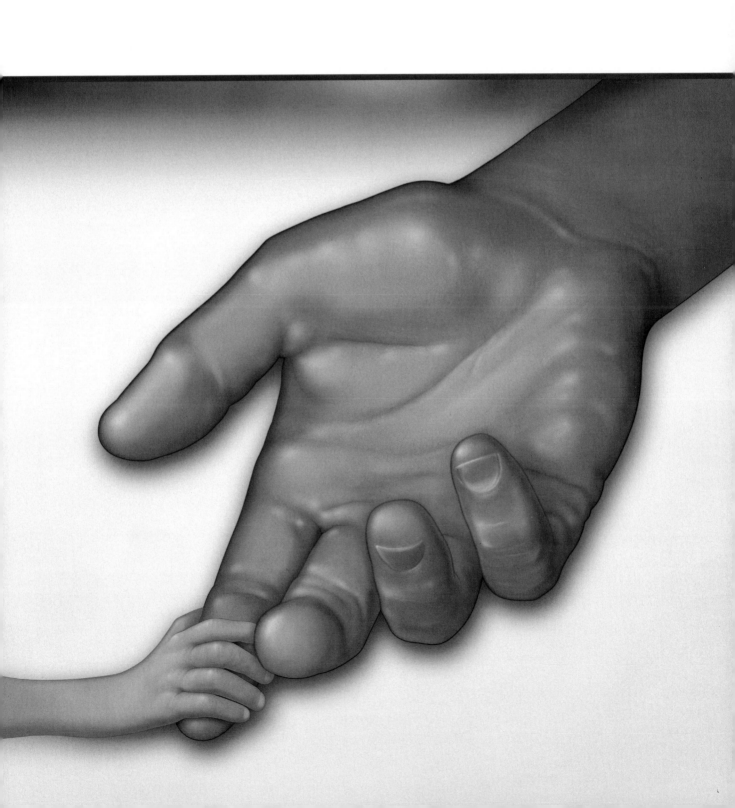

Chapter 58

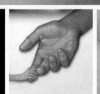

Disorders of the Breast

Mary L. Brandt

Development of the breast begins at around 35 days' gestation, when the ectoderm on the anterior body wall thickens into a ridge known as the milk line, milk ridge, or Hughes line.[20] This ridge of tissue extends from the area of the developing axilla to the area of the developing inguinal canal. In term infants, the milk line extends into the axilla and inferior to the inguinal area onto the medial thigh. The ridge above and below the area of the pectoralis muscle recedes around the 10th week of gestation, leaving the mammary primordium, which is the origin of the lactiferous ducts.[12,41] The initial ducts form between weeks 10 and 20 and become interspersed through the developing mesenchyma, which becomes the fibrous and fatty portions of the breast.[12] The breast bud becomes palpable at 34 weeks' gestation.[12] The nipple appears much later, at 8 months' gestation. It is initially a depression and later becomes elevated.[41]

Thelarche, or the onset of pubertal breast development, occurs between the ages of 8 and 13 years, at an average 11 to 11.5 years.[50] Lack of development by age 13 is considered delayed and warrants endocrinologic evaluation.[48] Normal breast development is hormonally mediated.[19] Adipose tissue and the lactiferous ducts grow in response to estrogen. Progesterone stimulation results in lobular growth and alveolar budding.[19,50] The normal development of the breast, which occurs over a period of 2 to 4 years after thelarche, is classified by the Tanner system into five stages (Table 58-1). Menarche usually occurs approximately 2 years after Tanner stage 2.

PREMATURE THELARCHE

Although normal thelarche occurs between 8 and 13 years of age, breast buds can appear in those as young as 1 to 3 years and have been reported to be present at birth.[47] Although the vast majority of patients with premature thelarche have no associated medical problems, hypothyroidism is a rare cause of premature thelarche that should be considered.[19] Premature thelarche is often an isolated condition but may be the first symptom of precocious puberty, particularly in girls older than 2 years.[47] Precocious puberty has been reported to occur in up to

18% of girls with premature thelarche who are followed over time.[44] Serial examinations, with particular emphasis on growth velocity and secondary sexual characteristics such as pubic hair and pigmentation of the labia or areola, are usually sufficient to identify precocious puberty in girls with premature thelarche.[12,47] Radiographs to estimate bone age may be indicated in some patients if precocious puberty is suspected.[44] Unless a patient with thelarche has associated signs of precocious puberty, the parents should be reassured and the child followed.[50] Ninety percent of patients with isolated premature thelarche have resolution of the breast enlargement 6 months to 6 years after diagnosis.[46] In asymmetrical premature thelarche, the resolution may also be asymmetrical.[47] Long-term follow-up has shown that patients with isolated premature thelarche develop normal breasts at puberty and are at no increased risk for disorders or tumors of the breast.[46]

TABLE 58–1 Tanner Stages of Breast Development

Tanner Stage	Description
1 (preadolescent)	Elevation of breast papilla only
2	Elevation of breast bud and papilla as small mound
	Enlargement of areola diameter
	Areola becomes more pink
3	Further enlargement of breast and areola, with no separation of their contours
	Montgomery's tubercles appear
4	Further enlargement, with projection of areola and papilla to form a secondary mound above the level of the breast
5 (mature stage)	Projection of papilla only, resulting from recession of areola to general contour of breast
	Erectile areolar tissue

From Duflos D, et al: Breast diseases in adolescents. In Sultan C (ed): Pediatric and Adolescent Gynecology. Basel, Karger, 2004; and Templeman C, Hertweck SP: Breast disorders in the pediatric and adolescent patient. Obstet Gynecol Clin North Am 2000;27:19-34.

CONGENITAL ANOMALIES OF THE BREAST

Amastia and Hypomastia

Complete absence of the breast, or amastia, is rare and is thought to occur from lack of formation or obliteration of the milk line.[41] Amastia can be associated with syndromes of more diffuse ectodermal anomalies such as congenital ectodermal dysplasia.[29,41] It can also be associated with anomalies of the underlying mesoderm, such as the abnormal pectoralis muscle seen in Poland's syndrome.[14,41] Bilateral amastia is associated with other congenital anomalies in 40% of patients.[29] Athelia is defined as presence of breast tissue with absence of the nipple. This is not infrequent in accessory breasts but is very rare in the normal location.[41] Amastia or hypomastia can also result from injuries sustained during thoracotomy, chest tube placement, inappropriate biopsy of the breast bud, radiotherapy, or severe burns.[12] Because the nipple complex does not normally develop until the eighth month of gestation, it can be difficult to identify in premature infants. As a result, placement of chest tubes or central lines can inadvertently injure the developing breast (Fig. 58-1).

Polymastia and Polythelia

Supernumerary breast tissue, most commonly accessory nipples, occurs in approximately 1% to 2% of the population.[19,20,41] The abnormally placed tissue is almost universally located in the axilla or just inferior to the normally positioned breast along the embryonic milk line.[41] The normal axillary extension of breast tissue (the tail of Spence) should not be confused with supernumerary breast tissue. Sixty-five percent of children with supernumerary breast tissue have a single accessory nipple or breast, and 30% to 35% have two.[41] The largest number of reported supernumerary structures is 10.[41] A complete accessory breast is termed polymastia (Fig. 58-2). Supernumerary nipples are referred to as polythelia. Some studies have suggested an association between polythelia and abnormalities of the urinary tract and

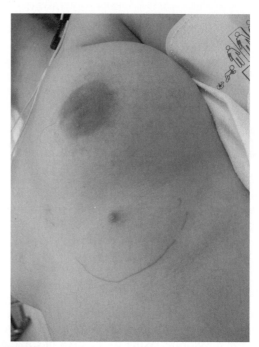

Figure 58–2 Polymastia. This complete breast, with nipple complex, is located in the most common position, just below the normal breast.

congenital heart disease, although this is debated by others.[12,20,29,45] True ectopic breast tissue, or breast tissue found outside the normal milk line, is exceedingly rare but has been reported on the face, back, and perineum and in the midline of the anterior torso.[24,26,41] Polymastia warrants surgical excision in girls to prevent painful swelling during pregnancy. Resection of accessory nipples is usually warranted for cosmetic reasons.

Congenital Anomalies of the Nipple

Inverted nipples may predispose patients to infection, which can usually be prevented by careful attention to hygiene of the recessed area.[19] Surgical correction is possible, but elevation of the nipple inevitably divides the lactiferous ducts and makes future breast-feeding problematic if not impossible.[19] Other anomalies of the nipple that have been described include bifid nipples and intra-areolar polythelia, which is also called dysplastic divided nipples (Fig. 58-3).[19,29]

Breast Asymmetry and Hypomastia

Some degree of asymmetry is normal in women and may be more pronounced during puberty, while the breasts are developing.[19,44] Significant hypomastia may be associated with connective tissue disorders or mitral valve prolapse.[19] Hypomastia is frequently familial.[12] Unilateral hypoplasia has been reported in association with a Becker's nevus of the breast, which on examination appears as a clear brown stain.[12] This nevus has been reported to have increased androgenic receptors, which may explain the hypomastia.[12] Hypomastia can also occur after radiation therapy to

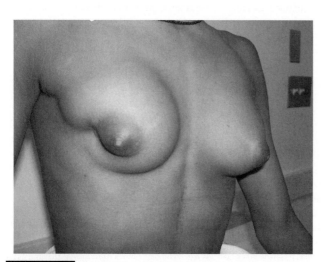

Figure 58–1 Breast deformity from placement of a neonatal chest tube.

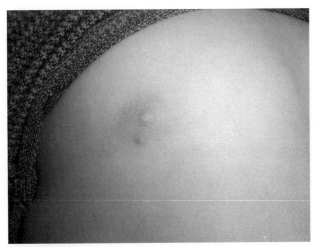

Figure 58–3 Intra-areolar polythelia, which is also called a dysplastic divided nipple.

the chest wall. Girls with bilateral breast hypoplasia should be evaluated for ovarian dysfunction, hypothyroidism, or androgen-producing tumors.[19] Hypoplastic breast tissue is also associated with a tuberous breast anomaly. In this condition, the base of the breast is limited, and the hypoplastic breast tissue "herniates" into the areolar complex.[19,44] Plastic surgery to correct the areolar complex and augment the hypoplastic breast may be indicated.

BREAST ENLARGEMENT

Macromastia

Excessively large breasts are referred to as macromastia. The differential diagnosis of macromastia in adolescents includes juvenile hypertrophy, pregnancy, tumors of the breast, and excessive endogenous or exogenous levels of estrogen or progesterone or both (Table 58-2).[32]

TABLE 58–2 Differential Diagnosis of Macromastia

Juvenile hypertrophy
Tumors of the breast
   Giant fibroadenoma
   Hamartoma[49]
   Cystosarcoma phyllodes
   Carcinoma
Hormonally active tumors
   Ovarian granulosa cell tumor
   Ovarian follicular cyst
   Adrenal cortical tumor
Exogenous hormones
   Estrogen
   Testosterone
   Gonadotropins
   Corticosterone
Medications
   D-Penicillamine
   Marijuana

D-Penicillamine and marijuana have also been reported as exogenous causes of macromastia.[32]

Juvenile or Virginal Hypertrophy

Spontaneous massive growth of the breast in an adolescent, which may be unilateral or bilateral, is thought to be the result of excessive end-organ sensitivity to gonadal hormones.[32] The number of hormonal receptors in the hypertrophic breast tissue is normal, as are serum estradiol levels.[12,32] An autoimmune cause has been suggested by some authors because of the occasional association with autoimmune disorders such as Hashimoto's thyroiditis, rheumatoid arthritis, and myasthenia.[12] The breast growth in patients with juvenile hypertrophy is rapid, begins shortly after thelarche, and can be dramatic, resulting in breasts that weigh up to 50 pounds each.[19,44] Spontaneous resolution is very rare.[32] Skin changes, such as peau d'orange and even necrosis, may occur during phases of rapid growth.[32] Treatment depends on whether breast growth has been completed. If the patient is still growing, progesterone or antiestrogen medications can be used to control breast growth.[44] If this is unsuccessful, or if breast growth is complete, breast reduction surgery is necessary.[32] Patients should be counseled that lactation may be affected by juvenile hypertrophy, particularly after breast reduction surgery, but there is no increased risk of breast cancer.[32]

INFECTIONS OF THE BREAST

Neonatal mastitis is an uncommon infection that usually occurs in term or near-term infants.[13] It affects female infants twice as often as male infants.[13] Approximately 50% of infants with neonatal mastitis develop a breast abscess.[13] Adolescents may develop nonpuerperal mastitis or a breast abscess as a result of irritation of the skin, a foreign body, or infection of an epidermal cyst.[44] The initial therapy of all breast infections is antibiotics and analgesics.[13] Adolescent girls with mastitis may have symptomatic relief with breast support.[44] Although *Staphylococcus aureus* is the offending organism in almost all cases, in infants, infections with *Shigella, Escherichia coli,* and *Klebsiella* have been reported.[13] In most communities, the incidence of methicillin-resistant *S. aureus* has become significant enough to warrant using clindamycin or vancomycin for up to 10 days. Gram-negative coverage may be indicated until culture results are obtained. Whether in an infant or an older child, small abscesses should be aspirated with a needle, using ultrasound guidance if necessary, and followed as antibiotic therapy is continued.[44] Larger abscesses may need incision and drainage, although some authors recommend needle aspiration initially, with surgery reserved for aspiration failure.[44] If incision and drainage are performed, a small, periareolar incision is indicated. Probing and disrupting of the tissue should be kept to a minimum to avoid injury to the underlying breast bud in a prepubertal child.

NIPPLE DISCHARGE

Bloody Discharge

The differential diagnosis of bloody discharge in children and adolescents includes mammary duct ectasia, chronic cystic mastitis, intraductal cysts, and intraductal papillomas. Mammary duct ectasia is a condition of benign dilatations of the subareolar ducts that results in inflammation and fibrosis. This is thought to be an anomaly of duct development that results from "pleats" of obstructing epithelium in the lumen of the duct.[12,42] This obstruction can lead to bacterial overgrowth and abscess, most commonly with *S. aureus*.[50] Other proposed causes include chronic inflammation of the periductal stroma with duct obliteration, trauma, and autoimmune reaction.[42] Infants with mammary duct ectasia typically present with a bloody discharge.[42] Adolescents typically present with a retroareolar mass, often bluish in color. There may be a bloody or brownish discharge. All children with bloody discharge should have the discharge cultured and appropriate antibiotics started.[50] Ductal ectasia often resolves spontaneously.[12,30,50] There may be recurrences, but these usually respond to conservative therapy. Surgical excision may be indicated for persistent or recurrent symptoms or for an associated persistent cyst.[50] In girls, the excision should be limited to any identified cyst, with great care taken not to injure the underlying breast bud. In boys with this condition, a simple mastectomy is curative.[50]

Intraductal papillomas are rare subareolar lesions that are often difficult to palpate.[19] They are bilateral in 25% of patients.[19] Cytology of the bloody discharge shows ductal cells.[19] Local excision, through a circumareolar incision, is curative.[19] Adenoma of the nipple, which is very rare, may also present with erosion of or discharge from the nipple.[43] In adolescent athletes, bloody discharge may be due to chronic nipple irritation (jogger's nipple) or cold trauma (cyclist's nipple).[27]

Galactorrhea

Milky discharge from the neonatal breast is a normal response to fetal prolactin levels, which peak at birth (Fig. 58-4).[38] In an adolescent, nonpuerperal lactation can be classified as neurogenic, hypothalamic, pituitary, endocrine, drug-induced, or idiopathic in origin.[38] Neurogenic lactation occurs as a result of disorders of the chest wall, thorax, or breast. Neurogenic lactation has been reported after thoracotomy, burns or injuries of the chest wall, herpes zoster, or chronic stimulation of the nipple.[38] Pituitary tumors, especially prolactinomas, are the most common hypothalamic or pituitary cause of galactorrhea.[38] The most common cause of galactorrhea in adolescents is hypothyroidism.[38] A wide variety of drugs has been implicated in causing galactorrhea, including dopamine receptor blockers and catecholamine-depleting agents.[38,44] Patients with galactorrhea require a careful history and physical examination directed at the possible causes of galactorrhea. If there is a question whether the discharge is true galactorrhea, it should be sent for fat staining. Laboratory studies should

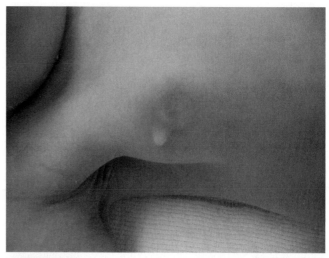

Figure 58–4 Normal breast bud and milky discharge in a neonate.

include serum prolactin, follicle-stimulating hormone, luteinizing hormone, and thyroid function studies.[38] Discharge from the areolar glands of Montgomery in an adolescent may be normal and should not be confused with galactorrhea.[19]

BREAST MASSES

Prepubertal Breast Masses

Neonatal breast hypertrophy is a normal response to maternal estrogen and occurs in both boys and girls in the first weeks of life.[19] Stimulation, such as attempting to squeeze the breast to promote discharge, may result in persistence of the hypertrophied tissue. Neonatal breast hypertrophy resolves spontaneously, and no treatment is necessary.

Breast development at the onset of thelarche starts with a firm, disklike area of tissue under the areolar complex that can be mistaken for a mass. It is often unilateral initially.[50] This is almost universally a normal physiologic process, but unilateral thelarche has been reported as a side effect of cimetidine administration and is reversible with stoppage of the drug.[6] Biopsy is contraindicated, as this can result in injury to the developing breast.[48]

Hemangiomas and lymphangiomas can involve the developing breast (Fig. 58-5). Although hemangiomas may involute after an initial growth spurt, compression of the breast bud during rapid growth can lead to injury and subsequent breast deformity. The diagnosis is usually made on physical examination but can be confirmed with ultrasonograpy or magnetic resonance imaging (MRI). If there is doubt about the diagnosis, a fine-needle biopsy may be indicated. Rapid growth of hemangiomas may require resection (if technically possible) or treatment with steroids.[1,50] In girls, the risk of injuring the breast bud by resection must be weighed against injury to the breast bud from the enlarging hemangioma or lymphangioma. MRI may aid in determining the resectability of the lesion and hence the risk-benefit ratio of surgical

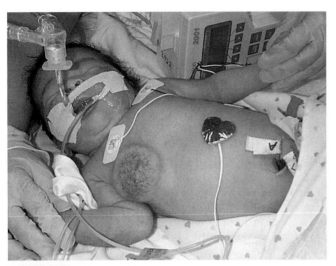

Figure 58–5 Hemangioma of the breast in a newborn infant.

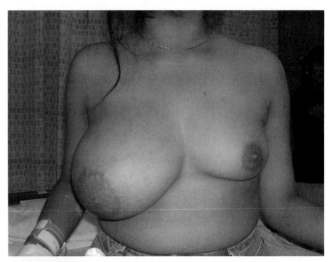

Figure 58–6 Giant fibroadenoma, mimicking juvenile hypertrophy, in an adolescent girl.

resection. Surgical resection of the lesion, with protection of the normal breast tissue, is indicated for complications such as ulceration or hemorrhage.[50]

Other soft tissue or metastatic tumors of the breast are rare but can present in prepubertal children (Table 58-3). The majority of lesions are benign, but if the diagnosis is uncertain, fine-needle or open biopsy may be indicated.[50]

Masses in Adolescent Girls

Fibroadenomas

The most common mass seen in adolescent girls is fibroadenoma. These masses usually occur in late adolescence but can occur as early as 1 to 2 years before menarche.[19] Fibroadenomas are most often located in the upper outer quadrant of the breast and are more common in African American patients.[50] The average size is 2 to 3 cm, but they can become massive (Fig. 58-6).[44] Ten percent of patients have bilateral lesions.[44] Up to 25% of patients have multiple fibroadenomas, a condition called fibroadenomatosis.[12,19] The lesions may enlarge slightly during the menstrual cycle.[50] The physical examination is usually diagnostic; these lesions are well circumscribed, "rubbery," mobile, and nontender. In equivocal cases, ultrasonography may be helpful in

TABLE 58–3 Differential Diagnosis of Prepubertal Breast Masses

Unilateral breast bud development (premature thelarche)
Hemorrhagic cyst[50]
Abscess[50]
Lymphangioma[50]
Hemangioma[50]
Lipoma[50]
Metastatic tumor
Galactocele[4]

making the diagnosis.[15] Mammography is not indicated in adolescent patients because the large amount of fibroglandular tissue makes interpretation difficult.[50]

Fibroadenomas are thought to develop because of a local exaggerated response to estrogen stimulation.[50] The natural history of these lesions is usually an initial period of growth, during which the mass doubles in size over 6 to 12 months, and then stabilization. Only 5% of fibroadenomas grow more rapidly.[21] Fibroadenomas have been reported to resolve spontaneously.[7,50] This is supported by findings of sclerotic vestiges of these lesions in women over the age of 40.[10] In 99 women aged 14 to 55 years (median age, 20) followed over 7 to 9 years, 38% of 107 clinically diagnosed fibroadenomas resolved spontaneously.[7] One group reported that up to 40% of presumed fibroadenomas in adults decreased in size over a 2-year period.[33] Even if some of these lesions were not true fibroadenomas, these findings support observation of presumed fibroadenomas as an alternative to early resection. All presumed fibroadenomas less than 5 cm can be safely observed for at least one or two menstrual cycles. If there is growth of the lesion, excisional biopsy is warranted.[33] If the lesion remains stable, there are two options that should be discussed with the patient and family:

1. Observation with or without fine-needle aspiration. Approximately 200 cases of carcinoma of the breast have been reported in adults with fibroadenomas.[36] There are no reports of malignant fibroadenomas in adolescents. The risk of malignancy in an adolescent girl with a typical fibroadenoma on examination is exceedingly low. In the setting of a classic examination and no tumor growth, there is essentially no risk in observing these lesions.
2. Excisional biopsy. Many authors recommend excision of all lesions that persist to adulthood, so a case could be made to excise all fibroadenomas that persist during adolescence.[50] Patients should be counseled that the biopsy may result in cosmetic changes to the breast. Persistent local pain following removal of a fibroadenoma has also been reported.[40]

Giant Fibroadenomas

Fibroadenomas greater than 5 cm are termed giant fibroadenomas. On examination, these may be softer than typical fibroadenomas and may even resemble the normal surrounding breast tissue.[44] There may also be dilated veins over the surface, and the skin overlying the mass may be warm to the touch (see Fig. 58-6).[44] Giant fibroadenomas should be excised because they cannot be distinguished from cystosarcoma phyllodes by physical examinination, mammography, or sonography.[8] In addition, these tumors have been reported to double in size in as little as 3 months in rare patients.[19] Fine-needle aspiration and core needle biopsy can be helpful for planning the operative approach if the histology leads to a definitive diagnosis of cystosarcoma phyllodes. However, it is very difficult to distinguish between fibroadenoma and cystosarcoma phyllodes by aspiration or needle biopsy, so a negative result should not affect the decision to operate.[8]

Incisions for giant fibroadenoma removal can be problematic. Whenever possible, a periareolar incision should be used. Large lesions can be removed through a periareolar incision by placing them in a bag and morcellating them before removal.[39] If the mass is close to the inframammary crease, this offers a second, cosmetically appropriate approach. Excision of large fibroadenomas can result in significant deformity of the breast. Placing a drain is not recommended because this results in adherence of skin to the chest wall. However, leaving the space to fill with serum or blood is also suboptimal; this too may result in contraction of the space and skin adherence. I distend the space with a mixture of saline and local anesthetic by inserting an intravenous catheter using a "Z" puncture. In most patients, this prevents the rapid influx of serum and decreases the risk of skin adherence.

Phyllodes Tumors

Phyllodes tumors were first described by Muller in 1838, who coined the term cystosarcoma phyllodes. This term is misleading, however, because these tumors are rarely cystic and do not have the malignant potential of most sarcomas.[33] For that reason, they are better termed phyllodes tumors.

Phyllodes tumors are stromal tumors that are histologically classified as benign, intermediate, or malignant.[50] The distinction is largely semantic, because benign phyllodes lesions can metastasize and may recur locally. The median age of presentation of phyllodes tumors is 45 years; however, they have been reported to occur in girls as young as 10 years.[2,33] These tumors may occur more frequently in African American adolescents.[19]

The diagnosis is difficult to make without a biopsy. On examination, the tumor may resemble a giant fibroadenoma. Large tumors may cause skin stretching and ulceration and venous distention.[19] If the nipple complex is involved, there may be a bloody discharge.[19] Ultrasound findings that are suggestive, but not diagnostic, of phyllodes tumors include lobulations, a heterogeneous echo pattern, and the absence of microcalcifications.[8]

The treatment of benign phyllodes tumors is total surgical excision with a 1-cm margin of normal tissue.[34] Patients with histologically malignant phyllodes tumors should undergo mastectomy.[8] Some authors have reported that adolescents with malignant phyllodes tumors have a more "benign" course than adults and suggest that the breast can be preserved in these patients.[33] Only clinically palpable nodes, which are present in approximately 20% of patients, should be resected.[28] The role of sentinel node biopsy has not been clarified for this tumor. The majority of nodes are enlarged in response to tumor necrosis and inflammation; metastases occur by hematogenous, not lymphatic, dissemination.[19] Re-excision is indicated if adequate margins were not obtained at the first surgery.[28] If an adequate margin cannot be achieved on the chest wall, local radiation therapy should be considered.[28]

Local recurrence occurs in up to 20% of patients with phyllodes tumors and is treated with re-excision or mastectomy.[33] Systemic recurrence has been reported in 14% to 15% of patients.[28] Metastases can occur in the lung, pleura, soft tissue, bone, pancreas, and central nervous system and usually occur without lymph node involvement.[28,33] There have been isolated reports of palliation from single or multiple chemotherapeutic agents, but in general, adjuvant therapy plays a limited role in the successful treatment of phyllodes tumors.[33]

The 5-year survival rate in adults with benign, borderline, and malignant phyllodes tumors is 96%, 74%, and 66%, respectively.[33] Overall, the 5-year survival rate for malignant phyllodes tumors in adults is approximately 80%.[33] Because adolescents with phyllodes tumors may have a biologically less aggressive tumor than adults, their prognosis may be better.[33]

Retroareolar Cysts

Montgomery's tubercles are the small papular projections on the edge of the areola and are related to the glands of Montgomery, which may play a role during lactation.[44] In adolescents, these glands can obstruct and present as either acute inflammation (62%) or an asymptomatic mass (38%).[22] The diagnosis of retroareolar cysts, also referred to as cysts of Montgomery, is primarily clinical but can be confirmed with ultrasonography, which most commonly demonstrates a single cystic lesion, usually unilocular, located in the expected retroareolar location. The most common presentation of patients with retroareolar cysts is acute inflammation with localized tenderness, erythema, and swelling under the areola and extending into the breast tissue.[22] Treatment with oral antibiotics directed at *Staphyloccocus* and nonsteroidal anti-inflammatory agents usually results in resolution of the acute inflammation within 7 days.[22] Only rarely is drainage of a persistent abscess necessary. Following this nonoperative treatment, an asymptomatic mass is usually present. Patients with retroareolar cysts may describe a brownish discharge from one of Montgomery's tubercles, particularly with compression of the mass. In the absence of persistent infection or other complications, retroareolar cysts should be observed with serial physical examinations and, if needed, repeat ultrasonography.

More than 80% of these cysts resolve spontaneously, although this can take up to 2 years.[22] Patients should be instructed not to compress the area, as this may prevent resolution of the mass. Resection may be indicated if the mass persists or if the diagnosis is in question.[44]

Fibrocystic Changes

Fibrocystic changes in the breast can result in both localized masses and pain in the breast, or mastalgia. Patients should be reassured that this is a normal variant of female physiology, with these changes reported in 50% of women of reproductive age and 90% of women on autopsy.[44] Physical examination alone usually suffices to make this diagnosis because there is usually significant change with serial examinations done at different points in the menstrual cycle. Ultrasonography may be helpful if the diagnosis is equivocal, but mammography is not indicated. The treatment of mastalgia is a firm brassiere and nonsteroidal anti-inflammatory drugs.[19] Oral contraceptives have been reported to improve symptoms in 70% to 90% of women.[44] Treatment with vitamin E or evening primrose oil and the avoidance of caffeine are unproved but popular methods.[19,44]

Other Benign Breast Masses

A variety of benign tumors of the breast have been described in adolescents and young adults (Table 58-4). Hamartomas of the breast are rare tumors composed of normal breast components that can present as unilateral macromastia.[49] They have also been called lipofibromas, adenolipomas, and fibroadenolipomas.[49] Only eight cases have been reported in women younger than 20 years.[49] The treatment of hamartomas is total excision.

Adenomas of the nipple are very rare but have been reported to occur in children and adolescents. They are treated by local excision.[43] Tubular adenomas cannot be distinguished from fibroadenomas by history or examination, and the diagnosis is usually made by pathologic evaluation.[10] No further treatment is necessary after local excision.

TABLE 58–4 Differential Diagnosis of Postpubertal Breast Masses in Girls

Fibroadenoma
Cyst of Montgomery
Duct ectasia
Fat necrosis
Vascular lipoma[50]
Subareolar neuroma[50]
Hamartoma[49]
Abscess[50]
Lymphangioma[50]
Hemangioma[50]
Lipoma[50]
Juvenile secretory carcinoma
Ductal carcinoma
Metastatic disease

Erosive adenomatosis is a rare benign tumor that presents with erythema, erosion, and crusting of the nipple.[3] Serosanguineous discharge may occur, and a nodule may or may not be palpable.[3] Treatment is local excision of the lesion, which may be delayed until breast growth is complete; successful treatment with cryosurgery has also been reported.[3]

Juvenile papillomatosis is a benign, localized, proliferative lesion usually seen in girls older than 10 years, although it has been reported in prepubertal boys as well.[35] Juvenile papillomatosis usually presents with a mass, similar on examination to a fibroadenoma, in one breast. When resected, this is a well-demarcated mass with multiple cysts separated by fibrous stroma, giving it a "swiss cheese" appearance.[10] Juvenile papillomatosis is considered a marker for increased breast cancer risk in family members but not necessarily in the patient, unless it is recurrent.[35] However, in situ and invasive carcinoma (usually juvenile secretory carcinoma) have been reported in up to 15% of patients with juvenile papillomatosis.[10] The treatment of juvenile papillomatosis is total resection, with preservation of the normal breast.[35]

Trauma can result in lesions that resemble either an infection or a mass in adolescents. In particular, fat necrosis that occurs after trauma can resemble a solid mass in the breast.[19] This has been reported following seat-belt injury and other direct blows to the breast.[51]

Malignant Tumors of the Breast

Primary carcinoma of the breast has been reported in 39 children 3 to 19 years of age.[31,50] More than 80% of these patients were diagnosed with juvenile secretory carcinoma, with the remainder having intraductal carcinoma. Juvenile secretory carcinoma has been reported in association with juvenile papillomatosis.[50] Juvenile secretory carcinoma often has a thick-walled capsule, which may cause the lesion to appear cystic on ultrasonography.[31] The treatment of primary breast cancer in children is complete surgical excision, usually by mastectomy.[50] The role of sentinel node mapping has not been determined in children. Estrogen and progesterone receptors should be determined. Local recurrence is treated by re-excision or completion mastectomy. Adjuvant therapy for juvenile secretory carcinoma is rarely used, and the prognosis for these patients is excellent following local excision. Adjuvant therapy for intraductal carcinoma is based on the node status and hormone receptors, with most oncologists using modified adult protocols for the treatment of children with this tumor.

Chest wall radiation, usually given to treat Hodgkin's lymphoma, increases the lifetime risk for breast cancer. This is particularly true for girls who are 10 to 16 years old when they receive radiation therapy, because this is a period of rapid breast growth.[18] Girls with Hodgkin's disease who require radiotherapy of the chest have an 82 times increased risk of breast cancer, with almost 40% of patients ultimately developing breast cancer.[18] The median time from radiation therapy to diagnosis of breast cancer is 20 years. The risk of breast cancer is also increased if there is a significant family history. Mutations in the *BRCA1* and *BRCA2* genes have been identified in 7% to 9% of all breast cancers.[44] Girls who have mutations in one of these genes have a 3.2% risk of breast cancer at age 30 and an 85% risk by age 70.[44]

Sarcoma of the breast is rare in all age groups and exceedingly rare in children. Rhabdomyosarcoma can occur as a primary tumor of the breast, usually in adolescent girls.[5] These tumors are typically rapidly growing mobile masses with no skin involvement; histologically, they are usually alveolar rhabdomyosarcomas.[5] Angiosarcoma of the breast has been reported in adult women following external beam radiation for breast conservation.[2] This rare tumor has also been reported in adolescents.[34] The treatment is mastectomy without routine axillary dissection.[34] Liposarcoma has been reported within a phyllodes tumor of the breast in an adolescent patient.[23] These tumors may appear encapsulated but should be treated by wide local excision.[2] Fibrosarcoma and malignant fibrous histiocytoma may be the most common soft tissue sarcomas of the breast; other rare primary sarcomas of the breast include leiomyosarcoma and osteogenic sarcoma.[2] Primary non-Hodgkin's lymphoma of the breast has been reported in children.[37] Treatment of these rare primary malignancies of the breast is based on established protocols for more common tumors of childhood.

Cancer metastatic to the breast has been reported in children with primary hepatocellular carcinoma, Hodgkin's lymphoma, non-Hodgkin's lymphoma, neuroblastoma, and rhabdomyosarcoma, particularly the alveolar variant.[9,37,50] Other less common tumors that have been reported to metastasize to the breast in children include histiocytosis, medulloblastoma, renal carcinoma, and neuroblastoma.[9] Bilateral breast disease occurs in 30% of children with rhabdomyosarcoma metastatic to the breast.[9] Ultrasonography is the diagnostic tool of choice because it can often differentiate these lesions from more common benign lesions.[9]

GYNECOMASTIA

Gynecomastia occurs in up to 70% of boys at the time of puberty.[19,25] The majority of boys have bilateral gynecomastia, with only 10% having unilateral breast enlargement.[11] A history of drug ingestion should be obtained, because gynecomastia has been reported to occur secondary to anabolic steroids, digitalis, isoniazid, tricyclic antidepressants, spironolactone, and marijuana.[50] Gynecomastia can be classified using a scale defined by Nydick, which is similar to the Tanner stages of breast development in girls. Stage 1 is limited to the subareolar area but does not reach the edge of the areola; stage 2 extends to the edge of the areola (B2) or beyond the edge (B3). In stage 4 and 5 gynecomastia, the breast assumes the characteristics of a female breast.[11] Examination of the testes is important as well. The combination of gynecomastia with hypogonadism suggests the diagnosis of Klinefelter's syndrome. In the vast majority of boys, physiologic gynecomastia resolves spontaneously as puberty progresses, although it may take several years. Some boys, however, suffer from

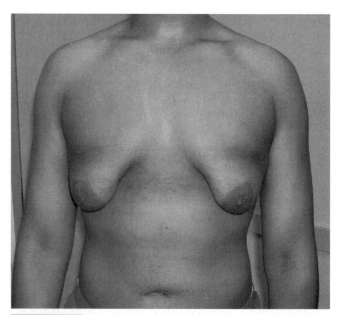

Figure 58–7 Stage 5 gynecomastia in an adolescent boy.

low self-esteem because of their large breasts (Fig. 58-7). These boys require surgery to allow normal psychological growth and development. Although plastic surgeons have promoted liposuction as an alternative to resection, an open approach is favored by most pediatric surgeons.[16,17] A simple mastectomy is performed through a periareolar incision. Drains are often necessary in cases of a significant breast tissue to prevent postoperative seromas. A "pad" of breast tissue should be left underneath the nipple to avoid adherence of the nipple to the chest wall.[50]

REFERENCES

1. Akyuz C, et al: Management of cutaneous hemangiomas: A retrospective analysis of 1109 cases and comparison of conventional dose prednisolone with high-dose methylprednisolone therapy. Pediatr Hematol Oncol 2001;18:47-55.
2. Alabassi A, Fentiman IS: Sarcomas of the breast. Int J Clin Pract 2003;57:886-889.
3. Albers SE, et al: Erosive adenomatosis of the nipple in an eight-year-old girl. J Am Acad Dermatol 1999;40:834-837.
4. Al Salem AH, Al Nazer M: An unusual cause of breast enlargement in a 5-year-old boy. Pediatr Pathol Mol Med 2002;21:485-489.
5. Binokay F, et al: Primary and metastatic rhabdomyosarcoma in the breast: Report of two pediatric cases. Eur J Radiol 2003;48:282-284.
6. Bosman JM, Bax NM, Wit JM: Premature thelarche: A possible adverse effect of cimetidine treatment. Eur J Pediatr 1990;149:534-535.
7. Cant PJ, et al: Non-operative management of breast masses diagnosed as fibroadenoma. Br J Surg 1995;82:792-794.
8. Chao TC, et al: Sonographic features of phyllodes tumors of the breast. Ultrasound Obstet Gynecol 2002;20:64-71.
9. Chateil JF, et al: Breast metastases in adolescent girls: US findings. Pediatr Radiol 1998;28:832-835.
10. Dehner LP, Hill DA, Deschryver K: Pathology of the breast in children, adolescents, and young adults. Semin Diagn Pathol 1999;16:235-247.

11. De Sanctis V, et al: Pubertal gynecomastia. Minerva Pediatr 2002;54:357-361.
12. Duflos D, et al: Breast diseases in adolescents. In Sultan C (ed): Pediatric and Adolescent Gynecology. Basel, Karger, 2004.
13. Efrat M, et al: Neonatal mastitis—diagnosis and treatment. Isr J Med Sci 1995;31:558-560.
14. Fokin AA, Robicsek F: Poland's syndrome revisited. Ann Thorac Surg 2002;74:2218-2225.
15. Fornage BD, Lorigan JG, Andry E: Fibroadenoma of the breast: Sonographic appearance. Radiology 1989;172:671-675.
16. Fruhstorfer BH, Malata CM: A systematic approach to the surgical treatment of gynaecomastia. Br J Plast Surg 2003;56:237-246.
17. Gabra HO, et al: Gynaecomastia in the adolescent: A surgically relevant condition. Eur J Pediatr Surg 2004;14:3-6.
18. Gold DG, Neglia JP, Dusenbery KE: Second neoplasms after megavoltage radiation for pediatric tumors. Cancer 2003;97:2588-2596.
19. Greydanus DE, Parks DS, Farrell EG: Breast disorders in children and adolescents. Pediatr Clin North Am 1989;36:601-638.
20. Grossl NA: Supernumerary breast tissue: Historical perspectives and clinical features. South Med J 2000;93:29-32.
21. Hanna RM, Ashebu SD: Giant fibroadenoma of the breast in an Arab population. Australas Radiol 2002;46:252-256.
22. Huneeus A, et al: Retroareolar cysts in the adolescent. J Pediatr Adolesc Gynecol 2003;16:45-49.
23. Jimenez JF, et al: Liposarcoma arising within a cystosarcoma phyllodes. J Surg Oncol 1986;31:294-298.
24. Koltuksuz U, Aydin E: Supernumerary breast tissue: A case of pseudomamma on the face. J Pediatr Surg 1997;32:1377-1378.
25. Lazala C, Saenger P: Pubertal gynecomastia. J Pediatr Endocrinol Metab 2002;15:553-560.
26. Leung W, Heaton JP, Morales A: An uncommon urologic presentation of a supernumerary breast. Urology 1997;50:122-124.
27. Loud KJ, Micheli LJ: Common athletic injuries in adolescent girls. Curr Opin Pediatr 2001;13:317-322.
28. Mangi AA, et al: Surgical management of phyllodes tumors. Arch Surg 1999;134:487-492.
29. Merlob P: Congenital malformations and developmental changes of the breast: A neonatological view. J Pediatr Endocrinol Metab 2003;16:471-485.
30. Miller JD, Brownell MD, Shaw A: Bilateral breast masses and bloody nipple discharge in a 4-year-old boy. J Pediatr 1990;116:744-747.
31. Murphy JJ, et al: Breast cancer in a 6-year-old child. J Pediatr Surg 2000;35:765-767.
32. O'Hare PM, Frieden IJ: Virginal breast hypertrophy. Pediatr Dermatol 2000;17:277-281.
33. Parker SJ, Harries SA: Phyllodes tumours. Postgrad Med J 2001;77:428-435.
34. Rainwater LM, et al: Angiosarcoma of the breast. Arch Surg 1986;121:669-672.
35. Rice HE, et al: Juvenile papillomatosis of the breast in male infants: Two case reports. Pediatr Surg Int 2000;16:104-106.
36. Rivera-Hueto F, et al: Long-term prognosis of teenagers with breast cancer. Int J Surg Pathol 2002;10:273-279.
37. Rogers DA, et al: Breast malignancy in children. J Pediatr Surg 1994;29:48-51.
38. Rohn RD: Galactorrhea in the adolescent. J Adolesc Health Care 1984;5:37-49.
39. Rojananin S, Ratanawichitrasin A: Limited incision with plastic bag removal for a large fibroadenoma. Br J Surg 2002;89:787-788.
40. Siegal A, Kaufman Z, Siegal G: Breast masses in adolescent females. J Surg Oncol 1992;51:169-173.
41. Skandalakis J, et al: The anterior body wall. In Gray S (ed): Embryology for Surgeons: The Embryologic Basis for the Treatment of Congenital Anomalies. Baltimore, Williams & Wilkins, 1994, pp 539-593.
42. Stringel G, Perelman A, Jimenez C: Infantile mammary duct ectasia: A cause of bloody nipple discharge. J Pediatr Surg 1986;21:671-674.
43. Sugai M, et al: Adenoma of the nipple in an adolescent. Breast Cancer 2002;9:254-256.
44. Templeman C, Hertweck SP: Breast disorders in the pediatric and adolescent patient. Obstet Gynecol Clin North Am 2000;27:19-34.
45. Urbani CE, Betti R: Accessory mammary tissue associated with congenital and hereditary nephrourinary malformations. Int J Dermatol 1996;35:349-352.
46. Van Winter JT, et al: Natural history of premature thelarche in Olmsted County, Minnesota, 1940 to 1984. J Pediatr 1990;116:278-280.
47. Verrotti A, et al: Premature thelarche: A long-term follow-up. Gynecol Endocrinol 1996;10:241-247.
48. Weinstein SP, et al: Spectrum of US findings in pediatric and adolescent patients with palpable breast masses. Radiographics 2000;20:1613-1621.
49. Weinzweig N, Botts J, Marcus E: Giant hamartoma of the breast. Plast Reconstr Surg 2001;107:1216-1220.
50. West KW, et al: Diagnosis and treatment of symptomatic breast masses in the pediatric population. J Pediatr Surg 1995;30:182-186.
51. Williams HJ, et al: Imaging features of breast trauma: A pictorial review. Breast 2002;11:107-115.

Chapter 59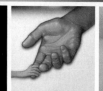

Congenital Chest Wall Deformities

Robert C. Shamberger

Congenital chest wall deformities are usually divided into five categories: pectus excavatum, pectus carinatum, Poland's syndrome, sternal defects, and the miscellaneous dysplasias or the thoracic deformities seen in diffuse skeletal disorders. Most are not life-threatening lesions and produce limited functional abnormalities. Rare lesions such as thoracic ectopia cordis and Jeune's asphyxiating thoracic dystrophy are, however, almost uniformly fatal.

DEPRESSION DEFORMITIES: PECTUS EXCAVATUM

Pectus excavatum (funnel chest, trichterbrust, or thorax *en entonnoir*) is the most common anterior chest wall deformity, involving posterior depression of the sternum and the lower costal cartilages. It occurs more frequently in boys than in girls by a greater than 3:1 ratio. In 90% of cases, it is noted within the first year of life.[125] Although cases of spontaneous resolution occur, they are infrequent, and the advice that a child will "grow out" of the pectus depression should be offered cautiously. Children with pectus excavatum, in addition to the central chest depression, are often noted to be tall and lanky, with poor posture, and to have an overall decrease in anteroposterior (AP) chest depth.[100,118]

Cause

The cause of pectus excavatum has not been established. Purported theories include intrauterine pressure, rickets, and abnormalities of the diaphragm resulting in posterior traction on the sternum.[15,16,22] Some support for this last theory has been provided by reports of pectus excavatum occurring after repair of agenesis of the diaphragm or congenital diaphragmatic hernia.[136] The association between pectus excavatum and other musculoskeletal abnormalities, particularly scoliosis (15% incidence) and Marfan's syndrome (Table 59-1), suggests that abnormal connective tissue plays a role. Studies have demonstrated abnormalities in the costal cartilage, including decreased levels of zinc and increased levels of magnesium and calcium.[6] Biomechanical analysis has suggested increased flexibility of costal cartilages in individuals with pectus excavatum, but abnormalities in the proteoglycan or collagen distribution between affected individuals and controls were not demonstrated.[35] A family history of chest wall deformity, identified in 37% of cases, supports a genetic predisposition.[125]

Clinical Presentation

Children present with a wide spectrum of depression deformities (Fig. 59-1), from a mildly depressed sternum to a severe case in which the sternum almost abuts the vertebral bodies. The depression is created by two components: (1) posterior angulation of the body of the sternum, generally beginning just below the insertion of the second costal cartilage, and (2) posterior angulation of the costal cartilages to meet the sternum. In older teenagers and adults, posterior angulation of the most anterior portion of the osseous ribs occurs. The depression may be deeper on the right than on the left, and the

TABLE 59-1 Musculoskeletal Abnormalities Identified in 704 Patients with Pectus Excavatum

Abnormality	No. of Patients
Scoliosis	107
Kyphosis	4
Myopathy	3
Poland's syndrome	3
Marfan's syndrome	2
Pierre Robin syndrome	2
Prune-belly syndrome	2
Neurofibromatosis	3
Cerebral palsy	4
Tuberous sclerosis	1
Congenital diaphragmatic hernia	2

From Shamberger RC, Welch KJ: Surgical repair of pectus excavatum. J Pediatr Surg 1988;23:615-622.

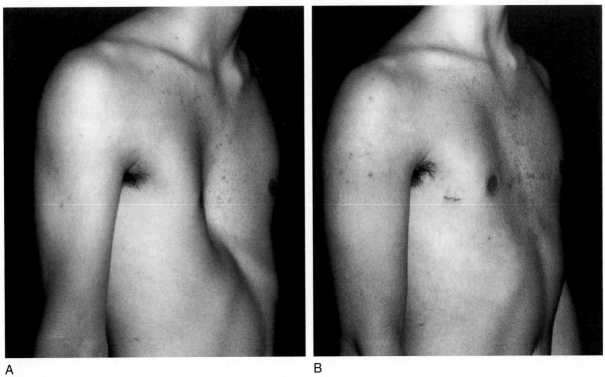

Figure 59–1   *A,* Preoperative clinical photograph of a 14½-year-old boy with a symmetrical pectus excavatum deformity. *B,* Postoperative clinical photograph a year after repair using retrosternal struts shows full correction of the deformity.

sternum may be rotated as well. The AP depth of the ribs may be different between the two sides, and in many children, the AP depth of the chest is narrower than normal.[100] Children may have a broad, shallow defect or a narrow central pocket. An asthenic build and slumped posture are frequently associated findings. Congenital heart disease was identified in 1.5% of children undergoing chest wall correction in one series, and the frequency of chest wall deformities among children with congenital heart disease was 0.17%.[126]

Many methods of assessing the severity of the depression have been developed. Most include the distance between the sternum and the spine as a primary factor. Willital[148] and Klinke et al.[72] used a ratio between the depth of the depression and the AP diameter of the chest. Welch[143] employed a ratio of the sternovertebral distance divided by the AP depth of the chest at the angle of Louis and added additional increments of severity if the cardiothoracic ratio was greater than 50% or the rib angles were greater than 25 degrees from horizontal. Backer et al.[5] used a ratio between the vertebral body diameter and the distance between the xiphosternal junction and the posterior border of the vertebral body to express the severity of the depression. Haller et al. proposed a method of grading that uses transverse and AP measurements obtained from computed tomography (CT) of the chest, but similar measurements can be obtained from standard chest radiographs.[50]

Pectus excavatum is well tolerated in infancy and childhood. Chronic upper airway obstruction because of tonsillar and adenoidal hypertrophy may accentuate the depression in an infant with a flexible chest but is not causative. Older children may complain of pain in the area of the deformed cartilages or of precordial pain after sustained exercise. Occasionally, palpitations occur, which presumably are the result of transient atrial arrhythmias and may be associated with mitral valve prolapse. A systolic ejection murmur is frequently identified in individuals with pectus excavatum. It is attributed to the close proximity between the posterior aspect of the sternum and the pulmonary artery, which results in transmission of a flow murmur.[45]

The physiologic impact of pectus excavatum has been the topic of many reports and much debate. Some authors contend that no cardiovascular or pulmonary impairment results from pectus excavatum. This position contrasts with the clinical impression that many patients have increased stamina and exercise tolerance after surgical repair. The cardiopulmonary impact of pectus excavatum has been extensively studied, with variable results. Despite 6 decades of work in the field, no consensus has been achieved on what degree of cardiopulmonary impairment, if any, this common chest wall deformity produces. Early pathologic studies of patients with pectus excavatum demonstrated compression of the heart between the vertebral column and the depressed sternum. The left lung was also compressed more than the right because of the frequent asymmetry of the deformity. Translation of these anatomic findings into their physiologic components has been the goal of many subsequent studies. A 1988 review tabulated this long series of studies.[123]

Pulmonary Function Evaluation

Deformity of the chest wall led many early authors to attribute the symptomatic improvement after pectus surgery to an improvement in pulmonary function. In an early work, Brown[17] performed respiratory studies on patients before and after surgical repair. Vital capacity was normal in these patients, but maximal breathing capacity was markedly diminished (50% or more) in 9 of 11 cases. Maximal breathing capacity increased an average of 31% after surgical repair.

Orzalesi and Cook[102] performed studies in 12 children with severe pectus excavatum deformities. The data for individual patients were within two standard deviations of normal values based on height except for three patients with low vital capacity and one with low maximal breathing capacity. In the aggregate, however, the group showed a significant ($P < 0.001$) decrease in vital capacity, total lung capacity, and maximal breathing capacity compared with height-matched normal children. Weg et al.[141] evaluated 25 Air Force recruits referred for respiratory symptoms and pectus excavatum and compared them with 50 unselected basic trainees. Although the lung compartments of both groups were equal, as were mean vital capacity and maximal voluntary ventilation, which best reflects chest wall function, muscular ability and patient effort showed a significant deviation from predicted normal values ($P = 0.005$).

Liese and Bühlmann[81] determined preoperative and postoperative lung volume and physical work capacity in an upright position on a bicycle ergometer in 12 adults with severe funnel chest. Postoperative studies were performed 3 to 11 years (mean, 8 years) after surgical correction. Absolute lung volume increased only in patients who had grown in height after surgery. Work capacity increased in 9 of 10 patients but was difficult to assess, given the interval between testing. Godfrey[44] reported on a select group of five patients with pectus excavatum and segmental bronchomalacia involving the left mainstem bronchus. Radionuclide pulmonary scans demonstrated severe gas trapping in the left lung in two patients and underventilation and underperfusion of the left lung in a third patient. This appeared to be a clinically distinct group of patients with bronchomalacia demonstrated at bronchoscopy in all cases. It is not clear that the bronchomalacia was caused by the pectus deformity.

Castile et al.[21] extensively evaluated eight patients, seven with pectus excavatum and one with pectus carinatum deformity. Five patients were symptomatic with exercise but were asymptomatic at rest. Complete pulmonary mechanics studies were performed, including standard lung volume, forced vital capacity (FVC), static pressure-volume curve, and progressive steady-state exercise testing on a bicycle ergometer. Flow and volume for the one patient with pectus carinatum were normal. The mean total lung capacity as a percentage of predicted in the pectus excavatum patients was 79%, a mild restrictive deficit. Flow volume configurations were normal and did not suggest airway obstruction. Workload tests revealed a normal dead-space response to exercise; tidal volume ratio and alveolar-arterial oxygen difference did not

suggest a significant ventilation-perfusion abnormality in the symptomatic patients. However, the measured oxygen uptake increasingly exceeded predicted values as the workload approached maximum; this was a strikingly different pattern when compared with normal subjects, who exhibit a linear response. The mean oxygen uptake at maximal effort exceeded the predicted values by 25.4% in the symptomatic patients. The three asymptomatic patients demonstrated normal linear oxygen uptake during exercise. Increased oxygen uptake suggests increased work of breathing in these symptomatic individuals, despite normal or mildly reduced vital capacity. Increases in tidal volume with exercise were uniformly depressed in those with pectus excavatum. No postoperative studies were performed in these subjects.

Cahill et al.[19] performed pre- and postoperative studies (3 to 9 months postoperatively) in 19 children and adolescents with pectus carinatum (5) and excavatum (14) ranging from 6 to 17 years of age. No preoperative abnormalities or postoperative changes were demonstrated in the pectus carinatum patients. The pectus excavatum patients demonstrated low-normal vital capacity that was unchanged by operation. Surgical correction did, however, result in a small improvement in their total lung capacity (3.21 ± 1.12 to 3.49 ± 1.07; $P < 0.02$) and a significant improvement in maximal voluntary ventilation (65.1 ± 31.5 to 78.9 ± 31.5 L/minute; $P < 0.001$). Exercise tolerance was also improved after surgery, as determined by both total exercise time and maximal oxygen consumption (1.26 ± 0.44 to 1.46 ± 0.42 mL/kg per minute; $P < 0.01$), although both these factors are clearly effort related. The heart rates at three identical work rates were assessed for each patient in the preoperative and postoperative workload study. There was a consistent decrease in heart rate at a given power output in the postoperative study ($P < 0.02$ by paired t-test) of the excavatum patients, but no decrease was observed in the carinatum patients. No difference in oxygen consumption at each work rate after surgery could be defined to support an improved efficiency of work. The observed decrease in heart rate at each workload level supported the hypothesis that some of the improvement in exercise capacity was a result of increased cardiac stroke volume. Mead et al.[90] studied rib cage mobility by assessing intra-abdominal pressure. The finding of normal abdominal pressure tracings in subjects with pectus excavatum suggested normal rib cage mobility.

Derveaux et al.[30] used pulmonary function tests to evaluate 88 subjects with pectus excavatum and carinatum before and 1 to 20 years (mean, 8 years) after repair involving a fairly extensive chest wall dissection. Preoperative studies were within the normal range (i.e., >80% predicted values) except in those subjects with both scoliosis and pectus excavatum. The postoperative values for forced expiratory volume in 1 second (FEV_1) and vital capacity were decreased in all groups when expressed as a percentage of predicted values, although the absolute values at follow-up may have been greater than at the preoperative evaluation. Radiologic evaluation of these individuals confirmed improved chest wall configuration, so the deterioration in pulmonary function was not the result of recurrence of the pectus deformity. An inverse relationship was found between preoperative and postoperative function. Those with less than 75% of predicted function preoperatively had improved function after surgery, whereas postoperative results were worse if the preoperative values were greater than 75%. Almost identical results were found in a study by Morshuis et al.,[95] who evaluated 152 subjects before and a mean of 8 years after surgery for pectus excavatum. These physiologic results were in contrast to the subjective improvement in symptoms reported by the subjects and their improved chest wall configurations. The decline in pulmonary function in the postoperative studies was attributed to the surgery, because the preoperative defect appeared to be stable on sequential studies regardless of the age at initial repair. Both these studies were marred by the obvious lack of an age-matched and severity-matched control group without surgery.

Derveaux et al.[31] evaluated transpulmonary and transdiaphragmatic pressures at total lung capacity in 17 individuals with pectus excavatum. Preoperative and long-term follow-up evaluations were performed a mean of 12 years apart. Reduced transpulmonary and transdiaphragmatic pressures showed that the increased restrictive defect was produced by extrapulmonary rather than pulmonary factors, suggesting that surgery produced increased rigidity of the chest wall.

Wynn et al.[150] assessed 12 children with pectus excavatum by pulmonary function tests and exercise testing. Eight had repair and were evaluated preoperatively and postoperatively. Four had two sets of evaluations but no surgery. A decline in total lung capacity was identified in the repaired children, whereas values were stable in the control group. Cardiac output and stroke volume increased appropriately with exercise before and after operation in both groups, and operation was thought to have no physiologically significant effect on the response to exercise.

Kaguraoka et al.[71] evaluated pulmonary function in 138 individuals before and after repair of pectus excavatum. A decrease in vital capacity occurred during the initial 2 months after surgery, with recovery to preoperative levels by 1 year after surgery. At 42 months, the values were maintained at baseline, despite a significant improvement in chest wall configuration. Tanaka et al.[132] had similar results and demonstrated that individuals with a more extensive sternal turnover procedure had more significant and long-term decreases in vital capacity.

Morshuis et al.[96] evaluated 35 subjects with pectus excavatum repaired as teenagers or young adults (age 17.9 ± 5.6 years). Preoperative evaluations were performed and repeated 1 year after surgery. Preoperative total lung capacity ($86.0 \pm 14.4\%$ of predicted) and vital capacity ($79.7 \pm 16.2\%$) were significantly lower than predicted values and decreased further after surgery ($-9.2 \pm 9.27\%$ and $-6.6 \pm 10.7\%$, respectively). The efficiency of breathing at maximal exercise improved significantly after operation. Ventilatory limitation of exercise occurred in 43% of the subjects after surgery, and there was a tendency toward improvement after operation. The group with no ventilatory limitation, however, initially demonstrated a limitation after operation, with a significant increase in oxygen consumption.

Haller et al.[51] evaluated 36 patients with pectus excavatum and 10 normal controls. Six months after surgery, the studies were repeated on 15 patients and 6 controls. Before surgical correction, a decrease in FVC was seen in the excavatum cohort, and no change occurred after repair. Although 58% of patients had subjective complaints of exercise limitation that improved after surgery in 66%, they exercised at similar workloads as controls. The respiratory parameters during exercise were similar between the two groups, suggesting that exercise was not limited by restrictive disease. After surgery, the subjects could exercise longer and had higher pulse oxygen levels than before surgery, with no change in the controls. The enhanced exercise tolerance was attributed to improved cardiac function, as demonstrated by increased pulse oxygen levels and no change in pulmonary function parameters.

Borowitz et al.[12] performed an early evaluation of patients undergoing the minimally invasive repair of pectus excavatum (MIRPE) technique. In that study of 10 patients, normal pulmonary function was demonstrated both before and after surgical repair. Sigalet et al.[129] also reported on the early effects of MIRPE in 11 patients, based on an evaluation of pulmonary function, exercise tolerance, and cardiac function as assessed by echocardiography. Although patients reported a subjective improvement in their exercise tolerance, pulmonary function (FVC and vital capacity) was significantly reduced at 3 months; similarly, maximal oxygen uptake was reduced. In contrast, cardiac function was enhanced, with an increase in stroke volume.

Malek et al.[84] evaluated 21 physically active patients with pectus excavatum. The observed values for FVC, FEV_1, maximal voluntary ventilation, and diffusing capacity of the lung for carbon monoxide were significantly lower than normal values, but those for total lung capacity and residual volume were not. Exercise testing revealed that the maximal oxygen uptake and oxygen tension were significantly lower than in normal controls. It was thought that the subjects' limitation in maximal exercise had a cardiovascular rather than a pulmonary cause, as demonstrated by an abnormally low metabolic threshold for lactate accumulation. This impairment was greatest in those with the most severe pectus deformities.

In composite, these studies of pulmonary function over the last 4 decades have failed to document consistent improvement in pulmonary function resulting from surgical repair. In fact, many studies demonstrated deterioration in pulmonary function at long-term evaluation, attributable to increased chest wall rigidity after surgery. Despite this finding, several workload studies have shown improvement in exercise tolerance after repair.

Cardiovascular Function

Posterior displacement of the sternum can produce deformity of the heart, particularly anterior indentation of the right ventricle. Garusi,[42] using angiography, showed displacement of the heart to the left side, with a sternal imprint on the anterior wall of the right ventricle.

Bevegård[9] in 1962 studied 16 patients with pectus excavatum using right heart catheterization and workload studies. The physical work capacity at a given heart rate was significantly lower in the sitting than in the supine position. Those with a 20% or greater decrease in physical work capacity from the supine to the sitting position had a shorter sternovertebral distance than did those with a less than 20% decrease. Measured stroke volume at rest decreased from the supine to the sitting position a mean of 40.3%, similar to normal subjects. In the supine position, stroke volume increased 13.2% with exercise. In the sitting position, the increase in stroke volume from rest to exercise was 18.5%, significantly lower ($P < 0.001$) than the 51% increase measured in normal subjects. Thus, increased cardiac output can be achieved primarily by increased heart rate, despite a limited stroke volume. This explains the lower work capacity achieved at any given heart rate in the sitting position. Intracardiac pressures were normal in all subjects measured at rest and with exercise, despite the apparent limitation of ventricular volume.

Beiser et al.[8] provided further evidence that cardiac function is impaired during upright exercise yet is relatively normal in the supine position. Cardiac catheterization was performed in six subjects with moderate pectus excavatum. Normal right atrial, right ventricular, pulmonary artery, and pulmonary capillary wedge pressures were obtained at rest in the supine position. The cardiac index during moderate exercise was normal, although the response to upright exercise was below that predicted in two subjects and at the lower limit of normal in three. The difference in cardiac performance in an upright position was produced primarily by a smaller stroke volume in subjects with pectus excavatum. Stroke volume was 31% lower and cardiac output was 28% lower during upright exercise compared with supine exercise. Postoperative studies were performed in three subjects; two achieved a higher level of exercise after repair. The cardiac index increased an average of 38%. An enhanced stroke volume response produced this increase, because heart rate at maximal exercise was not higher after repair.

Radionuclide angiography was used by Peterson et al.[104] to assess cardiac volume and output in 13 subjects with pectus excavatum. Eleven subjects were symptomatic before surgical repair, but the degree of symptoms could not be correlated with the severity of the anatomic deformity. Upright exercise was performed with a bicycle ergometer at progressive workloads until 85% of the age-predicted maximal heart rate was achieved or the patient could not continue because of fatigue or shortness of breath. Ten of the 13 subjects were able to reach the target heart rate before surgical repair, yet only 4 did so without symptoms. After operation, all but one subject reached the target heart rate during the exercise protocol, and 9 of 13 subjects did so without becoming symptomatic. This documentation of a marked decrease in symptoms after surgical correction of pectus excavatum in a regulated exercise protocol substantiated many anecdotal reports in the early literature regarding symptomatic improvement. The role of conditioning and subjective response to surgery is difficult to assess. Radionuclide injections were performed on subjects at rest and then at the target heart rate or exercise end point. This study

failed to demonstrate any significant change after pectus repair in the left ventricular ejection fraction either at rest or during exercise. The left ventricular end-diastolic volume was consistently increased after repair at rest, and the mean stroke volume increased 19% after repair but did not consistently increase with exercise. The cardiac index did not increase significantly after operation at rest or during exercise. Kowalewski et al.[73] performed a similar study with echocardiographic evaluation of cardiac function in 42 patients both before and 6 months after repair of pectus excavatum. Statistically significant changes were seen in the right ventricular volume indices (systolic, diastolic, and stroke volume) after surgery. No correlation could be defined between the changes in the pectus index and the cardiac changes. These results support those cited earlier by Haller et al.,[51] Sigalet et al.,[129] and Malek et al.,[84] which all suggest that limitations in the stroke volume result from right ventricular compression.

Additional studies are needed to further define the relationship between pectus excavatum and cardiopulmonary function. Dynamic or exercise studies have been most promising in this area. Methods to better evaluate preoperative cardiopulmonary function are needed to identify which children may achieve symptomatic and physiologic improvement after surgical repair.

Echocardiographic Studies

Prospective echocardiographic studies in adults with pectus excavatum demonstrated mitral valve prolapse in 6 of 33 subjects (18%) studied by Udoshi et al.[134] and in 11 of 17 subjects (65%) studied by Saint-Mezard et al.[113] Anterior compression of the heart by the depressed sternum may deform the mitral valve annulus or the ventricular chamber and produce mitral valve prolapse in these subjects. Resolution of mitral valve prolapse was seen in 10 of 23 children and adolescents after repair.[127]

Treatment

Meyer[90] in 1911 and Sauerbruch[115] in 1913 first achieved surgical repair of pectus excavatum. Significant changes in the method of repair have evolved as experience has increased and the primary components of the deformity have been identified. In 1939 Ochsner and DeBakey[98] summarized the early, sometimes fatal experience with a variety of repairs. Ravitch[108] in 1949 reported a technique that involved excision of all deformed costal cartilages with the perichondrium, division of the xiphoid from the sternum, division of the intercostal bundles from the sternum, and transverse sternal osteotomy displacing the sternum anteriorly with Kirschner wires in the first two patients and silk sutures in later patients. His technique was later modified to preserve the perichondrial sheaths, but he continued to separate the intercostal bundles and the sheaths from the sternum.[109] In 1957 and 1958 Baronofsky[7] and Welch,[142] respectively, reported similar techniques that emphasized total preservation of the perichondrial sheaths of the costal cartilage, preservation of the upper intercostal bundles, sternal osteotomy, and anterior fixation of the sternum with silk sutures. Haller et al.[52] subsequently developed a technique called *tripod fixation* in which subperichondrial resection of the abnormal cartilages is followed by a posterior sternal osteotomy. The most cephalad normal cartilages are then divided obliquely in a posterolateral direction. When the sternum is elevated, the sternal ends of the cartilage rest on the costal ends, providing further anterior support of the sternum.

Several authors used rib or cartilage placed posterior to the sternum for support, but this technique was never widely accepted.[27,109] A variation on this technique uses a vascularized rib.[54] Support of the sternum by an external brace secured to the mobilized sternum with sutures or wire has also been employed by numerous authors, but the duration of its use must be limited to avoid infection of the surgical wound.[16,80,98,149,151] Support of the sternum by metal struts has also been promoted by multiple authors.[36,53] Rehbein[110] developed struts that could be placed into the marrow cavity of the ribs at the costochondral junction. The struts were secured anterior to the sternum to create an arch, and the sternum was attached to this arch. Paltia[103] placed a transverse strut through the caudal end of the sternum with the two ends of the strut supported laterally by the ribs, firmly fixing its location. Adkins and Blades[1] and later Jensen et al.[66] used retrosternal elevation by a metal strut. Willital[148] employed a similar retrosternal strut after creating multiple chondrotomies in the costal cartilages to provide flexibility to the sternum and the chest wall. Innovations in these methods include the use of bioabsorbable struts, Marlex mesh or a Dacron vascular graft as a strut, or miniature metallic plates. There is no evidence, however, that any of these are preferable to traditional methods.[29,43,76,78,87,90,97]

In 1954 and 1956 Judet[69] and Jung,[70] respectively, proposed the sternal turnover in the French literature. This method has been used primarily in Japan, where a large series was reported by Wada et al.[138] This technique uses a free graft of sternum, which is rotated 180 degrees and then secured back to the costal cartilages from which it was divided. This method has a significant incidence of severe complications, including wound infection, dehiscence, and necrosis of the sternum. Taguchi[131] modified this method by preserving the internal mammary artery in an effort to prevent osteonecrosis and wound infection. Others have described microvascular anastomosis of one set of internal mammary vessels to preserve perfusion of the sternum.[133] Sternal turnover is a radical approach for children with pectus excavatum deformity, given the acceptable alternatives for repair.

A final method of repair is implantation of a Silastic mold into the subcutaneous space to fill the deformity.[2,34,140] Although this approach may improve the contour of the chest, it achieves no increase in intrathoracic volume and is often complicated by early seroma or hematoma formation.

The MIRPE technique described by Nuss is presented in the addendum to this chapter.

Surgical Technique

The surgical technique is depicted in Figure 59-2. In females, particular care is taken to place the incision within the projected inframammary crease to avoid injury to the breast bud or the creation of a scar extending onto the breast.[60] I currently use a retrosternal strut to secure the sternum firmly in an anterior position. I avoid skeletonizing the sternum; however, this may be required to achieve adequate mobility of the sternum for suture fixation. Preservation of the connections between the intercostal bundles, the perichondrium, and the rectus muscles provides a more normal chest contour.

Perioperative antibiotics are used, giving one dose immediately before surgery and three doses postoperatively. All patients are warned not to take aspirin or ibuprofen-containing compounds for 2 weeks before surgery to avoid abnormalities of platelet function. The Hemovac drain is removed when the drainage is less than 15 mL for an 8-hour shift. Rehbein or retrosternal struts are removed 6 months after repair to allow solid fixation of the sternum. The retrosternal struts are removed through a small incision over one end of the strut.

Complications

Complications of surgical repair should be limited, including wound infection and pneumothorax. Use of electrocautery can avoid the need for blood transfusion in most cases. Most pneumothoraces can be simply observed, unless they are large enough to produce pulmonary impairment. Recurrence is the bane of this procedure and can occur regardless of the technique used. I have shifted to strut fixation of the sternum to optimize early results, and I delay repair until the child is well into his or her pubertal growth spurt. Growth of the chest may produce the opportunity for remodeling of the chest wall and subsequent recurrence. No randomized study of strut fixation versus no strut fixation has been performed, and it is doubtful that such a study could ever be completed. In large series with adequate follow-up, recurrence is reported to occur in 5% to 15% of cases.[56,107,128,137,148] Progressive deterioration of the repair over time is well described, particularly during the interval of rapid growth at puberty.[11,62,74] Rigid fixation is fairly uniformly applied to patients with Marfan's syndrome because of their well-recognized high risk of recurrence.[117]

One serious complication has been noted in children who undergo repair at an early age, generally younger than 4 years: impaired growth of the ribs after resection of the costal cartilages, which produces a bandlike narrowing of the midchest (Fig. 59-3). In some cases, the first and second ribs have relative overgrowth, producing anterior protrusion of the upper sternum. In 1990 Martinez[86] first described this deficiency in thoracic growth after repair of pectus excavatum during the preschool years. In 1995 Haller[48] reported this occurrence in three boys who presented in their teens after resection of the costal cartilages at an early age, labeling this complication

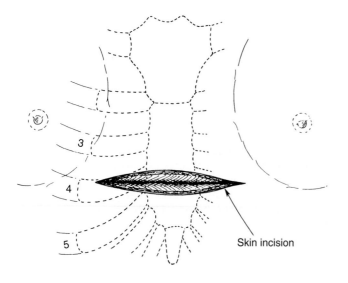

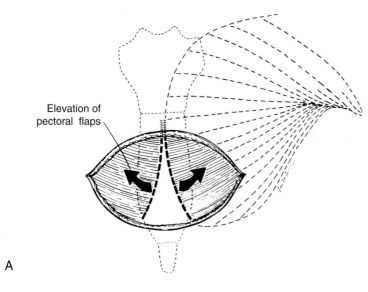

Skin incision

Elevation of
pectoral flaps

A

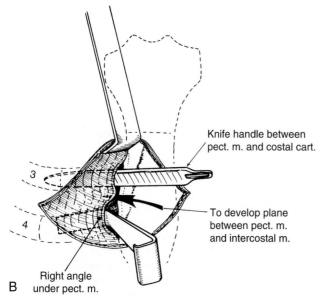

Knife handle between
pect. m. and costal cart.

To develop plane
between pect. m.
and intercostal m.

Right angle
under pect. m.

B

Figure 59–2 Surgical technique for pectus excavatum repair. *A,* A transverse incision is placed below and well within the nipple lines at the site of the future inframammary crease. Skin flaps are mobilized using electrocautery, primarily in the midline to the angle of Louis superiorly and to the xiphoid inferiorly. The pectoralis major muscle is elevated from the sternum, along with portions of the pectoralis minor and serratus anterior muscles. *B,* The correct plane of dissection of the pectoral muscle flap is defined by passing an empty knife handle directly anterior to a costal cartilage after the medial aspect of the muscle is elevated with electrocautery. The knife handle is then replaced with a right-angle retractor, which is pulled anteriorly. The process is then repeated anterior to an adjoining costal cartilage. The lateral extent of muscle dissection and elevation is to the costochondral junctions of the third to fifth ribs. Anterior distraction of the muscles during the dissection facilitates identification of the avascular areolar plane and avoids entry into the intercostal muscle bundles.

Continued

Figure 59-2 Cont'd *C,* Subperichondrial resection of the costal cartilages is achieved by incising the perichondrium anteriorly. It is then dissected away from the costal cartilages in the bloodless plane between the perichondrium and the costal cartilage. Cutting back the perichondrium 90 degrees in each direction at its junction with the sternum (*inset*) facilitates visualization of the back wall of the costal cartilage. *D,* The cartilages are divided at the junction of the sternum with a knife. A Welch perichondrial elevator is held posterior to the cartilage to protect the mediastinum (*inset*). The divided cartilage can then be held with an Allis clamp and elevated, and the costal cartilage is excised, preserving a 5- to 10-mm margin on the rib to protect the costochondral junction and the longitudinal growth plate. Segments of the sixth and seventh costal cartilages are resected to the point where they flatten to join the costal arch. Familiarity with the cross-sectional shape of the medial ends of the costal cartilages facilitates their removal. The second and third cartilages are broad and flat, the fourth and fifth are circular, and the sixth and seventh are narrow and deep.

Continued

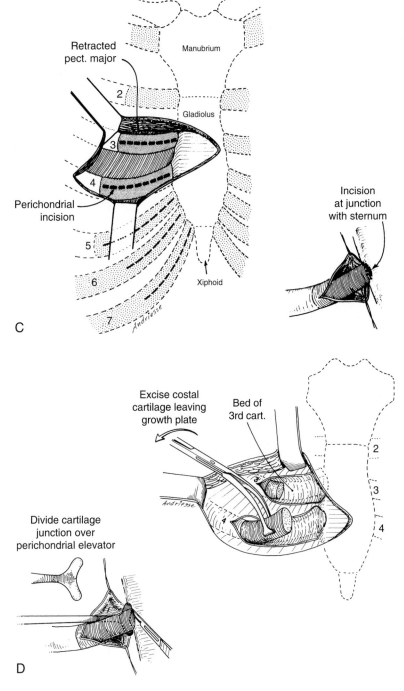

acquired Jeune's disease. Haller et al.[48] attributed this complication to injury during surgical repair of the costochondral junctions, the longitudinal growth centers for the ribs.

Martinez[86] demonstrated experimentally in 6-week-old normal rabbits that resection of the costal cartilage produced a marked impairment in chest growth, particularly the AP diameter, during a 5.5-month period of observation. Less severe impairment occurred if only the medial three fourths of the costal cartilage was resected, preserving the growth centers at the costochondral junction. This impairment was attributed to fibrosis and scarring within the perichondrial sheaths. Perichondrial sheaths, bone, or other prosthetic tissues that cannot grow should not be joined posterior to the sternum, because they will form a bandlike stricture across the chest. This complication can be avoided by delaying surgery until the children are older. Preservation of the costochondral junction by leaving a segment of the cartilage on the osseous portion of the rib may partially minimize growth impairment. Weber[139] described a method of improving the severe pulmonary impairment encountered in one patient with acquired Jeune's syndrome. A sternotomy was performed and wedged open permanently with rib struts.

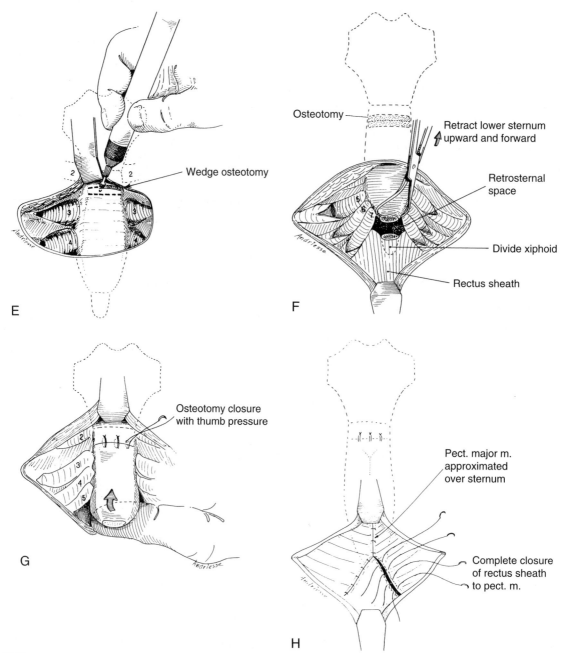

Figure 59–2 Cont'd *E,* The sternal osteotomy is created above the last deformed cartilage at the point of posterior angulation of the sternum. This is generally above the insertion of the third cartilage, or occasionally the second. Two transverse sternal osteotomies are created through the anterior cortex with a Hall air drill (Zimmer USA, Inc., Warsaw, Ind.) 2 to 4 mm apart. The short intervening segment of anterior cortex is then removed, along with the underlying cancellous bone. *F,* The base of the sternum and the rectus muscle flap are elevated with two towel clips, and the posterior plate of the sternum is fractured. The xiphoid can be divided from the sternum with electrocautery, allowing entry into the retrosternal space. This step is not necessary with the use of a retrosternal strut. Preservation of the attachment of the sheaths and xiphoid avoids an unsightly depression, which can occur below the sternum. *G,* When a strut is not used, the osteotomy is closed with several heavy silk sutures as the sternum is elevated to an overcorrected position with the assistant's thumb. *H,* A single-limb medium Hemovac drain (Snyder Laboratories, Inc., New Philadelphia, Ohio) is brought through the inferior skin flap to the left of the sternum and placed in a right parasternal position to the level of the highest costal cartilage resection. The pectoral muscle flaps are secured to the midline of the sternum, advancing the flaps to achieve coverage of the entire sternum. The rectus muscle flap, if divided, is joined to the pectoral muscle flaps.

Continued

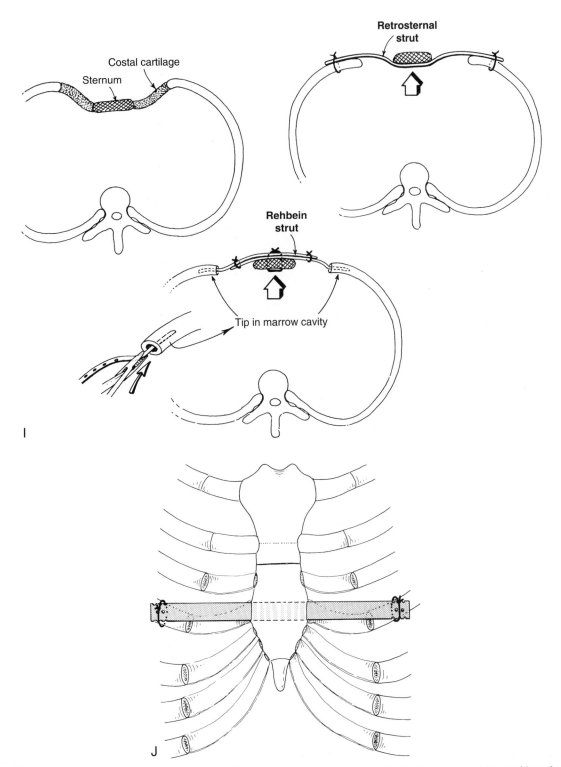

Figure 59–2 Cont'd *I,* Use of both retrosternal struts and Rehbein struts is demonstrated. The Rehbein struts are inserted into the marrow cavity (*inset*) of the third or fourth ribs and are then joined to each other medially to create a metal arch anterior to the sternum. The sternum is sewn to the arch to secure it in a forward position. The retrosternal strut is placed behind the sternum and is secured to the rib ends laterally to prevent migration. *J,* Anterior depiction of the retrosternal strut. The perichondrial sheath to either the third or fourth rib is divided at its junction with the sternum, and the retrosternal space is bluntly dissected to allow passage of the strut behind the sternum. An adequate space must be created to avoid injury to the pericardium. The strut is secured with two pericostal sutures laterally to prevent migration. (*A* to *H,* From Shamberger RC, Welch KJ: Surgical repair of pectus excavatum. J Pediatr Surg 1988;23:615-622. *I* and *J,* From Shamberger RC: Chest wall deformities. In Shields TW [ed]: General Thoracic Surgery, 5th ed. Philadelphia, Lippincott Williams & Wilkins, 2000.)

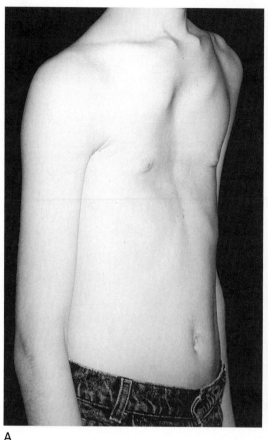

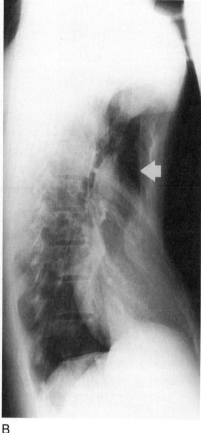

A   B

Figure 59–3 *A,* Eighteen-year-old man 15 years after pectus excavatum repair with a central broad recurrence and relative overgrowth of the upper unresected costal cartilages and ribs. *B,* Lateral radiograph demonstrates the sternum *(arrow)* lying parallel to the spine and the relative protrusion of the upper ribs.

The pleura was opened bilaterally, along with subperichondrial resection of six ribs. Pulmonary function was improved after the procedure.

Fracture of struts left in place for extended periods has been reported, with erosion of the strut into the myocardium.[101] For this reason, most struts should be removed after an adequate interval to allow complete healing of the chest wall.

PROTRUSION DEFORMITIES: PECTUS CARINATUM

Pectus carinatum consists of a spectrum of deformities that are less frequent than pectus excavatum by a ratio of 1:5.[122] It occurs more frequently in boys than in girls (4:1), as does pectus excavatum. In almost half the children, the deformity is not appreciated until after the 11th birthday. A mild deformity noted at birth or in early childhood often worsens as the child grows, particularly at puberty. As a result, most children present for repair as teenagers.

Cause

The origin of pectus carinatum is no better established than that of pectus excavatum. Early investigators implicated abnormal development of the diaphragm, but this has never been confirmed.[14,22] Others proposed that excessive growth of the ribs or costal cartilages produces either

pectus carinatum or pectus excavatum.[128] Two associations provide some clues to its origin: (1) a family history of chest wall deformity has been identified in 26% of patients, suggesting some genetic predisposition,[122] and (2) scoliosis in 15% of patients implies a diffuse abnormality in connective tissue development.

Clinical Presentation

The most frequent form of pectus carinatum is symmetrical protrusion of the body of the sternum (gladiolus) and costal cartilages, termed chondrogladiolar protrusion (Fig. 59-4). An associated lateral depression of the ribs (runnels or Harrison's grooves) is often present. It has been likened to a giant hand crushing the chest from each side.[61] Protrusion can also be asymmetrical, limited to one side of the sternum, with the costal cartilages producing a keel-like protrusion (Fig. 59-5). A mixed deformity also occurs with components of both protrusion and depression. The sternum is often rotated posteriorly toward the depressed side. This variant is most frequently seen in conjunction with Poland's syndrome. The rarest form of pectus carinatum, chondromanubrial protrusion, is produced by protrusion of the manubrium and the superior costal cartilages, with a relative depression of the body of the sternum (Fig. 59-6). It is frequently associated with premature fusion of the sternal sutures and a broad comma-shaped or Z-shaped sternum. An increased incidence of congenital heart

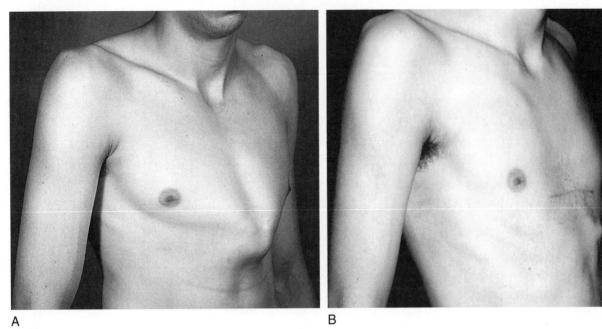

A   B

Figure 59–4 *A,* Nineteen-year-old man with symmetrical chondrogladiolar pectus carinatum. *B,* Postoperative photograph shows correction of the protruding sternum and costal cartilages.

disease has been identified in these children.[25] Lees and Caldicott[79] identified anomalies of sternal fusion in 135 of 1915 children. Twenty percent of those with sternal fusion had congenital heart disease.

Treatment

Surgical repair of pectus carinatum has a colorful past that has been reviewed elsewhere.[122] In 1973 Welch and Vos[144] reported their approach to these deformities in

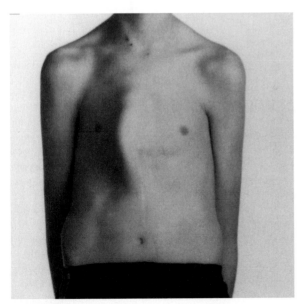

Figure 59–5 Twelve-year-old boy with asymmetrical pectus carinatum has protrusion of the costal cartilages on only the right side, producing a keel-like deformity.

26 children. They stressed the need to preserve the perichondrial sheaths and to tailor the osteotomies to achieve the appropriate position of the sternum. A similar method was used by Pickard et al.[105] Attempts to treat pectus carinatum by orthotic bracing have been reported, and success in younger children has been achieved.[33,46,93] In older children, poor compliance with bracing programs is common, presumably due to the discomfort.

Surgical Technique

Initial exposure for repair of pectus carinatum is through a transverse incision, identical to that for pectus excavatum repair, followed by mobilization of skin and pectoral muscle flaps. Many authors stress the need to remove all deformed or partially deformed cartilages,[114,122] because with continued growth, mild deformities worsen and become apparent. In the chondrogladiolar deformity, a single or occasionally a double osteotomy allows the posterior plate of the sternum to be fractured, returning the sternum to a normal position (Fig. 59-7A). The wound is drained and closed in a fashion identical to that for pectus excavatum repair.

In the mixed deformity, the oblique position of the sternum must be corrected, as well as the position of the depressed and protruding costal cartilages. After subperichondrial resection of the abnormal costal cartilages is completed, a wedge-shaped osteotomy is created in the anterior sternal plate, with the broad portion of the wedge on the depressed side of the sternum (Fig. 59-7B). Closure of the osteotomy both elevates and rotates the sternum into a corrected position. It is secured with sutures to close the osteotomy or with a strut.

With chondromanubrial and mixed deformities, management of the sternum requires special consideration.

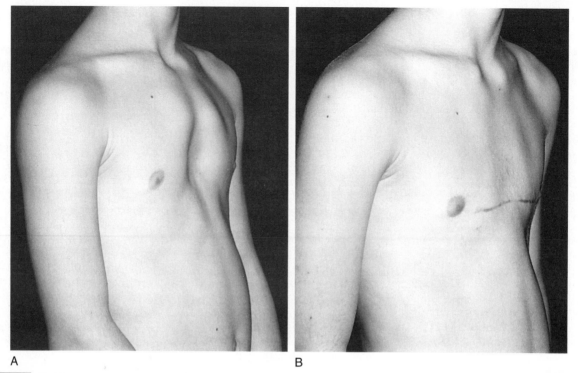

Figure 59-6 *A,* Fifteen-year-old boy with chondromanubrial deformity. Note the posterior depression of the lower sternum accentuated by the anterior bowing of the second and third costal cartilages. *B,* After repair, the sternal contour is improved, and costal cartilages reform in a more appropriate position.

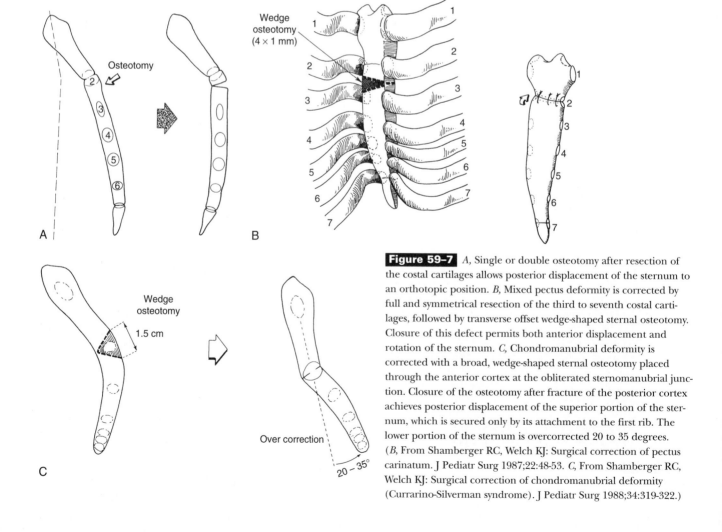

Figure 59-7 *A,* Single or double osteotomy after resection of the costal cartilages allows posterior displacement of the sternum to an orthotopic position. *B,* Mixed pectus deformity is corrected by full and symmetrical resection of the third to seventh costal cartilages, followed by transverse offset wedge-shaped sternal osteotomy. Closure of this defect permits both anterior displacement and rotation of the sternum. *C,* Chondromanubrial deformity is corrected with a broad, wedge-shaped sternal osteotomy placed through the anterior cortex at the obliterated sternomanubrial junction. Closure of the osteotomy after fracture of the posterior cortex achieves posterior displacement of the superior portion of the sternum, which is secured only by its attachment to the first rib. The lower portion of the sternum is overcorrected 20 to 35 degrees. (*B,* From Shamberger RC, Welch KJ: Surgical correction of pectus carinatum. J Pediatr Surg 1987;22:48-53. *C,* From Shamberger RC, Welch KJ: Surgical correction of chondromanubrial deformity (Currarino-Silverman syndrome). J Pediatr Surg 1988;34:319-322.)

In the chondromanubrial form, the upper position of the sternum protrudes, and the lower body is angled toward the spine. In Ravitch's[108] first description of the repair of this deformity, he removed a wedge of the anterior plate of the sternum at its point of maximal protrusion and created a second osteotomy at the site of the second angle of the Z-shaped sternum. In my experience, the sternum has been comma shaped and truncated, so a second osteotomy was not required (Fig. 59-7C).[124] When the osteotomy is closed, both the posterior depression of the lower portion of the sternum and the anterior angulation of the manubrium are corrected as the manubrium rotates posteriorly on its attachment to the first costal cartilage.

Complications

Complications of repair should be infrequent, including infection, pneumothorax, pneumonia, or wound separation. Blood transfusions are rarely required with the use of electrocautery. Results from correction are overwhelmingly successful, and recurrence is rare. Incomplete correction of the deformity and repair at an early age before complete development of the deformity are the primary reasons for reoperation.[114,122]

POLAND'S SYNDROME

The initial description of Poland's syndrome appeared in the English literature in 1841,[106] although German and French cases had been described earlier.[41,128] Poland reported a case in which he performed an anatomic dissection while still a medical student. He described a constellation of anomalies, including absence of the pectoralis major and minor muscles and syndactyly. Subsequent reports added other components of the syndrome, including absence of ribs, chest wall depression, athelia or amastia, absence of axillary hair, and limited subcutaneous fat. Thompson first summarized the full spectrum of anomalies in 1895.[128] Although described previously by others, this syndrome has been labeled Poland's syndrome since 1962, when Clarkson[23] first applied this eponym to a group of patients.

Embryology

Poland's syndrome has a sporadic occurrence estimated at 1 in 30,000 to 32,000 live births; it is rarely familial.[40,88] Various causes have been suggested, including abnormal migration of the embryonic tissues forming the pectoral muscles, hypoplasia of the subclavian artery, and in utero injuries from attempted abortion, but none of these theories has been uniformly accepted.[13,28] Although some forms of syndactyly have been described as autosomal dominant traits, a similar pattern has not been demonstrated in patients with Poland's syndrome, which is generally sporadic. Poland's syndrome is associated with a second rare syndrome, Möbius' syndrome, involving bilateral or unilateral facial palsy and abducens oculi palsy. Fontaine and Ovlaque[39] identified 19 such cases, but a unifying cause was

lacking. Boaz et al.[10] reported an unusual association between Poland's syndrome and childhood leukemia.

Clinical Presentation

Children demonstrate remarkable diversity in this syndrome (Fig. 59-8). The predominant defect varies, depending on the extent of involvement of the different components. By definition, all children with Poland's syndrome have aplasia or hypoplasia of the sternocostal portion of the pectoralis major muscle and at least one other associated lesion. The degree of abnormality of the hand, breast, or chest wall can be quite variable. Thompson,[128] in his early summary of this syndrome, found the pectoralis major muscle entirely absent in 20 cases and partially defective in 63; generally, the sternocostal component is the missing portion. The pectoralis minor was described as absent in 53 cases and defective in many others. In no case was it described as normal. Children do not present with functional deficiency of the ipsilateral arm, however, because they compensate well for the missing pectoral muscles. Hand anomalies vary widely. In the report by Ireland et al.,[64] all their patients had syndactyly and a variable degree of brachydactyly, an obvious result of the authors' patient selection and referral patterns. In another series of 75 children with Poland's syndrome, 50 had anomalies of the hand, and 37 had absence or hypoplasia of the breast or nipple.[120] In many, the nipple was lightly pigmented and higher on the chest than the normal contralateral nipple. There was no correlation between the severity of chest wall and hand anomalies. A broad range of thoracic deformities was seen in these children, ranging from a normal configuration of the ribs to aplasia of two to three ribs (Table 59-2; Fig. 59-9). Few children have a chest wall deformity so severe that it requires surgery.

CT scans have proved helpful in assessing the configuration of the chest wall and its need for reconstruction (Fig. 59-10).[6] CT scans can also evaluate the extent of muscular involvement. In one case, failure of a latissimus dorsi myocutaneous flap was attributed to unrecognized hypoplasia of the latissimus dorsi muscle.[24]

All patients with absent ribs should be considered candidates for repair. The aplastic ribs are generally some combination of the second to the fifth, with the second being least frequently involved.[128] Only two cases have

TABLE 59-2 Chest Wall Deformities in 75 Patients with Poland's Syndrome

Deformity	No. of Patients
None	41
Hypoplasia of ribs without depression	10
Depression deformity of ribs	
Major	11
Minor	5
Aplasia of ribs	8

From Shamberger RC, Welch KJ, Upton J III: Surgical treatment of thoracic deformity in Poland's syndrome. J Pediatr Surg 1989;24:760.

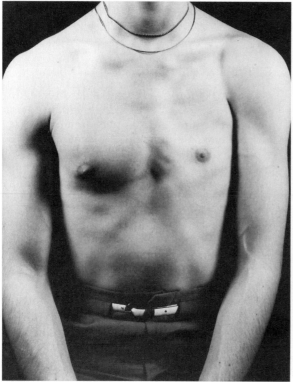

A

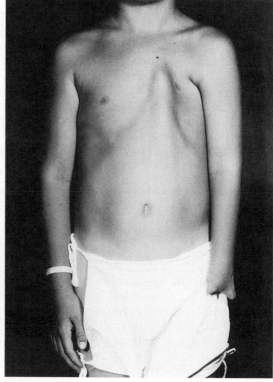

B

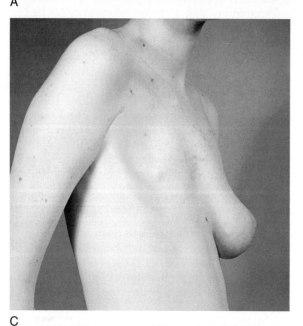

C

Figure 59–8 Poland's syndrome. *A*, Muscular 15-year-old boy with a mildly hypoplastic left chest and absent pectoralis minor muscle and costomanubrial component to the pectoralis major muscle, causing loss of the anterior axillary fold. *B*, Eight-year-old boy with aplasia of the third to fifth ribs on the left, rotation of the sternum to the left, and concave deformity of the remaining ribs on the left. Note also the hypoplastic left nipple and ectromelia of the hand. *C*, Fourteen-year-old girl with moderate depression of the chest wall on the right side in conjunction with a hypoplastic high-riding nipple and amastia. The second to fourth ribs were aplastic anteriorly. (From Shamberger RC, Welch KJ, Upton J III: Surgical treatment of thoracic deformity in Poland's syndrome. J Pediatr Surg 1989;24:760.)

been published in which there was involvement of all the ribs inserting into the sternum below the first. Patients with a severe ipsilateral concave deformity of the chest wall should also be considered for repair.

Treatment

Ravitch[109] and others have described reconstruction of aplastic ribs with autologous rib grafts. Use of the latissimus

dorsi muscle to provide coverage for the ribs produces an improved appearance but involves the possibility of functional loss when the pectoralis major muscle is also hypoplastic.[37,58,99] Use of the latissimus dorsi flap may be justified in females to optimize breast reconstruction, but its use in males—in whom arm strength is more important—is subject to debate, although it has been combined with implants in males to correct hypoplasia of the chest wall.[85] Haller et al.[49] and Urschel et al.,[135] in separate reports published in 1984, combined simultaneous latissimus dorsi

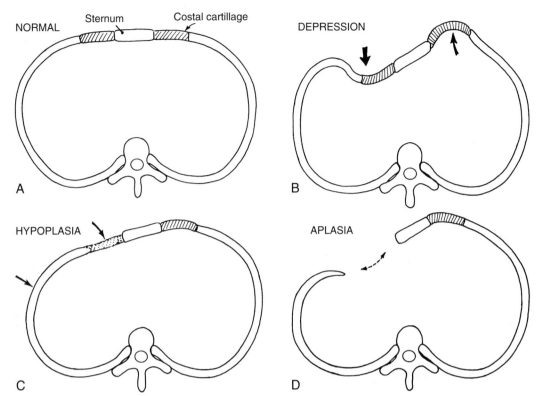

Figure 59–9 Spectrum of rib cage abnormalities seen in Poland's syndrome. *A,* Most frequently, the rib cage is normal, with only absent pectoral muscles. *B,* Depression of the involved side of the chest wall, with rotation and often depression of the sternum. A carinate protrusion of the contralateral side is frequently present. *C,* Hypoplasia of ribs on the involved side but without significant depression. This usually does not require surgical correction. *D,* Aplasia of one or more ribs is usually associated with depression of adjacent ribs on the involved side and rotation of the sternum. (From Shamberger RC, Welch KJ, Upton J III: Surgical treatment of thoracic deformity in Poland's syndrome. J Pediatr Surg 1989;24:760.)

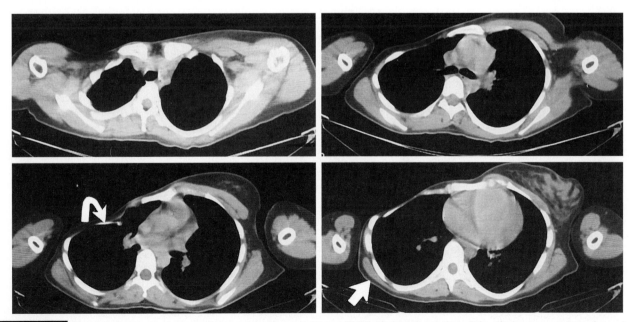

Figure 59–10 Computed tomography scan of the patient shown in Figure 59-8C. Marked depression of the ribs is apparent *(curved arrow),* as well as aplasia of the ribs in the lower two frames. Hypoplasia of the latissimus dorsi muscle is also noted on the lower right frame *(straight arrow).* (From Shamberger RC, Welch KJ, Upton J III: Surgical treatment of thoracic deformity in Poland's syndrome. J Pediatr Surg 1989;24:760.)

muscle flaps with placement of rib grafts or Marlex mesh. The vital components of chest wall repair include correction of the abnormal position and rotation of the sternum, as well as replacement of the aplastic ribs. Haller et al.[47] described the frequent carinate deformity of the contralateral ribs, which require resection to optimize results. Resection also allows correction of the depression and rotation of the sternum. Hypoplasia of the ribs without localized depression is not surgically correctable (see Fig. 59-9C).

Surgical Technique

Initial exposure of the chest wall is obtained through a transverse incision, as for pectus excavatum repair (Fig. 59-11A). In patients requiring surgical correction, there is invariably severe depression of the involved side (occasionally with absent ribs) and rotation of the sternum, often producing a carinate protrusion on the contralateral side (Fig. 59-11B). Caution must be used

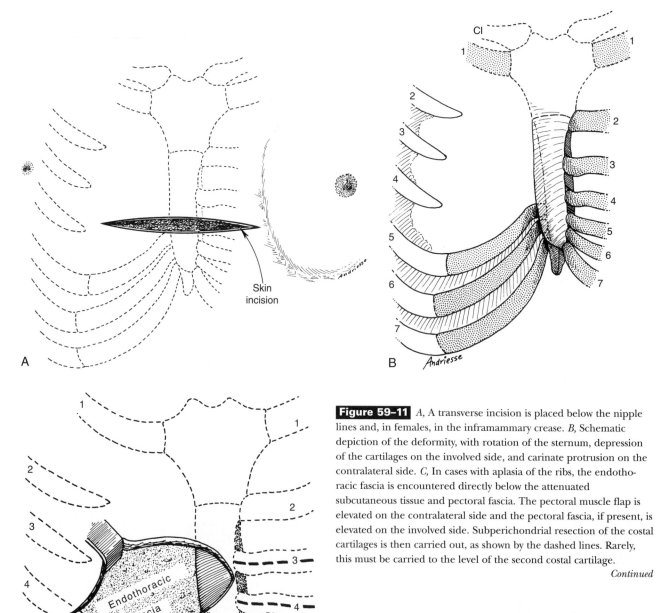

Figure 59–11 *A,* A transverse incision is placed below the nipple lines and, in females, in the inframammary crease. *B,* Schematic depiction of the deformity, with rotation of the sternum, depression of the cartilages on the involved side, and carinate protrusion on the contralateral side. *C,* In cases with aplasia of the ribs, the endothoracic fascia is encountered directly below the attenuated subcutaneous tissue and pectoral fascia. The pectoral muscle flap is elevated on the contralateral side and the pectoral fascia, if present, is elevated on the involved side. Subperichondrial resection of the costal cartilages is then carried out, as shown by the dashed lines. Rarely, this must be carried to the level of the second costal cartilage.

Continued

Figure 59-11 Cont'd *D*, A transverse offset wedge-shaped sternal osteotomy is created below the second costal cartilage. Closure of this defect with heavy silk sutures or by strut support corrects both the posterior displacement and the rotation of the sternum. *E*, In cases with rib aplasia, split rib grafts are harvested and secured medially with wire sutures into previously created sternal notches and with wire to the hypoplastic ribs laterally. Ribs are split as shown along their short axis to maintain maximal mechanical strength. (From Shamberger RC, Welch KJ, Upton J III: Surgical treatment of thoracic deformity in Poland's syndrome. J Pediatr Surg 1989;24:760.)

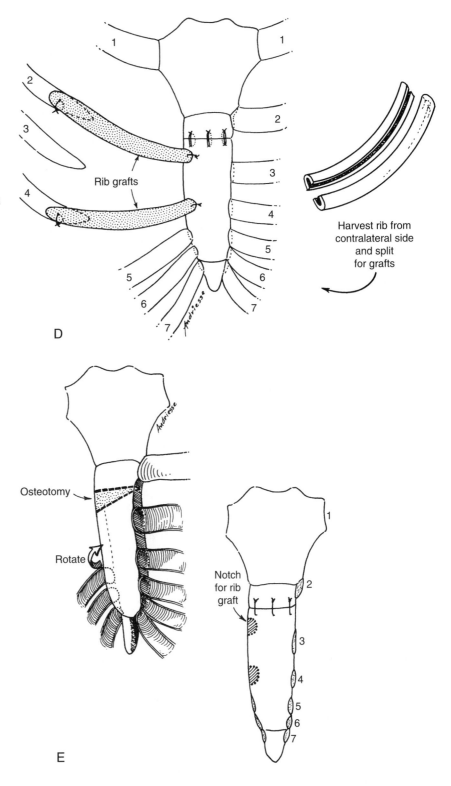

during this dissection when ribs are absent, because there is only a thin layer of attenuated pectoral fascia between the skin flaps and the endothoracic fascia (Fig. 59-11C). Violation of this layer should be avoided to prevent entry into the thoracic cavity. Subperichondrial resection of the costal cartilages is performed on both sides, removing the entire third, fourth, and fifth cartilages up to the costo-chondral junctions, which are preserved. Segments of the

sixth and seventh costal cartilages are resected to the point where they flatten to join the costal arch. To correct the rotational deformity of the sternum and the depression of the involved ribs, a transverse wedge-shaped osteotomy is placed, as for the mixed pectus carinatum deformity (Fig. 59-11D). Closure of this osteotomy corrects both components of the abnormal sternal position. In patients with absence of the second, third, and fourth ribs, a rib graft is harvested from the contralateral fifth or sixth rib through the anterior incision used for the repair; the periosteum is left in situ to allow regeneration of the rib. A split rib graft is generally used to facilitate revascularization of the graft through the marrow cavity. This often achieves correction of the defect with only one harvested rib (Fig. 59-11E). The graft is secured to notches created in the sternum before bringing the sternum anteriorly and to the involved ribs laterally with wire sutures placed through drill holes in the native rib and the graft. The rib grafts can be covered with a prosthetic mesh if further support is needed.

Breast reconstruction is required in most girls but is best delayed until late puberty to optimize the match between the contralateral and reconstructed breasts. Implants are generally required, often in conjunction with a latissimus dorsi flap. Customized implants have been used that correct both the hypoplasia of the chest wall and the absent breast tissue, but they have not been uniformly successful.[59,119]

Complications and Outcome

The patient, his or her parents, and the surgeon must enter into correction of this deformity with appropriate expectations. The components of the chest wall deformity must be well defined to identify the correctable factors. Diffuse hypoplasia of the ribs without depression is not correctable. Ipsilateral depression and contralateral protrusion with rotation of the sternum can generally be improved, as can aplasia of the ribs. The concavity below the clavicle created by the hypoplastic pectoralis major muscle is frequently bothersome in girls, because this area is apparent when wearing a bathing suit or gown. It can be partially corrected with rotation of the latissimus dorsi muscle flap at the time of breast reconstruction, but these flaps have been noted to atrophy with time.[85]

STERNAL DEFECTS

Sternal defects are rare compared with pectus excavatum and pectus carinatum, yet they have received a great deal of attention in the medical literature. Indeed, documentation of their occurrence dates to the ancient cuneiform tablets that made up the Royal Library of Nineveh.[125] Translations of those tablets reveal that the ancients believed that births with "the heart open, and that has no skin" predicted calamity. Dramatic presentations of such defects since that time, particularly involving the naked heart, have led to many isolated case reports in the modern medical literature, as well as several excellent reviews.

Weese[128] provided the first anatomic classification of sternal defects in 1818, dividing them into *ectopia cordis cum sterni fissura, ectopia suprathoracica,* and *ectopia subthoracica.* Breschet[128] in 1826 provided three comparable divisions: *l'ectopie thoracique du coeur, l'ectopie abdominale,* and *l'ectopie céphalique.* Roth[128] in 1939 divided these lesions into *ectopia cordis thoracalis extrathoracica, ectopia cordis ventralis,* and *ectopia cordis suprathoracica (cervicalis);*

the first division was further subdivided into defects in the manubrium, defects in the body of the sternum, and *ectopia cordis pectoralis sternoepigastrica.* Similarly, Shao-tsu[128] divided sternal defects into *ectopia cordis cervicalis,* with the heart in the neck; *ectopia cordis thoracalis,* with the heart outside the thorax and a sternal fissure; *ectopia cordis thoracoabdominalis;* and *ectopia cordis abdominalis.* Despite these classifications, subsequent case reports often blurred the divisions and confused the field that had been so well defined by early authors. One sternal defect that was not accounted for in these classifications was the bifid or cleft sternum. In this deformity, the heart is in an orthotopic position in the thoracic cavity, but the sternum is cleft or only partially fused overlying the heart. Skin coverage is normal or with only a small superficial ulceration.

More than a century after these descriptions and classifications, Cantrell and Ravitch[20] summarized a group of patients with ectopia subthoracica or *ectopia abdominale* deformity, along with its associated defects of the diaphragm, pericardium, abdominal wall, and heart. Subsequently, these patients were often referred to as having Cantrell's pentalogy, adding to the confusion. A more recent report summarized the world literature and tabulated the associated anomalies that occur in these infants and children.[121] Review of this topic provides four basic types of sternal defects based on tissue coverage of the heart, with limited overlap between categories. Further divisions seem artificial and do not clarify the anatomy or have prognostic significance.

Thoracic Ectopia Cordis

Thoracic ectopia cordis consists of the *ectopia cordis cum sterni fissura* of Weese and the *ectopie thoracique du coeur* of Breschet. These lesions constitute the classic naked heart with no overlying somatic structures. The orientation of the apex of the heart is anterior and often superior (Fig. 59-12). Intrinsic cardiac anomalies are frequent, and associated lesions have been summarized.[121] Many case reports do not provide information on the intrinsic cardiac anatomy owing to the striking external appearance of the heart. The sternum may be intact superiorly at the manubrium or entirely split; in rare cases, the heart may protrude through a defect in the central portion of the sternum. There is a severe lack of midline somatic tissues, and many attempts at primary closure have failed. Evaluation by CT has confirmed that the intrathoracic cavity is small in these infants.[55] Most successful repairs have not been achieved in true thoracic ectopia cordis but rather in thoracoabdominal ectopia cordis. Cutler and Wilens[26] first attempted repair in 1925 by skin flap coverage, but this failed because of cessation of cardiac function, presumably from pressure on the heart. In more than 29 attempts, only four survivors have been recorded.[32,77,94,116]

The first successful repair of ectopia cordis was achieved by Koop in 1975, as reported by Saxena.[116] An infant with a normal heart had skin flap coverage at 5 hours of age, with inferior mobilization of the anterior attachments of the diaphragm. The sternal bands were

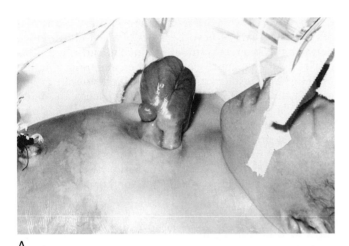

A

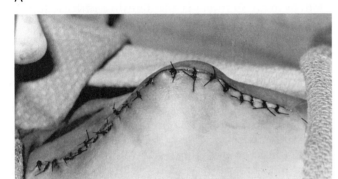

B

Figure 59–12 *A*, Infant with thoracic ectopia cordis with no significant abdominal wall defect. *B*, Repair via skin flap coverage was achieved by extensive mobilization of the skin flaps laterally on the day of birth. Repair of the intracardiac defect—tetralogy of Fallot with long-gap pulmonary atresia—was achieved later through the skin flaps. (Courtesy of Craig W. Lillehei, MD.)

2 inches apart and could not be approximated primarily without cardiac compression and compromise. At 7 months of age, an acrylic resin of Dacron and Marlex mesh was inserted to widen the sternal cleft, with primary skin closure. Necrosis of the skin flaps complicated the postoperative course, and infection of the prosthetic material necessitated its removal. This child has survived to age 18 years and is reported to be entirely well. The case of Dobell et al.[32] is notable because surgical correction was performed in two stages: skin flap coverage was provided as a newborn, and at 19 months of age, rib strut grafts were placed over the sternal defect and covered with pectoral muscle flaps. The pericardium was divided from its anterior attachments to the chest wall, allowing the heart to fall back partially into the thoracic cavity. Only Amato et al.[4] and Morales et al.[94] achieved complete soft tissue coverage in one stage. The unifying theme of successful management is the construction of a partial anterior chest cavity surrounding the heart and the avoidance of attempts to return the heart to an orthotopic

location (see Fig. 59-12B). Of note, in the successful cases, intrinsic cardiac lesions and associated abdominal defects were absent, except for a muscular ventricular septal defect and a ventricular diverticulum in the case of Morales[94]; these characteristics distinguish the successful cases from the failures rather than any differences in surgical technique. In cases repaired with autologous tissue grafts (bone or cartilage) or synthetic materials, infection and extrusion of the graft invariably occur. Ultimate success can be achieved only with tissue coverage over the displaced heart that avoids posterior compression of the heart into an already limited thoracic space. This type of coverage may require the use of tissues from sites distant from the anterior chest wall or extensive mobilization of local tissues. The severe intracardiac defects associated with thoracic ectopia cordis also make ultimate survival difficult. Regrettably, the only advancement in management of this lesion has been prenatal ultrasonographic identification, including definition of the intracardiac lesions and termination of the pregnancy if desired by the parents.[145]

Upper abdominal wall defects are also frequent in these patients, including upper abdominal omphalocele, diastasis recti, and rarely, eventration of the abdominal viscera. The presence of abdominal wall defects in conjunction with thoracic ectopia cordis should not, however, lead to the classification of these lesions as thoracoabdominal ectopia cordis; this term should be reserved for cases in which the heart is covered at birth.

Cervical Ectopia Cordis

Cervical ectopia cordis (*ectopia suprathoracica* of Weese and *ectopie céphalique* of Breschet) has historically been defined as a separate entity from thoracic ectopia cordis, based on the extent of superior displacement of the heart. Fusion between the apex of the heart and the mouth is often present, as are severe craniofacial anomalies. This lesion is relatively rare compared with thoracic ectopia cordis, but patients share the same dismal prognosis. In the summary of Shao-tsu,[128] only five infants were classified with cervical ectopia cordis, whereas 121 infants had the thoracic variety. No survivors or attempts at closure in this group of severely deformed infants have been reported.

Thoracoabdominal Ectopia Cordis

Thoracoabdominal ectopia cordis includes those lesions classified as *ectopia subthoracica* by Weese and *ectopie abdominale* by Breschet. It combines the rather artificial divisions of *ectopia cordis thoracalis extrathoracica sternoepigastrica* and *ectopia cordis ventralis* of Roth and the *ectopia cordis thoracoabdominalis* and *ectopia cordis abdominalis* of Shao-tsu. In this group, the heart is covered by a membrane of thin, often pigmented skin with an overlying, inferiorly cleft sternum (Fig. 59-13). The heart lacks the severe anterior rotation present in thoracic ectopia cordis. A 1798 report of this lesion by Wilson[77] clearly defined the associated somatic defects of the abdominal

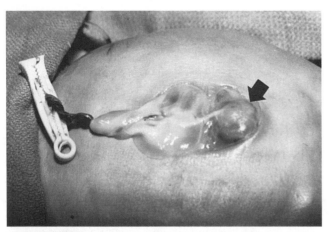

Figure 59–13 Infant with thoracoabdominal ectopia cordis demonstrating a small abdominal wall defect covered by an omphalocele below the costal arch. The infant's head is to the right, and the heart *(arrow)* is visible just below the superior margin of the defect, covered by a thin membrane. Primary skin closure was achieved during the initial operation, with subsequent repair of the cardiac defect.

wall, diaphragm, and pericardium, as well as the intrinsic cardiac anomalies, more than 150 years before the reviews by Major[83] and Cantrell and Ravitch.[20] These patients almost invariably have associated abdominal wall defects (omphalocele, diastasis recti, or ventral hernia), along with anterior semilunar defects in the diaphragm and pericardium. Intrinsic cardiac lesions are frequently present in these patients and have been summarized.[121] The position of the heart varies; it may lie within the thoracic cavity, with only the diaphragmatic and pericardial defect below it, or it may reside entirely within the abdominal cavity, with the major vessels extending through the defect in the diaphragm. Diverticula of the left ventricle occur with surprising frequency in this anomaly. In many cases, the diverticulum protrudes through the diaphragmatic and pericardial defect into the abdominal cavity.

Successful repair and long-term survival are more frequent in thoracoabdominal ectopia cordis than in thoracic ectopia cordis. Arndt[3] attempted the first repair in 1896, but return of the heart to the thoracic cavity resulted in death. Wieting[146] performed the first successful surgical repair with primary closure of the diaphragm and abdominal wall fascia in 1912. Initial surgical intervention must address the skin defects overlying the heart and abdominal cavity. Primary excision of the omphalocele with skin closure is preferred to avoid infection and mediastinitis, although several cases have been managed successfully by local application of topical astringents, allowing secondary epithelialization to occur. Several early cases document the viability of individuals with thoracoabdominal ectopia cordis when there is intact skin coverage over an intra-abdominal heart.

Advances in pediatric cardiac surgery now allow correction of the intrinsic cardiac lesions that were often fatal in the past. An aggressive approach in these infants is appropriate. Closure of the abdominal wall defect or diastasis can be managed by either primary closure of the

defect or prosthetic mesh closure. Primary closure is often difficult to achieve because of the wide distance between the two rectus muscles, which are attached superiorly to the splayed costal arches, limiting midline mobility. The costal cartilages are divided laterally in one modification of closure, allowing them to rotate medially.[68] Complete repair of the intracardiac defect is best performed before placement of any prosthetic material over the heart. Once skin coverage is achieved, closure of this defect is important, primarily for mechanical protection of the heart. Fatal pulmonary hypoplasia has occurred in some infants with this anomaly.[121]

Cleft or Bifid Sternum

Cleft or bifid sternum is the fourth and least severe anomaly of the sternum. Infants in this group have an orthotopic heart, normal skin coverage, an intact pericardium, and a partially or completely cleft sternum (Fig. 59-14). Omphalocele is not associated with cleft sternum. The sternal defect, if partial, involves the upper sternum and manubrium, in contrast with the sternal defect in thoracic or thoracoabdominal ectopia cordis, in which partial defects involve primarily the lower sternum. Most cases are partially split (Table 59-3), with an intact xiphoid or lower third of the body of the sternum.

The bifid or cleft sternum is distinct from the other three categories of sternal defects, in that intrinsic cardiac defects are rare. Several distinct somatic associations are seen, including bandlike scars extending from the umbilicus to the inferior aspect of the sternal defect. Other children have superior scarlike extensions to the neck or mandible; rarely, a split mandible occurs (gnathoschisis). Fischer[36] reported an unexplained association with cervicofacial hemangiomas in 1879, and Ingelrans and Debeugny[63] later reported the occurrence of fatal postoperative hemorrhage from presumed hemangioma of the trachea after repair of a sternal defect.

In most cases, these infants' sternal defects are asymptomatic. Repair is performed to provide protective coverage for the heart. It may also improve respiratory mechanics, which are compromised by the paradoxical motion of the defect. Lannelongue[77] in 1888 was allegedly the first to repair a cleft sternum, but his intervention was limited to excision of a small circular ulcer overlying

TABLE 59–3 Sternal Defects in 109 Patients with Cleft Sternum	
Defect	**No. of Patients**
Upper cleft	46
Upper cleft to xiphoid	33
Complete cleft	23
Lower defect with manubrium or midsegment intact	5
Central defect with manubrium and xiphoid intact	2
Skin ulceration noted in only	3 cases

From Shamberger R, Welch KJ: Sternal defects. Pediatr Surg Int 1990;5:156-164.

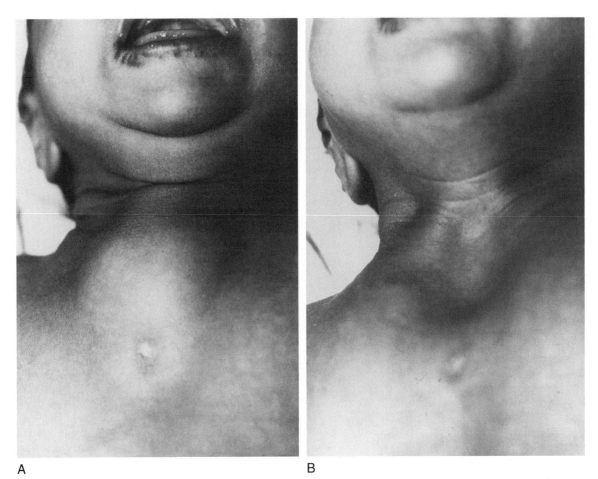

A   B

Figure 59–14 Six-week-old infant with bifid sternum. Note the marked protrusion from the defect when crying *(A)* and depression of the defect with inhalation *(B)*. Capillary hemangiomas are also visible on the lips.

the sternal defect. He created two relaxing incisions later-ally, allowing primary closure of the skin, but ignored the underlying sternal separation. The first complete repair of a cleft sternum was accomplished by placing a cartilage graft from the costal arch over the defect.[18] Maier and Bortone[82] achieved the first primary closure in 1949 in a 6-week-old infant. Subsequent methods have included bilateral oblique incisions through the costal cartilages to produce greater length and allow midline approxima-tion of the sternal halves (sliding chondrotomies of Sabiston[112]); division of the cartilages laterally, swinging them medially to cover the defect (door-wing plasty of Meissner[91]); coverage with various autologous grafts (costal cartilage, rib, parietal skull); and coverage with prosthetic materials. Maier and Bortone[82] first stressed the importance of early repair in infancy, when the chest is most flexible, to achieve primary closure (Fig. 59-15). In most reported cases of primary repair, correction took place within the first 3 months of life (18 of 22 cases) and rarely after 1 year of age (2 cases).[121] In contrast, some form of chondrotomy was required in 22 patients, 8 of whom were older than 1 year. Often a wedge of cartilage must be excised from the point where the two sternal halves unite to allow approximation without tension.

THORACIC DEFORMITIES IN DIFFUSE SKELETAL DISORDERS

Asphyxiating Thoracic Dystrophy: Jeune's Syndrome

In 1954 Jeune et al.[67] described a newborn with a narrow, rigid chest and multiple cartilage anomalies. The patient died early in the perinatal period because of respiratory insufficiency. Subsequent authors further characterized this form of osteochondrodystrophy, which has variable skeletal involvement. It is inherited in an autosomal recessive pattern and is not associated with chromosomal abnormalities. Its most prominent feature is a narrow, bell-shaped thorax and protuberant abdomen. The thorax is narrow in both the transverse and the sagittal axes and has little respiratory motion because of the hor-izontal direction of the ribs (Fig. 59-16). The ribs are short and wide, and the splayed costochondral junctions barely reach the anterior axillary line. The costal carti-lage is abundant and irregular, similar to a rachitic rosary. Microscopic examination of the costochondral junction reveals disordered, poorly progressing endo-chondral ossification resulting in decreased rib length.

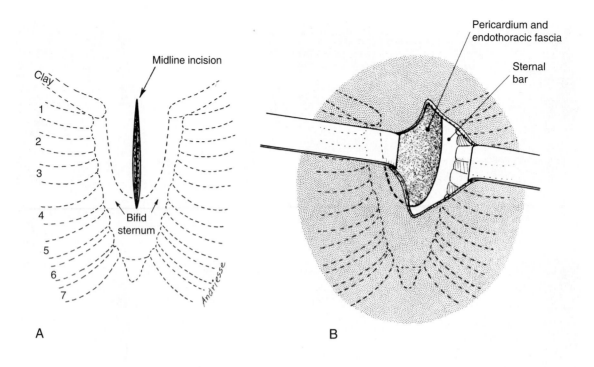

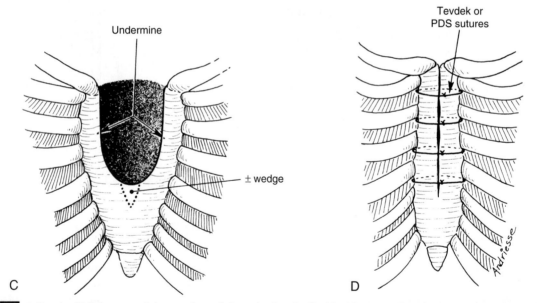

Figure 59–15 *A,* Repair of bifid sternum is best performed through a longitudinal incision extending the length of the defect. *B,* Directly beneath the subcutaneous tissues, the sternal bars are encountered, with pectoral muscles present lateral to the bars. The endothoracic fascia and pericardium are just below these structures. *C,* The endothoracic fascia is mobilized off the sternal bars posteriorly with blunt dissection, to allow safe placement of the sutures. Approximation of the sternal bars may be facilitated by excising a wedge of cartilage inferiorly. Repair is best accomplished in the neonatal period, when there is greatest flexibility of the chest wall. *D,* Closure of the defect is achieved with nonabsorbable sutures. (From Shamberger RC, Welch KJ: Sternal defects. Pediatr Surg Int 1990;5:156-164.)

Associated skeletal abnormalities that occur with this syndrome include short, stubby extremities with relatively short and wide bones. The clavicles are in a fixed and elevated position, and the pelvis is small and hypoplastic, with square iliac bones.

This syndrome has variable expression and extent of pulmonary impairment. Although the initial cases reported resulted in neonatal deaths, subsequent reports document a wide range of survival in patients with this syndrome.[75] The pathologic findings at autopsy are variable, showing a spectrum of abnormal pulmonary development. In most cases, however, bronchial development is normal, with fewer alveolar divisions, as described by Williams et al.[147] Surgical attempts to enlarge the

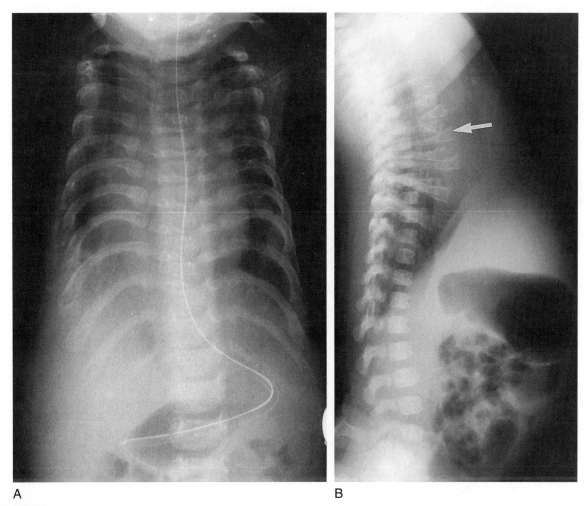

Figure 59–16   *A,* Anteroposterior radiograph shows the short horizontal ribs and narrow chest of an infant with Jeune's syndrome (asphyxiating thoracic dystrophy). *B,* Lateral radiograph demonstrates the short rib ends ending at the midaxillary line *(arrow)* and abnormal flaring at the costochondral junction. The infant died of progressive respiratory insufficiency at 1 month of age, and postmortem examination revealed alveolar hypoplasia.

thoracic cavity are generally unsuccessful and result in prolonged hospitalization and ultimate respiratory failure and death.

Spondylothoracic Dysplasia: Jarcho-Levin Syndrome

Spondylothoracic dysplasia is an autosomal recessive deformity described by Jarcho and Levin[65] in 1938 that is associated with multiple vertebral and rib malformations. Death often occurs in early infancy from respiratory failure and pneumonia. Patients have multiple alternating hemivertebrae that affect most if not all of the thoracic and lumbar spine. The vertebral ossification centers rarely cross the midline. Multiple posterior fusions of the ribs and remarkable shortening of the thoracic spine result in a crablike radiographic appearance of the chest (Fig. 59-17). One third of patients with this syndrome have associated malformations, including congenital heart disease and renal anomalies. Heilbronner and Renshaw[57]

reported its occurrence primarily in Puerto Rican families. Bone formation is normal in these patients.

The thoracic deformity is secondary to the spinal anomaly, which results in close posterior approximation of the origin of the ribs. Most infants with this entity succumb before 15 months of age, and no surgical efforts have been proposed or attempted.[111]

Cerebrocostomandibular Syndrome

The association of severe rib defects, micrognathia, and other anomalies was first described by Smith et al.[130] in 1966 and later by McNicholl et al.[89] Infants with this constellation of anomalies have ossified ribs with an aplastic segment a short distance beyond the posterior rib angles. They also have micrognathia, abnormal tracheal cartilage, and defects of the soft and hard palates. Mild to moderate mental retardation occurs in 50% of infants surviving beyond the first year of life.[130] The extent of rib defects is variable, both in the number of involved ribs

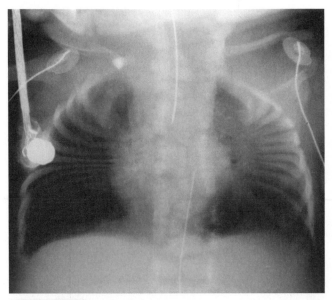

Figure 59–17 Chest radiograph of an infant with spondylothoracic dysplasia. Severe abnormality of the spine is apparent, with multiple alternating hemivertebrae and the crablike ribs.

and in the extent of the defect, ranging from a narrow gap to a rudimentary rib. The third to seventh ribs are most frequently involved. The rib gap may contain fibrous tissue, skeletal muscle, or cartilage with variable calcification. The rib gaps produce a flail chest, and the prognosis for these infants is poor. Forty percent die from respiratory failure during the first year of life.[130] The underlying cause and the inheritance pattern are not known, and chromosomal studies are normal.

REFERENCES

1. Adkins PC, Blades B: A stainless steel strut for correction of pectus excavatum. Suvr Med (Sofiia) 1961;113:111-113.
2. Allen RG, Douglas M: Cosmetic improvement of thoracic wall defects using a rapid setting Silastic mold: A special technique. J Pediatr Surg 1979;14:745-749.
3. Arndt C: Nabelschnurbruch mit Herzhernie. Operation durch Laparotomie mit Tödlichern Ausgang. Centralbl Gynäkol 1896;20:632-633.
4. Amato JT, Cotroneo JV, Gladiere R: Repair of complete ectopia cordis (film). Presented at the American College of Surgeons Clinical Congress, Chicago, October 23-28, 1988.
5. Backer OG, Brünner S, Larsen V: The surgical treatment of funnel chest: Initial and follow-up results. Acta Chir Scand 1961;121:253-261.
6. Bainbridge LC, Wright AR, Kanthan R: Computed tomography in the preoperative assessment of Poland's syndrome. Br J Plast Surg 1991;44:604-607.
7. Baronofsky I: Technique for the correction of pectus excavatum. Surgery 1957;42:884-890.
8. Beiser GD, Epstein SE, Stampfer M, et al: Impairment of cardiac function in patients with pectus excavatum, with improvement after operative correction. N Engl J Med 1972;287:267-272.
9. Bevegård S: Postural circulatory changes at rest and during exercise in patients with pectus excavatum. Acta Med Scand 1962;171:695-713.
10. Boaz D, Mace J, Gotlin RW: Poland's syndrome and leukemia. Lancet 1971;1:349-350.
11. Borgeskov S, Raahave D: Long-term result after operative correction of funnel chest. Thorax 1971;26:74-76.
12. Borowitz D, Cerny F, Zallen G, et al: Pulmonary function and exercise response in patients with pectus excavatum after Nuss repair. J Pediatr Surg 2003;38:544-547.
13. Bouvet J: Vascular origin of Poland syndrome? A comparative rheographic study of the vascularization of the arms in eight patients. Eur J Pediatr 1978;128:17-26.
14. Brodkin H: Congenital chondrosternal prominence (pigeon breast): A new interpretation. Pediatrics 1949;3:286-295.
15. Brodkin HA: Congenital anterior chest wall deformities of diaphragmatic origin. Dis Chest 1953;24:259-277.
16. Brown A: Pectus excavatum (funnel chest): Anatomic basis; surgical treatment of the incipient stage in infancy; and correction of the deformity in the fully developed stage. J Thorac Surg 1939;9:164-184.
17. Brown A: Cardio-respiratory studies in pre and postoperative funnel chest. Dis Chest 1951;20:378-391.
18. Burton JF: Method of correction of ectopia cordis. Arch Surg 1947;54:79-84.
19. Cahill JL, Lees GM, Robertson HT: A summary of preoperative and postoperative cardiorespiratory performance in patients undergoing pectus excavatum and carinatum repair. J Pediatr Surg 1984;19:430-433.
20. Cantrell HJ Jr, Ravitch MM: A syndrome of congenital defects involving the abdominal wall, sternum, diaphragm, pericardium, and heart. Surg Gynecol Obstet 1958; 107:602-614.
21. Castile RG, Staats BA, Westbrook PR: Symptomatic pectus deformities of the chest. Am Rev Respir Dis 1982;126: 564-568.
22. Chin E: Surgery of funnel chest and congenital sternal prominence. Br J Surg 1957;44:360-376.
23. Clarkson P: Poland's syndactyly. Guy Hosp Rep 1962; 111:335-346.
24. Cochran JH Jr, Pauly TJ, Edstrom LE, et al: Hypoplasia of the latissimus dorsi muscle complicating breast reconstruction in Poland's syndrome. Ann Plast Surg 1981;6:402-404.
25. Currarino G, Silverman FN: Premature obliteration of the sternal sutures and pigeon-breast deformity. Radiology 1958;70:532-540.
26. Cutler GD, Wilens G: Ectopia cordis: Report of a case. Am J Dis Child 1925;30:76-81.
27. Dailey JE: Repair of funnel chest using sub-sternal osteoperiosteal rib graft strut: Report of a case with four year follow-up. JAMA 1952;150:1203-1204.
28. David TJ: Nature and etiology of the Poland anomaly. N Engl J Med 1972;287:487-489.
29. de Agustin-Asensio JC, Banuelos C, Vazquez JJ: Titanium miniplates for the surgical correction of pectus excavatum. J Am Coll Surg 1999;188:455-458.
30. Derveaux L, Clarysse I, Ivanoff I, et al: Preoperative and postoperative abnormalities in chest x-ray indices and in lung function in pectus deformities. Chest 1989;95:850-856.
31. Derveaux L, Ivanoff I, Rochette F, et al: Mechanism of pulmonary function changes after surgical correction for funnel chest. Eur Respir J 1988;1:823-825.
32. Dobell ARC, Williams H, Long R: Staged repair of ectopia cordis. J Pediatr Surg 1982;17:353-358.
33. Egan JC, DuBois JJ, Morphy M, et al: Compressive orthotics in the treatment of asymmetric pectus carinatum: A preliminary report with an objective radiographic marker. J Pediatr Surg 2000;35:1183-1186.

34. Erbella J Jr, Behmand R, Cederna PS: Endoscopically assisted pectus excavatum repair. Surg Laparosc Endosc Percutan Tech 2001;11:213-216.

35. Feng J, Hu T, Liu W, et al: The biomechanical, morphologic, and histochemical properties of the costal cartilages in children with pectus excavatum. J Pediatr Surg 2001; 36:1770-1776.

36. Fischer H: Fissura sterno congenita mit partieller Bauchspalte. Dtsch Z Chir 1879;12:367-369.

37. Fodor PB, Khoury F: Latissimus dorsi muscle flap in reconstruction of congenitally absent breast and pectoralis muscle. Ann Plast Surg 1980;4:422-425.

38. Fonkalsrud EW, Salman T, Guo W, et al: Repair of pectus deformities with sternal support. J Thorac Cardiovasc Surg 1994;107:37-42.

39. Fontaine G, Ovlaque S: Le syndrome de Poland-Mobius. Arch Fr Pediatr 1984;41:351-352.

40. Freire-Maia N, et al: The Poland syndrome: Clinical and geneaological data, dermatoglyphic analysis, and incidence. Hum Hered 1973;23:97-104.

41. Froriep R: Beobachtung eines Falles Von Mangel der Brustdruse. Notizen aus dem Gebiete der Naturund Heilkunde 1839;10:9-14.

42. Garusi G: Angiocardiographic patterns in funnel chest. Cardiologia 1964;45:312-330.

43. Genc A, Mutaf O: Polytetrafluoroethylene bars in stabilizing the reconstructed sternum for pectus excavatum operations in children. Plast Reconstr Surg 2002;110:54-57.

44. Godfrey S: Association between pectus excavatum and segmental bronchomalacia. J Pediatr 1980;96:649-652.

45. Guller B, Hable K: Cardiac findings in pectus excavatum in children: Review and differential diagnosis. Chest 1974;66:165-171.

46. Haje SA, Bowen JR: Preliminary results of orthotic treatment of pectus deformities in children and adolescents. J Pediatr Orthop 1992;12:795-800.

47. Haller JA Jr: Severe chest wall construction from growth retardation after too extensive and too early (<4 years) pectus excavatum repair: An alert. Ann Thorac Surg 1995; 60:1857-1858.

48. Haller JA Jr, Colombani PM, Humphries CT, et al: Chest wall constriction after too extensive and too early operations for pectus excavatum. Ann Thorac Surg 1996;61:1618-1624.

49. Haller JA Jr, Colombani PM, Miller D, et al: Early reconstruction of Poland's syndrome using autologous rib grafts combined with a latissimus muscle flap. J Pediatr Surg 1984;19:423-429.

50. Hallen JAJ Jr, Kramen SS, Lietman SA: Use of CT scans in selection of patients for pectus excavatum surgery: a preliminary report. J Pediatr Surg 1987;22:904-906.

51. Haller JA Jr, Loughlin GM: Cardiorespiratory function is significantly improved following corrective surgery for severe pectus excavatum: Proposed treatment guidelines. J Cardiovasc Surg (Torino) 2000;41:125-130.

52. Haller JA Jr, Peters GN, Mazur D, et al: Pectus excavatum: A 20 year surgical experience. J Thorac Cardiovasc Surg 1970;60:375-383.

53. Haller JA Jr, Scherer LR, Turner CS, et al: Evolving management of pectus excavatum based on a single institutional experience of 664 patients. Ann Surg 1989;209:578-582.

54. Hayashi A, Maruyama Y: Vascularized rib strut technique for repair of pectus excavatum. Ann Thorac Surg 1992; 53:346-348.

55. Haynor DR, Shuman WP, Brewers DK, et al: Imaging of fetal ectopia cordis: Roles of sonography and computed tomography. J Ultrasound Med 1984;3:25-27.

56. Hecker WC, Procher G, Dietz HG: [Results of operative correction of pigeon and funnel chest following a modified procedure of Ravitch and Haller]. Z Kinderchir 1981;34:220-227.

57. Heilbronner DM, Renshaw TS: Spondylothoracic dysplasia: A case report. J Bone Joint Surg Am 1984;66:302-303.

58. Hester TR Jr, Bostwick J 3rd: Poland's syndrome: Correction with latissimus muscle transposition. Plast Reconstr Surg 1982;69:226-233.

59. Hochberg J, Ardenghy M, Graeber GM, et al: Complex reconstruction of the chest wall and breast utilizing a customized silicone implant. Ann Plast Surg 1994;32:524-528.

60. Hougaard K, Arendrup H: Deformities of the female breasts after surgery for funnel chest. Scand J Thorac Cardiovasc Surg 1983;17:171-174.

61. Howard R: Pigeon chest (protrusion deformity of the sternum). Med J Aust 1958;45:664-666.

62. Humphreys GH 2nd, Jaretzki A 3rd: Pectus excavatum: Late results with and without operation. J Thorac Cardiovasc Surg 1980;80:686-695.

63. Ingelrans P, Debeugny P: [Case of bifidity of the sternum associated with tracheal angiomatosis]. Ann Chir Infant 1965;6:123-128.

64. Ireland DC, Takayama N, Flatt AE: Poland's syndrome. J Bone Joint Surg Am 1976;58:52-58.

65. Jarcho S, Levin P: Hereditary malformation of the vertebral bodies. Bull Johns Hopkins Hosp 1938;62:216-262.

66. Jensen NK, Schmidt WR, Garamella JJ, et al: Pectus excavatum and carinatum: The how, when, and why of surgical correction. J Pediatr Surg 1970;5:4-13.

67. Jeune M, Carron R, Beraud C, et al: Polychondrodystrophie avec blocage thoracique d'evolution fatale. Pediatrie 1954;9:390-392.

68. Jona JZ: The surgical approach for reconstruction of the sternal and epigastric defects in children with Cantrell's deformity. J Pediatr Surg 1991;26:702-706.

69. Judet J: Thorax en entonnoir: Un procede operatoire. Rev Orthop 1954;40:248-257.

70. Jung A: Le traitement du thorax en entoinnoir par le "retournement pedicule" de la cuvette sterno-chondrale. Mem Acad Chir 1956;82:242-249.

71. Kaguraoka H, Ohnuki T, Itaoka T, et al: Degree of severity of pectus excavatum and pulmonary function in preoperative and postoperative periods. J Thorac Cardiovasc Surg 1992;104:1483-1488.

72. Klinke F, Dittrich H, Kujat R: [Scoring system for indication for operative correction of funnel chest]. Z Kinderchir 1981;33:237-243.

73. Kowalewski J, Brocki M, Dryjanski T, et al: Pectus excavatum: Increase of right ventricular systolic, diastolic, and stroke volumes after surgical repair. J Thorac Cardiovasc Surg 1999;118:87-92.

74. Kowalewski J, Brocki M, Zolynski K: Long-term observation in 68 patients operated on for pectus excavatum: Surgical repair of funnel chest. Ann Thorac Surg 1999;67:821-824.

75. Kozlowski K, Masel J: Asphyxiating thoracic dystrophy without respiratory disease: Report of two cases of the latent form. Pediatr Radiol 1976;5:30-33.

76. Lane-Smith DM, Gillis DA, Roy PD: Repair of pectus excavatum using a Dacron vascular graft strut. J Pediatr Surg 1994;29:1179-1182.

77. Lannelongue: De l'ectocardie et de sa cure par l'autoplastie. Ann Medico-Chirurgicales 1888;4:101-107.

78. Lansman S, Serlo W, Linna O, et al: Treatment of pectus excavatum with bioabsorbable polylactide plates: Preliminary results. J Pediatr Surg 2002;37:1281-1286.

79. Lees RF, Caldicott JH: Sternal anomalies and congenital heart disease. Am J Roentgenol Radium Ther Nucl Med 1975;124:423-427.

80. Lester C: The surgical treatment of funnel chest. Ann Surg 1946;123:1003-1022.
81. Liese W, Bühlmann A: Arbeitskapazitat und lungenvolumina vor und nach chirurgischer korrektur einer trichterbruszt. Schweiz Med Wochenschr 1974;104:83-86.
82. Maier HC, Bortone F: Complete failure of sternal fusion with herniation of pericardium. J Thorac Surg 1949;18:851-859.
83. Major JW: Thoracoabdominal ectopia cordis. J Thorac Surg 1953;26:309-317.
84. Malek MH, Fonkalsrud EW, Cooper CB: Ventilatory and cardiovascular responses to exercise in patients with pectus excavatum. Chest 2003;124:870-882.
85. Marks MW, Argenta LC, Izenberg PH, et al: Management of the chest-wall deformity in male patients with Poland's syndrome. Plast Reconstr Surg 1991;87:674-678.
86. Martinez D: The effect of costal cartilage resection on chest wall development. Pediatr Surg Int 1990;5:170-173.
87. Matsui T, Kitano M, Nakamura T, et al: Bioabsorbable struts made from poly-L-lactide and their application for treatment of chest deformity. J Thorac Cardiovasc Surg 1994;108:162-168.
88. McGillivray BC, Lowry RB: Poland syndrome in British Columbia: Incidence and reproductive experience of affected persons. Am J Med Genet 1977;1:65-74.
89. McNicholl B, Egan-Mitchell B, Murray JP, et al: Cerebro-costo-mandibular syndrome: A new familial developmental disorder. Arch Dis Child 1970;45:421-424.
90. Mead J, Sly P, Le Souef P, et al: Rib cage mobility in pectus excavatum. Am Rev Respir Dis 1985;132:1223-1228.
91. Meissner F: Fissura sterni congenita. Zentralbl Chir 1964;89:1832-1839.
92. Meyer L: Zur chirurgischen behandlung der angeborenen trichterbrust. Verh Berliner Med Gesellschaft 1911;42:364-373.
93. Mielke CH, Winter RB: Pectus carinatum successfully treated with bracing: A case report. Int Orthop 1993;17:350-352.
94. Morales JM, Patel SG, Duff JA, et al: Ectopia cordis and other midline defects. Ann Thorac Surg 2000;70:111-114.
95. Morshuis W, Folgering H, Barentsz J, et al: Pulmonary function before surgery for pectus excavatum and at long-term follow-up. Chest 1994;105:1646-1652.
96. Morshuis WJ, Folgering HT, Barentsz JO, et al: Exercise cardiorespiratory function before and one year after operation for pectus excavatum. J Thorac Cardiovasc Surg 1994;107:1403-1409.
97. Nakajima H, Chang H: A new method of reconstruction for pectus excavatum that preserves blood supply and costal cartilage. Plast Reconstr Surg 1999;103:1661-1666.
98. Ochsner A, Debakey M: Chone-chondrosternon: Report of a case and review of the literature. J Thorac Surg 1939;8:469-511.
99. Ohmori K, Takada H: Correction of Poland's pectoralis major muscle anomaly with latissimus dorsi musculocutaneous flaps. Plast Reconstr Surg 1980;65:400-404.
100. Ohno K, Nakahira M, Takeuchi S, et al: Indications for surgical treatment of funnel chest by chest radiograph. Pediatr Surg Int 2001;17:591-595.
101. Onursal E, Toker A, Vostanci K, et al: A complication of pectus excavatum operation: Endomyocardial steel strut. Ann Thorac Surg 1999;68:1082-1083.
102. Orzalesi MM, Cook CD: Pulmonary function in children with pectus excavatum. J Pediatr 1965;66:898-900.
103. Paltia V: Operative technique in funnel chest: Experience in 81 cases. Acta Chir Scand 1958;116:90-98.
104. Peterson RJ, Young WG Jr, Godwin JD, et al: Noninvasive assessment of exercise cardiac function before and after pectus excavatum repair. J Thorac Cardiovasc Surg 1985;90:251-260.
105. Pickard LR, Tepas JJ, Shermeta DW, et al: Pectus carinatum: Results of surgical therapy. J Pediatr Surg 1979;14:228-230.
106. Poland A: Deficiency of the pectoralis muscles. Guys Hosp Rep 1841;6:191-193.
107. Prevot J: Treatment of sternocostal wall malformations of the child: A series of 210 surgical corrections since 1975. Eur J Pediatr Surg 1994;4:131-136.
108. Ravitch M: The operative treatment of pectus excavatum. Ann Surg 1949;129:429-444.
109. Ravitch MM: Operative treatment of congenital deformities of the chest. Am J Surg 1961;101:588-597.
110. Rehbein F: The operative treatment of the funnel chest. Arch Dis Child 1957;32:5-8.
111. Roberts A: Spondylothoracic and spondylocostal dysostosis: Hereditary forms of spinal deformity. J Bone Joint Surg Br 1988;70:123-126.
112. Sabiston DC Jr: The surgical management of congenital bifid sternum with partial ectopia cordis. J Thorac Surg 1958;35:118-122.
113. Saint-Mezard G, Duret JC, Chanudet X, et al: Mitral valve prolapse and pectus excavatum: Fortuitous association or syndrome? Presse Med 1986;15:439.
114. Sanger PW, Taylor FH, Robicsek F: Deformities of the anterior wall of the chest. Surg Gynecol Obstet 1963;116:515-522.
115. Sauerbruch F: Die Chirurgie der Brustorgane. Berlin, Springer, 1920.
116. Saxena NC: Ectopia cordis child surviving: Prosthesis fails. Pediatr News 1976;10:3.
117. Scherer LR, Arn PH, Dressel DA, et al: Surgical management of children and young adults with Marfan syndrome and pectus excavatum. J Pediatr Surg 1988;23:1169-1172.
118. Schoenmakers MA, Gulmans VA, Bax NM, et al: Physiotherapy as an adjuvant to the surgical treatment of anterior chest wall deformities: A necessity? A prospective descriptive study in 21 patients. J Pediatr Surg 2000;35:1440-1443.
119. Seyfer AE, Icochea R, Graeber GM: Poland's anomaly: Natural history and long-term results of chest wall reconstruction in 33 patients. Ann Surg 1988;208:776-782.
120. Shamberger R: Surgical treatment of thoracic deformity in Poland's syndrome. J Pediatr Surg 1989;24:760-765.
121. Shamberger R, Welch KJ: Sternal defects. Pediatr Surg Int 1990;5:156-164.
122. Shamberger RC, Welch KJ: Surgical correction of pectus carinatum. J Pediatr Surg 1987;22:48-53.
123. Shamberger RC, Welch KJ: Cardiopulmonary function in pectus excavatum. Surg Gynecol Obstet 1988;166:383-391.
124. Shamberger RC, Welch KJ: Surgical correction of chondromanubrial deformity (Currarino-Silverman syndrome). J Pediatr Surg 1988;23:319-322.
125. Shamberger RC, Welch KJ: Surgical repair of pectus excavatum. J Pediatr Surg 1988;23:615-622.
126. Shamberger RC, Welch KJ, Castaneda AR, et al: Anterior chest wall deformities and congenital heart disease. J Thorac Cardiovasc Surg 1988;96:427-432.
127. Shamberger RC, Welch KJ, Sanders SP: Mitral valve prolapse associated with pectus excavatum. J Pediatr 1987;111:404-407.
128. Shao-tsu L: Ectopia cordis congenita. Thoraxchirurgie 1957;5:197-212.
129. Sigalet DL, Montgomery M, Harder J: Cardiopulmonary effects of closed repair of pectus excavatum. J Pediatr Surg 2003;38:380-385.

130. Smith KG, Sekar KC: Cerebrocostomandibular syndrome: Case report and literature review. Clin Pediatr (Phila) 1985;24:223-225.

131. Taguchi K: A new plastic operation for pectus excavatum: Sternal turnover surgical procedure with preserved internal mammary vessels. Chest 1975;67:606-608.

132. Tanaka F, Kitano M, Shindo T, et al: [Postoperative lung function in patients with funnel chest]. Nippon Kyobu Geka Gakkai Zasshi 1993;41:2161-2165.

133. Tang Chen YB, Chen JS, Lee YC, et al: Revascularization of turnover sternum: A definitive treatment for intractable funnel chest. Microsurgery 1999;19:296-302.

134. Udoshi MB, Shah A, Fisher VJ, et al: Incidence of mitral valve prolapse in subjects with thoracic skeletal abnormalities—a prospective study. Am Heart J 1979;97:303-311.

135. Urschel HC Jr, Byrd HS, Sethi SM, et al: Poland's syndrome: Improved surgical management. Ann Thorac Surg 1984;37:204-211.

136. Vanamo K, Peltonen J, Rintala R, et al: Chest wall and spinal deformities in adults with congenital diaphragmatic defects. J Pediatr Surg 1996;31:851-854.

137. von der Oelsnitz G: [Anomalies of the chest]. Z Kinderchir 1981;33:229-236.

138. Wada J, Ikeda K, Ishida T, et al: Results of 271 funnel chest operations. Ann Thorac Surg 1970;10:526-532.

139. Weber TR, Kurkchubasche AG: Operative management of asphyxiating thoracic dystrophy after pectus repair. J Pediatr Surg 1998;33:262-265.

140. Wechselberger G, Ohlbauer M, Haslinger J, Schoeller T: Silicone implant correction of pectus excavatum. Ann Plast Surg 2001;47:489-493.

141. Weg JG, Krumholz RA, Harkleroad LE: Pulmonary dysfunction in pectus excavatum. Am Rev Respir Dis 1967;96:936-945.

142. Welch K: Satisfactory surgical correction of pectus excavatum deformity in childhood: A limited opportunity. J Thorac Surg 1958;36:697-713.

143. Welch K: Chest Wall Deformities. Philadelphia, WB Saunders, 1980.

144. Welch KJ, Vos A: Surgical correction of pectus carinatum (pigeon breast). J Pediatr Surg 1973;8:659-667.

145. Wicks JD, Levine MD, Mettler FA Jr: Intrauterine sonography of thoracic ectopia cordis. AJR Am J Roentgenol 1981;137:619-621.

146. Wieting R: Eine operative behandelte Herzmissbildung. Dtsch Z Chir 1912;114:293-295.

147. Williams AJ, Vauter G, Reid LM: Lung structure in asphyxiating thoracic dystrophy. Arch Pathol Lab Med 1984;108:658-661.

148. Willital GH: [Indication and operative technique in chest deformities]. Z Kinderchir 1981;33:244-252.

149. Wolf WM, Fischer MD, Saltzman DA, et al: Surgical correction of pectus excavatum and carinatum. Minn Med 1987;70:447-453.

150. Wynn SR, Driscoll DJ, Ostrom NK, et al: Exercise cardiorespiratory function in adolescents with pectus excavatum: Observations before and after operation. J Thorac Cardiovasc Surg 1990;99:41-47.

151. Yamaguchi M, Tsukube T, Ohashi H, et al: [Early and long-term results of sternocostal elevation combined with bridge external traction for funnel chest in children]. Nippon Kyobu Geka Gakkai Zasshi 1993;41:2341-2348.

The Nuss Procedure for Pectus Excavatum

Donald Nuss and Robert E. Kelly, Jr.

MINIMALLY INVASIVE REPAIR

The minimally invasive repair of pectus excavatum consists of a two-pronged approach: the surgical repair and an exercise and posture program.

Surgical correction of pectus excavatum is accomplished by inserting a convex steel bar under the sternum with the convexity facing posteriorly. When the bar is in position, it is turned over 180 degrees, thereby correcting the deformity (see Figs. 59-18 to 59-27). The technique is possible because of the malleability and flexibility of the anterior chest wall; it requires no cartilage incision or resection and no sternal osteotomy. Because most of these patients lead sedentary lives and

have the classic "pectus posture," which aggravates the deformity, they are also given a set of breathing and posture exercises to do on a daily basis and are encouraged to participate in aerobic sports activities.

CLASSIFICATION AND TREATMENT ALGORITHM

When pectus excavatum patients are evaluated for the first time, they are classified as having mild, moderate, or severe deformities. Patients with mild or moderate deformities are started on the exercise and posture program and re-evaluated at 12-month intervals to ensure that they have developed an exercise routine and are

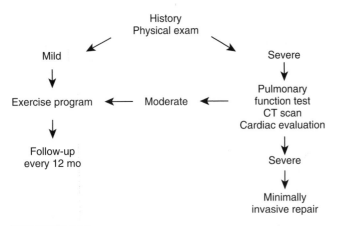

History
Physical exam

Mild   Severe

Exercise program ← Moderate ← Pulmonary function test
CT scan
Cardiac evaluation

Follow-up every 12 mo   Severe

Minimally invasive repair

Figure 59-18 Clinical pathway for management of patients with pectus excavatum.

doing the exercises correctly. Approximately 66% of patients are treated conservatively. Patients with severe deformities undergo a workup to determine whether they are candidates for surgery. The workup includes pulmonary function studies; a cardiology evaluation, including an electrocardiogram and echocardiogram; and a CT scan. For consistency, radiologists have suggested that the chest CT be performed during quiet respiration, not during maximal inspiration. Surgical correction is warranted if the patient has two or more of the following criteria: (1) progressive or symptomatic pectus excavatum; (2) restrictive disease, as determined by pulmonary function studies; (3) CT scan showing cardiac compression or displacement, pulmonary atelectasis, and a Haller CT index greater than 3.25; (4) cardiac abnormalities, including mitral valve prolapse or bundle branch block; (5) recurrent pectus excavatum after a failed repair.

SURGICAL TECHNIQUE

Preoperative Checklist: Day before Surgery

1. Review studies and check for allergies, including allergy to metallic objects.
2. To calculate the length of the pectus bar required, measure the distance from the right to the left midaxillary line and subtract 2 cm from this measurement. The bar takes a shorter course than the tape measure and therefore needs to be shorter than the measurement (Fig. 59-19).

Patient Anesthesia, Preparation, and Positioning

1. General endotracheal anesthesia.
2. Insertion of thoracic epidural catheter by the anesthesiologist. Epidural analgesia is continued for 3 to 5 days (average, 3 days).
3. Insertion of indwelling bladder catheter. Catheter is removed on the first postoperative day when the patient is awake and oriented.

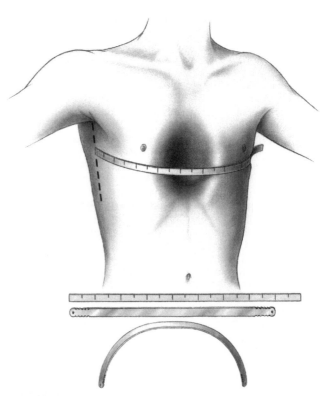

Figure 59-19 Measure the distance from the right to the left midaxillary line. The bar should be 2 cm shorter than the measurement. Bend the bar into the desired configuration, leaving a 2- to 4-cm flat section in the middle to support the sternum.

4. Nasogastric or orogastric tube is inserted during surgery and removed at the end of the procedure.
5. Antibiotic coverage (e.g., cefazolin × 5 days) is essential to minimize the risk of pneumonia with subsequent bar infection.
6. Both arms are abducted at the shoulder, and gel pads are used to prevent brachial plexus injury (see Fig. 59-19). Allow slight flexing at the elbows.
7. After draping, the Lorenz pectus support bar is bent into a semicircle, leaving the central 2-cm section flat to support the sternum (see Fig. 59-19). Bending the bar into an arch shape allows sustained load bearing of the bar. If the central flat section of the bar is too long, there will be undercorrection.

Patient Marking

1. The deepest point of the pectus excavatum is marked with a circle using a marking pen (Fig. 59-20). If the deepest point of the pectus is inferior to the sternum, the inferior end of the sternum is marked instead. This point sets the horizontal plane for bar insertion.
2. The intercostal spaces that are in the same horizontal plane as the deepest point of the pectus excavatum are marked with an X. These entry and exit points on each side of the sternum should be medial to the top of the pectus (costochondral) ridge (see Fig. 59-20).

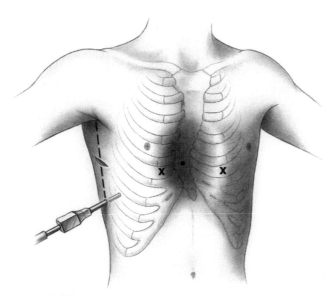

Figure 59–20 Mark the deepest point of the depression with a circle, mark the intercostal space medial to the top of the ridge with an X, and mark the incision site with a line. These marks should all be in the same horizontal plane. The thoracoscope is inserted two intercostal spaces below the incision site.

3. Lines are drawn for the proposed incision sites on each lateral chest wall in the same horizontal plane (see Fig. 59-20).

Thoracoscopy and Tunnel Creation

1. A thoracoscope is inserted through the right lower lateral chest wall approximately two interspaces inferior to the proposed skin incision (see Fig. 59-20).

Figure 59–21 On each side, a deep subcutaneous tunnel is created from the anterior aspect of the lateral thoracic incisions to the intercostal spaces marked with an X, medial to the top of the ridge.

A thorough inspection of the right hemithorax and mediastinum is performed, ensuring that there is no contraindication for repair. Then pressure is applied to the intercostal spaces marked for bar insertion to ensure that the external markings line up well with the internal anatomy.

2. After confirming by thoracoscopy that the internal and external anatomy match up well, bilateral thoracic skin incisions are made, and a deep subcutaneous tunnel is raised anteriorly toward the intercostal space marked with an X, medial to the top of the pectus ridge (Fig. 59-21). Also, a pocket is created for the distal end of the pectus bar and stabilizer.

3. Under thoracoscopic control, the appropriate size Lorenz introducer is inserted through the right intercostal space at the top of the pectus ridge at the previously marked X (Fig. 59-22). The electrocardiogram volume is turned up so that the heartbeat is clearly audible.

4. The pericardium is gently dissected off the undersurface of the sternum (see Fig. 59-22). The introducer is *slowly* advanced across the mediastinum under thoracoscopic guidance, with the point always facing anteriorly and in contact with the sternum.

5. When the substernal tunnel has been completed, the tip of the introducer is pushed through the contralateral intercostal space at the previously marked X and advanced out of the skin incision (Fig. 59-23).

Sternal Elevation and Bar Insertion

1. The introducer is used to elevate the sternum. The surgeon lifts the introducer on the right side, and the assistant lifts on the left side (see Fig. 59-23). The lifting is repeated until the sternum has been elevated out of its depressed position and the pectus excavatum has been corrected. An umbilical tape is attached to the

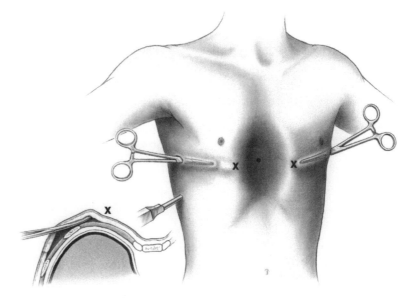

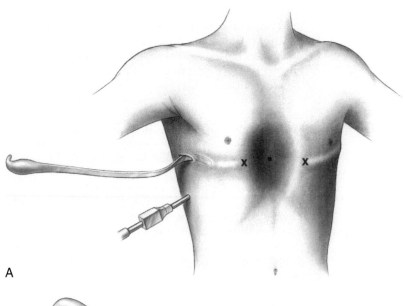

Figure 59–22 *A,* A Lorenz introducer is inserted into the subcutaneous tunnel on the right. Under thoracoscopic guidance, it is pushed through the right intercostal space marked with an **X**. *B,* Under thoracoscopic guidance, a transthoracic substernal tunnel is created by dissecting the pleura and pericardium off the undersurface of the sternum with the introducer. The introducer is pushed through the left intercostal space marked with an **X** and advanced out of the left lateral thoracic incision.

A

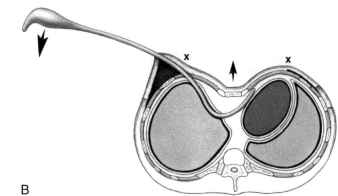

B

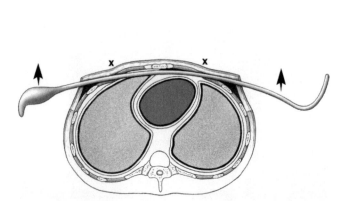

Figure 59–23 The sternum is elevated out of its depressed position by lifting the introducer on each side while applying pressure to the lower costal margin. The lifting is repeated until the pectus excavatum is corrected.

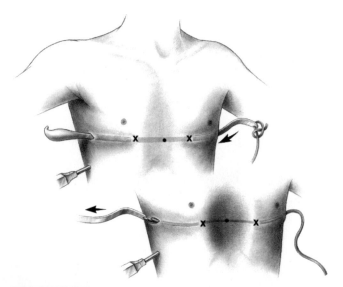

Figure 59–24 After correcting the pectus excavatum, umbilical tape is attached to the end of the introducer, which is then slowly withdrawn from the chest, thereby pulling the umbilical tape through the transthoracic tunnel.

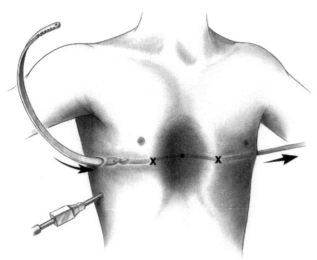

Figure 59–25 The previously prepared pectus support bar is tied to the umbilical tape and, under thoracoscopic guidance, is pulled through the substernal tunnel with the convexity facing posteriorly.

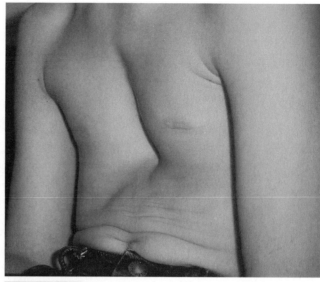

Figure 59–27 Severe pectus excavatum before surgery.

introducer, which is slowly extracted, pulling the umbilical tape through the substernal tunnel (Fig. 59-24).

2. The previously prepared pectus bar is tied to the umbilical tape and guided through the substernal tunnel using the tape for traction and the thoracoscope for vision. The bar is inserted with the convexity facing posteriorly (Fig. 59-25).

3. When the bar is in position, it is rotated 180 degrees using the bar flipper (Fig. 59-26).

4. If the bar requires further bending, it is turned over and molded where required, using the small Lorenz bar bender.

5. If one bar is not enough, a second bar is inserted one interspace above or below the first one. Two bars give

better and more stable correction, especially in older patients.

6. Slight overcorrection is necessary to prevent recurrence after the bar is removed (Figs. 59-27 and 59-28).

7. Some surgeons prefer to approach the mediastinal tunneling from the left rather than the right side. Other surgeons make a third incision over the xiphoid and then apply a towel clip to elevate the

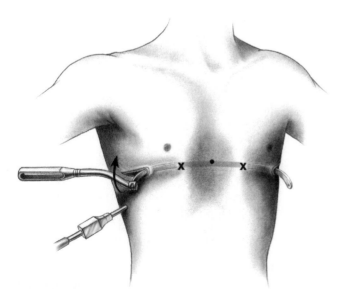

Figure 59–26 When the bar is in position, it is rotated 180 degrees using the bar flipper.

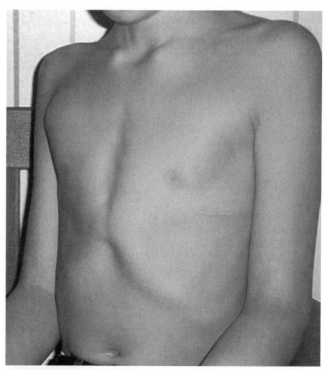

Figure 59–28 The patient in Figure 59-27 after repair, showing slight overcorrection.

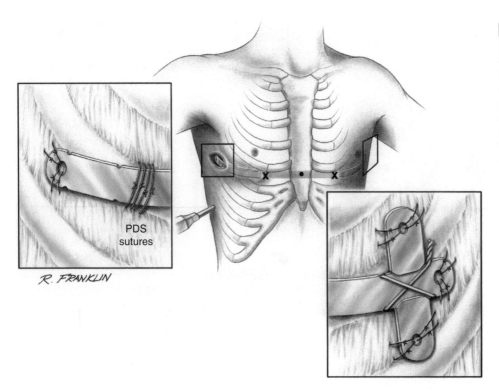

R. FRANKLIN

Figure 59–29 To prevent bar displacement, a stabilizer with wire fixation suture is applied on the left. On the right side, heavy absorbable sutures (0 or 1 PDS) are placed around the bar and underlying rib. In addition, sutures are placed through the holes in the bar and stabilizer and in the underlying fascia.

PDS sutures

sternum; others do a finger dissection under the sternum before inserting the introducer.

Bar Stabilization

1. Stabilization of the bar is absolutely essential for success. A stabilizer is inserted onto the left end of the bar and wired to the bar with No. 3 surgical steel wire (Fig. 59-29). If the bar does not seem stable, a second bar rather than a second stabilizer is probably required.
2. Heavy absorbable 0 or 1 PDS sutures are placed around the bar and underlying rib using an "endo-close" laparoscopic needle under thoracoscopic vision on the right side (see Fig. 59-29). Hebra et al.[5] advocate placing a suture adjacent to the sternum.
3. Once the bar is stabilized, the incisions are closed in layers, and the pneumothorax is evacuated using the trocar and attached tubing or a chest tube with a "water-seal" system.
4. A chest radiograph is obtained before the patient is taken out of the operating room, to check for residual pneumothorax.

Postoperative Management

1. In the recovery room, the patient is kept well sedated for 1 to 2 hours to provide a smooth emergence from anesthesia.
2. The epidural catheter is left in place for 3 to 5 days.

3. The patient is discharged home on the fourth or fifth postoperative day.
4. Patients may return to school after 2 weeks but may not participate in sports for 6 weeks after surgery.
5. After 6 weeks, patients are encouraged to resume their pectus breathing and posture exercises and to participate in aerobic sports activities (e.g., soccer, basketball, swimming).
6. Heavy contact sports (e.g., boxing, football, ice hockey) are prohibited until bar removal.

Technique of Bar Removal (2 to 4 Years after Insertion)

1. General endotracheal anesthesia with 5 to 6 cm of positive end-expiratory pressure.
2. Position the patient supine, with both arms abducted at the shoulder.
3. Check radiographs to see where the stabilizers are.
4. Palpate to see whether the bar and stabilizers are palpable and close to the old scar. If they are not palpable, use C-arm fluoroscopy to determine the exact site of the hardware.
5. Use old scars for the incision site if possible. In most patients, only one incision is necessary if only one stabilizer was used.
6. Mobilize the bar end and stabilizers. Cut the wire in two places and remove it.
7. When the bar and stabilizer have been freed from the surrounding scar tissue, insert a bone hook through the hole in the inferior wing of the stabilizer and

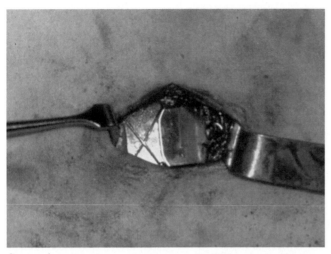

A

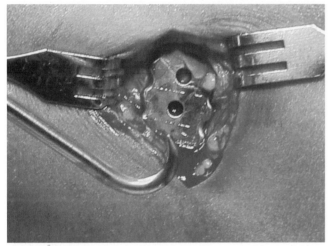

B

Figure 59–30 *A,* The bar and stabilizer are mobilized and delivered out of the incision. *B,* The stabilizer is removed by sliding it off the bar.

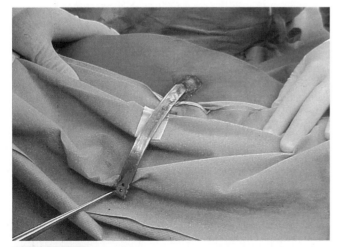

Figure 59–31 The bar is removed by turning the patient onto his side (lateral decubitus position), inserting an orthopedic hook through the hole in the bar, and pulling it down over his spine.

extract it from the incision. Then extract the end of the bar, followed by the superior wing of the stabilizer. Slide the stabilizer off the bar.

8. Insert an orthopedic bone hook through the hole in the end of the bar and apply gentle traction (Figs. 59-30 and 59-31). If the bar moves, turn the patient into the decubitus position and pull the bar out in a downward direction over the patient's back. Return the patient to the supine position, and close the incision.

9. Keep the patient on positive end-expiratory pressure until the incision is closed.

10. Bar "unbenders" have recently been developed and are useful in patients who have two stabilizers and require both right and left incisions.

Timing of Bar Removal

We advise that the pectus bar be left in place for 2 to 4 years (average age, 3 years). Patients are evaluated on an annual basis, and their growth and activity level are monitored. They are encouraged to do their pectus exercises and to participate in aerobic sports. Patients between the ages of 6 and 10 years often do not grow rapidly, and they tolerate the bar well for 3 or even 4 years. In contrast, teenagers who undergo a massive growth spurt may require bar removal after 2 years.

We consider the exercise programs to be just as important as the surgery. Many children and adults have sedentary lifestyles and never perform aerobic activities; it is thus necessary to stimulate their cardiopulmonary systems because tidal volume is only 10% of total lung capacity. Deep breathing with breath-holding for 10 to 15 seconds and aerobic activities such as running (e.g., soccer, basketball) and swimming are vigorously encouraged.

RESULTS

Demographics

As of December 2005, 785 patients had undergone primary Nuss procedures at our institution; 473 patients have had the bar removed, and 387 are more than 1-year post bar removal (Fig. 59-32). Since the original presentation,[14] numerous important modifications have been made[3] both to the surgical technique (e.g., routine use of thoracoscopy) and to the instruments to minimize risk and facilitate insertion and stabilization of the substernal support bar. These have markedly reduced the risks and complications and have been well documented in other publications.[7,13]

A total of 1511 patients were evaluated for chest wall deformities in the 17-year period from 1987 through December 2005 (Table 59-4); 785 had their initial minimally invasive procedure performed at our facility (primary repairs), and 67 had redo operations (initial operations done elsewhere).

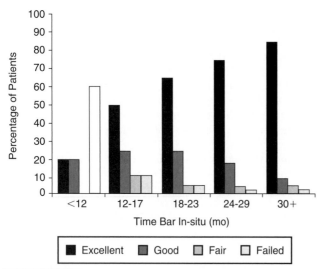

Figure 59–32 Results based on the amount of time the bar was left in place for patients 1 or more years post bar removal (*N* = 387).

The male-female ratio in patients undergoing repair was 4.7:1. The median age was 14.2 years, with a range of 22 months to 29 years. The median Haller CT index was 4.6 (range, 2.4 to 31). Cardiac compression was noted on echocardiography or CT scan in 654 of 785 patients (83%). Mitral valve prolapse was noted in 117 of 785 patients (14.9%). Resting pulmonary function testing was completed in 692 patients and demonstrated abnormalities in up to 42.3% of them.[1]

Operative Procedure, Analgesia, and Length of Stay

In 584 patients (74.4%), a single bar was inserted; two bars were inserted in 197 patients (25.1%). Blood loss in most patients was minimal (≤10 mL), with the exception of one patient who developed a hemothorax but did not require transfusion.[12] Epidural analgesia was used for 3 days in the vast majority of patients. The median length of stay was 5 days.[10]

TABLE 59–4 Demographics of Patients Undergoing Nuss Procedures

Total number of patients evaluated	1278
Total number of minimally invasive (Nuss) procedures	685
Total number of primary surgeries	633
Total number of redo surgeries	52
Prior Ravitch procedure	28
Prior Nuss procedure	24
Prior Leonard procedure	2*

*Prior Leonard procedures were also prior Ravitch procedures and were counted only once in the analysis.

TABLE 59–5 Early Postoperative Complications of the Nuss Procedure

Complication	No. of Patients (%)
Death	0
Cardiac perforation	0
Pneumothorax	481 (51.2)
Requiring chest tube	20 (2.5)
Requiring aspiration	3 (0.3)
Pleural effusion requiring drainage	3 (0.3)
Pericarditis	4 (0.5)
Hemothorax (surgical)	7 (0.9)
Pneumonia	2 (0.2)
Drug reaction	32 (4.0)
Horner's syndrome	166 (21.1)

COMPLICATIONS

Early Complications[4,6,7]

There were no deaths and no cardiac perforations during the 785 repairs performed at our institution (Table 59-5). Pneumothorax requiring chest tube drainage occurred in 20 repairs (2.5%); percutaneous aspiration only was required in 3 repairs (0.3%). Hemothorax requiring drainage occurred after 7 repairs (0.9%). Three pleural effusions required treatment by either chest tube or aspiration (0.3%).

Pericarditis requiring treatment with indomethacin occurred after 4 repairs (0.5%), with one requiring pericardiocentesis. Pneumonia occurred after 2 repairs (0.2%), and medication reactions occurred following 32 repairs (4.0%). A total of 166 patients had transient Horner's syndrome at varying times during the thoracic epidural administration.

TABLE 59–6 Late Postoperative Complications of the Nuss Procedure

Complication	No. of Patients (%)
Bar displacement	51/785 (6.5%)
Requiring revision	28/785 (3.5%)
Before stabilizer	10/113 (8.8%)
With stabilizers	18/672 (2.6%)
With wired stabilizers	9/360 (2.5%)
With PDS sutures	1/237 (0.4%)
Hemothorax	2/785 (0.2%)
Wound infection	7/785 (0.9%)
Bar infection	6/785 (0.7%)
Requiring early removal	2/785 (0.2%)
Bar allergy	19/785 (2.4%)
Overcorrection	22/785 (2.8%)
Recurrence	8/785 (1.0%)

Late Complications

Fifty-one patients (6.5%) experienced bar displacement (Table 59-6); however, only 28 displacements (3.5%) warranted repositioning. Of these 28 displacements, 10 occurred before stabilizers were available, a period covering our first 113 repairs. After the introduction of stabilizers, the incidence of bar displacement dropped from 8.8% to 2.6%. When the bar and stabilizers were wired together, the incidence of bar displacement dropped to 2.5%. There has been only one bar displacement (0.4%) since we started combining the placement of a stabilizer on the left and the placement of PDS sutures around the bar and the underlying rib on the right. Bar infection occurred in six patients (0.7%), requiring early bar removal in two (0.2%).

Nineteen patients had allergies to the bars.[16] These presented as rashes in the area of the bar or the stabilizer, sterile abscesses at the incision site, pleural and/or pericardial effusions.

Of 785 patients, 22 (2.8%) developed a moderate overcorrection of their deformity, and 4 (0.5%) developed a true carinatum deformity.

OVERALL RESULTS AND LONG-TERM FOLLOW-UP

Patients are re-examined at 6 months postoperatively and then annually. Long-term assessments classify the postoperative results as excellent, good, fair, or failed. A result is considered excellent if the patient experiences total repair of the pectus as well as resolution of any associated symptoms. A good result is distinguished by a markedly improved but not totally normal chest wall appearance and resolution of any associated symptoms. A fair result indicates a mild residual pectus excavatum without complete resolution of associated symptoms. A failed repair indicates recurrence of the pectus and associated symptoms or the need for another repair after bar removal.

The initial cosmetic and functional results were excellent in 718 patients (91%), good in 64 (8%), fair in 1 (0.2%), and failed in 2 (0.25%). A total of 385 have had their bars out for more than 1 year, and 88 have had their bars out for less than 1 year. Among those whose bars were removed 1 or more years ago, the results were excellent in 79.8%, good in 14.9%, fair in 2.3%, and failed in 2.0%. Patients who did not comply with the exercise program and had their bars removed before puberty had a higher recurrence rate. The length of time the bar was left in situ had a direct effect on the long-term outcome. The longer the bar stayed in, the better the results (see Fig. 59-32). The age of the patient also affected the long-term outcome, with the best results occurring in those 7 to 12 years old and 13 to 18 years old (Fig. 59-33).[2] In addition to the 785 primary operations, there were 67 successful remedial minimally invasive pectus repairs.[11]

CONCLUSION

The minimally invasive procedure provides good to excellent correction of pectus excavatum in more than 90% of

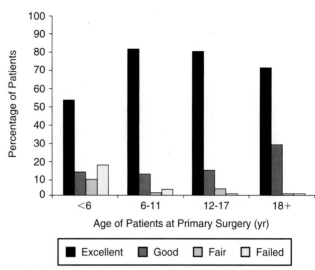

Figure 59–33 Results based on age at surgery for patients 1 or more years post bar removal (*N* = 276).

patients with no rib resection, no sternal osteotomy, minimal blood loss, and rapid return to normal activity.[2,4,6,10-12] Studies have shown marked improvement in the patient's body image[8,15] and have also shown improvement in pulmonary function studies.[1,9]

REFERENCES

1. Borowitz D, Cemy F, Zallen G, et al: Pulmonary function and exercise response in patients with pectus excavatum after Nuss repair. J Pediatr Surg 2003;38:544-547.
2. Coln D, Gunning T, Ramsey M: Early experience with the Nuss minimally invasive procedure. World J Surg 2002;26:1217-1221.
3. Croitoru DP, Kelly RE Jr, Nuss D, et al: Experience and modification update for the minimally invasive Nuss technique for pectus excavatum repair in 303 patients. J Pediatr Surg 2002;37:437-445.
4. Fonkalsrud EW, Beanes S, Hebra A, et al: Comparison of minimally invasive and modified Ravitch pectus excavatum repair. J Pediatr Surg 2002;37:413-417.
5. Hebra A, Gauderer MW, Tagge EP: A simple technique for preventing bar displacement with the Nuss repair of pectus excavatum. J Pediatr Surg 2001;36:1266-1268.
6. Hebra A, Swoveland B, Egbert M, et al: Outcome analysis of minimally invasive repair of pectus excavatum: Review of 251 cases. J Pediatr Surg 2000;35:252-257.
7. Hyung JP, Seock Y, Cheol SL: Complications associated with the Nuss procedure: Analysis of risk factors and suggested measures for prevention of complications. J Pediatr Surg 2004;39:391-395.
8. Lawson ML, Cash TF, Akers RA, et al: A pilot study of the impact of surgical repair on disease-specific quality of life among patients with pectus excavatum. J Pediatr Surg 2003;38:916-918.
9. Lawson M, Mellins R, Tabangin M, et al: Impact of pectus excavatum on pulmonary function before and after repair with the Nuss procedure. J Pediatr Surg (submitted for publication).

10. Miller KA, Woods RK, Sharp RJ, et al: Minimally invasive repair of pectus excavatum: A single institution's experience. Surgery 2001;130:652-657.

11. Miller RA: Minimally invasive bar repair for redo correction. J Pediatr Surg 2002;37:1090-1092.

12. Molik KA, Engum SA, Rescorla FJ, et al: Pectus excavatum repair: Experience with standard and minimally invasive techniques. J Pediatr Surg 2001;36:324-328.

13. Nuss D, Kelly RE Jr, et al: Repair of pectus excavatum. Pediatr Endosurg Innovat Techn 1998;2:205-221.

14. Nuss D, Kelly RE Jr, et al: A 10-year review of a minimally invasive technique for the correction of pectus excavatum. J Pediatr 1998;33:545-552.

15. Roberts J, Hayashi A, Anderson JO, et al: Quality of life of patients who have undergone the Nuss procedure for pectus excavatum: Preliminary findings. J Pediatr Surg 2003;38:779-783.

16. Saitoh C, Yamada A, Kosaka K, et al: Allergy to pectus bar for funnel chest. Plast Reconstr Surg 2002;110:719-721.

Chapter 60

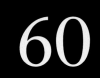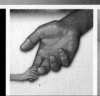

Congenital Diaphragmatic Hernia and Eventration

Charles J. H. Stolar and Peter W. Dillon

HISTORY

The earliest English language description of the gross anatomy and pathophysiology associated with congenital diaphragmatic hernia (CDH) in a newborn was by McCauley, an associate of Hunter, as reported in the *Proceedings of the Royal College of Physicans,* 1754[203]:

> The child was born in the lying-in-hospital in Brownlow Street on the 24th of August, 1752: and was a fully grown boy, remarkably fat and fleshy. He was the fifth child of a healthy young woman who was well during her pregnancy. The child, when first born, started and shuddered; so that the nurse apprehended his going into fits. He breathed also with difficulty and it was some time before he could cry; which when he did, there was something peculiar in its note.
> He seemed to revive a little in about half an hour and breathed more freely: but soon relapsed and died before he was quite an hour and a half old. Being informed of these particulars by the mother, the matron, and the nurse, I was desirous of examining the body.... I laid open the abdomen and found none of the intestines were contained in that cavity except part of the colon which was distended with meconium. Before I proceeded further with the dissection I sent to acquaint my ingenious friend, Dr. Hunter. We together dissected and examined this curious subject: and at the same time committed to writing the most remarkable appearances.
> When the sternum was raised, the stomach with the greatest part of the intestines, with the spleen, and part of the pancreas were found in the left cavity of the thorax; having been protruded through a discontinuation, or rather an aperture of the diaphragm, about an inch from the natural passage of the esophagus.
> From the extraordinary bulk of the parts contained in the left side of the thorax, the mediastinum, the heart, the esophagus, and the descending aorta were forced a considerable way to the right side of the thorax; because there was not the least mark of rupture or inflammation about the edges of the chasm: and because it is probable that

> the diminished size of the left lobes of the lungs, and the heart and mediastinum being pushed to the right side, were gradually affected by the bulk and increase of the viscera.
> As the esophagus was pushed to the right side by the stomach and the bowels, in the cavity of the thorax it kept the same course and pierced the diaphragm not in the usual place, but considerably further to the right side: and the aperture through which it passed was backwards and to the right side with respect to that for the vena cava.
> I have preserved the heart and lungs to show the disproportioned sizes of the lobes. And I have dried and prepared the diaphragm with its connections to the vertebrae and sternum to show the preternatural aperture through which the bowels passed into the thorax; as also the passage of the esophagus to the right side of the diaphragm. These preparations were at the same time shown to the Society.

Cooper,[59] in 1827, and Laennec,[177] in 1834, not only reported clinical descriptions and gross pathology of CDH but also suggested that laparotomy might be the proper approach for reduction and correction of the hernia. Bowditch,[34] in 1847, was the first to make the bedside diagnosis of CDH and further emphasized the clinical criteria for diagnosis. Although Bochdalek's understanding of the embryology was incorrect, this congenital defect continues to carry his name.[23] He speculated that the hernia resulted from a posterolateral rupture of the membrane separating the pleuroperitoneal canal into two cavities. He also incorrectly speculated that the best way to repair the defect was through the bed of the 12th rib. The record is not clear as to whether this was actually attempted. The earliest, although unsuccessful, efforts to repair CDHs were by Nauman,[220] in 1888, and O'Dwyer, in 1890.[227] The first reports of successful repairs were in an adult by Aue,[12] in 1901, and a child by Heidenhain,[132] in 1905.

The groundwork for treating CDH in the newborn period was laid by Hedblom,[128] whose review of the reported cases as of 1925 showed that 75% of 44 infants diagnosed in the newborn period died. He suggested that

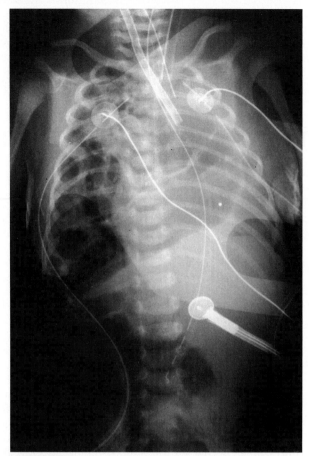

Figure 60–1 Chest radiograph of an infant with a right-sided congenital diaphragmatic hernia demonstrating air-filled loops of intestine in the right hemithorax with contralateral displacement of the mediastinum. The infant has been cannulated for venoarterial extracorporeal membrane oxygenation.

earlier intervention might improve survival. Successful repair of CDH remained rare until 1940, when Ladd and Gross[176] reported 9 of 16 patients surviving operative repair, the youngest being 40 hours old. It was not until 1946 that Gross[113] reported survival of the first infant younger than 24 hours old after operative repair of the defect. Until the 1980s, the standard of care remained immediate neonatal surgery followed by postoperative resuscitative therapy (Fig. 60-1).

EPIDEMIOLOGY AND GENETICS

The reported incidence of CDH is estimated to be between 1 in 2000 to 5000 births.[46,107,120,238] In the United States, approximately 1000 infants a year are affected with this condition, and in a recent study from Atlanta the birth prevalence was found to be 2.4 per 10,000 births.[84] The incidence in stillborns is less well documented. Approximately one third of infants with CDH are stillborn, but these deaths are usually due to associated fatal congenital anomalies.[110,238,312] When stillborns are counted with live births, females appear to be more commonly afflicted than males.[46,104,238]

Defects are more common on the left side, with approximately 80% being left sided and 20% right sided.

Bilateral CDH defects are rare and have a high incidence of associated anomalies.[222] Infants with isolated CDH are more likely to be premature, macrosomic, and male; and about one third of affected infants may have associated major defects.[84] Women who are thin or underweight for their height may have an increased risk of having an infant with an isolated CDH.[305] CDH is thought to represent a sporadic developmental anomaly, although a number of familial cases have been reported.[46,111,208] The expected recurrence risk in a first-degree relative has been estimated to be 1 in 45 or approximately 2%.[193] Structural chromosomal abnormalities have been identified in 9% to 34% of CDH infants and include trisomies, deletions, and translocations.[140,321] Specific chromosomes with deleted or translocated genes may be candidate loci for CDH development.[13,42,197] The combination of CDH and an abnormal karyotype has been associated with a poor outcome.[134,141,321]

The cause of a CDH is unknown. As with other embryopathies there is increasing evidence that CDH may be due to the exposure of genetically predisposed or susceptible individuals to environmental factors. Exposure to a number of pharmacologic agents and environmental hazards has been implicated in its development. These include insecticides and drugs such as phenmetrazine, thalidomide, quinine, cadmium, lead, and nitrofen.[65,138,149,232,307] The clinical findings of vitamin A deficiency in CDH infants and the effects of vitamin A administration in nitrofen-induced pulmonary hypoplasia have strengthened the evolving hypothesis that alterations in retinoid-regulated target genes may be responsible for CDH development.[112]

ASSOCIATED ANOMALIES

Any newborn with a major congenital anomaly, including infants with CDH, has an increased incidence of an additional malformation compared with the general population. Although previously thought to be low, the incidence of associated malformations in infants with a CDH ranges from 10% to 50%.[65,95,110,194,207,226,296,312] Skeletal defects have been noted in as many as 32% of CDH infants and include limb reduction and costovertebral defects.[207,226,285] Cardiac anomalies have been found in 24% of infants. Cardiac hypoplasia involving the left ventricle and often associated with hypoplasia of the aortic arch is frequently described and can be confused with hypoplastic heart syndromes. However, the clinical significance is limited. Most cardiovascular malformations involve the cardiac outflow tract such as ventricular septal defects, tetralogy of Fallot, transposition of the great vessels, double outlet right ventricle, and aortic coarctation.[88,206,284] Anatomic anomalies of the tracheobronchial tree have been found in 18% of patients with CDH and include congenital tracheal stenosis, tracheal bronchus, and trifurcated trachea.[226] The incidence of associated malformations in stillborn infants with CDH is even higher. In one study 100% of stillborn infants with CDH had associated lethal anomalies.[238] Abnormalities noted in this stillborn group were predominantly neural tube defects and included anencephaly, myelomeningocele, hydrocephalus, and encephaloceles. Even in infants who survive to birth but die shortly thereafter, neural tube defects were the most common malformations noted. Cardiac defects were the second most common group and included ventriculoseptal defects, vascular rings, and coarctation of the aorta.[284] Other midline developmental anomalies have also been reported and include esophageal atresia, omphalocele, and cleft palate. A number of syndromes have a CDH as a pathologic finding. These syndromes include trisomy 21, trisomy 18, trisomy 13, Frey's syndrome, Beckwith-Wiedemann syndrome, Goldenhar's syndrome, Coffin-Siris syndrome, Fryns syndrome, Meacham syndrome, and Kabuki syndrome.[71,83,134,166,223]

EMBRYOLOGY

Diaphragmatic Development

The embryologic development of the diaphragm remains incompletely understood and involves multiple, complex cellular and tissue interactions. The fully developed diaphragm is derived from four distinct components: (1) the anterior central tendon forms from the septum transversum, (2) the dorsolateral portions form from the pleuroperitoneal membranes, (3) the dorsal crura evolve from the esophageal mesentery, and (4) the muscular portion of the diaphragm develops from the thoracic intercostal muscle groups. The precursors of diaphragmatic structure begin to form during the fourth week of gestation with the appearance of the peritoneal fold from the lateral mesenchymal tissue. At the same time, the septum transversum forms from the inferior portion of the pericardial cavity. The septum transversum serves to separate the thoracic from the abdominal cavities and eventually forms the central tendinous area of the fully developed diaphragm. It defines the rudimentary pleuroperitoneal canals and allows for the establishment of mesenchymal tissue within these canals that ultimately results in pulmonary parenchymal development.

Closure of the pleuroperitoneal canals with the formation of a pleuroperitoneal membrane occurs during the eighth week of gestation. Several theories have been proposed to explain the formation of this membrane and the subsequent development of a diaphragmatic structure. Progressive growth of the pleuroperitoneal membrane has been one mechanism proposed for canal closure.[62,152] Other researchers have postulated that concurrent hepatic and adrenal organogenesis is crucial to this process.[41,43,311] The involvement of a posthepatic mesenchymal plate in diaphragmatic formation has been proposed.[149]

The pleuroperitoneal folds extend from the lateral body wall and grow medially and ventrally until they fuse with the septum transversum and dorsal mesentery of the esophagus during gestational week 6. Complete closure of the canal takes place during week 8 of gestation. Anatomically, the right side closes before the left.[212] Muscularization of the diaphragm appears to develop from the innermost muscle layer of the thoracic cavity, although it has been proposed that the posthepatic mesenchymal plate is a possible source of muscular tissue.[41,149] Posterolaterally, at the junction of the lumbar and costal muscle groups, the fibrous lumbocostal trigone remains as a small remnant of the pleuroperitoneal membrane

and relies on the fusion of the two muscle groups in the final stages of development for its strength. Delay or failure of muscular fusion leaves this area weak, perhaps predisposing to herniation. Bochdalek first described this area of the posterolateral diaphragm in 1848, and it is for this reason that the most common site for CDH bears his name.

Lung Development

Fetal lung development is divided into five stages: embryonic, pseudoglandular, canalicular, saccular, and alveolar.[79] Embryonic lung development begins during the third week of gestation as a derivative of the foregut and is marked by the formation of a diverticulum off of the caudal end of the laryngotracheal groove.[35] The trachea and the two primary lung buds form from this diverticulum by the fourth week of gestation. At 6 weeks, these lung buds have further developed into defined lobar structures. The pseudoglandular phase of lung development takes place during the 7th to 16th weeks of gestation and involves lung airway differentiation. It is during this period that all bronchial airways develop. From the 16th to the 24th weeks of gestation, fetal lung development enters the canalicular phase of growth. During this period, airspace development occurs, as crude alveolar air sacs begin to take shape. Type 1 pneumocytes begin to differentiate, and the precursors of type 2 pneumocytes ultimately responsible for surfactant production begin to appear. Gas exchange becomes functionally possible at this stage.

Continued maturation of the crude alveolar airspaces takes place during the saccular phase of development that extends from 24 weeks' gestation to term. During this time period there is continued remodeling of the airspace dimensions and a maturation of surfactant synthesis capabilities.[115] Mature, adult-like alveoli begin to appear shortly after birth.[36,37] Extensive alveolar maturation and multiplication then takes place from birth until approximately 8 years of age, with a 10-fold increase in the number of functioning alveoli.[66,87,309] Investigators have proposed that alveolar formation may be completed by 2 years of age.[290]

Pulmonary vascular development follows the stages of airway and alveolar growth and can be divided into two anatomic units based on associated airway structure. The term *acinus* describes the functional unit of the lung that includes the respiratory bronchioli, alveolar ducts, and alveoli—all structures that evolve during or after the canalicular phase of lung development. Vascular development in this region proceeds concurrently with alveolar growth and multiplication. The preacinar structures include the trachea, major bronchi, and lobar bronchi up to the terminal bronchioles. Preacinar vascular development is completed by 16 weeks' gestational age.[136,137,243]

It is now recognized that pulmonary development is marked by a series of programmed events regulated by master genes such as the homeobox genes, nuclear transcription factors, hormones, and growth factors. These processes involve genes regulating epithelial and endothelial interactions as well as temporal and spatial interactions of several hormones and growth factors. Early developmental transcription factors such as hepatocyte nuclear factor-3β and thyroid transcription factor-1 regulate pulmonary development from the foregut mesenchyme. Additional stimuli of pulmonary development involve the transforming growth factor-β pathway, sonic hedgehog pathway, Notch-delta pathway, Wingless-Int pathway, and cytokine receptor pathways. Subsequent signal transduction control of organogenesis includes the apoptotic pathways, nuclear receptor pathways, and interleukin pathways. Hormones such as the glucocorticoids, thyroid hormone, and retinoic acid have been shown to regulate several of the crucial cellular interactions required for proper pulmonary organogenesis and differentiation.[49]

Although the pathways of normal pulmonary development have become clearer, little is known about the alterations in gene expression, growth factor interactions, and hormone levels associated with the pulmonary maldevelopment of the CDH lung. A number of factors have been found to be elevated in CDH lung specimens including epidermal growth factor, transforming growth factor-α, vascular endothelial growth factor, insulin-like growth factor, tumor necrosis factor-α, and glucocorticoid receptor gene expression.[114,210,229,263,272] Other factors such as sonic hedgehog expression, heme oxygenase-1, and endothelial nitric oxide levels reportedly are decreased. The importance of these findings remains to be determined.[271,294]

Recently, advances in understanding the developmental defects in mammalian lung formation associated with CDH have come in the murine nitrofen model.[50] The adoption of the nitrofen model of experimental CDH coincides with the theory that many developmental defects, including CDH, are embryopathies caused by toxin exposure. Nitrofen is an environmental toxicant, and its administration to pregnant mice results in offspring with pulmonary hypoplasia, diaphragmatic hernia defects, reduced airway branching, excessive muscularization of pulmonary vessels, surfactant deficiency, and respiratory failure at birth. The pulmonary hypoplasia induced by nitrofen is associated with alterations in a number of growth factors and developmental pathways in embryonic mice.[49,50] The nitrofen model of CDH formation has dramatically changed the perception of this disease process as a simple mechanical defect in the diaphragm resulting in pulmonary compression and respiratory failure. Multiple studies now indicate that lung hypoplasia may precede diaphragmatic hernia formation and involves a number of pathways fundamental to the embryonic development of the lung.[153]

A number of physical factors may also affect pulmonary growth and development.[79] Adequate intrathoracic space is a prerequisite for normal pulmonary growth. Any intrathoracic or extrathoracic process that results in diminishment of the intrathoracic space and pulmonary parenchymal compression can lead to the development of structurally immature lungs.[69,78,121,190,235,315] Other physical factors important in lung growth include the maintenance of normal fetal lung liquid and amniotic fluid dynamics.[4,75,76,96,211]

PATHOLOGY

Although the cause of CDH is uncertain, its consequences on pulmonary development and function are well documented. During the early development of the diaphragm, the midgut is herniated into the yolk sac. If closure of the pleuroperitoneal canal has not occurred by the time the midgut returns to the abdomen during gestational weeks 9 and 10, the abdominal viscera herniate through the lumbocostal trigone into the ipsilateral thoracic cavity. The resulting abnormal position of the bowel prevents its normal counterclockwise rotation and fixation. No hernia sac is present if the event occurs before complete closure of the pleuroperitoneal canal, but a nonmuscularized membrane forms a hernia sac in 10% to 15% of CDH patients.[189] Although some claim the herniation can occur late in gestation or be intermittently present as a dynamic process, in most cases the defect is established by gestational week 12.[3] The subsequent postnatal problems relate to the effects of the herniated viscera on the developing heart and lungs.

The classic left-sided CDH features a 2.0- to 4.0-cm posterolateral defect in the diaphragm through which the abdominal viscera have been translocated into the hemithorax (Fig. 60-2). Herniated contents often include the left lobe of the liver, the spleen, and almost the entire gastrointestinal tract. The stomach is frequently in the chest, which results in some degree of obstruction at the

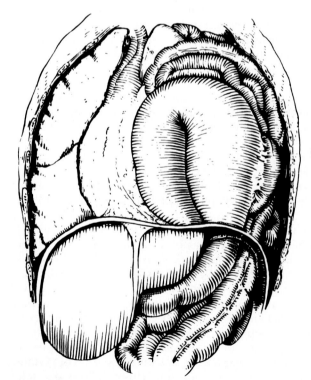

Figure 60–2 Schematic illustration of a left congenital diaphragmatic hernia showing translocation of abdominal viscera through a posterolateral aperture into the chest. (From Spitz L, Coran AG (eds): Rob & Smith's Pediatric Surgery. London, Chapman & Hall, 1996.)

gastroesophageal junction. This obstruction, in turn, causes dilatation and ectasia of the esophagus. Occasionally, the kidney may be in the chest tethered by the renal vessels. In instances of a right-sided defect, the large right lobe of the liver can occupy much of the hemithorax in addition to other abdominal viscera. The hepatic veins may drain ectopically into the right atrium, and fibrous fusion between the liver and the lung has been reported. Both of these anatomic findings can significantly complicate attempted surgical repair of the diaphragmatic defect.[158,163]

The diaphragmatic defect usually features a completely open space between the chest and abdomen, although some infants have a membrane of parietal pleura and peritoneum acting as a hernia sac. This finding is to be distinguished from an eventration of the diaphragm, which results from phrenic nerve or anterior horn cell degeneration. The muscle fibers of the diaphragm are usually present.

Elegant animal models by de Lorimier and Harrison have shown that long-term compression on the developing fetal lungs by the herniation of abdominal contents into the thoracic cavity results in pulmonary maldevelopment and lung hypoplasia[69,121] (Fig. 60-3). Unilateral visceral herniation affects both ipsilateral and contralateral pulmonary development, although hypoplasia is predictably more severe on the ipsilateral side. This is confirmed by an analysis of lung volumes and weights in human autopsy specimens and animal models.[10,69,121,235] Because the process of CDH herniation occurs at the time of bronchial subdivision, it is at this stage that lung development becomes compromised. Although all major bronchial buds are present in a CDH lung, the number of bronchial branches in the affected lung is greatly reduced. This finding was noted in both ipsilateral and contralateral pulmonary specimens.[10] Alveolar development is severely affected, and it has been reported that few normal alveoli exist in the lungs at term.[234] In addition, the changes in airway structure are quite variable. Infants requiring low ventilatory assistance during treatment had the same airway muscle mass as controls, whereas infants with prolonged ventilatory support had significantly greater muscle thickness throughout the conducting airways.[44]

The pulmonary vascular bed is distinctly abnormal in lungs from patients with CDH. A reduction in the total number of arterial branches in both the ipsilateral and the contralateral pulmonary parenchyma has been reported.[170,187] Structurally, significant adventitial and medial wall thickening has been noted in pulmonary arteries of all sizes in CDH lungs in association with abnormal muscularization of the small preacinar and intra-acinar arterioles.[26,216,325] The physiologic consequence of this abnormal arterial muscularization may be an increased susceptibility to the development of fixed and intractable pulmonary hypertension. No significant changes in pulmonary venous structure have been identified resulting from CDH development. Increased adventitial thickness of pulmonary veins has been noted in CDH infants but appears to be postnatally derived perhaps as a result of treatment or secondary to the pathology of pulmonary hypertension.[206]

Pulmonary blood flow accounts for only 7% of cardiac output during normal fetal development, and pulmonary vascular resistance remains high. The fetus preferentially shunts oxygenated blood from the placenta through the foramen ovale and ductus arteriosus in a right-to-left direction into the systemic circulation. At birth, a number of hemodynamic changes take place that dramatically alter this circulatory profile. With the institution of breathing, pulmonary vascular resistance falls, as does pulmonary artery pressure allowing for an increase in pulmonary blood flow. Systemic vascular resistance and left atrial pressure rise causing the foramen ovale to close. Increased arterial oxygen tension induces spontaneous closure of the ductus arteriosus. Transition from a fetal to an adult-type circulatory pattern is accomplished. Persistent fetal circulation may develop if this process is interrupted. After birth and interruption of placental circulatory support, persistently elevated pulmonary vascular resistance results in increased pulmonary artery pressures and decreased pulmonary vascular blood flow. The increased vascular resistance results in right-to-left shunting of blood at either the atrial or the ductal levels with the delivery of unsaturated blood into the systemic circulation. As the blood flow in the shunt increases, the oxygen saturation in the systemic circulation falls and the mixed venous return to the right side of the heart becomes progressively desaturated. The resulting hypoxia further increases pulmonary vascular resistance and compromises pulmonary blood flow while increasing the right-to-left shunt flow. Severe and progressive respiratory failure ensues.

Factors that contribute to the persistence of high pulmonary vascular resistance in CDH lungs are thought to

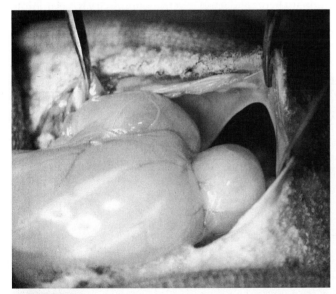

Figure 60-3 Operative photograph of a left congenital diaphragmatic hernia created in a fetal lamb. The posterolateral defect can be seen looking from the abdomen into the chest. (From Spitz L, Coran AG (eds): Rob & Smith's Pediatric Surgery. London, Chapman & Hall, 1996.)

be the structural changes in decreased total arteriolar cross-sectional area in the involved lungs and the increased muscularization of the arterial structures that are present. In the postnatal period there is failure of the normal arterial remodeling process further maintaining the abnormal vascular resistance that may be only partly reversed by treatment interventions.[264] Additional exacerbations of pulmonary vascular resistance may be induced by the known stimulators of pulmonary hypertension, including hypoxia, acidosis, hypothermia, and stress.[295] Alterations in the levels of various prostaglandins, leukotrienes, catecholamines, and the renin-angiotensin system have been implicated as mediators of this complex process.[99,280] It can only be surmised at this time whether there is an exaggerated response to these stimuli by the abnormal vascular structures of CDH lungs.[60]

DIAGNOSIS

The diagnosis of a CDH is often made on a prenatal ultrasound (US) examination and is accurate in 40% to 90% of cases.[188] Although considerable variation in detection rates have been reported, the mean gestational age at discovery is 24 weeks and has been reported as early as 11 weeks.[105] The US may be obtained for routine obstetric care or because of suspicion concerning the presence of polyhydramnios. Polyhydramnios has been reported present in up to 80% of pregnancies with associated CDH.[3] The mechanism of polyhydramnios is thought to be due to kinking of the gastroesophageal junction by translocation of the stomach into the thorax with resultant foregut obstruction. The US diagnosis of a CDH is suggested by observing the stomach or fluid-filled loops of intestine in the fetal thorax at the same cross-sectional level as the heart (Fig. 60-4A, B). Additional US findings suggestive of a CDH include the absence of the stomach in the abdomen and the presence of the liver or other solid viscera in the thorax. The stomach may be small because of interference with fetal swallowing. If the diaphragmatic defect is on the right side, the liver can tamponade the hernia site and obscure the diagnosis. The diagnosis of CDH may be missed because intermittent herniation of abdominal viscera into the thoracic cavity has been reported.[3] The misinterpretation of the fetal US scan can be caused by other diagnoses such as esophageal atresia and cystic lung anomalies. Functional information concerning fetal breathing can be obtained by duplex Doppler examination of amniotic flow at the fetal nares at the time of fetal US. A fetal tidal volume/minute ventilation can be determined that may have a bearing on prognosis.[15]

In addition to diagnosis, prenatal US may also be of benefit in predicting outcome by utilizing quantitative techniques to estimate the severity of pulmonary hypoplasia of the fetal CDH lung. Three-dimensional estimation of the fetal lung volume, calculation of the right lung area to thoracic area ratio, and calculation of the lung to thoracic circumference ratio are three different measurements that appear to correlate with neonatal outcome.[17,218,250] US can be limited by the poor acoustic contrast between fetal lung and herniated viscera, position of the fetus, and operator experience. As a result, prenatal magnetic resonance imaging (MRI) evaluation is being used with increasing frequency when obstetric sonography has detected a complex fetal anomaly and is ideally suited for fetuses with a diaphragmatic hernia.[142,186] MRI can readily determine liver position in relation to the diaphragm and detect herniated liver into either hemithorax. It may also be used to more accurately assess lung volume to determine pulmonary hypoplasia with subsequent correlation to outcome.[199,230,306]

After birth, the spectrum of respiratory symptoms in an infant with a CDH is determined by the degree of pulmonary hypoplasia and reactive pulmonary hypertension. The most severely affected infants develop respiratory

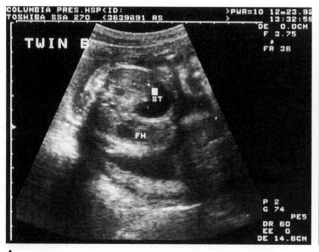

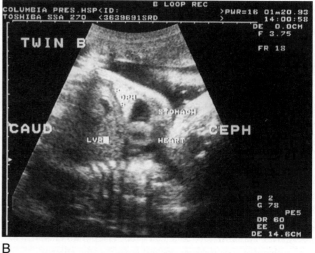

Figure 60–4 *A,* Ultrasound examination of a 28-week gestation fetus (twin B) in cross section demonstrating the fetal heart (FH) and stomach (ST) in the same plane. *B,* Ultrasound examination of the same fetus but in a sagittal plane demonstrating relationship of the stomach, liver, and heart.

distress at birth, whereas a majority demonstrates respiratory symptoms within the first 24 hours of life. Classically, these infants have a scaphoid abdomen and an asymmetrical distended chest. The chest may become more distended as swallowed air passes into the stomach and intestines. Gastrointestinal distention further compresses pulmonary parenchyma and affects parenchymal ventilatory characteristics. It may lead to additionl mediastinal compression with impairment of the contralateral lung. Because of the small size of the neonate's chest, breath sounds may or may not be present on the side of the defect. Mediastinal compression with shift into the contralateral thorax may cause deviation of the trachea away from the side of the hernia and also result in obstruction to venous return with the hemodynamic consequences of hypotension and inadequate peripheral perfusion. The signs of respiratory distress may include cyanosis, gasping, sternal retractions, and poor respiratory effort.

The diagnosis of a CDH can be confirmed by a plain chest radiograph that demonstrates loops of intestine in the chest. The location of the gastric bubble should also be noted, and its position can be confirmed by placement of an orogastric tube. Rarely, a contrast study of the upper gastrointestinal tract is required. The chest radiograph shows angulation of the mediastinum and a shifting of the cardiac silhouette into the contralateral thorax. Although minimal aeration of the ipsilateral parenchyma may be noted, chest radiographs are unreliable for estimating the degree of pulmonary hypoplasia.[52,140]

Once the diagnosis of a CDH is confirmed, additional radiographic and US examinations should be carried out to search for associated anomalies. Echocardiography and both renal and cranial US scans should be obtained.

Although most CDHs present in the first 24 hours of life, 10% to 20% of the infants with this defect present later.[201] These latter infants present with recurrent mild respiratory illnesses, chronic pulmonary disease, pneumonia, effusion, empyema, or gastric volvulus.

DIFFERENTIAL DIAGNOSIS

The diagnosis of a CDH can be confused with a number of other congenital thoracic conditions, including eventration of the diaphragm, anterior diaphragmatic hernia of Morgagni, congenital esophageal hiatal hernia, congenital cystic disease of the lung, and primary agenesis of the lung. Diaphragmatic eventration has many causes but is seen in the newborn with birth trauma or Werdnig-Hoffmann disease. The eventrated diaphragm can rise as high as the third intercostal space and have the same physiologic consequences as CDH. It can also be completely asymptomatic. The diagnosis is made by fluoroscopy or real-time US with the demonstration of paradoxic movement of the diaphragm. MRI is also useful in determining diaphragmatic structure. Morgagni hernias occur at the hiatus for the internal mammary arteries and are much less common than Bochdalek hernias. Affected infants can present as a gastrointestinal crisis because of incarceration or volvulus of the colon or small bowel and require immediate operative intervention.

PROGNOSTIC FACTORS

The search to determine clinically relevant prognostic factors that predict the outcome of infants with CDH has been frustratingly complex, contradictory, and for the most part unsuccessful. Many studies have attempted to examine both anatomic and physiologic parameters that relate to survival, but each has been hampered by its retrospective analysis in the presence of the continuing evolution of new therapies. Whereas consideration of multiple factors may influence one's clinical impression regarding survival potential of an infant with CDH, such an impression cannot be derived from one measurement alone.

Anatomic Factors

With the ability to establish the diagnosis of CDH in utero as a result of the increased use of prenatal US, studies suggested that the antenatal diagnosis of a CDH before 24 weeks' gestational age was associated with a high mortality. Others have shown that antenatal diagnosis, regardless of timing, of an isolated CDH without other associated anomalies is not an indicator of outcome.[317] A CDH associated with another significant anomaly still has a dismal prognosis. If a CDH is not detected by prenatal US but is subsequently diagnosed after birth, survival rates may be excellent. It was also reported that the presence of polyhydramnios was indicative of poor survival.[119] A number of studies, however, have refuted this observation and have shown that the presence of polyhydramnios has no predictive value on the eventual outcome of an infant with CDH.[61,261,278]

The position of the stomach has been proposed as a prognostic indicator by a number of investigators. Survival rates of infants with CDH with the stomach properly located below the diaphragm at the time of diagnosis have been reported to be as high as 100% but is only 30% when the stomach had herniated into the chest.[45,61,125] Other studies have shown no predictive value of such positioning.[289] The side of the diaphragmatic defect may be somewhat predictive of outcome. It has been reported that patients with right-sided defects have a worse prognosis than those with left-sided defects.[106,291] A recent study reported no differences in outcomes between the two sides.[129] However, right-sided defects may not become evident in the newborn period and may present with very mild respiratory symptoms at a later age.[64]

A prenatal anatomic parameter that appears to have predictive correlation is the determination of the lung-to-head ratio (LHR). The ratio is determined from simultaneous sonographic measurements of the lung and head, and ratios less than 1.0 have been associated with poor outcomes.[164,183,192] Correlation with outcome was independent of gestational age. Not all perinatal groups have found the LHR to be clinically helpful.[133]

Analysis of cardiopulmonary structure including ventricular and great vessel dimensions in either the prenatal or postnatal period as well as determining function in the postnatal period may also be of prognostic importance.[61,124] A number of indices have been reported, including calculation of the cardioventricular index (left ventricle/right ventricle), the cardiovascular index (Ao/PA), and a modified McGoon index (the combined diameter of hilar pulmonary arteries indexed to the descending aorta).[282,287] A modified McGoon index less than or equal to 1.3 predicted mortality with a sensitivity of 85% and a specificity of 100%. An analysis of left ventricular mass combined with the simultaneous determination of fractional shortening has also been used to predict outcome with an index of 1.2 associated with nonsurvival.[273] These measurements may be difficult to obtain either in utero or postnatally and are heavily observer dependent. In addition, no single measurement may give enough information to completely assess cardiopulmonary status in a CDH neonate.[288]

Physiologic Parameters

Unfortunately, there are few physiologic parameters that can be measured in the neonate to assess pulmonary function other than Po_2, Pco_2, and pH. Thus, arterial blood gas analysis has been the cornerstone for attempting to establish clinical predictive criteria. Early studies showed differences in pH and Pco_2 between survivors and nonsurvivors in response to therapeutic interventions available at that time.[30,209] Infants with a low Pco_2 and a Po_2 that was initially normal or improved with mechanical ventilation had an excellent outcome, whereas those infants who had high Pco_2 levels unresponsive to mechanical ventilation did poorly. These authors noted the importance of measuring both preductal and postductal blood gases to assess the degree of right-to-left shunting.

Since these initial reports, investigators have derived a number of formulas using various blood gas components to predict outcome. The most basic concept is the alveolar-arterial oxygen gradient ($Aado_2$) It is calculated by the formula:

$$Aado_2 = [((713 \times Fio_2) - Paco_2)/0.8] - Pao_2$$

Although initially used to determine entry criteria for extracorporeal membrane oxygenation (ECMO), its use has been superseded by the development of other indices.

Using blood gas analysis and Pco_2 levels in combination with ventilatory data, parameters were determined to predict outcome in CDH infants managed with conventional ventilatory techniques.[24,26-28] To do this, a ventilatory index (VI) was calculated:

$$VI = (RR \times MAP \times Paco_2)$$

When the Pco_2 could be reduced to less than 40 mm Hg with a ventilatory index less than 1000, all patients survived. A modified ventilatory index (MVI) was calculated by using peak inspiratory pressure (PIP) rather than mean airway pressure (MAP):

$$MVI = (RR \times PIP \times Paco_2) \div 1000$$

In infants with an MVI less than 40, the survival rate was 96% using conventional therapy. All infants died if the MVI was greater than 80.[225]

The most commonly used calculation is the oxygenation index (OI). It is calculated by the formula:

$$OI = (MAP \times Fio_2/Pao_2)$$

With conventional ventilatory therapy an OI less than 0.06 had a survival rate of 98%, whereas an OI greater than 0.175 had no survivors.[225] The predictive powers of these factors with such therapies as ECMO, high-frequency oscillation (HFO), surfactant, and nitric oxide (NO) have not been determined.

Pulmonary Function Tests

The analysis of preoperative and postoperative pulmonary function tests has been reported to have predictive value in identifying infants that might require ECMO therapy as well as identifying survivors. Initial studies of respiratory function in infants with CDH uncovered the detrimental changes in compliance measurements resulting from surgical repair and helped support the hypothesis of medical stabilization and delayed surgical intervention.[219,252] Using the treatment strategies of delayed surgical repair and ECMO when necessary, infants did not require ECMO when their initial preoperative compliance measurement was greater than 0.25 mL/cm H_2O/kg and initial tidal volume was greater than 3.5 mL/kg. An improvement in the tidal volume of 4 mL/kg after repair correlated with survival.[292]

Studies have indicated that preoperative measurement of functional residual capacity may predict fatal pulmonary hypoplasia.[8] In addition, serial measurements of total pulmonary compliance have been found useful in predicting outcome in high-risk infants.[159]

Although no single parameter has proven sufficient as a prognostic factor in managing CDH infants, recent multicenter studies have shown that significant independent predictors of total mortality include prenatal diagnosis, birth weight, low 1- and 5-minute Apgar scores, and right-sided defect.[56,267,274]

TREATMENT

Success in the management of CDH has improved dramatically from 1929 when Greenwald and Steiner[111] wrote, "For the patient in whom the hernia makes its appearance at birth, little or nothing can be done from a surgical standpoint." A number of innovative treatment strategies have been used, although consistent impact on overall survival is still difficult to obtain.

Prenatal Care

The diagnosis of a CDH is being made with increasing frequency by prenatal US examination. This study may be initiated when a discrepancy between size and dates is noted. The prenatal diagnosis of CDH should be complemented by a careful search for other congenital anomalies, particularly those affecting the cardiovascular and nervous systems. Evaluation of fetal karyotype should be accomplished by amniocentesis or chorionic villus or fetal blood sampling. Currently, the standard of care is to support the fetus and mother while bringing them to delivery as close as possible to term. The advantage of prenatal diagnosis is in being able to properly prepare and inform the parents about possible treatments and outcomes. The fetus and mother should be referred to an appropriate tertiary perinatal center where the full array of respiratory care strategies including NO, oscillating ventilators, and ECMO are immediately available. Anything less may potentially compromise the best possible outcome.[262] Spontaneous vaginal delivery is preferred unless obstetric issues supervene. The mere diagnosis of a CDH is not an indication for elective cesarean section.

At this time, fetal intervention with attempted in utero correction of the defect is investigational and highly experimental. Recent trials of fetal tracheal occlusion for CDH in an effort to promote antenatal lung growth have been abandoned because they did not show improved survival rates over contemporary conventional treatments.[73,98,122,123] Tracheal occlusion resulted in lung enlargement but did not reverse the pathologic process associated with pulmonary hypoplasia.[131] As discussed in the outcome section, the prognosis for isolated CDH is not as grave as popularly thought, and hence the rationale for jeopardizing the mother and fetus in the first place may need to be reevaluated.

Although prenatal corticosteroids are used to enhance lung development in premature infants, the role of antenatal corticosteroid therapy in CDH patients remains undetermined. The rationale for such therapy to induce pulmonary maturation in a hypoplastic lung is based on animal studies and isolated case reports.[100,161,200] Balanced against these observations is the growing evidence from premature infant studies that such drugs may also have adverse perinatal and long-term effects.[160,270] The true potential of this therapy in improving CDH outcomes awaits the results of a randomized prospective study.

Preoperative Care

Resuscitation

After the birth of the infant and confirmation of the diagnosis of CDH, all efforts should be made to stabilize the cardiorespiratory system while inducing minimal iatrogenic injury from therapeutic interventions. It is essential to consider that the CDH is a *physiologic* emergency and not a *surgical* emergency. The respiratory distress associated with a CDH in the newborns results from a combination of two factors previously discussed: uncorrectable pulmonary hypoplasia and potentially reversible pulmonary hypertension. The balance between these two factors determines the response to therapy and ultimately the outcome. Clinically, both are manifested by an increase in pulmonary vascular resistance and elevated pulmonary artery pressures, right-to-left shunting at the ductal and foramen levels, and progressive hypoxemia. Because there are no proven therapies to promote

pulmonary growth at this time, therapeutic interventions are aimed at governing pulmonary vascular tone.

Resuscitation begins with endotracheal intubation and nasogastric tube insertion. Ventilation by mask and Ambu bag is contraindicated to avoid distention of the stomach and intestines that may be in the thoracic cavity. Arterial and venous access should be acquired through the umbilicus. If the umbilical venous catheter can be passed across the liver into the right atrium, it can be useful for monitoring central venous pressures as well as obtaining mixed venous blood gas samples. Although the umbilical artery is excellent for monitoring systemic blood pressure and obtaining postductal arterial blood gas specimens, additional information can be obtained by monitoring arterial oxygen saturation in a *preductal* position either with a right radial arterial catheter or a transcutaneous saturation probe. An important part of the treatment algorithm is an attempted estimation as to whether the infant has enough lung capacity for meaningful gas exchange. It is important to consider this fact before exposing an infant and family to heroic treatment strategies.

As in any neonatal resuscitation, meticulous attention must be paid to maintaining proper temperature regulation, glucose homeostasis, and volume status in the neonate in an effort to maintain adequate oxygen delivery. Any stressful stimulus can further exacerbate already elevated pulmonary pressures and lead to increased shunt flow and further systemic desaturation. Infants should be properly sedated, and any combination of agents, including midazolam (Versed), fentanyl, or morphine can be used. Muscle paralysis is strongly discouraged because of its untoward consequences on ventilatory mechanics and potential morbidity. Infants not "cooperating" with ventilator strategies generally need attention to their discomfort, not muscle paralysis. Systemic hypotension and inadequate tissue perfusion may be observed and reversed with intravenous fluid administration including crystalloid, blood products, and colloid. Cardiotonic drugs such as dopamine or dobutamine may be required.

Metabolic acid-base disturbances are usually related to hypoperfusion and should be corrected by fluid management or bicarbonate administration. Metabolic acidosis can be reversed with bicarbonate administration if ventilation can be appropriately managed. Severe hypercapnia ($PCO_2 > 70$ mm Hg) should be managed by changing ventilator strategy.

Ventilation

The type of mechanical ventilator needed for the infant with a CDH is a matter of personal and institutional preference. Most infants can be successfully managed with a simple pressure-cycle ventilator using a combination of high rates (100 breaths per minute) and modest peak airway pressures (18 to 22 cm H_2O and no positive end-expiratory pressure [PEEP]) or lower rates (20 to 40 breaths per minute) and higher pressures (22 to 35 cm H_2O, 3 to 5 cm PEEP). The goal of such ventilatory support is to maintain minute ventilation while obtaining a preductal PO_2 greater than 60 mm Hg (SaO_2 90% to 100%) with a corresponding PCO_2 of less than 60 mm Hg.

pH and Pco_2 levels have been shown to be important in modifying pulmonary vascular tone.[251] The successful clinical manipulation of these parameters in therapeutic interventions in neonates with persistent pulmonary hypertension represents an initial treatment strategy.[86] It is now clear, however, that the extremes of hyperventilation with induced alkalosis should be avoided because such therapy compounds the pulmonary problems with serious iatrogenic injury.[162] A respiratory strategy based on permissive hypercapnea and spontaneous respiration has proven to be quite successful.[31] If conventional mechanical ventilatory techniques cannot reverse the hypoxemia or hypercarbia, high-frequency techniques using an oscillating ventilator may be required. This technique may be effective in removing carbon dioxide and temporarily stabilizing an infant in severe respiratory distress. When such techniques have been used as initial therapy, survival results have been quite good.[25]

Pharmacology

A broad spectrum of drugs and antihypertensive agents has been used in attempts to modify the pulmonary vascular resistance in infants with CDH and respiratory failure. Experience has been extrapolated from clinical trials of infants with persistent pulmonary hypertension of the newborn (PPHN) and other forms of neonatal respiratory failure.

In the past, agents such as tolazoline, which exerts its effects through α-receptor blockade, had been utilized to lower pulmonary vascular resistance in the face of hypoxemia and respiratory failure.[236,277] Its efficacy in CDH infants was marginal. Other drugs, such as nitroprusside, isoproterenol, nitroglycerin, and captopril, have not been effective.[38] The administration of various prostaglandin derivatives, including prostaglandin D_2 (PGD_2), prostaglandin E_1 (PGE_1), and prostacyclin, and of the cyclooxygenase inhibitor indomethacin has also been disappointing.[198,293]

New management strategies for treating persistent pulmonary hypertension now undergoing clinical evaluation include various calcium channel blockers, prostacyclin derivatives, endothelin receptor antagonists, and phosphodiesterase-5 inhibitors such as sildenafil.[92,240]

Surfactant

Animal models have demonstrated that experimentally induced CDH lungs are surfactant deficient, but such results have not been replicated in human studies. Early reports in infants with CDH demonstrated alterations in surfactant levels and composition.[277,314] However, recent studies have indicated that the surfactant pool in infants with CDH is no different than control patients even in infants requiring ECMO support.[54,147,151] There may be alterations in synthetic and metabolic kinetics for individual components.[53] In terms of improving respiratory function and outcomes, clinical and experimental investigations with surfactant administration have been mixed.[32,108,195,256] A multicenter review of surfactant administration in CDH patients showed no overall benefit to its use and demonstrated a lower survival rate in

preterm infants compared to full-term infants.[178] At this time, there are no clinical data to support the administration of surfactant in the management of CDH infants.

Nitric Oxide

NO is a potent mediator of vasodilatation and was originally identified as endothelial-derived relaxing factor.[145,289] Because it is a highly diffusible gas that is rapidly inactivated by binding to hemoglobin, it is particularly suited for administration to the pulmonary vasculature with mechanical ventilatory techniques. In clinical studies, NO was effective in improving oxygen saturation levels in neonates with respiratory failure due to PPHN.[169,247] In an animal model of PPHN, NO decreased pulmonary artery pressures and increased arterial oxygen saturation without discernable side effects.[103] Unfortunately, its effects in CDH infants with respiratory failure have been mixed.[1,80,91,157,167] There are no data to show that NO administration improves survival or decreases the requirement for ECMO.[97] The variable physiologic response to NO in these infants may be related to the method of its administration.[155] NO administered through a nasal cannula has been utilized for the treatment of late pulmonary hypertension following extubation.[168] The exact role of NO in the treatment of pulmonary hypertension and respiratory failure in CDH infants has not been defined despite its widespread use.

Surgical Management

Timing of Surgical Repair

Historically, CDH was considered a surgical emergency. Infants were rushed to the operating room as soon as possible after birth in the belief that reduction of the abdominal contents from the chest would relieve the compression of the lungs. Frequently, after a brief postoperative honeymoon period marked by adequate gas exchange, progressive deterioration in the infant's respiratory status ensued with elevated pulmonary vascular resistance, right-to-left shunting, hypoxemia, and ultimately death due to respiratory failure.

As management techniques for neonatal respiratory failure evolved, a period of medical stabilization and delayed surgical repair in an attempt to improve the overall condition of the infant with CDH was proposed.[26,181] At the same time there was increasing evidence of the potential detrimental effects of early surgical repair on respiratory function.[252] Since then, multiple single institutional studies have reported improved survival rates with delayed surgery as part of their treatment protocols, whereas others have found no changes in overall outcome.* Importantly, no study has shown a decrease in survival rates with this technique. Although delayed surgical repair is now widely practiced, there is no statistical evidence that supports this approach over immediate repair at this time.[214]

---

*See references 6, 31, 40, 48, 101, 109, 127, 224, 241, 246, 260, 313, and 320.

The optimal timing of operative repair when employing a strategy of delayed repair also remains undetermined. The period of preoperative stabilization has varied from several days to several weeks.[40,224,246,323] Some authors have reported waiting until the infant is successfully weaning off of mechanical ventilation and requiring low ventilator settings. Others follow the severity of pulmonary hypertension with serial echocardiographic examinations and wait until the hypertension has abated or at least stabilized.[81,126]

Operative Repair

Most surgeons approach the defect through a subcostal incision, although the repair can be done through a thoracotomy incision as well. For rare cases in which reduction of the herniated contents is difficult because of an abnormally shaped liver or spleen, a combined approach can be used. Both thoracoscopic and laparoscopic techniques have been used to repair these defects.[21,173,228,245,259,324] Ideally suited for older infants with delayed presentation, minimally invasive techniques may have a higher incidence of technical and physiologic consequences in the newborn.[9]

After division of the abdominal wall muscles and entrance into the abdominal cavity, the viscera are gently reduced from the defect and completely eviscerated for adequate visualization. The spleen on the left side and the liver on the right are usually the last organs to be mobilized from the chest cavity (Fig. 60-5A, B). Mobilization can be difficult and must be done without injury to either organ. On the right side, the kidney and adrenal gland

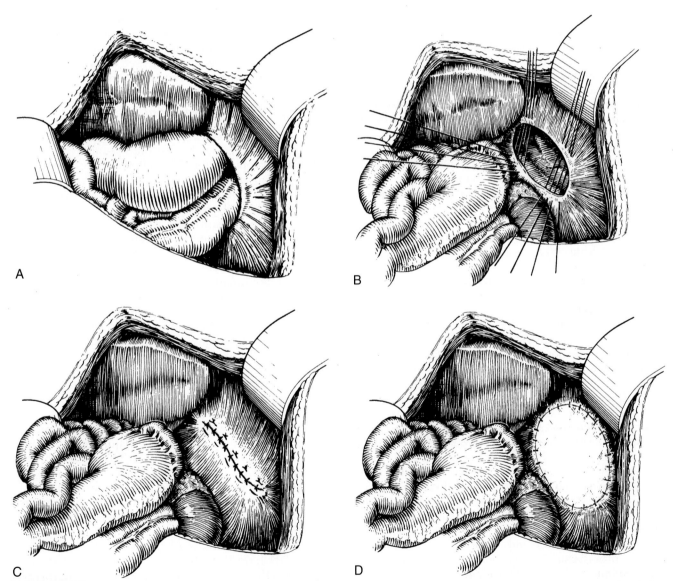

Figure 60–5   A, Schematic drawing of an unreduced left congenital diaphragmatic hernia as seen from the abdomen. B, The same hernia but now reduced, demonstrating that the spleen is usually the last organ to be reduced from the chest cavity. Sutures have been placed for a primary repair. C, Completed primary repair of a left congenital diaphragmatic hernia. D, Repaired left congenital diaphragmatic hernia using prosthetic material. (From Spitz L, Coran AG (eds): Rob & Smith's Pediatric Surgery. London, Chapman & Hall, 1996.)

may be found in the chest as well. Abnormal drainage of the hepatic veins on either side may complicate mobilization of the liver.

Once the abdominal contents are reduced, the defect in the diaphragm in the posterolateral position can be examined. In 20% of patients, a hernia sac formed by parietal pleura and peritoneum is present and must be excised to minimize chances of recurrence.[237] Usually, there is an anterior rim of diaphragm of varying size. The posterior rim of diaphragm must be searched for in the retroperitoneal tissue, because it may be rolled up like a window shade by the peritoneum. The peritoneum must be opened over this fold and the diaphragmatic tissue mobilized. When tissue is adequate, a primary repair with interrupted nonabsorbable suture material can be performed (see Fig. 60-5C). In some cases, the posterior rim of tissue may disappear along the lateral chest wall. If enough diaphragmatic tissue exists anteriorly, it can be sutured directly to the body wall with sutures placed around the ribs.

If the defect is too large to be closed in a primary fashion, a number of reconstructive techniques have been described using various nearby structures, such as prerenal fascia, rib structures, and various thoracic and abdominal wall muscle flaps.[22,139,255,266,304,310] If there is any chance that ECMO support might be required in the management of the infant, however, the use of complex reconstructive techniques requiring extensive tissue dissection is contraindicated because of the risk of bleeding. The use of prosthetic material to complete the diaphragmatic closure has gained widespread acceptance (see Fig. 60-5D). A floppy, tension-free diaphragmatic repair can be accomplished that may lessen the degree of intra-abdominal pressure when closing the abdominal wall.[19] Besides the risk of infection, the major drawback to using a prosthetic patch closure is the risk of dislodgment and subsequent reherniation.[11] Complications of prosthetic patch repair occur in approximately 10% to almost 50% of cases. Patients who develop a recurrent hernia present with bowel obstruction or respiratory distress or may be asymptomatic.[68,213]

With the loss of intra-abdominal domain, abdominal wall closure may not be possible at all or may result in unacceptable intra-abdominal pressure (i.e., abdominal compartment syndrome) even after extensively stretching the abdominal wall. In these situations, simple closure of the skin can be accomplished with repair of the resultant ventral wall defect some months later. If the skin cannot be closed successfully, temporary closure using prosthetic material such as a silo can be used. Biologic closure should then be obtained as soon as safely possible in the postoperative period. Drainage of the chest cavity on the repaired side with a tube thoracostomy is not indicated except for active bleeding or uncontrolled air leak. It has been proposed that such a tube with even a small degree of negative suction may add to the barotrauma and pulmonary hypertension imposed by mechanical ventilation on a hypoplastic lung.[323] Additional surgical procedures at the time of the repair such as correction of the nonrotation as well as appendectomy are not indicated and should be avoided if ECMO is to be considered.

The repair of recurrent defects can present a formidable surgical challenge. Since the most common organ involved in recurrent herniation is either the small or large bowel, intestinal adhesions to the disrupted diaphragm or intrathoracic organs may compromise attempted closure. Repair is most commonly approached through the abdomen but can be accomplished through a thoracotomy as well. If adequate diaphragmatic tissue is present, then primary reapproximation should be attempted. Otherwise, different techniques for mesh insertion have been tried.[68,248,254]

Anesthesia

To avoid the stresses of transport and sudden changes in ventilation parameters imposed by a trip to the operating room, a number of centers have adopted the policy of performing surgical repair of CDH infants in the neonatal intensive care unit. This change in location allows for the lowest degree of disruption in the neonate's environment. Anesthesia is achieved by intravenous narcotic and muscle relaxant techniques. With intravenous anesthetics, the infant ventilator can be used continuously rather than a conventional anesthesia machine.

Postoperative Management

Postoperative management should continue the trends and goals established before the operative procedure. Ventilator support should be tailored to keep preductal Po_2 levels at least above 80 mm Hg and Pco_2 levels less than 30 to 35 mm Hg. Echocardiograms should be obtained routinely to assess pulmonary hypertension, shunt flow, and ventricular performance. Therapeutic interventions discussed previously may be employed if respiratory decompensation develops. Weaning from ventilator support should be slow and deliberate as tolerated by the infant.

Meticulous attention to fluid status must be maintained, particularly in the immediate postoperative period. As a result of surgical intervention, these infants are often hypovolemic and frequently require extra volume administration over time.

Extracorporeal Membrane Oxygenation

Even with recent advancements in treatment strategies, overwhelming respiratory failure requiring ECMO support occurs in 15% to 45% of CDH infants.[14,57,81,241] Initially, infants were placed on ECMO after developing respiratory failure following the immediate repair of the diaphragmatic defect. With the evolution of delayed surgical repair, ECMO is now considered a part of the preoperative stabilization process.

Clinical criteria for determining ECMO use in infants with CDH have been based on factors predictive of at least an 80% mortality rate with mechanical ventilation. A number of parameters have been proposed, including the calculation of the oxygenation index (OI) and the alveolar-arterial oxygen difference [$(A - a)Do_2$]. For CDH patients the most common reason for the initiation of ECMO was an OI of 40 or greater, and it is often considered for an OI as low as 25.[57] Generally accepted criteria for initiating ECMO support for neonatal respiratory failure based on $[(A - a)DO_2]$ criteria include a value of 610 or greater despite 8 hours of maximal medical management. It must be realized that such criteria continue to be institutional specific and that no calculations can replace clinical judgment and frequent bedside assessment. Failure to improve in the setting of severe pulmonary hypertension and progressive hypoxemia despite maximum medical intervention remains a valid qualifying criterion for ECMO support.

Controversy still exists as to whether ECMO support should be offered to all infants with CDH and respiratory failure. The issue of severe pulmonary hypoplasia incompatible with life must be kept in mind when ECMO is being considered. This intervention is successful when used to support an infant with a reversible process of pulmonary hypertension. However, it is not a treatment for those infants with irreversible hypoplasia. Differentiating these infants on clinical parameters can be quite difficult. A newborn with a CDH who is unable to reach a preductal oxygen saturation level of at least 90% or a markedly elevated PCO_2 level unresponsive to any type of ventilatory intervention during the pre-ECMO course has a high likelihood of having irreversible hypoplasia.[278] On the other hand, others have proposed that all infants should be ECMO candidates.

Although widely accepted as a treatment for the respiratory failure associated with CDH, the impact of ECMO on improving overall survival continues to be debated. Over the past decade a number of studies have demonstrated improved survival rates in CDH infants with ECMO as part of the treatment strategy.[57,101,302] However, other institutions have either not noted any improvements resulting from ECMO or have been able to manage their infants without it with equivalent success.[6,25,165] Overall survival rates of infants treated with ECMO vary from 34% to 87% and are clearly dependent on a number of variables, including gestational age and birth weight, respiratory function, and the degree of pulmonary development and associated pulmonary hypertension.[81,90,165,185,276] As conventional treatment strategies continue to improve, ECMO utilization and concomitant survival rates may decrease.[14]

A number of surgical issues are involved in the management of CDH infants while on ECMO. Both venovenous and venoarterial techniques have been reported to be equally effective in supporting patients while on bypass.[82,174] With venovenous bypass, severe right-sided heart failure can be managed temporarily with a PGE_1 infusion to keep the ductus open until the pulmonary hypertension resolves or by converting to venoarterial support. The timing of the surgical repair of the defect in relation to ECMO support remains variable. As a result of the acceptance of delayed surgical repair as a treatment strategy, more than 90% of CDH infants requiring ECMO support are placed on bypass before undergoing surgical repair.[180] Surgical repair of the defect while on ECMO can then be accomplished but has been associated with hemorrhagic

complications in 60% of the patients.[179,301] Survival rates after surgery on ECMO have varied from 43% to 80%.[58,313,316] To minimize the risk of hemorrhagic complications a number of techniques have been proposed, including the use of heparin-bonded ECMO circuits, performance of the surgical repair just before expected decannulation, and aggressive management of the anticoagulant status of the infant, including the use of antifibrinolytic therapy. Because of the coagulation problems, less than 20% of infants are reportedly repaired while on ECMO.[51] The majority undergo repair after the completion of ECMO. This delayed operative approach sometimes not occurring until several days after decannulation has been extremely successful, with survival rates of almost 80% and higher.[1,81,265] However, there are currently no acceptable studies comparing either pathway.

Outcome

Survival rates (discharge to home) for infants born with an isolated CDH have improved dramatically over the past decade when compared with the historical values of approximately 50%.[3,116,185,261,319] Survival rates as high as 80% to 93% are being reached with current treatment modalities.[7,31,85,182,308] Nevertheless, variation in survival rates remains high, representing significant institutional differences in management strategies and patient accrual.[14,275] Further complicating the interpretation of most studies has been the continued evolution of respiratory care and medical treatment strategies. In addition, the presence of associated anomalies such as congenital heart disease remains a significant risk factor for a poor outcome in these infants.[55,154,267] With improved overall survival rates, a greater number of physiologically compromised infants are surviving beyond the neonatal period, and late death in approximately 10% of initial survivors has been reported mostly due to the consequences of persistent pulmonary hypertension or iatrogenic complications.[150,248,257]

Before the widespread use of ECMO and newer treatment modalities, long-term survivors of conventional mechanical ventilation were reportedly healthy and without clinically evident respiratory disease.[18,102,242] Studies have now shown that CDH survivors may be at risk for a number of long-term morbidities such as chronic pulmonary problems, growth failure, neurodevelopmental delay, gastrointestinal problems, and orthopedic issues. The probability of respiratory, nutritional, and musculoskeletal morbidity is higher in CDH infants treated with ECMO.[50]

Pulmonary issues are by far the most common long-term problems in infants surviving beyond the neonatal period. Pulmonary developmental studies have shown that alveolar multiplication continues for several years after birth. A normal number, however, is never achieved in CDH hypoplastic lungs. Over time the alveoli become emphysematous, and there is gradual remodeling of the pulmonary bed.[20] Emphysematous changes may affect both lung fields, because the contralateral lung may herniate across the mediastinum. Studies have shown that even in infants with severe respiratory distress in the neonatal period lung volume will increase with time. However, pulmonary blood flow remains significantly decreased compared with the contralateral side, suggesting that vascular growth in severe cases does not match alveolar growth.[217] Pulmonary function tests have been most useful in managing long-term survivors, because chest radiographs and ventilation-perfusion studies are almost always abnormal and therefore have had little influence on medical therapy. Although a number of infants may demonstrate compromised compliance early in their course, serial pulmonary function testing has demonstrated improved compliance over time associated with real lung growth.[172] In long-term studies of survivors, many had normal pulmonary function tests even with exercise testing.[202,215,300,322] In 30% to 50% of survivors there may be either obstructive or restrictive ventilatory impairments.[215,242,300] Increased bronchial hyperreactivity has also been noted.[146,269] Treatment strategies for these patients have included the use of supplemental oxygen, bronchodilator therapy, corticosteroids, and diuretics.

Clinically, chronic lung disease has been reported in CDH survivors, particularly in those requiring ECMO.[63,196,215] Whether this finding is related to the pathology of the disease or has been induced iatrogenically owing to techniques of ventilation is unclear.[253] Regardless, prolonged elevation in pulmonary artery pressure whether it results from pulmonary hypoplasia or bronchopulmonary dysplasia impacts long-term survival. Pulmonary artery pressures normalize in approximately 50% of all patients by 3 weeks of age but can remain elevated for months in as many as one third of surviving infants.[81,148,258] This morbidity improves over time, and most survivors lead unaffected lives.[172,196]

Studies have identified a number of nonpulmonary morbidities in CDH survivors with neurodevelopmental abnormalities being the most common. Developmental delay has been reported in a number of surviving infants.[196] Abnormalities in both motor and cognitive skills have been identified.[63,279] Other neurologic problems reported include visual disturbances, hearing loss, seizures, abnormal cranial computed tomography (CT) and MRI, and abnormal electroencephalographic studies.[63,143,196] Most studies have implicated ECMO as a factor in these neurologic problems, but CDH survivors treated without ECMO are also at risk.[5,33,204,239]

A high incidence of gastroesophageal reflux and foregut dysmotility has been found in CDH survivors (Fig. 60-6).[63,93,196,281,299] Most infants have been managed with feeding regimen manipulations and prokinetic agents. Antireflux procedures have been reserved for medically unresponsive patients or those requiring gastrostomy tube placement for feeding purposes. Nutritional and growth-related problems have been found in a significant number of these survivors as well.[20] Long-term surveillance and aggressive nutritional management are required for these infants. Worrisome anecdotal reports are beginning to appear describing Barrett's esophagitis and chronic lung disease secondary to chronic gastroesophageal reflux.

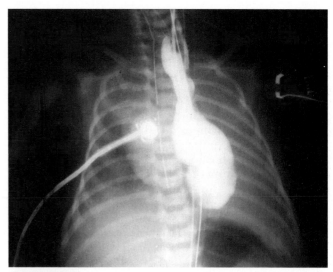

Figure 60–6 Barium sulfate esophagogram in an infant with a left congenital diaphragmatic hernia demonstrating a dilated, ectatic esophagus. The stomach was oriented vertically and emptied slowly.

A number of skeletal disorders have been reported, including chest wall defects (pectus anomalies) and scoliosis.[63,249,298] Treatment of these problems has included initial attempts at bracing followed by surgical correction.

As interventional therapies have evolved, a new group of survivors has emerged with different patterns of long-term morbidities. Sicker infants who are physiologically compromised to varying degrees are surviving in greater numbers. Resource management for these infants in the future will be crucial as we attempt to determine and justify the impact of treatment strategies on survival rates and quality of life.[231]

Future Therapies

Despite the advancements that have been made in treating infants with CDH, it still represents a frustrating and complex clinical problem. As the striking variance in survival rates attests, no currently employed therapeutic intervention or management strategy has emerged for widespread successful application. Even with the increasing success of current treatment strategies such as permissive hypercapnia, delayed operative repair, antihypertensive pharmacology, and advanced ventilatory techniques, a cohort of infants refractory to these interventions continue to be candidates for novel treatments.

The concept of fetal surgical intervention evolved from the experimental observation in lambs that reduction of compressive forces on the lung resulted in continued pulmonary growth and development.[2,118] Although technically and theoretically exciting, the clinical trial of fetal diaphragmatic repair was disappointing.[117]

Significant problems were encountered with patient selection and postoperative maternal management. A direct extension of these attempts at in utero repair was the observation that tracheal ligation accelerated fetal lung growth and reversed the alveolar hypoplasia and abnormal pulmonary vascular pattern in fetal lamb and rat models of CDH.[77,78,171,315] Tracheal occlusion or PLUG therapy (plug the lung until it grows) resulted in improved oxygenation and ventilation after birth when compared with untreated control animals.[130] These observations ultimately led to a randomized, clinical trial comparing fetal endoscopic tracheal occlusion to current standard postnatal care for severe congenital diaphragmatic hernia.[122] Fetuses qualified for enrollment if they were between 22 and 27 weeks' gestational age and had liver herniated into the left chest with an LHR below 1.4. The 90-day survival rate for the tracheal occlusion group was 73%, and it was 77% for the control group. Because there was no difference in survival between the two groups, the study was closed after 24 patients were treated. Nonetheless, there are reports of continued application of this intervention in European centers.[72] Future research will determine whether fetal intervention has a role in the treatment of CDH.

Liquid ventilation techniques have been attempted in CDH infants while on ECMO (Fig. 60-7).[233] After perfluorocarbon administration, significant increases were reported in PaO_2 levels and in static total pulmonary compliance measurements accompanied by a fall in $PaCO_2$ levels. No adverse side effects were noted. Extensive studies are required to examine this newest form of ventilation before its efficacy can be judged.

Based on the observations of fetal lung growth induced by tracheal occlusion, inducement of postnatal lung growth with static distention has also been investigated. During the course of the liquid ventilation experiments, pulmonary distention as a result of perfluorocarbon administration was observed. Its use as a potential treatment to induce postnatal lung growth in CDH patients was then reported.[94,135,303] Preliminary studies have shown significant radiographic enlargement of the lung and improved gas exchange. The same results have also been achieved using intra-alveolar albumin administration.[67,175] Further study of this potential intervention is required.

Lung transplantation has also been used anecdotally in the surgical treatment of CDH.[184,297] Both unilateral and bilateral transplants have been attempted. Currently, not enough experience exists to recommend this form of treatment.

The potential role of pharmacologic augmentation of pulmonary growth and development is currently being investigated. The combined administration of thyrotropin-releasing hormone and glucocorticoid therapy has been studied in a chemically induced rat model of CDH, with positive effects on lung growth.[283] It is also known that a number of growth factors are crucial to normal pulmonary development. It has been proposed that perhaps selected administration of one or several of these pharmacologic agents or growth factors may be able to reverse the pulmonary hypoplasia of CDH.[39,283] Continued experimental work using the nitrofen model of CDH may uncover new candidates to promote lung growth and development either prenatally or after birth.

Finally, given the current wide-ranging survival rates at various institutions, an in-depth study and evaluation of current management techniques and outcomes must be made. The efforts of the CDH Study Group to interpret very hetereogeneous data is an encouraging beginning. Such a study might result in the refinement and consolidation of current practices into a universally effective treatment strategy.

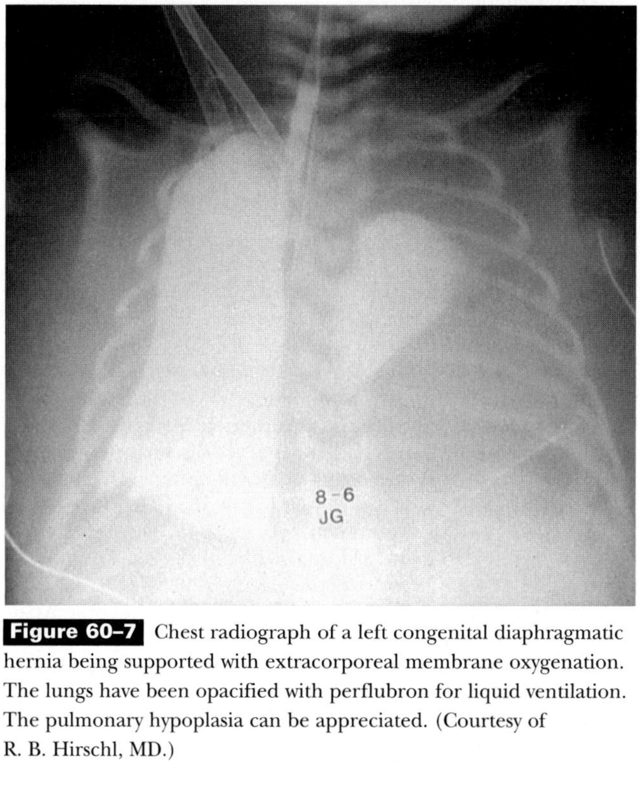

FORAMEN OF MORGAGNI HERNIA

The anterior diaphragmatic hernia of Morgagni is located anteromedially on either side of the junction of the septum transversum and the thoracic wall. The defect occurs through the embryologic space of Larrey. Occasionally, bilateral Morgagni hernias communicate in the midline, constituting a large anterior diaphragmatic defect extending all the way across the midline from right to left. Typically a sac is present, and herniation of the colon or small bowel is usually discovered to the right or left of the midline. Morgagni hernias account for less than 2% of diaphragmatic defects. Although this defect may be observed in neonates, it usually presents more commonly in older children or adults. Associated anomalies may be present and include malrotation. An anterior midline deficiency in the diaphragm with or without the other elements of the pentalogy of Cantrell with free pericardial and peritoneal communication may allow herniation of intestine into the pericardium. The hernia is often discovered incidentally as a mass or air-fluid level on a chest radiograph. A barium enema or a CT scan may confirm the diagnosis.

Operative correction is easily performed through an upper transverse abdominal incision. The diaphragm is

Figure 60–7 Chest radiograph of a left congenital diaphragmatic hernia being supported with extracorporeal membrane oxygenation. The lungs have been opacified with perflubron for liquid ventilation. The pulmonary hypoplasia can be appreciated. (Courtesy of R. B. Hirschl, MD.)

sutured to the underside of the posterior rectus sheath at the costal margin after reduction of the hernia and resection of the sac. Laparoscopic and thoracoscopic techniques have also been used to repair this defect.[70,144,191,221]

EVENTRATION OF THE DIAPHRAGM

Eventration of the diaphragm may be either congenital or acquired. The congenital form may be indistinguishable from a diaphragmatic hernia with a sac, and symptoms are usually similar. The acquired lesion is probably due to paralysis of the phrenic nerve that may occur from injury during repair of congenital heart defects, and some of the so-called congenital forms may be acquired through birth injury (Erb's palsy). The diaphragmatic muscle is usually present in its normal distribution, but it is attenuated and inactive. If a rim of diaphragm is present with a central defect to cover the pleural and peritoneal membrane, the lesion is probably a diaphragmatic hernia, although such a distinction may be moot.

There may be no symptoms whatsoever even in the presence of a large eventration, although the findings may range from wheezing, frequent respiratory infections, and exercise intolerance to extreme respiratory distress. Diagnosis is usually made on fluoroscopy of the chest. In such cases, the diaphragm moves paradoxically with respiratory motion. This paradoxic movement may be so marked that it results in severe compromise of gas exchange. Although pneumoperitoneum was used frequently in the past, CT or MRI is used more often today.

A small eventration may be left untreated. Repair is indicated when a large functional deficit in the function of the ipsilateral lung on ventilation/perfusion studies is found in an apparently asymptomatic patient. In such cases, the compressed lung will not grow well. For the same reason, a large eventration should be repaired even when asymptomatic. Repair may be performed either through the abdomen or the chest, but, in most cases, a low thoracotomy is recommended. Through this approach the diaphragm is best plicated with nonabsorbable interrupted 2-0 sutures. A radial or peripheral incision may also be made in the diaphragm and the edges overlapped and sutured. It is important to reef up and overlap the diaphragm so that it is taut, overcorrecting it somewhat, because invariably the muscle will stretch and the eventration will recur if this is not done. Diaphragmatic plication for acquired eventration is frequently necessary to wean infants from ventilatory support. Plication can also be accomplished by either a laparocoscopic or thoracoscopic approach.

REFERENCES

1. Adolph V, Flageole H, Perreault T, et al: Repair of congenital diaphragmatic hernia after weaning from extracorporeal membrane oxygenation. J Pediatr Surg 1995;30:349.
2. Adzick NS, Outwater KM, Harrison MR, et al: Correction of congenital diaphragmatic hernia in utero: IV. An early gestational fetal lamb model for pulmonary vascular morphometric analysis. J Pediatr Surg 1985;20:673.
3. Adzick NS, Harrison MR, Glick PL, et al: Diaphragmatic hernia in the fetus: Prenatal diagnosis and outcome in 94 cases. J Pediatr Surg 1985;20:357.
4. Adzick NS, Harrison MR, Glick PL, et al: Experimental pulmonary hypoplasia and oligohydramnios: Relative contributions of lung fluid and fetal breathing movements. J Pediatr Surg 1984;19:658.
5. Ahmad A, Gangitano E, Odell RM, et al: Survival, intracranial lesions, and neurodevelopmental outcome in infants with congenital diaphragmatic hernia treated with extracorporeal membrane oxygenation. J Perinatol 1999;19 (6 Pt 1):436.
6. Al-Hathal M, Crankson SH, al-Hargi F, et al: Congenital diaphragmatic hernia: Experience with preoperative stabilization and delayed surgery without ECMO and inhaled nitric oxide. Am J Perinatal 1998;15:487.
7. Al-Shanafey S, Giacomantonio M, Henteleff H: Congenital diaphragmatic hernia: Experience without extracorporeal membrane oxygenation. Pediatr Surg Int 2002;18:28.
8. Antunes MJ, Greenspan JS, Cullen JA, et al: Prognosis with preoperative pulmonary function and lung volume assessment in infants with congenital diaphragmatic hernia. Pediatrics 1995;96:1117.
9. Arca MJ, Barnhart DC, Lelli JL Jr, et al: Early experience with minimally invasive repair of congenital diaphragmatic hernias: Results and lessons learned. J Pediatr Surg 2003;38:1563.
10. Areechon W, Eid L: Hypoplasia of the lung with congenital diaphragmatic hernia. BMJ 1963;5325:230.
11. Atkinson JB, Poon MW: ECMO and the management of congenital diaghragmatic hernia with large diaphragmatic defects requiring a prosthetic patch. J Pediatr Surg 1992; 27:754.
12. Aue O: Uber angeborene Zwerfellhernien. Dtsch Z Chir 1920;160:14.
13. Aviram-Goldring A, Daniely M, Frydman M, et al: Congenital diaphragmatic hernia in a family segregating a reciprocal translocation t(5;15)(p15.3;q24). Am J Med Genet 2000;90:120.
14. Azarow K, Messineo A, Pearl R, et al: Congenital diaphragmatic hernia—a tale of two cities: Toronto experience. J Pediatr Surg 1997;32:395.
15. Badalian SS, Fox HE, Chao CR, et al: Fetal breathing characteristics and postnatal outcome in cases of congenital diaphragmatic hernia. Am J Obstet Gynecol 1994;171:970.
16. Bae JO, Wung JT, Stolar CJ: ECMO is unlikely to rescue CDH inborn CDH infants refractory to permissive hypercapnea/spontaneous ventilation. Pediatrics, in press.
17. Bahlmann F, Merz E, Hallermann C, et al: Congenital diaphragmatic hernia: Ultrasonic measurement of fetal lungs to predict pulmonary hypoplasia. Ultrasound Obstet Gynecol 1999;14:162.
18. Bartlett RH, Gazzaniga AB, Toomasian J, et al: Extracorporeal membrane oxygenation (ECMO) in neonatal respiratory failure: 100 cases. Ann Surg 1986;204:236.
19. Bax NM, Collins DL: The advantages of reconstruction of the dome of the diaphragm in congenital posterolateral diaphragmatic defects. J Pediatr Surg 1984;19:484.
20. Beals DA, Schloo BL, Vacanti JP, et al: Pulmonary growth and remodeling in infants with high-risk congenital diaphragmatic hernia. J Pediatr Surg 1992;27:997.
21. Becmeur F, Jamali RR, Moog R, et al: Thoracoscopic treatment for delayed presentation of congenital diaphragmatic hernia in the infant: A report of three cases. Surg Endosc 2001;15:1163.
22. Bianchi A, Doig CM, Cohen SJ: The reverse latissimus dorsi flap for congenital diaphragmatic hernia repair. J Pediatr Surg 1983;18:560.

23. Bochdalek VA: Einige Betrachtungen uber die Enstehung des angeborenen Zwerfekkbruches. Als Bietrag Zur pathologischen Anatomie der Hernien vjscher. Prakt Heilk 1848;18:89.

24. Bohn D: Blood gas and ventilatory parameters in predicting survival in congenital diaphragmatic hernia. Pediatr Surg Int 1987;2:336.

25. Bohn D: Congenital diaphragmatic hernia. Am J Respir Crit Care Med 2002;166:911.

26. Bohn D, Tamura M, Perrin D, et al: Ventilatory predictors of pulmonary hypoplasia in congenital diaphragmatic hernia, confirmed by morphologic assessment. J Pediatr 1987; 111:423.

27. Bohn DJ: Ventilatory management of blood gas changes in congenital diaphragmatic hernia. In Puri P (ed): Congenital Diaphragmatic Hernia. New York, Karger, 1989.

28. Bohn DJ, James I, Filler RM, et al: The relationship between $PaCO_2$ and ventilation parameters in predicting survival in congenital daphragmatic hernia. J Pediatr Surg 1984;19:666.

29. Bohn DJ, Pearl R, Irish M, et al: Postnatal management of congenital diaphragmatic hernia. Clin Perinatol 1996; 23:843.

30. Boix-Ochoa J, Peguero G, Seijo G, et al: Acid-base balance and blood gases in prognosis and therapy of congenital diaphragmatic hernia. J Pediatr Surg 1974;9:49.

31. Boloker J, Bateman DA, Wung JT, et al: Congenital diaphragmatic hernia in 120 infants treated consecutively with permissive hypercapnea/spontaneous respiration/elective repair. J Pediatr Surg 2002;37:357.

32. Bos AP, Tibboel D, Hazebroek FW, et al: Surfactant replacement therapy in high-risk congenital diaphragmatic hernia. Lancet 1991;338:1279.

33. Bouman NH, Koot HM, Tibboel D, et al: Children with congenital diaphragmatic hernia are at risk for lower levels of cognitive functioning and increased emotional and behavioral problems. Eur J Pediatr Surg 2000;10:3.

34. Bowditch HI: Peculiar case of diaphragmatic hernia. Buffalo Med J 1853;9:65.

35. Boyden EA: Development and growth of the airways. In Hodson WA (ed): Development of the Lung. New York, Marcel Dekker, 1977.

36. Boyden EA: The pattern of terminal air spaces in a premature infant of 30-32 weeks that lived nineteen and a quarter hours. Am J Anat 1969;126:31.

37. Boyden EA: The terminal air sacs and their blood supply in a 37-day infant lung. Am J Anat 1965;116:413.

38. Brands W, Kachel W, Wirth H, et al: Indication for using extracorporeal membrane oxygenation in congenital diaphragmatic hernias and pulmonary hypoplasia. Eur J Pediatr Surg 1992;2:81.

39. Brandsma AE, Tenbrinck R, Ijsselstijn H, et al: Congenital diaphragmatic hernia: New models, new ideas. Pediatr Surg Int 1995;10:10.

40. Breaux CW Jr, Rouse TM, Cain WS, et al: Improvement in survival of patients with congenital diaphragmatic hernia utilizing a strategy of delayed repair after medical and/or extracorporeal membrane oxygenation stabilization. J Pediatr Surg 1991;26:333.

41. Bremer JL: The diaphragm and diaphragmatic hernia. Arch Pathol 1943;36:539.

42. Brennan P, Croaker GD, Heath M: Congenital diaphragmatic hernia and interstitial deletion of chromosome 3. J Med Genet 2001;38:556.

43. Broman I: Uber die entwicklung der swerchfells beim menschen. Verh Anat Gres 1902;21:9.

44. Broughton AR, Thibeault DW, Mabry SM, Truog WE: Airway muscle in infants with congenital diaphragmatic

45. hernia: Response to treatment. J Pediatr Surg 1998; 33:1471.

45. Burge DM, Atwell JD, Freeman NV: Could the stomach site help predict outcome in babies with left sided congenital diaphragmatic hernia diagnosed antenatally? J Pediatr Surg 1989;24:567.

46. Butler N, Claireaux AE: Congenital diaphragmatic hernia as a cause of perinatal mortality. Lancet 1962;1:659.

47. Cacciari A, Ruggeri G, Mordenti M, et al: High frequency oscillatory ventilation versus conventional mechanical ventilation in congenital diaphragmatic hernia. Eur J Pediatr Surg 2001;11:3.

48. Charlton AJ, Bruce J, Davenport M: Timing of surgery in congenital diaphragmatic hernia: Low mortality after pre-operative stabilization. Anaesthesia 1991;46:820.

49. Chinoy MR: Lung growth and development. Front Biosci 2003;8:d392.

50. Chinoy MR: Pulmonary hypoplasia and congenital diaphragmatic hernia: Advances in the pathogenetics and regulation of lung development. J Surg Res 2002;106:209.

51. Clark RH, Hardin WD Jr, Hirschl RB, et al: Current surgical management of congenital diaphragmatic hernia: A report from the congenital diaphragmatic hernia study group. J Pediatr Surg 1998;33:1004.

52. Cloutier R, Allard V, Fournier L, et al: Estimation of lungs' hypoplasia on postoperative chest x-rays in congenital diaphragmatic hernia. J Pediatr Surg 1993;28:1086.

53. Cogo PE, Zimmerman LJ, Meneghini L, et al: Pulmonary surfactant disaturated-phosphatidylcholine (DSPC) turnover and pool size in newborn infants with congenital diaphragmatic hernia (CDH). Pediatr Res 2003;54:653.

54. Cogo PE, Zimmerman LJ, Rosso F, et al: Surfactant synthesis and kinetics in infants with congenital diaphragmatic hernia. Am J Respir Crit Care Med 2002;166:154.

55. Cohen MS, Rychik J, Bush DM, et al: Influence of congenital heart disease on survival in children with congenital diaphragmatic hernia. J Pediatr 2002;141:25.

56. Congenital Diaphragmatic Hernia Study Group: Estimating disease severity of congenital diaphragmatic hernia in the first 5 minutes of life. J Pediatr Surg 2001; 36:141.

57. Congenital Diaphragmatic Hernia Study Group: Does extracorporeal membrane oxygenation improve survival in neonates with congenital diaphragmatic hernia? J Pediatr Surg 1999;34:720.

58. Connors RH, Tracy T Jr, Bailey PV, et al: Congenital diaphragmatic hernia repair on ECMO. J Pediatr Surg 1990;25:1043.

59. Cooper AP: The Anatomy and Surgical Treatment of Abdominal Hernia. London, Longman, Rees, Orme, Brown and Green, 1827.

60. Coppola CP, Gosche JR: Oxygen-induced vasodilatation is blunted in pulmonary arterioles from fetal rats with nitrofen-induced congenital diaphragmatic hernia. J Pediatr Surg 2001;36:593.

61. Crawford DC, Wright VM, Drake DP, et al: Fetal diaphragmatic hernia: The value of fetal echocardiography in the prediction of postnatal outcome. Br J Obstet Gynaecol 1989;96:705.

62. Crosser O, Ottmann R: Grundiss der Entwicklungsgenchickle des Manchen, 7th ed. Berlin, Springer, 1970.

63. D'Agostino JA, Bernbaum JC, Gerdes M, et al: Outcome for infants with congenital diaphragmatic hernia requiring extracorporeal membrane oxygenation: The first year. J Pediatr Surg 1995;30:10.

64. Daher P, Zeidan S, Azar E, et al: Right congenital diaphragmatic hernia: A well-known pathology? Pediatr Surg Int 2003;19:293.

65. David TJ, Illingsworth CA: Diaphragmatic hernia in the south-west of England. J Med Genet 1976;13:253.

66. Davies G, Reid L: Growth of the alveoli and pulmonary arteries in childhood. Thorax 1970;25:669.

67. Davis C, et al: Post-natal trophic effects of perfluorcarbons on lung growth with congenital diaphragmatic hernia. J Pediatr Surg, in press.

68. de Kort LM, Bax KM: Prosthetic patches used to close congenital diaphragmatic defects behave well: A long-term follow-up study. Eur J Pediatr Surg 1996;6:136.

69. de Lorimier AA, Tierney DF, Parker HR: Hypoplastic lungs in fetal lambs with surgically produced congenital diaphragmatic hernia. Surgery 1967;62:12.

70. Del Castillo D, Sanchez J, Hernandez M, et al: Morgagni's hernia resolved by laparoscopic surgery. J Laparoendosc Surg Tech A 1998;8:105.

71. Delvaux V, Moerman P, Fryns JP: Diaphragmatic hernia in the Coffin-Siris syndrome. Genet Couns 1998;9:45.

72. Deprest J, Gratacos E, Nicolaides KH: The FETO Task Group. Fetoscopic tracheal occlusion (FETO) for severe congenital diaphragmatic hernia: Evolution of a technique and preliminary results. Obstet Gynecol Surv 2005;60:85.

73. Deprest J, Gratacos E, Nicolaides KH, et al: FETO Task Group: Fetoscopic tracheal occlusion (FETO) for severe congenital diaphragmatic hernia: Evolution of a technique and preliminary results. Ultrasound Obstet Gynecol 2004; 24:121.

74. Desfrere L, Jarreau PH, Dommergues M, et al: Impact of delayed repair and elective high-frequency oscillatory ventilation on survival of antenatally diagnosed congenital diaphragmatic hernia: First application of these strategies in the more "severe" subgroup of antenatally diagnosed newborns. Intensive Care Med 2000;26:934.

75. Dickson KA, Harding R: Decline in lung liquid volume and secretion rate during oligohydramnios in fetal sheep. J Appl Physiol 1989;67:2401.

76. Dickson KA, Maloney JE, Berger PJ: State-related changes in lung liquid secretion and tracheal flow rate in fetal lambs. J Appl Physiol 1987;62:34.

77. DiFiore JW, Fauza DO, Slavin R, et al: Experimental fetal tracheal ligation and congenital diaphragmatic hernia: A pulmonary vascular morphometric analysis. J Pediatr Surg 1995;30:917.

78. DiFiore JW, Fauza DO, Slavin R, et al: Experimental fetal tracheal ligation reverses the structural and physiological effects of pulmonary hypoplasia in congenital diaphragmatic hernia. J Pediatr Surg 1994;29:248.

79. DiFiore JW, Wilson JM: Lung development. Semin Pediatr Surg 1994;3:221.

80. Dillon PW, Cilley RE, Hudome SM, et al: Nitric oxide reversal of recurrent pulmonary hypertension and respiratory failure in an infant with CDH after successful ECMO therapy. J Pediatr Surg 1995;30:743.

81. Dillon PW, Cilley RE, Mauger D, et al: The relationship of pulmonary artery pressure and survival in congenital diaphragmatic hernia. J Pediatr Surg 2004;39:307.

82. Dimmitt RA, Moss RL, Rhine WD, et al: Venoarterial versus venovenous extracorporeal membrane oxygenation in congenital diaphragmatic hernia: The extracorporeal life support organization registry, 1990-1999. J Pediatr Surg 2001;36:1199.

83. Donadio A, Garavelli L, Banchini G, et al: Kabuki syndrome and diaphragmatic defects: A frequent association in non-Asian patients? Am J Med Genet 2000;91:164.

84. Dott MM, Wong LY, Rasmussen SA: Population-based study of congenital diaphragmatic hernia: Risk factors and survival in Metropolitan Atlanta, 1968-1999. Birth Defects Res A Clin Mol Teratol 2003;67:261.

85. Downard CD, Jaksic T, Garza JJ, et al: Analysis of an improved survival rate for congenital diaphragmatic hernia. J Pediatr Surg 2003;38:729.

86. Drummond WH, Gregory GA, Heymann MA, et al: The independent effects of hyperventilation, tolazoline and dopamine in infants with persistent pulmonary hypertension. J Pediatr Surg 1981;98:603.

87. Dunhill MS: Postnatal growth of the lung. Thorax 1962;17:329.

88. Eghtesady P, Skarsgard ED, Smith BM, et al: Congenital diaphragmatic hernia associated with aortic coarctation. J Pediatr Surg 1998;33:943.

89. Erenberg A, Rhodes ML, Weinstein MM, et al: The effect of thyroidectomy on ovine fetal lung maturation. Pediatr Res 1979;13(4 pt 1):230.

90. Extracorporeal Life Support Organization: 2004 ECMO Registry Data. Ann Arbor, Extracorporeal Life Support Organization, 2004.

91. Fackler JC, et al: Nitric oxide has no effect on hypoxia associated with congenital diaphragmatic hernia: Preliminary data. Children's National Medical Center ECMO Symposium 1993;9:35.

92. Farber HW, Loscalzo J: Pulmonary arterial hypertension. N Engl J Med 2004;351:1655.

93. Fasching G, Huber A, Uray E, et al: Gastroesophageal reflux and diaphragmatic motility after repair of congenital diaphragmatic hernia. Eur J Pediatr Surg 2000; 10:360.

94. Fauza DO, Hirschl RB, Wilson JM: Continuous intrapulmonary distension with perfluorocarbon accelerates lung growth in infants with congenital diaphragmatic hernia: Initial experience. J Pediatr Surg 2001;36:1237.

95. Fauza DO, Wilson JM: Congenital diaphragmatic hernia and associated anomalies: Their incidence, identification, and impact on prognosis. J Pediatr Surg 1994;29:1113.

96. Fewell JE, Hislop AA, Kitterman JA, et al: Effect of tracheostomy on lung development in fetal lambs. J Appl Physiol 1983;55:1103.

97. Finer NN, Barrington KJ: Nitric oxide for respiratory failure in infants born at or near term. Cochrane Database Syst Rev 2001;(4):CD 000399.

98. Flake AW, Crombleholme TM, Johnson MP, et al: Treatment of severe congenital diaphragmatic hernia by fetal tracheal occlusion: Clinical experience with fifteen cases. Am J Obstet Gynecol 2000;183:1059.

99. Ford WD, James MJ, Walsh JA: Congenital diaphragmatic hernia: Association between pulmonary vascular resistance and plasma thromboxane concentrations. Arch Dis Child 1984;59:143.

100. Ford WD, Kirby CP, Wilkinson CS, et al: Antenatal betamethasone and favourable outcomes in fetuses with 'poor prognosis' diaphragmatic hernia. Pediatr Surg Int 2002;18:244.

101. Frenckner B, Ehren H, Granholm T, et al: Improved results in patients who have congenital diaphragmatic hernia using preoperative stabilization, extracorporeal membrane oxygenation, and delayed surgery. J Pediatr Surg 1997;32:1185.

102. Frenckner B, Freyschsuss U: Long-term effects on lung function after repair of congenital diaphragmatic hernia. In Puri P (ed): Congenital Diaphragmatic Hernia. New York, Karger, 1989.

103. Frostell C, Fratacci MD, Wain JC, et al: Inhaled nitric oxide: A selective pulmonary vasodilator reversing hypoxic pulmonary vasoconstriction. Circulation 1991;83:2038.

104. Furuta Y, Nakamura Y, Miyamoto K: Bilateral congenital posterolateral diaphragmatic hernia. J Pediatr Surg 1987; 22:182.

105. Garne E, Haeusler M, Barisic I, et al: Congenital diaphragmatic hernia: Evaluation of prenatal diagnosis in 20 European regions. Ultrasound Obstet Gynecol 2002; 19:329.

106. Gibson C, Fonkalsrud EW: Iatrogenic pneumothorax and mortality in congenital diaphragmatic hernia. J Pediatr Surg 1983;18:555.

107. Gleeson F, Spitz L: Pitfalls in the diagnosis of congenital diaphragmatic hernia. Arch Dis Child 1991;66:670.

108. Glick PL, Leach CL, Besner GE, et al: Pathophysiology of congenital diaphragmatic hernia: III. Exogenous surfactant therapy for the high-risk neonate with CDH. J Pediatr Surg 1992;27:866.

109. Goh DW, Drake DP, Brereton RJ, et al: Delayed surgery for congenital diaphragmatic hernia. Br J Surg 1992; 79:644.

110. Green PW, Kreismer PT: Registry of fetal defects in Minnesota, incidence of congenital diaphragmatic hernia. Presented at annual meeting of the Extracorporeal Life Support Organization, Ann Arbor, Michigan, September 1990.

111. Greenwald HM, Steiner M: Diaphragmatic hernia in infancy and childhood. Am J Dis Child 1929;38:361.

112. Green JJ, Babiuk RP, Thebaud B: Etiology of congenital diaphragmatic hernia: The retinoid hypothesis. Pediatr Res 2003;53:726.

113. Gross RE: Congenital hernia of the diaphragm. Am J Dis Child 1946;71:579.

114. Guarino N, Solari V, Shima H, et al: Upregulated expression of EGF and TGF-alpha in the proximal respiratory epithelium in the human hypoplastic lung in congenital diaphragmatic hernia. Pediatr Surg Int 2004; 19:755.

115. Hallman M, Kulovich M, Kirkpatrick E, et al: Phosphatidylinositol and phosphatidylgylcerol in amniotic fluid: Indices of lung maturity. Am J Obstet Gynecol 1976;125:613.

116. Harrison MR, Adzick NS, Estes JM, et al: A prospective study of the outcome for fetuses with diaphragmatic hernia. JAMA 1994;271:382.

117. Harrison MR, Adzick NS, Flake AW, et al: Correction of congenital diaphragmatic hernia in utero: VI. Hard-earned lessons. J Pediatr Surg 1993;28:1411.

118. Harrison MR, Bressack MA, Churg AM, et al: Corrections of congenital diaphragmatic hernia in utero: II. Simulated correction permits fetal lung growth with survival at birth. Surgery 1980;88:260.

119. Harrison MR, Adzick NS, Nakayama DK, et al: Fetal diaphragmatic hernia: Fatal but fixable. Semin Perinatol 1985;9:103.

120. Harrison MR, de Lorimier AA: Congenital diaphragmatic hernia. Surg Clin North Am 1981;61:1023.

121. Harrison MR, Jester JA, Ross NA: Correction of congenital diaphragmatic hernia in utero: I. The model: Intrathoracic balloon produces fatal pulmonary hypoplasia. Surgery 1980;88:174.

122. Harrison MR, Keller RL, Hawgood SB, et al: A randomized trial of fetal endoscopic tracheal occlusion for severe fetal congenital diaphragmatic hernia. N Engl J Med 2003;349:1916.

123. Harrison MR, Sydorak RM, Farrell JA, et al: Fetoscopic temporary tracheal occlusion for congenital diaphragmatic hernia: Prelude to a randomized, controlled trial. J Pediatr Surg 2003;38:1012.

124. Hasegawa S, Kohno S, Sugiyama T, et al: Usefulness of echocardiographic measurement of bilateral pulmonary artery dimensions in congenital diaphragmatic hernia. J Pediatr Surg 1994;29:622.

125. Hatch EI Jr, Kendall J, Blumhagen J: Stomach position as in utero predictor of neonatal outcome in left sided diaphragmatic hernia. J Pediatr Surg 1992;27:778.

126. Haugen SE, Linker D, Eik-Nes S, et al: Congenital diaphragmatic hernia: Determination of the optimal time for operation by echocardiographic monitoring of the pulmonary arterial pressure. J Pediatr Surg 1991;26:560.

127. Hazebroek FW, Tibboel D, Bos AP, et al: Congenital diaphragmatic hernia: Impact of preoperative stabilization. A prospective pilot study in 13 patients. J Pediatr Surg 1988;23:1139.

128. Hedblom CA: Diaphragmatic hernia: A study of 378 cases in which an operation was performed. JAMA 1925;85:947.

129. Hedrick HL, Crumbleholme TM, Flake AW, et al: Right congenital diaphragmatic hernia: Prenatal assessment and outcome. J Pediatr Surg 2004;39:319.

130. Hedrick MH, Estes JM, Sullivan KM, et al: Plug the lung until it grows (PLUG): A new method to treat congenital diaphragmatic hernia in utero. J Pediatr Surg 1994; 29:612.

131. Heerema AE, Rabban JT, Sydorak RM, et al: Lung pathology in patients with congenital diaphragmatic hernia treated with fetal surgical intervention, including tracheal occlusion. Pediatr Dev Pathol 2003;6:536.

132. Heidenhain L: Geisichte eines Falles von chronisher: Incarceration des Mageus in einer angehorenen Zwerchfellhernie welcher durcher Laparotomie geheilt wurde, mitansheissenden Bermerkungen uber die Moglichkot, das Kardiacarconom der Speiserhre zzu reseciren. Dtsch Z Chir 1905;76:394.

133. Heling KS, Wauer RR, Hammer H, et al: Reliability of the lung-to-head ratio in predicting outcome and neonatal ventilation parameters in fetuses with congenital diaphragmatic hernia. Ultrasound Obstet Gynecol 2005; 25:112.

134. Hilfiker ML, Karamanoukian HL, Hudak M, et al: Congenital diaphragmatic hernia and chromosomal abnormalities: Report of a lethal association. Pediatr Surg Int 1998;13:550.

135. Hirschl RB, Philip WF, Glick L, et al: A prospective, randomized pilot trial of perfluorocarbon-induced lung growth in newborns with congenital diaphragmatic hernia. J Pediatr Surg 2003;38:283.

136. Hislop A, Reid L: Intra-pulmonary arterial development during fetal life: Branching pattern and structure. J Anat 1972;113:35.

137. Hislop A, Reid L: Pulmonary arterial development during childhood: Branching pattern and structure. Thorax 1973;28:129.

138. Hobolth N: Drugs and congenital abnormalities. Lancet 1962;2:1332.

139. Holcomb GW Jr: A new technique for repair of congenital diaphragmatic hernia with absence of the left hemidiaphragm. Surgery 1962;51:534.

140. Holt PD, Arkovitz MS, Berdon WE, et al: Newborns with diaphragmatic hernia: Initial chest radiography does not have a role in predicting clinical outcome. Pediatr Radiol 2003;34:462.

141. Howe DT, Kilby MD, Sirry H, et al: Structural chromosome anomalies in congenital diaphragmatic hernia. Prenat Diagn 1996;16:1003.

142. Hubbard AM, Crombleholme TM, Adzick NS, et al: Prenatal MRI evaluation of congenital diaphragmatic hernia. Am J Perinatol 1999;16:407.

143. Hunt RW, Kean MJ, Stewart MJ, et al: Patterns of cerebral injury in a series of infants with congenital diaphragmatic hernia utilizing magnetic resonance imaging. J Pediatr Surg 2004;39:31.

144. Hussong RL Jr, Landreneau RJ, Cole FH Jr: Diagnosis and repair of a Morgagni hernia with video-assisted thoracic surgery. Ann Thorac Surg 1997;63:1474.

145. Ignarro LJ, Buga GM, Wood KS, et al: Endothelium-derived relaxing factor produced and released from artery and vein is nitric oxide. Proc Natl Acad Sci U S A 1987;84:9265.

146. Ijsselstijn H, Tibboel D, Hop WJ, et al: Long-term pulmonary sequelae in children with congenital diaphragmatic hernia. Am J Respir Crit Care Med 1997;155:174.

147. Ijsselstijn H, Zimmerman LJ, Bunt JE, et al: Prospective evaluation of surfactant composition in bronchoalveolar lavage fluid of infants with congenital diaphragmatic hernia and of age-matched controls. Crit Care Med 1998;26:573.

148. Iocono JA, Cilley RE, Mauger DT, et al: Postnatal pulmonary hypertension after repair of congenital diaphragmatic hernia: Predicting risk and outcome. J Pediatr Surg 1999; 34:349.

149. Iritani I: Experimental study on embryogenesis of congenital diaphragmatic hernia. Anat Embryol (Berl) 1984; 169:133.

150. Jaillard SM, Pierrat V, Dubois A, et al: Outcome at 2 years of infants with congenital diaphragmatic hernia: A population-based study. Ann Thorac Surg 2003;75:250.

151. Janssen DJ, Tibboel D, Carnielli VP, et al: Surfactant phosphatidylcholine pool size in human neonates with congenital diaphragmatic hernia requiring ECMO. J Pediatr 2003;142:247.

152. Jenkinson EL: Absence of half of the diaphragm (thoracic stomach; diaphragmatic hernia). AJR Am J Roentgenol 1931;26:899.

153. Jesudason EC: Challenging embryological theories on congenital diaphragmatic hernia: Future therapeutic implications for paediatric surgery. Ann R Coll Surg Engl 2002;84:252.

154. Kaiser JR, Rosenfeld CR: A population-based study of congenital diaphragmatic hernia: Impact of associated anomalies and preoperative blood gases on survival. J Pediatr Surg 1999;34:1196.

155. Karamanoukian HL, Glick PL, Wilcox DT, et al: Pathophysiology of congenital diaphragmatic hernia: VIII. Inhaled nitric oxide requires exogenous surfactant therapy in the lamb model of congenital diaphragmatic hernia. J Pediatr Surg 1995;30:1.

156. Karamanoukian HL, Glick PL, Wilcox DT, et al: Pathophysiology of congenital diaphragmatic hernia: X: Localization of nitric oxide synthase in the intima of pulmonary artery trunks of lambs with surgically created congenital diaphragmatic hernia. J Pediatr Surg 1995;30:5.

157. Karamanoukian HL, Glick PL, Zayek M, et al: Inhaled nitric oxide in congenital hypoplasia of the lungs due to diaphragmatic hernia or oligohydramnios. Pediatrics 1994; 94:715.

158. Katz S, Kidron D, Litmanovitz I, et al: Fibrous fusion between the liver and the lung: An unusual complication of right congenital diaphragmatic hernia. J Pediatr Surg 1998;33:766.

159. Kavvadia V, Greenough A, Laubscher B, et al: Perioperative assessment of respiratory compliance and lung volume in infants with congenital diaphragmatic hernia: Prediction of outcome. J Pediatr Surg 1997;32:1665.

160. Kay HH, Bird IM, Coe CL, et al: Antenatal steroid treatment and adverse fetal effects: What is the evidence? J Soc Gynecol Invest 2000;7:269.

161. Kay S, Laberge JM, Flageole H, et al: Use of antenatal steroids to counteract the negative effects of tracheal occlusion in the fetal lamb model. Pediatr Res 2001;50:495.

162. Kays DW, Langham MR Jr, Ledbetter DJ, et al: Detrimental effects of standard medical therapy in congenital diaphragmatic hernia. Ann Surg 1999;230:340.

163. Keller RL, Aaroz PA, Hawgood S, et al: MR Imaging of hepatic pulmonary fusion in neonates. AJR Am J Roentgenol 2003;180:438.

164. Keller RL, Glidden DV, Paek BW, et al: The lung-to-head ratio and fetoscopic temporary tracheal occlusion: Prediction of survival in severe left congenital diaphragmatic hernia. Ultrasound Obstet Gynecol 2003;21:244.

165. Keshen TH, Gursoy M, Shew SB, et al: Does extracorporeal membrane oxygenation benefit neonates with congenital diaphragmatic hernia? Application of a predictive equation. J Pediatr Surg 1997;32:818.

166. Killeen OG, Kelehan P, Reardon W: Double vagina with sex reversal, congenital diaphragmatic hernia, pulmonary and cardiac malformations—another case of Meacham syndrome. Clin Dysmorphol 2002;11:25.

167. Kinsella JP, Neish SR, Ivy DD, et al: Clinical responses to prolonged treatment of persistent pulmonary hypertension with low doses of inhaled nitric oxide. J Pediatr 1993;123:103.

168. Kinsella JP, Parker TA, Ivy DD, et al: Noninvasive delivery of inhaled nitric oxide therapy for late pulmonary hypertension in newborn infants with congenital diaphragmatic hernia. J Pediatr 2003;142:397.

169. Kinsella JP, Neish SR, Shaffer E, et al: Low-dose inhalational nitric oxide in persistent pulmonary hypertension of the newborn. Lancet 1992;340:819.

170. Kitagawa M, Hislop A, Boyden EA, et al: Lung hypoplasia in congenital diaphragmatic hernia: A quantitative study of airway, artery, and alveolar development. Br J Surg 1971;58:342.

171. Kitano Y, Kanai M, Davies P, et al: Lung growth induced by prenatal tracheal occlusion and its modifying factors: A study in the rat model of congenital diaphragmatic hernia. J Pediatr Surg 2001;36:251.

172. Koumbourlis AC, Stolar CJ, Stylianos S: Lung function in infants after repair of congenital diaphragmatic hernia [abstract]. Am Rev Respir Dis 1994;148:A548.

173. Krishna A, Zargar N: Laparoscopic repair of a congenital diaphragmatic hernia. Pediatr Surg Int 2002;18:491.

174. Kugelman A, Gangitano E, Pincros J, et al: Venovenous versus venoarterial extracorporeal membrane oxygenation in congenital diaphragmatic hernia. J Pediatr Surg 2003; 38:1131.

175. Kunaisaki SM, Chanh R, Fauza D, et al: Hypertonic enhancement of fetal pulmonary growth after tracheal occlusion. J Pediatr Surg, in press.

176. Ladd WE, Gross RE: Congenital diaphragmatic hernia. N Engl J Med 1940;223:917.

177. Laennec RTH, 1834, cited in Ravitch MM: Congenital diaphragmatic hernia. In Nyhus LM (ed): Hernia. Philadelphia, JB Lippincott, 1964.

178. Lally KP, Lally PA, Langham MR, et al: Congenital Diaphragmatic Hernia Study Group: Surfactant does not improve survival rate in preterm infants with congenital diaphragmatic hernia. J Pediatr Surg 2004;39:829.

179. Lally KP, Paranka MS, Roden J, et al: Congenital diaphragmatic hernia: Stabilization and repair on ECMO. Ann Surg 1992;216:569.

180. Lally KP, The CDH Study Group. The use of ECMO for stabilization of infants with congenital diaphragmatic hernia—a report of the CDH Study Group. Presented at the 20th annual meeting of the Surgical Section of the American Academy of Pediatrics, Boston, October 2002.

181. Langer JC, Filler RM, Bohn DJ, et al: Timing of surgery for congenital diaphragmatic hernia: Is emergency operation necessary? J Pediatr Surg 1988;23:731.

182. Langham MR Jr, Kays DW, Beierle EA, et al: Twenty years of progress in congenital diaphragmatic hernia at the University of Florida. Am Surg 2003;69:45.

183. Laudy JA, Van Gucht M, Van Dooren MF, et al: Congenital diaphragmatic hernia: Evaluation of the prognostic value of the lung-to-head ratio and other prenatal parameters. Prenat Diagn 2003;23:634.

184. Lee R, Mendeloff EN, Huddleston C, et al: Bilateral lung transplantation for pulmonary hypoplasia caused by congenital diaphragmatic hernia. J Thorac Cardiovasc Surg 2003;126:295.

185. Lessin MS, Thompson IM, Deprez MF, et al: Congenital diaphragmatic hernia with or without extracorporeal membrane oxygenation: Are we making progress? J Am Coll Surg 1995;181:65.

186. Leung JW, Coakley FV, Hricak H, et al: Prenatal MR imaging of congenital diaphragmatic hernia. AJR Am J Roentgenol 2000;174:1607.

187. Levin DL: Morphologic analysis of the pulmonary vascular bed in congenital left-sided diaphragmatic hernia. J Pediatr 1978;92:805.

188. Lewis DA, Reickert C, Bowerman R, et al: Prenatal ultrasonography frequently fails to diagnose congenital diaphragmatic hernia. J Pediatr Surg 1997;32:352.

189. Lewis WH: The development of the muscular system. In Keibel F, Mall FP (eds): Manual of Human Embryology. Philadelphia, JB Lippincott, 1910.

190. Liggins GC, Vilos GA, Campos GA, et al: The effect of bilateral thoracoplasty on lung development in fetal sheep. J Dev Physiol 1981;3:275.

191. Lima M, Domini M, Libri M, et al: Laparoscopic repair of Morgagni-Larrey hernia in a child. J Pediatr Surg 2000; 35:1266.

192. Lipshutz GS, Albanese CT, Feldstein VA, et al: Prospective analysis of lung-to-head ratio predicts survival for patients with prenatally diagnosed congenital diaphragmatic hernia. J Pediatr Surg 1997;32:1634.

193. Lipson AH, Williams G: Congenital diaphragmatic hernia in half sibs. J Med Genet 1985;22:145.

194. Losty PD, Vanamo K, Rintala RJ, et al: Congenital diaphragmatic hernia—does the side of the defect influence the incidence of associated malformations? J Pediatr Surg 1998;33:507.

195. Lotze A, Knight GR, Anderson KD, et al: Surfactant (beractant) therapy for infants with congenital diaphragmatic hernia on ECMO: Evidence for persistent surfactant deficiency. J Pediatr Surg 1994;29:407.

196. Lund DP, Mitchell J, Kharasch V, et al: Congenital diaphragmatic hernia: The hidden morbidity. J Pediatr Surg 1994;29:258.

197. Lurie IW: Where to look for genes related to diaphragmatic hernia? Genet Couns 2003;14:75.

198. Lyrene RK, Phillips JB 3rd: Control of pulmonary vascular resistance in the fetus and the newborn. Clin Perinatol 1984;11:551.

199. Mahieu-Caputo D, Sonigo P, Dommergues M, et al: Fetal lung volume measurement by magnetic resonance imaging in congenital diaphragmatic hernia. Br J Obstet Gynaecol 2001;108:863.

200. Mann O, Huppertz C, Langwieler TE, et al: Effect of prenatal glucocorticoids and postnatal nitric oxide inhalation on survival of newborn rats with nitrofen-induced congenital diaphragmatic hernia. J Pediatr Surg 2002; 37:730.

201. Manning PB, Murphy JP, Raynor SC, et al: Congenital diaphragmatic hernia presenting due to gastrointestinal complications. J Pediatr Surg 1992;27:1225.

202. Marven SS, Smith CM, Claxton D, et al: Pulmonary function, exercise performance, and growth in survivors of congenital diaphragmatic hernia. Arch Dis Child 1998;78:137.

203. McCauley G: An account of viscera herniation. Phil Trans R Coll Phys 1754;6:25.

204. McGahren ED, Malik K, Rodgers BM: Neurologic outcome is diminished in survivors of congenital diaphragmatic hernia requiring extracorporeal membrane oxygenation. J Pediatr Surg 1997;32:1216.

205. Metkus AP, Filly RA, Stringer MD, et al: Sonographic predictors of survival in fetal diaphragmatic hernia. J Pediatr Surg 1996;31:148.

206. Migliazza L, Otten C, Xia H, et al: Cardiovascular malformations in congenital diaphragmatic hernia: Human and experimental studies. J Pediatr Surg 1999;34:1352.

207. Migliazza L, Xia H, Diez-Pardo JA, et al: Skeletal malformations associated with congenital diaphragmatic hernia: Experimental and human studies. J Pediatr Surg 1999; 34:1624.

208. Mishalany H, Gordo J: Congenital diaphragmatic hernia in monozygotic twins. J Pediatr Surg 1986;21:372.

209. Mishalany HG, Nakada K, Wooley MM: Congenital diaphragmatic hernias: Eleven years' experience. Arch Surg 1979;114:1118.

210. Miyazaki E, Ohshiro K, Tiara Y, et al: Altered insulin-like growth factor I mRNA expression in human hypoplastic lung in congenital diaphragmatic hernia. J Pediatr Surg 1998;33:1476.

211. Moessinger AC, Harding R, Adamson TM, et al: Role of lung fluid volume in growth and maturation of the fetal sheep lung. J Clin Invest 1990;86:1270.

212. Moore KL: The Developing Human: Clinically Oriented Embryology, 3rd ed. Philadelphia, WB Saunders, 1982.

213. Moss RL, Chen CM, Harrison MR: Prosthetic patch durability in congenital diaphragmatic hernia: A long term follow-up study. J Pediatr Surg 2001;36:152.

214. Moyer V, Moya F, Tibboel R, et al: Late versus early surgical correction for congenital diaphragmatic hernia in newborn infants. Cochrane Database Syst Rev 2002;CD001695.

215. Muratore CS, Kharasch V, Lund DP, et al: Pulmonary morbidity in 100 survivors of congenital diaphragmatic hernia monitored in a multidisciplinary clinic. J Pediatr Surg 2001; 36:133.

216. Naeye RL, Shochat SJ, Whitman V, et al: Unsuspected pulmonary vascular abnormalities associated with diaphragmatic hernia. Pediatrics 1976;58:902.

217. Nagaya M, Akatsuka H, Kato J, et al: Development in lung function of the affected side after repair of congenital diaphragmatic hernia. J Pediatr Surg 1996;31:349.

218. Nakata M, Sase M, Anno K, et al: Prenatal sonographic chest and lung measurements for predicting severe pulmonary hypoplasia in left-sided congenital diaphragmatic hernia. Early Hum Dev 2003;72:75.

219. Nakayama DK, Motoyama EK, Tagge EM: Effect of preoperative stabilization on respiratory system compliance and outcome in newborn infants with congenital diaphragmatic hernia. J Pediatr 1991;118:793.

220. Nauman G: Hernia diaphragmatic: Laparotomie dod. Hygeia 1888;50:524.

221. Nawaz A, Matta H, Jacobsz A, et al: Congenital Morgagni's hernia in infants and children. Int Surg 2000;85:158.

222. Neville HL, Jaksic T, Wilson JM, et al: Congenital Diaphragmatic Hernia Study Group: Bilateral congenital diaphragmatic hernia. J Pediatr Surg 2003;38:522.

223. Neville HL, Jaksic T, Wilson, JM, et al: Congenital Diaphragmatic Hernia Study Group: Fryns syndrome in children with congenital diaphragmatic hernia. J Pediatr Surg 2002;37:1685.

224. Nio M, Haase G, Kennaugh J, et al: A prospective randomized trial of delayed versus immediate repair of congenital diaphragmatic hernia. J Pediatr Surg 1994;29:618.

225. Norden MA, Butt W, McDougall P: Predictors of survival for infants with congenital diaphragmatic hernia. J Pediatr Surg 1994;29:1442.

226. Nose K, Kamata S, Sawai T, et al: Airway anomalies in patients with congenital diaphragmatic hernia. J Pediatr Surg 2000;35:1562.

227. O'Dwyer J: Operation for relief of congenital diaphragmatic hernia. Ann Surg 1890;11:124.

228. Ochoa de Castro A, Ramos MR, Calonge WM, et al: Congenital left-sided Bochdalek diaphragmatic hernia thoracoscopic repair—case report. Eur J Pediatr Surg 2003;13:407.

229. Ohshiro K, Miyazaki E, Taira Y, et al: Upregulated tumor necrosis factor-alpha gene expression in the hypoplastic lung in patients with congenital diaphragmatic hernia. Pediatr Surg Int 1998;14:21.

230. Paek BW, Coakley FV, Lu Y, et al: Congenital diaphragmatic hernia: Prenatal evaluation with MR lung volumetry—preliminary experience. Radiology 2001;220:63.

231. Poley MJ, Stolk EA, Tibboel D, et al: The cost-effectiveness of treatment for congenital diaphragmatic hernia. J Pediatr Surg 2002;37:1245.

232. Powell PD, Johnstone JM: Phenmetrazine and fetal abnormalities. BMJ 1962;17:1327.

233. Pranikoff T, Gauger PG, Hirschl RB: Partial liquid ventilation in newborn patients with congenital diaphragmatic hernia. J Pediatr Surg 1996;31:613.

234. Pringle KC: Lung development in congenital diaphragmatic hernia. In Puri P (ed): Congenital Diaphragmatic Hernia. Basel, Karger, 1989.

235. Pringle KC, Turner JW, Schofield JC, et al: Creation and repair of diaphragmatic hernia in the fetal lamb: Lung development and morphology. J Pediatr Surg 1984;19:131.

236. Purohit DM, Pais S, Levkoff AH: Effect of tolazoline on hypoxemia in neonatal respiratory distress. Crit Care Med 1978;6:14.

237. Puri P: Congenital diaphragmatic hernia. Curr Probl Surg 1994;31:787.

238. Puri P, Gorman WA: Natural history of congenital diaphragmatic hernia: Implication for management. Pediatr Surg Int 1987;2:327.

239. Rasheed A, Tindall S, Cueny DL, et al: Neurodevelopmental outcome after congenital diaphragmatic hernia: Extracorporeal membrane oxygenation before and after surgery. J Pediatr Surg 2001;36:539.

240. Rashid A, Ivy D: Severe paediatric pulmonary hypertension: New management strategies. Arch Dis Child 2005;90:92.

241. Reickert CA, Hirschl RB, Schumacher R, et al: Effect of very delayed repair of congenital diaphragmatic hernia on survival and extracorporeal life support use. Surgery 1996;120:766.

242. Reid IS, Hutcherson RJ: Long-term follow-up of patients with congenital diaphragmatic hernia. J Pediatr Surg 1976;11:939.

243. Reid L: Structural and functional reappraisal of the pulmonary artery system. In Scientific Basis of Medicine Annual Reviews. University of London, Athlone Press, 1968.

244. Reyes C, Chang LK, Waffarn F, et al: Delayed repair of congenital diaphragmatic hernia with early high-frequency oscillatory ventilation during preoperative stabilization. J Pediatr Surg 1998;33:1010.

245. Richardson WS, Bolton JS: Laparoscopic repair of congenital diaphragmatic hernias. J Laparoendosc Adv Surg Tech A 2002;12:277.

246. Roberts JP, Burge DM, Griffiths DM: High-risk congenital diaphragmatic hernia: How long should surgery be delayed? Pediatr Surg Int 1994;9:555.

247. Roberts JD, Polaner DM, Lang P: Inhaled nitric oxide in persistent pulmonary hypertension of the newborn. Lancet 1992;340:818.

248. Rowe DH, Stolar CJ: Recurrent diaphragmatic hernia. Semin Pediatr Surg 2003;12:107.

249. Roye DP: Personal communication, 1992.

250. Ruano R, Benachi A, Martinovic J, et al: Can three-dimensional ultrasound be used for the assessment of the fetal lung volume in cases of congenital diaphragmatic hernia? Fetal Diagn Ther 2004;19:87.

251. Rudolph AM, Yuan S: Response of the pulmonary vasculature to hypoxia and H$^+$ ion concentration changes. J Clin Invest 1966;45:399.

252. Sakai H, Tamura M, Hosokawa Y, et al: Effect of surgical repair on respiratory mechanics in congenital diaphragmatic hernia. J Pediatr 1987;111:432.

253. Sakurai Y, Azarow K, Cutz E, et al: Pulmonary barotrauma in congenital diaphragmatic hernia: A clinicopathological correlation. J Pediatr Surg 1999;34:1813.

254. Saltzman DA, Ennis JS, Mehall JR, et al: Recurrent congenital diaphragmatic hernia: A novel repair. J Pediatr Surg 2001;36:1768.

255. Scaife ER, Johnson DG, Meyers RL, et al: The split abdominal wall muscle flap—a simple, mesh-free approach to repair large diaphragmatic hernia. J Pediatr Surg 2003;38:1748.

256. Scheffers EC, Ijsselstijn H, Tenbrinck R, et al: Evaluation of lung function changes before and after surfactant application during artificial ventilation in newborn rats with congenital diaphragmatic hernia. J Pediatr Surg 1994;29:820.

257. Schoeman L, Pierro A, Macrae D, et al: Late death after extracorporeal membrane oxygenation for congenital diaphragmatic hernia. J Pediatr Surg 1999;34:357.

258. Schwartz IP, Bernbaum JC, Rychik J, et al: Pulmonary hypertension in children following extracorporeal membrane oxygenation therapy and repair of congenital diaphragmatic hernia. J Perinatol 1999;19:220.

259. Shah AV, Shah AA: Laparoscopic approach to surgical management of congenital diaphragmatic hernia in the newborn. J Pediatr Surg 2002;37:548.

260. Shanbhogue LK, Tam PK, Ninan G, et al: Preoperative stabilisation in congenital diaphragmatic hernia. Arch Dis Child 1990;65(10 spec no):1043.

261. Sharland GK, Lockhart SM, Heward AJ, et al: Prognosis in fetal diaphragmatic hernia. Am J Obstet Gynecol 1992;166(1 pt 1):9.

262. Shaw KS, Filiatrault D, Yazbeck S, et al: Improved survival for congenital diaphragmatic hernia, based on prenatal ultrasound diagnosis and referral to a combined obstetric-pediatric surgical center. J Pediatr Surg 1994;29:1268.

263. Shehata SM, Mooi WJ, Okazaki T, et al: Enhanced expression of vascular endothelial growth factor in lungs of newborn infants with congenital diaphragmatic hernia and pulmonary hypertension. Thorax 1999;54:427.

264. Shehata SM, Sharma HS, van der Staak FH, et al: Remodeling of pulmonary arteries in human congenital diaphragmatic hernia with or without extracorporeal membrane oxygenation. J Pediatr Surg 2000;35:208.

265. Sigalet DL, Tierney A, Adolph V, et al: Timing of repair of congenital diaphragmatic hernia requiring extracorporeal membrane oxygenation support. J Pediatr Surg 1995;30:1183.

266. Simpson JS, Gossage JD: Use of abdominal wall muscle flap in repair of large congenital diaphragmatic hernia. J Pediatr Surg 1971;6:42.

267. Skari H, Bjornland K, Frenckner B, et al: Congenital diaphragmatic hernia in Scandinavia from 1995 to 1998: Predictors of mortality. J Pediatr Surg 2002;37:1269.

268. Skari H, Bjornland K, Haugen G, et al: Congenital diaphragmatic hernia: A meta-analysis of mortality factors. J Pediatr Surg 2000;35:1187.

269. Skousgaard SG: Severe bronchial hyperreactivity as a sequel to congenital diaphragmatic hernia. Paediatr Anaesth 1998; 8:503.

270. Smith GN, Kingdom JC, Penning DH, et al: Antenatal corticosteroids: Is more better? Lancet 2000;355:25l.

271. Solari V, Piotrowska AP, Puri P: Expression of heme oxygenase-1 and endothelial nitric oxide synthase in the lung of newborns with congenital diaphragmatic hernia and persistent pulmonary hypertension. J Pediatr Surg 2003;38:808.

272. Solari V, Puri P: Glucocorticoid receptor gene expression in the hypoplastic lung of newborns with congenital diaphragmatic hernia. J Pediatr Surg 2002;37:715.

273. Springer SC, Fleming D, Hulsey TC: A statistical model to predict nonsurvival in congenital diaphragmatic hernia. J Perinatol 2002;22:263.

274. Sreenan C, Etches P, Osiovich H: The western Canadian experience with congenital diaphragmatic hernia: Perinatal factors predictive of extracorporeal membrane oxygenation and death. Pediatr Surg Int 2001;17:196.

275. Stege G, Fenton A, Jaffray B: Nihilism in the 1990s: The true mortality of congenital diaphragmatic hernia. Pediatrics 2003;112:532.

276. Stevens TP, Chess PR, McConnochie KM, et al: Survival in early and late-term infants with congenital diaphragmatic hernia treated with extracorporeal membrane oxygenation. Pediatrics 2002;110:590.

277. Stevens DC, Schreiner RL, Bull MJ, et al: An analysis of tolazoline therapy in the critically-ill neonate. J Pediatr Surg 1980;15:964.

278. Stolar C, Dillon P, Reyes C: Selective use of extracorporeal membrane oxygenation in the management of congenital diaphragmatic hernia. J Pediatr Surg 1988;23:207.

279. Stolar CJ, Crisafi MA, Discoll YT: Neurocognitive outcome for infants treated with extracorporeal membrane oxygenation: Are infants with congenital diaphragmatic hernia different? J Pediatr Surg 1995;30:366.

280. Stolar CJ, Dillon PW, Stalcup SA: Extracorporeal membrane oxygenation and congenital diaphragmatic hernia: Modification of the pulmonary vasoactive profile. J Pediatr Surg 1985;20:681.

281. Stolar CJ, Levy JP, Dillon PW, et al: Anatomic and functional abnormalities of the esophagus in infants surviving congenital diaphragmatic hernia. Am J Surg 1990; 159:204.

282. Suda K, Bigras JL, Bohn D, et al: Echocardiographic predictors of outcome in newborns with congenital diaphragmatic hernia. Pediatrics 2000;105:1106.

283. Suen HC, Losty P, Donahoe PK, et al: Combined antenatal thyrotropin-releasing hormone and low-dose glucocorticoid therapy improves the pulmonary biochemical immaturity in congenital diaphragmatic hernia. J Pediatr Surg 1994;29:359.

284. Sweed Y, Puri P: Congenital diaphragmatic hernia: Influence of associated malformations on survival. Arch Dis Child 1993;69(1 spec no):68.

285. Swietlinski J, Swist-Szulik K, Maruniak-Chudek I, et al: Spondylothoracic dysostosis associated with diaphragmatic hernia and camptodactyly. Genet Couns 2002; 13:309.

286. Taira Y, Yamataka T, Miyazaki E, et al: Comparison of the pulmonary vasculature in newborn and stillborns with congenital diaphragmatic hernia. Pediatr Surg Int 1998;14:30.

287. Thebaud B, Azancot A, de Lagausie P, et al: Congenital diaphragmatic hernia: Antenatal prognostic factors. Does cardiac ventricular disproportion in utero predict outcome and pulmonary hypoplasia? Intensive Care Med 1997;23:10062.

288. Thibeault DW, Olsen SL, Truog WE, Hubbell MM: Pre-ECMO predictors of nonsurvival in congenital diaphragmatic hernia. J Perinatol 2002;22:682.

289. Thorpe-Beeston JG, Gosden CM, Nicolaides KH: Prenatal diagnosis of congenital diaphragmatic hernia: Associated malformations and chromosomal defects. Fetal Ther 1989;4:21.

290. Thurlbeck WM: Postnatal human lung growth. Thorax 1982;37:564.

291. Touloukian RJ, Markowitz RI: A preoperative x-ray scoring system for risk assessment of newborns with congenital diaphragmatic hernia. J Pediatr Surg 1984;19:252.

292. Tracy TF Jr, Bailey PV, Sadiq F, et al: Predictive capabilities of preoperative and postoperative pulmonary function tests in delayed repair of congenital diaphragmatic hernia. J Pediatr Surg 1994;29:265.

293. Turner GR, Levin DL: Prostaglandin synthesis inhibition in persistent pulmonary hypertension of the newborn. Clin Perinatol 1984;11:581.

294. Unger S, Copland I, Tibboel D, et al: Down-regulation of sonic hedgehog expression in pulmonary hypoplasia is associated with congenital diaphragmatic hernia. Am J Pathol 2003;162:547.

295. Vacanti JP, Crone RK, Murphy JD, et al: The pulmonary hemodynamic response to perioperative anesthesia in the treatment of high-risk infants with congenital diaphragmatic hernia. J Pediatr Surg 1984;19:672.

296. van Dooren MF, Brooks AS, Tibboel D, et al: Association of congenital diaphragmatic hernia with limb-reduction defects. Birth Defects Res A Clin Mol Teratol 2003;67:578.

297. Van Meurs KP, Rhine WD, Benitz WE, et al: Lobar lung transplantation as a treatment for congenital diaphragmatic hernia. J Pediatr Surg 1994;29:1557.

298. Vanamo K, Peltonen J, Rintala R, et al: Chest wall and spinal deformities in adults with congenital diaphragmatic defects. J Pediatr Surg 1996;31:851.

299. Vanamo K, Rintala RJ, Lindahl H, et al: Long-term gastrointestinal morbidity in patients with congenital diaphragmatic defects. J Pediatr Surg 1996;31:551.

300. Vanamo K, Rintala R, Sovijarvi A, et al: Long-term pulmonary sequelae in survivors of congenital diaphragmatic defects. J Pediatr Surg 1996;31:1096.

301. Vazquez WD, Cheu HW: Hemorrhagic complications and repair of congenital diaphragmatic hernias: Does timing of the repair make a difference? Data from the Extracorporeal Life Support Organization. J Pediatr Surg 1994;29:1002.

302. von Staak FH, de Haan AF, Geven WB, et al: Improving survival for patients with high-risk congenital diaphragmatic hernia by using extracorporeal membrane oxygenation. J Pediatr Surg 1995;30:1463.

303. Walker GM, Kasem KF, O'Toole SJ, et al: Early perfluorodecalin lung distension in infants with congenital diaphragmatic hernia. J Pediatr Surg 2003;38:17.

304. Wallace CA, Roden JS: Reverse, innervated latissimus dorsi flap reconstruction of congenital diaphragmatic absence. Plast Reconstr Surg 1995;96:761.

305. Waller DK, Tita AT, Werler MM, et al: Association between prepregnancy maternal body mass index and the risk of having an infant with a congenital diaphragmatic hernia. Birth Defects Res A Clin Mol Teratol 2003;67:73.

306. Walsh DS, Hubbard AM, Olutoye OO, et al: Assessment of fetal lung volumes and liver herniation with magnetic resonance imaging in congenital diaphragmatic hernia. Am J Obstet Gynecol 2000;183:1067.

307. Warkany J, Roth CB: Malformations induced in rats by maternal vitamin A deficiency. J Nutr 1948;35:1.

308. Weber TR, Kountzman B, Dillon PA, et al: Improved survival in congenital diaphragmatic hernia with evolving therapeutic strategies. Arch Surg 1998;133:498.

309. Weibel ER, Gomez DM: A principle for counting tissue structures on random sections. J Appl Physiol 1962;17:343.

310. Weinberg J: Diaphragmatic hernia in infants: Surgical treatment with use of renal fascia. Surgery 1938;3(4):78.

311. Wells LJ: Development of the human diaphragm and pleural sacs. Contr Embryol Carnegie Inst 1954;35:107.

312. Wenstrom KD, Weiner CP, Hanson JW, et al: A five year statewide experience with congenital diaphragmatic hernia. Am J Obstet Gynecol 1991;165:838.

313. West KW, Bengston K, Rescorla FJ, et al: Delayed surgical repair and ECMO improves survival in congenital diaphragmatic hernia. Ann Surg 1992;216:454.

314. Wigglesworth JS, Desai R, Guerrini P: Fetal lung hypoplasia: Biochemical and structural variations and their possible significance. Arch Dis Child 1981;56:606.

315. Wilson JM, Difiore JW, Peters CA: Experimental fetal tracheal ligation prevents the pulmonary hypoplasia associated with fetal nephrectomy: Possible application for congenital diaphragmatic hernia. J Pediatr Surg 1993;28:1433.

316. Wilson JM, Bower LK, Lund DP: Evolution of the technique of congenital diaphragmatic hernia repair on ECMO. J Pediatr Surg 1994;29:1109.

317. Wilson JM, Fauza DO, Lund DP, et al: Antenatal diagnosis of isolated congenital diaphragmatic hernia is not an indicator of outcome. J Pediatr Surg 1994;29:815.

318. Wilson JM, Lund DP, Lillehei CW, et al: Congenital diaphragmatic hernia—a tale of two cities: Boston experience. J Pediatr Surg 1997;32:401.

319. Wilson JM, Lund DP, Lillehei CW, et al: Congenital diaphragmatic hernia: Predictors of severity in the ECMO era. J Pediatr Surg 1991;26:1028.

320. Wilson JM, Lund DP, Lillehei CW, et al: Delayed repair and preoperative ECMO does not improve survival in high-risk congenital diaphragmatic hernia. J Pediatr Surg 1992;27:368.

321. Witters I, Legius E, Moerman P, et al: Associated malformations and chromosomal anomalies in 42 cases of prenatally diagnosed diaphragmatic hernia. Am J Med Genet 2001;103:278.

322. Wohl ME, Griscom NT, Streider DJ, et al: The lung following repair of congenital diaphragmatic hernia. J Pediatr 1977;90:405.

323. Wung JT, Sahni R, Moffitt ST, et al: Congenital diaphragmatic hernia: Survival treated with very delayed surgery, spontaneous respiration, and no chest tube. J Pediatr Surg 1995;30:406.

324. Yamaguchi M, Kuwano H, Hashizume M, et al: Thoracoscopic treatment of Bochdalek hernia in the adult: Report of a case. Ann Thorac Cardiovasc Surg 2002;8:106.

325. Yamataka T, Puri P: Pulmonary artery structural changes in pulmonary hypertension complicating congenital diaphragmatic hernia. J Pediatr Surg 1997;32:387.

Chapter 61

Cysts of the Lungs and Mediastinum

N. Scott Adzick and Diana L. Farmer

Familiarity with normal variations and potential pathologic abnormalities in the lung and mediastinum is necessary because questions frequently arise on evaluation of chest radiographs. The possibility of infection, respiratory difficulty, and airway obstruction from space-occupying lesions makes mandatory the expeditious evaluation and treatment of children with a mediastinal or pulmonary cystic mass. The prognosis of mediastinal and lung cysts in most children is good.

EMBRYOLOGY

Mediastinal and lung cysts are developmental in origin. Embryologic development pertinent to mediastinal masses is mostly related to the foregut and the thymus. The foregut is first recognizable as an epithelial-lined tube late in the third postconceptual week, by which time the respiratory groove *(tracheal bud)* is visible. Septation of the esophagus and the trachea occurs over the ensuing 2 weeks by a process of cephalocaudal growth of both structures, lateral infolding of the foregut, and caudocranial septation of the trachea and esophagus. During this interval, there is proliferation of foregut epithelium that almost completely obliterates the esophageal lumen before subsequent tubularization. Differentiation of both esophageal and tracheal epithelium is recognizable in the fourth week. The process is largely completed by day 32 to 34. It is presumed that incomplete tubularization after the epithelial proliferative phase results in foregut duplication cysts.[117]

The thymus develops as paired primordia from the ventral third pharyngeal pouch. During the seventh postconceptual week, the primordia elongate caudad and ventromedially to their normal position anterior to the aortic arch. At that time, the two thymic lobes attach to each other by connective tissue but not parenchyma. Before complete descent, thymic primordia contain a thymopharyngeal duct, which is obliterated after complete descent. Incomplete descent may result in solid or cystic masses in the neck. Lack of obliteration of the thymopharyngeal duct results in congenital cysts of the thymus.[118]

Prenatal lung development is described in Chapter 60, "Congenital Diaphragmatic Hernia and Eventration." A mixed lung lesion consisting of a combination of bronchogenic cyst, bronchopulmonary sequestration, and congenital cystic adenomatoid malformation suggests a common embryologic link for these malformations, but the precise embryologic causes are unknown.[81]

CYSTIC LUNG LESIONS

Diagnosis and Treatment

The true incidence of cystic lung lesions is unknown because there are no population-based studies in the literature. Congenital cystic adenomatoid malformation was first described as a distinct pathologic entity by Chin and Tang in 1949.[27] Before then, congenital cystic adenomatoid malformation was grouped under the general diagnosis of congenital cystic lung disease, along with bronchopulmonary sequestration, congenital lobar emphysema, and bronchogenic cyst.

Prenatal diagnosis provides insight into the in utero evolution of fetal lung lesions such as congenital cystic adenomatoid malformation (CCAM), bronchopulmonary sequestration (BPS), and congenital lobar emphysema. Serial sonographic study of fetuses with lung lesions has helped define the natural history of these lesions, determine the pathophysiologic features that affect clinical outcome, and formulate management based on prognosis.[1,34,86,112,128,131] A series of more than 175 prenatally diagnosed cases from the Children's Hospital of Philadelphia and the University of California, San Francisco, found that the overall prognosis depends on the size of the lung mass and the secondary physiologic derangement: a large mass causes mediastinal shift, hypoplasia of normal lung tissue, polyhydramnios, and cardiovascular compromise leading to fetal hydrops and death (Fig. 61-1).[2]

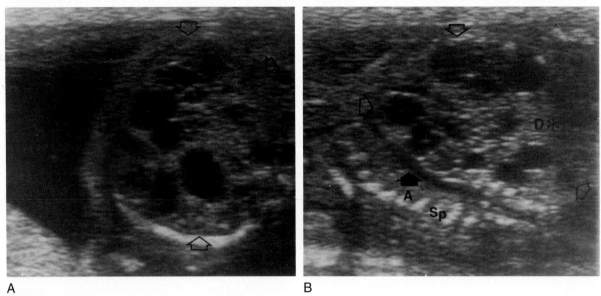

A   B

Figure 61-1 *A,* Transverse ultrasonographic scan of the fetal thorax at 22 weeks' gestation. A large multicystic mass in the left hemithorax *(open arrows)* displaces the mediastinum to the right. H, heart. *B,* Sagittal ultrasonographic scan of the fetal thorax and abdomen shows an echogenic mass *(open arrows)* of the left hemithorax that flattens the left hemidiaphragm (D). A, aorta; Sp, spine. This lesion grew and resulted in fetal hydrops. Fetal surgical resection of the affected lobe was performed successfully at 23 weeks' gestation, delivery occurred at 35 weeks' gestation, and the infant survived.

Huge fetal lung lesions have reproducible pathophysiologic effects on the developing fetus. Esophageal compression by the thoracic mass causes interference with fetal swallowing of amniotic fluid and results in polyhydramnios. Polyhydramnios is a common obstetric indication for ultrasonography, so a prenatal diagnostic marker exists for many large fetal lung tumors. Support for this concept comes from the absence of fluid in the fetal stomach in some of these cases, and the alleviation of polyhydramnios after effective fetal treatment.[2] The hydrops is secondary to vena caval obstruction and cardiac compression from large tumors causing an extreme mediastinal shift. Like CCAMs, a fetal BPS can also cause fetal hydrops, either from the mass effect or from a tension hydrothorax that is the result of fluid or lymph secretion from the BPS.[2] Hydrops is a harbinger of fetal or neonatal demise and manifests as fetal ascites, pleural and pericardial effusions, and skin and scalp edema. Although there is some association of both polyhydramnios and hydrops with fetal lung lesions, experience indicates that either can occur independently of the other.

Smaller thoracic lesions can cause respiratory distress in the newborn period, and the smallest masses may be asymptomatic until later in childhood when infection, pneumothorax, or malignant degeneration may occur. Large fetal lung tumors may regress in size on serial prenatal sonography illustrating that improvement can occur during fetal life.[70,80,113] In particular, many noncystic BPSs dramatically decrease in size before birth and may not need treatment after birth.[2] However, fetal lung lesions that seem to disappear on prenatal ultrasound and are not seen on neonatal chest radiograph still require evaluation by chest CT scan, which will frequently detect a lesion.[135]

Recently, fetal CCAM volume has been determined by sonographic measurement using the formula for a prolate ellipse (length × height × width × 0.52). A CCAM volume ratio (CVR) is obtained by dividing the CCAM volume by head circumference to correct for fetal size. A CVR greater than 1.6 is predictive of increased risk of hydrops, with 80% of these CCAM fetuses developing hydrops. The CVR may be useful in selecting fetuses at risk for hydrops and thus needing close ultrasound observation and possible fetal intervention.[30] Serial CVR measurements have shown that CCAM growth usually reaches a plateau by 28 weeks' gestation. For fetuses at less than 28 weeks' gestation, the recommendation is twice-weekly ultrasound surveillance if the CYR is greater than 1.6 and initial weekly surveillance for fetuses with smaller CVR values.

The finding that fetuses with hydrops are at very high risk for fetal or neonatal demise led to the performance of either fetal surgical resection of the massively enlarged pulmonary lobe (fetal lobectomy) for cystic/solid lesions or thoracoamniotic shunting for lesions with a dominant cyst.[2,3,52] Lesions with associated hydrops that are diagnosed late in gestation may benefit from resection using an ex utero intrapartum therapy approach.[53] The fetus with a lung mass but without hydrops has an excellent chance for survival with maternal transport, planned delivery, and neonatal evaluation and surgery.

Neonates with respiratory compromise due to a cystic lung lesion require prompt surgical resection, usually by lobectomy. In the most severe cases, ventilatory support with high-frequency ventilation or extracorporeal membrane oxygenation may be required. In asymptomatic neonates with a cystic lung lesion, we believe that elective resection is warranted because of the risks of infection and occult malignant transformation.[71] Malignancies consist mainly of pulmonary blastoma and rhabdomyosarcoma in infants and young children and bronchioloalveolar carcinoma in older children and adults.[15,31,89,106,132] After confirmation of CCAM location by postnatal chest computed tomography (CT) with intravenous contrast, we recommend elective resection at 1 month of age or older. An experienced pediatric surgeon can safely perform a thoracotomy and lobectomy in infants with minimal risk of morbidity, and thoracoscopic resection has been performed.[4] Early resection also maximizes compensatory lung growth; long-term follow-up has shown normal pulmonary function.[66,71] In contrast, we have usually followed patients with a tiny, asymptomatic, noncystic extralobar bronchopulmonary sequestration if we are confident of the diagnosis based on postnatal imaging studies. We do not favor the approach of catheterization and embolization for the treatment of larger bronchopulmonary sequestration lesions but instead opt for surgical resection.

Congenital Cystic Adenomatoid Malformation

CCAM is characterized by an "adenomatoid" increase of terminal respiratory bronchioles that form cysts of various sizes. Grossly, a CCAM is a discrete, intrapulmonaiy mass that contains cysts ranging in diameter from less than 1.0 mm to over 10.0 cm. Histologically, CCAM is distinguished from other lesions and normal lung by (1) polypoid projections of the mucosa, (2) an increase in smooth muscle and elastic tissue within cyst walls, (3) an absence of cartilage (except that found in "entrapped" normal bronchi), (4) the presence of mucus-secreting cells, and (5) the absence of inflammation.[122] Although the tissue within these malformations does not function in normal gas exchange, there are connections with the tracheobronchial tree, as evidenced by air trapping that can develop during postnatal resuscitative efforts. Cha has identified two histologic patterns of fetal CCAM: pseudoglandular and canalicular.[26] Stocker defined three types of CCAM (types I to III) based primarily on cyst size,[122,123] but this categorization has little clinical relevance. Prenatally diagnosed CCAMs are divided into two categories based on gross anatomy and ultrasound findings.[1] Macrocystic lesions contain single or multiple cysts that are 5.0 mm in diameter or larger on prenatal ultrasound, whereas microcystic lesions appear as a solid echogenic mass on sonography.

The overall prognosis for prenatally diagnosed lesions depends primarily on the *size* of the CCAM rather than on the lesion type, and the underlying growth characteristics are likely to be important. Resected large fetal CCAM specimens demonstrate increased cell proliferation and markedly decreased apoptosis compared with gestational-age–matched normal fetal lung tissue.[24] Examination of factors that enhance cell proliferation or down-regulate apoptosis in CCAM may provide further insights into the pathogenesis of this tumor and may suggest new therapeutic approaches. Fetal CCAMs that grew rapidly, progressed to hydrops, and required in utero resection showed increased platelet-derived growth factor (PDGF) gene expression and PDGF protein production

compared with either normal fetal lung or term CCAM specimens.[76]

CCAM usually arises from one lobe of the lung, with the lower lobes being the most common site. Bilateral lung involvement is rare. CCAM lesions have an equal left- and right-sided incidence. For those children who are not diagnosed as a fetus or newborn, the usual clinical presentation is with infection in the CCAM area, probably due to failure of clearance of environmental bacterial pathogens. Other presentations include pneumothorax, reactive airway disease, and failure to thrive. There is no gender predominance. Associated anomalies in our experience are very uncommon.

Bronchopulmonary Sequestration

A BPS is a mass of nonfunctioning lung tissue that is supplied by an anomalous systemic artery and does not have a bronchial connection to the native tracheobronchial tree. There are two forms of sequestration: extralobar and intralobar. Extralobar sequestrations are completely separate from the normal lung and are surrounded by a separate pleural covering, whereas intralobar sequestrations are incorporated into the normal surrounding lung. An extralobar sequestration may reside in the chest, within the diaphragm, or in a subdiaphragmatic location. Intralobar and extralobar sequestrations can occur simultaneously. An entire lung can be sequestered, and bilateral sequestrations have been reported but are very rare.[89] Because of the foregut derivation, communication between the esophagus or the stomach and a BPS may occur and, if suspected, should be delineated preoperatively by upper gastrointestinal series.[121] Arterial blood supply to the BPS can arise from below or above the diaphragm, and venous drainage can be to either the pulmonary or the systemic venous circulation. The anomalous blood supply can result in high-output cardiac failure because of substantial arteriovenous shunting through the BPS[104] or bleeding with massive hemoptysis or hemothorax.[109]

On prenatal ultrasonography, a BPS appears as a well-defined echodense, homogeneous mass. Detection by color flow Doppler of a systemic artery or arteries from the aorta to the fetal lung lesion is a pathognomonic feature of fetal BPS (Fig. 6l-2).[55] However, if this Doppler finding is not detected, then an echodense microcystic CCAM and a BPS can have an identical prenatal sonographic appearance. Ultrafast fetal magnetic resonance imaging (MRI) may help differentiate CCAM from BPS.[102] Furthermore, there are prenatally diagnosed lung masses that display clinicopathologic features of both CCAM and sequestration—hybrid lesions—which suggests a shared embryologic basis for some of these lung masses.[25,29,56] The ability to differentiate intralobar and extralobar sequestration before birth is limited unless an extralobar sequestration is highlighted by a pleural effusion or is located in the abdomen (usually close to the left adrenal gland). There are no diagnostic hallmarks for the specific prenatal diagnosis of an intralobar sequestration.

Extralobar BPS has a predominance in males (3:1), is more common on the left side, and can be associated

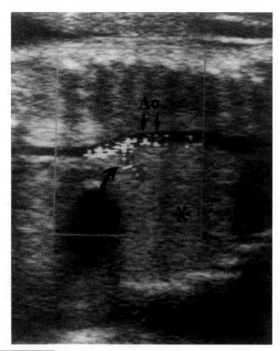

Figure 61-2 By Doppler studies, a systemic artery *(curved arrow)* from the descending aorta (Ao) supplies the mass (*), consistent with the prenatal diagnosis of pulmonary sequestration.

with conditions such as congenital diaphragmatic hernia, vertebral deformities, and congenital heart disease. Approximately 5% of neonates with a congenital diaphragmatic hernia will have an extralobar BPS, which is usually an incidental intraoperative finding. An isolated, tiny noncystic extralobar BPS rarely requires treatment. An intralobar BPS is most commonly seen in the medial basal or posterior basal segments of the lower lobes, left side more frequent than the right side. Upper lobe involvement is present in only 10% to 15% of cases. For those cases that are not prenatally diagnosed, the usual postnatal presentation of an intralobar BPS is recurrent pneumonia and even abscess formation within the BPS; thus resection (usually by lobectomy) is warranted. It is mandatory to identify and ligate the feeding systemic arterial vessel(s), which usually is found within the inferior pulmonary ligament.

Congenital Lobar Emphysema

Several causes for congenital lobar emphysema have been described,[79] but the fundamental mechanism is that the affected bronchus allows passage of air on inspiration but only limited expulsion of air on expiration leading to lobar overexpansion. Air trapping in the emphysematous lobe may be due to (1) dysplastic bronchial cartilages creating a ball-valve effect or a complete bronchial atresia[35,133]; (2) endobronchial obstruction from inspissated mucus[130] or extensive mucosal proliferation and infolding[54]; (3) extrinsic compression of the bronchi from aberrant cardiopulmonary vasculature or enlarged cardiac chambers[44]; and (4) diffuse bronchial abnormalities that may or may not be related to infection.[74]

Careful preoperative bronchoscopy may help delineate an intrinsic obstructive lesion.[35] The most common site of involvement for congenital lobar emphysema is the left upper lobe (40% to 50%), followed by the right middle lobe (30% to 40%), right upper lobe (20%), lower lobes (1%), and multiple sites for the remainder.

Barotrauma associated with the treatment of bronchopulmonary dysplasia in preterm infants can result in acquired emphysema in which multiple areas of hyperinflation may be present.[11] Because of endotracheal tube positioning, right lower lobe involvement is common in these cases, which helps to differentiate acquired from congenital disease. Polyalveolosis or the polyalveolar lobe first described by Hislop and Reid has been found in some cases of congenital lobar emphysema.[57] The total alveolar number is increased severalfold in this condition, but the airways and arteries are normal for age in number, size, and structure. The polyalveolar lobe becomes overinflated and hyperlucent on chest radiography because of impaired air exchange in the affected lobe.

Congenital lobar emphysema can be distinguished prenatally from other cystic lung lesions on ultrasonography by increased echogenicity and reflectivity compared with a microcystic CCAM and the absence of systemic arterial blood supply compared with a BPS.[8,92] Progressive enlargement of these lesions prior to 28 weeks' gestation may be due to fetal lung fluid trapping in the lobe analogous to the air trapping seen postnatally. Late in gestation, lobar emphysema may regress in the size and the character of the mass, rendering it indistinguishable from adjacent normal fetal lung.[92] Postnatal assessment is important because of the risk of postnatal air trapping in the emphysematous lobe. At the time of birth, the affected lobe may be radiopaque on chest radiography because of delayed clearance of fetal lung fluid. Prenatally diagnosed mainstem bronchial atresia results in massive lung enlargement, hydrops, and fetal death; ultrafast fetal MRI demonstrates that the entire lung is involved and that there are dilated bronchi distal to the mainstem atresia.[65]

Congenital lobar emphysema is diagnosed at birth in about 25% of cases and by age 1 month in about 50%. The diagnosis is sporadic after 6 months of age. The earlier the onset of symptoms, the more likely the progression of lobar emphysema and the need for resection. Nevertheless, some infants have very mild symptoms that do not progress, and the emphysematous lobe remains stable and does not encroach on adjacent lung, so resection is not required in these cases.[93] Besides chest radiography and CT (Fig. 61-3), a ventilation-perfusion scan can demonstrate delayed uptake and washout of the xenon radioisotope from the affected lobe and little blood flow through it. If the presentation is respiratory distress and pulmonary lobar hyperinflation, then the mainstay of management is resection of the emphysematous lobe. Positive-pressure ventilation may result in abrupt exaggerated air trapping in the lobe with sudden cardiopulmonary decompensation, so it is important for the surgeon to be present during anesthetic induction in the event that urgent thoracotomy is needed. At operation, the affected lobe will characteristically "pop out" through the thoracotomy wound. High-frequency ventilation,[45] selective bronchial intubation,[42] and endoscopic decompression

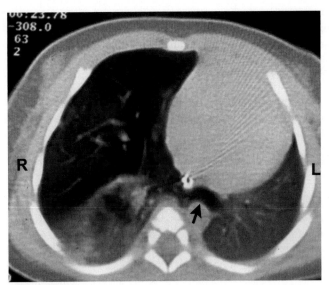

Figure 61–3 Chest CT scan from a neonate with congenital lobar emphysema involving the right middle lobe. There are dilated airspaces in the right middle lobe with compressive atelectasis of the right lower lobe. The mediastinum is shifted to the left, and a portion of the emphysematous lobe herniates across the midline posterior to the heart (*arrow*).

of the emphysematous lobe[96] may be useful adjuncts in the preoperative management of patients with respiratory distress. Long-term pulmonary growth and function after lobectomy for congenital lobar emphysema is excellent.[41]

CYSTIC MEDIASTINAL LESIONS

Clinical Features

The clinical manifestations of mediastinal lesions are the result of mass effects and are influenced by the location of the lesion within the chest. Many are asymptomatic, although the most important symptom of anterior and middle mediastinal masses is respiratory distress, particularly in infants when noisy, stridorous breathing or cyanosis while feeding is observed.[67] In older children, cough, chest pain, dyspnea, orthopnea, or, rarely, hemoptysis occurs.[20] Respiratory distress may be life threatening in all age groups.[9,10,67,98,108] Rapid onset of respiratory distress or symptoms of superior vena caval obstruction suggest lymphoma.[67,100] Although rare, infected teratomas have been reported to rupture into the bronchus, pleura, pulmonary artery, and pericardium.[20,94,110] Posterior mediastinal masses can be quite large and yet asymptomatic, often discovered incidentally on a chest radiograph taken for other indications. Less frequently, pain or symptoms of spinal cord compression lead to recognition.[75,115]

Reports from individual institutions regarding mediastinal masses may be biased by selection. If more recent series are compared with those published before 1967 (Table 61-1), an increase in malignancy, particularly of lymphomas and neuroblastoma, is evident.[19,48,49,51,67,100,110,114,115] Such is the case in a single large institutional series from Walter Reed Army Hospital[28] in

which a retrospective review compared the 60-year experience before and after 1970. The best estimate of prevalence of mediastinal masses is provided by a retrospective pathology study of mediastinal masses from Victoria in Australia, which had an estimated pediatric population of 900,000. In that series, 50% of mediastinal masses were lymphoma followed by 20% of neurogenic origin, 8% foregut duplication cysts, and 6% teratomas.[116] This prevalence is similar to the recent U.S. series (see Table 61-1).

Anatomic Considerations

A clear understanding of the anatomic subdivisions of the mediastinum is useful in differential diagnosis and selection of diagnostic studies. The mediastinum is the central thoracic space bounded laterally by the right and left parietal pleura, anteriorly by the sternum, posteriorly by the vertebral bodies to include the transverse processes, superiorly by the thoracic inlet, and inferiorly by the diaphragm. Although several classifications for subdividing the mediastinum exist, the classic anatomic description is used here.[82] The value of any system of anatomic subdivision is to provide insight into the contents of that region, which simplifies differential diagnosis.

The superior mediastinum is delimited by the thoracic inlet superiorly and the plane between the sternomanubrial junction and the inferior limit of the fourth thoracic vertebra inferiorly. The lateral boundaries are the parietal pleurae. Normal anatomic contents of this subdivision are the thymus, other lymphatic structures, and mesenchymal derivatives, including vasculature, diffusely found throughout the entire mediastinum.

The anterior mediastinum is the zone posterior to the sternum, anterior to the pericardium, superior to the diaphragm, and inferior to the plane through the sternomanubrial junction. This space normally contains mesenchymal derivatives, fat, and connective tissue.

The middle mediastinum is delimited by the pericardium and origins of the great vessels. Therefore, its normal contents are the pericardium, heart, great vessels, lymphatics, and mesenchymal derivatives.

The posterior mediastinum is outlined by the pericardium and great vessels anteriorly, the vertebral column posteriorly, and, as in each of the prior subdivisions, the parietal pleurae laterally. Its contents include the trachea and main bronchi, esophagus, widely distributed lymphatic structures, sympathetic nervous ganglia, descending aorta, azygous venous system, and thoracic duct.

Large masses or diffuse processes may transgress multiple subdivisions. An additional caveat to aid in differential diagnosis is age. With the exception of posterior mediastinal neuroblastoma, mediastinal masses in young children are most likely to be developmental in origin. Mediastinal masses that are not cystic will also be mentioned.

Diagnosis and Treatment

Recognition of cystic mediastinal masses may first occur on fetal ultrasound.[69,83,88] The fetus who develops progressive

TABLE 61-1 Incidence of Various Mediastinal Tumors

Cyst/Neoplasm	King et al., 1982[67]	Simpson and Campbell, 1991[116]	Saenz et al., 1993[111]	Cohen et al., 1991[28]	Grosfeld, 1994[47]	Total	%
Neurogenic Tumors							
Neuroblastoma/ganglioneuroblastoma	20	16	32	13	50	227	33
Ganglioneuroma	17	9	14	8	14		
Neurofibroma	4	4	3		2		
Neurilemoma/schwannoma	6	1	3	1	5		
Paraganglioma (pheochromocytoma)	1		2				
Primitive neuroectodermal tumor/neurosarcoma			2				
Lymphomas							
Hodgkin's disease	33	29	34	1	49	281	41
Non-Hodgkin's lymphoma	54	34	6	3	38		
Germ Cell Tumors							
Teratodermoid							
Benign	8	7	2	4	18	50	7
Malignant	7						
Seminoma/embryonal carcinoma	1				3		
Mesenchymal Tumors							
Lymphangioma/cystic hygroma	3	3	1	3	11	50	7
Hemangioma	2				1		
Fibroma/fibrosarcoma	1				1		
Lipoma/liposarcoma/sarcoma	12		3	1	3		
Rhabdomyosarcoma	5						
Cysts							
Pericardial		1		1		35	7
Bronchogenic	6	7		7			
Enteric	2	3		5			
Neurenteric/misc. cyst				3			
Thymic Lesions							
Thymic cyst	2	1		2		17	2.5
Hyperplasia				3			
Thymoma	2			2	3		
Thymic carcinoma		1		1			
Miscellaneous							
Granulomas, abscess, fibrosis	2	5	3	4	3	17	
Total	188	121	105	62	201	677	

nonimmune hydrops, cardiac failure, or mediastinal shift with compression of developing lung tissue may benefit from in utero decompression or resection of a cystic mediastinal lesion.[84]

For cystic mediastinal masses, the initial postnatal diagnostic study should be anteroposterior and lateral chest radiographs. A presumptive diagnosis can often be made based on the location of the lesion on the plain radiograph. CT has now largely replaced endoscopy and esophagograms as part of the preoperative evaluation. Several studies comparing contrast medium–enhanced CT to MRI suggest that CT is superior, given its ability to define calcification within a mass.[13,59] MRI is useful if spinal involvement is in question or if vascular lesions are being considered. An esophagogram reveals the characteristic extrinsic mass effect of a foregut duplication cyst, but CT is probably the most useful study for this diagnosis. Echocardiography has value in defining the rare

intrapericardial teratoma in the neonate with an enlarged pericardial silhouette[47] and can detect congenital heart disease if present.

The goal of the preoperative diagnostic workup is to help define the optimal surgical approach. When the nature of a mediastinal mass is uncertain or if the potential of malignancy exists, a preoperative serum sample should be drawn for determination of alpha fetoprotein or β-human chorionic gonadotropin levels, particularly in the case of anterior mediastinal tumors. Similarly, urinary catecholamine catabolites should be obtained in suspect posterior mediastinal masses.

Surgical resection at the time of diagnosis is the preferred treatment of benign mediastinal cysts and tumors. When indicated, thoracoscopic resection or biopsy can be performed with adequate results and minimal morbidity.[32,64,78] Large anterior mediastinal masses are best approached through median sternotomy, and middle and posterior mediastinal masses are best approached through posterolateral thoracotomy.

ANTERIOR AND SUPERIOR MEDIASTINUM

The anterior and superior mediastinum contains the thymus, great vessels, and a network of lymphatic structures, as well as connective and adipose tissue. Lymphomas are the most common tumors, followed by teratomas, germ cell tumors, cystic hygromas, and thymic lesions (Fig. 61-4). Anterior mediastinal masses in infants are usually either a teratoma or a thymic enlargement.

Foremost in evaluation of masses of the anterior mediastinum is assessment of the risk of malignancy. Malignant disease such as lymphoma generally presents in the older child, is often associated with systemic symptoms and adenopathy elsewhere, and is frequently associated with symptoms of airway compromise. When possible, the diagnosis should be sought from nonmediastinal sources, such as bone marrow, pleural fluid, or other nodal tissues, thus avoiding a general anesthetic.[6,49,84] If a diagnosis is still lacking in the presence of airway compromise, corticosteroid administration reduces the risk of open biopsy yet does not affect diagnostic accuracy. Lymphomas are discussed in Chapter 35.

Thymus

Thymic cysts are seen in the anterior mediastinum and the neck (Figs. 61-5 and 61-6). They are usually asymptomatic but can become infected or hemorrhagic or produce symptoms owing to mass effects and can create a cosmetically unacceptable appearance. The cysts are lined with ciliated, respiratory epithelium; contain lymphocytes as well as normal thymic tissue; and often show inflammatory and granulomatous changes. Thymolipoma is a benign tumor, possibly hamartoma, of mixed fatty and thymic tissue. Resection results in diagnosis and cure.

Thymomas are rare in children, accounting for less than 1% of mediastinal tumors, with only 20 well-documented cases of malignant thymoma in children in the literature.[61,72,103,126] These tumors originate in the thymic epithelium and are usually aggressive.[21] Treatment is multimodal, but outcome is poor.

Although the thymus is located in the anterior and superior mediastinum, ectopic thymic tissue can be found in the neck and posterior mediastinum as well.[7,12,119] Benign thymic hyperplasia is a physiologic enlargement of the thymus gland no longer believed to cause respiratory embarrassment, although rapid enlargement has led some authors to recommend resection.[77,107] If necessary, a short course of prednisone shrinks the normal thymus gland and helps differentiate it from nonlymphoid mediastinal masses. MRI can also be helpful.[17,119] Mediastinal radiation is of historical interest only because it had an unacceptably high association with thyroid carcinoma. Exploration is recommended only when malignancy cannot be ruled out, as in benign nodular thymic hyperplasia. Nodular thymic hyperplasia is usually asymptomatic and is usually recognized as a superior mediastinal mass on an incidental chest film. CT reveals a solid, asymmetrical, nonenhancing mass within a thymic lobe. Peripheral blood and bone marrow studies are normal. Operation in these instances reveals a lymphoid mass within one lobe of the thymus with histologic compression of adjacent normal thymus. Analysis of lymphocytes in the mass reveals a

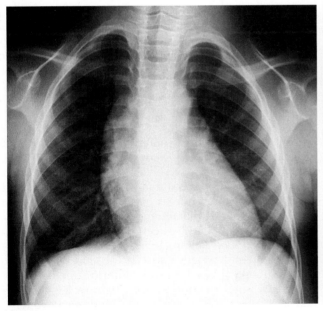

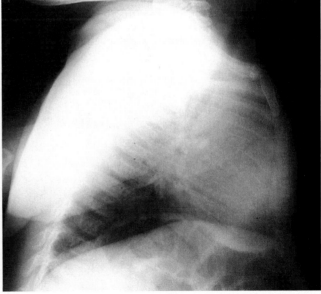

A   B

Figure 61–4 A 5-year-old boy presented with a superoanterior mediastinal mass noted to be separate from the pericardial silhouette on an anteroposterior chest film (*A*). Lateral chest radiograph (*B*) reveals sternomanubrial prominence and a mass anterior to the trachea. This mass turned out to be a teratoma.

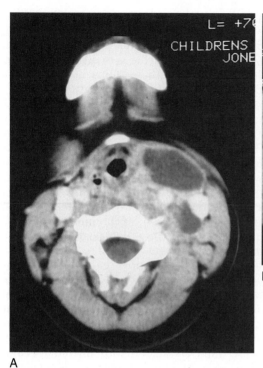

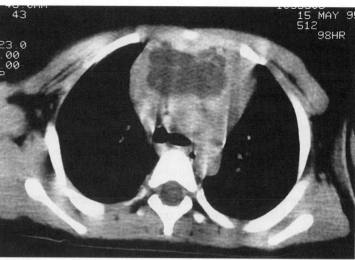

Figure 61–5 Fullness in the left neck led to these CT scans, which delineated a left thymic cyst anterior to neck vessels with extension into anterior mediastinum (*A*) at and below the level of the carina (*B*).

A

normal ratio of T and B lymphocytes. Today, most thymic lesions can be resected using thoracoscopic techniques.

Teratomas, Dermoid Cysts, and Germ Cell Tumors

After lymphoma, teratomas are the most common tumors of the anterior mediastinum. They also have been reported in other subdivisions of the mediastinum.[62] Teratomas characteristically have both cystic and solid components and are derived from at least two and, most often, all three germ cell layers.[22] Some controversy exists about the origin of teratomas because they may occur near or at the midline from brain to anus. One view is that they

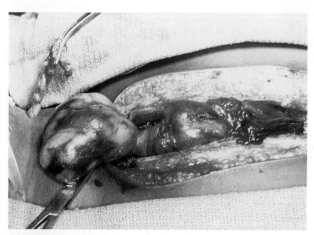

Figure 61–6 Thymic cyst mobilized from the mediastinum in the same patient as in Figure 61-5 through sternotomy before removal of the cervical extension.

represent a mature form of extragonadal germ cell tumor.[32] The other is that they arise from undifferentiated embryonic cells. The World Health Organization classifies teratomas as germ cell variants.[75] Dermoids are, by definition, composed of ectodermal and mesodermal derivatives only. They are mature, benign masses often encased in a fibrous, thick cyst wall containing various skin appendages including hair or teeth. True teratomas can be some of the largest and most unusual tumors with malignant elements, particularly when diagnosis is delayed.

In the young patient, teratomas are usually benign. Only 25% are malignant in all age groups.[129] Because it is not always possible to determine if a tumor is fully mature preoperatively, alpha-fetoprotein and β-human chorionic gonadotropin levels should be obtained in all patients. When malignant elements are present, they are most commonly yolk sac in origin, currently termed *endodermal sinus tumors*.[36]

The signs and symptoms of extrapericardial teratomas are that of any compressive, anterior mediastinal mass, such as tachypnea or stridor. Although rupture of teratomas into adjacent structures has been reported, this is a rare event.[94,129] Intrapericardial tumors are more common in neonates and young infants and present as low cardiac output.[6] Intrapericardial teratomas are invariably benign and arise in the sulcus between the origins of the aortic root and the main pulmonary artery.

On chest radiograph and CT, the mass is generally asymmetrically placed in the anterior mediastinum, commonly with extension into the right or left hemithorax. Flocculent calcifications are often seen. Anterior mediastinal teratomas are generally best approached through a sternum-splitting incision. Despite their large size, the vascular supply is often scant. Exceptions are those tumors with malignant elements, in which preoperative aortography may reveal a posterior mediastinal teratoma with arterial supply from the aorta.[60,62]

MIDDLE MEDIASTINUM

In the classic anatomic description, the middle mediastinum is circumscribed by the pericardium.[82] As such, pericardial cysts may be the only true common middle mediastinal cysts. Pericardial cysts are benign, thin-walled, fluid-containing cysts lined with mesothelium. It is postulated that the pericardium forms from a series of disconnected lacunae in the mesenchyme that later coalesce to form the pericardial sac. Occasionally, one of these lacunae persists as a pericardial cyst. They are nearly always asymptomatic and are often discovered on routine chest films or at autopsy. The classic description is that of a cystic mass lying anteriorly in the chest at either cardiophrenic sulcus, although the right side is more common. Historically, thoracotomy was recommended to establish a definitive diagnosis. Currently, CT provides a sufficiently characteristic appearance to allow accurate diagnosis, thus allowing nonintervention unless the cyst is large. If the diagnosis is uncertain, these can be excised or unroofed thoracoscopically as well.

POSTERIOR MEDIASTINUM

The posterior mediastinum lies behind a plane passing in front of the tracheal bifurcation and extending posteriorly to the paravertebral sulci.[82] The posterior mediastinum is the site of a heterogeneous group of cysts, neoplasms, and inflammatory processes in children. Most common of these lesions is the spectrum of benign to malignant neurogenic tumors of the sympathetic nervous system. In the young, the most common tumor is a malignant neuroblastoma, and in the older child, the most common tumors are benign ganglioneuromas; both of these lesions are discussed in Chapter 28.

Foregut Duplication Cysts

Foregut duplication cysts are reasonably common in pediatric specialty centers. The nomenclature of these lesions varies considerably. They can be subdivided clinically and pathologically into (1) enteric duplications and cysts (lined by intestinal epithelium), (2) bronchogenic cysts (lined by respiratory epithelium), and (3) neurenteric cysts (associated with vertebral anomalies or having a connection with the nervous system). *Enterogenous* is a confusing historical term and in various reports has included each of the aforementioned categories. The generic term *foregut duplication cyst* is a more accurate embryologic description with subdivision into bronchogenic or enteric cysts determined by the histology of the mucosa lining the cyst wall. In fact, all three endodermal derivatives may be found in the occasional foregut duplication, supporting a common embryologic derivation for foregut duplication cysts.

Bronchogenic Cysts

Bronchogenic cysts (Fig. 61-7) develop from abnormal budding of the tracheal diverticulum or ventral portion

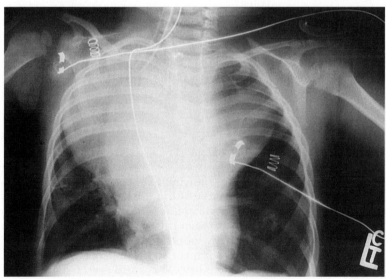

A

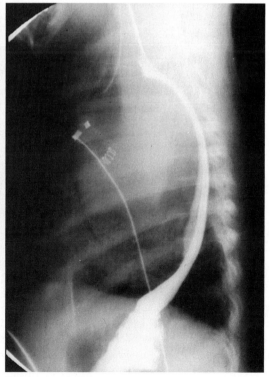

B

Figure 61–7 *A,* Bronchogenic cyst. Central tracheobronchial compression with respiratory distress was demonstrated in this 15-month-old boy transferred to the intensive care unit in critical condition. He had been treated for a year for symptoms of asthma. *B,* Lateral view shows remarkable tracheal compression with tracheoesophageal separation confirmed by contrast agent in the esophagus.

of the foregut. These cysts can be found in a variety of locations from paraesophageal to paratracheal, perihilar, or intraparenchymal,[91] depending on the level at which the abnormal budding occurred in the development of the foregut or tracheobronchial tree. It has been reported that about two thirds of bronchogenic cysts are located within the lung parenchyma, with the remainder in the mediastinum; but this distribution varies between different reports. Rarely, they can be found in remote locations, such as the tongue, neck, back, and even below the diaphragm.[18,40,51,101,127]

Histologically, bronchogenic cysts are thin walled, lined with bronchial epithelium, and filled with mucus. They can be single or multiple and are white or pinkish. Cartilage has been reported in the wall of these cysts, and air-fluid levels may be present. The cysts have no predilection for the right or left side. Although they do not usually communicate with the tracheobronchial tree, they may do so from inception or the communication may be acquired from superinfection.

Diagnosis in older children often results from identification of an incidental mass on chest radiograph obtained for an unrelated reason. Infants usually present with respiratory symptoms, and the mass may be obscured on plain film by associated atelectasis and infection (Figs. 61-8 and 61-9).[37,73,120] In this case, the diagnosis can be delayed, but CT usually confirms the diagnosis. Bronchogenic cysts have also been recognized on antenatal ultrasound[5] and on esophagogram for other indications. The differential diagnosis includes foreign body, lobar emphysema, pneumonia, bronchial stenosis, and pneumothorax.

Bronchogenic cysts should be excised to avoid the complications of infection, hemorrhage, or sudden death from rapid expansion under tension. A risk of malignant

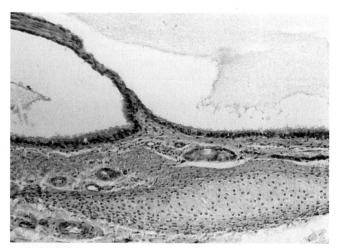

Figure 61–9 Microscopically, this bronchogenic cyst wall is lined by ciliated respiratory epithelium and contains bronchial cartilage, characteristic of bronchogenic cysts and evidence that they are central bronchial developmental anomalies (in contrast to cystic adenomatoid malformation, which is a peripheral parenchymal anomaly).

transformation does exist, as malignancy has been reported in two adult patients with bronchogenic cysts and adenocarcinoma has been reported arising from a bronchogenic cyst in an 8-year-old girl.[125] Excision should be accomplished without injury to the bronchial or esophageal wall. Small cysts in the pulmonary hilum may not be visualized until the mediastinal pleura is opened. Cyst resection is usually straightforward, but occasionally limited parenchymal lung resection or lobectomy may be required. In the majority of patients, bronchogenic cysts are amenable to thoracoscopic resection.[33,64] An error in recognition may lead to unnecessary resection of *emphysematous* lung tissue rather than removal of a cyst producing bronchial obstruction. Complete excision is recommended; recurrence 25 years after incomplete resection has been reported.[105] Although there are reports of transbronchial drainage, we do not recommend that approach.[95]

Enteric Duplication Cysts

Enteric cysts arise from failure of coalescence of vacuoles early in development of the foregut. They are lined by esophageal or gastric epithelium surrounded by smooth muscle. They have been called variously enterogenic or enterogenous cysts, esophageal cysts, enteric cysts, and esophageal duplications. Gastric mucosa is often seen, and intramural adrenal cortical rests have been reported.[136] Enteric cysts may be located throughout the posterior mediastinum and in the neck. Although most commonly integral to the wall of the esophagus, they may communicate with the lumen of the esophagus or exist completely separate from the structure of origin. A number of large thoracoabdominal enteric cysts have been reported, either ending blindly in the abdomen or

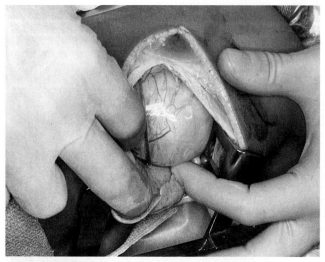

Figure 61–8 Urgent thoracotomy in the same patient as in Figure 61-7 showed a large unilocular cyst. It was aspirated of infected mucus to relieve bradycardia and then removed from its attachment to the posterior trachea. The microscopic appearance is shown in Figure 61-9.

connecting with the lumen of the stomach, jejunum, ileum, or pancreatic duct.[51,99] Biliary reflux during bronchoscopy was reported in a case of an enteric duplication cyst that penetrated the diaphragm and connected the carina with the biliary tree.[73] There is a 12% incidence of associated malformations. Most of these are additional enteric duplications.[58] Two cases of prenatally diagnosed intrathoracic enteric duplication cyst associated with hydrops have been treated with placement of a thoracoamniotic shunt in utero.[39]

In most series, enteric cysts are asymptomatic at presentation. Chest radiograph and CT are the mainstays of diagnosis (Figs. 61-10 to 61-12). Although ^{99m}Tc pertechnetate, abdominal ultrasound, barium swallow, or MRI may occasionally be useful adjunctive procedures, the goal of preoperative studies is less an attempt to make a definitive diagnosis than to provide information to aid in operative planning. Treatment consists of complete surgical excision either by thoracotomy or thoracoscopy. If necessary, as in long tubular duplications, the mucosal lining of a foregut duplication may be stripped, leaving the common muscular wall intact.[124]

Marsupialization is no longer recommended. These are benign lesions, and esophageal integrity should be preserved.

Neurenteric Cysts

Neurenteric cysts are rare foregut duplications that also have connections to the spinal canal, sometimes with the dura. Although they most commonly present as intrathoracic masses, they may also present as an intraspinal mass. The coexistence of a cystic posterior mediastinal mass with adjacent hemivertebrae should raise suspicion of a neurenteric cyst as well as anterior myelomeningocele.[14] Neurenteric cysts are thought to form early in development when the notochord and foregut are in apposition, either by failure of complete separation or by herniation of foregut endoderm into the dorsal ectoderm.[68,97]

Histologically, neurenteric cysts have alimentary tract mucosa, well-developed muscle walls, and no serosa. Gastric mucosa may be present, so signs of inflammation and ulceration may occur.[68] Symptoms often include pain

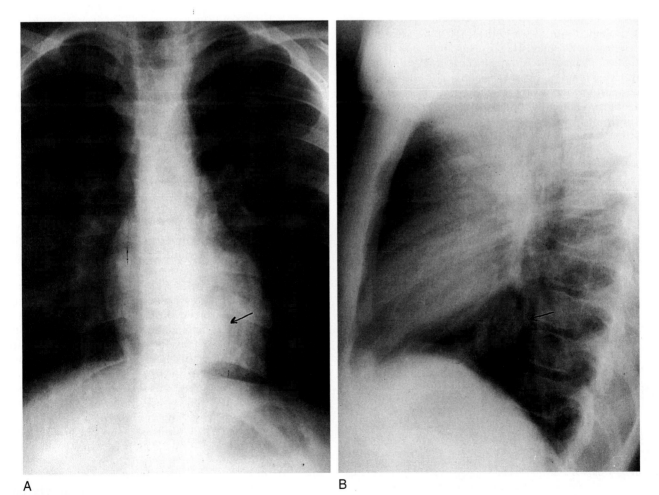

A   B

Figure 61–10 *A,* Incidental finding of an asymptomatic mediastinal mass behind the cardiac silhouette on anterior chest radiograph *(arrow).* *B,* On lateral film, the lesion was located just inferior and posterior to the base of the heart *(arrow)* and adjacent to the esophagus.

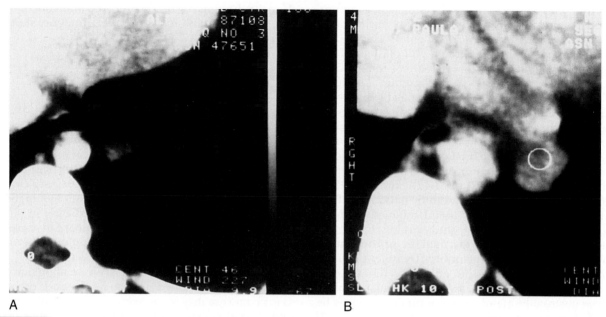

Figure 61–11   *A* and *B*, CT scan further delineates the lesion in the patient shown in Figure 61-10 *(ring marker)*. CT is probably the most useful imaging approach for patients with mediastinal tumors.

or neurologic findings (or both). MRI is suggested when a posterior mediastinal mass is associated with vertebral anomalies. Prompt excision is indicated. Paraplegia and death owing to meningitis have been reported.[97] Although some authors report leaving the neural connections intact, most recommend total excision with simultaneous laminectomy if necessary.[14,16,38]

Other miscellaneous entities enter into the differential diagnosis of rare posterior mediastinal cystic masses. Anterior thoracic meningoceles are seen in older children and are thought to be progressive degenerative lesions associated with vertebral anomalies.[134] MRI should distinguish this lesion from a neurenteric cyst.

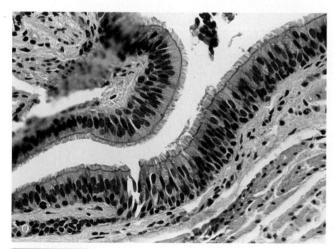

Figure 61–12   Operative findings revealed a single cyst with esophageal mucosal lining, and microscopic examination confirmed the presence of esophageal mucosa.

Miscellaneous Mesenchymal Cystic Tumors

Mesenchymal tumors may occur throughout the mediastinum and may compromise the airway. They originate from connective tissue, lymphatic tissue, smooth and striated muscle, fat, and blood vessels. As a group, they constitute less than 5% of mediastinal masses in children.

Mesenchymal tumors derived from blood and lymph vessels are the most common varieties in children, especially lymphangiomas (cystic hygroma). In most patients, lymphangioma presents as a superior or posterior mediastinal extension of a cervical lesion; however, primary mediastinal lymphangiomas do occur.[43,87] These tumors grow by proliferation of endothelial cell–lined buds within tissue planes. Symptoms relate to the size and invasiveness of the tumors or relate to infection.[85,87] Hemorrhage into these tumors can cause obstruction from rapid increase in size. Diagnostic steps include CT with intravenous contrast material or MRI. Fibrous reaction and neovascularization may make surgical resection tedious, although it remains the best therapy. Sclerotherapy with OK-432 is under investigational use in the United States and has been shown to have dramatic results in other countries. The most common complication after surgical resection of mediastinal lymphangioma is lymphatic fluid leak. Treatment of this complication by aspiration, chest tube drainage, and fibrin glue application (if drainage alone fails) is usually effective. Lymphangiomas recur in at least 15% of cases after resection, so long-term follow-up is important. There have been rare reports of mediastinal hemangiomas. The preferred treatment of hemangiomas is nonoperative when possible, including the use of pulse corticosteroids or interferon-α.

REFERENCES

1. Adzick NS, Harrison MR, Glick PL, et al: Fetal cystic adenomatoid malformation: Prenatal diagnosis and natural history. J Pediatr Surg 1985;20:483-488.
2. Adzick NS, Harrison MR, Crombleholme TM, et al: Fetal lung lesions: Management and outcome. Am J Obstet Gynecol 1998;179:884-889.
3. Adzick NS, Harrison MR, Flake AW, et al: Fetal surgery for cystic adenomatoid malformation of the lung. J Pediatr Surg 1993;28:806-812.
4. Albanese CT, Sydorak RM, Tsao K: Thoracoscopic lobectomy for prenatally diagnosed lung lesions. J Pediatr Surg 2003;38:553-555.
5. Albright EB, Crane JP, Shackelford GD: Prenatal diagnosis of a bronchogenic cyst. J Ultrasound Med 1988;7:91-95.
6. Aldousany AW, Joyner JC, Priam RA, et al: Diagnosis and treatment of intrapericardial teratoma. Pediatr Cardiol 1987;8:51-53.
7. al-Salem AH: Ectopic thymic tissue simulating a posterior mediastinal mass. Eur J Pediatr Surg 1992;2:106-107.
8. Ankermann T, Oppermann HC, Engler S, et al: Congenital masses of the lung, cystic adenomatoid malformation versus congenital lobar emphysema. J Ultrasound Med 2004;23:1379-1384.
9. Azarow KS, Pearl RH, Zurcher R, et al: Primary mediastinal masses. J Thorac Cardiovasc Surg 1993;106:67-72.
10. Azizkhan RG, Dudgeon DL, Buck JR, et al: Life-threatening airway obstruction as a complication to the management of mediastinal masses in children. J Pediatr Surg 1985;20:816-819.
11. Azizkhan RG, Grimmer DL, Askin FB, et al: Acquired lobar emphysema (over-inflation): Clinical and pathologic evaluation of infants requiring lobectomy. J Pediatr Surg 1992;27:1145-1151.
12. Bale PM, Sotelo-Avila C: Maldescent of the thymus: 34 necropsy and 10 surgical cases, including 7 thymuses medial to the mandible. Pediatr Pathol 1993;13:889-892.
13. Batra P, Brown K, Collins JD, et al: Mediastinal masses: Magnetic resonance imaging in comparison with computed tomography. J Natl Med Assoc 1991;83:969-974.
14. Beardmore HE, Wigglesworth FW: Vertebral anomalies and alimentary duplication. Pediatr Clin North Am 1958;5:457-462.
15. Benjamin DR, Cahill JL: Bronchoalveolar carcinoma of the lung and congenital cystic adenomatoid malformation. Am J Clin Pathol 1991;95:889-892.
16. Bilik R, Ginzberg H, Superina RA: Unconventional treatment of neurenteric cyst in a newborn. J Pediatr Surg 1995;30:115-117.
17. Boothroyd AE, Hall-Craggs MA, Dicks-Mireaux C, et al: The magnetic resonance appearances of the normal thymus in children. Clin Radiol 1992;45:378-381.
18. Boue DR, Smith GA, Krous HF: Lingual bronchogenic cyst in a child: An unusual site of presentation. Pediatr Pathol 1994;14:201-202.
19. Bower RJ, Kiesewetter WB: Mediastinal masses in infants and children. Arch Surg 1977;112:1003-1008.
20. Burgner DP, Carachi R, Beattie TJ: Foregut duplication cyst presenting as neonatal respiratory distress and hemoptysis. Thorax 1994;49:287-290.
21. Cajal SR, Suster S: Primary thymic epithelial neoplasm in children. Am J Surg Pathol 1991;15:466-467.
22. Carney JA, Thompson DP, Johnson CL, et al: Teratomas in children: Clinical and pathologic aspects. J Pediatr Surg 1972;7:271-282.
23. Cartagena AM: Pericardial effusion and cardiac hemangioma in the neonate. Pediatr Radiol 1993;23:384-385.
24. Cass DL, Quinn TM, Yang EY, et al: Increased cell proliferation and decreased apoptosis characterizes congenital cystic adenomatoid malformation. J Pediatr Surg 1998;33:1043-1047.
25. Cass DL, Crombleholme TM, Howell LJ, et al: Cystic lung lesions with systemic arterial blood supply: A hybrid of congenital cystic adenomatoid malformation and bronchopulmonary sequestration. J Pediatr Surg 1997;32:986-990.
26. Cha I, Adzick NS, Harrison MR, et al: Fetal congenital cystic adenomatoid malformations of the lung: A clinicopathologic study of eleven cases. Am J Surg Pathol 1997;21:537-544.
27. Chin KY, Tang MY: Congenital adenomatoid malformation of one lobe of a lung with general anasarca. Arch Pathol 1949;48:221-229.
28. Cohen AJ, Thompson L, Edwards FH, et al: Primary cysts and tumors of the mediastinum. Ann Thorac Surg 1991;51:378-384.
29. Conran RM, Stocker JT: Extralobar sequestration with frequently associated congenital cystic adenomatoid malformation, type 2: Report of 50 cases. Pediatr Dev Pathol 1999;2:454-463.
30. Crombleholme TM, Coleman BG, Howell LJ, et al: Elevated cystic adenomatoid malformation volume ratio (CVR) predicts outcome in prenatal diagnosis of cystic adenomatoid malformation of the lung. J Pediatr Surg 2002;37:331-338.
31. d'Agostino S, Bonoldi E, Dante S, et al: Embryonal rhabdomyosarcoma of the lung arising in cystic adenomatoid malformation. J Pediatr Surg 1997;32:1381-1383.
32. Dehner LP: Germ cell tumors of the mediastinum. Semin Diagn Pathol 1990;7:266-270.
33. Dillon PW, Cilley RE, Krummel TM: Video-assisted thoracoscopic excision of intrathoracic masses in children: Report of two cases. Surg Laparosc Endosc 1993;3:433-435.
34. Dommergues M, Louis-Sylvestre C, Mandelbrot L, et al. Congenital adenomatoid malformation of the lung: When is active fetal therapy indicated? Am J Obstet Gynecol 1997;177:953-958.
35. Doull IJ, Connett GJ, Warner JO: Bronchoscopic appearances of congenital lobar emphysema. Pediatr Pulmonol 1996;21:195-198.
36. Englund AT, Geffner ME, Nagel RA, et al: Pediatric germ cell and human chorionic gonadotropin producing tumors. Am J Dis Child 1991;145:1294-1297.
37. Eraklis AL, Griscom NT, McGovern JB: Bronchogenic cysts of the mediastinum in infancy. N Engl J Med 1969;281:1150-1153.
38. Fallon M, Gordon ARG, Lendrum AD: Mediastinal cysts of foregut origin associated with vertebral anomalies. Br J Surg 1954;41:520-524.
39. Ferro MM, Milner R, Cannizzaro C, et al: Intrathoracic alimentary tract duplication cysts treated in utero by thoracoamniotic shunting. Fetal Diagn Ther 1998;13:343-347.
40. Fischbach R, Benz-Bohm G, Berthold F, et al: Infradiaphragmatic bronchogenic cyst with high CT numbers in a boy with primitive neuroectodermal tumor. Pediatr Radiol 1994;24:504-505.
41. Frenckner B, Freyschuss U: Pulmonary function after lobectomy for congenital lobar emphysema and congenital

cystic adenomatoid malformation: A follow-up study. Scand J Thorac Cardiovasc Surg 1982;16:293-297.

42. Gienski JA, Thibeault DW, Hall FK, et al: Selective bronchial intubation in infants with lobar emphysema: Indications, complications, and long-term outcome. Am J Perinatol 1986;3:199-204.

43. Goetch E: Hygroma colli cysticum and hygroma axillae. Arch Surg 1938;36:395-399.

44. Gordon I, Dempsey JE: Infantile lobar emphysema in association with congenital heart disease. Clin Radiol 1990; 41:48-53.

45. Goto H, Boozalis ST, Benson KI, et al: High-frequency jet ventilation for resection of congenital lobar emphysema. Anesth Analg 1987;66:684-686.

46. Granata C, Gambini C, Balducci T, et al: Bronchioloalveolar carcinoma arising in a congenital cystic adenomatoid malformation in a child: Case report and review of the literature. Pediatr Pulmonol 1996;25:62-66.

47. Grosfeld JL: Primary tumors of the chest wall and mediastinum in children. Semin Thorac Cardiovasc Surg 1994; 6:235-239.

48. Grosfeld JL, Billmire DF: Teratomas in infancy and childhood. Curr Probl Cancer 1985;11:3-34.

49. Grosfeld JL, Skinner MA, Rescorla FJ, et al: Mediastinal tumors in children: Experience with 196 cases. Ann Surg Oncol 1994;1:121-127.

50. Gross RE: The Surgery of Infancy and Childhood: Its Principles and Techniques. Philadelphia, WB Saunders, 1953.

51. Gross RE, Neuhauser ED, Longino LA: Thoracic diverticula which originate from the intestine. Ann Surg 1950; 131:363-365.

52. Harrison MR, Adzick NS, Jennings RW, et al: Antenatal intervention for congenital cystic adenomatoid malformation. Lancet 1990;336:965-966.

53. Hedrick HL, Flake AW, Crombleholme TM, et al: The EXIT procedure for high risk fetal lung lesions. J Pediatr Surg 2005;40:1038-1043.

54. Hendren WH, McKee DM: Lobar emphysema in infancy. J Pediatr Surg 1966;1:24-32.

55. Hemanz-Schulman M, Stein SM, Neblett WW, et al: Pulmonary sequestration: Diagnosis with color Doppler sonography and a new theory of associated hydrothorax. Radiology 1991;180:817-821.

56. Hirose R, Suita S, Taguchi T, et al: Extralobar pulmonary sequestration mimicking cystic adenomatoid malformation in prenatal sonographic appearance and histologic findings. J Pediatr Surg 1995;30:1390-1394.

57. Hislop A, Reid L: New pathologic findings in emphysema of childhood: I. Polyalveolar lobe with emphysema. Thorax 1970;25:682-690.

58. Holcomb GW III, Gheissari A, O'Neill JA Jr, et al: Surgical management of alimentary tract duplications. Ann Surg 1989;209:167-174.

59. Ikezoe J, Takeuch N, Johkoh T, et al: MRI of anterior mediastinal tumors. Radiat Med 1992;10:176-183.

60. John LC, Kingston J, Edmondson ST: Teratoma associated with endodermal sinus tumor. Pediatr Hematol Oncol 1993; 10:49-53.

61. Kaplinsky C, Mor C, Cohen IJ, et al: Childhood malignant thymoma: Clinical, therapeutic, and immunohistochemical considerations. Pediatr Hematol Oncol 1992;9: 261-268.

62. Karl SR, Dunn J: Posterior mediastinal teratomas. J Pediatr Surg 1985;5:508-511.

63. Keon TP: Death on induction of anesthesia for cervical node biopsy. Anesthesiology 1981;55:471-473.

64. Kern JA, Daniel TM, Tribble C, et al: Thoracoscopic diagnosis and treatment of mediastinal masses. Ann Thorac Surg 1993;56:92-96.

65. Keswani SG, Crombleholme TM, Pawel BR, et al: Prenatal diagnosis and management of mainstem bronchial atresia. Fetal Diagn Ther 2005;20:74-78.

66. Khosa JK, Leong SL, Borzi PA: Congenital cystic adenomatoid malformation of the lung: Indications and timing of surgery. Pediatr Surg Int 2004;20:505-508.

67. King RM, Telander RL, Smithson KA, et al: Primary mediastinal tumors in children. J Pediatr Surg 1982;5:512-520.

68. Kropp J, Emons D, Winkler C: Neurenteric cyst diagnosed by technetium-99m pertechnetate sequential scintigraphy. J Nucl Med 1987;28:1218-1221.

69. Kuller JA, Laifer JA, Martin JG, et al: Unusual presentations of fetal teratoma. J Perinatol 1991;11:294-296.

70. Laberge JM, Flageole H, Pugash D, et al: Outcome of the prenatally diagnosed congenital cystic adenomatoid lung malformation: A Canadian experience. Fetal Diagn Ther 2001;16:178-186.

71. Laberge JM, Bratu I, Flageole H: The management of asymptomatic congenital lung malformations. Paediatr Respir Rev 2004;5(Suppl):S305-S312.

72. Lam WW, Chan FL, Lau YL, et al: Paediatric thymoma: Unusual occurrence in two siblings. Pediatr Radiol 1993;23: 124-126.

73. Lazar RH, Younis RT, Bassila MN: Bronchogenic cysts: A cause of stridor in the neonate, Am J Otolaryngol 1991; 12:117-120.

74. Leape LL, Longino LA: Infantile lobar emphysema. Pediatrics 1964;34:246-251.

75. Lemoine G, Montupet P: Mediastinal tumors in infancy and childhood. In Fallis JC, Filler FM, Lemoine G (eds): Pediatric Thoracic Surgery. New York, Elsevier, 1991, pp 103-110.

76. Liechty KW, Quinn TM, Cass DL, et al: Elevated PDGF-β in congenital cystic adenomatoid malformations requiring fetal resection. J Pediatr Surg 1999;34:805-810.

77. Linegar AG, Odell JA, Fennell WM, et al: Massive thymic hyperplasia. Ann Thorac Surg 1993;55:1197-1199.

78. Lobe TE: Pediatric thoracoscopy. Semin Thorac Cardiovasc Surg 1993;5:298-302.

79. Mani H, Suarez E, Stocker JT: The morphologic spectrum of infantile lobar emphysema: A study of 33 cases. Paediatr Respir Rev 2004;5(Suppl):S313-S320.

80. MacGillivray TE, Harrison MR, Goldstein RB, et al: Disappearing fetal lung lesions. J Pediatr Surg 1993;28: 1321-1324.

81. MacKenzie TC, Guttenberg ME, Nissenbaum HL, et al: A fetal lung lesion consisting of bronchogenic cyst, bronchopulmonary sequestration, and congenital cystic adenomatoid malformation: The missing link? Fetal Diagn Ther 2001;16:193-195.

82. McVay CB: Mediastinum. In Anson BJ, McVay CB (eds): Surgical Anatomy, 6th ed. Philadelphia, WB Saunders, 1984, pp 296-308.

83. Meizner I, Levy A: A survey of non-cardiac fetal intrathoracic malformations diagnosed by ultrasound. Arch Gynecol Obstet 1994;255:31-37.

84. Merchant AM, Hedrick HL, Crombleholme TM, et al: Management of fetal mediastinal teratoma: A report of two cases. J Pediatr Surg 2005;40:228-231.

85. Messineo A, Wesson DE, Filler RA, et al: Juvenile hemangiomas involving the thoracic trachea in children: Report of two cases. J Pediatr Surg 1992;27:1291-1295.

86. Miller JA, Corteville JE, Langer JC: Congenital cystic adenomatoid malformation in the fetus: Natural history and predictors of outcome. J Pediatr Surg 1996;31:805-808.

87. Moran CA, Suster S: Mediastinal hemangiomas: A study of 18 cases with emphasis on the spectrum of morphological features. Hum Pathol 1995;26:416-420.

88. Muraskas JK, Gianopoulos JG, Husain A, Black PR: Mediastinal cystic hygroma: Prenatal decompression with neonatal resection and recurrence at 19 months of age. J Perinatol 1993;13:381-383.

89. Murphy JJ, Blair GK, Fraser GC, et al: Rhabdomyosarcoma arising within congenital pulmonary cysts: Report of three cases. J Pediatr Surg 1992;27:1364-1367.

90. Murray ME: Bilateral communicating bronchopulmonary foregut malformation in an infant with multiple congenital anomalies. Pediatr Radiol 1994;24:128-132.

91. Nuchtern JG, Harberg FJ: Congenital lung cysts. Semin Pediatr Surg 3:233, 1994.

92. Olutoye O, Coleman B, Hubbard AM, et al: Prenatal diagnosis and management of congenital lobar emphysema. J Pediatr Surg 2000;35:792-795.

93. Ozcelik U, Gocmen A, Kiper N, et al: Congenital lobar emphysema: Evaluation and long-term followup of thirty cases at a single center. Pediatr Pulmonol 2003;35:384-391.

94. Paterson IM, Cockburn JS: Acute pericarditis due to perforation of a benign mediastinal teratodermoid into the pericardial sac. Thorax 1982;37:863-865.

95. Philippart AI: On foregut duplications. J Pediatr Pulm 1994;18:45.

96. Phillipos EZ, Libsekal K: Flexible bronchoscopy in the management of congenital lobar emphysema in the neonate. Can Resp J 1998;5:219-221.

97. Piramoon AN, Abbassioun K: Mediastinal enterogenic cyst with spinal cord compression. J Pediatr Surg 1974;9: 543-545.

98. Pokorny WJ: Mediastinal tumors. In Ashcraft KW, Holder TM (eds): Pediatric Surgery, 2nd ed. Philadelphia, WB Saunders, 1993, pp 218-227.

99. Pokorny WJ, Goldstein IR: Enteric thoracoabdominal duplications in children. J Thorac Cardiovasc Surg 1984; 87:821-825.

100. Pokorny WJ, Sherman JO: Mediastinal masses in infants and children. J Thorac Cardiovasc Surg 1974;68: 869-873.

101. Pul N, Pul M: Bronchogenic cyst of the scapular area in an infant: Case report and review of the literature. J Am Acad Dermatol 1994;3:120-122.

102. Quinn TM, Hubbard AM, Adzick NS: Prenatal magnetic resonance imaging enhances prenatal diagnosis. J Pediatr Surg 1998;33:312-316.

103. Ramon Y, Cajal S, Suster S: Primary thymic epithelial neoplasms in children. Am J Surg Pathol 1991;15:466-471.

104. Ransom JM, Norton JB: Pulmonary sequestration presenting as congestive heart failure. J Thorac Cardiovasc Surg 1978;76:378-381.

105. Read CA, Moront M, Carangelo R, et al: Recurrent bronchogenic cyst: An argument for complete surgical excision. Arch Surg 1991;126:1306-1308.

106. Ribet ME, Copin MC, Soots JG, et al: Bronchioloalveolar carcinoma and congenital cystic adenomatoid malformation. Ann Thorac Surg 1995;60:1126-1128.

107. Rice HE, Flake AW, Hori T, et al: Massive thymic hyperplasia: Characterization of a rare mediastinal mass. J Pediatr Surg 1994;29:1561-1564.

108. Robie DK, Gursoy MH, Pokorny WJ: Mediastinal tumors: Airway obstruction and management. Semin Pediatr Surg 1994;3:259-263.

109. Rubin EM, Garciatt C, Horowitz MD, et al: Fatal massive hemoptysis secondary to intralobar sequestration. Chest 1994;106:954-955.

110. Rubush JL, Gardner IR, Boyd WC, et al: Mediastinal tumors: Review of 186 cases. J Thorac Cardiovasc Surg 1973;65:216-222.

111. Saenz NC, Schnitzer JJ, Eraklis AE, et al: Posterior mediastinal masses. J Pediatr Surg 1993;28:172-176.

112. Sakala EP, Perrott WS, Grube GL: Sonographic characteristics of antenatally diagnosed extralobar pulmonary sequestration and congenital cystic adenomatoid malformation. Obstet Gynecol Surv 1994;49:647-655.

113. Saltzman DH, Adzick NS, Benacerraf BR: Fetal cystic adenomatoid malformation of the lung: Apparent improvement in utero. Obstet Gynecol 1988;71:1000-1003.

114. Shamberger RC, Holzman RS, Griscom NT, et al: CT quantification of tracheal cross-sectional area as a guide to the surgical and anesthetic management of children with anterior mediastinal masses. J Pediatr Surg 1991;26: 138-142.

115. Shields TW: Primary Tumors and Cysts of the Mediastinum. Philadelphia, Lea & Febiger, 1972, p 32.

116. Simpson I, Campbell PE: Mediastinal masses in childhood: A review from a paediatric pathologist's point of view. Prog Pediatr Surg 1991;27:92-96.

117. Skandalakis JE, Gray SW, Ricketts R: The esophagus. In Skandalakis JE, Gray SW (eds): Embryology for Surgeons. Philadelphia, WB Saunders, 1994, pp 65-112.

118. Skandalakis JE, Gray SW, Todd NW: The pharynx and its derivatives. In Skandalakis JE, Gray SW (eds): Embryology for Surgeons. Philadelphia, WB Saunders, 1994, pp 17-64.

119. Slovis TL, Meza M, Kuhn JP: Aberrant thymus––MR assessment. Pediatr Radiol 1992;22:490-494.

120. Snyder ME, Luck SR, Hernandez R, et al: Diagnostic dilemmas of mediastinal cysts. J Pediatr Surg 1985;20: 810-815.

121. Srikanth MS, Ford EG, Stanley P, et al: Communicating bronchopulmonary foregut malformations: Classification and embryogenesis. J Pediatr Surg 1992;27:732-736.

122. Stocker JT, Manewell JE, Drake RM: Congenital cystic adenomatoid malformation of the lung: Classification and morphologic spectrum. Hum Pathol 1977;8:155-161.

123. Stocker JT: Congenital pulmonary airway malformation: A new name and an expanded classification of congenital cystic adenomatoid malformations of the lung. Histopathology 2002;41:424-431.

124. Stringer MD, Spitz L, Abel R, et al: Management of alimentary tract duplications in children. Br J Surg 1995; 82:74-78.

125. Suen HC, Mathisen DJ, Grillo HC, et al: Surgical management and radiological characteristics of bronchogenic cysts. Ann Thorac Surg 1993;55:476-481.

126. Suster S, Rosai J: Thymic carcinoma. Cancer 1991;67: 1025-1028.

127. Swanson SJ 3d, Skoog SJ, Garcia V, et al: Pseudoadrenal mass: Unusual presentation of bronchogenic cyst. J Pediatr Surg 1991;26:1401-1403.

128. Taguchi T, Suita S, Yamanouchi T, et al: Antenatal diagnosis and surgical management of congenital cystic adenomatoid malformation of the lung. Fetal Diagn Ther 1995;10:400-404.

129. Thompson DP, Moore TC: Acute thoracic distress in childhood due to spontaneous rupture of a large mediastinal teratoma. J Pediatr Surg 1969;4:416-419.

130. Thompson J, Forfar JO: Regional obstructive emphysema in infancy. Arch Dis Child 1958;33:97-101.

131. Thorpe-Veeston JG, Nicolaides KH: Cystic adenomatoid malformation of the lung: Prenatal diagnosis and outcome. Prenat Diagn 1994;14:677-681.

132. Ueda K, Gruppo R, Martin L, et al: Rhabdomyosarcoma arising in a congenital cystic adenomatoid malformation. Cancer 1977;40:383-388.

133. Warner JO, Rubin S, Heard BE: Congenital lobar emphysema: A case with bronchial atresia and abnormal bronchial cartilages. Br J Dis Chest 1982;76:177-181.

134. Weimann RB, Hallman GL, Bahar D, et al: Intrathoracic meningocele: A case report and review of the literature. J Thorac Cardiovasc Surg 1963;46:40-49.

135. Winters WD, Effmann EL, Nghien HV, et al: Disappearing fetal lung masses: Importance of postnatal imaging studies. Pediatr Radiol 1997;27:535-539.

136. Wright JR Jr, Gillis DA: Mediastinal foregut cyst containing an intramural adrenal cortical rest: A case report and review of supradiaphragmatic adrenal rests. Pediatr Pathol 1993;13:407-409.

Chapter 62

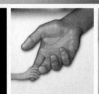

Laryngoscopy, Bronchoscopy, and Thoracoscopy

Bradley M. Rodgers and Eugene D. McGahren III

The ability to view the larynx and tracheobronchial tree directly in living subjects has long intrigued physicians. Bozzini, in 1806, is credited with being the first to design an instrument specially to visualize the larynx and upper airway.[5] His hollow tube was illuminated by a wax candle whose light was reflected with a mirror down the axis of the instrument. Babington, in 1829, devised the laryngeal mirror, which used reflected light. Several physicians subsequently developed rigid tubes with reflected light for observation of the esophagus and proximal part of the stomach. The major breakthrough, however, in the evolution of endoscopy came in 1879 when Nitze developed a cystoscope with a distal lens illuminated by a heated platinum coil.[40] Shortly thereafter, Nitze adapted Thomas Edison's discovery of the incandescent light bulb to his telescopic instrument by placing a bulb with a miniature filament at the end of the tube. Kirstein developed a laryngoscope with a blade, similar to our modern Miller blade, that was illuminated by an incandescent bulb in the handle, and Chevalier Jackson modified this instrument by placing the bulb on the distal portion of the blade and adding a removable floor to the laryngoscope.[27]

The final significant advance in rigid endoscopic technology was development of the Hopkins rod-lens system. Hopkins constructed a rigid endoscopic telescope with a series of lenses separated by quartz glass that enormously improved transmission of light through the instrument and allowed more magnification and better image resolution than had ever before been possible. In turn, this development allowed for miniaturization of endoscopes, applicable for use in children, and recording of high-resolution images on film and television.

Hopkins was also instrumental in development of the early flexible fiber-optic endoscopes. In 1930 Lamm discovered that images could be transmitted through thin fiberglass threads that were oriented and bound tightly together.[29] A prototype flexible gastroscope using this fiber-optic technology was developed by Hopkins in 1954 and was first used clinically by Hirschowitz et al. in 1958.[18] Ikeda adapted this same technology to the development of a flexible fiber-optic bronchoscope in 1970.[21]

Subsequent refinement in this technology allowed the development of truly miniaturized flexible fiber-optic laryngoscopes and bronchoscopes, suitable for use in infants and children of any size.

The history of the development of thoracoscopy, in significant measure, parallels that of airway and gastrointestinal endoscopy. In 1910 Hans Jacobaeus used Nitze's cystoscope to visualize the pleural space in patients with pulmonary tuberculosis.[22] In that era, artificial pneumothorax was known to be effective in treating many patients with cavitary tuberculosis, and Jacobaeus quickly perfected techniques to perform "closed intrapleural pneumolysis" with the cystoscope and a galvanic cautery. Jacobaeus coined the term "thoracoscopy" and by 1921 was able to show the utility of this procedure for the diagnosis of intrathoracic carcinoma by observation and direct biopsy.[23] Rodgers and Talbert used the Hopkins rod-lens telescope for thoracoscopy and suggested the use of this technique for lung biopsy for the diagnosis of pulmonary infiltrates in immunocompromised children and reported its successful application in this clinical setting in 1976.[59]

LARYNGOSCOPY

Indications

Laryngoscopy is used for both diagnostic and therapeutic purposes in pediatric patients. The most common indication for laryngoscopy in infants and children is for the evaluation of stridor.[17,32] The term *stridor* refers to a high-pitched respiratory sound created by turbulence of airway gases. Laryngeal and supraglottic pathology usually creates inspiratory stridor, which may change in nature with different positions or certain activities. Tracheal narrowing is generally manifested as expiratory stridor. Most infants and children with persistent inspiratory stridor should undergo laryngoscopy to establish a precise anatomic diagnosis. Other common indications for diagnostic laryngoscopy in children include a change in cry or voice, acute respiratory distress, or repeated episodes of aspiration. Indications for therapeutic laryngoscopy in children include the treatment of congenital or acquired subglottic stenosis, laryngeal webs, laryngoesophageal clefts, and laryngeal papilloma. Laryngeal foreign bodies, though uncommon, can be a cause of sudden respiratory distress and are thus an important indication for emergency laryngoscopy.

Instrumentation

A surgeon performing laryngoscopy in infants and children must be skilled in the use of both flexible and rigid endoscopes and must have a broad array of instrumentation available. Often, rigid and flexible instruments are used in conjunction with each other because each has advantages and disadvantages in certain clinical situations. The standard rigid laryngoscopes used in pediatric practice are open sided with blades varying between 8 and 13.5 cm in length. Illumination is provided by a high-intensity light source aimed down the blade from a prism in the handle of the instrument (Fig. 62-1). Certain specialized laryngoscopes, such as the pediatric Dedo laryngoscope, allow suspension laryngoscopy for more complex operative procedures. The anterior commissure endoscope has an 11-cm-long blade with a keel configuration of the distal portion (Fig. 62-2). This endoscope is helpful in exposing

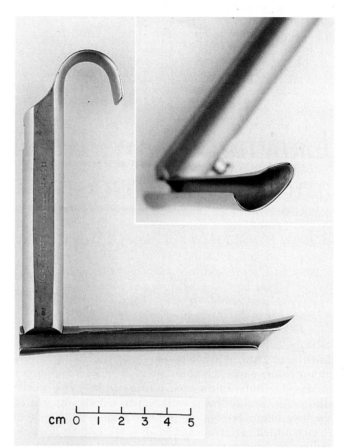

Figure 62–2 Anterior commissures endoscope. This instrument has an 11-cm-long blade with a keel configuration of the distal portion (*inset*). Illumination is provided by a prism in the handle. This instrument may be suspended.

the anterior aspect of the larynx in small infants. In addition, the configuration of the blade allows abduction of the vocal cords for the diagnosis of a laryngoesophageal cleft.

The flexible instruments used for laryngoscopy in infants and children vary in size from the 2.0-mm-outer-diameter ultrathin bronchoscope to the 3.6-mm-outer-diameter pediatric bronchoscope. The ultrathin endoscope does not have an instrument or suction channel and has only two-way deflection of the tip, thus limiting its use to diagnostic examinations. The standard pediatric flexible bronchoscope has two-way tip deflection and a suction or instrument channel. This endoscope can be used satisfactorily to visualize the larynx in all but very small premature infants (<1000 g) and may be used to obtain biopsy samples.[10] The flexible fiber-optic nasopharyngoscope is an instrument specifically designed for evaluation of the larynx and pharynx. This instrument has a 3.9-mm outer diameter and a length of only 25 cm.[66] In view of the cost of flexible instruments, however, most physicians prefer to use the small bronchoscopes for laryngeal evaluation despite their length.[11]

A surgeon preparing to perform a laryngoscopic examination must be certain that all these instruments are in functional order and that accessory instrumentation such as biopsy and foreign body forceps is available and functioning.

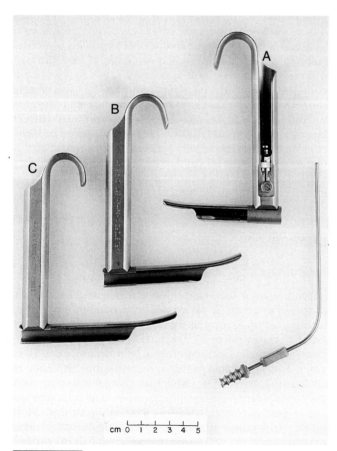

Figure 62–1 Pediatric rigid laryngoscopes. These instruments have blades ranging from 8 cm (A) through 13.5 cm (C) in length. Illumination is provided by a light prism in the handle of the instrument. These instruments may be suspended.

Procedure

Diagnostic laryngoscopy in infants and children may be performed either with sedation and topical anesthesia or with general anesthesia. Usually, patients undergoing rigid laryngoscopy are administered general anesthesia. All patients must be thoroughly monitored during the endoscopic procedures. Continuous electrocardiographic (ECG) and pulse oximeter monitoring should be performed to detect the hypoxia or bradycardia that is occasionally precipitated by these procedures. Anesthesia is induced with the mask, and if possible, the patient is not intubated before direct laryngoscopy. The patient is then positioned with the neck extended and the jaw slightly flexed. All the instruments anticipated for examination of the airway are sterilized and available in the operating room. The rigid laryngoscope is passed along the right border of the tongue until the epiglottis is visualized. The blade of the laryngoscope is passed under the epiglottis and used to elevate this structure to visualize the supraglottic larynx and vocal cords. Often, subglottic pathology can be appreciated from this vantage. With the endoscope in this position, movement of the larynx with respiratory effort is observed. In patients with laryngomalacia, the base of the epiglottis is often narrow ("omega shaped"), and the arytenoid processes coapt in the midline with inspiratory effort (Fig. 62-3). Frequently, visualization of the vocal cords is completely lost during inspiration in these patients. In cases of vocal cord paralysis, the affected cord will be noted to be in the midposition and will not abduct with inspiration. After the cords have been evaluated, the glottic airway may be sprayed with lidocaine (4 mg/kg) to minimize laryngospasm as the rest of the examination proceeds. Use of the anterior commissure endoscope often allows for better visualization of the anterior aspect of the larynx, particularly in small infants. Passage of the narrow tip of this endoscope into the glottic opening allows forced abduction of the cords and visualization of the cords and the

posterior laryngeal membrane, the area of a laryngoesophageal cleft.

For many therapeutic procedures on the larynx, use of the suspension laryngoscope is essential because it allows binocular magnification of the larynx and unimpeded use of laryngeal surgical instruments. The square blade of the suspension laryngoscope is passed beneath the epiglottis, and the tip is elevated to expose the larynx and supraglottic airway. The suspension apparatus is supported on a Mayo stand placed over the patient's chest. For procedures involving the anterior aspect of the larynx, the anterior commissure endoscope may be suspended in similar fashion.

If the preoperative diagnosis is laryngomalacia, the examination is often initiated with the flexible endoscope. This instrument is passed through the nose into the posterior of the pharynx. It is slowly advanced until the epiglottis is identified. Positioning the tip of the endoscope just beyond the epiglottis on the posterior pharyngeal wall allows excellent visualization of the laryngeal airway and assessment of its dynamic function with respiratory effort. Assessment of laryngeal motion with the flexible endoscope is superior to that obtained with the rigid endoscope because there is no distortion of the larynx or supraglottic airway with the instrument itself.[15] The flexible endoscope may be passed through the laryngeal mask airway (LMA) to visualize the glottis in patients under general anesthesia.[2] In most instances, after complete evaluation of the larynx and supraglottic airway, a bronchoscopic examination is performed to rule out associated distal pathology.

Complications

Complications of diagnostic laryngoscopy are rare, with the exception of exaggerated airway obstruction secondary to laryngeal edema. In situations in which diagnostic laryngoscopy is being performed in patients with severe airway obstruction, equipment should be available for emergency tracheostomy. Likewise, preoperative discussions with the anesthesiologist should emphasize the potential need for intubation with a small (2.5 mm) endotracheal tube for emergency ventilation. The complications resulting from therapeutic laryngoscopy depend on the procedure being performed. Perforation of the larynx or pharynx is a potential but uncommon complication after vigorous laryngeal dilation or the use of lasers or cryotherapy for the treatment of laryngeal or subglottic stenosis. The potential for hypoxia developing during the performance of laryngoscopy may be minimized by insufflating oxygen through the suction channel of the flexible laryngoscope or through a tube placed in the corner of the mouth while using the rigid scope. Hoeve et al. recorded an overall complication rate of 1.9% in children undergoing rigid laryngobronchoscopy.[19] There was a 0.5% complication rate in infants younger than 3 months. Complications included hemorrhage (0.5%), cardiac arrhythmias (0.6%), subglottic edema (0.3%), and pneumothorax (1.2%). The complication of cardiac arrhythmia was eliminated with the use of pulse oximetry to monitor patients. Wood has reported a 2.9% complication rate with no mortality in a large series of children undergoing flexible laryngobronchoscopy.[74]

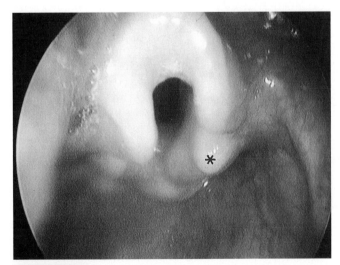

Figure 62–3 Endoscopic appearance of the supraglottic area in a child with laryngomalacia. Note the "omega-shaped" epiglottis with a very narrow base. The arytenoids (*asterisk*) collapsed in the midline with inspiration.

BRONCHOSCOPY

Indications

Bronchoscopy is used for both diagnostic and therapeutic purposes in the care of infants and children. Indications include stridor, persistent atelectasis, persistent cough, recurrent or persistent pneumonia, suspicion of an airway foreign body, assistance in intubation, assessment of endotracheal tube placement, bronchial toilet, airway bleeding, and postoperative or postextubation hoarseness or wheezing.[47,56,76] Interventions undertaken with bronchoscopy may include removal of a foreign body or secretions, tracheostomy care, bronchoalveolar lavage, instillation of medications, laser therapy, balloon dilation or placement of stents for obstructing lesions, and transbronchial biopsy.[8,39,51,57,63,77] Relative contraindications to bronchoscopy may include a bleeding diathesis, hemodynamic instability, arrhythmias, hypoxemia, pulmonary hypertension, or potential airway obstruction.[37,42] The value of the information to be gained from the bronchoscopic examination must always be weighed against the potential risks of the procedure.

Instrumentation

Pediatric bronchoscopes are available as both flexible and rigid instruments. The initial and still standard pediatric flexible bronchoscope has an outer diameter of 3.5 to 3.7 mm with a 1.2-mm suction instrument port. Movement of the tip is bidirectional and has a range of 180 to 220 degrees. The suction port allows either instillation of fluids or oxygen or suctioning of airway mucus. However, the small size of the suction channel makes suctioning of tenacious mucus difficult and does not easily allow transbronchial biopsy. The smallest endotracheal tube that this bronchoscope can pass through is 4.5 mm. In patients without endotracheal tubes, however, this bronchoscope can usually be passed transnasally, even in infants as small as 700 g.[10,74,75,77] There is also a 2.8-mm flexible bronchoscope with a 1.2-mm suction port that has the capabilities of the 3.5-mm scope and is therefore preferable in smaller children.[77] Smaller, ultrathin bronchoscopes with outer diameters of 2.7, 2.2, 2.0, and 1.8 mm are now commonly used. Suction channels of 0.7 to 0.8 mm are available in the 2.7- and 2.2-mm endoscopes.[16,65,77,78] The 1.8-mm scope lacks a bidirectional tip. Endoscopes 2.2 mm and smaller can pass through a 2.5-mm endotracheal tube.[41]

The rigid pediatric bronchoscope consists of a rigid rod-lens telescope that is passed through an outer sheath. The sheath has an inner diameter of 3.5 to 7.5 mm and a length of 23 or 30 cm (Fig. 62-4). The telescope size used for any particular sheath must be chosen to maximize visualization while minimizing airway resistance.[35] A special adapter allows for ventilation directly through the sheath. In addition, an instrument port allows passage of a catheter for irrigation or suctioning. Grasping and biopsy instruments are coupled directly to rigid telescopes

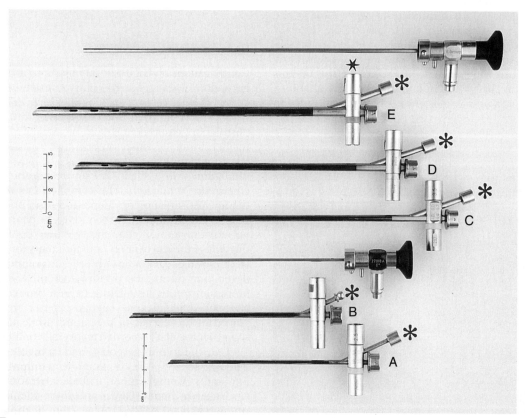

Figure 62-4 Pediatric rigid bronchoscopes. These instruments vary in size between 2.5 × 20 cm (A) and 6 × 30 cm (E). The rod-lens telescope is passed directly through the shaft of these instruments. The operative side channel (*asterisks*) allows passage of suction and surgical instruments. The ventilator side channel (*star*) allows continuous ventilation during the procedure.

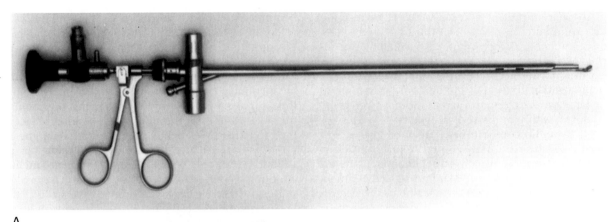

A

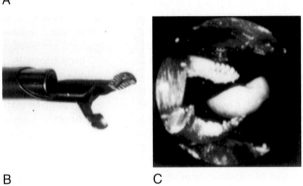

B   C

Figure 62–5 *A,* Optical forceps. *B,* The peanut grasper is coupled to a long endoscopic telescope for direct, magnified vision for foreign body extraction. *C,* The magnified image allows precise positioning of the grasping forceps for safe foreign body removal.

to create optical forceps that can be passed through the sheath (Fig. 62-5). Even though rigid bronchoscope sheaths are labeled according to their minimal inner diameter, these sizes do not necessarily correlate with actual working sizes. Actual sizes for the Storz rigid bronchoscopes are included in Table 62-1. Care must be taken to choose a bronchoscope that is the appropriate size for the infant or child to be examined and that allows enough room within the sheath for the placement of telescopic instruments or catheters if necessary.

TABLE 62-1 Storz Bronchoscope Dimensions

Nominal Size	Inside Diameter (mm)	Outside Diameter (mm)	Length (cm)
2.5 × 20	3.5	4.2	20
3.0 × 20/26/30	4.3	5.0	20/26/30
3.5 × 20/26/30	5.0	5.7	20/26/30
4.0 × 30	6.0	6.7	30
5.0 × 30	7.1	7.8	30
6.0 × 30	7.5	8.2	30

Adapted from Marzo SJ, Hotaling AJ: Trade-off between airway resistance and optical resolution in pediatric rigid bronchoscopy. Ann Otol Rhinol Laryngol 1995;104:282.

Procedure

Before any bronchoscopic examination, a thorough history and physical examination should be performed. Particular attention should be paid to any abnormalities of the neck or spine that might make passage of the bronchoscope difficult, the position of the trachea in the neck, and any asymmetry in breath sounds. Frontal and lateral chest radiographs should be obtained in all patients to define the intrathoracic anatomy and pathology. A barium swallow may be helpful if vascular compression of the airway or gastroesophageal reflux is suspected. Cinefluoroscopy or inspiratory-expiratory chest radiographs may help confirm the presence and identify the location of a suspected airway foreign body. In some instances, computed tomography (CT) of the chest may aid in evaluation of the intrathoracic airway and surrounding structures. Once the bronchoscopic procedure begins, one must be prepared for emergency access to the airway by either endotracheal intubation or tracheostomy.

A surgeon preparing to perform bronchoscopy must be familiar with all the available equipment, and the equipment must be in working order. Care must be taken in the maintenance of bronchoscopic equipment as well because inadequate cleaning or the development of cracks in the equipment may predispose to bacterial contamination.[39] The appropriate-sized equipment must be available for the size and needs of the child. If a foreign body is to be removed, it may be valuable to test the grasping equipment on a sample of the suspected object before commencing the procedure.[71] Virtually all bronchoscopic examinations are now undertaken with the use of video monitoring and recording with magnification. This facilitates visualization of the anatomy, documentation for later review, comparisons of findings over time, and discussion with parents and caretakers.[39]

Flexible bronchoscopy can be performed at the bedside in an intensive care unit setting. Preoxygenation is imperative. Sedation is usually supplemented with an antisialagogue such as atropine to minimize reflex bradycardia, a topical anesthetic such as lidocaine to anesthetize the pharynx and upper airway, and anxiolytics. Steroids may be helpful to minimize postprocedure edema.[37,41,47] The bronchoscope is passed transnasally in a nonintubated patient. In a ventilated patient, an appropriately sized bronchoscope can be passed directly through the endotracheal tube. In some instances, the flexible bronchoscope may be introduced through a T-adapter, thus allowing continuation of ventilation or administration of supplemental oxygen during the procedure. Ventilation cannot be accomplished through the flexible bronchoscope; therefore, the patient must be able to breathe spontaneously around the scope or must be mechanically ventilated while the bronchoscope is manipulated though the T-adapter. This is not an insignificant limitation because the normal infant airway is only approximately 5 mm in diameter and resistance to airflow increases inversely with the fourth power of the radius. In addition, the normal ventilatory cycle allows twice the time for expiration as for inspiration.

The LMA has proved to be a particularly useful adjunct to flexible bronchoscopy, although rigid bronchoscopy may be accomplished through the LMA as well. The LMA provides a leakless anesthesia circuit for bronchoscopic examination. It allows airway support with positive pressure, CO_2 monitoring, assisted ventilation, and anesthetic delivery without leakage into the surrounding environment. The LMA also allows the use of larger fiber-optic instruments than would be possible with a transnasal or endotracheal tube approach. This, in turn, allows the use of larger suction chambers. Finally, the LMA facilitates examination in patients with anatomic limitations such as micrognathia or a rigid neck and may facilitate securing of a difficult airway by allowing easier passage of a flexible bronchoscope over which an endotracheal tube may be placed. Potential contraindications to use of the LMA for bronchoscopy include gastroesophageal reflux, a full stomach, or poor pulmonary compliance.[2,43,64,70]

In the presence of a partially occluding bronchoscope, "breath stacking" may occur with an accumulation of carbon dioxide.[25] Thus, examinations with the flexible bronchoscope, including suctioning of mucus, should be limited to 30 to 45 seconds.[76] ECG, pulse oximetry, and possibly end-expiratory CO_2 monitoring should be performed during the entire procedure.[39] To compensate for the occlusive effects of the flexible bronchoscope, supplemental oxygen can be administered through the suction port or through a catheter in the opposite nares when an ultrathin scope without a suction port is

being used. In the setting in which mucus is being removed, saline or mucolytic agents may be instilled through the suction port to allow removal of thicker secretions. If a mucous plug is particularly tenacious and cannot be suctioned through the port, it can sometimes be suctioned against the tip of the bronchoscope and then removed by carefully withdrawing the scope from the airway. It is important that team members, other than the bronchoscopist, be involved in monitoring the child's progress because "bronchoscopist hypnosis" (i.e., preoccupation with the bronchoscopic findings and lack of attention to the patient's status) may be a hazard.[75]

Despite increasingly widespread use of the flexible bronchoscope, the rigid bronchoscope remains an important instrument for evaluation of the pediatric airway and for treatment of various airway disorders. Many centers still use the rigid bronchoscope almost exclusively in infants and children, and the pediatric surgeon should be familiar with its capabilities and limitations.[12,50] Rigid bronchoscopy is particularly indicated for the removal of foreign bodies. Use of the flexible bronchoscope as an adjunct in assessing for the presence of foreign bodies has been reported.[34,79] In these instances, flexible bronchoscopy has been used to rule in or out the presence of a foreign body. Rigid bronchoscopy is then used if a foreign body is found. There are limited reports of the use of flexible bronchoscopy to actually retrieve foreign bodies.[68,73] However, rigid bronchoscopy remains the preferred technique for retrieving aspirated airway foreign bodies.[8,77]

Rigid bronchoscopy in children is generally performed in the operating room with the patient under general anesthesia. The anesthesiologist should be fully aware of the plans for the procedure. The importance of the anesthesiologist's role in maintaining a proper level of anesthesia and being fully familiar with all of the planned manipulations by the surgeon cannot be stressed enough. The patient's breathing may be spontaneous or controlled, depending on the indications for the examination. Spontaneous breathing is usually desired to assess laryngeal, cord, and tracheal wall movement. It is also desired when removing a foreign body because positive-pressure ventilation can cause a foreign body to impact into distal bronchi. In the case of a severely ill infant or child, rigid bronchoscopy can be performed in the intensive care unit setting safely with the appropriate personnel and equipment.[38]

After induction of anesthesia, the patient is positioned with a small roll under the shoulders and the neck slightly extended. The larynx is visualized with a laryngoscope held in the left hand. A Miller blade is the most useful because it holds the epiglottis out of the way as the bronchoscope is advanced. The larynx and cords may be visualized through the bronchoscope as it is passed along the right side of the laryngoscope and advanced gently into the trachea. Because the pediatric airway is quite pliable, an appropriately sized rigid bronchoscope can usually be passed far enough distally to evaluate each of the lobar bronchi with a straight telescope. Straightening of the right or left mainstem bronchus can be facilitated by turning the head to the side opposite the bronchus being accessed during the examination. The use of angled telescopes is rarely necessary, although they may be helpful for specific lower airway evaluations.[71] After the airway is inspected, any appropriate manipulations are completed. Should ventilation become difficult, the telescope may be removed and ventilation can continue through the unobstructed bronchoscope sheath. Images may be projected onto a monitor by placing a video camera on the telescope eyepiece. During the course of the procedure, care must be taken to evaluate the dynamics of the airway and anatomic variations.

Removal of various sizes and types of foreign bodies requires the availability of a variety of grasping instruments.[4] Generally, removal of the object from the airway requires removal of the entire bronchoscope apparatus because most foreign bodies will not pass through the bronchoscope sheath. If a foreign body is particularly friable, such as an aspirated peanut, it may be helpful to pass a Fogarty balloon catheter through the access port or through the sheath and beyond the object. Care must be taken to not break the balloon. The balloon is then inflated, the object is withdrawn into the sheath, and the entire apparatus is removed.[28] The airway should always be reexamined to rule out any residual foreign body fragment and to suction any mucus and secretions that have accumulated in the airway beyond the foreign body.

Although all procedures should be performed in an efficient manner, time is usually not as limiting a factor during rigid bronchoscopy as it is during flexible bronchoscopy because of the ability to ventilate through the sheath. At the end of the procedure, the endoscope is removed under direct vision. An endotracheal tube can then be placed if necessary, a preexisting tracheostomy may be replaced, or the patient may be observed breathing spontaneously.

Complications

Significant complications of flexible and rigid bronchoscopy are uncommon but may include hypoxia, hypercapnia, bradycardia, laryngospasm, pneumothorax, subglottic or other airway edema, bleeding, fever, and nosocomial infection.[42,48,71,75] The most serious complications appear to occur in small infants undergoing bronchoscopy. In one series of 132 infants younger than 1 month undergoing rigid bronchoscopy, pneumothorax developed in 5, bronchial disruption in 1, and pulmonary artery disruption in 1. Each of these injuries was treated successfully.[31]

THORACOSCOPY

Indications

When originally described for use in children, thoracoscopy was proposed as a method for obtaining pulmonary biopsy samples in patients who were immunocompromised.[59] With further refinements in the technique and the development of better instrumentation, there are now many diagnostic and therapeutic indications for thoracoscopy in children. In our own series, the most common indication for thoracoscopy has become pleural débridement

for empyema.[14,26,55] The procedure remains our technique of choice for biopsy of mediastinal lesions, particularly lymphomas.[52] Certain mediastinal lesions, such as bronchogenic or duplication cysts, can be completely excised via thoracoscopy, thus avoiding a thoracotomy in these patients.[46,55] The technique remains quite useful for pulmonary biopsy, both in immunocompromised and in otherwise normal children with undiagnosed pulmonary infiltrates or nodules.[6] It is also useful in the treatment of many pleural disorders, such as spontaneous pneumothorax and chylothorax.[13,44] Recent reports have demonstrated its usefulness and safety in performing anatomic lobectomies in children.[61] Several authors have now described repair of esophageal atresia, with and without tracheoesophageal fistula, with thoracoscopic techniques.[3,33,62] Techniques have been developed for closure of diaphragm hernias and for occlusion of the ductus arteriosus.[30,62] Pericardial windows may be created to drain chronic pericardial effusions. Thoracoscopy has been used to achieve exposure for spinal diskectomy in children with thoracic scoliosis.[49] The role of the robot in pediatric thoracoscopy is in the early stages of definition.[9,20] The range of motion of the instruments with the robot may facilitate working in very small spaces.

Instrumentation

For thoracoscopy in children, 3-, 5-, or 10-mm Hopkins rod-lens telescopes may be used. We have preferred the 0-degree telescopes, although other authors have described using the 30- and 70-degree telescopes in certain circumstances.[54] In small infants, the 3-mm endoscopic telescope may be useful (Fig. 62-6). The telescopes and operating instruments are passed through transthoracic trocars, which may be valved, as those used for laparoscopy, or unvalved. We have found the Innerdyne expandable trocar useful in children because its radial expansion allows placement of a 5- or 10-mm trocar in small children without the hazard of intercostal vessel or nerve injury (Fig. 62-7). The operating instruments are, for the most part, 3 or 5 mm in diameter with insulated shafts for the use of cautery. We have preferred the reusable instruments and have chosen them to duplicate the types of instruments that we would use for an open thoracotomy (Fig. 62-8). The endoscopic GIA stapler is useful for obtaining lung biopsy samples and for excising cysts of the lung, but this instrument must be passed through a 12-mm trocar and must have 5 cm within the pleural space to fully open the anvil, thus limiting the usefulness of this instrument in small children.

Procedure

Successful performance of thoracoscopy in children requires careful attention to patient selection and preoperative imaging. In children with mediastinal pathology, special imaging studies such as CT or magnetic resonance imaging are helpful in defining the relationship of the pathology to other mediastinal structures and determining the most direct approach to the lesion. For lung

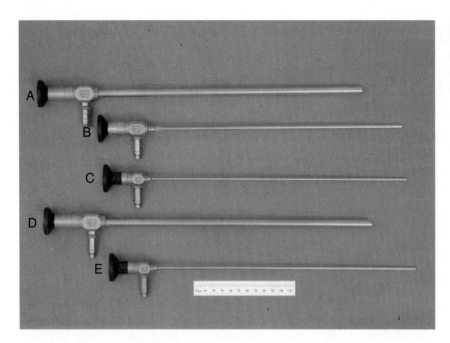

Figure 62-6 Endoscopic telescopes. An array of endoscopic telescopes from 3 to 10 mm in diameter is available: A, 10 mm, 0 degree; B, 5 mm, 0 degree; C, 3 mm, 0 degree; D, 10 mm, 30 degree; E, 3 mm, 30 degree.

biopsy, frontal and lateral radiographs usually suffice to localize the area of pathology. Patients undergoing thoracoscopy for biopsy of parenchymal nodules must be carefully selected on the basis of preoperative CT scans. Nodules further than 1 cm from the visceral pleura may be difficult to identify at the time of thoracoscopy, and preoperative localization techniques such as transthoracic wire placement or tattooing may be very helpful.[45,59,72] In patients with pleural effusions or empyema who are being considered for thoracoscopic drainage and débridement, transthoracic ultrasound or thoracic CT can help localize the area of largest loculation, into which the initial trocar should be placed.

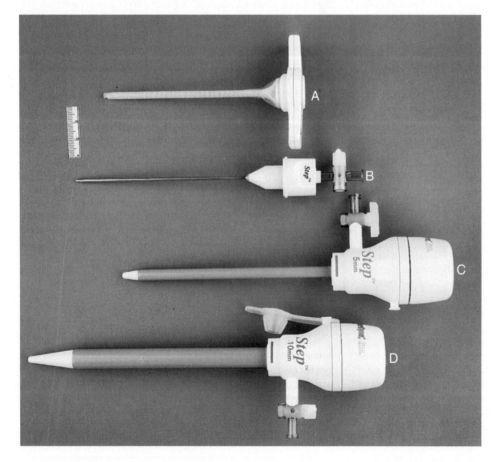

Figure 62-7 Expandable trocar set. The expandable trocar (A) is passed through the chest wall with a Veress needle (B) inserted through it. The trocar can then be expanded to 5 mm (C) or 10 mm (D) by passing the sleeves through the expandable sheath.

Figure 62–8 Thoracoscopic instruments. *A,* All of the following instruments have 5-mm shafts that are insulated: A, Babcock forceps; B, Right-angle dissector; C, Metzenbaum scissors; D, Allis forceps. *B,* Different handle configurations are available for all these instruments, depending on their expected use and operator preference.

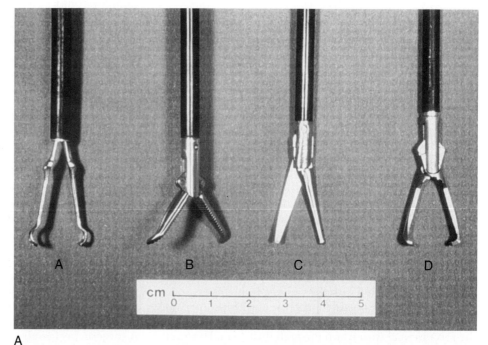

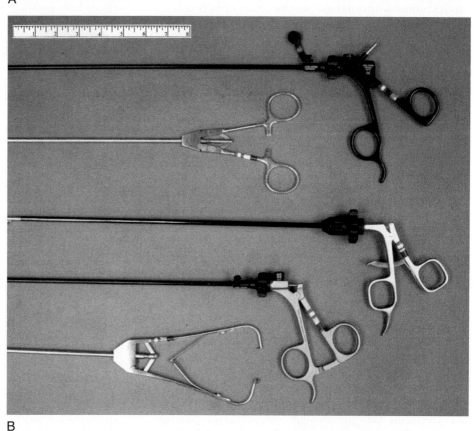

Thoracoscopic procedures in children may be performed with the use of either intravenous sedation and regional anesthesia or general anesthesia.[36] Procedures that may be performed rapidly and with little manipulation of the visceral pleura, such as talc pleurodesis or lung biopsy, may be successfully completed with regional anesthesia induced by intercostal nerve blocks.

More prolonged and complicated procedures are best performed with general anesthesia. Unilateral ventilation, with contralateral mainstem intubation, is helpful for cases requiring extensive mediastinal dissection. Patients should be monitored thoroughly during these procedures with continuous ECG monitoring as well as pulse oximetry. Instruments should be available in the operating room for performing an emergency thoracotomy if needed for control of bleeding.

The patient is positioned on the operating table to facilitate the approach to the area of pathology. Procedures involving lung biopsy or pulmonary resection are performed with the patient in a full lateral decubitus position to allow access to all pulmonary lobes and fissures. Lesions in the posterior mediastinum are best accessed by rolling the patient forward from the true lateral decubitus position, whereas anterior mediastinal lesions are best approached by rolling the patient posteriorly. The initial trocar is usually placed in the midaxillary line in the fifth or sixth intercostal space. Placement of subsequent trocars then depends on the accessibility of the pathology. Generally, the trocars for the operating instruments are placed on either side of the telescope in a triangular configuration, with the telescope at the apex.

Pleural débridement for empyema is accomplished with large grasping forceps and pressure irrigation. Denser adhesions are divided with the cautery. Lung biopsy specimens were initially obtained with the cup biopsy forceps, with a fragment of pulmonary parenchyma sheared off as the forceps were withdrawn through the trocar. However, this technique provided no pneumostasis or hemostasis. Tissue coagulation instruments are now available in 5-mm diameters and appear to provide excellent pneumostasis and hemostasis for lung biopsy.[69] In larger children, use of the endoscopic GIA stapler allows large wedge biopsy specimens to be obtained safely. Mediastinal lesions may be biopsied or resected by opening the parietal pleura overlying the lesion and dissecting the lesion with blunt and sharp techniques. Exposure of mediastinal lesions being considered for resection may be improved by instilling CO_2 into the chest under low pressure (4 to 6 mm Hg) to collapse the ipsilateral lung. Hemostasis is usually achieved with the electrocautery, although metallic clips may be used for larger vessels. We have used a core biopsy needle passed directly across the chest wall and positioned under direct vision to obtain deeper specimens after biopsy of the superficial portion of mediastinal lymph nodes with the cup forceps. Patients with chylothorax may be treated by ligation or clipping of the thoracic duct along with the adjacent tissue behind the esophagus at the aortic hiatus.[7,24,67] The duct may also be dissected individually and occluded with metallic clips. In the event of more diffuse lymphatic leakage, ligation of the thoracic duct may be followed by the application of fibrin glue to the region of leak.[13] Patients undergoing thoracoscopy for pneumothorax may have a complete pleural abrasion after division of pleural adhesions with the cautery. We have used a piece of Marlex mesh held in grasping forceps to perform the abrasion. In some cases an apical pleurectomy may be performed by incising the parietal pleura over the sixth rib laterally and bluntly dissecting the pleura from the upper half of the hemithorax. Talc pleurodesis may be performed in selected patients by dusting USP pure talc on the visceral and parietal pleural surfaces throughout the entire hemithorax. We have preferred to leave a chest tube in place after removal of the trocars, although some authors have not used tubes if the visceral pleura has not been violated during the procedure.[58]

Complications

Complications of thoracoscopy are in large part determined by the procedure performed and the medical condition of the patient. The majority of the complications, as well as all of the mortality, reported in children undergoing thoracoscopy has occurred in mechanically ventilated patients undergoing thoracoscopic lung biopsy for diffuse pulmonary infiltrates.[53] The incidence of prolonged bronchopleural fistula is highest in this group of patients, and this may complicate their respiratory management. Hemorrhage requiring transfusion is a rare complication of thoracoscopy, even in patients who are thrombocytopenic as a result of chemotherapy. Preoperative correction of coagulation abnormalities minimizes the risk for this complication. As with any biopsy procedure, false-negative biopsy results are occasionally reported with thoracoscopy. We believe that the addition of visually directed core needle biopsy to superficial nodal biopsy has minimized the frequency of this problem. Occasionally, lesions visible by radiographic studies cannot be localized by thoracoscopy. This appears to be particularly true for pulmonary parenchymal nodules. A surgeon performing thoracoscopy has limited ability to "palpate" the pulmonary surface, and it is often difficult to locate lesions situated deep within the pulmonary parenchyma. Occasionally, collapsing the ipsilateral lung with unilateral pulmonary ventilation will make these deeper lesions more evident. Various techniques of preoperative marking of these lesions have been described to aid in their localization. In general, thoracoscopy has proved to be a highly accurate and very safe procedure. The overall results are quite comparable to those with open thoracotomy, but with less postoperative morbidity.

Endoscopic techniques for visualization of the airway and intrathoracic structures have assumed a critically important role in the management of children. Newer uses of these techniques have been developed as the technology has been refined. It is incumbent on pediatric surgeons to be familiar with these techniques and facile in their performance.

REFERENCES

1. Arca MJ, Barnhart DC, Lelli JL, et al: Early experience with minimally invasive repair of congenital diaphragmatic hernias: Results and lessons learned. J Pediatr Surg 2003;38:1563.
2. Badr A, Tobias J, Rasmussen GE, et al: Bronchoscopic evaluation facilitated by the laryngeal mask airway in pediatric patients. Pediatr Pulmonol 1996;21:57.
3. Bax KN, van der Zee DC: Feasibility of thoracoscopic repair of esophageal atresia with distal fistula. J Pediatr Surg 2002;37:192.
4. Black RE, Johnson DG, Matlak ME: Bronchoscopic removal of aspirated foreign bodies in children. J Pediatr Surg 1994;29:682.
5. Bozzini PH: Lichteiter, eine Erfindung zur Anschauung innerer Teile und Krankheiten. J Prak Heilk 1806;24:107.
6. Burns RC, McGahren ED, Rodgers BM: Thoracoscopic approach to pulmonary parenchymal lesions. Pediatr Endosurg Innov Tech 2001;5:141.

7. Burns RC, McGahren ED, Rodgers BM: Thoracoscopy in the management of chylothorax. Pediatr Endosurg Innov Tech 2001;5:153.

8. Cohen S, Pine H, Drake A: Use of rigid and flexible bronchoscopy among pediatric otolaryngologists. Arch Otolaryngol Head Neck Surg 2001;127:505.

9. Drasin T, Gracia C, Atkinson J: Pediatric applications of robotic surgery. Pediatr Endosurg Innov Tech 2003; 7:377.

10. Fan LL, Sparks LM, Fix EJ: Flexible fiberoptic endoscopy for airway problems in a pediatric intensive care unit. Chest 1988;93:556.

11. Gaafar HA: The fiberoptic bronchoscope in the diagnosis and investigation of laryngeal disorders. Clin Otolaryngol 1983;8:103.

12. Godfrey S, Springer C, Maayan C, et al: Is there a place for rigid bronchoscopy in the management of pediatric lung disease? Pediatr Pulmonol 1987;3:179.

13. Graham DD, McGahren ED, Tribble CG, et al: Use of video-assisted thoracic surgery in the treatment of chylothorax. Ann Thorac Surg 1994;57:1507.

14. Grewal H, Jackson RJ, Wagner CW, Smith SD: Early video-assisted thoracic surgery in the management of empyema. Pediatrics 1999;103:63.

15. Handler SD: Direct laryngoscopy in children: Rigid and flexible fiberoptic. Ear Nose Throat J 1995;74:100.

16. Hasagawa S, Hitomi S, Murakawa M, et al: Development of an ultrathin fiberscope with a built-in channel for bronchoscopy in infants. Chest 1996;110:1543.

17. Hawkins DB, Clark RW: Flexible laryngoscopy in neonates, infants, and young children. Ann Otol Rhinol Laryngol 1987;96:81.

18. Hirschowitz BI, Curtis LE, Peters CW, et al: Demonstration of a new gastroscope, the fibergastroscope. Gastroenterology 1958;35:50.

19. Hoeve LJ, Rombout J, Meursing AEE: Complications of rigid laryngobronchoscopy in children. Int J Pediatr Otorhinolaryngol 1993;26:47.

20. Hollands CM, Dixey LN: Robotic-assisted esophago-esophagostomy. J Pediatr Surg 2002;37:983.

21. Ikeda S: Flexible bronchofiberscope. Ann Otol Rhinol Laryngol 1970;79:916.

22. Jacobaeus HC: Über die Moglichkeit die Zystoskopie bei Untersuchung seroser hohzungen Anzuwenden. Munch Med Wochenschr 1910;40:2090.

23. Jacobaeus HC, Key E: Some experiences of intrathoracic tumors, their diagnosis and their operative treatment. Acta Chir Scand 1921;53:573.

24. Kent RB III, Pinson TW: Thoracoscopic ligation of the thoracic duct. Surg Endosc 1993;7:52.

25. Keohane JD, Forte V, MacPherson B: Pressure, flow, and resistance characteristics of the pediatric Storz-Hopkins bronchoscopes. Otology 1991;20:155.

26. Kern JA, Rodgers BM: Thoracoscopy in the management of empyema in children. J Pediatr Surg 1993;28:1128.

27. Koltai PJ, Nixon RE: The story of the laryngoscope. Ear Nose Throat J 1989;68:494.

28. Kosloske AM: The Fogarty balloon technique for the removal of foreign bodies from the tracheobronchial tree. Surg Gynecol Obstet 1982;155:72.

29. Lamm H: Biegsame optische Cerate. Z Instrumentenkunde 1930;30:579.

30. LeBret E, Folliquet TA, Laborde F: Videothoracoscopic surgical interruption of patent ductus arteriosus. Ann Thorac Surg 1997;64:1492.

31. Lindahl H, Rintala R, Malinen L, et al: Bronchoscopy during the first month of life. J Pediatr Surg 1992;27:548.

32. Lis G, Szczerbinski T, Cichocka-Jarosz E: Congenital stridor. Pediatr Pulmonol 1995;20:220.

33. Lobe TE, Rothenberg SS, Waldschmidt J, et al: Thoracoscopic repair of esophageal atresia in an infant: A surgical first. Pediatr Endosurg Innov Tech 1999;3:141.

34. Martinot A, Closset M, Marquette CH, et al: Indications for flexible versus rigid bronchoscopy in children with suspected foreign-body aspiration. Am J Respir Crit Care Med 1997;155:1676.

35. Marzo SJ, Hotaling AJ: Trade-off between airway resistance and optical resolution in pediatric rigid bronchoscopy. Ann Otol Rhinol Laryngol 1995;104:282.

36. McGahren ED, Kern JA, Rodgers BM: Anesthetic techniques for pediatric thoracoscopy. Ann Thorac Surg 1995; 60:927.

37. Mehrishi S, Raoof S, Mehta AC: Therapeutic flexible bronchoscopy. Chest Surg Clin North Am 2001;11:657.

38. Muntz HR: Therapeutic rigid bronchoscopy in the neonatal intensive care unit. Ann Otol Rhinol Laryngol 1985;94:462.

39. Nicolai T: Pediatric bronchoscopy. Pediatr Pulmonol 2001; 31:150.

40. Nitze M: Eine neue Boebachtungs und Untersuchungs-methode fur Harnblase. Wien Med Wochenschr 1879; 24:650.

41. Nussbaum E: Usefulness of miniature flexible fiberoptic bronchoscopy in children. Chest 1994;106:1438.

42. Nussbaum E: Pediatric fiberoptic bronchoscopy. Clin Pediatr (Phila) 1995;34:430.

43. Nussbaum E, Zagnoev M: Pediatric fiberoptic bronchoscopy with a laryngeal mask airway. Chest 2001;120:614.

44. Ozcan C, McGahren ED, Rodgers BM: Thoracoscopic treatment of spontaneous pneumothorax in children. J Pediatr Surg 2003;38:1459.

45. Partrick DA, Bensard DD, Teitelbaum DH, et al: Successful thoracoscopic lung biopsy in children utilizing preoperative CT-guided localization. J Pediatr Surg 2002;37:970.

46. Partrick DA, Rothenberg SS: Thoracoscopic resection of mediastinal masses in infants and children: An evaluation of techniques and results. J Pediatr Surg 2001;36:1165.

47. Perez CR, Wood RE: Update on pediatric flexible bronchoscopy. Pediatr Clin North Am 1994;41:85.

48. Picard E, Schwartz S, Goldberg S, et al: A prospective study of fever and bacteremia after flexible fiberoptic bronchoscopy in children. Chest 2000;117:573.

49. Pollock ME, O'Neal KO, Picetti G, Blackman R: Results of video-assisted exposure of the anterior thoracic spine in idiopathic scoliosis. Ann Thorac Surg 1996;62:818.

50. Puhakka H, Kero P, Valli P, et al: Pediatric bronchoscopy—a report of methodology and results. Clin Pediatr (Phila) 1989;28:253-257.

51. Rimell FL, Shapiro AM, Mitskavich MT, et al: Pediatric fiberoptic laser rigid bronchoscopy. Otol Head Neck Surg 1996;114:413.

52. Rodgers BM: Thoracoscopy. In Holcomb GE (ed): Pediatric Endoscopic Surgery. Norwalk, CT, Appleton & Lange, 1993.

53. Rodgers BM: Pediatric thoracoscopy: Where have we come and what have we learned. Ann Thorac Surg 1994;56:704.

54. Rodgers BM: Instrumentation and technique for pediatric thoracoscopy. Pediatr Endosurg Innov Tech 2001;5:93.

55. Rodgers BM: The role of thoracoscopy in pediatric surgical practice. Semin Pediatr Surg 2003;12:62.

56. Rodgers BM, McGahren ED: Endoscopy in children. Chest Surg Clin North Am 1993;3:405.

57. Rodgers BM, Moazam R, Talbert JL: Endotracheal cryotherapy in the treatment of refractory airway strictures. Ann Thorac Surg 1983;35:52.

58. Rogers DA, Philippe PG, Lobe TE, et al: Thoracoscopy in children: An initial experience with an evolving technique. J Laparoendosc Surg 1992;2:7.

59. Rodgers BM, Talbert JL: Thoracoscopy for diagnosis of intrathoracic lesions in children. J Pediatr Surg 1976; 11:703.

60. Rothenberg SS: Thoracoscopic repair of tracheoesophageal fistula in newborns. J Pediatr Surg 2002;37:869.

61. Rothenberg SS: Experience with thoracoscopic lobectomy in infants and children. J Pediatr Surg 2003;38:102.

62. Rothenberg SS, Chang JH, Toews WH, Washington RL: Thoracoscopic closure of patent ductus arteriosus: A less traumatic and more cost-effective technique. J Pediatr Surg 1995;30:1057.

63. Schellhase D: Pediatric flexible airway bronchoscopy. Curr Opin Pediatr 2002;14:327.

64. Selim M, Mowafi H, Al-Ghamdi A, et al: Intubation via LMA in pediatric patients with difficult airways. Can J Anaesth 1999;46:891-893.

65. Shinwell ES: Ultrathin fiberoptic bronchoscopy for airway toilet in neonatal pulmonary atelectasis. Pediatr Pulmonol 1992;13:48.

66. Silberman HD: The use of flexible fiberoptic nasopharyngolaryngoscope in the pediatric upper airway. Otolaryngol Clin North Am 1978;11:365.

67. Stringel G, Teixcira JA: Thoracoscopic ligation of the thoracic duct. J Soc Laparoendosc Surg 2000;4:239.

68. Swanson KL, Prakash UB, Midthun DE, et al: Flexible bronchoscopic management of airway foreign bodies in children. Chest 2002;121:1695.

69. Tirabassi MV, Banever GT, Tashjian DB, et al: Use of energy devices in thoracoscopy: Quantification of lung-sealing capacity. Pediatr Endosurg Innov Tech 2003;7:267.

70. Tunkel DE, Fisher QA: Pediatric flexible fiberoptic bronchoscopy through the laryngeal mask airway. Arch Otolarygol Head Neck Surg 1996;122:1364.

71. Wain G: Rigid bronchoscopy: The value of a venerable procedure. Chest Surg Clin North Am 2001;11:691.

72. Waldhausen JH, Shaw DW, Hall DG, et al: Needle localization for thoracoscopic resection of small pulmonary nodules in children. J Pediatr Surg 1997;32:1624.

73. Wong K, Lai S, Lien R, et al: Retrieval of bronchial foreign body with central lumen using a flexible bronchoscope. Int J Pediatr Otorhinolaryngol 2002;28:253.

74. Wood RE: Spelunking in the pediatric airways: Explorations with the flexible fiberoptic bronchoscope. Pediatr Clin North Am 1984;31:785.

75. Wood RE: Pitfalls in the use of the flexible bronchoscope in pediatric patients. Chest 1990;97:99.

76. Wood RE: Flexible bronchoscopy in infants. Int Anesthesiol Clin 1992;30:125.

77. Wood RE: The emerging role of flexible bronchoscopy in infants. Clin Chest Med 2001;22:311.

78. Wood RE, Azizkhan RG, Lacey SR, et al: Surgical applications of ultrathin flexible bronchoscopes in infants. Ann Otol Rhinol Laryngol 1991;100:116.

79. Wood RE, Gauderer MWL: Flexible fiberoptic bronchoscopy in the management of tracheobronchial foreign bodies in children: The value of a combined approach with open tube bronchoscopy. J Pediatr Surg 1984;19:693.

Chapter 63

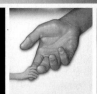

Lesions of the Larynx, Trachea, and Upper Airway

Dana Mara Thompson and Robin T. Cotton

Lesions of the upper airway, namely, the larynx and trachea, can cause life-threatening airway obstruction. The etiology of obstructive airway disease is often multifactorial and includes anatomic, congenital, and inflammatory problems, many of which are managed by surgical intervention. A variety of clinical signs and symptoms are associated with airway obstruction. Signs of acute airway obstruction are stridor, respiratory distress, apnea, cyanosis, pallor, tachypnea, use of accessory muscles of respiration and retractions, and mental status changes. Chronic airway obstruction may have similar signs and symptoms, and long-term complications of airway obstruction and hypoxia, such as failure to thrive, poor weight gain, pulmonary hypertension, and pectus excavatum, may develop. Regardless of whether the airway is acutely or chronically obstructed, stridor is the most useful noninvasive clinical examination finding for determining the location of the obstruction in the airway. Stridor occurs as a result of turbulent airflow through a narrowed lumen and is present in virtually all children with airway obstruction, except those on the brink of complete asphyxia. The phase of respiration in which stridor is heard will help an astute examiner better determine the location of the lesion. Inspiratory stridor typically occurs with obstructive lesions above the glottis, such as laryngomalacia and vocal cord paralysis. Biphasic stridor is heard with a fixed obstruction below the glottis, in the subglottis or trachea. Expiratory stridor usually represents an obstruction in the intrathoracic airway, such as tracheomalacia. Obstructive lesions of the airway may be mistakenly diagnosed as asthma on the basis of a respiratory "wheeze"; therefore, a high index of suspicion and correlation with other clinical examination findings are essential to not overlook a potentially critical or surgically correctable cause of airway obstruction.

Endoscopic evaluation of the airway has revolutionized the diagnosis and management of an obstructed airway. Endoscopic evaluations are divided into those done with the patient awake and those done under sedation or general anesthesia. Flexible fiber-optic nasopharyngoscopy and laryngoscopy are performed with the child awake. This technique permits safe, rapid examination of the nose, hypopharynx, supraglottis, and glottis in virtually all children, despite age or lack of cooperation. The awake state allows for evaluation of the dynamics of supraglottic tone, vocal fold mobility, and the impact of fixed obstructing lesions of the larynx. Examination under the influence of sedation or general anesthesia can alter the findings, and therefore a significant cause of airway obstruction, particularly pharyngomalacia, laryngomalacia, and vocal cord paralysis, could be overlooked. Direct examination of the airway under general or sedated anesthesia remains the mainstay for diagnosis and confirmation of lesions that obstruct the airway, especially those below the glottis that cannot be accurately evaluated by awake fiber-optic examination. Airway endoscopy confirms the presence of suspected laryngotracheal pathology such as subglottic stenosis and tracheal stenosis.

The goal of evaluation and management of any airway obstruction caused by laryngeal or tracheal disease is to establish and maintain a safe and stable airway. The number of children who require surgical intervention for airway obstruction has increased, in part because of the development of long-term intubation and ventilation techniques in the 1960s that allowed increased survival rates in critically ill premature newborns. As a result of long-term intubation, these infants were able to survive, but an entirely new spectrum of long-term health problems developed, including those of the airway and in particular the larynx and trachea.

AIRWAY PATHOPHYSIOLOGY AND DIAGNOSTIC CONSIDERATIONS

The larynx is the entry point for air into the trachebronchial tree and respiratory system. Without a functioning larynx, the remainder of the respiratory system is compromised. The phylogenetic purposes of the larynx are respiration and protection of the lower airway from aspiration. Voice is an evolutionary and secondary function of the larynx. The pediatric airway differs from the adult airway in structure and function. An infant's larynx is about a third its adult size and measures approximately 7 mm in the sagittal dimension and 4 mm in the coronal plane. The vocal cords are 6 to 8 mm long. The subglottic space is approximately 4.5 mm across; it is bounded by cricoid cartilage, the only complete ring of cartilage in the upper airway, and is the narrowest portion of the upper airway. Therefore, only 1 mm of mucosal edema in this portion of an infant's airway can obstruct the airway by 40%. As the airway space and dimensions grow with age, mucosal edema causes less compromise of the airway. The cartilaginous framework of the larynx and trachea is softer and more pliable in infancy. This can lead to a tendency to collapse under external compression or air pressure gradients and may result in airway obstruction as seen in laryngomalacia and tracheomalacia. As the infant grows and the cartilage matures, symptoms of these conditions often spontaneously improve and resolve without intervention. In an infant, the larynx sits high in the neck at the level of vertebrae C2 and C3, directly behind the nose, with approximation of the velum, tongue, and epiglottis functionally separating respiration from swallowing. Because neuromuscular function for airway protection is not fully developed at this stage, this intended anatomic relationship allows the infant to safely breathe and feed at the same time without aspirating. As a result of this anatomic relationship, however, any obstruction of the nasal cavity can cause significant obstruction of the airway, which also causes feeding difficulty. In conjunction with neuromuscular maturation, the position of the larynx descends in the neck. By the age of 2 years, the larynx descends to C4, thereby creating less of a functional separation between the functions of breathing and swallowing. By 6 years of age, the larynx has descended to its adult location directly behind C6. Airway and swallowing symptoms tend to be exaggerated if neuromuscular function is compromised or has not matured in conjunction with descent of the larynx.

TRACHEOTOMY

Tracheotomy is a means of managing severe airway obstruction caused by nearly all of the airway lesions discussed in this chapter. As mentioned earlier, the number of children who require surgical intervention for airway obstruction has increased, partly as a result of the development of long-term intubation and ventilation techniques in the 1960s that allowed critically ill premature newborns to survive. Because it is the sine qua non procedure for bypassing an obstruction in the upper airway, indications, technique, and complications will be discussed before the review of specific obstructive laryngotracheal lesions. The three major indications for long-term tracheotomy in children are airway obstruction, ventilatory support, and pulmonary toilet. Most children with tracheotomy tubes in place for airway obstruction undergo the procedure as very young infants, either for acquired subglottic stenosis related to prolonged endotracheal intubation or for congenital lesions that compromise the airway. Because of the morbidity and the psychosocial and developmental implications of tracheotomy in a child, all alternative interventions should be explored before proceeding to tracheotomy.

Tracheotomy Technique

The technique of pediatric tracheotomy preferred by the authors is as follows. The patient is taken to the operating room and the airway secured with an endotracheal tube. Because the typical landmarks for tracheotomy may be difficult to identify as a result of the small size of the larynx and cricoid, tracheotomy in the emergency setting is best done with a secured airway either by intubation or by rigid bronchoscopy. A vertical incision is made over the midline of the neck, its superior extent at the cricoid cartilage. Subcutaneous fat is removed with electrocautery, and the fascia is divided in layers in the midline. The strap muscles are separated at the raphe, and the thyroid isthmus is divided with electrocautery. Vertical 4-0 nonabsorbable "stay sutures" are placed through the third and fourth tracheal cartilage rings on the right and left sides just off the midline and tied loosely. Gentle tension is applied to these sutures to elevate the tracheal rings, and then the airway is entered with a blade in the midline between the third and fourth rings. As seen in Figure 63-1, the stoma is created by placing 4-0 chromic gut sutures through the cut edge of the trachea and sewing them to skin. The suggestion by some authors that this

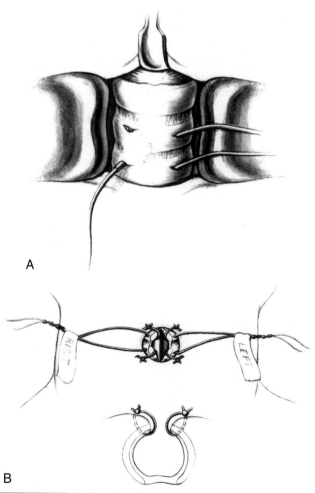

A

B

Figure 63-1   *A,* Placement of stay suture. *B,* Creation of immediate stoma.

technique fashions a more "permanent" stoma and may result in a persistent tracheocutaneous fistula after decannulation has not been substantiated. Because the major sources of mortality in pediatric patients undergoing tracheotomy are accidental decannulation or inability to replace an obstructed tube, the authors believe that the added margin of safety, particularly in the first few days, is justification for the approach outlined. In addition, pediatric tracheotomies are rarely short term, and even without the skin sutures, the tract tends to epithelialize over time.

The endotracheal tube (or bronchoscope) is withdrawn, an appropriately sized tracheotomy tube is inserted, and ventilation is ensured bilaterally. As seen in Figure 63-2, the previously placed stay sutures are labeled for each of the right and left sides and then taped to the anterior chest wall to serve as emergency traction lines in the event of accidental decannulation. The tracheotomy tube is secured around the neck with cotton twill ties. A tracheotomy tube, particularly if it does not have an inner cannula, should not be directly sewn to the skin of a child. If a significant life-threatening mucous plug obstructs the tracheotomy tube, particularly in the immediate postoperative period when the tract has not been fully established, having a tube secured to the skin presents a delay in urgent removal and replacement with a patent clean tube. Ideally, the position of the tracheotomy tube is evaluated by passing a telescope through the glottis, alongside the tracheotomy tube. This allows the surgeon to ensure that the tip of the tracheotomy tube is proximal to the carina. This technique also permits the surgeon to evaluate the fit of the tracheotomy tube within the lumen of the trachea. This relationship is ideally collinear and concentric without any rubbing or encroachment on the anterior or posterior tracheal wall. If assessment by this method is not possible, a flexible bronchoscope can be passed through the tracheotomy tube to ensure that the tip is proximal to the carina. The tracheotomy tube is changed and the stay sutures are removed in 5 days once the tract has been established. These patients should be managed in a monitored hospital setting, at least until

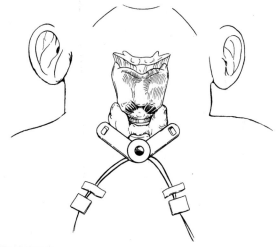

Figure 63–2 Labeling stay sutures.

the tract has been established, a successful change of the tracheotomy tube has occurred, and appropriate education is given and understood by at least two caregivers.

Tracheotomy Complications

Perioperative, postoperative, and long-term complications of tracheotomy may develop, many of which can occur whenever a tracheotomy tube is in place. Perioperative complications after tracheotomy tube placement include pneumothorax and major vessel bleeding, particularly from the innominate artery. A chest radiograph should be performed at the end of the procedure to assess for the possibility of pneumothorax or pneumomediastinum. The most common immediate postoperative complications can be life threatening and include mucous plugging and accidental decannulation. The diameter of tracheotomy tubes for children is significantly smaller than those for adults, so any occlusion of the tube by mucus easily leads to complete airway obstruction, particularly in a child who is totally dependent on the tracheotomy to breathe. Likewise, the stoma into the airway for the tracheotomy tube is much smaller in a child. If the tube accidentally dislodges, the increased work of breathing causes further collapse and a "sucking" in closure at the stoma that makes it both difficult to breathe through and challenging to replace the tube. This effect is particularly dramatic in the immediate postoperative period, when the stoma has not fully matured. Because these complications are life threatening, every precaution should be taken to ensure that the tracheotomy tube is patent, carefully suctioned, and at the same time secure around the neck to prevent accidental decannulation.

Any child with a tracheotomy tube for a prolonged period is at risk for a minor or major complication. As in the immediate postoperative period, mucous plugging and accidental decannulation are the most serious and life-threatening complications that can occur. Accidental decannulation remains a major concern throughout the time that a child has a tracheotomy tube. It is particularly concerning when a young child develops the manual dexterity to remove the tracheotomy tube. Accidental removal could prove to be a fatal event in a child with nearly total obstruction of the airway above the tracheotomy tube. Though not universally adopted, many caregivers recommend a home apnea monitor or a pulse oximeter to assist caregivers in detecting such a situation. In some cases the child will still be able to breathe comfortably through the stoma, and care should be taken to replace the tube rapidly, but safely. Hastily performed insertion of the tracheotomy tube may result in placement of the tube in a false tract and lead to airway compromise when none existed. We recommend that a tracheotomy tube one size smaller be readily available to the caregiver.

Complications related to local infection of either the skin or soft tissue surrounding the stoma (cellulitis), tracheal mucosa (tracheitis), or tracheal cartilage (chondritis) may occur. By adapting the skin directly to the cut edge of the tracheal cartilage, epithelialization of the tract is accelerated and healing promoted. Nevertheless, local infections may develop in some patients after the perioperative period. Typically, these individuals have some underlying predisposition to breakdown and bacterial invasion, such as drug-induced immunosuppression, primary immunopathy, or diabetes. Treatment consists of local antimicrobial packing, frequent dressing and cannula changes, and systemic antibiotics. The choice of antibiotics is dictated by culture results. Staphylococcal and pseudomonal infections are frequently seen in the intensive care unit setting. Aggressive infections leading to chondritis with breakdown of the wound, exposure of the great vessels, and extension of infection into the mediastinum are rare.

Suprastomal collapse and granuloma formation are nearly universal consequences of the presence of a tracheotomy tube, but the degree of obstruction caused is quite variable. Although some authors recommend routine removal of this tissue at regular intervals, this is not necessary in all patients. Overly aggressive removal of granulomas leads to more frequent recurrence, further arguing against routine excision.[82] Granulomas that completely obstruct the suprastomal airway require removal because of the potential for complete airway obstruction if the tube becomes blocked or displaced, as well as to preserve phonation. Parents are usually the first to note symptoms or findings that may suggest significant suprastomal granuloma formation. Most common are progressive loss of voice and difficulty changing the tracheotomy tube. Voice loss occurs because the granuloma prevents the passage of air around the tracheotomy tube that is required to vibrate the vocal cords for voice production.

The most lethal of late tracheotomy complications is erosion of the innominate artery at the level where the artery crosses the anterior tracheal wall. This complication can occur as a result of increased pressure from the tip of the tracheotomy tube against the anterior tracheal wall, which leads to the formation of granulation tissue, weakening of cartilage, and eventual erosion if not identified. Rigid and inappropriately curved tubes may contribute to this complication, thus emphasizing the importance of appropriate tracheotomy tube selection. Often, sentinel bleeding of bright red blood will alert the clinician to impending arterial rupture. For this reason, even small amounts of suctioned blood should be evaluated fully by flexible endoscopy.

In the same manner that the anterior wall of the trachea can erode from the continued pressure of a tracheal cannula, the posterior wall can break down as well. This is rare as a late complication, although the presence of an indwelling nasogastric tube worsens the situation by trapping the posterior wall between two rigid foreign bodies. The diagnosis is suspected in patients with unexplained recurrent pneumonia or pneumomediastinitis. In a ventilated patient, eructation will occur with each inspiratory breath. This complication is traditionally managed by an open surgical procedure with the interposition of healthy muscle between the trachea and esophagus.

With increased surgical experience, improved surgical techniques, identification and management of comorbid conditions that affect outcomes, and improvement in postoperative care, the indications for airway expansion surgery have been extended to patients with laryngotracheal stenosis as the primary definitive operation, thus avoiding tracheotomy for many of the airway lesions that may have traditionally required a tracheotomy for initial management.[29,34,101,105]

LESIONS OF THE LARYNX AND SUBGLOTTIS

Laryngomalacia

Laryngomalacia is the most common laryngeal anomaly and cause of stridor in infancy. The clinical manifestation is inspiratory stridor that is worse with feeding, agitation, and supine position. The symptoms are usually present at birth or shortly thereafter. Symptoms peak at 6 to 8 months and usually resolve between 18 and 24 months of age.[44] Mild forms of the disease are characterized by inspiratory stridor only. Those with moderate disease usually have feeding problems because it can be difficult for infants to coordinate the "suck-swallow-breathe" sequence in the setting of airway obstruction. Many of these infants have gastrointestinal reflux disease (GERD) and benefit from antireflux treatment and measures.[30,79] Several factors account for this. First, the increased intrathoracic airway pressure from the proximal airway obstruction promotes reflux. Second, the immature reflexes that regulate esophageal motility cause poor esophageal clearance. Third, GERD in this patient population, like other infant populations with airway problems and apnea, may be related to frequent relaxation events of the lower esophageal sphincter.[83]

Infants with severe laryngomalacia experience life-threatening complications of airway obstruction that can lead to pectus formation, failure to thrive, chronic hypoxia, pulmonary hypertension, and cor pulmonale. These patients require surgical intervention.[43,77,81,110]

The diagnosis is suspected by auscultation of the stridor, but it must be confirmed by flexible laryngoscopy. This examination must be done with the infant awake to demonstrate the cyclic collapse of supraglottic tissues into the laryngeal inlet. The influence of general anesthesia can obscure these findings. Other typical findings are an omega-shaped epiglottis and forward-prolapsing arytenoid cartilage obstructing airflow and complete view of the vocal folds. This examination is also done to exclude other significant supraglottic pathology. The etiology of this condition is multifactorial. Proposed theories include abnormal airway anatomy,[6,65] immature cartilage formation, and neurologic disorders.

Laryngomalacia is usually a self-limited disease that rarely requires surgical intervention. Surgical intervention is recommended for infants in whom life-threatening episodes of airway obstruction or complications of hypoxia develop. Tracheotomy was the treatment of choice for this condition until the mid-1980s, when techniques of supraglottoplasty were introduced.[54,87,110] Tracheotomy bypasses the site of laryngeal obstruction until the condition resolves spontaneously, generally after 18 to 24 months. Tracheotomy can be avoided by performing supraglottoplasty. This is accomplished by microsurgical removal of

Figure 63–3 Laryngomalacia before (*A*) and after (*B*) supraglottoplasty.

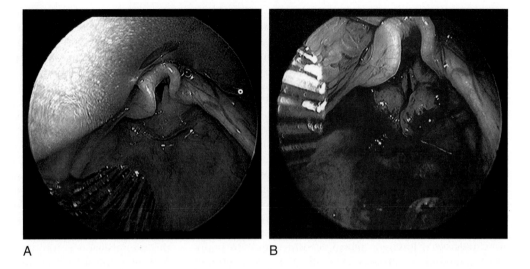

A   B

the redundant prolapsing tissue seen in the area of the cuneiform cartilage and release of the aryepiglottic folds tethering the position of the epiglottis (Fig. 63-3).[110] Long-term results with this approach have generally been excellent, with symptom reversal in 80% to 100% of cases.[43,51,61,63,81,96,110] Some authors report that as many as 50% of patients will require additional airway procedures, either revision supraglottoplasty or tracheotomy.[63,96] Supraglottic stenosis is the most severe complication of this operation and can occur after overzealous removal of tissue or failure to control for acid reflux disease. Although supraglottoplasty is a superior alternative to tracheotomy, in most circumstances some children with multiple medical comorbid conditions, particularly those with severe neurologic impairment or syndromes that involve the airway, are better initially managed with a tracheotomy.[22]

Laryngeal Atresia and Webs

Laryngeal webs are congenital (Fig. 63-4) or acquired (Fig. 63-5). Congenital laryngeal webs and atresia are rare and may be associated with velocardiac facial syndrome. The embryologic origin is failure of recanalization of the larynx during prenatal development. An atresia or web of sufficient size will be manifested at birth as aphonia and rapid asphyxiation if not immediately addressed. A thin web with a small residual airway may be ruptured by intubation. Thick webs and atresia make emergency intubation by standard techniques difficult, if not impossible. In this setting, survival of the infant may be dependent on securing the airway with urgent tracheotomy. Surgical management of thick webs and atresia requires a tracheostomy tube until surgical intervention is performed.[67] Surgical correction usually requires laryngofissure with open airway division of the atretic region and resection of excess cartilage of the cricoid ring if present. A costal cartilage graft to the anterior cricoid may be necessary, similar to laryngotracheal reconstruction for subglottic stenosis. Timing of reconstruction is dependent on many factors, including the age of the child and surgeon experience.

Thin and moderate anterior webs are manifested as aphonia or a weak cry at birth without obstructive

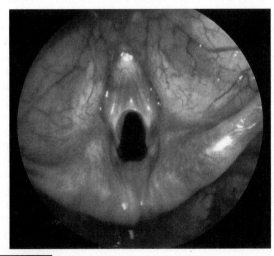

Figure 63–4 Congenital web.

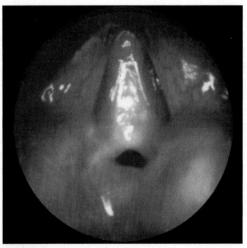

Figure 63–5 Acquired web.

airway symptoms. The primary goals of management are to provide a patent airway and achieve good voice quality. This is challenging because the vocal cords have a tendency for fibrosis and granulation tissue formation after surgical interventions. Traditionally, the treatment of choice for these thin and moderate laryngeal webs is laryngofissure and placement of a stent or keel when the surgeon believes that the child has grown appropriately, generally after 12 months of age. A recent report suggests that select laryngeal webs can be managed with endoscopic lysis and off-label (Food and Drug Administration) topical mitomycin C application, even in infants younger than 1 year.[100] This technique may allow congenital webs to be successfully managed at a younger age. However, long-term outcomes of this technique are not available, and it is unknown whether infants treated by this method eventually need laryngotracheal reconstruction to maintain a patent airway. Long-term results of the management of webs depend on the severity of the original lesion. Surgically treated thin webs often heal with minimal disruption of phonation, whereas thicker plates with associated subglottic stenosis have less satisfactory results.[7]

Acquired laryngeal webs are also uncommon. Such webs are usually caused by direct laryngeal trauma in which the medial surfaces of both vocal cords are disrupted and they heal together and form a web. This is most commonly encountered in the management and treatment of laryngeal papillomas, particularly in the setting of laryngopharyngeal reflux.[42]

Vocal Cord Immobility: Vocal Cord Paralysis and Vocal Cord Fixation

Vocal cord movement requires intact neurologic function of the vagus nerve and free rotation of the cricoarytenoid joint. The action of abduction of the vocal cords from the midline opens the glottic inlet for airflow into the tracheobronchial tree. Airflow is restricted if vocal cord abduction does not occur. Vocal cord immobility is caused by failure of the vocal cords to abduct. The two primary causes of vocal cord immobility are vocal cord paralysis and vocal cord fixation. Both can be congenital or acquired. Injury to the vagus nerve anywhere along its course from the cranial nucleus to the thoracic cavity causes neurogenic vocal cord paralysis. Acquired immobility is usually caused by a stretch injury, pressure encroachment, an inflammatory insult, or trauma or sectioning of the nerve itself; the cricoarytenoid joint is mobile, but neuromuscular function is compromised. A congenital, traumatic, or inflammatory process in the cricoarytenoid joint causes vocal cord fixation; the cricoarytenoid joint is fixed, but neuromuscular function is intact. Fixation and paralysis can coexist. Regardless of the etiology of immobility, failure of one or both of the vocal cords to abduct can lead to stridor and airway obstruction.

Unilateral vocal cord immobility causes stridor but not often airway obstruction. Bilateral vocal cord immobility limits airflow through the glottis and frequently causes severe airway obstruction requiring an artificial airway. Some infants and children have mild symptoms that occur only during periods of upper respiratory tract infection and may not require a tracheotomy. Most children with bilateral vocal cord immobility require tracheotomy early in the course of the disease, before definitive surgical therapy. Because it is bilateral immobility that most commonly leads to airway obstruction, the discussion of surgical treatment is limited to management of bilateral immobility.

Management of airway symptoms of bilateral vocal cord paralysis (BVCP) is based on the etiology and site of involvement along the vagus nerve. In neonates and infants, BVCP may have a central etiology and is most commonly associated with a Chiari malformation or hydrocephalus. The caudal displacement of the brainstem seen in a Chiari malformation causes pressure on the brainstem and on the vagus nerve and its nucleus. Recognition plus diagnosis of this compression is important to prevent other complications of a Chiari malformation. BVCP may be relieved once the Chiari malformation is decompressed. Hydrocephalus leads to increased compression of the fourth ventricle, as well as compression of the vagus nerve and nucleus. Decreasing intracranial pressure by shunt placement is often curative.[76,106] Infants with a central etiology of BVCP who fail to improve with central decompressive procedures require a tracheotomy for airway safety. These groups of patients are also often prone to the eventual development of other lower cranial nerve problems and aspiration that keep them tracheotomy tube dependent and not good candidates for surgical procedures to achieve decannulation. If the vagal nerve is intact and the cause of BVCP is a localized insult to the vagal nerve such as a stretch injury from obstetric trauma, infection, or extrinsic compression, an observational period is often warranted if there are no acute symptoms of airway obstruction. The paralysis is frequently transient in these patients, who are otherwise healthy. If the cause of vocal cord paralysis is traumatic as a result of direct nerve injury and function is not expected to return, a tracheotomy is required until another procedure can be performed to expand the glottic opening. This situation may be seen in "fixed wire" neck trauma[57] with nerve injury or in patients with injury as a complication of thyroid or cardiothoracic surgery.

Bilateral vocal fold immobility secondary to fixation occurs when the synovial joint surfaces of the cricoarytenoid joint become fixed, thereby preventing vocal fold abduction or adduction. In this setting, the vagal nerve is usually fully functional and physically intact. The most common cause of fixation of the joint is some type of direct trauma to the joint area itself, such as intubation or neck trauma in which the cricoarytenoid joint is dislocated. Once the joint is injured, an inflammatory process occurs and causes fixation of the joint. Juvenile rheumatoid arthritis can also result in bilateral immobility. Rarely is it congenital.

Regardless of the cause of vocal fold immobility, surgical approaches for treatment in children are similar. The fact that a wide variety of surgical approaches are available suggests that no single procedure is ideal. The goal is to open the posterior glottic airway enough to allow for adequate airflow without exposing the patient to an increased risk for the complications of aspiration or a debilitating change in voice. The procedures described are often performed after the airway has been secured and is stable with a tracheotomy tube, although surgery can be primary with the goal of avoiding a tracheotomy. The decision to perform definitive primary surgery depends on the acuity of the airway obstruction, the age of the child, and the ability to protect the airway against aspiration.

Repositioning and removal of structures and tissue in the posterior glottis, namely, the arytenoid cartilage and mucosa, are well-described techniques of opening the airway in the setting of bilateral vocal cord immobility. Such techniques include arytenoid lateralization, arytenoidopexy, partial arytenoidectomy, and cordotomy.[10,28,73,97] These procedures can be performed alone or in combination. The surgical approach can be external through a laryngofissure, endoscopic with the use of a CO_2 laser, or a combination of both. Endoscopic CO_2 laser removal of the vocal process of the arytenoid and a portion of the posterior vocal cord has been successfully used in some series.[28] The management challenge with this technique is treatment of postoperative granulation tissue formation, which may lead to airway obstruction.[80] Recent meta-analysis and retrospective studies evaluating the outcomes of surgically managed BVCP in children suggest that laryngofissure with partial arytenoidectomy combined with a vocal cord lateralization procedure results in the highest decannulation rates when compared with CO_2 arytenoidectomy and cordotomy procedures or arytenoidopexy procedures alone.[11,39] These same studies conclude that open external procedures appear to be more effective as first-line treatment of pediatric BVCP, with arytenoidopexy with or without partial arytenoidectomy offering an attractive first-line surgical option. They also conclude that CO_2 laser procedures, though being less successful as a primary procedure, are effective for revision. Although these procedures have been effective in achieving decannulation and maintaining airway patency, long-term outcomes on aspiration and voice are not documented.

Posterior graft laryngotracheoplasty is another effective technique to open the posterior glottis.[32,108] Through a laryngofissure with extension into the first two rings of the trachea, the posterior cricoid lamina is incised and distracted to separate the arytenoid cartilage. Inserting a costal cartilage graft into the distracted posterior cricoid lamina stabilizes the position of the arytenoid cartilage. Although published series of this procedure are small, the decannulation rate after posterior approaches is near 100%.[39] Endoscopic posterior cricoid split and rib graft insertion has been successfully accomplished in a few children with posterior glottic and subglottic stenosis.[47]

Recurrent Respiratory Papillomatosis

Recurrent respiratory papillomatosis (RRP) is the expression of human papillomavirus (HPV) infection in the mucosa of the upper aerodigestive tract. Papillomas involving the larynx are the most common laryngeal tumor in children, and the larynx is the most frequent site of occurrence in the aerodigestive tract (Fig. 63-6). RRP of childhood tends to occur in clusters and has an

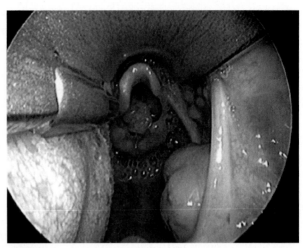

Figure 63-6 Laryngeal papilloma obstructing the glottis.

incredible propensity for recurrence. The clinical manifestation of laryngeal papilloma is progressive airway obstruction and dysphonia that may progress to aphonia. RRP is most commonly associated with HPV-6 and HPV-11. Subtypes 16 and 18 are only rarely associated with RRP but, if present, have a higher risk for malignant transformation. These viral particles are present in adjacent and clinically normal sites of the respiratory tract but are expressed primarily in anatomic locations of juxtaposed epithelium, hence the high predilection for the vocal cords.[53] The other common location is at an area of mucosal injury, such as a tracheotomy site.[53] The vector of transmission is controversial. Pediatric RRP and vaginal condyloma acuminatum are both caused by HPV subtypes 6 and 11, thus leading the majority of researchers to believe that vertical transmission from mother to child is taking place in most cases. Though unusual, vertical transmission to children born by cesarean section of mothers with vaginal warts has also been documented.[90]

The natural course of RRP is extremely variable, with no obvious patient-related risk factors to aid in prognosis. The estimated mean number of procedures per child for the disease is 19.7, with an average of 4.4 procedures per year. Many cases have been seen to regress spontaneously in adolescence, but others progress to extensive disease involving the trachea and pulmonary parenchyma, with a high fatality rate from untreatable airway obstruction or pulmonary complications. Even more uncommonly, the papilloma may undergo malignant degeneration to squamous cell carcinoma. For this reason, interval histologic examination of the removed tissue is important.

Pediatric RRP continues to be an extremely difficult management problem. The goal of surgical treatment is to maintain a patent airway while providing a usable voice and to prevent spread of disease into the distal airway.

Although the mainstay of surgical management has traditionally been the CO_2 laser, newer surgical techniques have demonstrated efficacy in the management of pediatric RRP, including powered instrumentation, the laryngeal shaver,[75] and the pulsed dye laser.[23] Regardless of the surgical technique used, scarring, stenosis, and web formation in the larynx are complications that occur despite careful endoscopic removal of the disease.

The papilloma should be removed down to the level of the vocal cord mucosa, but the cords themselves should not be incised. When working in the anterior commissure, bilateral resection should not be done to avoid web formation. Even in experienced hands, the incidence of minor scarring in the anterior glottis may be as high as 25%.[104] Aggressive resection beyond that necessary to maintain a safe airway will not improve the long-term prognosis for remission but may contribute to late morbidity.

The role of tracheotomy in the surgical management of laryngeal papilloma is controversial. Most surgeons try to avoid tracheotomy if possible. The mucosal injury at the tracheotomy site encourages the growth of papilloma outside the larynx, possibly increasing the probability of distal spread of the disease. The rate of tracheal spread in patients requiring tracheotomy has been reported to be as high as 50%.[16] It is quite possible, given the variable degree of aggressiveness of RRP, that patients who have distal spread of disease represent a subset with a predetermined propensity for dissemination beyond the larynx and would require a tracheotomy regardless. Patients in whom life-threatening airway obstruction develops as a result of aggressive disease within or beyond the larynx that cannot be managed by endoscopic procedures should have a tracheotomy placed until the disease can be controlled with further surgical intervention and adjunctive therapy. If a tracheotomy is placed, the clinician should make an effort to decannulate whenever possible.

None of the many adjunctive therapies described for the management of RRP has convincingly changed the outcome of the disease course. The most common adjuvant medical therapies used for pediatric RRP are interferon alfa-2a, retinoic acid, and indol-3-carbinol/diindolylmethane (I3C/DIM). The most recently introduced adjunctive therapy is cidofovir, an acyclic nucleoside phosphonate derivative with antiviral activity that is used for the treatment of cytomegalovirus retinitis in patients with acquired immunodeficiency syndrome. Off-label use of cidofovir injected directly into the region after removal of laryngeal papilloma has demonstrated efficacy in selected patients. In addition, promising research is being conducted to develop a vaccination for pediatric RRP.

Laryngotracheal and Subglottic Stenosis

Laryngotracheal stenosis may be characterized by etiology and area involved. Areas of involvement include the supraglottis, glottis, subglottis, and upper part of the trachea. A single area or multiple areas can be involved. Stenosis of the larynx is congenital (Fig. 63-7) or acquired (Fig. 63-8). Congenital stenoses are believed to be the result of failure or incomplete recanalization of the laryngeal lumen by the 10th week of gestation. Congenital subglottic stenosis is histopathologically divided into membranous and cartilaginous stenosis (Table 63-1).

Congenital stenosis is considered to exist when the lumen of the cricoid region of the airway measures less than 4 mm in a full-term infant or 3 mm in a premature infant with no previous history of intubation. As seen in Figure 63-7, the typical appearance of a congenital cartilaginous stenosis is that of an elliptically shaped

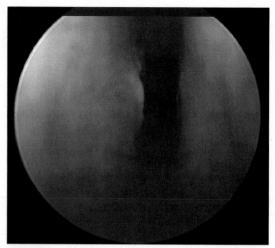

Figure 63-7 Congenital subglottic stenosis with an elliptically shaped cricoid.

cricoid cartilage. The definition of what may be congenital or acquired stenosis can be somewhat arbitrary because secondary soft tissue stenosis and scarring from injury may develop in children with congenital subglottic stenosis and thereby result in an acquired stenosis. This most commonly occurs with prolonged intubation, so the true incidence of congenital subglottic stenosis is difficult to determine. Of the areas involved in stenosis, the subglottis is the most common. Most subglottic stenoses that require surgical management are acquired. An example of acquired stenosis is seen in Figure 63-8. The principles of surgical management discussed are applicable to congenital and acquired disease.

Acquired subglottic stenosis became much more common after 1965 with the introduction of prolonged endotracheal intubation and ventilation of neonates.[64] As the survival of very-low-birth-weight infants increased, so did the number of patients with secondary laryngotracheal stenosis. It was recognized that acquired stenosis was more severe than congenital subglottic stenosis and a much more difficult management problem.[45] Fortunately, advances in the technique of endotracheal intubation and tube stabilization along with the implementation of softer

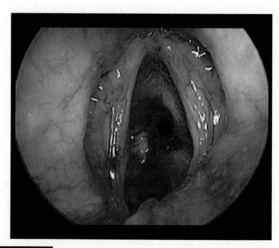

Figure 63-8 Acquired subglottic stenosis.

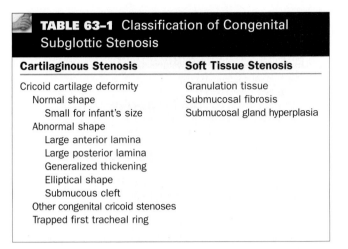

TABLE 63-1 Classification of Congenital Subglottic Stenosis

Cartilaginous Stenosis	Soft Tissue Stenosis
Cricoid cartilage deformity	Granulation tissue
Normal shape	Submucosal fibrosis
Small for infant's size	Submucosal gland hyperplasia
Abnormal shape	
Large anterior lamina	
Large posterior lamina	
Generalized thickening	
Elliptical shape	
Submucous cleft	
Other congenital cricoid stenoses	
Trapped first tracheal ring	

materials for endotracheal tubes have decreased the incidence of tracheal/laryngotracheal stenosis in surviving neonates to 0.9% to 8.3%.[78] With the proliferation of lifesaving advancements in medicine and surgery, children survive disease processes in which survival was not likely 20 years ago. Other chronic diseases also develop as a result of treatment, with subglottic stenosis being one of them. The numbers of toddlers, children, and adolescents in whom stenosis of the larynx is now developing has increased, but the exact percentages are unknown. The stenosis can be soft or firm and is commonly a combination of both. Causes of soft tissue stenosis are submucosal mucous gland hyperplasia, ductal cysts, fibrous and granulation tissue, and laryngopharyngeal reflux of gastric acid causing mucosal edema. Firm stenoses are usually associated with an abnormally shaped or thickened cricoid cartilage or mature scar tissue. The Cotton-Myer grading system is most widely used for documentation of the degree of obstruction (Fig. 63-9). Endotracheal tube sizing has become the most widely used means of grading and assessing the degree of stenosis.[71]

Successful laryngotracheal reconstructive surgery requires a carefully formulated plan that includes identification

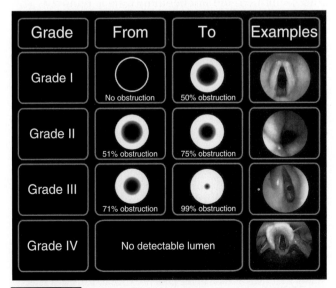

Grade	From	To	Examples
Grade I	No obstruction	50% obstruction	
Grade II	51% obstruction	75% obstruction	
Grade III	71% obstruction	99% obstruction	
Grade IV	No detectable lumen		

Figure 63-9 Cotton-Myer subglottic stenosis grading system.

and management of significant medical comorbid conditions that have the potential to contribute to poor outcomes. The plan also requires accurate identification of the type of stenosis and all areas of the larynx and upper trachea involved because the stenosis can be multilevel and require more than one type of intervention. The treatment plan is custom tailored to the specific patient and that patient's medical comorbid conditions and anatomic problems. The treatment plan is best formulated by a multidisciplinary team approach, including the pediatric otolaryngologist, pediatric surgeon, pulmonologist, gastroenterologist, anesthesiologist, intensivist, and appropriate allied health personnel.

Any laryngeal stenosis can be effectively managed by placement of a tracheotomy. The morbidity plus mortality associated with tracheotomy tube placement has encouraged advancements in laryngotracheal reconstructive procedures to either avoid tracheotomy tube placement or achieve decannulation.

Associated medical comorbid conditions, particularly cardiopulmonary disease and GERD, must be addressed, stabilized, and managed before considering surgical intervention. Children who require significant ventilatory or medical support are not good candidates for laryngotracheal reconstruction. Evaluation of swallowing function is essential to help determine the ability to protect the airway and the risk for aspiration so that preoperative and perioperative accommodations can be made to minimize the complications of aspiration. Patients with significant aspiration are not usually good candidates for laryngotracheal reconstruction.

The influence of gastroesophageal reflux on laryngotracheal stenosis and wounds cannot be overemphasized. GERD is an etiologic factor in acquired subglottic stenosis. Clinical and animal studies demonstrate that the presence of acid in the region of the larynx negatively affects healing.[31,36,58,62,95,107] Perioperative and postoperative aggressive medical and sometimes even surgical antireflux therapy[95] is recommended in the setting of laryngotracheal reconstructive surgery. Prospective and retrospective studies evaluating long-term outcomes of reflux control in such surgery are not available.

Surgical management of laryngotracheal stenosis is individualized to the patient, and no operative approach is exactly the same for all cases. Each individual patient has multiple variables that must be considered, including the location and extent of the stenotic area, medical comorbidity, airway protection and swallowing function, age, and weight. Surgical options include endoscopic techniques, expansion surgery, and resection surgery. The methods used are dependent on the degree and location of the stenosis. In general, grade I stenosis is usually managed by endoscopic techniques. Grade II stenosis may be approached with either endoscopic or open techniques, depending on the location and extent of the lesion. Grade III and IV lesions almost always require open surgical reconstruction.

Grade I and II stenosis can be approached with endoscopic techniques. CO_2 and potassium-titanyl-phosphate (KTP) lasers, because of their precise tissue characteristics, are the most widely used modalities. The laser is useful for treating early intubation injury with granulation tissue formation, subglottic cysts, thin circumferential webs, and crescent-shaped bands. Factors predisposing to failure of endoscopic laser treatment of subglottic stenosis are previous failed endoscopic procedures, significant loss of the cartilaginous framework, thick circumferential cicatricial scarring greater than 1 cm in vertical dimension, and posterior commissure involvement. A complication of laser treatment of subglottic stenosis is exposure of perichondrium or cartilage and subsequent perichondritis and chondritis, which may lead to further scar formation.

Open surgical reconstruction is recommended when endoscopic methods to establish a patent airway are inappropriate or have failed. An anterior cricoid split is considered one of the expansion surgical techniques. It is used predominantly in a neonate with anterior subglottic narrowing who fails multiple attempts at extubation despite adequate pulmonary reserve. In this setting the laryngotracheal problem is due to narrowing at the level of the cricoid cartilage, and the airway lumen expands and decompresses once the anterior cricoid cartilage is divided in the midline. The endotracheal tube is left in place for 5 to 10 days. Dexamethasone sodium phosphate is initiated 24 hours before extubation and continued for 5 days after extubation. This technique leads to successful extubation in 66% to 78% of patients.[19] As seen in Table 63-2, before considering the use of this technique in a neonate, several clinical criteria must be met to increase the probability of successful extubation after an anterior cricoid split.

In the authors' hands, this technique has been replaced by an anterior cricoid split with the placement of a small auricular cartilage graft followed by endotracheal intubation for 7 days. Outcomes comparing decannulation rates of cricoid split versus cricoid split with placement of an auricular cap graft have not been formally reviewed.

Multiple open procedures to expand a stenosed airway have been described. These procedures and their applications have evolved over the past 30 years. Since the introduction of laryngotracheal reconstruction with cartilage interpositional grafting in 1972 with placement of a cartilage graft between a split anterior cricoid and upper trachea,[19] this method has become one of the most common techniques of expanding stenotic airway segments. Anterior grafting alone is typically used for grade II

TABLE 63-2 Criteria for Performing an Anterior Cricoid Split
Extubation failure on at least two occasions secondary to subglottic laryngeal pathology
Weight greater than 1500 g
No ventilator support for at least 10 days before repair
Supplemental O$_2$ requirement less than 30%
No congestive heart failure for 1 month before repair
No acute respiratory tract infection
No antihypertensive medication for 10 days before repair

and III stenosis that does not involve the posterior glottis or subglottis. If there is posterior glottic or subglottic involvement in addition to the anterior stenosis, the posterior cricoid plate lamina is split with or without placement of an interpositional graft, depending on the degree of stenosis. This problem is more commonly seen in grade III and IV stenosis.

Partial cricotracheal resection has evolved into another option for the surgical management of selected grade III and IV stenosis.[38,69,85,93,98,102] In this operation the stenotic region of the anterior cricoid plate and any involved tracheal stenotic segment are resected, and the trachea is mobilized to allow for an end-to-end anastomosis. The posterior trachea and trachealis muscle are anastomosed to the posterior cricoid plate and its mucosa. The anterior mobilized trachea is then sewn into the removed segment of the cricoid and secured to the thyroid cartilage (Figs. 63-10 and 63-11).[38,85,93,98]

The traditional approach to laryngotracheal reconstructive surgery involves several stages of reconstruction[17,18,20,109] when an expansion operation is performed, and a stent (Silastic sheeting or Teflon) is placed to stabilize the reconstruction. The stent is left in place above the tracheotomy tube (suprastomal stent) for 1 to 6 weeks. After removal of the stent and once the surgical site has healed with a patent subglottis, the tracheotomy tube is downsized until the child tolerates and is able to breathe around a plugged tracheotomy tube. Once this is accomplished, the tracheotomy tube is removed. This process of reconstruction and decannulation can take weeks to several months. The morbidity and potential mortality associated with a tracheotomy tube are well

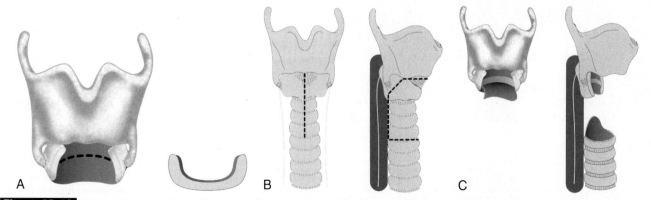

Figure 63-10 Cricotracheal resection. *A,* Resection of the anterior cricoid with a mucosal incision in the posterior cricoid. *B,* View of resection of a scarred airway with preservation of the recurrent laryngeal nerve. *C,* Resection complete with a cuff of posterior tracheal mucosa.

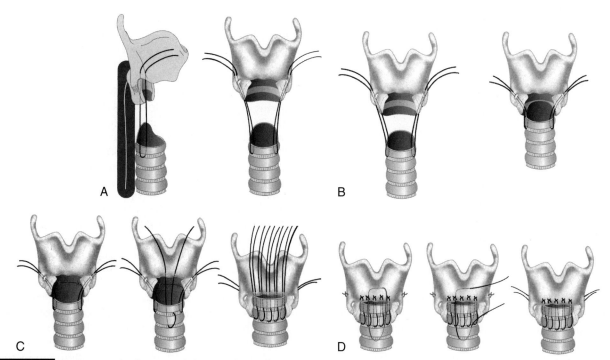

Figure 63–11 Reanastomosis of a resected airway. *A,* Detensioning suture. *B,* Mobilization of the trachea. *C,* Posterior anastomosis complete; anterior anastomotic sutures placed. *D,* Anastomosis complete.

recognized in children and have been discussed earlier in this chapter. With staged reconstruction and stent placement the child is left with little or no airway above the tracheotomy tube, which is life threatening if the tube accidentally falls out or is occluded. Long-term stenting carries the additional morbidity of granulation tissue formation, infection, dislodgment of the stent, dysphagia, and aspiration. To address these risks and circumvent some of these problems, single-stage laryngotracheal reconstruction (SSLTR) evolved. In the authors' hands, staged procedures are still performed in children with compromised pulmonary reserve, in those with complex multilevel stenosis that requires prolonged stenting, or in children in whom sedation is likely to be problematic.

SSLTR involves surgical correction of the stenotic airway with a short period of endotracheal intubation, thus avoiding the need for prolonged laryngotracheal stenting and tracheotomy tube dependency. The airway must have adequate cartilaginous support to consider SSLTR as a surgical option. SSLTR requires comprehensive understanding of the principles of airway reconstruction and extensive experience on the part of the surgeon, anesthesiologist, intensivist, and nursing staff. Postoperative care of these patients can be complicated.[34,37,48] The experience at our institution with 200 SSLTR cases showed that reintubation was required in 29% and postoperative tracheostomy in 15%. The overall decannulation rate was 96%. It was also found that the use of anterior and posterior costal cartilage grafting, age younger than 4 years, sedation for more than 48 hours, leak pressure around the endotracheal tube greater than 20 cm H_2O, and moderate/severe tracheomalacia significantly increased the rate of reintubation. The duration of stenting did not affect outcomes. Children with anterior and posterior grafts and those

with moderate or severe tracheomalacia were more likely to need a postoperative tracheostomy. SSLTR can be effectively used for the treatment of pediatric laryngotracheal stenosis; however, diligent preoperative assessment of the patient's comorbid conditions and airway, meticulous postoperative care, and surgical skill and experience are important to the success of this operation.

The ultimate goal of laryngotracheal reconstruction is tracheotomy decannulation or prevention. The rate of decannulation varies with the severity of stenosis and the method of reconstruction. Surgical management of pediatric subglottic stenosis is challenging. Multiple operations may be required to achieve eventual extubation or decannulation, and there is no specific model to predict the outcome of pediatric airway reconstructive surgery. Review of the experience at our institution shows that decannulation rates for double-staged laryngotracheal reconstruction for Cotton-Myer grades II, III, and IV are 95%, 74%, and 86%, respectively. SSLTR decannulation rates for Cotton-Myer grades II, III, and IV are 100%, 86%, and 100%. Our experience is that children with Cotton-Myer grade III or IV disease represent a significant challenge, and refinements of technique are needed to address this subset of children.

Children with grade IV stenosis are the most difficult group to obtain good results with surgical management. We have found that refinements in surgical technique plus the application of cricotracheal resection as the primary operation for grade IV stenosis has improved decannulation rates from 67% in the 1980s to 86% in the 1990s.[33] Our experience also shows that patients who undergo cricotracheal resection have higher decannulation rates than do those who undergo laryngotracheal reconstruction with anterior and posterior costal cartilage grafting (92% versus 81%). Cricotracheal resection patients are less likely to need additional open procedures to achieve decannulation (18% versus 46%).[33] Patients with grade IV stenosis and involvement of other areas of the larynx and trachea often require extended cricotracheal resection with the application of cartilage grafting or posterior cricoid and arytenoid procedures.

Hemangioma

Subglottic and tracheal hemangiomas are benign congenital vascular malformations derived from mesodermal rests. The lesions are relatively uncommon and account for 1.5% of all congenital laryngeal anomalies, with a 2:1 female preponderance.[44] Patients are usually asymptomatic at birth but have stridor within the first few months of life; 85% are identified in the first 6 months,[14] and 50% have cutaneous hemangiomas present at the time of diagnosis.[56] Asymmetric subglottic narrowing is the classic finding on soft tissue neck radiographs. Endoscopic diagnosis is usually made without biopsy because of the lesion's typical appearance of a compressible, asymmetric, submucosal mass with bluish or reddish discoloration most often found in the posterolateral region of the subglottis (Fig. 63-12).

Subglottic and tracheal hemangiomas have a rapid growth phase that slows by 12 months, followed by slow resolution over the subsequent months to years. Most show complete resolution by 5 years. However, subglottic hemangiomas are associated with 30% to 70% mortality when left untreated.[56] Therapeutic and surgical management of this problem is directed at maintaining the airway while minimizing potential long-term sequelae of the treatment itself. Current management options include partial laser excision, open surgical resection, systemic or intralesional steroids, systemic interferon alfa-2a, and tracheotomy.

Bypassing the obstructing lesion with a tracheotomy plus waiting for the expected involution provides the optimal anatomic result and is considered by many to be the standard of care by which all other treatment options need to be measured. However, as previously discussed in this chapter, there are risks associated with a tracheotomy, as well as the delay in speech and language that is routinely encountered when children require a tracheotomy at a young age. Early methods of treatment that are no longer used because of associated morbidity include external beam radiation, radium and gold implants, and sclerosing agents.

Systemic corticosteroids for the treatment of subglottic hemangiomas were introduced in 1969 by Cohen[15] and are used as both primary and adjuvant therapy. Steroids decrease the size of the hemangioma and accelerate involution by an unknown mechanism. They are thought to decrease hemangioma size by blocking estradiol-induced growth[40] or by directly increasing capillary sensitivity to vasoconstrictors. Corticosteroid therapy, with or without tracheotomy, has been shown to be successful in 82% to 97% of cases. However, whether the period of tracheotomy cannulation is decreased is unknown.[91] The risks associated with long-term steroid use include growth retardation, a cushingoid face, and increased susceptibility to infection, including life-threatening *Pneumocystis carinii* pneumonia.[3] Using an alternate-day dosing regimen in the smallest possible doses may reduce these effects. Recent reports suggest that systemic steroids followed by short-term intubation after diagnostic bronchoscopy can be used as a safe and effective alternative in the management of obstructive pediatric subglottic hemangiomas.[2] Others[66] report successful avoidance of tracheotomy by endoscopic intralesional injection of corticosteroids into the hemangioma, with or without short-term intubation.

Endoscopic surgical management with the CO_2 laser was first reported in 1980 by Healy and colleagues.[41] Since its introduction, the CO_2 laser alone or in combination with steroids or tracheotomy has become a standard therapy. Isolated unilateral subglottic hemangiomas are usually the best type and location for CO_2 laser treatment. In carefully selected patients, partial resection of the hemangioma with the CO_2 laser, with or without the addition of systemic corticosteroids, is successful.[92] Recent reports show that the KTP laser is a good tool for the management of subglottic hemangiomas and has a low incidence of complications.[52,60] The KTP laser is preferentially absorbed by hemoglobin, thus making this laser system well suited for the treatment of vascular tumors such as a hemangioma. Long-term outcomes of this technique are not available.

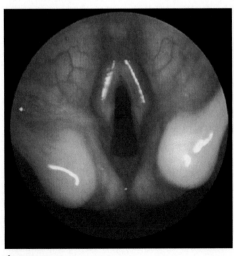
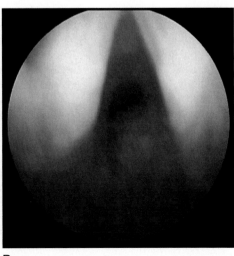

Figure 63-12 Subglottic hemangioma.

A

B

Interferon alfa-2a has been used recently in children with obstructing hemangiomas that were unresponsive to laser or corticosteroid therapy (or both), and it has achieved 50% or greater regression of the lesion in 73% of patients.[74] Interferon alfa-2a requires prolonged therapy because it does not promote involution but inhibits proliferation by blocking various steps in angiogenesis. The potential side effects, which include neuromuscular impairment, skin slough, fever, and liver enzyme elevation,[74] limit its use to larger, potentially fatal lesions.

Despite the more widespread use of steroids and other treatment modalities, the requirement for tracheostomy has remained unchanged over the last 20 years. The use of laser therapy does not appear to confer any additional therapeutic benefit over and above tracheostomy alone in bringing about resolution of subglottic hemangioma. Systemic steroids may reduce the size of the hemangioma but are associated with multiple adverse effects. The decision to use the aforementioned techniques must therefore be made in light of these observations.[13] To avoid the complications and provide more definitive treatment, the topic of open surgical excision has been revisited.[13,29,72,88,89,101,105] The surgical technique is similar to SSLTR. The airway is opened at the level of the cricoid cartilage, followed by submucosal dissection with excision of the hemangioma. Because an associated moderate subglottic stenosis is often present, an anterior cartilage graft is usually placed and the patient is intubated for 2 to 3 days. A recent study concluded that surgery for severe subglottic hemangioma is a reliable technique in selected patients and should be considered for corticoresistant or corticodependent, circular or bilateral hemangiomas[101] and large life-threatening hemangiomas.[29] The early experience of single-stage excision suggests that this technique is an exciting and promising surgical alternative, and more widespread adoption of it may be the best way of further improving the outcome of patients with subglottic hemangioma.[13]

Laryngeal and Laryngotracheoesophageal Clefts

Congenital laryngeal and laryngotracheoesophageal clefts (LTECs) are rare conditions that can be characterized by a posterior midline deficiency in separation of the larynx and trachea from the hypopharynx and esophagus (Fig. 63-13). The incidence is less than 0.1%, and the majority of cases may be sporadic or associated with a syndrome. There is a strong association with other anomalies (56%), most commonly tracheoesophageal fistula in 20% to 27%.[26] Six percent of children with a tracheoesophageal fistula have a coexisting laryngeal cleft. Of the children with a tracheoesophageal fistula, the laryngeal cleft goes undetected in three quarters until persistent aspiration, despite successful tracheoesophageal fistula repair, prompts further investigation.[26] Laryngeal clefts or LTECs are often associated with a syndrome, most commonly Opitz-G syndrome, the VATER association (vertebral defects, imperforate anus, tracheoesophageal fistula, radial and renal dysplasia), the VACTERL association (vertebral, anal, cardiac, tracheal, esophageal, renal, and limb anomalies), and Pallister-Hall syndrome.[25]

The degree of clefting may be relatively minor and involve only failure of interarytenoid muscle development,

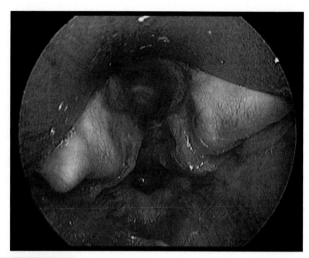

Figure 63-13   Laryngeal cleft.

or it can extend to the carina and even into the mainstem bronchi. Multiple classification systems have been used to describe laryngeal clefts. Independent of the numbering system used, it is useful to differentiate the length of the cleft as laryngeal (interarytenoid only, partial cricoid, or complete cricoid) and laryngotracheoesophageal (extending into the cervical trachea or the intrathoracic trachea).

Patients with a laryngeal cleft or LTEC have congenital inspiratory stridor, cyanotic attacks associated with feeding, aspiration, and recurrent pulmonary infections. As the length of the cleft increases, so does the severity of symptoms, with aspiration present in 100% of patients with LTECs. Although radiographic contrast studies may suggest aspiration, the best single study for identifying a laryngeal cleft is careful endoscopic examination with a high degree of suspicion on the part of the endoscopist. The arytenoids need to be parted to obtain adequate visualization because the clefts may be obscured by redundant esophageal mucosa prolapsing into the glottic and subglottic lumen. Most clefts that are limited to the supraglottic larynx do not require surgical intervention. The anatomic depth of these small clefts reaches to the interarytenoid level and stops at the vocal processes. Treatment methods include evaluation and treatment of gastroesophageal reflux and swallowing therapy.[26] When surgical intervention is required for these smaller clefts, the authors prefer an open repair, although some advocate endoscopic reapir.[8,26]

Surgical repair is required for all laryngeal clefts that extend below the vocal cords. An anterior approach through a laryngofissure is the standard technique, and it provides excellent exposure of the entire defect without risk to the laryngeal innervation. Complete LTECs that extend to the carina may require a posterolateral approach to allow for two-layer closure or an anterior approach with the use of either cardiopulmonary bypass or extracorporal circulation. In most circumstances, a tracheotomy is present before or placed at the time of reconstructive surgery. However, single-stage repair with endotracheal intubation used as a short-term stent is increasingly being performed and preferred by the authors for clefts extending to the midtrachea.

TRACHEAL LESIONS

Tracheomalacia

Tracheomalacia is a condition in which the tracheal wall cartilage is soft and pliable. The cardinal symptom of tracheomalacia is stridor with increased respiratory effort that leads to dynamic collapse of the airway. Tracheomalacia is primary or secondary, with the etiology of primary tracheomalacia being unknown. It is a common cause of stridor in infancy. Primary tracheomalacia differs from laryngomalacia in that the phase of stridor occurs during expiration; however, laryngomalacia and tracheomalacia can coexist, and the child may have both inspiratory and expiratory stridor. Most infants with primary or isolated tracheomalacia outgrow the condition by 18 months of age. Secondary tracheomalacia occurs as a result of another coexisting condition. The most common congenital conditions that cause secondary tracheomalacia are extrinsic compression of a vascular anomaly, such as a vascular ring or innominate artery (Fig. 63-14), and tracheoesophageal fistula, in which the malacia is opposite the fistula site located on the posterior tracheal wall. Tracheomalacia may also develop in infants who require long-term ventilatory support with high-pressure endotracheal tubes or cuffed tracheotomy tubes. There is no good treatment for severe or life-threatening tracheomalacia other than bypassing and stenting the area with a tracheotomy tube. Methods of endotracheal stenting with angioplasty and Palmaz stents have been attempted with varied success, and the authors prefer the use of a tracheotomy tube.

Congenital Tracheal Stenosis

Congenital tracheal stenosis is a rare, potentially life-threatening anomaly that usually involves complete cartilaginous tracheal rings and over the years has proved to be difficult to treat. In 1964, Cantrell and Guild[12] classified congenital tracheal stenosis into three categories: long-segment stenosis with generalized hypoplasia (22%), funnel-like stenosis (37%), and segmental stenosis (41%). Associated anomalies in children with congenital tracheal stenosis are common, with 24% having coexistent cardiovascular anomalies, including a pulmonary artery sling.[9]

Children with congenital tracheal stenosis usually have a history of biphasic stridor and possibly acute respiratory distress. Anteroposterior radiographs are strongly recommended at the initial evaluation, but a definitive diagnosis is best obtained with endoscopy (Fig. 63-15). Recent advances in three-dimensional magnetic resonance imaging provide an alternative for diagnosis and follow-up. Additionally, magnetic resonance imaging, contrast-enhanced computed tomography, or echocardiography is frequently needed to identify associated cardiovascular abnormalities. Over recent years, tremendous progress has been made in the treatment of congenital tracheal stenosis. Segmental resection with primary anastomosis has been shown to be the treatment of choice for stenoses involving up to 50% of the trachea. However, the large number of procedures advocated for the treatment of long-segment stenosis indicates that none has proved to be universally successful. Findings from our institution reiterate that nonoperative management of complete tracheal rings may be appropriate in selected patients. A retrospective study[86] estimated that up to 10% of patients with complete tracheal rings will not require tracheoplasty. Selected patients must be asymptomatic or have minimal symptoms and demonstrate tracheal growth over serial examinations; the rate of growth, however, is left to be determined. Anterior tracheoplasty with pericardium was first described by Idriss and colleagues in 1984.[46] Since then, reported results of this technique reveal survival rates of 47% to 76% in larger series.[24] Costal cartilage grafting for augmentation has had similar results[103] in a

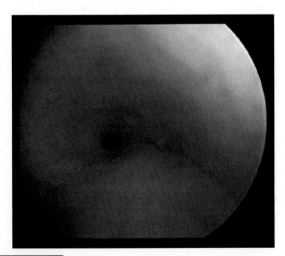

Figure 63–14 Secondary tracheomalacia from compression of the innominate artery.

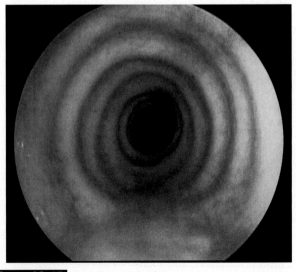

Figure 63–15 Complete tracheal rings.

smaller number of patients. Other augmentation materials that have been tried include esophageal wall, rib, dura, and periosteum.

Slide tracheoplasty, as described by Tsang and colleagues,[99] involves transverse division of the trachea in the middle of the stenosis and longitudinal incisions of the anterior portion on one end and the posterior portion on the other; the two ends slide over each other, thereby halving the length and doubling the diameter. In its original description, slide tracheoplasty was used for funnel-shaped stenoses. This technique has evolved and has now become the preferred surgical approach for tracheal stenosis regardless of the length of narrowing (Fig. 63-16).[21,84] Tracheal homograft reconstruction should be considered only if other methods are not applicable The 83% success and survival rate reported with this technique[49,50] has not stood the test of time.

Tracheobronchial Vascular Compression

Vascular compression of the tracheobronchial tree has been the subject of much discussion since 1945, when the first successful operation for a double aortic arch was described. A 1963 report[27] reviewed 104 cases and coined the term "reflex apnea" to describe the episodic apnea associated with airway vascular compression. This series was reviewed and updated in 1969,[70] with successful medical management reported in 86.3% of 285 cases.

Initial indications for surgical management included reflex apnea and recurrent bronchopulmonary infections, and these indications were expanded into absolute and relative criteria.[59] Relative criteria included failure of medical management, greater than 50% compression of the tracheal lumen, and associated airway and lung abnormalities. Further definition of indications was reported in 1975, when 60 children who were operated on for innominate artery compression of the trachea were compared with 30 children who did not undergo surgery; it should be noted that the appropriateness of surgical intervention was based not on the severity of compression seen at endoscopy or radiographically but on the severity of symptoms.[68] Discontinuation of the word "anomalous" was recommended in 1981 when it was reported that an origin of the innominate artery partially or totally to the left of the trachea was a normal finding in children, as seen on aortography in 96% of patients.[94]

Vascular compression of the tracheobronchial tree has an overall incidence of 3%. The most common symptomatic true vascular ring is a double aortic arch, which occurs if the fourth branchial arches and the dorsal aortic root persist on both sides. In 1 in 2500 persons, the left arch has an atretic segment, but the right arch persists. A right-sided arch with a descending right aorta does not cause airway compromise. However, if there is an associated left ductus or an aberrant left subclavian artery, a loose vascular ring is formed that generally results in less airway compromise than a true double aortic arch does. Because of the associated airway compression of the lower trachea and right main bronchus, a pulmonary artery sling is the most symptomatic of the noncircumferential vascular anomalies and occurs when the left sixth arch resorbs and the left pulmonary artery arises as a large collateral artery from the right pulmonary artery and passes between the esophagus and trachea to perfuse the left lung. This anomaly commonly results in significant compromise of the right mainstem bronchus and airway symptoms. In addition, 30% of patients with pulmonary artery slings have associated complete tracheal rings.[4] The aberrant right subclavian artery is the most common mediastinal vascular anomaly. However, because of its retroesophageal course, affected individuals may have dysphagia, but rarely symptomatic airway compromise. Innominate artery compression of the trachea is not associated with a true vascular anomaly. The innominate artery normally passes from its origin on the aortic arch left of midline, across the anterior surface of the trachea, to the right side. It has been hypothesized that in patients who are symptomatic, the innominate artery is more taut than normal and the tracheal cartilage is unusually compliant and more easily compressed or that dilatation of other structures, such as the heart, esophagus, or thymus, causes mediastinal crowding.

Respiratory compromise from tracheobronchial vascular compression is potentially life threatening but can cause subtle symptoms. A high index of suspicion is required to make the diagnosis. Patients with significant vascular compression are usually identified early because of the presence of stridor, chronic cough, recurrent bronchitis and pneumonia, difficulty feeding and failure to thrive, and occasionally reflex apnea. Reflex apnea has

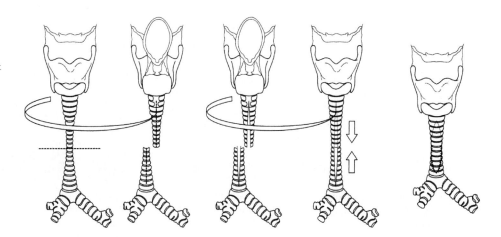

Figure 63–16 Slide tracheoplasty: transverse section of the trachea, with a proximal segment of the rings split posteriorly and the distal segment split anteriorly. Sliding of the two portions together doubles the circumference and halves the length.

been described as a reflexive respiratory arrest of variable duration that is secondary to the stimulation of vagal afferent nerve fibers during swallowing and other forms of transient intrathoracic pressure changes, and it can be fatal.

Chest radiographs may provide some evidence of tracheal compression, and a barium esophagogram can show relatively characteristic filling defects that correspond to the various types of vascular compression. However, once vascular compression is suspected, the diagnostic modality of choice is magnetic resonance imaging, which will clearly demonstrate the mediastinal vascular anatomy, as well as the size of the lower airway. Spiral computed tomography may be a useful adjunct or alternative to magnetic resonance imaging.[35,55] Although today the diagnosis of vascular compression is usually known before undergoing endoscopy, bronchoscopy also reveals characteristic findings of compression, depending on the type of vascular ring or sling. Bronchoscopy provides immediate visual assessment of the surgical results that can be achieved with relief of the compression and the degree of residual tracheomalacia present.

Nonsurgical management may be effective for the majority of cases of innominate artery compression and loose vascular rings and slings that are mildly symptomatic. In contrast, moderately to severely symptomatic patients usually require surgical repair. Absolute indications for surgical treatment include reflex apnea, failure of medical management of severe respiratory distress after 48 hours, and prolonged intubation. Relative criteria include repeated episodes of lower respiratory tract infection, exercise intolerance, significant dysphagia with failure to thrive, or coexisting subglottic stenosis, asthma, cystic fibrosis, or previous tracheoesophageal repair.

Innominate artery compression is relieved by aortopexy or reimplantation, with success rates of 93% to 100% and no reports of operative mortality or long-term morbidity.[1] Occasionally, aortopexy sutures can loosen and the procedure needs to be revised.

The results of surgical treatment of vascular rings are also encouraging, with 70% to 92% obtaining complete resolution of symptoms.[5] A double aortic arch requires surgical division of the smaller of the two arches. The ductus arteriosus or aberrant subclavian artery is divided in the case of a right aortic arch with a left ductus arteriosus or an aberrant left subclavian artery. In patients with severe tracheobronchial compression, residual tracheomalacia may persist for a variable period, and occasionally a tracheotomy is required to stent the malacic segment.

A pulmonary artery sling is corrected by dividing the aberrant left pulmonary artery at its origin and reimplanting it anterior to the trachea. Coexisting complete tracheal rings need to be addressed at the same operation either by resection and end-to-end anastomosis or with a slide tracheoplasty.

REFERENCES

1. Adler SC, Isaacson G, Balsara RK: Innominate artery compression of the trachea: Diagnosis and treatment by anterior suspension. A 25-year experience. Ann Otol Rhinol Laryngol 1995;104:924-927.

2. Al-Sebeih K, Manoukian J: Systemic steroids for the management of obstructive subglottic hemangioma. J Otolaryngol 2000;29:361-366.

3. Aviles R, Boyce TG, Thompson DM: *Pneumocystis carinii* pneumonia in a 3-month-old infant receiving high-dose corticosteroid therapy for airway hemangiomas. Mayo Clin Proc 2004;79:243-245.

4. Backer CL: Vascular rings, slings, and tracheal rings. Mayo Clin Proc 1993;68:1131-1133.

5. Backer CL, Ilbawi MN, Idriss FS, et al: Vascular anomalies causing tracheoesophageal compression. Review of experience in children. J Thorac Cardiovasc Surg 1989;97:725-731.

6. Baxter MR: Congenital laryngomalacia. Can J Anaesth 1994; 41:332-339.

7. Benjamin B: Chevalier Jackson Lecture. Congenital laryngeal webs. Ann Otol Rhinol Laryngol 1983;92:317-326.

8. Bent JP 3rd, Bauman NM, Smith RJ: Endoscopic repair of type IA laryngeal clefts. Laryngoscope 1997;107:282-286.

9. Blumer JR, Bauman NM, Kearns DP, et al: Distal tracheal stenosis in neonates and infants. Otolaryngol Head Neck Surg 1992;107:583-590.

10. Bower CM, Choi SS, Cotton RT: Arytenoidectomy in children. Ann Otol Rhinol Laryngol 1994;103:271-278.

11. Brigger MT, Hartnick CJ: Surgery for pediatric vocal cord paralysis: A meta-analysis. Otolaryngol Head Neck Surg 2002; 126:349-355.

12. Cantrell JR, Guild HG: Congenital stenosis of the trachea. Am J Surg 1964;108:297-305.

13. Chatrath P, Black M, Jani P, et al: A review of the current management of infantile subglottic haemangioma, including a comparison of CO_2 laser therapy versus tracheostomy. Int J Pediatr Otorhinolaryngol 2002;64:143-157.

14. Choa DI, Smith MC, Evans JN, et al: Subglottic haemangioma in children. J Laryngol Otol 1986;100:447-454.

15. Cohen SR: Unusual lesions of the larynx, trachea and bronchial tree. Ann Otol Rhinol Laryngol 1969;78: 476-489.

16. Cole RR, Myer CM 3rd, Cotton RT: Tracheotomy in children with recurrent respiratory papillomatosis. Head Neck 1989;11:226-230.

17. Cotton RT: Pediatric laryngotracheal stenosis. J Pediatr Surg 1984;19:699-704.

18. Cotton RT, Myer CM 3rd: Contemporary surgical management of laryngeal stenosis in children. Am J Otolaryngol 1984;5:360-368.

19. Cotton RT, Myer CM 3rd, Bratcher GO, et al: Anterior cricoid split, 1977-1987. Evolution of a technique. Arch Otolaryngol Head Neck Surg 1988;114:1300-1302.

20. Cotton RT, Gray SD, Miller RP: Update of the Cincinnati experience in pediatric laryngotracheal reconstruction. Laryngoscope 1989;99:1111-1116.

21. Cunningham MJ, Eavey RD, Vlahakes GJ, et al: Slide tracheoplasty for long-segment tracheal stenosis. Arch Otolaryngol Head Neck Surg 1998;124:98-103.

22. Denoyelle F, Mondain M, Gresillon N, et al: Failures and complications of supraglottoplasty in children. Arch Otolaryngol Head Neck Surg 2003;129:1077-1080, discussion 1080.

23. Derkay CS, Darrow DH: Recurrent respiratory papillomatosis of the larynx: Current diagnosis and treatment. Otolaryngol Clin North Am 2000;33:1127-1142.

24. Dunham ME, Holinger LD, Backer CL, et al: Management of severe congenital tracheal stenosis. Ann Otol Rhinol Laryngol 1994;103:351-356.

25. Eriksen C, Zwillenberg D, Robinson N: Diagnosis and management of cleft larynx. Literature review and case report. Ann Otol Rhinol Laryngol 1990;99:703-708.

26. Evans KL, Courteney-Harris R, Bailey CM, et al: Management of posterior laryngeal and laryngotracheoesophageal clefts. Arch Otolaryngol Head Neck Surg 1995;121:1380-1385.

27. Fearon B, Shortreed R: Tracheobronchial compression by congenital cardiovascular anomalies in children. Syndrome of apnea. Ann Otol Rhinol Laryngol 1963;72:949-969.

28. Friedman EM, de Jong AL, Sulek M: Pediatric bilateral vocal fold immobility: The role of carbon dioxide laser posterior transverse partial cordectomy. Ann Otol Rhinol Laryngol 2001;110:723-728.

29. Froehlich P, Seid AB, Morgon A: Contrasting strategic approaches to the management of subglottic hemangiomas. Int J Pediatr Otorhinolaryngol 1996;36:137-146.

30. Giannoni C, Sulek M, Friedman EM, et al: Gastroesophageal reflux association with laryngomalacia: A prospective study. Int J Pediatr Otorhinolaryngol 1998;43:11-20.

31. Gilger MA: Pediatric otolaryngologic manifestations of gastroesophageal reflux disease. Curr Gastroenterol Rep 2003;5:247-252.

32. Gray SD, Kelly SM, Dove H: Arytenoid separation for impaired pediatric vocal fold mobility. Ann Otol Rhinol Laryngol 1994;103:510-515.

33. Gustafson LM, Hartley BE, Cotton RT: Acquired total (grade 4) subglottic stenosis in children. Ann Otol Rhinol Laryngol 2001;110:16-19.

34. Gustafson LM, Hartley BE, Liu JH, et al: Single-stage laryngotracheal reconstruction in children: A review of 200 cases. Otolaryngol Head Neck Surg 2000;123:430-434.

35. Gustafson LM, Liu JH, Link DT, et al: Spiral CT versus MRI in neonatal airway evaluation. Int J Pediatr Otorhinolaryngol 2000;52:197-201.

36. Halstead LA: Gastroesophageal reflux: A critical factor in pediatric subglottic stenosis. Otolaryngol Head Neck Surg 1999;120:683-688.

37. Hartley BE, Gustafson LM, Liu JH, et al: Duration of stenting in single-stage laryngotracheal reconstruction with anterior costal cartilage grafts. Ann Otol Rhinol Laryngol 2001;110:413-416.

38. Hartley BE, Rutter MJ, Cotton RT: Cricotracheal resection as a primary procedure for laryngotracheal stenosis in children. Int J Pediatr Otorhinolaryngol 2000;54:133-136.

39. Hartnick CJ, Brigger MT, Willging JP, et al: Surgery for pediatric vocal cord paralysis: A retrospective review. Ann Otol Rhinol Laryngol 2003;112:1-6.

40. Hawkins DB, Crockett DM, Kahlstrom EJ, et al: Corticosteroid management of airway hemangiomas: Long-term follow-up. Laryngoscope 1984;94:633-637.

41. Healy GB, Fearon B, French R, et al: Treatment of subglottic hemangioma with the carbon dioxide laser. Laryngoscope 1980;90:809-813.

42. Holland BW, Koufman JA, Postma GN, et al: Laryngopharyngeal reflux and laryngeal web formation in patients with pediatric recurrent respiratory papillomas. Laryngoscope 2002;112:1926-1929.

43. Holinger LD, Konior RJ: Surgical management of severe laryngomalacia. Laryngoscope 1989;99:136-142.

44. Holinger PH, Brown WT: Congenital webs, cysts, laryngoceles and other anomalies of the larynx. Ann Otol Rhinol Laryngol 1967;76:744-752.

45. Holinger PH, Kutnick SL, Schild JA, et al: Subglottic stenosis in infants and children. Ann Otol Rhinol Laryngol 1976;85:591-599.

46. Idriss FS, DeLeon SY, Ilbawi MN, et al: Tracheoplasty with pericardial patch for extensive tracheal stenosis in infants and children. J Thorac Cardiovasc Surg 1984;88:527-536.

47. Inglis AF Jr, Perkins JA, Manning SC, et al: Endoscopic posterior cricoid split and rib grafting in 10 children. Laryngoscope 2003;113:2004-2009.

48. Jacobs BR, Salman BA, Cotton RT, et al: Postoperative management of children after single-stage laryngotracheal reconstruction. Crit Care Med 2001;29:164-168.

49. Jacobs JP, Elliott MJ, Haw MP, et al: Pediatric tracheal homograft reconstruction: A novel approach to complex tracheal stenoses in children. J Thorac Cardiovasc Surg 1996;112:1549-1558, discussion 1559-1560.

50. Jacobs JP, Haw MP, Motbey JA, et al: Successful complete tracheal resection in a three-month-old infant. Ann Thorac Surg 1996;61:1824-1826, discussion 1827.

51. Jani P, Koltai P, Ochi JW, et al: Surgical treatment of laryngomalacia. J Laryngol Otol 1991;105:1040-1045.

52. Kacker A, April M, Ward RF: Use of potassium titanyl phosphate (KTP) laser in management of subglottic hemangiomas. Int J Pediatr Otorhinolaryngol 2001;59:15-21.

53. Kashima H, Mounts P, Leventhal B, et al: Sites of predilection in recurrent respiratory papillomatosis. Ann Otol Rhinol Laryngol 1993;102:580-583.

54. Lane RW, Weider DJ, Steinem C, et al: Laryngomalacia. A review and case report of surgical treatment with resolution of pectus excavatum. Arch Otolaryngol 1984;110:546-551.

55. Lee KH, Yoon CS, Choe KO, et al: Use of imaging for assessing anatomical relationships of tracheobronchial anomalies associated with left pulmonary artery sling. Pediatr Radiol 2001;31:269-278.

56. Leikensohn JR, Benton C, Cotton R: Subglottic hemangioma. J Otolaryngol 1976;5:487-492.

57. Link DT, Cotton R: The laryngotracheal complex in pediatric head and neck trauma: Securing the airway and management of external laryngeal injury. Facial Plast Surg Clin North Am 1999;7:133-144.

58. Little FB, Koufman JA, Kohut RI, et al: Effect of gastric acid on the pathogenesis of subglottic stenosis. Ann Otol Rhinol Laryngol 1985;94:516-519.

59. Macdonald RE, Fearon B: Innominate artery compression syndrome in children. Ann Otol Rhinol Laryngol 1971;80:535-540.

60. Madgy D, Ahsan SF, Kest D, et al: The application of the potassium-titanyl-phosphate (KTP) laser in the management of subglottic hemangioma. Arch Otolaryngol Head Neck Surg 2001;127:47-50.

61. Marcus CL, Crockett DM, Ward SL: Evaluation of epiglottoplasty as treatment for severe laryngomalacia. J Pediatr 1990;117:706-710.

62. Maronian NC, Azadeh H, Waugh P, et al: Association of laryngopharyngeal reflux disease and subglottic stenosis. Ann Otol Rhinol Laryngol 2001;110:606-612.

63. McClurg FL, Evans DA: Laser laryngoplasty for laryngomalacia. Laryngoscope 1994;104:247-252.

64. McDonald IH, Stocks JG: Prolonged nasotracheal intubation. A review of its development in a paediatric hospital. Br J Anaesth 1965;37:161-173.

65. McSwiney PF, Cavanagh NP, Languth P: Outcome in congenital stridor (laryngomalacia). Arch Dis Child 1977;52:215-218.

66. Meeuwis J, Bos CE, Hoeve LJ, et al: Subglottic hemangiomas in infants: Treatment with intralesional corticosteroid injection and intubation. Int J Pediatr Otorhinolaryngol 1990;19:145-150.

67. Milczuk HA, Smith JD, Everts EC: Congenital laryngeal webs: Surgical management and clinical embryology. Int J Pediatr Otorhinolaryngol 2000;52:1-9.

68. Moes CA, Izukawa T, Trusler GA: Innominate artery compression of the trachea. Arch Otolaryngol 1975;101:733-738.

69. Monnier P, Lang F, Savary M: Partial cricotracheal resection for pediatric subglottic stenosis: A single institution's experience in 60 cases. Eur Arch Otorhinolaryngol 2003;260:295-297.

70. Mustard WT, Bayliss CE, Fearon B, et al: Tracheal compression by the innominate artery in children. Ann Thorac Surg 1969;8:312-319.

71. Myer CM 3rd, O'Connor DM, Cotton RT: Proposed grading system for subglottic stenosis based on endotracheal tube sizes. Ann Otol Rhinol Laryngol 1994;103: 319-323.

72. Naiman AN, Ayari S, Froehlich P: Controlled risk of stenosis after surgical excision of laryngeal hemangioma. Arch Otolaryngol Head Neck Surg 2003;129:1291-1295.

73. Narcy P, Contencin P, Viala P: Surgical treatment for laryngeal paralysis in infants and children. Ann Otol Rhinol Laryngol 1990;99:124-128.

74. Ohlms LA, Jones DT, McGill TJ, et al: Interferon alfa-2a therapy for airway hemangiomas. Ann Otol Rhinol Laryngol 1994;103:1-8.

75. Parsons DS, Bothwell MR: Powered instrument papilloma excision: An alternative to laser therapy for recurrent respiratory papilloma. Laryngoscope 2001;111:1494-1496.

76. Pollack IF, Kinnunen D, Albright AL: The effect of early craniocervical decompression on functional outcome in neonates and young infants with myelodysplasia and symptomatic Chiari II malformations: Results from a prospective series. Neurosurgery 1996;38:703-710, discussion 710.

77. Polonovski JM, Contencin P, Francois M, et al: Aryepiglottic fold excision for the treatment of severe laryngomalacia. Ann Otol Rhinol Laryngol 1990;99:625-627.

78. Ratner I, Whitfield J: Acquired subglottic stenosis in the very-low-birth-weight infant. Am J Dis Child 1983;137: 40-43.

79. Remacle M, Bodart E, Lawson G, et al: Use of the CO_2-laser micropoint micromanipulator for the treatment of laryngomalacia. Eur Arch Otorhinolaryngol 1996;253:401-404.

80. Rimell FL, Dohar JE: Endoscopic management of pediatric posterior glottic stenosis. Ann Otol Rhinol Laryngol 1998; 107:285-290.

81. Roger G, Denoyelle F, Triglia JM, et al: Severe laryngomalacia: Surgical indications and results in 115 patients. Laryngoscope 1995;105:1111-1117.

82. Rosenfeld RM, Stool SE: Should granulomas be excised in children with long-term tracheotomy? Arch Otolaryngol Head Neck Surg 1992;118:1323-1327.

83. Rudolph CD, Mazur LJ, Liptak GS, et al: Guidelines for evaluation and treatment of gastroesophageal reflux in infants and children: Recommendations of the North American Society for Pediatric Gastroenterology and Nutrition. J Pediatr Gastroenterol Nutr 2001;32(Suppl 2): S1-S31.

84. Rutter MJ, Cotton RT, Azizkhan RG, et al: Slide tracheoplasty for the management of complete tracheal rings. J Pediatr Surg 2003;38:928-934.

85. Rutter MJ, Hartley BE, Cotton RT: Cricotracheal resection in children. Arch Otolaryngol Head Neck Surg 2001;127: 289-292.

86. Rutter MJ, Willging JP, Cotton RT: Nonoperative management of complete tracheal rings. Arch Otolaryngol Head Neck Surg 2004;130:450-452.

87. Seid AB, Park SM, Kearns MJ, et al: Laser division of the aryepiglottic folds for severe laryngomalacia. Int J Pediatr Otorhinolaryngol 1985;10:153-158.

88. Seid AB, Pransky SM, Kearns DB: The open surgical approach to subglottic hemangioma. Int J Pediatr Otorhinolaryngol 1991;22:85-90.

89. Seid AB, Pransky SM, Kearns DB: The open surgical approach to subglottic hemangioma. Int J Pediatr Otorhinolaryngol 1993;26:95-96.

90. Shah K, Kashima H, Polk BF, et al: Rarity of cesarean delivery in cases of juvenile-onset respiratory papillomatosis. Obstet Gynecol 1986;68:795-799.

91. Shikhani AH, Jones MM, Marsh BR, et al: Infantile subglottic hemangiomas. An update. Ann Otol Rhinol Laryngol 1986;95:336-347.

92. Sie KC, McGill T, Healy GB: Subglottic hemangioma: Ten years' experience with the carbon dioxide laser. Ann Otol Rhinol Laryngol 1994;103:167-172.

93. Stern Y, Gerber ME, Walner DL, et al: Partial cricotracheal resection with primary anastomosis in the pediatric age group. Ann Otol Rhinol Laryngol 1997;106:891-896.

94. Strife JL, Baumel AS, Dunbar JS: Tracheal compression by the innominate artery in infancy and childhood. Radiology 1981;139:73-75.

95. Suskind DL, Zeringue GP 3rd, Kluka EA, et al: Gastroesophageal reflux and pediatric otolaryngologic disease: The role of antireflux surgery. Arch Otolaryngol Head Neck Surg 2001;127:511-514.

96. Toynton SC, Saunders MW, Bailey CM: Aryepiglottoplasty for laryngomalacia: 100 consecutive cases. J Laryngol Otol 2001;115:35-38.

97. Triglia JM, Belus JF, Nicollas R: Arytenoidopexy for bilateral vocal fold paralysis in young children. J Laryngol Otol 1996;110:1027-1030.

98. Triglia JM, Nicollas R, Roman S: Primary cricotracheal resection in children: Indications, technique and outcome. Int J Pediatr Otorhinolaryngol 2001;58:17-25.

99. Tsang V, Murday A, Gillbe C, et al: Slide tracheoplasty for congenital funnel-shaped tracheal stenosis. Ann Thorac Surg 1989;48:632-635.

100. Unal M: The successful management of congenital laryngeal web with endoscopic lysis and topical mitomycin-C. Int J Pediatr Otorhinolaryngol 2004;68:231-235.

101. Van Den Abbeele T, Triglia JM, Lescanne E, et al: Surgical removal of subglottic hemangiomas in children. Laryngoscope 1999;109:1281-1286.

102. Walner DL, Stern Y, Cotton RT: Margins of partial cricotracheal resection in children. Laryngoscope 1999;109: 1607-1610.

103. Weber TR, Eigen H, Scott PH, et al: Resection of congenital tracheal stenosis involving the carina. J Thorac Cardiovasc Surg 1982;84:200-203.

104. Wetmore SJ, Key JM, Suen JY: Complications of laser surgery for laryngeal papillomatosis. Laryngoscope 1985;95: 798-801.

105. Wiatrak BJ, Reilly JS, Seid AB, et al: Open surgical excision of subglottic hemangioma in children. Int J Pediatr Otorhinolaryngol 1996;34:191-206.

106. Yamada H, Tanaka Y, Nakamura S: Laryngeal stridor associated with the Chiari II malformation. Childs Nerv Syst 1985;1:312-318.

107. Yellon RF, Goldberg H: Update on gastroesophageal reflux disease in pediatric airway disorders. Am J Med 2001;111(Suppl 8A):78S-84S.

108. Younis RT, Lazar RH, Astor F: Posterior cartilage graft in single-stage laryngotracheal reconstruction. Otolaryngol Head Neck Surg 2003;129:168-175.

109. Zalzal GH, Cotton RT, McAdams AJ: Cartilage grafts—present status. Head Neck Surg 1986;8:363-374.

110. Zalzal GH, Anon JB, Cotton RT: Epiglottoplasty for the treatment of laryngomalacia. Ann Otol Rhinol Laryngol 1987;96:72-76.

Chapter 64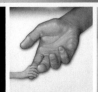

Infections and Diseases of the Lungs, Pleura, and Mediastinum

Pramod S. Puligandla and Jean-Martin Laberge

LUNG INFECTIONS

Pulmonary infections affect children of all ages. Although the majority of mild to moderate infections can be treated effectively on an outpatient basis, there are still those patients who require hospitalization for treatment. The availability of vaccines and the use of a larger arsenal of antibiotics have decreased the incidence of severe lung infections and their complications. Indeed, empyema and lung abscess are presently less common sequelae of pulmonary infections. However, there has been a concurrent increase in the use of immunosuppressive medications and intensive chemotherapy that predisposes this population of patients to increased risk. Adjunctive techniques, including bronchoalveolar lavage and lung biopsy, are being required more frequently in immunocompromised patients to guide therapy and direct management.

Epidemiology

Previous estimates of the incidence of respiratory infections were based on studies from the 1980s and early 1990s from Europe and the United States.[160,208,265] These reports indicated that the incidence of respiratory infections was highest for younger children (6 months to 5 years) and decreased with age. More recent data support these previous findings.[25,247,253,408] The incidence of respiratory infections for children younger than 5 years of age is 3.0 to 3.6/100. From an etiologic standpoint, several studies have identified both *Streptococcus pneumoniae* and viral agents as the most common causes of respiratory infections.[247,341] In terms of age, respiratory syncytial virus (RSV) prevails in young children (<2 years) with a larger proportion of community-acquired pneumonia being attributable to *S. pneumoniae* for children older than 2 years of age.[247,253,341] No causative agent may be identified in up to 40% to 60% of community-acquired pneumonia.[158]

Community-Acquired Bacterial Pneumonia

Streptococcus pneumoniae

Streptococcus pneumoniae is a major cause of morbidity and mortality around the world. It is the most common pathogen in infants and children and is responsible for approximately 500,000 cases of pneumonia per year in the United States.[356] Worldwide, up to 3 million deaths per year occur as a result of pneumonia, with the majority of these cases occurring in developing countries and as a result of *S. pneumoniae* infection.[116,143] The increasing antibiotic resistance of this species over the past several years has led to changes in empirical therapy that may not be as effective.[185,260,358]

S. pneumoniae is a gram-positive coccus that is part of the normal flora in children and adults. Colonization rates, particularly of the nasopharyngeal mucosa, appear to decrease with age and are an important factor in the development of infection.[356] The symptoms of infection include fever, productive cough, tachypnea, dyspnea, malaise, and occasional emesis. On physical examination, patients have hypoxia and decreased breath sounds with crackles over the affected area. Radiographically, pneumococcal infections can be lobar, multilobar, or sometimes segmental (Fig. 64-1), and up to 40% of these patients will also have pleural fluid. The treatment of this infection, most often performed on an outpatient basis, is complicated by bacterial resistance.[37,185,358] For patients infected with a strain demonstrating low to intermediate resistance, penicillin and other β-lactam antibiotics are still effective. Cephalosporins may be used in cases of high resistance or if there is no clinical improvement with conventional therapy.[185,358] The introduction of new heptavalent conjugate vaccines has impacted on the severity of disease.[60,287] These vaccines appear to be safe and effective, potentially reducing the number of cases of pneumococcal pneumonia by 50,000 to 300,000 per year.[357]

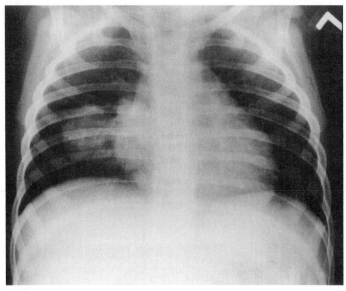

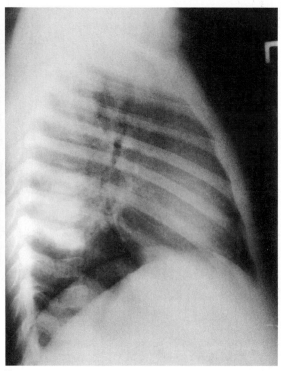

A

Figure 64–1 Chest radiograph of a 1.5-year old boy with fever and dyspnea shows a typical round pneumonia of the superior segment of the lower lobe; an air bronchogram can be seen within the opacity. *A,* Anteroposterior view. *B,* Lateral view.

B

Haemophilus influenzae

This small, encapsulated gram-negative bacillus is a common cause of community-acquired pneumonia.[137,253,408] Over 95% of invasive cases of *Haemophilus* are caused by the type B strain. Infections with *Haemophilus* usually occur in the winter and spring. The clinical presentation includes fever, tachypnea, elevated white blood cell count, and the presence of unilateral consolidation with pleural effusion on chest radiographs. Extrapulmonary manifestations, such as meningitis and epiglottitis, are more common with this organism. Treatment is based on the susceptibility of these bacteria to β-lactam antibiotics. Cephalosporins can be used for those strains producing β-lactamase.[277] The overall incidence of this species causing significant infections has been dramatically reduced with the introduction of the *Haemophilus* vaccine, although a recent report has linked this immunization with the development of type 1 diabetes in children.[75] Secondary transmission of invasive *Haemophilus* may still be significant in the household or day-care setting.[81] In such cases, prophylaxis with rifampin may be needed for high-risk children or if elimination of nasopharyngeal carriage is desired.[81]

Staphylococcus aureus

These ubiquitous gram-positive cocci are commonly found on the skin and nasal mucosa, with 20% to 30% of the population being normal carriers of this bacterium.[81] *S. aureus* produces toxins and enzymes that form the basis of the lesions produced by this pathogen—a pyogenic exudate or an abscess.[81,114] Staphylococcal infections

are usually progressive, occurring in infancy and early childhood. Primary pneumonias occur during the winter and spring. Patients often present with fever and rapidly develop respiratory symptoms. Clinical and radiologic deterioration quickly ensues if the infection is left untreated. Radiographically, primary pneumonias display unilateral lobar consolidation. Secondary infection/pneumonia usually involves a prolonged febrile illness and is often accompanied by positive blood cultures.[81] These infections usually present as diffuse bilateral infiltrates on chest radiographs. Staphylococcal pneumonias are often associated with pleural effusions,[58,319] empyemas,[63,175,182] lung abscesses,[114,405] or pneumatoceles[203,405] during the healing phase. Such lesions require follow-up until complete resolution (see later). Treatment involves the use of appropriate antistaphylococcal antibiotics. If penicillin allergy exists, other agents, including vancomycin, clindamycin, and macrolides, may be used.[126,220,240] The duration of treatment is usually 3 to 4 weeks, with fevers persisting for up to 2 weeks after the institution of therapy.

Mycoplasma and Chlamydia

Mycoplasma pneumoniae and *Chlamydia pneumoniae* are unique pathogens that can cause respiratory infections in children of all ages. However, such infections are usually found in children of school age or older.[153,267,297] These organisms represent clinically significant causes of atypical pneumonia. *M. pneumoniae* and *C. pneumoniae* have similar seroepidemiologic characteristics.[267,296,383] Infection is spread by person-to-person contact and usually involves a 1- to 2-week incubation period. The presentation of atypical pneumonias is very similar to that of an RSV infection. There is gradual onset of symptoms, including sore throat, hoarseness, and rhinitis, with or without fever. These upper respiratory tract symptoms progress to the lower respiratory tract over several days and include cough, pleuritic chest pain, rales, and rhonchi. *Mycoplasma* can also produce fever, chills, headache, and myalgias. Classically, these infections display interstitial infiltrates with unilateral subsegmental distribution, but this can be highly variable.[121] The diagnosis is usually made on clinical grounds based on the history and physical examination. Other adjunctive tests including polymerase chain reaction (PCR), culture, and serology can also be used to confirm the diagnosis.[82,133,156] Macrolides (erythromycin, clarithromycin) are the mainstay of therapy for these infections.[135,153,267] New azalide (azithromycin) medications have been shown in a number of studies to be as effective as standard macrolide antibiotics but with a much shorter course of therapy, usually 5 days.[157,219]

Mycobacterium tuberculosis

Tuberculosis infection in childhood almost invariably results from infection spread by an adult with active pulmonary disease.[99,100,183] When adult tuberculosis is properly controlled, the incidence of childhood tuberculosis is significantly reduced as well.[100,146] Indeed, the aggressive treatment of infection during the early stages of disease can have a major impact on morbidity and disseminated infection in the future.[183,354] In North America, surgical complications of tuberculosis have been dramatically reduced secondary to effective medical therapy and intensive follow-up. Recent reports[120,136,191] on the epidemiology of tuberculosis in developed nations have common themes: (1) immigrants and their children have the highest incidence of tuberculosis, (2) more serious disease is occurring in young children, and (3) skin testing and screening play an important role in identifying children with tuberculosis. The emergence of antibiotic-resistant strains of tuberculosis is a problem for the future and reflects the changes in the organism within the community as a whole.[4,190,272,328]

Childhood tuberculosis differs from the adult form because primary pulmonary tuberculosis is a disease of the lymphatic system, the "primary complex."[99] Primary tuberculosis results in secondary damage to the lungs through obstruction or damage to the large airways leading to atelectasis, chronic infection, and bronchiectasis.[173] Most primary infections heal without residual lesions in the lung other than the Ghon complex (calcium deposit in a mediastinal or hilar lymph node). The healing of the primary lesion is believed to be associated with a positive host-organism balance, which has been attributed to either a strong natural host resistance or to a small initial inoculating dose.[173] If defense mechanisms are unable to control the primary infection, tuberculous pneumonia progresses with caseation, often accompanied by pleural effusion.[173] The clinical manifestations include fever, dyspnea, and cough. Suspicion for tuberculosis should be raised in any child with chronic cough, history of contact with an adult with tuberculosis, failure to thrive, or inability to recover from infection despite adequate treatment.[100,171]

The diagnosis of tuberculosis is established by cultures of *M. tuberculosis*, obtained from sputum, bronchial washings, gastric aspirates, or other infected material.[230,231,320] Recently, a reliable urine test for tuberculosis using PCR has also been introduced.[231,302] In children, a positive tuberculin skin test indicates disease requiring anti-tuberculous therapy.[115] The tuberculin test may be negative in immunosuppressed children, in those who are severely malnourished, or in those who have disseminated tuberculosis, who often are anergic.[115,250] Other factors that may lead to misdiagnosis include the interobserver reliability of test interpretation, repeated skin testing, particularly in high incidence populations, and the use of corticosteroids at the time of testing.[99,173] Anti-tuberculous therapy may be indicated when the disease is suspected in such patients, because cultures may take several weeks to become positive. It is now evident that the absorption of anti-tuberculous drugs in adults may be impaired by a number of factors, including food consumption, regardless of the immune status of the patient.[138,284,304] There is a paucity of this type of data for children, but drug monitoring may be indicated to ensure that proper tissue levels are being delivered. Furthermore, standard medications, such as rifampin, isoniazid, ethionamide, ethambutol, and pyrazinamide can cause hepatotoxicity.[173]

Currently, surgery is required only for pulmonary tuberculosis in which significant damage to a localized area of the lung has occurred. In contrast to adults, this usually involves the lower lobes in children. The operation should be conservative, usually consisting of a wedge resection, segmental resection, or lobectomy.[129,130,162,294] The indications for surgical intervention in childhood tuberculosis include (1) major airway obstruction by extraluminal lymph nodes, (2) chronic airway compromise, (3) airway obstruction by intraluminal material, (4) post-tuberculosis pulmonary destruction with or without fungal superinfection, (5) chronic cavitary lesions, and (6) tuberculosis-induced bronchiectasis.

Atypical Mycobacteria

Atypical mycobacterial species were first identified in the 1950s.[72] The incidence of these infections was relatively stable until the 1980s, when an increase in incidence concurred with the human immunodeficiency virus (HIV) epidemic.[243] Many more organisms are being identified owing to more sophisticated culture techniques as well as to the increased number of immunocompromised patients.[2,316] The most common presentation of atypical mycobacterial infections is cervical lymphadenitis.[2,22,313] The incidence of pulmonary infections with atypical mycobacteria in immunocompetent patients is low,[103,273] but it is frequently observed in patients with cystic fibrosis[110,145,239,278] and in patients infected with HIV[96,180,184,295] (see later). The most common subtypes responsible for pulmonary infection include *Mycobacterium avium* complex. Other important species include *M. kansasii*, *M. abscessus*, *M. xenopi*, and *M. malmoense*.[2] Clinically, immunocompetent patients may have minimal symptoms or present with fatigue and chronic cough with wheezing. The diagnosis may be suspected on chest radiographs and high-resolution computed tomography (CT),[2,154,178] which demonstrate fibrocavitary lung disease, particularly at the apices of the lung. Nodular, interstitial lung disease and even bronchiectasis[154] may also be present. The laboratory diagnosis of atypical mycobacteria can be made with sputum samples using PCR,[57] high-performance liquid chromatography,[61] or DNA probe techniques.[69,345] The relapse of infection after treatment was a common occurrence in the pre-macrolide era because anti-tubercular medications are less potent against atypical mycobacteria than tuberculosis. Thus, many patients required surgical excision of affected regions of the lung. However, with the development of macrolides (erythromycin, clarithromycin), azalides (azithromycin), and newer nonmacrolide antibiotics (ciprofloxacin), surgery is rarely indicated for pulmonary disease.[2] In contrast, atypical mycobacterial cervical lymphadenitis is best treated by surgical excision of the affected lymph nodes, with antibiotic treatment reserved for patients with unresectable lesions or disseminated disease.

Viral Infections

Bronchiolitis

Bronchiolitis is a major cause for hospital admission in young children. The most common cause of bronchiolitis is RSV, which accounts for up to 125,000 admissions and 200 to 500 deaths per year in the United States.[333] Other pathogens that have been implicated with bronchiolitis include parainfluenza viruses, influenza viruses, and adenoviruses.[347] Peak times for infection occur during the early winter through the spring, with the mode of transmission being direct contact. The peak incidence of infection occurs between the ages of 2 and 6 months.[392] Initially starting as an upper respiratory tract infection with rhinorrhea, cough, and low-grade fever, lower respiratory symptoms progress rapidly over the next 24 to 48 hours. At this time, patients may demonstrate tachypnea, retractions, and wheezing. High fever is not uncommon, and young infants may also present with apnea. Transcutaneous oxygen saturations may fall below 95%, but these measurements may not necessarily correlate with clinical findings. Radiographically, patients exhibit hyperinflation, interstitial pneumonitis, and occasionally pleural thickening. Acquired lobar emphysema occasionally develops (Fig. 64-2). Lung resection rarely may be indicated, but in most patients the hyperinflation resolves with time.

Several patient populations are at increased risk for RSV.[392] These include premature infants, patients younger than 6 weeks of age, and children with chronic lung or congenital heart disease. Aboriginal populations are also at increased risk of the disease.[236] RSV is shed by both symptomatic and asymptomatic children,[152] with the rate of shedding decreasing with age.[151] However, immunocompromised patients can shed virus for even longer periods of time, regardless of age.[199] Overall, the mortality from RSV is approximately 1% but can rise to 4% for those patients at risk.[167,333,347] A presumptive diagnosis of

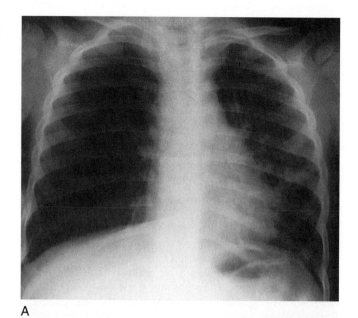

A

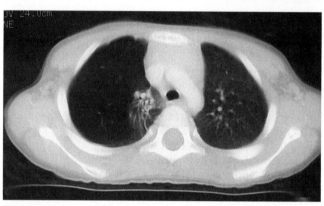

B

Figure 64–2 *A,* Chest radiograph in a 3-year-old child with acquired lobar emphysema secondary to pneumonia with respiratory syncytial virus. *B,* CT scan of chest reveals collapsed upper lobe and emphysematous middle lobe.

bronchiolitis can often be made on the clinical presentation and is supported by radiographic impressions. Confirmation of infections requires a nasopharyngeal aspirate using a rapid immunosorbent assay.[19,49,163] Treatment for bronchiolitis is generally supportive with supplemental oxygen, maintenance of hydration, and close monitoring.[198,281] In severe infection, particularly in at-risk populations, mechanical ventilation may be required. Interruption of transmission is paramount to prevent epidemics on the hospital wards[246]; thus, strict hand washing and the segregation of affected patients is also very important. Bronchodilators and inhaled corticosteroid medications have a limited role in the overall treatment plan but may provide temporary symptomatic relief.[322] Antiviral therapies have not been as successful as anticipated but are still used for treatment in immunocompromised patients.[176,202,393] Vaccinations against RSV should be provided to high-risk children.[288] Most infections are self-limited, but there is increasing evidence to support a link between previous RSV infections and the development of childhood asthma.[244,369]

Parasitic Infections

Echinococcus

Echinococcus hydatid disease is a parasitic tapeworm infection of sheep and dogs that is transmissible to humans. Infections are common in Egypt, the Middle East, and Australia. Once rare in North America, hydatid disease has been diagnosed in several patients living in the southwestern United States[102] and northern Canada.[216,258] Cysts occur in the liver, spleen, and lungs. Most patients who present with pulmonary disease are children. These cysts should be removed because 30% of these lesions may eventually rupture,[35] producing pleural effusions,[18] bronchial seeding, and occasionally acute anaphylaxis.[186,196,365] Some children with hydatid lung disease are asymptomatic, whereas others experience a nonproductive cough. Chest radiographs typically demonstrate a single large pulmonary nodule or a large cyst(s) with an air-fluid level (Fig. 64-3). CT and magnetic resonance imaging (MRI) are also being used to provide more detail or to identify occasional lesions that are not apparent with conventional radiography despite the presence of symptoms. A serum enzyme-linked

immunosorbent assay can also be used to confirm cases that are equivocal after radiologic investigations. Medical therapy with mebendazole has been recommended for patients with small cysts or asymptomatic disease.[192] Patients with secondarily infected or symptomatic/ enlarging cysts will usually require pulmonary resection.[35,196,317,372] There is some evidence that primary surgical resection of large or complicated hydatid cysts may decrease postoperative complications and shorten hospital stay.[192] For the surgical management of hydatid cysts, gentle manipulation of lung tissue, careful control of cyst contents to avoid spillage, and a parenchyma-sparing approach is recommended. Percutaneous drainage of these cysts has been described but with only partial success.[21]

The Immunocompromised Patient

Pediatric Cancer Patient

Overall, cure rates for all types of childhood cancers have exceeded 60%.[269] This significant improvement has been the result of improved chemotherapy regimens, improved agents, and increased intensity of therapy. A persistent obstacle for these patients, however, is the threat of infectious complications. Indeed, the single most important factor contributing to the risk of infection is the degree of neutropenia. Neutrophil counts below $0.5 \times 10^9/L$ place

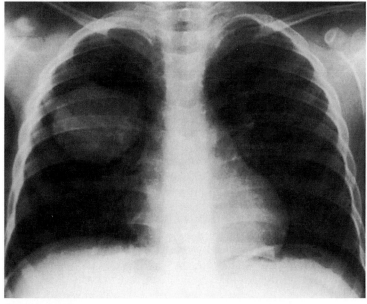

A

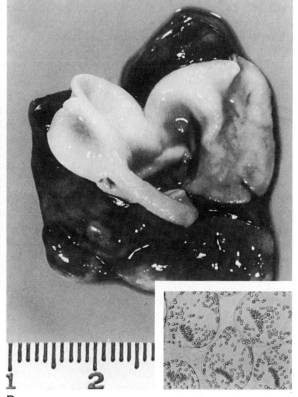

B

Figure 64–3 Echinococcal cyst in a 4-year-old American Indian boy whose family lived in a sheep-herding area and owned several dogs. Large, homogeneous, spherical mass is visible in the right lung in the posteroanterior radiograph (*A*). At wedge resection (*B*), the opened cyst contained proglottids with scolices and hooklets. The boy recovered without complications. (*Inset,* ×400.)

patients at significantly increased risk of bacterial infection.[181,318] If the duration of neutropenia is prolonged, the incidence of fungal infections is also increased.[290,388,389]

The lung is the most common site of opportunistic infection in the immunocompromised cancer patient.[269] The incidence of pneumonia in this population ranges from 0.5% to 10%.[123] The mechanism of infection is either from the aspiration of pathogens from the upper airway into the tracheobronchial tree or by hematogenous spread. The immune system can be affected in many different ways depending on the type, duration, and intensity of chemotherapy. Indeed, combination chemotherapy can impair multiple different facets of the immune response as a result of the different mechanisms of action of these medications.

Bacterial Infections

Bacterial infections represent the most common cause of pulmonary infection early in the course of chemotherapy. Several factors, including bacteremia, aspiration, ciliary dysfunction, decreased pulmonary toilet, impaired mucosal barriers, and endotracheal intubation may predispose pediatric cancer patients to pulmonary infections.[70,380] Deficiencies in immunoglobulins as a result of immunosuppression also place these patients at risk of infection by encapsulated bacteria, such as *S. pneumoniae* and *Haemophilus*, owing to improper opsonization.[225] The risk of infection in bone marrow transplant patients has been reported to be in the range of 12% to 15% within the first 100 days after transplant.[54,87,235]

Overall, gram-negative bacilli are the most common pathogens responsible for pulmonary infection in pediatric cancer patients. The most common gram-negative species include *Pseudomonas, Klebsiella,* and *Enterobacter.* Patients with gram-negative infections present with early pulmonary infiltrates, which can be sufficiently treated with β-lactams, cephalosporins, and/or aminoglycosides. *Pseudomonas* infections generally require double antibiotic coverage. Infiltrates persisting longer than 7 days of treatment are usually due to these same species that possess intrinsic antibiotic resistance, necessitating a change to the treatment protocol. Gram-positive infections usually involve *Staphylococcus, S. pneumoniae,* and streptococcal (group A) species[389] for which β-lactams, cephalosporins, and vancomycin are usually sufficient for treatment. *Listeria* usually produces late and refractory infiltrates. Nocardial infections are uncommon but can be very severe, with a propensity for spread to the central nervous system.[289] Sulfonamides are the treatment of choice for this organism.

Fungal Infections

Fungal infections represent a common cause of mortality in highly immunocompromised patients. Indeed, there has been an increase in the incidence of invasive fungal infections, particularly in those patients with protracted neutropenia and in those patients receiving prolonged corticosteroid or antibiotic therapy.[226,291] There are two major patterns to fungal infection: (1) opportunistic infections with *Aspergillus* and *Candida,* the two most common

mycoses in immunocompromised patients, and (2) reactivation of latent infections with *Histoplasma, Coccidioides,* and *Blastomyces.*[79]

The lung is the most common site for an invasive infection with *Aspergillus.*[291,335] The most common portal of entry for this fungus is the upper airway. Indeed, hospital epidemics have occurred secondary to the inhalation of shed spores from contaminated air-conditioning units and from nearby building construction or renovation sites.[20] However, the incidence of such infections can be reduced with the use of laminar flow and high-efficiency filters.[44]

Aspergillus infections can be rapidly invasive. Necrosis and hemorrhage result from the invasion and thrombosis of pulmonary arteries and veins. This in turn leads to the development of cavitary lesions. Plain chest radiographs are not as sensitive for *Aspergillus* as CT scans because these infections may present as either diffuse infiltrates or nodular disease (Fig. 64-4).[74] Amphotericin B is the treatment of choice,[350] and the effectiveness of therapy may be gauged by the recovery of white blood cells and granulocytes. Because the response of pulmonary aspergillosis to amphotericin B alone can be as low as 5%,[70] the surgical resection of localized disease may be required if no clinical improvement is observed.[95,404] New lipophilic amphotericin may have improved efficacy over the standard preparation.[228] In bone marrow transplant patients, the incidence of *Aspergillus* infection can be as high as 10%.[384] The diagnosis of aspergillosis may be difficult in these patients because of concurrent problems such as graft-versus-host disease (GVHD). The presence of *Aspergillus* in sputum samples of bone marrow transplant patients is highly suggestive of infection,

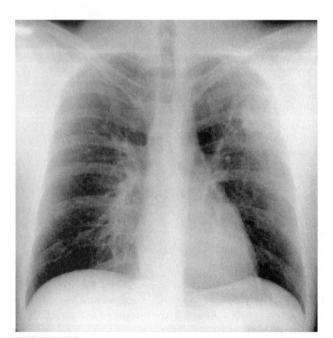

Figure 64–4 Left upper lobe aspergilloma with diffuse bilateral lung infiltrates in a 17-year-old patient with acute lymphoblastic leukemia undergoing intensive chemotherapy.

but in equivocal cases a lung biopsy may be required to confirm the diagnosis.

Candida is the most common fungal organism responsible for infection in immunocompromised patients.[291] The oral cavity is the major site of infection. Although the lung is not usually involved with *Candida,* it is the most common site of invasive infections.[113,161,344] Spread to the lung may occur hematogenously or from the aspiration of contaminated oropharyngeal secretions. Plain chest radiographs are usually nonspecific. Bronchoalveolar lavage can be useful in confirming the diagnosis, but often a lung biopsy is required. The treatment of invasive candidal infections is evolving.[283] The azoles fluconazole and itraconazole are the standards of therapy against most species of *Candida,*[282] yet certain strains of *Candida* have specific, intrinsic resistance to either the azoles and/or amphotericin. Newer classes of antifungal agents such as the echinocandins (caspofungin), which affect fungal wall synthesis, are effective in cases of resistance, if standard therapies are ineffective or if the side effects of standard medications are limiting treatment.[94,282] However, it is clear that if the candidal infection is left untreated the prognosis of patients is uniformly poor.[289]

Viral Infections

Viral infections are uncommon in cancer patients except if the patients are severely immunocompromised. The susceptibility to viral infection depends on the extent to which host defense mechanisms have been affected. For example, cellular immunity can predispose patients to infection with the herpesvirus family, such as cytomegalovirus (CMV). The incidence of CMV infection varies with the underlying disease process. It is more prevalent in patients with allogeneic rather than autologous bone marrow transplant.[269] This infection is usually the result of the reactivation of a latent infection and presents as fever, headache, malaise, and myalgias and may precede the pneumonitis by 1 or 2 weeks. Radiographs are nonspecific, demonstrating diffuse, nodular, or atelectatic changes within the lung.[79] The diagnosis of CMV may be confirmed by bronchoalveolar lavage with cytology or PCR on the recovered specimens.[361,374] Treatment includes the use of ganciclovir and immunoglobulins.[374,411] In bone marrow transplant patients, interstitial pneumonias are caused by CMV up to 50% of the time.[252] The risk of CMV infection appears to be increased in patients who have concurrent GVHD, who receive frequent transfusions, or who receive methotrexate or antithymocyte medications.[79]

Varicella pneumonia is rare in immunocompetent patients. Thirty percent of patients who have visceral involvement may develop pneumonia.[269] This can increase to 80% if they are receiving concurrent chemotherapy. Radiographically, these patients will present with diffuse bilateral fluffy infiltrates. If patients have been exposed to varicella, chemotherapy should be stopped for the period of incubation (up to 21 days). Passive immunization with varicella-zoster immune globulin should be administered at this time. The treatment of active infection includes acyclovir. Herpesvirus infections are usually rare unless there is concomitant

gingivostomatitis. RSV infection can be very problematic in bone marrow transplant patients owing to their decreased T-cell–mediated immunity. Up to 80% of immunocompromised patients with RSV infections can progress to life-threatening infection. Only supportive treatment can be offered; therefore, preventive immunization is recommended for high-risk patients.[393]

Pneumocystis jiroveci (carinii)

This unusual organism has properties of protozoa (susceptible to trimethoprim) as well as fungi (based on RNA studies) and is seen almost exclusively in patients who are immunocompromised. Routine prophylaxis has dramatically reduced the incidence of this infection.[79] Infection with *Pneumocystis* is usually the result of the reactivation of latent disease. The risk of infection is dependent on the level of immunosuppression, but bone marrow transplant patients and patients receiving corticosteroids are at particular risk. Patients usually complain of a fever, dry cough, and dyspnea. Progressive disease may present as hypoxia and respiratory distress. Radiographically, fulminant disease presents as bilateral hilar infiltrates that extend to the periphery of the lung (Fig. 64-5). The diagnosis is confirmed by histology and cytology that identifies trophozoite cysts recovered by bronchoalveolar lavage.[289] Trimethoprim/sulfamethoxazole (TMP/SMX) is the mainstay of treatment and prophylaxis.[172] Corticosteroids and supplemental oxygen are also useful for patients with severe infections. If no response occurs within 72 hours, a lung

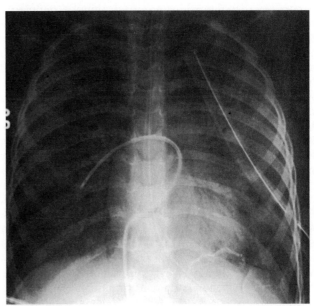

Figure 64–5 *Pneumocystis jiroveci (carinii)* pneumonia in a 5-year-old girl receiving chemotherapy for acute lymphocytic leukemia. Diffuse interstitial infiltrates are seen in both lungs. Biopsy of the lingula *(note staples)* demonstrated *P. jiroveci (carinii)*. A Swan-Ganz catheter is positioned in the right inferior pulmonary artery. Although her leukemia was in remission, the child died of respiratory failure from the pulmonary disease. (Currently with antibiotic prophylaxis, early institution of empirical therapy, and diagnostic confirmation by bronchoalveolar lavage, such an outcome would be unusual.)

biopsy is indicated. Mortality approaches 100% for untreated patients. Aerosolized pentamidine may also be used if myelosuppression or rash occurs secondary to TMP/SMX administration.[266]

Pediatric HIV Patient

The early diagnosis of HIV infection has translated into prolonged survival.[286] Acute pneumonia is the most common severe infection in HIV-infected children in the United States.[286] In developing countries, particularly in sub-Saharan Africa, respiratory infections are one of the most common causes of illness, hospitalization, and mortality in HIV-infected children.[141] The introduction of highly active antiretroviral therapy (HAART) in 1997 has dramatically improved the survival of HIV-infected adult patients[8] in developed nations through the "reconstitution of the immune system."[223] The efficacy of this therapy in children has also been demonstrated, particularly for those patients with severe immunosuppression.[375] Interestingly, despite the effect of HAART on the natural history of HIV infection, there is conflicting evidence regarding its impact on the risk of developing bacterial pneumonia.[353,403]

The most common organisms responsible for bacterial pneumonia in HIV-infected patients are *S. pneumoniae*, *S. aureus*, group A β-hemolytic *Streptococcus*, *H. influenzae* type b, *Salmonella*, and *Pseudomonas*.[141] The clinical features of respiratory infections in children with HIV are similar to those with normal immune systems. However, patients with decreasing CD4+ counts, severe immunosuppression, and previous acquired immune deficiency syndrome (AIDS)-defining respiratory infections are more likely to develop acute pneumonias.[14,256] Furthermore, these patients may be predisposed to recurrent infection and its sequelae, including bronchiectasis, abnormal lung parenchymal architecture, and bullous lung disease.[286] The diagnosis of pneumonia in HIV-infected children is based on clinical and radiographic findings. However, it is very important that opportunistic and atypical infections be excluded in this population of patients. Furthermore, the differential diagnosis of pulmonary infiltrates for these patients also includes noninfectious causes such as non-Hodgkin's lymphoma, the incidence of which may be increased with the institution of HAART.[141,403] A lung biopsy may be required to confirm a diagnosis in these patients. The prevention of infection plays a key role in the management of these patients and includes the routine immunization against *Haemophilus* and pneumococci as well as prophylactic TMP/SMX for *Pneumocystis*.[5,7] Treatment should be initiated against the specific pathogen as soon as possible, but empirical therapy (cefotaxime or ceftriaxone) may be instituted while waiting for culture results.

Pneumocystis jiroveci (carinii)

Pneumocystis jiroveci (carinii) infection is the most common AIDS-defining illness in children younger than 1 year of age.[340] The mortality with this infection is higher in children than in adults despite higher CD4+ levels.[13]

The incidence of *Pneumocystis* pneumonia, however, has decreased with the introduction of TMP/SMX prophylactic therapy.[1] Although there are currently insufficient data for children, recent adult series have demonstrated minimal recurrence of *Pneumocystis* pneumonia with the discontinuation of prophylaxis in patients with a good response to HAART therapy.[323,395] Currently, *Pneumocystis* prophylaxis is still recommended for (1) HIV-exposed infants, starting at 4 to 6 weeks of age until infection is disproven; (2) for all HIV-infected infants younger than 1 year of age regardless of CD4+ count; and (3) all HIV-infected children if their CD4+ counts are below age-specific thresholds.[1] The clinical presentation of *Pneumocystis* pneumonia includes the rapid onset of dyspnea, tachypnea, and hypoxemia with cough and fever. Increases in serum lactate dehydrogenase may support the diagnosis. Radiographs commonly demonstrate hyperinflation and peribronchial thickening that can progress to diffuse alveolar infiltrates. Bronchoalveolar lavage or deep tracheal suctioning with balloon urinary catheters often confirms the diagnosis of *Pneumocystis* pneumonia, but lung biopsy may sometimes be required. TMP/SMX, in conjunction with corticosteroids and supplemental oxygen in severe cases, is the mainstay of treatment.

Lymphoid Interstitial Pneumonitis

Lymphocytic or lymphoid interstitial pneumonitis (LIP) is a chronic lymphocytic infiltrative process seen in children with HIV older than 2 years of age and represents another AIDS-defining illness. Epstein-Barr virus has been implicated in its pathogenesis. LIP has been estimated to occur in 20% to 30% of vertically transmitted cases of HIV in the United States and Europe.[331] Patients often present with an insidious onset of respiratory symptoms that may be confused with tuberculosis. Other clinical findings include fever, digital clubbing, asymptomatic parotid swelling, symmetrical lymphadenopathy, and hepatomegaly. The clinical course is benign but may predispose patients to bacterial and viral pneumonias, bronchiectasis, and bullous lung disease.[141,286] Plain radiographs can demonstrate persistent reticulonodular infiltrates and hilar adenopathy that can be better appreciated by CT (Fig. 64-6). Lung biopsy is usually necessary to confirm the diagnosis and demonstrates significantly altered pulmonary architecture with an infiltration of CD8+ cells.[141] Systemic corticosteroid administration over 4 to 6 weeks usually leads to resolution of the infiltrates. HAART has been shown to improve the clinical course of LIP and may reduce the prevalence of chronic lung disease associated with it.

Tuberculosis

The increase in the incidence of tuberculosis in children in developed countries has paralleled the increase of the disease in HIV-infected adults, the primary source of transmission to children.[349] The clinical features of tuberculosis in HIV-infected children are similar to those in immunocompetent patients but with a predilection for rapid progression and extrapulmonary and/or disseminated disease.[66] Radiographs often demonstrate lobar or

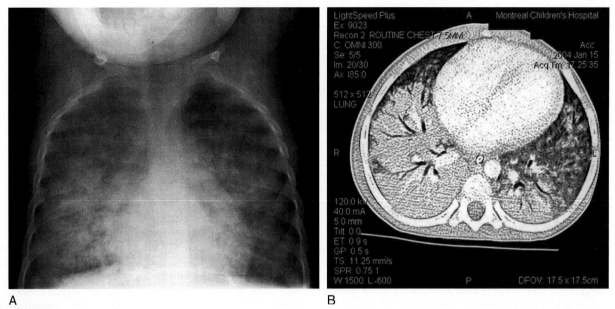

Figure 64–6 A 3-year-old child who recently immigrated from Africa presented with a history of weakness and coughing, having been treated for pulmonary tuberculosis 2 years previously. Respiratory distress worsened, and intubation was required. *A,* Plain radiograph demonstrates a lung infiltrate with an alveolar pattern. *B,* Diffuse consolidation with air bronchogram especially in the right lower lobe can be appreciated on CT. HIV was suspected and later confirmed. Bronchoscopy and bronchoalveolar lavage were not diagnostic. Lung biopsy revealed lymphoid interstitial pneumonitis. He was treated with corticosteroids and triple antiretroviral therapy and rapidly recovered.

diffuse infiltrates and atelectasis from bronchi compressed by hilar adenopathy. If a child is found to have tuberculosis, HIV testing should be undertaken. The diagnosis of tuberculosis is based on the clinical, epidemiologic, and radiographic data available.[6] The early morning gastric aspirate of retained overnight secretions is the best non-invasive culture technique for tuberculosis and may provide a better yield than more invasive procedures, such as bronchoalveolar lavage and bronchoscopy.[11] The tuberculin skin test is still a valuable diagnostic aid in all HIV-infected children and should be performed every 9 to 12 months.[5,115] Prevention is key, and a clear determination of the tuberculosis status of all adults in the household is essential. Currently, vaccination of HIV-infected children with bacille Calmette-Guérin is contraindicated in the United States owing to the risk of disseminated disease.[40] However, in endemic areas, the World Health Organization has recommended the vaccine for asymptomatic HIV-infected children.[286] For patients with significant exposure, isoniazid, regardless of skin test result, is indicated. If a repeat PPD test in 3 months is negative, the medication can be stopped. Treatment of active infections includes a multiple-agent regimen.[337,348] Care must be taken to watch for interactions between antiretroviral and antituberculous medications.[9]

Atypical Mycobacterial Infections

Several species of atypical mycobacteria are clinically significant in patients with HIV. These include *M. avium,* *M. intracellulare, M. lepraemurium,* and *M. scrofulaceum.* These bacteria represent a major source of morbidity for HIV-infected children and usually cause systemic infection later in the course of AIDS. Previously, patients infected

with atypical mycobacteria had a 9- to 11-month life expectancy,[170,312] but with the advent of more effective treatments for HIV and atypical mycobacteria the disease is less common and the prognosis is better. Indeed, the incidence of disseminated nontuberculous mycobacterial infections appears to be decreasing in the era of HAART in adults.[96,218,370] Controversy exists as to whether prophylactic therapy against opportunistic infections should be discontinued for patients responsive to this therapy.[200,370] In the pediatric population, clinical trials evaluating the effects of HAART on atypical mycobacteria infection have yet to be conducted. Thus, prophylaxis is still recommended for pediatric patients with disseminated disease.[3]

The clinical presentation of these patients usually involves failure to thrive, abdominal pain, and fatigue rather than respiratory symptoms. Patients may also have leukopenia, thrombocytopenia, and an increased serum lactate dehydrogenase. The diagnosis is made through blood culture or biopsy of a normally sterile site, including bone marrow and lymph nodes. Investigations must also eliminate the possibility of tuberculosis infection. Prevention of infection is accomplished through protection of the immune system with effective antiretroviral therapy. Primary prophylaxis with clarithromycin or azithromycin is based on CD4+ counts specific for age.[5] Treatment of active infections can be accomplished with clarithromycin, ethambutol, ciprofloxacin, or azithromycin. Macrolides inhibit the metabolism of many antiretroviral medications.

Viral Infections

CMV infection can present as chronic interstitial pneumonitis and is usually accompanied by retinitis, hepatitis, or colitis. It often occurs in severely immunosuppressed patients. Respiratory symptoms include nonproductive cough, dyspnea, and hypoxemia. Pneumonitis may be associated with concurrent *Pneumocystis* infection. Radiographic findings include diffuse interstitial infiltrates. The diagnosis of CMV infection is made by identifying viral inclusions in urine, bronchoalveolar lavage, or biopsy specimens. However, the differentiation between active infection and asymptomatic viral shedding in HIV-infected patients is difficult and may complicate management regimens.[396] The preferred treatment is ganciclovir, particularly if gastrointestinal or retinal involvement is also identified.

Fungal Infections

Systemic fungal infections are uncommon in HIV, because, more commonly, these infections involve the skin or mucosa. Pulmonary mycoses are being identified with some frequency in children with HIV owing to impaired T-cell immunity. Histoplasmosis is uncommonly reported in this group of patients. A primary pulmonary focus may progress rapidly to disseminated disease and become fatal if left untreated. Severe disease presents as fever, hepatosplenomegaly, pancytopenia, reticulonodular lobar infiltrates, and the occasional progression to septic shock. The diagnosis is based on cultures of bronchoalveolar lavage samples or lung biopsy. Treatment involves the use of intravenous amphotericin B. Children with primary pulmonary disease should receive itraconazole for prophylaxis in the hopes of preventing disseminated disease.

Cryptococcus and *Coccidioides* infections are usually associated with disseminated infection, and 50% of these patients have concurrent pulmonary infection. Cryptococcal infections present as fever, headache, pulmonary infiltrates, and confusion in disseminated disease. The diagnosis is made through sputum, blood, or cerebrospinal fluid cultures and the direct examination of cerebrospinal fluid with India ink or latex agglutination. Treatment includes amphotericin B followed by fluconazole after 2 weeks. Coccidioidomycosis usually presents as disseminated disease affecting the lungs, brain, and skin. Fever, weight loss, cough, and an altered level of consciousness are often present. The diagnosis is made from sputum, bronchoalveolar lavage, or lung biopsy specimens. Acute infections are managed with amphotericin B, but recurrence is common, thus mandating prophylactic therapy with fluconazole. Aspergillosis is another uncommon infection that usually presents as pulmonary disease and sinusitis. These patients experience fever, cough, dyspnea, and pleuritic chest pain. Sputum analysis, bronchoalveolar lavage, and occasionally lung biopsy are required to confirm the diagnosis. Amphotericin B is the treatment of choice, although newer azoles and the echinocandins have also been shown to be effective.[188,305] Long-term suppressive therapy with itraconazole may also be required.[335,336]

The immunocompromised pediatric patient is under the constant threat of infection. These patients require constant surveillance and aggressive management strategies. For patients with pulmonary infiltrates, broad-spectrum antibiotics should be started promptly. If no response is observed over the next 48 to 72 hours, a change in the antibiotic regimen and possibly the addition of amphotericin B and TMP/SMX may be indicated. For persistent lung infiltrates, either bronchoalveolar lavage, but more likely lung biopsy, should be performed. The results of lung biopsy for patients with persistent lung infiltrates have been shown to impact on the management of these patients up to 90% of the time.[206]

Cystic Fibrosis

Cystic fibrosis (CF) is the most common autosomal recessive disease affecting whites and occurs in approximately 1 in 3,400 live births.[259] Almost 30,000 people are affected in the United States.[298] The prognosis for this disease has improved considerably over the past 30 years but has plateaued since the mid 1990s. The current life expectancy for patients with CF is over 30 years of age. It is characterized by thick, inspissated mucus, chronic infection, and neutrophil-dominated inflammation of the airways.[298] The cystic fibrosis transmembrane conductance regulator (CFTR) is a cyclic adenosine monophosphate–dependent chloride channel located on chromosome 7q21-31.[193] Mutations in *CFTR* are responsible for the clinical manifestations of the disease. Several hypotheses have been proposed. One hypothesis suggests that the loss of *CFTR* as an ion channel in CF decreases fluid production and enhances sodium absorption.[51] This leads to impaired ciliary function and mucus transport. Others believe increased sodium in the air-surface layer inactivates antimicrobial defensins and impairs lung defenses, including intraluminal killing of ingested bacteria.[147] Sodium is also thought to allow for increased bacterial binding to the airway epithelia, particularly *Pseudomonas*, in homozygous patients. Furthermore, there also appears to be dysregulation of the inflammatory cascade in CF patients, leading to chronic inflammation.[26]

The clinical signs and symptoms of CF can vary widely. Patients may be relatively asymptomatic, present with chronic illness and failure to thrive, or complain of acute, recurrent exacerbations of pulmonary disease. However, the usual presentation is with the progression of a nonproductive cough to a loose productive cough with copious, purulent secretions. Classic physical findings include a barrel chest, rales, rhonchi, and digital clubbing with occasional cyanosis. Although initial pulmonary function tests demonstrate obstructive patterns, disease progression leads to the development of restrictive lung disease. The diagnosis of CF is confirmed with sweat tests (elevated chloride) or with the identification of mutations in *CFTR*, the most common being $\Delta F508$.

In the first decade of life, the most common organism isolated from CF patients is *S. aureus* (40%), followed by *H. influenzae* (15%).[299] *Pseudomonas* is usually the first pathogen isolated in children younger than 1 year of age, and over 80% are infected with this organism by 18 years of age.[59] Clinically, *Pseudomonas* is the most important pathogen in CF. These bacteria are able to form biofilms that enable them to avoid normal clearance mechanisms and the penetration of antibiotics.[59] *Pseudomonas* also produces exotoxins that contribute to its virulence, increasing the viscosity of secretions and further impairing ciliary transport.[346] *Burkholderia cepacia* is an organism with intrinsic antibiotic resistance. Patients infected with this organism present with high fevers, rapid pulmonary deterioration, and sometimes death. Viral infections may pose a special problem, particularly in young children, in whom they may predispose to secondary infection, the need for mechanical ventilation, and oxygen dependence.[12] RSV prophylaxis has been recommended for these infants.[31]

The cornerstone of medical therapy for pulmonary disease in CF patients is the aggressive use of intravenous, oral, and nebulized antibiotics. Indeed, the increased life span of CF patients can be attributed directly to the development of effective antipseudomonal medications. Maintenance therapy is designed to prolong the period between pulmonary exacerbations with *Pseudomonas*. Recent phase III clinical trials have demonstrated the effectiveness of nebulized tobramycin.[301] Macrolides are also effective because they possess anti-inflammatory properties and help to prevent biofilm formation.[134,326] The clearance of abnormal secretions is of paramount importance and includes regular chest physiotherapy and postural drainage. Mucolytic agents such as *N*-acetylcysteine and DNase can help mobilize thick inspissated secretions in CF patients.[299,300] Attempts to reduce the inflammatory response with corticosteroids or other anti-inflammatory medications have been complicated by the side effects of these medications.

Adequate nutritional support and early treatment of pancreatic insufficiency is another critical area for the medical therapy of patients with CF. Significant malnutrition may already be evident at the time of diagnosis in neonates and young children, even if they are asymptomatic. The imbalance between the increased energy needs of infants for growth and their impaired ability to achieve adequate nutritional intake can predispose to pulmonary complications.[205,324] Indeed, long-term gains in both height and weight have been demonstrated in infants treated earlier for their pancreatic insufficiency,[119] and recommendations are in place to help guide clinicians with regard to nutritional requirements and surveillance for children with cystic fibrosis.[50]

Pediatric surgeons may be involved in the care of these patients in several ways as they get older. Implantable Infuse-A-Ports are useful to provide intravenous access for patients who frequently require antibiotics for pulmonary exacerbations. Nutritional management may require the use of a gastrostomy. Pulmonary complications of CF such as bronchiectasis, massive hemoptysis, and pneumothorax are discussed later in this chapter, and gastrointestinal and hepatic complications are discussed in other chapters.

Lung transplantation remains the ultimate resort for patients with end-stage pulmonary disease. Approximately 1200 patients from the United States, Canada, England, and France have undergone transplant for this reason.[298] Bilateral, sequential lung transplantation is the preferred approach for children with CF. Although long-term survival is still a problem for most patients, 1- and 2-year survival rates between 65% and 85% have been reported.[32,112,249,351] However, the optimal time to provide the maximal benefit from transplant is still unclear. Gene therapy, unfortunately, has not progressed beyond phase 1 trials despite the gene being identified over 10 years ago.[193] The main limitation to progress has been due to the development of inflammatory reactions to the lipid and viral vectors used to transmit the functioning *CFTR* gene to airway epithelial cells.[189] More research to appropriately deliver such a therapy is being actively undertaken.

Chronic and Recurrent Pneumonia

Pneumonias are a common cause of illness and hospitalization in children. The difference between recurrent or persistent pneumonias is often difficult to make. Indeed, there is no uniform definition for these types of pneumonias, and radiographic abnormalities may persist for several weeks to months before true resolution is observed. Optimally, the diagnosis of recurrent pneumonia should only be made after complete resolution of the index infection, but this is often difficult. By definition, recurrent pneumonias are pulmonary infections that occur twice in 1 year or as three episodes over any time frame.[385] Several authors have tried to identify the most common causes of recurrent pneumonia in children.[16,159,232,279] Interestingly, unlike acute pneumonias, an underlying cause may be identified in chronic or recurrent pneumonias up to 92% of the time. To many, asthma is the most common cause of recurrent pneumonia, followed by aspiration.

Broadly, pneumonias may be classified into those that affect a single region of the lung and those that affect multiple areas.[379] Abnormalities that affect single regions of the lung include those processes causing intraluminal obstruction (foreign body, bronchial tumor), extraluminal compression (tuberculosis, sarcoidosis, tumors, and vascular rings), or structural abnormalities of the lung (tracheal bronchus, localized bronchiectasis, congenital cystic adenomatoid malformation).[379] Abnormalities causing pneumonia in several regions of the lung include recurrent micro-aspiration, asthma, immune deficiency syndromes, mucociliary dysfunction (cystic fibrosis), structural abnormalities (bronchomalacia, Williams-Campbell syndrome), bronchopulmonary dysplasia, and other rare diseases such as Wegener's granulomatosis and idiopathic pulmonary fibrosis.[379] Other causes of recurrent lung infiltrates exist, such as the acute chest syndrome in patients with sickle cell disease (Fig. 64-7).

Clinical evaluation of patients with chronic or recurrent pneumonias requires a thorough history and physical examination. The frequency, duration, and severity of previous infections, and the circumstances surrounding them, must be fully detailed. Associated symptoms such as wheezing, weight loss, and fever are also important details. The timing of the onset of symptoms, especially in the context of congenital malformations or genetic diseases such as cystic fibrosis can help narrow the differential diagnosis. The family history also provides valuable information. During the physical examination, a thorough assessment of the growth and development of the

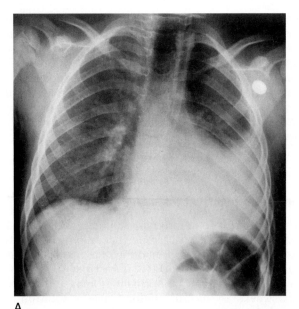

A

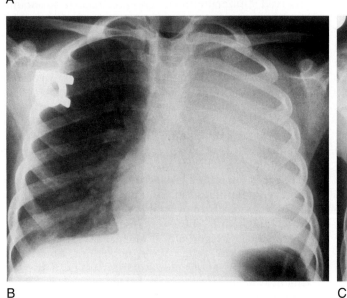

B

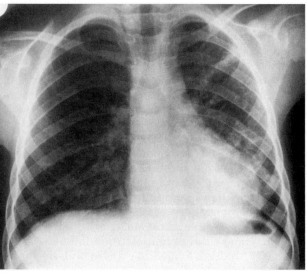

C

Figure 64–7 Acute chest syndrome in sickle cell disease. A 5-year-old girl known to have hemoglobin S/β-thalassemia presented with nasal congestion, cough, and chest pain. The initial chest radiograph was normal (not shown); she was admitted for intravenous hydration and analgesia. Antibiotics were started when she became febrile. She became increasingly tachypneic and hypoxic. *A*, Two days after admission, the chest radiograph shows airspace disease mostly in the left lower lobe. *B*, On day 5 of the admission there is a complete opacification of the left hemithorax, with increased airspace disease in the right base. *C*, Four days later, after exchange transfusion, there is marked improvement.

child is necessary. Evaluation of a recent chest radiograph and the review of radiographs surrounding previous episodes of pneumonia may provide some details that may help direct management and investigations. The clinical status of the child will dictate the urgency of subsequent examinations. The need for supplemental oxygen or respiratory support can often be assessed by the physical examination in conjunction with pulse oximetry and blood gas analysis. Patients with a localized pneumonia may require bronchoscopy for foreign body removal or to assess for bronchial tumors and structural abnormalities. High-resolution CT of the chest may help to identify parenchymal lung lesions as well as intrinsic and extrinsic causes of bronchial obstruction. Patients with multifocal pneumonias may require an upper gastrointestinal series and pH probe to rule out aspiration, pulmonary function tests to assess for asthma,

or investigation for immunodeficiencies and other systemic diseases.

Bronchiectasis

First described by Laënnec in 1819,[56] bronchiectasis is the irreversible dilatation of the airways secondary to the inflammatory destruction of bronchial and peribronchial tissue. In the 1940s and 1950s, bronchiectasis was a leading cause of pulmonary resection in children.[306] Currently, it has become an uncommon disease in developed countries and predominantly limited to the pediatric population. However, the incidence of and morbidity secondary to bronchiectasis is still a problem in developing countries and certain indigenous populations in developed nations (aboriginal peoples of Alaska and Australia and Samoans).[303] The overall decrease in morbidity and mortality from this disease is the result of improvements in antibiotic therapy and vaccinations against common pathogens such as *S. pneumoniae*.

Pathogenesis and Etiology

The pathogenesis of bronchiectasis follows three progressive stages. Initially, there is destruction of the ciliary epithelium, which is replaced with cuboidal squamous epithelium. In the early stages of disease (cylindrical bronchiectasis), there is localized damage to the elastic tissue of the airway in addition to edema and inflammation. Later in the disease (saccular bronchiectasis), the damage involves the muscle layers and cartilage of the airways, with anastomoses forming between pulmonary and bronchial arteries in the areas of saccular dilation. There is also evidence to support a host-mediated component to local tissue damage.

Numerous different hypotheses regarding the development of bronchiectasis have been proposed.[91,398] It is clear that infection is the most common cause of bronchiectasis and is the only theory that has been supported by animal studies (Fig. 64-8).[56] Bronchiectasis may not result from the index infection but is usually the result of concomitant or subsequent infection with many agents such as tuberculosis and histoplasmosis,[309] viruses,[41,330] certain fungi,[262] and, occasionally, *Mycoplasma*.[397] Historically, measles and pertussis infections were also linked to the subsequent development

of bronchiectasis.[187,330] Cystic fibrosis is the most common genetic cause of bronchiectasis; here it occurs secondary to infection and bronchial obstruction with inspissated mucus. Other causes include congenital absence of supportive airway cartilage (Williams-Campbell syndrome),[400] tracheomegaly, Marfan syndrome,[406] α_1-antitrypsin deficiency,[378] foreign body aspiration,[212] ciliary abnormalities (Kartagener's syndrome),[43,368] immunodeficiencies (IgA),[164] asthma,[108] and right middle lobe syndrome.[33,382]

Clinical Manifestations and Investigation

Most patients present during the preschool years with cough, profuse sputum, wheezing, and chest pain. Up to 50% may have digital clubbing, which is reversible. Bronchiectasis, demonstrated by bronchial dilation, bronchial thickening, or a signet-ring sign, may be apparent on plain radiographs. Lung scintigraphy has been suggested as a valuable adjunctive test for patients with bronchiectasis.[29,377] This technique allows for the identification of diseased areas of the lung that may not have been apparent on plain chest radiographs and could be used to plan surgical resections instead of bronchography.[257] However, high-resolution CT of the chest has replaced bronchography to document the pattern and severity of disease.[155,343] Findings include cylindrical or saccular dilatation of bronchi, pooling of secretions, and bronchial thickening (Fig. 64-9). However, acute suppurative infections of the lung may cause *reversible* dilatation of the bronchi that may be confused with bronchiectasis.[306] The distribution of bronchiectasis may give insight into the underlying cause. Patients with tuberculosis have generally unilateral involvement, whereas patients with CF and viral-induced disease have involvement of the upper lobes and lower lobes, respectively.

Therapy

The treatment of bronchiectasis focuses on identifying and treating the underlying causes in addition to postural

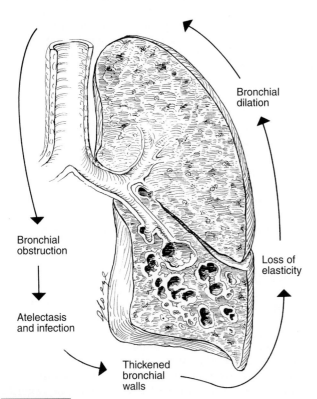

Figure 64–8 Diagrammatic representation of factors influencing the pathogenesis of bronchiectasis.

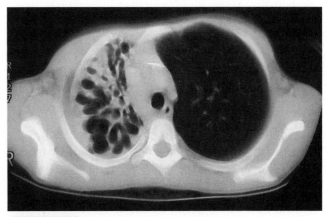

Figure 64–9 CT scan of the chest of a 10-year-old girl with cystic fibrosis. Preoperative ventilation-perfusion scanning revealed no function of this bronchiectatic lobe. The patient underwent an upper lobectomy.

drainage techniques and chest physiotherapy. Antibiotic therapy is essential for acute exacerbations, whereas adequate nutritional support, with pancreatic enzyme replacement for patients with cystic fibrosis, is needed to prevent failure to thrive from recurrent infections and pulmonary exacerbations. Bronchoscopy has also been used to temporarily help alleviate bronchial obstruction due to foreign bodies[97] and inspissated secretions[342] or to aid in the preoperative or diagnostic evaluation of chronic lung infection.[68,131]

Although the frequency of surgical therapy for bronchiectasis has declined over the past several years, there are still those patients who do not respond to medical therapy and would benefit from surgical resection. The main indications for surgery include[401]: (1) localized disease with severe and debilitating symptoms, such as profuse sputum, fetid breath, and severe cough that significantly impacts quality of life; (2) life-threatening hemorrhage from localized disease; (3) resectable disease in the context of failure to thrive; and (4) resectable disease in an area of recurrent lower respiratory tract infections. Lesser indications for surgery include bilateral or nonlocalized disease or patients with only mild-to-moderate symptoms.

The outcome of pediatric patients undergoing surgical resection has generally resulted in the cessation or improvement of clinical symptoms in the majority of patients. Indeed, data from older pediatric series demonstrated that almost three fourths of patients improved after surgery and experienced minimal morbidity.[355,390,401] This success has also been reflected in recent combined reports assessing both children and adults and those patients with nonlocalized and bilateral disease.[30,36,131,213] In these series, segmentectomy, lobectomy, and pneumonectomy (with or without additional segmentectomy or lobectomy) were performed. In a combined total of 581 patients among these series, over 80% were asymptomatic or improved after a median follow-up of 4 years. Mortality ranged from 0% to 1.7%, and the surgical morbidity, including atelectasis, persistent air leak, empyema, bronchopleural fistula, and postoperative hemorrhage, ranged from 8% to 17%. In one pediatric series of 33 patients,[150] the mortality and morbidity rates for similar types of operations were 2.8% and 17.6%, respectively. Only 11.7% of patients in this series did not benefit from the surgical procedure. In 2003, Rothenberg reported on his experience of thoracoscopic lung resection in 45 infants and children[311] over a 7-year period. Twelve of these patients had localized but severe bronchiectasis. No mortality and only one intraoperative complication (in a patient with left lower lobe bronchiectasis) occurred in this series, indicating the feasibility of such techniques in children. The common themes for the successful operative management of bronchiectasis are careful patient selection, preoperative evaluation, and surgical technique, as well as an attempt to completely resect all diseased lung tissue.

Pulmonary Hemorrhage and Hemoptysis

The causes of pulmonary hemorrhage and hemoptysis are wide ranging and may be classified according to the age of the patient or on the basis of underlying lung disease.[46] In neonates, prematurity, pulmonary edema, respiratory distress syndrome, intracerebral bleeding, coagulopathy, and metabolic disorders can lead to pulmonary hemorrhage. For patients with chronic lung disease, bronchiectasis secondary to cystic fibrosis is the most common cause in the pediatric population. However, cavitary lung lesions, tuberculosis, neoplasms, retained foreign bodies, and frequent airway manipulation can lead to symptomatic hemorrhage. In otherwise normal patients, massive hemoptysis may be secondary to hemangiomas, congenital arteriovenous malformations, intralobar pulmonary sequestration, bronchopulmonary foregut malformations, unilateral pulmonary artery agenesis (due to the development of collaterals), and Ehlers-Danlos syndrome.

Massive hemoptysis is defined in children as the expectoration of at least 240 mL of blood in 24 hours or recurrent episodes involving substantial amounts of blood (>100 mL/day) over days to weeks.[362] It occurs in approximately 1% of patients with CF and is more frequent in those patients with severe lung disease.[124] Most of these patients are older than the age of 10 years. The pathogenesis is related to the enlargement and tortuosity of the bronchial arteries and the multiple anastomoses that form between these vessels and the pulmonary arteries (Fig. 64-10).[407] Nonbronchial arteries may also form collaterals with the bronchial circulation or enter the lung through granulation tissue. Most episodes of major hemoptysis resolve spontaneously, but sedation and the discontinuation of medications that impair coagulation should be initiated. Hemoptysis usually indicates deteriorating lung function, and thus antibiotics may be used at this time to treat underlying infection. Vasopressin, endobronchial balloon tamponade, selective mainstem intubation, and topical α-adrenergic agonists have also been used.[321]

Bronchial artery embolization has emerged as a highly successful nonsurgical intervention for the short-term control of hemoptysis.[177] Several series have demonstrated that this technique is safe and effective for the control of massive hemoptysis.[39,86,410] However, up to 20% of these patients require repeated embolization. Failure of embolization is mainly attributable to nonbronchial collaterals.[85,409] Bronchoscopy can be used to help with the preoperative localization of bleeding. Surgery with lobectomy may be lifesaving for patients who fail embolization or for those patients with fulminant, massive hemoptysis.

Complications of Pneumonia

Pneumatocele

Pneumatoceles are small, thin-walled structures consisting of single or multiple cysts within an air-lined cavity secondary to alveolar and bronchiolar necrosis. These abnormalities are seen frequently as a consequence of infection by S. aureus, group A Streptococcus, and occasionally H. influenzae. Pneumatoceles secondary to S. aureus infections may be identified early in the disease process and occur in up to 80% of patients.[203] Pneumothorax and pyopneumothorax are complications resulting from the

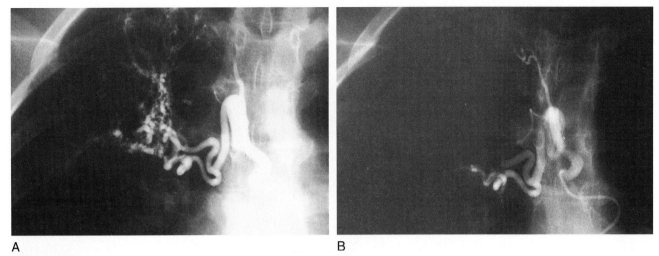

A B

Figure 64–10 *A,* Arteriogram obtained to identify the cause of hemoptysis in a 10-year-old girl with cystic fibrosis. Note the tortuous bronchial artery. *B,* After successful Gelfoam embolization, the peripheral branches of the artery are not visualized.

rupture of infected pneumatoceles.[334] These lesions can be difficult to distinguish from congenital cysts of the lung. However, pneumatoceles are prone to spontaneous resolution whereas congenital abnormalities should not involute. Follow-up of chest radiographs are required until the resolution of the pneumatocele, and a CT scan may be useful in suspicious instances (Fig. 64-11).

Lung Abscess

A pulmonary abscess develops when a localized infection in the lung parenchyma becomes necrotic and then cavitates. Classically, pulmonary abscesses were classified into primary (occurring in healthy children) or secondary (occurring in otherwise compromised children).[242] However, it is now clear that lung abscesses occur almost exclusively in areas of pneumonia.[27] When appropriate antibiotic therapy is administered early, the frequency of lung abscesses decreases considerably. Abscesses developing in immuno-compromised, severely ill, or occasionally very young patients have recently become a more frequent problem. Occasionally, congenital bronchogenic or pulmonary cysts may become secondarily infected. These lesions may be indistinguishable from lung abscess on chest radiographs (see Fig. 64-11C and Fig. 64-12).

History

In the 17th century, Bonet described two patients whom he cured of lung abscess by external drainage.[165] In the 1930s, Neuhoff and Touroff[268] reported good results with one-stage surgical drainage of acute putrid abscess of the lung. A two-stage procedure, the first step to induce pleural symphysis, was used by Welch,[391] with a mortality rate of 40%. The treatment of lung abscess by resection in the early 1940s gave way to almost total reliance on antibiotics, which is still the approach now.[306]

Pathogenesis

The aspiration of gastric contents is a leading cause of chronic pneumonia and lung abscess in children,[27]

particularly in those with neurologic deficits.[360] Aspiration may occur acutely during trauma, anesthesia, or epileptic seizures or in those children with severe gastroesophageal reflux. Patients with repaired esophageal atresia or esophageal dysmotility are also at risk of aspiration.[306] The aspiration of foreign bodies, including blood or tissue after tonsillectomy, were previously common antecedents of lung abscess.[27,306] Such abscesses are now infrequent because they are prevented by prompt bronchoscopic removal of foreign objects[97] and by endotracheal intubation and pharyngeal packing, which protects against aspiration during operations on the oropharynx.

Lung abscess is an occasional complication of bacterial pneumonia and is much less frequent in the pediatric population than in adults.[360] The most common causative organisms are anaerobes,[55] followed by *S. aureus, Pseudomonas,* streptococcal species, pneumococci, and occasionally *H. influenzae.* Other bacteria implicated in lung abscess include *Klebsiella, Escherichia coli, Peptostreptococcus,* and *Peptococcus.* Children with cellular or humoral immune deficiencies, either congenital or acquired, are occasionally unable to eradicate a pulmonary infection despite appropriate antibiotics, leading to inflammation, the breakdown of pulmonary parenchyma, and eventual abscess formation. Histologically, a lung abscess may be identified 18 to 36 hours after the inciting event but may only be apparent on chest radiographs after 7 days.[27] When a lung abscess occurs in infants, an underlying congenital anomaly, such as a bronchogenic cyst or congenital cystic adenomatoid malformation, should be suspected (see Fig. 64-11).[84] These lesions require resection but initial treatment with antibiotics with or without drainage is usually indicated.

The position of the child at the moment of aspiration determines the location of the lung abscess.[306] In supine patients, the superior segments of the lower lobes are most often involved. If the child is on the right side, the right upper lobe is at risk; if the child is on the left side, the apical posterior segment of the left upper lobe may be the site. The upright child aspirates into basilar segments of the lower lobes. The distribution of lung abscesses in various lobes and segments in children is similar to

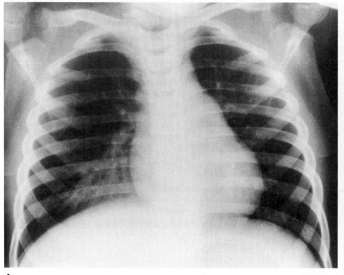

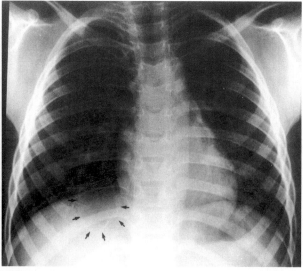

A

B

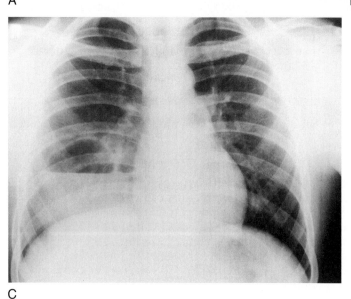

C

Figure 64–11 *A,* A 5-year-old child presented with a right lower lobe pneumonia that responded to intravenous antibiotics. *B,* During outpatient monitoring, small cysts were noted 6 weeks later and appeared to coalesce in a larger pneumatocele on this radiograph, taken 11 weeks after the initial study. Follow-up was recommended. *C,* At 14 years of age, the patient presented with a new episode of infection with a large air-fluid level and some smaller ones. Intravenous antibiotics were required for more than 2 weeks. CT confirmed the presence of three cysts. Six weeks later a right lower lobectomy was performed and microscopic examination confirmed a type I congenital cystic adenomatoid malformation.

that in adults. Lung abscesses often occur at the periphery of a segment or lobe, making them amenable to external drainage procedures.

Diagnosis

The most common symptoms caused by lung abscess include fever, cough, chest pain, anorexia, productive sputum, weight loss, malaise, hemoptysis, and chills. Purulent sputum may be easily obtained from older children to help with a bacteriologic diagnosis; younger patients usually swallow their secretions. Putrid sputum is characteristic of an anaerobic abscess. The affected area of the chest may be dull to percussion and have decreased breath sounds. Leukocytosis is common. Patients may also present with restrictive lung disease patterns from the enlarging abscess or secondary to pleuritic chest pain.

The diagnosis of lung abscess is established by a chest radiograph that shows a cavity, commonly with an air-fluid level (see Fig. 64-12). An abscess should be distinguished

from pneumatocele, a localized collection of intrapulmonary air that usually does not have an air-fluid level, and from empyema with an air-fluid level. CT has become a valuable adjunct in the diagnosis and characterization of lung disease in complicated pneumonia, revealing pathology that may not be apparent on plain chest radiographs.[101]

Treatment

A specific bacteriologic diagnosis should be established before treatment whenever possible. Diagnostic bronchoscopy with direct aspiration of purulent fluid from the parent bronchus should be performed, except in those older children who are able to induce a satisfactory sputum sample. The needle aspiration of a peripheral abscess cavity under imaging guidance to isolate bacterial species and drain collections has been used with moderate success.[285] Isolation of the causative organism is possible with this technique even if patients are concurrently receiving antibiotic therapy.

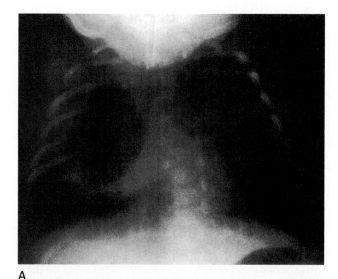

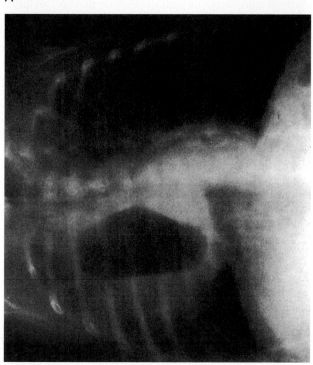

Figure 64–12 Lung abscess after aspiration in an infant. *A,* A thick-walled cavity is present on the anteroposterior supine view. *B,* An air-fluid level is visible on the lateral decubitus view.

The preferred treatment of lung abscess is appropriate intravenous antibiotic therapy and drainage. Satisfactory drainage can usually be accomplished by chest physiotherapy with postural drainage and percussion and by occasional bronchoscopic aspiration. For children who are unable to cough adequately, therapeutic bronchoscopy or transbronchial drainage may be necessary. Intravenous antibiotics are recommended for 2 to 4 weeks, followed by oral antibiotics for a total treatment period of 6 to 8 weeks. Antibiotics are discontinued when the child is symptom free and the chest radiographs are clear.

This may take from 1 to 6 months.[28] The most effective antibiotic for the treatment of lung abscess has been clindamycin. Aminoglycosides are usually recommended for coliform bacteria. If *Pseudomonas* is strongly suspected, then an appropriate β-lactam with an aminoglycoside is recommended.[360]

Medical therapy for lung abscesses is frequently unsuccessful in neonates and immunocompromised children, in whom the mortality approaches 20%.[391] Percutaneous catheter drainage of the abscess may be helpful in acutely ill children,[38,209,386,412] particularly for those who experience rapid progression of the disease despite maximal antibiotic therapy. The complications related to percutaneous techniques occur occasionally and include pneumothorax, hemothorax, incomplete drainage, and bronchopleural fistulas.[201,386] Surgical resection of the lung abscess by segmental resection or lobectomy is recommended for the chronic, large, and thick-walled abscesses or for those few patients who do not respond to intensive antibiotic therapy or percutaneous drainage.[84,274] Other indications for resection include chronic abscesses lasting longer than 3 months, persistent significant hemoptysis, bronchial stenosis, significant bronchiectasis, and massive pulmonary necrosis.

Empyema

History

Even during the ancient times of Hippocrates, Paul of Aegina, and Fabricius, empyema was a known complication that followed pulmonary infections and required external drainage for cure. In the 16th century, Paré manually evacuated a putrid hematoma from the pleural cavity of a French soldier.[165] Formal decortications were performed by Kuster in 1889 and Fowler in 1891.[125] Until the antibiotic era, discussions of therapy for empyema largely centered on the relative advantages of open drainage, various types of closed drainage, and the optimal time for the use of these measures.[93]

Definition and Pathogenesis

An empyema is the accumulation of purulent fluid in the pleural cavity and complicates pneumonia in up to 30% of children.[359] It may also occur after trauma, neoplastic processes, intrathoracic esophageal perforation, or surgeries on the chest. Normally, the pleural membranes are permeable to liquid and a small amount of fluid exists between the visceral and parietal pleura to minimize friction during respiration. When the adjacent lung is healthy, the pleural cavity is generally resistant to infection. Empyema, once established, exhibits three characteristic stages[67,314]: (1) an exudative or early stage when the fluid is thin and of low cellular content; (2) an intermediate or fibrinopurulent stage during which large numbers of polymorphonuclear cells and fibrin are deposited in the pleural space, progressively impairing lung expansion and leading to the formation of fluid loculations; and (3) a final stage or organizing empyema during which a thick exudate forms and fibroblasts invade the fibrinous peel. The empyema may be diffuse and involve the entire pleural space, or it may be localized and encapsulated in an interlobar, diaphragmatic, or paramediastinal location.

Currently, the most common organisms in childhood empyema are *S. pneumoniae, S. aureus,* and *H. influenzae.*[128] Other streptococci, mixed oral flora, and anaerobes have also been classically associated with the development of empyema. The changes in bacteriology are likely due to changing antibiotic resistance patterns. However, the incidence of empyema may be increasing,[109,292] and the virulence of the causative organisms appears to impact the natural course and, ultimately, the management of these patients.[241] Tuberculous empyema is much more rare than effusion and is associated with a high bacterial load within the pleural space. Mycobacterial resistance is a problem in this situation owing to the poor pleural penetration of standard chemotherapeutic agents.[174]

Clinical Manifestations and Diagnosis

The symptoms of empyema in a child are usually those of a short history of pulmonary infection followed by respiratory distress, fever, and cough. Chest or shoulder pain coupled with abdominal pain, distention, and ileus may intensify the respiratory difficulty. The radiographic appearance often includes bilateral pulmonary involvement with pneumatoceles occasionally identified within the lung. Haziness of a hemithorax may represent either pulmonary consolidation or pleural fluid. In the early exudative phase, the pleural fluid flows freely along the lateral chest wall on decubitus views (Fig. 64-13). In advanced empyema, the exudate is a solid mass of fibrin and does not move with changes in position. In the intermediate fibrinopurulent stage, loculations typically develop (see Fig. 64-13C). Air-fluid levels within the loculations suggest the presence of anaerobes in the pleural contents. Thoracentesis may provide valuable information on the quality of pleural fluid. The progression to advanced-stage empyema may be suspected if the fluid demonstrates any of the following characteristics after diagnostic thoracentesis: (1) gross pus, (2) pH < 7.0, (3) lactate dehydrogenase > 1000 U/mL, (4) glucose < 40 mg/dL, and (5) bacteria visible on Gram stain.

Treatment

Primary therapy for empyema is the administration of high-dose intravenous antibiotics. Effective drainage of the pleural space also speeds the resolution of the empyema. Fluid that layers in the decubitus position may be amenable to chest tube drainage alone. Loculated fluid collections may not be sufficiently drained in such a manner, and the optimal management of these patients is still debated. Fibrinolytic therapy was recommended as early as the 1940s to improve the drainage of pleural fluid.[364] Currently, the use of fibrinolytics remains controversial. Cameron and Davies[64] reviewed the four randomized trials involving patients aged over 14 years conducted to date[52,53,88,371] and concluded that fibrinolytic therapy conferred significant benefit (shorter lengths of stay, increased chest tube drainage) without morbidity when compared with saline controls. However, routine use of this therapy could not be recommended owing to

the small numbers of patients involved in this meta-analysis. Several retrospective case series in children have also demonstrated increased pleural drainage with the use of urokinase[207,211] and streptokinase,[76,280] with an average 20% failure rate of therapy. Recombinant tissue plasminogen activator (alteplase) may provide even more effective drainage but has not been extensively evaluated thus far.[394] Thomson and colleagues, in the only randomized trial in children to date, assessed the efficacy of urokinase in 60 children with empyema.[363] Although a significantly shorter length of stay was noted in the treatment group, control group patients had a much longer duration of prehospital illness (9 versus 5 days). Interestingly, this study also demonstrated a shorter length of stay for those patients receiving smaller-caliber chest tubes. In the end, there is evidence to support the use of fibrinolysis as an adjunctive therapy for children with complicated pleural effusions or empyema. The major reported complications with fibrinolytic therapy, including anaphylactic/allergic reactions (with streptokinase), chest pain, hemorrhage, and bronchopleural fistula occurred rarely in these reports. Urokinase is no longer available on the market, whereas alteplase is very expensive.

Decortication has been recommended in the treatment of complicated pleural effusions and empyema not responsive to medical therapy and attempts at pleural drainage. Indeed, using an empyema score, Hoff and colleagues demonstrated shorter and less complicated hospital stays for patients undergoing thoracotomy, particularly in severe disease.[166] Video-assisted thoracoscopic surgery (VATS) is an excellent alternative to thoracotomy for this purpose and has been advocated by many as a primary intervention in pediatric patients.[77,104,144,204,229,352] Given that patients with nonloculated effusions (stage 1) tend to recover with appropriate antibiotic therapy and chest tube drainage,[67] VATS may play more of a role in late-stage empyema. Chen and colleagues[71] noted that 70% of these patients eventually required surgery and that delay to surgical treatment increased length of stay. Patients in this series who were treated with VATS experienced the shortest lengths of stay, despite later intervention. Gates and colleagues systematically reviewed the English and Spanish language literature from 1987 to 2002 to determine the most effective treatment strategy for pediatric patients with empyema.[132] In their analysis of 44 studies involving 1369 patients, only the length of stay could be shown to be statistically shorter for those patients treated by either thoracotomy or VATS.

Unlike in adults for whom the American College of Chest Physicians has established guidelines,[78] treatment algorithms for pediatric patients with empyema vary widely and are often institution based. Interestingly, in a study from the Arkansas Children's Hospital,[122] a clinical pathway for the appropriate management of childhood empyema has been developed (Fig. 64-14). In this protocol, if an empyema is identified on chest radiographs it is then assessed by ultrasound for the presence of loculations. If loculations are identified, early VATS is advocated. The results of this pathway have demonstrated significantly reduced lengths of stay and hospital costs when compared with the national children's database. However, others maintain that antibiotics and chest tube drainage

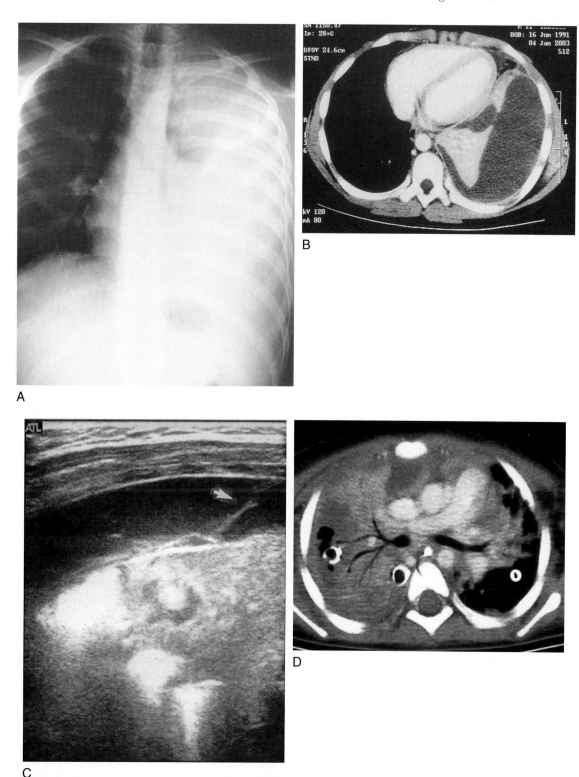

Figure 64–13 *A* and *B,* An 11-year-old boy presented with left-sided pleuritic pain and fever. *A,* Chest radiograph shows a large left-sided effusion with mediastinal shift. *B,* Because of concern about an underlying malignancy, a CT scan was obtained that showed a large nonloculated fluid collection, with a collapsed lower lobe; fluid can be seen in the fissure. A chest tube was inserted and drained 400 mL of serous fluid, with a lactate dehydrogenase of 4000 U/L, thus qualifying it as a fibrinopurulent empyema. There were no bacteria on Gram stain, but cultures grew *Streptococcus.* The patient improved with intravenous antibiotics, and the chest tube was removed 8 days later. *C* and *D,* A 3-year-old girl had a more fulminant course. Loculations *(arrow)* and debris in the pleural fluid were evident on ultrasound in *C.* Despite early thoracoscopic drainage, she developed lung necrosis (seen on CT with intravenous contrast in *D*) with a persistent air leak, requiring 10 days in the intensive care unit and 1 month in hospital.

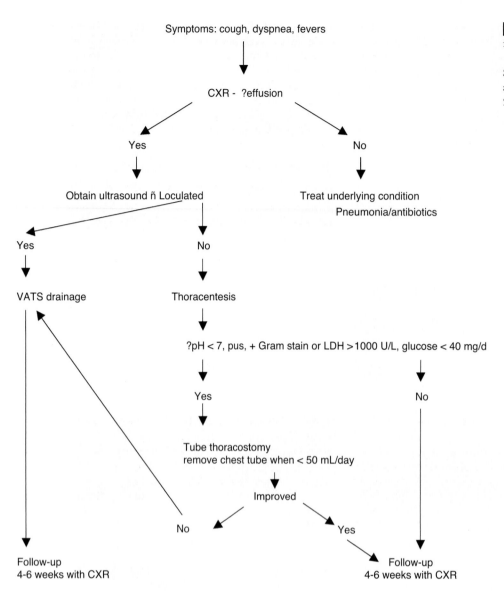

Symptoms: cough, dyspnea, fevers

CXR - ?effusion

Yes — No

Obtain ultrasound ñ Loculated — Treat underlying condition
Pneumonia/antibiotics

Yes — No

VATS drainage — Thoracentesis

?pH < 7, pus, + Gram stain or LDH >1000 U/L, glucose < 40 mg/d

Yes — No

Tube thoracostomy
remove chest tube when < 50 mL/day

Improved

No — Yes

Follow-up
4-6 weeks with CXR

Follow-up
4-6 weeks with CXR

Figure 64–14 Critical pathway for management of empyema in children. (From Finck C, Wagner C, Jackson R, Smith S: Empyema: Development of a critical pathway. Semin Pediatr Surg 2002;11:25-28, with permission.)

are still the most cost-effective strategies for the treatment of empyema.[248] Because of the lack of any prospective studies, there is a need for a multicenter, prospective, and randomized trial to answer ongoing questions regarding the best treatment of pediatric patients with empyema.

PEDIATRIC SPONTANEOUS PNEUMOTHORAX

Primary spontaneous pneumothorax is defined as a pneumothorax occurring secondary to apical blebs or bullae without evidence of other lung pathology.[293,332,399] It can also occur in term neonates without any risk factors. In contrast, secondary spontaneous pneumothoraces occur in the context of underlying lung disease, such as cystic fibrosis or *P. jiroveci (carinii)* pneumonia. Other lung infections, bronchiolitis, asthma (even mild), connective tissue disorders, congenital cystic adenomatoid malformations, and traumatic lung contusions are risk factors.[89,214,332] The incidence of primary spontaneous pneumothorax is estimated to be 7.4 to 18 per 100,000 boys

and 1.2 to 6.0 per 100,000 girls in the United States.[149,315] Typically, the patient is a thin, lean adolescent who presents with an acute onset of ipsilateral pleuritic chest pain and nonproductive cough. Most patients are clinically stable on initial assessment. However, a small number may present in fulminant distress, including hypotension and respiratory failure, secondary to a tension pneumothorax. Other clinical findings in patients with pneumothorax include tachypnea and tachycardia. Chest radiographs confirm the diagnosis and may identify a secondary pathologic process within the lung. Expiratory films may be helpful to identify small pneumothoraces. Different methods are available to quantitate the size of the pneumothorax, because this factor is most likely to influence subsequent management. Indeed, a Light Index has been described that compares the diameter of the lung to the ipsilateral hemithorax as a means of quantitating the size of the pneumothorax.[227,275]

Patients who present with an acute pneumothorax require supplemental oxygen and intravenous access. For those few patients presenting with a tension pneumothorax, immediate needle decompression in the second intercostal space (midclavicular line) is necessary even before chest radiograph confirmation, followed by the prompt placement of a chest tube. A pneumothorax of less than 15% can often be managed by observation with or without supplemental oxygen, especially if the initial symptoms occurred more than 24 hours before presentation. Needle aspiration and the insertion of small pleural drains has also been used,[293] but the Delphi Consensus Statement (2001) does not support the routine use of needle decompression in this instance.[10] Heimlich valves connected to the pleural drain allow for outpatient management of small pneumothoraces in compliant patients. Large pneumothoraces require the placement of a chest tube with underwater seal and drainage. An air leak that persists for more than 5 to 7 days may require further intervention, or at least confirmation that the chest tube in place is functioning properly.[245] For most young children (<8 years), and those with asthma as a predisposing factor, chest tube drainage is sufficient for treatment. However, adolescents with spontaneous pneumothorax have been reported to have a recurrence rate of up to 40% to 60%.[80,293,332] Interestingly, in one adult series, small drains were associated with a higher recurrence rate of pneumothorax (33%) than either observation alone (17%) or large-bore chest tubes (6%).[381] In the end, symptomatology should direct further investigation and treatment. CT is more sensitive at detecting blebs and bullae than normal radiographs, but it is unclear if its routine use for spontaneous pneumothorax ultimately changes management.[255,332,338] Some authors advocate the use of CT after the index presentation, whereas others wait for a recurrence before further investigation.[197] No firm consensus has been established for the role of imaging in spontaneous pneumothorax.

The indications for surgical management include recurrence, persistent air leak, bilateral disease, and possibly the presence of large bullae. VATS appears to be superior to standard thoracotomy with respect to postoperative pain and complications in several series.[168,387] Transaxillary mini-thoracotomy is a viable alternative to VATS and has certain advantages, particularly in the context of poor visualization and the presence of dense adhesions.[169,332,339] For pleurodesis, thoracoscopic pleural abrasion and talc poudrage are effective techniques.[65,367] Apical pleurectomy can be easily performed through a transaxillary incision. For bilateral disease, both VATS and transaxillary mini-thoracotomy are effective and can be used as a single-stage operation.[217,332] Despite similar results in outcome, VATS has become more popular among surgeons for the treatment of spontaneous pneumothorax even though some controversy persists.[98,111,197,387] The recurrence rate with VATS ranges from 2% to 14%, although this does appear to decrease with increasing experience.[105,169,179,263] For transaxillary mini-thoracotomy, the recurrence rate has been reported to be as low as 2%.[105,197] All in all, both VATS and transaxillary thoracotomy are effective in the treatment of spontaneous pneumothorax. Furthermore, the guidelines for the treatment of spontaneous pneumothorax are often extrapolated from adult series, and randomized trials in the pediatric population are clearly warranted.

Pneumothoraces in patients with cystic fibrosis are more difficult to treat because the air leak frequently persists. The use of a higher negative pressure (20 to 25 cm H_2O) may be helpful. If this fails, thoracoscopic talc poudrage[367] or other sclerosing agents[238] are required to achieve pleurodesis and prevent recurrence. Pleurectomy is usually avoided to facilitate pneumonectomy should lung transplantation become necessary.

INTRATHORACIC ACCESS AND PROCEDURES

Chest Tube Insertion in the Newborn for Pneumothorax

In preparation of chest tube insertion, the infant is placed in an oxygen hood or, if intubated, maintained on ventilator support, restrained, and monitored via pulse oximetry and electrocardiography. A surgical headlamp or an overhead light source of similar quality should be available. The procedure is performed with sterile technique (mask, cap, gown, and gloves). In addition to sterile instruments (scalpel, mosquito clamps, Adson forceps, needle holder, fine scissors) and drapes, No. 8 and No. 10 French catheters, a sterile connector, 3-0 and 4-0 nonabsorbable suture on curved swedged-on needles, and an infant-sized underwater seal drainage system should be readily available. The chest wall is prepared with an iodophor solution and draped with sterile towels. The skin is infiltrated with lidocaine via a 25-gauge needle placed lateral to the nipple in the anterior axillary line over the fourth rib. Injury to the nipple and underlying breast tissue should be avoided. A 3- to 4-mm incision is made with a No. 11 scalpel blade. A mosquito clamp is placed through the incision and used to spread the subcutaneous tissues. It is advanced upward over the rib and used to spread the intercostal muscles above the incision, which requires firm pressure, and then passed into the pleural cavity. This method produces a "tunnel" so that the entrance into the pleural cavity is superior to the level of the skin incision. Entry into the pleural space is heralded by reduced resistance and is usually followed by the sound of escaping air. The tip of the No. 8 French chest tube is placed in the end of the curved mosquito clamp, and the tube is advanced into the pleural cavity (Fig. 64-15). An alternative is to use a trocar inside the chest tube to guide the latter through the tunnel. With this technique, it is safer to withdraw the tip of the trocar by a few millimeters and to place a large clamp on the tube 5 cm proximal to the tip to avoid uncontrolled penetration and injury to the mediastinal structures. The tube is advanced superiorly and anteriorly 3 to 4 cm, being certain that all of the holes in the tube are intrapleural, yet avoiding a tube that is too far and kinks after reaching the mediastinum. The tube is then sutured in place with a 3-0 nonabsorbable purse-string suture. Povidone-iodine (Betadine) ointment is placed at the tube-skin interface, and the tube is secured. The connecting tube is attached to an underwater seal, and the water level is observed to ensure fluctuation with respiration. The system may be set at 10 cm H_2O of negative

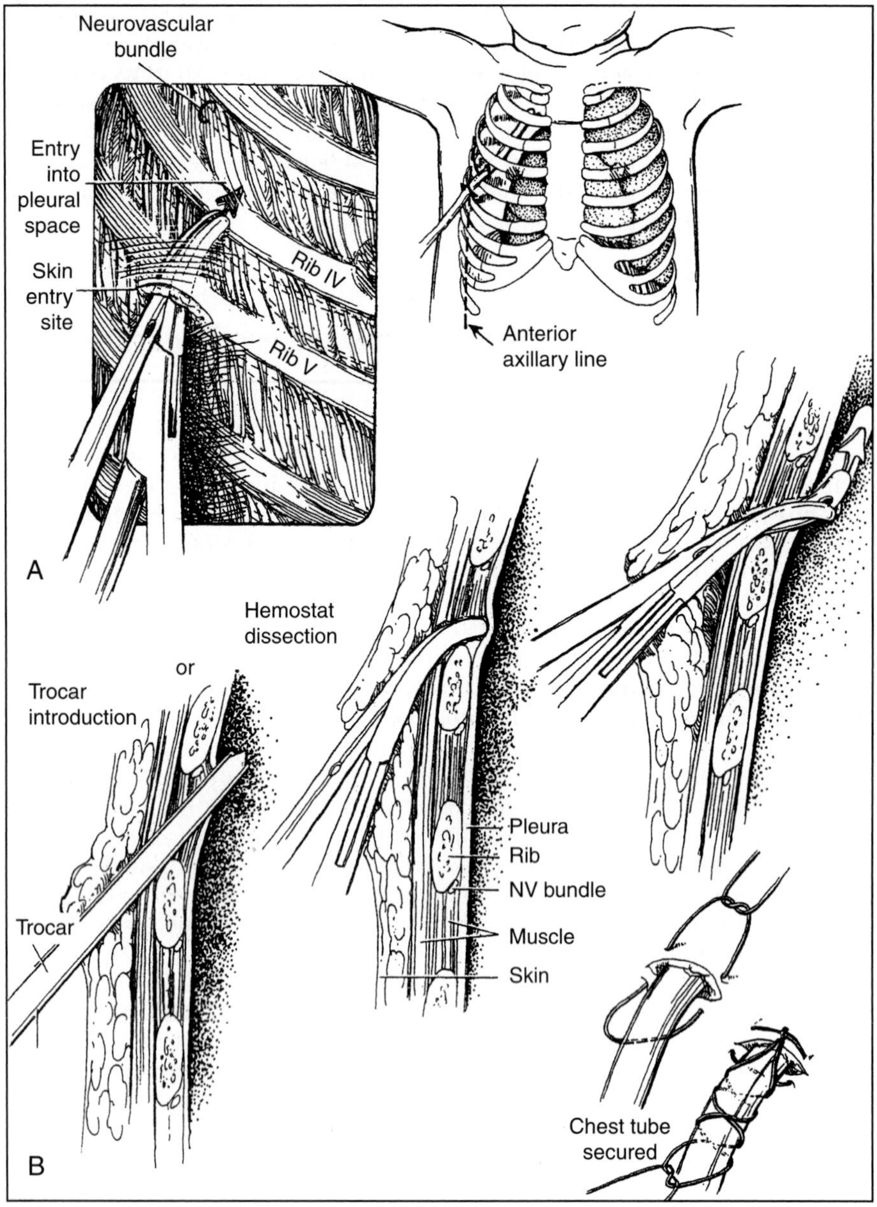

Figure 64–15 Chest tube insertion in the newborn for pneumothorax. *A,* Preferably a small hemostat is inserted through a small incision in the anterior or midaxillary line and is tunneled upward, entering the chest above the next rib. The chest tube is inserted and secured with a suture ligature. Several knots should be placed after each circumferential pass of the thread to avoid any slippage. *B,* A trocar can be used as an alternative method of tube insertion, as long as the trocar is withdrawn by a few millimeters within the tube; this technique allows easier guidance of the tube, for example, if it has to be placed posteriorly and inferiorly to drain an effusion.

pressure if necessary, remembering that a high negative pressure will add to the positive pressure applied by a ventilator and may lead to barotrauma. A disposable infant Pleur-Evac system is highly effective and easily managed in the neonatal intensive care unit.

A chest radiograph is obtained to determine the location of the tube, to ensure that all the holes are intrapleural, and to check that tube placement was effective in expanding the collapsed lung. A lateral chest radiograph may be obtained to determine whether the tube is in an anterior or a posterior location. A superior and anteriorly placed tube most effectively evacuates pneumothorax. Excessive bubbling indicates a continued source of air leak from the injured lung, a bronchopulmonary fistula, or most commonly a leak in the system.

The most frequent complications related to chest tube insertion are (1) injury to the intercostal vessels during insertion and (2) lung perforation caused by the clamp or tube. If there is excessive bleeding and continued significant air leak, surgical correction is required. Injury to mediastinal lymphatic, venous, and nervous structures has also been described.

Kits are available that allow the Seldinger technique to be used to rapidly and safely place a small chest tube in infants. A needle is inserted in the pleural cavity and a guidewire passed. The needle is removed, and a dilator is passed over the wire, followed by a pigtail catheter.

Chest Tube Care and Removal

After insertion for pneumothorax a chest tube usually drains little fluid after the air is evacuated. In infants who do not require mechanical ventilation, when there is no further bubbling in the water seal chamber and the lung is fully expanded for 24 to 48 hours, the suction, if utilized, is removed and the tube left only on an underwater seal. If the pneumothorax does not reaccumulate in 12 to 24 hours, it is probably safe to remove the tube. The tube should be removed rapidly and the tube site sealed with petroleum gauze dressing to prevent air from entering the chest. An additional chest radiograph is usually obtained to be sure that there is no recurrence of the pneumothorax. It is probably safer to leave the chest tube in place for longer periods if the infant requires mechanical ventilation, especially if high peak inspiratory pressure and/or positive end-expiratory pressure is necessary.

Chest Tube Insertion in Older Children

Pneumothorax in older children is usually encountered in patients with spontaneous rupture of an emphysematous bleb, asthma, cystic fibrosis, and after blunt, or, occasionally, penetrating chest wall trauma. A tube thoracostomy is required in symptomatic patients. Chest tube insertion in older infants and children may also be required for pleural effusions from a variety of causes, including chylothorax; traumatic hemothorax; lymphoma; inflammation as a result of bacterial, fungal, and viral pneumonia; empyema; and other causes.

Insertion of a chest tube in these patients follows the same pattern of sterile techniques and preparation described in the management of neonates. Infants and toddlers can be premedicated with intravenous fentanyl (1.0 μg/kg) and midazolam (0.1 mg/kg) as part of a conscious sedation protocol. Alternatively, ketamine (1.0 mg/kg) with or without midazolam provides excellent analgesia and sedation while preserving respiration reflexes and cardiac parameters throughout the duration of the procedure. Children are kept in the supine position with a small roll under the affected hemithorax to elevate the area. The ipsilateral arm is positioned superiorly and laterally. The chest tube size is determined by the child's weight and whether the problem is a pneumothorax, a transudate, or an exudate (Table 64-1). After sterile preparation, a local anesthetic, and placement of a small skin incision, the appropriate-sized tube is inserted in the third or fourth interspace in the anterior to midaxillary line and positioned upward and anteriorly for pneumothorax. If the patient has an effusion, the location should be determined by correlating the physical examination (e.g., dullness to percussion and diminished tactile fremitus) with the findings on chest radiograph,

ultrasound, and/or chest CT. A 20-gauge needle or angiocatheter may be inserted just at the level of transition of percussion sounds (from tympanic to dull) to locate the effusion. The chest tube can then be inserted as noted earlier and positioned inferiorly and posteriorly. The chest tube should not be placed below the level of the seventh rib to avoid injury to the spleen, liver, or diaphragm.

Lung Biopsy

Open-lung biopsy is usually obtained early in the diagnostic evaluation of diffuse pulmonary disorders in children and is generally preferred to a percutaneous transthoracic needle biopsy for establishing the diagnosis. Needle lung biopsies are fairly reliable and accurate; however, pneumothorax or hemothorax occur in approximately one third of patients. Larger specimens are obtained by open lung biopsy for cultures and histologic study as well as special staining and occasionally for electron microscopy. It is easier to avoid air leaks and to secure complete hemostasis with open wedge biopsy. Pneumothorax is prevented by the routine use of a chest tube. The mortality after surgery is rarely a result of the procedure; death, when it occurs, is almost always caused by the patient's underlying disease. A tissue diagnosis is established in almost all patients after open-lung biopsy and influences subsequent therapy in over 90%.[206] The preoperative diagnosis is confirmed in approximately 60% of patients and corrected in over 35%. Moreover, the differential diagnosis is often between infectious, neoplastic, or inflammatory processes such as bronchiolitis obliterans with organizing pneumonia (BOOP) or lymphoid interstitial pneumonitis. Because inflammatory processes require tissue for diagnosis and are treated with corticosteroids, a lung biopsy is essential to confirm the diagnosis (Fig. 64-16; see also Fig. 64-6).

Children who must undergo open-lung biopsy may be poor risks for surgery and anesthesia. They are often immunosuppressed with spreading pulmonary infiltrates and impending respiratory failure. Biopsy should be performed early, when indicated, rather than after respiratory failure has supervened and the child is dependent on a ventilator. However, even for patients with persisting or undiagnosed respiratory failure, lung biopsy still leads to significant changes in management despite a higher incidence of complications, mainly as air leak (45%). Careful preoperative review of chest radiographs is essential to identify the optimal site for biopsy; sometimes two different areas should be sampled, one heavily infiltrated and the other less involved. Preoperative discussion with the pathologist is invaluable. A small anterior thoracotomy incision with the biopsy performed using a stapler device is safe and expeditious; in smaller children, a Lahey clamp allows an adequate biopsy specimen through a smaller incision, especially if the lung parenchyma is stiff and cannot be brought out through the incision (Fig. 64-17). Alternatively, a transaxillary incision may provide adequate access to lung tissue desired for lung biopsy. In experienced hands there is minimal mortality or morbidity from open-lung biopsy in spite of the patient population. In patients large enough

TABLE 64-1 Guide for Chest Tube Selection			
Patient Weight (kg)	**Size (French)**		
	Pneumothorax	**Transudate**	**Exudate**
<3	8-10	8-10	10-12
3-8	10-12	10-12	12-16
8-15	12-16	12-16	16-20
16-40	16-20	16-20	20-28
>40	20-24	24-28	28-36

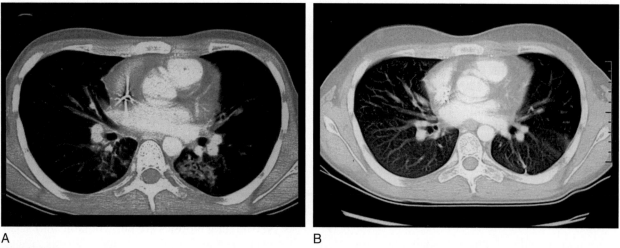

Figure 64–16 A 17-year-old boy with stage IV Hodgkin's disease underwent radiotherapy and autologous bone marrow transplantation. *A*, On routine surveillance CT, bilateral focal airspace disease was seen, mostly in the superior segments of the lower lobes. Lung biopsy revealed bronchiolitis obliterans. He was treated with corticosteroids, and a repeat scan 3 months later (*B*) showed a near-complete resolution.

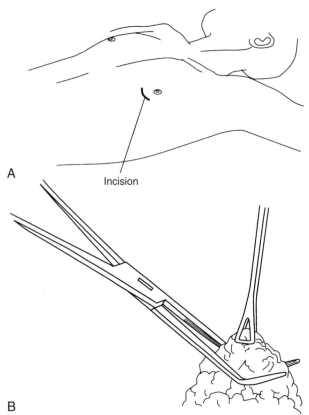

Figure 64–17 *A*, An open-lung biopsy can be done with minimal morbidity using a small anterior thoracotomy. *B*, The lingula can be grasped easily and provides an adequate specimen in patients with diffuse lung infiltrate; in small children (or when a stiff lung cannot be brought outside the chest wall) a Lahey clamp is used to obtain the biopsy specimen instead of a linear stapler. After the lung tissue above the Lahey clamp is cut sharply with a scalpel, a continuous U suture is passed underneath the clamp, the clamp is released, and the suture is tightened and brought back as a simple continuous stitch. This provides excellent hemostasis and prevents air leaks.

to allow the use of endoscopic stapling devices, lung biopsy can also be performed by thoracoscopy, with similar risks and complications to the open procedures (see Chapter 62).

CHYLOTHORAX

The escape of chyle into the mediastinum from a defective thoracic duct and thence into one or both pleural spaces is a well-described entity. Historical perspectives on chylothorax and its management include the evolution of the knowledge of anatomy and physiology of the thoracic duct, the development of the science of nutrition, and progress in thoracic surgery. Of note, Blalock reported in 1937 the experimental occlusion of the superior vena cava could produce chylothorax, which was prevented by prior ligation of the thoracic duct.[45] A decade later, Lampson was the first to use this treatment clinically.[215] Considerations of therapy focus on causative factors and include dietary modification and octreotide to decrease thoracic duct flow, thoracentesis and/or thoracostomy drainage to relieve respiratory embarrassment and promote pleural sealing, and surgical ligation of the disrupted duct or pleuroperitoneal shunting when conservative measures fail.

Etiology

Effusion of chylous fluid into the thorax may occur spontaneously in newborns and has usually been attributed to congenital abnormalities of the thoracic duct or trauma from delivery.[47] However, the occurrence of chylothorax in most cases cannot be related to the type of labor or delivery and lymphatic effusions may be discovered prenatally.[118,233] Chylothorax is the leading cause of pleural effusions in neonates.[92]

Chylothorax in older children is rarely spontaneous and occurs almost invariably after trauma or cardiothoracic

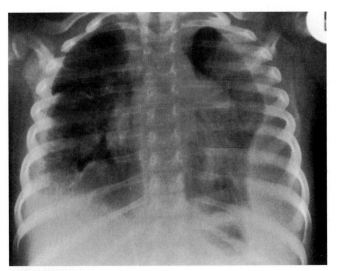

Figure 64–18 Chest radiograph of 4-year-old girl with bilateral extensive lymphangioma and chylothorax. Note hazy appearance of fluid and major compression of the left lung.

surgery; however, some patients with thoracic lymphangioma may present in this older age group (Fig. 64-18).[42,48,215,261] Operative injury may be in part a result of anatomic variations of the thoracic duct. Trauma leading to hyperextension of the spine with rupture of the duct from stretching has been reported with high diving, wrestling, and other such activities.[215,327] Extensive bouts of coughing have been reported to cause rupture of the thoracic duct, which is particularly vulnerable when full following a fatty meal.[310] Neoplasms, particularly lymphomas and neuroblastomas, have occasionally been noted to cause obstruction of the thoracic duct.[107,254] Lymphangiomatosis or diffuse lymphangiectasia may produce chylous effusion in the pleural space and peritoneal cavity. Other causes include mediastinal inflammation, subclavian vein or superior vena caval thrombosis, misplaced central venous catheters, and child abuse.[42,62,92,148,251,373]

Anatomy and Pathophysiology

The thoracic duct develops from outgrowths of the jugular lymphatic sacs and the cisterna chyli. During embryonic life, bilateral thoracic lymphatic channels are present, each attached in the neck to the corresponding jugular sac. As development progresses, the upper third of the right duct and the lower two thirds of the left duct involute and close. The wide variation in the final anatomic structure of the main ductal system attests to the multiple communications of the small vessels comprising the lymphatic system. The thoracic duct originates in the abdomen at the cisterna chyli located over the second lumbar vertebra (Fig. 64-19). The duct extends into the thorax through the aortic hiatus and then passes upward into the posterior mediastinum on the right before shifting toward the left at the level of the fifth thoracic vertebra. It then ascends posterior to the aortic

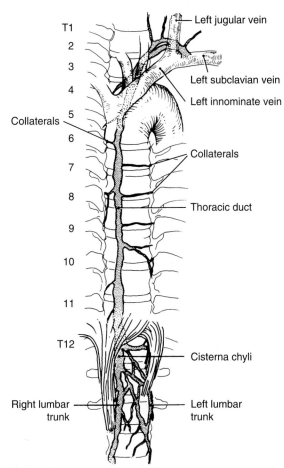

Thoracic duct

Figure 64–19 Schematic representation of most common anatomic arrangement of the thoracic duct. (From DeMeester R, Lafontaine E: The pleura. In Sabiston DC, Spencer FC [eds]: Gibbon's Surgery of the Chest, 4th ed. Philadelphia, WB Saunders, 1983, reprinted with permission.)

arch and into the posterior neck to the junction of the subclavian and internal jugular veins.

Many variations are present in the entire ductal system, and the typical course of the thoracic duct is present in only approximately 50% of individuals.[90,310] The most common variations are a double system originating from the cisterna or a multiple ductal pattern at the level of the diaphragm. In the chest a rich collateral system originates from intercostal spaces, the posterior mediastinum, and visceral lymphatics, which communicate freely with the main duct via collecting trunks.

The thoracic duct contains smooth muscle in the wall that is capable of contracting with sufficient force to propel lymph upward toward the jugular venous junction at a rate of 50 to 200 mL/hr.[15] The rate of lymph flow in the thoracic duct varies widely and relates to the volume of fat ingestion, scar tissue in the mediastinum, presence of portal hypertension, and other factors. The flow of chyle superiorly into the subclavian vein is enhanced by the presence of valves in the thoracic duct, portal pressure, and the differential gradient between the negative intrapleural pressure and the positive intra-abdominal pressure.[45,139] Conversely, increasing the intrathoracic pressure through the use of positive end-expiratory pressure has been shown to decrease by half the flow of chyle in the thoracic duct.

The chyle contained in the thoracic duct conveys approximately three fourths of the ingested fat from the intestine to the systemic circulation. The fat content of chyle varies from 0.4 to 4.0 g/dL.[45,310] The large fat molecules absorbed from the intestinal lacteals flow through the cisterna chyli and superiorly through the thoracic duct.[127] Total protein content of thoracic duct lymph is also high. Nutritional complications were a major source of mortality from chylothorax in the era preceding parenteral nutrition. Other than nutrients, the thoracic duct carries white blood cells (primarily lymphocytes [T cells])—2000 to 20,000 cells/mL. Eosinophils are also present in higher proportion than in circulating blood. Loss of lymphocytes through a thoracic duct fistula may lead to an immunocompromised state[139]; in fact, external drainage of the thoracic duct was used as an adjunct to immunosuppression in the early era of organ transplantation. Chyle appears to have a bacteriostatic property, which accounts for the rare occurrence of infection complicating chylothorax.

Clinical Manifestations

Birth trauma was formerly thought to be the cause of many neonatal chylothoraces, but the increasing use of prenatal ultrasonography has changed the perspective. Non-iatrogenic chylothorax occurring in young children is usually related to congenital anomalies of the chyliferous vessels, cisterna chyli, or the thoracic duct itself. Most of these chylothoraces result from intrapleural leakage from dilated and thin-walled intercostal, diaphragmatic, or accessory mediastinal lymphatics. When there is lymphatic overload, these alternate lymphatics may dilate considerably to eventually become transudative lymphatic varices. In other cases, subpleural lymphatics may rupture into the pleural cavity, as in certain cardiac anomalies (e.g., total anomalous pulmonary venous return).

The accumulation of chyle in the pleural space from a thoracic duct leak may occur rapidly and produce pressure on other structures in the chest, causing acute respiratory distress, dyspnea, and cyanosis with tachypnea. In the fetus, a pleural effusion may be secondary to generalized hydrops but a primary lymphatic effusion (idiopathic, secondary to subpleural lymphangiectasia, pulmonary sequestration, or associated with syndromes such as Down, Turner's, and Noonan's) can cause mediastinal shift and result in hydrops or lead to pulmonary hypoplasia.[118,233] Postnatally, the effects of chylothorax and the prolonged loss of chyle may include malnutrition, hypoproteinemia, fluid and electrolyte imbalance, metabolic acidosis, and immunodeficiency.

In a neonate, symptoms of respiratory embarrassment observed in combination with a pleural effusion strongly suggest chylothorax. The involved side presents characteristic findings of intrapleural fluid with respiratory lag, dullness on percussion, diminished breath sounds, and

shift of the mediastinum. Fever is not common. Chest radiographs typically show massive fluid effusion in the ipsilateral chest with pulmonary compression and mediastinal shift. Bilateral effusions may also occur. Aspiration of the pleural effusion reveals a clear straw-colored fluid in the fasting patient, which becomes milky after feedings. Analysis of the chyle generally reveals a total fat content of more than 400 mg/dL (or triglyceride level greater than 110 mg/dL) and a protein content of more than 5 g/dL. In a fetus or a fasting neonate, the most useful and simple test is to perform a complete blood cell count and differential on the fluid; when lymphocytes exceed 80% or 90% of the white blood cells, a lymphatic effusion is confirmed; the differential can be compared with that obtained from the blood cell count, in which lymphocytes rarely represent more than 70% of white blood cells.

Most cases of traumatic chylothorax develop after thoracic operations, in particular, repair of patent ductus arteriosus, coarctation of the aorta, and Blalock-Taussig shunt.[271] Injury to the thoracic duct in the left chest is particularly common during secondary thoracotomies for correction of lesions in the descending aorta or esophagus just inferior to the arch. If lymphatic drainage is noted at operation, the proximal and distal ends of the thoracic duct should be ligated.[271] A period of days or weeks may elapse between trauma or surgery and the development of a symptomatic chylothorax.

As chyle accumulates in the pleural space from a thoracic duct leak, progressively more pronounced respiratory symptoms develop as pulmonary compression becomes more severe. Dyspnea, tachypnea, and eventually arterial desaturation with cyanosis can develop. Nutritional deficiency is a late manifestation of chyle depletion and occurs when dietary intake is insufficient to replace the thoracic duct fluid loss.

Therapy

Whereas small quantities of short-chain fatty acids are absorbed through the portal venous circulation, 80% to 90% of all fat absorbed from the gut is transported by way of the thoracic duct in the form of chylomicrons. Thus, feedings restricted to medium- or short-chain triglycerides theoretically result in reduced lymph flow in the thoracic duct and may enhance spontaneous healing of a thoracic duct fistula.[168,210] However, it has been shown that any internal feeding, even with clear fluids, significantly increases thoracic duct flow.[221] Therefore, for patients who experience large chylous fluid losses, withholding oral feedings and providing total parenteral nutrition is preferred.[24] For patients who are already on mechanical ventilation, the addition of positive end-expiratory pressure can further decrease the lymphatic flow. Recently, somatostatin or its analogue octreotide have been found useful in several reports.[73,83,221] These agents decrease gastric, pancreatic, and intestinal secretions and have become an important tool in the management of pancreatic and intestinal fistulas. Because of its short half-life, somatostatin requires a continuous intravenous infusion, whereas the synthetic analogue octreotide can be given subcutaneously every 8 hours, starting at a dose of 10 to 20 μg/kg/day.[73] Continuous infusions of octreotide at 1 to 4 μg/kg/hour may be more effective. It has been used as a rescue after failed surgery[83] and even as the first-line treatment without diet modification.[224] If nonoperative management is effective, external intake should be reinstituted first with medium-chain triglycerides, followed by a normal diet for age after 2 weeks. Cultures of chylous fluid are rarely positive; providing long-term antibiotics during the full course of chest tube drainage is not considered necessary.

Thoracentesis is used for diagnosis and may be sufficient to relieve spontaneous chylothorax in occasional infants with the dietary measures described; however, chest tube drainage will be necessary for the majority. Furthermore, tube drainage allows quantification of the daily chyle leak and promotes pulmonary reexpansion, which may enhance healing. Chylothorax in newborns usually ceases spontaneously.[233,329,376] Because identifying the actual site of the fluid leak is difficult, surgery is often deferred for several weeks. Similarly, most cases of traumatic injury to the thoracic duct can be managed successfully by chest tube drainage and replacement of the protein and fat loss.[271] If drainage persists in quantities beyond the tolerance of the infant or child and shows no evidence of diminishing, or if it persists after 2 to 3 weeks without decreasing, ligation of the thoracic duct on the side of the effusion may be necessary. Standard contrast lymphangiography has been abandoned, but isotope lymphangiography using technetium-99m colloid, or other markers, may be helpful in identifying the site of the fistula.[194]

Occasionally the chylous fluid may enter the pericardial sac and cause chylopericardial tamponade, in which case pericardiocentesis should provide immediate relief. Although bilateral spontaneous chylothorax in newborns is uncommon, it can produce fatal respiratory distress unless recognized and drained promptly.

When chylothorax remains resistant despite prolonged chest tube drainage and total parenteral nutrition, thoracotomy or thoracoscopy on the ipsilateral side may be necessary.[48,329] The decision whether to continue with conservative management or to undertake surgical intervention should be based on the nature of the underlying disorder, the duration of the leak, the daily volume of fluid drainage, and the severity of nutritional and/or immunologic depletion. Several authors have suggested that patients in whom the chest tube drains more than 100 mL/year of age/day or 10 mL/kg/day without slowing down after 10 to 20 days should undergo surgery. Although this is not an absolute indication, one should remember that loss of lymphocytes may lead to overwhelming bacterial or fungal infections, thus explaining the majority of deaths from chylothorax in the current era.[23,221,222] The ingestion of 60 mL of cream 30 minutes before surgery may facilitate the identification of the thoracic duct and the fistula. When identified, the draining lymphatic vessel should be suture ligated above and below the leak with reinforcement by a pleural or intercostal muscle flap. Meticulous dissection of the thoracic duct with isolation of the fistula is often not feasible. When a leak cannot be identified with certainty, or when multiple leaks originate from the mediastinum, ligation of all the tissues surrounding the aorta at the level of the hiatus provides the best results. Fibrin glue and argon-beam coagulation have also been used as an adjunct for ill-defined areas of leakage or incompletely resected lympangiomas.[270]

Thoracoscopy has been used in larger patients to avoid thoracotomy.[140] The leak, if visualized, can be ligated, clipped, or sealed with fibrin glue. If the leak cannot be identified, pleurodesis can be accomplished with talc or other sclerotic agents under direct vision through the thoracoscope, but this technique should probably be avoided in infancy because of the consequences on lung and chest wall growth. If there is concomitant chyloperi-cardium, a pericardial window can be fashioned. Because thoracoscopy is less invasive, some surgeons advocate early intervention, as early as 5 to 10 days. This approach may be indicated in conditions where the failure rate of conservative management is higher, such as superior vena cava thrombosis or problems associated with increased right-sided heart pressures.

Pleuroperitoneal shunts have been used for refractory chylothorax in which a leak has not been identified and in those patients who do not respond to initial nonoperative management, especially if they have a higher operative risk.[264] This approach has been used with occasional success both in patients with congenital anomalies of the thoracic duct or lymphangiomas or in patients who have persistent drainage after cardiac surgery.[307] A Denver double-valve shunt system is the type most commonly employed; it may be totally implanted under local anesthesia and allows the patient or parent to pump the valve to achieve decompression of the pleural fluid into the abdominal cavity, where it is reabsorbed. An externalized pumping chamber was found to be superior in smaller infants.[402] It may offer the least invasive treatment for neonates or infants who develop a refractory chylothorax after surgery for complex cardiac malformations, as long as right-sided heart pressures are below 25 cm H_2O.

Overall, most patients with chylothorax can be cured with conservative measures, nutritional support, and occasional operative intervention. Patients with diffuse lymphatic malformations remain a challenge.

MEDIASTINAL INFECTIONS

Acute Mediastinitis

Acute mediastinitis occurs as a result of contamination and/or soilage of the mediastinal space secondary to the trauma or perforation of either the trachea or esophagus. Rarely, mediastinitis can develop from a descending retropharyngeal or cervical abscesses[195] or the rupture of suppurative mediastinal lymph nodes. Infection within the mediastinum can disseminate quickly because this space contains no anatomic barriers to the spread of infection. Clinically, acute mediastinitis is heralded by high fever, chest pain, dyspnea, cyanosis, and marked tachycardia as well as a significant leukocytosis. In neonates, the signs and symptoms may be subtle, including lethargy, fever, apnea, temperature instability, and leukopenia. The management of mediastinitis includes hemodynamic support, the prompt administration of intravenous antibiotics, and mediastinal drainage. Drainage may be particularly important in the context of a mediastinal abscess or continued leak/contamination from a perforated esophagus. Cervical, transthoracic, retropleural, or anterior approaches may be utilized to facilitate drainage, depending on the location of abscess or leakage.

Infections After Median Sternotomy

Although the incidence of sternal wound and mediastinal infections after median sternotomy is low, these infections can have devastating implications on the postoperative course of these patients. In adult series, sternal wound infections have been shown to occur in up to 20% of patients,[234] whereas the incidence of mediastinitis ranges from 1% to 2%.[308] Tortoriello and colleagues reviewed their experience with mediastinitis after pediatric cardiac surgery over 15 years at the Texas Children's Hospital.[366] Only 15 pediatric patients in their series of 7616 patients developed mediastinitis (0.2%). The only mortality in this series was secondary to a fulminant fungal mediastinitis after orthotopic heart transplantation. The most common infective organism was *S. aureus,* a finding supported by other reviews.[237] Other organisms included *Pseudomonas* and *Candida.* Deep sternal infections may also be caused by gram-negative enteric flora and anaerobes.

The early identification and aggressive treatment of mediastinal infections is required. Clinically, patients present with local erythema, fluctuance, purulent drainage, sternal instability, fever, and leukocytosis. These features may only be apparent after the first postoperative week. Indeed, the median time for diagnosis of sternal wound complications was 14 days postoperatively in the Texas Children's series.[366] CT and gallium scanning has been useful in identifying deep sternal infections as well as sternal osteomyelitis. Controversy still exists regarding the optimal modalities that may be used to treat mediastinitis in sternotomy patients. Standard management strategies including débridement and antibiotic irrigation have evolved to the liberal use of omental[17] and rotational muscle flaps.[34,117,142] The results with these new techniques have generally been good, and an aggressive approach to the management of sternal wound complications is recommmended.[366]

Granulomatous and Sclerosing Mediastinitis

This invasive and compressive process results from the enlargement of mediastinal and hilar lymph nodes secondary to tuberculosis or fungal diseases such as histoplasmosis.[106] In a review of 180 cases, Schowengerdt demonstrated that ongoing enlargement or suppuration of these lymph nodes would lead to the compression, invasion, and fibrosis of mediastinal structures.[325] The superior vena cava syndrome and pulmonary vascular and bronchial obstruction have also been ascribed to this process. CT and MRI are often used to fully delineate the extent of disease,[276] but biopsy is often required to confirm the diagnosis. The course of this disease is generally mild and may be treated medically. Symptoms related to the compression of mediastinal structures usually subside with control of the underlying tubercular or fungal infection.

REFERENCES

1. 1995 Revised guidelines for prophylaxis against *Pneumocystis carinii* pneumonia for children infected with or perinatally exposed to human immunodeficiency virus. MMWR Recomm Rep 1995;44:1.
2. Diagnosis and treatment of disease caused by nontuberculous mycobacteria. Am J Respir Crit Care Med 1997;156 (Suppl):S1.
3. Antiretroviral therapy and medical management of pediatric HIV infection. Pediatrics 1998;102:1005.
4. Guidelines for surveillance of drug resistance in tuberculosis. Int J Tuberc Lung Dis 1998;2:72.
5. 1999 USPHS/IDSA guidelines for the prevention of opportunistic infections in persons infected with human immunodeficiency virus. MMWR Recomm Rep 1999;48:1.
6. Diagnostic standards and classification of tuberculosis in adults and children. Am J Respir Crit Care Med 2000; 161:1376.
7. Policy statement: Recommendations for the prevention of pneumococcal infections, including the use of pneumococcal conjugate vaccine (Prevnar), pneumococcal polysaccharide vaccine, and antibiotic prophylaxis. Pediatrics 2000;106:362.
8. Survival after introduction of HAART in people with known duration of HIV-1 infection. Lancet 2000;355:1158.
9. Updated guidelines for the use of rifabutin or rifampin for the treatment and prevention of tuberculosis among HIV-infected patients taking protease inhibitors or non-nucleoside reverse transcriptase inhibitors. Centers for Disease Control and Prevention. MMWR 2000;49:185.
10. American College of Chest Physicians Delphi consensus statement on management of spontaneous pneumothorax. Chest 2001;119:148.
11. Abadco DL, Steiner P: Gastric lavage is better than bronchoalveolar lavage for isolation of *Mycobacterium tuberculosis* in childhood pulmonary tuberculosis. Pediatr Infect Dis J 1992;11:735.
12. Abman SH, Ogle JW, Butler-Simon N, et al: Role of respiratory syncytial virus in early hospitalizations for respiratory distress of young infants with cystic fibrosis. J Pediatr 1988; 113:826.
13. Abrams EJ: Opportunistic infections and other clinical manifestations of HIV disease in children. Pediatr Clin North Am 2000;47:79.
14. Abuzaitoun OR, Hanson IC: Organ-specific manifestations of HIV disease in children. Pediatr Clin North Am 2000;47:109.
15. Acevedo D: Motor control of the thoracic duct. Am J Physiol 1943;139:600.
16. Adam KA: Persistent or recurrent pneumonia in Saudi children seen at King Khalid University Hospital, Riyadh: Clinical profile and some predisposing factors. Ann Trop Paediatr 1991;11:129.
17. Aeba R, Katogi T, Moro K, et al: Omental flap for mediastinitis after median sternotomy in asplenia syndrome and gut malrotation. Thorac Cardiovasc Surg 2000;48:243.
18. Agrawal RL, Jain SK, Gupta SC, et al: Hydropneumothorax secondary to hydatid lung disease. Indian J Chest Dis Allied Sci 1993;35:93.

19. Ahluwalia GS, Hammond GW: Comparison of cell culture and three enzyme-linked immunosorbent assays for the rapid diagnosis of respiratory syncytial virus from nasopharyngeal aspirate and tracheal secretion specimens. Diagn Microbiol Infect Dis 1988;9:187.

20. Aisner J, Schimpff SC, Bennett JE, et al: *Aspergillus* infections in cancer patients: Association with fireproofing materials in a new hospital. JAMA 1976;235:411.

21. Akhan O, Ozmen MN, Dincer A, et al: Percutaneous treatment of pulmonary hydatid cysts. Cardiovasc Intervent Radiol 1994;17:271.

22. Albright JT, Pransky SM: Nontuberculous mycobacterial infections of the head and neck. Pediatr Clin North Am 2003;50:503.

23. Allen EM, van Heeckeren DW, Spector ML, et al: Management of nutritional and infectious complications of postoperative chylothorax in children. J Pediatr Surg 1991;26:1169.

24. Alvarez JRF, Kalache KD, Grauel EL: Management of spontaneous congenital chylothorax: Oral medium-chain triglycerides versus total parenteral nutrition. Am J Perinatal 1999;16:415.

25. Andrews J, Nadjm B, Gant V, et al: Community-acquired pneumonia. Curr Opin Pulm Med 2003;9:175.

26. Armstrong DS, Grimwood K, Carlin JB, et al: Lower airway inflammation in infants and young children with cystic fibrosis. Am J Respir Crit Care Med 1997;156:1197.

27. Asher MI, Leversha AM: Lung abscess. In Chernick V, Boat TF (eds): Kendig's Disorders of the Respiratory Tract in Children, 6th ed. Philadelphia, WB Saunders, 1998.

28. Asher MI, Spier S, Beland M, et al: Primary lung abscess in childhood: The long-term outcome of conservative management. Am J Dis Child 1982;136:491.

29. Ashford NS, Buxton-Thomas MS, Flower CD, et al: Aerosol lung scintigraphy in the detection of bronchiectasis. Clin Radiol 1988;39:29.

30. Ashour M, Al Kattan K, Rafay MA, et al: Current surgical therapy for bronchiectasis. World J Surg 1999;23:1096.

31. Aujard Y, Fauroux B: Risk factors for severe respiratory syncytial virus infection in infants. Respir Med 2002; 96(Suppl B):S9.

32. Aurora P, Whitehead B, Wade A, et al: Lung transplantation and life extension in children with cystic fibrosis. Lancet 1999;354:1591.

33. Ayed AK: Resection of the right middle lobe and lingula in children for middle lobe/lingula syndrome. Chest 2004; 125:38.

34. Backer CL, Pensler JM, Tobin GR, et al: Vascularized muscle flaps for life-threatening mediastinal wounds in children. Ann Thorac Surg 1994;57:797.

35. Balci AE, Eren N, Eren S, et al: Ruptured hydatid cysts of the lung in children: Clinical review and results of surgery. Ann Thorac Surg 2002;74:889.

36. Balkanli K, Genc O, Dakak M, et al: Surgical management of bronchiectasis: Analysis and short-term results in 238 patients. Eur J Cardiothorac Surg 2003;24:699.

37. Ball P: Therapy for pneumococcal infection at the millennium: Doubts and certainties. Am J Med 1999;107(Suppl):77S.

38. Ball WS Jr, Bisset GS III, Towbin RB: Percutaneous drainage of chest abscesses in children. Radiology 1989; 171:431.

39. Barben J, Robertson D, Olinsky A, et al: Bronchial artery embolization for hemoptysis in young patients with cystic fibrosis. Radiology 2002;224:124.

40. Bass JB Jr, Farer LS, Hopewell PC, et al: Treatment of tuberculosis and tuberculosis infection in adults and children. American Thoracic Society and the Centers for Disease Control and Prevention. Am J Respir Crit Care Med 1994;149:1359.

41. Bateman ED, Hayashi S, Kuwano K, et al: Latent adenoviral infection in follicular bronchiectasis. Am J Respir Crit Care Med 1995;151:170.

42. Beghetti M, La Scala G, Belli D, et al: Etiology and management of pediatric chylothorax. J Pediatr 2000;136:653.

43. Berdon WE, Willi U: Situs inversus, bronchiectasis, and sinusitis and its relation to immotile cilia: History of the diseases and their discoverers—Manes Kartagener and Bjorn Afzelius. Pediatr Radiol 2004;34:38.

44. Bergen GA, Shelhamer JH: Pulmonary infiltrates in the cancer patient: New approaches to an old problem. Infect Dis Clin North Am 1996;10:297.

45. Blalock A, Robinson CS, Cunningham RS: Experimental studies in lymphatic blockage. Arch Surg 1937;34:1049.

46. Boat TF: Pulmonary hemorrhage and hemoptysis. In Chernick V, Boat TF (eds): Kendig's Disorders of the Respiratory Tract in Children, 6th ed. Philadelphia, WB Saunders, 1998.

47. Boles ET, Izant RJ: Spontaneous chylothorax in the neonatal period. Am J Surg 1960;99:870.

48. Bond S, et al: Management of pediatric postoperative chylothorax. Ann Thorac Surg 1993;56:469.

49. Bordley WC, Viswanathan M, King VJ, et al: Diagnosis and testing in bronchiolitis: A systematic review. Arch Pediatr Adolesc Med 2004;158:119.

50. Borowitz D, Baker RD, Stallings V: Consensus report on nutrition for pediatric patients with cystic fibrosis. J Pediatr Gastroenterol Nutr 2002;35:246.

51. Boucher RC: Human airway ion transport: II. Am J Respir Crit Care Med 1994;150:581.

52. Bouros D, Schiza S, Patsourakis G, et al: Intrapleural streptokinase versus urokinase in the treatment of complicated parapneumonic effusions: A prospective, double-blind study. Am J Respir Crit Care Med 1997;155:291.

53. Bouros D, Schiza S, Tzanakis N, et al: Intrapleural urokinase versus normal saline in the treatment of complicated parapneumonic effusions and empyema: A randomized, double-blind study. Am J Respir Crit Care Med 1999; 159:37.

54. Breuer R, Lossos IS, Berkman N, et al: Pulmonary complications of bone marrow transplantation. Respir Med 1993; 87:571.

55. Brook I, Finegold SM: Bacteriology of aspiration pneumonia in children. Pediatrics 1980;65:1115.

56. Brown RA, Lemen RJ: Bronchiectasis. In Chernick V, Boat TF (eds): Kendig's Disorders of the Respiratory Tract in Children, 6th ed. Philadelphia, WB Saunders, 1998.

57. Brown-Elliott BA, Griffith DE, Wallace RJ Jr: Diagnosis of nontuberculous mycobacterial infections. Clin Lab Med 2002;22:911.

58. Buckingham SC, King MD, Miller ML: Incidence and etiologies of complicated parapneumonic effusions in children, 1996 to 2001. Pediatr Infect Dis J 2003;22:499.

59. Burns JL, Emerson J, Stapp JR, et al: Microbiology of sputum from patients at cystic fibrosis centers in the United States. Clin Infect Dis 1998;27:158.

60. Butler JC, Shapiro ED, Carlone GM: Pneumococcal vaccines: History, current status, and future directions. Am J Med 1999;107(Suppl):69S.

61. Butler WR, Guthertz LS: Mycolic acid analysis by high-performance liquid chromatography for identification of *Mycobacterium* species. Clin Microbiol Rev 2001;14:704.

62. Buttiker V, Fanconi S, Burger R: Chylothorax in children: Guidelines for diagnosis and management. Chest 1999; 116:682.

63. Caksen H, Ozturk MK, Uzum K, et al: Pulmonary complications in patients with staphylococcal sepsis. Pediatr Int 2000;42:268.

64. Cameron R, Davies HR: Intra-pleural fibrinolytic therapy versus conservative management in the treatment of parapneumonic effusions and empyema. Cochrane Database Syst Rev 2004;CD002312.

65. Cardillo G, Facciolo F, Giunti R, et al: Videothoracoscopic treatment of primary spontaneous pneumothorax. Ann Thorac Surg 2000;69:357.

66. Chan SP, Birnbaum J, Rao M, et al: Clinical manifestation and outcome of tuberculosis in children with acquired immunodeficiency syndrome. Pediatr Infect Dis J 1996;15:443.

67. Chan W, Keyser-Gauvin E, Davis GM, et al: Empyema thoracis in children: A 26-year review of the Montreal Children's Hospital experience. J Pediatr Surg 1997;32:870.

68. Chang AB, Boyce NC, Masters IB, et al: Bronchoscopic findings in children with non-cystic fibrosis chronic suppurative lung disease. Thorax 2002;57:935.

69. Chang CT, Wang LY, Liao CY, et al: Identification of nontuberculous mycobacteria existing in tap water by PCR-restriction fragment length polymorphism. Appl Environ Microbiol 2002;68:3159.

70. Chanock SJ, Pizzo PA: Infectious complications of patients undergoing therapy for acute leukemia: Current status and future prospects. Semin Oncol 1997;24:132.

71. Chen CF, Soong WJ, Lee YS, et al: Thoracic empyema in children: Early surgical intervention hastens recovery. Acta Paediatr Taiwan 2003;44:93.

72. Chesney PJ: Nontuberculous mycobacteria. Pediatr Rev 2002;23:300.

73. Cheung Y, Leung MP, Yip M: Octreotide for treatment of postoperative chylothorax. J Pediatr 2001;139:157.

74. Choi YH, Leung AN: Radiologic findings: Pulmonary infections after bone marrow transplantation. J Thorac Imaging 1999;14:201.

75. Classen JB, Classen DC: Clustering of cases of insulin dependent diabetes (IDDM) occurring three years after *Haemophilus influenzae* B (HiB) immunization support causal relationship between immunization and IDDM. Autoimmunity 2002;35:247.

76. Cochran JB, Tecklenburg FW, Turner RB: Intrapleural instillation of fibrinolytic agents for treatment of pleural empyema. Pediatr Crit Care Med 2003;4:39.

77. Cohen G, Hjortdal V, Ricci M, et al: Primary thoracoscopic treatment of empyema in children. J Thorac Cardiovasc Surg 2003;125:79.

78. Colice GL, Curtis A, Deslauriers J, et al: Medical and surgical treatment of parapneumonic effusions: An evidence-based guideline. Chest 2000;118:1158.

79. Collin BA, Ramphal R: Pneumonia in the compromised host including cancer patients and transplant patients. Infect Dis Clin North Am 1998;12:781.

80. Cook CH, Melvin WS, Groner JI, et al: A cost-effective thoracoscopic treatment strategy for pediatric spontaneous pneumothorax. Surg Endosc 1999;13:1208.

81. Correa AG, Starke JR: Bacterial pneumonias. In Chernick V, Boat TF (eds): Kendig's Disorders of the Respiratory Tract in Children, 6th ed. Philadelphia, WB Saunders, 1998.

82. Corsaro D, Valassina M, Venditti D, et al: Multiplex PCR for rapid and differential diagnosis of *Mycoplasma pneumoniae* and *Chlamydia pneumoniae* in respiratory infections. Diagn Microbiol Infect Dis 1999;35:105.

83. Coulter DM: Successful treatment with octreotide of spontaneous chylothorax in a premature infant. J Perinatol 2004;24:194.

84. Cowles RA, Lelli JL Jr, Takayasu J, et al: Lung resection in infants and children with pulmonary infections refractory to medical therapy. J Pediatr Surg 2002;37:643.

85. Cowling MG, Belli AM: A potential pitfall in bronchial artery embolization. Clin Radiol 1995;50:105.

86. Cremaschi P, Nascimbene C, Vitulo P, et al: Therapeutic embolization of bronchial artery: A successful treatment in 209 cases of relapse hemoptysis. Angiology 1993;44:295.

87. Cunningham I: Pulmonary infections after bone marrow transplant. Semin Respir Infect 1992;7:132.

88. Davies RJ, Traill ZC, Gleeson FV: Randomised controlled trial of intrapleural streptokinase in community acquired pleural infection. Thorax 1997;52:416.

89. Davis AM, Wensley DF, Phelan PD: Spontaneous pneumothorax in pediatric patients. Respir Med 1993;87:531.

90. Davis H: A statistical study of the thoracic duct in man. Am J Anat 1915;17:211.

91. Davis PB, Hubbard VS, McCoy K, et al: Familial bronchiectasis. J Pediatr 1983;102:177.

92. de Beer HG, Mol MJ, Janseen JP: Chylothorax. Neth J Med 2000;56:25.

93. de la Rocha AG: Empyema thoracis. Surg Gynecol Obstet 1982;155:839.

94. Denning DW: Echinocandin antifungal drugs. Lancet 2003;362:1142.

95. Denning DW, Stevens DA: Antifungal and surgical treatment of invasive aspergillosis: Review of 2,121 published cases. Rev Infect Dis 1990;12:1147.

96. Desimone JA Jr, Babinchak TJ, Kaulback KR, et al: Treatment of *Mycobacterium avium* complex immune reconstitution disease in HIV-1–infected individuals. AIDS Patient Care STDS 2003;17:617.

97. Dikensoy O, Usalan C, Filiz A: Foreign body aspiration: Clinical utility of flexible bronchoscopy. Postgrad Med J 2002;78:399.

98. Donahue DM, Wright CD, Viale G, Mathisen DJ: Resection of pulmonary blebs and pleurodesis for spontaneous pneumothorax. Chest 1993;104:1767.

99. Donald PR: Childhood tuberculosis. Curr Opin Pulm Med 2000;6:187.

100. Donald PR: Preventing tuberculosis in childhood. Indian J Pediatr 2000;67:383.

101. Donnelly LF, Klosterman LA: The yield of CT of children who have complicated pneumonia and noncontributory chest radiography. AJR Am J Roentgenol 1998;170:1627.

102. Donovan SM, Mickiewicz N, Meyer RD, et al: Imported echinococcosis in southern California. Am J Trop Med Hyg 1995;53:668.

103. Dore ND, LeSouef PN, Masters B, et al: Atypical mycobacterial pulmonary disease and bronchial obstruction in HIV-negative children. Pediatr Pulmonol 1998;26:380.

104. Doski JJ, Lou D, Hicks BA, et al: Management of parapneumonic collections in infants and children. J Pediatr Surg 2000;35:265.

105. Dumont P, Diemont F, Massard G, et al: Does a thoracoscopic approach for surgical treatment of spontaneous pneumothorax represent progress? Eur J Cardiothorac Surg 1997;11:27.

106. Dunn EJ, Ulicny KS Jr, Wright CB, et al: Surgical implications of sclerosing mediastinitis: A report of six cases and review of the literature. Chest 1990;97:338.

107. Easa D, Balaraman V, Ash K, et al: Congenital chylothorax and mediastinal neuroblastoma. J Pediatr Surg 1991;26:96.

108. Eastham KM, Fall AJ, Mitchell L, et al: The need to redefine non-cystic fibrosis bronchiectasis in childhood. Thorax 2004;59:324.

109. Eastham KM, Freeman R, Kearns AM, et al: Clinical features, aetiology and outcome of empyema in children in the north east of England. Thorax 2004;59:522.

110. Ebert DL, Olivier KN: Nontuberculous mycobacteria in the setting of cystic fibrosis. Clin Chest Med 2002;23:655.

111. Efeldt RJ, Shroder DW, Thies J: Long-term follow up of different therapy procedures in spontaneous pneumothorax. J Cardiovasc Surg 1994;35:229.

112. Egan TM, Detterbeck FC, Mill MR, et al: Long term results of lung transplantation for cystic fibrosis. Eur J Cardiothorac Surg 2002;22:602.

113. Eggimann P, Garbino J, Pittet D: Management of *Candida* species infections in critically ill patients. Lancet Infect Dis 2003;3:772.

114. Emanuel B, Shulman ST: Lung abscess in infants and children. Clin Pediatr (Phila) 1995;34:2.

115. Enarson DA: Use of the tuberculin skin test in children. Paediatr Respir Rev 2004;5(Suppl A):S135.

116. English M: Impact of bacterial pneumonias on world child health. Paediatr Resp Rev 2000;1:21.

117. Erez E, Katz M, Sharoni E, et al: Pectoralis major muscle flap for deep sternal wound infection in neonates. Ann Thorac Surg 2000;69:572.

118. Farmer DL, Albanese CT: Fetal hydrothorax. In Harrison MR, Evans MI, Adzick NS, Holzgreve W (eds): The Unborn Patient, 3rd ed. Philadelphia, WB Saunders, 2001.

119. Farrell PM, Mischler EH: Newborn screening for cystic fibrosis. The Cystic Fibrosis Neonatal Screening Study Group. Adv Pediatr 1992;39:35.

120. Felten MK, Rath T, Magdorf K, et al: Childhood tuberculosis in Germany between 1985 and 1994: Comparison of three selected patient groups. Int J Tuberc Lung Dis 1998;2:797.

121. Fernald GW: Infections of the Respiratory Tract due to *Mycoplasma pneumoniae*. In Chernick V, Boat TF (eds): Kendig's Disorders of the Respiratory Tract in Children, 6th ed. Philadelphia, WB Saunders, 1998.

122. Finck C, Wagner C, Jackson R, et al: Empyema: Development of a critical pathway. Semin Pediatr Surg 2002;11:25.

123. Fishman JA, Rubin RH: Infection in organ-transplant recipients. N Engl J Med 1998;338:1741.

124. FitzSimmons SC: The changing epidemiology of cystic fibrosis. J Pediatr 1993;122:1.

125. Fowler GR: A case of thoracoplasty for removal of a large cicatricial fibrous growth from the interior chest, the result of an old empyema. Med Rec 1893;44:838.

126. Frank AL, Marcinak JF, Mangat PD, et al: Clindamycin treatment of methicillin-resistant *Staphylococcus aureus* infections in children. Pediatr Infect Dis J 2002;21:530.

127. Frazer A: Differentiation in the absorption of olive oil and oleic acid in the rat. J Physiol 1943;102:306.

128. Freij BJ, Kusmiesz H, Nelson JD, et al: Parapneumonic effusions and empyema in hospitalized children: A retrospective review of 227 cases. Pediatr Infect Dis J 1984;3:578.

129. Freixinet J: Surgical indications for treatment of pulmonary tuberculosis. World J Surg 1997;21:475.

130. Freixinet J, Varela A, Lopez RL, et al: Surgical treatment of childhood mediastinal tuberculous lymphadenitis. Ann Thorac Surg 1995;59:644.

131. Fujimoto T, Hillejan L, Stamatis G: Current strategy for surgical management of bronchiectasis. Ann Thorac Surg 2001;72:1711.

132. Gates RL, Caniano DA, Hayes JR, et al: Does VATS provide optimal treatment of empyema in children? A systematic review. J Pediatr Surg 2004;39:381.

133. Gaydos CA, Roblin PM, Hammerschlag MR, et al: Diagnostic utility of PCR-enzyme immunoassay, culture, and serology for detection of *Chlamydia pneumoniae* in symptomatic and asymptomatic patients. J Clin Microbiol 1994;32:903.

134. Gaylor AS, Reilly JC: Therapy with macrolides in patients with cystic fibrosis. Pharmacotherapy 2002;22:227.

135. Gendrel D: Antibiotic treatment of *Mycoplasma pneumoniae* infections. Pediatr Pulmonol Suppl 1997;16:46.

136. Gessner BD: Incidence rates, clinical features and case identification of pediatric tuberculosis in Alaska. Int J Tuberc Lung Dis 1998;2:378.

137. Gilbert K, Fine MJ: Assessing prognosis and predicting patient outcomes in community-acquired pneumonia. Semin Respir Infect 1994;9:140.

138. Gilljam M, Berning SE, Peloquin CA, et al: Therapeutic drug monitoring in patients with cystic fibrosis and mycobacterial disease. Eur Respir J 1999;14:347.

139. Glenn W: The lymphatic system, some surgical considerations. Arch Surg 1981;116:989.

140. Graham DD, McGahren ED, Tribble CG, et al: Use of video-assisted thoracic surgery in the treatment of chylothorax. Ann Thorac Surg 1994;57:1507.

141. Graham SM: HIV and respiratory infections in children. Curr Opin Pulm Med 2003;9:215.

142. Grant RT, Breitbart AS, Parnell V: Muscle flap reconstruction of pediatric poststernotomy wound infections. Ann Plast Surg 1997;38:365.

143. Greenwood B: The epidemiology of pneumococcal infection in children in the developing world. Philos Trans R Soc Lond B Biol Sci 1999;354:777.

144. Grewal H, Jackson RJ, Wagner CW, et al: Early video-assisted thoracic surgery in the management of empyema. Pediatrics 1999;103:e63.

145. Griffith DE: Emergence of nontuberculous mycobacteria as pathogens in cystic fibrosis. Am J Respir Crit Care Med 2003;167:810.

146. Grzybowski S: Tuberculosis. Chest 1983;84:756.

147. Guggino WB: Cystic fibrosis and the salt controversy. Cell 1999;96:607.

148. Guleserian KJ, Gilchrist BF, Luks FI, et al: Child abuse as a cause of traumatic chylothorax. J Pediatr Surg 1996;31:1696.

149. Gupta D, Hansell A, Nichols T, et al: Epidemiology of pneumothorax in England. Thorax 2000;55:666.

150. Haciibrahimoglu G, Fazlioglu M, Olcmen A, et al: Surgical management of childhood bronchiectasis due to infectious disease. J Thorac Cardiovasc Surg 2004;127:1361.

151. Hall CB, Douglas RG Jr, Geiman JM: Quantitative shedding patterns of respiratory syncytial virus in infants. J Infect Dis 1975;132:151.

152. Hall CB, Douglas RG Jr, Geiman JM: Respiratory syncytial virus infections in infants: Quantitation and duration of shedding. J Pediatr 1976;89:11.

153. Hammerschlag MR: Pneumonia due to *Chlamydia pneumoniae* in children: Epidemiology, diagnosis, and treatment. Pediatr Pulmonol 2003;36:384.

154. Han D, Lee KS, Koh WJ, et al: Radiographic and CT findings of nontuberculous mycobacterial pulmonary infection caused by *Mycobacterium abscessus*. AJR Am J Roentgenol 2003;181:513.

155. Hansell DM: Bronchiectasis. Radiol Clin North Am 1998;36:107.

156. Hardegger D, Nadal D, Bossart W, et al: Rapid detection of *Mycoplasma pneumoniae* in clinical samples by real-time PCR. J Microbiol Methods 2000;41:45.

157. Harris JA, Kolokathis A, Campbell M, et al: Safety and efficacy of azithromycin in the treatment of community-acquired pneumonia in children. Pediatr Infect Dis J 1998;17:865.

158. Heath PT: Epidemiology and bacteriology of bacterial pneumonias. Paediatr Resp Rev 2000;1:4.

159. Heffelfinger JD, Davis TE, Gebrian B, et al: Evaluation of children with recurrent pneumonia diagnosed by World Health Organization criteria. Pediatr Infect Dis J 2002;21:108.

160. Heiskanen-Kosma T, Korppi M, Jokinen C, et al: Etiology of childhood pneumonia: Serologic results of a prospective, population-based study. Pediatr Infect Dis J 1998;17:986.

161. Heurlin N, Bergstrom SE, Winiarski J, et al: Fungal pneumonia: The predominant lung infection causing death in children undergoing bone marrow transplantation. Acta Paediatr 1996;85:168.

162. Hewitson JP, Von Oppell UO: Role of thoracic surgery for childhood tuberculosis. World J Surg 1997;21:468.

163. Hierholzer JC, Bingham PG, Coombs RA, et al: Comparison of monoclonal antibody time-resolved fluoroimmunoassay with monoclonal antibody capture-biotinylated detector enzyme immunoassay for respiratory syncytial virus and parainfluenza virus antigen detection. J Clin Microbiol 1989;27:1243.

164. Hilton AM, Doyle L: Immunological abnormalities in bronchiectasis with chronic bronchial suppuration. Br J Dis Chest 1978;72:207.

165. Hochberg LA: Thoracic Surgery Before the 20th Century. New York, Vantage Press, 1960.

166. Hoff SJ, Neblett WW, Edwards KM, et al: Parapneumonic empyema in children: Decortication hastens recovery in patients with severe pleural infections. Pediatr Infect Dis J 1991;10:194.

167. Holman RC, Shay DK, Curns AT, et al: Risk factors for bronchiolitis-associated deaths among infants in the United States. Pediatr Infect Dis J 2003;22:483.

168. Holt P: Studies of medium chain triglycerides in patients with differing mechanisms for fat malabsorption. In Senior JR (ed): Medium Chain Triglycerides. Philadelphia, University of Pennsylvania Press, 1968.

169. Horio H, Nomori H, Fuyuno G, et al: Limited axillary thoracotomy vs video-assisted thoracoscopic surgery for spontaneous pneumothorax. Surg Endosc 1998;12:1155.

170. Horsburgh CR Jr, Caldwell MB, Simonds RJ: Epidemiology of disseminated nontuberculous mycobacterial disease in children with acquired immunodeficiency syndrome. Pediatr Infect Dis J 1993;12:219.

171. Huebner RE, Castro KG: The changing face of tuberculosis. Annu Rev Med 1995;46:47.

172. Hughes WT, Rivera GK, Schell MJ, et al: Successful intermittent chemoprophylaxis for *Pneumocystis carinii* pneumonitis. N Engl J Med 1987;316:1627.

173. Inselman LS, Kendig EL: Tuberculosis. In Chernick V, Boat TF (eds): Kendig's Disorders of the Respiratory Tract in Children, 6th ed. Philadelphia, WB Saunders, 1998.

174. Iseman MD, Madsen LA: Chronic tuberculous empyema with bronchopleural fistula resulting in treatment failure and progressive drug resistance. Chest 1991;100:124.

175. Jaffe A, Cohen G: Thoracic empyema. Arch Dis Child 2003;88:839.

176. Jafri HS: Treatment of respiratory syncytial virus: Antiviral therapies. Pediatr Infect Dis J 2003;22(Suppl):S89.

177. Jean-Baptiste E: Clinical assessment and management of massive hemoptysis. Crit Care Med 2000;28:1642.

178. Jeong YJ, Lee KS, Koh WJ, et al: Nontuberculous mycobacterial pulmonary infection in immunocompetent patients: Comparison of thin-section CT and histopathologic findings. Radiology 2004;231:880.

179. Jimenez-Mercàn R, Garcia-Diaz F, Arenas-Linàres C, et al: Comparative retrospective study of surgical treatment of spontaneous pneumothorax. Surg Endosc 1997;11:919.

180. Jones D, Havlir DV: Nontuberculous mycobacteria in the HIV infected patient. Clin Chest Med 2002;23:665.

181. Jones GR, Konsler GK, Dunaway RP, et al: Infection risk factors in febrile, neutropenic children and adolescents. Pediatr Hematol Oncol 1996;13:217.

182. Joosten KF, Hazelzet JA, Tiddens HA, et al: Staphylococcal pneumonia in childhood: Will early surgical intervention lower mortality? Pediatr Pulmonol 1995;20:83.

183. Kabra SK, Lodha R, Seth V: Tuberculosis in children—what has changed in last 20 years? Indian J Pediatr 2002;69(Suppl 1):S5.

184. Kaplan JE, Hanson D, Dworkin MS, et al: Epidemiology of human immunodeficiency virus-associated opportunistic infections in the United States in the era of highly active antiretroviral therapy. Clin Infect Dis 2000; 30(Suppl 1):S5.

185. Kaplan SL: Review of antibiotic resistance, antibiotic treatment and prevention of pneumococcal pneumonia. Paediatr Respir Rev 2004;5(Suppl A):S153.

186. Karaoglanoglu N, Kurkcuoglu IC, Gorguner M, et al: Giant hydatid lung cysts. Eur J Cardiothorac Surg 2001;19:914.

187. Kaschula RO, Druker J, Kipps A: Late morphologic consequences of measles: A lethal and debilitating lung disease among the poor. Rev Infect Dis 1983;5:395.

188. Keating G, Figgitt D: Caspofungin: A review of its use in oesophageal candidiasis, invasive candidiasis and invasive aspergillosis. Drugs 2003;63:2235.

189. Kennedy MJ: Current status of gene therapy for cystic fibrosis pulmonary disease. Am J Respir Med 2002;1:349.

190. Kent JH: The epidemiology of multidrug-resistant tuberculosis in the United States. Med Clin North Am 1993;77:1391.

191. Kenyon TA, Driver C, Haas E, et al: Immigration and tuberculosis among children on the United States–Mexico border, county of San Diego, California. Pediatrics 1998;104:103.

192. Keramidas D, Mavridis G, Soutis M, et al: Medical treatment of pulmonary hydatidosis: Complications and surgical management. Pediatr Surg Int 2004;19:774.

193. Kerem B, Rommens JM, Buchanan JA, et al: Identification of the cystic fibrosis gene: Genetic analysis. Science 1989;245:1073.

194. Kettner BI, Aurisch R, Ruckert JC, et al: Scintigraphic localization of lymphatic leakage site after oral administration of iodine-123 IPPA. J Nucl Med 1998;39:2141.

195. Kiernan PD, Hernandez A, Byrne WD, et al: Descending cervical mediastinitis. Ann Thorac Surg 1998;65:1483.

196. Kilani T, El Hammami S: Pulmonary hydatid and other lung parasitic infections. Curr Opin Pulm Med 2002;8:218.

197. Kim J, Kim K, Shim YM, et al: Video-assisted thoracic surgery as a primary therapy for primary spontaneous pneumothorax. Surg Endosc 1998;12:1290.

198. Kimpen JL: Management of respiratory syncytial virus infection. Curr Opin Infect Dis 2001;14:323.

199. King JC Jr, Burke AR, Clemens JD, et al: Respiratory syncytial virus illnesses in human immunodeficiency virus- and noninfected children. Pediatr Infect Dis J 1993;12:733.

200. Kirk O, Reiss P, Uberti-Foppa C, et al: Safe interruption of maintenance therapy against previous infection with four common HIV-associated opportunistic pathogens during potent antiretroviral therapy. Ann Intern Med 2002;137:239.

201. Klein JS, Schultz S, Heffner JE: Interventional radiology of the chest: Image-guided percutaneous drainage of pleural effusions, lung abscess, and pneumothorax. AJR Am J Roentgenol 1995;164:581.

202. Kneyber MC, Kimpen JL: Current concepts on active immunization against respiratory syncytial virus for infants and young children. Pediatr Infect Dis J 2002;21:685.

203. Knight GJ, Carman PG: Primary staphylococcal pneumonia in childhood: A review of 69 cases. J Paediatr Child Health 1992;28:447.

204. Knudtson J, Grewal H: Pediatric empyema—an algorithm for early thoracoscopic intervention. JSLS 2004;8:31.

205. Koletzko S, Reinhardt D: Nutritional challenges of infants with cystic fibrosis. Early Hum Dev 2001;65(Suppl):S53.

206. Kornecki A, Shemie SD: Open lung biopsy in children with respiratory failure. Crit Care Med 2001;29:1247.

207. Kornecki A, Sivan Y: Treatment of loculated pleural effusion with intrapleural urokinase in children. J Pediatr Surg 1997;32:1473.

208. Korppi M, Heiskanen-Kosma T, Kleemola M: *Mycoplasma pneumoniae* causes over 50% of community-acquired pneumonia in school-aged children. Scand J Infect Dis 2003;35:294.

209. Kosloske AM, Ball WS Jr, Butler C, et al: Drainage of pediatric lung abscess by cough, catheter, or complete resection. J Pediatr Surg 1986;21:596.

210. Kosloske A, Martin L, Schubert W: Management of chylothorax in children by thoracentesis and medium-chain triglyceride feedings. J Pediatr Surg 1974;9:365.

211. Krishnan S, Amin N, Dozor AJ, et al: Urokinase in the management of complicated parapneumonic effusions in children. Chest 1997;112:1579.

212. Kurklu EU, Williams MA, Le Roux BT: Bronchiectasis consequent upon foreign body retention. Thorax 1973;28:601.

213. Kutlay H, Cangir AK, Enon S, et al: Surgical treatment in bronchiectasis: Analysis of 166 patients. Eur J Cardiothorac Surg 2002;21:634.

214. Laberge J-M, Bratu I, Flageole H: The management of asymptomatic congenital lung malformations. Paediatr Resp Rev 2004;5(Suppl):S305.

215. Lampson RS: Traumatic chylothorax—a review of the literature and report of a case treated by mediastinal ligation of the thoracic duct. J Thorac Surg 1948;17:778.

216. Lamy AL, Cameron BH, LeBlanc JG, et al: Giant hydatid lung cysts in the Canadian northwest: Outcome of conservative treatment in three children. J Pediatr Surg 1993;28:1140.

217. Lang-Lazdunski L, Kerangal X, Pons F, et al: Primary spontaneous pneumothorax: One-stage treatment by bilateral video-thoracoscopy. Ann Thorac Surg 2000;70:412.

218. Lange CG, Woolley IJ, Brodt RH: Disseminated mycobacterium avium-intracellulare complex (MAC) infection in the era of effective antiretroviral therapy: Is prophylaxis still indicated? Drugs 2004;64:679.

219. Langtry HD, Balfour JA: Azithromycin: A review of its use in paediatric infectious diseases. Drugs 1998;56:273.

220. Langtry HD, Brogden RN: Clarithromycin: A review of its efficacy in the treatment of respiratory tract infections in immunocompetent patients. Drugs 1997;53:973.

221. Le Coultre C: Chylothorax. In Ziegler MM, Azizkhan RG, Weber TR (eds): Operative Pediatric Surgery. New York, McGraw-Hill, 2003.

222. Le Coultre C, Oberhänsli I, Mossaz A, et al: Postoperative chylothorax in children: Differences between vascular and traumatic origin. J Pediatr Surg 1991;26:519.

223. Lederman MM, Valdez H: Immune restoration with antiretroviral therapies: Implications for clinical management. JAMA 2000;284:223.

224. Leelahanon S, Petlek W, Sontimuang W, et al: Can octreotide be the first line treatment for chylothorax? J Med Assoc Thai 2003;86(Suppl 3):S741.

225. Lehrnbecher T, Foster C, Vazquez N, et al: Therapy-induced alterations in host defense in children receiving therapy for cancer. J Pediatr Hematol Oncol 1997;19:399.

226. Lehrnbecher T, Groll AH, Chanock SJ: Treatment of fungal infections in neutropenic children. Curr Opin Pediatr 1999;11:47.

227. Light PW, O'Hara VS, Moritz TE, et al: Intrapleural tetracycline or the prevention of recurrent spontaneous pneumothorax. JAMA 1990;264:2224.

228. Linden PK: Amphotericin B lipid complex for the treatment of invasive fungal infections. Expert Opin Pharmacother 2003;4:2099.

229. Liu HP, Hsieh MJ, Lu HI, et al: Thoracoscopic-assisted management of postpneumonic empyema in children refractory to medical response. Surg Endosc 2002;16:1612.

230. Lobato MN, Loeffler AM, Furst K, et al: Detection of *Mycobacterium tuberculosis* in gastric aspirates collected from children: Hospitalization is not necessary. Pediatrics 1998;102:E40.

231. Lodha R, Kabra SK: Newer diagnostic modalities for tuberculosis. Indian J Pediatr 2004;71:221.

232. Lodha R, Puranik M, Natchu UC, et al: Recurrent pneumonia in children: Clinical profile and underlying causes. Acta Paediatr 2002;91:1170.

233. Longaker MT, Laberge J-M, Danserau J, et al: Primary fetal hydrothorax: Natural history and management. J Pediatr Surg 1989;24:573.

234. Loop FD, Lytle BW, Cosgrove DM, et al: J. Maxwell Chamberlain memorial paper. Sternal wound complications after isolated coronary artery bypass grafting: Early and late mortality, morbidity, and cost of care. Ann Thorac Surg 1990;49:179.

235. Lossos IS, Breuer R, Or R, et al: Bacterial pneumonia in recipients of bone marrow transplantation: A five-year prospective study. Transplantation 1995;60:672.

236. Lowther SA, Shay DK, Holman RC, et al: Bronchiolitis-associated hospitalizations among American Indian and Alaska Native children. Pediatr Infect Dis J 2000;19:11.

237. Lowy FD, Waldhausen JA, Miller M, et al: Report of the National Heart, Lung and Blood Institute-National Institute of Allergy and Infectious Diseases working group on antimicrobial strategies and cardiothoracic surgery. Am Heart J 2004;147:575.

238. Luck SR, Raffensperger JG, Sullivan HJ, et al: Management of pneumothorax in children with chronic pulmonary diseases. J Thorac Cardiovasc Surg 1997;74:834.

239. Maiz-Carro L, Navas-Elorza E: Nontuberculous mycobacterial pulmonary infection in patients with cystic fibrosis: Diagnosis and treatment. Am J Respir Med 2002;1:107.

240. Marcinak JF, Frank AL: Treatment of community-acquired methicillin-resistant *Staphylococcus aureus* in children. Curr Opin Infect Dis 2003;16:265.

241. Margenthaler JA, Weber TR, Keller MS: Predictors of surgical outcome for complicated pneumonia in children: Impact of bacterial virulence. World J Surg 2004;28:87.

242. Mark PH, Turner JA: Lung abscess in childhood. Thorax 1968;23:216.

243. Marras TK, Daley CL: Epidemiology of human pulmonary infection with nontuberculous mycobacteria. Clin Chest Med 2002;23:553.

244. Martinez FD: Respiratory syncytial virus bronchiolitis and the pathogenesis of childhood asthma. Pediatr Infect Dis J 2003;22(Suppl):S76.

245. Mathur R, Cullen J, Kinnear WJ, et al: Time course of resolution of persistent air leak in spontaneous pneumothorax. Respir Med 1995;89:129.

246. McCarthy CA, Hall CB: Respiratory syncytial virus: Concerns and control. Pediatr Rev 2003;24:301.

247. McCracken GH Jr: Etiology and treatment of pneumonia. Pediatr Infect Dis J 2000;19:373.

248. Meier AH, Smith B, Raghavan A, et al: Rational treatment of empyema in children. Arch Surg 2000;135:907.

249. Mendeloff EN: Lung transplantation for cystic fibrosis. Semin Thorac Cardiovasc Surg 1998;10:202.

250. Menzies D: Interpretation of repeated tuberculin tests: Boosting, conversion and reversion. Am J Respir Crit Care Med 1999;159:15.

251. Merrigan BA, Winter DC, O'Sullivan GC: Chylothorax. Br J Surg 1997;84:15.

252. Meyers JD, McGuffin RW, Bryson YJ, et al: Treatment of cytomegalovirus pneumonia after marrow transplant with combined vidarabine and human leukocyte interferon. J Infect Dis 1982;146:80.

253. Michelow IC, Olsen K, Lozano J, et al: Epidemiology and clinical characteristics of community-acquired pneumonia in hospitalized children. Pediatrics 2004;113:701.

254. Miller JI Jr: Diagnosis and management of chylothorax. Chest Surg Clin North Am 1996;6:139.

255. Mitlehner W, Friedrich M, Dissmann W: Value of computed tomography in the detection of bullae and blebs in patients with primary spontaneous pneumothorax. Respiration 1992;59:221.

256. Mofenson LM, Yogev R, Korelitz J, et al: Characteristics of acute pneumonia in human immunodeficiency virus-infected children and association with long term mortality risk. National Institute of Child Health and Human Development Intravenous Immunoglobulin Clinical Trial Study Group. Pediatr Infect Dis J 1998;17:872.

257. Mohamadiyeh MK, Ashour M, el Desouki M, et al: Contribution of ventilation and perfusion lung imaging to the management of patients with bronchiectasis. Clin Nucl Med 1994;19:292.

258. Moore RD, Urschel JD, Fraser RE, et al: Cystic hydatid lung disease in northwest Canada. Can J Surg 1994;37:20.

259. Morgan WJ, Butler SM, Johnson CA, et al: Epidemiologic study of cystic fibrosis: Design and implementation of a prospective, multicenter, observational study of patients with cystic fibrosis in the U.S. and Canada. Pediatr Pulmonol 1999;28:231.

260. Moroney JF, Fiore AE, Harrison LH, et al: Clinical outcomes of bacteremic pneumococcal pneumonia in the era of antibiotic resistance. Clin Infect Dis 2001;33:797.

261. Morphis GL, Arcinne EL, Krause JR: Generalized lymphangioma in infancy with chylothorax. Pediatrics 1970;46:566.

262. Morrissey BM, Evans SJ: Severe bronchiectasis. Clin Rev Allergy Immunol 2003;25:233.

263. Moureux J, Elkaim D, Padovani B, et al: Video-assisted thoracoscopic treatment of spontaneous pneumothorax: Technique and results of one hundred cases. J Thorac Cardiovasc Surg 1996;112:385.

264. Murphy MC, Newman BM, Rodgers BM: Pleuroperitoneal shunts in the management of persistent chylothorax. Ann Thorac Surg 1989;48:195.

265. Murphy TF, Henderson FW, Clyde WA Jr, et al: Pneumonia: An eleven-year study in a pediatric practice. Am J Epidemiol 1981;113:12.

266. Mustafa MM, Pappo A, Cash J, et al: Aerosolized pentamidine for the prevention of *Pneumocystis* pneumonia in children with cancer intolerant or allergic to trimethoprim/sulfamethoxazole. J Clin Oncol 1994;12:258.

267. Nelson CT: *Mycoplasma* and *Chlamydia* pneumonia in pediatrics. Semin Respir Infect 2002;17:10.

268. Neuhoff H, Touroff ASW: Acute putrid abscess of the lung: Principles of operative treatment. Surg Gynecol Obstet 1936;63:353.

269. Neville K, Renbarger J, Dreyer Z: Pneumonia in the immunocompromised pediatric cancer patient. Semin Respir Infect 2002;17:21.

270. Nguyen D, Tchervenkov CI: Successful management of postoperative chylothorax with fibrin glue in a premature neonate. Can J Surg 1994;37:158.

271. Nguyen DM, Shum-Tim D, Dobell AR, et al: The management of chylothorax/chylopericardium following pediatric cardiac surgery: A 10-year experience. J Card Surg 1995; 10:302.

272. Nolan CM, Goldberg SV: Treatment of isoniazid-resistant tuberculosis with isoniazid, rifampin, ethambutol, and pyrazinamide for 6 months. Int J Tuberc Lung Dis 2002;6:952.

273. Nolt D, Michaels MG, Wald ER: Intrathoracic disease from nontuberculous mycobacteria in children: Two cases and a review of the literature. Pediatrics 2003;112:e434.

274. Nonoyama A, Tanaka K, Osako T, et al: Surgical treatment of pulmonary abscess in children under ten years of age. Chest 1984;85:358.

275. Noppen M, Alexander P, Driesen P, et al: Quantification of primary spontaneous pneumothorax: Accuracy of the Light index. Respiration 2001;68:396.

276. Odev K, Ozer F, Ceran S, et al: CT diagnosis of granulomatous mediastinitis due to tuberculosis. Eur J Radiol 1996;23:241.

277. Olivier C: Clinical use of cefuroxime in paediatric community-acquired pneumonia. Paediatr Drugs 2000; 2:331.

278. Olivier KN, Weber DJ, Wallace RJ Jr, et al: Nontuberculous mycobacteria: I: Multicenter prevalence study in cystic fibrosis. Am J Respir Crit Care Med 2003;167:828.

279. Owayed AF, Campbell DM, Wang EE: Underlying causes of recurrent pneumonia in children. Arch Pediatr Adolesc Med 2000;154:190.

280. Ozcelik C, Inci I, Nizam O, et al: Intrapleural fibrinolytic treatment of multiloculated postpneumonic pediatric empyemas. Ann Thorac Surg 2003;76:1849.

281. Panitch HB: Respiratory syncytial virus bronchiolitis: Supportive care and therapies designed to overcome airway obstruction. Pediatr Infect Dis J 2003;22(Suppl):S83.

282. Pappas PG, Rex JH: Therapeutic approach to *Candida* sepsis. Curr Infect Dis Rep 1999;1:245.

283. Pappas PG, Rex JH, Sobel JD, et al: Guidelines for treatment of candidiasis. Clin Infect Dis 2004;38:161.

284. Peloquin CA: Therapeutic drug monitoring in the treatment of tuberculosis. Drugs 2002;62:2169.

285. Pena GN, Munoz LF, Vargas RJ, et al: Yield of percutaneous needle lung aspiration in lung abscess. Chest 1990;97:69.

286. Perez MS, Van Dyke RB: Pulmonary infections in children with HIV infection. Semin Respir Infect 2002;17:33.

287. Peters TR, Edwards KM: The pneumococcal protein conjugate vaccines. J Pediatr 2000;137:416.

288. Piedra PA: Clinical experience with respiratory syncytial virus vaccines. Pediatr Infect Dis J 2003;22(Suppl):S94.

289. Pizzo PA: Infectious complications in the child with cancer: II. Management of specific infectious organisms. J Pediatr 1981;98:513.

290. Pizzo PA, Rubin M, Freifeld A, et al: The child with cancer and infection: II. Nonbacterial infections. J Pediatr 1991;119:845.

291. Pizzo PA, Walsh TJ: Fungal infections in the pediatric cancer patient. Semin Oncol 1990;17:6.

292. Playfor SD, Smyth AR, Stewart RJ: Increase in incidence of childhood empyema. Thorax 1997;52:932.

293. Poenaru D, Yazbeck S, Murphy S: Primary spontaneous pneumothorax in children. J Pediatr Surg 1994;29:1183.

294. Pomerantz M, Brown J: The surgical management of tuberculosis. Semin Thorac Cardiovasc Surg 1995;7:108.

295. Pozniak A: Mycobacterial diseases and HIV. J HIV Ther 2002;7:13.
296. Principi N, Esposito S: Emerging role of *Mycoplasma pneumoniae* and *Chlamydia pneumoniae* in paediatric respiratory-tract infections. Lancet Infect Dis 2001;1:334.
297. Principi N, Esposito S: *Mycoplasma pneumoniae* and *Chlamydia pneumoniae* cause lower respiratory tract disease in paediatric patients. Curr Opin Infect Dis 2002;15:295.
298. Rajan S, Saiman L: Pulmonary infections in patients with cystic fibrosis. Semin Respir Infect 2002;17:47.
299. Ramsey BW: Management of pulmonary disease in patients with cystic fibrosis. N Engl J Med 1996;335:179.
300. Ramsey BW, Dorkin HL: Consensus conference: Practical applications of Pulmozyme. September 22, 1993. Pediatr Pulmonol 1994;17:404.
301. Ramsey BW, Pepe MS, Quan JM, et al: Intermittent administration of inhaled tobramycin in patients with cystic fibrosis. Cystic Fibrosis Inhaled Tobramycin Study Group. N Engl J Med 1999;340:23.
302. Rattan A: Diagnosis of tuberculosis by polymerase chain reaction. Indian J Pediatr 1990;57:673.
303. Redding G, Singleton R, Lewis T, et al: Early radiographic and clinical features associated with bronchiectasis in children. Pediatr Pulmonol 2004;37:297.
304. Reid J, Marciniuk D, Peloquin CA, et al: Pharmacokinetics of antituberculosis medications delivered via percutaneous gastrojejunostomy tube. Chest 2002;121:281.
305. Rex JH, Walsh TJ, Sobel JD, et al: Practice guidelines for the treatment of candidiasis. Infectious Diseases Society of America. Clin Infect Dis 2000;30:662.
306. Reynolds M: Disorders of the thoracic cavity and pleura and infections of the lung, pleura and mediastinum. In O'Neill JAJ, Rowe MI, Grosfeld JL, et al (eds): Pediatric Surgery, 5th ed. St. Louis, Mosby–Year Book, 1998.
307. Rheuban KS, Kron IL, Carpenter MA, et al: Pleuroperitoneal shunts for refractory chylothorax after operation for congenital heart disease. Ann Thorac Surg 1992;53:85.
308. Ridderstolpe L, Gill H, Granfeldt H, et al: Superficial and deep sternal wound complications: Incidence, risk factors and mortality. Eur J Cardiothorac Surg 2001;20:1168.
309. Rosenzweig DY, Stead WW: The role of tuberculosis and other forms of bronchopulmonary necrosis in the pathogenesis of bronchiectasis. Am Rev Respir Dis 1966;93:769.
310. Ross JK: A review of the surgery of the thoracic duct. Thorax 1961;16:12.
311. Rothenberg SS: Experience with thoracoscopic lobectomy in infants and children. J Pediatr Surg 2003;38:102.
312. Rutstein RM, Cobb P, McGowan KL, et al: *Mycobacterium avium-intracellulare* complex infection in HIV-infected children. AIDS 1993;7:507.
313. Saggese D, Compadretti GC, Burnelli R: Nontuberculous mycobacterial adenitis in children: Diagnostic and therapeutic management. Am J Otolaryngol 2003;24:79.
314. Sahn SA: Management of complicated parapneumonic effusions. Am Rev Respir Dis 1993;148:813.
315. Sahn SA, Heffner JE: Spontaneous pneumothorax. N Engl J Med 2000;342:868.
316. Saiman L: The mycobacteriology of non-tuberculous mycobacteria. Paediatr Respir Rev 2004;5(Suppl A):S221.
317. Salih OK, Topcuoglu MS, Celik SK, et al: Surgical treatment of hydatid cysts of the lung: Analysis of 405 patients. Can J Surg 1998;41:131.
318. Santolaya ME, Alvarez AM, Aviles CL, et al: Prospective evaluation of a model of prediction of invasive bacterial infection risk among children with cancer, fever, and neutropenia. Clin Infect Dis 2002;35:678.
319. Sarihan H, Cay A, Aynaci M, et al: Empyema in children. J Cardiovasc Surg (Torino) 1998;39:113.
320. Schaaf HS, Shean K, Donald PR: Culture confirmed multidrug resistant tuberculosis: Diagnostic delay, clinical features, and outcome. Arch Dis Child 2003;88:1106.
321. Schidlow DV, Taussig LM, Knowles MR: Cystic Fibrosis Foundation consensus conference report on pulmonary complications of cystic fibrosis. Pediatr Pulmonol 1993;15:187.
322. Schlesinger C, Koss MN: Bronchiolitis: Update 2001. Curr Opin Pulm Med 2002;8:112.
323. Schneider MM, Borleffs JC, Stolk RP, et al: Discontinuation of prophylaxis for *Pneumocystis carinii* pneumonia in HIV-1-infected patients treated with highly active antiretroviral therapy. Lancet 1999;353:201.
324. Schoni MH, Casaulta-Aebischer C: Nutrition and lung function in cystic fibrosis patients: Review. Clin Nutr 2000;19:79.
325. Schowengerdt CG, Suyemoto R, Main FB: Granulomatous and fibrous mediastinitis: A review and analysis of 180 cases. J Thorac Cardiovasc Surg 1969;57:365.
326. Schultz MJ: Macrolide activities beyond their antimicrobial effects: Macrolides in diffuse panbronchiolitis and cystic fibrosis. J Antimicrob Chemother 2004;54:21.
327. Schumacker HP, Moore TC: Surgical management of traumatic chylothorax. Surg Gynecol Obstet 1951;93:46.
328. Schwoebel V, Lambregts-van Weezenbeek CS, Moro ML, et al: Standardization of antituberculosis drug resistance surveillance in Europe. Recommendations of a World Health Organization (WHO) and International Union Against Tuberculosis and Lung Disease (IUATLD) Working Group. Eur Respir J 2000;16:364.
329. Selle JG, Snyder WH, Schreiber JT: Chylothorax: Indications for surgery. Ann Surg 1973;177:245.
330. Severien C, Teig N, Riedel F, et al: Severe pneumonia and chronic lung disease in a young child with adenovirus and *Bordetella pertussis* infection. Pediatr Infect Dis J 1995;14:400.
331. Sharland M, Gibb DM, Holland F: Respiratory morbidity from lymphocytic interstitial pneumonitis (LIP) in vertically acquired HIV infection. Arch Dis Child 1997;76:334.
332. Shaw KS, Prasil P, Nguyen LT, et al: Pediatric spontaneous pneumothorax. Semin Pediatr Surg 2003;12:55.
333. Shay DK, Holman RC, Roosevelt GE, et al: Bronchiolitis-associated mortality and estimates of respiratory syncytial virus-associated deaths among US children, 1979-1997. J Infect Dis 2001;183:16.
334. Shen HN, Lu FL, Wu HD, et al: Management of tension pneumatocele with high-frequency oscillatory ventilation. Chest 2002;121:284.
335. Shenep JL, Flynn PM: Pulmonary fungal infections in immunocompromised children. Curr Opin Pediatr 1997;9:213.
336. Shetty D, Giri N, Gonzalez CE, et al: Invasive aspergillosis in human immunodeficiency virus-infected children. Pediatr Infect Dis J 1997;16:216.
337. Shingadia D, Novelli V: Diagnosis and treatment of tuberculosis in children. Lancet Infect Dis 2003;3:624.
338. Sihoe AD, Yim APC, Lee TW, et al: Can CT scanning be used to select patients with unilateral primary spontaneous pneumothorax for bilateral surgery? Chest 2000;118:380.
339. Simansky DA, Yellin A: Pleural abrasion via axillary thoracotomy in the era of video-assisted thoracic surgery. Thorax 1994;49:922.
340. Simonds RJ, Orejas G: *Pneumocystis carinii* pneumonia and toxoplasmosis. In Pizzo PA, Wilfert C (eds): Pediatric AIDS: The Challenge of HIV Infection in Infants, Children and Adolescents, 3rd ed. Baltimore, Williams & Wilkins, 1998.
341. Sinaniotis CA: Viral pneumoniae in children: Incidence and aetiology. Paediatr Respir Rev 2004;5(Suppl A):S197.

342. Slattery DM, Waltz DA, Denham B, et al: Bronchoscopically administered recombinant human DNase for lobar atelectasis in cystic fibrosis. Pediatr Pulmonol 2001;31:383.

343. Smevik B: Complementary investigations in bronchiectasis in children. Monaldi Arch Chest Dis 2000;55:420.

344. Sobel JD, Vazquez J: Candidemia and systemic candidiasis. Semin Respir Infect 1990;5:123.

345. Somoskovi A, Mester J, Hale YM, et al: Laboratory diagnosis of nontuberculous mycobacteria. Clin Chest Med 2003;23:585.

346. Sorensen RU, Waller RL, Klinger JD: Cystic fibrosis: Infection and immunity to *Pseudomonas*. Clin Rev Allergy 1991;9:47.

347. Staat MA: Respiratory syncytial virus infections in children. Semin Respir Infect 2002;17:15.

348. Starke JR: Childhood tuberculosis: Treatment strategies and recent advances. Paediatr Respir Rev 2001;2:103.

349. Starke JR, Jacobs RF, Jereb J: Resurgence of tuberculosis in children. J Pediatr 1992;120:839.

350. Stevens DA, Kan VL, Judson MA, et al: Practice guidelines for diseases caused by *Aspergillus*. Infectious Diseases Society of America. Clin Infect Dis 2000;30:696.

351. Stillwell PC, Mallory GB Jr: Pediatric lung transplantation. Clin Chest Med 1997;18:405.

352. Subramaniam R, Joseph VT, Tan GM, et al: Experience with video-assisted thoracoscopic surgery in the management of complicated pneumonia in children. J Pediatr Surg 2001;36:316.

353. Sullivan JH, Moore RD, Keruly JC, et al: Effect of antiretroviral therapy on the incidence of bacterial pneumonia in patients with advanced HIV infection. Am J Respir Crit Care Med 2000;162:64.

354. Swaminathan S: Basic concepts in the treatment of tuberculosis. Indian J Pediatr 2002;69(Suppl 1):S44.

355. Tabachnik NF: Surgical treatment and the patient with cystic fibrosis. Surg Gynecol Obstet 1981;152:837.

356. Tan TQ: Pneumococcal infections in children. Pediatr Ann 2002;31:241.

357. Tan TQ: Update on pneumococcal infections of the respiratory tract. Semin Respir Infect 2002;17:3.

358. Tan TQ: Antibiotic resistant infections due to *Streptococcus pneumoniae*: Impact on therapeutic options and clinical outcome. Curr Opin Infect Dis 2003;16:271.

359. Tan TQ, Mason EO Jr, Wald ER, et al: Clinical characteristics of children with complicated pneumonia caused by *Streptococcus pneumoniae*. Pediatrics 2002;110:1.

360. Tan TQ, Seilheimer DK, Kaplan SL: Pediatric lung abscess: Clinical management and outcome. Pediatr Infect Dis J 1995;14:51.

361. Tendero DT: Laboratory diagnosis of cytomegalovirus (CMV) infections in immunodepressed patients, mainly in patients with AIDS. Clin Lab 2001;47:169.

362. Thompson AB, Teschler H, Rennard SI: Pathogenesis, evaluation, and therapy for massive hemoptysis. Clin Chest Med 1992;13:69.

363. Thomson AH, Hull J, Kumar MR, et al: Randomised trial of intrapleural urokinase in the treatment of childhood empyema. Thorax 2002;57:343.

364. Tillet WS, Sherry S: The effect in patients of streptococcal fibrinolysin (streptokinase) and streptococcal deoxyribonuclease on fibrinous, purulent and sanguineous pleural exudations. J Clin Invest 1949;23:173.

365. Tor M, Atasalihi A, Altuntas N, et al: Review of cases with cystic hydatid lung disease in a tertiary referral hospital located in an endemic region: A 10 years' experience. Respiration 2000;67:539.

366. Tortoriello TA, Friedman JD, McKenzie ED, et al: Mediastinitis after pediatric cardiac surgery: A 15-year experience at a single institution. Ann Thorac Surg 2003;76:1655.

367. Tribble CG: Talc poudrage in the treatment of spontaneous pneumothoraces in patients with cystic fibrosis. Ann Surg 1986;204:677.

368. Tsang KW, Zheng L, Tipoe G: Ciliary assessment in bronchiectasis. Respirology 2000;5:91.

369. Tuffaha A, Gern JE, Lemanske RF Jr: The role of respiratory viruses in acute and chronic asthma. Clin Chest Med 2000;21:289.

370. Tumbarello M, Tacconelli E, de Donati KG, et al: Changes in incidence and risk factors of *Mycobacterium avium complex* infections in patients with AIDS in the era of new antiretroviral therapies. Eur J Clin Microbiol Infect Dis 2001;20:498.

371. Tuncozgur B, Ustunsoy H, Sivrikoz MC, et al: Intrapleural urokinase in the management of parapneumonic empyema: A randomised controlled trial. Int J Clin Pract 2001;55:658.

372. Turna A, Yilmaz MA, Haciibrahimoglu G, et al: Surgical treatment of pulmonary hydatid cysts: Is capitonnage necessary? Ann Thorac Surg 2002;74:191.

373. Vain NE, Swarner OW, Cha CC: Neonatal chylothorax. J Pediatr Surg 1980;15:261.

374. van der Meer JT, Drew WL, Bowden RA, et al: Summary of the International Consensus Symposium on Advances in the Diagnosis, Treatment and Prophylaxis of Cytomegalovirus Infection. Antiviral Res 1996;32:119.

375. van Rossum AM, Fraaij PL, de Groot R: Efficacy of highly active antiretroviral therapy in HIV-1 infected children. Lancet Infect Dis 2002;2:93.

376. van Straaten HL, Gerards LJ, Krediet TG: Chylothorax in the neonatal period. Eur J Pediatr 1993;152:2.

377. Vandevivere J, Spehl M, Dab I, et al: Bronchiectasis in childhood: Comparison of chest roentgenograms, bronchography and lung scintigraphy. Pediatr Radiol 1980;9:193.

378. Varpela E, Koistinen J, Korhola O, et al: Deficiency of alpha1-antitrypsin and bronchiectasis. Ann Clin Res 1978;10:79.

379. Vaughan D, Katkin JP: Chronic and recurrent pneumonias in children. Semin Respir Infect 2002;17:72.

380. Vento S, Cainelli F: Infections in patients with cancer undergoing chemotherapy: Aetiology, prevention, and treatment. Lancet Oncol 2003;4:595.

381. Vernejoux JM, Raherison C, Combe P, et al: Spontaneous pneumothorax: Pragmatic management and long-term outcome. Respir Med 2001;95:857.

382. Wagner RB, Johnston MR: Middle lobe syndrome. Ann Thorac Surg 1983;35:679.

383. Waites KB: New concepts of *Mycoplasma pneumoniae* infections in children. Pediatr Pulmonol 2003;36:267.

384. Wald A, Leisenring W, van Burik JA, et al: Epidemiology of *Aspergillus* infections in a large cohort of patients undergoing bone marrow transplantation. J Infect Dis 1997;175:145.

385. Wald ER: Recurrent and nonresolving pneumonia in children. Semin Respir Infect 1993;8:46.

386. Wali SO, Shugaeri A, Samman YS, et al: Percutaneous drainage of pyogenic lung abscess. Scand J Infect Dis 2002;34:673.

387. Waller DA, Forty J, Morritt GN: Video-assisted thoracoscopic surgery versus thoracotomy for spontaneous pneumothorax. Ann Thorac Surg 1994;58:372.

388. Walsh TJ, Lee JW, Roilides E, et al: Recent progress and current problems in management of invasive fungal infections in patients with neoplastic diseases. Curr Opin Oncol 1992;4:647.

389. Walsh TJ, Rubin M, Pizzo PA: Respiratory diseases in patients with malignant neoplasms. In Shelhammer J,

Pizzo PA, Parillo JE (eds): Respiratory Disease in the Immunocompromised Host. Philadelphia, JB Lippincott, 1991.

390. Welch KJ: Bronchiectasis. In Ravitch MM, Welch KJ, Benson CA, et al (eds): Pediatric Surgery, 3rd ed. Chicago, Year Book Medical Publishers, 1979.

391. Welch KJ: Lung abscess. In Ravitch MM, Welch KJ, Benson CA, et al (eds): Pediatric Surgery, 3rd ed. Chicago, Year Book Medical Publishers, 1979.

392. Welliver RC: Review of epidemiology and clinical risk factors for severe respiratory syncytial virus (RSV) infection. J Pediatr 2003;143(Suppl):S112.

393. Welliver RC: Respiratory syncytial virus infection: Therapy and prevention. Paediatr Respir Rev 2004;5(Suppl A):S127.

394. Wells RG, Havens PL: Intrapleural fibrinolysis for parapneumonic effusion and empyema in children. Radiology 2003;228:370.

395. Weverling GJ, Mocroft A, Ledergerber B, et al: Discontinuation of *Pneumocystis carinii* pneumonia prophylaxis after start of highly active antiretroviral therapy in HIV-1 infection. EuroSIDA Study Group. Lancet 1999; 353:1293.

396. Whitley RJ, Jacobson MA, Friedberg DN, et al: Guidelines for the treatment of cytomegalovirus diseases in patients with AIDS in the era of potent antiretroviral therapy: Recommendations of an international panel. International AIDS Society-USA. Arch Intern Med 1998;158:957.

397. Whyte KF, Williams GR: Bronchiectasis after mycoplasma pneumonia. Thorax 1984;39:390.

398. Wigglesworth FW: Bronchiectasis: An evaluation of present concepts. McGill Med J 1955;24:189.

399. Wilcox DT, Glick PL, Karamanoukian HL, et al: Spontaneous pneumothorax: A single-institution, 12-year experience in patients under 16 years of age. J Pediatr Surg 1995;30:1452.

400. Williams HE, Landau LI, Phelan PD: Generalized bronchiectasis due to extensive deficiency of bronchial cartilage. Arch Dis Child 1972;47:423.

401. Wilson JF, Decker AM: The surgical management of childhood bronchiectasis: A review of 96 consecutive pulmonary resections in children with nontuberculous bronchiectasis. Ann Surg 1982;195:354.

402. Wolff AB, Silen ML, Kokoska ER, et al: Treatment of refractory chylothorax with externalized pleuroperitoneal shunts in children. Ann Thorac Surg 1999;68:1053.

403. Wolff AJ, O'Donnell AE: Pulmonary manifestations of HIV infection in the era of highly active antiretroviral therapy. Chest 2001;120:1888.

404. Wong K, Waters CM, Walesby RK: Surgical management of invasive pulmonary aspergillosis in immunocompromised patients. Eur J Cardiothorac Surg 1992;6:138.

405. Wong KS, Chiu CH, Yeow KM, et al: Necrotising pneumonitis in children. Eur J Pediatr 2000;159:684.

406. Wood JR, Bellamy D, Child AH, et al: Pulmonary disease in patients with Marfan syndrome. Thorax 1984;39:780.

407. Wood RE: Hemoptysis in cystic fibrosis. Pediatr Pulmonol 1992;8:82.

408. Wubbel L, Muniz L, Ahmed A, et al: Etiology and treatment of community-acquired pneumonia in ambulatory children. Pediatr Infect Dis J 1999;18:98.

409. Yoon W, Kim JK, Kim YH, et al: Bronchial and nonbronchial systemic artery embolization for life-threatening hemoptysis: A comprehensive review. Radiographics 2002;22:1395.

410. Yu-Tang GP, Lin M, Teo N, et al: Embolization for hemoptysis: A six-year review. Cardiovasc Intervent Radiol 2002;25:17.

411. Zaia JA: Prevention and management of CMV-related problems after hematopoietic stem cell transplantation. Bone Marrow Transplant 2002;29:633.

412. Zuhdi MK, Spear RM, Worthen HM, et al: Percutaneous catheter drainage of tension pneumatocele, secondarily infected pneumatocele, and lung abscess in children. Crit Care Med 1996;24:330.

Chapter 65

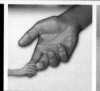

Esophagoscopy and Diagnostic Techniques

Harry Lindahl

HISTORY

The first person to perform esophagoscopy was Kussmaul in 1870, who used a hollow rigid tube with a reflected light for illumination. His patient was a professional sword swallower.[22]

Mikulicz introduced the gastroscope in 1881. His instrument consisted of several small optical units coupled with articulated joints. In 1897, Kelling invented a flexible metal esophagoscope; and in 1898 he invented a gastroscope, the lower third of which could be flexed to 45 degrees. The gastroscope also featured an objective window that could be rotated 360 degrees. Kelling used a miniature electric bulb and a prism for lighting. In 1936, Schindler worked with Wolf, an optical physicist and manufacturer, to design a semi-flexible gastroscope that incorporated a rubber finger at the working end. The system contained more than 48 lenses and used an electric bulb for illumination.[22]

Hirschowirz and coworkers developed flexible fiberglass gastroscopes in 1958 for endoscopy of the upper gastrointestinal tract. During the past 10 to 15 years flexible video endoscopes have surpassed the use of fiber endoscopes. Video endoscopes are at present available from major manufacturers in sizes enabling upper gastrointestinal endoscopy even in small premature infants.[22]

EVALUATION OF ESOPHAGEAL ANATOMY AND FUNCTION

Radiographic Imaging

Esophageal length, diameter, and contour are best evaluated by radiographic imaging with intraluminal barium. Whenever esophageal perforation is suspected, however, a water-soluble contrast medium such as Hypaque or an iso-osmotic agent such as Omnipaque (Amersham Health, Buckinghamshire, UK) is preferred over barium. The possibility of leaking barium into the mediastinum through an esophageal perforation should be avoided.

The esophagogram provides limited accuracy for locating the junction of esophagus and stomach in relation to the diaphragmatic hiatus. Esophagoscopy is more useful in determining the presence or absence of an intra-abdominal length of esophagus, and esophageal manometry is necessary for evaluating function of the lower esophageal sphincter.

Esophagoscopy

Direct visualization and mucosal biopsy through an esophagoscope are the only accurate means of evaluating mucosal changes in the esophagus. The normal esophageal mucosa has a flat, shiny surface with a pattern of fine vessels.

Esophageal contour can be inspected during endoscopic examination because the normal curvature of the thoracic spine is reflected in the curvature of the esophagus. Extrinsic pulsations from the aortic arch are usually seen easily in the upper third of the esophagus. With slight air insufflation, the point of diaphragmatic closure is easily identified at the lower end, and the junction between the flat esophageal and the more reddish and velvety gastric mucosa is normally below the level of diaphragmatic closure. This gastroesophageal junction forms an undulating circle that is usually easy to identify.

Mucosal biopsy is necessary to evaluate submucosal and subtle surface changes. Advanced degrees of inflammation are obvious by visual inspection, and the deeper changes can often be inferred.

The usefulness of open-channel esophagoscopy, the forerunner of all upper gastrointestinal endoscopy, is now limited almost exclusively to the removal of esophageal foreign bodies.

Pressure Monitoring

Intraluminal recording of esophageal pressure dynamics is currently the most accurate way to evaluate esophageal motility. Observation of peristalsis during radiographic contrast study is less reproducible and certainly less quantifiable, although information about coordination of peristalsis, esophageal spasm, and completely uncoordinated esophageal contractions is easily seen radiographically. Early pressure recording techniques used intraesophageal balloons. Water-perfused catheters with multiple pressure recording ports that are pulled back through the length of the esophagus during the recording have supplanted this technique. More sophisticated techniques incorporate circular ports to calculate radial pressure vectors during the pull-back.[23]

Esophageal manometry is considered essential for the study of several esophageal disorders in adults. Achalasia, diffuse esophageal spasm, and nonspecific motor disorders are conditions identified by manometry, and some surgeons think that manometry is an important means in the selection of patients for antireflux surgery.[24]

Manometry has been applied much less widely in infants and children. Patient cooperation is required for a good study. Infants and children seldom tolerate esophageal-pressure recording probes without sedation, and the sedation itself may alter interpretation of the study results. Moreover, the motility disorders identified by manometry in adults are much less common in children. Finally, data from motility studies in children, with the exception of the few with achalasia, have seldom produced significant changes in surgical management.[18]

Eighteen to 24-Hour pH Monitoring

Reflux of gastric acid into the esophagus is thought to be the most common cause of esophageal inflammation, and evaluation of the presence and severity of reflux esophagitis is the most common reason for esophagoscopy in children. In situations in which some quantification of reflux is important, the 24-hour esophageal pH study is suggested.[14] Several authors have described the technical aspects of performing esophageal pH studies in children.[3,29] Normal values for infants and children have also been documented.[11,28] However, pH monitoring only measures acid reflux, and, recently, there has been a study showing the irreproducibility of serial pH measurings.[17]

Esophageal pH studies seldom provide the major basis for decisions on esophageal reflux surgery in children, but esophageal pH data can provide important corroboration for complex clinical situations that are suggestive but not diagnostic of reflux disease. These situations are primarily associated with respiratory complications of presumed reflux, which is not confirmed by barium esophagogram or by esophagoscopy with biopsy. Whereas esophagitis is the most common complication of gastroesophageal reflux in adults, respiratory complications of reflux without significant esophagitis are much more common in infants and children. Thus, esophageal pH monitoring is often important in the management of such children.[10]

Bile Reflux Detection

Reflux of bile into the esophagus has been implicated as a synergistic factor in the development of reflux esophagitis,[26] and convincing data suggest that bile, combined with acid reflux, is the critical factor in the development of Barrett's mucosal dysplasia in the lower esophagus.[25]

Esophageal bile detection is difficult and uncertain with pH monitoring because the mixture of acid with alkaline bile is often recorded in the neutral range by pH monitoring. The presence of bile and acid reflux is thus masked unless bile acids are measured directly from gastric aspirates. Technical improvements have allowed the direct and continuous measurement of bile in the esophagus independent of pH.[2]

INDICATIONS AND APPLICATIONS OF ESOPHAGOSCOPY

Esophagoscopy is performed for either diagnostic or therapeutic indications. For diagnostic endoscopy the flexible adequate-size video endoscope is superior. For some therapeutic procedures the open-tube rigid esophagoscope still has its advantages. Esophagoscopy is an unpleasant procedure and should preferably be performed in children under general anesthesia with endotracheal intubation. Therapeutic esophagoscopy should always be performed under general anesthesia with endotracheal intubation. In units where safe anesthesia cannot be guaranteed, therapeutic esophagoscopy should not be done.

Diagnostic Evaluation

Suspicion of Gastroesophageal Reflux

The suspicion of gastroesophageal reflux is probably the most common cause of diagnostic esophagoscopy in children. The examination is performed to evaluate the presence or severity of reflux esophagitis. However, inflammation of the esophageal mucosa and submucosa is not reliably diagnosed endoscopically in the absence of mucosal ulcerations or erosions. The macroscopic appearance of the esophageal mucosa is difficult to interpret, and therefore the diagnosis and grading of esophagitis depends on mucosal biopsy.[20]

The more advanced degrees of esophagitis are easily recognized. Normally, a fine vascular pattern can be seen just below the mucosal surface (Fig. 65-1). Loss of this superficial vascular pattern, along with erythema, erosions, ulcerations, or nodularity, is associated with varying degrees of biopsy-proven esophagitis. Additional signs of esophagitis include mucosal bleeding on contact, white plaques of various configurations surrounded by an erythematous border, and a cobblestone appearance of the mucosa. Narrowing of the lumen caused by stricture is a complication of long-standing untreated severe esophagitis.

Esophagoscopy for suspicion of gastroesophageal reflux must include gastroduodenoscopy to evaluate possible gastric mucosal lesions and to rule out pyloric or duodenal obstruction. Retrograde view of the cardia gives information of hiatal hernia and the angle of His,

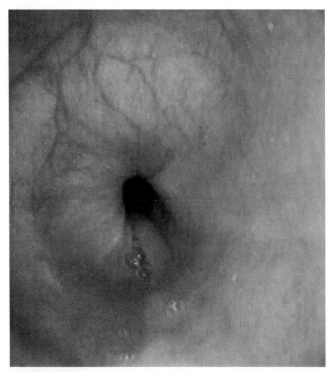

Figure 65–1 Normal cardia of a 7-month old boy as seen from above. Normal esophageal mucosa: a pattern of fine vessels can be seen under the mucosa.

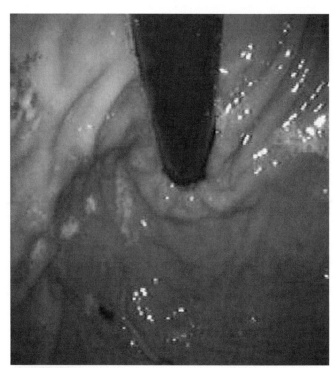

Figure 65–2 Cardia of a 10-year-old boy with portal vein thrombosis 3 months after a successful Rex shunt. The His angle is normal. Submucous veins are still prominent after 10 years of portal vein hypertension.

which are factors affecting gastroesophageal reflux (Figs. 65-2 and 65-3).

Dysphagia

Dysphagia may be associated with esophagitis, esophageal foreign body, congenital or acquired stricture, congenital malformations, benign tumors, structural disease of the esophageal wall, or functional disorders. Endoscopic evaluation gives information of anatomic defects (e.g., stricture) but nothing of functional disorders.

Corrosive Injury

Indications for esophagoscopy after caustic ingestion are controversial in children. Also, the preferred timing of endoscopy varies. I prefer to perform esophagoscopy within 24 hours of ingestion of caustic liquid in symptomatic patients. Patients without symptoms, that is, those who can swallow without difficulties and pain, do not need endoscopy.

Flexible endoscopes instead of rigid instruments should be used to assess the severity of mucosal injury. In severe cases even in older children the use of a neonatal video endoscope of 5 to 6 mm in diameter can be useful because it causes less trauma than a larger instrument. Endoscopy should always be performed with complete visual control. The instrument must never be pushed blindly forward because this may cause esophageal perforation, especially in cases with full-thickness injury. Circumferential damage is not a

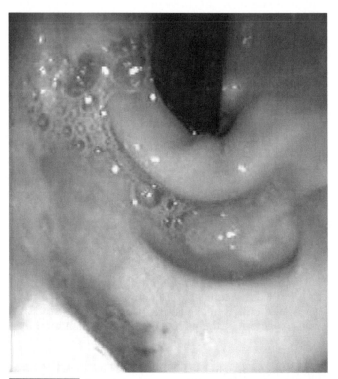

Figure 65–3 Inversion endoscopy of the cardia of a 6-year-old boy with esophageal atresia and fundoplication. The fundoplication has partially slipped into the chest.

contraindication of passing the endoscope, provided it can be done in full visual control. In circular damage it is advisable to pass a silicone tube to the stomach because this enables enteral feeding and also facilitates dilatation of the following stricture.

The diagnosis of full-thickness injury cannot be made with endoscopy. It is a clinical diagnosis, in which the knowledge of the nature and amount of ingested material, the patient's clinical condition, and the laboratory parameters are more important than endoscopic findings.

Upper Gastrointestinal Bleeding

Upper gastrointestinal bleeding is rare in children. Severe esophagitis, variceal bleeding, Mallory-Weiss lesion, or bleeding from mucosal lesions of the stomach or duodenum are the causes. The best way to diagnose these is upper gastrointestinal endoscopy.

Endoscopy for acute upper gastrointestinal hemorrhage is technically demanding and should only be performed by an experienced endoscopist. Bleeding from esophageal varices can be anticipated from a palpable large spleen. The cause can be either portal vein thrombosis or liver cirrhosis, which in children is usually caused by biliary atresia. If variceal bleeding is suspected, preparation for acute sclerotherapy or ligation of the varices should be made.

Severe esophagitis causing significant blood loss is very rare but easily detected in endoscopy. Mallory-Weiss tear occurs even in neonates and is best seen in inversion endoscopy from the stomach side of the cardia. Often Mallory-Weiss tear appears as a local hematoma in the cardia, which hides the actual tear.

Trauma

The most common cause of esophageal disruption is iatrogenic. Most often it results from esophageal dilatation or other therapeutic instrumentation.[15] If the dilatation is performed under endoscopic control, the perforation is usually easily diagnosed in the same endoscopy. There should be no perforations associated with diagnostic esophagoscopy.

Both blunt and penetrating forces can cause esophageal disruption or perforation. Compression injuries to the chest more commonly disrupt the airway, but an air-filled esophagus may also be disrupted. In these cases esophagography with water-soluble contrast medium provides the best approach to diagnosis of esophageal perforation if the patient is conscious and a swallowing study can be performed. Flexible esophagoscopy can identify major tears or complete disruption, but a small crack in the wall after stricture dilatation may not be apparent without contrast radiographic imaging.

Anatomic Abnormalities

Anatomic abnormalities of the esophagus, such as congenital stenoses, cartilaginous rings in the esophageal wall, leiomyomas, and cystic duplications are usually first identified radiographically and then confirmed endoscopically.

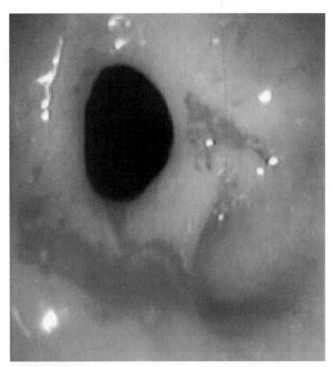

Figure 65–4 Anastomotic stricture of a 6-month-old boy with esophageal atresia.

The unyielding, ribbed esophageal wall associated with cartilaginous rings is striking to view with a flexible scope. Tracheoesophageal fistulas are best seen with tracheoscopy and are usually invisible from the esophageal side. Figure 65-4 shows the anastomotic stricture of a patient with esophageal atresia.

Follow-up of Congenital Upper Gastrointestinal Anomalies

Operated congenital upper gastrointestinal anomalies carry a significant risk of late esophageal pathology. Complications of gastroesophageal reflux, esophagitis, gastric metaplasia, and even adenocarcinoma have been reported. Many of the patients are asymptomatic, even when harboring gastric metaplasia. To prevent irreversible premalignant mucosal changes, routine follow-up esophagoscopy of corrected upper gastrointestinal anomalies should be considered.[12,13,19,27] Follow-up endoscopy of a 3-year-old boy with esophageal atresia and gastric tube is shown in Figure 65-5. Esophageal atresia anastomosis is evident in a 22-year-old woman in Figure 65-6.

Therapeutic Applications

Stricture Dilatation

Balloon dilatation with or without a guidewire and with either fluoroscopic or endoscopic control is the treatment of choice for strictures. Localized anastomotic strictures are commonly managed with balloon dilatation either under fluoroscopic control or using direct endoscopic

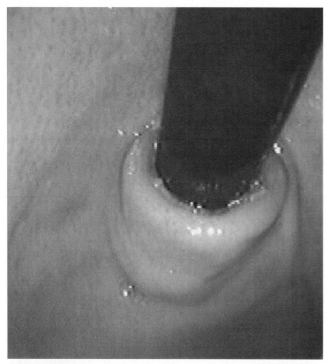

Figure 65–5 Pseudocardia of a patient with esophageal atresia. The esophagus has been reconstructed with retrosternal reversed gastric tube.

visualization. Long or tight and tortuous strictures require the passage of a guidewire either endoscopically or under fluoroscopic control. The choice whether to dilate under fluoroscopic or endoscopic control depends on the preference and experience of the unit. The use of

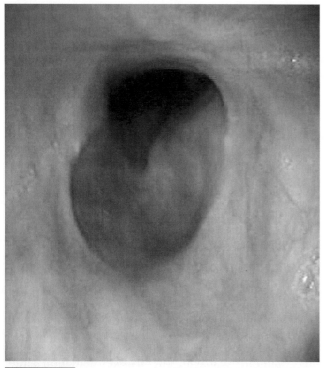

Figure 65–6 Esophageal atresia anastomosis in a 22-year-old woman.

hard metal dilatators or rubber bougies or retrograde dilatation has very little to offer anymore.

Balloon Dilatation with Fluoroscopic Control

The high-pressure balloons used with this technique have a precisely controlled maximum diameter and were originally developed for angioplasty. The dilating balloon is passed over a small slippery wire, which is positioned through the esophagus and into the stomach by fluoroscopy. A balloon of appropriate diameter is selected and passed over the wire to a point at which the balloon straddles the stricture. In simple, not too tight strictures a soft-tipped balloon without a guidewire can also be used. The balloon is then filled with water-soluble contrast agent so that the waist-like indentation on the balloon can be visualized under fluoroscopy as the stricture is stretched.

This technique offers the advantage of direct visualization during dilatation, and the radial forces generated during dilatation are thought to be safer and more localized than the shearing forces generated by longitudinal tapered dilators.[16]

Balloon Dilatation with Direct Endoscopic Visualization

The balloon dilatator can also be introduced with endoscopic control. Small-caliber dilatators fit the endoscope working channel and can be directly pushed into the stricture. Larger caliber balloons usually require separate passing of the guidewire through the working channel of the scope into the stricture. After that, the endoscope is removed and the dilator is passed over the wire as in fluoroscopic assisted dilatation. The dilatation procedure can be inspected if the endoscope is passed beside the dilator to have a direct view of the stricture. The advantage of this method is that the extent of inflammation can be assessed and biopsy can be done, balloon dilatation can be monitored through the flexible esophagoscope, and any cracking or mucosal damage can be evaluated after the balloon is withdrawn. Figure 65-4 shows the anastomotic stricture of a patient with esophageal atresia.

Dilatation with a Guidewire Left In Situ

In difficult strictures requiring multiple dilatations this technique is helpful. A gastrostomy is required. A guidewire is passed from the upper esophagus through the flexible scope into the stomach. The intragastric portion is then recovered with an endoscope through the gastrostomy opening. With the use of this guidewire, balloon dilators can be pushed to the stricture either from below or from above. After dilatation the guidewire can be replaced with a nasogastric tube, which is tied to the gastrostomy tube. In the next session the nasogastric tube can be used to lead the guidewire from the nose through the gastrostomy, making repeated dilatations easy and safe.

Gastrostomy Tube or Button Insertion

Flexible gastroscopy is an essential component of the retrograde "pull" technique for percutaneous placement of gastrostomy tubes or gastrostomy buttons.[5] Details of the technique are well described in the supply kits for these devices. Previous upper-abdominal surgery is a relative contraindication to endoscopic placement of gastrostomy devices because adhesions may prevent apposition of the stomach with the anterior abdominal wall when it is filled with air through the gastroscope. Tubes have actually traversed the colon or small bowel en route to the stomach because of adhesions limiting direct contact between the stomach and parietal peritoneum.

With the "pull" technique, a percutaneously placed guide string or flexible wire is endoscopically retrieved from the stomach. The use of a basket snare through the instrument channel of the gastroscope is the simplest way to retrieve the guidewire up through the esophagus and out the mouth. The tube is then attached at its tapered, muscle-penetrating end and pulled retrograde down the esophagus, across the stomach, and out the anterior abdominal wall. The final position of the flared end in the stomach should be monitored by direct inspection through the gastroscope to make certain the gastric wall is pulled up snugly against the parietal peritoneum.

I prefer to make the first tube or button change with endoscopic control to ensure that the end of the tube or button is inside the stomach. Separation of the stomach and anterior peritoneum has happened, resulting in feeding into the peritoneal cavity, which is a potentially lethal complication.

Foreign-Body Removal

Effective management of esophageal foreign bodies requires familiarity and skill in the use of several different extraction techniques.

Many esophageal foreign bodies that are not sharp and not embedded in the mucosa as a result of long-term residence can be removed with a contrast medium–filled balloon catheter under fluoroscopic control. Coins account for most of these problems. In a series of 415 cases,[21] 76% were caused by coins; the catheter removal technique was successful in 91%. Foreign bodies that are stuck at the cricopharyngeus sphincter can often be removed using a long-bladed laryngoscope and Magill forceps.[9] There are also other minimally invasive techniques for removing coins.[4] Esophagoscopic removal is considered necessary when the foreign body seems imbedded, has sharp points or corners, or is soft and fragmented and may present a risk for aspiration during balloon extraction. However, depending on the experience of the unit, esophagoscopic removal using an open channeled esophagoscope can also be used in simple coin removals.

Impacted organic matter is best removed using the rigid open-channel esophagoscope. Chunks of meat and other debris are usually lodged above a stricture, making advancement into the stomach with a bougie difficult or even dangerous. Large extraction forceps can be introduced through the rigid scope, allowing several passes of the instrument without removal of the scope sheath with each fragment. Large, sharp objects also are more safely manipulated into the protecting sheath of the open-channel scope. This prevents contact with the esophageal wall during extraction of the foreign body and scope as a unit. In all extractions with the open-channel esophagoscope the use of optical forceps from a rigid pediatric bronchoscope can be helpful, because it provides a magnified view.

Small, imbedded objects can sometimes be handled with the flexible scope and the appropriate alligator, cup, or tack forceps or various grasping wires or baskets. Open safety pins pointing upward are easily extracted by grasping the spring loop with a tack forceps, passing the entire pin into the stomach for a turnaround, and then extracting the pin with the open point downward as it is removed as a unit with the scope.

Injection Sclerotherapy

Injection sclerotherapy for esophageal varices is done with the flexible esophagoscope and the flexible needle injector. We have used intravariceal injection with 3% sodium tetradecyl sulfate. The injection volume has been 0.5 to 1.0 mL per varicose vein, with a total volume of 2.0 to 3.0 mL per session. In more than 25 years of experience I have seen no complications associated with the sclerosant, nor has there been any need for blood transfusions because of the injection. There are few randomized controlled trials of the effect of injection sclerotherapy. In a series of 100 children with varices, randomized for prophylactic sclerotherapy, good elimination of varices was achieved in the sclerotherapy group, but this did not improve survival.[7]

Endoscopic variceal ligation with small rubber bands has been developed as an alternative to endoscopic variceal sclerosis, and the effectiveness and complication rates for the two techniques were similar in a randomized trial in adults.[6] Ligation of varices is gaining popularity also in the pediatric age group.[1,8]

Intraluminal Laser Therapy

Intraluminal laser ablation of esophageal lesions is used in adults.[30] Flexible optical fibers for cutting, sclerosing, or ablating lesions are available for passage through the instrument channel of a fiberscope, but clinical applications in infants and children are currently so rare that most pediatric surgical units do not maintain the necessary equipment or expertise. Endoscopic laser applications can be a possibility for future development.

INSTRUMENTATION

Flexible Fiberoscopy

The flexible video end-viewing gastroscope is the instrument of choice for esophagoscopy in infants and children. Excellent videoscopes in pediatric sizes are now available from several major manufacturers of endoscopic equipment. For routine diagnostic and therapeutic applications, the endoscopes are equipped with at least one channel for suction and instrumentation. The gastroscopes also include positive-pressure insufflation and the capability to flush and clear the lens without withdrawal of the scope. Four-way directional controls for the viewing tip are standard. The video picture can be tape recorded, and both paper and digital pictures can be obtained with modern equipment. The external diameter of most pediatric videoscopes with these features ranges from 6.0 to 9.0 mm.

Guidelines for sterilization of fiberscopes are now fairly rigid. Automatic sterilizers are available from the manufacturers to facilitate cleaning and decontamination. Accessory instrumentation for passage through the long working channel of the scopes includes various biopsy and foreign-body forceps, graspers, baskets, flexible injectors, magnets, diathermy loops, and laser optical fibers.

Rigid, Open-Channel Endoscopy

The use of a rigid, open-channel instrument in the esophagus still has a few specific indications. The large working channel of the open, rigid scope allows safe removal of large, sharp, pointed foreign bodies because the sharp edges of the foreign body can be partially drawn into the scope for protection during withdrawal. Large organic foreign bodies are also more easily removed. The large working channel allows several passes with much larger extractors than could be used otherwise, and the larger graspers lessen the break up and fragmentation that complicate manipulation with flexible instruments. For better visualization, the rigid Hopkins optical rod of the rigid bronchoscope can be used. The use of rigid optical foreign-body forceps of the bronchoscope often facilitates foreign-body removal.

PATIENT PREPARATION, SEDATION, AND PAIN CONTROL

Even flexible esophagoscopy is an unpleasant procedure in children. Therefore, I prefer general anesthesia with airway intubation. It provides a more controlled and, in many cases, a safer environment for esophagoscopy than sedation. General anesthesia is mandatory in children for the management of foreign-body extraction, stricture dilatation, injection sclerotherapy, or variceal ligation. It might seem that general anesthesia would involve increased risk, but the reverse is usually the case. Intravenous sedation and a forceful endoscopy in an agitated or uncooperative child without airway control can invite disaster from respiratory depression and cardiovascular collapse. Aspiration is also an increased risk in procedures such as injection sclerotherapy or evaluation of acute bleeding, in which irrigation fluid or blood may reflux back into an unprotected airway. General anesthesia minimizes psychic trauma, increases the safety of the manipulation, and makes endoscopy much easier for the surgeon.

I have no personal experience with esophagoscopy under conscious sedation without general anesthesia. However, some clinicians still use this approach. The usual agents for intravenous sedation include a short-acting central nervous system depressant of the benzodiazepine class combined with a narcotic. Dosages are titrated to effect, within predetermined limits. A topical anesthetic spray of the hypopharynx is helpful before introduction of the endoscope. Continuous monitoring of heart rate and oxygen saturation and intermittent monitoring of blood pressure during the procedure and for an appropriate interval afterward are mandatory. Oxygen, bag, mask, and an intravenous narcotic antagonist should be available at the bedside during the procedure. Esophagoscopy under sedation should not be performed outside of an endoscopy suite that is equipped for resuscitation and cardiorespiratory support. An exception can be made, of course, for procedures required in an intensive care unit where similar supportive facilities are available. Trained personnel, as well as appropriate facilities and equipment, are essential for making the procedure maximally productive and safe.

Some cooperative teenagers can undergo endoscopy without sedation, using only topical anesthetic spray of the pharynx. In selected patients this provides better cooperation than endoscopy under sedation.

TECHNICAL CONSIDERATIONS

Before use, all equipment must be checked to ensure that it is in working order. The lens focus on the flexible endoscope must also be adjusted before insertion, and the video endoscope must be white balanced. The control element of the flexible scope is held in the notch between thumb and fingers of the left hand. The upward-pointing second and third fingers operate the suction and insufflation controls, and the fourth and fifth fingers stabilize the endoscope. The left thumb is used to control the north and south movement, and the right hand stabilizes the distal scope at the mouth, controls insertion, and provides lateral movement by rotational changes. Fine adjustments in east and west orientation of the tip can be made with the lateral adjustment control wheel. To protect the flexible scope, a mouthpiece is inserted between the anterior teeth.

Flexible Endoscopy with General Anesthesia

Flexible videoendoscopy under general anesthesia is simpler in every respect except for insertion of the scope through the cricopharyngeus. The anesthetized patient does not swallow, either voluntarily or involuntarily. The patient is placed supine. The endoscopist stands at the head of the patient on the right side of the table. The endoscope is passed under visual control behind the larynx to the esophagus. If the larynx lies tightly against the back wall of the hypopharynx, the anesthetist can be asked to gently lift the angle of the jaw. A small jet of air can be introduced from the level of the pyriform sinus to open the cricopharyngeus. The tip of the endoscope is then advanced under vision into the orifice that comes into view. Once through the cricopharyngeus, the endoscope is adjusted so that the lumen of the esophagus is straight ahead. Observations are made during advancement and withdrawal of the endoscope. In evaluation of esophagitis or caustic injury, it is important to record the condition of the mucosa before the endoscope has passed over it.

Flexible Endoscopy with Intravenous Sedation or Without Sedation

Intravenous sedation rarely provides total cooperation of the child undergoing endoscopy. The examination must be comprehensive but brief. This requires gentleness, precise manipulation, no unnecessary or false maneuvers, and considerable experience on the part of the endoscopist.

In larger patients without sedation and those only lightly sedated, the introduction of the endoscope is best performed when the patient is sitting. After the introduction of the endoscope through the cricopharyngeus sphincter, the patient is usually placed in the left lateral position with the head slightly extended. A smooth introduction greatly reduces fear of and resistance to the procedure. Many endoscopists prefer blind intubation of the cricopharyngeus, accomplished by pressing the tongue forward with the index and middle fingers of the left hand while the right hand advances the scope during a swallow. However, introduction under direct vision through the scope offers more precise placement. A swallow can sometimes be initiated in a child by squirting water into the pharynx through the lens-washing system.

Rigid Endoscopy with Open-Channel Viewing

Rigid endoscopy in a child should always involve general intubation anesthesia to minimize trauma and the risk for perforation. The supine position, with the neck forward and the head extended, is satisfactory for most examinations.

The open-channel rigid esophagoscope is introduced under direct vision into the back of the pharynx with the lip of the beveled portion anterior. This lip is then used to elevate the larynx gently and to open the cricopharyngeus. The patient's mandible and maxilla are supported with the endoscopist's left hand; the thumb and index finger hold the esophagoscope as if holding a billiard cue. The right hand manipulates the scope as it would a cue. The scope should not be advanced unless the lumen of the pharynx or esophagus is clearly visualized straight ahead. If the cricopharyngeus does not open up with elevation by the lip of the scope against the posterior portion of the larynx, the esophageal lumen should be identified by passage of a soft suction catheter through the scope as a lumen finder. The scope is then passed over this catheter into the upper esophagus under direct vision. A view of the esophageal lumen should be maintained as the scope is advanced through the gastroesophageal junction into the stomach. More detailed inspection can then be obtained as the scope is withdrawn.

COMPLICATIONS

Esophagoscopy involves risks associated with sedation or anesthesia in addition to the risk for direct instrumental perforation of the pharynx, esophagus, or stomach. Drug reactions, tracheobronchial aspiration, and hypoxic brain damage are all potential and almost entirely preventable complications associated with upper gastrointestinal endoscopy. Instrumental perforation should be entirely preventable; unfortunately, this complication still occurs.

Before flexible endoscopy, the more common sites for perforation involved the posterior pharynx in children who were restrained and were examined while awake. Esophagoscopy associated with the dilatation of tight strictures still carries a greater risk for perforation than does a purely diagnostic procedure, but reliable figures on the incidence of instrumental perforation are not available for children. Even for simple diagnosis, the risk for perforation in the presence of severe esophagitis, whether from reflux or from caustic ingestion, must be greater than that in a patient with an esophagus that is not inflamed. The predominant use of flexible instruments in recent years is a major factor in reducing and almost eliminating instrumental perforation in children. As long as a magnified view of the esophageal lumen is maintained throughout the procedure, perforation remains unlikely.

During the 10-year period 1994-2003 there were 6418 esophagoscopies or upper gastrointestinal endoscopies performed by pediatric surgeons in Helsinki University Children's Hospital. Esophageal dilatation was performed in 386 sessions. There were two perforations, both related to dilatation of anastomotic stricture after esophageal atresia repair. Both required surgical correction. There was no mortality associated with the perforations, but in one patient several operations were required to preserve the patient's esophagus. During the same period, esophagoscopy and extraction of esophageal foreign body was performed on 140 patients and sclerotherapy of esophageal varices was performed in 102 sessions. There were no surgical complications associated with these procedures, nor have there been esophageal perforations associated with diagnostic esophagoscopies.

REFERENCES

1. Celinska-Cedro D, Teisseyre M, Woynarowski M, et al: Endoscopic ligation of esophageal varices for prophylaxis of first bleeding in children and adolescents with portal hypertension: Preliminary results of a prospective study. J Pediatr Surg 2003;38:1008-1011.
2. Champion G, Richter JE, Vaezi MF, et al: Duodenogastroesophageal reflux: Relationship to pH and importance in Barrett's esophagus. Gastroenterology 1994;107:747.
3. Evans DF, Haynes J, Jones JA, et al: Ambulatory esophageal pH monitoring in children as an indicator for surgery. J Pediatr Surg 1986;21:221.
4. Gauderer MW, DeCou JM, Abrams RS, et al: The penny pincher: A new technique for fast and safe removal of esophageal coins. J Pediatr Surg 2000;35:276-278.
5. Gauderer MW: Percutaneous endoscopic gastrostomy 20-years later: A historical perspective. J Pediatr Surg 2001;36:217-219.

6. Gimson AE, Ramage JK, Panos MZ, et al: Randomised trial of variceal banding ligation versus injection sclerotherapy for bleeding oesophageal varices. Lancet 1993;342:391.

7. Gonçalves MEP, Cardoso SR, Maksoud JG: Prophylactic sclerotherapy in children with esophageal varices: Long-term results of a controlled prospective randomized trial. J Pediatr Surg 2000;35:401-405.

8. Hall RJ, Lilly JR, Stiegmann GV: Endoscopic esophageal varix ligation: Technique and preliminary results in children. J Pediatr Surg 1988;23:1222.

9. Janik JE, Janik JS: Magill forceps extraction of upper esophageal coins. J Pediatr Surg 2003;38:227-229.

10. Johnson DG, Syme WC, Matlak ME, et al: Gastro-oesophageal reflux and respiratory disease: The place of the surgeon. Aust NZ J Surg 1984;54:405.

11. Jolley SG, Johnson DG, Herbst JJ, et al: An assessment of gastroesophageal reflux in children by extended pH monitoring of the distal esophagus. Surgery 1978;84:16.

12. Koivusalo A, Rintala R, Lindahl H: Gastroesophageal reflux in children with a congenital abdominal wall defect. J Pediatr Surg 1999;34:1127-1129.

13. Lindahl H, Rintala R, Sariola H: Chronic esophagitis and gastric metaplasia are frequent complications of esophageal atresia. J Pediatr Surg 1993;28:1178-1180.

14. Meyers WF, Roberts CC, Johnson DG, et al: Value of tests for evaluation of gastroesophageal reflux in children. J Pediatr Surg 1985;20:515.

15. Moghissi K, Pender D: Instrumental perforations of the oesophagus and their management. Thorax 1988;43:642.

16. Myer CM III, Ball WS Jr, Bisset GS III: Balloon dilatation of esophageal strictures in children. Arch Otolaryngol Head Neck Surg 1991;117:529.

17. Nielsen RG, Kruse-Andersen S, Husby S: Low reproducibility of 2 × 24-hour continuous esophageal pH monitoring in infants and children: A limiting factor for interventional studies. Dig Dis Sci 2003;48:1495-1502.

18. Opie JC, Chaye H, Fraser GC: Fundoplication and pediatric esophageal manometry: Actuarial analysis over 7 years. J Pediatr Surg 1987;22:935.

19. Schalamon J, Lindahl H, Saarikoski H, et al: Endoscopic follow-up in esophageal atresia—for how long is it necessary? J Pediatr Surg 2003;38:702-704.

20. Schapiro M: Flexible fiberoptic esophagoscopy. In Berci G (ed): Endoscopy. New York, Appleton-Century-Crofts, 1976.

21. Schunk JE, Harrison AM, Corneli HM, et al: Fluoroscopic Foley catheter removal of esophageal foreign bodies in children: Experience with 415 episodes. Pediatrics 1994;94:709.

22. Spaner SJ, Warnock GL: A brief history of endoscopy, laparoscopy and laparoscopic surgery. J Laparoendosc Adv Surg Tech A 1997;7:369-373.

23. Stein HJ, DeMeester TR, Naspetti R, et al: Three-dimensional imaging of the lower esophageal sphincter in gastro-esophageal reflux disease. Ann Surg 1991;214:374.

24. Stein HJ, DeMeester TR: Indications, technique, and clinical use of ambulatory 24-hour esophageal motility monitoring in a surgical practice. Ann Surg 1993;217:128.

25. Stein HJ, Hoeft S, DeMeester TR: Functional foregut abnormalities in Barrett's esophagus. J Thorac Cardiovasc Surg 1993;105:107.

26. Stoker DL, Williams JG: Alkaline reflux oesophagitis. Gut 1991;32:1090.

27. Vanamo K, Rintala RJ, Lindahl H, et al: Long-term gastrointestinal morbidity in patients with congenital diaphragmatic defects. J Pediatr Surg 1996;31:551-554.

28. Vandenplas Y, Goyvaerts H, Helven R, et al: Gastroesophageal reflux, as measured by 24-hour pH monitoring, in 509 healthy infants screened for risk of sudden infant death syndrome. Pediatrics 1991;88:834.

29. Vandenplas Y: Esophageal pH monitoring: Methodology, indication and interpretation. Eur J Pediatr Surg 1991;1:67.

30. Weston AP: Use of lasers in Barrett's esophagus. Gastrointest Endosc Clin North Am 2003;13:467-481.

Chapter 66

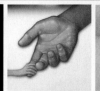

Esophageal Rupture and Perforation

Thomas R. Weber

Boerhaave's classic postmortem description of a patient, Baron Wassenaer, is recognized to be the first report of a case of spontaneous, postemetic esophageal rupture. In 1952, Fryfogle[12] reported spontaneous rupture of the esophagus in a neonate that was successfully repaired surgically. In 1968, Eklof et al.[8] first emphasized iatrogenic perforation of the cervical esophagus by catheters in the newborn. These authors suggested that nonsurgical therapy might be appropriate in many cases.

CLASSIFICATION AND INCIDENCE

Abnormal communications of the esophagus into the pleural cavity or mediastinum are classified as either esophageal rupture or esophageal perforation. Esophageal rupture is also labeled spontaneous perforation, Boerhaave's syndrome, effort perforation, and esophageal apoplexy. In these conditions, no instrumentation or intubation of the esophagus has occurred, thus implying that an intrinsic anatomic abnormality or dysfunction is present within the esophageal wall.[1,6,7,15,17] Esophageal perforation, on the other hand, is produced by the introduction of an object into the esophageal lumen. These lesions are traumatic and, in many cases, result from diagnostic or therapeutic manipulation.[2,9,10,13,18,23,24] Esophageal perforation can also be caused by the ingestion of foreign bodies[5,16] and caustic substances or by blunt and penetrating trauma.[4,22]

Spontaneous rupture of the esophagus in neonates and infants is rare and accounts for only 4% of all reported cases.[13] In contrast, iatrogenic perforation of the upper part of the esophagus by attempted passage of a nasogastric or endotracheal tube is not uncommon and probably occurs more frequently than reported in the literature.[18,19] In addition, esophageal perforation complicates 0.4% to 1.2% of esophagoscopy and esophageal dilatation procedures,[23] thus making this an important risk factor in the use of these procedures.

CLINICAL FINDINGS

Neonatal spontaneous esophageal rupture occurs most frequently in full-term babies after uncomplicated pregnancies. Respiratory distress with cyanosis may be present immediately or may be delayed for several hours.[15] Respiratory distress is caused by a pneumothorax that is usually located on the right side and in which tension may rapidly develop. The predilection for neonatal Boerhaave's syndrome to be manifested as right-sided pneumothorax, as opposed to rupture into the left pleural cavity (most commonly found in adults), is explained by the close adherence of the aorta to the left side of the esophagus in infants. This adherence provides additional support to that side of the esophagus.[11] If the perforation remains undiagnosed, respiratory distress usually worsens with the first feeding. Vomiting, coughing, choking episodes, and mild hematemesis have been observed in several cases. Thoracentesis or tube thoracostomy may reveal serosanguineous or grossly bloody pleural fluid or the contents of previous feedings. Formula promptly appears if feeding is again attempted.

In contrast, esophageal perforation is most frequently associated with difficulty passing a nasogastric tube in premature infants (63% of cases).[18,19] At least 75% of patients with perforation have difficulty swallowing, characterized by drooling, increased oral secretions, and feeding problems. In older children, severe pleuritic or substernal pain is the hallmark of perforation as a result of esophagoscopy or dilatation procedures. Fever, often high, and rapid, toxic progression to shock may occur in any age group but seems to be more prevalent in older children after mediastinal or free pleural perforation. Subcutaneous emphysema, often present in adults with esophageal perforation, is rare in infants unless massive pneumomediastinum occurs.

DIAGNOSIS

The early diagnosis of esophageal rupture or perforation is indicated by clinical findings and confirmed by radiographic procedures. The typical appearance of spontaneous rupture or extensive traumatic injury of the esophagus includes right-sided tension pneumothorax or hydropneumothorax on an upright radiograph or pneumomediastinum (Fig. 66-1). Plain chest radiographs in children with iatrogenic catheter perforation frequently show malpositioning of a nasogastric tube, usually into the right pleural cavity (Fig. 66-2).

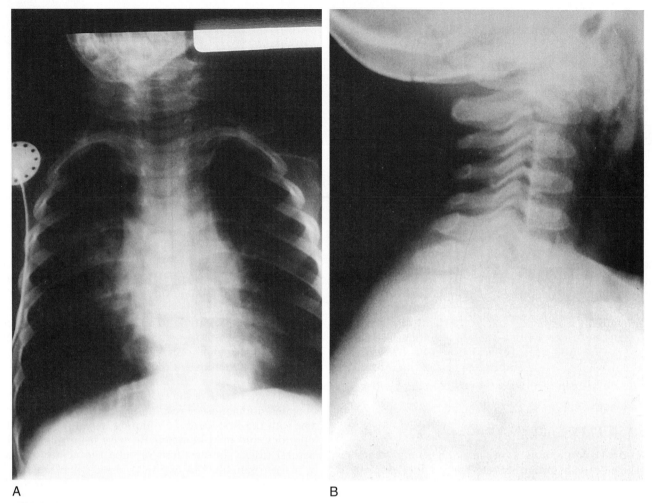

A   B

Figure 66–1 *A,* The esophagus was injured when the patient fell while holding a pencil in his mouth. Note the large amount of mediastinal air on each side of the mediastinum. *B,* Air is also seen in the soft tissues of the neck, indicative of injury to the cervical esophagus. Lateral views are particularly helpful for demonstration of air in the neck or chest.

In other cases, the perforating tube may be located in a submucosal or mediastinal position and cause the formation of a "pseudodiverticulum" of the esophagus. In cases of perforation caused by esophageal dilatation, pneumomediastinum or left chest pneumothorax is frequently present (Fig. 66-3). A lateral chest radiograph may be needed to demonstrate mediastinal air early.

In all cases of esophageal perforation, esophagography is necessary to establish the diagnosis, localize the perforation, and direct therapy.[10] If perforation of the upper part of the esophagus is suspected to have been caused by a nasogastric tube, the tube can be left in place and a small amount of water-soluble contrast can be injected through it. If the tube has been removed or if the perforation was suspected after other procedures such as laryngoscopy or endotracheal intubation, esophagography may be performed by carefully injecting soluble contrast material into the upper part of the esophagus through a small tube. Patients with suspected lower esophageal perforation secondary to instrumentation frequently show extravasation of contrast into the

pleural space or mediastinum during esophagography. If questions remain after water-soluble contrast esophagography or if anatomic definition is inadequate, the study may be repeated with barium. However, most surgeons consider extravasation of barium into the thorax undesirable. Esophagoscopy offers no diagnostic advantages and may actually enlarge the perforation, thus making subsequent repair more difficult.

TREATMENT

The decision about the most appropriate therapy after the diagnosis of esophageal rupture and perforation depends on the site of perforation, whether the perforation is free or contained, the interval from injury to diagnosis, and the systemic response to injury.[3,21] Spontaneous rupture not related to instrumentation usually results in substantial contamination of the mediastinum or pleural space and elicits a severe systemic response of fever, sepsis, pleuritic pain, and occasionally shock. This group of patients needs rapid

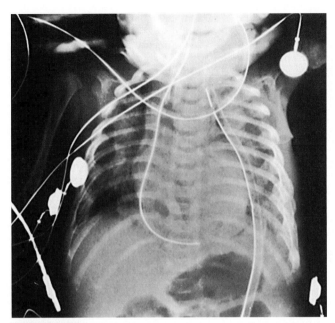

Figure 66–2 Upper esophageal perforation in a premature infant. Note the position of the presumed nasogastric tube in the right side of the chest. The tube was withdrawn, and nonsurgical therapy resulted in complete recovery.

preoperative preparation, including intravenous fluids, antibiotics, thoracentesis, tube thoracostomy (if pneumothorax or hydrothorax is present), and cessation of oral intake. Esophagography should be performed to define the location of the perforation, followed immediately by

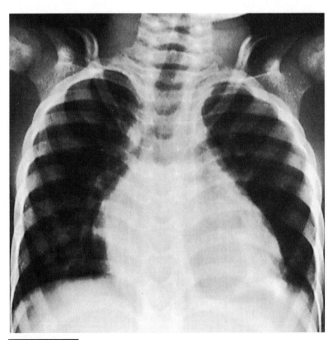

Figure 66–3 This collection of gas in the mediastinum behind the heart occurred 1 hour after an esophageal dilatation procedure. Subsequent esophagography demonstrated distal esophageal perforation.

thoracotomy, irrigation of the pleural space, and suture or patch of the laceration if it can be found. Flexible esophagoscopy during the exploration may help localize the perforation. A flap of pleura or pericardium can also be used to reinforce the esophageal closure.[14] Placement of several large chest tubes completes the procedure.

Free pleural perforation secondary to instrumentation should be managed in an identical manner. Because most of these latter perforations are diagnosed early, little reaction is generally present, and primary repair of the perforation or esophageal resection with primary anastomosis is usually possible. The pleural cavity should be generously irrigated and drained with one or two chest tubes. Ancillary procedures, such as diverting or tube cervical esophagostomy, esophageal division without anastomosis, gastrostomy, and feeding jejunostomy, also have a role in selected cases. These techniques, however, have not been used extensively in children.

Upper esophageal perforation caused by attempted placement of a nasogastric or endotracheal tube can generally be managed nonsurgically.[18,20] These perforations may affect the mediastinum only or may extend into the pleural space (usually the right side). The perforating tube should be withdrawn, a new nasogastric tube should be inserted under fluoroscopic guidance, and contrast should be injected to confirm placement of the tube in the stomach. A chest tube is placed if a pneumothorax is present. The infant is given broad-spectrum antibiotics and intravenous nutrition, and oral feedings are withheld. After several days, feedings through the nasogastric tube may be started. If gastroesophageal reflux occurs, the nasogastric tube can be advanced through the pylorus so that duodenal feedings can be initiated. If sepsis occurs at any time during nonsurgical therapy, formation of a mediastinal abscess must be suspected. Computed tomography of the chest should be done and surgical drainage performed.

Regardless of the therapy used, contrast esophagography is performed 7 to 10 days after injury or repair. If the perforation has completely healed, the chest or mediastinal tubes are removed and oral feeding is resumed. If extravasation is observed, continued conservative therapy generally results in healing within another 7 to 10 days. Persistent esophageal fistula is unusual and suggests distal esophageal or gastric outlet obstruction.

RESULTS OF THERAPY

Because of the rarity of spontaneous esophageal rupture in childhood, it is difficult to assess the success of surgical repair. In a review of 13 patients, Aaronson et al.[1] noted that 3 patients treated by chest tube drainage alone died, whereas 7 of 8 infants treated by thoracotomy and suture repair survived. Late stricture was occasionally encountered at the site of the repair; this complication responded well to dilatation. Other case reports have emphasized the uniform mortality with nonsurgical therapy[9] and the satisfying results obtained with thoracotomy and repair.[6] Similar results can be expected with aggressive surgical repair of esophageal perforation secondary to instrumentation and foreign bodies in which the perforation has entered the pleural space.

Many authors advocate the use of nonsurgical therapy for upper esophageal perforations.[2,8,13,17,18,20,21,24] When selectively applied to infants with no systemic symptoms of perforation, the survival rate approaches 100%. This is usually the case when the perforation is submucosal or well contained in the mediastinum, the so-called pseudo-diverticulum of the esophagus. When free perforation into a pleural space has occurred, conservative therapy can still be used if the baby does not appear ill; however, vital signs must be monitored closely and thoracotomy performed if signs of sepsis appear.

REFERENCES

1. Aaronson IA, Cywes S, Louw JH: Spontaneous esophageal rupture in the newborn. J Pediatr Surg 1975;10:459.
2. Astley R, Roberts KD: Intubation perforation of the oesophagus in the newborn baby. Br J Radiol 1970;43:219.
3. Attar S, Hankins JR, Suter CM, et al: Esophageal perforation: A therapeutic challenge. Ann Thorac Surg 1991; 50:45.
4. Beal SL, Pottmeyer EV, Pisso S: Esophageal perforation following external blunt trauma. J Trauma 1988;28:1425.
5. Benda TJ: Perforating foreign body of the esophagus. Laryngoscope 1969;79:470.
6. Chunn UD, Geppert LJ: Spontaneous rupture of the esophagus in the newborn. J Pediatr 1962;60:404.
7. Dorsey JM, Hohf RP, Lynn TE: Relationship of peptic esophagitis to spontaneous rupture of the esophagus. Arch Surg 1959;78:878.
8. Eklof O, Lohr G, Okmian L: Submucosal perforation of the esophagus in the neonate. Acta Radiol 1969;8:187.
9. Engum SA, Grosfeld JL, West KW, et al: Improved survival in children with esophageal perforation. Arch Surg 1996; 131:604.
10. Fadoo F, Ruiz DE, Dawn SK, et al: Helical CT esophagography for the evaluation of suspected esophageal perforation or rupture. AJR Am J Roentgenol 2004;182:1177.
11. Fleming PJ, Venugopal S, Lewins M, et al: Esophageal perforation into the right pleural cavity in a neonate. J Pediatr Surg 1980;15:335.
12. Fryfogle JD: Discussion of paper by Anderson RL: Rupture of the esophagus. J Thorac Surg 1952;24:369.
13. Grunebaum M, Horodniceanu C, Wilunsky E, et al: Iatrogenic transmural perforation of the oesophagus in the preterm infant. Clin Radiol 1980;31:257.
14. Grillo HC, Wilkins EW: Esophageal repair following late diagnosis of intrathoracic perforation. Ann Thorac Surg 1975;20:387.
15. Harrell GS, Friedland GW, Daily WJ, et al: Neonatal Boerhaave's syndrome. Radiology 1970;95:665.
16. Kerschner JE, Beste DJ, Conley SF, et al: Mediastinitis associated with foreign body erosion of the esophagus in children. Int J Pediatr Otorhinolaryngol 2001;59:89.
17. Kimura K, Kubo M, Okasora T, et al: Esophageal perforation in a neonate associated with gastroesophageal reflux. J Pediatr Surg 1984;19:191.
18. Krasna IH, Rosenfeld D, Benjamin BG, et al: Esophageal perforation in the neonate: An emerging problem in the newborn nursery. J Pediatr Surg 1987;22:784.
19. Lee HB, Kuhn JP: Esophageal perforation in the neonate. Am J Dis Child 1976;130:325.
20. Lynch FP, Coran AG, Cohen SR, et al: Traumatic esophageal pseudodiverticula in the newborn. J Pediatr Surg 1974;9:675.
21. Martinez L, Rivas S, Hernandez F, et al: Aggressive conservative treatment of esophageal perforations in children. J Pediatr Surg 2003;38:685.
22. Sartorelli KH, McBride WJ, Vane DW: Perforation of the intrathoracic esophagus from blunt trauma in a child: Case report and review of the literature. J Pediatr Surg 1999;34:495.
23. Wychulis AR, Fontana RS, Payne WS: Instrumental perforation of the esophagus. Dis Chest 1969;55:184.
24. Zorzi C, Perale R, Piovesan A, et al: Esophageal perforation in the newborn. Eur J Pediatr 1981;13:113.

Chapter 67

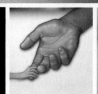

Congenital Anomalies of the Esophagus

Carroll M. Harmon and Arnold G. Coran

HISTORICAL BACKGROUND

The documented history of esophageal atresia (EA) began in the year 1670 with William Durston's published description of "A Narrative of a Monstrous Birth in Plymouth..." in which he described a blind-ending upper esophageal pouch in the right infant of a set of female thoracopagus-conjoined twins.[66] The first description of EA with the typical form of tracheoesophageal fistula (EA-TEF) appeared in 1697 in the fifth edition of Thomas Gibson's *The Anatomy of Humane Bodies Epitomized*.[91] Isolated case reports of EA-TEF surfaced in the 19th century, including one by Thomas Hill in 1840. Published in the *Boston Medical and Surgical Journal*, this report described an infant with EA-TEF and associated rectal agenesis with a rectourinary fistula.[106] In 1861, Harald Hirschsprung of Copenhagen reported 4 cases of his own and collected 10 cases of EA and distal TEF from the literature.[108] In 1880, Morell Mackenzie,[165] another prominent medical figure of the 19th century, reported 57 cases of congenital esophageal malformation with 37 examples of tracheal or bronchial esophageal fistula. He also discussed at length the embryology, pathology, and clinical diagnosis of these anomalies, including a description of associated anomalies such as spina bifida, horseshoe kidney, and imperforate anus. E. D. Plass, an instructor in obstetrics at the Johns Hopkins University, surveyed the literature in 1919 and reported 136 verifiable cases of EA, including 92 with an associated TEF.[199] By 1931, Rosenthal had collected data on 255 patients[215] and indicated, as Ladd emphasized in 1944,[143] "that atresia of the esophagus is a much more frequent anomaly than it has usually been considered to be."

The history of the surgical treatment of EA-TEF is remarkable and covers 270 years linking the first description and the first survivor. In 1869, Timothy Holmes of London, the author of *Surgical Management of Children's Diseases*, was the first to suggest the possibility of a surgical esophageal anastomosis in infants who had EA without TEF; however, he added that "the attempt ought not, I think, be made."[113] The first operative attempt to correct EA without TEF was undertaken in 1888 by Charles Steele of London, and his report titled "Case of Deficient Oesophagus" was published in *The Lancet*.[257] Using chloroform anesthesia, Steele performed a gastrotomy and attempted to perforate through what he suspected was an esophageal membrane by pushing a long, slender steel probe through the gastrotomy site and up the lower esophageal pouch into the upper pouch, which was simultaneously pushed down with a bougie.[257] The attempt was unsuccessful, and at autopsy, the esophagus was found "to terminate above and below in blind rounded ends an inch and a half apart and there was no cord or connection between the parts."[257] In 1899, Hoffman performed the first permanent gastrostomy in an infant with EA.[111] In 1913, H. M. Richter of Chicago described two infants with EA-TEF, on whom he operated without success. Despite his results, Richter was optimistic about the eventual success of primary esophageal repair and stated, "I do not wish to dismiss the idea of immediate union of the two ends of the esophagus."[214] In the same year, however, J. Brennemann, a prominent pediatrician working in Chicago with Richter, referred to the fatal outcome of the two infants who underwent attempted surgical repair by stating that "the physician who, after making his diagnosis of congenital atresia of the esophagus, decides to let his little patient die undisturbed can amply justify his course."[26] Despite Richter's optimism, primary esophageal anastomosis and a myriad of other operations continued to fail; the mortality rate for EA remained 100%. In a 1925 textbook of thoracic surgery, Lilienthal proposed that operative treatment might include "division of the tracheoesophageal fistula and 'anastomosis' of the atretic esophagus by tying each pouch over a rubber tube stent."[151] In 1936, Mims Gage and Alton Oschner of New Orleans, Louisiana, proposed early transabdominal ligation of the cardiac end of the esophagus and gastrostomy with early secondary cervical esophagostomy.[86] Like Richter, they noted that "the ideal operation would be the separation of the esophagus from the trachea and an end-to-end anastomosis of the upper to the lower segment."[86] They added that "such an extensive intrathoracic procedure is not justified in a newborn infant, however, and the operation would always be finished as a postmortem procedure."

The first published report of a case of EA-TEF treated by fistula ligation and primary esophageal anastomosis was presented by Robert Shaw of Dallas, Texas. Shaw performed the operation on September 25, 1938, and reported it in December 1939.[234] In his report, Shaw referred to a personal communication from Paul C. Samson, who had also performed "an operation very similar" to the one Shaw described. Samson's patient died 12 hours after the operation. Shaw's patient died on the 12th day after the operation, apparently as the result of a transfusion reaction. Shaw performed the operation without knowing that Thomas Lanman in Boston had performed four primary esophageal repairs for EA-TEF between January 2, 1936, and July 27, 1937, with the use of an extrapleural approach.[146] In November 1940, Lanman reported these 4 cases, 1 other case of primary esophageal repair, and 27 other cases of EA seen at Boston Children's Hospital between September 1929 and February 1940. All 32 patients in the series died. However, Lanman's fourth patient treated by fistula ligation and primary esophageal repair lived 9 days and at autopsy was found to have died of overhydration, not of mediastinitis or pneumonia. Remarkably, Lanman summarized: "In spite of the fatal outcome in all the 30 operative cases, it is felt that considerable progress along rational lines is being made. The successful operative treatment of a patient with this anomaly is only a question of time."

According to Humphreys and Ferrer,[115] the first survivor of congenital atresia of the esophagus without TEF was a boy born in New York on February 16, 1935. The patient was initially treated by gastrostomy alone, with his "first thoracic operation performed in 1946."[115] The first survivors of EA-TEF were a boy born in Minnesota on November 26, 1939, and a girl born in Massachusetts on the next day. After many failures in caring for infants with EA, N. Logan Leven of the University of Minnesota performed a gastrostomy on a 2500-g male infant with EA-TEF on November 29, 1939. After a failed attempt to close the TEF bronchoscopically with a coagulation electrode, extrapleural ligation of the fistula was accomplished on January 5, 1940. When the infant's weight increased to 4630 g, a cervical esophagostomy was performed on March 27, 1940. The child thrived, and Leven proposed that a subsequent antethoracic esophagoplasty be performed to re-establish continuity of the gastrointestinal tract. In Boston, William Ladd performed a gastrostomy on a female infant on November 28, 1939; on March 15, 1940, he closed the TEF and created a cervical esophagostomy. Although both these patients survived, esophagogastric continuity was achieved only after multiple operations to create an anterior skin-lined thoracic neoesophagus.

In 1935, Cameron Haight began caring for infants with EA at the University of Michigan (Fig. 67-1). His first patient was managed unsuccessfully by a gastrostomy alone. In 1939, Haight attempted his first primary repair of EA, which was unsuccessful. Four subsequent attempts at primary repair also failed; however, on March 15, 1941, the first successful primary repair of EA was performed. The infant girl was an "unusually robust"

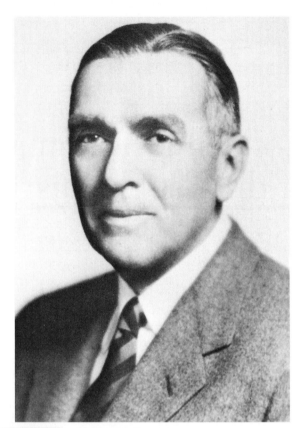

Figure 67-1   Cameron Haight, MD, performed the first successful primary repair of esophageal atresia with a tracheoesophageal fistula on March 15, 1941.

12-day-old child who weighed 8 lb, 4 oz and had been transferred from Marquette, Michigan, to the care of the Chief of Pediatrics, Harry A. Towsley. Dr. Towsley, in turn, consulted Dr. Haight.

The first successful primary repair of EA-TEF was accomplished by using a left extrapleural approach with fistula ligation and a single-layered esophageal anastomosis. An anastomotic leak developed on postoperative day 6 but was managed without surgical intervention. A stricture later developed at the anastomosis and responded to a single dilatation. Drs. Haight and Towsley presented this case in February 1942 at the Central Surgical Association meeting in Chicago and published the report in 1943.[101] In 1943, Haight revised his procedure to a right extrapleural approach because he believed that better exposure of the distal segment was obtained from this side. He also moved to a modified two-layer, "telescoping" anastomosis in the hope of decreasing the risk for leak. Between 1939 and 1969, Dr. Haight cared for more than 284 infants with EA and reported a 52% overall survival rate.[100] After Haight's first success in 1941, reports of survival after direct esophageal anastomosis were sporadic; however, many centers soon began reporting series of successes. One interesting report by Longmire in 1947 describes four consecutive successful primary esophageal anastomoses, including success in a baby who weighed only 1.4 kg.[162]

The history of attempts to classify EA reflects differences in the terminology, but not in the types of

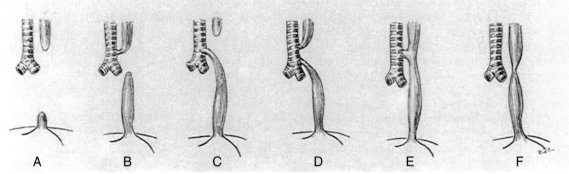

Figure 67–2 Gross classification of anatomic patterns of esophageal atresia. *A*, Esophageal atresia without a tracheoesophageal fistula. This malformation is almost invariably associated with a "long gap." *B*, Atresia with a proximal tracheoesophageal fistula. It is an uncommon anomaly; the abdomen is airless, and the diagnosis may be missed unless contrast studies or endoscopy is performed. *C*, Esophageal atresia with a distal tracheoesophageal fistula, the most frequently encountered form of esophageal anomaly. *D*, Atresia with a double (proximal and distal) fistula. Though rare, this form is found more often than originally thought. *E*, Tracheoesophageal fistula without atresia (H-type fistula). This anomaly may be missed in the newborn period because swallowing is possible. It is associated with recurrent cough, pneumonia, and abdominal distention. *F*, Esophageal stenosis. (From Gross RE: Surgery of Infancy and Childhood. Philadelphia, WB Saunders, 1953.)

anomalies encountered. In 1929, E. C. Vogt, a radiologist, recognized and classified the following types of anomalies[290]: *type 1*, absent esophagus; *type 2*, EA without accompanying TEF; *type 3*, EA accompanied by TEF; *type 3a*, EA with proximal TEF; *type 3b*, EA with distal TEF; *type 3c*, EA with TEF between both esophageal segments and the trachea; and *type 4*, isolated TEF with an intact esophagus. With the success of operative repair, many other anatomic classifications were proposed. In 1944, Ladd introduced a numeric form of classification that consisted of five types with Roman numerals.[143] Gross altered the numeric system in 1953 to an alphabetic system that is still frequently used (Fig. 67-2).[97] In 1962, Swenson returned to a numeric classification and used Arabic numbers instead of Roman numerals.[179] In a 1976 report, Kluth published a complete listing of all described variations of EA, including 10 separate classes and additional subclasses.[131]

In addition to anatomic classifications, in 1962 D. J. Waterston, R. E. Bonham Carter, and Eoin Aberdeen of the Hospital for Sick Children in London developed a classification system related to risk factors in infants with EA.[293] This risk stratification allowed comparison of case outcomes over time and between hospitals. The use of

this classification scheme—which was based on birth weight, the presence of pneumonia, and associated congenital anomalies—allowed the identification of factors that predicted survival and guided operative treatment. This approach to the classification of EA anomalies has been an important contribution to the care of these infants (Table 67-1).

EMBRYOLOGY

The pathogenesis of congenital EA malformations remains unknown. Although many theories have been offered to explain the etiology of EA, EA-TEF, and TEF, no single unifying theory has been proposed that addresses all the variations seen with this group of anomalies. Because most EA malformations occur sporadically, it is highly unlikely that a simple, inheritable genetic mechanism is responsible. The pathogenesis is therefore most likely heterogeneous and multifactorial and involves multiple genes and complex gene-environment interactions.

A clear understanding of the pathogenesis of the EA malformation is hindered by the fact that normal foregut embryology is still obscure. Wilhelm His, Sr., the founder of human embryology, was the first to describe normal development of the respiratory system.[109] He believed that division of the foregut was the result of fusion of invaginating lateral longitudinal ridges that created a septum dividing the foregut into a dorsal digestive tract and a ventral respiratory system. Formation of the so-called tracheoesophageal septum is believed to begin caudally and end cranially.[215] Many of the theories concerning the pathogenesis of EA malformations have been based on this description.[98,215,240,242,258] However, several investigators have more recently found little evidence to support this theory of normal foregut separation and development. Reinvestigation of human specimens from the Collection of Embryos at the Carnegie Institute suggests that ingrowth of lateral foregut wall ridges and

Group	Survival (%)	Waterston Classification
A	100	Birth weight >2500 g and otherwise healthy
B	85	Birth weight 2000-2500 g and well or higher weight with moderate associated anomalies (noncardiac anomalies plus patent ductus arteriosus, ventricular septal defect, and atrial septal defect)
C	65	Birth weight <2000 g or higher with severe associated cardiac anomalies

TABLE 67-1 Waterston Risk Groups and Current Survival Figures

cranial development of a tracheoesophageal septum do not occur in the human embryo.[188,302] In addition, Kluth et al.[133] studied staged chicken embryos via scanning electron microscopy in an attempt to clarify normal foregut development. In this model they also found no evidence of lateral ridges or an epithelial tracheoesophageal septum.

A summary of the major theories to explain the embryopathology of the foregut has recently been presented by Kluth and Fiegel.[132] Several categories of theories include esophageal occlusion, theories that deal with spontaneous deviation of the tracheoesophageal septum, mechanical theories, and new theories generated by the study of a recently described teratogen (doxorubicin [Adriamycin])-induced EA malformations in a rat model.[132]

Theories of foregut occlusion and failure of recanalization of the intestinal lumen have been historically prominent in discussions regarding the pathogenesis of intestinal atresias, including EA.[139,265] Overwhelming proliferation of esophageal epithelium may play a role in the development of rare membranous EA, but it falls short as a comprehensive theory of typical EA malformations.[131] As noted, pathogenic theories of abnormal migration of the putative tracheoesophageal septum have been prominent.[98,215,240,242,258] However, as suggested earlier, the lack of evidence that this structure exists in normal foregut development has lessened the importance of this theory. Theories of EA embryogenesis based on mechanical pressure on the developing foregut continue to be discussed.

Yet another theory has been put forth by Cozzi et al.[50,176] and others[192] in which it is suggested that EA is a component of cephalic neurocristopathy. The observation that there is a clear association of neural crest–implicated cardiovascular anomalies (aortic arch, conotruncal and membranous ventricular septal defects), as well as thymic, thyroid, parathyroid, and facial malformations with EA, as seen with the DiGeorge syndrome, suggests that the pathogenesis of EA may be related to defective pharyngeal arch development.

An animal model in which Adriamycin is used as a teratogen and results in embryos with a variety of malformations, including EA and TEF, has been described and promises to provide new insight into EA pathogenesis.[60,269] Merei and Hutson have used this model to develop a theory suggesting that the primitive foregut develops into the trachea, with subsequent EA-TEF anomalies.[173] Gittes has recently used this model, as well as human TEF tissue samples, to investigate the molecular mechanisms that may play a role in the pathogenesis of EA-TEF. He has proposed that the distal fistula tract and esophagus are of respiratory origin and that defects in lung morphogenesis account for this aspect of the EA-TEF anomaly.[51,245]

Several candidate molecules and pathways have been proposed to play a role in the pathogenesis of EA-TEF. Spitz has suggested that the HOX D group of genes involved in pattern formation of the limbs and foregut may be linked to the VACTERL association (vertebral, anorectal, cardiac, tracheoesophageal, renal, and limb abnormalities).[249] Gittes has reported that a defect in the signaling pathway of the extracellular, organ differentiation–promoting glycoprotein sonic hedgehog (Shh) plays an important role in the development of the TEF in the rat

model[244] and in human TEF tissue.[244] Insight into the cellular, biochemical, and genetic signals responsible for normal cell-cell and cell-matrix interactions, migration, and subsequent organogenesis is required to more clearly understand the pathogenesis of esophagotracheal and associated anomalies.

EPIDEMIOLOGY

The reported incidence of EA, with or without TEF (EA±TEF), varies widely from 1 in 2440 births in Finland[142] to 1 in 4500 births in the United States[101] and Australia.[180] More recently, according to data from the California Birth Defects Monitoring Program database, from 1983 to 1988 the total prevalence of EA, EA-TEF, and TEF alone was reported to be 2.82 per 10,000 live births and stillbirths.[274] In Europe, the prevalence rate of EA-TEF during 1980 to 1988 was 2.86 per 10,000 births, although this rate appeared to be decreasing over time.[57] In this European study, 62% of infants with EA-TEF were male, whereas the California database found that male-to-female ratios varied considerably between types of EA-TEF defects, with ratios of 2.29 for TEF alone, 1.44 for EA-TEF, and 1.33 for EA alone.[274] Nonwhite populations have a lower prevalence of EA-TEF and TEF than white populations do.[102,274] An increased risk for EA-TEF with a first pregnancy,[102] mothers younger than 20 years,[57] and increasing maternal age[19,274] has been reported.

The rate of multiple births is high for each type of EA-TEF anomaly (TEF, 3.7%; EA-TEF, 4.9%; and EA alone, 8.8% in a control population).[102,274] Chromosomal anomalies are also frequent and occur in 6% to 10% of infants with some form of EA.[57,102] These anomalies include trisomy 13 and 18 syndromes and the well-described concurrence of anomalies in the VACTERL association.[102]

As suggested by the Adriamycin rat model for EA-TEF described earlier, environmental teratogens have also been implicated in the pathogenesis of EA±TEF. EA has occurred in infants born to mothers with prolonged exposure to contraceptive pills[263] and exposure to progesterone and estrogen during a pregnancy.[184] In addition, EA has been reported in some infants of hyperthyroid[228] and diabetic mothers and after intrauterine exposure to thalidomide.[36]

Although EA defects are typically sporadic, they have also been described as occurring in infants with a variety of known genetic syndromes, including the DiGeorge sequence,[125] polysplenia sequence, Holt-Oram syndrome, Pierre Robin sequence,[200] and Feingold syndrome.[31] Many studies have described transverse and vertical familial cases of all varieties of EA. Empirical risk figures based on the literature to date give a 0.5% to 2% recurrent risk in parents of one affected child; the risk increases to 20% if more than one sibling is affected.[200] The empirical risk for an affected child born to an affected parent is 3% to 4%.[200]

ASSOCIATED ANOMALIES

The early disturbance in organogenesis that results in EA deformities, whatever the exact cause, also affects other

TABLE 67-2 Incidence of Associated Anomalies

Cardiovascular	≈35%
Genitourinary	≈24%
Gastrointestinal	≈24%
Neurologic	≈12%
Musculoskeletal	≈20%
VACTERL association	≈20%
Overall incidence	50%-70%

VACTERL, vertebral, anorectal, cardiac, tracheoesophageal, renal, and limb abnormalities.

organ systems. Other congenital anomalies are frequently associated with EA, and the associated anomaly often significantly alters treatment and affects survival (Table 67-2). Numerous reports have suggested that between 50% and 70% of infants with EA have at least one associated congenital malformation. The anomalies are most common in cases of EA without TEF and are least common in cases of H-type TEF.[112] Cardiovascular anomalies occur most frequently (11% to 49%),[59,62,148,176] followed by genitourinary (24%),[14] gastrointestinal (24%),[253] and musculoskeletal (13% to 22%)[89,285] anomalies. Associated neurologic anomalies include neural tube defects (2.3%), hydrocephalus (5.2%), holoprosencephaly (2.3%), and anophthalmia or microphthalmos (3.7%).[102] Other anomalies are choanal atresia (5.2%), facial cleft (7.2%), abdominal wall defects (4.3%), and diaphragmatic hernia (2.9%).[102] A recent report suggests that the incidence of certain associated anomalies may vary by world region in that genitourinary anomalies were found in 26% of a European cohort of patients versus only 4% of an Asian cohort.[285]

Complex cardiac deformities may account for most of the deaths associated with EA malformations. The relative risk for death in infants with EA malformations associated with a major cardiac anomaly is reported to be 3.47 (95% confidence interval [CI], 1.51 to 7.96).[62,248] In a series of 153 patients with EA, Leonard et al. reported that the 1-year survival rate of infants with congenital heart disease (CHD) was 67% versus 95% in those without CHD.[148] Interestingly, these authors concluded that although CHD is associated with higher mortality in EA patients, it is not the direct cause of it.[148] The most common single defects identified are ventricular septal defects (19%), which have reportedly been associated with a mortality rate of 16%,[172] and atrial septal defects (20%).[59] Other common cardiac anomalies include the tetralogy of Fallot (5%) and patent ductus arteriosus (13%).[59] Coarctation of the aorta is found in 1% to 4% of infants with EA malformations.[59,278] A descending aorta on the right side has been reported in 4% of infants with EA.[59]

Some gastrointestinal anomalies associated with EA±TEF are anorectal malformations (14%),[59] duodenal atresia (2%),[59] intestinal malrotation (4%),[41] ileal atresia, annular pancreas, and pyloric stenosis. Genitourinary defects are varied and include renal agenesis or hypoplasia (1%), hypospadias, undescended testes, cystic renal

disease, hydronephrosis, vesicoureteral reflux, ureteric duplication, pelvic ureteral and vesicoureteral obstruction, urachal anomalies, ambiguous genitalia, and cloacal or bladder exstrophy.[14,47,102] Typical musculoskeletal malformations include limb (15%) and vertebral (17%) anomalies.[59]

In 1973, Quan and Smith[207] suggested a broad spectrum of associated malformations that are associated with EA malformations. They arranged this association into the acronym VATER: vertebral defects, anal atresia, tracheoesophageal fistula, esophageal atresia, and renal defects. The term "association" is defined as "a nonrandom occurrence in two or more individuals of multiple congenital anomalies not known to be a polytopic defect, sequence or syndrome."[48] Affected patients have no family history of malformations, no recognizable teratogen is involved, and no chromosomal abnormality is observed. As the phenotype expanded, the acronym was changed to the VACTERL association, which includes vertebral, anorectal, cardiac, tracheoesophageal, renal, and limb abnormalities.[12] The incidence of the VACTERL association in the EA population is approximately 20%.[62] Infants specifically with EA-TEF frequently have VACTERL anomalies (vertebral, 17%; anal, 12%; cardiac, 20%; renal, 16%; limb, 10%), as well as other midline defects (cleft lip and palate, 2%; sacral dysgenesis, 2%; urogenital anomalies, 5%).[28] The "renal" category should include urinary tract anomalies such as megalourethra, urethral duplication, urethral valves, stricture, and hypospadias. Recently, the VACTERL-H association has been described and includes congenital hydrocephalus.[161] Infants with EA malformations in association with the VACTERL association have a high mortality rate. Iuchtman et al.[116] analyzed the results of 46 infants born with EA and features of the VACTERL association among 313 patients with EA, TEF, or both. In this series, the mortality rate was 24%. Cardiovascular anomalies were present in 78% of the patients and were the principal cause of death. More recently, Driver et al. reported that the relative risk for mortality in patients with VACTERL associations was 2.54 (95% CI, 1.14 to 4.86).[62]

EA malformations are increasingly being described in association with other polytopic defects, sequences, syndromes, and associations. Some of these include Down's syndrome,[18] the DiGeorge sequence,[125] the polysplenia sequence, Holt-Oram syndrome, the Pierre Robin sequence,[200] Feingold's syndrome,[31] Fanconi's syndrome, Townes-Brock syndrome, Bartsocas-Papas syndrome, McKusick-Kaufman syndrome,[70,105,194,200,205] the CHARGE association (coloboma, heart defects, atresia choanae, developmental retardation, genital hypoplasia, and ear deformities),[141] and the schisis association (omphalocele, neural tube defects, cleft lip and palate, and genital hypoplasia).[38,250] Other serious or lethal associations are trisomy 18 syndrome, cerebral hypoplasia, and Potter's syndrome (bilateral renal agenesis).[201,254] In addition to the well-described anomalies associated with EA just discussed, many recent reports describe significant malformations and associated conditions that may become more frequently recognized. Unilateral pulmonary agenesis associated with EA-TEF is a rare condition; only 37 cases have been reported since 1874.[35,110,130,160,222,246,256]

Usui et al.[281] reported a 47% incidence of tracheobronchial abnormalities, such as ectopic or absent right upper lobe bronchus, congenital bronchial stenosis, and a decreased ratio of circumferential cartilaginous trachea to membranous trachea; these abnormalities could play an important role in such respiratory conditions as tracheomalacia and atelectasis associated with EA.[281] Several reports also suggest that EA is associated with abnormalities in vagal nerve innervation that are not related to surgical intervention to repair the esophageal defect.[54]

CLASSIFICATION

Derived from more than 2200 cases of various esophageal anomalies from six large series, the incidence of the various types of anomalies is shown in Table 67-3.

As noted previously, numerous classification schemes have been proposed and used to describe EA. The most useful and practical classifications are perhaps simple anatomic descriptions, such as that listed in Table 67-3, even though many institutions and surgeons still use the Gross classification. It is important to note, however, that there are many variations to the fairly straightforward anatomic descriptions given in the table. In 1976, Kluth[131] summarized and diagrammed many of the anatomic variants not described by the many classifications mentioned here.

Waterston's 1962 classification, which was based on risk factors, placed infants with EA-TEF into groups according to birth weight, pneumonia, and associated congenital anomalies (see Table 67-1). The classification affected the surgical care of these patients. Infants in the "good"-risk category (A) were typically treated with immediate operative repair, "moderate"-risk infants (B) were managed by delayed repair, and "high"-risk infants (C) were treated by staged repair. Although the Waterston classification continues to be used to compare results between centers, many investigators have questioned its current validity in caring for these infants.[201,209,253] With modern neonatal critical care, more low-birth-weight infants are surviving and more treatment options are available for infants with multiple congenital anomalies. As a result, a search for modern criteria for survival has produced several new classification schemes.

TABLE 67-3 Incidence of Anomalies

Type	Incidence (%)	Gross Type
1. Esophageal atresia with a distal tracheoesophageal fistula	85.8	C
2. Esophageal atresia without tracheoesophageal fistula	7.8	A
3. Tracheoesophageal fistula without esophageal atresia	4.2	E
4. Esophageal atresia with a fistula to both pouches	1.4	D
5. Esophageal atresia with a proximal tracheoesophageal fistula	0.8	B

TABLE 67-4 Spitz Classification: Predictors of Survival in Cases of Esophageal Anomalies

Group	Survival Rate (%)
I. Birth weight >1500 g without major congenital heart disease	97
II. Birth weight <1500 g or major congenital heart disease	59
III. Birth weight <1500 g and major congenital heart disease	22

In 1989, Randolph et al.[209] suggested a refinement in Waterston's classification based on the overall physiologic status of an infant with EA. According to a report analyzing the results of 39 infants managed with the physiologic status criteria, more and earlier primary repairs were performed, and excellent survival rates were maintained in stable infants in comparison to 87 infants previously managed by using Waterston's criteria.[209]

Other prognostic classifications have recently been proposed. Poenaru et al.[201] suggested that only severe pulmonary dysfunction with a preoperative mechanical ventilation requirement and severe associated anomalies were independent predictors of survival. Brown and Tam[29] suggested that the measured length of the esophageal gap provides a method of classification to predict morbidity and long-term outcome. In a review of 357 cases of EA treated at the Hospital for Sick Children on Great Ormond Street in London between 1980 and 1992, Spitz et al.[254] found that birth weight and major cardiac disease were important predictors of survival. The results are given in Table 67-4.[116] The Spitz classification is currently the system most commonly used.[62,135] Recently, a new classification system has been put forward that adds preoperative respiratory distress syndrome and pneumonia to the Spitz risk factors.[299]

DIAGNOSIS AND CLINICAL FINDINGS

Unlike many congenital pediatric surgical problems, prenatal EA is rarely diagnosed. Prenatal detection of EA by ultrasonography relies on the finding of a small or absent stomach bubble and associated maternal polyhydramnios.[76] However, with these criteria, the predictive value of prenatal ultrasonography in the diagnosis of EA is only 20% to 40%.[243,259] The ultrasonographic finding of an anechoic area in the middle of the fetal neck in association with polyhydramnios and a small stomach may increase the accuracy of prenatal diagnosis of EA.[223] Recent reports suggest that fetal magnetic resonance imaging may be a useful adjunct in the prenatal diagnosis of EA anomalies suspected on ultrasound.[145,170]

Most infants with EA are symptomatic in the first few hours of life. The earliest clinical sign of EA is usually excessive salivation that results from pooling of secretions in the posterior of the pharynx. Typically, the first feeding is followed by regurgitation, choking, and coughing. Other features are cyanosis with or without feeding, respiratory distress, inability to swallow, and inability to pass a feeding or suction catheter through the mouth or nose into the stomach. If a distal fistula is present, the abdomen distends as inspired air passes through the fistula into the stomach. Pulmonary compromise can become significant as gastric fluid passes upward through the TEF, spills into the trachea and lungs, and subsequently leads to chemical pneumonitis. As the abdomen distends with air, the diaphragms (the principal muscles of respiration in the newborn) elevate and pulmonary status worsens. Aspiration of saliva from the upper pouch into the trachea further exacerbates the pulmonary compromise.

The diagnosis of EA can be confirmed by passing a firm catheter through the mouth into the esophagus to the point at which resistance is met. A few milliliters of air can be injected through the tube and used as a contrast agent to distend the upper esophageal pouch as frontal and lateral films are obtained (Fig. 67-3). If necessary, 0.5 to 1.0 mL of diluted barium can be used as a contrast agent and injected into the upper pouch to confirm the diagnosis (Fig. 67-4). Under carefully controlled fluorography, barium may also detect a proximal TEF; in the usual circumstance of a portable film performed in the neonatal unit, however, barium identified in the tracheobronchial tree is more likely to represent contrast aspirated through the larynx rather than through a proximal TEF. A small upper blind pouch may suggest the presence of a proximal TEF. Air in the stomach and bowel confirms the presence of a distal TEF. Absence of air in the abdomen typically represents isolated EA without TEF (Fig. 67-5). However, reports have described narrow or occluded distal fistulas found at thoracotomy

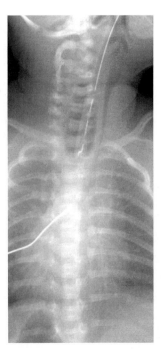

Figure 67–3 Plain radiograph demonstrating the "Replogle" tube in the upper esophageal pouch after the injection of 2 mL of air.

in the absence of intestinal air.[93,193] The diagnosis of TEF without EA is more difficult and requires a high index of suspicion based on clinical symptoms. The diagnosis can be made by barium esophagography in the prone position (Fig. 67-6); however, bronchoscopy or esophagoscopy is often required to confirm the diagnosis.

Figure 67–4 The upper esophageal pouch is outlined by 0.5 to 1.0 mL of thin barium in the frontal (*A*) and lateral (*B*) projections.

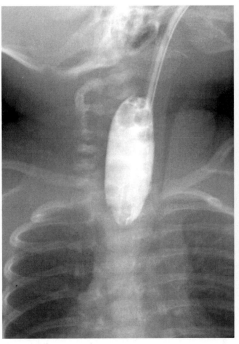

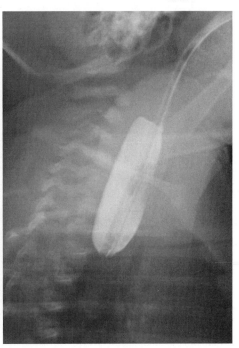

A

B

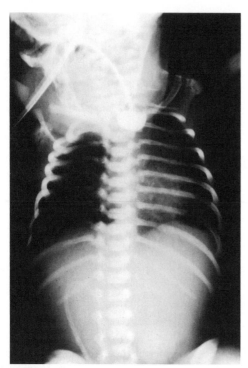

Figure 67–5   Absence of intestinal air suggests isolated esophageal atresia without a tracheoesophageal fistula. Dilute barium fills the upper esophageal pouch.

As previously discussed, the incidence of recognizable congenital defects associated with EA is between 50% and 70%. The clinical evidence of these other anomalies should therefore be considered in the diagnostic evaluation for EA. In addition to a physical examination focused on seeking known associated defects (such as those of the

VACTERL association), additional testing usually includes echocardiography, renal ultrasonography, and chromosomal analysis. In fact, it is not unusual for the finding of an anorectal malformation, for example, to precede the clinical signs and symptoms of a concomitant EA.

PREOPERATIVE TREATMENT

Pneumonitis from aspiration of upper pouch secretions and reflux of gastric acid through the TEF are the most critical preoperative problems for an infant with EA-TEF. Immediate management includes measures to prevent further aspiration and treatment of pneumonitis. A sump catheter should be positioned in the upper esophageal pouch to continuously aspirate saliva under low-pressure suction. The double-lumen Replogle type of catheter is best for this purpose because the perforations along the side of the catheter are located only near the tip, which minimizes the possibility of suctioning oxygenated air away from the larynx. The infant should be positioned to minimize reflux of gastric fluid up through the TEF. An upright sitting position has traditionally been advocated (Fig. 67-7), but some authors argue that the head-up, prone position is most effective at minimizing reflux. Broad-spectrum antibiotic coverage and pulmonary physiotherapy are also initiated. Intravenous fluid therapy with 10% dextrose and hypotonic saline should be started to maintain fluid, electrolyte, and glucose balance. Vitamin K analogue should also be administered before surgery. Routine endotracheal intubation should be avoided because of the risk for gastric perforation and worsening respiratory distress as the abdomen becomes distended from ventilation through the TEF.

OPERATIVE REPAIR

The operative approach to an infant with EA depends greatly on the specific type of anomaly present and the occurrence of associated anomalies.

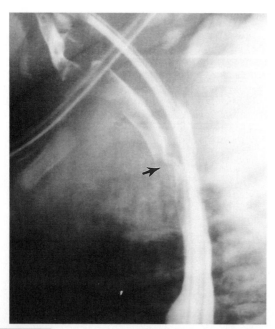

Figure 67–6   An H-type tracheoesophageal fistula is shown as contrast is injected through a nasoesophageal tube. Contrast is noted passing from the esophagus, through the fistula *(arrow)*, and filling the upper part of the trachea and larynx.

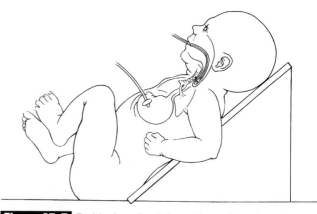

Figure 67–7   Positioning of an infant with esophageal atresia–tracheoesophageal fistula to minimize gastric reflux and tracheal aspiration of upper esophageal pouch secretions. A double-lumen sump catheter is placed in the upper pouch. On rare occasion, a gastrostomy tube is placed before esophageal atresia–tracheoesophageal fistula repair.

Esophageal Atresia with Distal Tracheoesophageal Fistula

Immediate surgery for EA with distal TEF is seldom necessary, and a period of 24 to 48 hours between diagnosis and surgery permits full assessment of the infant and treatment of pulmonary insufficiency, including atelectasis and pneumonitis. In most of these infants, division of the fistula with primary anastomosis of the esophagus is possible and is the operative procedure of choice.

Current anesthetic techniques include minimal use of premedication drugs, careful positioning of the endotracheal tube to allow adequate ventilation with minimal gas flow through the fistula, and typically, manual control of ventilation until the fistula is ligated. The infant is usually positioned for a standard right posterolateral thoracotomy, with the right arm extended above the head and the head slightly flexed. If a right-sided aortic arch (2.5%) is identified on a preoperative echocardiogram, a left-sided thoracotomy is preferred; however, a double aortic arch is not unusual and makes a left thoracic approach difficult as well.[9] A curved skin incision is made around the lower border of the scapula and extends from the anterior axillary line posteriorly to the paravertebral region (Fig. 67-8). Subcutaneous tissue and chest wall muscles are either divided or spared by using electrocautery; this allows elevation of the scapula and identification of the fourth intercostal space. The thorax is entered through the fourth intercostal space by dividing the intercostal muscles, with care taken to avoid incising the pleura. Most pediatric surgeons continue to advocate the extrapleural approach for EA-TEF repair because a substantial anastomotic leak does not result in empyema but merely causes an esophagocutaneous fistula, which typically closes in 1 to 2 weeks. Surgeons who use the transpleural route argue that the operative time is shorter and, with current antibiotic options, the risk for empyema after a leak is minimal. With the extrapleural approach, the pleura is gently pushed away from the chest wall; this in turn allows insertion of a rib-spreading retractor. Moist pledgets, tissue applicators, or gauze can be used to dissect the pleura anteromedially as the rib spreader is sequentially opened (Fig. 67-9). With further retropleural

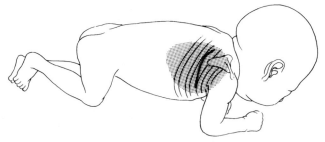

Figure 67–8 Positioning of an infant for repair of esophageal atresia with or without a tracheoesophageal fistula. The thorax is entered through the fourth interspace, and extrapleural dissection is begun.

dissection, the azygos vein is exposed and divided between ties as the lung and pleura are gently retracted medially. When the posterior mediastinum is exposed, the upper pouch, distal TEF, trachea, and vagus nerve are identified. The lower part of the esophagus is dissected circumferentially at the level of the fistula, and every effort is made to preserve the vagal fibers that supply the distal portion of the esophagus. Traction on a heavy silk, tape, or vessel loop passed around the distal end of the esophagus controls gas flow through the fistula into the stomach and allows exposure for fistula closure. The latter is usually performed with 5-0 or 6-0 silk or polypropylene suture placed in interrupted fashion (Fig. 67-10). It is important to leave 1 to 2 mm of esophagus on the tracheal end of the fistula to minimize the risk for postoperative tracheal stricture. The airtightness of the tracheal closure can be tested by filling the thoracic cavity with saline and watching for bubbles with positive-pressure ventilation.

A small tube should be passed through the distal end of the esophagus to ensure that the lumen is adequate and open and to aspirate air distending the stomach. Two fine stay sutures on the distal esophageal opening allow gentle traction for dissection. The extent of distal mobilization should be minimized to avoid damaging vagal branches and the segmental blood supply. However, distal mobilization should be undertaken if it is necessary to ensure a primary anastomosis. Identification of the

Figure 67–9 Extrapleural dissection is facilitated by using moistened tissue applicators or pledgets to push the parietal pleura away from the chest wall and subsequently away from the posterior mediastinum.

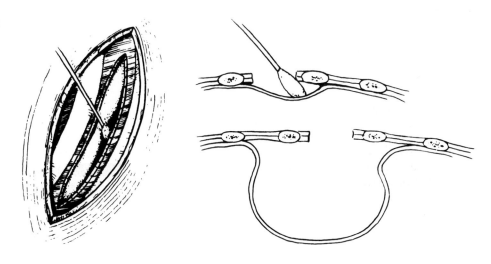

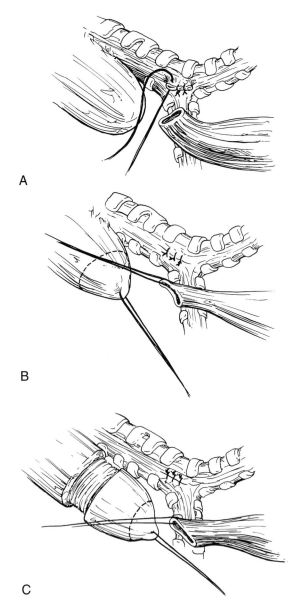

A

B

C

proximal esophageal pouch can be facilitated if the anesthesiologist gently pushes on the suction catheter, which is passed through the mouth into the pouch. A traction suture can be placed through the tip of the pouch, and even through the suction catheter, to assist in proximal dissection and avoid the trauma caused by repeatedly applying forceps to the proximal pouch. Mobilization of the upper pouch should be sufficient to bring the upper pouch down to the distal esophageal segment. This usually necessitates dissection up to the thoracic inlet. Extensive circumferential dissection of the proximal pouch also allows for identification of an undiagnosed proximal TEF (1.4% of cases). Because the cervical

blood supply to the proximal part of the esophagus is excellent, this type of extensive dissection does not run a risk for ischemic injury. Great care must be taken during the dissection between the esophagus and the membranous trachea, however, to avoid inadvertently opening the trachea. Unfortunately, the more extensive the proximal dissection, the greater the likelihood of disturbance to the vagal branches.

The tip of the upper esophageal pouch is excised at its lowest point to a diameter corresponding to the distal esophageal lumen. Traction sutures are placed at the corners, and an end-to-end anastomosis is begun by placing interrupted 5-0 or 6-0 sutures in the back wall with the knots tied on the inside of the lumen; great care should be taken to include full-thickness esophageal wall, including the mucosa and muscularis (Fig. 67-11). The upper pouch mucosa often retracts and can easily be missed if the surgeon is not vigilant. Unless the two ends of the esophagus are very close, it is best to insert the entire back row of sutures before tying them. A small feeding tube can then be passed and advanced across the anastomosis

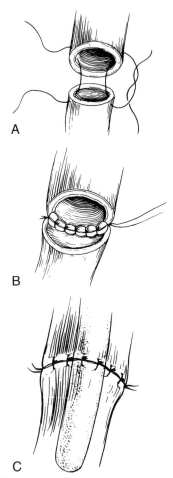

A

B

C

into the stomach to ensure distal esophageal patency and the potential for early postoperative enteral feeding if desired.[175,230,262] The anterior layer of the anastomosis is then completed over the tube, with the knots tied on the outside. The effect of the type of suture material used in the esophageal anastomosis on subsequent stricture formation has been a point of debate. In a review of patients in whom anastomotic strictures developed, Chittmittrapap et al.[39] reported a statistically significant increased rate of stricture when braided silk was used versus polypropylene or polyglycolic acid suture.

Once the anastomosis is complete, the position of the tube should be confirmed if it is to remain in place for postoperative gastric decompression and feeding. A chest tube or closed suction drain is usually placed in the retropleural space and secured to the lateral chest wall by a loose absorbable suture. The drain should be placed away from the anastomosis. Some surgeons leave no chest tube or drain in the chest after a retropleural dissection.[196]

In infants with EA and distal TEF, another technique for handling the fistula and uniting the esophageal ends is the end-to-side anastomosis developed by Sulamaa et al.[260] and championed by Duhamel and others.[64,198,275] With this technique, a single ligature is used to ligate the fistula; the upper pouch is mobilized down to the lower esophageal segment, and a wide, oblique end-to-side anastomosis is performed. Because of concern for recurrent TEF formation, this method has not been widely accepted. However, in a series of 68 infants treated with this technique, Touloukian et al.[275] reported a TEF recurrence rate of 7%, a rate similar to or lower than that seen in large series of end-to-end reconstructions. In addition, the rate of other complications, such as stricture (5%), anastomotic leak (8%), and gastroesophageal reflux (GER) (6%), was lower than in most other series using end-to-end esophageal reconstruction.

In recent years, as pediatric minimally invasive endosurgical techniques have improved, a number of surgeons have developed and advocated thoracoscopic repair of EA-TEF.[13,217,218] This technique typically uses three 2.5- to 5-mm transpleural access trocars, an angled telescope, a video camera, and small-diameter (2.5 to 5 mm) instruments to identify and ligate the TEF, mobilize the proximal esophageal pouch, and perform an end-to-end esophagoesophagostomy in a fashion that is similar to the open thoracotomy approach (Fig. 67-12). To date, several small series of infants who underwent thoracoscopic EA-TEF repair have been published, and a number of pediatric surgeons worldwide have used this approach.[13,217,218] Advocates of this approach have suggested that its benefits include superior visualization, improved cosmesis, and elimination of the morbidity of neonatal thoracotomy, including scoliosis, winged scapula, chronic pain, shoulder weakness, chest wall asymmetry, and maldevelopment. However, the thoracoscopic EA-TEF repair is technically demanding and requires advanced endosurgical skills. The thoracoscopic end-to-end esophageal anastomosis is challenging because of limited working space, lack of articulation at the end of the instruments (the needle driver in particular), and the necessity of tying sutures under tension. The limited published results of endosurgical repair of EA-TEF to date suggest the following: 2- to 4-hour operative times, 30% to 50% esophageal stenosis rates, 12% to 15% leak rates, and 30% to 50% postoperative GER rates requiring fundoplication.[13,218] As pediatric endosurgical skills improve and technology advances to allow for more precise esophageal anastomosis techniques, thoracoscopic EA-TEF repair may well become the standard surgical approach. However, at present, clear outcome benefits of this newer access approach to the posterior mediastinum over the tradiional thoracotomy have not been determined.

Particular attention must be given to infants with EA and a large distal TEF with severe respiratory distress syndrome. Under these circumstances, preoperative endotracheal intubation is often necessary. However, high-pressure ventilation may worsen lung ventilation and abdominal distention as inspired air is diverted through the TEF into the stomach, thus exacerbating respiratory compromise. Affected infants may require emergency surgical intervention to stabilize the pulmonary status and avoid gastric perforation, which is typically fatal in these circumstances.

Several operative approaches have been described to manage this problem, including gastric division,[210] banding of the gastroesophageal junction,[147] and positioning the tip of the endotracheal tube below the fistulous orifice.[221] Bronchoscopic placement of a Fogarty balloon catheter through the fistula has been successfully used to ablate the flow of ventilated air through the fistula.[80] This approach may be used to stabilize a rapidly deteriorating infant; however, concern has been raised about potential technical difficulties with this approach and problems with injury to the distal end of the esophagus in which the balloon is inflated.[268] Emergency gastrostomy to decompress the air-filled stomach and small bowel has also been used in this situation. This approach, however, places the infant at risk for pulmonary collapse because each ventilator breath volume bypasses the lung by preferentially passing through the TEF and escaping via the low-resistance gastrostomy tube. The use of a gastrostomy tube with an underwater seal may increase air resistance and decrease runoff through the fistula.

We, as well as Templeton et al.[268] and Spitz,[249] recommend early thoracotomy and fistula division in an infant with severe respiratory distress syndrome who requires high-pressure ventilation; we believe that these techniques provide the most expeditious and effective approach to improving pulmonary failure. In many circumstances, the infant remarkably improves after emergency fistula ligation; this improved condition allows primary repair of the esophagus and thus eliminates the need for a second operation.

Long-Gap Esophageal Atresia

Occasionally in infants with EA-TEF and usually in infants with isolated EA, the upper pouch is high and the distance between the upper and lower esophageal segments limits the ability to easily complete a tension-free, end-to-end esophagoesophagostomy. Although much has been said and written about the subject, there is no precise definition

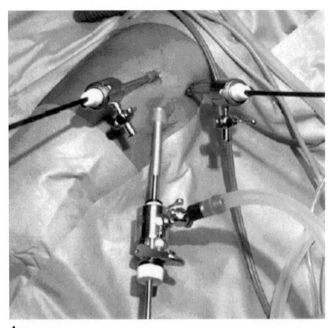

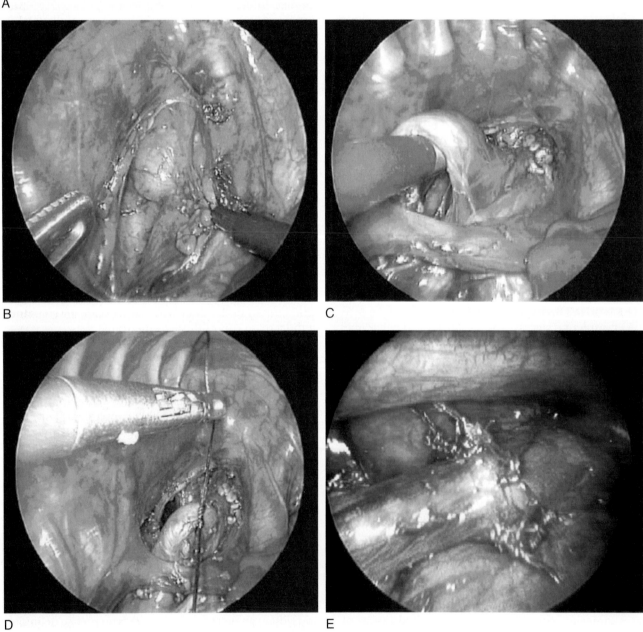

Figure 67–12 Thoracoscopic repair of esophageal atresia with a distal tracheoesophageal stricture. *A,* Position of the trocars, a 6-mm trocar for the telescope and two 4-mm trocars for instruments. *B,* The posterior pleura has been incised and the upper pouch is being mobilized. *C,* The distal fistula has been dissected free with the azygos vein left intact. *D,* Fistula being ligated close to the trachea. *E,* Completed end-to-end esophagoesphagostomy. (From Bax KMA, Van der Zee DC: Feasibility of thoracoscopic repair of esophageal atresia with distal fistula. J Pediatr Surg 2002;37:192.)

A

B

C

D

E

of "long-gap" EA. What is amenable to primary anastomosis by some surgeons may be considered "long gap," "very long gap," or "ultralong gap" by others. In addition, measurement of gap length can be biased by the method used to measure the distance between the proximal and distal ends of the esophagus. Some reports describe preoperative measurement of the gap by inserting a radiopaque tube or bougie into the upper pouch and placing contrast or a flexible endoscope into the distal pouch through a previously placed gastrostomy tube.[33] Other definitions of gap length are based on intraoperative measurements obtained before or after mobilization of the proximal pouch and, on occasion, the proximal and distal pouches. These variations on the method of determining gap length contribute to the confusion and debate about how long is long.[45]

In the case of isolated EA, in which a "long gap" is expected, most pediatric surgeons would proceed with the operative placement of a gastrostomy tube, a period of observation, and an attempted delayed primary repair (Fig. 67-13). It is well documented that during the first several months of life, the gap between the two ends of the esophagus tends to lessen because of spontaneous growth, which makes primary repair more feasible.[68,206] In addition, many preoperative mechanical techniques have been described as a means to facilitate narrowing of the esophageal gap. The most commonly used method is that of upper pouch bougienage, first described by Howard

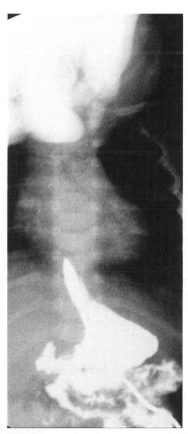

Figure 67–13 Isolated esophageal atresia with a long gap is shown by upper esophageal pouch contrast, together with injection of contrast through a gastrostomy tube to fill the stomach and distal esophageal segment.

and Myers[114] in 1965, in which a weighted bougie is passed through the mouth into the upper pouch, with forward pressure applied daily or twice daily for 6 to 12 weeks before attempting delayed primary repair.[168] The use of preoperative upper and lower pouch bougienage to decrease gap length has also been described.[249] In 1975, Hendren and Hale[103,104] reported using an electromagnetic field to pull together metallic "bullets" placed in the two ends of the esophagus in order to shorten the gap.

Various innovative operative techniques designed to narrow the long gap before attempted surgical esophageal anastomosis have been advocated. In 1971, Rehbein and Schweder[212] described the use of a nylon thread bridging the gap between the two ends of the esophagus and attached to silver olives[249] residing within each lumen. The olives were pushed toward each over time until the two ends of the esophagus pressed together and created a fistula. Shafer and David[229] used a similar technique to create a fistula between the two ends of the esophagus by simply connecting the two ends of the mobilized esophagus with a bridging silk suture. Another method that facilitates esophageal lengthening is a multistaged, extrathoracic elongation technique in which the upper part of the esophagus is mobilized and initially brought out as an end cervical esophagostomy. Every 2 to 3 weeks, the esophagus and its cutaneous stoma are surgically mobilized and translocated down the anterior chest wall until enough length is achieved to perform an end-to-end esophageal anastomosis.[127,128]

More recently, Foker has described a novel technique in which traction sutures on both the proximal and distal esophageal pouches exit through the chest wall and are serially pulled in opposite directions until the pouches approximate (Fig. 67-14). The external traction technique is reported to expedite approximation of the pouches, thus allowing for earlier primary repair (10 to 14 days).[4,82]

In addition to preoperative attempts to elongate the esophagus, many intraoperative techniques have been used to establish a primary esophageal anastomosis, either at an initial operation in the newborn period or at the time of a delayed operation after the elongation methods previously described have been used. Livaditis et al.[157,159] described the use of a circular myotomy of the upper part of the esophagus to decrease the tension on an end-to-end esophageal anastomosis in a piglet model of EA and, in 1973, reported the clinical use of this technique to lengthen the upper esophageal segment in order to allow for a primary anastomosis in an infant with long-gap EA (see Fig. 67-10).[158] Since that time, proximal esophageal circular myotomy to lengthen the upper esophageal pouch and achieve a primary anastomosis in long-gap EA has been widely used. The use of balloon catheters inflated in the upper esophageal pouch to facilitate mobilization and subsequent circular myotomy seems to be a useful modification of this method.[55,73,152,226] We have occasionally made an additional right cervical incision to mobilize the upper esophageal pouch up and out of the neck and perform a more proximal second or third circular myotomy.[45]

However, complications of circular myotomy have been described and have created a debate among surgeons regarding its safety. Complications include esophageal

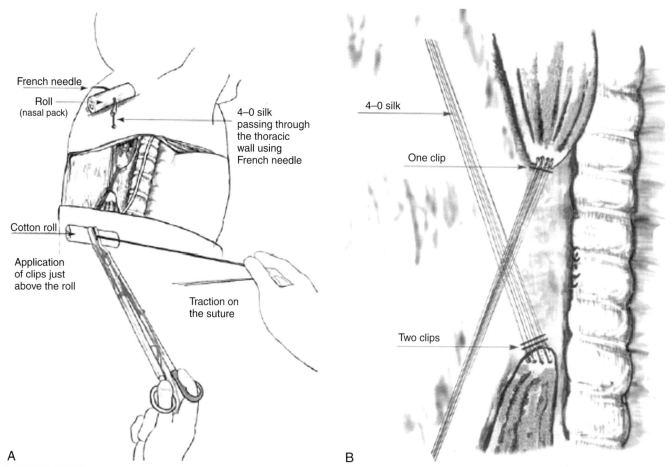

Figure 67–14 Foker technique for lengthening the upper and lower esophageal pouches by external traction sutures. *A,* External view of crossed traction sutures and bolsters. *B,* Internal view. (From Foker JE, Linden BC, Boyle EM Jr, et al: Development of a true primary repair for the full spectrum of esophageal atresia. Ann Surg 1997;226:533.)

leak, impaction of food particles in the myotomized segment,[241] and mild ballooning of the myotomized segment. Severe ballooning resulting in an esophageal pseudodiverticulum has been reported to be a potentially serious complication in only a few patients; we recently saw this effect in one of our patients with isolated long-gap EA. Several reports have noted the formation of a pseudodiverticulum with a distal anastomotic stricture, as might be expected.[73,191,241] If the stricture is not treated, the pseudodiverticulum can enlarge so much that it causes complications such as dysphagia and life-threatening respiratory obstruction.[191]

In addition to the formation of a pseudodiverticulum, circular myotomy may also worsen esophageal dysmotility, which can be expected in any infant with EA.[65,190,236,296] However, this issue has been a point of debate, with various investigators arguing for[237,241,266] and against[150,261] the procedure. Several reports have suggested the use of a distal esophageal pouch circular myotomy in addition to proximal myotomy to achieve a primary esophageal anastomosis.[90,144] Many technical modifications have been suggested to minimize the risk for potential serious complications from circular myotomy. The use of a spiral upper pouch myotomy with oblique suture closure of the muscular layer has been advocated as a technique that

minimizes the chance of diverticulum formation and, theoretically, improves motility.[126,216] Another modification of the esophageal myotomy is circumferential incision of the upper pouch muscle layer by means of short horizontal myotomies placed in rows so that when pulled distally, the upper pouch lengthens and narrows. This technique allows a better fit for the smaller distal esophageal segment.[154]

Another method used to elongate the upper pouch involves the creation of a full-thickness anterior flap of the upper pouch wall as described by Gough; when folded distally, the flap can be rolled into a tube and attached to the lower esophageal segment.[94] In 1989, Bar-Maor et al.[11] emphasized the technical details of this method to elongate the upper pouch. Davenport and Bianchi[53] reported good follow-up results in 25 infants with EA treated by this method over a 5-year period. Variations of this technique have been described and consist of the creation of a 5-mm posterior flap[233] or anterior esophageal flap,[239] followed by an end-to-end oblique anastomosis with a spatulated distal esophagus.

At the time of attempted initial or delayed primary repair, the esophageal segments sometimes do not reach together even though one or more of the methods just presented have been tried. Several additional techniques have been described to facilitate an esophageal anastomosis. Despite the long-held opinion that the blood supply to the distal end of the esophagus is tenuous and may be compromised by mobilization, many surgeons have found that the distal esophagus can be, and often is, mobilized to facilitate a primary anastomosis.[149] We have successfully achieved primary end-to-end esophageal anastomosis by completely mobilizing the distal esophagus down to and even through the esophageal hiatus of the diaphragm. With this approach, some of the fundus of the stomach can be brought up into the chest to facilitate anastomosis.[45]

Taking this concept further, Schärli described a combined abdominal and thoracic procedure in which distal esophageal elongation was achieved by ligation and division of the left gastric artery, transverse or diagonal division of the lesser curvature of the stomach, and mobilization of the gastric cardia and upper fundus into the chest to achieve primary esophageal anastomosis.[77,225] A partial fundoplication is recommended to treat the anticipated GER. Not surprisingly, postoperative GER has been reported to be a significant problem after this procedure.[284] By use of a similar approach, a Collis gastroplasty with Nissen fundoplication has also been described as a means of lengthening the distal end of the esophagus to avoid esophageal replacement.[75,122]

In addition to the surgical techniques used to facilitate saving the native esophagus as the conduit of choice for the repair of long-gap EA, the use of postoperative head flexion, paralysis, and mechanical ventilatory support has been strongly advocated by some to minimize the risk for anastomotic disruption when the esophageal anastomosis is under substantial tension.[5,166,249,253]

The rationale for this approach is the prevention of disruptive force at the anastomotic site by flexion of the neck and paralysis of the striated muscles in the proximal part of the esophagus.[164,249]

Esophageal Replacement

For an extensive discussion of esophageal replacement see Chapter 69. Despite the many methods and innovations developed to achieve esophageal continuity in infants with EA, the esophagus may need to be replaced if these methods fail. Numerous operative procedures have been described for esophageal replacement in infants with EA, as well as children with caustic injury.

The choice of esophageal substitute depends on many factors. Colon replacement, or ileocolon, has been widely practiced for many years as a method of esophageal replacement.[74,84,203,292] Either the right or left colon can be placed substernally or behind the hilum of the lung on the right or left side. Vagotomy and a gastric drainage procedure are typically performed to avoid stricture or ulceration at the cologastric anastomosis. Several complications occur after colonic interposition, including cervical anastomotic leak (30% to 50% of cases), stricture, and intrathoracic redundant colon with stasis, gastric reflux, respiratory problems, and diarrhea. Some surgeons favor a reversed gastric tube as a substitute; in this procedure, a tubularized portion of the greater curvature is

brought up to the cervical esophagus in the substernal or retrohilar position.[23,69,204] Complications are similar to those described for colonic interposition. A modified gastric tube has also been described in which a portion of the greater curve is fashioned into a "free" tube graft based on the right gastroepiploic artery.[30] The jejunum has also been used for esophageal replacement both in a Roux-en-Y fashion and as a free graft with microvascular anastomosis.[52]

Gastric transposition has more recently become a well-established and successful esophageal substitute in infants with EA.[107,249,255] Spitz et al. have reported good to excellent outcomes in 90% of more than 173 (127 with EA) infants and children in whom this method of replacement was used.[255] The survival rate was 94.8%, the incidence of anastomotic leak was 12%, the incidence of strictures requiring dilation was 19.6%, and there was no deterioration in function over a 10-year follow-up.[257]

Esophageal Atresia Without Tracheoesophageal Fistula

Infants born with isolated EA have almost no esophagus in their thorax. It is important to be aware of this fact in order to institute an appropriate treatment plan and avoid fruitless exploratory thoracotomy. The preoperative and operative treatment of this lesion has been discussed extensively in the previous section of this chapter on long-gap EA. In a review of 69 infants with isolated EA treated over a period of 50 years, Ein and Shandling[67] reported a 52% incidence of prematurity, a 10% to 20% incidence of Down's syndrome, and a 10% incidence of duodenal atresia; all these rates are higher than typically reported in patients with EA-TEF.

The clinical manifestations of an infant with isolated EA are similar to those of an infant with EA-TEF in terms of inability to swallow; in the former, however, the abdomen is typically scaphoid, and plain radiographs of the abdomen show no air in the gastrointestinal tract. A gastrostomy tube should be placed within the first 24 to 48 hours of life, and delayed primary repair using the various methods previously discussed should be attempted. Placement of the gastrostomy tube allows the early institution of enteral feedings, which leads to subsequent enlargement of the diminutive stomach (see Fig. 67-13). Enlargement permits the stomach to be used as an esophageal substitute if necessary. At the time of placement, a contrast imaging study can be performed to evaluate the unusual possibility of an occluded, but present distal esophageal fistula to the trachea, which might suggest the potential for early esophageal repair.[93,193] A period of observation and enteral nutritional support is instituted with or without daily upper pouch bougienage. Over an 8- to 12-week period, the process of esophageal elongation can be monitored by imaging studies that use contrast material, metallic probes, or bougies placed in the upper and lower esophageal segments.

When no further elongation progress is evident or when the two ends of the esophagus can be brought to close proximity, surgery is performed. Thoracotomy with retropleural dissection and mobilization of the proximal and distal esophageal segments is done and primary anastomosis is attempted. If these efforts do not allow primary anastomosis, circular myotomy, hiatal mobilization, proximal pouch flap esophagoplasty, or the addition of an abdominal approach to mobilize some or all of the stomach to pull it up into the chest (or neck) can be undertaken. When the two ends of the esophagus are clearly too distant for primary esophageal anastomosis despite preoperative attempts at elongation, we have proceeded with a primary gastric transposition to the cervical esophagus, typically without a thoracotomy. In these latter circumstances, some surgeons proceed to a cervical esophagostomy, preferably on the left side, with plans for a future esophageal replacement procedure. Postoperative complications are similar to those in infants with repaired EA-TEF (see the later section "Outcomes"); these adverse effects primarily include anastomotic leak and stricture, dysphagia, and GER. Perhaps surprisingly, infants with EA but without TEF have been reported to have significant tracheomalacia. This finding is consistent with reports that tracheobronchial anomalies occur in association with EA.[67,281]

Isolated (H-Type) Tracheoesophageal Fistula

Congenital TEF without EA or the "H" type of TEF (perhaps more anatomically accurately called the "N" type) occurs in approximately 4% of esophageal anomalies reported. This anomaly is usually manifested in the first few days of life when the neonate chokes on attempting to feed or has unexplained cyanotic spells.[120] When the infant is coughing or crying, intermittent abdominal distention can occur as air passes through the fistula into the stomach. Older infants and children are more likely to have recurrent bouts of pneumonia, typically involving the right upper lobe. A high index of suspicion is necessary in considering this diagnosis.

The diagnosis of isolated TEF can be suspected if plain radiographs of the chest show evidence of aspiration pneumonitis with gastric distention. A reliable way to establish the diagnosis is by tube video esophagography performed while the infant is prone; a small nasogastric tube is passed into the distal end of the esophagus, and contrast medium is gradually injected as the tube is slowly withdrawn. The radiologist performing the study must be familiar with this diagnostic approach because more than 50% of H-type fistulas may be missed on routine esophageal contrast swallow studies (see Fig. 67-6). Bronchoscopy with esophagoscopy can typically confirm the diagnosis and, if done immediately before surgery to divide the fistula, allows for the passage of a fine catheter or guidewire through the fistula to aid in subsequent identification at surgical exploration.[87]

Most isolated TEFs can be successfully divided through a cervical approach.[134] The site of a right-sided, low cervical incision is determined, and the infant is placed with the head extended and turned to the left. The sternocleidomastoid muscle is retracted posteriorly, with division of the sternal head if necessary; dissection then proceeds medially to the carotid sheath. Identification of the trachea and esophagus is facilitated by palpating the endotracheal and nasogastric tubes. Division of the inferior

thyroid artery and middle thyroid vein may be necessary to expose the plane between the trachea and esophagus. The recurrent laryngeal nerve must be identified and preserved. Identification of the fistula is facilitated by encircling the esophagus with slings, but it is important to be aware that the contralateral recurrent laryngeal nerve can be damaged during this maneuver. Once the fistula is identified (it is often higher than expected), traction stitches should be placed close to the esophagus through the superior and inferior extent of the fistula to avoid rotation of the esophagus after division of the fistula. On the tracheal side, 5-0 polypropylene or silk sutures are placed at the superior and inferior limits of the fistula. The fistula is now divided close to the esophagus, and interrupted 5-0 polypropylene or silk sutures are placed on the tracheal side to close the fistula. The esophageal end of the fistula is closed with interrupted fine silk or absorbable polyglycolic acid sutures (Fig. 67-15). Some surgeons advocate interposing muscle tissue between the two opposing suture lines to reduce the likelihood of recurrence of the fistula. A right thoracotomy is best used on the rare occasion when the fistula is located well within the thorax or when a recurrent fistula from a previous EA repair is being approached. Recently, a thoracoscopic approach to the repair of a thoracic isolated TEF has been reported.[2]

Postoperative complications include respiratory distress secondary to edema of the trachea or injury to the recurrent laryngeal nerves. The degree of preexisting lung disease and concerns about tracheal edema may warrant leaving the endotracheal tube in place for several days after the operation. Esophageal leak and recurrence of isolated TEF are rare.

Esophageal Atresia with an Upper Pouch Fistula

Several reports have cited varying incidences of a fistula between the upper esophageal pouch and the trachea. The exact incidence of this type of fistula has probably been underestimated because some initially unrecognized proximal pouch fistulas have been reported as recurrent TEFs after repair of EA with distal TEF[117] and some of these cases have been diagnosed as pure EA because the upper TEF was missed. There are two versions of this anomaly: (1) proximal pouch fistula in association with distal TEF (double fistula) (incidence, 1.4%) and (2) proximal pouch fistula without distal TEF (incidence, 0.8%). These incidences represent averages from several large reports. Although this type of fistula is rare, it must be identified and treated early so that ongoing pulmonary aspiration with recurrent pneumonia is avoided.

The diagnosis can be made by a preoperative proximal pouch contrast study, preferably performed by a skilled pediatric radiologist under optimum conditions in the radiology suite using fluoroscopy and video recording. This study usually shows a small upper pouch in addition to identifying the fistula. However, a frequent point of confusion during this study and in the interpretation of results is the occurrence of spillover of contrast from the pouch up into the larynx and down into the trachea. Because of the potential for inaccurate interpretation, some surgeons rely on preoperative bronchoscopy with

Figure 67–15 H-type tracheoesophageal fistula. *A,* Anatomic relationship between the fistula and the recurrent laryngeal nerve. *B,* After division, the fistula is closed by interrupted suture on both the trachea and esophagus.

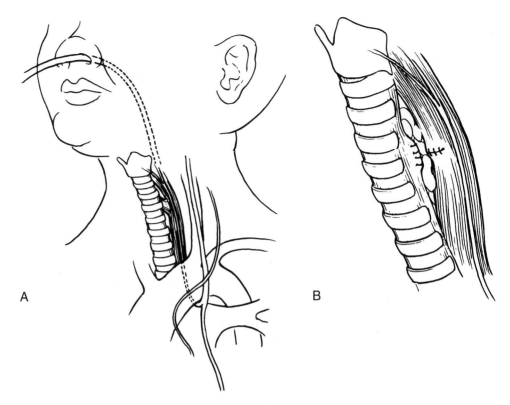

esophagoscopy to make or confirm the diagnosis of a proximal pouch fistula. Unfortunately, a small proximal fistula can also be missed when endoscopy is used. Another common approach to the diagnosis of this anomaly is complete mobilization of the upper pouch during repair of the EA in order to localize and repair an unsuspected upper pouch fistula. As with the other diagnostic methods mentioned, proximal pouch fistulas may also be unrecognized during surgical exploration, in part because of the extreme proximal nature of some of these fistulas. A proximal pouch fistula should be suspected and specifically looked for if the upper pouch is unusually narrow or short at the time of preoperative imaging studies or at surgical exploration because such findings suggest decompression through a fistula.

Once identified, a proximal fistula should be surgically ligated and divided as with a distal TEF. If an upper pouch fistula is diagnosed after the initial repair of EA with or without distal TEF, a cervical approach can often be used as previously described for an H-type TEF.

OUTCOMES

Survival rates for infants who have EA with or without TEF have improved dramatically in the past 50 years. Recent reviews reported 85% to 95% overall survival as compared with rates less than 40% before the 1950s.[40,59,62,135,189,232,273] However, subsets of infants with EA still have a worse prognosis. Waterston's risk classification scheme historically helped identify infants with EA who were at particular risk for a poor outcome and as such helped direct treatment options.[293] In recent years, other risk

classification schemes have been proposed. Infants with EA who appear to be at increased risk for death and long-term morbidity include those with (1) lower birth weight (<1500 g)/prematurity,[59,249] (2) major CHD,[40,148,273] (3) severe associated anomalies and ventilator dependency,[201] and (4) a long gap length between the two ends of esophagus.[29]

COMPLICATIONS

Despite excellent long-term survival for infants with EA, many significant complications can occur. Complications can generally be classified as early (including anastomotic leak, anastomotic stricture, and recurrent tracheoesophageal stricture) and late (including GER, tracheomalacia, and disordered esophageal peristalsis).

Early Complications

Anastomotic Leak

Anastomotic leak at the esophagoesophagostomy occurs in approximately 14% to 16% of patients with EA. Most leaks are clinically insignificant and can be managed with adequate drainage and nutritional support (Fig. 67-16). When a retropleural approach is undertaken and a patent mediastinal drain is in place, up to 95% of anastomotic leaks close spontaneously.[169] Even when transthoracic repair is followed by disruption and the pleural space is contaminated, adequate drainage can usually be achieved. This in turn allows spontaneous closure of the leak.

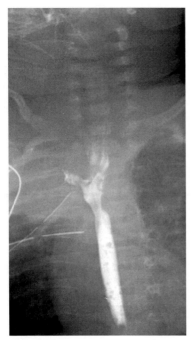

Figure 67–16 Anastomotic leak at the esophagoesophagostomy. The leak is contained and adequately drained. Right upper lobe atelectasis is common.

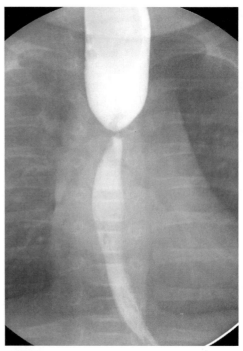

Figure 67–17 Barium esophagogram showing an anastomotic stricture.

Breakdown of the anastomosis is frequently followed by the formation of a stricture at the site of the leak and is sometimes associated with a recurrent TEF. Major disruptions of the esophageal anastomosis account for only 3% to 5% of postoperative leaks and are typically recognized early (24 to 48 hours) after the initial repair. The infant frequently deteriorates from tension pneumothorax or mediastinitis uncontrolled by drainage and antibiotics. Factors that probably contribute to anastomotic leak include poor surgical technique, ischemia of the esophageal ends, use of myotomy, and excessive tension at the anastomotic site.[288,300] In this critical setting, reoperation for control of sepsis with adequate drainage and attempted repair of the anastomotic leak are warranted. A pleural or pericardial patch, with or without an intercostal muscle flap buttress, may help secure anastomotic closure.[34,297] If the esophageal anastomosis is not repairable, cervical esophagostomy and delayed esophageal replacement may be required.

Esophageal Stricture

Esophageal stricture is a common complication of anastomosis of the esophagus in EA, but the reported incidence varies widely depending on the criteria used to define a stricture. In recent large series, stricture requiring dilatation is reported to occur in as many as 80% of patients.[10,72,135,253,273] Spitz and Hitchcock[250] proposed that stricture be defined as the presence of symptoms (dysphagia and recurrent respiratory problems from aspiration or foreign body obstruction) and narrowing noted on endoscopy or contrast esophagography (Fig. 67-17). Factors that have been implicated in the pathogenesis of

esophageal stricture include poor anastomotic technique (excessive tension, two-layered anastomosis, silk suture material), ischemia at the ends of the esophagus, GER, and anastomotic leak. Up to 13% of infants and children will have an esophageal foreign body after repair of EA with or without TEF.[303]

Clinically significant narrowing at the site of the esophageal anastomosis is traditionally treated by dilation performed via antegrade or retrograde bougienage. We have found that passing Savory-type dilators prograde over a guidewire has many advantages: this method allows fluoroscopic assessment during sequential dilations, enables the use of contrast injection during the dilation session, and typically eliminates the need for rigid esophagoscopy. The use of Gruntzig-type balloon catheters to dilate esophageal strictures, including those occurring after repair of EA, has recently been reported. This technique has the theoretical advantage of producing a uniform and radial force at the site of the stricture rather than the shearing axial force applied with traditional bougienage.[3,92,220,264] Many strictures respond to one to three dilatations (53%) in the first months after esophageal repair. However, a recalcitrant stricture resistant to repeated dilations will require resection and reanastomosis or even esophageal replacement. It is crucial to determine whether the esophageal stricture is associated with GER by investigation with contrast esophagography, endoscopy, pH monitoring, or any combination of these studies. Many strictures do not respond to dilation attempts if severe GER continues to bathe the stricture with acid.[220] The stricture is often successfully treated with dilations after an antireflux operation.

Recurrent Tracheoesophageal Fistula

Recurrent TEF occurs in 3% to 14% of patients after initial operative division or ligation.[71,72,135,163,169,171,275] Recurrent TEF has been attributed to anastomotic leak with local inflammation and erosion through the previous site of TEF repair. Techniques that have minimized the likelihood of recurrent TEF include the use of a pleural flap,[72] vascularized pericardial flap,[24,44,298] and azygos vein flap[136] interposed between the esophageal and tracheal suture lines. Although recurrent TEF typically occurs in the early postoperative period, it may not be recognized for months to years. Symptoms can be typical of those seen with a congenital H-type TEF, including coughing and choking or cyanosis with feedings; however, less obvious symptoms such as recurrent pulmonary infections are more common. The diagnosis may be suggested by an air-filled esophagus on plain radiographs of the chest. Routine contrast swallow studies will miss as many as 50% of recurrent fistulas. As with a congenital H-type fistula, esophagography performed in the prone position under video fluoroscopy is a reliable method of establishing the diagnosis. Bronchoscopy with cannulation of the fistula with a 2- to 3-French catheter is also a reliable diagnostic approach and is invaluable in locating the fistula during the operative procedure. A recurrent TEF rarely closes spontaneously and typically requires surgical repair. Thoracotomy with fistula ligation and division is the operation of choice. To minimize the chance of recurrent fistulization, which has been reported in 10% to 20% of patients with a first-time TEF recurrence, pleura, intercostal muscle, or pericardium should be interposed between the esophagus and trachea.[251] Endoscopic eradication of TEF by means of various chemicals or diathermy has been reported.[88,202,211] Fibrin glue has recently been successfully used for this purpose in a single case report[99]; however, others continue to report failure with chemical techniques.[27]

Late Complications

Gastroesophageal Reflux Disease

Gastroesophageal reflux disease (GERD) in infants and children with repaired EA is common, and the incidence seems to be increasing as suspicion and diagnostic investigation have become more common. In addition, the trend to preserve the native esophagus with many of the techniques described earlier in this chapter also promotes GERD. The magnitude of the problem is reflected in the findings that GERD occurs in 30% to 70% of patients after repair of EA.[10,72,135,155,169,276,298] The cause of GER in this group of infants probably relates to shortening of the intra-abdominal portion of the esophagus because of anastomotic tension or esophageal motor dysfunction, either acquired as a result of operative manipulation or intrinsic to the congenital anomaly itself.[8,119,276] The consequences of GERD are then magnified by the poor or absent esophageal peristaltic pump, thus exposing the esophagus to prolonged acid contact. Esophagitis is frequently observed in older children and adolescents on long-term follow-up of patients with EA.[43,195,270,276,277] In several recent long-term follow-up studies, it appears that adults who had EA repaired as infants continue to be at risk for GERD and its complications,[58,140] including an apparent increased risk for the development of Barrett's esophagus, perhaps as high as 9%.[58,140] One case of esophageal adenocarcinoma was reported in a 20-year-old patient in whom a TEF had been repaired during infancy.[1]

The diagnosis of pathologic GERD is suspected in patients with symptoms of vomiting, dysphagia, and recurrent anastomotic stenosis, which is occasionally associated with the impaction of a foreign body or food bolus. In addition, respiratory symptoms such as stridor, cyanotic spells, recurrent pneumonia, and reactive airways disease may indicate GERD rather than other conditions such as tracheomalacia.

The diagnosis of pathologic GERD in infants and children after repair of EA is suggested by upper gastrointestinal contrast study. Twenty-four-hour pH probe data, though not as standardized for children as they are for adults, typically document pathologic reflux.[276] Extensive esophageal manometric studies have consistently documented abnormal esophageal peristalsis and decreased lower esophageal sphincter pressures after EA repair; as a result, this test is probably not helpful in diagnosing GERD.[272]

In infants and children with pathologic GER, aggressive medical management typically consists of thickening of feedings, positioning of the infant in a prone or upright posture, and administration of acid reduction agents such as histamine-2 blockers (e.g., cimetidine or ranitidine), proton pump inhibitors (e.g., omeprazole), and prokinetic agents (e.g., metoclopramide). However, 45% to 75% of these infants ultimately undergo antireflux operations because of failed medical management, chronic pulmonary infection, refractory anastomotic stricture, or the development of a distal esophageal stricture.[72,169,298] The choice of antireflux operation is controversial. The Nissen fundoplication has typically been considered the best option.[17,83,119,252] However, debilitating dysphagia and significant complications, including wrap disruption and recurrent GERD in a third of patients, have been frequent after the 360-degree wrap.[46,153,169,298] Because of the generally poor results with Nissen fundoplication in this setting, some surgeons have been using the anterior Thal partial-wrap fundoplication in these patients. However, as other surgeons have modified the Nissen fundoplication to create a very short, floppy wrap (1.0 to 1.5 cm over a large dilator), this operation continues to be commonly used.[17] In addition, because the esophagus is frequently shortened in the setting of repair of EA, some surgeons have used the Collis-Nissen fundoplication to gain intraesophageal length.[122]

Tracheomalacia

Substantial respiratory symptoms occurring after repair of EA-TEF can be due to tracheomalacia. Tracheomalacia has been noted to affect up to 75% of pathologic specimens from patients suffering from EA-TEF; however, the condition is symptomatic in approximately 10% to 25% of infants after repair of EA-TEF, approximately half of whom require surgical correction.[72,79,137,187] It is often difficult to clinically distinguish these symptoms from those of recurrent TEF, anastomotic leak, or GER.[56] Tracheomalacia is defined as generalized or localized weakness of the trachea that allows the anterior and posterior tracheal walls to come together during expiration or coughing. In infants with associated TEF, structural anomalies of the trachea were identified in 75% of 40 infants at autopsy, thus suggesting that embryologic events leading to TEF may contribute to the development of tracheomalacia.[291] The cartilage was shorter than normal and thereby failed to provide the support necessary to maintain a patent airway.[291] In infants, the trachea may also be easily compressed between the aorta anteriorly and the often dilated upper esophagus posteriorly after repair of EA-TEF; such compression has been considered a significant contributor to the pathophysiology of tracheomalacia. Kimura et al.[129] studied tracheomalacia with cine computed tomography and suggested that the primary cause of tracheomalacia is related to intrinsic tracheal weakness. One series showed no evidence of tracheomalacia in infants with EA alone, which suggests that EA-tracheomalacia has a separate pathogenesis.[215] This has been confirmed in the Adriamycin-induced EA-TEF rat model and may also provide more insight into the pathogenesis of the anomaly. The level of tracheal collapse is usually in the region of or just above the original site of the TEF in the distal third of the trachea, generally at the level of the aortic arch.

The clinical manifestations of tracheomalacia are broad and range from a "brassy" or "barking" cough in mild cases to recurrent pneumonia or acute, life-threatening apneic spells. Infants with tracheomalacia are often reluctant to feed because of difficulty breathing during feeding or cyanotic attacks. These symptoms usually appear when the infant is a few months of age.[124] Life-threatening apneic spells were noted in 27 of 32 children with tracheomalacia described by Filler et al. in 1992.[78] These spells occur during or within 5 to 10 minutes of a meal and are characterized by cyanosis progressing to apnea, bradycardia, and ultimately, cardiorespiratory arrest if not interrupted. The diagnosis is established by bronchoscopy with spontaneous ventilation, which reveals a slitlike lumen of the trachea at the involved area (Fig. 67-18).

Treatment of tracheomalacia remains controversial. Most infants with mild to moderate symptoms of tracheomalacia do not require operative intervention because the symptoms tend to improve with time. In infants with severe symptoms, including acute life-threatening events, the operative treatment of choice is aortopexy.[97,227,287,294] This operation is usually performed through a left anterolateral thoracotomy, and the ascending aorta and arch are sutured up to the posterior surface of the sternum. Lifting the aorta up in this fashion raises the anterior wall of the trachea and opens the tracheal lumen.[16,42,124] A proposed modification of this operation has been the use of a flap of pericardium based at the root of the aorta to be sutured to the sternum in cases in which the aortic arch would not reach the posterior aspect of the sternum without undue tension.[7,138] An anterior mediastinal

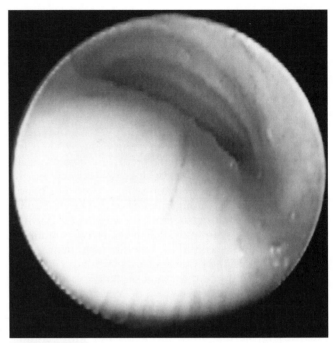

Figure 67–18 Tracheomalacia after repair of esophageal atresia–tracheoesophageal fistula. A bronchoscopic view of the tracheal lumen during spontaneous respirations shows almost complete collapse of the trachea during expiration.

approach via a low transverse cervical incision for aortopexy and tracheopexy has recently been advocated.[174] Many surgeons use intraoperative bronchoscopy to document the adequacy of aortopexy with regard to opening the tracheal lumen as sutures are being tied. Recently, the use of endosurgical thoracoscopic techniques to perform aortopexy has produced good results.[224]

Other surgical treatment options for tracheomalacia associated with EA have been suggested. The role of various stents in the treatment of tracheomalacia after repair of EA, though successful in case reports, has yet to be validated as a standard treatment method.[25,118,267,289] Filler et al.[78] recommend that an airway stent be considered for children in whom aortopexy fails to relieve tracheal collapse. Recently, glossopexy has been suggested as an early alternative to aortopexy to treat infants with suspected retrodisplacement of the tongue (glossoptosis).[49] Tracheostomy is a final treatment option.

Other Long-Term Quality-of-Life Issues

As previously discussed, the esophagus of an infant with EA has abnormal peristaltic activity that is secondary to the congenital defect itself, as well as secondary to operative repair of the lesion. The incidence of the problem approaches 75% to 100% in children and adults who have been studied with esophageal manometry. Dysphagia is worse after intestinal interposition for esophageal replacement. Occasional dysphagia has been reported to occur in as many as 50% to 90% of adults, with 30% having additional problems with choking.[20,37,137] This disorder is clinically significant in that it is responsible for many long-term symptoms after EA repair, including dysphagia, esophageal foreign body obstruction, GERD, and recurrent respiratory problems. Although these symptoms may improve with time, early problems with feeding intolerance and food bolus obstruction can lead to failure to thrive. Many children must eat slowly and be selective with food choices.

CONGENITAL STENOSIS OF THE ESOPHAGUS

True congenital esophageal stenosis (CES) is a rare condition that has historically been confused with esophageal strictures secondary to inflammation, especially GER. CES has been reported to occur once in every 25,000 to 50,000 births[182,283]; as of 2004, fewer than 600 cases have been described in the world literature. For unknown reasons, the incidence of CES seems to be higher in Japan than in other parts of the world.[121,183] The incidence of other anomalies associated with CES is reported to be 17% to 33%; these anomalies include EA with or without TEF; H-type TEF; cardiac anomalies; intestinal atresia; midgut malrotation; anorectal malformations; hypospadias; malformations of the head, face, and limbs; and chromosomal anomalies.[182] In addition, a recent report by Vasudevan et al. noted that 5% of their patients with tracheoesophageal anomalies had CES (three with tracheobronchial remnants), whereas Kawahara et al. have reported that 14% of their patients with EA had associated CES.[121,286]

Classification schemes for CES have been numerous and confusing, in part because of the difficulty in differentiating congenital from acquired lesions. The definition and classification proposed by Nihoul-Fekete et al.[182] are perhaps the most clear. CES is defined as an intrinsic stenosis of the esophagus, present at birth, that is caused by congenital malformation of esophageal wall architecture.[182] This classification delineates three forms of CES: (1) a membranous web or diaphragm, (2) fibromuscular thickening, and (3) stricture secondary to tracheobronchial remnants in the wall of the esophagus.

A congenital membranous web or diaphragm is reported as the rarest of the three forms of CES.[178] It has been considered to represent a missed form of EA[131] and may be analogous to membranes in other parts of the gastrointestinal tract. It is usually a partially obstructing lesion located in the middle or lower portions of the esophagus. The membrane is covered on both sides with squamous epithelium and often has an eccentric opening. Symptoms typically occur at several months of age as the infant begins consuming solid food.

The second type of CES has been called idiopathic muscular hypertrophy or fibromuscular stenosis and in some reports has been the most common form of CES.[182] Its histologic characteristics are submucosal proliferation of smooth muscle fibers and fibrous connective tissue with normal overlying squamous epithelium.[182] A resemblance to hypertrophic pyloric stenosis has been suggested,[182,271] but no clear embryologic or pathogenic factors explain these lesions.

CES caused by tracheobronchial remnants is described as the most common type of CES in some reports and is certainly the most described and understood of the three types of CES. It is believed that CES caused by tracheobronchial remnants occurs as part of a spectrum of anomalies, including EA-TEF, related to separation of the foregut from the respiratory tract around the 25th embryonic day.[275] Tracheobronchial tissue is believed to become sequestered in the wall of the esophagus and comes to reside in the typical distal location because of the faster growth rate of the esophagus than the tracheobronchial tree.

CES secondary to tracheobronchial remnants was first reported in 1936 by Frey and Dusche[85] in a 19-year-old woman who died with the diagnosis of achalasia.[275] In 1964, Holder et al.[112] noted three cases of distal esophageal stenosis in their review of 1058 infants with EA, TEF, or both. After several additional reports,[167,279] Spitz, in 1973, first demonstrated a clear congenital basis for this disorder.[247] As of 1991, fewer than 50 cases of CES caused by tracheobronchial remnants had been reported in the English and German language literature.[301] In addition, 71 cases of CES have been reported in the Japanese literature as of 1981[183]; 6 cases were reported in the Chinese literature (out of 76 total cases of CES in 1987).[156] An additional three cases of CES have recently been reported, one of each type described earlier.[208]

Diagnosis

Symptoms of CES usually begin in infancy with progressive dysphagia and vomiting, generally after the introduction of semisolid or solid foods around the age of 6 months. Some case reports, however, describe severe symptoms of regurgitation and respiratory distress in the newborn.[182] In some patients, a foreign body in the esophagus may be the first symptom noted.[21] The correct diagnosis is frequently difficult to establish. Contrast esophagography typically reveals an abrupt distal esophageal narrowing, most often interpreted as a stricture related to GER. Stenosis secondary to fibromuscular hypertrophy can result in a more tapered narrowing (Fig. 67-19). CES caused by webs or fibromuscular hypertrophy can be manifested as midesophageal or even upper esophageal stenosis.[95] Over time, the esophagus proximal to the stenosis can dilate, and contrast study results can be interpreted as achalasia.[181] Additional studies helpful in differentiating CES from achalasia and strictures caused by GER include esophageal manometry and pH monitoring. Esophagoscopy typically shows esophageal narrowing with normal-appearing mucosa at the level of the stenosis in cases of CES. Recently, high-frequency endoscopic ultrasonography has been reported to be helpful in the diagnosis of CES.[282]

Treatment

Treatment of CES should relieve the symptoms of stenosis and maintain the antireflux mechanism of the gastroesophageal junction. Bougienage has been successful in treating CES secondary to fibromuscular hypertrophy and, occasionally, esophageal webs. Antegrade and

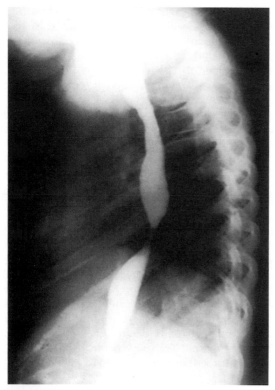

Figure 67–19 Barium esophagogram showing narrowing of the midesophagus as a result of congenital esophageal stenosis.

retrograde tapered dilators have been the traditional form of bougienage, but more recent use of hydrostatic balloon dilation has been successful.[6,181,182] A series of dilatations may be required for resolution of the stenosis. Membranous webs have sometimes been adequately treated with dilation, and one report described successful endoscopic excision of a congenital web.[208,231,286]

Most membranous webs and CES secondary to tracheobronchial remnants must be treated by surgical excision, either as the primary approach or after failed attempts at dilation.[6] It is important to clearly identify the location of the stenosis before surgery by contrast esophagography in order to plan the operative approach. A right thoracotomy is typically used for stenosis in the midesophagus and a left thoracotomy for stenosis in the lower part of the esophagus. An abdominal approach should be used for CES in the abdominal portion of the esophagus. At exploration, the extent of the stenosis can be difficult to determine; the use of a balloon catheter passed beyond the stenosis, inflated, and pulled back against the stenosis has been suggested as a helpful technique.[186] In most cases, the stenosis is less than 3 cm in length, and segmental resection and end-to-end esophageal anastomosis can be accomplished. Care should be taken to preserve the vagus nerves. In cases of long fibromuscular hypertrophy unresponsive to dilation, resection and esophageal replacement with the colon, stomach, or jejunum may be necessary. If the stenosis is near the gastroesophageal junction, most surgeons advocate segmental resection with esophageal anastomosis and an antireflux procedure to prevent postoperative reflux.

Modified Hill gastropexy and Nissen fundoplication, with or without pyloroplasty, have been most commonly used[182,186]; however, Collis gastroplasty in combination with Nissen fundoplication has been reported to be effective for managing esophageal shortening and postoperative GER.[6,32,121]

Results

Good long-term results have been reported for dilation and operative resection.[182] In patients who have undergone distal esophageal CES resection without an antireflux procedure, significant GER has developed and required a subsequent antireflux operation.[123] Reported complications from treatment by dilatation include esophageal leakage and failure of therapy. Complications of resection and anastomosis include esophageal leak with mediastinitis, which can be successfully treated by mediastinal drainage.[121,286]

LARYNGOTRACHEOESOPHAGEAL CLEFT

A laryngotracheoesophageal cleft (LTEC) is a rare congenital anomaly consisting of midline communication between the larynx, trachea, and esophagus. The malformation was possibly first described in 1792 by Richter in his doctoral thesis, in which he described an infant who choked and vomited upon feeding.[213] The infant died, but because no autopsy was performed, the diagnosis was unconfirmed. An infant with LTEC was next described in 1949 by Finlay.[81] In 1955, Pettersson[197] performed the first successful correction of a laryngotracheal cleft.

As with EA-TEF, the embryogenesis of LTEC is not completely understood. The long-held theory is that there is an arrest of the cranial extension of the tracheoesophageal septum that permits the persistence of an esophagotrachea.[22,109,242] More recent studies have suggested that as with TEF, initial normal development is followed by a far-reaching fusion of the trachea and esophagus.[188] Although no consistent pattern of inheritance has been seen, sporadic familial associations have occurred; LTEC is reported with the "G" syndrome and the Pallister-Hall syndrome.[96] The incidence of LTEC favors males by a ratio of 5:3.63.

Various associated congenital anomalies occur in the setting of LTEC, including gastrointestinal, genitourinary, and cardiac malformations.[63] EA with TEF occurs in 20% to 37% of patients with LTEC.[61,63,295] Other associated gastrointestinal malformations include anal defects (21%), anomalies of rotation and fixation (13%), and meconium ileus (8%).[63,280] Genitourinary anomalies occur with an incidence of 14% to 44% and include hypospadias, inguinal hernias, undescended testes, and renal agenesis.[63,280] Cardiovascular anomalies, identified in 16% to 33% of patients, include ventricular septal defects, coarctation of the aorta, and transposition of the great vessels.[63]

To more adequately delineate therapy, several classification schemes have been described. In reporting the first surgical repair in 1955, Pettersson described three types of clefts: type I, limited to the larynx and involving part or all of the cricoid plate; type II, extending beyond the cricoid lamina to the cervical trachea; and type III, involving the entire trachea down to the carina. In 1991, Ryan et al.[219] suggested a type IV in which the cleft extends beyond the carina to involve one or both mainstem bronchi.

Symptoms of LTEC vary depending on the extent of the cleft, but most patients immediately after birth exhibit respiratory distress aggravated by feeding. Additional symptoms can include a characteristic toneless or hoarse cry, cyanosis, choking, increased secretions, and recurrent aspiration pneumonia. It is not unusual for the severity of associated anomalies to obscure the presence of LTEC, especially if it is a minimal type I or II lesion. On the basis of the common symptoms of LTEC, the diagnostic evaluation typically proceeds along the line of the more commonly suspected diagnosis of EA-TEF or tracheomalacia. Contrast esophagography demonstrates rapid confluence of contrast material in the upper part of the esophagus and trachea; however, it is often difficult to know whether this is secondary to spillover at the level of the larynx or passage of contrast through a cleft. Endoscopy is the definitive method for diagnosis of LTEC, but it can still be difficult to identify a cleft unless the index of suspicion is high and unless the frequent mucosal infolding at the level of the subglottic region is pushed open to reveal the cleft (Fig. 67-20).

Management of infants with LTEC begins by maneuvers to minimize aspiration and stabilize the airway. Ryan et al.[219,238] recommended avoiding endotracheal intubation before surgery if possible, but it is often necessary to intubate the trachea and perform tube gastrostomy before definitive surgical repair. Operative procedures for repair of LTEC vary depending on the severity of the cleft. Asymptomatic type I clefts may require no operative intervention, and symptomatic clefts have been successfully repaired endoscopically.[63] Type II LTEC can be approached through a lateral pharyngotomy, posterior pharyngotomy, or anterior laryngofissure. The lateral

exposure has been most often reported; this method permits easy access to the cleft and allows asymmetric incisions in the mucosa, thereby avoiding contiguous suture lines. The major disadvantage to this approach is risk to the recurrent laryngeal nerves. The anterior laryngeal approach exposes the larynx and upper part of the trachea and has no risk for recurrent laryngeal nerve injury. Concern about postoperative laryngeal stability has been raised, and some surgeons recommend the use of stents during the healing process.[15,63]

Operative management for types III and IV LTEC requires a combined cervical and thoracic approach. Donahoe et al.[61,219,238] have described the use of a specifically designed bifurcated endotracheal tube with flanged ends that can be positioned during bronchoscopy to suspend the trachea anteriorly with a ureteral catheter sling (Fig. 67-21). The endotracheal tube allows for confident airway control during the multiple position changes frequently required during the operation. A right thoracotomy is performed and the tracheoesophageal cleft is exposed retropleurally. The tracheoesophageal groove is incised on the right and opened from the carina to the thoracic inlet. Separation of the two tubes is completed by incising along the left side of the common esophagotracheal wall, and an approximately 1.0-cm flap of esophagus running the length of the trachea should be left to help create the neomembranous portion of the trachea. It is important to size the esophageal flap correctly in order to avoid stenosis or a floppy posterior wall, which can result in tracheal obstruction. As the dissection proceeds, it is also important to push away and thus protect the left vagus and recurrent laryngeal nerves. Closure of the trachea and esophagus is accomplished in a caudal-to-cranial fashion with running polypropylene suture for the esophagus and interrupted polypropylene for the trachea. A right cervical incision is then made to expose the upper portion of the esophagus, trachea, pharynx, and larynx; the repair is continued with inclusion of a three-layer repair of the larynx and placement of a

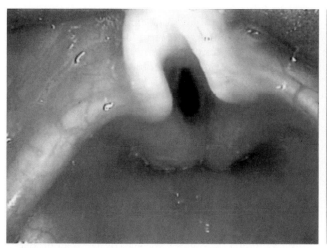
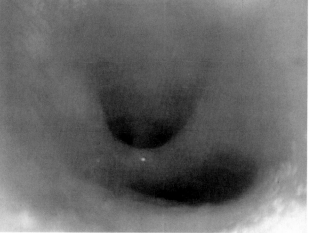

A   B

Figure 67–20   Endoscopic view of a type III laryngotracheoesophageal cleft. *A,* The proximal end of the cleft may be difficult to appreciate at first glance. *B,* The distal end of the cleft ends just proximal to the tracheal bifurcation.

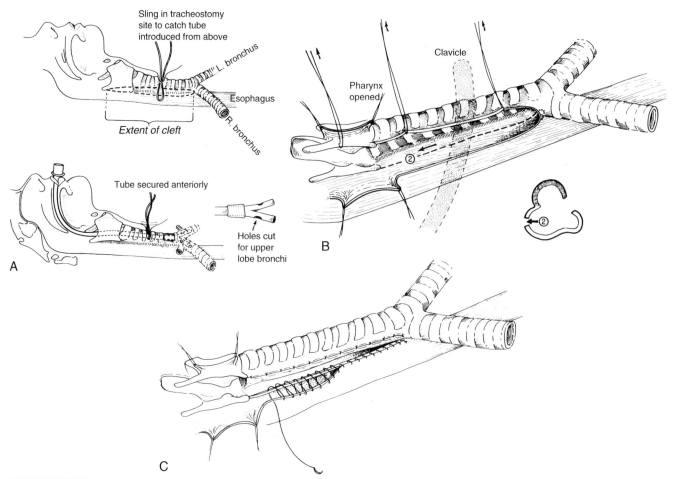

Figure 67–21 Repair of a type III laryngotracheoesophageal cleft. *A,* Stabilization of a bifurcated endotracheal tube is done at bronchoscopy with a loop passed through a tracheotomy, which draws the endotracheal tube forward. *B,* A cervical and thoracic approach allows retropleural exposure of the cleft. A longitudinal incision is made in the right tracheoesophageal groove below the tracheal rings. The incision is extended inferiorly and across the esophagus and up the left side, with approximately 1 cm of esophageal wall left attached to the trachea to allow adequate tissue to close the trachea. *C,* The trachea has been closed with interrupted sutures, and the esophagus is closed in running fashion up to the thoracic inlet. Closure of the laryngeal portion of the cleft and the lateral pharyngeal wall is not yet accomplished. (From Donahoe PK, Gee PE: Complete laryngotracheal cleft: Management and repair. J Pediatr Surg 1984;19:143.)

tracheostomy tube, which can be custom-designed to avoid undue pressure against the posterior tracheal repair. Some surgeons prefer an anterior approach and divide the larynx and trachea in the midline, as described for type II defects.[185] Cardiopulmonary bypass has been used both as a supporting technology during the anterior approach[177] to repair a type IV cleft and as support in the form of extracorporeal membrane oxygenation for one patient treated via a lateral thoracic and cervical approach.

Few patients with these complex anomalies are treated at any single institution.[185,235,238] Postoperative survival rates continue to be rather poor and range from 50% to 75%, depending on the severity of the malformation. Anastomotic leakage is reported to occur in approximately 50% of repairs and typically requires reoperation via a different approach.[63] In addition, an inability to wean patients from the ventilator, pharyngoesophageal dysfunction, and GER are common postoperative complications. A reduction in morbidity

and mortality depends, in part, on earlier recognition so that secondary complications can be prevented. At present there is no clear consensus about the best surgical approach; however, treatment is clearly complex and should be undertaken at centers with multidisciplinary expertise.

REFERENCES

1. Adzick NS, Fisher JH, Winter HS, et al: Esophageal adenocarcinoma 20 years after esophageal atresia repair. J Pediatr Surg 1989;24:741.
2. Allal H, Montes-Tapia F, Andina G, et al: Thoracoscopic repair of H-type tracheoesophageal fistula in the newborn: A technical case report. J Pediatr Surg 2004;39:1568.
3. Allmendinger N, Hallisey MJ, Markowitz SK, et al: Balloon dilation of esophageal strictures in children. J Pediatr Surg 1966;31:334.

4. Al-Qahtani AR, Yazbeck S, Rosen NG, et al: Lengthening technique for long gap esophageal atresia and early anastomosis. J Pediatr Surg 2003;38:737.

5. Al-Salem AH, Qaisaruddin S, Abu Srair H, et al: Elective, postoperative ventilation in the management of esophageal atresia and tracheoesophageal fistula. Pediatr Surg Int 1997;12:261.

6. Amae S, Nio M, Kamiyama T, et al: Clinical characteristics and management of congenital esophageal stenosis: A report on 14 cases. J Pediatr Surg 2003;38:565.

7. Applebaum H, Wosley MM: Pericardial flap aortopexy for tracheomalacia. J Pediatr Surg 1990;25:30, discussion 31.

8. Ashcraft KW, Goodwin C, Amoury RA, Holder TM: Early recognition and aggressive treatment of gastroesophageal reflux following repair of esophageal atresia. J Pediatr Surg 1977;12:317.

9. Babu R, Pierro A, Spitz L, et al: The management of oesophageal atresia in neonates with right-sided aortic arch. J Pediatr Surg 2000;35:56.

10. Bagolan P, Iacobelli Bd B, De Angelis P, et al: Long gap esophageal atresia and esophageal replacement: Moving toward a separation? J Pediatr Surg 2004;39:1084.

11. Bar-Maor JA, Shoshany G, Sweed Y: Wide gap esophageal atresia: A new method to elongate the upper pouch. J Pediatr Surg 1989;24:882.

12. Baumann W, Greinacher I, Emmrich P, Sprenger J: [VATER oder VACTERL syndrome.] Klin Padiatr 1976;188:328.

13. Bax KMA, Van der Zee DC: Feasibility of thoracoscopic repair of esophageal atresia with distal fistula. J Pediatr Surg 2002;37:192.

14. Beasley SW, Phelan E, Kelly JH, et al: Urinary tract abnormalities in association with oesophageal atresia: Frequency, significance, and influence on management. Pediatr Surg Int 1992;7:94.

15. Bell DW, Christiansen TW, Smith TE Jr, Stucker FJ: Laryngotracheoesophageal cleft: The anterior approach. Ann Otol Rhinol Laryngol 1977;86:616.

16. Benjamin B, Cohen D, Glasson M: Tracheomalacia in association with congenital tracheoesophageal fistula. Surgery 1976;79:504.

17. Bergmeijer JH, Tibboel D, Hazebroek FW: Nissen fundoplication in the management of gastroesophageal reflux occurring after repair of esophageal atresia. J Pediatr Surg 2000;35:573.

18. Bianca S, Bianca M, Ettore G: Oesophageal atresia and Down syndrome. Down Syndr Res Pract 2002;8:29.

19. Bianca S, Ettore G: Isolated esophageal atresia and perinatal risk factors. Dis Esophagus 2003;16:39.

20. Biller JA, Allen JL, Schuster SR, et al: Long-term evaluation of esophageal and pulmonary function in patients with repaired esophageal atresia and tracheoesophageal fistula. Dig Dis Sci 1987;32:985.

21. Bluestone CD, Kerry R, Sieber WK: Congenital esophageal stenosis. Laryngoscope 1969;79:1095.

22. Blumberg JB, Stevenson JK, Lemire RJ, Boyden EA: Larynogotracheo-esophageal cleft, the embryologic implications: Review of the literature. Surgery 1965;57:559.

23. Borgnon J, Tounian P, Auber F, et al: Esophageal replacement in children by an isoperistaltic gastric tube: A 12-year experience. Pediatr Surg Int 2004;20:829.

24. Botham MJ, Coran AG: The use of pericardium for the management of recurrent tracheoesophageal fistula. J Pediatr Surg 1986;21:164.

25. Bousamra M 2nd, Tweddell JS, Wells RG, et al: Wire sent for tracheomalacia in a five-year-old girl. Ann Thorac Surg 1996;61:1239.

26. Brennemann J: Am J Dis Child 1913;5:143.

27. Broto J, Asensio M, Vernet JM, et al: [Endoscopic treatment of tracheo-esophageal fistulas: Fact or fiction?] Cir Pediatr 2003;16(2):69.

28. Brown AK, Roddam AW, Spitz L, et al: Oesophageal atresia, related malformations, and medical problems: A family study. Am J Med Genet 1999;85:31.

29. Brown AK, Tam P: Measurement of gap length in esophageal atresia: A simple predictor of outcome. J Am Coll Surg 1996;182:41.

30. Burge DM: Gastric tube interposition: A new technique for the management of long-gap oesophageal atresia. Pediatr Surg Int 1995;10:279.

31. Celli J, van Bokhoven H, Brunner HG: Feingold syndrome: Clinical review and genetic mapping. Am J Med Genet 2003;122A:294.

32. Chahine AA, Campbell AB, Hoffman MA: Management of congenital distal esophageal stenosis with combined Collis gastroplasty–Nissen fundoplication. Pediatr Surg Int 1995;10:23.

33. Chan KL, Saing H: Combined flexible endoscopy and fluoroscopy in the assessment of the gap between the two esophageal pouches in esophageal atresia without fistula. J Pediatr Surg 1995;30:668.

34. Chavin K, Field G, Chandler J, et al: Save the child's esophagus: Management of major disruption after repair of esophageal atresia. J Pediatr Surg 1996;31:48.

35. Chen CY, Tsao PN, Chou HC, et al: Esophageal atresia associated with tracheal stenosis and right lung agenesis: Report of one case. Acta Paediatr Taiwan 2002;43:348.

36. Chen H, Goei GS, Hertzler JH: Family studies in congenital esophageal atresia with or without tracheoesophageal fistula. Birth Defects Orig Artic Ser 1979;15(5C):117.

37. Chetcuti P, Myers NA, Phelan PD, Beasley SW: Adults who survived repair of congenital oesophageal atresia and tracheo-oesophageal fistula. BMJ 1988;297:344.

38. Chittmittrapap S, Spitz L, Kiely EM, Bereton RJ: Oesophageal atresia and associated anomalies. Arch Dis Child 1989;64:364.

39. Chittmittrapap S, Spitz L, Kiely EM, Bereton RJ: Anastomotic stricture following repair of esophageal atresia. J Pediatr Surg 1990;25:508.

40. Choudhury SR, Ashcraft KW, Sharp RJ, et al: Survival of patients with esophageal atresia: Influence of birth weight, cardiac anomaly, and late respiratory complications. J Pediatr Surg 1999;34:70, discussion 74.

41. Cieri MV, Arnold GL, Torfs CP: Malrotation in conjunction with esophageal atresia/tracheo-esophageal fistula. Teratology 1999;60(3):114.

42. Cohen D: Tracheopexy—aorto-tracheal suspension for severe tracheomalacia. Aust Paediatr J 1981;17:117.

43. Cooper JE, Spitz L, Wilkins BM: Barrett's esophagus in children: A histologic and histochemical study of 11 cases. J Pediatr Surg 1987;22:191.

44. Coran AG: Pericardioesophagesoplasty. A new operation for partial esophageal replacement. Am J Surg 1973;125:294.

45. Coran AG: Ultra-long gap esophageal atresia: How long is long? Ann Thorac Surg 1994;57:528.

46. Corbally MT, Muftah M, Gunney EJ: Nissen fundoplication for gastro-esophageal reflux in repaired tracheo-esophageal fistula. Eur J Pediatr Surg 1992;2:332.

47. Cord-Udy CL, Wright VM, Drake DP: Association of ambiguous genitalia with VATER anomalies and its significance in management. Pediatr Surg Int 1996;11:50.

48. Corsello G, Maresi E, Corrao AM, et al: VATER/VACTERL association: Clinical variability and expanding phenotype including laryngeal stenosis. Am J Med Genet 1992:44:813.

49. Cozzi F, Morini F, Casati A, et al: Glossopexy as an alternative to aortopexy in infants with repaired esophageal atresia and upper airway obstruction. J Pediatr Surg 2002; 37:202.

50. Cozzi F, Myers NA, Piacenti S, et al: Maturational dysautonomia and facial anomalies associated with esophageal atresia: Support for neural crest involvement. J Pediatr Surg 1993;28:798.

51. Crisera CA, Connelly PR, Marmureanu AR, et al: TTF-1 and HNF-3beta in the developing tracheoesophageal fistula: Further evidence for the respiratory origin of the distal esophagus. J Pediatr Surg 1999;34:1322.

52. Cusick EL, Batchelor AA, Spicer RD: Development of a technique for jejunal interposition in long-gap esophageal atresia. J Pediatr Surg 1993;28:990.

53. Davenport M, Bianchi A: Early experience with oesophageal flap oesophagoplasty for repair of oesophageal atresia. Pediatr Surg Int 1990;5:332.

54. Davenport M, Mughal M, McCloy RF, Doig CM: Hypogastrinemia and esophageal atresia. J Pediatr Surg 1992;27:568.

55. De Carvalho JL, Maynard J, Hadley GP: An improved technique for in situ esophageal myotomy and proximal pouch mobilization in patients with esophageal atresia. J Pediatr Surg 1989;24:872.

56. Delius RE, Wheatley MJ, Coran AG: Etiology and management of respiratory complications after repair of esophageal atresia with tracheoesophageal fistula. Surgery 1992;112:527.

57. Depaepe A, Dolk H, Lechat MF: The epidemiology of tracheo-oesophageal fistula and oesophageal atresia in Europe. EUROCAT Working Group. Arch Dis Child 1993; 68:743.

58. Deurloo JA, Ekkelkamp S, Bartelsman JF, et al: Gastroesophageal reflux: Prevalence in adults older than 28 years after correction of esophageal atresia. Ann Surg 2003; 238:686.

59. Deurloo JA, Ekkelkamp S, Schoorl M, et al: Esophageal atresia: Historical evolution of management and results in 371 patients. Ann Thorac Surg 2002;73:267.

60. Diez-Pardo JA, Bao-Quan Q, Navarro C, Tovar JA: A new rodent experimental model of esophageal atresia and tracheoesophageal fistula: Preliminary report. J Pediatr Surg 1996;31:498.

61. Donahoe PK, Hendren WH: The surgical management of laryngotracheoesophageal cleft with tracheoesophageal fistula and esophageal atresia. Surgery 1972;71:363.

62. Driver CP, Shankar KR, Jones MO, et al: Phenotypic presentation and outcome of esophageal atresia in the era of the Spitz classification. J Pediatr Surg 2001;36:1419.

63. DuBois JJ, Pokorny WJ, Harberg FJ, et al: Current management of laryngeal and laryngotracheoesophageal clefts. J Pediatr Surg 1990;25:855.

64. Duhamel B: Technique Chirurgicale Infantile. Paris, 1957.

65. Duranceau A, Fisher SR, Flye M, et al: Motor function of the esophagus after repair of esophageal atresia and tracheoesophageal fistula. Surgery 1977;82:116.

66. Durston W: A Narrative of a Monstrous Birth in Plymouth. Philosophical Transactions of the Royal Society. 1670.

67. Ein SH, Shandling B: Pure esophageal atresia: A 50-year review. J Pediatr Surg 1994;29:1208.

68. Ein SH, Shandling B, Heiss K: Pure esophageal atresia: Outlook in the 1990s. J Pediatr Surg 1993;28:1147.

69. Ein SH, Shandling B, Stephens CA: Twenty-one year experience with the pediatric gastric tube. J Pediatr Surg 1987; 22:77.

70. Ein SH, Shandling B, Wesson D, et al: Esophageal atresia with distal tracheoesophageal fistula: Associated anomalies and prognosis in the 1980s. J Pediatr Surg 1989;24:1055.

71. Ein SH, Stringer DA, Stephens CA, et al: Recurrent tracheoesophageal fistulas—seventeen-year review. J Pediatr Surg 1983;18:436.

72. Engum SA, Grosfeld JL, West KW, et al: Analysis of morbidity and mortality in 227 cases of esophageal atresia and/or tracheoesophageal fistula over two decades. Arch Surg 1995; 130:502, discussion 508.

73. Eraklis AJ, Rossello PJ, Ballantine TV: Circular esophagomyotomy of upper pouch in primary repair of long-segment esophageal atresia. J Pediatr Surg 1976;11:709.

74. Erdogan E, Emir H, Eroglu E, et al: Esophageal replacement using the colon: A 15-year review. Pediatr Surg Int 2000;16:546.

75. Evans M: Application of Collis gastroplasty to the management of esophageal atresia. J Pediatr Surg 1995;30:1232.

76. Farrant P: The antenatal diagnosis of oesophageal atresia by ultrasound. Br J Radiol 1980;53:1202.

77. Fernandez MS, Gutierrez C, Ibanez V, et al: Long-gap esophageal atresia: Reconstruction preserving all portions of the esophagus by Scharli's technique. Pediatr Surg Int 1998;14:17.

78. Filler RM, Messineo A, Vinograd I: Severe tracheomalacia associated with esophageal atresia: Results of surgical treatment. J Pediatr Surg 1992;27:1136, discussion 1140.

79. Filler RM, Rossello PJ, Lebowitz RL: Life-threatening anoxic spells caused by tracheal compression after repair of esophageal atresia: Correction by surgery. J Pediatr Surg 1976;11:739.

80. Filston HC, Chitwood WR Jr, Schkolne B, et al: The Fogarty balloon catheter as an aid to management of the infant with esophageal atresia and tracheoesophageal fistula complicated by severe RDS or pneumonia. J Pediatr Surg 1982;17:149.

81. Finlay HVL: Familial congenital stridor. Arch Dis Child 1949;24:219.

82. Foker JE, Linden BC, Boyle EM Jr, et al: Development of a true primary repair for the full spectrum of esophageal atresia. Ann Surg 1997;226:533, discussion 541.

83. Fonkalsrud EW: Gastroesophageal fundoplication for reflux following repair of esophageal atresia. Experience with nine patients. Arch Surg 1979;114:48.

84. Freeman NV, Cass DT: Colon interposition: A modification of the Waterston technique using the normal esophageal route. J Pediatr Surg 1982;17:17.

85. Frey EK, Dusche L: The cardiospasms. Ergeb Chirur Orthop 1936;29:637.

86. Gage M, Oschner A: The surgical treatment of congenital tracheoesophageal fistula in the new-born. Ann Surg 1936;103:725.

87. Garcia NM, Thompson JW, Shaul DB: Definitive localization of isolated tracheoesophageal fistula using bronchoscopy and esophagoscopy for guide wire placement. J Pediatr Surg 1998;33:1645.

88. Gdanietz K, Krause I: Plastic adhesives for closing esophagotracheal fistulae in children. Z Kinderchir 1975;17:137.

89. German JC, Mahour GH, Woolley MM: Esophageal atresia and associated anomalies. J Pediatr Surg 1976;11:299.

90. Giacomoni MA, Tresoldi M, Zamana C, et al: Circular myotomy of the distal esophageal stump for long gap esophageal atresia. J Pediatr Surg 2001;36:855.

91. Gibson T: The Anatomy of Humane Bodies Epitomized. London, Awnsham & Churchill, 1697.

92. Gilchrist BF, Scriven R, Sanchez J, et al: The application of vascular technology to esophageal and airway strictures. J Pediatr Surg 2002;37:47.

93. Goh DW, Brereton RJ: Success and failure with neonatal tracheo-oesophageal anomalies. Br J Surg 1991;78:834.

94. Gough MH: Esophageal atresia—use of an anterior flap in the difficult anastomosis. J Pediatr Surg 1980;15:310.

95. Grabowski ST, Andrews DA: Upper esophageal stenosis: Two case reports. J Pediatr Surg 1996;31:1438.

96. Greenberg CR, Schnaufnagel D: The G syndrome: A case report. Am J Med Genet 1979;3:59.

97. Gross RE: The Surgery of Infancy and Childhood. Philadelphia, WB Saunders, 1953.

98. Grosser O, Lewis FT, McMurrich JP: The development of the intestinal tract and respiratory organs. In Keibel F, Mall FP (eds): Manual of Human Embryology. Philadelphia, JB Lippincott.

99. Gutierrez, C, Barrios JE, Lluna J, et al: Recurrent tracheoesophageal fistula treated with fibrin glue. J Pediatr Surg 1994;29:1567.

100. Haight C: Congenital esophageal atresia and tracheoesophageal fistula. In Mustard W (ed): Pediatric Surgery. Chicago, Year Book.

101. Haight C, Towsley H: Congenital atresia of the esophagus with tracheoesophageal fistula: Extrapleural ligation of fistula and end-to-end anastomosis of esophageal segments. Surg Gynecol Obstet 1943;76:672.

102. Harris J, Kallen B, Robert E: Descriptive epidemiology of alimentary tract atresia. Teratology 1995;52:15.

103. Hendren WH: Esophageal atresia treated by electromagnetic bougienage and subsequent repair. J Pediatr Surg 1975;11:719.

104. Hendren WH, Hale JR: Electromagnetic bougienage to lengthen esophageal segments in congenital esophageal atresia. N Engl J Med 1975;293:428.

105. Hennekam RC, Huber J, Variend D: Bartsocas-Papas syndrome with internal anomalies: Evidence for a more generalized epithelial defect or new syndrome? Am J Med Genet 1994;53:102.

106. Hill TP: Bost Med Surg J 1840;21:320.

107. Hirschl RB, Yardeni D, Oldham K, et al: Gastric transposition for esophageal replacement in children: Experience with 41 consecutive cases with special emphasis on esophageal atresia. Ann Surg 2002;236:531, discussion 539.

108. Hirschsprung H: Den medfordte tillerkning of spieseroret. Medico-Chirurg Rev 31;1861:437.

109. His W: Zur Bildungsgechischte der Lungen beim menschlischen Embryo. Arch Anat 89, 1887.

110. Hoffman MA, Superina R, Wesson DE: Unilateral pulmonary agenesis with esophageal atresia and distal tracheoesophageal fistula: Report of two cases. J Pediatr Surg 1989;24:1084.

111. Hoffman W: Atresia oesophogi congenital et communicato inter oesapgaiu et tracheoni. Griefswald, (Dissertation). University of Griefswald, Germany, 1899.

112. Holder TM, Clout DT, Lewis JE Jr, Pilling GP 4th: Esophageal atresia and tracheoesophageal fistula: A survey of its members by the surgical section of the American Academy of Pediatrics. Pediatrics 1964;34:542.

113. Holmes T: Surgical Management of Children's Diseases. London, Longmans, Green, Reader, & Dyer, 1869.

114. Howard R, Myers N: Esophageal atresia: A technique for elongating the upper pouch. Surgery 1965;58:725.

115. Humphreys GH II, Ferrer JM Jr: Management of esophageal atresia. Am J Surg 1964;107:406.

116. Iuchtman M, Brereton R, Spitz L, et al: Morbidity and mortality in 46 patients with the VACTERL association. Isr J Med Sci 1992;28:281.

117. Johnson AM, Rodgers BM, Alford B, et al: Esophageal atresia with double fistula: The missed anomaly. Ann Thorac Surg 1984;38:195.

118. Johnston MR, Loebner N, Hillyer P, et al: External stent for repair of secondary tracheomalacia. Ann Thorac Surg 1980;30:291.

119. Jolley SG, Johnson DG, Roberts CC, et al: Patterns of gastroesophageal reflux in children following repair of esophageal atresia and distal tracheoesophageal fistula. J Pediatr Surg 1980;15:857.

120. Karnak I, Senocak ME, Hicsonmez A, et al: The diagnosis and treatment of H-type tracheoesophageal fistula. J Pediatr Surg 1997;32:1670.

121. Kawahara H, Imura K, Yagi M, Kubota A: Clinical characteristics of congenital esophageal stenosis distal to associated esophageal atresia. Surgery 2001;127:29.

122. Kawahara H, Imura K, Yagi M, et al: Collis-Nissen procedure in patients with esophageal atresia: Long-term evaluation. World J Surg 2002;26:1222.

123. Kawahara H, Oue T, Okuyama H, et al: Esophageal motor function in congenital esophageal stenosis. J Pediatr Surg 2003;38:1716.

124. Kiely E, Spitz L, Brereton R: Management of tracheomalacia. Pediatr Surg Int 1987;2:13.

125. Kilic SS, Gurpinar A, Yakut T, et al: Esophageal atresia and tracheo-esophageal fistula in a patient with DiGeorge syndrome. J Pediatr Surg 2003;38:E21.

126. Kimura K, Nishijima E, Tsugawa C, et al: A new approach for the salvage of unsuccessful esophageal atresia repair: A spiral myotomy and delayed definitive operation. J Pediatr Surg 1987;22:981.

127. Kimura K, Nishijima E, Tsugawa C, et al: Multistaged extrathoracic esophageal elongation procedure for long gap esophageal atresia: Experience with 12 patients. J Pediatr Surg 2001;36:1725.

128. Kimura K, Soper RT: Multistaged extrathoracic esophageal elongation for long gap esophageal atresia. J Pediatr Surg 1994;29:566.

129. Kimura K, Soper RT, Kao SC, et al: Aortosternopexy for tracheomalacia following repair of esophageal atresia: Evaluation by cine-CT and technical refinement. J Pediatr Surg 1990;25:769.

130. Kitagawa H, Nakada K, Fujioka T, et al: Unilateral pulmonary agenesis with tracheoesophageal fistula: A case report. J Pediatr Surg 1995;30:1523.

131. Kluth D: Atlas of esophageal atresia. J Pediatr Surg 1976; 11:901.

132. Kluth D, Fiegel DH: The embryology of the foregut. Semin Pediatr Surg 2003;12:3.

133. Kluth D, Steding G, Seidl W: The embryology of foregut malformations. J Pediatr Surg 1987;22:389.

134. Ko BA, Frederic R, DiTirro PA, et al: Simplified access for division of the low cervical/high thoracic H-type tracheoesophageal fistula. J Pediatr Surg 2000;35:1621.

135. Konkin DE, O'Hali AW, Webber EM, Blair GK: Outcomes in esophageal atresia and tracheoesophageal fistula. J Pediatr Surg 2003;38:1726.

136. Kosloske AM: Azygous flap technique for reinforcement of esophageal closure. J Pediatr Surg 1990;25:793.

137. Kovesi T, Rubin T: Long-term complications of congenital esophageal atresia and/or tracheoesophageal fistula. Chest 2004;126:915.

138. Koyluoglu G, Gunay I, Ceran C, Berkan O: Pericardial flap aortopexy: An easy and safe technique in the treatment of tracheomalacia. J Cardiovasc Surg (Torino) 2002; 43:295.

139. Kreuter E: Die angeborenen Verschliebungen und Verengungen des Darmkanals im Lichte der Entwicklungsgeschichte. Dtsch Z Chir 1905;79:1.

140. Krug E, Bergmeijer JH, Dees J, et al: Gastroesophageal reflux and Barrett's esophagus in adults born with esophageal atresia. Am J Gastroenterol 1999;94:2825.

141. Kutiyanawala M, Wyse RK, Brereton RJ, et al: CHARGE and esophageal atresia. J Pediatr Surg 1992;27:558.

142. Kyyronen P, Hemminki K: Gastro-intestinal atresias in Finland in 1970-79, indicating time-place clustering. J Epidemiol Commun Health 1988;42:257.

143. Ladd WE: The surgical treatment of esophageal atresia and tracheoesophageal fistulas. N Engl J Med 1944;230:625.

144. Lai JY, Sheu JC, Chang PY, et al: Experience with distal circular myotomy for long-gap esophageal atresia. J Pediatr Surg 1996;31:1503.

145. Langer JC, Hussain H, Khan A, et al: Prenatal diagnosis of esophageal atresia using sonography and magnetic resonance imaging. J Pediatr Surg 2001;36:804.

146. Lanman TH: Congenital atresia of the esophagus: A study of thirty-two cases. Arch Surg 1940;7:1060.

147. Leininger BJ: Silastic banding of esophagus with subsequent repair of esophageal atresia and tracheosesophageal fistula. J Pediatr Surg 1972;7:404.

148. Leonard H, Barrett AM, Scott JE, et al: The influence of congenital heart disease on survival of infants with oesophageal atresia. Arch Dis Child Fetal Neonat Ed 2001;85:F204.

149. Lessin MS, Wesselhoeft CW, Luks FI, et al: Primary repair of long-gap esophageal atresia by mobilization of the distal esophagus. Eur J Pediatr Surg 1999;9:369.

150. Levine JJ, Shoshany G, Davidson M, et al: Manometric variations following spiral myotomy for long-gap esophageal atresia. J Pediatr Gastroenterol Nutr 1990;10:380.

151. Lilienthal H: Thoracic Surgery. Philadelphia, WB Saunders, 1925.

152. Lindahl H: Esophageal atresia: A simple technical detail aiding the mobilization and circular myotomy of the proximal segment. J Pediatr Surg 1987;22:113.

153. Lindahl H, Rintala R, Louhimo I: Failure of the Nissen fundoplication to control gastroesophageal reflux in esophageal atresia patients. J Pediatr Surg 1989;24:985.

154. Lindell-Iwan L: Modification of Livaditis' myotomy for long gap oesophageal atresia. Ann Chir Gynaecol 1990;79:101.

155. Little DC, Rescorla FJ, Grosfeld JL, et al: Long-term analysis of children with esophageal atresia and tracheoesophageal fistula. J Pediatr Surg 2003;38:852.

156. Liu YX, Xue F: Congenital esophageal stenosis due to tracheo-bronchial cartilage. Int J Pediatr Otorhinolaryngol 1987;14:95.

157. Livaditis A: End-to-end anastomosis in esophageal atresia. A clinical and experimental study. Scand J Thorac Cardiovasc Surg Suppl 1969;2:7-20.

158. Livaditis A: Esophageal atresia. A method of over-bridging long segmental gaps. Z Kinderchir 1973;13:298.

159. Livaditis A, Radberg L, Odensjo G: Esophageal end-to-end anastomosis. Reduction of anastomotic tension by circular myotomy. Scand J Thorac Cardiovasc Surg 1972;6:206.

160. Lokare RV, Manvi RS: Esophageal atresia with right pulmonary agenesis. Indian Pediatr 1998;35:555.

161. Lomas FE, Dahlstrom JE, Ford JH: VACTERL with hydrocephalus: Family with X-linked VACTERL-H. Am J Med Genet 1998;76:74.

162. Longmire WP: Congenital atresia and tracheo-esophageal fistula. Arch Surg 1947;55:330.

163. Louhimo IH, Lindahl H: Esophageal atresia: Primary results of 500 consecutively treated patients. J Pediatr Surg 1983;18:217.

164. Lyall P, Bao-Quan Q, Beasley S: The effect of neck flexion on oesophageal tension in the pig and its relevance to repaired oesophageal atresia. Pediatr Surg Int 2001;17:193.

165. Mackenzie M: Malformation of the esophagus. Arch Laryngol 1880;1:301.

166. MacKinlay GA, Burtles R: Oesophageal atresia: Paralysis and ventilation in management of the wide gap. Pediatr Surg Int 1987;2:10.

167. Mahour GH, Johnston PW, Gwinn JL, et al: Congenital esophageal stenosis distal to esophageal atresia. Surgery 1971;69:936.

168. Mahour GH, Woolley MM, Gwinn JL: Elongation of the upper pouch and delayed anatomic reconstruction in esophageal atresia. J Pediatr Surg 1974;9:373.

169. Manning PB, Morgan RA, Coran AG, et al: Fifty years' experience with esophageal atresia and tracheoesophageal fistula. Beginning with Cameron Haight's first operation in 1935. Ann Surg 1986;204:446.

170. Matsuoka S, Takeuchi K, Yamanaka Y, et al: Comparison of magnetic resonance imaging and ultrasonography in the prenatal diagnosis of congenital thoracic abnormalities. Fetal Diagn Ther 2003;18:447.

171. McKinnon LJ, Kosloske AM: Prediction and prevention of anastomotic complications of esophageal atresia and tracheoesophageal fistula. J Pediatr Surg 1990;25:778.

172. Mee RBB, Beasley SW, Auldist AW, et al: Influence of congenital heart disease on management of oesophageal atresia. Pediatr Surg Int 1992;7:90.

173. Merei JM, Hutson JM: Embryogenesis of tracheoesophageal anomalies: A review. Pediatr Surg Int 2002;18:319.

174. Morabito A, MacKinnon E, Alizai N, et al: The anterior mediastinal approach for management of tracheomalacia. J Pediatr Surg 2000;35:1456.

175. Moriarty KP, Jacir NN, Harris BH, et al: Transanastomotic feeding tubes in repair of esophageal atresia. J Pediatr Surg 1996;31:53, discussion 54.

176. Morini F, Cozzi DA, Ilari M, et al: Pattern of cardiovascular anomalies associated with esophageal atresia: Support for a caudal pharyngeal arch neurocristopathy. Pediatr Res 2001;50:565.

177. Moukheiber AK, Camboulives J, Guys JM, et al: Repair of a type IV laryngotracheoesophageal cleft with cardiopulmonary bypass. Ann Otol Rhinol Laryngol 2002;111:1076.

178. Murphy SG, Yazbeck S, Russo P: Isolated congenital esophageal stenosis. J Pediatr Surg 1995;30:1238.

179. Myers NA: The history of oesophageal atresia and tracheo-oesophageal fistula—1670-1984. Prog Pediatr Surg 1986;20:106.

180. Myers NA: Oesophageal atresia: The epitome of modern surgery. Ann R Coll Surg Engl 1974;54:277.

181. Neilson IR, Croitoru DP, Guttman FM, et al: Distal congenital esophageal stenosis associated with esophageal atresia. J Pediatr Surg 1991;26:478, discussion 481.

182. Nihoul-Fekete C, Backer A, Lortat-Jacob S, et al: Congenital esophageal stenosis. Pediatr Surg Int 1987;2:86.

183. Nishina T, Tsuchida Y, Saito S: Congenital esophageal stenosis due to tracheobronchial remnants and its associated anomalies. J Pediatr Surg 1981;16:190.

184. Nora AH, Nora JJ: A syndrome of multiple congenital anomalies associated with teratogenic exposure. Arch Environ Health 1975;30:17.

185. Obatake M, Tanaka T, Muraoka M, et al: Anterior approach bilateral musculomucosal flaps repair for laryngotracheoesophageal clefts. J Pediatr Surg 2003;38:1720.

186. Ohi R, Tseng SW: Congenital oesophageal stenosis. In Newborn Surgery. Oxford, Butterworth-Heinemann.

187. Okada A, Usui N, Inoue M, et al: Esophageal atresia in Osaka: A review of 39 years' experience. J Pediatr Surg 1997;32:1570.

188. O'Rahilly R, Muller F: Chevalier Jackson lecture. Respiratory and alimentary relations in staged human embryos. New embrological data and congenital anomalies. Ann Otol Rhinol Laryngol 1984;93:421.

189. Orford J, Cass DT, Glasson MJ: Advances in the treatment of oesophageal atresia over three decades: The 1970s and the 1990s. Pediatr Surg Int 2004;20:402.

190. Orringer MB, Kirsh MM, Sloan H: Long-term esophageal function following repair of esophageal atresia. Ann Surg 1977;186:436.

191. Otte JB, Gianello P, Wese FX, et al: Diverticulum formation after circular myotomy for esophageal atresia. J Pediatr Surg 1984;19:68.

192. Otten C, Migliazza L, Xia H, et al: Neural crest–derived defects in experimental esophageal atresia. Pediatr Res 2000;47:178.

193. Pandit SK, Rattan KN, Budhiraja S: Esophageal atresia with blocked distal tracheo-esophageal fistula. Indian J Pediatr 1998;65:763.

194. Parent P, Bensaid M, Le Guern H, et al: [Clinical heterogeneity of Townes-Brock syndrome.] Arch Pediatr 1995;2:551.

195. Parker AF, Christie DL, Cahill JL: Incidence and significance of gastroesophageal reflux following repair of esophageal atresia and tracheoesophageal fistula and the need for anti-reflux procedures. J Pediatr Surg 1979;14:5.

196. Patel SB, Ade-Ajayi N, Kiely EM: Oesophageal atresia: A simplified approach to early management. Pediatr Surg Int 2002;18:87.

197. Pettersson G: Inhibited separation of the larynx and the upper part of the trachea from the esophagus in a newborn: Report of a case successfully operated upon. Acta Chir Scand 1955;10:250.

198. Pietsch JB, Stokes KB, Beardmore HE: Esophageal atresia with tracheoesophageal fistula: End-to-end version versus end-to-side repair. J Pediatr Surg 1978:13;677.

199. Plass E: Congenital atresia of the esophagus with tracheoesophageal fistula: Associated with fused kidney. A case report and a survey of the literature on congenital anomalies of the esophagus. Johns Hopkins Hosp Rep 1919;18:259.

200. Pletcher BA, Friedes JS, Breg WR, et al: Familial occurrence of esophageal atresia with and without tracheoesophagel fistula: Report of two unusual kindreds. Am J Med Genet 1991;39:380.

201. Poenaru D, Laberge JM, Neilson IR, et al: A new prognostic classification for esophageal atresia. Surgery 1993; 113:426.

202. Pompino HJ: Endoscopic closure of tracheo-esophageal fistulae. Z Kinderchir 1979;27:90.

203. Postlethwait R: Clonic interposition for esophageal substitution. Surg Gynecol Obstet 1983;156:377.

204. Postlethwait RW: Technique for isoperistaltic gastric tube for esophageal bypass. Ann Surg 1979;189:673.

205. Pul N, Pul M, Gedik Y: McKusick-Kaufman syndrome associated with esophageal atresia and distal tracheoesophageal fistula: A case report and review of the literature. Am J Med Genet 1994;49:341.

206. Puri P, Ninan GK, Blake NS, et al: Delayed primary anastomosis for esophageal atresia: 18 months' to 11 years' follow-up. J Pediatr Surg 1992;27:1127.

207. Quan LD, Smith W: The VATER association. Vertebral defects, Anal atresia, T-E fistula with esophageal atresia, Radial and Renal dysplasia: A spectrum of associated defects. J Pediatr 1973;82:104.

208. Ramesh JC, Ramanujam TM, Jayaram G: Congenital esophageal stenosis: Report of three cases, literature review, and a proposed classification. Pediatr Surg Int 2001; 17:188.

209. Randolph JG, Newman KD, Anderson KD: Current results in repair of esophageal atresia with tracheoesophageal fistula using physiologic status as a guide to therapy. Ann Surg 1989;209:526, discussion 530.

210. Randolph JG, Tunell WP, Lilly JR: Gastric division in the critically ill infant with esophageal atresia and tracheoesophageal fistula. Surgery 1968;63:496.

211. Rangecroft L, Bush GH, Lister J, et al: Endoscopic diathermy obliteration of recurrent tracheoesophageal fistulae. J Pediatr Surg 1984;19:41.

212. Rehbein F, Schweder N: Reconstruction of the esophagus without colon transplantation in cases of atresia. J Pediatr Surg 1971;6:746.

213. Richter CF: Dissertatio Medica de Infanticido in Artis Obstericae. Leipzig, Germany, 1792.

214. Richter HM: Congenital atresia of the esophagus: An operation designed for its cure. Surg Gynecol Obstet 1913;17:397.

215. Rosenthal AH: Congenital atresia of the esophagus with tracheoesophageal fistula: Report of eight cases. Arch Pathol 1931;12:756.

216. Rossello PJ, Lebron H, Franco AA: The technique of myotomy in esophageal reconstruction: An experimental study. J Pediatr Surg 1980;15:430.

217. Rothenberg S: Thoracoscopic repair of a tracheoesophageal fistula in a newborn infant. Pediatr Surg Innov Tech 2000;4:289.

218. Rothenberg S: Thoracoscopic repair of tracheoesphageal fistula in newborns. J Pediatr Surg 2002;37:869.

219. Ryan DP, Meuhrcke DD, Doody DP, et al: Laryngotracheoesophageal cleft (type IV): Management and repair of lesions beyond the carina. J Pediatr Surg 1991;26:962, discussion 969.

220. Said M, Mekki M, Golli M, et al: Balloon dilatation of anastomotic strictures secondary to surgical repair of oesophageal atresia. Br J Radiol 2003;76:26.

221. Salem M, Wong AY, Lin YH, et al: Prevention of gastric distention during anesthesia for newborns with tracheoesophageal fistulas. Anesthesiology 1973;38:82.

222. Sarin YK: Esophageal atresia and tracheo-esophageal fistula with right pulmonary agenesis. Indian Pediatr 1996; 33:595.

223. Satoh S, Takashima T, Takeuchi H, et al: Antenatal sonographic detection of the proximal esophageal segment: Specific evidence for congenital esophageal atresia. J Clin Ultrasound 1995;23:419.

224. Schaarschmidt K, Kolberg-Schwerdt A, Bunke K, Strauss J: A technique for thoracoscopic aortopericardiosternopexy. Surg Endosc 2002;16:1639.

225. Schärli AF: Esophageal reconstruction in very long atresias by elongation of the lesser curvature. Pediatr Surg Int 1992;7:101.

226. Schwartz MZ: An improved technique for circular myotomy in long-gap esophageal atresia. J Pediatr Surg 1983;18:833.

227. Schwartz MZ, Filler RM: Tracheal compression as a cause of apnea following repair of tracheoesophageal fistula: Treatment by aortopexy. J Pediatr Surg 1980;15:842.

228. Seoud M, Nassar A, Usta I, et al: Gastrointestinal malformations in two infants born to women with hyperthyroidism untreated in the first trimester. Am J Perinatol 2003;20:59.

229. Shafer AD, David TE: Suture fistula as a means of connecting upper and lower segments in esophageal atresia. J Pediatr Surg 1974;9:669.

230. Shandling B: The insertion of a soft Silastic nasogastric tube at an operation for an esophageal atresia. J Pediatr Surg 1993;28:280.

231. Sharma AK, Sharma KK, Sharma CS, et al: Congenital esophageal obstruction by intraluminal mucosal diaphragm. J Pediatr Surg 1991;26:213.

232. Sharma AK, Shekhawat NS, Agrawal LD, et al: Esophageal atresia and tracheoesophageal fistula: A review of 25 years' experience. Pediatr Surg Int 2000;16:478.

233. Sharma AK, Wakhlu A: Simple technique for proximal pouch mobilization and circular myotomy in cases of

esophageal atresia with tracheoesophageal fistula. J Pediatr Surg 1994;29:1402.

234. Shaw R: Surgical correction of congenital atresia of the esophagus with tracheo-esophageal fistula. J Thorac Surg 1939;9:213.

235. Shehab ZP, Bailey CM: Type IV laryngotracheoesophageal clefts—recent 5 year experience at Great Ormond Street Hospital for Children. Int J Pediatr Otorhinolaryngol 2001;60:1.

236. Shepard R, Fenn S, Sieber WK: Evaluation of esophageal function in postoperative esophageal atresia and tracheoesophageal fistula. Surgery 1966;59:608.

237. Siegel MJ, Shackelford GD, McAlister WH, et al: Circular esophageal myotomy simulating a pulmonary or mediastinal pseudocyst. Radiology 1980;136:365.

238. Simpson BB, Ryan DP, Donahoe PK, et al: Type IV laryngotracheoesophageal clefts: Surgical management for long-term survival. J Pediatr Surg 1996;31:1128.

239. Singh S, Shun JA: A new technique of anastomosis to avoid stricture formation in oesophageal atresia. Pediatr Surg Int 2001;17:575.

240. Skandalakis JE, Gray SW: Embrology for Surgeons. Philadelphia, WB Saunders, 1994.

241. Slim MS: Circular myotomy of the esophagus: Clinical application in esophageal atresia. Ann Thorac Surg 1977;23:62.

242. Smith EI: The early development of the trachea and esophagus in relation to atresia of the esophagus and tracheoesophageal fistula. Embryol Carnegie Inst 1957;36:41.

243. Sparey C, Jawaheer G, Barrett AM, et al: Esophageal atresia in the Northern Region Congenital Anomaly Survey, 1985-1997: Prenatal diagnosis and outcome. Am J Obstet Gynecol 2000;182:427.

244. Spilde T, Bhatia A, Ostlie D, et al: A role for sonic hedgehog signaling in the pathogenesis of human tracheoesophageal fistula. J Pediatr Surg 2003;38:465.

245. Spilde TL, Bhatia AM, Marosky JK, et al: Complete discontinuity of the distal fistula tract from the developing gut: Direct histologic evidence for the mechanism of tracheoesophageal fistula formation. Anat Rec 2002;267:220.

246. Spilde TL, Bhatia AM, Mehta S, et al: Defective sonic hedgehog signaling in esophageal atresia with tracheoesophageal fistula. Surgery 2003;134:345.

247. Spitz L: Congenital esophageal stenosis distal to associated esophageal atresia. J Pediatr Surg 1973;8:973.

248. Spitz L: Esophageal atresia and tracheoesophageal fistula in children. Curr Opin Pediatr 1993;5:347.

249. Spitz L: Esophageal atresia: Past, present, and future. J Pediatr Surg 1996;31:19.

250. Spitz L, Hitchcock R: Oesophageal atresia and tracheoesophageal fistula. In Burge DM, Griffiths M, Freeman NV (eds): Surgery of the Newborn. New York, Churchill Livingstone.

251. Spitz L, Hitchcock R: Recurrent tracheoesophageal fistula. In Spitz L, Coran AG (eds): Pediatric Surgery. London, Chapman & Hall.

252. Spitz L, Kiely E, Brereton RJ: Esophageal atresia: Five years' experience with 148 cases. J Pediatr Surg 1987;22:103.

253. Spitz L, Kiely E, Brereton RJ, Drake D: Management of esophageal atresia. World J Surg 1993;17:296.

254. Spitz L, Kiely EM, Morecroft JA, Drake DP: Esophageal atresia: At-risk groups for the 1990s. J Pediatr Surg 1994;29:723.

255. Spitz L, Kiely E, Pierro A: Gastric transposition in children—a 21-year experience. J Pediatr Surg 2004;39:276, discussion 276.

256. Steadland KM, Langham MR Jr, Greene MA, et al: Unilateral pulmonary agenesis, esophageal atresia, and distal tracheoesophageal fistula. Ann Thorac Surg 1995;59:511.

257. Steele C: Case of deficient oesophagus. Lancet 1888;2:764.

258. Streeter GL: Development horizons in human embryos: Description of age groups XV, XVI, XVII, XVIII. Contr Embryol Carnegie Inst 1945;32:133.

259. Stringer MD, McKenna KM, Goldstein RB, et al: Prenatal diagnosis of esophageal atresia. J Pediatr Surg 1995;30:1258.

260. Sulamaa MGL, Alvenainen EK: Prognosis and treatment of congenital atresia of the esophagus. Acta Chir Scand 1951;102:141.

261. Sumitomo K, Ikeda K, Nagasaki A: Esophageal manometrical assessment after esophageal circular myotomy for wide-gap esophageal atresia. Jpn J Surg 1988;18:218.

262. Sweed Y, Bar-Maor JA, Shoshany G: Insertion of a soft Silastic nasogastric tube at operation for esophageal atresia: A new technical method. J Pediatr Surg 1992;27:650.

263. Szendrey T, Danyi G, Czeizel A: Etiological study on isolated esophageal atresia. Hum Genet 1985;70:51.

264. Tam PK, Sprigg A, Cudmore RE, et al: Endoscopy-guided balloon dilatation of esophageal strictures and anastomotic strictures after esophageal replacement in children. J Pediatr Surg 1991;26:1101.

265. Tandler J: Entwicklungsgeschichte des menschlichen Duodenum in frühen Embryonalstadien. Morph JB 1902;29:187.

266. Tannuri U, Teodoro WR, de Santana Witzel S, et al: Livaditis' circular myotomy does not decrease anastomotic leak rates and induces deleterious changes in anastomotic healing. Eur J Pediatr Surg 2003;13:224.

267. Tazuke Y, Kawahara H, Yagi M, et al: Use of a Palmaz stent for tracheomalacia: Case report of an infant with esophageal atresia. J Pediatr Surg 1999;34:1291.

268. Templeton JM Jr, Templeton JJ, Schnaufer L, et al: Management of esophageal atresia and tracheoesophageal fistula in the neonate with severe respiratory distress syndrome. J Pediatr Surg 1985;20:394.

269. Thompson DJ, Molello JA, Strebing RJ, et al: Teratogenicity of Adriamycin and daunomycin in the rat and rabbit. Teratology 1978;17:151.

270. Tibboel D, Pattenier JW, Krugten RJ, et al: Prospective evaluation of postoperative morbidity in patients with esophageal atresia. Pediatr Surg Int 1988;4:252.

271. Todani T, Watanabe Y, Mizuguchi T, et al: Congenital oesophageal stenosis due to fibromuscular thickening. Z Kinderchir 1984;39:11.

272. Tomaselli V, Volpi ML, Dell'Agnola CA, et al: Long-term evaluation of esophageal function in patients treated at birth for esophageal atresia. Pediatr Surg Int 2003;19:40.

273. Tonz M, Kohli S, Kaiser G: Oesophageal atresia: What has changed in the last 3 decades? Pediatr Surg Int 2004.

274. Torfs CP, Curry CJ, Bateson TF: Population-based study of tracheoesophageal fistula and esophageal atresia. Teratology 1995;52:220.

275. Touloukian RJ, Seashore JH: Thirty-five-year institutional experience with end-to-side repair for esophageal atresia. Arch Surg 2004;139:371, discussion 374.

276. Tovar JA, Diez Pardo JA, Murcia J, et al: Ambulatory 24-hour manometric and pH metric evidence of permanent impairment of clearance capacity in patients with esophageal atresia. J Pediatr Surg 1995;30:1224.

277. Tovar JA, Gorostiaga L, Escheverry J, et al: Barrett's esophagus in children and adolescents. Pediatr Surg Int 1993; 8:389.

278. Tsang TM, Tam PKH, Westaby S: Management of coexisting coarctation of the aorta and oesophageal atresia. Pediatr Surg Int 1996;11:107.

279. Tuqan NA: Annular stricture of the esophagus distal to the congenital tracheoesophageal fistula. Surgery 1962;52:394.

280. Tyler DC: Laryngeal cleft: Report of eight patients and review of the literature. Am J Genet 1990;21:61.

281. Usui N, Kamata S, Ishikawa S, et al: Anomalies of the tracheobronchial tree in patients with esophageal atresia. J Pediatr Surg 1996;31:258.

282. Usui N, Kamata S, Kawahara H, et al: Usefulness of endoscopic ultrasonography in the diagnosis of congenital esophageal stenosis. J Pediatr Surg 2002;37:1744.

283. Valerio D, Jones PF, Stewart AM: Congenital oesophageal stenosis. Arch Dis Child 1977;52:414.

284. Van Biervliet S, Van Winckel M, Robberecht E, et al: High-dose omeprazole in esophagitis with stenosis after surgical treatment of esophageal atresia. J Pediatr Surg 2001; 36:1416.

285. van Heurn LW, Cheng W, de Vries B, et al: Anomalies associated with oesophageal atresia in Asians and Europeans. Pediatr Surg Int 2002;18:241.

286. Vasudevan SA, Kerendi F, Lee H, Ricketts RR: Management of congenital esophageal stenosis. J Pediatr Surg 2002;37:1024.

287. Vazquez-Jimenez JF, Sachweh JS, Liakopoulos OJ, et al: Aortopexy in severe tracheal instability: Short-term and long-term outcome in 29 infants and children. Ann Thorac Surg 2001;72:1898.

288. Villegas-Alvarez F, Olvera-Duran J, Rodriguez-Aranda E: et al: Esophageal anastomotic failure: An experimental study. Arch Med Res 2003;34:171.

289. Vinograd I, Filler RM, Bahoric A: Long-term functional results of prosthetic airway in tracheomalacia and bronchomalacia. J Pediatr Surg 22:38, 1987.

290. Vogt EC: Congenital atresia of the esophagus. AJR Am J Roentgenol 1929;22:463.

291. Wailoo MP, Emery JL: The trachea in children with tracheo-oesophageal fistula. Histopathology 1979;3:329.

292. Waterston D: Colonic replacement of esophagus (intrathoracic). Surg Clin North Am 1964;44:1441.

293. Waterston DJ, Bonham Carter RE, Aberdeen E: Esophageal atresia: Tracheo-oesophageal fistula. A study of survival in 218 infants. Lancet 1962;1:819.

294. Weber TR, Keller MS, Fiore A: Aortic suspension (aortopexy) for severe tracheomalacia in infants and children. 2002;184:573, discussion 577.

295. Welch RG, Husain OAN: Atresia of the oesophagus with common tracheo-oesophageal tube. Arch Dis Child 1958;33:367.

296. Werlin SL, Dodds WJ, Hogan WJ, et al: Esophageal function in esophageal atresia. Dig Dis Sci 1981;26:796.

297. Wheatley MJ, Coran AG: Pericardial flap interposition for the definitive management of recurrent tracheo-esophageal fistula. J Pediatr Surg 1992;27:1122.

298. Wheatley MJ, Coran AG, Wesley JR: Efficacy of the Nissen fundoplication in the management of gastroesophageal reflux following esophageal atresia repair. J Pediatr Surg 1993;28:53.

299. Yagyu M, Gitter H, Richter B, et al: Esophageal atresia in Bremen, Germany—evaluation of preoperative risk classification in esophageal atresia. J Pediatr Surg 2000; 35:584.

300. Yanchar NL, Gordon R, Cooper M, et al: Significance of the clinical course and early upper gastrointestinal studies in predicting complications associated with repair of esophageal atresia. J Pediatr Surg 2001;36:815.

301. Yeung CK, Spitz L, Brereton RJ, et al: Congenital esophageal stenosis due to tracheobronchial remnants: A rare but important association with esophageal atresia. J Pediatr Surg 1992;27:852.

302. Zaw-Tun HA: The tracheo-esophageal septum—fact or fantasy? Origin and development of the respiratory primordium and esophagus. Acta Anat 1982;114:1.

303. Zigman AS, Yazbeck: Esophageal foreign body obstruction after esophageal atresia repair. J Pediatr Surg 2002; 37:776.

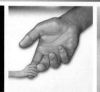
Caustic Strictures of the Esophagus

Alastair J. W. Millar, Alp Numanoglu, and Heinz Rode

HISTORICAL NOTE

Corrosive ingestion is a disease of the industrial age.[75] The tragic consequences of ingesting caustic substances and the evolution of treatment methods have been well summarized by Tucker et al.[119] Esophageal dilatation of the resulting stricture, initially using blind bougie dilatation through the mouth, has changed little in principle but greatly in practice as a result of technologic advances.[95,96] Development of the distally lighted esophagoscope, introduction of string-guided retrograde dilatation via gastrostomy, and improvements in general medical and nutritional support have nearly eliminated early mortality.[60,103,119,127] Based on experimental evidence, the use of steroids and antibiotics became widespread in the 1950s and 1960s in an attempt to reduce the incidence of stricture by inhibiting inflammation, scar formation, and infection.[16,18,21,24,52,56,67,70,80,99] However, mortality still occurs from pharyngeal and laryngeal burns resulting in edema and airway obstruction, massive ingestion with perforation, and complications after stricture dilatation or surgical bypass of an irreversibly damaged esophagus.[4,9,31,32,48,49,79]

EPIDEMIOLOGY

The ingestion of corrosive substances remains a major health hazard in children, despite aggressive educational programs aimed at both children and adults, preventive labeling and packaging, and even legislation limiting the strength and availability of caustic substances.[26,75,103,112,119,122,123] In rural areas and in developing countries, caustic soda in both crystal and liquid form is used in home industry for soap making, fruit drying, and container cleaning on farms. In addition, the availability of innumerable over-the-counter caustic cleaning agents virtually ensures that children will continue to be at risk. The most distressing aspect is that the majority of ingestions occur in children younger than 3 years and are entirely preventable. Boys are more frequently involved.[26,32,75] Toxic ingestion in children older than 5 years is suspect, and ingestion in adolescents (where girls predominate) is usually intentional[54,75]; in these cases, larger volumes and more potent corrosive and caustic materials tend to be used. Although mortality is rare, morbidity is often devastating and can be associated with lifelong consequences. Comprehensive statistics dating back to the 1970s indicate a decrease in the incidence of ingestion; however, in developing countries, the many reports of esophageal replacement procedures bear witness to this serious worldwide public health problem.[2,11,48,75,86] This is particularly true in areas where corrosive substances are available in containers that are not childproof or where such substances have been decanted from larger containers for use in homes.[75] There is still a great need for adult education and for legislation to ensure correct labeling and safe packaging and to restrict the strength and availability of caustic agents.[26,122,123]

Approximately 20% of ingestions of caustic substances result in some degree of esophageal injury.[54,70,77] Early management strategies for ingestion are now well defined, particularly the use of fiber-optic endoscopy to assess the extent and severity of injury.[1,40,128] However, controversy still surrounds the use of steroids, antibiotics, and esophageal stents and the timing, frequency, and method of esophageal dilatation in the prevention and management of caustic strictures. Indications for definitive esophageal surgery or bypass and the type of procedure to use are also subjects of ongoing debate.[31]

CAUSE

Strong alkalis that are sold in both liquid and granular form are the principal cause of severe injury (Table 68-1).[26] Household bleach, dishwasher detergents, and other cleaning agents, all of which are moderately alkaline, are the most frequent corrosive material ingested. However, these burns are usually limited to the esophageal mucosa, without extensive necrosis or subsequent stricture formation.[26,72] A wide variety of caustic substances can cause direct injury to living tissues and particularly to moist mucous membranes, including corrosives such as potassium and sodium hydroxide (lye) and phenols; reducing agents such as hydrochloric and nitric acids; desiccants such as sulfuric acid; oxidizing agents such as chromic acid, sodium hypochlorite, and potassium permanganate; and protoplasmic poisons such as acetic and formic acids.[61,103,126] The physical form of the substance ingested and its pH play a

TABLE 68-1 Common Caustic Substances Ingested

Caustic Substance	Type	Commercially Available From
Acids	Sulfuric	Batteries
		Industrial cleaning agents
		Metal plating
	Oxalic	Paint thinners, strippers
		Metal cleaners
	Hydrochloric	Solvents
		Metal cleaners
		Toilet and drain cleaners
		Antirust compounds
	Phosphoric	Toilet cleaners
Alkali	Sodium hydroxide	Drain cleaners
	Potassium hydroxide	Oven cleaners
		Washing powders
	Sodium carbonate	Soap manufacturing
		Fruit drying on farms
Ammonia	Commercial ammonia	Household cleaners
	Ammonium hydroxide	
Detergents, bleach	Sodium hypochlorite	Household bleach, cleaners
	Sodium polyphosphate	Industrial detergents
Condy's crystals	Potassium permanganate	Disinfectants, hair dyes

substantial role in the site and type of postingestion esophageal injury, with a pH greater than 12 or less than 1.5 being associated with severe corrosive injuries.[10,52,53,61,75] Crystalline drain cleaners in the form of concentrated sodium hydroxide tend to adhere to the oropharynx or become lodged in the upper esophagus, where injury is most severe.[52,64,66,90,127] Highly concentrated caustic liquids usually pass rapidly through the oropharynx and cause injury to the entrance of the esophagus, the midesophagus, and immediately proximal to the esophagogastric junction.

Unlike alkaline solutions, which do not have much taste, strong acids are bitter, burn on contact, and are usually expectorated. However, when swallowed, they pass rapidly through the esophagus and cause the most substantial damage in the antrum of the stomach. The injury tends to be worse when the stomach is empty.[51] The duodenum and proximal small intestine are relatively protected by pylorospasm.[25,62,98,103] Ferrous sulfate as tablets (Clinitest) or capsules may also induce caustic injury to the esophagus or stomach.[19] Disk batteries contain concentrated potassium or sodium hydroxide, but they rarely lodge in the esophagus because of their small size.[76] If charged, these batteries may also cause injury to adjacent mucosa because of hydrolysis at the negative electrode.

PATHOPHYSIOLOGY

Much of what is known about the pathology of caustic injury in children has been derived from adult experience with self-inflicted injury and experimental studies in animals.[38,53,57,64,66,69,78,97,106] Injury to mucosal surfaces occurs within seconds after contact with a strong acid or alkali.[53,66] The nature of the injury caused by acidic

and alkaline substances differs considerably. With acid ingestion, coagulation necrosis of the musoca, hard eschar formation, and usually limitation of acid penetration through the mucosa occur. With alkali ingestion, tissue penetration with liquefactive necrosis is followed by destruction of the epithelium and submucosa, which may extend through the muscle layer.[16,53,61] A friable discolored eschar develops, under which tissue destruction continues until the alkali is neutralized. The esophagus is damaged principally at the areas of holdup: the cricopharyngeal area, the midesophagus where it is crossed by the aortic arch and left mainstem bronchus, and immediately above the esophagogastric junction. Immediate spasm and disorganized motility occur; these events may result in delayed emptying and even gastric regurgitation.[47] Hemorrhage, thrombosis, and marked inflammation with edema may be seen in the first 24 hours after injury. Depending on the degree of burn, inflammation may extend through the muscle layer until perforation occurs. After 48 hours, there is evidence of thrombosis of submucosal vessels, which gives rise to local necrosis and gangrene. Bacterial contamination leads to the development of small intramural abscesses, which may extend to the mediastinum with full-thickness injury.[18] After several days, necrotic tissue is sloughed, edema decreases, and neovascularization begins. This early reparative or subacute phase is evident from the end of the first week through the second week after injury. Scar formation begins in the third week, when fibroblast proliferation replaces the submucosa and muscularis and stricture formation commences. Mucosal re-epithelialization begins during the third week and is usually complete by the sixth week. It is during this period that adhesions may form, narrowing or obliterating the esophageal lumen. The end result may be a fibrotic stricture and a shortened esophagus.[16] If the injury is transmural, necrosis may extend to the surrounding mediastinum, leading to mediastinitis, or in an anterior direction into the trachea, giving rise to tracheoesophageal or even aortoesophageal fistulas.[9,20,79,87]

Steroids have been used to modify the inflammatory response both at the site of the burn and in the deeper tissues, with the ultimate goal of less extensive scarring.[18,30,52,53,90,109] However, the extent of the initial injury largely determines the outcome of the healed injury; this can range from mucosal re-epithelialization, with loss of esophageal glands and some submucosal fibrosis but preservation of the muscularis, to complete replacement of the esophageal wall by fibrous tissue.[66,81] Once the muscle of the esophagus has been destroyed, it cannot regenerate; at that point, maturation of the fibrous replacement with epithelialization of the luminal surface is the only "positive" outcome.[24] Reduction of scar tissue formation by induced inhibition of intermolecular covalent bonding of collagen with lathyrogens and mitomycin C has been demonstrated experimentally but not clinically.[21,34,35,44]

CLINICAL PRESENTATION

Most infants and children who ingest caustic substances present with few symptoms or signs.[1,29,40,77] Only approximately one quarter have substantial objective evidence of corrosive ingestion.[43,77] The extent and severity of injury depend on the concentration and form of the ingested substance. Crystalline alkalis tend to adhere to moist surfaces and cause immediate pain; in this case, oropharyngeal burns and primarily upper esophageal injury result. Esophageal burns in the absence of objective oropharyngeal evidence may occur in a small percentage ($\leq 10\%$) of patients and should not deter the clinician from taking the appropriate diagnostic steps. However, most patients with extensive oropharyngeal injury present with substantial esophageal damage; esophageal injury is unlikely if only the tongue and soft palate are involved.[1,40,43,77]

The viscosity and specific gravity of corrosive acids are lower than those of liquid alkalis. As a result, acid ingestion is associated with rapid transit through the esophagus; thus, this organ may be largely spared. Damage occurs primarily in the antrum of the stomach because of the pooling of swallowed acid proximal to the pylorus, which goes into spasm on contact with the ingested acid.[49,62,97,113]

Obvious signs and symptoms of injury may be evident, with inflammatory mucosal edema in the oropharyngeal area and severe pain in the mouth and in a retrosternal direction.[29,43] This is often associated with agitation and tachycardia. Drooling and inability to swallow indicate severe posterior pharyngeal or upper esophageal injury.[30,90] Acute obstruction of the upper airway may result from posterior pharyngeal and laryngeal edema caused by spillage of the caustic agent into the upper airway.[54,116]

Concentrated ammonia fumes may be inhaled, causing nasopharyngeal edema and leading to respiratory injury.[54] Although rare, esophageal perforation with mediastinitis, peritonitis, and shock may occur.[9,90]

INITIAL MANAGEMENT AND DIAGNOSIS

Initial management is directed at maintaining an adequate airway and oxygenation and ensuring cardiovascular stability. A few patients may require immediate intervention to maintain the airway. Once respiratory and hemodynamic stability has been achieved, the noxious agent, its composition and concentration, and the circumstances of ingestion should be investigated. Although the caregiver should be able to identify the ingested substance, this information is often lacking. Many health regions have poison centers where detailed product information is available.[117] In cases of caustic ingestion, inducing vomiting or encouraging the ingestion of any liquid is contraindicated because the alkali is mostly neutralized by gastric acids, and the consequences of acid regurgitation may cause further injury. Also, inhaled or aspirated vomitus may introduce corrosive matter into the upper airway, leading to acute inflammation and edema with airway obstruction.

Because the history and physical examination are unreliable in assessing the degree of esophageal involvement, endoscopic examination of the oropharynx and upper gastrointestinal tract is crucial.[1] Fiber-optic endoscopy is both accurate and safe, especially when done within 24 to 48 hours after ingestion.[38,40,95,127,128] Unnecessary treatment is avoided when esophageal injury can be excluded; however, there is still debate about which

Grade	Description
0	Normal
I	Edema and hyperemia of mucosa
IIa	Friability: hemorrhage; erosion blisters, exudates, or whitish membranes; superficial ulcers
IIb	Grade IIa plus deep, discrete or circumferential ulceration
IIIa	Small scattered areas of necrosis; areas of brownish black or gray discoloration
IIIb	Extensive necrosis

TABLE 68–2 Endoscopic Grading of Injury Severity

patients with a history of ingestion require endoscopy. Some advocate endoscopy only in symptomatic patients.[50,74]

Technetium-labeled sucralfate radioisotope scanning of the esophagus has been used successfully as a screening device, with lack of sucralfate adherence indicating the absence of significant injury.[83] Using endoscopy findings to grade the severity of the injury, one can predict the long-term outcome, particularly with regard to subsequent stricture formation; however, it is sometimes difficult in practice to obtain an accurate assessment (Table 68-2).[37,38,54] An attempt is made to visualize the entire upper gastrointestinal tract, but identifying circumferential or grade III injuries provides sufficient information to initiate treatment protocols; attempts at further visualization are unnecessary and potentially dangerous.[54,81] Perforation in this situation is a severe complication that may be accompanied by mediastinitis and even mortality. In the presence of visual evidence of a pharyngeal burn with stridor, early esophagoscopy is contraindicated because of the risk of aggravating the airway obstruction.[123] Indirect fiber-optic laryngoscopy is useful to assess the upper airway.[90] Esophagoscopy may be done at the same time if intubation is required, or it may be done later, when edema of the upper airway has resolved. Initial radiographic studies should be restricted to the neck, chest, and abdomen if aspiration or respiratory burn is suspected. If fever, systemic sepsis, and upper abdominal signs are present, perforation may have occurred, and a water-soluble contrast esophagogram may be useful to provide evidence of perforation.[40] A contrast esophagogram is usually done after 10 to 14 days, when an assessment of the entire esophagus and upper gastrointestinal tract can identify the extent of injury and may help in choosing the appropriate therapy (Fig. 68-1).[71]

TREATMENT

If a known mild irritant, such as hypochlorite bleach, has been ingested without evidence of injury, treatment can be expectant.[43,96,128] If the substance ingested is not known and symptoms are apparent, endoscopy is indicated.[36,37,92,96] For patients with first-degree burns (grade I injury), no specific treatment is necessary. Liquid oral intake is initiated and extended to solids. If solid foods are tolerated, the child can be discharged. Clinical follow-up at 2 to

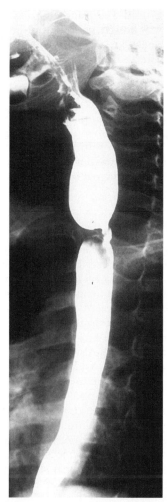

Figure 68–1 Localized stricture from ingestion of caustic crystals in a 4-year-old. The patient was managed successfully by local resection and primary esophageal anastomosis.

3 weeks is indicated, and contrast examination is done if residual clinical symptoms of dysphagia are noted.

Patients with moderate (grade IIa) or severe (grade IIb and III) injuries require further treatment aimed at the prevention of stricture formation.[89] Although most patients with grade IIa injuries recover completely, close follow-up is required, and endoscopy and dilatation must be done as prophylactic measures.[95,96] Major controversy surrounds the treatment options for severe injuries— namely, the use of steroids and antibiotics, esophageal stents, and esophageal dilatation.[112] Grade IIIb injuries are rare in the pediatric age group and usually occur in adolescents attempting suicide. These injuries may require immediate and aggressive surgery if extensive necrosis and perforation are present, especially if the stomach is also involved.[3,38,78]

The use of systemic steroids is based on the knowledge that they inhibit the inflammatory response, which is backed by animal experiments.[16,18,52,53,111] However, in clinical trials using a variety of dosing regimens, no statistical difference in the prevention of stricture formation was evident.[5,120] Extensive retrospective reviews have also failed to show any significant benefit of steroid therapy for patients with severe injuries.[38,90] More recently, the

use of very high dose steroids (dexamethosone 1 mg/kg for 4 to 6 weeks) has been advocated.[22,24,30] However, the number of patients in these studies was small, and morbid conditions, such as mycotic infection of the esophagus, osteitis, peptic ulceration, and osteoporosis, were significant.

For patients with severe injuries, a nasogastric tube may be passed for early feeding purposes. In patients who are unable to swallow, the tube can be used for enteral feeding, to serve as a guide for prograde dilatation, and, to some degree, to maintain patency of the esophageal lumen.

In most cases, oral feeding commences as soon as the patient is able to swallow saliva. If dysphagia occurs, an esophagogram can identify the extent of involvement. Concomitant use of antifungal agents, antacids, and acid-secreting inhibitors (H_2 receptor blockers or proton pump inhibitors) is widespread, but their efficacy has not been proved.[95,96,103,123]

COMPLICATIONS OF INJURY AND TREATMENT

If a stricture is demonstrated on contrast radiography done 10 to 14 days after injury, a program of dilatation is commenced (Fig. 68-2).[96] Various methods can be used,

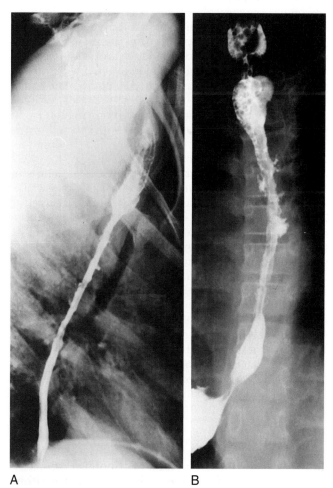

A   B

Figure 68–2 *A,* Early esophagogram after caustic ingestion. *B,* Several areas of full-thickness ulceration progressed to extensive strictures, which required esophageal bypass.

ranging from mercury-filled bougies, flexible-graded bougie dilatation, guidewire-directed metal olives (Eder-Puestow system), or various balloon dilators.* Dilatation should always be attempted with great care. Initial passing of bougies for prograde dilatation should never be done blindly. If there are several strictures and visualization is difficult, it is much safer to place a transesophageal string, which is then used to guide the dilators either retrograde through the gastrostomy or antegrade through the mouth.[119] This is best done by initially passing a soft-tipped, flexible guidewire into the distal esophagus through a gastrotomy.[80,114] Easy access to the gastroesophageal orifice is gained by advancing a polyvinyl chloride endotracheal tube up the lesser curve through the gastrotomy.[82] For satisfactory dilatation of a stricture, a general anesthetic is required in the early stages to protect the airway.

To be effective, dilatations should be done at least once a week, commencing with catheters that are one or two French sizes smaller than the estimated diameter of the stricture. It is generally prudent not to dilate more than two to three sizes larger than the size of the first dilator meeting resistance. Initially, dilatation should be continued as long as esophageal healing and a progressive increase in esophageal caliber are noted, along with re-establishment of normal feeding. Poor prognostic factors are delay in presentation, extensive grade III injury, ongoing esophageal ulceration, a densely fibrotic stricture that cracks on dilatation, a stricture longer than 5 cm, and inadequate lumen patency despite repeated dilatations over a 9- to 12-month period.[9,32] No data support the routine use of prophylactic antibiotics; however, if systemic infection or transmural necrosis occurs, appropriate antibiotic therapy should be commenced.[41,43,53] During recovery, it is essential to provide adequate nutrition; in most cases, the gastrointestinal tract can be used, with access through the nasogastric tube or by placement of a feeding gastrostomy or jejunostomy tube.

If dilatation fails and a dense stricture develops, it requires treatment.[17] As with other benign esophageal strictures, the incidence and severity of gastroesophageal reflux must be investigated and excluded as a contributing cause of the persisting stricture.[23,32,88] Gastroesophageal reflux should be managed surgically, if necessary, before definitive procedures are attempted.[101] Localized strictures may be resected with an end-to-end anastomosis. However, the whole esophagus must first be carefully assessed endoscopically to confirm that the stricture is localized, because the fibrotic injury may be much more extensive than is evident on radiography.[32,86] A healthy color of the esophageal mucosa and distensibility with air insufflation at esophagoscopy are useful signs when assessing the esophagus. Local injection of steroids (1% triamcinolone acetate) into short strictures has had some success when combined with dilatation but has not been assessed prospectively.[13,20,42,56,68,80]

Some investigators advocate the use of esophageal stenting by means of an indwelling nasogastric tube.[27,39,55] The lumen is maintained, and adhesion of de-epithelialized areas of the esophagus is prevented; simultaneously, tube feedings can be given. Over the years, various types of stents have been used (e.g., silicone, polytetrafluoroethylene).[14,27,39,84,88,125] If used, stents should remain in place for at least 6 weeks, at which time epithelial healing should be complete and fibrosis will have begun to mature. However, in many cases, these tubes are not well tolerated; they may promote gastroesophageal reflux, and if an extensive inflammatory response through the muscle occurs, the stent must be in place for much longer to be effective. Stents have also been used in the management of esophageal fistulas resulting from caustic injury or dilatation therapy, mainly as a temporizing measure before surgical repair or esophageal bypass (Fig. 68-3).[87]

LONG-TERM OUTCOME

Extensive caustic injury may heal without stricture or may respond to the various prophylactic and therapeutic measures outlined. However, residual motility dysfunction can be expected, and an achalasia-like picture has been described.[33,45,85]

Carcinoma of the previously injured esophagus is a real risk, but the disease has a latency period of 15 to 40 years.[8,12,15,46,58,69,73,96,118] Also, Barrett's esophagus has

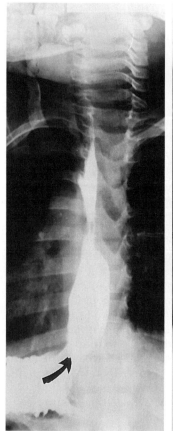
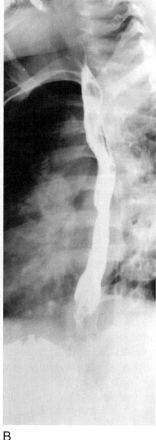

A   B

Figure 68–3 *A,* Contrast esophagogram of a persistent caustic stricture of the midesophagus, with esophageal shortening and marked gastroesophageal reflux *(arrow). B,* This resolved after antireflux surgery and dilatation.

*See references 17, 28, 32, 36, 41, 63, 95, 96, 104, 105, 108, 114, 122, 124.

been observed following lye-induced injury.[89,110] Thus, long-term surveillance with esophagoscopy is advocated. In this regard, two prudent questions arise: To what extent should the clinician try to preserve the damaged esophagus? When should attempts at dilatation be abandoned?[59,94]

Currently, there is a trend toward earlier esophageal bypass in a severely injured esophagus, with the addition of resection of the damaged esophagus.[9,95,109,111] Complications such as abscess or cyst formation in the bypassed but retained esophagus are rare, and carcinoma has not been reported.[9,32]

Esophageal perforation, as evidenced by pain, fever, and tachycardia, is a life-threatening iatrogenic complication of esophageal dilatation (Fig. 68-4).[65,82] With immediate recognition by endoscopy or contrast swallow, many patients with a perforated esophagus can be treated conservatively with systemic antibiotics and parenteral nutrition.[93,107,121] Established methods of management with either thoracostomy drainage or primary repair with proximal and distal esophageal and gastric diversion are reserved for patients with delayed recognition or extensive disruption. Transesophageal water irrigation with or without chest drainage as a supplement to conservative measures has also been advocated.[93] If dilatation has failed or if the esophagus cannot be salvaged, esophageal bypass or substitution is indicated. Operations currently used are colonic interposition, gastric tube esophagoplasty, jejunal interposition, and gastric advancement (see Chapter 69).[32,86,92,100,111,115] Colonic patch procedures have also been used for less extensive but persistent strictures.[92] Deciding which procedure to use and whether to bypass or resect the injured esophagus is influenced by local practice and the morbidity and mortality from esophageal resection. Clearly, the risks associated with resection must be less than the risk of cancer in the retained but bypassed esophagus.[6,8,91,92,102]

RESULTS

Between 1957 and 2003, 327 children with caustic injuries of the esophagus were treated at the University of Cape Town teaching hospitals (Red Cross Water Memorial Children's Hospital and Groote Schuur Hospital). The average age was 35 months, with a range of 9 to 144 months. Forty-eight percent were younger than 2 years. In recent years (1990 to 2003) there has been a trend toward an increasing number of caustic ingestions (832), but only 305 patients (36%) required hospitalization, and of these, only 24 (8%) developed strictures. The mean age was 3.1 years, with a slight male predominance (58%). Most children ingested household cleaners or disinfectants (Table 68-3).

Overall, 82 of the 327 (25%) patients developed fibrous strictures of the esophagus. Caustic soda was the most common corrosive agent (78 of 82 patients) and was taken in the crystal form by 31 children. This form of caustic soda was used extensively on orchards and sheep farms. Acid burns were responsible for only four strictures.

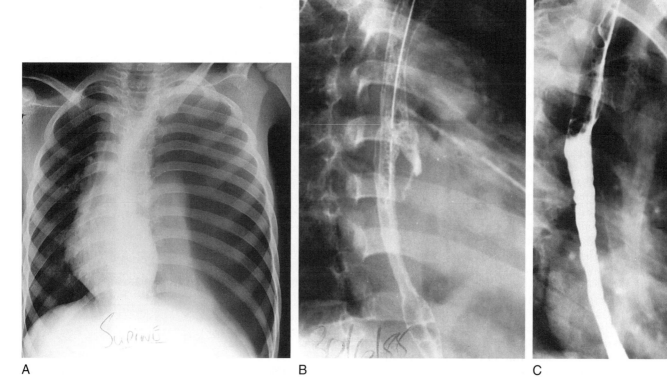

A   B   C

Figure 68–4 Left-sided tension pneumothorax secondary to perforation after dilatation of an upper esophageal caustic stricture. *A*, Treatment by thoracotomy drainage. *B*, Contrast study 10 days later shows that the leak has been contained. *C*, Healed esophagus 12 weeks after perforation. Esophageal replacement was not required in this case.

TABLE 68–3 Caustic Substances Ingested Requiring Admission, 1990-2003 (*N* = 305)

Substance	No. of Patients
Acids (toilet bowl cleaner, soldering flux, antirust compounds, battery acid)	7
Anionic surfactants and polyphosphates (household cleaning agents)	9
Sodium hydroxide (drain and oven cleaners)	52
Ammonium hydroxide (bleach, cleaning agents)	5
2% to 3.5% sodium hypochlorite (bleach)	154
3.2% phenols, 2% alkali (household cleaners and disinfectants)	19
Permanganate crystals	44
Dishwasher detergent granules*	1
Unknown	14

*Very corrosive because of granular form and alkalinity of binders.

One patient with an acid burn who had extensive esophageal injury developed a severe stricture of the stomach antrum and upper jejunum; another patient presented 8 months after ingesting soldering acid with a near-complete antral stricture. Early management did not include steroids or the routine use of antibiotics; antibiotics were administered only in cases of infection, usually of the respiratory tract. Recently, we have empirically used an antifungal agent (nystatin [Mycostatin]) prophylactically and an antacid coating agent (sucralfate) to protect the esophagus from fungal infection and gastroesophageal reflux. Most patients had endoscopy only as far as the first grade II lesion encountered.

A nasogastric tube was inserted into the stomach for feeding purposes and to prevent total occlusion of the esophageal lumen. Strictures were initially treated by regular prograde dilatation. Bougienage commencing 10 to 14 days after injury was performed with the patient under general anesthesia. Antegrade dilatation was initially performed through a rigid esophagoscope using gum elastic bougies; for the last 2 decades, however, this has been done using a fiber-optic endoscope with balloon dilators, the Eder-Puestow wire-guided dilator system, or string-guided dilatation with a transesophageal string and gastrostomy. Successful dilatation was usually accompanied by a steady lengthening of the interval between successive treatments and was confirmed by contrast-swallow radiography. Over the past decade, we have been using the string-guided system through the mouth because we found that the gastrostomy aperture is often too small for the larger-diameter bougies. The Eder-Puestow system is useful on occasion, but for the most part, it is too rigid and does not allow sufficient "feel" for safe dilatation. The esophageal balloon dilator was ineffective for established fibrotic strictures. Patients with an ulcerated esophagus requiring repeated dilatations were given prophylactic antibiotics with each dilatation as a precaution against dissemination of bacteria, after a brain abscess occurred in one of our patients.[7] Two patients received a local injection of the steroid 1% triamcinolone—one into a very scarred supraglottic area, and the other into a fairly localized esophageal stricture—but neither patient had

sustained effects. An esophageal stent was used for 6 weeks in one patient with an extensive grade III injury, but within weeks of removal, complete obliteration of the lumen recurred.

Of the 82 patients with strictures, 38 (46%) responded to repeated dilatations, whereas the other 44 required operative management. Ten of the 44 had severe oropharyngeal burns in addition to the scarred esophagus, and 6 of these patients required tracheostomy. The 82 patients had an average of 18 dilatations (range, 1 to 38). The 38 who responded to dilatation had an average of 17 dilatations over a period of 15 months (range, 0.5 to 20 months); the 44 children with strictures who required esophageal replacement were dilated an average of 12 times (range, 1 to 31) over a 13-month period (range, 0.5 to 87 months). The outcome was poor when presentation was delayed for more than 1 month, with 8 of 10 such patients requiring esophageal bypass. Length of stricture greater than 5 cm was another adverse factor; 17 of 18 patients with this finding did not respond to dilatation.

The most significant complication was esophageal perforation, which occurred in 11 patients (Table 68-4). Perforation occurred after an average of six dilatations. Two perforations occurred during the first dilatation, and others occurred after as many as 14 dilatations, indicating that perforation can occur at any stage. With early recognition, perforation was associated with minimal morbidity, and some patients could be treated conservatively with intravenous antibiotics alone. If extension of the inflammatory process or perforation into the mediastinum or pleura occurred, these areas were drained. One patient developed a tracheoesophageal fistula and had esophagectomy of an extensively scarred esophagus, followed by retrosternal left colonic interposition; no complications such as cyst or abscess formation have occurred in the retained esophagus. Seven patients developed gastroesophageal reflux, six of whom underwent antireflux surgery. Four subsequently responded to dilatations, whereas the other three required esophageal replacement. Since 1969, we have performed an isoperistaltic retrosternal left transverse and left descending colon interposition based on the ascending branches of the left colonic vessels in 35 cases and local resection with end-to-end anastomosis in 1 case. Details of the operative procedure have been reported.[32] Colonic interposition has proved to be a successful conduit for all nutritional needs, with satisfactory long-term results (Fig. 68-5; Table 68-5).

TABLE 68–4 Complications of Caustic Strictures of the Esophagus (*N* = 82)

Complication	No. of Patients
Perforation	11
Tracheoesophageal fistula	1
Gastroesophageal reflux	7
Pneumonia	8
Cerebral abscess	1
Hemorrhage	1
Tracheostomy	6

Some practical aspects of the operation are worthy of mention and should be emphasized, because most complications can be prevented. The feeding vessels of the conduit must be carefully selected and preserved with some adjacent mesentery. Usually, two of the ascending branches of the left colic artery can be retained. The colonic segment required to reach the upper esophagus and pharynx should be measured on the mesenteric border while the pedicle is being pulled taut. As this is being done, the bowel contracts circumferentially and shrinks in length after decompression and irrigation. Care must be taken to avoid entering the pleura when tunneling digitally in a substernal direction, because a tear into the pleural cavity sucks the colon into the adjacent thorax and may result in tortuosity of the graft. Redundancy of the lower end of the conduit should be avoided by resecting any distal redundancy before cologastric anastomosis is performed. The upper anastomosis is performed as a primary procedure in a meticulous manner with an inverted U-shaped inlay of colon into the anterolateral proximal esophagus or pharynx, thereby extending the length of the anastomosis and reducing the incidence of stricture. Pyloroplasty should be done as an adjunct to ensure adequate gastric emptying, thus preventing gastrocolonic reflux or reflux into the retained distal esophagus. Tight closure of the abdominal sheath in the epigastrium should be avoided.[30,32] At the end of the procedure it is useful to hitch the stomach to the anterior abdominal wall with sutures or by placing a gastrostomy to avoid a posteriorly directed "bow" of the inferior aspect of the graft.

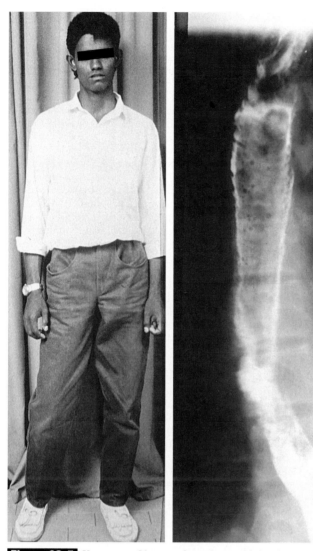

Figure 68–5 Young man 21 years after substernal left colonic esophageal replacement for caustic injury, with accompanying esophagogram. He recently developed fatal squamous carcinoma of the cricopharynx nearly 30 years after caustic ingestion.

TABLE 68–5 Complications After Left Colonic Interposition for Corrosive Esophageal Strictures, 1969-1995 (N = 33)

Complication	No. of Patients
Early	
Death	2 (1 small bowel volvulus; 1 cardiac tamponade of PVC central line)
Leaks (upper anastomosis)	2
Recurrent laryngeal nerve palsy	1
Late	
Stricture (upper anastomosis)	4 (2 revisions)
Significant gastrocolonic reflux	1
Intestinal obstruction (adhesions)	1
Peptic ulceration (distal cologastric)	1

REFERENCES

1. Adams JS, Brick HG: Pediatric caustic ingestion. Ann Otol Rhinolaryngol 1982;91:656.
2. Aghaji MAC, Chuklwu OC: Oesophageal replacement in pediatric patients. J R Coll Surg Edinb 1992;37:101.
3. Allen RE, et al: Corrosive injuries of the stomach. Arch Surg 1970;100:409.
4. Amoury RA, et al: Tracheoesophageal fistula after lye ingestion. J Pediatr Surg 1975;10:273.
5. Anderson KD, Rouse TM, Randolph JG: A controlled trial of corticosteroids in children with corrosive injury of the esophagus. N Engl J Med 1990;323:637.
6. Anderson KD, et al: Long-term follow-up of children with colon and gastric tube interposition for esophageal atresia. Surgery 1992;111:131.
7. Angel C, Wrenn E, Lobe T: Brain abscess: An unusual complication of multiple esophageal dilatations. Pediatr Surg Int 1991;6:42.
8. Appelqvist P, Salmo M: Lye corrosion carcinoma of the esophagus: A review of 63 cases. Cancer 1980;43:2655.
9. Ashcraft KW: Chemical esophageal injuries. In Ashcraft KW, Holder TM (eds): Pediatric Surgery, 2nd ed. Philadelphia, WB Saunders, 1993.
10. Ashcraft KW, Padula RT: The effect of dilute corrosives on the esophagus. Pediatrics 1974;53:226.
11. Bahnassy AF, Bassiouny IE: Esophagocoloplasty for caustic stricture of the esophagus: Changing concepts. Pediatr Surg Int 1993;8:103.
12. Benirschke T: Time bomb of lye ingestion? Am J Dis Child 1981;135:17.

13. Berenson GA, et al: Intralesional steroids in the treatment of refractory esophageal strictures. J Pediatr Gastroenterol Nutr 1994;18:250.

14. Berkovits RN, et al: Caustic injury of the esophagus: Sixteen years' experience, an introduction of a new model oesophageal stent. J Laryngol Otol 1996;110:1041.

15. Bigelow NH: Carcinoma of the esophagus developing at the site of lye stricture. Cancer 1953;6:1159.

16. Bosher LJ Jr, Burford TH, Ackerman L: The pathology of experimentally produced lye burns and strictures of the esophagus. J Thorac Surg 1951;21:483.

17. Broor SL, et al: Long term results of endoscopic dilatation for corrosive oesophageal strictures. Gut 1993;34:1498.

18. Burford TH, Webb WR, Ackerman L: Caustic burns of the esophagus and their surgical management: A clinico-experimental correlation. Ann Surg 1953;138:453.

19. Burrington JD: Clinitest burns of the esophagus. Ann Thorac Surg 1975;20:400.

20. Burrington JD, Raffensberger JG: Surgical management of tracheoesophageal fistula complicating caustic ingestion. Surgery 1978;84:329.

21. Butler C, et al: Morphologic aspects of experimental esophageal lye strictures. II. Effect of steroid hormones, bouginage and induced lathyrism on acute lye burns. Surgery 1977;81:431.

22. Cadranel S, et al: Treatment of esophageal caustic injuries: Experience with high-dose dexamethasone. Pediatr Surg Int 1993;8:97.

23. Capella M, et al: Persistence of corrosive esophageal stricture due to gastroesophageal reflux in children. Pediatr Surg Int 1992;7:180.

24. Cardona JC, Daly JF: Management of corrosive esophagitis: Analysis of treatment, methods and results. N Y State J Med 1964;4:2307.

25. Chodak GW, Paesaro E Jr: Acid ingestion, need for gastric resection. JAMA 1978;239:225.

26. Christensen HBT: Epidemiology and prevention of caustic ingestion. Acta Pediatr 1994;83:212.

27. Coln D, Chang JHT: Experience with esophageal stenting for caustic burns in children. J Pediatr Surg 1986;21:588.

28. Cox JGC, et al: Balloon or bougie for dilatation of benign esophageal stricture. Dig Dis Sci 1994;39:776.

29. Crain EF, Gershel JC, Mezey AP: Caustic ingestions: Symptoms as prediction of esophageal injury. Am J Dis Child 1984;138:863.

30. Curtis JA, et al: Endocrine complications of topical and intralesional corticosteroid therapy. Arch Dis Child 1982;57:204.

31. Cywes S: Challenges and dilemmas for a pediatric surgeon. J Pediatr Surg 1994;29:957.

32. Cywes S, et al: Corrosive strictures of the esophagus in children. Pediatr Surg Int 1993;8:8.

33. Dantas RO, Mamede RC: Esophageal motility in patients with esophageal caustic injury. Am J Gastroenterol 1996;91:1157.

34. Davis WM, Madden JW, Peacock EE Jr: A new approach to control of esophageal stenosis. Ann Surg 1972;176:469.

35. Demitbilek S, et al: Effects of estradiol and progesterone on the synthesis of collagen in corrosive esophageal burns in rats. J Pediatr Surg 1994;29:1425.

36. De Peppo F, et al: Conservative treatment of corrosive esophageal strictures: A comparative study of endoscopic dilatations and esophageal stenting. Pediatr Surg Int 1993;8:2.

37. DiConstanzo J, et al: New therapeutic approach to corrosive burns of the upper gastrointestinal tract. Gut 1980;21:370.

38. Estrera A, et al: Corrosive burns of esophagus and stomach: A recommendation for an aggressive surgical approach. Ann Thorac Surg 1986;41:276.

39. Fell SC, et al: The effect of intraluminal splinting in the prevention of caustic stricture of the esophagus. J Thorac Cardiovasc Surg 1966;52:675.

40. Ferguson MK, et al: Early evaluation and therapy for caustic esophageal injury. Am J Surg 1989;157:116.

41. Fyfe AH, Auldist AW: Corrosive ingestion in children. Z Kinderchir 1984;39:229.

42. Gandhi RP, Cooper A, Barlow BA: Successful management of esophageal strictures without resection or replacement. J Pediatr Surg 1989;24:745.

43. Gaudreault P, et al: Predictability of esophageal injury from signs and symptoms: A study of caustic ingestion in 378 children. Pediatrics 1983;71:767.

44. Gehanno P, Guedon C: Inhibition of experimental esophageal lye strictures by penicillamine. Arch Otolaryngol 1981;107:145.

45. Genc A, Mutaf O: Esophageal motility changes in acute and late periods of caustic esophageal burns and their relation to prognosis in children. J Pediatr Surg 1998;37:1526.

46. Gerzic Z, et al: Post corrosive stricture and carcinoma of the esophagus. In Siewert JR, Holsher AH (eds): Diseases of the Esophagus. New York, Springer Verlag, 1988.

47. Guelrud M, Ardeha M: Motor function abnormalities in acute caustic esophagitis. J Clin Gastroenterol 1980;2:247.

48. Gundogdu HZ, et al: Colonic replacement for the treatment of caustic esophageal strictures in children. J Pediatr Surg 1992;27:771.

49. Gupta S: Total obliteration of esophagus and hypopharynx due to corrosives. J Thorac Cardiovasc Surg 1970;60:264.

50. Gupta SK, Croffie JM, Fitzgerald JF: Is esophagogastroduo-denoscopy necessary in all caustic ingestions? J Pediatr Gastroenterol Nutr 2001;32:50.

51. Hall RJ, Lilly JR: Treatment of acid burns of the stomach in children by pedicle pyloroplasty. Surg Gynecol Obstet 1988;167:153.

52. Haller JA Jr, Bachman K: The comparative effect of current therapy on experimental burns of the esophagus. Pediatrics 1964;34:236.

53. Haller JA Jr, et al: Pathophysiology and management of acute corrosive burns of the esophagus: Results and treatment of 285 children. J Pediatr Surg 1971;6:578.

54. Hawkins DB, Demerer MJ, Barnett TE: Caustic ingestion: Controversies in management. A review of 214 cases. Laryngoscope 1980;90:98.

55. Hill JL, et al: Clinical technique and success of the esophageal stent to prevent corrosive strictures. J Pediatr Surg 1976;11:443.

56. Holder TM, Ashcraft KW, Leape L: The treatment of patients with esophageal strictures by local steroid injections. J Pediatr Surg 1969;4:646.

57. Holinger PH: Management of esophageal lesions caused by chemical burns. Ann Otol Rhinolaryngol 1968;77:819.

58. Hopkins RA, Postlethwaite RW: Caustic burns and carcinoma of the esophagus. Ann Surg 1981;194:146.

59. Imre J, Kopp M: Arguments against long term conservative treatment of esophageal strictures due to corrosive burns. Thorax 1972;27:594.

60. Jackson C: Esophageal stenosis following swallowing of caustic alkalis. JAMA 1971;77:22.

61. Jelenko C: Chemicals that "burn." J Trauma 1974;14:65.

62. Jena GP, Lazarus C: A case report: Acid corrosive gastritis. S Afr Med J 1985;67:473.

63. Johnsen A, Jensen LI, Mauritzen K: Balloon-dilatation of esophageal strictures in children. Pediatr Radiol 1986;16:388.

64. Johnson EE: A study of corrosive esophagitis. Laryngoscope 1963;73:1651.

65. Kim I-O, et al: Perforation complicating balloon dilatation of esophageal strictures in infants and children. Radiology 1993;189:741.

66. Kirsch MM, Ritter F: Caustic ingestion and subsequent damage to the oropharyngeal and digestive passages. Ann Thorac Surg 1976;21:74.
67. Kirsch MM, et al: Treatment of caustic injuries of the esophagus. Ann Surg 1978;188:675.
68. Kirsch MM, et al: Intralesional steroid injections for peptic oesophageal strictures. Gastrointest Endosc 1991;37:180.
69. Kiviranta UK: Corrosion carcinoma of the esophagus. Acta Otolaryngol 1952;42:88.
70. Krey H: Treatment of corrosive lesions of the esophagus. Acta Otolaryngol 1952;102(Suppl):1.
71. Kuhn JR, Tunell WP: The role of initial cine-esophagography in caustic esophageal injury. Am J Surg 1983;146:804.
72. Landau G, Saunders W: The effect of chlorine bleach on the esophagus. Laryngol Rhinol Otol 1978;92:499.
73. Lansing PB, Ferrante WA, Ochsner JL: Carcinoma of the esophagus at the site of lye stricture. Am J Surg 1969;118:108.
74. Larimeau T, et al: Accidental caustic injury in children: Is endoscopy always mandatory? J Pediatr Gastroenterol Nutr 2001;33:81.
75. Leape LL, et al: Hazard to health—liquid lye. N Engl J Med 1971;284:578.
76. Litovitz R, Schmitz BF: Ingestion of cylindrical and button batteries: An analysis of 2382 cases. Pediatrics 1992;89:747.
77. Mansson I: Diagnosis of acute corrosive lesions of the esophagus. J Laryngol Otol 1978;92:499.
78. Marshall F: Caustic burns of the esophagus: Ten-year results of aggressive care. South Med J 1979;72:1236.
79. McCabe RE, Scott JR, Knox WC: Fistulation between the esophagus, aorta and trachea as a complication of acute corrosive esophagitis: Report of a case. Ann Surg 1969;35:450.
80. Mendelsohn HJ, Maloney WH: The treatment of benign strictures of the esophagus with cortisone injection. Ann Rhinol Laryngol 1970;79:85.
81. Middlekamp JN, et al: The management and problems of caustic burns in children. J Thorac Cardiovasc Surg 1969;57:341.
82. Millar AJW, et al: Negotiating the "difficult" oesophageal stricture. Pediatr Surg Int 1993;8:445.
83. Millar AJW, et al: Detection of caustic oesophageal injury with technetium 99m-labelled sucralfate. J Pediatr Surg 2001;36:262.
84. Mills LJ, Estrera SA, Platt MR: Avoidance of esophageal stricture following severe caustic burns by use of an intraluminal stent. Ann Thorac Surg 1979;28:60.
85. Moody FG, Garrett JM: Esophageal achalasia following lye ingestion. Ann Surg 1969;17:775.
86. Mutaf O: Esophagoplasty for caustic esophageal burns in children. Pediatr Surg Int 1992;7:106.
87. Mutaf O, et al: Management of tracheoesophageal fistula as a complication of esophageal dilatations in caustic esophageal burns. J Pediatr Surg 1995;30:823.
88. Mutaf O, et al: Gastroesophageal reflux: A determinant in the outcome of caustic esophageal burns. J Pediatr Surg 1996;31:1494.
89. Naef AP, Savary M, Ozzello L: Columnar lined lower esophagus: An acquired lesion with malignant predisposition: Report of 140 cases of Barrett's esophagus with 12 adenocarcinomas. J Thorac Cardiovasc Surg 1975;70:826.
90. Oakes DD, Sherck JP, Mark JBD: Lye ingestion: Clinical patterns and therapeutic implications. J Thorac Cardiovasc Surg 1982;83:194.
91. Orringer MB, Orringer JS, Arbor A: Esophagectomy without thoracotomy: A dangerous operation? J Thorac Cardiovasc Surg 1983;85:72.
92. Othersen BH Jr, Parker EP, Smith CD: The surgical management of esophageal stricture in children. Ann Surg 1988;207:590.
93. Panieri E, et al: Iatrogenic esophageal perforation in children: Patterns of injury, presentation, management and outcome. J Pediatr Surg 1996;31:890.
94. Panieri E, et al: Oesophageal replacement in the management of corrosive strictures: When is surgery indicated? Pediatr Surg Int 1998;13:336.
95. Pintus C, et al: Caustic ingestion in childhood: Current treatment possibilities and their complications. Pediatr Surg Int 1993;8:109.
96. Rappert P, et al: Diagnosis and therapeutic management of oesophageal and gastric caustic burns in childhood. Eur J Pediatr Surg 1993;3:202.
97. Ray JF, et al: The natural history of liquid lye ingestion. Arch Surg 1974;109:436.
98. Ritter F, Newman MH, Newman DE: A clinical and experimental study of corrosive burns of the stomach. Ann Otol Rhinol Laryngol 1968;77:830.
99. Rivosecchi M: Lye strictures (part 1) [editorial]. Pediatr Surg Int 1993;8:1.
100. Rode H, et al: Colonic oesophageal replacement in children—functional results. Z Kinderchir 1986;41:201.
101. Rode H, et al: Reflux strictures of the esophagus in children. J Pediatr Surg 1992;27:462.
102. Rodgers BM, Ryckman FC, Talbert JL: Blunt transmediastinal esophagectomy with simultaneous substernal colon interposition for esophageal strictures in children. J Pediatr Surg 1981;16:184.
103. Rothstein FC: Caustic injuries to the esophagus in children. Pediatr Clin North Am 1986;33:665.
104. Saeed ZA, Graham DY: Treatment of benign esophageal stricture: Where do we go from here? Dig Dis Sci 1994;39:2099.
105. Sato Y, et al: Balloon dilatation of esophageal stenosis in children. AJR Am J Roentgenol 1988;150:639.
106. Sellars SL, Spence RAJ: Chemical burns of the oesophagus. J Laryngol Otol 1987;101:1211.
107. Shaffer HA, Valenzuela G, Mittal RK: Esophageal perforation: A reassessment of the criteria for choosing medical or surgical therapy. Arch Intern Med 1992;152:757.
108. Shemesh E, Czerniak A: Comparison between Savary-Gilliard and balloon dilatation of benign esophageal stricture. World J Surg 1990;14:518.
109. Spain DM, Molomut N, Haber A: The effect of cortisone on the formation of granulation tissue in mice. Am J Pathol 1957;26:710.
110. Spechler SJ, et al: Barrett's epithelium complicating lye ingestion with sparing of the distal esophagus. Gastroenterology 1981;81:580.
111. Spitz L: Gastric transposition via the mediastinal route for infants with long-gap esophageal atresia. Pediatr Surg 1984;19:149.
112. Spitz L, Lakhoo K: Caustic ingestion. Arch Dis Child 1993;68:157.
113. Symbas PN, Vlasis SE, Hatcher CR Jr: Esophagitis secondary to ingestion of caustic material. Ann Thorac Surg 1983;36:73.
114. Tanyel FC, Buyukpamukcu NB, Hicsonmez A: An improved stringing method for retrograde dilatations of caustic esophageal strictures. Pediatr Surg Int 1987;2:57.
115. Thomas AN, Dedo HH: Pharyngogastrostomy for treatment of severe stricture of the pharynx and esophagus. J Thorac Cardiovasc Surg 1977;73:817.
116. Thomas AN, et al: Pharyngoesophageal caustic stricture. Am J Surg 1976;132:195.
117. Thompson DF, et al: Evaluation of regional and nonregional poison centers. N Engl J Med 1983;308:191.
118. Ti TK: Esophageal carcinoma associated with corrosive injury—prevention and treatment by esophageal resection. Br J Surg 1983;70:223.

119. Tucker JA, et al: Tucker retrograde esophageal dilatation 1924-1974: A historical review. Ann Otol Rhinol Laryngol 1974;83(Suppl 16):1.

120. Ulman I, Mutaf O: A critique of systemic steroids in the management of esophageal burns in children. Eur J Pediatr Surg 1998;8:71.

121. Van der Zee DC, et al: Management of pediatric esophageal perforation. J Thorac Cardiovasc Surg 1988;95:692.

122. Walton WW: An evaluation of the poison prevention packaging act. Pediatrics 1982;69:363.

123. Wasserman RL, Ginsburg CM: Caustic substance injuries. J Pediatr 1985;107:169.

124. Webb WA: Esophageal dilatation: Personal experience with current instruments and techniques. Am J Gastroenterol 1988;83:471.

125. Wijburg FA, Heymans HAS, Urbanus NAM: Caustic esophageal lesions in childhood: Prevention of stricture formation. J Pediatr Surg 1989;24:171.

126. Yarrington CT Jr: The experimental causticity of sodium hypochloride in the esophagus. Ann Otol Rhinol 1970; 179:895.

127. Zarger SA, et al: Ingestion of strong corrosive alkalis: Spectrum of injury to upper gastrointestinal tract and natural history. Gastroenterology 1989;97:276.

128. Zarger SA, et al: The role of fibreoptic endoscopy in the management of corrosive ingestion and modified endoscopic classification of burns. Gastrointest Endosc 1991; 37:165.

Chapter 69

Esophageal Replacement

Lewis Spitz

The need to replace the esophagus is becoming increasingly rare, mainly because of improved methods of retaining the native esophagus in infants born with long-gap esophageal atresia. In addition, general awareness of the damage that can occur as a consequence of intractable gastroesophageal reflux has resulted in more aggressive approaches in antireflux surgery, and with the introduction of childproof containers, fewer lye and caustic injuries to the esophagus occur. Nevertheless, there continue to be instances in which substitution of the esophagus is required, and it is therefore important for the pediatric surgeon to be aware of the various options available for replacement.

INDICATIONS FOR ESOPHAGEAL REPLACEMENT

Esophageal Atresia

Infants with long-gap esophageal atresia constitute the main group that requires esophageal replacement because of failure to achieve end-to-end anastomosis. Numerous maneuvers have been adopted to overcome the long gap and achieve a primary anastomosis to allow retention of the infant's native esophagus. A list of these techniques is presented in Table 69-1. For isolated esophageal atresia, it is important to exclude an upper pouch tracheo-esophageal fistula. When only a small nubbin of distal esophagus is present above the hiatus or there is no intrathoracic esophagus at all, a replacement is clearly going to be required, and it is best to perform a cervical esophagostomy at an early stage and allow the infant to go home pending a later replacement procedure. The infant is now free of the danger of aspiration, and appropriate bonding with the family can take place at home. If an anastomosis cannot be achieved even under extreme tension, current opinion favors an attempt at delayed primary repair. The infant is fed by gastrostomy while suction is applied to the upper esophageal pouch for a period of 6 to 12 weeks. During this time, the gap between the two ends of the esophagus gradually diminishes. If primary anastomosis is impossible at this stage, further delay is unproductive and esophageal substitution is required. It is

now possible to perform a primary interposition procedure, or if circumstances do not permit, a cervical esophagostomy is performed with a later replacement procedure. Although it is obvious that the patient's own esophagus is the best esophagus, persisting with futile attempts to retain the native esophagus in the presence of major complications (such as empyema, intractable stricture, and repeated recurrent fistulas) is occasionally detrimental to the well-being of the infant. In such situations, it is clearly in the patient's best interest and safety to abandon the esophagus and perform a replacement procedure at a later stage.

Peptic Strictures

Antireflux surgery is usually performed for pathologic gastroesophageal reflux before intractable strictures develop. However, in children with severely scarred and

---

TABLE 69-1 Surgical Maneuvers for Correction of Long-Gap Esophageal Atresia

During the Initial Procedure
Anastomosis under tension[40,69,112]
Tension-relieving procedures[26,50,65,96]
Flap technique[25,36]
Suture fistula[48,100,103,104]

Delayed Primary Anastomosis
With bougienage: proximal,[51,70] proximal and distal,[43] magnetic[47]
Without bougienage[89]
Esophageal-lengthening techniques (e.g., flap,[22,36] spiral myotomy,[123] gastric division[101])

Transmediastinal "Thread"
With and without "olives"[80,91]
Kato technique[57]

Esophageal Replacement
Colonic interposition[29,115,127]
Gastric tube esophagoplasty[5,45]
Jejunal interposition[93]
Gastric transposition[73,114]

inflamed strictures of the esophagus, most of these strictures resolve with effective antireflux surgery followed by regular postoperative esophageal dilatation. A small percentage requires limited "sleeve" resection of the strictured area, but some fail to respond and require esophageal replacement.

Caustic Strictures

Though uncommon in developed countries as a result of legislation mandating childproof containers for caustic substances, many children in developing countries continue to sustain caustic esophageal injuries. Most cases are mild and respond to repeated dilatation. Full-thickness injury to more than a very short segment of the esophagus invariably results in an intractable stricture that fails to respond to dilatation and usually requires substitution. Continuing with dilatation at regular intervals for longer than 6 to 12 months is unproductive. The need to resect the damaged esophagus continues to be disputed. The risk for malignant conditions and the ease with which esophagectomy can be performed in children favor resection and substitution rather than bypass procedures. Caustic strictures are discussed extensively in Chapter 68.

Miscellaneous Indications

The need for replacement because of bleeding esophageal varices is virtually obsolete as a result of the success of alternative techniques, particularly sclerotherapy and portosystemic shunts. Tumors of the esophagus may require resection of extensive length of the esophagus. Examples of such tumors in children are diffuse leiomyoma and inflammatory pseudotumor. The esophagus may be extensively damaged by prolonged impaction of foreign bodies, such as aluminum ring pull-tabs, which are radiolucent and may escape detection on conventional radiography. Other unusual indications for esophageal replacement include intractable achalasia, diffuse candidiasis in children with immune deficiency, scleroderma,[71] and epidermolysis bullosa.[118]

CHARACTERISTICS OF AN IDEAL ESOPHAGEAL SUBSTITUTION

1. The substitute must function as an efficient conduit from mouth to stomach to satisfy the nutritional needs of the child.
2. Gastric acid reflux into the conduit must be minimal; if reflux does occur, the substitute should be resistant to gastric acid.
3. The substitute should not impair respiratory or cardiac function.
4. The operative technique should be technically unchallenging and adaptable to small children.
5. The conduit should not produce any external deformity.
6. The conduit must grow with the child and continue to function into adult life.[13]

TYPES OF ESOPHAGEAL REPLACEMENT

Although the colon continues to be the most frequently used organ for esophageal substitution in children, dissatisfaction by some surgeons has led to the use of alternatives. The methods most commonly used are shown in Figure 69-1.

The advantages and disadvantages of the various substitution procedures are outlined in Table 69-2.

Several artificial prostheses have been used as substitutes for the esophagus; however, all of them have functioned for only very short periods.[100]

ROUTE FOR POSITIONING THE ESOPHAGEAL SUBSTITUTE

The posterior mediastinum is the shortest distance between the cervical region and the abdomen for esophageal replacement.[77] Colonic interpositions were originally placed subcutaneously on the anterior chest wall, but the cosmetic appearance of this method is unacceptable and it

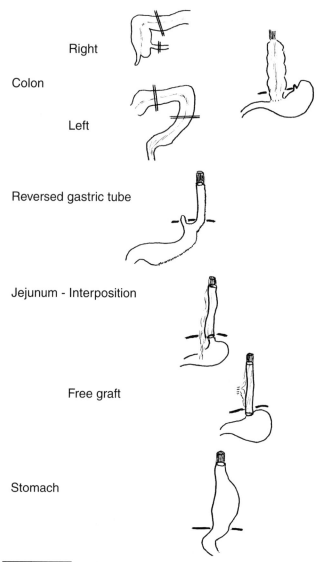

Right

Colon

Left

Reversed gastric tube

Jejunum - Interposition

Free graft

Stomach

Figure 69-1 Methods of esophageal replacement.

TABLE 69-2 Substitution Procedures

Method	Advantages	Disadvantages
Colon	Adequate length Reflux seldom occurs	Precarious blood supply Graft necrosis High incidence of leaks and strictures Multiple anastomoses Redundancy over the long term Slow transit of food
Gastric tube	Adequate length Good blood supply Size of conduit appropriate Rapid transit	Very long suture line High incidence of leaks and strictures Reflux leading to Barrett's syndrome
Jejunum	Appropriate size	Very precarious blood supply Retention of peristaltic activity Length can be a problem Three anastomoses
Free jejunal graft	Appropriate size Good peristaltic activity	Specialized technique for microvascular anastomosis Prolonged operating time Precarious blood supply High failure rate
Stomach	Adequate length easily attained Excellent blood supply Single anastomosis Ease of procedure	Bulk of stomach in thorax Reflux common early on Poor gastric emptying Affects pulmonary function? Affects growth?

has been abandoned. The advantages and disadvantages of the other routes are outlined in Table 69-3.

TIMING

Although esophageal replacement is possible in newborns, the procedure should generally be delayed until the infant is thriving and weighs at least 5 kg. In the interim, it is important to stimulate the swallowing reflex by offering sham oral feedings during regular gastrostomy feedings. Infants who achieve good sham feeding will undoubtedly rapidly accept oral nutrition when the esophageal substitute has been successfully connected. In all cases, adequate mechanical preparation of the intestine is essential because the organ that has been selected for esophageal replacement may be unsuitable and an alternative technique may be required.

Excellent comprehensive reviews of the history of esophageal replacement have been documented by May and Samson in 1969[74] and by Postlethwait in 1983.[87]

COLONIC INTERPOSITION

Colonic interposition continues to be the most widely used procedure for esophageal replacement in children. In adults with carcinoma of the esophagus, the currently preferred technique is gastric transposition, with colonic interposition being reserved as a secondary procedure.

History

In 1911, Kelling[58] used a segment of transverse colon to bypass the esophagus. Because the mesentery was too short for the planned jejunal interposition, he based the colon on the left colic artery. However, the patient died before an attempt could be made to join the cervical esophagostomy to the upper end of the colon. In 1911, Vulliet[125] preserved the mesenteric pedicle to the right end of the colon transplant in a cadaver. In 1914, Von Hacker carried out the first successful colonic interposition in an adult.[124] The first successful colonic bypass in a child was reported by Lundblad in 1921.[68] The patient underwent the procedure for an esophageal stricture at 3 years of age and lived until he was 37 years old, at which time he died accidentally. Ochsner and Owens[79] reviewed the literature in 1934 and could find only 20 reported cases of colonic esophagoplasty. In 1951, Rudler and Monod-Broca[98] described the retrosternal ileocolonic graft. In 1955, Dale and Sherman[20] described two infants with esophageal atresia who underwent

TABLE 69-3 Routes for Positioning the Esophageal Substitute

Route	Advantages	Disadvantages
Retrosternal	Ease of procedure Useful when the transpleural and mediastinal routes are inflamed or surgery has previously been performed	Longest route from neck to abdomen Angulation of the graft unavoidable Problems with access if cardiac surgery is required
Transpleural	Convenience and ease of the procedure	Displacement of the lung Requires thoracotomy
Posterior mediastinal	Most direct route Organ contained in the mediastinum Little or no lung compression Thoracotomy not always required	Mediastinum may be unavailable because of previous surgery, fibrosis, or inflammation

reconstruction of the esophagus with a right colonic retrogastric anterior mediastinal interposition at 2 years of age. Four years later, Battersby and Moore[10] reported five cases of right colon replacement for congenital atresia of the esophagus. The three children who underwent substernal placement of the colon survived. They recommended delaying the procedure until the infant was at least 9 months of age. Major advances in use of the colon for esophageal replacement were documented by Sherman and Waterston in 1957,[106] by Waterston in 1961 and 1964,[126] and by Belsey in 1965.[12] Waterston and Belsey were strong proponents of the transpleural route and use of the left colon supplied by the left colic vessels. In 1967, Othersen and Clatworthy[83] stated that the colon was the best organ for esophageal replacement in children and recommended delaying the operation until the child was 18 to 24 months old so that gravity in the erect position would assist in food passage through the colonic interposition. Freeman and Cass,[29] in 1982, advocated placing the transposed colon in the route of the native esophagus in the posterior mediastinum and reported an impressively low rate of complications.

Surgical Technique

Colonic interposition entails use of either the right colon based on the ileocolic vessels placed in the retrosternal position or the left colon based on the left colic vessels positioned in a retrohilar position in the left pleural cavity or in the posterior mediastinum (Fig. 69-2).

Right Colon Retrosternal Technique

The abdomen is opened through either a midline upper abdominal incision or a transverse upper abdominal muscle-cutting incision that transects both rectus abdominis muscles. The entire colon must be mobilized and exposed to provide detailed and accurate assessment of its blood supply. In a study of 600 specimens, Sonneland et al.[108] reported that only 24% of specimens showed the typical textbook picture of three vessels to the right side of the colon arising from the superior mesenteric artery. The middle colic artery was absent in 3.6% of cases. The marginal artery was occasionally absent. In individual children, the anatomy of the vascular supply determines the section of colon most appropriate for the interposition procedure. The blood supply for the right colonic interposition is based on the middle colic artery. However, if a segment of terminal ileum is to be used for the interposition,[119] the ileocolic vascular supply to the graft must be preserved if possible. The length of intestine to be used is carefully estimated, and bulldog clamps are placed across all vessels that require division. The clamps are left in position for at least 10 minutes to ensure that the blood supply is adequate, that the marginal vessels continue to pulsate, and that the color of the section of colon selected for the interposition remains normal. The blood supply can be further evaluated by removing the appendix and observing the flow of blood in the appendicular artery. If the blood supply seems to be satisfactory, the vessels that require division are carefully and securely ligated and divided. It is important to preclude hematoma formation

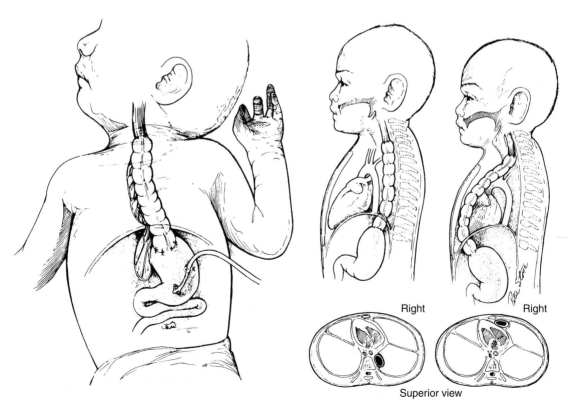

Right

Right

Superior view

Figure 69–2 Colon esophagoplasty. The colon may be placed in a retrosternal or retrohilar position with equal success. (From Randolph JG: Surgical problems of the esophagus. In Sabiston D, Spencer F [eds]: Gibbon's Surgery of the Chest, 3rd ed. Philadelphia, WB Saunders, 1976.)

in the mesentery. The ileum is divided between the clamps, and the distal stump is closed in preparation for relocation into the neck. The transverse colon is then divided to the left of the middle colic artery, and intestinal continuity is restored by an end-to-end ileotransverse colostomy.

A transverse cervical incision that encircles the previously constructed cervical esophagostomy is made. The incision should extend to the midline of the neck approximately 1 cm above the manubrium sterni. The upper border and posterior surface of the manubrium are exposed by dividing the cervical fascia and the origin of the sternomastoid muscle. It may be necessary to enlarge the opening into the retrosternal space by removing the upper part of the manubrium, sternoclavicular joint, or both.

The retrosternal tunnel is developed from above through a cervical incision in a plane directly posterior to the sternum and anterior to the thymus and pericardium, and the anterior attachments of the diaphragm are divided from below. The tunnel must be wide enough to accommodate at least two to three fingers.

The stomach is then mobilized to allow the colon and its vascular pedicle to pass behind the stomach, over the anterior surface of the liver, and through the retrosternal tunnel into the neck. It is vital to ensure that there are no kinks or twists in the graft that may impair the blood supply. The distal end of the colonic interposition is anastomosed to the anterior wall of the stomach close to the lesser curvature. An antireflux submucosal gastric tunnel has been devised as a method of preventing reflux of gastric acid into the colon graft.[39] The proximal end of the graft, which will comprise the ascending colon or the terminal ileum, is anastomosed in end-to-end fashion to the distal end of the cervical esophagus. During preparation of the esophagus for anastomosis, it is imperative to preserve the blood supply and to meticulously mobilize the full thickness of the esophagus. The length of the colonic interposition must be just sufficient to bridge the gap between the esophagus and the stomach. Excess intestine should be resected before anastomosis while the blood supply to the remaining graft is preserved. Redundancy is a problem that increases with time and can lead to stasis. Pyloroplasty is generally recommended to prevent this complication.

Left Colon Transpleural Technique

The left colon transpleural technique was originally described by Waterston.[126] In this method the left transverse colon based on the ascending branch of the left colic artery is placed isoperistaltically in the retrohilar position. In the original description, the entire procedure was performed through a left thoracic incision with access to the abdomen provided by detaching the diaphragm peripherally from the chest wall. An alternative approach is to use separate abdominal and thoracic incisions or a thoracoabdominal incision.[12] The left colon graft is based on the ascending branch of the left colic artery. Intestinal continuity is restored by an end-to-end colocolic anastomosis. The colon graft is passed in a retrogastric and retropancreatic direction and then through a separate lateral incision in the posterior diaphragm into the left pleural cavity. The colon is passed behind the hilum of the left lung and into

the neck by tunneling through Sibson's fascia in a posterior direction to the subclavian vessels and lateral to the carotid sheath. The proximal end of the colonic interposition is anastomosed in end-to-end fashion to the cervical esophagus, and the distal end is anastomosed either to the distal stump of esophagus (in cases of esophageal atresia) or preferably to the posterior wall of the stomach. Pyloroplasty is again recommended. Freeman and Cass[29] modified the procedure by placing the colon in the posterior mediastinum in the site of the normal esophagus.

Results

With modern anesthetic techniques and postoperative management, the mortality from colonic interposition alone should be negligible.[52] Graft necrosis should also be very rare, particularly if meticulous attention is paid to ensuring that the graft has an adequate blood supply and that the vessels do not kink as the graft is passed behind the stomach. Venous obstruction may result in gradual infarction of the colonic interposition weeks or months after surgery. The most common complications are anastomotic leakage, particularly leakage involving the esophagocolonic anastomosis in the neck, and stricture formation. Leaks are attributed to a poor blood supply to the proximal end of the colon or to damage to or impairment of the blood supply to the esophageal wall. Most leaks resolve spontaneously within a few weeks, but some progress to stricture formation. Strictures at the cervical anastomosis generally resolve with dilatations, but resection of the strictured area and revision of the anastomosis are occasionally necessary.

The incidence of complications subsequent to colonic interposition in various large series in the literature is shown in Table 69-4.

Gastric reflux into the colonic interposition may occur and occasionally results in peptic ulceration of the colon. This may progress to hemorrhage or, on rare occasion, perforation with resultant empyema. Late deaths from perforation and empyema have been reported.

Complications after bypass procedures have also been described in the retained esophagus.[46,81] Shamberger et al.[105] reported eight patients in whom chronic inflammation developed in the esophageal remnant, including three cases of Barrett's syndrome. Others have documented mucocele and empyema developing in the retained esophagus.[56]

Peristalsis in the colonic segment is usually absent, and food is conducted through the colon by gravity.[53,67,95] The intrathoracic colon may become increasingly redundant with time,[64] and this redundancy may result in delayed emptying and stasis, which increases the risk for regurgitation and aspiration. It may be necessary to resect the redundant portion of colon, but in so doing, care must be taken to avoid damage to the blood supply to the remaining colon.

The nutritional state of children after colonic interposition seems to be satisfactory.[42] Children who originally had esophageal atresia tend to be in the lower percentiles for height and weight, whereas those who underwent esophageal replacement for caustic stricture fall into a normal growth curve.[6,7,34,38,59] Nearly half the patients with colonic interposition have depleted stores of iron.[95]

TABLE 69-4 Results of Colon Interposition

Year	Author	No. of Patients	Deaths	Leaks (%)	Strictures (%)
1967	Gross and Firestone[38]	47	4	6 (13)	7 (15)
1967	Othersen and Clatworthy[83]	11	0	4 (36)	3 (27)
1971	Azar et al.[9]	60	5	15 (25)	18 (30)
1972	Soave[107]	32	5	28 (87)	—
1972	Martin[72]	21	2	4 (19)	6 (28)
1978	Rodgers et al.[95]	13	0	5 (38)	3 (23)
1976	German and Waterston[34]	32	1	7 (21)	7 (21)
1982	Freeman and Cass[29]	33	2	2 (6)	2 (6)
1982	Campbell et al.[15]	23	1	8 (34)	4 (17)
1985	Hendren and Hendren[48]	32	1	2 (6)	0
1986	Rode et al.[94]	35	4	8 (23)	5 (14)
1986	West et al.[127]	25	0	10 (40)	11 (44)
1986	Ahmed and Spitz[2]	112	15	54 (48)	34 (30)
1989	Mitchell et al.[76]	79	9	23 (29)	17 (22)
1993	Carneiro and Doig[16]	11	2	5 (45)	2 (18)
1995	Raffensperger et al.[90]	59	2	11 (19)	13 (22)
1998	Khan et al.[60]	25	0	10 (40)	7 (28)
2000	Erdogan et al.[27]	18	4	11 (61)	3 (17)
2003	Hamza et al.[41]	475	5	47 (10)	25 (5)

GASTRIC TUBE ESOPHAGOPLASTY

History

In 1905, Beck and Carrel[11] constructed tubes of the greater curvature of the stomach in dogs and cadavers; the tubes were brought antethoracically into the neck. In 1912, Jianu[55] successfully used this tube intrathoracically in two patients with strictures. In 1948, Mes[75] showed that a tube of the greater curvature of the stomach could reach the neck. Later, researchers Gavriliu in Hungary[31-33] and Heimlich[44,45] in the United States popularized this method of esophageal replacement. More recent advocates for gastric tube esophagoplasty include Burrington and Stephens,[14] Cohen,[18] Ein et al.,[24] and Anderson et al.[5-7]

Surgical Technique

The abdomen is opened through a transverse supraumbilical incision, and the gastrocolic omentum is divided at a safe distance from the gastroepiploic arcade (Figs. 69-3 and 69-4).[3] The right gastroepiploic artery is divided at the point of origin of the gastric tube; the site of division must be chosen carefully to avoid narrowing the pyloric outlet. The optimum location is usually approximately 2 cm proximal to the pylorus, where a vertical incision is made through the anterior and posterior walls of the stomach. An 18 to 24 French chest tube is placed in the stomach along the greater curvature to act as a guide to ensure the construction of an appropriately sized gastric tube, and a GIA stapler is applied 1.5 to 2.0 cm from the greater curvature and oriented so that both the anterior and posterior gastric walls are encompassed. The staple line is placed, and the stomach is cut parallel to the greater curvature. Three to four applications of the stapler are usually required. The short gastric vessels are divided, and the spleen is protected during construction of the tube. Splenectomy is *never* necessary. The staple lines on the gastric tube and the native stomach are reinforced simultaneously with interrupted Lembert sutures of 4-0 nonabsorbable material. If the left gastroepiploic artery has been previously ligated and is unavailable to supply the antiperistaltic tube, an isoperistaltic tube based on the right gastroepiploic artery can be constructed.

The route to the neck is selected at this point, and either a retrosternal tunnel is created or a left thoracotomy is performed in the sixth intercostal space. The neck incision is placed in the suprasternal notch for a substernal tube and in the left anterior triangle for the transthoracic route. Finger dissection from cervical and thoracic approaches facilitates selection of the safest place to incise Sibson's fascia. This position may be anterior or posterior to the subclavian vessels, depending on which space is larger. An incision is made in the diaphragm in a medial and anterior direction to the aortic hiatus, and the gastric tube is drawn into the chest and passed in a proximal direction into the neck. The orientation of the pedicle is maintained to prevent twisting or kinking of vessels. Anastomosis with the cervical esophagus is done with a single layer of nonabsorbable suture. A few sutures placed between tube and diaphragm anchor the tube in the chest. The gastrostomy is re-established in the remnant of the stomach. The chest and neck are drained, and the abdomen is closed without drainage. If the left gastroepiploic artery was damaged during a previous operation, the right gastroepiploic artery can be used to support the vascular pedicle, and the tube would be constructed in the reverse (isoperistaltic) direction. In this instance, after creation of the gastric tube, the stomach is rotated in a posterior direction so that the tube can be brought to the neck.

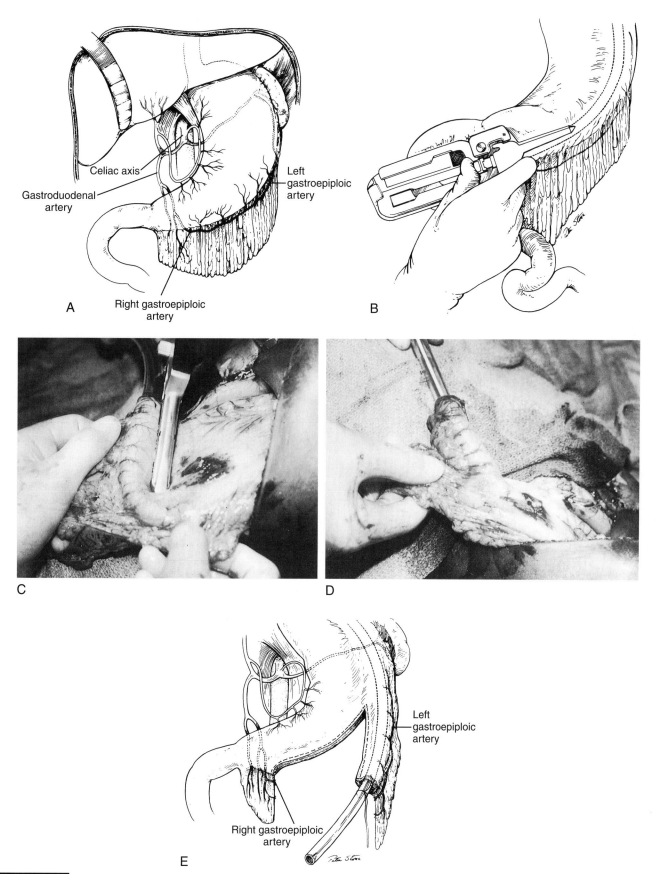

Figure 69–3 Reverse gastric tube construction. *A*, The tube is vascularized by the left gastroepiploic artery. The right gastroepiploic artery is divided where shown, and the arcade is carefully preserved. *B* through *E*, Step-by-step division of the stomach with the GIA stapler. A chest tube along the greater curvature is used as a guide to ensure uniform size of the gastric tube. Oversewing of the staple line on the tube and stomach is also shown.

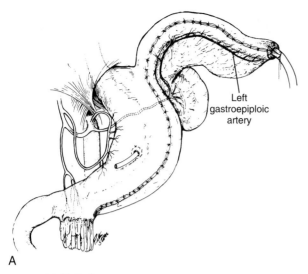

Left
gastroepiploic
artery

A

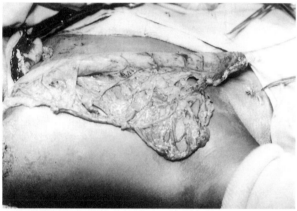

B

Figure 69–4 Reverse gastric tube. *A,* The spleen has been preserved; staple closure of the tube and stomach has been reinforced with interrupted sutures. *B,* The tube is placed over the chest and reaches the cervical esophagostomy, to which the clamp is pointing. The intrathoracic course is even shorter.

Results

The gastric tube tends to retain its shape without the redundancy and dilatation that is apt to occur in colon grafts. Reflux is almost always present and may cause Barrett's changes in the proximal esophageal stump.[63] Peptic ulceration has been reported as a long-term complication associated with gastric tubes.[120,121] Nocturnal coughing is a common problem that can be alleviated by elevating the head of the bed and avoiding fluids shortly

before bedtime. The gastric tube supports nutrition well. Children with lye strictures fall into normal growth curves, whereas those with esophageal atresia tend to fall in lower percentiles for weight and height but grow satisfactorily and maintain good nutrition.[4]

The mortality associated with gastric tube esophagoplasty is low, but leaks and strictures are common. Perforation of the gastric tube occurs occasionally.[102] Peristalsis is generally absent, and the tube empties by gravity (Table 69-5).

JEJUNAL INTERPOSITION

History

In 1906, Roux[97] used the jejunum in an antethoracic direction to bypass a caustic stricture in a 12-year-old child. Follow-up of this patient was published by Pirot-Roux and Hase in 1950.[85] The patient did well until 1940, when a large fistula developed subsequent to trauma, and in 1941, an epithelioma was found in the cutaneous portion of the esophagus; this disorder was successfully treated with radiation therapy. The patient died of unrelated causes at 53 years of age. In 1913, Lexer[62] combined the Roux isolated jejunal loop with a cutaneous skin tube when the jejunum was not long enough to reach the neck. Approximately 20 years later, Ochsner and Owens[79] reviewed the literature of antethoracic esophageal replacement and found that of 240 patients, 56% had tubes constructed of jejunum. In 1946, Reinhoff[92] performed the first intrathoracic jejunal replacement of the esophagus. He recommended the shorter intrathoracic route and stated that the jejunum was long enough to reach the neck. Longmire[66] in 1951 reported a jejunal interposition for caustic stricture in which the inadequate blood supply to the upper end of the jejunum was supplemented by an anastomosis between the internal mammary artery and the mesenteric artery of the jejunum.

The advantages of the jejunum as an esophageal substitute are that peristaltic activity is preserved and its caliber is similar to that of a normal esophagus (see Table 69-2).

Surgical Technique

Two methods of jejunal replacement of the esophagus are used[28,93]: (1) jejunal interposition—transection of the jejunum distal to the ligament of Treitz, in which the proximal end of the loop is brought up through the

TABLE 69–5 Results of Gastric Tube Esophagoplasty

Year	Author	No. of Patients	Deaths	Leaks (%)	Strictures (%)
1968	Burrington and Stephens[14]	8	1	3 (37)	—
1973	Ein et al.[24]	15	—	7 (47)	9 (60)
1978	Anderson and Randolph[6]	15	—	5 (33)	5 (33)
1985	Goon et al.[35]	46	1	35 (76)	27 (59)
1987	Ein et al.[25]	36	3	24 (67)	15 (42)
1998	Ein[23]	11	—	9 (81)	8 (72)

TABLE 69-6 Results of Jejunal Interposition					
Year	Author	No. of Patients	Deaths	Leaks (%)	Strictures (%)
1958	Jezioro and Kus[54]	14	2	3 (21)	1 (7)
1982	Ring et al.[93]	16	0	4 (25)	2 (12)
1988	Saeki et al.[99]	19	2	3 (15)	2 (10)
1993	Cusick et al.[19]	6	2	1 (17)	2 (33)

thorax into the neck to join the esophagus, the distal end is anastomosed to the stomach, and intestinal continuity is restored by a jejunojejunal anastomosis, and (2) free jejunal interposition—interposition of an isolated jejunal segment, in which case microvascular anastomosis of the jejunal pedicle is performed. The results of jejunal interposition in a small number of series reported are shown in Table 69-6.

GASTRIC TRANSPOSITION

History

In 1922, Kummell reported mobilization of the esophagus in two patients by bluntly freeing the esophagus with fingers introduced from cervical and abdominal wounds.[61,78] The stomach was then transplanted into the esophageal bed and the esophagus was anastomosed to the stomach. Although both patients died, this was the first attempt at gastric transposition by means of the mediastinal route. In 1938, Adams and Phemister[1] successfully resected a carcinoma in the lower thoracic esophagus of a 53-year-old patient and restored continuity by esophagogastrostomy. In 1944, Garlock's successful re-establishment of esophagogastric continuity after resection of the esophagus for carcinoma of the middle third in a 58-year-old man was reported.[30] At follow-up, the only complication was regurgitation in the recumbent position, and this problem was controlled by sleeping on two pillows. In 1945, Sweet[116] recorded 12 esophageal resections with esophagogastric anastomosis above the arch of the aorta, and in 1948,[117] he described the successful application of his technique after resection of a carcinoma of the upper thoracic esophagus with anastomosis of the stomach to the cervical esophagus. Soon thereafter, successful pharyngogastrostomy was described. Replacement of the esophagus by gastric transposition is currently the procedure of choice in adults with carcinoma, but its use in children has been limited.[88] Atwell and Harrison[8] reported six children who underwent gastric transposition; two died, but good long-term results were achieved in the other four patients.

Surgical Technique

Transhiatal gastric transposition without thoracotomy is the procedure of choice (Fig. 69-5).[82,88,109,111,114] It is contraindicated in the presence of extensive scarring from previous surgery or mediastinal inflammation.[110]

To preserve the vascular arcades of the gastroepiploic vessels, the initial feeding gastrostomy should ideally be sited on the anterior surface of the body of the stomach well away from the greater curvature.

The stomach is exposed through an upper midline abdominal incision. Alternatively, a left oblique muscle-cutting incision that may extend into a left thoracotomy may be used, particularly if resection of a fibrotic esophagus or previous colonic interposition is required.

The gastrostomy is carefully mobilized, and the defect in the stomach is closed in two layers with interrupted 4-0 polyglycolic acid suture.

Adhesions between the stomach and the left lobe of the liver are lysed while care is taken to preclude damage to the major blood vessels. The greater curvature of the stomach is mobilized by ligating and dividing the vessels in the gastrocolic omentum and the short gastric vessels. These vessels should be ligated well away from the stomach wall to preserve the vascular arcades of the right gastroepiploic vessels. Meticulous care must be taken to avoid damaging the spleen. The lesser curvature of the stomach is freed by dividing the lesser omentum from the pylorus to the diaphragmatic hiatus. The right gastric artery is carefully identified and preserved, whereas the left gastric vessels are ligated and divided close to the stomach (Fig. 69-5A).

The lower portion of the esophagus is exposed by dividing the phrenoesophageal membrane, and the margins of the esophageal hiatus in the diaphragm are defined. The inevitably short blind-ending lower esophageal stump in patients with isolated esophageal atresia is dissected out of the posterior mediastinum by a combination of blunt and sharp dissection through the diaphragmatic hiatus. The vagal nerves are usually divided during this part of the procedure. The body and fundus of the stomach are now free of all attachments and can be delivered into the wound. The esophagus is transected at the gastroesophageal junction, and the defect is closed in two layers with 4-0 polyglycolic acid suture. A Heineke-Mickulicz pyloroplasty is usually performed, although whether it is necessary continues to be controversial.[17] The second part of the duodenum is kocherized to obtain maximum mobility of the pylorus.

The highest part of the fundus of the stomach is identified, and stay sutures of different material are inserted to the left and the right of the area selected for the anastomosis. These sutures help avoid torsion of the stomach as it is drawn through the posterior mediastinum into the neck (Fig. 69-5B).

Attention is now turned to the neck, where a previously constructed cervical esophagostomy is mobilized through a 3- to 4-cm transverse incision. Care must be taken to not damage the muscular coat of the esophagus. The recurrent laryngeal nerve that courses upward on the posterolateral

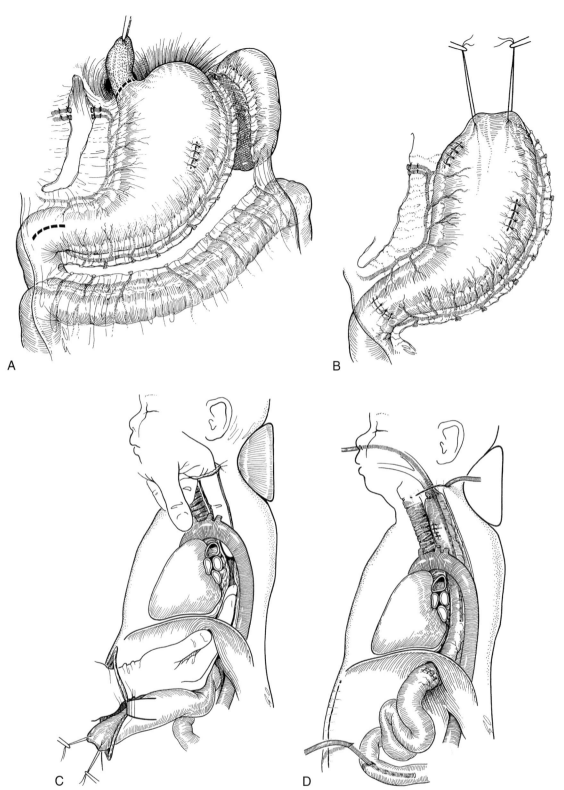

Figure 69–5 *A,* Technique of gastric tube esophagoplasty. The stomach is mobilized along the greater and lesser curvatures, with preservation of the right gastric epiploic and right gastric vessels. The short gastric vessels are carefully divided, with care taken to avoid trauma to the spleen. The left gastric vessels have been ligated and divided; the duodenum (to which the Kocher technique has been applied) and the site of pyloroplasty are indicated. The short stump of esophagus in a case of isolated atresia is shown being mobilized from within the esophageal hiatus of the diaphragm. The gastrostomy site has been sutured. *B,* Pyloroplasty has been completed, the distal esophageal stump has been resected, and the two sutures on the fundus of the stomach indicate the highest point of the stomach at the proposed site for the esophagogastric anastomosis. *C,* Fashioning of the posterior mediastinal tunnel by blunt dissection from above by means of a cervical incision to mobilize the esophagostomy or expose the esophagus in the case of caustic injury and from below by means of the esophageal hiatus in the diaphragm. The dissection is done strictly in the midline in the prevertebral plane. *D,* The final position of the stomach in the posterior mediastinum with the esophagogastric anastomosis in the lower part of the neck and the pyloroplasty situated immediately within the peritoneal cavity below the esophageal hiatus. A jejunostomy tube has been placed for postoperative enteral feeding.

surface of the trachea is identified and preserved. A plane of dissection between the membranous posterior surface of the trachea and the prevertebral fascia is established, and a tunnel is created into the superior mediastinum by blunt dissection immediately in the midline. A similar tunnel is fashioned from below in the line of the normal esophageal hiatus in the tissues posterior to the heart and anterior to the prevertebral fascia.[37] When continuity of the superior and inferior posterior mediastinal tunnels has been established, the space to be occupied by the stomach is developed into a tunnel the width of two to three fingers (Fig. 69-5C).

If thoracotomy was required for resection of a fibrotic esophagus (e.g., in cases of caustic or reflux esophagitis) or a nonfunctioning previous interposition or when blunt dissection would be hazardous because of fibrosis from previous surgery or infection, the transthoracic part of the procedure is carried out under direct vision and the remainder of the operation is done in the same manner as described for the mediastinal procedure.

A long, blunt hemostat is passed into the posterior mediastinal tunnel from the cervical incision, and the two stay sutures on the fundus of the stomach are grasped. Gentle withdrawal of the hemostat pulls the stomach up through the esophageal hiatus and the posterior mediastinal tunnel into the cervical incision. The orientation of the fundus is checked by realigning the stay sutures in their correction position. The end of the esophagus is anastomosed to the highest part of the stomach with a single layer of interrupted 4-0 polyglycolic acid suture.

A large-caliber (12-gauge) nasogastric tube is inserted into the stomach through the esophagogastric anastomosis. The tube remains in place to allow free drainage and is aspirated at regular intervals to prevent acute gastric dilatation in the early postoperative period. A soft rubber drain is placed at the site of the anastomosis, and the wound is closed in layers.

The surgeon then returns to the abdomen, where the margins of the diaphragmatic hiatus are sutured to the antrum of the stomach with a few interrupted sutures so that the pylorus lies immediately below the diaphragm in the midline. A fine-bore feeding jejunostomy has been found to be of considerable value in providing enteral nutrition in the first few weeks after gastric transposition before full oral nutrition is established (Fig. 69-5D).

Postoperative Management

Careful monitoring of vital functions is essential in the early postoperative period. Extensive dissection of the soft tissues in a posterior direction to the trachea has been performed, and the resulting edema may cause respiratory compromise. Elective nasotracheal intubation with or without assisted ventilation for a few days may simplify the postoperative course and reduce the incidence of respiratory problems.

Jejunal feedings are instituted on the second or third day after surgery. The safest technique for delivery of nutrition by this method is a slow, continuous infusion rather than a bolus technique, which can provoke a "dumping" effect. A contrast swallow is performed 7 days after surgery, and if no leak is identified at the anastomosis, careful oral feeding may begin. The cervical drain is removed when integrity of the anastomosis has been demonstrated.

Since 1981, 173 gastric transpositions have been performed at Great Ormond Street Hospital, London.[113] The most common indication for esophageal replacement was esophageal atresia in 127 patients, 70 of whom had failed primary repair and 43 had isolated atresia without a fistula. Twenty-three children had intractable caustic strictures. More than 80% of patients were referred from abroad or from other centers within the United Kingdom. The method of replacement was via the posterior mediastinum without thoracotomy in 90 patients (52%). In the remainder a thoracotomy was necessary because of dense mediastinal scarring secondary to the original injury (caustic, perforation) or as a result of previous failed attempts at esophageal reconstruction. All patients are currently routinely paralyzed and mechanically ventilated for at least 48 to 72 hours postoperatively.

There have been nine deaths (5.2%), eight of whom had had complex courses before the transposition. Anastomotic leakage at the esophagogastric connection occurred in 12% of cases, all except one of which closed spontaneously. Strictures developed in 19.6% of patients, all but three of which responded to endoscopic dilatation.[84] In these three cases, stricture resection plus reanastomosis was successfully carried out through a cervical approach. Strictures were more common after caustic injury (38%). Swallowing problems postoperatively were encountered in 30% of cases.

Establishing oral feeding can be extremely difficult, particularly in infants with esophageal atresia who have not been properly sham-fed. The jejunal feeding tube greatly simplifies postoperative nutrition and avoids the need for parenteral nutrition. Vomiting, which may be bilious in nature as a consequence of pyloroplasty, is common in the early postoperative period, especially when the child is recumbent.

A follow-up of 17 patients who underwent gastric transposition more than 5 years previously has shown

TABLE 69-7 Results of Gastric Transposition

Year	Author	No. of Patients	Deaths (%)	Leaks (%)	Strictures (%)
1980	Atwell and Harrison[8]	6	2 (33)	—	—
1987	Valente et al.[122]	21	1 (4.7)	4 (19)	3 (14)
1991	Marujo et al.[73]	21	1 (4.7)	4 (17)	3 (14)
1995	Spitz[111]	83	6 (7.2)	10 (12)	10 (12)
2002	Hirschl[49]	41	0	15 (36)	20 (49)
2004	Spitz et al.[113]	173	9 (5.2)	21 (12)	34 (19.6)

that the intrathoracic stomach functions as a conduit as opposed to a reservoir for both liquids and solids.[21] Rapid emptying (>50%) of both liquids and solids occurred within 5 minutes of ingestion in 82% of patients. Dumping symptoms are occasionally an early feature, but these symptoms resolve within a few weeks in most cases. Of 17 children, 13 were within normal percentiles for height and 11 were within normal percentiles for weight. Low iron stores is a feature in all types of esophageal replacement and was documented in all patients who had undergone gastric transposition. All but one child had restricted pulmonary function, with a mean total lung capacity of 68% and a mean forced vital capacity of 64% of expected values. It is uncertain at present whether these reduced values are a consequence of the primary condition or a direct result of gastric transposition.[22]

In 90% of our patients, the long-term outcome was judged to be good to excellent in terms of absence of swallowing difficulties and other gastrointestinal symptoms such as dumping or diarrhea. There has been no deterioration in function of the transposed stomach over time.

The outcome of gastric transposition in children is shown in Table 69-7.

REFERENCES

1. Adams WE, Phemister DB: Carcinoma of the lower thoracic esophagus: Report of a successful resection and esophagogastrostomy. J Thorac Surg 1938;7:621.
2. Ahmed A, Spitz L: The outcome of colonic replacement of the esophagus in children. Prog Pediatr Surg 1986;19:37.
3. Anderson KD: Progress in pediatric surgery. In Wurnick P (ed): Long-Gap Esophageal Atresia—Prenatal Diagnosis of Congenital Malformations. Berlin, Springer-Verlag, 1986.
4. Anderson KD, Noblett H, Belsey R: Long-term follow-up of children with colon and gastric tube interposition for esophageal atresia. Surgery 1992;111:131.
5. Anderson KD, Randolph JG: The gastric tube for esophageal replacement in infants and children. J Thorac Cardiovasc Surg 1973;66:333.
6. Anderson KD, Randolph JG: Gastric tube interposition: A satisfactory alternative to the colon for esophageal replacement in children. Ann Thorac Surg 1978;25:521.
7. Anderson KD, Randolph JG, Lilley JR: Peptic ulcer in children with gastric tube interposition. J Pediatr Surg 1975;10:701.
8. Atwell JD, Harrison GSM: Observations on the role of esophagogastrostomy in infancy and childhood with particular reference to the long-term results and operative mortality. J Pediatr Surg 1980;15:303.
9. Azar H, Chrispin AR, Waterston DJ: Esophageal replacement with transverse colon in infants and children. J Pediatr Surg 1971;6:3.
10. Battersby JS, Moore TC: Esophageal replacement and bypass with the ascending and right half of transverse colon for the treatment of congenital atresia of the esophagus. Surg Gynecol Obstet 1959;109:207.
11. Beck C, Carrel A: Demonstration of specimens illustrating a method of formation of a prethoracic esophagus. Illinois Med J 1905;7:463.
12. Belsey R: Reconstruction of the esophagus with left colon. J Thorac Cardiovasc Surg 1965;49:33.
13. Belsey R: Reconstruction of the oesophagus. Ann R Coll Surg Engl 1983;65:360.
14. Burrington JD, Stephens CA: Esophageal replacement with a gastric tube in infants and children. J Pediatr Surg 1968;3:24.
15. Campbell JR, Webber BR, Harrison MW, Campbell TJ: Esophageal replacement in infants and children by colon interposition. Am J Surg 1982;144:29.
16. Carneiro PM, Doig CM: Colon interposition for wide gap oesophageal atresia. East Afr Med J 1993;70:682.
17. Cheung HC, Siu KG, Wong J: Is pyloroplasty necessary in esophageal replacement by stomach? A prospective randomised, controlled trial. Surgery 1987;102:19.
18. Cohen D: Oesophageal reconstruction using a gastric tube: A preliminary report. Aust Pediatr J 1970;6:22.
19. Cusick EL, Batchelor AAG, Spicer RD: Development of a technique for jejunal interposition in long-gap esophageal atresia. J Pediatr Surg 1993;28:990.
20. Dale WA, Sherman CD: Late reconstruction of congenital esophageal atresia by intrathoracic colon transplantation. J Thorac Surg 1955;29:344.
21. Davenport M, Bianchi A: Early experience with oesophageal flap esophagoplasty for repair of esophageal atresia. Pediatr Surg Int 1990;5:332.
22. Davenport M, Hosie GP, Tasker RC, et al: The long-term effects of gastric transposition in children: A physiological study. J Pediatr Surg 1996;31:588.
23. Ein SH: Gastric tubes in children with caustic esophageal injury. J Pediatr Surg 1998;33:1363.
24. Ein SH, Shandling B, Simpson JS, Stevens CA: A further look at the gastric tube as an esophageal replacement in infants and children. J Pediatr Surg 1973;8:859.
25. Ein SH, Shandling B, Stephens CA: Twenty-one year experience with the pediatric gastric tube. J Pediatr Surg 1987;22:77.
26. Eraklis AJ, Rosello PJ, Ballantine TVN: Circular esophagomyotomy of upper pouch in primary repair of long segment esophageal atresia. J Pediatr Surg 1976;11:709.
27. Erdogan E, Emir H, Eroglu E: Esophageal replacement using the colon: A 15-year review. Pediatr Surg Int 2000;16:546.
28. Foker JE, Ring WS, Varco RL: Technique of jejunal interposition for esophageal replacement. J Thorac Cardiovasc Surg 1982;83:928.
29. Freeman NV, Cass DT: Colon interposition: A modification of the Waterston technique using the normal esophageal route. J Pediatr Surg 1982;17:17.
30. Garlock JH: Reestablishment of esophagogastric continuity following resection of esophagus for carcinoma of middle third. Surg Gynecol Obstet 1944;78:23.
31. Gavriliu D: Etat actual de procede de reconstruction de l'oesophage par tube gastrique. Ann Chir 1965;19:219.
32. Gavriliu D: Aspects of esophageal surgery. Curr Probl Surg 1975;12:1.
33. Gavriliu D, Georgescue L: Esofagoplastie directa cu material gastric. Rev Stiintelor Medicale (Bucurest) 1951;3:33.
34. German JC, Waterston DJ: Colon interposition for replacement of the esophagus in children. J Pediatr Surg 1976;11:227.
35. Goon HK, Cohen DH, Middleton AW: Gastric tube oesophagoplasty—a long-term assessment. Z Kinderchir 1985;40:21.
36. Gough MH: Esophageal atresia—use of an anterior flap in the difficult anastomosis. J Pediatr Surg 1980;15:310.
37. Gross BH, Asha FP, Galzer GM, Orringer MB: Gastric interposition following transhiatal esophagectomy: CT evaluation. Radiology 1985;155:177.
38. Gross RE, Firestone N: Colonic reconstruction of the esophagus in infants and children. Surgery 1967;61:955.
39. Guzzetta PC, Randolph JG: Antireflux cologastric anastomosis following colonic interposition for esophageal replacement. J Pediatr Surg 1986;21:1137.

40. Hagberg S, Rubenson A, Sillen U, Werkmaster K: Management of long-gap esophagus: Experience with end-to-end anastomosis under maximal tension. Prog Pediatr Surg 1986;19:88-92.

41. Hamza AF, Abdelhay S, Sherif H, et al: Caustic esophageal strictures in children: 30 years' experience. J Pediatr Surg 2003;38:828.

42. Harju E, Isolauri J: Nutritional state after colon interposition for benign oesophageal disease. Eur J Clin Nutr 1988;42:351.

43. Hays DM, Woolley M, Synder WH: Esophageal atresia and tracheoesophageal fistula: Management of the uncommon types. J Pediatr Surg 1966;1:240.

44. Heimlich HJ: Peptic esophagitis with stricture treated by reconstruction of the esophagus with a reversed gastric tube. Surg Gynecol Obstet 1962;114:673.

45. Heimlich HJ: Elective replacement of esophagus. Br J Surg 1966;53:913.

46. Heiss K, Wesson D, Bohn D, et al: Respiratory failure due to retained esophagus: A complication of esophageal replacement. J Pediatr Surg 1991;26:1359.

47. Hendren WH, Hale JR: Electromagnetic bougienage to lengthen esophageal segments in congenital esophageal atresia. N Engl J Med 1975;293:428.

48. Hendren WH, Hendren WG: Colon interposition for esophagus in children. J Pediatr Surg 1985;20:829.

49. Hirschl RB: Gastric transposition for esophageal replacement in children: Experience with 41 consecutive cases with special emphasis on esophageal atresia. Ann Surg 2002;236:531.

50. Hoffman DG, Moazam F: Transcervical myotomy for wide-gap esophageal atresia. J Pediatr Surg 1984;19:680.

51. Howard R, Myers NA: Esophageal atresia: A technique for elongating the upper pouch. Surgery 1965;58:725.

52. Isolauri J: Colonic interposition for benign esophageal disease. Long-term clinical and endoscopic results. Am J Surg 1988;155:498.

53. Isolauri J, Reinikainen P, Markkula H: Functional evaluation of interposed colon in esophagus. Manometric and 24-hour pH observations. Acta Chir Scand 1987;44:84.

54. Jezioro Z, Kus H: Experiences with the retrosternal esophageal replacement employing jejunum or ileum. J Pediatr Surg 1958;44:275.

55. Jianu A: Gastrostomie und Oesophagoplastik. Dtsch Z Chir 1912;11:8.

56. Kamath MV, Ellison RG, Rubin JW, et al: Esophageal mucocele: A complication of blind loop esophagus. Ann Thorac Surg 1987;43:263.

57. Kato T, Hollmann G, Hopper F, et al: Ein neues Instrument zur Faden-legung ohne Thorakotomie in ausgewahlten Fallen von oesophagusatresie. Z Kinderchir 1980;29:20.

58. Kelling G: Oesophagoplastik mit Hilfe des Quercolon. Zentralbl Chir 1911;38:1209.

59. Kelly JP, Shackelford GD, Roper CL: Esophageal replacement with colon in children: Functional results and long-term growth. Ann Thorac Surg 1983;36:634.

60. Khan AR, Stiff G, Mohammed AR, et al: Esophageal replacement with colon in children. Pediatr Surg Int 1998; 13:79.

61. Kummell HJ: Ueber intrathorakale Oesophagus Plastik. Beitr Klin Chir 1922;126:264.

62. Lexer E: Oesophagoplastik. Zentralbl Chir 1914;40:1970.

63. Lindahl H, Louhimo I, Virkola K: Colon interposition or gastric tube? Follow-up study of colon-esophagus and gastric tube–esophagus patients. J Pediatr Surg 1983;18:58.

64. Lindahl H, Rintala R, Sariola H, Louhimo I: Long-term endoscopic and flow cytometric follow-up of colon interposition. J Pediatr Surg 1992;27:859.

65. Lividitis A: Esophageal atresia. A method of over-bridging large segment gaps. Z Kinderchir 1973;13:278.

66. Longmire WP: Antethoracic jejunal transplantation for congenital esophageal atresia with hypoplasia of the lower esophagus. Surg Gynecol Obstet 1951;93:310.

67. Louhimo I, Pasila M, Visa Koepi JK: Late gastrointestinal complications in patients with colonic replacement of the oesophagus. J Pediatr Surg 1969;4:663.

68. Lundblad O: Uber antethorakale Osophagoplastik. Acta Chir Scand 1921;53:535.

69. MacKinlay GA, Burtles R: Oesophageal atresia: Paralysis and ventilation in management of the wide gap. Pediatr Surg Int 1987;2:10.

70. Mahour GH, Woolley MM, Gwinn JL: Elongation of the upper pouch and delayed anatomic reconstruction in esophageal atresia. J Pediatr Surg 1974;9:373.

71. Mansour KA, Malone CE: Surgery for scleroderma of the esophagus: A 12-year experience. Ann Thorac Surg 1988; 46:513.

72. Martin LW: The use of colon for esophageal replacement in children. Aust N Z J Surg 1972;42:160.

73. Marujo WC, Tannuri U, Maksoud JG: Total gastric transposition: An alternative to esophageal replacement in children. J Pediatr Surg 1991;26:676.

74. May IA, Samson PC: Esophageal reconstruction and replacements. Ann Thorac Surg 1969;7:249.

75. Mes GM: New method of esophagoplasty. J Int Coll Surg 1948;11:270.

76. Mitchell IM, Goh DW, Roberts KD, Abrahms CD: Colon interposition in children. Br J Surg 1989;76:681.

77. Ngan SY, Wong J: Lengths of different routes for esophageal replacement. J Thorac Cardiovasc Surg 1986;91:790.

78. Ochsner A, De Bakey M: Surgical aspects of cancer of the esophagus. A review of the literature. J Thorac Surg 1940; 10:401.

79. Ochsner A, Owens N: Antethoracic esophagoplasty for impermeable stricture of the esophagus. Ann Surg 1934; 100:1055.

80. Okmian Z, Booss D, Ekelund I: An endoscopic technique for Rehbein's silver olive method. Z Kinderchir 1975; 16:212.

81. Orringer MB, Kirsh MM, Sloan H: New trends in esophageal replacement for benign disease. Ann Thorac Surg 1977; 23:409.

82. Orringer MB, Sloan H: Esophagectomy without thoracotomy. J Thorac Cardiovasc Surg 1978;76:643.

83. Othersen HB Jr, Clatworthy HW Jr: Functional evaluation of esophageal replacement in children. J Thorac Cardiovasc Surg 1967;53:55.

84. Pierie JP, de Graaf PW, Poen H, et al: Incidence and management of benign anastomotic stricture after cervical oesophagogastrostomy. Br J Surg 1993;80:471.

85. Pirot-Roux L, Hase O: Epicrise de la premiére operatian de l'oesophagoplastie prethoracique faite par le Dr. Cesar Roux en 1906. Rev Med Suisse Romande 1950;90:19.

86. Postlethwait RW: Technique for isoperistaltic gastric tube for esophageal bypass. Ann Surg 1979;189:673.

87. Postlethwait RW: Colonic interposition for esophageal substitution. Surg Gynecol Obstet 1983;156:377.

88. Postlethwait RW: Surgery of the Esophagus, 2nd ed. Norwalk, CT, Appleton-Century-Crofts, 1995.

89. Puri P, Blake N, O'Donnell B, Guiney EJ: Delayed primary anastomosis following spontaneous growth of esophageal segments in esophageal atresia. J Pediatr Surg 1981;6:180.

90. Raffensperger JG, Luck SR, Reynolds M, Schwartz D: Intestinal bypass of the esophagus. J Pediatr Surg 1996; 31:38.

91. Rehbein F, Schweder N: Reconstruction of the esophagus without colon transplantation in cases of atresia. J Pediatr Surg 1971;6:746.

92. Rienhoff WF: Intrathoracic esophagojejunostomy for lesions of the upper third of the esophagus. South Med J 1946;39:928.

93. Ring WS, Varco RL, L'Heureux PR, Foker JE: Esophageal replacement with jejunum in children: An 18 to 33 year follow-up. J Thorac Cardiovasc Surg 1982;83:918.

94. Rode H, Cywes S, Millar AJ, Davies MR: Colonic oesophageal replacement in children—functional results. Z Kinderchir 1986;41:201.

95. Rodgers BM, Talbert JL, Moazarn F, Felman AH: Functional and metabolic evaluation of colon replacement of the esophagus in children. J Pediatr Surg 1978; 13:35.

96. Rossello PJ, Lebron H: The technique of myotomy in esophageal reconstruction: An experimental study. J Pediatr Surg 1980;15:430.

97. Roux C: L'esophago-jejuno-gastrome: Nouvelle operation pour retrecessement infranchissable de l'esophage. Semin Med 1907;27:37.

98. Rudler JC, Monod-Broca P: Uncas d'esophagoplastie palliative retro-sternale avec l'ileocolon droit. Mem Acad Chir (Paris) 1951;77:747.

99. Saeki M, Tsuchida Y, Ogata T, et al: Long-term results of jejunal replacement of the esophagus. J Pediatr Surg 1988;23:483.

100. Salo JA, Heikkila L, Nemlander A, et al: Barrett's oesophagus and perforation of gastric tube ulceration into the pericardium: A late complication after reconstruction of oesophageal atresia. Ann Chir Gynaecol 1995;84:92.

101. Scharli AF: Esophageal reconstruction in very long atresias by elongation of the lesser curvature. Pediatr Surg Int 1992;7:101.

102. Schier F, Schier C, Hoppner D, Willital GH: [Esophageal replacement with resorbable vicryl tubes—an animal experiment study.] Osophagusersatz mit resorbierbaren Vicryl-Schlauchen—Eine tierexperimentelle Untersuchung. Z Kinderchir 1987;42:224.

103. Schullinger JN, Vinocur CD, Santulli T: The suture-fistula technique in the repair of selected cases of esophageal atresia. J Pediatr Surg 1982;17:234.

104. Shafer AD, David TE: Suture fistula as a means of connecting upper and lower segments in oesophageal atresia. J Pediatr Surg 1974;9:669.

105. Shamberger RC, Eraklis AJ, Kosakewich HP, Hendren WH: Fate of the distal esophageal remnant following esophageal replacement. J Pediatr Surg 1988;23:1210.

106. Sherman CD, Waterston DW: Oesophageal reconstruction in children using intrathoracic colon. Arch Dis Child 1957;32:11.

107. Soave F: Intrathoracic transposition of the transverse colon in complicated oesophageal atresia. Proc Pediatr Surg 1972; 4:91.

108. Sonneland J, Anson BJ, Beaton LE: Surgical anatomy of the arterial supply to the colon from the superior mesenteric artery based upon a study of 600 specimens. Surg Gynecol Obstet 1958;106:385.

109. Spitz L: Gastric transposition via the mediastinal route for infants with long-gap esophageal atresia. J Pediatr Surg 1984;19:149.

110. Spitz L: Gastric transposition for esophageal substitution in children. J Pediatr Surg 1992;27:252.

111. Spitz L: Gastric replacement of the esophagus. In Spitz L, Coran AG (eds): Pediatric Surgery, 5th ed. London, Chapman & Hall, 1995.

112. Spitz L, Kiely E, Brereton RJ, Drake D: Management of esophageal atresia. World J Surg 1993;17:296.

113. Spitz L, Kiely E, Pierro A: Gastric transposition in children—a 21-year experience. J Pediatr Surg 2004;39:276.

114. Spitz L, Kiely E, Sparnon T: Gastric transposition for esophageal replacement in children. Ann Surg 1987;206:69.

115. Stone MM, Fonkalsrud EW, Mahour GH, et al: Esophageal replacement with colon interposition in children. Ann Surg 1986;203:346-351.

116. Sweet RH: Transthoracic gastrectomy and esophagectomy for carcinoma of the stomach and esophagus. Clinics 1945;3:1288.

117. Sweet RH: A method of restoring continuity of the alimentary canal in cases of congenital atresia of the esophagus and with tracheo-esophageal fistula not treated by immediate primary anastomosis. Ann Surg 1948;127:757.

118. Touloukian RJ, Schonholz SM, Gryboski JD, et al: Perioperative considerations in esophageal replacement for epidermolysis bullosa: Report of two cases successfully treated by colon interposition. Am J Gastroenterol 1988; 83:857.

119. Touloukian RJ, Tellides G: Retrosternal ileocolic esophageal replacement in children revisited. Antireflux role of the ileocecal valve. J Thorac Cardiovasc Surg 1994;107:1067.

120. Tsujinaka T, Ogawa M, Kido Y, et al: A giant tracheogastric tube fistula caused by a penetrated peptic ulcer after esophageal replacement. Am J Gastroenterol 1988;83:862.

121. Uchida Y, Tomonari K, Murakami S, et al: Occurrence of peptic ulcer in the gastric tube used for esophageal replacement in adults. Jpn J Surg 1987;17:190.

122. Valente A, Brereton RJ, Mackersie A: Esophageal replacement with whole stomach in infants and children. J Pediatr Surg 1987;22:913.

123. Vizas D, Ein SH, Simpson JS: The value of circular myotomy for esophageal atresia. J Pediatr Surg 1978;13:357.

124. Von Hacker V: [On esophagoplasty in general and on the repair of the esophagus by antethoracic construction of a skin-colon tube in particular.] Uber Oesophagoplastic in allgemeinen unter uber den ersatz der Speuserohre durch antethorackle Hauntdickdarmschlauchbildung im besonderen. Arch Klin Chir 1914;105:973.

125. Vulliet H: De l'esophagoplastie et des diverses modifications. Semin Med 1911;31:529.

126. Waterson D: Colonic replacement of esophagus (intrathoracic). Surg Clin North Am 1964;44:1441.

127. West KW, Vane DW, Grosfeld JL: Esophageal replacement in children: Experience with thirty-one cases. Surgery 1986; 100:751.

Chapter 70

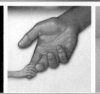

Disorders of Esophageal Function

Juan A. Tovar

The esophagus has no significant secretory or absorptive function and acts only as a conduit interposed between the pharynx and stomach. Its main function is therefore propulsive, and disorders of this function induce several pathologic conditions that in general mirror their adult counterparts, but with specific pediatric features. However, some of these disorders are related to malformations and become clinically evident during infancy and childhood. Most are incompletely understood, mainly because of our limited knowledge of the mechanisms of regulation of gastrointestinal motility, but also because of the inadequacy of the diagnostic tools available to apply in children as a result of problems with size or cooperation. In the present chapter these motor disorders of the esophagus are addressed.

HISTORY

Gastroesophageal reflux (GER) or chalasia has been recognized by pediatricians and pediatric surgeons for many years, and its history is addressed elsewhere in this book (Chapter 71). Conversely, the existence of other disorders of esophageal function in children has only recently been acknowledged. With the exception of achalasia[63,133] and "esophageal diverticulum," which probably correspond to cricopharyngeal achalasia,[133] they were not even mentioned in the first modern pediatric surgery textbooks.[63,133,134,164] The nature of the functional disturbances involved in their pathogenesis and their sometimes elusive symptoms have recently been elucidated, but only after the necessary diagnostic tools were developed and conveniently miniaturized. Since these conditions were investigated, new clinical manifestations in which dysmotility plays a role have been identified and examined.

EMBRYOLOGY

The esophagus is derived from the foregut or cranial part of the endodermal tube that runs longitudinally along the embryonal body within the coelomic space. Cranially, it starts at the lower end of the pharynx, and caudally, it is in continuity with the stomach, which is an expansion of the primitive foregut.[92] The endodermal lining of the foregut is surrounded by muscle fibers that originate from the mesoderm and progressively arrange themselves in two layers: an external layer in which the fibers are longitudinal and an internal layer in which they adopt a circular pattern.

On approximately day 26 of gestation an outgrowth appears on the ventral side of the upper part of the foregut, and this anlage progressively undergoes more branching until it has the configuration of the definitive tracheobronchial tree.[92] Interaction between the endoderm and the mesenchyme and the influence of various genes, transcription factors, and growth factors contribute to shaping of the lung with its multiple types of cells.[30,188] The endodermal lining undergoes changes leading to differentiation into either esophageal or tracheobronchial epithelia.[189] This period of tracheoesophageal separation is crucial for normal organogenesis, and several malformations or dysfunctions of the esophagus have their origin at this point. On completion of these phases, the esophagus in its final configuration has two muscular layers, a submucosa and a nonkeratinized mucosa. Some esophageal glands derived from the endoderm are formed in the submucosal layer of the organ, but their alkaline secretion is minimal in comparison to that noted in other parts of the gastrointestinal tract.[102]

On weeks 8 to 12 of embryonal life, the neuroblasts that originate in the cranial neural crest colonize the primitive foregut in a craniocaudal direction and settle in the intermuscular and submucosal layers, where they establish fibrillar connections that allow for neural control of esophageal function by the parasympathetic and sympathetic systems.[121] Nonadrenergic-noncholinergic, or nitrergic, innervation is present in the myenteric plexus in week 12 and in the submucosal plexus in week 14. It is fully developed by week 22[68] or 23.[19] Both the vagus nerves and the sympathetic paravertebral chains are of neural crest origin, and their development is synchronous with that of the intramural innervation.

When the coelom is divided into the pleural and peritoneal spaces, the diaphragm establishes a functional relationship with the distal part of the esophagus that is crucial for its physiology: the stomach and a portion of the esophagus are located below the diaphragm, whereas most of the organ remains intrathoracic. The muscle fibers of the diaphragm are contributed to by the truncal mesoderm, and a part of its myoblasts are probably of cervical origin.[2,3] The central tendon and other connective tissue structures derive from the post-hepatic mesenchymal plate that contributes to closure of the remaining pleuroperitoneal canals.[88]

ANATOMY

The upper end of the esophagus is in direct continuity with the pharynx. Its muscle fibers fuse with those of the cricopharyngeal muscle, the lower portion of the inferior pharyngeal constrictor, and it acts as an upper esophageal sphincter (UES). The esophageal body is located in the posterior mediastinum in close contact with the spine posteriorly, with the trachea and heart anteriorly and both pleural spaces on the sides. The vagal trunks run on the surface of the esophagus, where they give off numerous branches. Esophageal length is less than 10 cm in the newborn and reaches 35 to 40 cm in adults. The lower end of the esophagus traverses the hiatus to become intra-abdominal before entering into the stomach. On this end there are no anatomically distinct sphincteric fibers, but at the level of the gastroesophageal junction the circular layer adopts a horizontal U shape on the right side of the esophagus (clasp fibers). On the left side the fibers arrange themselves into a U-shaped structure that overrides the gastric incisura and extends downward onto the anterior and posterior surfaces of the stomach (sling fibers).[98] The diaphragmatic sling that forms the hiatus from the right crus overlaps the distal end of the esophagus and the sphincter. Its striated fibers are closely attached to the esophagus and separate the thoracic space, lined by pleura, from the abdominal cavity, lined by peritoneum. The ensemble of these structures constitutes a zone of high pressure in which the lower esophageal sphincter (LES) and the crural sling are the main functional structures. In contrast to other segments of the gastrointestinal tract, the esophagus is devoid of a serosal layer, although it is in part in close contact laterally with the right and left mediastinal pleurae in the thorax and anteriorly with the peritoneum in its short intra-abdominal portion. The muscle layers are quite similar to those of the intestine except for the nature of the muscle fibers, which are striated in the upper third and smooth for the remainder of the organ.

The intermuscular and submucosal plexuses contain ganglion cells and an extensive network of fibers that connect neurons among themselves and with the parasympathetic vagus, the sympathetic trunks, and the celiac plexus. The cholinergic and adrenergic mediators exert positive and negative motor effects, respectively, on the organ. Relaxation is mediated by nitrergic nerve endings that have their neurons in the intramural plexuses.[165] The c-kit–positive interstitial cells of Cajal are distributed among the muscle fibers and have a pacemaker role.[86,141,142,179] The extent to which these cells are regulated by neural control has not been clarified.[194]

PHYSIOLOGY

The function of the esophagus is primarily transportation of the alimentary (food) bolus from the pharynx to the stomach. Secondarily, this organ is responsible for the clearance of fluid that refluxes from the stomach.

To avoid aspiration of digestive juices into the larynx and insufflation of the esophagus by air during inspiration, the UES maintains a permanent tone that relaxes only during deglutition when the glottis is closed and respiration ceases.[77] The unfavorable pressure conditions imposed on the esophagus by its intrathoracic location require that the distal end normally be closed to prevent reflux. This function is ensured by the LES, which maintains its tone except during deglutition.[178] The balance between cholinergic and nitrergic mediators regulates closure of the sphincter and its relaxation.[171]

The intrathoracic location of most of the esophagus together with the intra-abdominal location of the stomach allows maintenance of a permanent abdominothoracic pressure gradient. As a consequence, the intermittent negative inspiratory thoracic pressure coupled with the permanently positive abdominal pressure tends to push the gastric contents back into the esophagus.[187] The normal resting tone of the LES opposes this gradient, assisted by the contribution of the rhythmic contractions of the diaphragmatic crural sling, which aids in closure of the lumen during inspiration. At this point the unfavorable gradient is more powerful and the sling displaces the cardia downward, thereby accentuating the angle of His and lengthening the intra-abdominal segment of the esophagus.[110] The synergistic play of these smooth and striated muscular structures has been studied extensively in animals[112,183,184] and bears some resemblance to the mechanism of anorectal continence, in which the normal resting tone is provided by the internal sphincter and the intermittently required additional closure is achieved by voluntary contraction of the striated muscle complex and the external sphincter.

Deglutition is possible only if the UES and LES relax. Such relaxation occurs whenever the pharyngeal muscles mount a propulsive wave, and the relaxation lasts until the peristalsis of the esophageal body triggered by pharyngeal contractions reaches the lower end of the organ. To effect these propulsive waves, the muscles of the esophagus contract in a coordinated craniocaudal manner along the entire length of the organ to push the esophageal contents into the stomach. These are *"primary"* waves. Normal muscle layers and neural control are necessary for achieving this complex function, and motor disorders of the esophagus are probably the result of abnormalities in these two entities.

Reflux is the retrograde passage of gastric contents into the esophagus, which to a certain extent is normal because the natural tone of the LES fails several times every day, particularly during meals, and allows the unwavering gastroesophageal pressure gradient to push gastric juice backward. This sphincter may be persistently insufficient in some patients, particularly in the neurologically impaired,[56] but it is presently acknowledged that most episodes of reflux in adults and children are due to nondeglutitory extemporaneous relaxation of the sphincter.[32,83,178,181] During these relaxations, the esophageal lumen is filled with a refluxate that contains acidic gastric juice and eventually other digestive material. The mucosa is not prepared for this chemical insult, and it must clear the fluid promptly to avoid permanent damage. To achieve this objective the esophagus initiates peristaltic contractions that may be independent of deglutition; they may arise at different levels of the organ and are progressive and therefore able to propel the refluxed material back into the stomach. These are *"secondary"* waves.[155] This motor action rids the esophagus of the bulk of the refluxed fluid, but the acid that adheres to the mucosa is completely cleared only after several deglutitions allow the buffering action of saliva (which is alkaline) and, to an unknown extent, the alkaline secretion of esophageal glands to neutralize the acid.[66,67] A normal esophagus may also produce a limited number of simultaneous non-propulsive motor waves that close the lumen of the esophagus along its entire length. These are known as *"tertiary"* waves and, when they occur too frequently, may contribute to some of the motor disturbances of the esophagus.[7,8,62,116,175]

METHODS USED FOR EVALUATING ESOPHAGEAL FUNCTION

For many years the barium meal has been the main tool for investigating the esophagus. It shows not only anatomic anomalies of the organ but also abnormal contractility and relaxation of the UES and LES. However, significant radiation exposure is unavoidable if prolonged assessment is required, and such exposure has progressively limited its use. However, this method remains necessary for some of the conditions mentioned in this chapter.

Scintigraphy with liquid or solid radionuclide-tagged meals has helped clarify the normal mechanisms of esophageal clearance and is useful for assessing esophageal transit and esophageal and gastric emptying. However, it is of relatively limited use in children.[42,146,168,177]

Endoscopy with suitable fiberscopes allows direct inspection of the esophageal lumen and mucosa. Some contractility disorders may be detected by this procedure, but its main usefulness resides in the information obtained by inspection and biopsy of the mucosa. Some functional disorders are related to esophagitis, and this condition can be adequately detected by endoscopy and biopsy.

Extended pH studies are primarily intended to quantitate the extent of acid exposure of the esophagus, but there are clear correlations between motor function and the clearance capacity of the organ; therefore, the information gained by pH probes may be crucial for understanding some of the motor disturbances.[29,31,32,139,146]

Manometry is the main tool for examining the motor function of the esophagus. This procedure is based on the principle of Pascal, which states that the pressure exerted on any point of a liquid is transmitted in all directions with similar strength. Using tip-occluded

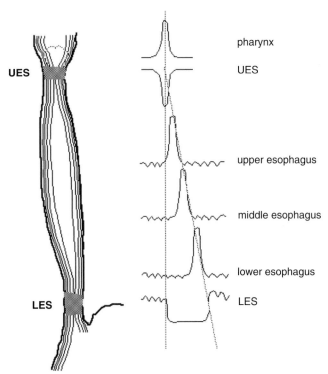

Figure 70–1   Schematic drawing of pressure recorded manometrically within the lumen of the esophagus during deglutition. Contraction of the pharyngeal constrictors is accompanied by relaxation of the cricopharyngeal muscle or upper esophageal sphincter (UES). Progressive peristaltic waves are generated in the body of the esophagus. The lower esophageal sphincter (LES) remains relaxed during the entire process and closes subsequently with a post-relaxation peak.

probes with lateral holes perfused at constant rates, the pressure at any point of the esophageal lumen can be recorded through pressure transducers connected in a "T" to the perfusion system. Assemblies of several probes with spaced holes can explore the progression of pressure waves along the organ (Fig. 70-1).* Solid-state sensors can replace the perfused probes, but fragility and high price limit their use.

Manometry is also helpful for assessing sphincteric function. Use of a single perfused probe or assemblies of several of them with radially arranged orifices and passage of the recording orifices through the gastroesophageal junction at constant speed allows recording of the pressure profile of both the UES and LES.[7,14,83,104,166] For the LES the profile shows the gastric pressure followed by a "plateau" corresponding to the overlapping LES pressure and the crural sling contractions.[69] Furthermore, it allows detection of the point at which the esophagus becomes intrathoracic because there is an "inversion point" when the positive-pressure inspiratory deflections become negative (Fig. 70-2). Stationary sphincter

---

*See references 7, 15, 32, 33, 59, 64, 83, 104, 138, 154, 158, 185.

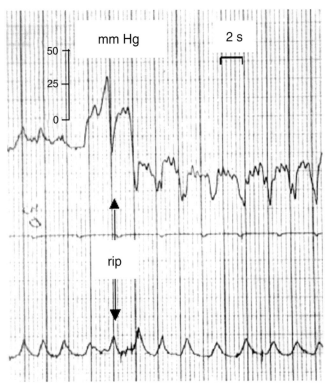

Figure 70–2 Pull-through manometric recording of the lower esophageal sphincter (LES) in a normal child (*upper tracing*) with simultaneous recording of abdominal pressure (*lower tracing*). Intragastric pressure is first recorded with positive inspiratory deflections. A "plateau" corresponds to the high-pressure zone of the LES. When the probe enters the thoracic esophagus, intraluminal inspiratory deflections become negative (respiratory inversion point [rip]). From then on the pressure baseline is lower and the inspirations are recorded by negative waves. Withdrawal speed is 1 mm/sec. The time between vertical marks is 2 seconds.

manometry with one of the orifices at the sphincteric level allows detection and assessment of the extent of relaxation.

However, because it is understood that reflux is possible with normal sphincteric pressure, more attention has been paid to the relaxations seen with continuous sphincteric recording probes with constantly perfused sleeves located at the appropriate level.[32,83,84,111,178] These recording probes, coupled with the availability of very finely extruded Silastic probes, have permitted the study of gastroesophageal physiology in small babies and premature infants over relatively long periods.[122,123]

Manometry requires bulky, expensive, and delicate equipment and some cooperation on the part of the patient, which may be difficult to obtain in children. In addition, sedation might change the registered pressures.[58,172]

The recently introduced 24-hour ambulatory manometry coupled with pH-metry has generated important information on several esophageal disorders in both adults[1,5,6,20,50,76,125,150,161] and children. However, the size of the solid-state sensor probes and the bulk of the equipment have limited these tests to older children for the present.[29,62,174,185] These techniques have allowed extended recordings of pressure or pH to be reduced to electrical signals that can be analyzed and measured in computers with the assistance of specifically designed software. It is likely that these diagnostic tools will be further miniaturized and adapted to use in children in the near future, thereby enlarging the scope of manometric studies.

DISORDERS OF THE UPPER ESOPHAGUS

The cricopharyngeus occasionally fails to maintain its normal tonus or to relax during deglutition. This leads to difficulty swallowing and consequent choking, which may be life threatening during early infancy.

Permanent *cricopharyngeal relaxation* is sometimes seen in neurologically impaired patients who undergo repeated episodes of aspiration.[159] *Delayed* or *incomplete relaxation* may be observed in children with the Chiari syndrome,[127,129] in those with 22q11.2 deletion,[48] or after diazepam medication.[99] Absence of relaxation (*cricopharyngeal achalasia*) occurs rarely as a primary phenomenon and is usually secondary to neuromuscular disorders.[135,159] In all these conditions the primary symptoms are choking during feeding and respiratory distress during early infancy, which often prompt urgent diagnostic workup. A barium meal or cineradiography depict simultaneous opacification of the respiratory and digestive tracts in cases of permanent relaxation and a dilated pharynx with permanent upper esophageal closure and occasional passage of contrast into the trachea in cases of delayed or absent relaxation.[89,135]

Manometry is useful for the diagnosis of cricopharyngeal disorders because it shows the incompleteness or absence of relaxation of the muscle during deglutition.[22,129,159] However, it is particularly difficult to perform in infants because the use of perfused catheters in the upper part of the esophagus is unpleasant for the baby, who chokes, coughs, and does not cooperate. Recordings with sphincteric sleeves depict the lack of relaxation better and are associated with less risk for fluid aspiration.[37]

Gastrostomy may be necessary for feeding babies with permanent cricopharyngeal relaxation and also for those with UES achalasia.[54,127] Achalasia of the muscle can be treated by balloon dilatation,[43,95] but extramucosal myotomy is more effective.[22,117] If reflux is present, concurrent fundoplication should be considered because insufficiency of both the upper and lower esophageal closure mechanisms may be devastating.[113] Some nonspecific histologic changes in the muscle obtained during myotomy have been reported in cricopharyngeal achalasia.[93]

DISORDERS OF THE ESOPHAGEAL BODY

Primary Motor Disorders

Abnormal motility of the body of the esophagus is a frequent cause of symptoms in adults, in whom *diffuse esophageal spasm,*[10,40,144,161,181] *nutcracker esophagus,*[21,82] or other abnormal motor patterns impairing propulsion of the food bolus are occasionally diagnosed after investigation for dysphagia, non–cardiac-related chest pain, or suspected reflux. Simultaneous, nonpropulsive contractions or an excessive proportion of long-duration waves alternating with normal ones are found in the first of these conditions, whereas extremely powerful, high-amplitude waves that can be peristaltic or retrograde are demonstrated in the second abnormality.[125,160,161] Nutcracker esophagus has been noted to evolve into achalasia.[4]

Manometry is the main diagnostic tool, and its accuracy has improved considerably since 24-hour ambulatory recordings have become available because the disturbances may not be permanent and appear only occasionally at some point in the circadian cycle. Because of the difficulties of performing this procedure in children, primary motor disorders of the esophageal body were practically unheard of until recently, although apnea, bradycardia,[57] and bizarre posturing[193] had been considered symptoms and signs of motor disturbances. However, the introduction of better manometric techniques has produced growing evidence of their existence in children. Food impaction in the absence of stenosis has been found in association with manometric patterns similar to those seen in adults with nutcracker esophagus (Fig. 70-3), but this disorder might not be primary because most patients have reflux as well and respond to treatment of esophagitis.[26,90,138,185]

Pharmacologic treatment of primary motor disorders with prokinetic agents or calcium channel blockers[17,61] is seldom indicated in children with these conditions.[65] Sildenafil, a drug that helps induce nitric oxide–related relaxation of the esophageal body and LES, has been introduced for the treatment of motor disorders in

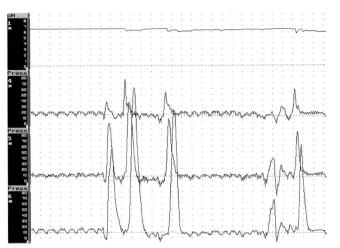

Figure 70–3 Nocturnal ambulatory manometric recording of intraluminal lower esophageal pH (1) and upper (4), middle (5), and lower (6) esophageal pressure in a 10-year-old boy with recurrent episodes of nonobstructive food impaction. The tracing demonstrates a nutcracker esophagus pattern of long duration, apparently peristaltic waves that are extremely powerful, particularly at the lower end of the esophageal body (more than 200 mm Hg or three to four times above normal). This occurs during sleep and without reflux as seen in the pH tracing.

adults,[94,136,196] but it has rarely been used in children. Balloon dilatation or extended myotomy, procedures occasionally performed in adults, have not been used in children.

Secondary Motor Disorders

Abnormal esophageal motility has been demonstrated in several syndromes and chromosomal disorders. Abnormal peristalsis sometimes associated with reflux has been observed in children with *Down's syndrome*,[169,195] *Cornelia de Lange syndrome*,[23,25,47,103,126] *scleroderma*,[55,191] *polymyositis-dermatomyositis*,[192] and *lupus*,[91] which are well-known causes of esophageal dysmotility in adults that rarely start during childhood. *Babies breast-fed by mothers with silicone implants*[96] may also have esophageal motor disturbances similar to those of scleroderma.

More relevant for pediatric surgeons are the motor disturbances of the esophagus experienced by survivors of neonatal operations for *esophageal atresia with tracheoesophageal fistula*.[44-46,168,170,173] In this malformation the structure of the muscle layers[198] and the extrinsic[38,130] and intrinsic[28,131] innervations are abnormal and impair the peristaltic pump, probably for life. This is particularly harmful in this condition because the function of the LES is also abnormal. Both these failures make GER a nearly constant aspect of the disease from birth, independent of the type of repair.[137,166] In addition, esophageal shortening secondary to the anastomosis,[114] an abnormal hiatus,[197] and perhaps operative denervation may influence dysmotility. Many studies have demonstrated that LES function is abnormal in survivors of operations for esophageal atresia.[45,166] Some authors have shown that peristalsis is permanently damaged even many years after the anastomosis.[170,173] The clinical relevance of these disorders is probably greater than was previously thought. Patients who undergo surgery for esophageal atresia have swallowing problems that are perceived by them as minor but are nearly always present when specifically searched for.[79,173] These esophagi cannot prevent reflux, and because of the structural basis of these dysfunctions, there is not much benefit from prokinetic medications. Furthermore, spontaneous improvement of the reflux with age, which is a part of the natural history of reflux in children without esophageal atresia, cannot be expected in patients operated on for esophageal atresia.

GER should be treated in patients with esophageal atresia when it is symptomatic or when it causes esophagitis. Dysmotility, a constant problem with this malformation, does not preclude complete fundoplication, which should be loose. Gravity is probably the main esophageal emptying force before or after the plication, and there should be no problem if the wrap is loose enough. However, the incidence of long-term failure of the plication is high in this group of patients because all the causes of GER and dysmotility remain active despite the new valve.[56,153]

Other relevant conditions involving esophageal motor disorders are *chronic intestinal pseudo-obstruction*, a heterogeneous group of gastrointestinal dysfunctions with a myogenic or neural basis that are characterized by distal esophageal dysmotility with simultaneous, short-lasting, low-amplitude waves.[18,109,145] However, the dysmotility is widespread and the esophageal part is not the most important. Patients with *Hirschsprung's disease* have simultaneous and double-peaked esophageal waves,[157] and children with *congenital central hypoventilation syndrome* (*Ondine's curse*)[53] or *Goldenhar's syndrome*[148] also have also esophageal dysmotility. Survivors of neonatal operations for *congenital diaphragmatic hernia* have radiologic and clinical evidence of abnormal esophageal motor function[105,162,163] that may be related to innervation anomalies. Esophageal dysfunction involving decreased sphincteric pressure or abnormal distal esophageal contractility has been described in children with *chronic renal failure*,[132] *Noonan's syndrome*,[147] and *Pierre Robin syndrome*.[12] The same anomalies have been observed in adults with *celiac disease*,[74] but to our knowledge, this issue has not been examined in children.

Children with *corrosive injuries* of the esophagus have impaired peristaltic activity both in the acute postinjury period[60] and when scars are established.[13] These manometric findings have been confirmed by radionuclide studies.[24] The contribution of dysmotility to the clinical course and prognosis of this condition is still unclear, although secondary esophagitis may aggravate the condition.

In the last few years we have treated a growing number of patients with *eosinophilic esophagitis*, a condition probably of allergic origin with symptoms of reflux or food impaction.[36,85,97,124] Reflux and stenosis are usually ruled out, but a typical type of Schatzki ring[120] or multiple rings[149] is seen on endoscopy (Fig. 70-4). Heavy infiltration of the mucosa by eosinophils is found on biopsy. Strictures are rarely observed in eosinophilic esophagitis, and the ones

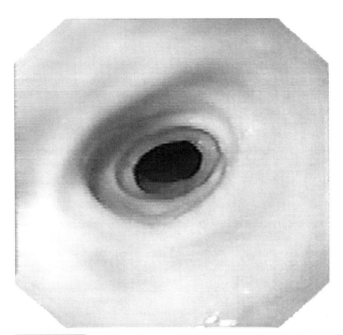

Figure 70–4 Typical "multiple ring" pattern of the esophagus on fiberoptic endoscopy in an 11-year-old girl with dysphagia secondary to eosinophilic esophagitis. On biopsy the mucosa was heavily infiltrated with eosinophils. pH levels were normal, and the patient did well after a course of treatment with steroids.

that do occur respond to conservative treatment.[11,39] Oral corticosteroids,[97] fluticasone,[167] or eosinophil stabilizers such as montelukast[9,151] are usually helpful in the management of this condition.[39]

Disorders of the Distal Esophagus

Primary gastroesophageal reflux involves both failure of the gastroesophageal barrier and abnormal esophageal motility. The etiology of the sphincteric failure is not completely understood, but there is increasing evidence of prolonged nondeglutitory relaxation as the main mechanism.[32,83,178] These abnormalities permit the creation of a "common cavity" phenomenon that negates the normal gastroesophageal pressure gradient between the stomach and the esophagus. The gastric fluid refluxed into the esophagus has to be cleared into the stomach by peristalsis, but this second defensive mechanism is also abnormal and increases the risk for esophagitis. The proportion of peristaltic contractions after deglutition or reflux and the amplitude of the waves are decreased, particularly at the lower end of the organ.[7,59,62] Whether dysmotility in GER disease is a primary phenomenon or secondary to esophageal inflammation is unclear. There is solid clinical and experimental evidence that chronic esophagitis adversely affects previously healthy peristalsis,[35,182] and at least in some cases, motor function remains abnormal even after medical or surgical cure of reflux and esophagitis.[7,33-35,108]

The success of prokinetic treatment used extensively in the last 2 decades illustrates the relevance of the dysmotility in GER disease. These drugs act by reinforcing the failing sphincter, by hastening gastric emptying, and by improving peristalsis.

The more characteristic motor disorder of the lower end of the esophagus is *achalasia*, in which the LES is hypertonic and does not relax during deglutition. In addition, dilation of the esophagus and primary hypoperistaltism create a propulsive function that is totally ineffective. This condition is relatively rare in young children, and although some cases have an early onset, most are diagnosed in late childhood or early adolescence. Only a few studies include more than a limited number of cases,[16,73,78,80,174,176,180] and the largest multicenter series involves only 175 patients.[118]

The etiology of achalasia is unknown, but there is increasing evidence of a progressive disturbance in the intrinsic innervation with reduced or absent nitric oxide synthase (NOS) activity.[86,165] This enzyme is responsible for the synthesis of nitric oxide, the nonadrenergic-noncholinergic neurotransmitter involved in smooth muscle relaxation.[165] nNOS(−/−)mice with absent NOS have a hypertensive, nonrelaxing LES.[152] The progressive degeneration of the intrinsic innervation has some similarity to that noted in Chagas' disease, a parasitic condition seen in South America that is caused by *Trypanosoma cruzi*; this disease produces degeneration of the neural structures leading to megaesophagus.[41]

Achalasia may be associated with Allgrove's syndrome, an autosomal recessive familial condition[128] caused by a mutation of the *AAAS* gene[81,143,194] that is characterized by adrenocortical insufficiency and alacrima, in addition to esophageal motor dysfunction. This association is called ALADIN syndrome (alacrima, achalasia, adrenal insufficiency, and neurologic disorder).[70] Achalasia is more frequent in boys, and it is occasionally associated with Down's syndrome.[195]

Achalasia patients complain of progressive dysphagia and regurgitation of food retained in the esophagus; these findings should not be confused with vomiting. Some have retrosternal pain, which may become distressing. Patients lose weight and often have foul breath and respiratory symptoms such as nocturnal cough or repeated pneumonia because of frequent microaspiration.[72,80] Patients with Allgrove's syndrome also have symptoms of adrenocortical insufficiency, such as progressive pigmentation and asthenia and eventually absence of tears (alacrima), but these symptoms and other manifestations of neurologic disease[70] may appear later after the full clinical picture of achalasia has developed.

The barium meal is often diagnostic: the esophagus is large (megaesophagus) and contains stagnant fluid above the barium column. There is marked aperistalsis, and the esophagogastric junction is filiform, with a classic "bird's beak" shape.[80] The contrast material progresses into the stomach after a considerable time, and most of it is retained in the esophagus for hours (Fig. 70-5).

Fiber-optic endoscopy rules out the presence of a stricture; the esophagoscope can usually be advanced into the stomach with relative ease. Esophagitis may be seen after aspiration of the retained fluid, but it is generally secondary to fermentation of the stagnant fluid. pH studies are not useful at this stage and can be misleading because this fluid is often acidic and the probe reading may suggest GER, which is in fact impossible. Radionuclide scintigraphy may depict the lack of progression of the esophageal content and allows more prolonged observation with less radiation exposure, but it is less informative than the barium meal in regard to evaluating the shape of the distal end of the esophagus.[27,195]

Manometry is the most useful diagnostic tool for achalasia: the sphincter is hypertonic and does not relax or relaxes incompletely during deglutition. Esophageal peristalsis is absent, and rare pressure is present, particularly during meals. Such pressure is recorded simultaneously at all points in the lumen, which is in fact a common chamber (Fig. 70-6).[16,78] Twenty-four-hour ambulatory recordings performed with probes equipped with multiple solid-state sensors show that the aperistalsis is constant during the entire circadian cycle, including meals, a time when motor waves are normally more active.[174]

Pharmacologic treatment, particularly calcium channel blockers such as nifedipine, may alleviate the spasm in some cases,[106] but they cannot be relied on as a long-term

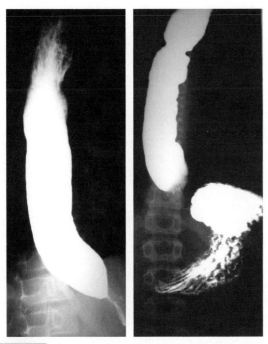

Figure 70–5 Barium meal in a 9-year-old patient with achalasia. The esophagus is enlarged and contained stagnant fluid before the contrast was administered. Emptying is very slow and the cardia has a typical "carrot" or "bird's beak" pattern (*left*). Some feeble esophageal contractions are seen (*right*), but peristalsis is impossible because the esophageal walls remain widely separated.

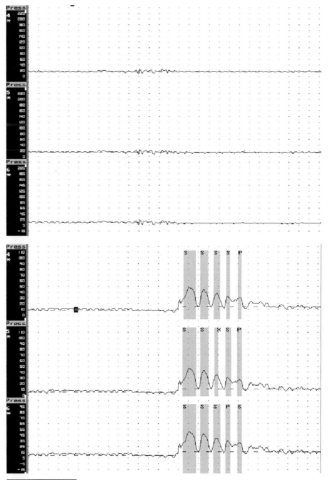

Figure 70–6 Ambulatory esophageal manometry in an 8-year-old boy with achalasia. In the upper tracing, the pressure at the upper (4), middle (5), and lower (6) levels of the esophagus is identical and no waves are seen. In the lower tracing, corresponding to a meal, some waves are generated, but they are simultaneous and nonpropulsive (time between vertical marks, 5 seconds).

treatment in children.[61] Forceful balloon dilation of the distal end of the esophagus is often successful in adults with achalasia, but such treatment is seldom permanently effective in children.[16,49,180] Local injection of botulinum toxin has also been attempted in children, but its success has been limited as well.[71,72,75,87,186] Extramucosal Heller myotomy remains the treatment of choice in children, and it can be performed through either the thorax or the abdomen.[16,78,80,118,174,180] The latter approach probably allows a more complete myotomy on the gastric side and an easier complementary fundoplication. In fact, if sought after, reflux is rather constant after a Heller myotomy, and some form of fundoplication is probably reasonable to consider in children, whose long life expectancy after the operation supports the use of this procedure to prevent the complications of GER.[72,73,78,115,140,174,180] A Nissen antireflux procedure may be inappropriate because of the often large diameter of the thickened esophagus; a posterior Toupet or anterior Thal-Dor hemifundoplication is preferred.[78,140,174] All these procedures can be performed laparoscopically, and this approach is presently the gold standard.[51,52,107,140]

Postoperatively, patients are relieved of their symptoms immediately and they can feed properly and regain weight. However, the esophagus remains dilated for months or even years, and its function only rarely returns to normal. Most patients maintain rare and ineffective peristalsis despite the decrease in sphincteric pressure provided by the myotomy (Fig. 70-7).[100,101,115,174,180] Some have low-level symptoms such as dysphagia and often require a few swallows of water during feeding, but esophagomyotomy allows a good quality of life. Esophageal replacement has been reported in some rare cases of achalasia in which all other treatments have failed.[119,156]

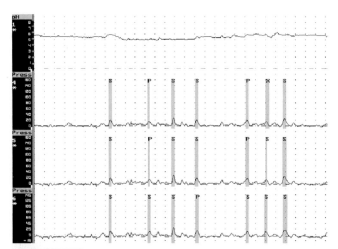

Figure 70–7 Ambulatory esophageal manometry during a meal in a 24-year-old woman 12 years after a Heller myotomy for achalasia. She was asymptomatic, but esophageal motility remained very poor. The motor waves at the upper (4), middle (5), and lower (6) levels of the esophagus showed peristaltic organization but were very weak (less than 25 mm Hg, roughly half normal). The time between vertical marks is 5 seconds.

This suggests that the myotomy relieves the obstruction but does not cure the condition. Long-term follow-up is essential.

REFERENCES

1. Adamek RJ, Wegener M, Wienbeck M, Gielen B: Long-term esophageal manometry in healthy subjects. Evaluation of normal values and influence of age. Dig Dis Sci 1994; 39:2069.
2. Allan DW, Greer JJ: Pathogenesis of nitrofen-induced congenital diaphragmatic hernia in fetal rats. J Appl Physiol 1997;83:338.
3. Allan DW, Greer JJ: Embryogenesis of the phrenic nerve and diaphragm in the fetal rat. J Comp Neurol 1997; 382:459.
4. Anggiansah A, Bright NF, McCullagh M, Owen WJ: Transition from nutcracker esophagus to achalasia. Dig Dis Sci 1990;35:1162.
5. Anggiansah A, Taylor G, Marshall RE, et al: Oesophageal motor responses to gastro-oesophageal reflux in healthy controls and reflux patients. Gut 1997;41:600.
6. Anggiansah A, Taylor G, Marshall RE, et al: What is normal oesophageal motility? An ambulatory study. Scand J Gastroenterol 1998;33:473.
7. Arana J, Tovar JA: Motor efficiency of the refluxing esophagus in basal conditions and after acid challenge. J Pediatr Surg 1989;24:1049.
8. Arana J, Tovar JA, Garay J: Abnormal preoperative and postoperative esophageal peristalsis in gastroesophageal reflux. J Pediatr Surg 1986;21:711.
9. Attwood SE, Lewis CJ, Bronder CS, et al: Eosinophilic oesophagitis: A novel treatment using montelukast. Gut 2003;52:181.
10. Barham CP, Gotley DC, Fowler A, et al: Diffuse oesophageal spasm: Diagnosis by ambulatory 24 hour manometry. Gut 1997;41:151.
11. Batres LA, Liacouras C, Schnaufer L, Mascarenhas MR: Eosinophilic esophagitis associated with anastomotic strictures after esophageal atresia repair. J Pediatr Gastroenterol Nutr 2002;35:224.
12. Baujat G, Faure C, Zaouche A, et al: Oroesophageal motor disorders in Pierre Robin syndrome. J Pediatr Gastroenterol Nutr 2001;32:297.
13. Bautista A, Varela R, Villanueva A, et al: Motor function of the esophagus after caustic burn. Eur J Pediatr Surg 1996; 6:204.
14. Berezin S, Halata MS, Newman LJ, et al: Esophageal manometry in children with esophagitis. Am J Gastroenterol 1993;88:680.
15. Berezin S, Medow MS, Glassman MS, Newman LJ: Esophageal chest pain in children with asthma. J Pediatr Gastroenterol Nutr 1991;12:52.
16. Berquist WE, Byrne WJ, Ament ME, et al: Achalasia: Diagnosis, management, and clinical course in 16 children. Pediatrics 1983;71:798.
17. Blackwell JN, Holt S, Heading RC: Effect of nifedipine on oesophageal motility and gastric emptying. Digestion 1981; 21:50.
18. Boige N, Faure C, Cargill G, et al: Manometrical evaluation in visceral neuropathies in children. J Pediatr Gastroenterol Nutr 1994;19:71.
19. Brandt CT, Tam PK, Gould SJ: Nitrergic innervation of the human gut during early fetal development. J Pediatr Surg 1996;31:661.

20. Bremner RM, Costantini M, DeMeester TR, et al: Normal esophageal body function: A study using ambulatory esophageal manometry. Am J Gastroenterol 1998;93:183.

21. Breumelhof R, Van Wijk HJ, Van Es CD, Smout AJ: Food impaction in nutcracker esophagus. Dig Dis Sci 1990; 35:1167.

22. Brooks A, Millar AJ, Rode H: The surgical management of cricopharyngeal achalasia in children. Int J Pediatr Otorhinolaryngol 2000;56:1.

23. Bull MJ, Fitzgerald JF, Heifetz SA, Brei TJ: Gastrointestinal abnormalities: A significant cause of feeding difficulties and failure to thrive in Brachmann–de Lange syndrome. Am J Med Genet 1993;47:1029.

24. Cadranel S, Di Lorenzo C, Rodesch P, et al: Caustic ingestion and esophageal function. J Pediatr Gastroenterol Nutr 1990;10:164.

25. Cates M, Billmire DF, Bull MJ, Grosfeld JL: Gastroesophageal dysfunction in Cornelia de Lange syndrome. J Pediatr Surg 1989;24:248.

26. Catto-Smith AG, Machida H, Butzner JD, et al: The role of gastroesophageal reflux in pediatric dysphagia. J Pediatr Gastroenterol Nutr 1991;12:159.

27. Chawda SJ, Watura R, Adams H, Smith PM: A comparison of barium swallow and erect esophageal transit scintigraphy following balloon dilatation for achalasia. Dis Esophagus 1998;11:181.

28. Cheng W, Bishop AE, Spitz L, Polak JM: Abnormal enteric nerve morphology in atretic esophagus of fetal rats with Adriamycin-induced esophageal atresia. Pediatr Surg Int 1999;15:8.

29. Chitkara DK, Fortunato C, Nurko S: Prolonged monitoring of esophageal motor function in healthy children. J Pediatr Gastroenterol Nutr 2004;38:192.

30. Costa RH, Kalinichenko VV, Lim L: Transcription factors in mouse lung development and function. Am J Physiol Lung Cell Mol Physiol 2001;280:L823.

31. Cucchiara S, Bortolotti M, Minella R, Auricchio S: Fasting and postprandial mechanisms of gastroesophageal reflux in children with gastroesophageal reflux disease. Dig Dis Sci 1993;38:86.

32. Cucchiara S, Campanozzi A, Greco L, et al: Predictive value of esophageal manometry and gastroesophageal pH monitoring for responsiveness of reflux disease to medical therapy in children. Am J Gastroenterol 1996;91:680.

33. Cucchiara S, Staiano A, Di Lorenzo C, et al: Esophageal motor abnormalities in children with gastroesophageal reflux and peptic esophagitis. J Pediatr 1986;108:907.

34. Cucchiara S, Staiano A, Di Lorenzo C, et al: Pathophysiology of gastroesophageal reflux and distal esophageal motility in children with gastroesophageal reflux disease. J Pediatr Gastroenterol Nutr 1988;7:830.

35. Cucchiara S, Staiano A, Paone FM, Basile P: Esophageal aperistalsis due to reflux esophagitis: A report of two cases. J Pediatr Gastroenterol Nutr 1989;9:388.

36. Cury EK, Schraibman V, Faintuch S: Eosinophilic infiltration of the esophagus: Gastroesophageal reflux versus eosinophilic esophagitis in children—discussion on daily practice. J Pediatr Surg 2004;39:e4.

37. Davidson GP, Dent J, Willing J: Monitoring of upper oesophageal sphincter pressure in children. Gut 1991; 32:607.

38. Davies MRQ: Anatomy of the extrinsic nerve supply of the oesophagus in oesophageal atresia of the common type. Pediatr Surg Int 1996;11:230.

39. De Agustin JC, Sanz N, Canals MJ, et al: Successful medical treatment of two patients with eosinophilic oesophagitis. J Pediatr Surg 2002;37:207.

40. de Caestecker JS, Blackwell JN, Brown J, Heading RC: The oesophagus as a cause of recurrent chest pain: Which patients should be investigated and which tests should be used? Lancet 1985;2:1143.

41. de Oliveira RB, Rezende Filho J, Dantas RO, Iazigi N: The spectrum of esophageal motor disorders in Chagas' disease. Am J Gastroenterol 1995;90:1119.

42. Di Lorenzo C, Piepsz A, Ham H, Cadranel S: Gastric emptying with gastro-oesophageal reflux. Arch Dis Child 1987; 62:449.

43. Dinari G, Danziger Y, Mimouni M, et al: Cricopharyngeal dysfunction in childhood: Treatment by dilatations. J Pediatr Gastroenterol Nutr 1987;6:212.

44. Duranceau A, Fisher SR, Flye M, et al: Motor function of the esophagus after repair of esophageal atresia and tracheoesophageal fistula. Surgery 1977;82:116.

45. Dutta HK, Grover VP, Dwivedi SN, Bhatnagar V: Manometric evaluation of postoperative patients of esophageal atresia and tracheo-esophageal fistula. Eur J Pediatr Surg 2001; 11:371.

46. Dutta HK, Rajani M, Bhatnagar V: Cineradiographic evaluation of postoperative patients with esophageal atresia and tracheoesophageal fistula. Pediatr Surg Int 2000;16:322.

47. DuVall GA, Walden DT: Adenocarcinoma of the esophagus complicating Cornelia de Lange syndrome. J Clin Gastroenterol 1996;22:131.

48. Eicher PS, McDonald-Mcginn DM, Fox CA, et al: Dysphagia in children with a 22q11.2 deletion: Unusual pattern found on modified barium swallow. J Pediatr 2000;137:158.

49. Emblem R, Stringer MD, Hall CM, Spitz L: Current results of surgery for achalasia of the cardia. Arch Dis Child 1993; 68:749.

50. Emde C, Armstrong D, Castiglione F, et al: Reproducibility of long-term ambulatory esophageal combined pH/manometry. Gastroenterology 1991;100:1630.

51. Esposito C, Cucchiara S, Borrelli O, et al: Laparoscopic esophagomyotomy for the treatment of achalasia in children. A preliminary report of eight cases. Surg Endosc 2000; 14:110.

52. Esposito C, Mendoza-Sagaon M, Roblot-Maigret B, et al: Complications of laparoscopic treatment of esophageal achalasia in children. J Pediatr Surg 2000;35:680.

53. Faure C, Viarme F, Cargill G, et al: Abnormal esophageal motility in children with congenital central hypoventilation syndrome. Gastroenterology 2002;122:1258.

54. Fernbach SK, McLone DG: Derangement of swallowing in children with myelomeningocele. Pediatr Radiol 1985; 15:311.

55. Flick JA, Boyle JT, Tuchman DN, et al: Esophageal motor abnormalities in children and adolescents with scleroderma and mixed connective tissue disease. Pediatrics 1988;82:107.

56. Fonkalsrud EW, Ament ME: Gastroesophageal reflux in childhood. Curr Probl Surg 1996;33:1.

57. Fontan JP, Heldt GP, Heyman MB, et al: Esophageal spasm associated with apnea and bradycardia in an infant. Pediatrics 1984;73:52.

58. Fung KP, Math MV, Ho CO, Yap KM: Midazolam as a sedative in esophageal manometry: A study of the effect on esophageal motility. J Pediatr Gastroenterol Nutr 1992; 15:85.

59. Ganatra JV, Medow MS, Berezin S, et al: Esophageal dysmotility elicited by acid perfusion in children with esophagitis. Am J Gastroenterol 1995;90:1080.

60. Genc A, Mutaf O: Esophageal motility changes in acute and late periods of caustic esophageal burns and their relation to prognosis in children. J Pediatr Surg 2002;37:1526.

61. Glassman MS, Medow MS, Berezin S, Newman LJ: Spectrum of esophageal disorders in children with chest pain. Dig Dis Sci 1992;37:663.

62. Godoy J, Tovar JA, Vicente Y, et al: Esophageal motor dysfunction persists in children after surgical cure of reflux: An ambulatory manometric study. J Pediatr Surg 2001; 36:1405.

63. Gross RE: The Surgery of Infancy and Childhood, 1st ed. Philadelphia, WB Saunders, 1953.

64. Gustafsson PM, Tibbling L: Gastro-oesophageal reflux and oesophageal dysfunction in children and adolescents with brain damage. Acta Paediatr 1994;83:1081.

65. Hegar B, de Pont S, Vandemaele K, Vandenplas Y: Effect of prokinetics in children with recurrent nocturnal retrosternal pain. Eur J Gastroenterol Hepatol 1998;10:565.

66. Helm JF: Esophageal acid clearance. J Clin Gastroenterol 1986;8(Suppl 1):5.

67. Helm JF, Dodds WJ, Riedel DR, et al: Determinants of esophageal acid clearance in normal subjects. Gastroenterology 1983;85:607.

68. Hitchcock RJ, Pemble MJ, Bishop AE, et al: The ontogeny and distribution of neuropeptides in the human fetal and infant esophagus. Gastroenterology 1992;102:840.

69. Hollwarth M, Uray E: Physiology and pathophysiology of the esophagus in childhood. Prog Pediatr Surg 1985; 18:1.

70. Houlden H, Smith S, De Carvalho M, et al: Clinical and genetic characterization of families with triple A (Allgrove) syndrome. Brain 2002;125:2681.

71. Hurwitz M, Bahar RJ, Ament ME, et al: Evaluation of the use of botulinum toxin in children with achalasia. J Pediatr Gastroenterol Nutr 2000;30:509.

72. Hussain SZ, Thomas R, Tolia V: A review of achalasia in 33 children. Dig Dis Sci 2002;47:2538.

73. Illi OE, Stauffer UG: Achalasia in childhood and adolescence. Eur J Pediatr Surg 1994;4:214.

74. Iovino P, Ciacci C, Sabbatini F, et al: Esophageal impairment in adult celiac disease with steatorrhea. Am J Gastroenterol 1998;93:1243.

75. Ip KS, Cameron DJ, Catto-Smith AG, Hardikar W: Botulinum toxin for achalasia in children. J Gastroenterol Hepatol 2000;15:1100.

76. Janssens J, Vantrappen G, Ghillebert G: 24-Hour recording of esophageal pressure and pH in patients with noncardiac chest pain. Gastroenterology 1986;90:1978.

77. Kahrilas PJ: Anatomy, physiology and pathophysiology of dysphagia. Acta Otorhinolaryngol Belg 1994;48:97.

78. Kalicinski P, Dluski E, Drewniak T, Kaminski W: Esophageal manometric studies in children with achalasia before and after operative treatment. Pediatr Surg Int 1997; 12:571.

79. Kapila L, Daniel RD: Foreign body impaction arising in adulthood: A result of neonatal repair of tracheo-oesophageal fistula and oesophageal atresia [letter]. Ann R Coll Surg Engl 1996;78:559.

80. Karnak I, Senocak ME, Tanyel FC, Buyukpamukcu N: Achalasia in childhood: Surgical treatment and outcome. Eur J Pediatr Surg 2001;11:223.

81. Katsumata N, Hirose H, Kagami M, Tanaka T: Analysis of the AAAS gene in a Japanese patient with triple A syndrome. Endocr J 2002;49:49.

82. Katz PO, Castell JA: Nonachalasia motility disorders. In Castell DO, Richter JE (eds): The Esophagus, 3rd ed. Philadelphia, Lippincott Williams & Wilkins, 1999, p 215.

83. Kawahara H, Dent J, Davidson G: Mechanisms responsible for gastroesophageal reflux in children. Gastroenterology 1997;113:399.

84. Kawahara H, Imura K, Yagi M, et al: Mechanisms underlying the antireflux effect of Nissen fundoplication in children. J Pediatr Surg 1998;33:1618.

85. Khan S, Orenstein SR, Di Lorenzo C, et al: Eosinophilic esophagitis: Strictures, impactions, dysphagia. Dig Dis Sci 2003;48:22.

86. Khelif K, De Laet MH, Chaouachi B, et al: Achalasia of the cardia in Allgrove's (triple A) syndrome: Histopathologic study of 10 cases. Am J Surg Pathol 2003;27:667.

87. Khoshoo V, LaGarde DC, Udall JN Jr: Intrasphincteric injection of botulinum toxin for treating achalasia in children. J Pediatr Gastroenterol Nutr 1997;24:439.

88. Kluth D, Keijzer R, Hertl M, Tibboel D: Embryology of congenital diaphragmatic hernia. Semin Pediatr Surg 1996;5:224.

89. Kohda E, Hisazumi H, Hiramatsu K: Swallowing dysfunction and aspiration in neonates and infants. Acta Otolaryngol Suppl 1994;517:11.

90. Lao J, Bostwick HE, Berezin S, et al: Esophageal food impaction in children. Pediatr Emerg Care 2003;19:402.

91. Lapadula G, Muolo P, Semeraro F, et al: Esophageal motility disorders in the rheumatic diseases: A review of 150 patients. Clin Exp Rheumatol 1994;12:515.

92. Larsen WJ: Human Embryology, 2nd ed. New York, Churchill Livingstone, 1997.

93. Laurikainen E, Aitasalo K, Halonen P, et al: Muscle pathology in idiopathic cricopharyngeal dysphagia. Enzyme histochemical and electron microscopic findings. Eur Arch Otorhinolaryngol 1992;249:216.

94. Lee JI, Park H, Kim JH, et al: The effect of sildenafil on oesophageal motor function in healthy subjects and patients with nutcracker oesophagus. Neurogastroenterol Motil 2003;15:617.

95. Lernau OZ, Sherzer E, Mogle P, Nissan S: Congenital cricopharyngeal achalasia treatment by dilatations. J Pediatr Surg 1984;19:202.

96. Levine JJ, Trachtman H, Gold DM, Pettei MJ: Esophageal dysmotility in children breast-fed by mothers with silicone breast implants. Long-term follow-up and response to treatment. Dig Dis Sci 1996;41:1600.

97. Liacouras CA, Wenner WJ, Brown K, Ruchelli E: Primary eosinophilic esophagitis in children: Successful treatment with oral corticosteroids. J Pediatr Gastroenterol Nutr 1998;26:380.

98. Liebermann-Meffert D, Allgöwer M, Schmid P, Blum AL: Muscular equivalent of the lower esophageal sphincter. Gastroenterology 1979;76:31.

99. Lim HC, Nigro MA, Beierwaltes P, et al: Nitrazepam-induced cricopharyngeal dysphagia, abnormal esophageal peristalsis and associated bronchospasm: Probable cause of nitrazepam-related sudden death. Brain Dev 1992; 14:309.

100. Liu HC, Huang BS, Hsu WH, et al: Surgery for achalasia: Long-term results in operated achalasic patients. Ann Thorac Cardiovasc Surg 1998;4:312.

101. Liu JF, Zhang J, Tian ZQ, et al: Long-term outcome of esophageal myotomy for achalasia. World J Gastroenterol 2004;10:287.

102. Long JD, Orlando RC: Esophageal submucosal glands: Structure and function. Am J Gastroenterol 1999; 94:2818.

103. Luzzani S, Macchini F, Valade A, et al: Gastroesophageal reflux and Cornelia de Lange syndrome: Typical and atypical symptoms. Am J Med Genet 2003;119A:283.

104. Mahony MJ, Migliavacca M, Spitz L, Milla PJ: Motor disorders of the oesophagus in gastro-oesophageal reflux. Arch Dis Child 1988;63:1333.

105. Makhoul IR, Shoshany G, Smolkin T, et al: Transient mega-esophagus in a neonate with congenital diaphragmatic hernia. Eur Radiol 2001;11:867.

106. Maksimak M, Perlmutter DH, Winter HS: The use of nifedipine for the treatment of achalasia in children. J Pediatr Gastroenterol Nutr 1986;5:883.

107. Mattioli G, Esposito C, Prato AP, et al: Results of the laparoscopic Heller-Dor procedure for pediatric esophageal achalasia. Surg Endosc 2003;17:1650.

108. McDougall NI, Mooney RB, Ferguson WR, et al: The effect of healing oesophagitis on oesophageal motor function as determined by oesophageal scintigraphy and ambulatory oesophageal motility/pH monitoring. Aliment Pharmacol Ther 1998;12:899.

109. Milla PJ: Intestinal motility during ontogeny and intestinal pseudo-obstruction in children. Pediatr Clin North Am 1996;43:511.

110. Mittal RK, Balaban DH: The esophagogastric junction. N Engl J Med 1997;336:924.

111. Mittal RK, Rochester DF, McCallum RW: Sphincteric action of the diaphragm during a relaxed lower esophageal sphincter in humans. Am J Physiol 1989;256:G139.

112. Mittal RK, Sivri B, Schirmer BD, Heine KJ: Effect of crural myotomy on the incidence and mechanism of gastroesophageal reflux in cats. Gastroenterology 1993;105:740.

113. Mondragon F, Arana J, Tovar JA, et al: Cricopharyngeal dysphagia and gastro-oesophageal reflux. Z Kinderchir 1985;40:361.

114. Montedonico S, Diez-Pardo JA, Possogel AK, Tovar JA: Effects of esophageal shortening on the gastroesophageal barrier: An experimental study on the causes of reflux in esophageal atresia. J Pediatr Surg 1999;34:300.

115. Morris-Stiff G, Khan R, Foster ME, Lari J: Long-term results of surgery for childhood achalasia. Ann R Coll Surg Engl 1997;79:432.

116. Motil KJ, Schultz RJ, Browning K, et al: Oropharyngeal dysfunction and gastroesophageal dysmotility are present in girls and women with Rett syndrome. J Pediatr Gastroenterol Nutr 1999;29:31.

117. Muraji T, Takamizawa S, Satoh S, et al: Congenital cricopharyngeal achalasia: Diagnosis and surgical management. J Pediatr Surg 2002;37:E12.

118. Myers NA, Jolley SG, Taylor R: Achalasia of the cardia in children: A worldwide survey. J Pediatr Surg 1994;29:1375.

119. Neville WE, Najem AZ: Colon replacement of the esophagus for congenital and benign disease. Ann Thorac Surg 1983;36:626.

120. Nurko S, Teitelbaum JE, Husain K, et al: Association of Schatzki ring with eosinophilic esophagitis in children. J Pediatr Gastroenterol Nutr 2004;38:436.

121. Okamoto E, Ueda T: Embryogenesis of intramural ganglia of the gut and its relationship to Hirschsprung's disease. J Pediatr Surg 1967;2:437.

122. Omari TI, Barnett C, Snel A, et al: Mechanisms of gastroesophageal reflux in healthy premature infants. J Pediatr 1998;133:650.

123. Omari T, Barnett C, Snel A, et al: Mechanism of gastroesophageal reflux in premature infants with chronic lung disease. J Pediatr Surg 1999;34:1795.

124. Orenstein SR, Shalaby TM, Di Lorenzo C, et al: The spectrum of pediatric eosinophilic esophagitis beyond infancy: A clinical series of 30 children. Am J Gastroenterol 2000;95:1422.

125. Paterson WG, Beck IT, Wang H: Ambulatory esophageal manometry/pH-metry discriminates between patients with different esophageal symptoms. Dig Dis Sci 1996;41:357.

126. Pei RS, Lin CC, Mak SC, et al: Barrett's esophagus in a child with de Lange syndrome: Report of one case. Acta Paediatr Taiwan 2000;41:155.

127. Pollack IF, Pang D, Kocoshis S, Putnam P: Neurogenic dysphagia resulting from Chiari malformations. Neurosurgery 1992;30:709.

128. Prpic I, Huebner A, Persic M, et al: Triple A syndrome: Genotype-phenotype assessment. Clin Genet 2003;63:415.

129. Putnam PE, Orenstein SR, Pang D, et al: Cricopharyngeal dysfunction associated with Chiari malformations. Pediatrics 1992;89:871.

130. Qi BQ, Merei J, Farmer P, et al: The vagus and recurrent laryngeal nerves in the rodent experimental model of esophageal atresia. J Pediatr Surg 1997;32:1580.

131. Qi BQ, Uemura S, Farmer P, et al: Intrinsic innervation of the oesophagus in fetal rats with oesophageal atresia. Pediatr Surg Int 1999;15:2.

132. Ravelli AM, Ledermann SE, Bisset WM, et al: Foregut motor function in chronic renal failure. Arch Dis Child 1992;67:1343.

133. Ravitch MM: Chalasia and achalasia of the esophagus. In Benson CD, Mustard WT, Ravitch MM, et al (eds): Pediatric Surgery, vol 1, 1st ed. Chicago, Year Book, 1962, p 299.

134. Rehbein F: Kinderchirurgische Operationen, 1st ed. Stuttgart, Germany, Hippokrates Verlag, 1976.

135. Reichert TJ, Bluestone CD, Stool SE, et al: Congenital cricopharyngeal achalasia. Ann Otol Rhinol Laryngol 1977;86:603.

136. Rhee PL, Hyun JG, Lee JH, et al: The effect of sildenafil on lower esophageal sphincter and body motility in normal male adults. Am J Gastroenterol 2001;96:3251.

137. Romeo G, Zuccarello B, Proietto F, Romeo C: Disorders of the esophageal motor activity in atresia of the esophagus. J Pediatr Surg 1987;22:120.

138. Rosario JA, Medow MS, Halata MS, et al: Nonspecific esophageal motility disorders in children without gastroesophageal reflux. J Pediatr Gastroenterol Nutr 1999;28:480.

139. Ross MN, Haase GM, Reiley TT, Meagher DP Jr: The importance of acid reflux patterns in neurologically damaged children detected by four-channel esophageal pH monitoring. J Pediatr Surg 1988;23:573.

140. Rothenberg SS, Partrick DA, Bealer JF, Chang JH: Evaluation of minimally invasive approaches to achalasia in children. J Pediatr Surg 2001;36:808.

141. Rumessen JJ, de Kerchove d'Exaerde A, Mignon S, et al: Interstitial cells of Cajal in the striated musculature of the mouse esophagus. Cell Tissue Res 2001;306:1.

142. Rumessen JJ, Vanderwinden JM: Interstitial cells in the musculature of the gastrointestinal tract: Cajal and beyond. Int Rev Cytol 2003;229:115.

143. Sandrini F, Farmakidis C, Kirschner LS, et al: Spectrum of mutations of the AAAS gene in Allgrove syndrome: Lack of mutations in six kindreds with isolated resistance to corticotropin. J Clin Endocrinol Metab 2001;86:5433.

144. Schima W, Stacher G, Pokieser P, et al: Esophageal motor disorders: Videofluoroscopic and manometric evaluation—prospective study in 88 symptomatic patients. Radiology 1992;185:487.

145. Schuffler MD, Pope CE 2nd: Studies of idiopathic intestinal pseudoobstruction. II. Hereditary hollow visceral myopathy: Family studies. Gastroenterology 1977;73:339.

146. Seibert JJ, Byrne WJ, Euler AR, et al: Gastroesophageal reflux—the acid test: Scintigraphy or the pH probe? AJR Am J Roentgenol 1983;140:1087.

147. Shah N, Rodriguez M, Louis DS, et al: Feeding difficulties and foregut dysmotility in Noonan's syndrome. Arch Dis Child 1999;81:28.

148. Shokeir MH: The Goldenhar syndrome: A natural history. Birth Defects Orig Artic Ser 1977;13:67.

149. Siafakas CG, Ryan CK, Brown MR, Miller TL: Multiple esophageal rings: An association with eosinophilic esophagitis: Case report and review of the literature. Am J Gastroenterol 2000;95:1572.

150. Singh S, Stein HJ, DeMeester TR, Hinder RA: Non-obstructive dysphagia in gastroesophageal reflux disease: A study with combined ambulatory pH and motility monitoring. Am J Gastroenterol 1992;87:562.

151. Sinharay R: Eosinophilic oesophagitis: Treatment using montelukast. Gut 2003;52:1228.

152. Sivarao DV, Mashimo HL, Thatte HS, Goyal RK: Lower esophageal sphincter is achalasic in nNOS(−/−) and hypotensive in W/W(v) mutant mice. Gastroenterology 2001;121:34.

153. Snyder CL, Ramachandran V, Kennedy AP, et al: Efficacy of partial wrap fundoplication for gastroesophageal reflux after repair of esophageal atresia. J Pediatr Surg 1997; 32:1089.

154. Sondheimer JM: Gastroesophageal reflux: Update on pathogenesis and diagnosis. Pediatr Clin North Am 1988; 35:103.

155. Sondheimer JM: Clearance of spontaneous gastroesophageal reflux in awake and sleeping infants. Gastroenterology 1989;97:821.

156. Spitz L: Gastric transposition for esophageal substitution in children. J Pediatr Surg 1992;27:252.

157. Staiano A, Corazziari E, Andreotti MR, Clouse RE: Esophageal motility in children with Hirschsprung's disease. Am J Dis Child 1991;145:310.

158. Staiano A, Cucchiara S, Del Giudice E, et al: Disorders of oesophageal motility in children with psychomotor retardation and gastro-oesophageal reflux. Eur J Pediatr 1991;150:638.

159. Staiano A, Cucchiara S, De Vizia B, et al: Disorders of upper esophageal sphincter motility in children. J Pediatr Gastroenterol Nutr 1987;6:892.

160. Stein HJ, DeMeester TR: Indications, technique, and clinical use of ambulatory 24-hour esophageal motility monitoring in a surgical practice. Ann Surg 1993;217:128.

161. Stein HJ, DeMeester TR, Eypasch EP, Klingman RR: Ambulatory 24-hour esophageal manometry in the evaluation of esophageal motor disorders and noncardiac chest pain. Surgery 1991;110:753.

162. Stolar CJ, Berdon WE, Dillon PW, et al: Esophageal dilatation and reflux in neonates supported by ECMO after diaphragmatic hernia repair. AJR Am J Roentgenol 1988; 151:135.

163. Stolar CJ, Levy JP, Dillon PW, et al: Anatomic and functional abnormalities of the esophagus in infants surviving congenital diaphragmatic hernia. Am J Surg 1990; 159:204.

164. Swenson O: Pediatric Surgery, vol 1, 3rd ed. London, Butterworths, 1969.

165. Takahashi T: Pathophysiological significance of neuronal nitric oxide synthase in the gastrointestinal tract. J Gastroenterol 2003;38:421.

166. Takano K, Iwafuchi M, Uchiyama M, et al: Evaluation of lower esophageal sphincter function in infants and children following esophageal surgery. J Pediatr Surg 1988; 23:410.

167. Teitelbaum JE, Fox VL, Twarog FJ, et al: Eosinophilic esophagitis in children: Immunopathological analysis and response to fluticasone propionate. Gastroenterology 2002; 122:1216.

168. Thomas EJ, Kumar R, Dasan JB, et al: Radionuclide scintigraphy in the evaluation of gastro-oesophageal reflux in post-operative oesophageal atresia and tracheo-oesophageal fistula patients. Nucl Med Commun 2003;24:317.

169. Thompson LD, McElhinney DB, Jue KL, Hodge D: Gastroesophageal reflux after repair of atrioventricular septal defect in infants with trisomy 21: A comparison of medical and surgical therapy. J Pediatr Surg 1999;34:1359.

170. Tomaselli V, Volpi ML, Dell'Agnola CA, et al: Long-term evaluation of esophageal function in patients treated at birth for esophageal atresia. Pediatr Surg Int 2003;19:40.

171. Tomita R, Tanjoh K, Fujisaki S, Fukuzawa M: Physiological studies on nitric oxide in the lower esophageal sphincter of patients with reflux esophagitis. Hepatogastroenterology 2003;50:110.

172. Tovar JA, Arana J, Tapia I: Effects of sedation on motor function of the refluxing esophagus. Pediatr Surg Int 1990;5:418.

173. Tovar JA, Diez Pardo JA, Murcia J, et al: Ambulatory 24-hour manometric and pH metric evidence of permanent impairment of clearance capacity in patients with esophageal atresia. J Pediatr Surg 1995;30:1224.

174. Tovar JA, Prieto G, Molina M, Arana J: Esophageal function in achalasia: Preoperative and postoperative manometric studies. J Pediatr Surg 1998;33:834.

175. Triadafilopoulos G, Castillo T: Nonpropulsive esophageal contractions and gastroesophageal reflux. Am J Gastroenterol 1991;86:153.

176. Tuck JS, Bisset RA, Doig CM: Achalasia of the cardia in childhood and the syndrome of achalasia alacrima and ACTH insensitivity. Clin Radiol 1991;44:260.

177. Vandenplas Y, Derde MP, Piepsz A: Evaluation of reflux episodes during simultaneous esophageal pH monitoring and gastroesophageal reflux scintigraphy in children. J Pediatr Gastroenterol Nutr 1992;14:256.

178. Vandenplas Y, Hassall E: Mechanisms of gastroesophageal reflux and gastroesophageal reflux disease. J Pediatr Gastroenterol Nutr 2002;35:119.

179. Vanderwinden JM: Role of interstitial cells of Cajal and their relationship with the enteric nervous system. Eur J Morphol 1999;37:250.

180. Vane DW, Cosby K, West K, Grosfeld JL: Late results following esophagomyotomy in children with achalasia. J Pediatr Surg 1988;23:515.

181. Vantrappen G, Janssens J, Hellemans J, Coremans G: Achalasia, diffuse esophageal spasm, and related motility disorders. Gastroenterology 1979;76:450.

182. Vicente Y, da Rocha C, Perez-Mies B, et al: Effect of reflux and esophagitis on esophageal volume and acid clearance in piglets. J Pediatr Gastroenterol Nutr 2004;38:328.

183. Vicente Y, Da Rocha C, Yu J, et al: Architecture and function of the gastroesophageal barrier in the piglet. Dig Dis Sci 2001;46:1899.

184. Vicente Y, Da Rocha C, Yu J, et al: Individual inactivation of the sphincteric component of the gastroesophageal barrier causes reflux esophagitis in piglets. J Pediatr Surg 2002;37:40.

185. Vicente Y, Hernandez-Peredo G, Molina M, et al: Acute food bolus impaction without stricture in children with gastroesophageal reflux. J Pediatr Surg 2001; 36:1397.

186. Walton JM, Tougas G: Botulinum toxin use in pediatric esophageal achalasia: A case report. J Pediatr Surg 1997; 32:916.

187. Wang WL, Tovar JA, Eizaguirre I, Aldazabal P: Airway obstruction and gastroesophageal reflux—an experimental study on the pathogenesis of this association. J Pediatr Surg 1993;28:995.

188. Warburton D, Schwarz M, Tefft D, et al: The molecular basis of lung morphogenesis. Mech Dev 2000;92:55.

189. Warburton D, Zhao J, Berberich MA, Bernfield M: Molecular embryology of the lung: Then, now, and in the future. Am J Physiol 1999;276:L697.

190. Watanabe Y, Ando H, Seo T, et al: Attenuated nitrergic inhibitory neurotransmission to interstitial cells of Cajal in the lower esophageal sphincter with esophageal achalasia in children. Pediatr Int 2002;44:145.

191. Weber P, Ganser G, Frosch M, et al: Twenty-four hour intraesophageal pH monitoring in children and adolescents with scleroderma and mixed connective tissue disease. J Rheumatol 2000;27:2692.

192. Weston S, Thumshirn M, Wiste J, Camilleri M: Clinical and upper gastrointestinal motility features in systemic sclerosis and related disorders. Am J Gastroenterol 1998;93:1085.

193. Wyllie E, Wyllie R, Rothner AD, Morris HH: Diffuse esophageal spasm: A cause of paroxysmal posturing and irritability in infants and mentally retarded children. J Pediatr 1989;115:261.

194. Yuksel B, Braun R, Topaloglu AK, et al: Three children with triple A syndrome due to a mutation (R478X) in the AAAS gene. Horm Res 2004;61:3.

195. Zarate N, Mearin F, Hidalgo A, Malagelada JR: Prospective evaluation of esophageal motor dysfunction in Down's syndrome. Am J Gastroenterol 2001;96:1718.

196. Zhang X, Tack J, Janssens J, Sifrim DA: Effect of sildenafil, a phosphodiesterase-5 inhibitor, on oesophageal peristalsis and lower oesophageal sphincter function in cats. Neurogastroenterol Motil 2001;13:325.

197. Zhou B, Hutson JM, Myers NA: Investigation of the intra-abdominal oesophagus and hiatus in fetal rats with oesophageal atresia and tracheo-oesophageal fistula. Pediatr Surg Int 2001;17:97.

198. Zuccarello B, Nicotina PA, Centorrino A, et al: Immuno-histochemical study on muscle actinin content of atresic esophageal upper pouch. J Pediatr Surg 1988;2:75.

Chapter 71

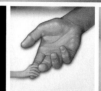

Gastroesophageal Reflux Disease

Keith E. Georgeson and Gonca Topuzlu Tekant

HISTORY

Symptoms of gastroesophageal reflux (GER) have been recognized for hundreds of years. Shakespeare described the infant "mewling and puking in the nurse's arms" as part of the first stage of human life. Anatomic dissections performed during the Renaissance provided a way to study the consequences of esophageal injury and stricture in patients who had GER. One of the first recorded descriptions of childhood gastroesophageal reflux disease (GERD) was in 1828 in Paris, where children with repeated vomiting were found to have esophageal ulcerations at autopsy.[25] In 1836, Bright described partial herniation of the stomach into the chest and associated this anatomic abnormality with GER.[37] In 1935, Winkelstein mentioned the term peptic esophagitis.[261] Allison defined the underlying causes of reflux esophagitis and presented an operative method of repair of hiatal hernia in 1943.[6] He also defined the anatomic problem as being a malfunctioning gastroesophageal valve and described heartburn as the primary symptom of GER.[5]

One of the first detailed publications about pediatric GER was by Neuhauser and Berenberg, who coined the term "chalasia" to describe physiologic GER in infants.[167] In the 1960s, Carré emphasized the self-limited nature of the disease in infants and suggested postural treatment to control the symptoms.[42,43]

Allison described and advocated hiatal hernia repair for the control of GER. Subsequently, Belsey and Nissen independently described fundoplication procedures that effectively controlled reflux in most patients.[20,168] Rossetti modified the Nissen repair to include only the anterior wall of the stomach in the wrap.[202] Lucius Hill emphasized the importance of keeping the gastroesophageal junction below the diaphragm.[103] Thal and Toupet popularized partial-wrap fundoplications to prevent the symptoms associated with a tight complete wrap.[231,237]

The development of improved diagnostic studies evolved about the same time as the surgical techniques were being devised. Barium esophagography,[66,205] pH monitoring,[119] endoscopy,[244] scintigraphy,[22] and manometry[61] were developed and refined over the last few decades. These investigations have provided a better, yet incomplete understanding of the underlying disease and evaluation of the effectiveness of treatment strategies.

All of the surgical techniques just described have been performed in children. Nissen fundoplication has emerged as the most frequently used procedure for refluxing children,[80,83,117,130] but there are many advocates of a partial-wrap fundoplication. Ashcraft popularized a modification of the Thal operation.[9,10] Boix-Ochoa performed a similar operation, which he described as an attempt to restore the anatomic and physiologic mechanisms that normally prevent GER.[27,29] In 1991, Dallemagne reported his initial experience with laparoscopic fundoplication in adults.[64] Two years later, Georgeson[88] and Lobe[147] independently reported laparoscopic fundoplication results in children. Today, minimally invasive techniques have become the standard for surgical correction of GERD in children.*

INTRODUCTION

Vomiting and regurgitation are common occurrences in childhood. Seventy percent of 4-month-old infants regurgitate daily, and only 25% of their parents consider it a problem.[165,246] The challenge for physicians is to differentiate the symptoms that are physiologic and will resolve spontaneously from those that need medical or surgical intervention. The spectrum of clinical signs in pathologic GER is variable, and recognition of these symptoms, followed by diagnostic evaluation and therapy, is important to prevent the serious sequelae of this pathologic process.

EMBRYOLOGY AND ANATOMY

The precise embryologic mechanisms that predispose infants and children to GER are unknown. Many explanations of the embryology of reflux have been proposed.[98,134,160,214,262,268] One of the more interesting concepts was offered by Mansfield, who believed that GER in *Homo sapiens* stems from alterations in embryogenesis

---

*See references 86, 87, 89, 146, 156, 163, 182, 203, 216, 225, 228, 255.

to support the extrauterine consequences of adopting the upright position and bipedal locomotion.[154] Adopting the upright posture leads to changes in structure and positional relationships of many intracavitary organs and systems. Rotation of the stomach, which alters the inferior relationship of the antrum to the fundus and causes the dorsal aspect of the stomach to move to the left and the ventral aspect to move to the right, may be a critical aspect in the etiology of reflux. These changes cause abnormalities in the intrinsic pinch valve mechanism and the gravitational pull on the stomach. The heart's vertical position places more stress on the human diaphragm. Mansfield believes that these changes are significant and may be the underlying reason why humans are so prone to the development of GERD and related disorders.

A high-pressure zone in the lower portion of the esophagus also plays an important role in the prevention of GER.[214,267] A critical length of intra-abdominal esophagus is necessary to prevent GERD.[267] Anatomic defects that affect the high-pressure zone of the gastroesophageal junction and interfere with rapid clearing of physiologic GER, such as esophageal atresia, diaphragmatic hernia, and motility disorders, are all associated with significant reflux pathology.*

DEFINITION

GERD is defined as the pathologic consequences of the involuntary passage of gastric contents into the esophagus.[209,249] In adults, GERD is primarily concerned with peptic esophagitis and its complications, including heartburn, esophageal stricture, and the formation of Barrett's esophagus. In children, pathologic reflux is

_____
*See references 14, 23, 49, 70, 78, 104, 111, 115, 124, 137, 222, 223.

considerably more complex.[165,166,179,209,246,249] Pathologic GER is most commonly seen in children with neurologic dysfunction. Neurologically impaired children with GER often have associated swallowing disorders, failure to thrive, primary aspiration, spasticity, increased intra-abdominal pressure, and central mechanisms for inducing gagging, choking, and retching. Additionally, they often have associated delayed gastric emptying, dysmotility of the esophagus and upper gastrointestinal tract, and a hiatal hernia and usually remain primarily in a supine position. Neurologically normal infants and children have reflux-associated reactive airways disease, aspiration, aspiration pneumonia, laryngeal symptoms, and apnea. Sometimes this apnea is prolonged and life threatening.[177,186,209,245,256] Children also have digestive symptoms, including frequent regurgitation with failure to thrive, irritability, food rejection, heartburn, hematemesis, melena, dysphagia, and the epithelial changes associated with Barrett's esophagus.[96,100,101,183,209,210]

PATHOPHYSIOLOGY

GERD occurs when refluxed contents produce clinical symptoms or result in histopathologic alterations. The pathogenesis of GERD is multifactorial and complex. The primary anatomic and physiologic factors that become dysfunctional and are associated with GER are discussed in the following sections (Fig. 71-1).[67,249]

Secretion of Saliva: Saliva is responsible for the lubrication of food and enhanced esophageal transport. It contributes to the neutralization of refluxed contents with its alkaline content and stimulates primary peristalsis of the esophagus. The secretion of saliva and frequency of swallowing are decreased during sleep. Salivary flow can be increased by gum chewing, which has been offered

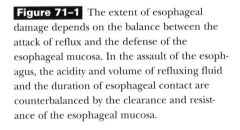

Figure 71-1 The extent of esophageal damage depends on the balance between the attack of reflux and the defense of the esophageal mucosa. In the assault of the esophagus, the acidity and volume of refluxing fluid and the duration of esophageal contact are counterbalanced by the clearance and resistance of the esophageal mucosa.

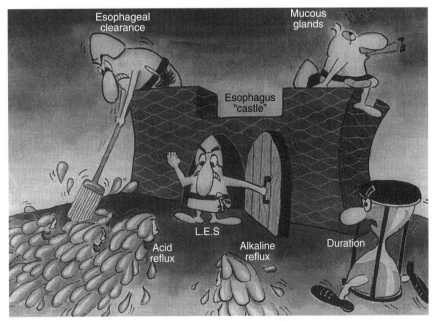

as a nonpharmacologic treatment for some patients with GERD.[125,249]

Esophageal Peristalsis: Esophageal contractions are classified as primary, secondary, and tertiary. Swallowing initiates primary waves. Secondary peristalsis is induced by reflux of material into the esophageal lumen and contributes to esophageal clearance.[125,142] Tertiary contractions are simultaneous, nonpropagated waves that occur spontaneously and are unrelated to swallowing or reflux. Swallowing induces contraction waves that begin at the pharynx and advance through the striated and smooth muscle to the cardia.[58,73,121] During daytime reflux episodes, swallowing frequency increases and is an effective mechanism for acid clearance.

Esophageal Clearance: Esophageal clearance is influenced by three primary factors: peristaltic waves, gravity, and saliva.[102,122] Delayed clearance of acid in the esophagus is a primary cause of esophagitis.[41,105] Swallowed saliva is responsible for neutralization of the refluxed material, and patients with GERD often have decreased salivary function. The efficacy of positional treatment may be partially related to gravity.[3,175,249,251] Different types of afferent neurons have been identified in the esophageal wall.[15,67,249] C unmyelinated fibers are responsible for deep, burning pain, and A delta fibers are responsible for sharp pain. Repeated noxious stimuli or one very strong stimulus can sensitize both types of fibers to respond to non-noxious stimuli. Visceral hyperalgesia may result in a disordered motility causing more reflux.[120,181] Thus, in some patients, GERD may initially be caused by an abnormal stimulus, which in turn induces an abnormal motility problem. The sensation of pain is transported to the brain via the neurotransmitters calcitonin gene–related peptide and substance P.[8,266] Substance P causes smooth muscle contractions and vasodilatation and stimulates increased mucosal permeability. It is released when there is tissue damage. With esophagitis, the more substance P released, the greater the noxious effect of the reflux material, which leads to a vicious cycle. Substance P also causes release of histamine from mast cells in the alveoli, thus contributing to bronchospasm. It has been speculated that substance P released in the esophagus may sometimes contribute to the initiation of reactive airways disease.[190,224]

Lower Esophageal Sphincter: The concept of a defective lower esophageal sphincter (LES) as the prominent cause of pathologic GER was first demonstrated in 1971.[53] The LES is a functional barrier 3 to 5 cm long in adults that manometry has defined as an area of elevated distal esophageal resting pressure; it serves as the barrier against abnormal regurgitation of gastric contents into the esophagus. Adult studies have demonstrated that mean LES pressure lower than 6 mm Hg and overall sphincter length less than 2 cm are likely to be associated with pathologic GER.[198,269] Studies by Boix-Ochoa and Canals have demonstrated that the length of the LES is only 0.5 to 1.0 cm in neonates and increases with age as seen in Figure 71-2.[30]

The LES relaxes 2 seconds after the initiation of a swallow and remains open for 10 to 12 seconds until

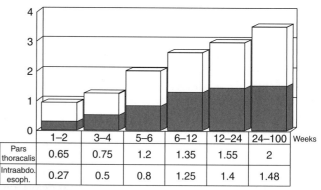

	1–2	3–4	5–6	6–12	12–24	24–100	Weeks
Pars thoracalis	0.65	0.75	1.2	1.35	1.55	2	
Intraabdo. esoph.	0.27	0.5	0.8	1.25	1.4	1.48	

Figure 71–2   Mean values of the lower esophageal sphincter in neonates and infants.

the bolus has passed through the region. Dodds et al. first described the phenomenon of transient lower esophageal sphincter relaxations (TLESRs), which are responses mediated via vagal reflexes.[71] TLESRs are initiated by stimulation of mechanoreceptors in the gastric fundus, or stretching of the gastric fundus.[107] LES pressure decreases postprandially. Gastric contractions, gastric alkalinization, and proteins increase LES pressure. Gastrin, motilin, and substance P also increase LES pressure, whereas cholecystokinin, glucagon vasoactive intestinal peptide, nitric oxide, dopamine, secretin, estrogen, nicotine, alcohol, mint, and chocolate all decrease LES pressure.[249] In children, most reflux episodes occur in relation to TLESRs, and they are the predominant mechanism of GER in healthy term infants, as well as those with chronic lung disease.[170,171] Large meals leading to increased secretory volume induce more TLESRs. Thus, the efficacy of proton pump inhibitors (PPIs) and histamine H_2 receptor antagonists (H2RAs) may be related to decreased secretory gastric volume, independent of its pH. The antireflux effects of surgery may be related to achievement of incomplete LES relaxation and a reduction in the number of TLESRs.[128,129]

Intra-abdominal Esophagus: The length of the intra-abdominal portion of the esophagus is an important part of the antireflux barrier. The intra-abdominal esophageal diameter is approximately a fifth the diameter of the stomach. According to the law of Laplace, GER in response to elevation of intra-abdominal pressure is prevented if there is adequate length of the intra-abdominal part of the esophagus with a significantly smaller luminal diameter than that of the stomach. If the intra-abdominal segment of the esophagus is short, less than 2.0 cm, or if the overall sphincter length is less than 2.0 cm, gastroesophageal reflux is much more likely to occur.[34,69,267] During the first year of life, the length of the intra-abdominal portion of the esophagus is physiologically short, which contributes to the increased incidence of regurgitation in this population.[30]

Angle of His: The angle of His is formed by the esophagus and the greater curvature of the stomach and is normally an acute angle.[11,28,144,189] The antireflux effect of this angle becomes obvious when the child attempts to vomit and the gastric contents strike the fundus, which closes the gastroesophageal junction. In cases in which the angle is obtuse, the stomach is converted into a funnel that directs its contents back into the esophagus with a sudden increase in abdominal pressure.[18] There is also a collection of convoluted folds of the esophageal mucosa at the gastroesophageal junction. With changes in intragastric pressure or with negative pressure in the thoracic esophagus, these mucosal folds squeeze together and act as a weak antireflux valve.[144,189]

Pinchcock Action: The esophageal hiatus at the diaphragm is formed by the sling shape of the right crus of the diaphragm. During deep inspiration, this sling pulls the esophagus toward the right and downward, which narrows the lumen of the distal end of the esophagus.[7,33,68,106,113,153,194,254] The pinchcock action of the diaphragm can be observed during awake endoscopy.[176]

Gastric Volume and Emptying: In children with significant GERD, gastric electrical abnormalities and delayed gastric emptying have often been documented.[59,201] Two important physiologic reflexes are involved in the gastric response to food intake. In adaptive relaxation, the fundus of the stomach dilates in response to food entering the stomach. In receptive relaxation, the gastric fundus dilates when food passes down the esophagus. Nitric oxide is involved in both pathways and causes relaxation of the circular muscle of the fundus.[196,229] Children with neurologic abnormalities often have abnormal gastric motility or delayed gastric emptying, or both.[2,40,141,178,196]

Gastric Acid: The majority of reflux patients have normal acid secretion, but some groups of pediatric patients with GERD have been shown to have gastric hypersecretion.[55,123] Acid combined with pepsin can cause injury to the esophageal mucosa.[180,199] In most cases, the volume secreted may be more important than the pH. Thus, PPIs decrease gastric secretion volume and are potent in the treatment of esophagitis despite nocturnal breakthrough of acid secretion.[36,45,90,93]

Helicobacter pylori Infection: In the past 3 decades, mortality rates related to gastric cancer, gastric ulcer, and duodenal ulcer have declined, whereas those of esophageal adenocarcinoma and GERD have risen.[133] Some studies suggest that *H. pylori* colonization may be protective against severe esophagitis and Barrett's esophagus.[52,265] These epidemiologic data have led some to suggest that *H. pylori* should not be eradicated in patients with GERD. However, *H. pylori* is a risk factor for the development of peptic ulcer and gastric cancer, which has caused many physicians to be uncomfortable with that recommendation. This issue remains under investigation.[92,140,151]

Pepsin, Trypsin, and Bile Salts: Pepsin and trypsin are proteolytic enzymes that have a traumatic effect on the esophageal mucosa. Pepsin causes its most significant damage at a pH of 2 to 3, whereas trypsin is most damaging at a pH between 5 and 8.[200,243] Bile salts increase the permeability of the esophageal mucosa to acid and are noxious to the esophageal mucosa in the presence of acid. Conjugated bile salts are injurious to the esophagus at an acid pH, whereas deconjugated bile salts and trypsin are harmful at a neutral pH.[193,234] With the development of intraluminal impedance and bilirubin-detecting technologies, studies have demonstrated bile salts in the refluxate of adults with GERD. Mixed refluxate may be more harmful to the esophageal mucosa than pure acid is.[240,241]

Intra-abdominal Pressure: The role of increased intra-abdominal pressure in children has not been well investigated, and reports are conflicting.[94] In adults, 17% of GER episodes were related to increases in abdominal pressure.[72] Obesity, ascites, and peritoneal dialysis have been shown to cause GER by increasing intra-abdominal pressure.[17,162,164] Abdominal wall defects in children have also been related to an increased incidence of GER, apparently caused by the associated increased intra-abdominal pressure after closure of the defect.[19,136]

Gastroesophageal Reflux Causing Gastroesophageal Reflux: GER is an important factor contributing to GER by initiating a positive feedback cycle. Contact of the refluxed acid with the esophageal mucosa increases regional blood flow and increases the secretion of prostaglandin E_2. Prostaglandin locally affects esophageal permeability, which increases the susceptibility of the mucosa to inflammation. Inflammation causes impairment in motility and decreases the resting pressure of the LES. It also leads to pylorospasm, which creates more reflux and esophagitis.[249] The presence of trypsin, pepsin, and bile may potentiate damage to the esophageal mucosa.

Respiratory Factors: Respiratory problems cause deeper inspiratory efforts and more negative intrathoracic pressure, which initiates GER.[127]

Medications and Hormones: Medications and hormones such as antihistamines, xanthines, theophyllines, chocolate, caffeine, calcium channel blockers, gastrin, dopamine, glucagons, and prostaglandins are associated with an increased incidence of GER.[139,192,226,230]

Underlying Congenital Problems: Children with esophageal atresia are prone to pathologic GER.[23,70,137,145,219,223] In these cases, esophageal peristalsis is impaired and the LES is incompetent. The incidence of reflux in these children declines as the children grow, but complications of GERD mandate antireflux surgery in 10% to 30% of children after esophageal atresia repair.[24,138,215] One of the common manifestations of GERD in children with esophageal atresia is recurrent esophageal anastomotic stenosis. Appropriate prophylactic medical treatment of reflux in these children may lead to diminished stricture formation. Children with congenital diaphragmatic hernia often have functional anatomic abnormalities of the esophagus leading to GER. The incidence of pathologic GER is reported to be greater than 20% in surviving infants. About 15% of children with congenital diaphragmatic hernia require an antireflux procedure.[78,115,124] Congenital abdominal wall defects such as gastroschisis and omphalocele are also associated with an increased incidence of GER, possibly because of increased intra-abdominal pressure.[19,136]

Neurologically Impaired Children: Neurologically impaired children are prone to the development of GER. The underlying cause is thought to be related to a foregut motility problem. Impaired esophageal motility and delayed gastric emptying are important factors contributing to reflux in these children.[49,227]

DIAGNOSIS

There are few objective studies that compare the value of the various diagnostic techniques used for the diagnosis of GER in children. Tests for GER are individually useful in documenting different aspects of GER and are valuable only when used in the appropriate clinical context.

History and Physical Examination: The history and physical examination are the most important components of the evaluation of an infant or child with possible GERD. Documentation of the growth rate and identification of the primary symptoms, such as failure to thrive, primary aspiration, recurrent coughing, reactive airways disease, stridor, apnea, recurrent pneumonia, irritability, heartburn, abdominal pain, and dysphagia, are helpful in guiding the remainder of the patient's workup.[209,250]

Upper Gastrointestinal Contrast Series: An upper gastrointestinal contrast series is neither specific nor sensitive for the diagnosis of GER.[1,47,187] It does, however, provide a detailed road map of the patient's anatomy to rule out other causes of vomiting. Problems such as pyloric stenosis, malrotation, partial duodenal outlet obstruction, hiatal hernia, and esophageal stricture are readily seen.

Esophageal pH Monitoring: Esophageal pH monitoring measures the duration and frequency of acid reflux episodes. It is most useful if used in conjunction with regular daily activities such as eating and sleeping. The presence of symptoms should be noted in parallel with the pH probe record. A reflux episode is defined as an esophageal pH of less than 4 for a period of 15 to 30 seconds. The percentage of total time that the esophageal pH is less than 4 is then converted into a reflux index, which reflects the cumulative exposure of the esophagus to acid.[56] It should be remembered that acid reflux is more common in the first year of life and that adult indices are not applicable to these patients. In children, the upper limit of normal is a pH below 4 less than 5.5% of the time. In infants younger than 1 year, the normal value increases to 12%.[31,75,209,221,248,266]

Endoscopic and histopathologic confirmation of esophagitis shows a strong correlation with abnormal pH monitoring. Ninety-five percent of adults with biopsy-documented esophagitis will have an abnormal pH probe reading.[26,191,223] However, esophagitis is not the only significant symptom seen in children with pathologic GER.[95,131,157] pH probe monitoring does not detect nonacid reflux episodes. In some studies, the presence of duodenal contents in the esophagus has been confirmed by monitoring for the presence of bilirubin in the gastroesophageal refluxate.[16,84,135,193,242] Orel and Markovic reported a study of 65 children with symptoms of GERD and noted that duodenal GER increased in relation to the severity of the esophagitis.[174] They also noted that some patients with esophagitis had pathologic duodenal-gastroesophageal reflux, but not pathologic reflux by pH probe analysis.

Multiple intraluminal electrical impedance technologies with the capacity to detect all types of reflux (acid, nonacid, liquid, and air) have been developed over the last 2 decades. This technique is useful for investigating nonacid reflux.[220,239,259] Belaji et al. reported that 59% of GER events were not conventional acid reflux and were not detected by the pH probe studies.[16] In infants, nonacid GER has been documented in association with respiratory symptoms such as apnea. Such findings have led investigators to hypothesize that apneic episodes in infants may be caused by a protective respiratory reflex. Further investigation will be required to determine the importance of impedance and other new technologies in identifying pathologic GERD in infants and children.[188,260]

Endoscopy: Endoscopy and biopsy are useful for determining the presence and degree of esophagitis and the presence of other problems such as strictures, webs, or infections. There is a poor correlation between endoscopic appearance and histopathology, so esophageal biopsy is recommended at the time of endoscopy.[26,148,207] The presence of intraepithelial eosinophils or neutrophils and increased morphometric measures of basal cell layer thickness and papillary height are valid indicators of reflux esophagitis.[26,46,209]

Nuclear Scintigraphy: In nuclear scintigraphy, technetium-labeled formula or food is orally ingested, and patients are scanned for evidence of GER or aspiration. This technology can demonstrate nonacid reflux and can provide information relative to gastric emptying.[169,185,218,232] Lack of standardized techniques and the short duration of the study limit the value of this test.[218]

Esophageal Manometry: Esophageal manometry studies evaluate the activity of the lower and upper esophageal sphincters and monitor the organized contractile activity of the esophagus. The technique is not used for the diagnosis of GER, but helps the clinician better understand the underlying pathophysiology. It is useful in the differential diagnosis of primary and secondary esophageal motility alterations but is used infrequently to diagnose GER in the pediatric population.[91,110,114] Other new technologies, including fiber-optic endoscopic evaluation of swallowing with sensory testing, are also being assessed for their value in the workup of GERD in children.[143,233]

EVALUATION OF PEDIATRIC PATIENTS WITH SUSPECTED GASTROESOPHAGEAL REFLUX DISEASE

GERD in infants and children is multifaceted and complex. The appropriate steps in the evaluation of a child suspected of having GER are controversial. The workup must include a careful history and physical examination. An upper gastrointestinal study to look for anatomic abnormalities, a 24-hour pH probe monitoring study, or an impedance study and, in some cases, endoscopy with biopsy of the distal esophageal mucosa are performed as a part of the workup. Please refer to Box 71-1 for the recommendations formulated by the Society of Pediatric Gastroenterology and Nutrition.[209]

TREATMENT

Conservative Therapy

Infants and children who have symptoms of GER can benefit from changes in lifestyle. Smaller and frequent feeding is encouraged in babies instead of larger feedings at infrequent intervals. Thickened feedings may be helpful in those with poor weight gain, and there is evidence to support a 1- to 2-week trial of hypoallergenic formula in formula-fed babies with vomiting.[97,209,235,246,249] Positioning therapy is a widely adopted, but controversial part of antireflux therapy. Although esophageal pH monitoring has demonstrated that infants have significantly less GER in the prone position than in the supine position, prone positioning has been associated with a higher rate of sudden infant death syndrome (SIDS).[76,161,184] In infants from birth to 12 months old with GERD, the risk for SIDS outweighs the benefits of prone sleeping. Therefore, the American Academy of Pediatrics recommends nonprone positioning during sleep.[126] Prone positioning is acceptable in an awake baby in the postprandial period. For older children,

Box 71-1 Evaluation of Children for Gastroesophageal Reflux Disease

1. *Recurrent vomiting.* Pediatric patients with recurrent vomiting should be evaluated with a detailed history and physical examination, with special attention paid to identify warning signals. These warning signals may be bilious or forceful vomiting, failure to thrive, gastrointestinal (GI) bleeding, fever, hepatosplenomegaly, signs of raised intracranial pressure, seizures, abdominal distention, diarrhea, constipation, feeding or respiratory problems, irritability, or genetic disorders. If none of these signs are present and the infant has a normal growth pattern, no diagnostic workup is necessary. Because vomiting in this group of patients will resolve by 12 months of age, conservative treatment, including supine positioning of the infant, a short trial of hypoallergenic formula, or thickening of feedings, may be recommended. If symptoms do not improve by 18 to 24 months of age, further evaluation with upper GI contrast studies should be considered. If an infant with recurring vomiting has additional symptoms, such as failure to thrive or irritability, or if the child is older than 2 years, an upper GI series, 24-hour pH monitoring, and in selected cases, upper endoscopy with biopsy to rule out the presence of esophagitis may be performed. If the infant has failure to thrive despite adequate calorie intake, tests to include a complete blood count, electrolytes, bicarbonate, urea nitrogen, creatinine, alanine aminotransferase, ammonia, glucose, urine analysis, and urine ketones and reducing substances and a review of newborn screening tests must be performed.

2. *Heartburn or chest pain.* These patients are older children and adolescents, and initially, a change in lifestyle, avoidance of precipitating factors, and a 2- to 4-week trial of histamine H_2 receptor antagonists (H2RAs) or proton pump inhibitors (PPIs) is recommended. If the symptoms do not resolve, an upper GI series to rule out esophageal motor disorders, such as achalasia, and upper endoscopy with biopsy to determine the presence and severity of esophagitis should be considered.

3. *Esophagitis.* This diagnosis can be confirmed with upper endoscopy and biopsy, and the initial treatment consists of lifestyle changes and H2RA or PPI therapy. In patients who do not respond to therapy, an incorrect diagnosis such as eosinophilic esophagitis or inadequate treatment should be considered. Esophageal pH monitoring is useful for determining the efficacy of the treatment being used.

4. *Dysphagia or odynophagia.* An upper GI study is recommended in children with difficult or painful swallowing and upper GI endoscopy with biopsy in those with suspected esophagitis.

5. *Apnea or apparent life-threatening event (ALTE).* ALTE can be identified as an episode of apnea or change in color and muscle tone in an infant requiring intervention. The first event genereally occurs around the first 2 months of life and rarely after the age of 8 months. These babies carry a high risk for sudden death and have a prevalence of vomiting of 60% to 70% and abnormal esophageal pH monitoring of 40% to 80%. Despite reports that demonstrate gastroesophageal reflux (GER) as a potential cause of apnea, investigations in unselected patients with ALTE have not demonstrated a relationship between esophageal acidification and apnea or bradycardia. If an infant's esophageal pH monitoring demonstrates gross emesis or oral regurgitation at the time of ALTE, this group of patients may benefit from antireflux therapy. In severe cases not responding to medical management, surgery may be considered. Caution is advised when diagnosing and treating GER as an underlying cause of ALTE.

6. *Asthma.* The prevalence of children with asthma and abnormal esophageal pH monitoring ranges between 25% and 75%. It is suggested that esophageal acid exposure in asthmatic patients may cause airway irritability and variable airway obstruction. Thus, esophageal pH monitoring plus a trial of vigorous medical therapy for GER is recommended for children with asthma who may have the following problems: GER disease, radiologic evidence of recurrent pneumonia, nocturnal asthma occurring more than once a week, need for a high or continuous dose of corticosteroids, and inability to wean from medical therapy.

7. *Recurrent pneumonia.* Clinical studies have demonstrated that GER can cause recurrent pneumonia and lead to pulmonary fibrosis. Flexible bronchoscopy with pulmonary lavage fluid demonstrating a large percentage of lipid-laden macrophages and nuclear scintigraphy can be used to detect aspiration, but both test results lack specificity. Neurologically impaired children may have abnormal swallowing leading to aspiration. In such cases, videofluoroscopic swallowing studies or fiber-optic endoscopic swallowing evaluation may be helpful in making the diagnosis.

recommended conservative treatment includes weight loss if the patient is overweight and avoidance of large meals, caffeine, chocolate, and spicy foods.[159,209]

Medical Therapy

The goals of antireflux medical treatment are to control symptoms, prevent complications, and facilitate the healing of esophagitis. Acid suppressants and prokinetic agents are the two major pharmacotherapies that can be used to prevent the symptoms and damage caused by GER. Antacids neutralize gastric acid, whereas antisecretory agents, H2RAs and PPIs, reduce the secretion of gastric acid.

Histamine H₂ Receptor Antagonists

H2RAs decrease acid secretion by inhibiting the H₂ receptor at the parietal cell of the stomach. Ranitidine at an oral dose of 5.0 mg/kg has been shown to control gastric pH for 9 to 10 hours in infants.[152] Different randomized controlled trials in adults have demonstrated that cimetidine, ranitidine, and famotidine are effective in controlling symptoms and treating esophagitis.[48,236]

Proton Pump Inhibitors

PPIs bond and deactivate H^+,K^+-ATPase, or proton pumps, by crossing parietal cell membranes and accumulating in secretory canaliculi.[263] These drugs are most effective if they are administered half an hour before a meal.[211] Some studies have demonstrated that omeprazole may be very effective in the treatment of esophagitis that has been refractory to different treatment regimens, including H2RAs.[4,155] The drug most often reported is omeprazole at dosages of 0.5 to 3.3 mg/kg daily.[57] There are potential concerns regarding prolonged use of PPIs in children and associated hypergastrinemia. Pathologists have described parietal cell hypertrophy and polyps in fundus biopsy samples from patients receiving long-term PPI treatment.[50] Additionally, because gastrin is a trophic hormone, patients maintained on long-term PPI therapy may have the potential for the development of colon cancer if they are genetically susceptible to do so.[36]

Antacids and Surface Agents

Antacids neutralize gastric acid and are preferred for the short-term relief of GER symptoms such as heartburn and esophagitis. Studies have shown that treatment with aluminum-containing antacids increases plasma aluminum levels in infants.[264] Because other safe alternatives are available, chronic use is not recommended. Sucralfate is a surface agent that adheres to damaged mucosal lesions on the esophagus. However, there are not enough data to determine the safety and efficacy of sucralfate in children.[209]

Prokinetic Agents

In recent studies, TLESRs are considered the most important component of GER. Prokinetic agents increase LES pressure, enhance esophageal peristalsis, and accelerate gastric emptying. Cisapride is a mixed serotonergic agent that reduces esophageal acid exposure. Studies have shown that cisapride improves symptom scores, esophagitis, and pulmonary function in patients with GER.[60,217,247] However, it has also been noted to potentially cause serious cardiac arrhythmias and has been withdrawn from the market in many countries.[13,63,74] Meta-analysis and randomized controlled trials have demonstrated no clinically important benefits of cisapride in children.[13,63] Metoclopramide, an antidopaminergic agent, is reported to give equivocal results in some studies.[149,209] Its adverse effects, such as dyskinesia, may be irreversible. In conclusion, the present evidence is not sufficient to support the use of prokinetic therapy for GER, although it is widely used.

Erythromycin

Reports have suggested that erythromycin has prokinetic effects on the gastrointestinal tract at doses lower than antimicrobial levels, but no randomized controlled trials have been performed.[62]

Endoscopic Treatment

Endoluminal therapy for GERD in adults as an alternative to other surgical therapies has been a new development. Two techniques are currently under active investigation. Internal gastroplication involves the placement of sutures just below the esophageal-gastric junction by way of an endoscope.[150,204]

The other endoluminal technique uses radiofrequency energy delivered to the distal LES tissues and gastric cardia. This technique, known as the Stretta procedure, decreases LES compliance and increases LES muscle mass, thereby limiting the TLESRs responsible for GERD.[238] It has shown positive clinical results in open-label prospective clinical trials.[77,238] Islam and associates have reported the use of radiofrequency to treat recurrent GERD in six children. The short-term follow-up results appear to be promising.[112]

Indications for Surgical Treatment

Surgical management is indicated in children under the following circumstances[117,137,209,223,249]:

1. Failure of medical therapy. In children who have continuing symptoms such as persistent pulmonary symptoms, life-threatening events, vomiting with failure to thrive, unremitting heartburn, or an inability to wean from medical treatment despite optimal medical therapy, surgery should be considered.
2. Presence of an associated anatomic defect such as a hiatal hernia, malrotation, or diaphragmatic hernia.
3. Esophageal stricture secondary to GERD.
4. Post–esophageal atresia repair status with a recurrent stricture that does not respond to conservative medical treatment.
5. Neurologically impaired children who have difficulty feeding and have serious reflux as an associated symptom.

Surgical Techniques

The aim of surgical treatment in GER is to prevent episodes of reflux while avoiding complications such as dysphagia and an inability to burp and vomit. Many operative techniques have been described for children. The main techniques currently used for children include the complete-wrap Nissen fundoplication, the modified complete-wrap Nissen-Rossetti fundoplication, and partial-wrap procedures, including the Thal-Ashcraft fundoplication, the Toupet fundoplication, and the Boix-Ochoa fundoplication.[32,82,216,223,250] All these techniques attempt to achieve a physiologic high-pressure zone at the distal end of the esophagus that will prevent reflux. Over the last decade, all of these procedures have been performed via a laparoscopic approach. Long-term results after laparoscopic fundoplication seem to be similar to those after the open procedure, but the laparoscopic procedures are less invasive and appear to have fewer complications.[158]

There are advocates for each of the techniques just mentioned. The authors prefer a floppy Nissen fundoplication under all circumstances when correcting GER. Other surgeons advocate for a complete-wrap fundoplication in neurologically impaired children and a partial-wrap fundoplication in neurologically normal children with GER.[54] Still other authors prefer a partial-wrap fundoplication in all patients.[44] No high-quality randomized studies have been conducted to determine which operation is best under what circumstances. The senior author has retrospectively reviewed the results after partial-wrap Toupet fundoplication in neurologically normal patients and complete-wrap Nissen fundoplication in a similar population and found the recurrence rate to be almost twice as high with the partial-wrap procedure.[51] This finding is consistent with results reported by Jobe and others, who also found a much higher recurrence rate in adult patients after a partial-wrap procedure.[116] However, many pediatric surgery groups have advocated the efficacy of partial-wrap procedures in children with acceptable recurrence rates.[32,44,54]

Open Operative Techniques

Nissen Fundoplication

The operation is best performed through an upper midline or left subcostal incision. The left lobe of the liver is mobilized, folded on itself, and retracted to the patient's right. Three or more upper short gastric vessels are divided to mobilize the fundus of the stomach. The anterior peritoneum over the gastroesophageal junction is incised transversely. The distal end of the esophagus is mobilized circumferentially. Dissection is continued up into the thorax when needed to achieve at least a 3.0-cm length of the intra-abdominal portion of the esophagus. The vagus nerves are mobilized with the esophagus. A Penrose drain is often looped around the esophagus and vagi to help mobilize the distal esophageal segment. The diaphragmatic crura are repaired posteriorly with nonabsorbable suture. The fundus is then fitted around the esophagus for 360 degrees. Usually, three to four interrupted sutures are placed in the fundus and esophagus

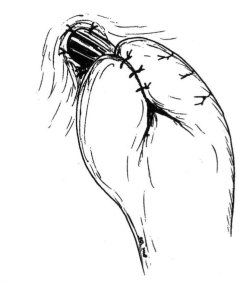

Figure 71–3 Nissen fundoplication.

to complete the wrap. Some surgeons also place four to six sutures to attach the esophagus to the crura circumferentially above the wrap to prevent herniation of the wrap or other intra-abdominal contents into the chest (Fig. 71-3). The wrap is performed over an appropriately sized bougie within the esophagus to prevent the creation of a tight wrap. Additionally, the fundoplication should be loose enough to allow a blunt-tipped clamp to pass between the fundal wrap and the esophagus containing the bougie.[81]

Thal-Ashcraft Fundoplication

In this technique, at least 2.0 cm of the distal intra-abdominal portion of the esophagus is mobilized circumferentially. The crural defect is closed posteriorly with a figure-of-eight suture that also passes through the posterior esophageal wall. Anteriorly, the fundus is folded over the anterior surface of the intra-abdominal part of the esophagus and held in place with running or interrupted nonabsorbable suture. The fundus is attached to the crura and to the esophagus to achieve a 270-degree anterior fundoplication. Some surgeons prefer interrupted sutures for this suture line, but most surgeons use a running suture. The anterior 270-degree surface of the intra-abdominal portion of the esophagus is wrapped by the fundus (Fig. 71-4).[206]

Toupet Fundoplication

In the Toupet technique, the esophagus is dissected in the same manner as for a Nissen fundoplication. The crura are approximated posteriorly to snug the hiatus. The fundus is mobilized either with or without division of the short gastric vessels. The fundus is then pulled through the retroesophageal space and secured to the left and right crura with interrupted sutures. The most cephalad sutures of the wrap incorporate all three structures: fundus, crus, and esophagus. The wrap is anchored posteriorly to the crura with two or three sutures.

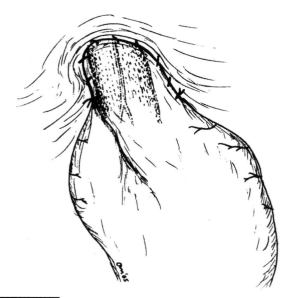

Figure 71–4 Thal-Ashcraft fundoplication.

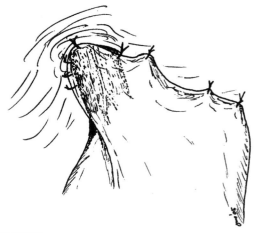

Figure 71–6 Boix-Ochoa fundoplication.

The fundus is sewn to the right and left lateral borders of the esophagus to create a 270-degree posterior wrap, with the anterior quadrant of the esophagus left free of the wrap (Fig. 71-5).[258]

Boix-Ochoa Technique

In this technique, a 2.0- to 3.0-cm length of the intra-abdominal portion of the esophagus is restored. The crural defect is repaired and the crura are sutured to the esophagus at the anterior and two lateral points. To restore the angle of His, a suture is passed through the fundus and the right rim of the hiatus. Multiple sutures are placed between the fundus and the anterior esophageal wall. The fundus is then tacked to the diaphragm with sutures that open the fundus like an umbrella (Fig. 71-6).[31]

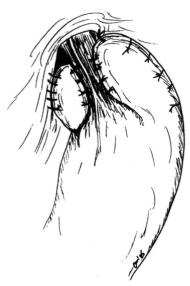

Figure 71–5 Toupet fundoplication.

Laparoscopic Nissen Fundoplication

Although all the aforementioned open techniques have been performed laparoscopically, the most commonly performed laparoscopic technique is the Nissen fundoplication. The laparoscopic approach has the technical advantages of enhanced visualization and magnification and is associated with less postoperative pain. For these reasons, laparoscopic fundoplication has become the treatment of choice in children with pathologic GER over the last decade. Safe and effective laparoscopic procedures in the treatment of GER in infants and children require advanced laparoscopic skills, as well as sophisticated electronic equipment and specialized laparoscopic instruments.

Positioning and Trocar Placement

The patient is placed at the end of the operating table with the lower extremities taped in a cross-legged position or, in the case of older children (>30 kg), with the legs supported in stirrups. Proper padding must be used to prevent pressures sores or peripheral neuropathy. The bladder is emptied with a Credé maneuver in infants. Catheterization is not usually necessary in older children. After the anesthesiologist has secured the airway, an appropriately sized dilator is placed. Because dysphagia is a common early postoperative problem unless carefully avoided, the authors prefer large dilators to fully distend the esophagus and avoid the formation of a tight wrap. The patient is placed in a reverse Trendelenburg position with the left side raised slightly. This position uses gravity to pull the small bowel loops and the transverse colon away from the upper part of the abdomen and establish better exposure of the gastroesophageal junction. The operating surgeon is positioned at the end of the table. An open technique is used to insert the first trocar. The authors prefer an expandable 5-mm trocar through the deepest aspect of the umbilicus. This expandable trocar helps keep air from leaking through the trocar site during the operative procedure. A 30-degree, 4- or 5-mm scope is then passed through the trocar after the pneumoperitoneum has been developed. The other four

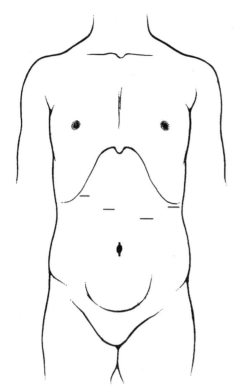

Figure 71–7 Trocar placement for laparoscopic Nissen fundoplication.

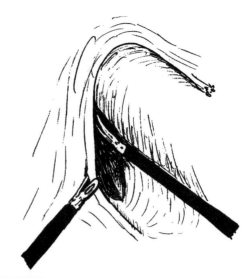

Figure 71–8 Laparoscopic Nissen fundoplication: a plane is developed between the right crus and the esophagus.

trocars are placed under laparoscopic surveillance as indicated in Figure 71-7. The trocars should be secured to the abdominal wall to avoid slippage in or out during insertion or withdrawal of instruments during the procedure. Three-millimeter and 4-mm trocars are used for most children up into adolescence. A segmented, multiarticulated retractor is used to hold the left lobe of the liver away from the esophageal hiatus. Fundoplication is begun by dividing the gastrohepatic ligament. A hook cautery or scissors can be used for this purpose. Dissection is continued up to the right crus. The small vessels and the hepatic branches of the vagus nerve in the gastrohepatic ligament are divided. If the left hepatic artery is encountered in the gastrohepatic ligament, it should be preserved. A plane between the right crus and the esophagus is identified and enlarged (Fig. 71-8). The dissection is continued over the top of the esophagus while taking care to not injure the anterior vagus nerve, which is usually adherent to the esophageal muscle. A hook cautery is used to divide the short gastric vessels (Fig. 71-9). The dissection is continued proximally along the fundus to the esophagus. The left side of the esophagus is freed from the crura. This circumesophageal dissection is continued until the entire esophagus has been freed from the crura. The window behind the esophagus is enlarged. The intra-abdominal portion of the esophagus should be freed until a tension-free, 3.0-cm length of esophagus is developed. The crura are approximated posteriorly with interrupted nonabsorbable sutures. The most cephalad of the sutures should also pass through the posterior wall of the esophagus while avoiding injury to the posterior vagus. Three to five more

sutures are then applied between the esophagus and the crura to prevent potential herniation of the wrap into the chest (Fig. 71-10). Additionally, it should be noted that the longer the intra-abdominal esophagus, the less likely the patient will suffer from migration of the fundoplication wrap into the chest. The fundus is wrapped around the esophagus after pulling it through the retroesophageal window (Fig. 71-11). The wrap is secured in position with interrupted nonabsorbable sutures (Fig. 71-12). The length of the wrap should be around 2.0 cm in children and 1.5 cm in infants. Longer wraps are associated with dysphagia and an inability to burp and vomit. The abdomen is inspected for bleeding and visceral injury. The instruments and trocars are removed

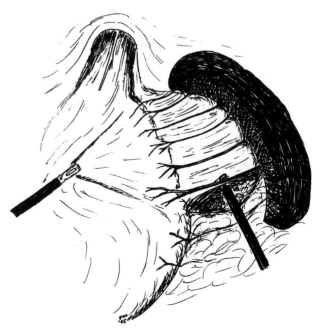

Figure 71–9 Laparoscopic Nissen fundoplication: the short gastric vessels are divided with a hook cautery.

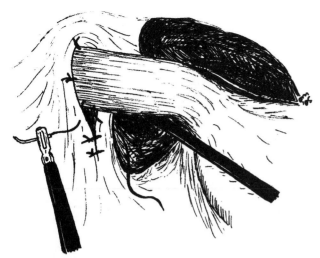

Figure 71–10 Laparoscopic Nissen fundoplication: the hiatus is closed posteriorly and the esophagus is attached to the crura with four to six sutures.

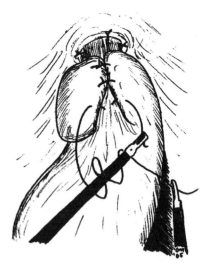

Figure 71–12 Laparoscopic Nissen fundoplication: the "floppy" fundoplication is secured to the esophagus for a distance of 1.5 to 2.0 cm.

and the wounds closed according to the preference of the operating surgeon.

Pyloroplasty or Antroplasty

The prevalence of foregut autonomic dysfunction is high in children with GER.[49,227] Approximately 50% of children with GER have delayed gastric emptying. Postfundoplication complications attributed to delayed gastric emptying include early satiety, gas bloating, and recurrent GER. Pediatric surgeons have often used pyloroplasty or a derivative pyloric operation with the intent to improve gastric emptying after fundoplication, and multiple studies have shown improved gastric emptying after fundoplication and pyloric surgery.[170,212] In 1997, Brown et al. reported a study in which children with delayed gastric

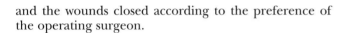

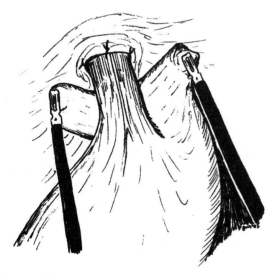

Figure 71–11 Laparoscopic Nissen fundoplication: the fundus is pulled through the retroesophageal window and evaluated for appropriate symmetry with the "shoeshine" maneuver.

emptying showed marked improvement of their gastric emptying with fundoplication alone.[38] Johnson et al. subsequently reported a small group of children with foregut autonomic dysfunction who did not show improvement of their gastric emptying after pyloroplasty alone.[118] Pyloroplasty or antroplasty to improve gastric emptying in children with gastrointestinal autonomic dysfunction remains controversial. It is likely that the fundoplication improves gastric emptying more than pyloroplasty does.

Gastrostomy

Gastrostomy is often performed in children with swallowing disorders, food refusal, chronic failure to thrive, and aspiration with swallowing. Obviously, patients with a short-term need for enteral feeding are benefited by nasogastric or nasoenteric tubes. However, patients with a long-term need for enteric feeding are best served by a gastrostomy or jejunostomy. Currently, there are multiple surgical options for enteral feeding devices, including open gastrostomy, percutaneous endoscopic gastrostomy, a gastrojejunostomy tube through the gastrostomy, laparoscopic gastrostomy, lesser curvature gastrostomy, simple jejunostomy, and Roux-en-Y jejunostomy.

It is controversial whether patients who need gastrostomy placement should undergo a workup for GER. Some authors believe that no workup is needed.[39,99] Their view is that either most patients with a gastrostomy will not vomit or the vomiting will resolve after gastrostomy feedings are initiated. This view is not shared by many pediatric surgeons who believe that a workup for GER should be performed before gastrostomy placement.[21,173] If significant reflux is identified, an antireflux procedure should be performed along with the gastrostomy. A third view is that patients with GER who need enteric feedings should have either a gastrojejunostomy or a jejunostomy tube placed. The disadvantage of this third view is that the patients must then be fed by drip methods, which is a much less attractive option for parents who are struggling to care for their child. Gastrojejunal tubes are frequently dislodged. Many patients live a long distance away from a medical facility for children, so dislodgement of the tube is a difficult logistic issue for them to cope with. Feeding into the stomach without an antireflux procedure also risks massive aspiration. In our experience, parental fatigue seems to be much greater as parents try to cope with the persistent vomiting and poor weight gain of their vomiting child. For these reasons, the authors prefer to rule out gross reflux before performing a gastrostomy. Patients with significant documented reflux or a predilection for post-gastrostomy reflux, such as those with a large hiatal hernia or spasticity associated with increased intra-abdominal pressure, are treated by simultaneous gastrostomy and fundoplication.

Richards et al. reported that two thirds of patients who gag and retch postoperatively can be identified preoperatively by a careful history. They characterized these patients as vomiters and not refluxers and advocated the avoidance of fundoplication in such patients.[197] On the other hand, Owings reviewed 138 neurologically impaired patients undergoing fundoplication. She found that 33% of these neurologically impaired patients were cured of their gagging and retching by fundoplication. Thirty-five percent did not retch either preoperatively or postoperatively. Twenty percent of the patients retched both preoperatively and postoperatively, and these symptoms developed postoperatively in 12% (Owings E, personal communication). Because two thirds of neurologically impaired patients do not have significant retching postoperatively, the authors do not withhold fundoplication from these patients.

When a patient needs chronic enteral feeding, several gastrostomy options are most frequently used. Open gastrostomy can be performed with a variety of techniques. The classic technique is a Stamm gastrostomy, which is usually performed by way of a small 4-cm midline incision located equidistant between the xiphoid and umbilicus.[12] The anterior wall of the stomach is identified and two purse-string sutures are placed. A tube is passed through the left upper quadrant in an appropriate position. A balloon or mushroom catheter is inserted into the stomach inside the purse-string sutures (Fig. 71-13). The purse-string sutures are tied snugly. The gastrostomy is tacked in two to four quadrants to the abdominal wall with absorbable sutures (Fig. 71-14). The gastrostomy tube is secured to the skin with a suture.

The percutaneous endoscopic gastrostomy (PEG) technique was first described by Michael Gauderer, a pediatric surgeon. Excellent descriptions of the PEG technique are available in the literature.[79,85,195] PEG is a minimally invasive technique that usually requires a general anesthetic in the pediatric population. Its disadvantages include an inability to choose the precise position on the stomach wall to site the gastrostomy and the fact that it is a blind technique that can lead to penetration of the colon or liver. Another common method for placement of a gastrostomy tube or button is laparoscopic gastrostomy. It is a minimally invasive technique that requires a general anesthetic. However, it is versatile and can easily be performed with other laparoscopic techniques. It allows precise placement of the gastrostomy

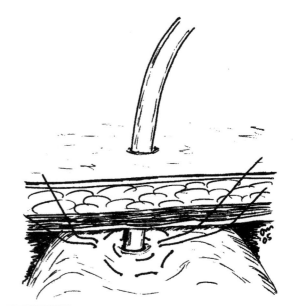

Figure 71-13 Stamm gastrostomy: one or two purse-string sutures are placed in the anterior wall of the stomach and tied snugly around the gastrostomy tube.

device at the chosen site on the stomach wall. Placement of a primary button is relatively easy with this technique.

Two methods are commonly used to place a gastrostomy laparoscopically.[213] The first method is the port site method in which a medial left upper quadrant port site is enlarged. The intra-abdominal stomach is grasped at the site of the intended gastrostomy site and pulled up through the abdominal wall. Two stabilizing sutures are then passed through the fascia, through the wall of the stomach, and back out through the fascia on the opposite side.

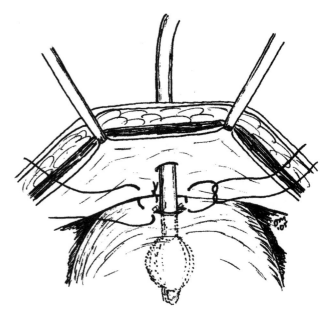

Figure 71-14 Stamm gastrostomy: the stomach is secured to the abdominal wall around the gastrostomy site with three or four sutures.

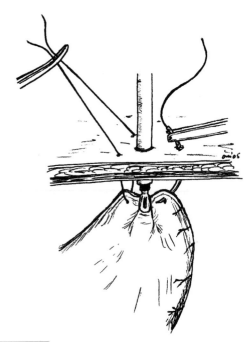

Figure 71-15 Laparoscopic U-stitch gastrostomy: the stomach is grasped and held near the abdominal wall while two U-stitches are placed for countertraction of the anterior stomach wall.

This stitch is repeated on the lower side of the gastrostomy wound. The stomach is pulled out through the enlarged port site and a purse-string suture applied. A hole is made in the stomach wall inside the purse-string suture. The button or catheter is inserted through the hole and the stomach is allowed to return to the abdominal cavity. The purse-string suture is tied snugly. The two stabilizing sutures are also tied snugly. The gastrostomy tube or button can be fixed externally with a suture, depending on the surgeon's preference. This port site technique is simple but has some drawbacks. The port site, which is enlarged, can break down and allow evisceration of the stomach wall through the skin site, particularly in thin-walled infants. The most common problem with this technique is that it is difficult to completely return the stomach wall back into the peritoneal cavity. The gastrostomy tract is lined with gastric mucosa, which has a greater tendency to leak and also creates a troublesome, nonclosing gastrocutaneous fistula when the gastrostomy tube or button is removed.[213]

The other commonly used laparoscopic gastrostomy technique is the U-stitch technique. In this technique, a U-stitch is passed through the abdominal wall adjacent and medial to a left upper quadrant port site, through the stomach wall, and back out through the abdominal wall. A second U-stitch is passed parallel to the first about 1 cm apart (Fig. 71-15). A needle is passed through the trocar site and directly into the stomach, which has been inflated with air through a Levine tube placed by the anesthetist. The needle is passed into the inflated stomach through the port site inside the two U-stitches. A guidewire is passed through this needle into the stomach (Fig. 71-16). The tract is dilated over the guidewire up to

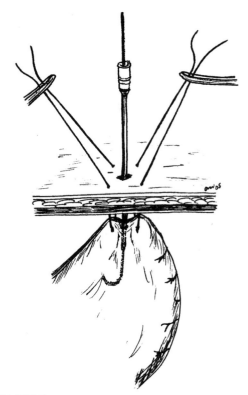

Figure 71-16 Laparoscopic U-stitch gastrostomy: a needle and guidewire are passed through the port site into the inflated stomach. Dilators are passed over the guidewire up to a size 20 French.

a size 20 French. A 14-French balloon button is passed over the guidewire into the stomach, with an 8-French dilator used to stiffen the stem of the button as it is passed into the stomach. The U-stitches are tied over the wings of the gastrostomy button or over bolsters if a gastrostomy tube is being placed (Fig. 71-17).[213] The primary disadvantage of this technique is that the stomach

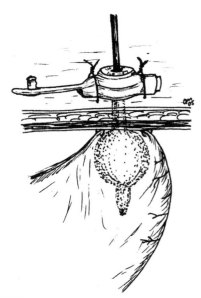

Figure 71-17 Laparoscopic U-stitch gastrostomy: the U-stitches are loosely tied over the wings of the gastrostomy button and removed on the second postoperative day.

is not directly secured to the abdominal wall. However, after placing over 1000 gastrostomy buttons in this manner, lack of site fixation does not seem to be a major problem, very much like a PEG tube does not usually lead to local leakage of gastric contents into the peritoneal cavity.[255]

Complications of Antireflux Procedures

Complications may be classified according to occurrence during surgery, early after surgery, or late. Complications during surgery include bleeding from the short gastric vessels, the spleen, or an aberrant left hepatic artery. In adult laparoscopic series, it has been reported that perforation of the esophagus or stomach occurs in about 1% of primary procedures.[257] We have seen only one gastric perforation and no esophageal perforations during primary fundoplication in over 1000 laparoscopic fundoplication procedures. Pneumothorax may occur with either open or laparoscopic techniques. The pneumothorax usually develops during dissection of the mediastinal esophagus in an effort to gain more esophageal length. The pneumothorax can be relieved by placing a small intravenous catheter in the ipsilateral chest and removing it at the end of the operation after the abdomen has been closed. Conversion rates from laparoscopic to open surgery should be less than 3% for primary operations. Many fundoplication patients experience early dysphagia when the wrap becomes edematous several days after completion of the surgical procedure. This dysphagia can be avoided by keeping the wrap loose and floppy, dividing the upper short gastric vessels, and placing the patient on a soft diet for 2 to 3 weeks postoperatively.[109] A tight hiatus can likewise cause dysphagia and must be carefully avoided. It is also important to not make the wrap too long. In the authors' experience, a wrap 3.0 cm in length is more likely to elicit dysphagia than a floppy 2.0-cm wrap. Patients with severe esophageal dysmotility can report dysphagia even with a loose wrap. Prokinetic agents may be helpful in treating this group of patients.

Recurrent reflux is a common complication after fundoplication in children.[82] It is often related to postoperative retching and gagging (Ngerncham M, personal communication). It is important to recognize that postfundoplication retching is most often initiated by central nervous system abnormalities and is not primarily a gastrointestinal symptom. The most common cause of postoperative gagging is overfeeding of the patient. Zealous parents are thrilled to have a reliable mechanism to feed their semi-starved child and often overfeed them. A careful history of the timing of the retching is essential in determining its underlying cause. Gagging and retching can be ameliorated by drip feedings, emptying the stomach of air before initiating feedings, treating constipation, and as previously mentioned, avoiding overfeeding of the patient. However, postfundoplication gagging and retching remain a major problem, especially in neurologically impaired children.

Other postfundoplication complications include gas-bloating syndrome and an inability to vomit. Most patients with a floppy Nissen fundoplication can burp and vomit within 6 months of the operative procedure (Owings E, personal communication). True gas-bloating syndrome is uncommon in these patients. It is usually seen in neurologically impaired patients who are aerophagic. More commonly, patients who seem bloated are constipated and have a distended, air-filled colon rather than air in their stomach. These gas-bloating symptoms can be ameliorated by treating their constipation with fiber and appropriate laxative administration.[35]

Dumping syndrome can also follow the formation of an antireflux wrap. The fundoplication streamlines the stomach and decreases the size and reservoir function of the stomach. The addition of a pyloroplasty is associated with an even higher incidence of dumping. Patients with sweating and diarrhea after feeding should be managed by restriction of food intake, reduction in carbohydrate intake, and drip feedings.[132] Small bowel obstruction is another complication that is relatively rare after laparoscopic fundoplication, but not uncommon in patients after open fundoplication. A rate of 2.6% has been reported after open surgery.[82]

Outcome and Results

The success rates of open and laparoscopic antireflux procedures are excellent. In a multicenter review of more than 7000 children over a 20-year period, good to excellent results were achieved in 95% of neurologically normal children and 84.6% of neurologically impaired children with the use of open surgical techniques.[82,159] Similar success rates can be achieved with laparoscopic fundoplication. Chung and Georgeson reported their success with both laparoscopic Nissen and Toupet fundoplication. They showed that of patients undergoing laparoscopic Nissen fundoplication, 3.5% had recurrent symptoms at 2 years versus 6.1% of those undergoing Toupet fundoplication.[51] The most common cause of fundoplication failure after laparoscopic repair is slippage of the wrap into the chest (Ngerncham M, personal communication). For this reason, great effort should be made to prevent slippage of the fundoplication wrap into the chest. A recent report assessing laparoscopic Thal antireflux procedures showed a silent reflux rate of 25% in symptom-free children.[108] As mentioned earlier, partial-wrap fundoplications appear to be associated with a higher recurrence of GER than complete-wrap fundoplications.

A common problem is knowing what to do with a child who has failed multiple fundoplications. Medical management of the reflux should be used to control the recurrent symptoms whenever possible. Radiofrequency ablation is another possibility, as suggested by Islam et al.[112] If redo surgery is necessary, Roux-en-Y esophagojejunostomy has been reported to be effective, but this technique is associated with a high rate of serious complications.[65] Another possibility is to redo the fundoplication with a Collis-Nissen technique[108] or hiatoplasty,[40] thereby lengthening the intra-abdominal portion of the esophagus. No reliable resolution to the problem of recurrent reflux after fundoplication in children has been reported thus far. The authors prefer performing a redo Nissen fundoplication after the first recurrence, followed by a laparoscopic Collis-Nissen procedure for a second recurrence of reflux symptoms.

SUMMARY

GER is a common disorder in children and often requires surgical correction. GER in infants and children is more complex than adult GER. Failure of medical management and an inability to wean from antireflux medications are the most common indications for the surgical treatment of reflux. A complete-wrap fundoplication appears to have better outcomes than partial-wrap fundoplication, although this contention is controversial. Postoperative retching and recurrent GER are the most common and vexing complications of antireflux surgery.

REFERENCES

1. Aksglaede K, Funch-Jensen P, Thommesen P: Radiological demonstration of gastroesophageal reflux: Diagnostic value of barium and bread studies compared with 24-hour pH monitoring. Acta Radiol 1999;40:652.
2. Alexander F, Wyllie R, Jirousek K: Delayed gastric emptying affects outcome of Nissen fundoplication in neurologically impaired children. Surgery 1997;122:690.
3. Allen ML, Zamani S, Dimarino AJ Jr: The effect of gravity on esophageal peristalsis in humans. Neurogastroenterol Motil 1997;9:71.
4. Alliet P, Raes M, Bruneel E, et al: Omeprazole in infants with cimetidine-resistant peptic esophagitis. J Pediatr 1998; 132:352.
5. Allison PR: Reflux esophagitis, sliding hiatus hernia and the anatomy of repair. Surg Gynecol Obstet 1951;92:419.
6. Allison PR, Johnston AS, Royce GB: Short esophagus with simple peptic ulceration. J Thorac Cardiovasc Surg 1943; 12:432.
7. Altorki NK, Skinner DB: Pathophysiology of gastroesophageal reflux. Am J Med 1989;86:685.
8. Andrews PL, Sanger GJ: Abdominal vagal afferent neurons: An important target for the treatment of gastrointestinal dysfunction. Curr Opin Pharmacol 2002;2:650.
9. Ashcraft KW, Goodwin CD, Amoury RW, et al: Thal fundoplication: A simple and safe operative treatment for gastroesophageal reflux. J Pediatr Surg 1978;13:643.
10. Ashcraft KW, Holder TM, Amoury RA: Treatment of gastroesophageal reflux in children by Thal fundoplication. J Thorac Cardiovasc Surg 1981;82:706.
11. Atkinson M, Summerling ME: The competence of the cardia after cardiomyotomy. Gastroenterologia 1959;92:123.
12. Au FC: The Stamm gastrostomy: A sound procedure. Am Surg 1993;59:674.
13. Augood C, MacLennan S, Gilbert R, et al: Cisapride treatment for gastro-oesophageal reflux in children. Cochrane Database Syst Rev (4):CD002300, 2003.
14. Axelrod FB, Schneider KM, Ament ME, et al: Gastroesophageal fundoplication and gastrostomy in familial dysautonomia. Ann Surg 1982;195:253.
15. Aziz Q, Thompson DG: Brain-gut axis in health and disease. Gastroenterology 1998;114:559.
16. Belaji NS, Blom D, DeMeester TR, et al: Redefining gastroesophageal reflux (GER). Surg Endosc 2003;17:1380.
17. Barak N, Ehrenpreis ED, Harrison JR, et al: Gastrooesophageal reflux disease in obesity: Pathophysiological and therapeutic considerations. Obes Rev 2002;3:9.
18. Bardaji C, Boix-Ochoa J: Contribution of the His angle to the gastroesophageal antireflux mechanism. Pediatr Surg Int 1986;1:172.
19. Beaudoin S, Kieffer G, Sapin E, et al: Gastroesophageal reflux in neonates with congenital abdominal wall defect. Eur J Pediatr Surg 1995;5:323.
20. Belsey R: Diaphragmatic hernia. In Modern Trends in Gastroenterology. London, Butterworth, 1952, p 134.
21. Berezin S, Schwartz SM, Halata MS, Newman LJ: Gastroesophageal reflux secondary to gastrostomy placement. Am J Dis Child 1986;40:649.
22. Berger D, Bischof-Delaloye A, Reinberg O, et al: Esophageal and pulmonary scintiscanning in gastroesophageal reflux in children. Prog Pediatr Surg 1985; 18:68.
23. Bergmeijer JH, Hazebroek FW: Prospective medical and surgical treatment of gastroesophageal reflux in esophageal atresia. J Am Coll Surg 1998;187:153.
24. Bergmeijer JH, Tibboel D, Hazebroek FW: Nissen fundoplication in the management of gastroesophageal reflux occurring after repair of esophageal atresia. J Pediatr Surg 2000;35:573.
25. Billiard MC: Traite des maladies des enfans nouveaux-nes et a la mamelle. In Billiard M (ed): Atlas D'Anatomie Pathologique pour Servir A L'Historie des Maladies des Enfants. Paris, Imprimerie de H Balzac, 1828, p 271.
26. Black DD, Haggitt RC, Orenstein SR, et al: Esophagitis in infants. Morphometric histological diagnosis and correlation with measures of gastroesophageal reflux. Gastroenterology 1990;98:1408.
27. Boix-Ochoa J: Diagnosis and management of gastroesophageal reflux in children. Surg Ann 1981;13:123.
28. Boix-Ochoa J: Gastroesophageal reflux. In Welch K, Randolph JG, Rautch M, et al (eds): Pediatric Surgery. St Louis, Mosby–Year Book, 1986.
29. Boix-Ochoa J: Gastroesophageal reflux in children. In Jemieson G (ed): Surgery of the Esophagus. Edinburgh, Churchill Livingstone, 1988.
30. Boix-Ochoa J, Canals J: Maturation of the lower esophagus. J Pediatr Surg 1976;11:749.
31. Boix-Ochoa J, Lafuenta JM, Gil-Vernet JM: Twenty-four hour esophageal pH monitoring in gastroesophageal reflux. J Pediatr Surg 1980;15:74.
32. Boix-Ochoa J, Rowe MI: Gastroesophageal reflux. In O'Neill JA (ed): Pediatric Surgery, vol 2. St Louis, Mosby–Year Book, 1998, p 1007.
33. Bombeck CT, Dillard NH, Nyhus LM: Muscular anatomy of the gastroesophageal junction and role of phrenoesophageal competence. Ann Surg 1966;164:643.
34. Bonavina L, Evander A, DeMeester TR, et al: Length of the distal esophageal sphincter and competency of the cardia. Am J Surg 1986;151:25-34.
35. Borowitz SM, Satphen JL: Recurrent vomiting and persistent gastroesophageal reflux caused by unrecognized constipation. Clin Pediatr (Phila) 2004;43:461.
36. Boyle JT: Acid secretion from birth to adulthood. J Pediatr Gastroenterol Nutr 2003;37(Suppl):S12.
37. Bright R: Account of a remarkable misplacement of the stomach. Guys Hosp Rep 1836;1:598.
38. Brown RA, Wynehank S, Rode H: Is a gastric drainage procedure necessary at the time of antireflux surgery? J Pediatr Gastroenterol Nutr 1997;25:377.
39. Burd RS, Price MR, Whalen TV: The role of protective antireflux procedures in neurologically impaired children: A decision analysis. J Pediatr Surg 2002;37:500.
40. Bustorff-Silva J, Moreira AP, Cavalsco MA, et al: Extended hiatoplasty: Early experience with a simple technique increases the intraabdominal esophageal length in complicated gastroesophageal reflux. J Pediatr Surg 2001; 35:555.

41. Cadiot G, Bruhat A, Rigaud D, et al: Multivariate analysis of pathophysiological factors in reflux oesophagitis. Gut 1997;40:167.

42. Carré IJ: Natural history of partial thoracic stomach ("hiatal hernia") in children. Arch Dis Child 1959;34:344.

43. Carré IJ: Postural treatment of children with partial thoracic stomach ("hiatus hernia"). Arch Dis Child 1960;35:569.

44. Ceriati E, Guarino N, Zaccara A, et al: Gastroesophageal reflux in neurologically impaired children: Partial or total fundoplication? Arch Surg 1998;383:317.

45. Cezard JP: Managing gastro-oesophageal reflux disease in children. Digestion 2004;69:3.

46. Chadwick LM, Kurinczuk JJ, Hallam LA, et al: Clinical and endoscopic predictors of histological oesophagitis in infants. J Paediatr Child Health 1997;33:388.

47. Chen MY, Ott DJ, Sinclair JW, et al: Gastroesophageal reflux disease: Correlation of esophageal pH testing and radiographic findings. Radiology 1992;185:483.

48. Chiba N, Gara CJ De, Wilkinson JM, et al: Speed of healing and symptom relief in grade II to IV gastroesophageal reflux disease: A meta-analysis. Gastroenterology 1997;112:1798.

49. Chong SK: Gastrointestinal problems in the handicapped child. Curr Opin Pediatr 2001;13:441.

50. Choudhry U, Boyce HW Jr, Coppola D: Proton pump inhibitor–associated gastric polyps: A retrospective analysis of their frequency, and endoscopic, histologic, and ultrastructural characteristics. Am J Clin Pathol 1998;110:615.

51. Chung DH, Georgeson KE: Fundoplication and gastrostomy. Semin Pediatr Surg 1998;7:213.

52. Clark GW: Effect of *Helicobacter pylori* infection in Barrett's esophagus and the genesis of esophageal adenocarcinoma. World J Surg 2003;27:994.

53. Cohen S, Harris LD: Does hiatus hernia affect competence of the gastroesophageal sphincter? N Engl J Med 1971; 284:1053.

54. Cohen Z, Fishman S, Yulevich A, et al: Nissen fundoplication and Boix-Ochoa antireflux procedure: Comparison between two surgical techniques in the treatment of gastroesophageal reflux disease in children. Eur J Pediatr Surg 1999;9:289.

55. Collen MJ, Ciarleglio CA, Stanczak VJ, et al: Basal gastric acid secretion in children with atypical epigastric pain. Am J Gastroenterol 1988;83:923.

56. Colletti RB, Christie DL, Orenstein SR: Statement of the North American Society for Pediatric Gastroenterology and Nutrition (NASPGN). Indications for pediatric esophageal pH monitoring. J Pediatr Gastroenterol Nutr 1995;21:253.

57. Colletti RB, Di Lorenzo C: Overview of pediatric gastroesophageal reflux disease and proton pump inhibitor therapy. J Pediatr Gastroenterol Nutr 2003;37(Suppl):S7.

58. Cook IJ, Dodds WJ, Dantos RO, et al: Opening mechanisms of the human upper esophageal sphincter. Am J Physiol 1989;257:G748.

59. Cucchiara S, Salvia G, Borrelli O, et al: Gastric electrical dysrhythmias and delayed gastric emptying in gastroesophageal reflux disease. Am J Gastroenterol 1997;92:1103.

60. Cucchiara S, Staiano A, Boccieri A, et al: Effects of cisapride on parameters of oesophageal motility and on the prolonged intraoesophageal pH test in infants with gastrooesophageal reflux disease. Gut 1990;31:21.

61. Cucchiara S, Staiano A, Di Lorenzo C, et al: Esophageal motor abnormalities in children with gastroesophageal reflux and peptic esophagitis. J Pediatr Gastroenterol Nurs 1986;108:907.

62. Curry JI, Lander TD, Stringer MD: Erythromycin as prokinetic agent in infants and children. Aliment Pharmacol Ther 2001;15:595.

63. Dalby-Payne JR, Morris AM, Craig JC: Meta-analysis of randomized controlled trials on the benefits and risks of using cisapride for the treatment of gastroesophageal reflux in children. J Gastroenterol Hepatol 2003;18:196.

64. Dallemagne B, Weerts JM, Jehaes C, et al: Laparoscopic Nissen fundoplication: Preliminary report. Surg Laparosc Endosc 1991;1:138.

65. Danielson PD, Emmers RW: Esophagogastric disconnection for gastroesophageal reflux in children with severe neurological impairment. J Pediatr Surg 1999;34:84.

66. Darling DB: Hiatal hernia and gastroesophageal reflux in infancy and childhood. AJR Am J Roentgenol 1975;123:724.

67. Davidson G: The role of lower esophageal sphincter function and dysmotility in gastroesophageal reflux in premature infants and in the first year of life. J Pediatr Gastroenterol Nutr 2003;37(Suppl):S17.

68. Delattre JF, Avisse C, Marcus C, et al: Functional anatomy of the gastroesophageal junction. Surg Clin North Am 2000;80:241.

69. DeMeester TR, Wernly JA, Bryant GH, et al: A clinical and in vitro analysis of determinants of gastroesophageal competence. A study of the principles of antireflux surgery. Am J Surg 1979;137(Suppl):39.

70. Deurloo JA, Ekkelkamp S, Bartelsman JF, et al: Gastroesophageal reflux: Prevalence in adults older than 28 years after correction of esophageal atresia. Ann Surg 2003;238:686.

71. Dodds WJ, Dent J, Hogan WJ, et al: Mechanisms of gastroesophageal reflux in patients with reflux esophagitis. N Engl J Med 1982;307:1547.

72. Dodds WJ, Stef JJ, Hogan WJ: Factors determining pressure measurement accuracy by intraluminal esophageal manometry. Gastroenterology 1976;70:117.

73. Duranceau A, Liebermann-Mefferret D: Physiology of the esophagus. In Zuidema G (ed): Shackelford's Surgery of the Alimentary Tract, 5th ed. Philadelphia, WB Saunders, 2002.

74. Enger C, Cali C, Walker AM: Serious ventricular arrhythmias among users of cisapride and other QT-prolonging agents in the United States. Pharmacoepidemiol Drug Saf 2002;11:477.

75. Euler AR, Byrne WJ: Twenty-four-hour esophageal intraluminal pH probe testing: A comparative analysis. Gastroenterology 1981;80:957.

76. Ewer AK, James ME, Tobin JM: Prone and left lateral positioning reduce gastro-oesophageal reflux in preterm infants. Arch Dis Child Fetal Neonatal Ed 1999;81:F201.

77. Fanelli RD, Gersin KS, Bakhsh A: The Stretta(r) procedure: Effective endoluminal therapy for GERD. Surg Technol Int 2003;11:129.

78. Fasching G, Huber A, Uray E, et al: Gastroesophageal reflux and diaphragmatic motility after repair of congenital diaphragmatic hernia. Eur J Pediatr Surg 2000;10:360.

79. Ferguson RD, Harig JM, Kozarek RA, et al: Placement of feeding button (One-Step Button) as the initial procedure. Am J Gastroenterol 1993;8:501.

80. Follette D, Fonkalsrud EW, Euler A, et al: Gastroesophageal fundoplication for reflux in infants and children. J Pediatr Surg 1976;11:757.

81. Fonkalsrud EW: Nissen fundoplication for pediatric gastroesophageal reflux disease. Semin Pediatr Surg 1998;7:110.

82. Fonkalsrud EW, Ashcraft KW, Coran AG, et al: Surgical treatment of gastroesophageal reflux in children: A combined hospital study of 7467 patients. Pediatrics 1998; 101:419.

83. Fonkalsrud EW, Foglia RP, Ament ME, et al: Operative treatment for the gastroesophageal reflux syndrome in children. J Pediatr Surg 1989;24:525.

84. Freedman J, Lindqvist M, Hellstrom PM, et al: Presence of bile in the oesophagus is associated with less effective oesophageal motility. Digestion 2002;66:42.

85. Gauderer MWL, Ponsky JL: A simplified technique for constructing a tube feeding gastrostomy. Surg Gynecol Obstet 1981;152:83.

86. Georgeson K: Results of laparoscopic antireflux procedures of neurologically normal infants and children. Semin Laparosc Surg 2002;9:172.

87. Georgeson K: Minimally invasive surgery in neonates. Semin Neonatal 2003;8:243.

88. Georgeson KE: Laparoscopic gastrostomy and fundoplication. Pediatr Ann 1993;92:675.

89. Georgeson KE: Laparoscopic fundoplication and gastrostomy. Semin Laparosc Surg 1998;5:25.

90. Gibbons TE, Gold BD: The use of proton pump inhibitors in children: A comprehensive review. Paediatr Drugs 2003;5:25.

91. Godoy J, Tovar JA, Vicente Y, et al: Esophageal motor dysfunction persists in children after surgical cure of reflux: An ambulatory manometric study. J Pediatr Surg 2001;36:1405.

92. Gold BD: Outcomes of pediatric gastroesophageal reflux disease: In the first year of life, in childhood, and in adults. oh, and should we really leave *Helicobacter pylori* alone? J Pediatr Gastroenterol Nutr 2003;37(Suppl):S33.

93. Gold BD, Freston JW: Gastroesophageal reflux in children: Pathogenesis, prevalence, diagnosis, and role of proton pump inhibitors in treatment. Paediatr Drugs 2002;4:673.

94. Goldani HA, Fernandes MI, Vicente YA, et al: Lower esophageal sphincter reacts against intraabdominal pressure in children with symptoms of gastroesophageal reflux. Dig Dis Sci 2002;47:2544.

95. Gorenstein A, Levine A, Boaz M, et al: Severity of acid gastroesophageal reflux assessed by pH metry: Is it associated with respiratory disease? Pediatr Pulmonol 2003;36:330.

96. Gorrotxategi P, Reguilon MJ, Arana J, et al: Gastroesophageal reflux in association with the Sandifer syndrome. Eur J Pediatr Surg 1995;5:203.

97. Gremse DA: Gastroesophageal reflux disease in children: An overview of pathophysiology, diagnosis, and treatment. J Pediatr Gastroenterol Nutr 2002;35(Suppl):S297.

98. Grosser O: The development of respiratory apparatus. In Keibel F, Mall F (eds): Manual of Human Embryology. Philadelphia, JB Lippincott, 1912, p 473.

99. Hamant JM, Bax NM, van der Zee DC, et al: Complications of percutaneous endoscopic gastrostomy with or without concomitant antireflux surgery in 96 children. J Pediatr Surg 2001;36:1412.

100. Hassall E: Co-morbidities in childhood Barrett's esophagus. J Pediatr Gastroenterol Nutr 1997;25:255.

101. Hassall E, Weinstein WM, Ament ME: Barrett's esophagus in childhood. Gastroenterology 1985;89:1331.

102. Helm JF: Esophageal acid clearance. J Clin Gastroenterol 1986;8:5.

103. Hill LD: An effective operation for hiatal hernia: An eight-year appraisal. Ann Surg 1967;166:681.

104. Hillemeier C, Buchin PJ, Gryboski J: Esophageal dysfunction in Down's syndrome. J Pediatr Gastroenterol Nutr 1982;1:101.

105. Ho SC, Chang CS, Wu CY, et al: Ineffective esophageal motility is a primary motility disorder in gastroesophageal reflux disease. Dig Dis Sci 2002;47:652.

106. Holloway RH: The anti-reflux barrier and mechanisms of gastro-oesophageal reflux. Baillieres Best Pract Res Clin Gastroenterol 2000;14:681.

107. Holloway RH, Hongo M, Berger K, et al: Gastric distention: A mechanism for postprandial gastroesophageal reflux. Gastroenterology 1985;89:779.

108. Hunter JG, Smith CD, Branum GD, et al: Laparoscopic fundoplication failures: Patterns of failure and response to fundoplication revision. Am Surg 1999;230:595.

109. Hunter JG, Swanstrom L, Waring JP: Dysphagia after laparoscopic antireflux surgery: The impact of operative technique. Ann Surg 1996;224:51.

110. Hussain SZ, Di Lorenzo C: Motility disorders. Diagnosis and treatment for the pediatric patient. Pediatr Clin North Am 2002;49:27.

111. Hyams JS: Functional gastrointestinal disorders. Curr Opin Pediatr 1999;11:375.

112. Islam S, Geiger JD, Coran AG, et al: Use of radiofrequency ablation of the lower esophageal sphincter to treat recurrent gastroesophageal reflux disease. J Pediatr Surg 2004;39:282.

113. Jackson C: The diaphragmatic pinchcock. Laryngoscope 1922;32:139.

114. Jadcherla SR: Manometric evaluation of esophageal-protective reflexes in infants and children. Am J Med 2003;115(Suppl):157S.

115. Jaillard SM, Pierrat V, Dubois A, et al: Outcome at 2 years of infants with congenital diaphragmatic hernia: A population-based study. Ann Thorac Surg 2003;75:250.

116. Jobe BA, Wallace J, Hansen PD, et al: Evaluation of laparoscopic Toupet fundoplication as a primary repair for all patients with medically resistant gastroesophageal reflux. Surg Endosc 1997;11:1080.

117. Johnson DG: Current thinking on the role of surgery in gastroesophageal reflux. Pediatr Clin North Am 1985;325:1165.

118. Johnson DG, Reid BS, Meyers RL, et al: Are scintiscans accurate in the selection of reflux patients for pyloroplasty? J Pediatr Surg 1998;33:573.

119. Johnson LF, DeMeester TH: Twenty-four hour pH monitoring of the distal esophagus: Quantitative measure of gastroesophageal reflux. Am J Gastroenterol 1974;63:325.

120. Kahrilas PJ: GERD pathogenesis, pathophysiology, and clinical manifestations. Cleve Clin J Med 2003;70(Suppl):S4.

121. Kahrilas PJ, Dodds WJ, Dent J, et al: Upper esophageal sphincter function during deglutition. Gastroenterology 1988;95:52.

122. Kahrilas PJ, Dodds WJ, Hogan WJ: Effect of peristaltic dysfunction on esophageal volume clearance. Gastroenterology 1988;94:73.

123. Kalach N, Badran AM, Jaffray P, et al: Correlation between gastric acid secretion and severity of acid reflux in children. Turk J Pediatr 2003;45:6.

124. Kamiyama M, Kawahara H, Okuyama H, et al: Gastroesophageal reflux after repair of congenital diaphragmatic hernia. J Pediatr Surg 2002;37:1681.

125. Kapila YV, Dodds WJ, Helm JF, et al: Relationship between swallow rate and salivary flow. Dig Dis Sci 1984;29:528.

126. Kattwinkel J, Brooks JG, Keenan ME, et al: Changing concepts of sudden infant death syndrome: Implications for infant sleeping environment and sleep position. Pediatrics 2000;105:650.

127. Kawahara H, Dent J, Davidson G, et al: Relationship between straining, transient lower esophageal sphincter relaxation, and gastroesophageal reflux in children. Am J Gastroenterol 2001;96:2019.

128. Kawahara H, Imura K, Nakajima K, et al: Motor function of the esophagus and the lower esophageal sphincter in children who undergo laparoscopic Nissen fundoplication. J Pediatr Surg 2000;35:1666.

129. Kawahara H, Imura K, Yagi M, et al: Mechanisms underlying the antireflux effect of Nissen fundoplication in children. J Pediatr Surg 1998;33:1618.

130. Kazerooni NL, VanCamp J, Hirschl RB, et al: Fundoplication in 160 children under 2 years of age. J Pediatr Surg 1994;29:677.

131. Khoshoo V, Le T, Haydel RM Jr: Role of gastroesophageal reflux in older children with persistent asthma. Chest 2003; 123:1008.

132. Khoshoo V, Reifen RM, Gold BD, et al: Nutritional manipulation in the management of dumping syndrome. Arch Dis Child 1991;66:1447.

133. Kleeff J, Friess H, Buchler MW: How *Helicobacter pylori* changed the life of surgeons. Dig Dis Sci 2003;20:93.

134. Kluth D, Fiegel H: The embryology of the foregut. Semin Pediatr Surg 2003;12:3.

135. Koek GH, Tack J, Sifrim D, et al: The role of acid and duodenal gastroesophageal reflux in symptomatic GERD. Am J Gastroenterol 2001;96:2033.

136. Koivusalo A, Rintala R, Lindahl H: Gastroesophageal reflux in children with a congenital abdominal wall defect. J Pediatr Surg 1999;34:1127.

137. Krug E, Bergmeijer JH, Dees J, et al: Gastroesophageal reflux and Barrett's esophagus in adults born with esophageal atresia. Am J Gastroenterol 1999;94:2825.

138. Kubiak R, Spitz L, Kiely EM, et al: Effectiveness of fundoplication in early infancy. J Pediatr Surg 1999;34:295.

139. Lagergren J, Bergstrom R, Adami HO, et al: Association between medications that relax the lower esophageal sphincter and risk for esophageal adenocarcinoma. Ann Intern Med 2000;133:165.

140. Levine A, Milo T, Broide E, et al: Influence of *Helicobacter pylori* eradication on gastroesophageal reflux symptoms and epigastric pain in children and adolescents. Pediatrics 2004;113:54.

141. Levy J: Use of electrogastrography in children. Curr Gastroenterol Rep 2002;4:259.

142. Liebermann-Mefferet D, Duranceau A, Stein HJ: Anatomy of the esophagus. In Zuidema G (ed): Shackelford's Surgery of the Alimentary Tract, 5th ed. Philadelphia, WB Saunders, 2002.

143. Link DT, Willging JP, Miller CK, et al: Pediatric laryngopharyngeal sensory testing during flexible endoscopic evaluation of swallowing: Feasible and correlative. Ann Otol Rhinol Laryngol 2000;109:899.

144. Little AG: Mechanisms of action of antireflux surgery: Theory and fact. World J Surg 1992;16:320.

145. Little DC, Rescorla FJ, Grosfeld JL, et al: Long-term analysis of children with esophageal atresia and tracheoesophageal fistula. J Pediatr Surg 2003;38:852.

146. Lobe TE: Pediatric laparoscopy 2003. Clin Obstet Gynecol 2003;46:98.

147. Lobe TE, Schropp KP, Lunsford K: Laparoscopic Nissen fundoplication in childhood. J Pediatr Surg 1993;28:358.

148. Lundell LR, Dent J, Bennett JR, et al: Endoscopic assessment of oesophagitis: Clinical and functional correlates and further validation of the Los Angeles classification. Gut 1999;45:172.

149. Machida HM, Forbes DA, Gall DG, et al: Metoclopramide in gastroesophageal reflux of infancy. J Pediatr 1988; 112:483.

150. Mahmood Z, McMahon BP, Arfin Q, et al: EndoCinch therapy for gastro-oesophageal reflux disease: A one year prospective follow up. Gut 2003;52:34.

151. Malfertheiner P: *Helicobacter pylori* eradication does not exacerbate gastro-oesophageal reflux disease. Gut 2004; 53:312.

152. Mallet E, Mouterde O, Dubois F, et al: Use of ranitidine in young infants with gastro-oesophageal reflux. Eur J Clin Pharmacol 1989;36:641.

153. Mann CV, Greenwood RK, Ellis FH: The esophagogastric junction. Surg Gynecol Obstet 1964;104:853.

154. Mansfield LE: Embryonic origins of the relation of gastroesophageal reflux disease and airway disease. Am J Med 2001;111(Suppl):3S.

155. Marchetti F, Gerarduzzi T, Ventura A: Proton pump inhibitors in children: A review. Dig Liver Dis 2003; 35:738.

156. Mattioli G: Italian multicenter survey on laparoscopic treatment of gastro-esophageal reflux disease in children. Surg Endosc 2002;16:1666.

157. Mattioli G, Sacco O, Repetto P, et al: Necessity for surgery in children with gastrooesophageal reflux and supraoesophageal symptoms. Eur J Pediatr Surg 2004;14:7.

158. Meehan JJ, Georgeson KE: Laparoscopic fundoplication in infants and children. Surg Endosc 1996;10:1154.

159. Meining A, Classen M: The role of diet and lifestyle measures in the pathogenesis and treatment of gastroesophageal reflux disease. Am J Gastroenterol 2000;95:2692.

160. Merei JM, Hutson JM: Embryogenesis of tracheoesophageal anomalies: A review. Pediatr Surg Int 2002; 18:319.

161. Meyers WF, Herbst JJ: Effectiveness of positioning therapy for gastroesophageal reflux. Pediatrics 1982;69:768.

162. Min F, Tarlo SM, Bargman J, et al: Prevalence and causes of cough in chronic dialysis patients: A comparison between hemodialysis and peritoneal dialysis patients. Adv Perit Dial 2000;16:129.

163. Montupet P: Laparoscopic Toupet's fundoplication in children. Semin Laparosc Surg 2002;9:163.

164. Navarro-Rodriguez T, Hashimoto CL, Carrilho FJ, et al: Reduction of abdominal pressure in patients with ascites reduces gastroesophageal reflux. Dis Esophagus 2003; 16:77.

165. Nelson SP, Chen EH, Syniar GM, Christoffel KK: Prevalence of symptoms of gastroesophageal reflux during infancy: A pediatric practice-based survey. Pediatric Practice Research Group. Arch Pediatr Adolesc Med 1997; 151:569.

166. Nelson SP, Chen EH, Syniar GM, et al: One-year follow-up of symptoms of gastroesophageal reflux during infancy. Pediatric Practice Research Group. Pediatrics 1998; 102:E67.

167. Neuhauser EBD, Berenberg W: Cardioesophageal relaxation as a cause of vomiting in infants. Radiology 1947; 48:480.

168. Nissen R: Eine einfache Operation zur Beeinflussung der Refluxoesophagitis. Schwiez Med Wochenschr 1956; 86:590.

169. O'Hara SM: Pediatric gastrointestinal nuclear imaging. Radiol Clin North Am 1996;34:845.

170. Okagami H, Urao M, Stan GA, et al: A comparison of the efficacy of pyloromyotomy and pyloroplasty in patients with gastroesophageal reflux and delayed gastric emptying. J Pediatr Surg 1997;32:316.

171. Omari TI, Barnett CP, Bennings MA, et al: Mechanisms of gastro-oesophageal reflux in preterm and term infants with reflux disease. Gut 2002;51:475.

172. Omari TI, Barnett C, Snell A, et al: Mechanisms of gastroesophageal reflux in healthy premature infants. J Pediatr 1998;133:650.

173. O'Neill JA, Grosfeld JL, Fonkalsrud EW, et al (ed): Nutritional support of the pediatric surgical patient. In Principles of Pediatric Surgery, 2nd ed. St Louis: Mosby, 2004, p 87.

174. Orel R, Markovic S: Bile in the esophagus: A factor in the pathogenesis of reflux esophagitis in children. J Pediatr Gastroenterol Nutr 2003;36:266.

175. Orenstein SR: Effects on behavior state of prone versus seated positioning for infants with gastroesophageal reflux. Pediatrics 1990;85:765.

176. Orenstein SR: Gastroesophageal reflux. Curr Probl Pediatr 1991;21:193.

177. Orenstein SR: An overview of reflux-associated disorders in infants: Apnea, laryngospasm, and aspiration. Am J Med 2001;111(Suppl):60S.

178. Orenstein SR, Di Lorenzo C: Postfundoplication complications in children. Curr Treat Options Gastroenterol 2001; 4:441.

179. Orenstein SR, Izadnia F, Khan S: Gastroesophageal reflux disease in children. Gastroenterol Clin North Am 1999; 28:947.

180. Orlando RC: Pathogenesis of gastroesophageal reflux disease. Gastroenterol Clin North Am 2002;31(Suppl):S35.

181. Orlando RC: Pathogenesis of gastroesophageal reflux disease. Am J Med Sci 2003;326:274.

182. Ostlie D, Holcomb GW: Laparoscopic fundoplication and gastrostomy. Semin Pediatr Surg 2002;11:196.

183. Othersen HB Jr, Ocampo RJ, Parker EF, et al: Barrett's esophagus in children: Diagnosis and management. Ann Surg 1993;217:676.

184. Oyen N, Markestad T, Skaerven R, et al: Combined effects of sleeping position and prenatal risk factors in sudden infant death syndrome: The Nordic Epidemiological SIDS Study. Pediatrics 1997;100:613.

185. Ozcan Z, Ozcan C, Erinc R, et al: Scintigraphy in the detection of gastro-oesophageal reflux in children with caustic oesophageal burns. A comparative study with radiography and 24-h pH monitoring. Pediatr Radiol 2001; 31:737.

186. Page M, Jeffery H: The role of gastro-esophageal reflux in the aetiology of SIDS. Early Hum Dev 2000;59:127.

187. Pan JJ, Levine MS, Refern RO, et al: Gastroesophageal reflux: Comparison of barium studies with 24-h pH monitoring. Eur J Radiol 2003;47:149.

188. Pandolfino JE, Richter JE, Ours T, et al: Ambulatory esophageal pH monitoring using a wireless system. Am J Gastroenterol 2003;98:740.

189. Paterson WG: The normal antireflux mechanism. Chest Surg Clin North Am 2001;11:473.

190. Patterson PE, Harding SM: Gastroesophageal reflux disorders and asthma. Curr Opin Pulm Med 1999;5:63.

191. Patwari AK, Bajaj P, Kashyp R, et al: Diagnostic modalities for gastroesophageal reflux. Indian J Pediatr 2002;69:133.

192. Pehl C, Pfeiffer A, Wendl B, et al: The effect of decaffeination of coffee on gastro-oesophageal reflux in patients with reflux disease. Aliment Pharmacol Ther 1997;11:483.

193. Penagini R: Bile reflux and oesophagitis. Eur J Gastroenterol Hepatol 2001;13:1.

194. Pettersson GB, Bombeck CT, Nyhus LM: The lower esophageal sphincter: Mechanisms of opening and closure. Surgery 1980;88:307.

195. Ponsky JL: Percutaneous endoscopic gastrostomy: Techniques of removal and replacement. Gastrointest Endosc Clin North Am 1992;2:215.

196. Ravelli AM, Milla PJ: Vomiting and gastroesophageal motor activity in children with disorders of the central nervous system. J Pediatr Gastroenterol Nutr 1998; 26:56.

197. Richards CA, Milla PJ, Andrews PL, et al: Retching and vomiting in neurologically impaired children after fundoplication: Predictive preoperative factors. J Pediatr Surg 2001;36:1401.

198. Richter J: Do we know the cause of reflux disease? Eur J Gastroenterol Hepatol 1999;11(Suppl):S3.

199. Richter JE: Importance of bile reflux in Barrett's esophagus. Dig Dis Sci 2001;18:208.

200. Richter JE: Duodenogastric reflux–induced (alkaline) esophagitis. Curr Treat Options Gastroenterol 2004;7:53.

201. Riezzo G, Chiloiro M, Guerra V: Comparison of gastric electrical activity and gastric emptying in healthy and dyspeptic children. Dig Dis Sci 2000;45:517.

202. Rossetti M, Hell K: Fundoplication for the treatment of gastroesophageal reflux in hiatal hernia. World J Surg 1977;1:439.

203. Rothenberg SS: Laparoscopic Nissen procedure in children. Semin Laparosc Surg 2002;9:146.

204. Rothstein RI, Filipi CJ: Endoscopic suturing for gastroesophageal reflux disease: Clinical outcome with the Bard EndoCinch. Gastrointest Endosc Clin North Am 2003; 13:89.

205. Rowen SJ, Gyepes MT: 'The trumpeting elephant' sign of gastroesophageal reflux. Radiology 1978;167:188.

206. Roy-Choudhung S, Ashcraft KW: Thal fundoplication for pediatric gastroesophageal reflux disease. Semin Pediatr Surg 1998;7:115.

207. Ruchelli E, Wenner W, Voytek T, et al: Severity of esophageal eosinophilia predicts response to conventional gastroesophageal reflux therapy. Pediatr Dev Pathol 1999;2:15.

208. Rudolph CD: Supraesophageal complications of gastroesophageal reflux in children: Challenges in diagnosis and treatment. Am J Med 2003;115(Suppl):150S.

209. Rudolph CD, Mazur LJ, Liptak GS, et al: Guidelines for evaluation and treatment of gastroesophageal reflux in infants and children. Recommendations of the North American Society for Pediatric Gastroenterology and Nutrition. J Pediatr Gastroenterol Nutr 2001;32(Suppl):S1.

210. Sacher P, Stauffer UG: The Herbst triad: Report of two cases. J Pediatr Surg 1990;25:1238.

211. Sachs G: Improving on PPI-based therapy of GERD. Eur J Gastroenterol Hepatol 2001;13(Suppl):S35.

212. Sampson LK, Georgeson KE, Royal SA: Laparoscopic gastric antroplasty in children with delayed gastric emptying and gastroesophageal reflux. J Pediatr Surg 1998; 33:282.

213. Sampson LK, Georgeson KE, Winters DC: Laparoscopic gastrostomy as an adjunctive procedure to laparoscopic fundoplication in children. Surg Endosc 1996;10:1106.

214. Sanudo JR, Domenech-Mateu JM: The laryngeal primordium and epithelial lamina: A new interpretation. J Anat 1990;171:207.

215. Schalamon J, Lindahl H, Saarikoski H, et al: Endoscopic follow-up in esophageal atresia—for how long is it necessary? J Pediatr Surg 2003;38:702.

216. Schier F: Indications for laparoscopic antireflux procedures in children. Semin Laparosc Surg 2002;9:139.

217. Scott RB, Ferreira C, Smith L, et al: Cisapride in pediatric gastroesophageal reflux. J Pediatr Gastroenterol Nutr 1997; 25:499.

218. Seibert JJ, Byrne WJ, Euler AR, et al: Gastroesophageal reflux—the acid test: Scintigraphy or the pH probe. AJR Am J Roentgenol 2001;140:1087.

219. Somppi E, Tammela O, Ruuska T, et al: Outcome of patients operated on for esophageal atresia: 30 years' experience. J Pediatr Surg 1998;33:1341.

220. Sondheimer J: Expanding the definition of GE reflux. J Pediatr Gastroenterol Nutr 2002;34:511.

221. Sondheimer JM: Continuous monitoring of distal esophageal pH: A diagnostic test for gastroesophageal reflux in infants. J Pediatr 1980;96:804.

222. Sondheimer JM, Morris BA: Gastroesophageal reflux among severely retarded children. J Pediatr 1979;94:710.

223. Spitz L, McLeod E: Gastroesophageal reflux. Semin Pediatr Surg 2003;12:237.

224. Stein MR: Possible mechanisms of influence of esophageal acid on airway hyperresponsiveness. Am J Med 2003; 115(Suppl):55S.

225. Steyaert H, Al Mohaidly M, Lembo MA, et al: Long-term outcome of laparoscopic Nissen and Toupet fundoplication in normal and neurologically impaired children. Surg Endosc 2003;17:543.

226. Sturdivant RA: Is gastrin the major regulator of lower esophageal sphincter pressure? Gastroenterology 1974; 67:551.

227. Sullivan PB: Gastrointestinal problems in the neurologically impaired child. Baillieres Clin Gastroenterol 1997; 11:529.

228. Sydorak RM, Albanese CT: Laparoscopic antireflux procedures in children: Evaluating the evidence. Semin Laparosc Surg 2002;9:133.

229. Takahashi T: Pathophysiological significance of neuronal nitric oxide synthase in the gastrointestinal tract. J Gastroenterol 2003;38:421.

230. Terry P, Lagergren J, Wolk A, et al: Reflux-inducing dietary factors and risk of adenocarcinoma of the esophagus and gastric cardia. Nutr Cancer 2000;38:186.

231. Thal AP: A modified approach to surgical problems of the esophagogastric portion. Ann Surg 1968;168:542.

232. Thomas EJ, Kumar R, Dasan JB, et al: Gastroesophageal reflux in asthmatic children not responding to asthma medication: A scintigraphic study in 126 patients with correlation between scintigraphic and clinical findings of reflux. Clin Imaging 2003;27:333.

233. Thompson DM: Laryngopharyngeal sensory testing and assessment of airway protection in pediatric patients. Am J Med 2003;115(Suppl):166S.

234. Todd JA, de Caestecker J, Jankowski J: Gastro-esophageal reflux disease and bile acids. J Pediatr Gastroenterol Nutr 2003;36:172.

235. Tolia V, Wuerth A, Thomas R: Gastroesophageal reflux disease: Review of presenting symptoms, evaluation, management, and outcomes in infants. Dig Dis Sci 2003; 48:1723.

236. Tougas G, Armstrong D: Efficacy of H_2 receptor antagonists in the treatment of gastroesophageal reflux disease and its symptoms. Can J Gastroenterol 1997;11:51B.

237. Toupet A: Technic of esophago-gastroplasty with phrenogastropexy used in radical treatment of hiatal hernia as a supplement to Heller's operation in cardiospasms. Mem Acad Chir (Paris) 1963;89:384.

238. Triadafilopoulos G: Stretta: An effective, minimally invasive treatment for gastroesophageal reflux disease. Am J Med 2003;115(Suppl):192S.

239. Tutuian R, Castell DO: Use of multichannel intraluminal impedance to document proximal esophageal and pharyngeal nonacidic reflux episodes. Am J Med 2003; 115(Suppl):119S.

240. Tutuian R, Vela MF, Shay SS: Multichannel intraluminal impedance in esophageal function testing and gastroesophageal reflux monitoring. J Clin Gastroenterol 2003; 37:206.

241. Vaezi MF, Richter JE: Duodenogastro-oesophageal reflux. Baillieres Best Pract Res Clin Gastroenterol 2000;14:719.

242. Vaezi MF, Richter JE: Duodenogastroesophageal reflux and methods to monitor nonacidic reflux. Am J Med 2001; 111(Suppl):160S.

243. Vaezi MF, Singh S, Richter JE: Role of acid and duodenogastric reflux in esophageal mucosal injury: A review of animal and human studies. Gastroenterology 1995; 108:1897.

244. Vandenplas Y: Reflux esophagitis in infants and children: A report from the working group on gastro-esophageal reflux disease of the European Society of Paediatric Gastroenterology and Nutrition. J Pediatr Gastroenterol Nurs 1994;18:413.

245. Vandenplas Y: Invited review: Asthma and gastroesophageal reflux. J Pediatr Gastroenterol Nutr 1997; 24:89.

246. Vandenplas Y: Diagnosis and treatment of gastroesophageal reflux disease in infants and children. Can J Gastroenterol 2000;14:26D.

247. Vandenplas Y, de Roy C, Sacre L: Cisapride decreases prolonged episodes of reflux in infants. J Pediatr Gastroenterol Nutr 1991;12:44.

248. Vandenplas Y, Goyvaerts H, Helven R, et al: Gastroesophageal reflux, as measured by 24-hour pH monitoring, in 509 healthy infants screened for risk of sudden infant death syndrome. Pediatrics 1991;88:834.

249. Vandenplas Y, Hassall E: Mechanisms of gastroesophageal reflux and gastroesophageal reflux disease. J Pediatr Gastroenterol Nutr 2002;35:119.

250. Vandenplas Y, Hegar B: Diagnosis and treatment of gastro-oesophageal reflux disease in infants and children. J Gastroenterol Hepatol 2000;15:593.

251. Vandenplas Y, Sacre-Smits L: Seventeen-hour continuous esophageal pH monitoring in the newborn: Evaluation of the influence of position in asymptomatic and symptomatic babies. J Pediatr Gastroenterol Nutr 1985;4:356.

252. van der Zee DC, Arendo NJ, Bax NM: The value of 24-hour pH study in evaluating the results of laparoscopic antireflux surgery in children. Surg Endosc 1999;13:918.

253. van der Zee DC, Bax KN, Ure BM, et al: Long-term results after laparoscopic Thal procedure in children. Semin Laparosc Surg 2002;9:168.

254. Vantrappen G, Texter EC Jr, Barborka CJ, et al: The closing mechanism at the gastroesophageal junction. Am J Med 1960;28:564.

255. Wadre GM, Lobe TE: Gastroesophageal reflux disease in neurologically impaired children: The role of the gastrostomy tube. Semin Laparosc Surg 2002;9:180.

256. Waring JP, Lacayo L, Hunter J, et al: Chronic cough and hoarseness in patients with severe gastroesophageal reflux disease: Diagnosis and therapy. Dig Dis Sci 1995;40:1093.

257. Watson DI, de Beaux AC: Complications of laparoscopic antireflux surgery. Surg Endosc 2001;15:344.

258. Weber TR:. Toupet fundoplication for gastroesophageal reflux disease. Semin Pediatr Surg 1998;7:121.

259. Wenzl TG, Moroder C, Trachterna M, et al: Esophageal pH monitoring and impedance measurement: A comparison of two diagnostic tests for gastroesophageal reflux. J Pediatr Gastroenterol Nutr 2002;34:519.

260. Wenzl TG, Schenke S, Peschgens T, et al: Association of apnea and nonacid gastroesophageal reflux in infants: Investigations with the intraluminal impedance technique. Pediatr Pulmonol 2001;31:144.

261. Winkelstein A: Peptic esophagitis: A new clinical entity. JAMA 1935;104:906.

262. Winter HS: Disorders of the Oesophagus. Philadelphia, WB Saunders, 1984.

263. Wolfe MM, Sachs G: Acid suppression: Optimizing therapy for gastroduodenal ulcer healing, gastroesophageal reflux disease, and stress-related erosive syndrome. Gastroenterology 2000;118(Suppl):S9.

264. Woodard-Knight L, Fudge A, Teubner J, et al: Aluminium absorption and antacid therapy in infancy. J Pediatr Child Health 1992;28:257.

265. Wu JC, Chan FK, Ching JY, et al: Effect of *Helicobacter pylori* eradication on treatment of gastro-oesophageal reflux disease: A double blind, placebo controlled, randomised trial. Gut 2004;53:174.

266. Yoshida Y, Tanaka Y, Hirano M, et al: Sensory innervation of the pharynx and larynx. Am J Med 2000;108(Suppl):51S.

267. Zaninotto G, DeMeester TR, Schwizer W, et al: The lower esophageal sphincter in health and disease. Am J Surg 1988;155:104.

268. Zaw-Tun HA: The tracheo-esophageal septum: Fact or fantasy? Origin and development of the respiratory primordium and esophagus. Acta Anat (Basel) 1982; 114:1.

269. Zwischenberger JB, Alpard SK, Orringer MB: Esophagus. In Townsend CM (ed): Sabiston Textbook of Surgery, 16th ed. Philadelphia, WB Saunders, 2001.

Index

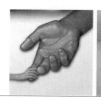

Note: Page numbers followed by the letter f refer to figures and those followed by t refer to tables. Page numbers followed by the letter b indicate boxed material.